Tenth Edition

# GHAI
# Essential Pediatrics

As per the latest NMC Guidelines | Competency Based Medical Education (CBME) Curriculum for the Indian Medical Graduate

Tenth Edition

# GHAI Essential Pediatrics

As per the latest NMC Guidelines | Competency Based Medical Education (CBME) Curriculum for the Indian Medical Graduate

*Editors*

**Vinod K Paul** MD, PhD, FAMS, FNASc, FASc, FNA
Member (Health), NITI Aayog
Government of India, and
Former Professor and Head, Department of Pediatrics
All India Institute of Medical Sciences, New Delhi

**Arvind Bagga** MD, FIAP, FISN, FAMS
Professor and Head
Department of Pediatrics
All India Institute of Medical Sciences, New Delhi

CBSPD

**CBS Publishers & Distributors** Pvt Ltd

New Delhi • Bengaluru • Chennai • Kochi • Kolkata • Lucknow • Mumbai
Gujarat • Hyderabad • Jharkhand • Nagpur • Patna • Pune • Uttarakhand

*Disclaimer*

Medical knowledge is constantly changing. As new information becomes available, changes in treatment, procedures, equipment and the use of drugs become necessary. The contributors, editors and the publishers, as far as possible, have taken care to ensure that the information given in this text is accurate and up-to-date. However, the readers are strongly advised to confirm that the information, especially with regard to drug usage, complies with the latest legislation and standards of practice.

*Notice*

Research in treatment and drug therapy is continually in progress throughout the world. Recommendations and contraindications in dosage schedules require constant updating and change, both from year-to-year and country-to-country. Different drugs may have a similar name in other countries or the same drugs may be packed in different strengths. It is, therefore, advisable to consult the product information sheet provided with each drug, particularly in the case of new, foreign or rarely used drugs, to ensure that changes have not been made in the recommended dosages.

Tenth Edition

**GHAI**

**Essential Pediatrics**

As per the latest NMC Guidelines | Competency Based Medical Education (CBME) Curriculum for the Indian Medical Graduate

**ISBN:** 978-93-5466-507-3



**Tenth Edition 2023**
**Reprint** 2024, 2025, 2026, **2027**
**First Edition 1982**
**Second Edition 1990**
**Third Edition 1993**
**Fourth Edition 1996**
**Fifth Edition 2000**
**Sixth Edition 2004**
**Seventh Edition 2009**
**Eighth Edition 2013**
**Ninth Edition 2019**



Published by Satish Kumar Jain and produced by Varun Jain for

**CBS Publishers & Distributors** Pvt Ltd

4819/XI Prahlad Street, 24 Ansari Road, Daryaganj, New Delhi 110 002, India
Ph: 011-23266838, 23289259 Website: www.cbspd.com
e-mail: delhi@cbspd.com

*Corporate Office:* 204 FIE, Industrial Area, Patparganj, Delhi 110 092, India
Ph: 011-49344934 Fax: 011-49344935
e-mail: publishing@cbspd.com; publicity@cbspd.com

***Branches***

- Bengaluru: Seema House 2975, 17th Cross, KR Road, Banasankari 2nd Stage, Bengaluru 560 070, Karnataka, India
  Ph: +91-80-26771678/79 Fax: +91-80-26771680 e-mail: bangalore@cbspd.com
- Chennai: 18/8B, Subbarayan Street, Shenoy Nagar, Chennai 600 030, Tamil Nadu, India
  Ph: +91-44-42032115, 45022115 e-mail: chennai@cbspd.com
- Kochi: 42/1325, 1326, Power House Road, Opposite KSEB, Kochi 682018, Kerala, India
  Ph: +91-484-4059061–65 Fax: +91-484-4059065 e-mail: kochi@cbspd.com
- Kolkata: 147, Hind Ceramics Compound, 1st Floor, Nilgunj Road, Belghoria, Kolkata 700056, West Bengal, India
  Ph: +91-33-25633055/56 e-mail: kolkata@cbspd.com
- Lucknow: Basement, Khushnuma Complex, 7 Meerabai Marg (behind Jawahar Bhawan), Lucknow 226001, UP, India
  Ph: +91-522-4000032 e-mail: tiwari.lucknow@cbspd.com
- Mumbai: PWD Shed, Gala No. 25/26, Ramchandra Bhatt Marg, Next JJ Hospital Gate No. 2, Opp. Union Bank of India, Noorbaug, Mumbai 400009, Maharashtra, India
  Ph: +91-22-66661880/89 e-mail: mumbai@cbspd.com

***Representatives***

**• Gujarat • Hyderabad • Jharkhand • Nagpur • Patna • Pune • Uttarakhand**

*For trade terms please contact* customercare@cbspd.com
*For general enquiries please contact* info@cbspd.com

*Printed at* Thomson Press India Private Ltd., Faridabad, Haryana, India

# Prof. Om Prakash Ghai

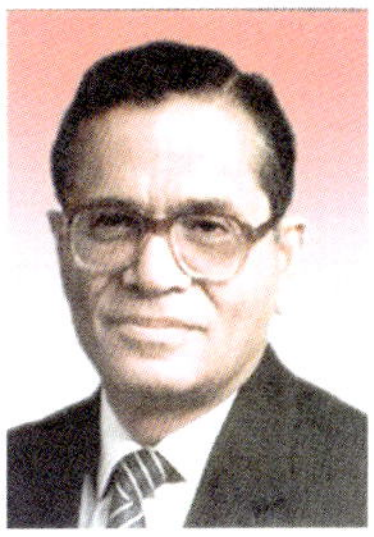

Prof. Om Prakash Ghai had a distinguished academic tenure at the All India Institute of Medical Sciences, New Delhi. He started the Department of Pediatrics in 1959 with six beds for children. Under his leadership, the department evolved into a multispecialty centre of international repute. After his retirement as Dean of the Institute and Professor and Head of the Department of Pediatrics, he chaired the Department of Pediatrics at the University College of Medical Sciences, Delhi, where he served until 1991.

Prof. Ghai was President of the Indian Academy of Pediatrics in 1978 and President of the International College of Pediatrics from 1987 to 1990. The International Pediatric Association presented him the prestigious 'Insignia of Merit Medallion' (1977) for his outstanding contributions to child welfare. The Indian Council of Medical Research awarded him the Dr Kamla Menon Prize (1983) and Amrut Mody Prize (1985). The Medical Council of India bestowed on him the Dr BC Roy Memorial Award for 'Eminent Medical Teacher' (1987). He was awarded honorary fellowships of the American Academy of Pediatrics, the National Academy of Medical Sciences and the Indian Academy of Pediatrics.

Prof. Ghai served as a short-term consultant to the World Health Organization and Asian Development Bank. He was a member of the Technical Advisory Group of the Control of Diarrheal Diseases Program of the World Health Organization (1987–89). He was member of the National Children's Board and several expert groups of the Government of India, UNICEF and Indian Council of Child Welfare. He was the editor of Indian Pediatrics and member of the editorial advisory boards of multiple journals.

Prof. Ghai was a teacher par excellence, an inspiring leader and a true visionary. His name shall always remain etched in the annals of pediatrics of our country.

# Preface to the Tenth Edition

We are excited to present to you the tenth edition of **Essential Pediatrics,** which is considered the reference standard for undergraduate teaching in pediatrics, and a primer for postgraduate students. Moreover, this edition is special because it marks **40 years** since the first edition of the textbook was published.

The present edition of **Essential Pediatrics** continues to maintain its focus on undergraduate medical students. We believe that the purpose of the book is threefold. The first aim is to impart up-to-date knowledge and concepts in pediatrics. In addition, the book endeavors to shape the reader's mind for a caring and gentle disposition toward the needs of children. And, finally we hope that the book sensitizes the future doctors with the all-important public health dimensions of child health and development.

A number of changes have been incorporated in the present edition, keeping in mind that **Essential Pediatrics** should remain the most trusted, contemporary and relevant resource for the students. The core chapters of growth, development, nutrition, neonatal care and integrated management of neonatal and childhood illnesses have been thoroughly revised and enhanced. Keeping in mind the recent global challenges, chapters on infectious disorders and immunization have been significantly updated. Several additional tables, figures and algorithms are included in the entire book to emphasize the current approach to diagnosis and management of systemic diseases. The list of suggested reading and online resources has been updated across all chapters.

The core competencies included in the Competency Based Undergraduate Curriculum for the Indian Graduate prescribed by the National Medical Commission are listed in the preliminary pages of the book. These competencies have also been enumerated and introduced in specific subsections of each chapter. This will allow the reader to appreciate the competence associated with the defined knowledge content.

We are truly proud of our authors for their insightful contributions, and gratefully acknowledge their devotion and partnership. They met timelines despite their intense involvement in the clinical and teaching responsibilities and the stresses of the pandemic. Their scholarly writings, characterized by the succinct expression and updated concepts, continue to meet the learning needs of the readers. Sadly in 2022 our community lost Dr Savitri Srivastava who, along with Dr Rajan Tandon, had left an indelible imprint on the chapter on cardiovascular diseases in previous editions. We welcome Dr Amanpreet Sethi, Dr Rakesh Pilania, Dr Georgie Mathew, Dr P Ashok Babu, Dr Sumita Ghosh and Dr Nitin Dhochak for their maiden contributions to this edition.

We feel privileged to offer this edition of **Essential Pediatrics** as a tribute to all sick children and their families who touched our professional lives. Even as they navigated their life through innumerable challenges, our patients granted us an opportunity to learn, serve and teach. Dr Paul dedicates the book to his wife, Dr Shashi Paul, for being a constant source of inspiration. Dr Bagga dedicates this book to his parents for constant motivation, and his wife, Subhita, and children for their unconditional support.

We thank our colleagues at CBS Publishers & Distributors, Mr YN Arjuna and his team (Ms Ritu Chawla | print production |, Mr Surinder Jha | editing/reading |, Ms Jyoti Kaur | typesetting/pagination |, Mr Sanjay Chauhan | graphics designing/preparation |, Mr Neeraj Prasad | cover designing |) for ensuring the high quality of the textbook across multiple editions. We continue to be indebted to our readers and teachers for enthusing their trust, lending the support and providing useful suggestions.

New Delhi
March 2023

**Vinod K Paul**
**Arvind Bagga**

# Preface to the First Edition

The health problems of the children in the third world are the most pressing. Physicians in these countries often have to work under constraints of poor resources and a lack of access to the modern diagnostic aids. They, therefore, of necessity require a more exhaustive training in clinical skills and a sharper clinical acumen than their counterparts more fortunately placed. The present textbook is primarily aimed to fulfil this need.

This book covers a broad spectrum of the subject, laying a special emphasis on the nutritional and infectious disorders. Rare diseases are referred to only briefly. This has helped to restrict the size of the book to a manageable level so that the undergraduate medical students may find it handy and useful.

The sections on the applied aspects of anatomy and physiology of the various body systems and pathophysiology of the disease processes affecting them will appeal to the postgraduate medical students. These may help them in understanding the biological basis of diagnosis and management. The sections on the use of drugs, clinical approach to the diagnosis and details of diagnostic and therapeutic procedures will be useful especially for the general practitioners and clinical residents.

Most references used in the preparation of the manuscript have been cited but if some have been left out through oversight, I offer my sincere apologies. I thank Prof MMS Ahuja for the permission to include some excerpts from the chapter on "Nutrition" written by Dr Tara Gopaldas and me from the book Progress in Clinical Medicine, Series IV, published by Arnold-Heinemann, New Delhi.

I acknowledge my gratitude to all my colleagues in the department who gave me unstinted support and stood solidly beside me in our joint endeavour for upgrading the status of pediatric services in India. The erudition and scholarship of Professors KL Wig and V Ramalingaswami have been a great source of inspiration to me. I am grateful to Professors PN Taneja and Harish Chandra, who encouraged me to write this book.

I take this opportunity to thank Dr PSN Menon, my erstwhile student, now a dear colleague, who helped me at every stage of preparation of this edition. The book bears an indelible imprint of his meticulous efforts. I am grateful to my colleague Dr HS Wasir for his valuable suggestions on the section on hypertension. Drs RK Menon, Vedanarayanan and Anil Gupta read through several sections and made helpful suggestions.

Many medical students, especially Mr Gurkirpal Singh, helped at several stages in the preparation of the book. I am grateful to Messrs Ganguly, Mitra, Ghosh and Awasthi for their help in artwork. Shri Suraj Bhan did the typing work with great patience. Shri JN Mathur of Mehta Offset Works toiled painstakingly to give the finishing touches to the book. Shri SN Mehta, our publisher, was very co-operative and took a special pride in publishing this volume.

**1982** **OP Ghai**

# Contributors

**Vinod K Paul**
Member (Health), NITI Aayog
Government of India, and
Former Professor and Head, Department of Pediatrics
All India Institute of Medical Sciences, New Delhi

**Arvind Bagga**
Professor and Head, Department of Pediatrics
Chief, Division of Pediatric Nephrology
All India Institute of Medical Sciences, New Delhi

**Ramesh Agarwal**
Professor, Division of Neonatology
Department of Pediatrics
All India Institute of Medical Sciences, New Delhi

**Anuja Agarwala**
Hon. Senior Advisor (Nutrition), INCLEN
Nutrition Consultant, Blossom Children Clinic
Former Senior Dietitian, Department of Pediatrics
All India Institute of Medical Sciences, New Delhi

**P Ashok Babu**
Joint Secretary (RCH)
Ministry of Health and Family Welfare
Government of India, New Delhi

**Anurag Bajpai**
Consultant Pediatrics and Adolescent Endocrinology
Regency Hospital Limited, Kanpur
Fortis Memorial Research Institute, Gurgaon

**Neetu Bhari**
Associate Professor
Department of Dermatology and Venereology
All India Institute of Medical Sciences, New Delhi

**Vijayalakshmi Bhatia**
Professor of Pediatric Endocrinology
Department of Endocrinology
Sanjay Gandhi Postgraduate Institute of Medical Sciences, Lucknow

**Biswaroop Chakrabarty**
Additional Professor, Division of Neurology
Department of Pediatrics
All India Institute of Medical Sciences, New Delhi

**Nitin Dhochak**
Assistant Professor, Division of Pulmonology and Intensive Care
Department of Pediatrics
All India Institute of Medical Sciences, New Delhi

**Sumita Ghosh**
Additional Commissioner (Child Health)
Ministry of Health and Family Welfare
Government of India, New Delhi

**Tushar R Godbole**
Associate Professor, Dr Vasantrao Pawar Medical College, Nashik
Pediatric Endocrinologist
Harmony Health Specialty Clinic, Nashik

**Neerja Gupta**
Additional Professor, Division of Genetics
Department of Pediatrics
All India Institute of Medical Sciences, New Delhi

**Sheffali Gulati**
Professor, Division of Neurology
Department of Pediatrics
All India Institute of Medical Sciences, New Delhi

**Barath Jagadisan**
Pediatric Hepatologist
King's College Hospital
Denmark Hill, London, UK

**Vandana Jain**
Professor, Division of Endocrinology
Department of Pediatrics
All India Institute of Medical Sciences, New Delhi

**Kana Ram Jat**
Additional Professor, Division of Pulmonology and Intensive Care
Department of Pediatrics
All India Institute of Medical Sciences, New Delhi

**Madhulika Kabra**
Professor, Division of Genetics
Department of Pediatrics
All India Institute of Medical Sciences, New Delhi

**Sushil K Kabra**
Professor, Division of Pulmonology and Intensive Care
Department of Pediatrics
All India Institute of Medical Sciences, New Delhi

**Neena Khanna**
Professor and Head
Department of Dermatology
Amrita Hospitals & Amrita Institute of Medical Sciences & Research
Faridabad

**R Krishna Kumar**
Clinical Professor and Head
Department of Pediatric Cardiology
Amrita Institute of Medical Sciences and Research Centre, Kochi

**Rashmi Kumar**
Consultant Pediatrician
Professor of Pediatrics and Former Head
King George Medical University, Lucknow

**Rakesh Lodha**
Professor, Division of Pulmonology and Intensive Care
Department of Pediatrics
All India Institute of Medical Sciences, New Delhi

**Georgie Mathew**
Associate Professor, Division of Nephrology
Department of Child Health
Christian Medical College and Hospital, Vellore

**PSN Menon**
Consultant and Head
Department of Pediatrics
Jaber Al-Ahmad Armed Forces Hospital, Kuwait

**Rakesh Kumar Pilania**
Associate Professor, Allergy Immunology Unit
Department of Pediatrics, Advanced Pediatrics Centre
Post Graduate Institute of Medical Education and Research, Chandigarh
WHO Collaborating Centre for Education, Research and Training in Pediatric Immunology

**Anu Thukral**
Additional Professor, Division of Neonatology
Department of Pediatrics
All India Institute of Medical Sciences, New Delhi

**Prem Sagar**
Additional Professor
Department of Otolaryngology and Head Neck Surgery
All India Institute of Medical Sciences, New Delhi

**Sandeep Samant**
Professor, Department of Otolaryngology and Head-Neck Surgery
Feinberg School of Medicine, Northwestern Memorial Hospital
Greater Chicago, IL, USA

**Jhuma Sankar**
Additional Professor, Division of Pulmonology and Intensive Care
Department of Pediatrics
All India Institute of Medical Sciences, New Delhi

**Naveen Sankhyan**
Professor, Pediatric Neurology Unit
Department of Pediatrics, Advanced Pediatrics Centre
Post Graduate Institute of Medical Education and Research, Chandigarh

**Rachna Seth**
Professor, Division of Oncology
Department of Pediatrics
All India Institute of Medical Sciences, New Delhi

**Rajeev Seth**
Medical Director, Child Health and Development Center
Chair, International Society for Prevention of Child Abuse and Neglect
New Delhi

**Tulika Seth**
Professor, Department of Hematology
All India Institute of Medical Sciences, New Delhi

**Amanpreet Sethi**
Assistant Professor, Neonatology
Department of Pediatrics
Guru Gobind Singh Medical College, Faridkot

**Rajni Sharma**
Additional Professor, Division of Endocrinology
Department of Pediatrics
All India Institute of Medical Sciences, New Delhi

**Surjit Singh**
Head, Department of Pediatrics and Chief, Allergy Immunology Unit
Advanced Pediatrics Centre
Post Graduate Institute of Medical Education and Research, Chandigarh
WHO Collaborating Centre for Education, Research and Training in Pediatric Immunology

**Tanu Singhal**
Consultant, Departments of Pediatrics and Infectious Disease
Kokilaben Dhirubhai Ambani Hospital and Medical Research Institute
Mumbai

**Aditi Sinha**
Additional Professor, Division of Nephrology
Department of Pediatrics
All India Institute of Medical Sciences, New Delhi

**Anshu Srivastava**
Professor, Department of Pediatric Gastroenterology
Sanjay Gandhi Postgraduate Institute of Medical Sciences
Lucknow, Uttar Pradesh

**RN Srivastava**
Senior Consultant, Pediatric Nephrology
Indraprastha Apollo Hospitals, New Delhi

**Radhika Tandon**
Professor, Department of Ophthalmology
Dr. Rajendra Prasad Centre for Ophthalmic Sciences
All India Institute of Medical Sciences, New Delhi

**Alok Thakar**
Professor and Head
Department of Otolaryngology and Head Neck Surgery
All India Institute of Medical Sciences, New Delhi

**Surender K Yachha**
Director and Head
Department of Pediatric Gastroenterology, Hepatology and Liver Transplantation
Sakra World Hospital, Bengaluru

# Contents


*Preface to the Tenth Edition* vii
*Preface to the First Edition* ix
*Contributors* xi

**1. Introduction to Pediatrics** 1
*Vinod K Paul*
Historical perspective 1
Challenge of child health 2
National programs on child health 3

**2. Growth** 6
*Ramesh Agarwal, Naveen Sankhyan, Vandana Jain*
Concept of growth 6
Biology of growth 6
Factors affecting growth 8
Assessment of physical growth 9
Growth charts 12
Disorders of growth 16
Failure of thrive 21

**3. Development** 22
*Ramesh Agarwal, Naveen Sankhyan*
Normal development 22
Domains of development 24
Developmental assessment 36
Nurturing care 39

**4. Developmental and Behavioral Disorders** 42
*Biswaroop Chakrabarty, Sheffali Gulati*
Global developmental delay, intellectual disability 42
Developmental deviance and dissociation 42
Autism spectrum disorder 42
Attention deficit hyperactivity disorder 44
Specific learning disability 44
Tic disorder and stereotypies 44
Other developmental and behavioral disorders 45
Mental health in children and adolescents 47

**5. Adolescent Health and Development** 48
*Tushar R Godbole, Vijayalakshmi Bhatia*
Physical aspects 48
Problems faced by adolescents 50
Role of the health care provider 52
Government interventions in adolescent health care 54

**6. Fluid and Electrolyte Disturbances** 55
*Georgie Mathew, Arvind Bagga*
Composition of body fluids 55
Normal maintenance fluid and electrolyte requirements 57
Sodium 59
Potassium 62
Calcium 65
Magnesium 68
Acid–base disorders 69

**7. Nutrition** 75
*Rakesh Lodha, Anuja Agarwala*
Food 75
Dietary standards 77
Balanced diet 81
Normal balanced diet for various age groups 81
Undernutrition 85
Management of malnutrition 88
Overnutrition and obesity 98

**8. Micronutrients in Health and Disease** 100
*Rajni Sharma*
Fat-soluble vitamins 100
Rickets 104
Water-soluble vitamins 110
Minerals and trace elements 114

**9. Newborn Care** 118
*Ramesh Agarwal, Amanpreet Sethi*
Definitions 118
Resuscitation 119
Level of newborn care 126
Care of normal neonates 127
Evaluation of newborn 131
Thermal protection 139
Breastfeeding 142
Care of low birth weight neonates 147
Kangaroo mother care 149
Fluid and electrolyte management 151
Feeding of LBW neonates 152
Respiratory distress 156
Cyanosis in newborn 160
Perinatal asphyxia 161
Neonatal seizures 164
Infections in neonates 166
Necrotizing enterocolitis 170
Jaundice 170
Neonatal cholestasis 175
Birth injury 175
Congenital malformations 175
Transport of neonates 179
Follow-up of high-risk neonates 179
Metabolic disorders 180
Effect of maternal conditions on fetus and neonates 181
Specialized newborn screening before discharge 183

**10. Immunization** 185
*Aditi Sinha*
Definitions and principles 185
Vaccination schedules and immunization programs 187
Commonly used vaccines 190
Adverse events following immunization (AEFI) 212
Immunization in special circumstances 215

## 11. Infections and Infestations 220

*Tanu Singhal, Rakesh Lodha, Sushil K Kabra*

Fever 220
Common viral infections 225
Common bacterial infections 254
Other bacterial infections 261
Fungal infections 272
Protozoal infections 274
Congenital and perinatal infections 284
Helminthic infections 286
Health care-associated infections 292
Rational antimicrobial therapy 293

## 12. Diseases of Gastrointestinal System and Liver 294

*Anshu Srivastava, Barath Jagadisan, Surender K Yachha*

Vomiting 294
Dysphagia 298
Constipation 300
Abdominal pain 303
Acute diarrhea 309
Persistent diarrhea 315
Chronic diarrhea 317
Gastrointestinal bleeding 325
Disorders of the hepatobiliary system 328
Jaundice 331
Liver failure 333
Chronic liver disease 334
Ascites 336
Portal hypertension 338
Autoimmune liver disease 340
Chronic hepatitis B infection 340
Hepatitis C infection 341
Metabolic liver disease 342
Hepatic manifestations of systemic diseases 344
Neonatal cholestasis 345
Liver transplantation 349

## 13. Hematological Disorders 350

*Tulika Seth*

Approach to anemia 350
Approach to hemolytic anemias 357
Hereditary spherocytosis 358
Abnormalities in red cell glycolysis 359
Autoimmune hemolytic anemia 359
Thalassemias 360
Sickle cell disease 364
Aplastic anemia 365
Hematopoietic stem cell transplantation 367
Approach to a bleeding child 369
Approach to thrombosis 375
White blood cells 377

## 14. Otorhinolaryngology 379

*Prem Sagar, Alok Thakar, Sandeep Samant*

Diseases of the ear 379
Diseases of nose and sinuses 385
Diseases of oral cavity and pharynx 389
Diseases of the larynx and trachea 391
Diseases of the salivary glands 394

## 15. Disorders of Respiratory System 395

*Sushil K Kabra*

Developmental physiology 395
Common respiratory symptoms 396
Diagnosis of respiratory illnesses 399
Respiratory tract infections 400
Acute lower respiratory tract infections 401
Acute bronchiolitis 406
Bronchial asthma 407
Management of acute exacerbation of asthma 415
Foreign body aspiration 416
Lung abscess 416
Bronchiectasis 416
Empyema thoracis 417
Cystic fibrosis 417
Acute respiratory distress syndrome (ARDS) 418
Chronic cough 419
Pulmonary manifestations of HIV infection 420

## 16. Disorders of Cardiovascular System 422

*R Krishna Kumar*

Epidemiology and disease burden of pediatric heart disease in India 422
Congestive cardiac failure 423
Congenital heart disease 427
Acyanotic congenital heart defects 437
Cyanotic heart disease 444
Obstructive lesions 453
Rheumatic fever and rheumatic heart disease 457
Infective endocarditis 466
Myocardial diseases 469
Cardiovascular manifestations of SARS-CoV-2 infection 473
Pericardial disease 473
Systemic hypertension 474
Pulmonary arterial hypertension 477
Rhythm disorders 480
Preventing adult cardiovascular disease 485

## 17. Disorders of Kidney and Urinary Tract 486

*Arvind Bagga, Aditi Sinha, RN Srivastava*

Renal anatomy and physiology 486
Diagnostic evaluation 489
Hematuria 493
Proteinuria 496
Acute glomerulonephritis 496
Nephrotic syndrome 500
Steroid-sensitive nephrotic syndrome 500
Steroid-resistant nephrotic syndrome 505
Chronic glomerulonephritis 506
Interstitial nephritis 507
Urinary tract infections 507
Vesicoureteric reflux 510
Acute kidney injury 511
Hemolytic uremic syndrome 517
Chronic kidney disease 518
Kidney replacement therapy 520
Disorders of tubular transport 521
Nephrolithiasis and nephrocalcinosis 525
Enuresis 527
Congenital abnormalities of kidney and urinary tract 528
Antenatal hydronephrosis 530
Cystic kidney diseases 531

## 18. Endocrine and Metabolic Disorders 533

*PSN Menon, Anurag Bajpai, Vandana Jain, Rajni Sharma*

General principles 533
Disorders of the pituitary gland 533
Disorders of the thyroid gland 537
Disorders of bone and mineral metabolism 541
Disorders of adrenal glands 543
Obesity 547
Disorders of the gonads 552
Differences in sex development 558
Diabetes mellitus 562

## 19. Diseases of Central Nervous System 571
*Rashmi Kumar*
Neurological diagnosis 571
Congonital malformations 574
Neurocutaneous syndromes 576
Cerebral palsy 578
Seizures and epilepsy 579
Epilepsy 580
Headache 583
Infections and acute encephalitis syndrome 583
Raised intracranial pressure, space occupying lesions and hydrocephalus 589
Coma 592
Hemiplegia 594
Paraplegia and quadriplegia 597
Ataxia 598
Movement disorders 600
Neurological regression 602

## 20. Neuromuscular Disorders 605
*Sheffali Gulati*
Approach to evaluation 605
Disorders affecting anterior horn cells 607
Peripheral neuropathies 609
Acute flaccid paralysis 611
Neuromuscular junction disorders 612
Muscle disorders 614

## 21. Childhood Malignancies 618
*Rachna Seth*
Acute leukemia 619
Chronic myeloid leukemia 627
Lymphoma 628
Retinoblastoma 634
Wilms tumor 636
Neuroblastoma 638
Malignant tumors of the liver 640
Soft tissue sarcoma 640
Bone tumors 641
Germ cell tumors 642
Brain tumors 642
Histiocytoses 644
Oncologic emergencies 646
Late effects and survivorship 647
Bone marrow transplantation (BMT) 649

## 22. Rheumatological Disorders 650
*Rakesh Kumar Pilania, Surjit Singh*
Arthritis 650
Systemic lupus erythematosus 654
Juvenile dermatomyositis 656
Scleroderma 657
Mixed connective tissue disease 658
Vasculitides 658

## 23. Genetic Disorders 662
*Neerja Gupta, Madhulika Kabra*
Chromosomes and genes 662
Chromosomal disorders 663
Down syndrome 666
Turner syndrome 668
Single gene disorders 670
Polygenic inheritance 674
Therapy for genetic disorders 674
Prevention of genetic disorders 675

## 24. Inborn Errors of Metabolism 677
*Neerja Gupta, Madhulika Kabra*
Classification 677
Principles of management 681
Specific disorders 681

## 25. Inborn Errors of Immunity 696
*Rakesh Kumar Pilania, Surjit Singh*
Immunity 696
Inborn errors of immunity 697
Treatment of IEI 701

## 26. Ophthalmic Disorders 702
*Radhika Tandon*
Pediatric eye screening 702
Congenital and developmental abnormalities 704
Acquired eye diseases 704

## 27. Skin Disorders 711
*Neena Khanna, Neetu Bhari*
Basic principles 711
Genodermatoses 714
Nevi 720
Dermatitis 723
Disorders of skin appendages 725
Papulosquamous disorders 727
Bullous disorders 730
Disorders of pigmentation 731
Abnormal vascular responses 732
Infections 733
Diseases caused by arthropods 741
Miscellaneous dermatoses 742

## 28. Poisonings, Injuries and Accidents 745
*Jhuma Sankar*
Road traffic accidents and falls 745
Burns, electrical and inhalational injuries 746
Drowning and near drowning 748
Choking and suffocation 748
Poisoning 749
Common poisonings 753
Envenomations 757
Injury control 760

## 29. Pediatric Critical Care 761
*Nitin Dhochak, Rakesh Lodha*
Assessment of a seriously ill child 761
Pediatric basic and advanced life support 762
Shock 767
Nutrition in the critically ill 770
Sedation, analgesia, paralysis 771
Healthcare-associated infections 772
Blood transfusions 772

## 30. Important Medical Procedures 776
*Nitin Dhochak, Arvind Bagga*

## 31. Rights of Children 787
*Rajeev Seth*
Child rights 787
Child maltreatment (abuse and neglect) 788
Adoption 791
Foster care 792

## 32. Integrated Management of Neonatal and Childhood Illness 793

*P Ashok Babu, Sumita Ghosh*

Integrated management of neonatal and childhood illness strategy 793
Outpatient management of young infants age up to 2 months 794
Outpatient management of sick child age 2 months to 5 years 797
IMNCI charts, 2022 802

## 33. Rational Drug Therapy 840

*Anu Thukral, Kana Ram Jat*

Introduction 840
Analgesics, antipyretics, non-steroidal 840
Anti-inflammatory drugs (NSAIDs) 840
Antiarrhythmics 841
Agents for myasthenia 842
Antimicrobials 842
Anticancer drugs 848
Anticoagulants 848
Anticonvulsants 848
Antidotes 848
Antiemetics and gastrointestinal medications 848
Antihistaminics 849
Antihypertensives 850
Antitoxins and immunoglobulins 850
Bronchodilators, respiratory stimulants and anti-asthma agents 851
Inotropic agents 852
Diuretics 852
Hormones 853
Micronutrients 855
Sedatives, hypnotics, antidepressants and antiepileptics 856
Vasodilators 858

## *Annexures* 859

## *Index* 877

# Index of Competencies

## Competency based Undergraduate Curriculum for the Indian Medical Graduate


| *Code* | *Competency* | *Chapter* | *Page no* |
|---|---|---|---|
| PE1.1 | Define the terminologies growth and development and discuss the factors affecting normal growth and development | 2 | 6, 8 |
| PE1.2 | Discuss and describe the patterns of growth in infants, children and adolescents | 2 | 6 |
| PE1.3 | Discuss and describe the methods of assessment of growth including use of WHO and Indian national standards. Enumerate the parameters used for assessment of physical growth in infants, children and adolescents | 2 | 8, 12 |
| PE1.4 | Perform anthropometric measurements, document in growth charts and interpret | 2 | 8, 12 |
| PE1.5 | Define development and discuss the normal developmental mile stones with respect to motor, behaviour, social, adaptive and language | 3 | 22 |
| PE1.6 | Discuss the methods of assessment of development | 3 | 24 |
| PE1.7 | Perform developmental assessment and interpret | 3 | 24, 36 |
| PE2.1 | Discuss the etiopathogenesis, clinical features and management of a child who fails to thrive | 2 | 21 |
| PE2.2 | Assessment of a child with failing to thrive including eliciting an appropriate history and examination | 2 | 21 |
| PE2.3 | Counselling a parent with failing to thrive child | 2 | 21 |
| PE2.4 | Discuss the etiopathogenesis, clinical features and management of a child with short stature | 2 | 16 |
| PE2.5 | Assessment of a child with short stature: Elicit history, perform examination, document and present | 2 | 16 |
| PE2.6 | Enumerate the referral criteria for growth related problems | 2 | 16, 21 |
| PE3.1 | Define, enumerate and discuss the causes of developmental delay and disability including intellectual disability in children | 4 | 42 |
| PE3.2 | Discuss the approach to a child with developmental delay | 3 | 36 |
| PE3.3 | Assessment of a child with developmental delay—elicit document and present history | 3 | 36 |
| PE3.4 | Counsel a parent of a child with developmental delay | 3 | 36 |
| PE3.5 | Discuss the role of the child developmental unit in management of developmental delay | 3 | 36 |
| PE3.6 | Discuss the referral criteria for children with developmental delay | 3 | 36 |
| PE3.8 | Discuss the etiopathogenesis, clinical presentation and multidisciplinary approach in the management of cerebral palsy | 19 | 578 |
| PE4.1 | Discuss the causes and approach to a child with scholastic backwardness | 4 | 42 |
| PE4.2 | Discuss the etiology, clinical features, diagnosis and management of a child with learning disabilities | 4 | 44 |
| PE4.3 | Discuss the etiology, clinical features, diagnosis and management of a child with attention deficit hyperactivity disorder (ADHD) | 4 | 44 |
| PE4.4 | Discuss the etiology, clinical features, diagnosis and management of a child with autism | 4 | 42 |
| PE4.5 | Discuss the role of child guidance clinic in children with developmental problems | 3 | 38 |
| PE4.6 | Visit to the child guidance clinic | 3 | 38 |
| PE5.1 | Describe the clinical features, diagnosis and management of thumb sucking | 4 | 45 |
| PE5.2 | Describe the clinical features, diagnosis and management of feeding problems | 4 | 45 |
| PE5.4 | Describe the clinical features, diagnosis and management of breath holding spells | 4 | 45 |
| PE5.5 | Describe the clinical features, diagnosis and management of temper tantrums | 4 | 45 |
| PE5.6 | Describe the clinical features, diagnosis and management of pica | 4 | 45 |
| PE5.8 | Discuss the etiology, clinical features and management of enuresis | 4 | 45 |
| PE5.9 | Discuss the etiology, clinical features and management of encopresis | 4 | 45 |
| PE5.10 | Discuss the role of child guidance clinic in children with behavioural problems and the referral criteria | 3 | 38 |
| PE5.11 | Visit to child guidance clinic and observe functioning | 3 | 38 |
| PE6.1 | Define adolescence and stages of adolescence | 5 | 48 |
| PE6.2 | Describe the physical, physiological and psychological changes during adolescence (Puberty) | 5 | 48 |
| PE6.3 | Discuss the general health problems during adolescence | 5 | 50 |
| PE6.4 | Describe adolescent sexuality and common problems related to it | 5 | 50 |
| PE6.5 | Explain the adolescent nutrition and common nutritional problems | 5 | 50 |
| PE6.6 | Discuss the common adolescent eating disorders (anorexia nervosa, bulimia) | 4, 5 | 45, 50 |
| PE6.7 | Describe the common mental health problems during adolescence | 5 | 50 |
| PE6.8 | Respecting patient privacy and maintaining confidentiality while dealing with adolescence | 5 | 52 |
| PE6.9 | Perform routine adolescent health check up including eliciting history, performing examination including SMR (sexual maturity rating), growth assessments (using growth charts) and systemic exam including thyroid and breast exam and the HEADSS screening | 5 | 48, 52 |
| PE6.10 | Discuss the objectives and functions of AFHS (adolescent friendly health services) and the referral criteria | 5 | 52 |

| Code | Competency | Chapter | Page no |
|---|---|---|---|
| PE6.11 | Visit to the adolescent clinic | 5 | 52 |
| PE6.12 | Enumerate the importance of obesity and other NCD in adolescents | 5 | 50 |
| PE6.13 | Enumerate the prevalence and the importance of recognition of sexual, drug abuse in adolescents and children | 5 | 50 |
| PE7.1 | Awareness on the cultural beliefs and practices of breastfeeding | 7, 9 | 81, 142 |
| PE7.2 | Explain the physiology of lactation | 9 | 142 |
| PE7.3 | Describe the composition and types of breast milk and discuss the differences between cow's milk and human milk | 9 | 142 |
| PE7.4 | Discuss the advantages of breast milk | 9 | 142 |
| PE7.5 | Observe the correct technique of breastfeeding and distinguish wrong right from techniques | 9 | 142 |
| PE7.7 | Perform breast examination and identify common problems during lactation such as retracted nipples, cracked nipples, breast engorgement, breast abscess | 9 | 142 |
| PE7.8 | Educate mothers on antenatal breast care and prepare mothers for lactation | 9 | 142 |
| PE7.9 | Educate and counsel mothers for best practices in breastfeeding | 9 | 142 |
| PE7.10 | Respects patient privacy | 9 | 142 |
| PE8.1 | Define the term complementary feeding | 7 | 81 |
| PE8.2 | Discuss the principles, the initiation, attributes, frequency, techniques and hygiene related to complementary feeding including IYCF | 7 | 81 |
| PE8.3 | Enumerate the common complimentary foods | 7 | 81 |
| PE8.4 | Elicit history on the complementary feeding habits | 7 | 81 |
| PE8.5 | Counsel and educate mothers on the best practices in complimentary feeding | 7 | 81 |
| PE9.1 | Describe the age related nutritional needs of infants, children and adolescents including micronutrients and vitamins | 7 | 75 |
| PE9.2 | Describe the tools and methods for assessment and classification of nutritional status of infants, children and adolescents | 7 | 77 |
| PE9.3 | Explain the calorific value of common Indian foods | 7 | 77 |
| PE9.4 | Elicit document and present an appropriate nutritional history and perform a dietary recall | 7 | 77 |
| PE9.5 | Calculate the age related calorie requirement in health and disease and identify gap | 7 | 77, 81 |
| PE9.6 | Assess and classify the nutrition status of infants, children and adolescents and recognize deviations | 7 | 85, 98 |
| PE9.7 | Plan an appropriate diet in health and disease | 7 | 85, 88 |
| PE10.1 | Define and describe the etiopathogenesis, classify including WHO classification, clinical features, complication and management severe acute malnourishment (SAM) and moderate acute malnutrition (MAM) | 7 | 88 |
| PE10.2 | Outline the clinical approach to a child with SAM and MAM | 7 | 88 |
| PE10.3 | Assessment of a patient with SAM and MAM, diagnosis, classification and planning management including hospital and community based intervention, rehabilitation and prevention | 7 | 88 |
| PE10.4 | Identify children with under nutrition as per IMNCI criteria and plan referral | 7, 32 | 88, 797 |
| PE10.5 | Counsel parents of children with SAM and MAM | 7 | 88 |
| PE10.6 | Enumerate the role of locally prepared therapeutic diets and ready to use therapeutic diets | 7 | 88 |
| PE11.1 | Describe the common etiology, clinical features and management of obesity in children | 7, 18 | 98, 547 |
| PE11.2 | Discuss the risk approach for obesity and discuss the prevention strategies | 18 | 547 |
| PE11.3 | Assessment of a child with obesity with regard to eliciting history including physical activity, charting and dietary recall | 18 | 547 |
| PE11.4 | Examination including calculation of BMI, measurement of waist hip ratio, identifying external markers like acanthosis, striae, pseudogynaecomastia, etc. | 18 | 547 |
| PE11.5 | Calculate BMI, document in BMI chart and interpret | 18 | 547 |
| PE11.6 | Discuss criteria for referral | 18 | 547 |
| PE12.1 | Discuss the RDA, dietary sources of vitamin A and their role in health and disease | 7, 8 | 77, 100 |
| PE12.2 | Describe the causes, clinical features, diagnosis and management of deficiency/excess of vitamin A | 8 | 100 |
| PE12.3 | Identify the clinical features of dietary deficiency / excess of vitamin A | 8 | 100 |
| PE12.4 | Diagnose patients with vitamin A deficiency, classify and plan management | 8 | 100 |
| PE12.5 | Discuss the vitamin A prophylaxis program and their recommendations | 8 | 100 |
| PE12.6 | Discuss the RDA, dietary sources of vitamin D and their role in health and disease | 7, 8 | 77, 102 |
| PE12.7 | Describe the causes, clinical features, diagnosis and management of deficiency/excess of vitamin D (rickets and hypervitaminosis D) | 8 | 102,104 |
| PE12.8 | Identify the clinical features of dietary deficiency of vitamin D | 8 | 102,104 |
| PE12.9 | Assess patients with vitamin D deficiency, diagnose, classify and plan management | 8 | 102,104 |
| PE12.10 | Discuss the role of screening for vitamin D deficiency | 8 | 102 |
| PE12.11 | Discuss the RDA, dietary sources of vitamin E and their role in health and disease | 7, 8 | 77, 109 |
| PE12.12 | Describe the causes, clinical features, diagnosis and management of deficiency of vitamin E | 8 | 109 |
| PE12.13 | Discuss the RDA, dietary sources of vitamin K and their role in health and disease | 7, 8 | 77, 109 |
| PE12.14 | Describe the causes, clinical features, diagnosis management and prevention of deficiency of vitamin K | 8 | 109 |
| PE12.15 | Discuss the RDA, dietary sources of vitamin B and their role in health and disease | 7, 8 | 77, 110 |

| Code | Competency | Chapter | Page no |
|---|---|---|---|
| PE12.16 | Describe the causes, clinical features, diagnosis and management of deficiency of B complex Vitamins | 8 | 110 |
| PE12.17 | Identify the clinical features of vitamin B complex deficiency | 8 | 110 |
| PE12.18 | Diagnose patients with vitamin B complex deficiency and plan management | 8 | 110 |
| PE12.19 | Discuss the RDA, dietary sources of vitamin C and their role in health and disease | 7, 8 | 77, 110 |
| PE12.20 | Describe the causes, clinical features, diagnosis and management of deficiency of vitamin C (scurvy) | 8 | 110 |
| PE12.21 | Identify the clinical features of vitamin C deficiency | 8 | 110 |
| PE13.1 | Discuss the RDA, dietary sources of iron and their role in health and disease | 7, 8 | 77, 115 |
| PE13.2 | Describe the causes, diagnosis and management of Fe deficiency | 13 | 354 |
| PE13.3 | Identify the clinical features of dietary deficiency of iron and make a diagnosis | 13 | 354 |
| PE13.4 | Interpret hemogram and iron panel | 13 | 354 |
| PE13.5 | Propose a management plan for Fe deficiency anemia | 13 | 354 |
| PE13.7 | Discuss the RDA, dietary sources of iodine and their role in health and disease | 7, 8 | 77, 116 |
| PE13.8 | Describe the causes, diagnosis and management of deficiency of Iodine | 8, 18 | 116, 540 |
| PE13.9 | Identify the clinical features of iodine deficiency disorders | 8, 18 | 116, 540 |
| PE13.11 | Discuss the RDA, dietary sources of calcium and their role in health and disease | 6, 7, 8 | 65, 70, 114 |
| PE13.12 | Describe the causes, clinical features, diagnosis and management of Ca deficiency | 6, 8, 18 | 65, 114 541 |
| PE13.13 | Discuss the RDA, dietary sources of magnesium and their role in health and disease | 6, 7, 8 | 68, 77, 114 |
| PE13.14 | Describe the causes, clinical features, diagnosis and management of magnesium deficiency | 6, 8 | 68, 114 |
| PE14.2 | Discuss the risk factors, clinical features, diagnosis and management of kerosene ingestion | 28 | 753 |
| PE14.3 | Discuss the risk factors, clinical features, diagnosis and management of organophosphorus poisoning | 28 | 755 |
| PE14.4 | Discuss the risk factors, clinical features, diagnosis and management of paracetamol poisoning | 28 | 756 |
| PE15.1 | Discuss the fluid and electrolyte requirement in health and disease | 6 | 57 |
| PE15.2 | Discuss the clinical features and complications of fluid and electrolyte imbalance and outline the management | 6 | 57, 59, 62 |
| PE15.3 | Calculate the fluid and electrolyte requirement in health | 6 | 57, 59, 62 |
| PE15.4 | Interpret electrolyte report | 6 | 57, 59, 62 |
| PE15.5 | Calculate fluid and electrolyte imbalance | 6 | 57, 59, 62 |
| PE16.1 | Explain the components of Integrated Management of Neonatal and Childhood Illnesses (IMNCI) guidelines and method of risk stratification | 32 | 793 |
| PE16.2 | Assess children <2 months using IMNCI guidelines | 32 | 794 |
| PE16.3 | Assess children >2 to 5 years using IMNCI guidelines and stratify risk | 32 | 797 |
| PE17.1 | State the vision and outline the goals, strategies and plan of action of NHM and other important national programs pertaining to maternal and child health including RMNCH A+, RBSK, RKSK, JSSK, mission Indradhanush and ICDS | 1 | 3 |
| PE17.2 | Analyse the outcomes and appraise the monitoring and evaluation of NHM | 1 | 3 |
| PE18.1 | List and explain the components, plan, outcome of Reproductive Child Health (RCH) program and appraise its monitoring and evaluation | 1 | 3 |
| PE18.2 | Explain preventive interventions for child survival and safe motherhood | 1 | 3 |
| PE19.1 | Explain the components of the Universal Immunization Program and the National Immunization Program | 10 | 187 |
| PE19.2 | Explain the epidemiology of vaccine preventable diseases | 10 | 190 |
| PE19.3 | Vaccine description with regard to classification of vaccines, strain used, dose, route, schedule, risks, benefits and side effects, indications and contraindications | 10 | 190 |
| PE19.4 | Define cold chain and discuss the methods of safe storage and handling of vaccines | 10 | 213 |
| PE19.5 | Discuss immunization in special situations – HIV positive children, immunodeficiency, pre-term, organ transplants, those who received blood and blood products, splenectomised children, adolescents, travellers | 10 | 215 |
| PE19.16 | Enumerate available newer vaccines and their indications including pentavalent pneumococcal, rotavirus, JE, typhoid IPV & HPV | 10 | 190, 211 |
| PE19.6 | Assess patient for fitness for immunization and prescribe an age appropriate immunization schedule | 10 | 187 |
| PE20.1 | Define the common neonatal nomenclatures including the classification and describe the characteristics of a normal term neonate and high risk neonates | 9 | 118 |
| PE20.2 | Explain the care of a normal neonate | 9 | 127 |
| PE20.3 | Perform neonatal resuscitation in a manikin | 9 | 119 |
| PE20.4 | Assessment of a normal neonate | 9 | 131 |
| PE20.5 | Counsel/educate mothers on the care of neonates | 9 | 127 |
| PE20.6 | Explain the follow up care for neonates including breastfeeding, temperature maintenance, immunization, importance of growth monitoring and red flags | 9 | 127 |

| Code | Competency | Chapter | Page no |
|---|---|---|---|
| PE20.7 | Discuss the etiology, clinical features and management of birth asphyxia | 9 | 161 |
| PE20.8 | Discuss the etiology, clinical features and management of respiratory distress in newborn including meconium aspiration and transient tachypnea of newborn | 9 | 156 |
| PE20.9 | Discuss the etiology, clinical features and management of birth injuries | 9 | 175 |
| PE20.10 | Discuss the etiology, clinical features and management of hemorrhagic disease of newborn | 8 | 109 |
| PE20.11 | Discuss the clinical characteristics, complications and management of low birth weight (preterm and small for gestation) | 9 | 147, 149 152 |
| PE20.12 | Discuss the temperature regulation in neonates, clinical features and management of neonatal hypothermia | 9 | 139 |
| PE20.13 | Discuss the temperature regulation in neonates, clinical features and management of neonatal hypoglycemia | 9 | 180 |
| PE20.14 | Discuss the etiology, clinical features and management of neonatal hypocalcemia | 6, 9 | 65, 180 |
| PE20.15 | Discuss the etiology, clinical features and management of neonatal seizures | 9 | 164 |
| PE20.16 | Discuss the etiology, clinical features and management of neonatal sepsis | 9 | 166 |
| PE20.17 | Discuss the etiology, clinical features and management of perinatal infections | 9 | 166 |
| PE20.18 | Identify and stratify risk in a sick neonate using IMNCI guidelines | 32 | 794 |
| PE20.19 | Discuss the etiology, clinical features and management of neonatal hyperbilirubinemia | 9 | 170 |
| PE20.20 | Identify clinical presentations of common surgical conditions in the newborn including TEF, esophageal atresia, anal atresia, cleft lip and palate, congenital diaphragmatic hernia and causes of acute abdomen | 9 | 175 |
| PE21.1 | Enumerate the etiopathogenesis, clinical features, complications and management of urinary tract infection in children | 17 | 507 |
| PE21.2 | Enumerate the etiopathogenesis, clinical features, complications and management of acute post-streptococcal glomerular nephritis in children | 17 | 496 |
| PE21.3 | Discuss the approach and referral criteria to a child with proteinuria | | |
| PE21.4 | Discuss the approach and referral criteria to a child with hematuria | 17 | 493 |
| PE21.5 | Enumerate the etiopathogenesis, clinical features, complications and management of acute renal failure in children | 17 | 511 |
| PE21.6 | Enumerate the etiopathogenesis, clinical features, complications and management of chronic renal failure in children | 17 | 518 |
| PE21.7 | Enumerate the etiopathogenesis, clinical features, complications and management of Wilms tumor | 21 | 636 |
| PE21.8 | Elicit, document and present a history pertaining to diseases of the genitourinary tract | 17 | 489, 527 |
| PE21.9 | Identify external markers for kidney disease, like failing to thrive, hypertension, pallor, icthyosis, anasarca | 17 | 489 |
| PE21.10 | Analyse symptom and interpret the physical findings and arrive at an appropriate provisional/ differential diagnosis | 17 | 489 |
| PE21.11 | Perform and interpret the common analytes in a urine examination | 17 | 489 |
| PE21.12 | Interpret report of plain X-ray of KUB | 17 | 491 |
| PE21.13 | Enumerate the indications for and interpret the written report of ultrasonogram of KUB | 17 | 489 |
| Pe21.14 | Recognize common surgical conditions of the abdomen and genitourinary system and enumerate The indications for referral including acute and subacute intestinal obstruction, appendicitis, pancreatitis, perforation intussusception, phimosis, undescended testis, chordee, hypospadiasis, torsion testis, hernia hydrocele, vulval synechiae | 12 | 303 |
| PE21.15 | Discuss and enumerate the referral criteria for children with genitourinary disorder | 17 | 493–531 |
| PE21.16 | Counsel/educate a patient for referral appropriately | 17 | 493–531 |
| PE21.17 | Describe the etiopathogenesis, grading, clinical features and management of hypertension in children | | |
| PE22.1 | Enumerate the common rheumatological problems in children. Discuss the clinical approach to recognition and referral of a child with rheumatological problem | 22 | 650, 654 656, 658 |
| PE22.3 | Describe the diagnosis and management of common vasculitic disorders including Henoch-Schonlein purpura, Kawasaki disease, SLE, JIA | 22 | 654, 658 |
| PE23.1 | Discuss the hemodynamic changes, clinical presentation, complications and management of acyanotic heart diseases—VSD, ASD and PDA | 16 | 427, 437 |
| PE23.2 | Discuss the hemodynamic changes, clinical presentation, complications and management of cyanotic heart diseases—Fallot's physiology | 16 | 444 |
| PE23.3 | Discuss the etiopathogenesis, clinical presentation and management of cardiac failure in infant and children | 16 | 423 |
| PE23.4 | Discuss the etiopathogenesis, clinical presentation and management of acute rheumatic fever in children | 16 | 457 |
| PE23.5 | Discuss the clinical features, complications, diagnosis, management and prevention of acute rheumatic fever | 16 | 457 |
| PE23.6 | Discuss the etiopathogenesis, clinical features and management of infective endocarditis in children | 16 | 466 |
| PE23.7 | Elicit appropriate history for a cardiac disease, analyse the symptoms, e.g. breathlessness, chest pain, tachycardia, feeding difficulty, failing to thrive, reduced urinary output, swelling, syncope, cyanotic spells, Suck rest cycle, frontal swelling in infants. Document and present | 16 | 423, 427 |

| Code | Competency | Chapter | Page no |
|---|---|---|---|
| PE23.8 | Identify external markers of a cardiac disease, e.g. cyanosis, clubbing, dependent edema, dental caries, arthritis, erythema rash, chorea, subcutaneous nodules, Oslers node, Janeway lesions and document | 16 | 423, 427 |
| PE23.9 | Record pulse, blood pressure, temperature and respiratory rate and interpret as per the age | 16 | 423, 427 |
| PE23.11 | Develop a treatment plan and prescribe appropriate drugs including fluids in cardiac diseases, anti-failure drugs, and inotropic agents | 16 | 423 |
| PE23.13 | Choose and interpret blood reports in cardiac illness | 16 | 457, 466 |
| PE23.14 | Interpret pediatric ECG | 16 | 437, 444, 453, 457, 469, 480 |
| PE23.15 | Use the ECHO reports in management of cases | 16 | 437, 444, 453, 457, 466, 469, 473, 477 |
| PE23.16 | Discuss the indications and limitations of cardiac catheterization | 16 | 427 |
| PE23.17 | Enumerate some common cardiac surgeries like BT shunt, Potts and Waterston's and corrective surgeries | 16 | 427, 474 |
| PE24.1 | Discuss the etiopathogenesis, classification, clinical presentation and management of diarrheal diseases in children | 12 | 309 |
| PE24.2 | Discuss the classification and clinical presentation of various types of diarrheal dehydration | 12 | 309 |
| PE24.3 | Discuss the physiological basis of ORT, types of ORS and the composition of various types of ORS | 12 | 309 |
| PE24.4 | Discuss the types of fluid used in pediatric diarrheal diseases and their composition | 12 | 309 |
| PE24.5 | Discuss the role of antibiotics, antispasmodics, antisecretory drugs, probiotics, antiemetics in acute diarrheal diseases | 12 | 309, 777 |
| PE24.6 | Discuss the causes, clinical presentation and management of persistent diarrhoea in children | 12 | 315 |
| PE24.7 | Discuss the causes, clinical presentation and management of chronic diarrhoea in children | 12 | 317 |
| PE24.8 | Discuss the causes, clinical presentation and management of dysentery in children | 12 | 309 |
| PE24.9 | Elicit, document and present history pertaining to diarrheal diseases | 12 | 309 |
| PE24.10 | Assess for signs of dehydration, document and present | 12 | 309 |
| PE24.11 | Apply the IMNCI guidelines in risk stratification of children with diarrheal dehydration and refer | 32 | 794, 797 |
| PE24.13 | Interpret RFT and electrolyte report | 6 | 57, 59, 62 |
| PE24.14 | Plan fluid management as per the WHO criteria | 12 | 309 |
| PE24.15 | Perform NG tube insertion in a manikin | 30 | 779 |
| PE24.17 | Perform interosseous insertion model | | |
| PE25.1 | Discuss the etiopathogenesis, clinical presentation and management of malabsorption in children and its causes including celiac disease | 12 | 317 |
| PE26.1 | Discuss the etiopathogenesis, clinical features and management of acute hepatitis in children | 11 | 237, 332 |
| PE26.2 | Discuss the etiopathogenesis, clinical features and management of fulminant hepatic failure in children | 12 | 333 |
| PE26.3 | Discuss the etiopathogenesis, clinical features and management of chronic liver diseases in children | 12 | 334 |
| PE26.4 | Discuss the etiopathogenesis, clinical features and management of portal hypertension in children | 12 | 334 |
| PE26.5 | Elicit document and present the history related to diseases of gastrointestinal system | 12 | 294, 298, 300, 303, 325, 328, 336 |
| PE26.6 | Identify external markers for GI and liver disorders, e.g. jaundice, pallor, gynecomastia, spider angioma, palmar erythema, icthyosis, caput medusa, clubbing, failing to thrive, vitamin A and D deficiency | 12 | 294, 298, 336 |
| PE26.7 | Perform examination of the abdomen, demonstrate organomegaly, ascites, etc. | 12 | 294, 304 |
| PE26.8 | Analyse symptoms and interpret physical signs to make a provisional/ differential diagnosis | 12 | 294, 328 |
| PE26.9 | Interpret liver function tests, viral markers, ultrasonogram report | 12 | 328 |
| PE26.11 | Enumerate the indications for upper GI endoscopy | 12 | 325 |
| PE26.12 | Discuss the prevention of Hep B infection—universal precautions and immunisation | 11 | 238 |
| PE27.1 | List the common causes of morbidity and mortality in the under five children | 29 | 761 |
| PE27.2 | Describe the etiopathogenesis, clinical approach and management of cardiorespiratory arrest in children | 1, 29 | 2, 761 |
| PE27.3 | Describe the etiopathogenesis of respiratory distress in children | 29 | 761 |
| PE27.4 | Describe the clinical approach and management of respiratory distress in children | 29 | 761 |
| PE27.5 | Describe the etiopathogenesis, clinical approach and management of shock in children | 29 | 767 |
| PE27.6 | Describe the etiopathogenesis, clinical approach and management of status epilepticus | 19 | 579 |
| PE27.7 | Describe the etiopathogenesis, clinical approach and management of an unconscious child | 19 | 583, 592 |
| PE27.8 | Discuss the common types, clinical presentations and management of poisoning in children | 28 | 749 |
| PE27.9 | Discuss oxygen therapy, in pediatric emergencies and modes of administration | 30 | 780 |
| PE27.10 | Observe the various methods of administering oxygen | 30 | 780 |

| Code | Competency | Chapter | Page no |
|---|---|---|---|
| PE27.11 | Explain the need and process of triage of sick children brought to health facility | 28, 29 | 749, 761 |
| PE27.12 | Enumerate emergency signs and priority signs | 28, 29 | 749, 761 |
| PE27.13 | List the sequential approach of assessment of emergency and priority signs | 28, 29 | 749, 761 |
| PE27.14 | Assess emergency signs and prioritize | 28, 29 | 749, 761 |
| PE27.15 | Assess airway and breathing: recognise signs of severe respiratory distress. Check for cyanosis, severe chest indrawing, grunting | 28, 29 | 749, 761 |
| PE27.16 | Assess airway and breathing. Demonstrate the method of positioning of an infant and child to open airway in a simulated environment | 29 | 762 |
| PE27.17 | Assess airway and breathing: administer oxygen using correct technique and appropriate flow rate | 29 | 762 |
| PE27.18 | Assess airway and breathing: perform assisted ventilation by bag and mask in a simulated environment | 29 | 762 |
| PE27.19 | Check for signs of shock i.e. pulse, blood pressure, CRT | 29 | 762 |
| PF27.21 | Choose the type of fluid and calculate the fluid requirement in shock | 6 | 57 |
| PE27.23 | Assess for signs of severe dehydration | 6, 12 | 57, 309 |
| PE27.24 | Monitoring and maintaining temperature: define hypothermia. Describe the clinical features, complications and management of hypothermia | 9 | 139 |
| PE27.25 | Describe the advantages and correct method of keeping an infant warm by skin to skin contact | 9 | 139, 149 |
| PE27.26 | Describe the environmental measures to maintain temperature | 9 | 139 |
| PE27.27 | Assess for hypothermia and maintain temperature | 9 | 139 |
| PE27.28 | Provide BLS for children in manikin | 29 | 762 |
| PE.27.29 | Discuss the common causes, clinical presentation, medicolegal implications of abuse | 31 | 788 |
| PE27.30 | Demonstrate confidentiality with regard to abuse | 31 | 788 |
| PE27.31 | Assess child for signs of abuse | 31 | 788 |
| PE28.1 | Discuss the etiopathogenesis, clinical features and management of nasopharyngitis | 14, 15 | 389, 400 |
| PE28.2 | Discuss the etiopathogenesis of pharyngotonsillitis | 14, 15 | 389, 400 |
| PE28.3 | Discuss the clinical features and management of pharyngotonsillitis | 14, 15 | 389, 400 |
| PE28.4 | Discuss the etiopathogenesis, clinical features and management of acute otitis media (AOM) | 14 | 379 |
| PE28.5 | Discuss the etiopathogenesis, clinical features and management of epiglottitis | 14 | 391 |
| PE28.6 | Discuss the etiopathogenesis, clinical features and management of acute laryngotracheobronchitis | 14, 15 | 391, 401 |
| PE28.7 | Discuss the etiology, clinical features and management of stridor in children | 14, 15 | 391, 397 |
| PE28.8 | Discuss the types, clinical presentation, and management of foreign body aspiration in infants and children | 14 | 391 |
| PE28.9 | Elicit, document and present age appropriate history of a child with upper respiratory problem including stridor | 14, 15 | 391, 396 |
| PE28.13 | Analyse the clinical symptoms and interpret physical findings and make a provisional/differential diagnosis in a child with ENT symptoms | 14, 15 | 385, 396 |
| PE28.14 | Develop a treatment plan and document appropriately in a child with upper respiratory symptoms | 14, 15 | 385, 400 |
| PE28.15 | Stratify risk in children with stridor using IMNCI guidelines | 32 | 797 |
| PE28.16 | Interpret blood tests relevant to upper respiratory problems | 15 | 399 |
| PE28.17 | Interpret X-ray of the paranasal sinuses and mastoid; and /or use written report in case of management Interpret CXR in foreign body aspiration and lower respiratory tract infection, understand the significance of thymic shadow in pediatric chest X-rays | 14, 15 | 385, 391, 399 |
| PE28.18 | Describe the etiopathogenesis, diagnosis, clinical features, management and prevention of lower respiratory infections including bronchiolitis, wheeze associated LRTI pneumonia and empyema | 15 | 399 |
| PE28.19 | Describe the etiopathogenesis, diagnosis, clinical features, management and prevention of asthma in children | 15 | 407 |
| PE28.20 | Counsel the child with asthma on the correct use of inhalers in a simulated environment | 15 | 407 |
| PE29.1 | Discuss the etiopathogenesis, clinical features, classification and approach to a child with anemia | 13 | 350 |
| PE29.2 | Discuss the etiopathogenesis, clinical features and management of iron deficiency anemia | 13 | 354 |
| PE29.3 | Discuss the etiopathogenesis, clinical features and management of vitamin $B_{12}$, folate deficiency anemia | 13 | 355 |
| PE29.4 | Discuss the etiopathogenesis, clinical features and management of Hemolytic anemia, Thalassemia Major, sickle cell anemia, hereditary spherocytosis, autoimmune hemolytic anemia and hemolytic uremic syndrome | 13 | 357 |
| PE29.6 | Discuss the cause of thrombocytopenia in children: describe the clinical features and management of idiopathic thrombocytopenic purpura (ITP) | 13 | 369, 371 |
| PE29.7 | Discuss the etiology, classification, pathogenesis and clinical features of hemophilia in children | 13 | 372 |
| PE29.8 | Discuss the etiology, clinical presentation and management of acute lymphoblastic leukemia in children | 21 | 619 |
| PE29.9 | Discuss the etiology, clinical presentation and management of lymphoma in children | 21 | 628 |
| PE29.10 | Elicit, document and present the history related to hematology | 13 | 350, 357, 369, 372, 375 |

| Code | Competency | Chapter | Page no |
|---|---|---|---|
| PE29.11 | Identify external markers for hematological disorders, e.g. jaundice, pallor, petechiae purpura, ecchymosis, lymphadenopathy, bone tenderness, loss of weight, mucosal and large joint bleed | 13, 21 | 350, 357, 360, 364, 365, 369, 375, 619, 628 |
| PE29.12 | Perform examination of the abdomen, demonstrate organomegaly | 21 | 619, 628, 640 |
| PE29.13 | Analyse symptoms and interpret physical signs to make a provisional/differential diagnosis | 13, 21 | 360, 364, 619, 628 |
| PE29.15 | Perform and interpret peripheral smear | 13 | 357 |
| PE29.16 | Discuss the indications for hemoglobin electrophoresis and interpret report | 13 | 360, 364 |
| PE29.18 | Enumerate the referral criteria for hematological conditions | 13 | 364 |
| PE30.1 | Discuss the etiopathogenesis, clinical features, complications, management and prevention of meningitis in children | 19 | 583 |
| PE30.2 | Distinguish bacterial, viral and tuberculous meningitis | 19 | 583 |
| PE30.3 | Discuss the etiopathogenesis, classification, clinical features, complication and management of hydrocephalus in children | 19 | 574, 589 |
| PE30.4 | Discuss the etiopathogenesis, classification, clinical features, and management of microcephaly in children | 19 | 574 |
| PE30.5 | Enumerate the neural tube defects. Discuss the causes, clinical features, types, and management of neural tube defect | 19 | 574 |
| PE30.6 | Discuss the etiopathogenesis, clinical features, and management of infantile hemiplegia | 19 | 594 |
| PE30.7 | Discuss the etiopathogenesis, clinical features, complications and management of febrile seizures in children | 19 | 580 |
| PE30.8 | Define epilepsy. Discuss the pathogenesis, clinical types, presentation and management of epilepsy in children | 19 | 579, 580 |
| PE30.9 | Define status epilepticus. Discuss the clinical presentation and management | 19 | 579 |
| PE30.10 | Discuss the etiopathogenesis, clinical features and management of mental retardation in children | 4, 19 | 42, 602 |
| PE30.11 | Discuss the etiopathogenesis, clinical features and management of children with cerebral palsy | 19 | 578 |
| PE30.12 | Enumerate the causes of floppiness in an infant and discuss the clinical features, differential diagnosis and management | 20 | 607 |
| PE30.13 | Discuss the etiopathogenesis, clinical features, management and prevention of poliomyelitis in children | 11, 20 | 235, 611 |
| PE30.14 | Discuss the etiopathogenesis, clinical features and management of Duchene muscular dystrophy | 20 | 614 |
| PE30.15 | Discuss the etiopathogenesis, clinical features and management of ataxia in children | 19 | 598 |
| PE30.16 | Discuss the approach to and management of a child with headache | 19 | 583 |
| PE30.17 | Elicit document and present an age appropriate history pertaining to the CNS | 19 | 571 |
| PE30.18 | Demonstrate the correct method for physical examination of CNS including identification of external markers. Document and present clinical findings | 19 | 571 |
| PE30.19 | Analyse symptoms and interpret physical findings and propose a provisional/differential diagnosis | 19 | 571 |
| PE30.20 | Interpret and explain the findings in a CSF analysis | 19 | 573, 583 |
| PE30.21 | Enumerate the indication and discuss the limitations of EEG, CT, MRI | 19 | 573, 582 |
| PE30.22 | Interpret the reports of EEG, CT, MRI | 19 | 573, 582 |
| PE30.23 | Perform in a mannequin lumbar puncture. Discuss the indications, contraindication of the procedure | 30 | 781 |
| PE31.1 | Describe the etiopathogenesis, management and prevention of allergic rhinitis in children | 14 | 386 |
| PE31.2 | Recognize the clinical signs of allergic rhinitis | 14 | 386 |
| PE31.3 | Describe the etiopathogenesis, clinical features and management of atopic dermatitis in children | 27 | 723 |
| PE31.4 | Identify atopic dermatitis and manage | 27 | 723 |
| PE31.5 | Discuss the etiopathogenesis, clinical types, presentations, management and prevention of childhood asthma | 15 | 407 |
| PE31.6 | Recognise symptoms and signs of asthma | 15 | 407 |
| PE31.7 | Develop a treatment plan for asthma appropriate to clinical presentation and severity | 15 | 407 |
| PE31.8 | Enumerate criteria for referral | 15 | 407 |
| PE31.9 | Interpret CBC and CX-ray in asthma | 15 | 407 |
| PE31.10 | Enumerate the indications for PFT | 15 | 409 |
| PE31.12 | Discuss etiopathogenesis, clinical features and complications and management of urticaria angioedema | 27 | 732 |
| PE32.1 | Discuss the genetic basis, risk factors, complications, prenatal diagnosis, management and genetic counselling in Down's syndrome | 23 | 666 |
| PE32.2 | Identify the clinical features of Down's syndrome | 23 | 666 |
| PE32.3 | Interpret normal karyotype and recognize Trisomy 21 | 23 | 663, 666 |
| PE32.4 | Discuss the referral criteria and multidisciplinary approach to management | 23 | 666 |
| PE32.5 | Counsel parents regarding: 1. Present child; 2. Risk in the next pregnancy | 23 | 666 |

| Code | Competency | Chapter | Page no |
|---|---|---|---|
| PE32.6 | Discuss the genetic basis, risk factors, clinical features, complications, prenatal diagnosis, management and genetic counselling in Turner's syndrome | 23 | 668 |
| PE32.7 | Identify the clinical features of Turner syndrome | 23 | 668 |
| PE32.8 | Interpret normal karyotype and recognize the Turner karyotype | 23 | 668 |
| PE32.9 | Discuss the referral criteria and multidisciplinary approach to management of Turner syndrome | 23 | 668 |
| PE32.10 | Counsel parents regarding: 1. Present child; 2. Risk in the next pregnancy | 23 | 668 |
| PE32.12 | Identify the clinical features of Klineferlter syndrome | 23 | 669 |
| PE33.1 | Describe the etiopathogenesis clinical features, management of hypothyroidism in children | 18 | 538 |
| PE33.2 | Recognize the clinical signs of hypothyroidism and refer | 18 | 538 |
| PE33.3 | Interpret and explain neonatal thyroid screening report | 9, 18 | 183, 538 |
| PE33.4 | Discuss the etiopathogenesis, clinical types, presentations, complication and management of diabetes mellitus in children | 18 | 562 |
| PE33.5 | Interpret blood sugar reports and explain the diagnostic criteria for type 1 diabetes | 18 | 562 |
| PE33.7 | Perform genital examination and recognize ambiguous genitalia and refer appropriately | 18 | 558 |
| PE33.8 | Define precocious and delayed puberty | 18 | 552, 558 |
| PE33.9 | Perform sexual maturity rating (SMR) and interpret | 5 | 48 |
| PE33.10 | Recognize precocious and delayed puberty and refer | 18 | 552 |
| PE33.11 | Identify deviations in growth and plan appropriate referral | 2 | 8, 16 |
| PE34.1 | Discuss the epidemiology, clinical features, clinical types, complications of tuberculosis in children and adolescents | 11 | 254 |
| PE34.2 | Discuss the various diagnostic tools for childhood tuberculosis | 11 | 254 |
| PE34.3 | Discuss the various regimens for management of tuberculosis as per National Guidelines | 11 | 254 |
| PE34.4 | Discuss the preventive strategies adopted and the objectives and outcome of the National Tuberculosis Control Program | 11 | 254 |
| PE34.5 | Able to elicit, document and present history of contact with tuberculosis in every patient encounter | 11 | 254 |
| PE34.7 | Interpret a Mantoux test | 11 | 254 |
| PE34.8 | Interpret a chest radiograph | 11 | 254 |
| PE34.9 | Interpret blood tests in the context of laboratory evidence for tuberculosis | 11 | 254 |
| PE34.10 | Discuss the various samples for demonstrating the organism, e.g. gastric aspirate, sputum, CSF, FNAC | 11 | 254 |
| PE34.13 | Enumerate the newer diagnostic tools for tuberculosis including BACTEC CBNAAT and their indications | 11 | 254 |
| PE34.14 | Enumerate the common causes of fever and discuss the etiopathogenesis, clinical features, complications and management of fever in children | 11 | 220 |
| PE34.15 | Enumerate the common causes of fever and discuss the etiopathogenesis, clinical features, complications and management of child with exanthematous illnesses like measles, mumps, rubella and chickenpox | 11 | 220, 224, 230, 232 235 |
| PE34.16 | Enumerate the common causes of fever and discuss the etiopathogenesis, clinical features, complications and management of child with diphtheria, pertussis, tetanus | 11 | 220, 264, 265, 269 |
| PE34.17 | Enumerate the common causes of fever and discuss the etiopathogenesis, clinical features, complications and management of child with typhoid | 11 | 220, 266 |
| PE34.18 | Enumerate the common causes of fever and discuss the etiopathogenesis, clinical features, complications and management of child with dengue, chikungunya and other vector-born diseases | 11 | 240, 241 |
| PE34.19 | Enumerate the common causes of fever and discuss the etiopathogenesis, clinical features, complications and management of children with common parasitic infections, malaria, leishmaniasis, filariasis, helminthic infestations, amebiasis, giardiasis | 11 | 274 |
| PE34.20 | Enumerate the common causes of fever and discuss the etiopathogenesis, clinical features, complications and management of child with ricketsial diseases | 11 | 270 |
| PE35.1 | Identify, discuss and defend medicolegal, socio-cultural and ethical issues as they pertain to health care in children (including parental rights and right to refuse treatment) | 31 | 788, 791 |

Chapter 1

# Introduction to Pediatrics

Vinod K Paul

The branch of medicine that deals with the care of children and adolescents is *pediatrics*. This term has roots in the Greek word *pedo pais* (a child) and *iatros* (healer). The goal of the specialty is to enable a child to survive, remain healthy, and attain the highest possible potential of growth, development and cognitive achievement. A physician who specializes in the health care of children and adolescents is a *pediatrician*.

Pediatrics covers the age group less than 18 years of age which constitutes roughly 30% of the population of the country. Children under 15 years of age comprise around 25% of the population. Childhood is the state when the human being is growing and developing. It is the age to acquire good habits, values and lifestyles that would make children, the future adults, fully fit, responsible and productive citizens. The family, society and nation are duty-bound to make children feel secure, cared for, and protected from exploitation, violence and societal ills. Female children face gender bias in access to nutrition, health care and opportunities. A civilized society nurtures all its children, girls and boys alike, with love, generosity and benevolence.

Child health is a broader term that encompasses approaches, interventions and strategies that preserve, protect, promote and restore health of children at individual and population level. Child health care may be provided by health professionals other than pediatricians and physicians, such as nurses, as well as community health workers.

Child is not a miniature adult. The principles of adult medicine cannot be directly adapted to children. Pediatric biology is unique and risk factors of disease are distinct. Clinical manifestations of childhood diseases may be different from adults. Indeed, many disorders are unique to children–these do not occur in adults. Drug dosages in children are specific and not a mathematical derivation of adult dosages. Wholesome nutrition is even more important for children not only to sustain life, but also to ensure their growth and development. Child psychology and mental health are distinct domains.

Medical students should possess competencies for the care of healthy and sick children. Understanding of childhood growth, development and nutrition is fundamentally important. As future doctors, you should be patient and gentle with children. You need to learn how to communicate with the mother and the family about the child.

Pediatrics is a fascinating specialty. It encompasses care of premature neonates on the one hand, and adolescents, on the other. The discipline of pediatrics has branched into well-developed specialities (such as neonatology, nephrology, pulmonology, infectious disease, critical care, neurology, hemato-oncology, gastroenterology, endocrinology and cardiology). Pediatrics encompasses intensive care of neonates and children using the most sophisticated technology, as well as providing home care to newborns and children at the end of care spectrum. Child health is thus a state-of-art clinical science as also a vital public health discipline.

## HISTORICAL PERSPECTIVE

Medical care of children finds place in the ancient Indian, Greek and Chinese systems of health. In Ayurveda, *Kaumarabhrtya*, based on *Kashyap Samhita*, is the branch that deals with child health and disease, *Charak Samhita* and *Sushruta Samhita* also have described health care of children. As a formal discipline in modern times, pediatrics took root in Europe and the US in the 19th century when some of the famous children hospitals were established. In India, the BJ Hospital for Children, Mumbai was the first children's hospital to be established in 1928. Postgraduate diploma in pediatrics was started there in 1944. MD degree programs began in the fifties. Pediatrics became an independent subject in MBBS course in mid-nineties. The first DM program in neonatology started in 1989 at PGIMER, Chandigarh, followed by one in pediatric neurology at AIIMS in 2004. Several institutions in the country now run DM programs in various pediatric specialties that include nephrology, pulmonology, critical care, hemato-oncology, immunology, oncology, cardiology and endocrinology.

*Competency:* **PE27.1**

## CHALLENGE OF CHILD HEALTH

India has the highest number of child births as well as child deaths for any single nation in the world. Each year, as many as 2.5 crore babies are born in India. This comprises about one-fifth of the global birth cohort. Of the 50 lakh under-5 child deaths in the world each year, 8 lakh occur in our country. Table 1.1 provides the most recent figures on the key child mortality indices.

There has been a steady decline in child deaths in Inda. U5MR has fell by 75% in three decades between 1990 and 2020 from 126 to 32 per 1000 live births. Since 2000, U5MR has declined by 65%, IMR by almost 60%, and NMR by 55% **(Fig. 1.1)**. Polio and neonatal tetanus have been eliminated. Presently, majority of under-5 deaths (63%) occur in the neonatal period (<28 days of life), and the neonatal deaths account for 71% infant deaths.

**Table 1.1:** Child mortality indices in India in 2020

| *Indices* | *Rate* |
|---|---|
| Under-5 mortality rate (U5MR) | 32 per 1000 live births |
| Infant mortality rate (IMR) | 28 per 1000 live births |
| Neonatal mortality rate (NMR) | 20 per 1000 live births |
| Early neonatal mortality rate (ENMR) | 15 per 1000 live births |
| Late neonatal mortality rate (LNMR) | 5 per 1000 live births |

U5MR Number of deaths under the age of 5 years per 1000 live births
IMR Number of deaths under the age of 1 year per 1000 live births
NMR Number of deaths under the age of 28 days per 1000 live births
ENMR Number of deaths under the age of 7 days per 1000 live births
LNMR Number of deaths after completing 7 days of age but before 28 days per 1000 live births

**Table 1.2:** Child mortality targets in the National Health Policy (2017)

| |
|---|
| Reduce under-five mortality rate (U5MR) to 23 per 1000 live births by 2025 |
| Reduce neonatal mortality rate (NMR) to 16 per 1000 live births by 2025 |

Despite progress, the under-5 mortality in the country is still unacceptably high given our stature as an economic, scientific and strategic power. Under-5 mortality rate (U5MR) in Japan (3), UK (4), USA (6), Sri Lanka (7), China (7) and Brazil (15) is worth comparing with that of India (35).

The U5MR and NMR targets enshrined in the National Health Policy 2017 are depicted in Table 1.2.

### Why do Children Die?

The seven important causes of under-5 mortality in children in India (with % contribution) are: (i) Prematurity (27%), (ii) neonatal infections (13%), (iii) birth asphyxia (11%), (iv) pneumonia (11%), (v) diarrhea (9%), (vi) congenital anomalies (9%), and (vii) injuries (3%) **(Fig. 1.2)**. The above causes are the proximate conditions that lead to life-threatening situations and death. Poverty, illiteracy, low caste, rural habitat and harmful cultural practices are important determinants of ill-health. Undernutrition is a critical underlying intermediate risk factor of child mortality, associated with about 45% of under-5 child deaths. Undernutrition causes stunting and wasting, predisposes to infections and is associated with adult disorders and low economic productivity.

The agenda of high child mortality due to pneumonia, neonatal infections, preterm birth complications, diarrhea, birth asphyxia and vaccine preventable diseases is still unfinished. Yet, systemic disorders and surgical conditions also have to be addressed. The benefits of pediatric care must reach all children. Care of children with developmental

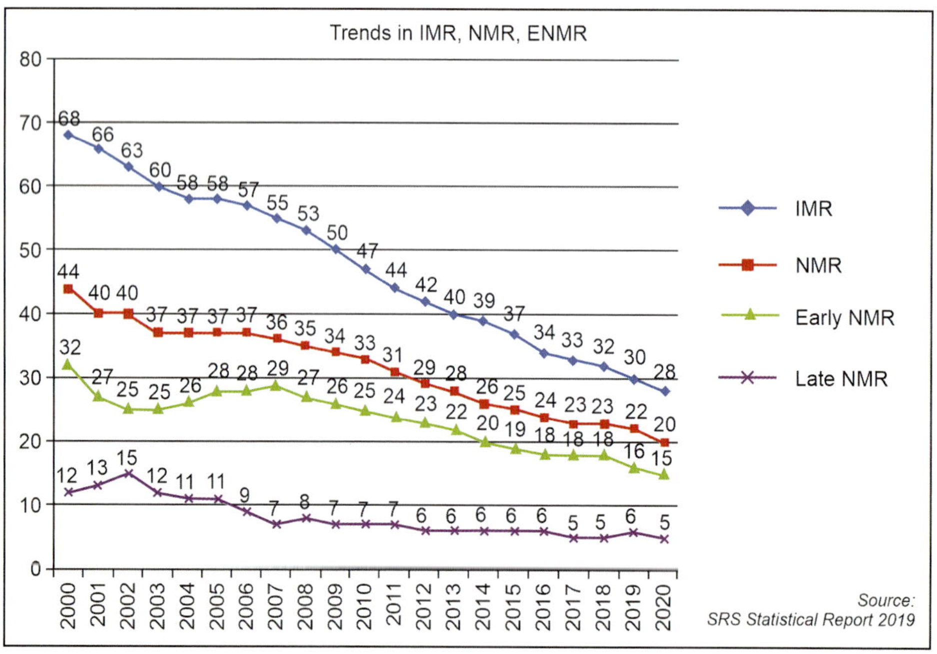


**Fig. 1.1:** Trends in neonatal and infant mortality, sample registration system. IMR infant mortality rate; NMR neonatal mortality rate

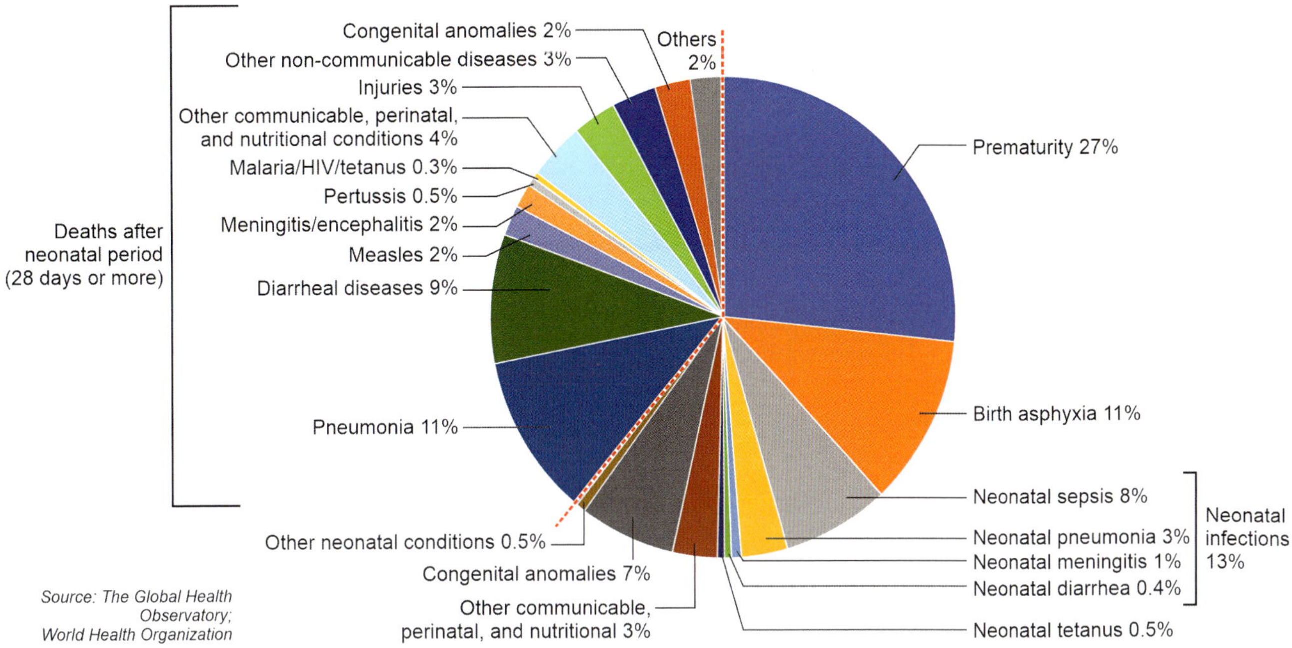


**Fig. 1.2:** Causes of deaths among children under 5 years of age. Area to the right of the dotted line indicates neonatal conditions and that on the left comprises deaths after the neonatal period

disorders, disability and mental illness deserve greater emphasis. Besides, an increasing body of knowledge on pediatric origins of non-communicable diseases of the adult is set to change the paradigm of child health. Primary prevention and early detection of future adult disorders is an important goal of pediatrics. Adolescence is associated with significant biological changes and a predilection for unique physical and behavioral challenges. This period offers a remarkable opportunity to shape positive lifestyles and prepare for adulthood.

*Competencies:* **PE17.1; PE17.2; PE18.1; PE18.2**

## NATIONAL PROGRAMS ON CHILD HEALTH

Child health has been at the core of our health policy. The Universal Immunization Program (UIP) launched in 1985 focused on immunization against six diseases (tuberculosis, poliomyelitis, diphtheria, pertussis, tetanus and measles). UIP now covers 2.67 crore newborns and 2.9 crore pregnant women annually providing free vaccines against 12 vaccine preventable diseases. The Diarrheal Disease Control Program was initiated in 1981 and Acute Respiratory Infections Control Program in 1990. In 1992, India launched the Child Survival and Safe Motherhood Program (CSSM) by combining interventions for child survival (immunization, control of diarrheal disease and respiratory infections, vitamin A supplementation, and essential newborn care) and maternal health (antenatal care, deliveries in institutions, emergency obstetric care). In 1997, the programs for family planning and the CSSM program were merged to create the Reproductive and Child Health (RCH) program. In phase 2 of the RCH program (2005), adolescent health component was also added.

The government launched the National Rural Health Mission (NRHM) in 2005. This mission included additional investments in public health, improvements in health systems, focus on communities, decentralization and demand-side interventions to improve effectiveness of the programs. The RCH program was integrated into the NRHM, with prime focus on child and maternal health. NRHM strategies include deployment of 10 lakh ASHAs; an increase in ANMs, nurses and doctors; setting up of village health and sanitation committees; strengthened primary health care infrastructure; strengthened program management capacity, establishment of patient-welfare committees at facilities, and creation of emergency transport networks. With the advent of the National Urban Health Mission, the NRHM evolved into National Health Mission (NHM).

All these efforts coupled with overall socioeconomic development are paying good dividends as evidenced by remarkable declines in child mortality referred to above. Swachh Bharat mission is further contributing toward saving lakhs of child lives.

India has attained institutional delivery rate of 89% (2019–20), a remarkable jump from just 39% in 2005–06. Over three-fourths (76.4%) of children are fully vaccinated. The use of oral rehydration solution (ORS) and zinc tablets for diarrhea has reached 61% and 31% (compared to 51% and 20% in 2015–16), respectively.

The summary of the major national programs for newborns and children is provided in Table 1.3. The roles of ASHA, AWW, ANM and CHO in maternal, newborn and child health in national programs are shown in Table 1.4.

The nation is addressing child health challenges with greater dynamism than ever before. Under Ayushman Bharat Health and Wellness Centre (HWC) program, primary care services including those for children are being strengthened nationwide. By end 2022, 1.5 lakh HWCs will become operational. Also, under Ayushman Bharat Pradhan

**Table 1.3:** Summary of newborn and child health programs

| *Pregnancy, childbirth and immediate newborn care* | *Interventions* |
|---|---|
| Skilled obstetric care and essential newborn care including resuscitation<br><br>Emergency Obstetric and Newborn care (EmONC)<br><br>Postpartum care for mother and baby | ***Package***<br>Facility deliveries by skilled birth attendants<br>Neonatal resuscitation (Navjat Shishu Suraksha Karyakram that aims to train nurses and doctors in neonatal resuscitation)<br>Essential newborn care (warmth, hygienic care, breastfeeding, extra care of small babies, kangaroo mother care, complication detection and management)<br>Linkages to facility-based newborn care for small and sick neonates<br>Linkages with home-based newborn care including postpartum care |
| *Newborn and child care* | |
| Home-based newborn care (HBNC) | Home visits by ASHAs (six for facility born babies, on days 3, 7, 14, 21, 28 and 42; an extra visit on day 1 for home births) ASHAs are paid incentive for the task.<br>***Interventions for infants:*** Examination; counsel for warmth; breastfeeding; hygiene; extra care of low birth weight babies including kangaroo mother care; detection of sickness, referral<br>***Interventions for mother:*** Postpartum care and counselling for family planning |
| Facility-based newborn care (FBNC) | ***Special newborn care units (SNCUs):*** These specialized newborn units at district hospitals with specialized equipment including radiant warmers. These units have a minimum of 12–16 beds with a staff of 3 physicians, 10 nurses and 4 support staff to provide round the clock services for newborn requiring special care, such as those with very low birth weight, neonatal sepsis/pneumonia and common complications.<br>***Newborn stabilization units (NBSUs):*** These are step down units providing facilities for neonates from the periphery where babies can be stabilized through effective care. These are set up in community health centres (CHCs) and provide services including resuscitation, provision of warmth, initiation of breastfeeding, prevention of infection and cord care, supportive care (oxygen, IV fluids, provision for monitoring of vital signs), and referral.<br>***Newborn care corners (NBCCs):*** These are special corners within the labor room at all public health facilities where deliveries occur. Services include resuscitation, provision of warmth, prevention of infections and early initiation of breastfeeding. |
| Integrated Management of Neonatal and Childhood Illness (IMNCI) | Integrated Management of Neonatal and Childhood Illness (IMNCI) by ANMs (community IMNCI) and at first level facility (PHC).<br>Facility – IMNCI at first referral level (e.g. CHC). Focuses on providing inpatient management of major causes of childhood mortality such as asphyxia, sepsis, low birth weight and pneumonia, diarrhea, malaria, meningitis and severe malnutrition |
| Universal Immunization Program (UIP) | Under UIP, immunization is provided free of cost against 12 vaccine preventable diseases. These include: Diphtheria, pertussis, tetanus, polio, measles, rubella, tuberculosis, hepatitis B; meningitis and pneumonia caused by *Hemophilus influenzae* type B; pneumonia caused by pneumococci; diarrhea caused by rotavirus; and Japanese encephalitis (in endemic areas). |
| Home Based Care for Young Child (HBYC) | Home visits by ASHAs in the 3rd, 6th, 9th, 12th and 15th month. The purposes are:<br>• Promoting good child nutrition, especially exclusive breastfeeding and appropriate and adequate complementary feeding from 6 months of age<br>• Ensuring age appropriate immunization<br>• Ensuring optimal early childhood development<br>• Promoting *swachh* practices<br>• Ensuring health care seeking behavior |
| Rashtriya Bal Swasthya Karyakram (RBSK) | Child health screening and early intervention services through mobile health teams at block level. Screening of all children (0–6 years old) enrolled at least twice a year for 30 disorders (4Ds).<br>***Defects*** (neural tube defect, Down syndrome, cleft lip/palate, club foot, dysplasia hip, congenital cataract or deafness, congenital heart diseases and retinopathy of prematurity)<br>***Deficiencies*** (anemia, vitamin A deficiency, vitamin D deficiency, severe acute malnutrition and goiter)<br>***Diseases*** (skin conditions, otitis media, rheumatic heart disease, reactive airway disease, dental caries and convulsions)<br>***Development delays and disabilities*** (vision or hearing impairment, neuromotor impairment, motor delay, cognitive delay, language delay, behavior disorder, learning disorders, attention deficit hyperactivity disorder)<br>***Optional*** (congenital hypothyroidism, sickle cell anemia, beta thalassemia) Free management of these children at district early interventions centres or identified tertiary level institutions |

Table 1.4: Roles of grassroot team members in child health

| Provider | Role in maternal, newborn and child health |
|---|---|
| **ASHA** (accredited social health activist) | • Mobilizing pregnant mother for antenatal check and care<br>• Accompanying pregnant mother to facility for delivery<br>• Home care of the newborns and postpartum mothers<br>• Home care of young children<br>• Facilitating immunization<br>• Promoting complementary feeding<br>• Home and community-based care of diarrhea and pneumonia<br>• Health education |
| **AWW** (Anganwari worker) | • Providing nutrition supplement to pregnant mothers and children<br>• Facilitating antenatal checks and immunization<br>• Promoting infant and young child feeding<br>• Growth monitoring of children<br>• Supplementary nutrition to children<br>• Managing malnourished children<br>• Non-formal pre-school education |
| **ANM** (auxiliary nurse midwife) | • Antenatal checks and care of pregnant mothers<br>• Immunization<br>• Supervising ASHAs and AWWs in all newborn and child care<br>• Providing IMNCI services for neonates and children<br>• Health education |
| **CHO** (community health officer) | As incharge of the health and wellness centre provides outpatient and preventive care to children (if required, by teleconsulting a physician) |

Mantri Jan Arogya Yojana (PMJAY), treatment up to 5 lakh per annum per family is available free for more than 40% of our population *including children,* in 25,000 public and private hospitals.

## EPILOGUE

The country is surging ahead with ever stronger economy and accelerated development in all spheres. The realization of the demographic dividend of the nation depends on ensuring good health, nutrition, development, education and opportunities for all our children. Child health, wellbeing and welfare is a paramount national and societal priority. India will ensure that none of her children is left behind.

### Suggested Reading

1. National Health Mission. https://nhm.gov.in/
2. National Family Health Survey 5 (2019–20), National Fact Sheet, 2021; http://rchiips.org
3. Registrar General of India (2019). Sample Registration System (SRS) statistical report 2020. New Delhi: Registrar General of India.
4. World Health Organization. Global Health Observatory. https://www.who.int/data/gho/data/countries

Chapter 2

# Growth

❍ Ramesh Agarwal ❍ Naveen Sankhyan ❍ Vandana Jain

*Competency:* **PE1.1**

## CONCEPT OF GROWTH

The term growth denotes a net increase in the size or mass of tissues. It is attributed mainly to the multiplication of cells and the increase in the intracellular substance. Hypertrophy or expansion of cell size contributes to a lesser extent to the process of growth. Growth is an essential feature that distinguishes a child from an adult. The growth process of a child starts from conception into a fully mature adult. The terms 'growth' and 'development' are often used together but are not interchangeable because they represent two different facets of change dynamics, i.e., quantity and quality.

Development specifies the maturation of functions. It is related to the maturation and myelination of the nervous system. It indicates the acquisition of various skills for the individual's optimal functioning.

Growth and development usually proceed concurrently. While they are discussed separately, growth and development are closely related; hence, factors affecting one tend to impact the other. During the early embryonic period of life, an exponential increase in the number of cells occurs. At the early embryonic stage, fetal cells divide and differentiate to form tissues and organs. In the latter half of pregnancy and early childhood, there is also an increase in cell size that manifests as an increase in the protein-to-DNA ratio. The cell size continues to enlarge until about 10 years of age. The body cells remain in dynamic equilibrium; hence aging cells are continuously replaced by new cells. The rate of turnover of cells in different tissues is variable.

*Competency:* **PE1.2**

## BIOLOGY OF GROWTH

### Laws of Growth

The growth and development of children is a continuous and orderly process. There are specific periods in a child's life when the growth rate is steady, accelerates, or decelerates (Table 2.1). The fetus grows fast in the first half of gestation. After that, the growth rate is slowed until the baby is born. The growth velocity is high in the early postnatal period, especially in the first few months. After that, there is a slower but steady growth during mid-childhood. The second phase of accelerated growth occurs at puberty. Growth decelerates after that for some time and then ceases altogether (Fig. 2.1).

**Table 2.1:** Periods of growth

| | |
|---|---|
| **Prenatal period** | |
| Ovum | 0 to 2 weeks |
| Embryo | 3 to 8 weeks |
| Fetus | 9 weeks to birth |
| Perinatal period | 22 weeks to 7 days after birth |
| **Postnatal period** | |
| Newborn | First 4 weeks after birth |
| Infant | Birth to <12 months (neonate: Birth to 28 days; post-neonate: 29 days to <1 year) |
| Toddler | 1 year to 36 months |
| Preschool child | 37–72 months |
| School-age child | 73 months–12 years |
| **Adolescence** | 10–19 years |
| Early | 10–13 years |
| Middle | 14–16 years |
| Late | 17–19 years |

***The growth pattern of every individual is unique:*** The order of growth is cephalocaudal and distal to proximal. During fetal life, the growth of the head occurs before that of the neck, and arms grow before the legs. Distal body parts, such as hands, increase in size before the upper arms. In postnatal life, the growth of the head slows down, but limbs continue to grow rapidly.

#### *Different Tissues Grow at Different Rates* (Fig. 2.2)

***Brain growth:*** The brain enlarges rapidly during the latter months of fetal life and early months of postnatal life. At

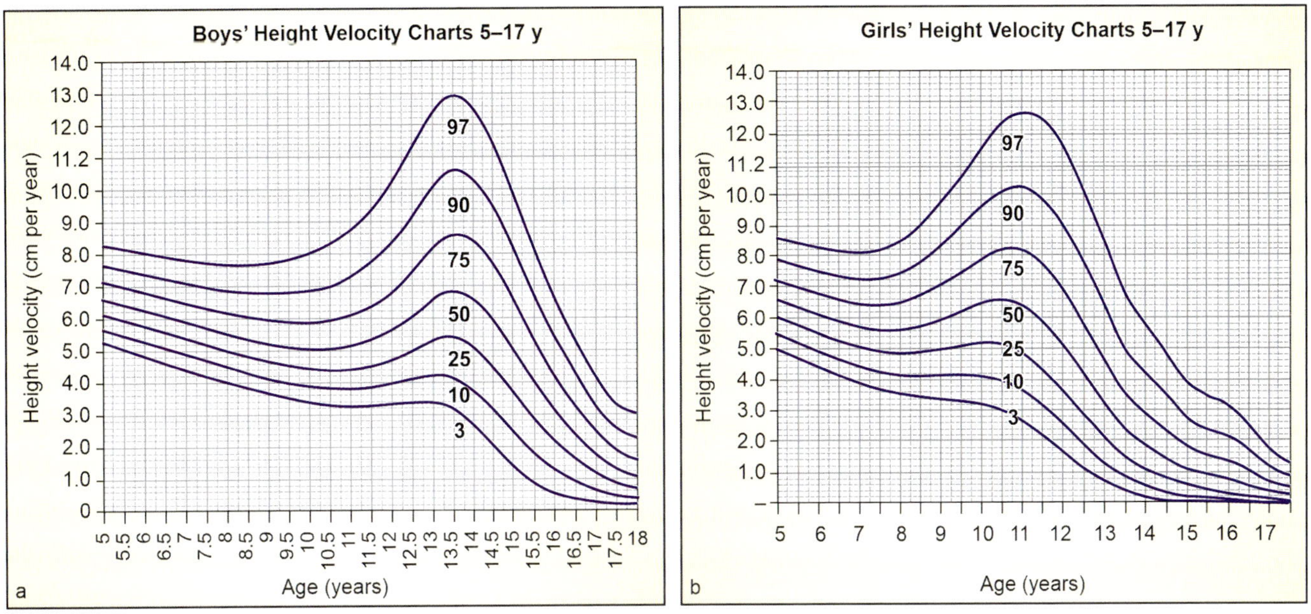


**Fig. 2.1:** (a) Height velocity percentiles for Indian boys aged 5–17 years; (b) Height velocity percentiles for Indian girls aged 5–17 years (Reference: Khadilkar V, Khadilkar A, Arya A, et al. Height velocity percentiles in Indian children aged 5–17 years. Indian Pediatr 2019;56:23–28)



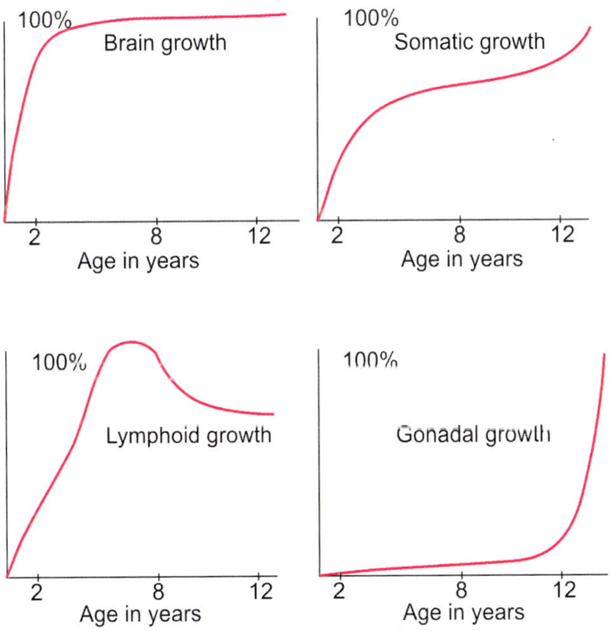


**Fig. 2.2:** Rates of growth of different tissues and organs

birth, the head size is about 65–70% of the expected head size in adults. It reaches 90% of the adult head size in two years. Thus, the fetal period and the first two years are a critical phase for brain development. Later periods are also important for acquiring neuromotor functions and cognitive abilities.

*Growth of gonads:* Gonadal growth is dormant during childhood and becomes conspicuous during puberty.

*Lymphoid growth:* The growth of lymphoid tissue is most notable during the mid-childhood. During this period, the lymphoid tissue is overgrown, and its mass may appear larger than that of a fully mature adult. A sign of accelerated lymphoid growth is the frequent finding of large tonsils and palpable lymph nodes in normal children between 4 and 8 years.

*Growth of body fat and muscle mass:* Body tissues can be divided into fat and fat-free (lean) components. The lean body mass includes muscle tissue, internal organs, and skeleton. The growth in lean body mass is primarily due to increased skeletal and muscle mass.

Lean body mass correlates closely with stature. Taller children have greater lean body mass than shorter children of the same age. After the pubertal growth spurt, boys have greater lean body mass than girls. Body fat, a storehouse of energy, is primarily deposited in the subcutaneous adipose tissue. Girls have more subcutaneous adipose tissue than boys. Moreover, the sites and quantity of adipose tissue differ in girls and boys. Girls tend to add adipose tissue to breasts, buttocks, thighs, and back of arms during adolescence.

*Skeletal growth:* Skeletal growth is a continuous process occurring throughout childhood and adolescence. It is steady until the pubertal growth spurt, when it accelerates and subsequently slows considerably. The skeleton matures once the epiphysis or growth plates at the end of long bones fuse to the shaft or diaphysis. This occurs by about 18 years in girls and 20–22 years in boys. The degree of skeletal maturation closely correlates with the degree of sexual maturation. Obesity/overweight is also associated with advancement in skeletal maturation. Skeletal maturation is assessed by noting the appearance and fusion of epiphysis at the ends of long bones.

### Bone Age Estimation

Assessment of bone age postnatally is based on (i) the number, shape, and size of epiphyseal centers, and (ii) the size, shape, and density of the ends of bones. Bone age is typically assessed on the radiograph of left hand and wrist, using bone age atlases (such as those by Gruelich and Pyle or Tanner and Whitehouse) or software such as BoneXpert.

Table 2.2: Timing of dentition

| Primary dentition | Time of eruption, months | | Time of fall, years | | |
|---|---|---|---|---|---|
| | Upper | Lower | Upper | Lower | |
| Central incisors | 8–12 | 6–10 | 6–7 | 6–7 | |
| Lateral incisors | 9–13 | 10–16 | 7–8 | 7–8 | |
| First molar | 13–19 | 14–18 | 9–11 | 9–11 | |
| Canine | 16–22 | 17–23 | 10–12 | 9–12 | |
| Second molar | 25–33 | 23–31 | 10–12 | 10–12 | |
| *Permanent teeth* | *Time of eruption, years* | | | | |
| | Upper | Lower | | Upper | Lower |
| First molar | 6–7 | 6–7 | First premolar | 10–11 | 10–12 |
| Central incisors | 7–8 | 6–7 | Second premolar | 10–12 | 10–12 |
| Lateral incisors | 8–9 | 7–8 | Second molar | 12–13 | 11–13 |
| Canine | 11–12 | 10–12 | Third molar | 17–21 | 17–21 |

*Eruption of teeth:* For primary teeth, the teeth in the upper jaw erupt earlier than those in the lower jaw, except for lower central incisors and second molar. At the same time, the first molars are the first permanent teeth to erupt (Table 2.2).

Competency: **PE1.1**

## FACTORS AFFECTING GROWTH

### Fetal Growth

Fetal growth is influenced primarily by fetal, placental, and maternal factors. The fetus has inherent growth potential and grows into a healthy, appropriate-sized newborn under normal circumstances. The maternal-placental-fetal unit acts harmoniously to provide for the needs of the fetus.

*Genetic potential:* Intrauterine growth is mainly determined by the genetic potential of the fetus, with environmental and nutritional factors acting as modulators. There is a strong correlation of maternal weight and height with the birth weight. This so-called 'maternal constraint' limits overgrowth of the fetus, thus preventing dystocia, and conserving mother's ability to have further pregnancies.

*Sex:* Boys are generally taller and heavier than girls at birth.

*Fetal hormones and growth factors:* The most important endocrine factors regulating growth in fetal life are insulin, insulin-like growth factor (IGF)-1 and IGF-2. Insulin is secreted by the fetal pancreas in response to the nutrient supply, whereas IGFs are chiefly produced by the placenta. An adequate supply of triiodothyronine ($T_3$) derived from maternal free thyroxine ($T_4$) is needed for fetal neurodevelopment. Fetal thyroid hormone production begins in the 12th week but is low, and maternal $T_4$ is important throughout gestation. Glucocorticoids also play an essential role, primarily towards the end of gestation, influencing the prepartum maturation of organs such as the liver, lungs, and gastrointestinal tract. Growth hormone, though present in high levels in fetuses, does not have a major influence on fetal growth.

*Placental factors:* As in most species, fetal weight directly correlates with placental weight at term. Fetal growth is highly dependent on the structural and functional integrity of the placenta. With advancing gestation, the weight of the placenta increases to cater to the baby's increased needs. Significant functional and structural changes in the placenta make this adaptation more efficient. The total villous surface area increases, the diffusion distance decreases, the fetal capillaries dilate, and the resistance in fetoplacental vasculature falls. This positive remodeling facilitates nutrient transport across the placenta.

*Maternal factors:* The mother's own fetal and childhood growth, her current height and weight, and her nutrient intake at the time of conception and during pregnancy play a vital role in determining fetal size. In India, half the women who enter pregnancy are anemic, while one in five women are undernourished. Teen or advanced age, recent pregnancy, high parity, and anemia negatively influence fetal size and health. Maternal intake of tobacco (smoked or chewed) and drug or alcohol abuse also retard fetal growth. Obstetric complications such as pregnancy-induced hypertension, pre-eclampsia, and multiple pregnancies produce fetal growth restriction. Pre-existing chronic systemic disease (chronic kidney disease, congestive heart failure) and acquired infections (rubella, syphilis, hepatitis B, HIV, CMV, toxoplasmosis) may influence fetal growth. Maternal obesity, by increasing the risk of gestational diabetes, hypertension and pre-eclampsia, can also adversely affect fetal outcome.

### Postnatal Period

The child's growth during postnatal life is determined by genetic potential and internal and external influences.

*Genetic factors:* Chromosomal disorders and mutations in specific genes can affect growth. Chromosomal defects like Turner syndrome and Down syndrome manifest as growth retardation. Certain single-gene disorders may also result in retardation of growth, e.g., Prader-Willi syndrome and Noonan syndrome. While most genetic disorders lead to short stature, some defects can also result in tall stature, e.g., Klinefelter syndrome and Sotos syndrome.

*Intrauterine growth restriction (IUGR):* IUGR resulting in low birth weight (LBW) constitutes a significant risk factor for postnatal malnutrition and poor growth. LBW increases the chances of being underweight, stunting, and wasting in the first five years of life. It is estimated that about 90% of infants born small for gestational age (SGA) catch-up in weight and length during first two years of life, but up to 10% remain short.

During early infancy, exclusive breastfeeding provides adequate nutrition, prevents infections, and protects infants from further undernourishment. However, at 3–5 months, the widespread practice of supplementing infants with animal milk increases morbidity due to infections leading to underweight and stunting. Subsequently, faulty complementary feeding practices (too late; too little; too less energy density; too less diversity of food items), poor hygiene, and frequent infections further increase underweight rates and stunting. On the other hand, overfeeding and cosumption of junk food or force-feeding of infants with calorie-dense formulae can lead to upward crossing of centiles and increase the risk of developing obesity in childhood.

*Hormonal influence:* Normal growth cannot proceed without the proper milieu of hormones in the body throughout childhood and adolescence. Absence of growth hormone or thyroxine results in poor linear growth, underscoring the importance of these factors in promoting growth. During adolescence, androgens and estrogens have an important influence on the growth spurt and final adult height.

*Sex:* The pubertal growth spurt occurs earlier in girls, but the peak height velocity attained in puberty is lower than boys. This, combined with the shorter duration of the pubertal spurt and the earlier onset, leads to a mean difference in adult height of about 13 cm between males and females.

*Nutrition:* The growth of children suffering from protein-energy malnutrition, anemia, and vitamin deficiency is retarded. Calcium, iron, zinc, iodine, and vitamins A and D are closely related to growth and development disorders. On the other hand, overeating and obesity accelerate somatic growth during childhood, but with no effect on the final height.

*Infections:* In low-resource settings, infections are among the commonest contributors to poor childhood growth. Persistent or recurrent diarrhea and respiratory tract infections are common causes of growth impairment. Systemic infections and parasitic infestations may also retard the velocity of growth. The risk of stunting at two years of age increases with each episode of diarrhea and each day of diarrhea before two years of age. The attributable risk for stunting for five or more bouts of diarrhea before 24 months of age is 25%.

*Trauma:* A fracture at the end of a bone may damage the growing epiphysis and thus hamper skeletal growth.

### Social Factors

*Socioeconomic level:* Children from families with high socioeconomic levels usually have a better nutritional state. They suffer from fewer infections because of better nutrition and hygienic living conditions.

*Poverty:* Hunger, undernutrition, and infections, often associated with poverty, cause poor growth.

*Natural resources:* Plentiful natural resources encourage industrial and agricultural enterprise in the country. Improved nutrition of children in the community is facilitated when there is a rise in gross national product and per capita income.

*Climate:* The growth velocity may alter in different seasons, usually higher in spring and low in summer months. Infections and infestations are common in a hot and humid climate. Weather also has a pivotal effect on agricultural productivity, ready availability of food, and capacity for strenuous labor by the population.

*Emotional factors:* Children from broken homes and orphanages do not grow and develop optimally. Anxiety, insecurity, and lack of emotional support and love from the family prejudice the neurochemical regulation of growth hormone release. Parents with a happy childhood and cheerful personalities are more likely to have children with similar countenances.

*Cultural factors:* The community's methods of child-rearing and infant feeding are determined by cultural habits and conventions. There may be religious taboos against the consumption of particular types of food. These affect the nutritional state and growth performance of children.

*Parental education:* Mothers with more education are more likely to adopt appropriate health-promoting behaviors, directly and indirectly influencing growth and development.

*Competencies:* **PE1.3; PE1.4; PE33.11**

## ASSESSMENT OF PHYSICAL GROWTH

*Weight:* The child's weight in the nude (for newborns or infants) or in minimal light clothing and without footwear, is recorded accurately on a lever or electronic weighing scale (Fig. 2.3). Spring balances are less accurate. The child must be placed in the middle of the weighing pan. Correct the zero error before weighing. Weigh a small baby with the mother/caregiver **(Panel 1)**.

*Length:* Length is recorded for children under two years of age. Hairpins are removed, and braids are undone. Bulky diapers should be removed. The child is placed supine on a rigid measuring table or an infantometer. One person holds the head firmly in position against a fixed

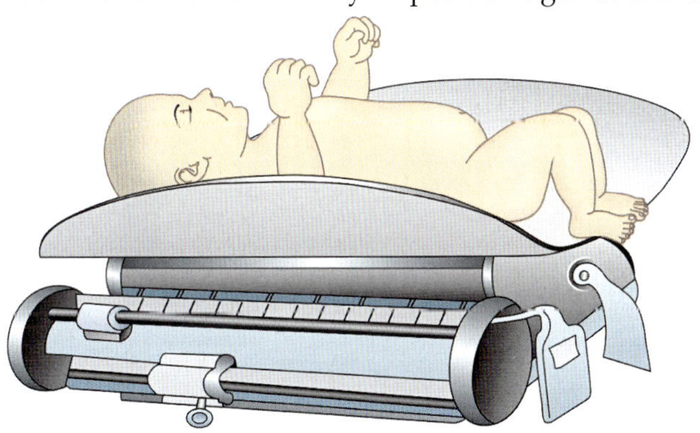

**Fig. 2.3:** Beam scale for accurate measurement of weight. The child should be nude or in minimal clothing

**Panel 1: Steps in weighing a small baby with the mother/caregiver (Fig. 2.4)**

1. Use an adult weighing scale.
2. Place the weighing scale on a flat, hard, and even surface. Correct the zero error.
3. Babies should be weighed naked or with minimal clothing.
4. Ask the mother/caregiver to take the baby in her lap and stand in the middle of the scale, feet slightly apart and to remain still. Take the measurement (W2)
5. Now weigh the mother alone without the baby (W1).
6. Calculate baby's weight: W2–W1

***Note:*** If the mother is very heavy (e.g. 100 kg), then a lighter person should hold the baby on the tared scale.

**Panel 2: Steps in measuring length (Fig. 2.5)**

1. Place the child on his back on a clean length board (use a clean cloth to make the board comfortable)
2. Ensure that the head is in firm contact with the headboard
3. Position the head such that the child is looking straight up (the line joining the external auditory meatus and the lower border of the eyeball is perpendicular to the board
4. The shoulders and the spine should be in touch with the board and the knees should be gently straightened.
5. The footboard should be moved to ensure that the feet are firmly against it.
6. Measure the length in this position.

***Note:*** Be gentle with newborns, their knees may not straighten fully. If it is not possible to position both knees, then measure with one leg in position.

*Reference:* World Health Organization. Training Course on Child Growth Assessment. Geneva, WHO, 2008.

upright headboard. Legs are straightened, keeping feet at right angles to legs, with toes pointing upward. The free footboard is brought into firm contact with the child's heels (Fig. 2.5). The baby's length is measured from a scale set on the measuring table. Measuring the length of a child lying on a mattress and using cloth tapes is inaccurate and not recommended **(Panel 2)**.

***Height:*** For height, the child stands upright. Heels are slightly separated, and the weight is borne evenly on both feet. Heels, buttocks, shoulder blades, and the back of the head are brought in contact with a vertical surface such as the wall, height measuring rod, or a stadiometer. The head is so positioned that the child looks directly forwards with the Frankfort plane (the line joining the root of the external auditory meatus to the lower margin of the orbit) and the biauricular plane being horizontal. The headpiece is kept firmly over the head to compress the hair (Fig. 2.6 and **Panel 3**).

***Head circumference:*** Hair ornaments are removed and braids undone. Using a nonstretchable tape, the maximum circumference of the head from the occipital protuberance to the supraorbital ridges on the forehead is recorded

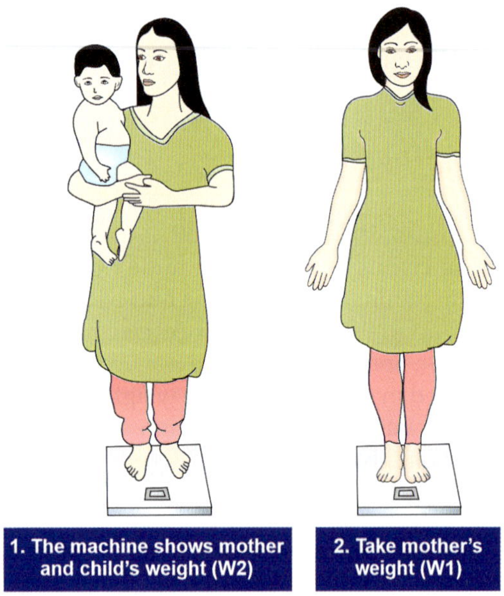


**Fig. 2.4:** Weighing a small child with mother on a weighing scale with taring facility

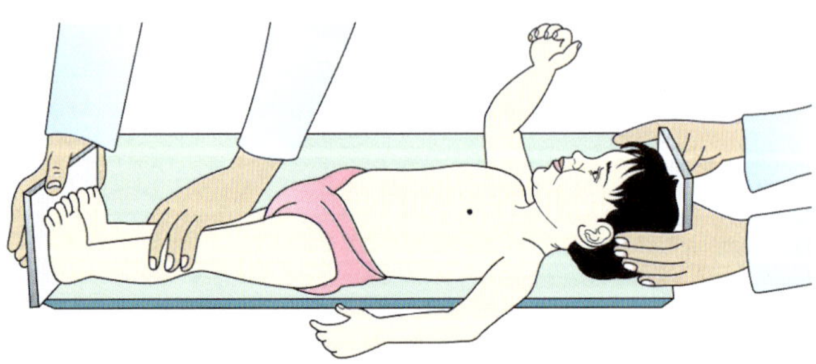

**Fig. 2.5:** Measurement of length on an infantometer. Note how the knees are gently straightened while the head and feet are aligned

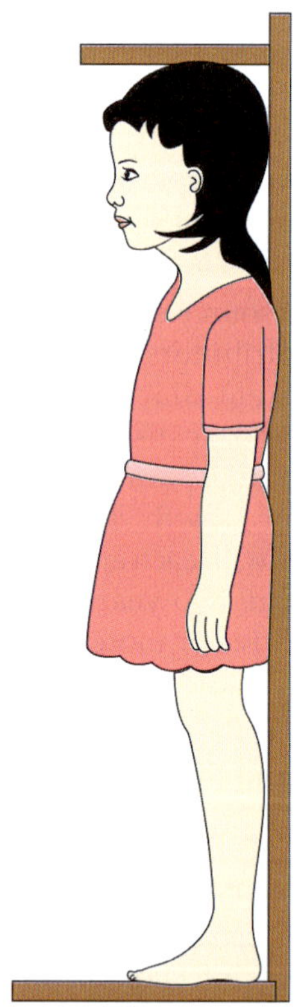

**Fig. 2.6:** Method of recording height. Note the erect posture and the bare feet placed flat on the ground. The back of heels, buttocks, shoulders and occiput are touching the wall

**Panel 3: Steps in measuring standing height (Fig. 2.6)**

1. The child's footwear and any hair tie-up should be removed.
2. The child should stand on the height board with the back of the head, shoulders, buttocks, calves, and heels touching the vertical board.
3. Position the head such that the child is looking straight ahead (the line joining the external auditory meatus and the lower border of the eyeball should be parallel to the floor)
4. With the child still in this position, the headboard is gently pulled down to rest firmly on the head.
5. Measure the height in this position.

*Reference:* World Health Organization. Training Course on Child Growth Assessment. Geneva, WHO, 2008.

(Fig. 2.7). A special head tape is now available and can be used to measure the head circumference accurately.

*Chest circumference:* The chest circumference is measured at the level of the nipples, midway between inspiration and expiration (Fig. 2.8).

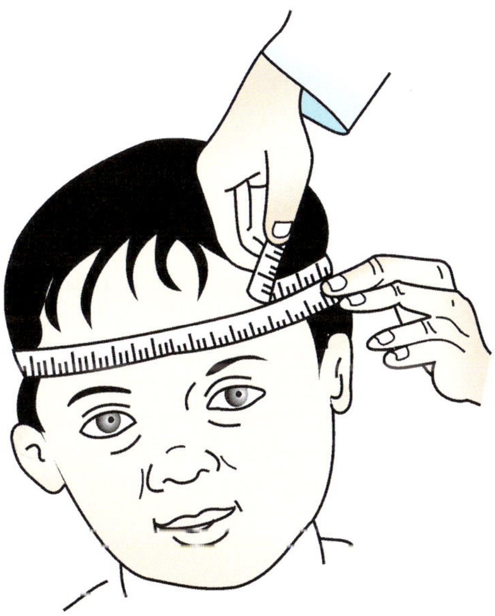

Fig. 2.7: Method of recording head circumference

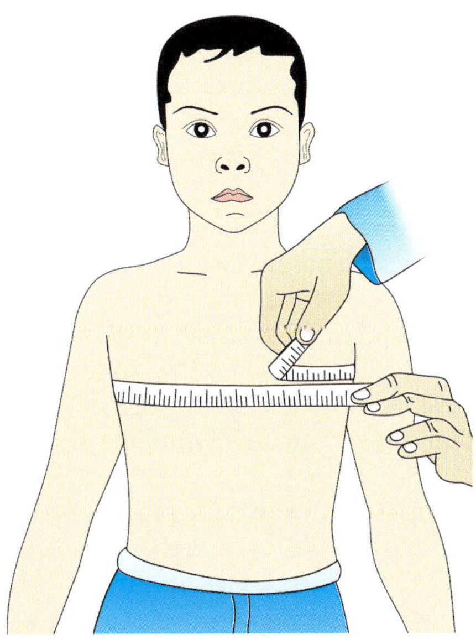

Fig. 2.8: Method of measurement of chest circumference at the level of nipples

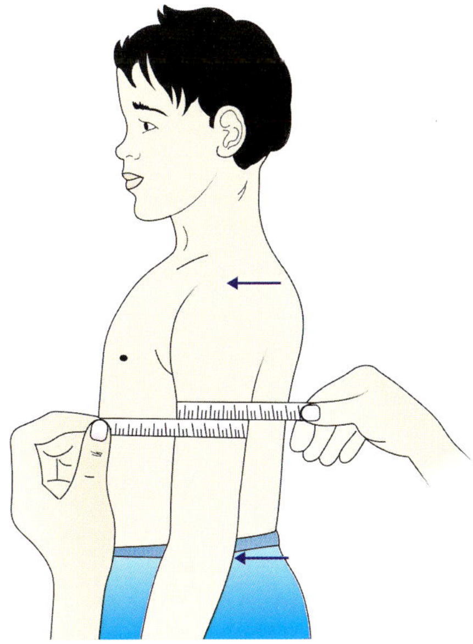

Fig. 2.9: Measurement of mid-upper arm circumference. Note how the anatomical landmarks are first located (arrows) to accurately measure the circumference

*Mid-upper arm circumference:* To measure the mid-upper arm circumference (MAC), first mark a point midway between the tip of the acromion process of the scapula and the olecranon of the ulna on the left side. Take the measurement while the child keeps the arm by his side, straight at the elbow (Fig. 2.9). Ensure the tape is tight enough to avoid any gap and compression of soft tissues.

## Normal Growth

It is difficult to define the normal pattern of growth precisely. Generally, it implies an average of readings obtained in a group of healthy individuals, along with a permissible range of variation, i.e., between the third and ninety seventh percentiles. Most healthy children maintain their growth percentile on the growth charts as the years pass. A significant deviation in a child's plotted position on the growth chart can be due to a recent illness or over- or undernutrition. It is also essential to consider the gestational age of infants born prematurely. The duration of prematurity is subtracted from the infant's chronological age (corrected age). This correction, however, is not required after two to three years of age.

*Weight:* The average birth weight of Indian neonates is about 3 kg. During the first few days after birth, the newborn loses extracellular fluid equivalent to about 7 to 10% of the body weight. Most infants regain their birth weight by the age of 10 days. Subsequently, they gain weight at approximately 20–40 g per day for the first three months of life. After that, they gain about 400 g of weight every month for the remaining part of the first year. An infant usually doubles his birth weight by the age of 5 months. The birth weight triples at one year and is four times at two years of age. Thus, the weight at five months, one year, and two years is approximately 6, 9, and 12 kg, respectively. A child's weight at the age of 3 years is about five times that of the birth weight. The expected weight can be calculated at five years by multiplying the birth weight by 6, 7 years

**Table 2.3:** Approximate anthropometric values by age

| Age | Weight (kg) | Length or height (cm) | Head circumference (cm) |
|---|---|---|---|
| Birth | 3 | 50 | 34 |
| 6 months | 6 (doubles) | 65 | 43 |
| 1 year | 9 (triples) | 75 | 46 |
| 2 years | 12 (quadruples) | 87 | 48 |
| 3 years | 15 | 95 | 49 |
| 4 years | 16 | 100 | 50 |

by 7, and 10 years by 10. The expected weight at 3, 5, 7, and 10 years is approximately 15, 18, 21, and 30 kg, respectively. On average, a child gains about 2 kg every year between the ages of 3 and 7 years and 3 kg per year until the pubertal growth spurt begins (Table 2.3).

*Length or height:* The infant measures approximately 50 cm at birth, 60 cm at three months, 65 cm at six months, 70 cm at nine months, 75 cm at one year, and 87 cm at two years. A normal child gains about 6 cm in height every year until 12 years. After this, height increments vary according to the age at the onset of puberty. There is a marked acceleration of growth during puberty.

*Head circumference (HC):* Head growth is rapid, especially in the first half of infancy. It reflects brain growth during this period. The head growth slows considerably after that. Thirty-four cm on average at birth, the head circumference increases approximately 2 cm per month for the first three months, 1 cm per month between 3 and 6 months, and 0.5 cm per month for the rest of the first year of life. The head circumference is approximately 40 cm at three months, 43 cm at six months, 46–47 cm at one year, and 48 cm at two years. By 12 years, it is 52 cm.

*Chest circumference:* The chest circumference is about 3 cm less than the head circumference at birth. The circumference of the head and chest are almost equal by the age of 1 year. After that, the chest circumference exceeds the head circumference.

*Body mass index (BMI):* The formula to calculate BMI is the weight (kg)/height (meter)$^2$. BMI is a better measurement than weight alone to assess obesity as well as undernutrition.

*Competencies:* **PE1.3; PE1.4**

## GROWTH CHARTS

Growth charts are a good tool for growth surveillance. If a child's growth measurements are plotted on a graph, the deviation in the child's growth from the normal pattern can be easily interpreted. The normal variation in growth is taken as values between the 3rd and 97th percentiles curves. Percentile curves represent frequency distribution curves. For example, the 25th percentile for height in a population would mean that the height of 75% of individuals is above, and 24% is below this value. One standard deviation score (SDS) above the mean coincides with the 84th percentile curve. Likewise, the 16th percentile curve represents one SDS below the mean. Values between the third and 97th percentile curves correspond to mean ±2 SDS.

*z-scores:* In a population with observations in a typical Gaussian (normal) distribution, any individual value can be expressed as how many SDS it lies above or below the mean. This is the z-score for that observation. Thus, if a child's weight is 2 SDS below the mean, it is equivalent to –2 z. If the value lies above the mean, z-score is positive; otherwise, it is negative. The formula for calculating the z-score is:

$$\text{z-score} = \frac{\text{Observed value} - \text{mean value}}{\text{Standard deviation}}$$

z-score allows the comparison of different observations between individuals. For example, one can compare the height and weight of two individuals by obtaining the respective z-scores.

### Growth Standards

Growth standards represent growth norms and can be presented in a tabular or graphical manner. These are obtained by either cross-sectional or longitudinal studies in large populations. Based on data obtained from US children, the National Center for Health Statistics (NCHS) developed growth charts in 1977. In the year 2000, revised growth charts provided by CDC offered an improved tool to assess child health. However, these charts were based on data obtained from formula-fed US children.

Sensing the need for more internationally applicable growth standards, the WHO conducted the Multicentre Growth Reference Study (MGRS) and published new growth charts for infants and children up to 5 years of age in 2006. The MGRS was a community-based, multi-country project conducted in Brazil, Ghana, India, Norway, Oman, and the United States. The children included in the study were raised in environments that minimized growth constraints such as poor nutrition and infection. In addition, their mothers followed healthy practices such as breastfeeding their children and did not smoke during and after pregnancy. These WHO child growth standards are unique on several counts. They provide data on 'how children should grow and go beyond the traditional descriptive references. The new standards make breastfeeding the biological norm and establish the breastfed infant as the normative growth model. The pooled sample from the six participating countries makes it a truly international standard. It reiterates that child populations grow similarly across the world's major regions when their needs for health and care are met. These standards also include new growth indicators beyond height and weight that are particularly useful for monitoring the increasing epidemic of childhood obesity, such as skinfold thickness. The study's longitudinal nature further allows the development of growth velocity standards, enabling the early identification of under or over-nourishment. **Annexures 1–8** provide curves of z-score for weight, length or height, weight for height, and head circumference for girls and boys up to 5 years of age based on WHO MGRS standards.

Growth standards are not available for children older than five years. The Indian Academy of Pediatrics (IAP) has provided updated growth reference charts for children aged 5 to 18 years based on data from 33148 children **(Annexures 9–12)**. The charts can also be downloaded from https://iapindia.org/iap-growth-charts/.

**Annexures 13–18** provide detailed tables for SDS for weight, height, weight for height or length, body mass index (BMI) and head circumference for children <5 years old, based on WHO-MGRS standards. **Annexures 19 and 20** provide tables for centiles for weight, height and BMI for children 5–18 years old, based on IAP charts.

There are consolidated charts that combine WHO-MGRS and IAP charts for monitoring children from 0 to 18 years. [doi.org/10.1515/jpem-2020-0573]

### Velocity of Growth

Plotting a child's height and weight on a growth chart helps determine, if he is within the normal range for their age. One-time measurement, however, does not indicate if the child's growth rate has been normal in the recent past. The position on the growth chart becomes abnormal only when the factors retarding growth are profound or have persisted for a long time. On the other hand, serial measurements provide the rate of growth. Plotting growth velocity is a valuable tool for the early identification of factors affecting growth. The velocity of growth more accurately helps in predicting the ultimate adult height.

***Interpretation of growth measurements:*** Table 2.4 provides details regarding the interpretation of growth charts.

### Growth Monitoring

During infancy, growth monitoring is conveniently done during visits for vaccination. Later it can be integrated into visits for vaccination, minor illnesses, or a school health program. After 7–8 years of age, sexual maturity rating (SMR) staging should also be monitored (Table 2.5).

### Software and Apps to Assist Anthropometric Analysis for Clinical and Research Use

The WHO provides software "*WHO-Anthro*" for anthropometric analysis. The software consists of three modules: An anthropometric calculator, an individual assessment, and a nutritional survey. The software is



**Table 2.4:** Interpretation of growth parameters in children 0–18 years old

| **Age**<br>*Reference/standard* | **≤5 years**<br>*MGRS* | **>5 years**<br>*IAP* | |
|---|---|---|---|
| ***Stature*** | **Height** | **Height** | |
| Stunting/short stature | <–2 SDS, or <3rd centile | –2 SDS or <3rd centile | |
| Severe stunting | <–3 SDS | Not applicable | |
| ***Undernutrition*** | **Weight for height**[1] | **Body mass index** | |
| Wasting | <–2 SDS or <3rd centile | Not applicable | |
| Severe wasting | <–3 SDS | Not applicable | |
| Thinness | Not applicable | <–1.88 SDS or <3rd centile | |
| | **Weight** | | |
| Underweight (very low weight) | <–2 SDS or <3rd centile | Not applicable | |
| Severely underweight | <–3 SDS | Not applicable | |
| ***Overnutrition*** | **Weight for height SDS** | **Body mass index SDS** | |
| *Sex* | *Either* | *Boys* | *Girls* |
| Overweight | ≥+2 to +3 | ≥+0.55 to +1.33[2] | ≥+0.67 to +1.63[2] |
| Obese | ≥±3 | >+1.34[3] | >+1.64[3] |

IAP Indian Academy of Pediatrics; MGRS multicenter growth reference study; SDS standard deviation score
[1]Alternatively, body mass index
[2]Corresponds to body mass index >23 kg/m$^2$ in adults
[3]Corresponds to body mass index >27 kg/m$^2$ in adults

**Table 2.5:** Suggested growth monitoring in children at different ages

| *Age* | *Height/length* | *Weight* | *Head circumference* | *Other* |
|---|---|---|---|---|
| Birth | ✓ | ✓ | ✓ | |
| 1½, 3½, 6, 9, 15 months | ✓ | ✓ | ✓ | |
| 18 months–3 years | ✓ (6 monthly) | ✓ (6 monthly) | ✓ (6 monthly) | |
| 3.5–5.5 years | ✓ (6 monthly) | ✓ (6 monthly) | | |
| 6–8 years | ✓ (6 monthly) | ✓ (6 monthly) | | BMI (yearly) |
| 9–18 years | ✓ (yearly) | ✓ (yearly) | | BMI and SMR (yearly) |

Adapted from guidelines of Indian Academy of Pediatrics (2006)
BMI body mass index, SMR sexual maturity rating

downloadable at https://www.who.int/tools/child-growth-standards/software. The page allows the download WHO-Anthro software for personal computers (PC) and mobile devices. In addition, there are macros for the statistical software packages to facilitate data analysis.

### Mobile Apps for Analysis of Anthropometric Data

Several mobile applications (apps) are now available for instant and quick analysis of anthropometric data (Table 2.6). While a few are paid, many of them are free for download. Some use the CDC charts, while others use WHO charts for analysis. A few apps allow users to choose charts for calculations and interpretation. Many of these apps have additional capabilities and calculators.

### Plotting on Growth Charts and Interpretation

Growth charts allow the plotting of growth parameters for an individual child against their age and allow monitoring of trends over time. Plotting a single value may indicate an abnormality if it is extreme (**Fig. 2.10a and b**) while trends help assess a child's growth trajectory against the median. Children growing normally will usually be between –2.0 and +2.0 z-scores (two standard deviations above and below the mean, or between 3rd and 97th percentiles). The growth of an individual child plotted over time is expected to track reasonably close to the same z-score. If the growth curve tends towards the median, it is usually not a problem. But if it tends away from the median, it may signal a problem or risk of a problem (Fig. 2.11).

The following situations may indicate a problem or suggest a risk:

- A child's growth curve crosses a major z-score line or two major centile lines.
- A sharp incline or decline in the child's growth curve.
- A growth curve that remains flat (stagnant) (**Fig. 2.12**).

Knowing if the above situations represent a problem or risk depends on when it started, the trend, and the medical history. For example, If a baby, born as small for gestational age, showing improvement in birth centiles of weight and length may indicate catch up growth with optimum nutritional practices (**Fig. 2.13**). Distinct from height, head circumference, and weight, BMI does not typically increase with age in children between 2 and 5 years of age, and the serial plotting of BMI is usually a flat curve (**Figs 2.14 and 2.15**).

### Interpretation of Growth Data in Children above 5 Years of Age

It is important to remember that in children, BMI is also a function of age and gender. For example, the median BMI in boys increases from 14.6 kg/m$^2$ at 5 years to 21.2 kg/m$^2$ at 18 years, as shown in the IAP 2015 growth charts (**Annexures 11 and 12**). In these charts, the 23rd adult equivalent centile, which corresponds to approximately 0.55 SDS (71st centile) for boys and 0.67 SDS (75th centile) for girls is considered as the threshold for defining *overweight*; while the 27th adult equivalent centile, which corresponds to 1.33 SDS (90th centile) for boys and 1.63 SDS (95th centile) for girls is considered as the threshold for defining *obesity*. BMI for age below the 3rd centile is considered as *thinness* (**Table 2.4**).

For children above 5 years of age, height for age and BMI for age are the most important parameters for defining normal and abnormal growth and nutritional status.

### Secular Trends in Growth

The final adult height attained by the child has been increasing worldwide for a century and a half. This secular trend has occurred in almost all industrialized countries. The increase occurs throughout childhood and adolescence. There is also a secular trend towards early onset of sexual maturation. The final height appears to have reached a plateau in Northern European countries, but it is still increasing in southern European countries and Japan. There is sparse long-term data from India, but the available data suggests a trend toward increasing final height and weight and a decreasing age at menarche in the Indian population. This secular trend in growth is a marker of public health. It is affected by income, social status, infections, and nutrition. It is postulated that epigenetic factors could link growth and the environment. The secular trends and variations in growth in various regions of the world have implications for using common child growth references and imply a need to update growth standards constantly.

**Table 2.6:** Examples of selected mobile apps to interpret anthropometric data

| *Name* | *Operating mobile system* | *Basis of calculation* |
|---|---|---|
| AnthroCal | Android | WHO and IAP |
| Growth percentiles | Android | WHO |
| Growth chart CDC WHO percentiles | Android | WHO, CDC |
| IAP growth charts | Android, iOS | WHO |
| Pediatric growth chart | iOS | WHO |
| Pediatric growth charts by Boston Children's Hospital | iOS | WHO, CDC |
| STAT growth charts Lite | iOS | WHO |
| Child growth chart | Windows | WHO |
| Ped (Z) | Windows, Android | WHO, CDC |

The authors provide this list only as example; they do not endorse these apps. Many other apps are continually being developed, user discretion is advised

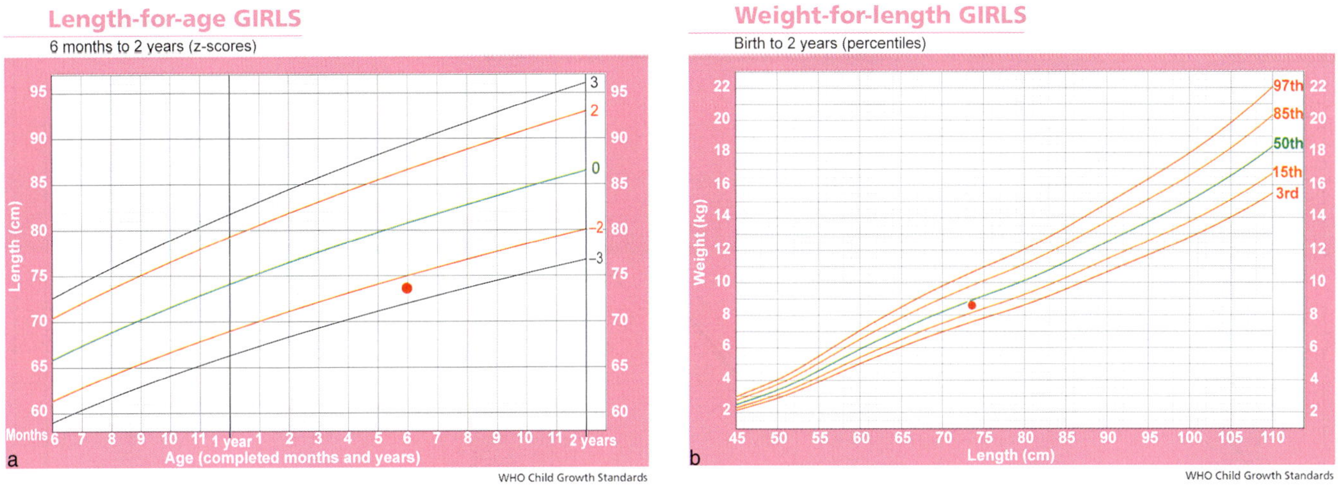


**Fig. 2.10:** Riya is an 18-month-old girl who weighs 8.5 kg and has a length of 73.5 cm. Note her plots on the WHO growth charts. Her weight-for-length (b), weight-for-age, and head circumference are within normal range, but her length-for-age (a) is below –2 z-score for age. Hence, she is stunted (but not wasted)

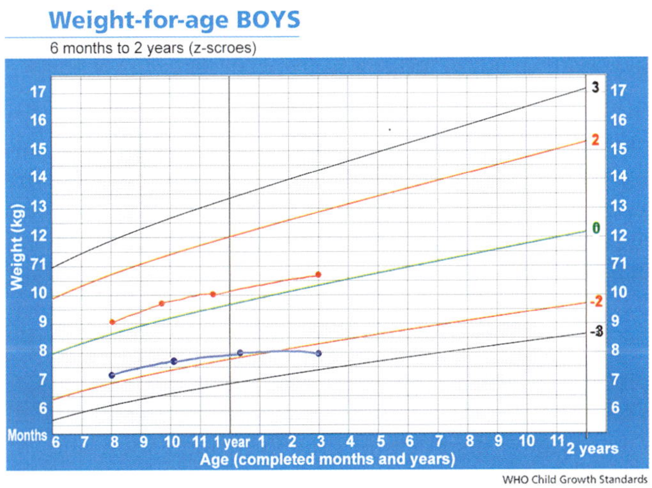


**Fig. 2.11:** The weight-for-age growth curve of two boys is plotted. The boy's weight in the top line (red dots) tracks just above the median, indicating a healthy trend. The bottom line (blue dots) shows a boy's weight falling from his expected growth track and crossing the z-scores line indicating risk

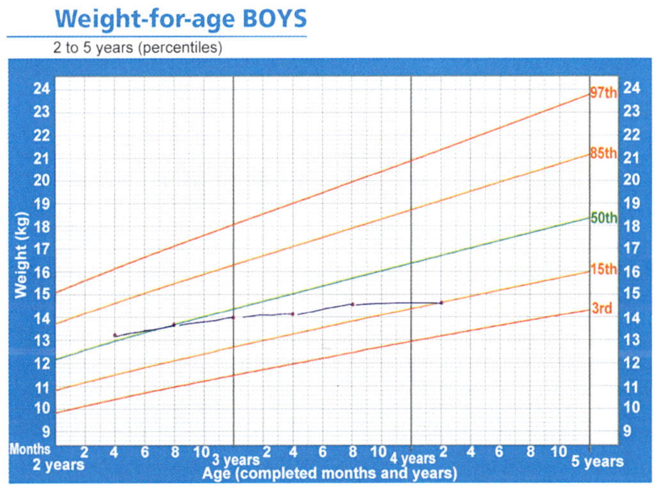


**Fig. 2.12:** Weight-for-age plot showing abnormal stagnation of weight. Some examples for such a trajectory are repeated infections and celiac disease

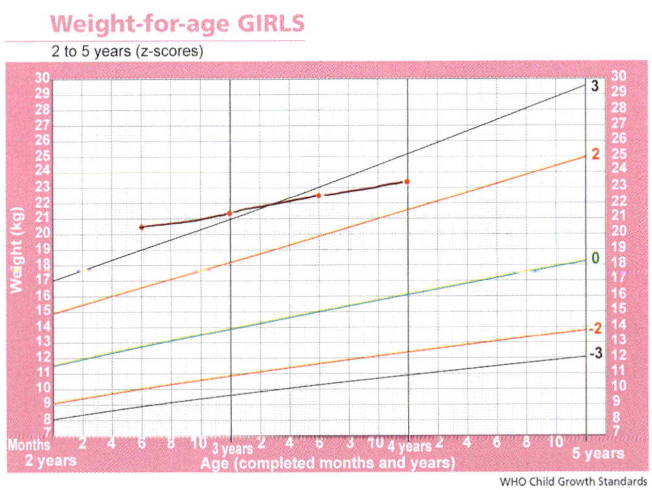


**Fig. 2.13:** Weight-for-age plot for an obese child, a slowly declining curve towards the median indicates a desirable "catch-down" after the nutritional intervention. The height and height increase was age-appropriate during the same period

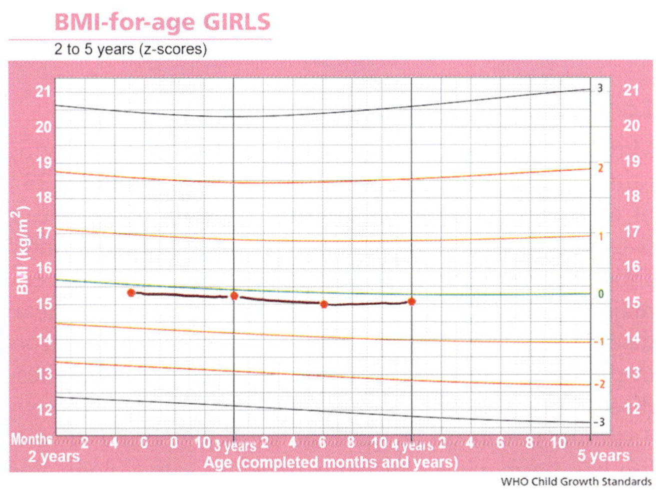


**Fig. 2.14:** A typical BMI plot for a girl from 2.5 to 4 years of age. Distinct from height and weight, BMI does not typically increase with age in children between 2 and 5 years of age, and the serial plotting of BMI is usually a flat curve

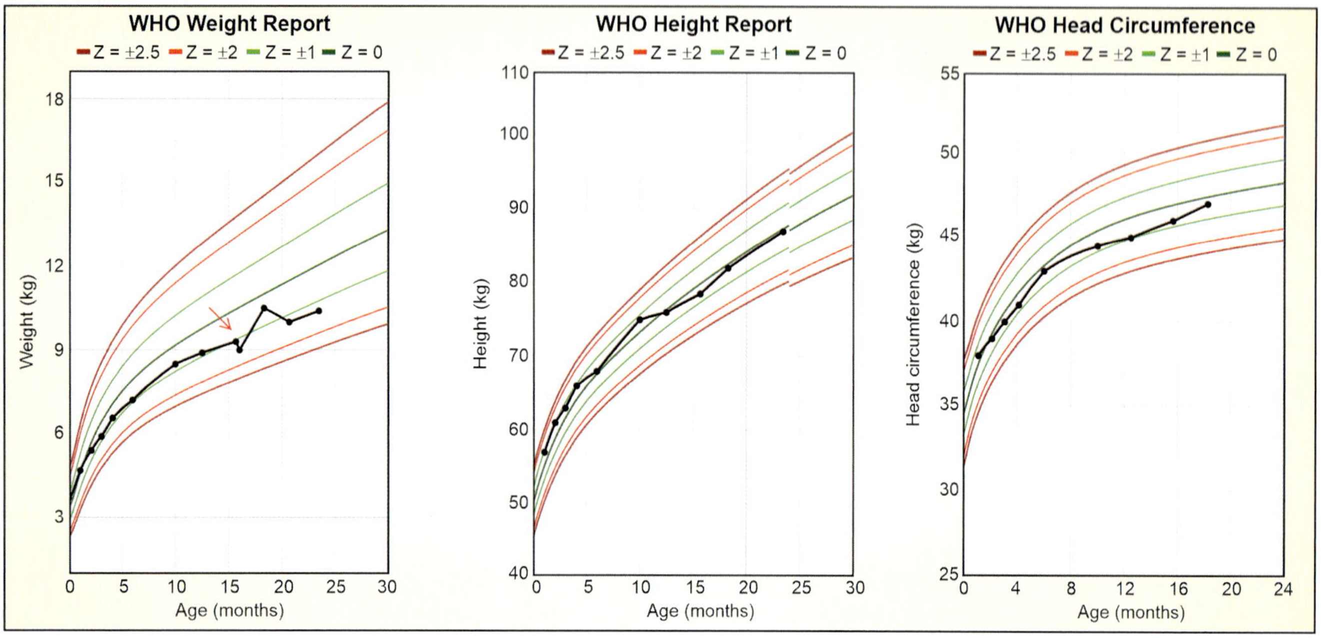


**Fig. 2.15:** Plotting of growth curves using a mobile app. Serial height, weight, and head circumference measurements in a boy indicate a healthy trend over the first two years. The sudden weight decline and catch-up (arrow) happened after an acute diarrheal illness

## Suggested Reading

1. Essential Nutrition Actions; Improving Maternal, Newborn, Infant and Young Child Health and Nutrition. Available at https://apps.who.int/iris/bitstream/handle/10665/84409/9789241505550_eng.pdf
2. Indian Academy of Pediatrics Growth Charts Committee, Khadilkar V, Yadav S, et al. Revised IAP growth charts for height, weight and body mass index for 5- to 18-year-old Indian children. Indian Pediatr 2015;52:47–55.
3. Khadilkar V, Khadilkar AV, Lohiya NN, et al. Extended growth charts for Indian children. J Pediatr Endocrinol Metab 2021;34(3):357–62.
4. Victora CG, Christian P, Vidaletti LP, et al. Revisiting maternal and child undernutrition in low-income and middle-income countries: variable progress towards an unfinished agenda. Lancet 2021;397:1388–99.
5. World Health Organisation. https://www.who.int/health-topics/nutrition; https://www.who.int/tools/child-growth-standards
6. World Health Organization. Training Course on Child Growth Assessment. Geneva, WHO, 2008.

## Consequences of Impaired Growth

Maternal and child undernutrition is the underlying cause of 3–5 million deaths annually. It accounts for 35% of the disease burden in children younger than five. It is estimated that India has more than 61 million stunted children, which amounts to 34% of the global total. Several major disorders of later life, including coronary heart disease, hypertension, and type 2 diabetes, originate from impaired intrauterine growth and development. These diseases may be consequences of 'programming,' whereby a stimulus or insult at a critical, sensitive period of early life has permanent effects on structure, physiology, and metabolism. The "Developmental Origins of Health and Diseases; (DOHaD); Barker hypothesis" proposes that alterations in fetal nutrition and endocrine status result in developmental adaptations that permanently change the structure, physiology, and metabolism, thereby predisposing individuals to cardiovascular, metabolic, and endocrine disease in adult life. As a result, infants born with low birth weight have an increased risk of diabetes, hypertension, coronary artery disease, and hyperlipidemia in adult life.

*Competencies:* **PE2.4; PE2.5; PE2.6; PE33.11**

# DISORDERS OF GROWTH

The common disorders of growth include short and tall stature, failure to thrive and obesity.

## Short Stature

### *Definition and Epidemiology*

Short stature is defined as height below the third centile or more than two standard deviation scores (SDS) below the median height for age and gender (<–2 SDS) according to the population standard. Two to 3% of children in any given population are short by this statistical definition. Children whose stature is more than 3 SDS below the population mean for age and gender (<–3 SDS) are more likely to be suffering from pathological short stature, as compared to those with stature between –2 and –3 SDS, who are more likely to have physiological, i.e., familial or constitutional short stature.

### *Etiology*

Short stature is attributable to several causes (Table 2.7). Undernutrition and chronic systemic illness are the common etiological factors, followed by growth hormone deficiency (GHD) and hypothyroidism.

### *Steps in Assessment*

***Accurate height measurement:*** For children below 2 years, the supine length should be measured using an infantometer

**Table 2.7:** Causes of short stature

| |
|---|
| **Physiological or normal variant short stature** |
| Familial |
| Constitutional |
| **Pathological short stature** |
| *Undernutrition* |
| *Chronic systemic illness* |
| • Cerebral palsy |
| • Congenital heart disease, cystic fibrosis, asthma |
| • Malabsorption, e.g. celiac disease, chronic liver disease, acquired immunodeficiency syndrome, other chronic infections |
| *Endocrine causes* |
| • Growth hormone deficiency or insensitivity |
| • Hypothyroidism |
| • Cushing syndrome |
| • Pseudohypoparathyroidism |
| • Precocious or delayed puberty |
| *Rickets* |
| *Psychosocial dwarfism* |
| *Children born small for gestational age with inadequate catch-up growth* |
| *Skeletal dysplasias*, e.g. achondroplasia |
| *Genetic syndromes*, e.g. Turner syndrome, Down syndrome |
| *Idiopathic short stature* |

with a rigid headboard on one side and a moveable footboard on the other side wile holding the infant straight on the horizontal board (Fig. 2.5). For older children, height should be measured with a stadiometer, as explained in the previous section (Fig. 2.6).

*Assessment of height velocity:* Height velocity is the rate of increase in height over time, expressed as cm/year. The average height velocity is 25 cm/yr in the first year, declines to 4–6 cm/yr in prepubertal children between 4 and 9 years of age, and increases during puberty to a peak height velocity of 8–12 cm/yr. If height velocity is lower than expected for age, the child is likely to be suffering from a pathological cause of short stature.

*Comparison with population norms:* The height should be plotted on appropriate growth charts and expressed in centile or as a standard deviation score.

*Comparison with child's genetic potential:* Parents' height significantly affects the child's height. Mid-parental height (MPH) gives an approximate estimate of the child's genetic potential.

$$\text{MPH for boys} = \frac{\text{Mother} + \text{Father height (cm)}}{2} + 6.5\text{ cm}$$

$$\text{MPH for girls} = \frac{\text{Mother} + \text{Father height (cm)}}{2} - 6.5\text{ cm}$$

This value is plotted on the growth chart at 18–20 years (adult equivalent). This gives an estimate of the target height for the child and the percentile that he/she is likely to follow.

*Assessment of body proportion:* Short stature can be proportionate or disproportionate. The proportionality is assessed by the upper segment (US): lower segment (LS) ratio and comparison of arm span with height. The US can be measured by taking the sitting height of the child. The child is made to sit on a square stool against the stadiometer's vertical rod. The headboard is brought down to the vertex, similarly to taking height. The height of the stool is subtracted from the reading to get the sitting height. LS can be obtained by subtracting the US from height. Alternatively, LS can be measured by taking the length from the upper border of the pubic symphysis to the ground while the child stands erect. For measuring arm span, the child is asked to stand straight with both arms extended outwards parallel to the ground. The length between the tips of the middle finger of the outstretched hands is the arm span.

Normally, the US:LS ratio is 1.7 at birth, 1.3 at three years, 1.1 by six years, one by 10 years, and 0.9 in adults. An increase in the US : LS ratio is seen in rickets, achondroplasia, and untreated congenital hypothyroidism. A decrease in the US: LS ratio is seen in spondyloepiphyseal dysplasia and vertebral anomalies. Arm span is shorter than the length by 2.5 cm at birth, equals height at 11 years, and after that is slightly (usually, <1 cm) greater than height.

*Sexual maturity rating (SMR):* SMR stage should be assessed in children above 7 years of age (*see* Chapter 5). Height spurt is seen in early puberty in girls and mid-puberty in boys. Precocious puberty can lead to an early height spurt followed by premature epiphyseal fusion and ultimate short stature. On the other hand, delayed puberty can also present with short stature in adolescents as the height spurt is also delayed.

### Differential Diagnosis

Diagnosis is based on a detailed history, examination, and laboratory evaluation. Careful history and examination can unravel many clues to the etiology of short stature (Tables 2.8 and 2.9). Clues from history and physical examination guide the investigative work-up.

Bone age assessment should be done in all children with short stature. The appearance of various epiphyseal centers and the fusion of epiphyses with metaphyses tell about the skeletal maturity of the child. Bone age is conventionally read from a radiograph of the left hand and wrist using standard atlases or softwares. It gives an idea as to what proportion of the adult height has been achieved by the child and what is the remaining potential for height gain. Bone age is delayed compared to chronological age in almost all causes of short stature. Exceptions to this are familial short stature, in which bone age equals chronological age, and precocious puberty, in which bone age exceeds chronological age. In constitutional delay, undernutrition and systemic illness, bone age is less than chronological age and corresponds to height age. In cases of growth hormone deficiency and hypothyroidism, bone age may be lower than height age, if the endocrine condition is diagnosed late.

In addition, all children with disproportionate short stature require a skeletal survey to rule out skeletal dysplasia and rickets. Essential screening investigations that should be done in children with short stature are listed in Table 2.10. If these investigations are normal and bone

**Table 2.8:** Clues to etiology of short stature from history

| *History* | *Etiology* |
|---|---|
| Low birth weight | Small for gestational age |
| Polyuria | Chronic renal failure, renal tubular acidosis |
| Chronic diarrhea, greasy stools | Malabsorption |
| Neonatal hypoglycemia, prolonged jaundice, micropenis | Congenital hypopituitarism |
| Headache, vomiting, visual problem | Pituitary or hypothalamic space occupying lesion, e.g. craniopharyngioma |
| History of cranial irradiation, trauma, tubercular meningitis | Acquired hypopituitarism |
| Lethargy, constipation, weight gain | Hypothyroidism |
| Inadequate dietary intake | Undernutrition |
| Social history | Psychosocial dwarfism |
| Delayed puberty in parent(s) | Constitutional delay of growth and puberty |

**Table 2.9:** Clues to etiology of short stature from examination

| *Examination finding* | *Etiology* |
|---|---|
| Disproportion | Skeletal dysplasia, rickets, hypothyroidism |
| Dysmorphism | Congenital syndromes |
| Pallor | Chronic anemia, chronic kidney disease, malabsorption |
| Hypertension | Chronic kidney disease, Turner syndrome |
| Frontal bossing, depressed nasal bridge, dental anomalies, small penis | Hypopituitarism |
| Goiter, coarse skin | Hypothyroidism |
| Central obesity, striae | Cushing syndrome |
| Low BMI for age | Undernutrition, malabsorption, chronic systemic illness |
| Rickets | Nutritional, renal tubular acidosis, chronic kidney disease |

age is delayed, level 2 investigations should be done. If these investigations are also normal, then growth hormone deficiency remains the major diagnostic possibility (*see* Chapter 18). If the child has borderline short stature, i.e., height between –2 and –3 SDS, then it is prudent to wait for 6–12 months and observe for height velocity. On the other hand, if the child is significantly short (≤3 SDS) or has documented poor height velocity over 6–12 months, one should proceed to level 3 investigations.

**Table 2.10:** Investigative work-up for short stature

**Level 1 (essential) investigations**
- Complete hemogram with ESR
- Bone age
- Urinalysis including microscopy, osmolality and pH
- Stool examination for parasites, steatorrhea and occult blood
- Blood urea, creatinine, bicarbonate, pH, calcium, phosphate, alkaline phosphatase, fasting glucose, albumin and transaminases

**Level 2 investigations**
- Serum thyroxine, thyroid stimulating hormone
- Karyotype in girls (to rule out Turner syndrome)
- Celiac serology

**Level 3 investigations**
- Serum insulin-like growth factor-1, and insulin-like growth factor binding protein-3 levels
- Provocative growth hormone testing
- MRI brain (focussed on pituitary and hypothalamus), if peak growth hormone level is low

### Specific Etiologies

***Familial short stature:*** The child is short as per definition (height <3rd centile) but is normal according to his genetic potential determined by the parent's height. These children show catch-down growth between birth and two years of age, so the height and weight lie on their target (mid-parental) centiles by age 2. Subsequently, the growth velocity remains normal throughout childhood and adolescence. The body proportion is appropriate, and bone age equals the chronological age. Puberty is achieved at an appropriate age, and the final height is within the target range (Fig. 2.16).

***Constitutional growth delay:*** These children are born with a normal length and weight and grow normally during the first year. Their growth then decelerates so that the height and weight gradually fall below the 3rd centile. By three years of age, normal height velocity is resumed, and they continue to grow just below and parallel to the 3rd centile with a normal height velocity. The onset of puberty and adolescent growth spurt is delayed in these children, but the final height is within normal limits. Bone age is lower than chronological age and corresponds to the height age. History of delayed puberty and delayed height spurt is usually present in one or both parents (Fig. 2.17). Table 2.11 lists features that help to distinguish between these two common causes of short stature.

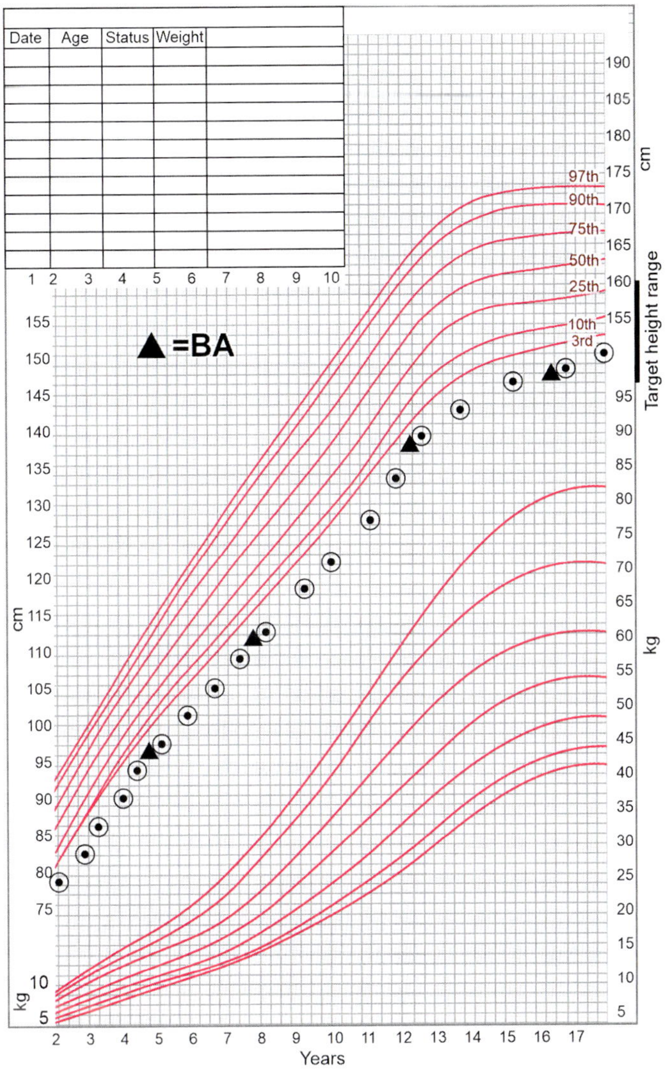


**Fig. 2.16:** Growth chart of a girl with familial short stature. The child is growing below and parallel to 3rd centile from early childhood till adulthood, height velocity is normal, bone age (BA) corresponds to chronological age and target height (range indicated by vertical bold bar) is low

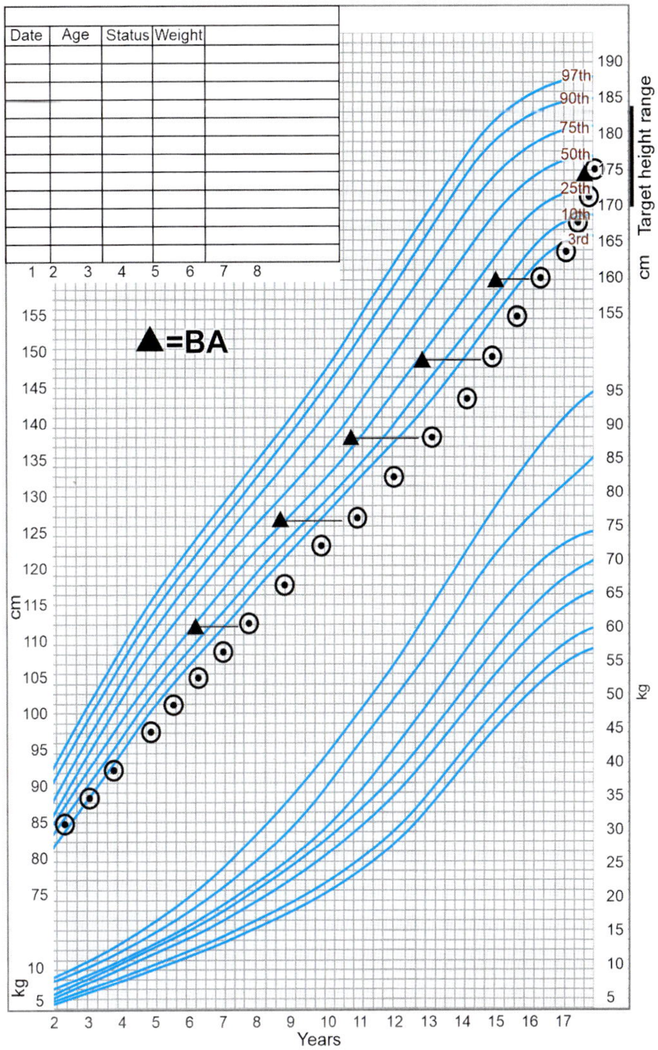


**Fig. 2.17:** Growth chart of a boy with constitutional delay of growth and puberty. The child falls to a lower centile in early childhood, grows below and parallel to 3rd centile in childhood, with an apparent downward deviation of growth curve during the normal time of pubertal growth, with later acceleration of growth and reaching target height (range indicated by vertical bold bar). Bone age (BA) is lower than chronological age by 2–3 years

**Table 2.11:** Distinction between constitutional delay in growth and familial short stature

| *Feature* | *Constitutional growth delay* | *Familial short stature* |
|---|---|---|
| Height | Short | Short |
| Height velocity | Normal | Normal |
| Family history | Delayed puberty | Short stature |
| Bone age | Less than chronological age | Normal |
| Puberty | Delayed | Normal |
| Final height | Normal | Low but normal for target height |

***Undernutrition:*** Stunted growth caused by chronic undernutrition is one of the commonest causes for short stature in our country. A detailed dietary history and the presence of other features of malnutrition, such as low mid-upper arm circumference and low weight for height or low body mass index (BMI) for age, suggest the diagnosis.

***Endocrine causes:*** These are discussed in detail in Chapter 18.

***Skeletal dysplasias:*** Inborn errors in the formation of cartilage and bone cause chondrodysplasias or skeletal dysplasias, which are usually associated with abnormal skeletal proportions and severe short stature (except hypochondroplasia, where growth retardation is mild). Careful elicitation of family history, measurement of body proportions, examination of the limbs and skull, and skeletal survey (radiographs of skull, thoracolumbar spine, chest, pelvis, one upper and one lower limb) are required for diagnosis.

***Genetic syndromes:*** Turner syndrome, with an incidence of 1:2000 live births, is a common cause of short stature in girls and should be considered as a diagnostic possibility and investigated for, even if the typical phenotypic features are absent. Elevated serum FSH levels in girls older than 8–9 years, and streak ovaries on ultrasound are helpful pointers to the diagnosis, with karyotype being the confirmatory test. Other syndromes associated with short stature are Down, Prader-Willi, Russell-Silver, and Seckel syndromes.

*Psychosocial dwarfism:* This condition, also known as emotional deprivation dwarfism, maternal deprivation dwarfism, or hyperphagic short stature, is seen in children in unhappy homes where the emotional needs of the child are neglected. It is characterized by functional hypopituitarism indicated by low IGF-1 levels and inadequate response of GH to stimulation. Therapy with GH is, however, not beneficial. Good catch-up growth is seen when the child is placed in a less stressful environment and nurtured with love and affection.

*Children born small for gestational age (SGA):* Birth weight below the 10th centile for gestational age can be caused by maternal, placental, or fetal factors. Most of these infants show catch-up growth by two years of age. However, an estimated 10–15% of babies born SGA fail to show catch-up growth and remain short. Subtle defects in the growth hormone and insulin-like growth factor (GH-IGF) axis are considered responsible for the short stature.

*Idiopathic short stature:* Children in whom no specific etiology for short stature, such as systemic illness, low birth weight, skeletal dysplasia, endocrine, nutritional or chromosomal abnormality is found are classified as idiopathic short stature (ISS). Up to 30–40% of all children with short stature may be given a diagnosis of ISS. These children may have subtle abnormalities of GH-IGF axis, or in several of the other regulatory pathways that control chondrogenesis in the growth plates.

#### Management

The general management principles for any child with short stature include counseling parents and dietary advice. Intake of a balanced diet containing the recommended amounts of macro- and micronutrients is recommended. The specific management depends on the underlying cause. For physiological causes, reassurance and annual monitoring of height and weight are sufficient. Parents should be counseled to highlight the positive aspects of their child's personality and not put undue emphasis on stature. Dietary rehabilitation for undernutrition and treatment of an underlying condition such as renal tubular acidosis or celiac disease is generally associated with good catch-up growth. With any form of therapy, regular and accurate monitoring of height velocity is mandatory for a satisfactory outcome.

Limb lengthening procedures are offered at a few orthopedic centers for skeletal dysplasias. For hypothyroidism, levothyroxine replacement is advised. Treatment with daily subcutaneous injections of GH is recommended for growth hormone deficiency. GH therapy is also approved for several other conditions though the doses required are generally higher, and improvement in final height is smaller and more variable than GH deficiency. These conditions include Turner syndrome, SGA with inadequate catch-up growth, and chronic kidney disease stage 4–5.

### Tall Stature

Height above two standard deviations for age and gender according to the population-specific growth reference is considered as tall stature. Although, the prevalence of tall stature in the population is expected to be approximately the same as short stature, the number of referrals for this complaint is much smaller, reflecting the societal perception of tall stature as a desirable trait.

#### Etiology

The causes of tall stature in children are summarized in Table 2.12. Majority of tall children have physiological tall stature, i.e., familial tall stature or constitutional acceleration of growth (CAG). CAG is like the mirror image of CDGP with tall stature, normal growth velocity and advanced bone age, generally associated with early puberty and final stature in the expected mid-parental range. Children with obesity are taller than their peers due to higher insulin and IGF-1 levels. However, their bone age is advanced and they typically have early adrenarche and puberty, so that final height is not increased.

Klinefelter syndrome (47,XXY) has a prevalence of 1 in 500 to 1 in 1000 boys. It is characterized by disproportionate tall stature (taller limbs). The phenotype is variable, but a majority of the affected boys have behavioral problems, delayed puberty, small testes and gynecomastia. Overgrowth syndromes (e.g., Sotos syndrome) are characterized by dysmorphic facies, large head and developmental delay or learning difficulties. Marfan syndrome is caused by mutations in fibrillin-1 (*FBN1*) gene, and inherited in an autosomal dominant manner. The main features are tall stature, ectopia lentis and aortic root dilatation. Homocystinuria has similar phenotype, along with increased predisposition to thromboembolism and psychiatric problems. It is diagnosed by measuring plasma homocysteine levels.

Excessive GH synthesis is rare in children and is usually caused by a GH-secreting pituitary adenoma. Children with precocious puberty are also tall for their age, but final height is compromised due to early epiphyseal fusion. Adolescents with sex steroid deficiency, as in hypogonadotropic

**Table 2.12:** Causes of tall stature in children

- Familial tall stature
- Constitutional acceleration of growth
- Obesity
- Syndromic
  - o Klinefelter syndrome
  - o Marfan syndrome
  - o Homocystinuria
  - o Overgrowth syndromes, e.g., Sotos syndrome
- Endocrine
  - o Growth hormone excess, e.g., GH-secreting pituitary adenoma, McCune-Albright syndrome
  - o Hyperthyroidism
  - o Precocious puberty
  - o Sex steroid deficiency or resistance, e.g., hypogonadotropic hypogonadism, aromatase deficiency

hypogonadism have tall stature with long legs and low upper segment ratio (eunuchoid proportions) due to delayed fusion of epiphyses.

### Management

Management of tall stature depends upon the specific underlying etiology. For most children with familial or constitutional tall stature, reassurance and explanation is sufficient and no intervention is required. However, in rare cases, if the tall stature is causing significant psychological impact, early induction of puberty in prepubertal children or use of high dose sex steroids in pubertal children may be used to hasten epiphyseal fusion.

*Competencies:* **PE2.1; PE2.2; PE2.3; PE2.6**

## Failure to Thrive

### Definition and Epidemiology

Failure to thrive (FTT) is a descriptive term rather than a diagnosis and is used for infants and children up to 5 years of age whose physical growth is significantly less than their peers of the same age and sex. FTT usually refers to weight below the 3rd or 5th centile, failure to gain weight over time, or a change in the rate of growth, such that weight for age or weight for length/ height has crossed two major centiles, e.g. 50th to 10th, over a period of time. The prevalence of FTT varies according to the population sampled.

### Etiology

Traditionally, FTT is classified as organic, where the child has some known underlying medical condition, and non-organic or psychosocial, where poor growth results from the inadequate caloric provision and emotional deprivation. Organic and non-organic etiological factors may coexist, e.g., in children with cerebral palsy or multiple congenital anomalies. FTT is non-organic in up to 80% of cases. The common etiological factors are listed in Table 2.13.

### Clinical Features

These children present with poor growth, often associated with poor development and cognitive functioning.

### Diagnosis

History, physical examination, and observation of parent–child interaction are important. Detailed laboratory investigations are needed only if history and physical examination suggest that an organic cause is responsible for FTT and to localize the systems involved. For an initial evaluation, the following investigations are adequate: (i) Complete blood count with ESR; (ii) urine and stool microscopy and culture; and (iii) kidney and liver function tests and serum electrolytes. Weight gain in response to adequate calorie feeding establishes the diagnosis of psychosocial FTT.

**Table 2.13:** Causes of failure to thrive

| |
|---|
| **Organic** |
| *Gastrointestinal:* Gastroesophageal reflux, malabsorption, inflammatory bowel disease, pyloric stenosis |
| *Neurological:* Mental retardation, cerebral palsy |
| *Renal:* Renal tubular acidosis, chronic kidney disease |
| *Cardiopulmonary:* Congenital heart disease, cystic fibrosis, asthma |
| *Endocrine:* Hypothyroidism, diabetes mellitus |
| *Infections:* Chronic parasitic infections of gastrointestinal tract, tuberculosis, human immunodeficiency virus |
| *Genetic:* Inborn errors of metabolism, chromosomal anomalies |
| *Miscellaneous:* Lead poisoning, malignancy |
| **Nonorganic** |
| Poverty |
| Misperceptions or lack of knowledge about diet and feeding |
| Lack of breastfeeding, feeding diluted formulae |
| Dysfunctional parent child relationship |

### Management

The goals of management are nutritional rehabilitation, treatment of organic causes, if present, and remedial measures for psychosocial factors. Important indications for hospitalization include: (i) Severe malnutrition; (ii) diagnostic and laboratory evaluation needed for organic cause; (iii) lack of catch-up growth during outpatient treatment; and (iv), suspected child abuse or neglect. The management of these patients depends on the underlying cause. Nutritional rehabilitation is necessary.

### Prognosis

If managed early and adequately, the prognosis for physical growth recovery is good. However, the outlook for cognitive, emotional and behavioral development is variable and less certain. The growth and development of these children should be monitored regularly.

## Protein-Energy Malnutrition

Being underweight, wasting, and other disorders resulting from poor intake of calories and proteins are discussed in detail in Chapter 7.

## Abnormalities in Head Size

Microcephaly and macrocephaly are discussed in Chapter 19.

## Suggested Reading


1. Lauffer P, Kamp GA, Menke LA, et al; on behalf of the Dutch Working Group on Triage and Diagnosis of Growth Disorders in Children. Towards a rational and efficient diagnostic approach in children referred for tall stature and/or accelerated growth to the general paediatrician. Horm Res Paediatr 2019;91:293–310.
2. Polidori N, Castorani V, Mohn A, Chiarelli F. Deciphering short stature in children. Ann Pediatr Endocrinol Metab 2020;25:69–79.

Chapter

3

# Development

❍ Ramesh Agarwal ❍ Naveen Sankhyan

*Competency:* **PE1.5**

## NORMAL DEVELOPMENT

Development refers to the maturation of functions and acquisition of various skills for optimal functioning of an individual. Developmental milestones are easily identifiable events during the continuous development process, e.g. turning over, sitting, reaching for objects, and speaking words. The sequential attainment of developmental milestones reflects maturation and myelination of the nervous system.

Over 80% of brain development occurs in the first three years of life. The fastest and most critical acquisition of sensory, cognitive, and linguistic capabilities occurs in this period of life.

Early childhood development (ECD) refers to the physical, motor, socio-emotional, cognitive, and linguistic development of a young child, especially in the first three years of life. ECD determines learning outcomes in school years and beyond. We must ensure that all our children acquire maximum developmental potential regardless of their socioeconomic background.

### Common Patterns of Development

There are some basic facts about the complex process of human development:

i. Development is a *continuous process*, starting *in utero* and progressing until maturity. The child must go through many developmental stages before achieving a milestone.

ii. Development *depends on the functional maturation of the nervous system*. Maturity of the central nervous system is essential for a child to learn a milestone or skill; no amount of practice can make a child learn new skills without the required maturation of the nervous system. However, without practice, the child may not learn skills despite neural maturation.

iii. The *sequence of attainment of milestones is the same in all children*. All infants babble before they speak words and sit before they stand. Variations may exist in the time and manner of their attainment.

iv. The *development progresses in a cephalocaudal direction*. Head control precedes trunk control, which precedes the ability to use lower limbs. The control of limbs happens from proximal to distal such that the child learns to use his hands before fingers.

v. *The attainment of certain milestones requires that relevant primitive reflexes disappear*. For example, the child can voluntarily hold an object once the palmar grasp reflex disappears. Similarly, a child can only turn over once the asymmetric tonic neck reflex disappears.

vi. *Specific actions replace the initial disorganized mass activity*. For example, on seeing a bright toy, a 3–4-month-old squeals and excitedly moves all the limbs, whereas a 3–4-year-old may smile and ask for it.

### Factors Affecting Development

Development depends on many factors, such as genetic potential, biological integrity, physical and psychosocial environment, and emotional stimulation. Infancy and early childhood are the most crucial ages for development.

Appropriate sensory inputs through hearing and vision, a secure environment, and responsive parenting provide the solid foundation for healthy learning and behavior. Poverty is a critical risk factor associated with poor development. Poverty exposes the child to many other risk factors, such as scarcity of opportunities, excessive stress, malnutrition, environmental toxins, and concurrent diseases.

#### *Prenatal Factors*

***Genetic factors:*** Parents' intelligence correlates to child's. Specific developmental patterns such as speech in children mimic that of their parents. Genetic disorders such as chromosomal abnormalities (e.g. Down syndrome), single-gene disorders (e.g. congenital deafness), and metabolic disorders (e.g. phenylketonuria) are important causes of developmental delay and subsequent mental retardation (MR).

*Maternal factors:* A host of factors that impair growth in utero can potentially affect brain growth, especially when severe or sustained:

i. *Maternal nutrition:* Maternal malnutrition (macro- and micronutrients) adversely affects birth weight and child development.
ii. *Exposure to drugs and toxins:* Maternal substance abuse, medications such as antiepileptic agents, and environmental toxins hurt child development.
iii. *Maternal diseases and infections:* Pregnancy-induced hypertension, hypothyroidism, and fetoplacental insufficiency can negatively influence brain development. Congenital infections (e.g. syphilis, toxoplasmosis, rubella, cytomegalovirus, herpes) impact the fetus' physical growth and brain development. Maternal chorioamnionitis can result in cerebral palsy and developmental impairment in the child.

### Neonatal Risk Factors

*Small for gestational age (SGA) status:* SGA is often a consequence of poor maternal nutrition and infections during the crucial period of brain development. Such infants are disadvantaged compared to their normal birth weight counterparts in neurocognitive development.

*Prematurity:* Babies born before 37 weeks of gestation are more likely to have developmental impairment compared to term counterparts, with babies born before 32 weeks at the highest risk.

*Perinatal asphyxia:* Significant asphyxia occurs in approximately 2% of total births. Major neurocognitive disabilities occur in the survivors of significant asphyxia.

*Hyperbilirubinemia:* High serum bilirubin levels can damage the developing brain, and children may have cerebral palsy and developmental delays.

### Postneonatal Factors

*Infant and child nutrition:* Severe calorie deficiency, as evident by stunting, is associated with apathy, depressed emotions, reduced activities, and poor interactions with caregivers. Concomitant deficiency of multiple micronutrients and vitamins also contributes to developmental impairment.

Linear growth retardation or stunting occurs in nearly one-third of children aged less than five years in low- and middle-income countries. There is a positive association between height for age and cognitive ability, academic performance in adolescence, and later formal employment at age 20–22.

Congenital hypothyroidism is the most common preventable cause of mental retardation. Children growing up in iodine-deficient areas have an IQ of 12.5 points lower than those in iodine-sufficient areas.

*Infectious diseases:* A variety of infectious morbidities such as diarrhea, malaria, other parasitic infections, and HIV are associated with poorer neurodevelopment.

*Environmental toxins:* Children exposed to toxins (lead, arsenic, pesticides, mercury, and polycyclic aromatic hydrocarbons) through maternal exposure, and postnatally through food, water, house dust, or soil can have an adverse influence on their neurocognitive development.

*Acquired insults to the brain:* Traumatic or infectious insults (meningitis, encephalitis, cerebral malaria) and other factors (near-drowning, trauma) in early life can have a permanent adverse effect on brain development.

*Associated impairments:* Sensory impairment such as diminished vision or hearing can significantly impact the development of children. Early detection and management of hearing and visual impairments are essential for promoting optimum child development.

### Psychosocial Factors

Several social factors influence the children's cognition, attitudes, social-emotional competence, and sensorimotor development.

*Parenting:* Suboptimal parenting, such as inadequate emotional warmth or responsiveness in conjunction with poverty and social factors, has a critical bearing on child development. Education and opportunities influence childhood development in a significant way.

*Lack of nurturing conditions:* Social and emotional deprivation and lack of adequate stimulation are important causes of developmental impairment, particularly evident in the setting of poverty.

*Violence and abuse:* Domestic and community violences are emerging threats to child development. Physical or sexual abuse has a profound psychological effect on the child.

*Maternal depression:* Low- and middle-income countries have a high incidence of maternal depression, negatively affecting early childhood development and quality of parenting through unresponsive caregiving.

*Institutionalization:* Institutional care (e.g. orphanages) during early life increases the risk of poor growth, ill-health, attachment and attention disorders, poor cognition, anxiety, and autistic-like behavior.

### Protective Factors

Breastfeeding, kangaroo mother care, optimum nutrition, absence of illness, nurturing family, secure home, exposure to stimulating environment, educated parents are some of the cardinal protective factors. These protective factors that can offset the disadvantages to relative poverty and pave way for optimum developmental outcomes including intelegence and scholastic achievements.

A variety of factors in early life determine the child's developmental trajectory (**Fig. 3.1**). In the presence of protective factors, children attain their developmental potential. In contrast, risk factors prevent this from happening. Timely intervention can make a big difference in the child's developmental potential.

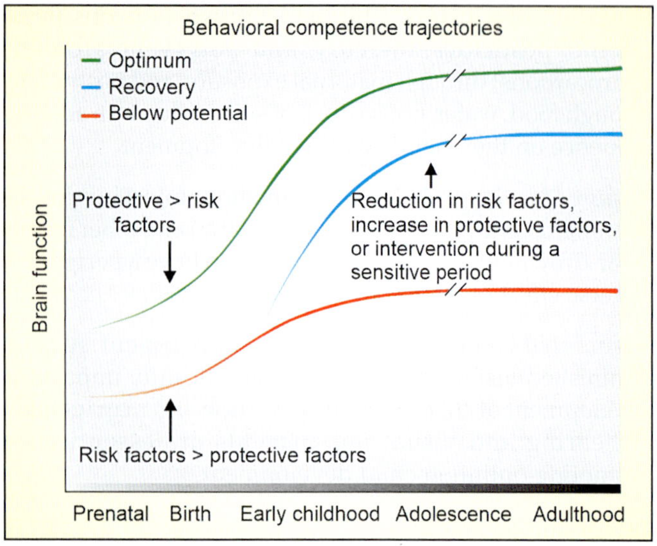


**Fig. 3.1:** Brain and behavioral development trajectories depending on risk and protective factors (*Reproduced with permission:* Lancet 2011;378:1325–38)

*Competencies:* **PE1.6; PE1.7**

## DOMAINS OF DEVELOPMENT

It is convenient to classify development under the following domains:

i. Gross motor
ii. Fine motor and skills
iii. Personal, social and general understanding
iv. Language
v. Vision and hearing

### Gross Motor

Motor development progresses in an orderly sequence to attain locomotion and the ability to do more complex motor tasks. In an infants, it is assessed and observed as follows:

***Supine and pull to sit:*** Observe the infant in the supine position. Pull her gently to a sitting position. Examine the control of the head and curvature of the spine. In the newborn period, the head completely lags with a rounded back **(Fig. 3.2)**. By four months, head lag is minimum, and the back is less rounded **(Fig. 3.3)**.

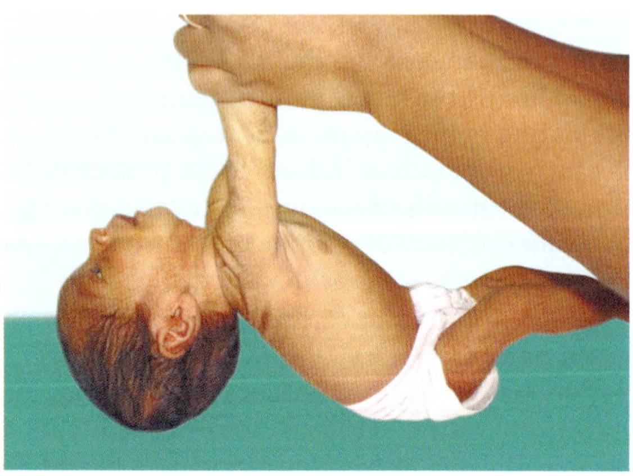

**Fig. 3.2:** Pull to sit: Complete head lag in a newborn

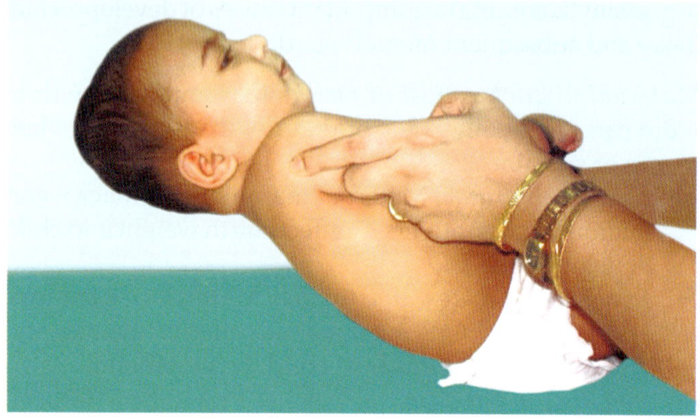

**Fig. 3.3:** Pull to sit: Minimal head lag at four months

The child achieves complete neck control by 20 weeks **(Fig. 3.4)**. The neck stays stable, even if the examiner sways the child gently. Infant lifts head from the supine position in anticipation when about to be pulled at five months. At this age, the baby loves to play with his feet and may take the foot to the mouth **(Fig. 3.5)**.

***Ventral suspension:*** The examiner lifts the infant off the couch by placing one hand under the infant's chest and abdomen. Up to four weeks of age, the head flops down **(Fig. 3.6)**. At eight weeks, the child holds his head up in the

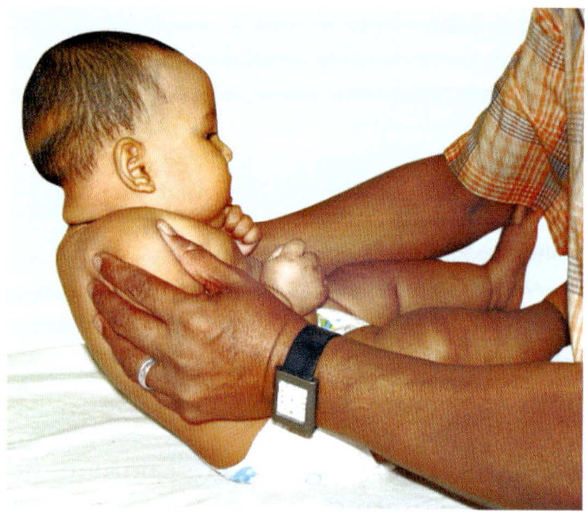

**Fig. 3.4:** Pull to sit: The child has complete neck control and is able to flex the head onto the chest at five months

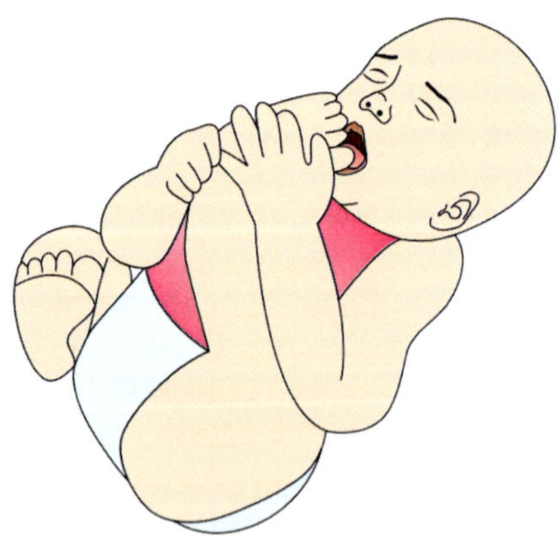

**Fig. 3.5:** Takes the foot to the mouth at 20 weeks

horizontal plane (Fig. 3.7). By 12 weeks, he can lift his head above the horizontal plane (Fig. 3.8).

***Prone position:*** At birth, the newborn turns the head to one side. At two weeks, the baby lies on the bed with

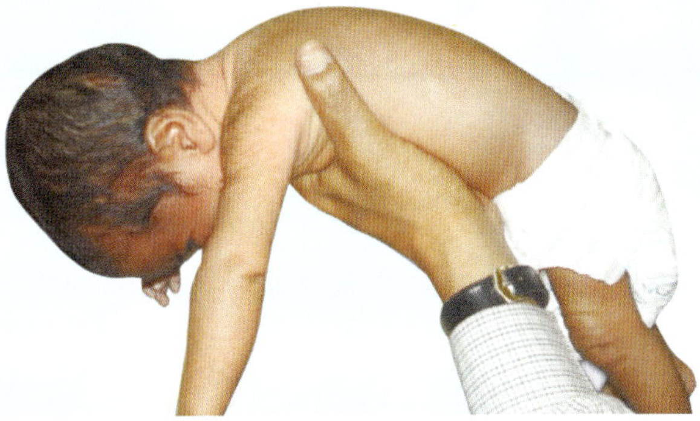

Fig. 3.6: Ventral suspension: Unable to hold the neck in line with the trunk at four weeks

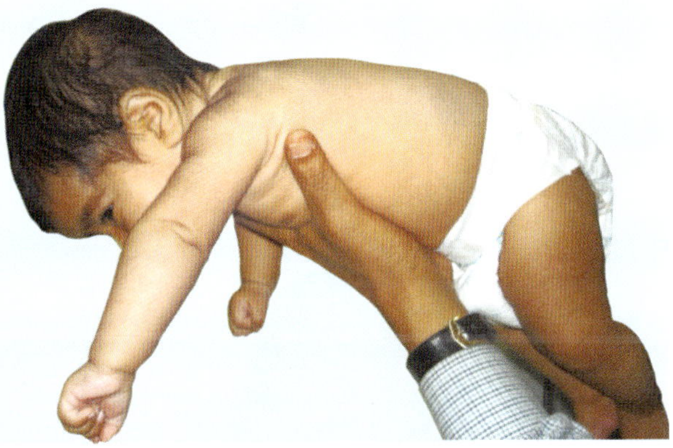

Fig. 3.7: Ventral suspension: Head in line with the trunk at 8 weeks

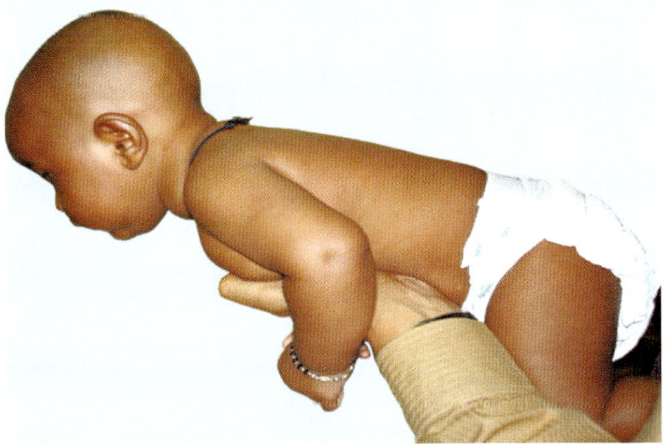

Fig. 3.8: Ventral suspension: Head in line with the trunk at 12 weeks

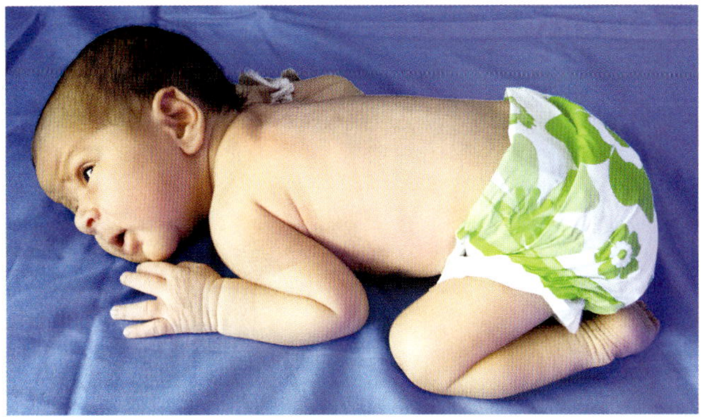

Fig. 3.9: The infant lies on the bed with high pelvis and knees drawn up at two weeks (*Courtesy:* Dr Vijay K Charchi)

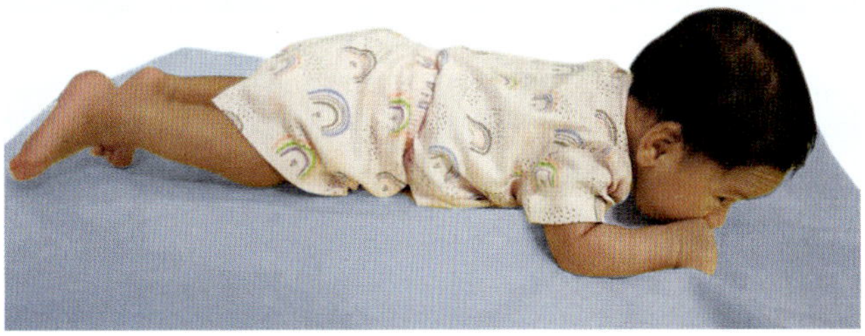

Fig. 3.10: Lies with flat pelvis and extended hip at six weeks

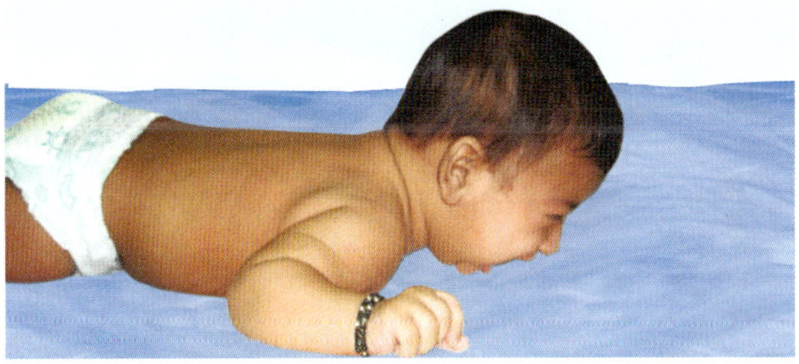

Fig. 3.11: In prone position, face at 45° at eight weeks

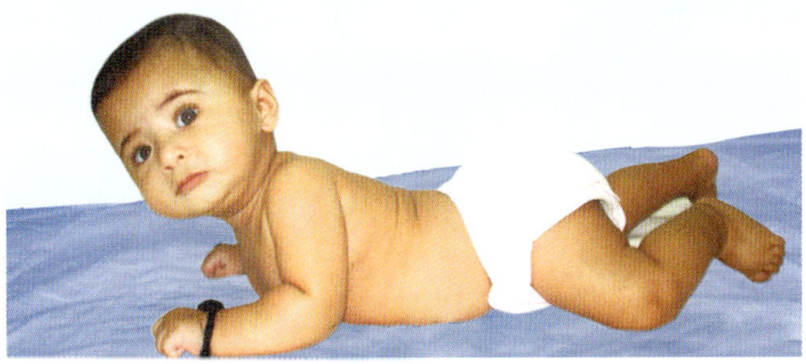

Fig. 3.12: In prone position, face, head, and chest off the couch at three months

knees drawn under the pelvis (Fig. 3.9). The infant lies with a flat pelvis and extended hips at six weeks (Fig. 3.10). By eight weeks, the infant lifts his face at 45° (Fig. 3.11). By 12 weeks, the child bears weight on the forearms with chin and shoulder off the couch (Fig. 3.12). By six months, the child supports his weight on the extended arms (Fig. 3.13). Between 4 and 6 months, he rolls over—at first back to side and then back to stomach. The infant crawls (abdomen on the ground) by eight months and creeps (abdomen off the ground) by ten months (Fig. 3.14) and bear walk at 12 months (Fig. 3.15).

***Sitting:*** The child can be made to sit with the support of pillows or examiner's hands—with rounded back at 8 weeks and straight back at 4 months (Figs 3.16 and 3.17).

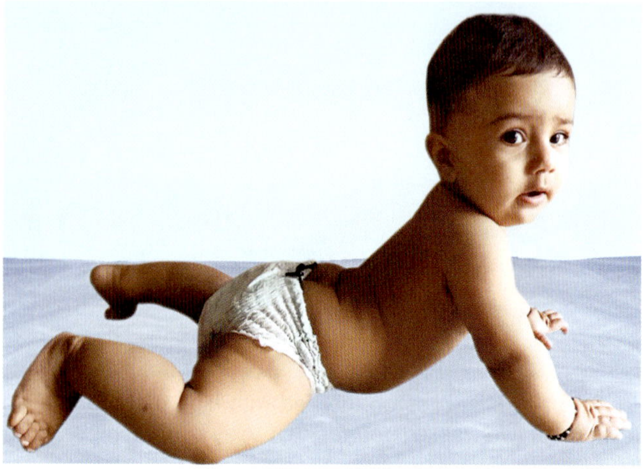

Fig. 3.13: In prone position, weight on hands with extended arms at six months (*Courtesy:* Dr Md Tousifullah)

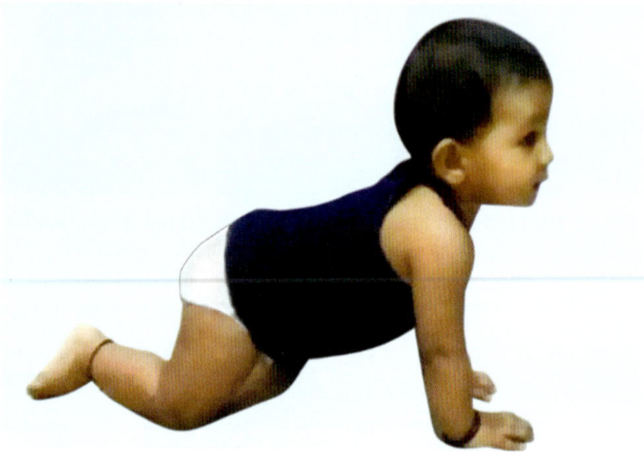

Fig. 3.14: Creeping at 10 months (*Courtesy:* Dr Vijay K Charchi)

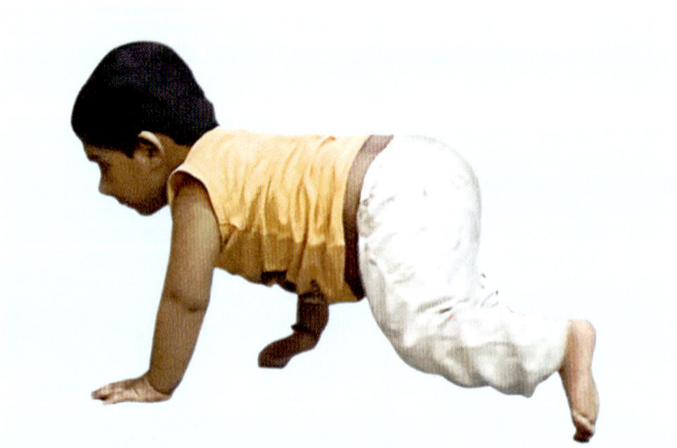

Fig. 3.15: Bear walk at 12 months (*Courtesy:* Dr Naveen Gowda)

He independently sits with his arms forward for support (tripod or truly 'sitting with support') at 6 months (Fig. 3.18).

Sitting without support develops at eight months (Fig. 3.19). By 10–11 months, he can pivot to reach an object (Fig. 3.20).

***Standing and walking:*** At six months, the child can bear weight and bounces actively when made to stand (Fig. 3.21).

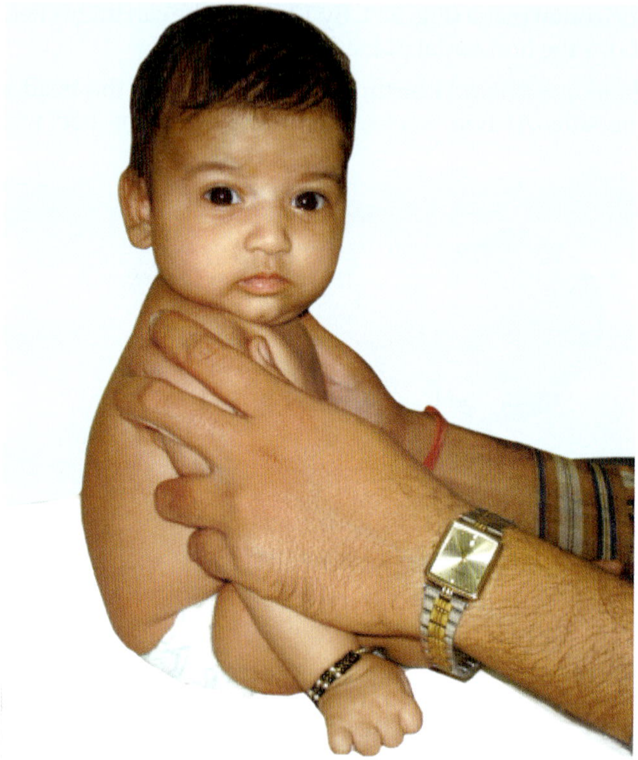

Fig. 3.16: Sitting: Back rounded but holding the head at eight weeks

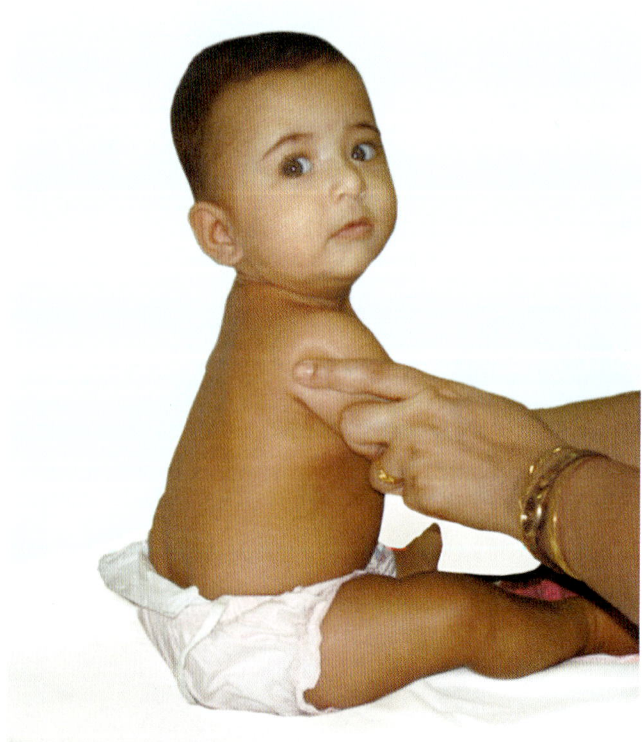

Fig. 3.17: Sitting: Back straight at four months

At nine months, the child can pull to stand and can stand holding furniture (Figs 3.22 and 3.23). By 10 and 11 months, the child starts cruising around furniture (Fig. 3.24). At about 12 months, the child can stand independently (Fig. 3.25) and walk with one hand held (Fig. 3.26). Between the ages of 13 and 15 months, the child starts walking

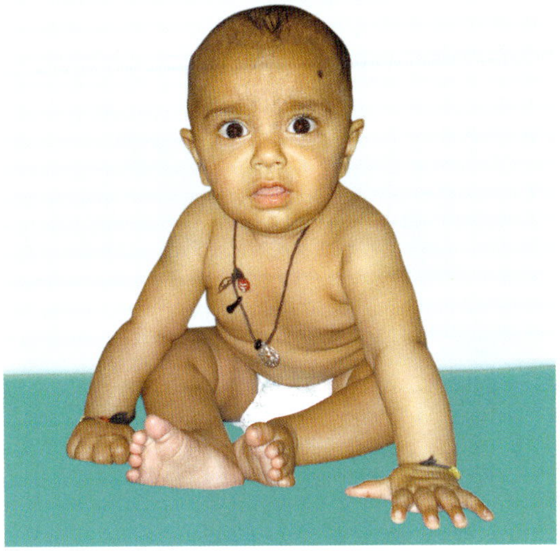

**Fig. 3.18:** Sitting with support at 6 months

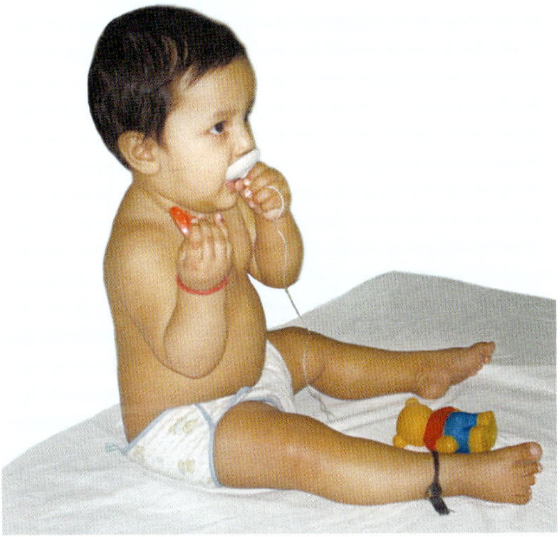

**Fig. 3.19:** Sitting without support at eight months

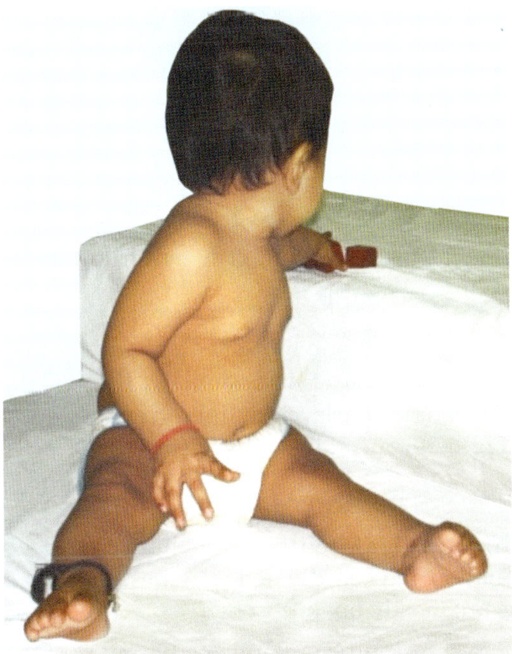

**Fig. 3.20:** Pivoting: Turns around to pick up an object at 11 months

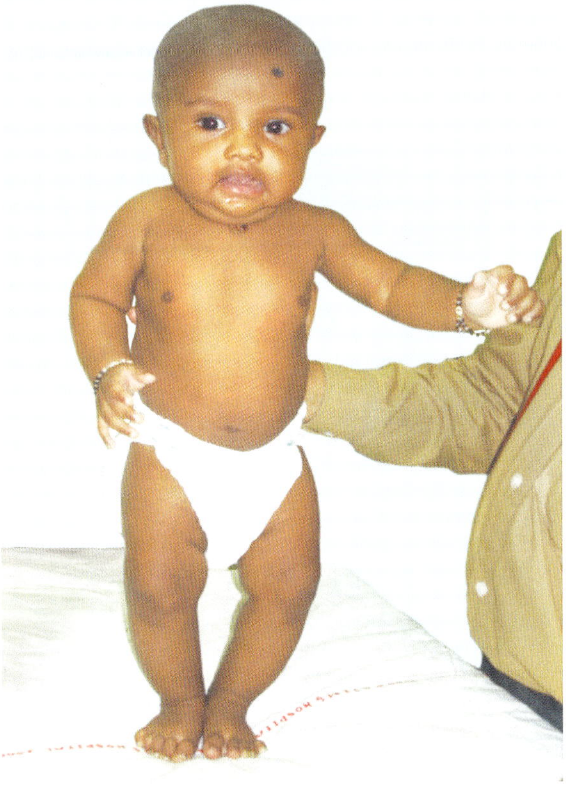

**Fig. 3.21:** Bears almost entire weight at six months

independently **(Fig. 3.27)**. At 18 months, he runs **(Fig. 3.28)**, crawls up and down the stairs, and pulls a doll or wheeled toy on the floor.

By two years, the child walks backward and climbs upstairs with both feet on one step. By three years, he can

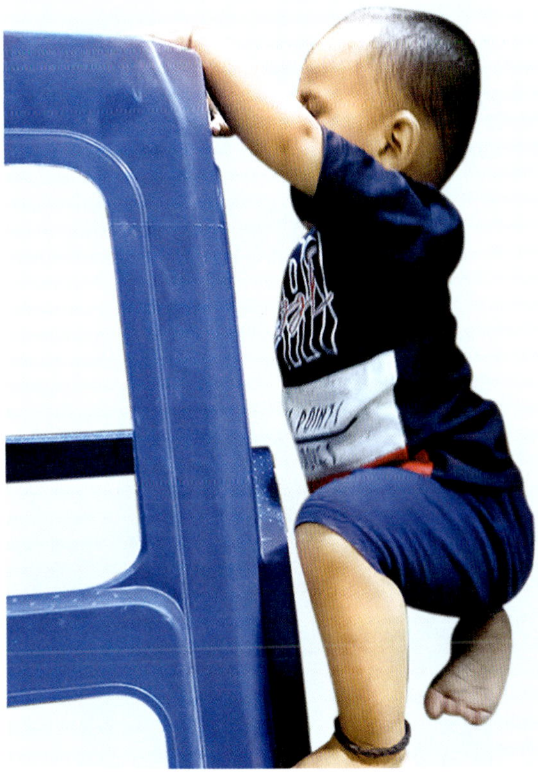

**Fig. 3.22:** Pulls to stand at nine months

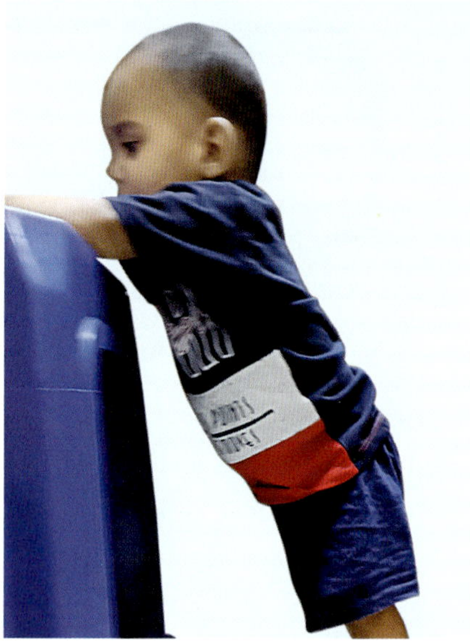

Fig. 3.23: Stands holding furniture at 9 months

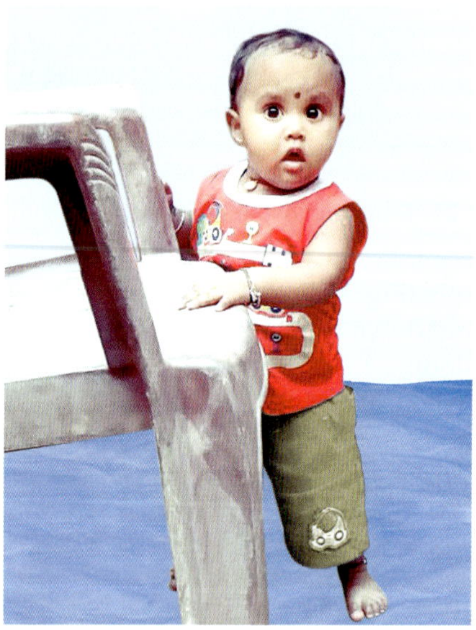

Fig. 3.24: Cruising around furniture at 10 to 11 months (*Courtesy:* Dr Vijay K Charchi)

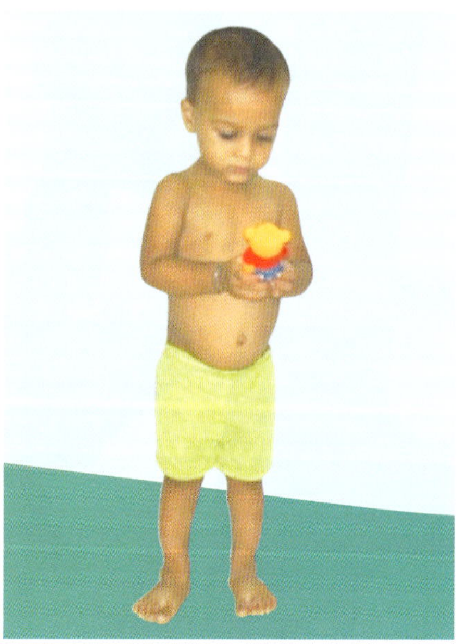

Fig. 3.25: Stands independently at 12 months

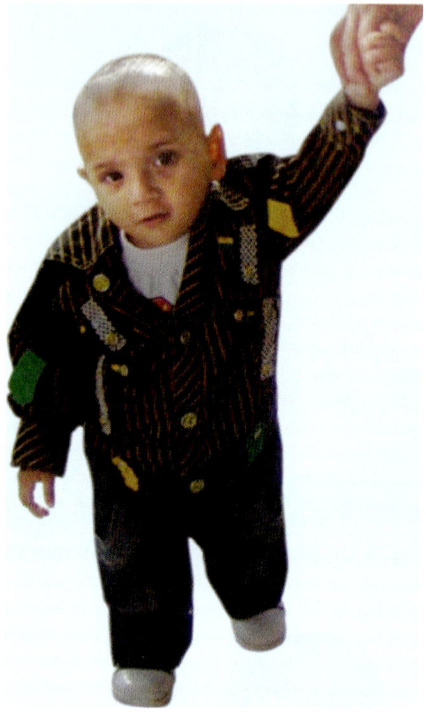

Fig. 3.26: Walking with one hand-held at 12–13 months

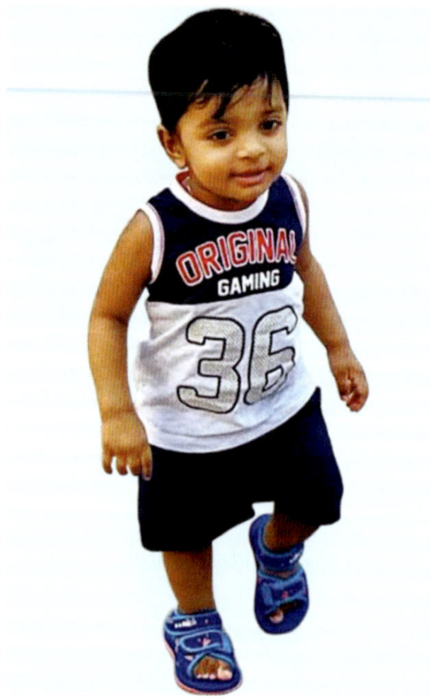


Fig. 3.27: Walks independently at 15 months (*Courtesy:* Dr Md Tousifullah)

climb upstairs with one foot per step, and by four years, she can move down the stairs similarly **(Fig. 3.29)**.

A child can ride a tricycle at three years. He hops at four years **(Fig. 3.30)** and skips at five years **(Table 3.1)**.

### *Fine Motor Skill Development*

This domain deals with using hands and eyes for manipulation and coordinated activities. At 2 to 3 months, the fists are mostly open.

***Hand-eye coordination:*** Between 12 and 20 weeks, the child observes his own hands very intently (hand regard;

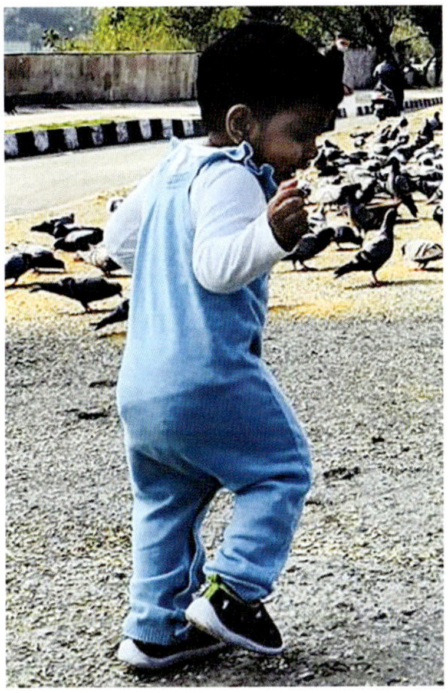

Fig. 3.28: Runs at 18 months (*Courtesy:* Dr Md Tousifullah)

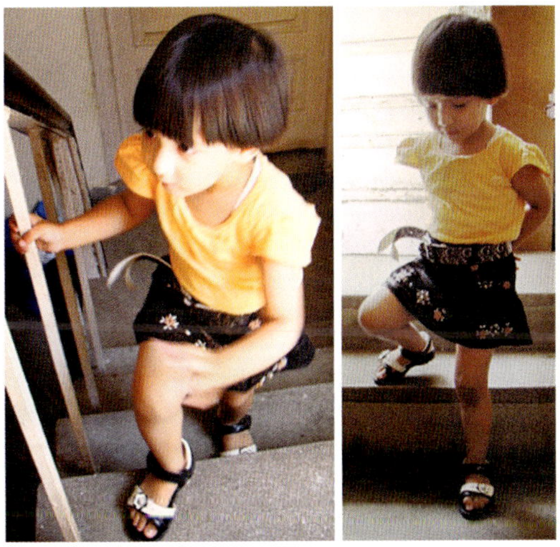

Fig. 3.29: Walking upstairs and downstairs one foot per step at 4 years

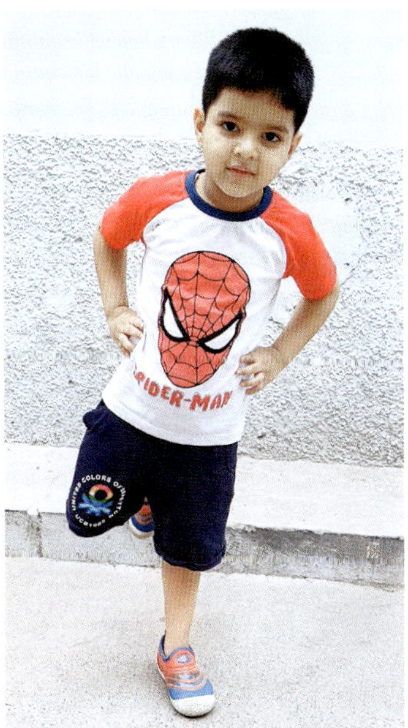

Fig. 3.30: Hops at four years (*Courtesy:* Dr Md Tousifullah)

**Table 3.1:** Key gross motor developmental milestones

| *Age* | *Milestone* |
|---|---|
| 3 months | Neck holding |
| 5 months | Rolls over |
| 6 months | Sits in tripod fashion (sitting with own support) |
| 8 months | Sitting without support |
| 9 months | Stands holding on (with support) |
| 12 months | Creeps well; walks but falls; stands without support |
| 15 months | Walks alone; creeps upstairs |
| 18 months | Runs; explores drawers |
| 2 years | Walks up and downstairs (2 feet/step); jumps |
| 3 years | Rides tricycle; alternate feet going upstairs |
| 4 years | Hops on one foot; alternate feet going downstairs |
| 5 years | Skips |

Fig. 3.31). Hand regard is even present in children without vision. Its persistence beyond 20 weeks is abnormal. At 3 to 4 months, the hands of the child come together in the midline as he plays (Fig. 3.32). On dangling a red ring in

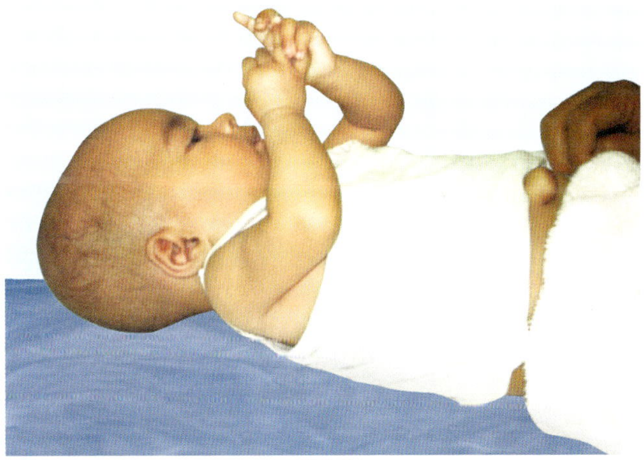

Fig. 3.31: Hand regard (between 12 and 20 weeks)

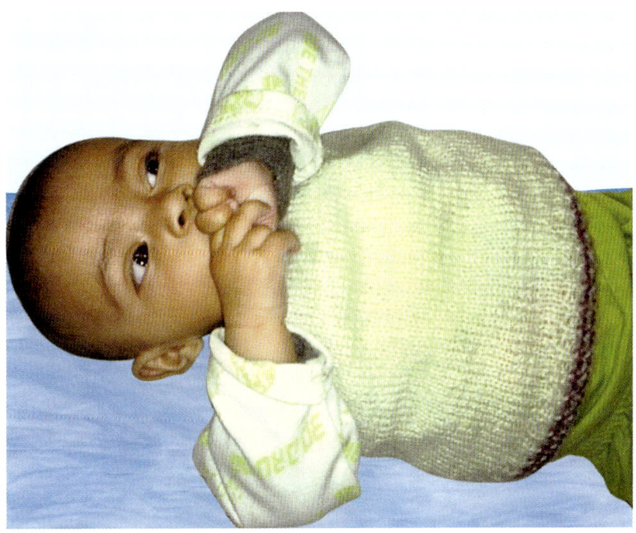

Fig. 3.32: The child brings hands in the midline as he plays at 3 to 4 months of age

front of him, he fixes his attention (Fig. 3.33) and then tries to reach for it (Fig. 3.34). Initially, he overshoots but eventually brings it to the mouth.

Assess the crude grasp by offering the child a red cube of one cubic inch dimension. At six months, the child grasps the cube from the ulnar side (crude ulnar grasp). He holds it in the middle of his palm at 8 to 9 months (crude intermediate grasp; Fig. 3.35) and with the radial side of his hand at 10 months (crude radial grasp; Fig. 3.36). By one year, a mature grasp (index finger and thumb) for a larger object like a cube appears (Fig. 3.37).

The child transfers the cube from one hand to the another at seven months, compares two cubes at eight months, and looks for the dropped cube at nine months (object permanence; Fig. 3.38).

Assess fine hand skills by offering a pellet (small objects; beware as the children take things to their mouth, risking choking at this age). By 9–10 months, the child pokes the pellet using his index finger (Fig. 3.39).

The infant picks up the pellet in the next few months using his index finger and thumb (pincer grasp). Initially,

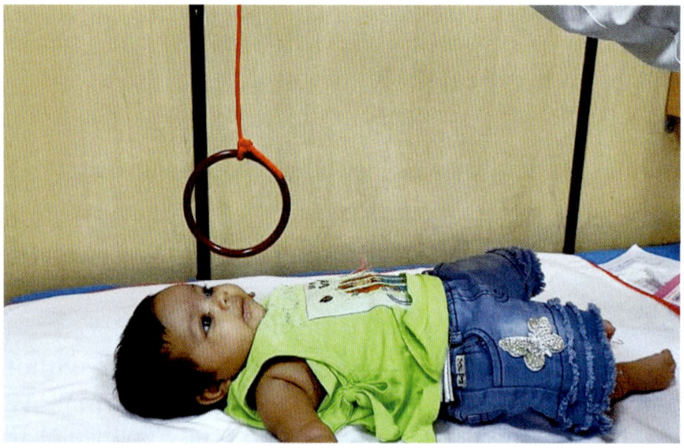

Fig. 3.33: Fixes attention on a red ring at 4 months (*Courtesy:* Dr Md Tousifullah)

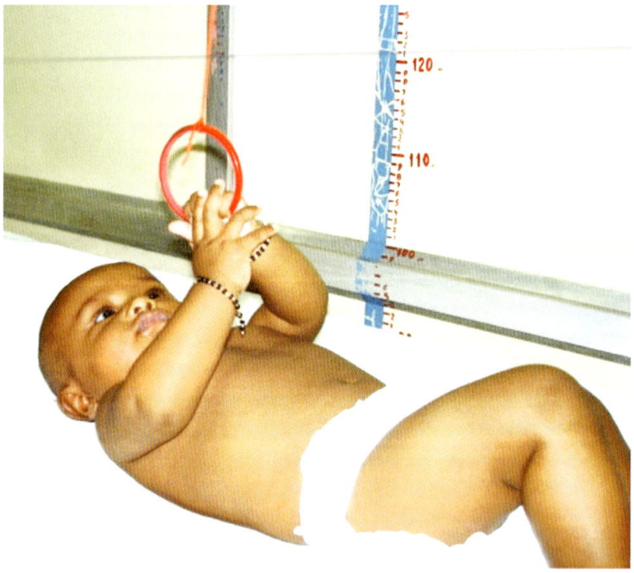


Fig. 3.34: Bidextrous grasp approach to a dangling ring at 4 months

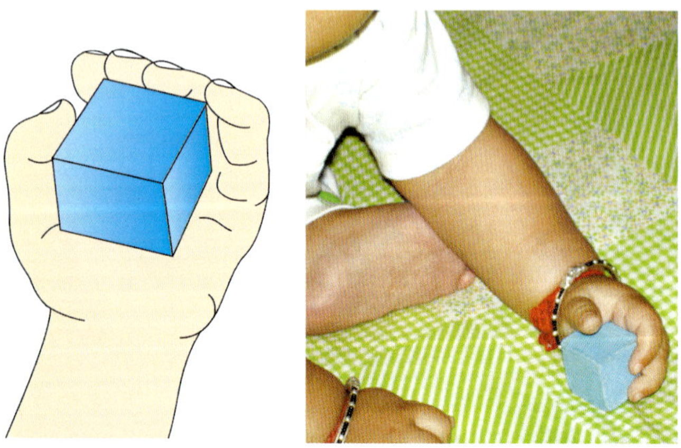

Fig. 3.35: Immature grasp at 6 months (palmar grasp)

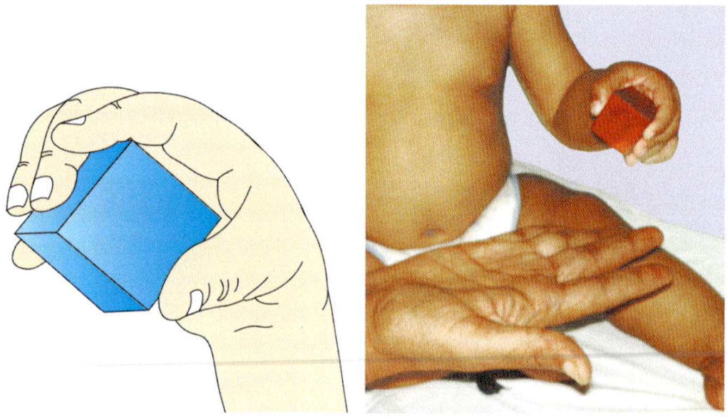

Fig. 3.36: Crude radial grasp at 8 to 10 months, beginning to use radial aspect of the hand

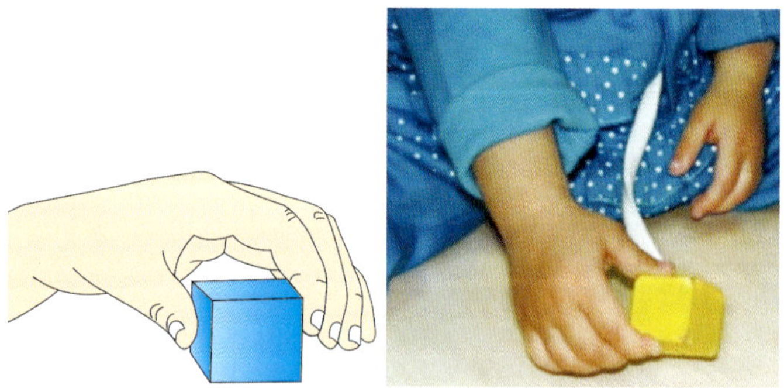

Fig. 3.37: Mature radial grasp at 1 year of age, note the use of thumb and index finger

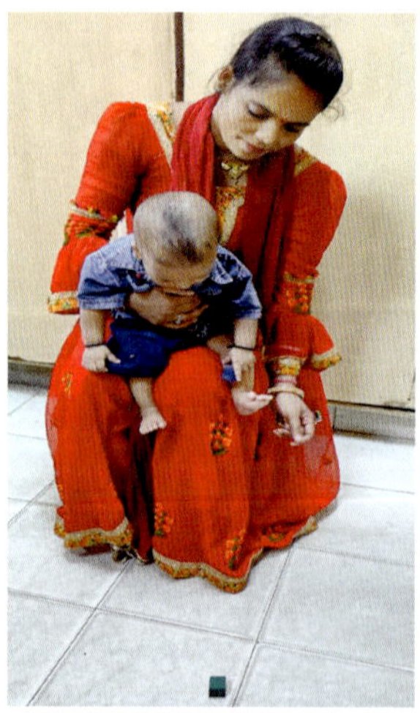

Fig. 3.38: Looks for dropped cube at 9 months (*Courtesy:* Dr Md Tousifullah)

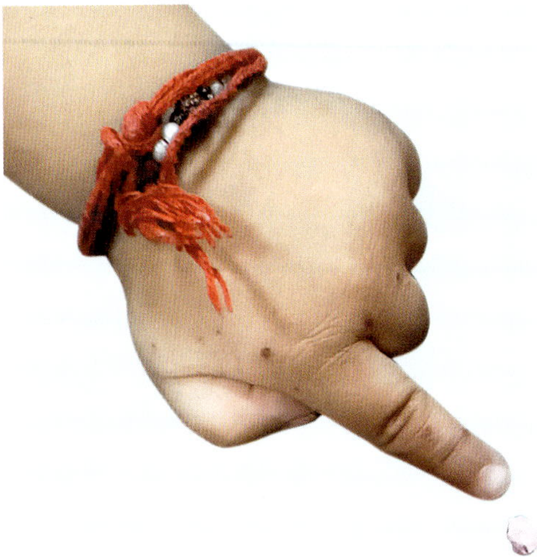

**Fig. 3.39:** Pokes at a small object at 9–10 months

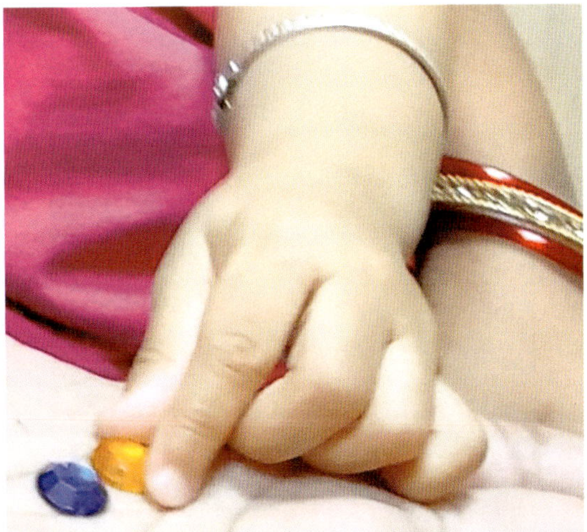

**Fig. 3.40:** Immature pincer grasp at 10 months (*Courtesy:* Dr Deepika Kainth)

the child supports his hand on the surface and picks up the object (immature pincer grasp; 10 and 11 months; Fig. 3.40). Later at 11 and 12 months, the child approaches the object directly and picks up the pellet (mature pincer grasp; Fig. 3.41).

***Hand-to-mouth coordination:*** At six months, as the ability to chew develops, the child brings the biscuit to his mouth and chews (Fig. 3.42). At this age, he tends to mouth all objects offered to him (Fig. 3.43). This tendency decreases by one year of age. By 12 months, he tries to feed himself from a cup with spilling. By 15 months, the child can pick up a cup and drink from it without much spilling (Fig. 3.44). By 18 months, he can feed himself well using a spoon (Fig. 3.45).

***Advanced hand skills:*** At 15 months, he turns 2–3 pages of a book at a time (Fig. 3.46) and scribbles on paper with a crayon (Fig. 3.47). By 18 months, he can build a tower of 2–3 cubes and draw a stroke with a pencil. He can unscrew lids at 18 months (Fig. 3.48) and turn doorknobs at two years, and his block skills have also advanced (Table 3.2 and Fig. 3.49). He now draws a circular stroke and turns pages of a book one at a time.

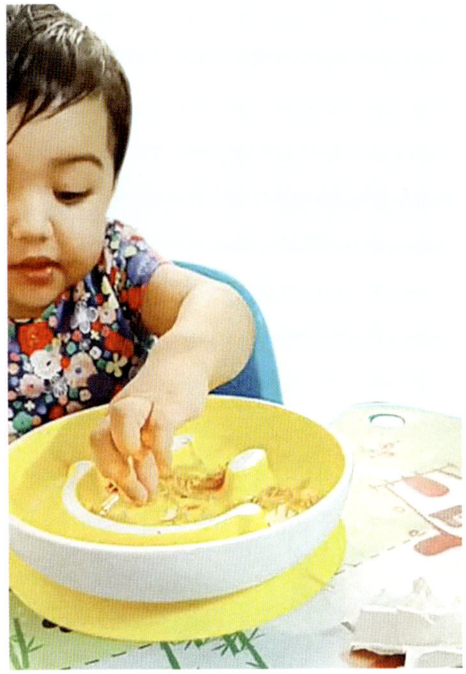

**Fig. 3.41:** Mature pincer grasp at 12 months (*Courtesy:* Dr Deepika Kainth)

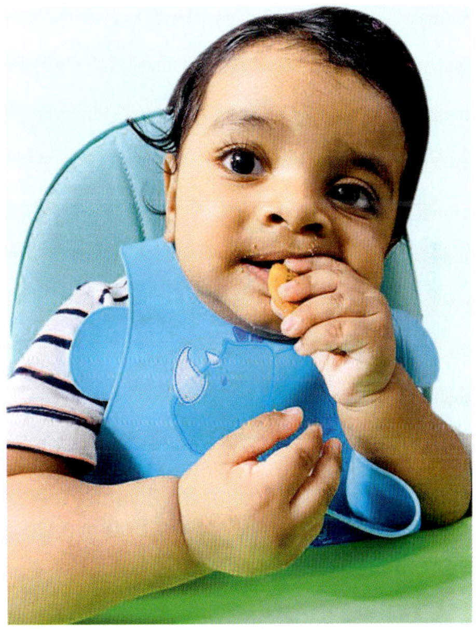

**Fig. 3.42:** Chews biscuit at six months (*Courtesy:* Dr Md Tousifullah)

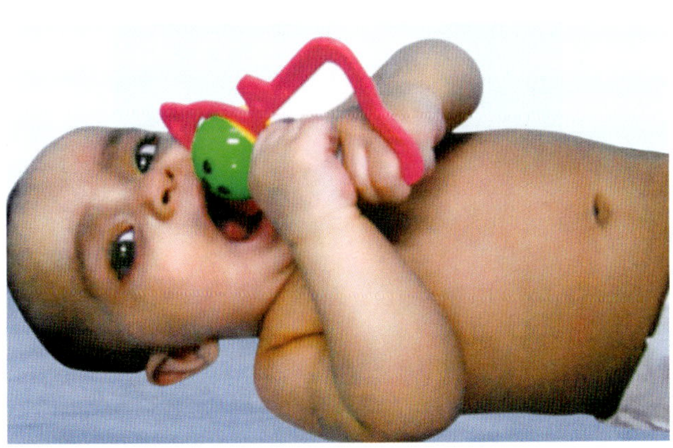

**Fig. 3.43:** A child mouthing an object at six months of age

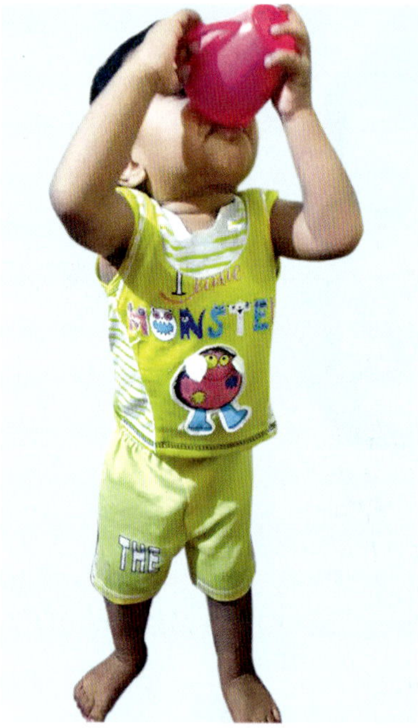

**Fig. 3.44:** Feeding from a cup without spilling at 15 months of age

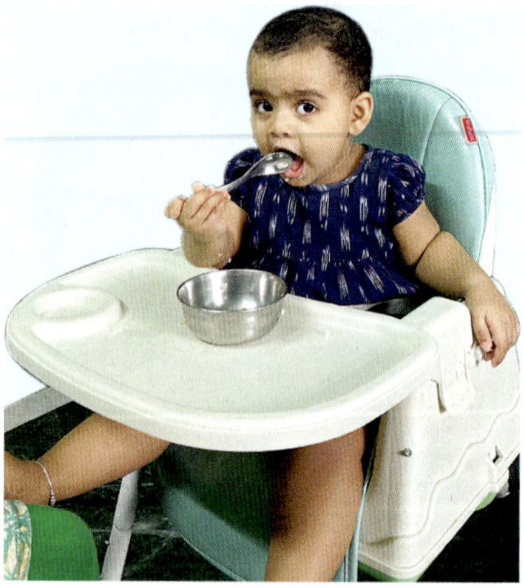

**Fig. 3.45:** Feeds herself well using spoon at 18 months. Note that child rotates the spoon at this age. By 2 years, the child is able to feed herself with spoon (*Courtesy:* Dr Soumya Devarapalli)

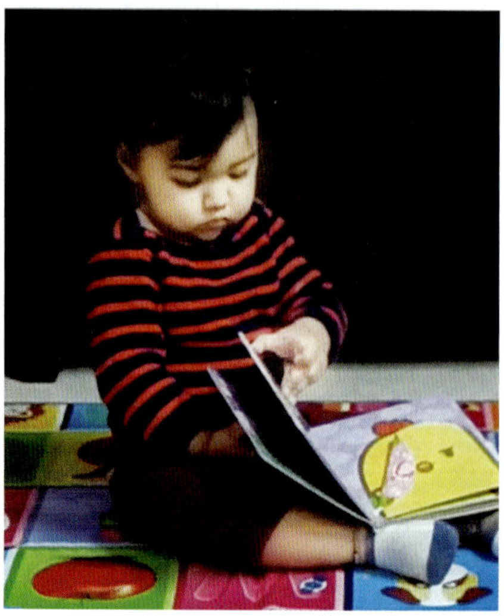

**Fig. 3.46:** Turns 2–3 pages of a book at 15 months (*Courtesy:* Dr Deepika Kainth)

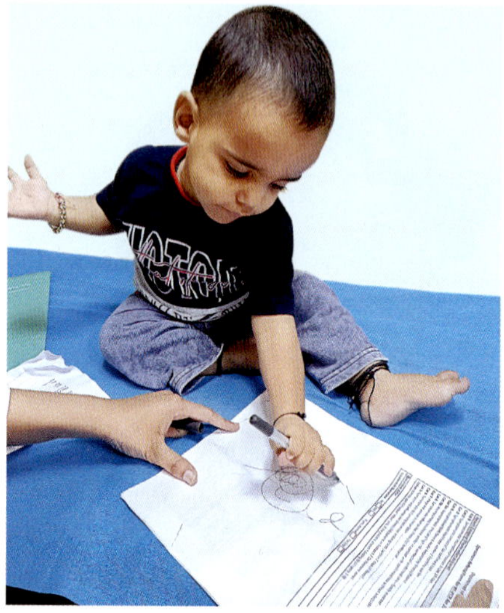

**Fig. 3.47:** Scribbles on the paper at 15 months

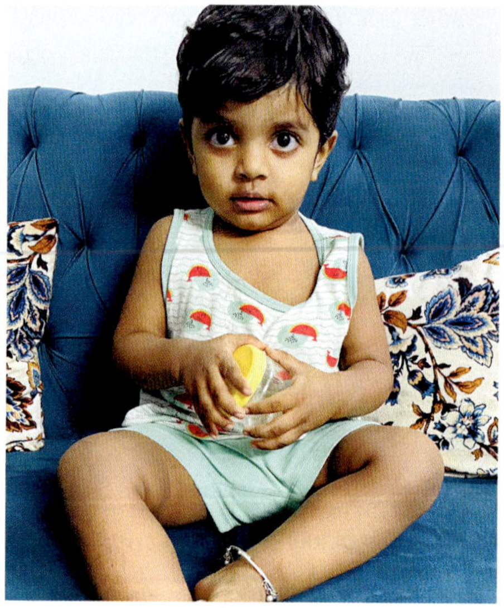

**Fig. 3.48:** Unscrews the lid at 18 months (*Courtesy:* Dr Md Tousifullah)

Figures 3.50 to 3.52 show drawing and block skills at various ages. In general, imitating a skill (seeing while

**Table 3.2:** Key fine motor milestones

| *Age* | *Milestone* |
|---|---|
| 4 months | Bidextrous reach (reaching out for objects with both hands) |
| 6 months | Unidextrous reach (reaching out for objects with one hand); transfers objects |
| 9 months | Immature pincer grasp; probes with forefinger |
| 12 months | Pincer grasp mature |
| 15 months | Imitates scribbling; tower of 2 blocks |
| 18 months | Scribbles; tower of 3 blocks |
| 2 years | Tower of 6 blocks; vertical and circular stroke |
| 3 years | Tower of 9 blocks; copies circle |
| 4 years | Copies cross; bridge with blocks |
| 5 years | Copies triangle; gate with blocks |

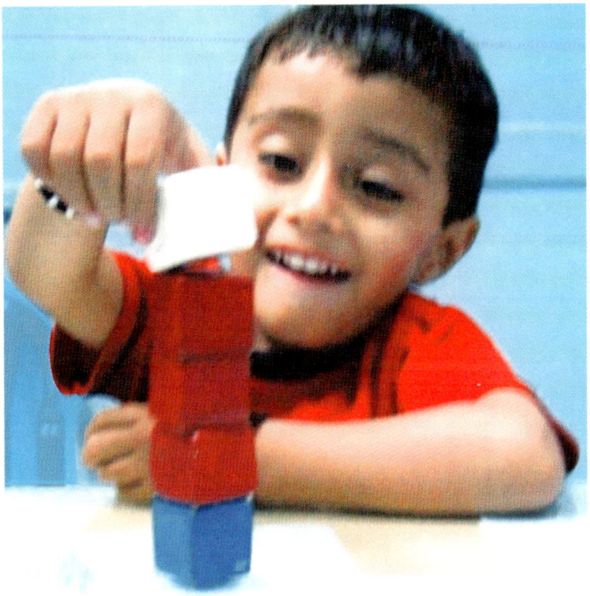

**Fig. 3.49:** Makes a tower of 5–6 cubes at two years of age

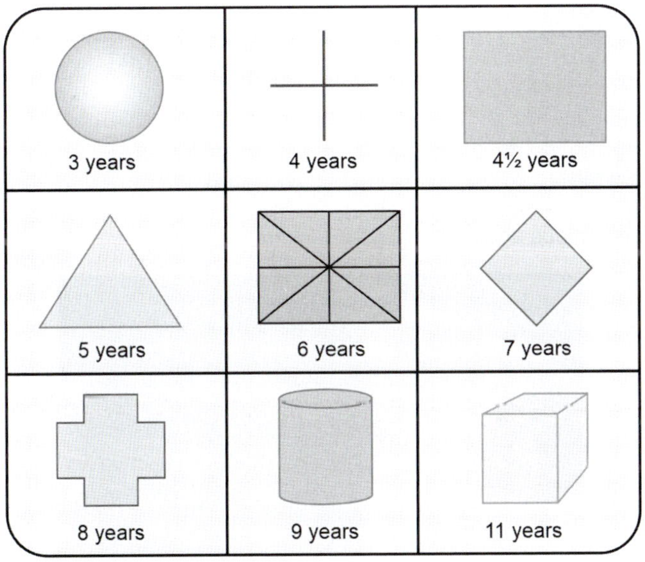


**Fig. 3.50:** Drawing skills at various ages

doing) comes 6 months before copying (first sees and then does it without noticing).

***Dressing:*** A child learns to undress before dressing. At one year, the child starts to pull off mittens, caps, and socks. At 18 months, he can unzip but fumbles with buttons. The child put on shoes or socks by two years. Dressing usually comes at three years but the child is able to button at 4 years. He can fully dress by himself at five years.

### Personal and Social Development and General Understanding

The child intently watches his mother when she talks to him at one month **(Fig. 3.53)**. He smiles back (social smile) when anyone talks or smiles at him at six weeks **(Fig. 3.54)**. A social smile is different from a spontaneous smile (without any social interaction), which is present even in neonates. By three months, he enjoys looking around and recognizes

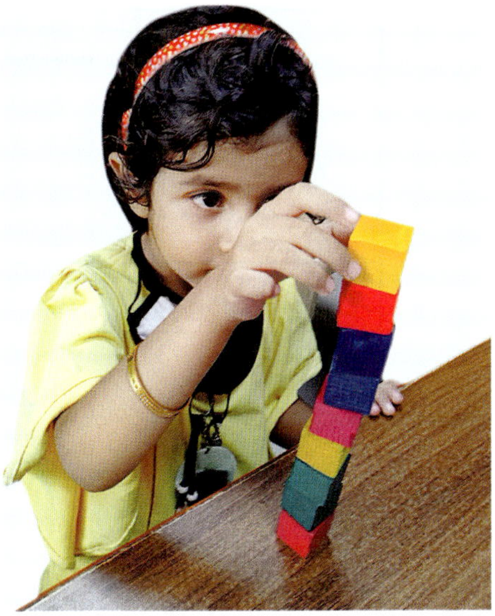

**Fig. 3.51:** Builds a tower of 9 cubes at 3 years (*Courtesy:* Dr Md Tousifullah)

his mother. By six months, he vocalizes and smiles at his mirror image **(Fig. 3.55)** and imitates acts such as coughing or tongue protrusion.

The child becomes anxious about meeting strangers (stranger anxiety) by 6–7 months **(Fig. 3.56)**. At this age, he inhibits to "no". At nine months, he waves "bye-bye" and repeats a performance that evokes an appreciative response from the observers. By one year, he can understand simple questions, such as "where is papa" ,"where is your ball", etc. By 15 months, he points to objects in which he is interested. By 18 months, he follows simple orders and indulges in domestic mimicry (imitates mother sweeping or cleaning) **(Fig. 3.57)**. At two years, he can point to 5–6 familiar objects, name at least 2–3 objects, and point to 3–4 body parts. By three years, the child begins to count, identifies 1–2 colors, and sings simple rhymes. The left and right discrimination comes by four years. At this age, play activities can be imaginative also called pretend play. For example, the child may pretend to bathe or feed a doll or attend to a doll pretending to be a nurse or doctor. By five years of age, children can follow 3-step commands, identify four colors and repeat four digits **(Table 3.3)**.

### Language

Throughout the development of language, understanding precedes the expressive skills. Following social smile at six weeks, the child begins to vocalize vowel sounds such as 'ah, and uh'. At 3–4 months, he squeals with delight and laughs loud. He begins to say 'ah-goo', 'gaga' by 5 months. By six months, he uses monosyllables (ba, da, pa). At nine months, he joins consonants to form bisyllables (mama, baba, dada).

Before developing meaningful speech, by 9–10 months, the child learns to imitate sounds of his native language. On his first birthday, he says 1–2 words with meaning. At 18 months, he has a vocabulary of 8–10 words. By two years, the vocabulary increases rapidly to around 100 words, and the child starts joining 2–3 words to form simple sentences.

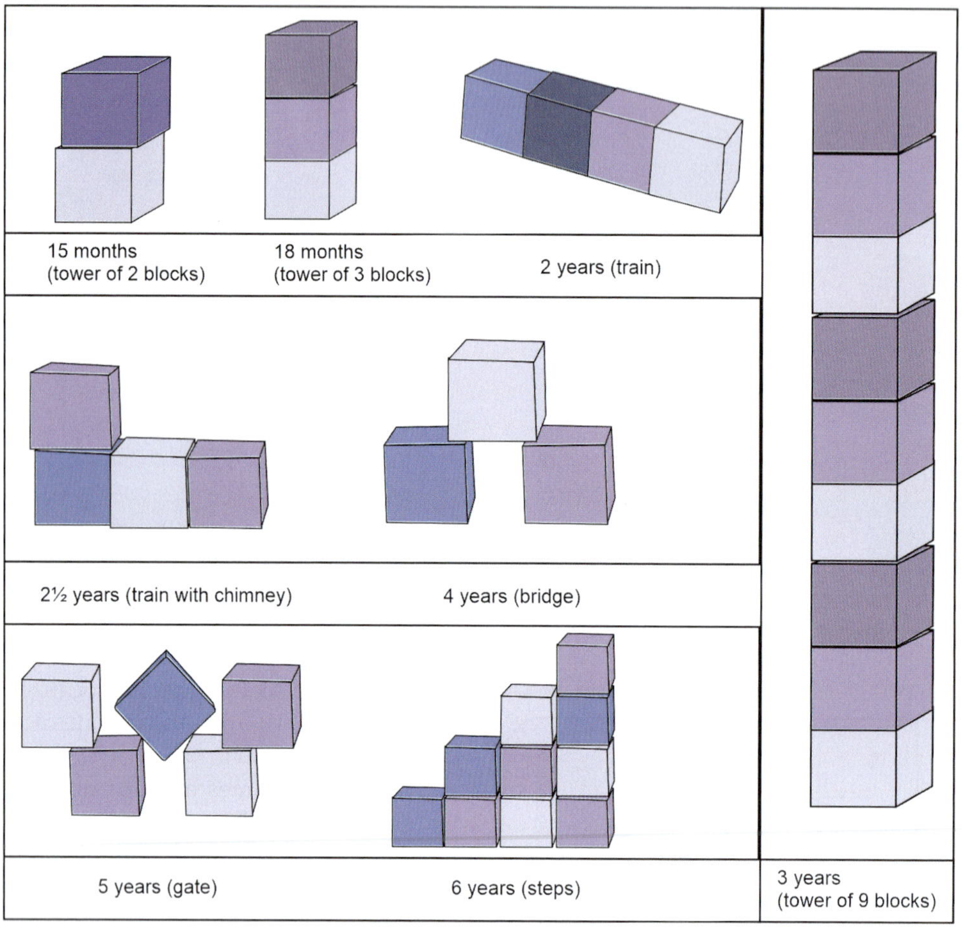


**Fig. 3.52:** Block skills at various ages

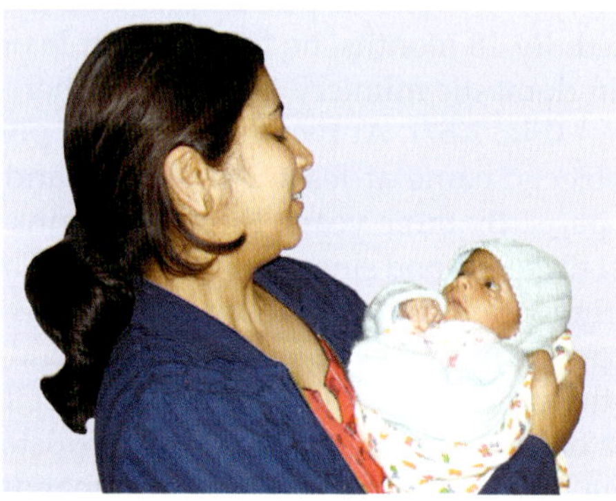

**Fig. 3.53:** At 1 month, the baby shows intent regard for his mother's face as she talks to him

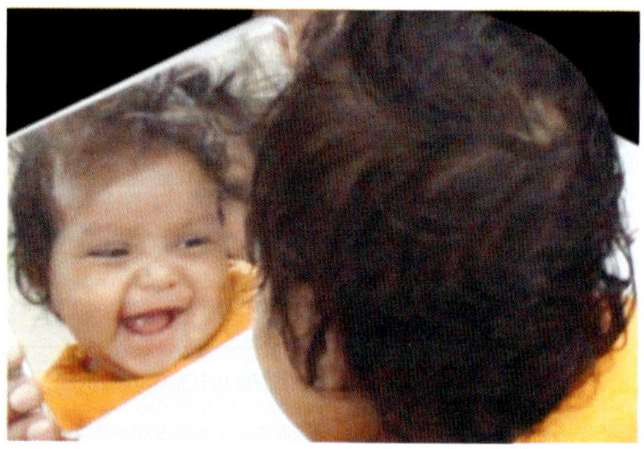

**Fig. 3.55:** A child smiles at himself in the mirror at 6 months of age

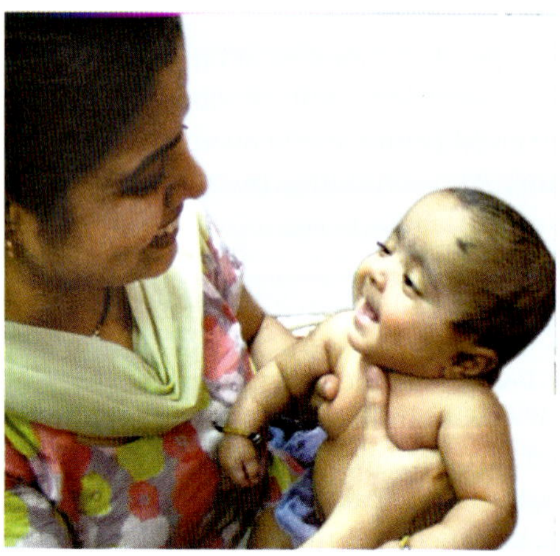

**Fig. 3.54:** Social smile

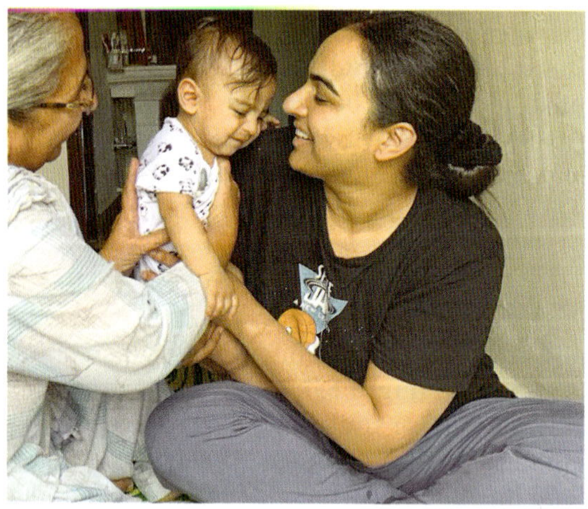

**Fig. 3.56:** Stranger anxiety at 6 to 7 months

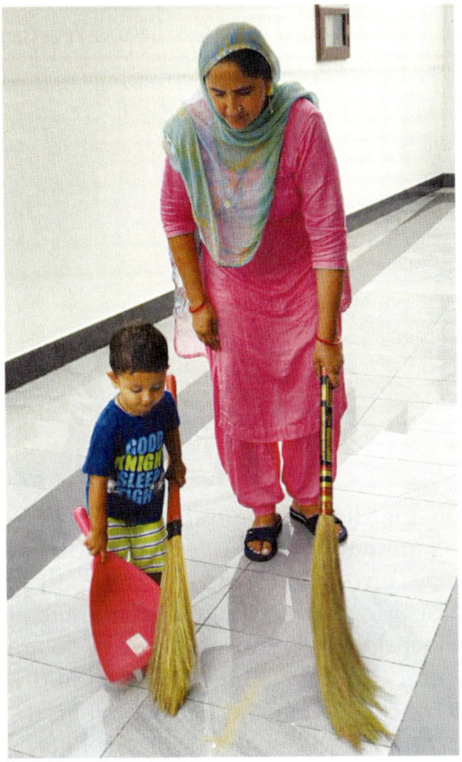

Fig. 3.57: Domestic mimicry at 18 months (*Courtesy:* Dr Md Tousifullah)

**Table 3.3:** Key social and adaptive milestones

| *Age* | *Milestone* |
|---|---|
| 2 months | Social smile (smile after being talked to) |
| 3 months | Recognizes mother; anticipates feeds |
| 6 months | Recognizes strangers, stranger anxiety |
| 9 months | Waves "bye bye" |
| 12 months | Comes when called; plays simple ball game |
| 15 months | Jargon |
| 18 months | Copies parents in task (e.g. sweeping) |
| 2 years | Asks for food, drink, toilet; pulls people to show toys |
| 3 years | Shares toys; knows full name and gender |
| 4 years | Plays cooperatively in a group; goes to toilet alone |
| 5 years | Helps in household tasks, dresses and undresses |

By three years, the toddler continually asks questions and knows his full name. He can give a coherent account of recent experiences and events by the age of 4 years (Table 3.4).

### *Vision and Hearing*

The ability to see and hear is apparent even in the newborn.

***Vision:*** The best stimulus to check visual behavior is the primary caretaker's face. At birth, a baby can fixate and follow a moving person or dangling ring held 8–10 inches away up to a range of 45 , which increases to 90 by four weeks and 180 by 12 weeks. At around one month, the baby can fixate on his mother as she talks to her (Fig. 3.58).

Binocular vision begins at around six weeks and is well established by four months. At about 3–4 months, the child fixates intently on an object shown to him (grasping with the eye) as if the child wants to reach for the object (Fig. 3.59). By six months, the child adjusts his position to follow objects of interest and can follow rapidly moving objects by one year.

***Hearing:*** Newborns respond to sounds by startling, blinking, crying, quieting, or changing activity. Make a sound of a bell kept 1½ feet away and out of the field of vision to test

**Table 3.4:** Key language milestones

| *Age* | *Milestone* |
|---|---|
| 1 month | Alerts to sound |
| 3 months | Coos (musical vowel sounds) |
| 4 months | Laugh loud |
| 6 months | Monosyllables (ba, da, pa), ah-goo sounds |
| 9 months | Bisyllables (mama, baba, dada) |
| 12 months | 1–2 words with meaning |
| 18 months | 8–10 word vocabulary |
| 2 years | 2–3 word sentences, uses pronouns " I", "me", "you" |
| 3 years | Asks questions; knows full name and gender |
| 4 years | Says song or poem; tells stories |
| 5 years | Asks meaning of words |

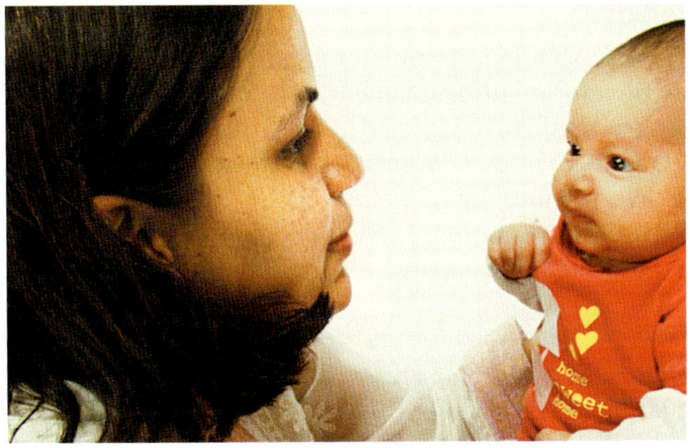

Fig. 3.58: Infant fixates on mother as she talks to her at one month

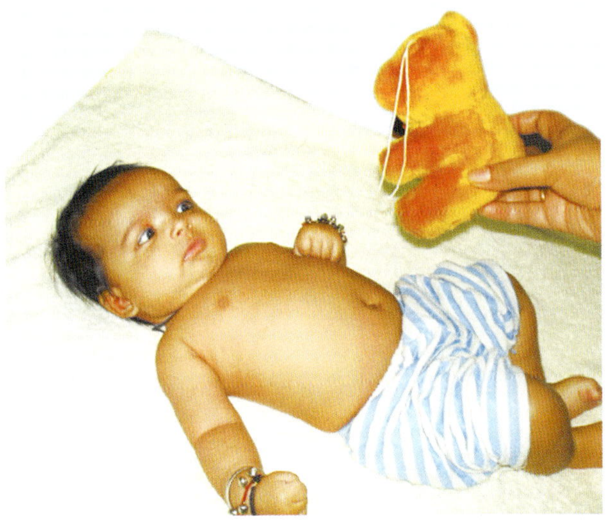

Fig. 3.59: Grasping 'with the 'eye' at 3 months

hearing. By 3 to 4 months, the child turns his head toward the sound. At 5 to 6 months, the child turns the head to the side and then downwards to the sound produced below the ear level. One month later, he can localize sounds made above the level of ears. By 10 months, the child directly looks at the source of sound diagonally (Fig. 3.60).

*Competencies:* **PE1.7; PE3.2; PE3.3; PE3.4; PE3.5; PE3.6**

## DEVELOPMENTAL ASSESSMENT

Developmental delay is estimated to be present in about 10% of children. Severe developmental disorders are recognizable early in infancy. Speech impairment, hyperactivity, and emotional disturbances are often not detected until 3–4 years. Learning disabilities may become evident once the child starts school.

### Prerequisites

The place should feel comfortable and free from distractions for development assessment. The child should not be hungry, tired, ill, or irritated and be in a playful mood with his mother. The development assessment of a sick child can be deferred until he recovers well.

The assessors must carry a development kit **(Box 3.1)** and the list of milestones.

#### *Steps*

***History:*** A well-taken history will provide information regarding (i) risk factors, (ii) rate of acquisition of milestones and differentiating the delay from the regression (loss of already achieved milestones), and (iii) approximate development age of the child, which helps to choose the appropriate tools for evaluation.

***Examination:*** Examine for (i) physical growth and head circumference, (ii) dysmorphic features (strange-looking face, abnormal orientation of ears or eyes), stigmata of intrauterine infections (microcephaly, cataract, etc.), and signs of hypothyroidism, (iii) vision and hearing, and (iv) neurological status including the presence of primitive reflexes.

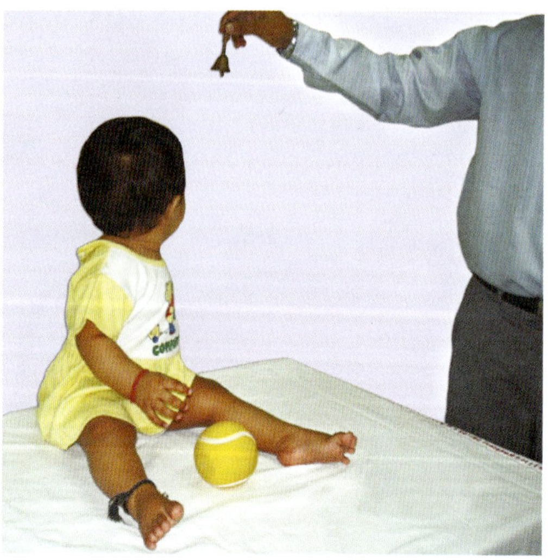

Fig. 3.60: Diagonal localization of the source of sound at 10 months

**Box 3.1: Equipment for Development Assessment**

- A red ring (diameter 6–7 cm) tied to a string
- Nine red cubes
- Paper pellets
- Spoon
- Cup with handle
- A book with thick pages
- Picture book
- Red pencil, paper
- Doll and mirror
- Red ball
- Red wool
- A bell

Perform the developmental assessment before the systemic examination. Observe the child for alertness, interest in the surroundings, and vocal responses. Assessing reflexes, measuring the head circumference, and performing ventral suspension or pull-to-sit should be done at the end.

By the end of the evaluation, one should be able to arrive at a conclusion whether the neurological status and cognitive status are within normal range or not. Significant delay on screening is an indication for a detailed formal assessment of development status. By assessment, one can assign developmental quotient (DQ) for any developmental sphere. It is calculated as:

$$\frac{\text{Average age at attainment}}{\text{Observed age at attainment}} \times 100$$

A DQ below 70% is taken as the delay that warrants detailed evaluation by a trained child psychologist. There are many tests to assess DQ giving different kinds of information.

IQ tests mainly assess the cognitive/adaptive behavior part of the development. Specific IQ tests (Stanford-Binet intelligence scales) are available to assess IQ starting from 2 years of age. However, in younger children (<5 years), it is more meaningful to have a global assessment of abilities; hence DQ testing is more comprehensive.

### Interpretation

Use corrected age for developmental status till two years of age in preterm-born children. For example, a child born at 32 weeks gestation (gestational age) seen at 12 weeks of age (postnatal age) should be considered a 4-week-old (corrected age). There are wide variations of normality in development. For example, in a WHO study, the average age for standing alone was 10.8 months (Fig. 3.61), with 3rd and 97th centiles being 7.7 and 15.2 months.

Single assessment or isolated examination findings should not be the basis for the diagnosis of retardation. Consider factors such as recent illness, significant malnutrition, emotional deprivation, sensory deficits, and neuromuscular disorders. Repeat the assessment, especially if there is no gross delay. Table 3.5 gives the upper age limits for milestones. A child who does not attain a milestone by the age limit should be evaluated for the cause of developmental delay.

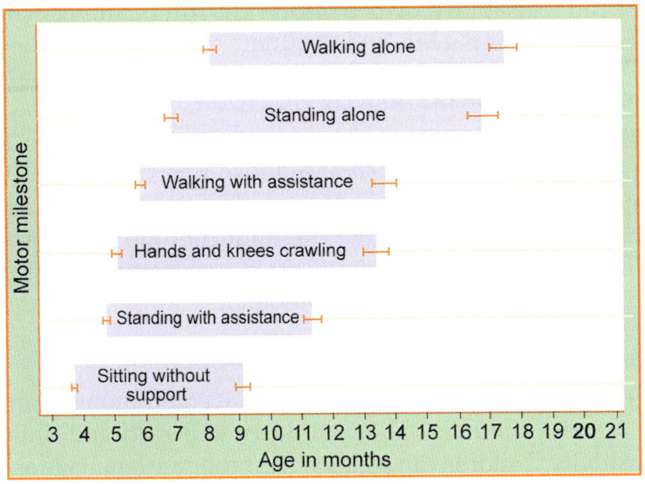


**Fig. 3.61:** Windows of achievement of six major motor milestones. The box denotes the age range for a given milestone between 3rd and 97th percentiles. The orange bars at both the ends of the boxes represent 95% confidence intervals of 3rd and 97th percentiles, respectively (WHO; Multicenter Growth Reference Study Group, 2006).

Significant variation in domains is known as dissociation, such as a 1-year-old child who speaks 2–3 words with meaning and has finger thumb opposition (10–12 months) but is unable to stand with support (less than 10 months). Such children may have a physical disorder affecting a particular developmental domain. Normal development in all domains except language may indicate a hearing deficit. Similarly, normal social and language but delayed motor milestones may indicate rickets or neuromuscular problem.

The predictive value of different domains of development for subsequent intelligence is not the same. Fine motor, personal-social and linguistic milestones predict intelligence far better than gross motor skills. In particular, an advanced language predicts high intelligence in a child.

## Development Screening Tests

Screening is a brief assessment procedure designed to identify children requiring detailed assessment. Screening tools require proper training and sound knowledge of interpreting the results. Some tools are parent-reported, while others require trained personnel.

**Table 3.5:** Upper limit of age for the attainment of milestones

| *Milestone* | *Age* |
|---|---|
| Visual fixation or following | 2 months |
| Vocalization | 6 months |
| Sitting without support | 10 months |
| Standing with assistance | 12 months |
| Hands and knees crawling | 14 months |
| Standing alone | 17 months |
| Walking alone | 18 months |
| Single words | 18 months |
| Imaginative play | 3 years |
| Loss of comprehension, single words or phrases at any age | |

Adapted from WHO; MGRS group, WHO motor development study. Acta Pediatr 2006;450:86–95

### Developmental Surveillance

Child development is dynamic, and it is challenging to quantify it on a one-time assessment. Developmental surveillance entails repeated evaluation to see the rate and pattern. It helps to detect emerging disabilities. The physician should choose a standardized developmental screening tool that is practical and easy to use in the office setting. Screening tests popular in the West include Parents' Evaluations of Development Status (PEDS) and Ages and Stages Questionnaires (ASQ).

***Phatak's Baroda screening test:*** This is India's best-known development testing system that Dr. Promila Phatak developed. It is meant to be used by child psychologists rather than physicians. It is the Indian adaptation of the Bayley development scale and is applied to children up to 30 months.

***Ages and stages questionnaire (ASQ-3):*** It consists of age-based, parent-completed questionnaires for children from one month to 5½ years of age. The questionnaire takes about 10–15 minutes for parents to complete and about 2–3 minutes to score. It assesses the following domains: Communication, gross motor, fine motor, problem-solving, and personal-social.

***Denver II:*** The revised Denver Development Screening Test (DDST) or Denver II was revised in 1992 and assesses child development in four domains, i.e. gross motor, fine motor adaptive, language, and personal-social behavior.

***Trivandrum Development Screening Chart (TDSC):*** It consists of 51 items for children of 0–6 years with items adapted from existing developmental charts/scales. It is primarily a screening tool for use in the community to identify children between 0 and 6 years with developmental delay.

***Clinical adaptive test and clinical linguistic and auditory milestone scale (CAT/CLAMS):*** This easy-to-learn scale assesses the child's cognitive and language skills. It uses parental reports and direct testing of the children from birth to 36 months.

***Goodenough-Harris drawing test:*** The child draws a man in the best possible manner, and the detail of the drawing determines the score of the child (Fig. 3.62; note the mature grip of pen, compare it with immatre grip in Fig. 3.47). One can determine the mental age by comparing scores obtained with a normative sample.

#### *Definitive Tests*

These tests are required once screening tests or clinical assessment is abnormal. They accurately define the impairments. For example, it gives domain-wise scores for verbal, motor, personal, and social skills domains (Table 3.6).

## Early Stimulation

Brain development is most rapid during pregnancy and early years (first 1000 days of life—fetal and postnatal).

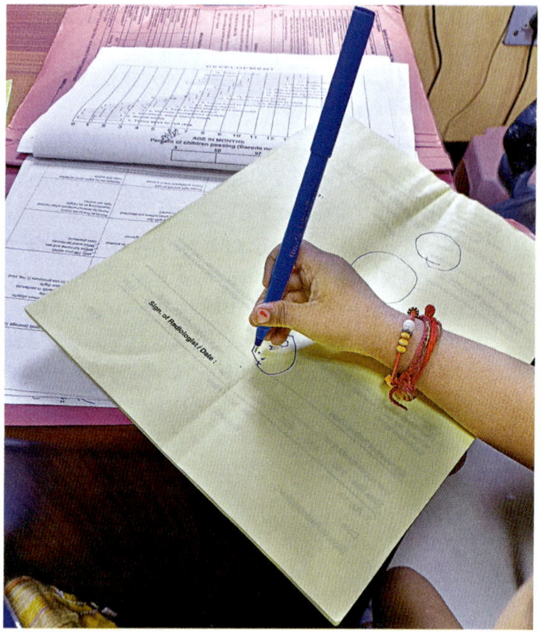

Fig. 3.62: Drawing a man at 4 years

On average, 1.8 million synapses are formed per second between 2 months gestation and two years of life. Early experiences greatly influence the architecture of the brain and the extent of adult capacity. A safe, nurturing, enabling, stimulating environment potentiates development, while stress, neglect, and abuse results in poor development and poor ability as an adult.

Infants with suspected or early developmental delays need additional support to develop motor skills, language or cognitive abilities. These extra efforts (early stimulation) include making the child sit or walk, giving toys to manipulate, playing and speaking with the child, etc.

*Competencies:* **PE4.5; PE4.6; PE5.10; PE5.11**

### Child Guidance Clinics

These multidisciplinary clinics provide diagnostic and therapeutic services to children with intellectual disability, learning disability or behavioral disorders, along with counseling for parents and children.

### Promoting Development by Effective Parenting

Parenting has an immense impact on emotional, social, and cognitive development and also plays a role in the later occurrence of mental illness, educational failure, and criminal behavior. Creating the right conditions for early childhood development is likely more effective and less costly than addressing problems later.

### Television, Mobile Devices and Development

Television viewing is a passive form of entertainment, and it impairs children's ability to learn and read and limits creativity. Children can pick up inappropriate language and habits by watching TV shows and commercials. Violence and sexuality on television can have a lasting impact on the child's mind.

Besides television, children and caregivers are increasingly getting exposed to mobile devices. Preliminary research suggests that exposure to mobile devices at a young age can impact language development, sleep, and social connectivity. Excessive and addictive use of mobile media in children can impair their executive functioning, impulse control, and emotional regulation. Screen time is also associated with obesity.

*World Health Organization recommends avoiding all screen time except video chatting in children up to 24 months.* Children between 2 and 5 years are limited to 1 hour of screen time involving high-quality programs in the presence of a parent.

Parents of children aged six years and older should place consistent limits on the time spent using media and types of media and ensure that it does not take the place of adequate sleep, physical activity, or other healthy behavior. Parents should avoid using screens as pacifiers, babysitters, or to stop tantrums.

Infants and children need attentive and accessible caregiving to meet their physical and psychological developmental needs. Inadequate parental attentiveness,

Table 3.6: Scales for definitive testing of intellect and neurodevelopment

| *Name of the test* | *Age range* | *Time taken to administer* | *Scoring details; comments* |
|---|---|---|---|
| Bayley Scale for Infant Development IV | 16 days to 42 months | 30–70 min | Assesses language, cognitive, adaptive behavior, motor, and social-emotional<br>Subtest level scaled scores, domain level composite scores, percentile ranks, confidence intervals, developmental age equivalents, and growth scale values |
| Wechsler Intelligence Scale for Children IV | 6 to 17 years | 65–80 min | Assesses verbal and performance skills, provides full-scale IQ and indices of verbal comprehension, perceptual reasoning, working memory and processing speed |
| Stanford-Binet Intelligence Scales, 5th edition | 2 to 85 years | 50–60 min | Provides full-scale IQ, verbal IQ, nonverbal IQ, 10 subset scores and 4 composite scores |
| Vineland Adaptive Behavior Scale III | 0 to 90 years | 20–60 min | Measures personal and social skills as reported by the caregiver or parent in 3 domains (communication, daily living skills, and socialization) |
| Development Assessment Scale for Indian Infants (DASII) | Birth–30 months | 45–60 min | The scale has motor (67 items) and mental domains (163 items) |

responsiveness, and poorly modeled behaviors can negatively impact child development. An emerging body of research also suggests that caregivers' excessive use of mobile devices reduces the attention and responsivity of caregivers to children.

More needs to be done to understand the effects of new modern technology and know how to best use it to benefit children and adolescents and improve their development and behavior. Mobile media can have positive effects with the right content and parental interaction. However, this requires parents to have media literacy and guidance.

## Early Childhood Development (ECD) as a High Public Health Priority

Early childhood development determines readiness for school learning, which in turn determines the productive capabilities of individuals as adults. According to estimates, 250 million children (43% of all children) under five in developing countries are at high risk of not reaching their developmental potential due to stunting, ill health, poverty, and a disadvantaged environment. SDG 4, target 4.2, aims to ensure by 2030 that all girls and boys have access to quality early childhood development, care, and pre-primary education so they are ready for primary education.

The National Education Policy (NEP 2020) calls for universal provisioning of quality early childhood development, care, and education, to ensure that all students entering Grade 1 are school ready.

## Nurturing Care

WHO has provided Nurturing Care (NC) framework as a pathway for ECD **(Box 3. 2)**. The five components of NC are Good health, Adequate nutrition, Responsive caregiving, Security and safety, and Opportunities for early learning.

*Responsive caregiving* is at the heart of nurturing care. Parents and grandparents should interact with the child. Father and other male members also have a significant role.

### Box 3.2: Nurturing Care

Nurturing care refers to that enabling environment of integrated and multisectoral care starting from fetal life through early childhood (up to age three). It ensures the children have optimum conditions for achieving their best potential in terms of health, well-being, growth, development, and overall learning experience. Nurturing care focuses on the elimination of adverse exposures and creating a facilitatory environment. Every interaction with a child is taken as a learning opportunity for him, however, big or small, formal, or informal, or structured or unstructured. Nurturing care provides a solid foundation for lifelong good health, well-being, and productivity.

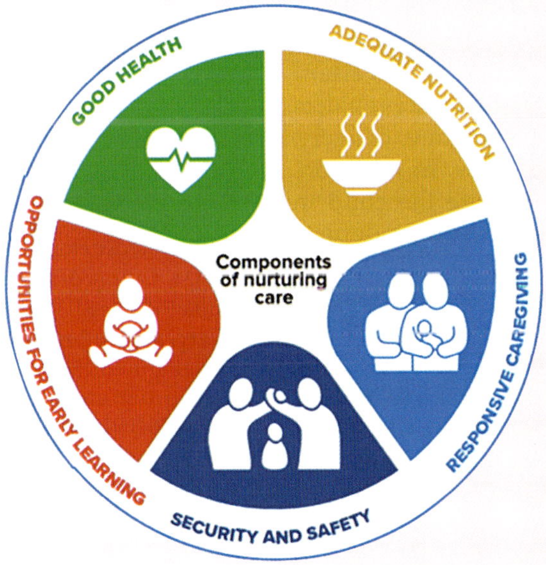


**Five components of nurturing child care**

1. **Good health:** Children should have optimum health and well-being to achieve their developmental potential. Also, the caregivers have good physical and mental health to take care of their children well.
2. **Adequate nutrition:** The adequate nutrition of the mother during pregnancy and the child is essential for a child's optimum health. Good nutrition of the mother during pregnancy ensures that her unborn child receives optimum nutrition. Subsequently, optimum nutrition of the mother makes her better capable of providing adequate care to her young child.
3. **Safety and security:** The community where the family lives must be free from physical dangers, emotional stress, and environmental risks (e.g. pollution and toxins). There must be optimum access to food and safe water.
4. **Opportunities for early learning:** The child learns from his environment—the people, objects, and places around him. A child should have optimum opportunities and enabling environment to ensure adequate learning opportunities.
5. **Responsive caregiving:** The caregivers should be able to notice and understand the needs of the children, and respond timely and adequately in a positive manner. Responsive caregiving lies at the heart of the other four components.

(*Reference:* World Health Organization, United Nations Children's Fund, World Bank Group. Nurturing care for early childhood development: A framework for helping children survive and thrive to transform health and human potential. Geneva: World Health Organization; 2018. Licence: CC BY-NC-SA 3.0 IGO; Reproduced with permission)

Learning opportunities should be created and used. The following are five key approaches by caregivers in engaging the child:

i. *Conversation:* Talk, explain, sing, tell a story, read a book.
ii. *Responsive feeding:* Interact, and converse while offering complementary feeds
iii. *Offering objects/toys:* Explain colors and shapes; encourage touch, holding, manipulation.
iv. *Facilitating motor activity:* Help with sitting, standing, walking, and running—at appropriate ages.
v. *Playing:* Play with the child, let the child play with other children.

Toys are an age-old tool for facilitating child development. Several household objects also serve as excellent toys (a steel glass, a spoon, a ball of wool, and a bangle). Home improvised and locally produced affordable toys may be employed.

Other useful adjuncts include child engagement video clips, flip charts, calenders, and child books. Child development Apps are also becoming popular.

Table 3.7 provides age-appropriate activities for promoting optimum development and red flag signs at different ages. The items to promote development should be explained to caregivers. The red flag signs should alert the provider to seek referral for investigation.

### Mother–Child Protection (MCP) Card

The Mother–Child Protection Card is an excellent monitoring-cum-counseling tool for families and providers alike. It provides information on antenatal care, delivery, immunization, nutrition, and milestones. In addition, it gives parental tips on how to engage the child in developmental stimulation **(Table 3.7)**. It also depicts indicators of developmental delay (red flag signs) that should alert the caregiver and family to seek expert help. *Mother–Child Protection Card should be used as a routine practice in tracking and counseling child development.*

Anganwari workers (AWW) have an vital role in child development in the community. Since 0–3 children do not come to Anganwari, AWW visits them at home for health, nutrition, and ECD counseling using appropriate tools.

ASHA workers play a role in child development through the Home-Based Young Child Program **(Box 3.3)**.

A critical approach to promote child development is to ensure community participation. AWW, ASHA, women self-help groups, and other stakeholders should organize community-based events for awareness generation and participatory learning.

**Box 3.3: Home-based Young Child (HBYC) Program**

HBYC program envisages home visits by ASHA in the 3rd, 6th, 9th, 12th and 15th month. The purpose is:

- Promoting good child nutrition
- Ensuring age appropriate immunization
- Ensuring optimal early childhood development (ECD)
- Promoting *swachh* practices
- Ensuring health care seeking behaviour

Under this program, ASHA counsels the family to promote child development using Mother-Child Protection Card and other tools.

At every contact with a child, a physician must always assess development and counsel the family on nurture care, and, in particular, give tips on engaging children for Early Childhood Development.

### Useful Internet Resources

- https://nhm.gov.in/New_Updates_2018/NHM_Components/Immunization/Guildelines_for_immunization/MCP_Card_English_version.pdf
- https://www.who.int/teams/maternal-newborn-child-adolescent-health-and-ageing/child-health/nurturing-care
- http://www.nlm.nih.gov/medlineplus/child development.html
- http://kidshealth.org/parent/growth/
- http://www.nichd.nih.gov/
- http://www.med.umich.edu/yourchild/
- http://www.bridges4kids.org/disabilities/SLI.html
- http://www.zerotothree.org/

### Suggested Reading

1. Black MM, Walker SP, Fernald LCH, et al; Lancet Early Childhood Development Series Steering Committee. Early childhood development coming of age: science through the life course. Lancet 2017;389(10064):77–90.
2. Britto PR, Lye SJ, Proulx K, et al; Early Childhood Development Interventions Review Group, for the Lancet Early Childhood Development Series Steering Committee. Nurturing care: promoting early childhood development. Lancet 2017; 389(10064):91–102.
3. Indian Academy of Pediatrics Position Paper on Nurturing Care for Early Childhood Development. Indian Pediatrics 2021 PII: S097475591600349.
4. Nair MK, Nair GS, George B, et al. Development and validation of Trivandrum development screening chart for children aged 0–6 years. Indian J Pediatr 2013; 80 Suppl2: S248–55.
5. Richter LM, Daelmans B, Lombardi J, et al; Paper 3 Working Group and the Lancet Early Childhood Development Series Steering Committee. Investing in the foundation of sustainable development: pathways to scale up for early childhood development. Lancet 2017;389(10064):103–18.

**Table 3.7:** Parenting tips to nurture development and red flag signs for developmental delay (Adapted from Mother and Child Protection card)

| *Age* | *Parenting tips for nurturing development* | *Warning signs of delay (red flag signs)* |
|---|---|---|
| 0 to 3 months | Encourage babies to lie on tummy for some time everyday<br>Massage gently; stretch and exercise arms and legs<br>Cuddle and play with babies daily<br>Respond to the cry<br>Talk to babies in your mother tongue<br>Hang colorful objects at 30 cm above them<br>*Avoid digital media in children <24 months of age* | **At 3 months**<br>No social smile<br>No eye contacts<br>Persistent squint<br>Does not startle or respond to sound<br>Head pushed back, with stiff arms and legs<br>Persistent fisting |
| 4 to 6 months | Communicate with babies; imitate their sound and praise them when they imitate yours<br>Put interesting things on the floor for babies to reach out and explore<br>Expose to outdoors<br>Thumb sucking is normal at this age | **At 6 months**<br>Lacks head control<br>Cannot sit even with help<br>Does not grasp things within reach<br>Does not vocalize<br>Head and eyes do not track objects<br>Unable to raise head when on tummy |
| 7 to 9 months | Give clean utensils and other item to play, bang and throw<br>Play games like peek a boo, play by hiding toys under cloth, or in a box | **At 9 months**<br>Cannot roll over or sit<br>Does not turn to sound<br>Does not utter bisyllables; pa-pa, ma- a, ba-ba<br>Tilt head always to one side when looking at objects |
| 10 to 12 months | Tell stories<br>Show picture books<br>Tell names of objects and body parts<br>Let them explore home safely | **At 12 months**<br>Does not stretch hands to be picked up<br>Does not pick small objects with finger and thumb<br>Does not respond to own name<br>Does not search for half hidden toys that the child sees you hide<br>Does not play social games (peek-a-boo) |
| 13 to 18 months | Provide push toys for babies to learn walking<br>Ask simple questions and encourage them to talk<br>Provide picture books and colorful toys<br>Let them explore indoor and outdoor safely under supervision | **At 18 months**<br>Cannot stand<br>Cannot put small objects in a container<br>Does not use both hands equally<br>Does not point finger at an object when named<br>Does not respond to mothers' gestures and seems to be in his/her own world<br>Does not say single words like "mama" or "dada" |
| 19 to 24 months | Provide opportunity for babies to walk, run, or climb in safe environments<br>Allow children to imitate and allow them to do simple home tasks<br>Read aloud stories from picture books<br>Provide books and paper, colors for scribbling<br>Encourage interactional play with peers | **At 24 months**<br>Does not walk steady while pulling a toy<br>Cannot scribble<br>Does not use two words pharases such as "give milk, amma come"<br>Does not respond to gesture like bye-bye or namaste<br>Does not point to body parts<br>Does not seem to understand and follow simple instructions |
| 25 to 36 months | Play outdoor games<br>Encourage interactional play with peers<br>Give more complex games like puzzles, blocks, jigsaw<br>Allow them to do simple household work safely | Cannot climb stairs<br>Cannot feed self<br>Continuous drooling, unclear speech<br>Does not communicate meaningfully and frequently repeats others' speech<br>Cannot speak simple sentences like "mummy give milk/water" |

Adapted from: https://nhm.gov.in/New_Updates_2018/NHM Components/Immunization/Guildelines_for_ immunization/MCP_Guide_Book.pdf

Chapter

4

# Developmental and Behavioral Disorders

❍ Biswaroop Chakrabarty ❍ Sheffali Gulati

The cognitive and behavioral phenotype of an individual reflects the growth and development of the body, particularly the brain, during early years. Nutrition, environment and social and emotional milieu are important determinants of the phenotype.

*Competencies:* **PE3.1; PE4.1; PE30.10**

## GLOBAL DEVELOPMENTAL DELAY, INTELLECTUAL DISABILITY

Global developmental delay is defined as delay in acquiring milestones in two or more of the following domains, namely gross and fine motor, speech and language, cognition, socio-personal and activities of daily living. Above 5 years of age, the term intellectual disability is used, replacing the previously used term mental retardation. The estimated prevalence is 2.5–5%.

*Competencies:* **PE3.1; PE4.1**

## DEVELOPMENTAL DEVIANCE AND DISSOCIATION

Deviance is the acquisition of milestones in a sequence that is different from usual. For example, children with cerebral palsy may show early standing with support secondary to increased extensor tone. Normally, developing children may not crawl and directly start walking from sitting and standing without support. Dissociation is defined as the acquisition of developmental milestones in various domains at differing rates, viz., isolated speech delay with normal development in other domains, as in patients with congenital hearing loss.

### Etiology

An etiology can be defined in 70% patients with developmental disorders (Table 4.1). In developed countries, antenatal factors predominate; whereas in the developing world, perinatal and postnatal factors are more common. Patients with developmental delay may have various comorbidities depending on the etiology (Table 4.2). Depending on the etiology, the yield of diagnostic tests varies from 10 to 80% (Table 4.3).

**Table 4.1:** Etiology of developmental delay according to the time of insult

| | |
|---|---|
| Antenatal | • Syndromes (fragile X, Rett syndrome)<br>• Chromosomal disorders (Down syndrome)<br>• Cortical malformations<br>• Intrauterine infections<br>• Inborn errors of metabolism (aminoacidopathy, organic acidemia, mitochondrial disorder, urea cycle disorder, disorders of glycosylation)<br>• Teratogen exposure<br>• Neuromuscular disorders (predominantly motor delay) |
| Perinatal, neonatal | • Hypoxic ischemic encephalopathy<br>• Kernicterus<br>• After meningitis or encephalitis<br>• Hypoglycemic brain injury<br>• Hypothyroidism<br>• After head trauma |
| Postnatal | Deficiency of vitamin $B_{12}$, iodine or $B_1$; toxins (lead) |

### Management

A child with developmental delay is managed by a multidisciplinary team comprising of a pediatric neurologist, geneticist, psychologist, psychiatrist, occupational and physiotherapist, speech therapist, audiologist, ophthalmologist, nutritionist and social worker. Early intervention is important to achieve maximum cognitive and developmental potential.

*Competency:* **PE4.4**

## AUTISM SPECTRUM DISORDER

Autism spectrum disorder (ASD) is characterized by the triad of qualitative impairment of social behavior,

**Table 4.2:** Comorbidities in patients with development disorders

| |
|---|
| *Developmental delay, intellectual disability*<br>• Seizures<br>• Vision abnormalities, hearing impairment, speech disorders Feeding problems<br>• Behavioral problems, sleep disturbances<br>• Contractures, bedsores |
| *Autism spectrum disorder*<br>• Seizures<br>• Feeding problem<br>• Behavioral problems: Aggression, impulsivity, hyperactivity, inattention, sleep-related problems<br>• Cognitive impairment |
| *Attention deficit hyperactivity disorder*<br>• Sleep problems<br>• Enuresis, encopresis; obesity<br>• Learning disability<br>• Behavioral comorbidities: Autism spectrum disorder, tics, conduct disorder, delinquency<br>• Anxiety, bipolar illness |
| *Specific learning disability*<br>• Epilepsy<br>• Attention deficit hyperactivity disorder, tics<br>• Obsessive compulsive disorder |
| *Tic disorder*<br>• Obsessive compulsive disorder; anxiety, depression<br>• Attention deficit hyperactivity disorder<br>• Learning disability<br>• Autism spectrum disorder |

communication (verbal and non-verbal) skills and associated stereotypic and restrictive behavioral patterns, with onset before 3 years of age (Table 4.4). The estimated global prevalence is 1–2%.

### Etiopathogenesis

The pathogenesis of autism is not clear. Abnormalities in neural connectivity and migration, dendritic and synaptic morphology and functioning of mirror neurons have been implicated. Genetic causes such as fragile X syndrome, tuberous sclerosis, Angelman syndrome and metabolic diseases like phenylketonuria and hypothyroidism account for 10% cases.

### Diagnostic Approach

The Diagnostic and Statistical Manual of Mental Disorders (DSM) IV required fulfillment of a minimum number of symptoms listed in the three domains (social interaction, communication and behavior) to label a child as having an ASD. Guidelines, according to DSM 5, have combined social interaction and communication domains into one. Thus, to be labeled as ASD, a child has to fulfill a minimum number of symptoms in two domains (social interaction and communication, and behavior). Common comorbidities are shown in Table 4.2.

### Management

The cornerstone is behavioral intervention with limited role of pharmacotherapy (Table 4.5).

**Table 4.3:** Diagnostic tests in evaluation of developmental delay

| *Investigation* | *Indication* |
|---|---|
| Neuroimaging (MRI preferred over CT) | Specifically if abnormal head size and/or abnormality on neurological examination |
| Metabolic tests (ammonia, bicarbonate, lactate, sugar; blood TMS; urine GCMS) | Clues on history or examination (recurrent encephalopathy, vomiting, seizures, regression of milestones, organomegaly, cataract, retinopathy) |
| Genetic studies (cytogenetic studies, karyotyping) | Developmental delay without a known cause, irrespective of dysmorphic features |
| Thyroid function tests; blood and urine lead; micronutrient levels | If indicated clinically |
| Electrophysiological tests | Where indicated: Electroencephalogram, visual evoked responses, brainstem evoked response, audiometry, nerve conduction studies, electromyography |

MRI magnetic resonance imaging; GCMS gas chromatography mass spectrophotometry; TMS tandem mass spectrophotometry

**Table 4.4:** Clinical features of autism, ADHD and specific learning disability

| *Disorder* | *Salient clinical features* |
|---|---|
| Autism spectrum disorder | • Onset before 3 years of age<br>• Impaired verbal and gestural communication<br>• Defect in social and emotional reciprocity<br>• Stereotypic and restrictive behavioral patterns |
| Attention deficit hyperactivity disorder (ADHD) | • Onset up to 12 years of age<br>• Present in at least 2 different social settings<br>• Interfering with social, academic and occupational functioning<br>• Inattention (difficulty sustaining attention, prone to careless mistakes, easily distracted)<br>• Hyperactivity (often on the go, fidgety)<br>• Impulsivity (intrusive, interruptive, cannot wait for turn) |
| Specific learning disability* | • Dyslexia (difficulty in reading)<br>• Dysgraphia (illegible handwriting, spelling mistakes)<br>• Dyscalculia (difficulty performing simple calculations) |

*Preserved intelligence, vision and hearing; persistent for at least 6 months despite interventions targeting specific disability

**Table 4.5:** Pharmacotherapy for autism spectrum disorder

| *Medication* | *Indication* |
|---|---|
| Antipsychotics (risperidone, olanzapine) | Anxiety, aggression, repetitive behavior |
| Methylphenidate | Inattention, hyperactivity, impulsivity |
| Alpha-2 agonists (clonidine, atomoxetine) | Hyperactivity |
| Melatonin | Sleep-related problems |
| Iron supplements | If deficiency is documented |

*Competency:* **PE4.3**

## ATTENTION DEFICIT HYPERACTIVITY DISORDER

Attention deficit hyperactivity disorder (ADHD) is the most common neurobehavioral disorder of childhood. Its prevalence in India is estimated at 1.3 per 1000. The American Academy of Pediatrics recommends evaluating any child between 4 and 18 years of age for ADHD, with academic or behavioral problems with symptoms of inattention, hyperactivity and impulsivity (Table 4.4).

### Diagnosis

ADHD is diagnosed clinically. The DSM 5 criteria require fulfillment of predefined criteria in inattention, hyperactivity and impulsivity domains. The onset of symptoms can be up to 12 years of age, and they should be present in at least two different settings interfering with social, academic and occupational functioning. The associated morbidities are summarized in Table 4.2.

### Management

The cornerstone of management is psychotherapy tailored for each individual and the family. In patients with inadequate response to psychological interventions, drugs like methylphenidate and atomoxetine are used.

*Competency:* **PE4.2**

## SPECIFIC LEARNING DISABILITY

Specific learning disability is defined as a persistent impairment in reading (dyslexia), writing (dysgraphia) and/or arithmetic (dyscalculia) skills in an individual with preserved cognition, vision, hearing and adequate opportunities (Table 4.4). It affects 5–15% of school-going children. Dyslexia accounts for 80% of all specific learning disabilities. These disorders are probably caused by functionally disrupted networks in the cerebral cortex with intact anatomy.

### Diagnosis

Features suggestive of specific learning disabilities include reading slowly and incorrectly, skipping lines while reading aloud, making repeated spelling mistakes, untidy/illegible hand-writing with poor sequencing, and inability to perform even simple mathematics. The DSM 5 diagnosis of SLD requires fulfilling of a predefined criteria in reading, writing and arithmetic skills, and these impairments should persist despite interventions targeting the specific disability for at least 6 months.

### Management

Management revolves around remedial education with active participation from both school and parents.

Clinical approach to common developmental and behavioral problems is summarized in Fig. 4.1.

## TIC DISORDER AND STEREOTYPIES

Tics are abrupt onset, fast, paroxysmal, non-rhythmic motor or vocal manifestations which may be simple or complex (Table 4.6). The age of onset is 4–6 years with peak at 10–12 years and significant attenuation by 18–20 years. The prevalence is around 10–15% with higher rates in boys.

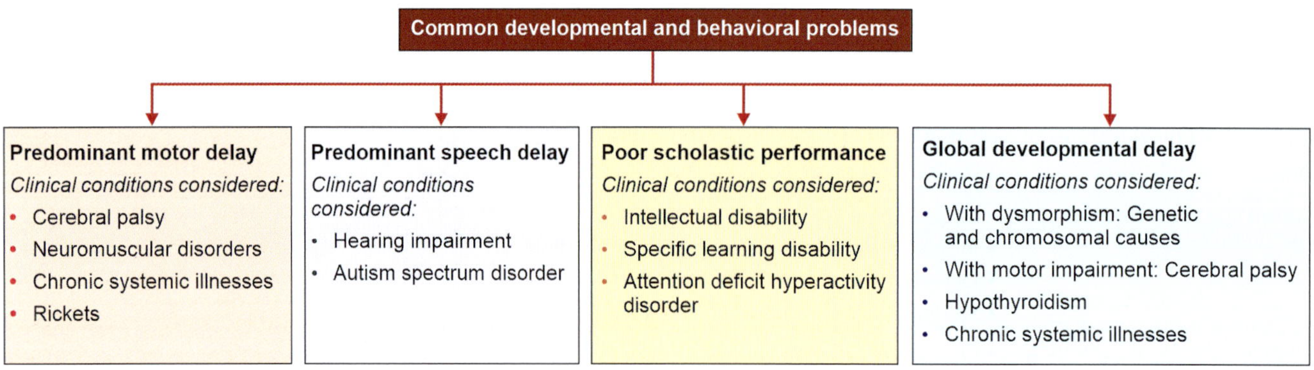


**Fig. 4.1:** Approach to common developmental and behavioral problems

**Table 4.6:** Common tics in children

| *Motor tics* | *Vocal tics* |
|---|---|
| **Simple:** Eye blinking, neck jerking, shoulder shrugging | **Simple:** Throat clearing, sniffing, coughing |
| **Complex:** Foot tapping, echopraxia (imitating others), copropraxia (obscene gestures) | **Complex:** Words out of context, coprolalia (obscene words), echolalia (repeating heard phrases or words), palilalia (repeating own words or phrases) |

Tourette syndrome is characterized by onset before 18 years of age, presence of both motor and vocal tics and persistence beyond 1 year, including the waning phase. Tics can be associated with neurological ailments like Huntington and Wilson disease, or with parainfectious illnesses, e.g. pediatric autoimmune neuropsychiatric disorders associated with streptococcal infection (PANDAS).

It is important to differentiate stereotypies from tics. Although stereotypies may have similar vocal and motor manifestations, classically they are rhythmic and distractable, and usually remain stable over a time period, unlike tics which may evolve temporally. Stereotypies usually have an early onset (before 3 years of age) and, along with neurodevelopmental disorders, may affect normal children, as well.

### Management

The essential component is behavioral therapy. Medications like haloperidol and clonidine are considered in situations where the tics are socially and functionally disabling despite adequate behavioral therapy.

*Competencies:* **PE5.1; PE5.2; PE5.4; PE5.5; PE5.6; PE5.8; PE5.9; PE6.6**

## OTHER DEVELOPMENTAL AND BEHAVIORAL DISORDERS

### Oppositional Defiant Disorder

Oppositional defiant disorder is a repetitive and persistent pattern of opposing, defiant, disobedient and disruptive behavior towards authority figures persisting for at least 6 months. Many children are later diagnosed with conduct disorders. Diagnostic criteria for labeling the condition have been developed. Oppositional defiant disorder results from interplay of factors in the child's characteristics, parental interactions and environmental factors. Family history of mental health problems such as depression, ADHD or antisocial personality is often seen. The management should focus on alleviating risk factors or stresses that might contribute to oppositional behavior. Use of stimulant medication is effective in patients with ADHD.

### Conduct Disorder

Conduct disorder is characterized by aggressive and destructive activities that cause disruption in the child's environments such as home, school or the neighborhood. The overriding feature is the repetitive and persistent pattern of behaviors that violate societal norms and the rights of other people, for a period of at least one year. Management consists of behavioral therapy and psychotherapy.

### Juvenile Delinquency

Children who show oppositional defiant behavior or conduct disorders and come into conflict with the juvenile justice system are called juvenile delinquents. The term refers to a person under 18 years of age who is brought to the attention of the juvenile justice system for committing a criminal act or displaying other illegal behaviors, like the use of alcohol or illicit drugs. Family and parenting interventions have been shown to reduce the risks of reincarceration and criminal behavior by juvenile delinquents. In some cases, placement in foster care is recommended with similar interventions administered by the foster family.

### Munchausen by Proxy

Munchausen syndrome by proxy is a disorder in which a caregiver, usually mother, deliberately makes up a history of illness in her child and/or harms the child to create illness. The name is derived from Munchausen syndrome in which a person self-induces or acts out illness to gain medical attention. In Munchausen by proxy, the abusing caregiver gains attention from the relationships formed with health care providers, or her family, as a result of the problems created.

Confirmation of diagnosis needs careful history and reviewing of past and current hospital records. Once the diagnosis is made, the offending caregiver should be confronted, separated from the child and provided psychotherapy.

### Parasomnias

Parasomnias are defined as abnormal behavioral and/or motor manifestations seen in sleep. During the first half of sleep, the non-rapid eye movement stage (NREM) parasomnias predominate, which are more common and consist of sleep walking (awake and ambulatory), confusional arousals (awake but not ambulatory) and sleep terrors (terrorized child, inconsolable and presence of a spine-chilling scream).

The relatively uncommon REM (rapid eye movement stage) parasomnias are seen in the second half of the sleep and comprise nightmares (unpleasant dreams) and bizarre movements and behavioral manifestations. The child is more likely to remember REM than NREM parasomnias on waking up. The conditions are self-limiting and management is targeted at reassurance and management of stress, if any; benzodiazepines may occasionally be used.

### Eating Disorders

This group consists of primarily two disorders, anorexia nervosa and bulimia that chiefly affect girls and have in common a disturbed body image perception. Anorexia nervosa usually affects 15–19 years old girls. Characteristic features are an intense fear of becoming fat even though the child is under-weight (body weight <85% of expected). Two subtypes are recognized, with either restricted eating or increased physical activity. Induced vomiting or use of laxatives and diuretics may be present. Complications include secondary amenorrhea and metabolic complications related to malnutrition.

Bulimia affects 10–19 years old children, chiefly girls. There are recurrent episodes of binge eating alternating with inappropriate compensatory behavior such as self-induced vomiting, misuse of laxatives, diuretics or enemas, each occurring at least twice a week for 3 months. Depression, anxiety, suicidal ideation and/or obsessive compulsive disorder are often present. Management of both conditions focuses on psychotherapy, along with nutritional rehabilitation and treating comorbidities and complications.

### Pica

Pica is the persistent ingestion of non-nutritive substances such as plaster, charcoal, paint and soil for at least 1 month, inappropriate to the child's development level and cultural practice. It is common in children less than 5 years of age. Poor socioeconomic status, malnutrition and iron deficiency are commonly associated. Developmental delay, psychosocial stress (maternal deprivation, parental neglect and abuse) and other behavioral disorders can predispose to pica. Children with pica are at increased risk for lead poisoning and parasitic infestations. Management comprises behavior modification, alleviating the psychosocial stress, screening for lead poisoning, deworming and iron supplementation.

### Temper Tantrums

Temper tantrums are a child's response to physical or emotional challenges by attention seeking tactics like yelling, biting, crying, kicking, pushing, throwing objects, hitting and head banging. Tantrums typically begin at 18–36 months of age and gradually subside by the age of 3–6 years. Parents are counseled to handle this behavioral problem strategically, by staying calm, firm and consistent so that the child is unable to take advantage from such behavior. The child should be protected from injuring himself or others. Distraction and 'time out' techniques are useful.

### Breath-Holding Spells

Breath-holding spells are reflex events typically initiated by a provocation that causes anger, frustration or pain making the child cry. The crying stops at full expiration, and the child becomes apneic and cyanotic or pale. In some cases, the child may become unconscious and hypotonic. In prolonged events, brief tonic-clonic movements may happen. Breath-holding spells are rare before 6 months of age, peak at 2 years and abate by 5 years of age. The differential diagnoses include seizures and cardiac arrhythmias. The history of a provoking event and stereotyped pattern of events help in distinguishing breath-holding spells from seizures. In relevant clinical scenarios, seizures and cardiac arrhythmias including long QT syndrome should be ruled out.

The essential component of management is parental reassurance. The family should be advised to be consistent in handling the child, to remain calm during the event, turn him sideways so that secretions can drain and avoid picking the child up (since this decreases blood flow to the brain). The family should avoid exhibiting undue concern nor give into the child's demands, if the spell was provoked by anger or frustration.

### Thumb Sucking

This entity is normal in infants and toddlers. It peaks by 18–21 months of age and usually disappears by the age of 4 years. Its persistence in older children is socially unacceptable and can lead to dental malalignment. In children below 4 years, parents should be reassured. Beyond 4 years of age, the child should be motivated to refrain from this habit. Both positive and negative reinforcements can be used.

### Stuttering

Stuttering is a defect in speech characterized by hesitation or spasmodic repetition of some syllables with pauses. There is difficulty in pronouncing the initial consonants caused by spasm of lingual and palatal muscles. It can affect up to 5% of children between 2 and 5 years of age. In this age group, parents should be reassured as most of them show resolution. If it persists beyond or appears after 5 years of age, expert opinion should be sought.

### Enuresis

Enuresis is defined as passage of urine in the clothes beyond an age when bladder control should be established (usually 5 years). Both psychological stressors and physiological dysfunction (hyposecretion of vasopressin) can be seen in affected individuals.

Enuresis may be primary or secondary (loss of control after an initial bladder control for 6 months or more), diurnal or nocturnal. Primary monosymptomatic nocturnal enuresis is the commonest variety. Before labeling as primary enuresis, diabetes, urinary tract anomalies, infection and bowel bladder dysfunction should be ruled out. The most important aspect of management is behavioral therapy with positive reinforcement. Bladder alarms or desmopressin is reserved for patients resistant to behavioral interventions (also *see* Chapter 17).

### Encopresis

Encopresis is defined as passage of stools in clothes beyond an age when bowel control should have been achieved (usually 4 years). It may be retentive (associated with constipation) or non-retentive, primary (never achieved bowel control) or secondary (loss of control after an initial phase of control for at least 6 months). Primary encopresis is usually associated with constipation, while secondary is associated with significant psychological stressors. Behavioral therapy with positive reinforcement and treatment of constipation are necessary (also *see* Chapter 12).

### Suggested Reading


1. American Academy of Pediatrics. Autism toolkit, physician fact sheet. 2012; available at www.autismsciencefoundation.org
2. American Psychiatric Association: Diagnostic and Statistical Manual of Mental Disorders, 5th edn. Arlington, VA, American Psychiatric Association, 2013.
3. Kotagal S. Parasomnias in childhood. Sleep Med Rev 2009; 13: 157–68.
4. Lord C, Brugha TS, Charman T, et al. Autism spectrum disorder. Nat Rev Dis Primers 2020;6:5.
5. McDowell M. Specific learning disability. J Pediatr Child Health 2018;54:1077–83.
6. Mithyantha R, Kneen R, McCann E, et al. Current evidence-based recommendations on investigating children with global developmental delay. Arch Dis Child 2017;102:1071–6.
7. Posner J, Polankzyk GV, Sonuga-Barke E. Attention-deficit hyperactivity disorder. Lancet 2020;395:450–62.

## MENTAL HEALTH IN CHILDREN AND ADOLESCENTS

The global burden of disease study recently reported that mental health disorders account for most years lived with disability in children and adolescents. The World Health Organisation (WHO) have urged for robust survey data in Mental Health Action Plan 2013-2020, however, only 7% countries in the world have such data.

In a recently concluded prospective cohort study in Caucasian population, the incidence of mental disorders under 18 years of age was estimated at 15%. Schizophrenia, mood, anxiety, obsessive compulsive, eating and personality disorders were more common in females whereas developmental and behavioral disorders like intellectual disability, ASD, ADHD, oppositional defiance/conduct disorders and tic disorders were more common in males. They also reported a trend of delayed detection of developmental and behavioral disorders in girls.

In a systematic review and meta-analysis from India, reporting prevalence of mental health disorders in children and adolescents, the estimate varied from 6.5% in the community to 23.3% in schools. Similar rates have also been observed in European and Latin American countries. The National Mental Health Survey 2016 estimated the prevalence of mental health disorders at 7.3% in adolescents (13–17 years) with urban population affected twice as much as the rural population. The most common disorders were anxiety, depression, intellectual disability and ASD. The survey reported tobacco and alcohol consumption in 7–8%. The WHO has reported high prevalence of suicide in Indian children and adolescents.

The economic burden of mental health disorders is more than other non-communicable diseases and can be as high as 4% of gross national product. Globally, there is a considerable gap between needs and services in mental health, more so in the low and middle income countries. Well-planned epidemiological studies will help in prioritising resources, research and public health decisions.

### Suggested Reading

1. Dalsgaard S, Thorsteinsson E, Trabjerg BB, et al. Incidence rates and cumulative incidences of the full spectrum of diagnosed mental disorders in childhood and adolescence. JAMA Psychiatry 2020;77:155–64.
2. Hossain MM, Purohit N. Improving child and adolescent mental health in India: Status, services, policies, and way forward. Indian J Psychiatry 2019;61:415–19.
3. Malhotra S, Patra BN. Prevalence of child and adolescent psychiatric disorders in India: A systematic review and meta-analysis. Child Adolesc Psychiatry Ment Health 2014;8:22.

Chapter 5

# Adolescent Health and Development

❍ Tushar R Godbole ❍ Vijayalakshmi Bhatia

Adolescence is a stage of transition from childhood to adulthood. During this stage of life, a youth undergoes rapid changes in body structure, mediated by the sex hormones. The appearance of sexual characters is coupled with changes in cognition and psychology. Whereas adolescence refers to this entire process, puberty refers to the physical aspect. The age group 10–19 years is considered as the period of adolescence, and puberty marks the early half of adolescence. Though it is a continuous process, adolescence is generally divided, for convenience, into three phases: Early (10–13 years), mid (14–16 years) and late (17–19 years) adolescence.

*Competencies:* **PE6.1; PE6.2; PE6.9; PE33.9**

## PHYSICAL ASPECTS

The onset of puberty is triggered by various genetic and environmental factors including the body fat stores. Activation of the hypothalamic–pituitary–gonadal axis leads to the production of gonadotropins (luteinizing hormone, follicle-stimulating hormone) and sex steroids (estrogen and testosterone) (Fig. 5.1). Gonadal sex steroids bring about secondary sexual characters (breast development, increase in penile size and menarche), whereas adrenal androgens cause development of sexual hair, acne and underarm odor.

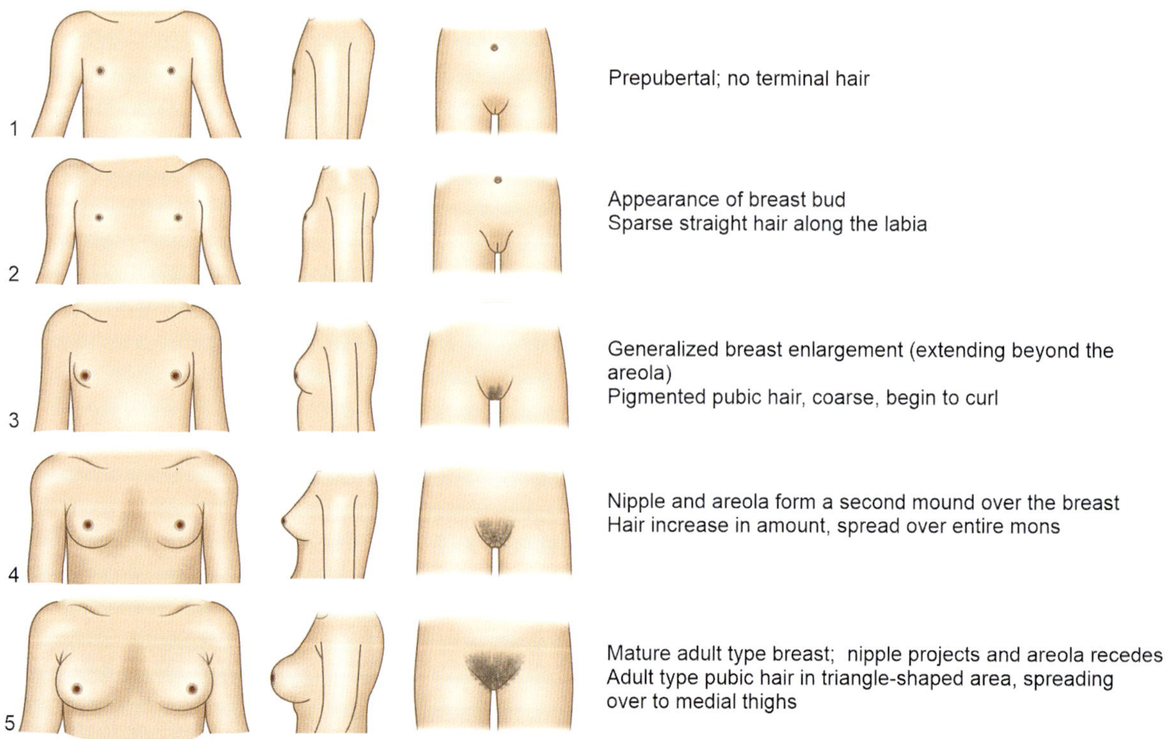


**Fig. 5.1:** Sexual maturity rating (1–5) in girls (*Courtesy:* Anil Kumar, Sanjay Gandhi Postgraduate Institute of Medical Sciences, Lucknow)

Details of hormonal mechanisms of onset and progression of puberty are dealt with in Chapter 18.

### Onset and Sequence of Puberty

Puberty in girls starts with breast development (thelarche) between 8 and 13 years (Fig. 5.1). This is followed by appearance of pubic hair (pubarche) and then, menstruation (menarche) occurring at an average of 12.6 years (range 10–16 years). The breast buds may be tender and there may be asymmetry in the breast size during early phases of puberty. Menarche usually occurs after 2–2½ years of thelarche. In boys, the earliest change is increase in testicular size (volume reaching 4 mL or length 2.5 cm) that occurs between 9 and 14 years (Fig. 5.2). This is followed by appearance of pubic hair and lengthening of the penis.

Spermarche or production of sperms starts during mid-adolescence. Laryngeal growth under androgenic stimulus, manifesting as cracking of voice, begins in mid-puberty in males and deepening of voice is complete by the end of puberty. Mild degree of breast enlargement is seen in more than half of boys (gynecomastia) in early puberty, which subsides spontaneously over several months. The onset of puberty is variable; thus in an age cohort (e.g. students of 7th class), many will have advanced puberty while others will be awaiting its onset.

### Physical Growth and Nutritional Requirements

During puberty, boys gain about 20–30 cm and girls about 16–28 cm. Peak growth velocity in girls occurs before attainment of menarche (stage 3), while boys show peak growth velocity during later stages of puberty (stages 4–5).The growth spurt affects the distal skeleton first, hence enlargement of limbs and extremities is followed by increase in trunk size. There is an exuberant increase in muscle mass and bone diameter, particularly in boys and total bone mass in both the sexes. Lean body mass increases during the early stages in both the sexes, fat mass increases in girls at later stages of puberty. Under the influence of sex steroids, rapid calcium accretion occurs during puberty, achieving almost 50% of adult bone mass. The recommended dietary allowance (RDA) for calcium is 800 mg/day and an intake of 500 mL milk is recommended in order to achieve this with a cereal-based Indian diet. With minimal sun exposure, the RDA for vitamin D is 600 IU/day. Since dietary vitamin D is mainly available from fatty fish, intake as a pharmacological supplement may be necessary. Increase in body structure is paralleled by increase in blood volume and muscle mass; both of these tissues have high iron content. With commencement of menstruation, nutritional requirements of iron are further increased. With predominantly cereal-based diet and poor bioavailability, an adolescent needs to have a daily intake of 25–30 mg iron in order to meet the daily requirements of 1.3 mg. The WHO recommends at least 60 minutes of daily physical activity with moderate to vigorous intensity to promote cardiovascular and muscular fitness, skeletal health along with other psychological benefits.

### Cognitive and Social Development

Volumetric and functional imaging techniques show that the adolescent brain undergoes subtle structural changes and differential growth. Though the exact implications of these changes are largely unknown, these indicate reorganizational or accommodating effort of

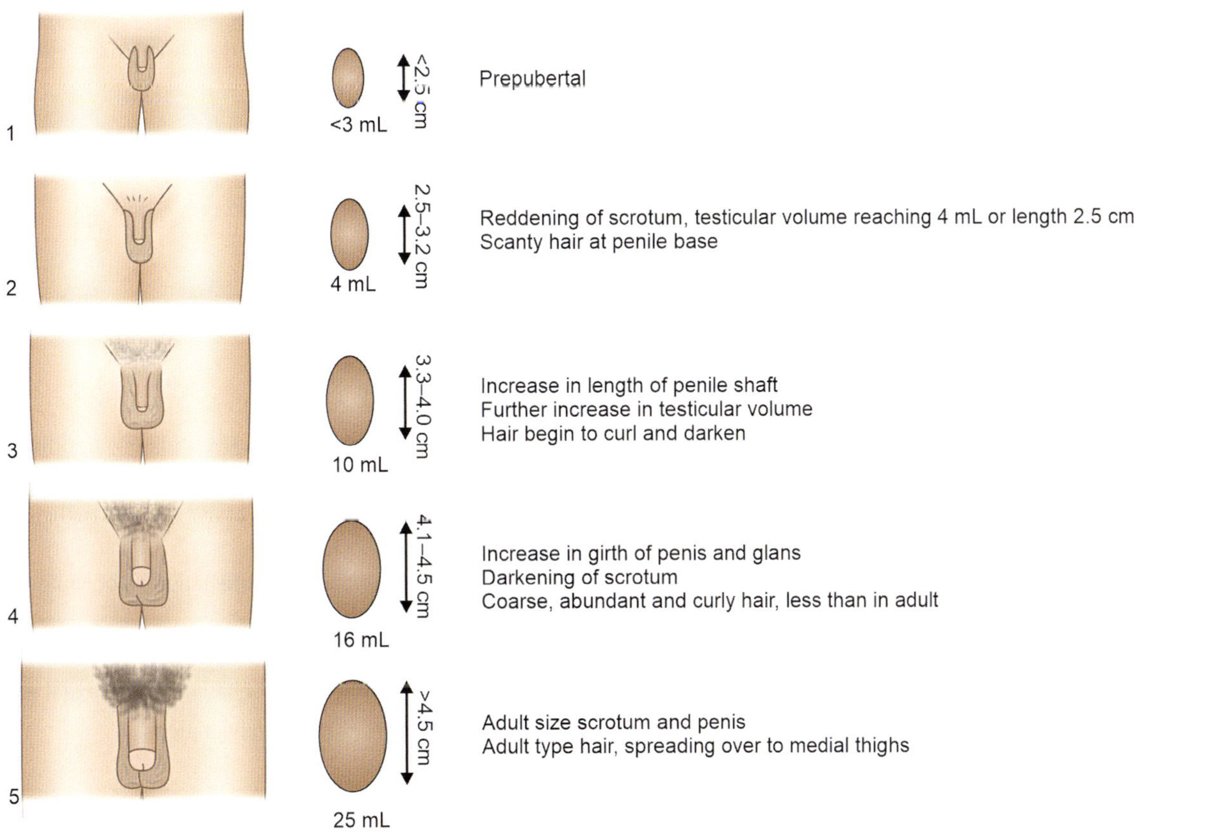


Fig. 5.2: Sexual maturity rating (1–5) in boys (*Courtesy:* Anil Kumar, Sanjay Gandhi Postgraduate Institute of Medical Sciences, Lucknow)

brain paralleling the multi-fold increase in its functional capabilities.

***Early phase:*** The 'concrete thinking model' of childhood persists into early adolescence, where the concepts are perceived more 'literally'. Teens are impulsive and have limited ability to perceive future implications of their current behavior. They prefer same sex peers. Many are excessively conscious of other people's concerns about their appearance and actions. Curiosity about sexual anatomy and comparison with peers is common.

***Mid-phase:*** This phase is marked by emotional autonomy; they might seem detached from their family. The youth starts to think beyond self and there is beginning of abstract reasoning. Acceptance by the peer group becomes important. Sexual experimentation, such as masturbation, starts at this age.

***Late phase:*** By this time, most of the pubertal changes are already achieved. Moral values and strong self-identity are now established. They are now able to suppress impulsivity and are less affected by peer pressure. Personal relations become more important than the peer group. The youth becomes career-oriented and starts short- and long-term planning for his or her goals in life. Many start engaging in sexual activity.

### Attitude Towards Health

Adolescents are considered to be at the peak of their health; yet, adolescence coincides with the onset of many health disorders. Girls are often unprepared for their first periods. High-risk behavior is common in mid-adolescent age group. The National Family Health Survey 4 (NFHS4) reported the median age of sexual debut in boys and girls to be 24 years and 19 years, respectively, but a significant proportion are sexually active much before. Knowledge about contraception is improving among adolescents. Though awareness about HIV is increasing among Indian youth, most of them lack comprehensive knowledge of the disease.

*Competencies:* **PE6.3; PE6.4; PE6.5; PE6.6; PE6.7; PE6.12; PE6.13**

## PROBLEMS FACED BY ADOLESCENTS

Adolescents are under immense pressure because of the rapid changes in their hormonal milieu, changing ideas and concepts about the world, having to cope up with the expectations from society and the need to establish their own identity. The problems faced by an adolescent in India are diverse (Table 5.1) and are often not addressed by the health care system.

### Health Problems

***Nutrition and eating disorders:*** There is increase in nutritional requirements during this period of rapid growth, micronutrients being as important as energy and protein (*see* Chapter 8). Data from the NFHS5 shows that 57% Indian adolescent girls (and 31% boys) are anemic; the prevalence of anemia has remained unchanged over the last three decades. There is lack of sun exposure due to clothing coupled with dark skin pigment. Insufficient intake of dairy products results in poor intake of calcium and vitamin $B_{12}$. The resulting low bone mineral density is more pronounced

**Table 5.1:** Problems faced by an adolescent

| | | |
|---|---|---|
| *Health problems* | Nutrition and eating disorders | Anemia, vitamin D, vitamin A deficiency, low bone mass, eating disorders |
| | Mental health problems | Anxiety, depression, suicides, delinquency, mood disorders |
| | Sleep disturbances | Poor sleep, daytime somnolence, poor academics, snoring |
| | Infections | Tuberculosis, HIV, sexually transmitted diseases, parasites |
| | Issues related to menstruation | Menstrual hygiene, polycystic ovary syndrome |
| *Lifestyle diseases* | Lifestyle diseases | Obesity, type 2 diabetes, hypertension |
| | Substance abuse | Tobacco, alcohol, others |
| *Vulnerability* | Abuse, violence, accidents | Physical, sexual violence, trauma, burns |
| | Migration | Child labor, trafficking, prostitution, HIV |
| | Adolescent pregnancy | Early marriages, sexual abuse, complications |
| | Lack of sex education | No formal education on masturbation, safe sex, dating, abortion, HIV and sexually transmitted diseases; untrusted information sources |
| *Environmental and social challenges* | Pollution | Asthma, skin conditions, endocrine disruptors, possible malignancies |
| | Media | Substance abuse, violence, unrealistic expectations, poor role models, social isolation, depression |
| | Peer pressure | High-risk behavior, addictions |
| | Poverty, illiteracy | Undernutrition, depression, anti-social behavior, early sexual activity |
| | Academic stress | Mental stress, discrimination, parental expectations |
| | Early marriage | Early pregnancy |
| | Discrimination | No decision-making power, gender discrimination in education and food distribution |

in underprivileged girls as they have low protein intake in addition to calcium and vitamin D deficiency. Vitamin A deficiency is also an important issue in economically deprived adolescents. Undernutrition often delays the onset of puberty and sexual maturation, results in stunting, poor bone mass accrual and reduced work capacity. Girls from poor families are likely to suffer from malnutrition due to gender discrimination in food distribution, whereas girls from urban upper socioeconomic group show malnutrition due to eating disorders. Anorexia nervosa and bulimia are increasingly reported.

*Mental health problems:* Adjustment and anxiety disorders, depression, suicide, delinquent behavior, poor body image and low self-esteem are major concerns, with onset at a median age of 14 years. Suicide rates are increasing, with higher number of completed suicide in boys and attempted suicides in girls. Adolescents are at high risk of committing suicide because of cognitive immaturity and impulsivity. Psychological disorders like depression or mood disorders, substance abuse, parent–child conflict, physical or sexual abuse and family history of suicide make them prone for such attempts.

*Sleep disturbances:* During the period of rapid growth, adolescents have increased sleep requirements. Under the effect of physiologic delay in melatonin secretion, adolescents have a delay in sleep onset and awakening by almost an hour. In urban adolescents, this may be compounded by increasing academic activity or watching electronic screens late into the night. Poor sleep habits are likely to reflect in school performance and cause daytime drowsiness, aggressive behavior, conduct disorders, anxiety, restless leg syndrome and depression.

*Infections:* With increased outdoor activity, teens are exposed to TB, HIV, skin and parasitic infections and sexually transmitted diseases. Early sexual activity is not uncommon. Various biological (immature, incompletely estrogenized mucosa) and psychosocial factors (lack of preparedness, knowledge regarding barrier contraceptives) make adolescents susceptible to these infections. Gonorrhea can cause vulvovaginitis, urethritis or proctitis. Chlamydia may cause intermenstrual or post-coital bleeds. Both may be asymptomatic in the majority or only cause vaginal discharge. Candidal infections become common with starting of menstruation and often have a cyclic nature. Pelvic inflammatory disease (PID) is a spectrum of inflammatory disorder of female genital tract, which occurs in sexually active females and can present with abdominal pain with vaginal discharge. Lower abdominal, cervical or adnexal tenderness is suggestive of the diagnosis (Table 5.2).

*Issues related to menstruation:* There are many social taboos about menstruation in Indian families. Many adolescent girls are found to miss school during their menstruation because of lack of access to safe sanitary products or lack of privacy. Poor menstrual hygiene may contribute to reproductive infections. With the introduction of government and private run 'Menstrual Hygiene Schemes', more young women are now able to access hygienic methods during menses (NHFS5).

It is common to have anovulatory and irregular menstrual cycles during first two years after menarche. The polycystic ovary syndrome (PCOS), a combination of menstrual irregularities and ovarian cysts with androgen excess like acne or hirsutism, occurs in ~9% adolescent girls. The condition is associated with other metabolic

**Table 5.2:** Sexually transmitted infections: Salient features and treatment

| *Disease* | *Salient features* | *Specific treatment* |
|---|---|---|
| Gonorrhea | Coinfection common | Ceftriaxone 125 mg IV or IM single dose |
| Chlamydia infection | Urethritis, vaginal discharge | Oral azithromycin 1 g single dose, or doxycycline 100 mg twice daily for 14 days |
| Herpes | Multiple painful vesicles and ulcers; tend to recur | Oral acyclovir 400 mg thrice daily for 7 days |
| Primary syphilis | Painless genital ulcer | Benzathine penicillin 2.4 MU IM (after test dose); oral doxycycline, if allergic to penicillin |
| Genital warts (papillomavirus) | Tend to recur | Local application of podophyllin weekly, cryotherapy or surgical removal; preventable with vaccination |
| Chancroid | Painful ulcer with lymphadenopathy | Oral azithromycin 1 g single dose, or ciprofloxacin 500 mg twice daily for 3 days |
| Trichomoniasis | Malodorous yellow green discharge | Oral metronidazole or tinidazole 2 g single dose |
| Candidiasis | Itching, redness, white discharge | Clotrimazole cream or pessary for 7 days, miconazole pessary for 3 days, or oral fluconazole 150 mg single dose |
| Pelvic inflammatory disease | Polymicrobial; varied disease spectrum | *Mild to moderate illness:* Oral cefixime 400 mg twice daily for 7 days, metronidazole 400 mg orally twice daily for 14 days and doxycycline 100 mg twice daily for 14 days; abstinence; symptomatic treatment<br>*Severe disease:* IV antibiotics |
| Pediculosis pubis | Pruritus | Local application of 1% permethrin, wash after 10 minutes |
| Scabies | Pruritus and rash | Local application of 5% permethrin; oral ivermectin 2 doses 14 days apart |

All patients should be screened for HIV infection; partners should be treated if affected. IM intramuscular; IV intravenous

derangements like obesity, insulin resistance and type 2 diabetes mellitus (T2DM).

### Lifestyle Diseases

Obesity is epidemic in the urban settings. Among Delhi school children, 5% obesity and 17–19% overweight have been reported, higher in boys than in girls. Obesity has strong association with asthma, sleep disorders, reflux disease, Blount disease, slipped femoral epiphysis, gallstones, fatty liver and metabolic derangements like T2DM, dyslipidemia, hypertension and PCOS. Essential hypertension is rising, with prevalence of 29% in obese and 7% in normal weight school children in a recent meta-analysis from India.

*Substance abuse:* NFHS5 showed that around 40% and 20% of men above the age of 15-yr consume tobacco and alcohol respectively, in both urban and rural India, starting as early as 10 years. The percentages in females are also increasing. The Global Youth Tobacco Survey 2019 showed that around 20% school children experiment with tobacco, but around 8% keep using it. Apart from tobacco, alcohol, cannabis and opium are most abused substances. Addicts are prone to accidents, injuries, violence, trading sex-for-drugs, HIV, hepatitis C, sexually transmitted diseases and tuberculosis.

### Vulnerability

*Abuse and violence (physical and sexual):* Physical and sexual violence is common in India, with 20–30% young females suffering from domestic violence; and 2% young females experience sexual violence before their 18th birthday (NFHS5). Road traffic and industrial accidents (in boys), burns (in girls) and poisoning are leading causes of traumatic mortality and disability in Indian youth.

*Migration:* Many adolescents migrate from rural to urban settings, for labor or educational opportunities. Trafficking of youth is a serious problem in India and happens for industrial or domestic labor, forced marriages and prostitution. In some states, 70% of new HIV infections are related to outward male migration.

*Adolescent pregnancy:* Unmarried adolescents are likely to resort to unsafe methods of abortion, which increase risk of septicemia and mortality. As compared to adult pregnancy, they are also at a higher risk for pre-eclampsia, preterm labor and postpartum hemorrhage. Prolonged and obstructed labor are common in adolescent pregnancies and they are 2–4 times more likely to die during childbirth as compared to adult females. Neonatal, infant and child mortality rates are higher in children delivered to adolescent mothers. Fortunately, the prevalence of adolescent pregnancy (8%) is lower in the results of NFHS 4 than in previous surveys, due to schooling and knowledge about contraception.

### Environmental and Social Challenges

*Media:* With easy availability of electronic media, adolescents are exposed to unsupervised information from all across the world. Adolescents often succumb to glamorous portrayal of tobacco or alcohol consumption, unrealistic expectations, physical aggression, destructive behavior and unprotected sex. Spending much of spare time indoors on social networking apps, teenagers are deprived of sunlight and physical activity and socially isolated.

*Peer pressure:* Peer formation is a part of adolescent social development. Pressure for conforming to norms drives many of their actions and decisions, including risk taking behavior and initiation of substance abuse.

*Academic and emotional stress:* Examinations cause significant physiological and psychological stress. Switching from vernacular to English medium schools, long hours of school and tuitions are additional stress factors that are unaddressed. Various other factors like peer acceptance, discrimination, academic burden, parental expectations and changing social environments cause stress among youth. While most adolescents have adequate coping skills, some have serious adjustment problems resulting in psychological and somatic effects.

*Early marriage:* Though the legal age for marriage in India is 18 years for girls (Table 5.3), the practice of childhood and early marriage is still quite common. Among late adolescent girls, 30% are married, more so in rural areas.

*Discrimination:* Young people are often treated as second class citizens, under the control of adults and often not involved in any decision making. Adolescent girls are often asked to limit their outdoor/extracurricular activities, confined to their houses and expected to do the household work. Gender discrimination is seen in education and even food distribution.

**Table 5.3:** Legal age definitions relevant to adolescence

| *Definition of child* | *Below 18 years* |
|---|---|
| Minimum age for marriage | Boys 21 years; girls 18 years |
| Responsibility for crime | 12 years |
| Juvenile criminal | 12–18 years |
| Compulsory free education | 6–14 years |
| Consumption of alcohol | Beyond 18–25 years in different states (illegal in some states and union territories) |
| Employment in hazardous occupation or hotels | 14 years |

*Competencies:* **PE6.8; PE6.9; PE6.10; PE6.11**

## ROLE OF THE HEALTH CARE PROVIDER

A checklist for the adolescent clinic visit is provided in Table 5.4. During each visit, the following are important.

*Identifying risks:* The physician needs to detect risk factors like obesity, hypertension, possible substance/drug abuse, behavioral and social problems and risky behavior. Subtle cues like sad or depressed mood, avoidance of eye contact, bruises or undue resistance to examination are the likely pointers towards physical or sexual abuse.

*Establishing rapport:* Being empathetic and non-judgemental is the key to effective communication. Direct questioning of the adolescent is as important as questioning the parents. Beginning the interview with icebreakers, use

**Table 5.4:** Checklist for adolescent health visit

| | |
|---|---|
| History from parents and adolescent | • History of presenting problems<br>• Parental concerns on growth, development<br>• Academic success; school absenteeism<br>• Diet including calcium, protein, iron, calorie-dense foods<br>• Menstrual history; sleep problems |
| Separate questioning of adolescent | • Emotional problems; relationship with family and peers<br>• Outlook towards physical and sexual changes<br>• Involvement in relationship or sexual activity<br>• Awareness about safe sex and contraception<br>• Specific problems related to sex organs<br>• Tobacco or other substance use<br>• Counsel and clear doubts on sensitive topics |
| Separate questioning of parents | • Relationship with family<br>• Level of communication on sensitive matters<br>• Unusual behavior noticed |
| Physical examination | • Anthropometry<br>• Blood pressure, markers of obesity, acanthosis<br>• Sexual maturity rating<br>• Signs of malnutrition, anemia and vitamin deficiencies<br>• Signs of skin and genital infections<br>• Level of general hygiene<br>• Signs of trauma; abuse<br>• Signs of drug abuse or tobacco use |
| Counseling | • Nutritional intervention<br>• Hygienic practices<br>• Building rapport between parents and adolescent<br>• Providing information and resources on sex education |
| Investigations | • Hemoglobin level<br>• Blood sugar, lipid profile<br>• Genital swabs<br>• Ultrasound of ovaries |
| Referrals | • Counselor<br>• Dietitian<br>• Psychiatrist<br>• Gynecologist<br>• Voluntary and confidential HIV testing<br>• Social services, child protection agencies, support groups |

of open-ended non-sensitive questions and then moving to sensitive/targeted questions is helpful.

*Confidentiality:* One may need to interview a young patient separately, as he/she may not want to discuss sensitive topics in the presence of parents. While examining the genitalia, the doctor can ask patient preference for presence of their parent inside the examination room. A boy may prefer his parents standing outside the exam room, whereas a girl may find it comforting, if her mother accompanies her during the examination.

*Consent:* For a child who is less than 12 years, consent for examination or medical/surgical procedure is obtained from the parent or guardian. While an adolescent aged 12–18 years can give consent for examination, consent for medical/surgical procedure can be given only after 18 years. This also includes consent for medical termination of pregnancy, blood and organ donation.

*Nutritional/ health intervention:* Improving the nutritional status of adolescent girls breaks the cycle of malnutrition and low birth weight babies, and prevents long-term complications of the latter in future generations.

*Providing health information:* The adolescent health visit is an excellent opportunity to talk to the parents and their adolescent about the pubertal changes. It is likely that they have not received any formal sex education in school and need to be provided correct educational resources for the same.

*Referral to social services, psychological evaluation and support:* The National Commission for Protection of Child Rights Act 2005 considers a person below 18 years as a 'child'. It is mandatory for a health care provider to report all cases of child abuse (even suspected) to the Commission, online or in writing. Doctors are protected in case of erroneous reporting but punishable, if they fail to report. Adolescents with special needs or victims of any kind of abuse need social and psychological support.

*Adolescent-friendly health services:* These services include provision of reproductive health services, nutritional counseling, sex education and life skill education. Confidentiality, easy accessibility, friendly attitude and quick comprehensive health care delivery have made a positive impact on adolescent clients. 'Adolescent reproductive and sexual health' has been identified as a key strategy under RCH II program. Adolescent friendly clinics are functional at many centers in the country. **Box 5.1** lists the key services and interventions that should be provided for comprehensive care for adolescents.

*Management of sexual violence:* This includes the following measures:

i. Forensic examination and collection of blood or body fluid samples by trained staff.
ii. Care of the injuries
iii. *Prophylaxis against pregnancy:* Two doses of levonorgestrel 12 hours apart, first dose being given within 72 hours of intercourse.
iv. Prophylaxis against sexually transmitted infections includes a single oral dose of azithromycin 1 g along with cefixime 400 mg and metronidazole or tinidazole 2 g, protects against syphilis, gonorrhea, Chlamydia and Trichomonas. Hepatitis B vaccination is recommended, if the person is not previously immunized.
v. Prophylaxis against HIV requires referral to the nearest integrated counseling and testing center.
vi. Psychological support includes counseling and referral to a psychiatrist. Informing concerned authorities or social services is important as patient may need shelter and legal help. A teen may not be willing to disclose this assault to his parents. Childline (1098) is a support service provided by Government of India focused on child care and protection.

**Box 5.1: Healthy Adolescence: Package of Interventions**

***Healthy lifestyle***
- Healthy food
- Exercise and yoga
- No to tobacco, alcohol, drugs
- Safe conduct on road
- Papillomavirus, rubella

***Anemia***
- Prevention, detection and management of anemia, especially for adolescent girls

***Sexual health***
- Sexuality education
- Menstrual hygiene
- Marriage after 18 years, childbirth after 20 years
- Counseling and services for comprehensive sexual and reproductive health, including contraception

***Mental health***
- Supportive family; counseling and peer/family support in anxiety, depression
- Prevention and management of hazardous and harmful substance use
- Prevention of suicide and management of self-harm/suicide risk

***Violence prevention***
- Prevention and management of unintentional injury
- Prevention of and response to sexual and other forms of gender-based violence

***Communicable and non-communicable diseases***
- Prevention, detection and treatment of communicable and non-communicable diseases

***Preparing for adulthood***
- Parenting skills, responsible husband, wife and father

*Protection of Children from Sexual Offenses [POCSO] Act 2012 (amended 2019):* The POCSO Act protects individuals below 18 years from sexual offense or harassment of any form, be it physical or pornographic. It also explicitly states that an event of abuse must be informed to legal authorities; failing which, the knowing person (including the health care provider) is liable to legal actions including imprisonment.

*Contraception:* A pediatrician should advocate for abstinence and delayed initiation of sex to adolescent patients. In case the adolescent is already sexually active, condom seems a better choice compared to other methods. Adolescents with disabilities or mental retardation are wrongly assumed to be at low risk for STIs and pregnancy. Parents of such children need to be counseled regarding these issues.

*Adolescent immunization:* India has low coverage for booster doses of TT at 10 and 16 years. Human papillomavirus (HPV) vaccine is recommended for peripubertal girls (before initiation of sexual activity) for prevention of infection with HPV and cervical cancer. Parents need to be counseled thoroughly as the principle behind giving the vaccine might alarm them (Table 5.5).

**Table 5.5:** Immunization during adolescence

| | |
|---|---|
| Tetanus and diphtheria toxoids and acellular pertussis (Tdap) vaccine | Tdap at 10–12 years, and Td every 10 years thereafter |
| [Td at 10 and 16 years as per national program] | |
| Papillomavirus | • 2 doses, if given between 9 and 14 years<br>• 3 doses, if given beyond age 15 years |
| Influenza | Annually |

Catch-up vaccination is discussed in Chapter 10

*Transition to adult care:* With better medical care, a large number of chronically ill or disabled children are surviving into adulthood. As the problems of these children are diverse, they need multidisciplinary care even in their adulthood. Transition to adult care is not mere transfer of the case to a different physician. It is a gradual and planned process; keeping in mind the abilities of the child to participate in self-care, taking responsibilities and decision making. The age at transfer is not fixed; a window of age 14–18 years is used in some countries for a gradual transfer.

## GOVERNMENT INTERVENTIONS IN ADOLESCENT HEALTH CARE

Kishori Shakti Yojana and SABLA Yojana aim to provide health, nutrition, education and vocational skills to adolescent girls. National Youth Policy believes in youth empowerment through education. Recognizing the contribution of adolescent care to maternal and child health, National Health Mission now follows Reproductive, Maternal, Neonatal, Child and Adolescent Health (RMNC+A) approach. Under this program, weekly iron and folic acid supplementation program provides 100 mg of iron and 500 μg folic acid with biennial deworming to all adolescents attending government schools. The Rashtriya Kishor Swasthya Karyakram (RKSK) under RMNC+A extends the spectrum of adolescent care from reproductive and sexual health to non-communicable diseases, violence, injuries, substance abuse and mental health.

### Suggested Reading


1. American Academy of Pediatrics Committee on Adolescence; Blythe MJ, Diaz A. Contraception and Adolescents: Committee on Adolescents, Pediatrics 2007;120:1135–48.
2. Juvenile Justice (Care and Protection of Children) Act, 2015. The Gazette of India, Ministry of Law and Justice.
3. National Guidelines on Prevention, Management and Control of RTIs/STIs. Ministry of Health and Family Welfare, Govt of India, 2007.
4. National Family Health Survey [NFHS4, 2015-16] and [NFHS5, 2019-21]. International Institute for Population Sciences, Mumbai.
5. National Non-communicable Disease Monitoring Survey (NNMS) 2017–18.
6. Nutrient requirements for Indian. ICMR–National Institute of Nutrition, 2020.
7. WHO Fact Sheet 2021. Adolescent and young adult health.

Chapter

6

# Fluid and Electrolyte Disturbances

❍ Georgie Mathew ❍ Arvind Bagga

## COMPOSITION OF BODY FLUIDS

Water is the single largest constituent of the human body. Total body water (TBW) declines from comprising 90% of body weight in early fetal life to nearly 75–80% at the time of birth; declining progressively to 60% by the end of the first year and remains so till puberty. Since adipose tissue has lower water content, adolescent females and overweight children have lower TBW as a percentage of body weight.

Total body water is distributed between intracellular fluid (ICF; 2/3rd) and extracellular fluid (ECF; 1/3rd). Nearly one-fourth of ECF is distributed in the extravascular (interstitial) and intravascular space (plasma water) in a 3:1 ratio. Preservation of intravascular volume is of paramount importance to homeostasis. The relative size of the two main compartments varies with age. Increase in ECF volume contributes to the increased TBW in neonates, especially in preterm babies.

The interstitial fluid component of ECF is actually a matrix, a collagen/gel substance that allows the interstitium to provide structural rigidity during extracellular volume depletion. The interstitial space, especially in skin and connective tissue, is an important reservoir of extracellular fluid.

### Water Balance

In the steady state, water balance represents the difference between water intake (including that generated from endogenous metabolism) and water losses (Fig. 6.1). Obligatory urine output (proportional to the amount of solutes requiring excretion) comprises two-thirds of the total water losses; stools, evaporation from the moist surfaces of the skin and respiratory tract (insensible losses) form the remainder. The evaporative losses play an important role in thermoregulation. In contrast to these insensible losses, sweat which is hypotonic ($Na^+$ concentration 35 to 65 mEq/L) is actually 'sensible loss', contributing to thermoregulation. When exposed to high heat environments (endogenous or ambient), sweat contributes to significant loss of water with electrolytes.

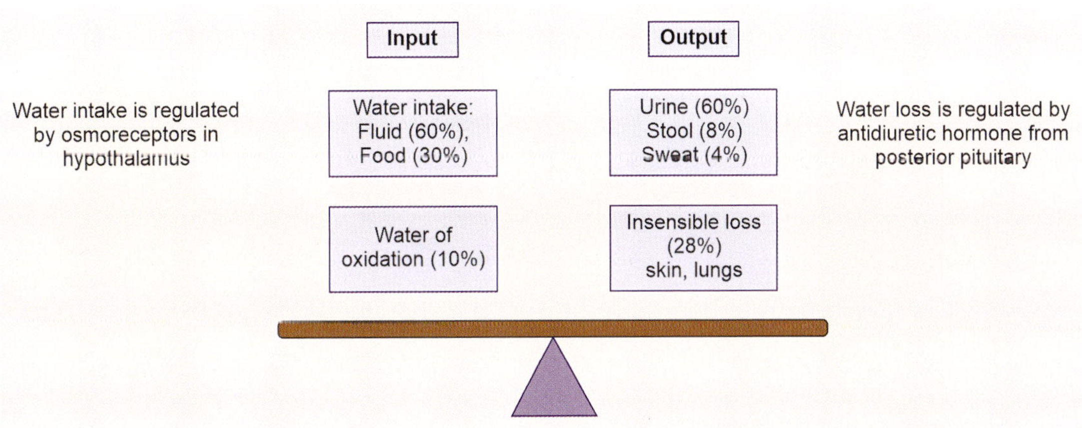


Fig. 6.1: Balance of water intake and losses maintains normal plasma osmolality. Only water intake and urinary losses can be regulated

Changes in $Na^+$ concentration in the ECF are tightly linked to ECF volume and are most commonly due to dysregulated water balance than primary $Na^+$ balance. The primary effectors for volume regulation, the renin–angiotensin–aldosterone system and atrial natriuretic peptide, work by affecting the $Na^+$ excretion. Besides this, regulation of body water is made possible by interplay of multiple other factors, including vasopressin, prostaglandins, dopaminergic receptors, α-adrenergic receptors, thirst mechanism and intrinsic renal properties.

### Electrolyte Composition of Body Compartments

The ECF compartment contains high concentration of $Na^+$, $Cl^-$, and bicarbonate (Fig. 6.2). Potassium, organic phosphates and proteins are the predominant ICF osmoles. As most electrolytes, in homeostasis, are distributed between ECF and ICF or bound to protein/tissues, the serum concentrations do not necessarily reflect the total body content of a particular electrolyte. Permeability to ions varies in each organ with the brain having the least and the liver the most permeability. However, water readily crosses cell membranes to achieve an osmotic equilibrium between the two compartments. The balance and appropriate distribution of fluid within these spaces is maintained by the colloid oncotic pressure, membrane permeability and hydrostatic pressure. Plasma and interstitial fluid are rich in proteins, which determine the oncotic pressure.

### Osmolality and Tonicity

Osmolality (mOsm/kg) is the solute concentration of a fluid. Changes in osmolality can produce grave neurologic consequences and even death, primarily due to water movement into and out of the brain. To prevent this, the plasma osmolality, primarily determined by the plasma $Na^+$ concentration, is normally maintained closely between 1 and 2% of the normal (285 to 295 mOsm/kg) by variations in water intake and water excretion. This regulatory system is governed by different osmoreceptors in the hypothalamus that influence both thirst and the secretion of antidiuretic hormone (ADH) (Fig. 6.3). Plasma osmolality can be measured directly using osmometers, as well as estimated indirectly as follows:

$$\text{Plasma osmolality} = 2 \times \text{Na (mEq/L)} + \text{Blood urea nitrogen (mg/dL)}/2.8 + \text{glucose (mg/dL)}/18$$

Measured values are generally higher than calculated values by up to 10 mOsm/kg and this difference is called osmolal gap. Increase in osmolal gap may occur due to increase in unmeasured osmoles.

Osmolality is distinct from tonicity (effective osmolality) in that tonicity relates to both the effect on a cell of a fluid (dependent on the selective permeability of the membrane) and the osmolality of the fluid. In the plasma, urea affects osmolality but not tonicity because urea moves freely across cell membranes with no effect on tonicity. The tonicity of intravenous fluids is primarily affected by the $Na^+$ and $K^+$ concentration. Although dextrose affects the osmolality of intravenous fluids, it is not a significant contributor to the plasma osmotic pressure or tonicity, because except in uncontrolled diabetes, it is rapidly metabolized after entering the bloodstream. Hence, a hypertonic fluid has high osmolality but the converse may not be true. Another important concept to be understood in this context is the free water content of IV fluids. Due to the above-mentioned reasons, any IV fluid containing only of glucose dissolved

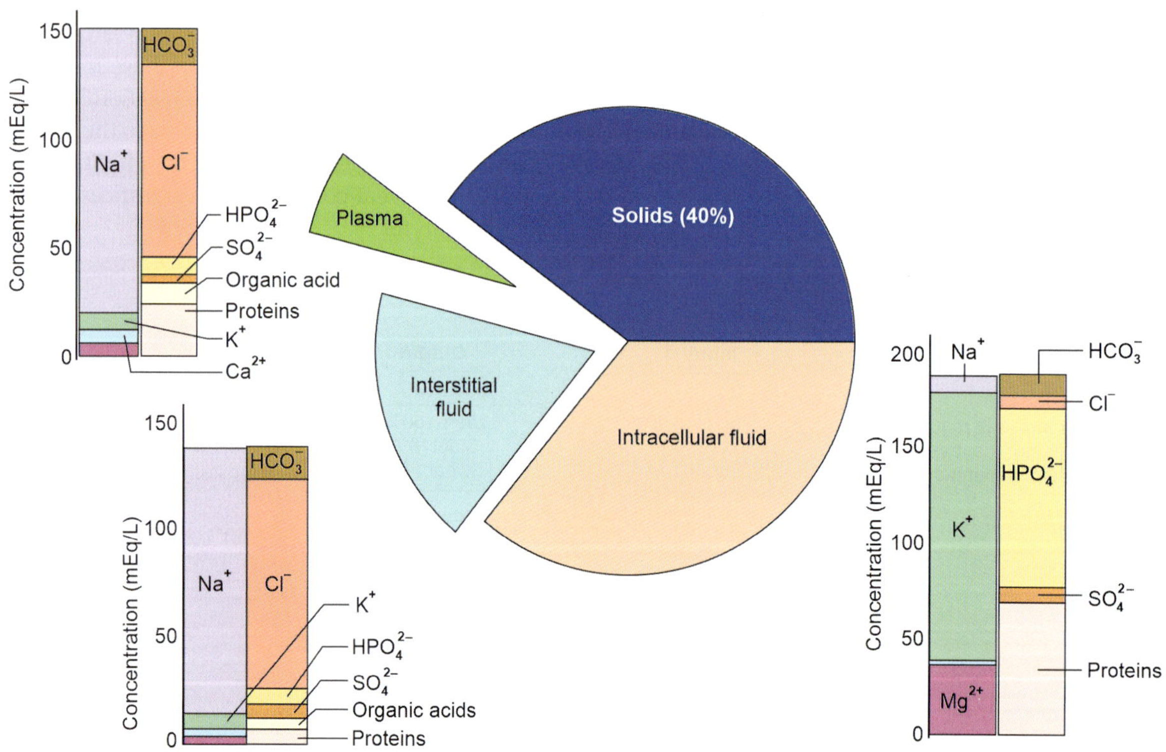


Fig. 6.2: Electrolyte composition of intracellular and extracellular fluid compartments. $Cl^-$ chloride; $HCO_3^-$ bicarbonate; $HPO_4^{2-}$ hydrogen phosphate; $K^+$ potassium; $Mg^{2+}$ magnesium; $Na^+$ sodium; $SO_4^{2-}$ sulfate

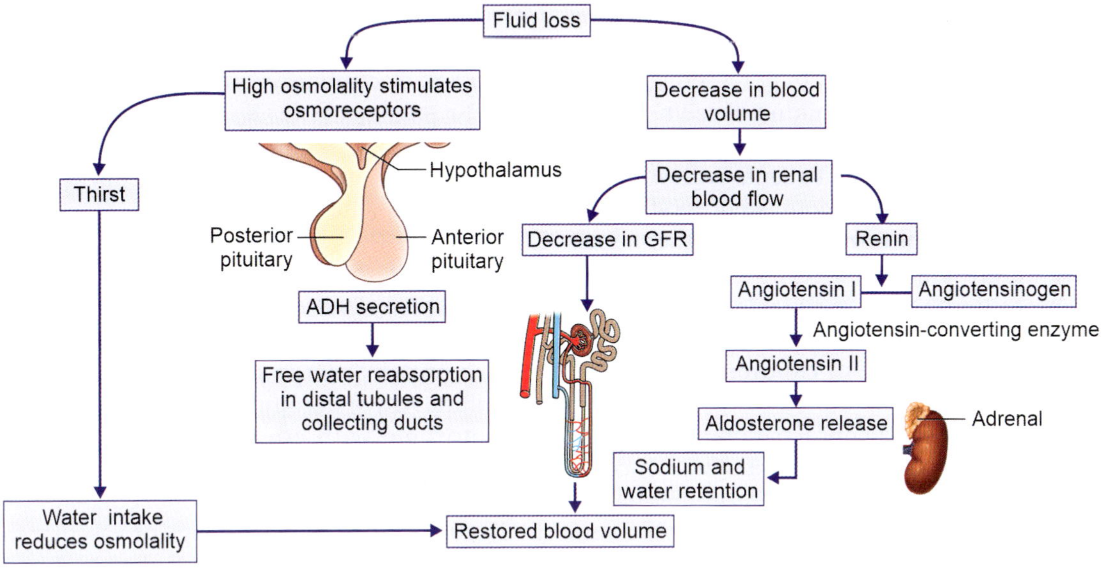


**Fig. 6.3:** Regulation of sodium and water balance

in water, acts as 100% free water per volume infused; half normal saline consists of 50% free water; and normal saline does not provide any free water for normonatremic children.

*Competencies:* **PE15.1; PE15.2; PE15.3; PE15.4; PE15.5; PE24.13; PE27.21; PE27.23**

## NORMAL MAINTENANCE FLUID AND ELECTROLYTE REQUIREMENTS

The normal maintenance water requirement is equal to the insensible and urinary water losses. Holliday and Segar guidelines (1957) calculate maintenance fluid volumes to match electrolyte-free water requirements from estimates of water of evaporation (heat dissipation) and caloric expenditure (heat production). They estimated a daily $Na^+$ requirement of 3 mEq/kg, $K^+$ and $Cl^-$ 2 mEq/kg each and daily glucose requirement as 5 g/kg based on the electrolyte composition of human and cow milk, and recommended 30 mEq/L sodium chloride (saline) for maintenance fluid in children.

Maintenance IV fluids in an unwell child were initiated with 0.2–0.45% normal saline along with 5% dextrose and 20 mEq/L of potassium chloride (provided urine output is adequate). This guideline for maintenance volume (Table 6.1) assumes average calorie expenditure in a healthy child, which does not concur with the deranged physiology with (critically or otherwise ill) hospitalized children who have significant non-osmotic stimuli for vasopressin release (e.g. stress, pain, hypoxia, etc.).

While using large volume hypotonic IV fluids, numerous cases of severe hyponatremia were observed around the world. Multiple studies conducted over the last 30 years showed that administration of isotonic fluids was effective and safe, and avoided the risk of moderate to severe hyponatremia in children. Current guidelines, therefore, recommend that children between the age of 28 days to 18 years requiring maintenance fluids, should receive ***isotonic fluids*** with appropriate potassium chloride and dextrose. This practice would significantly decrease the risk of developing hyponatremia and not increase the risk of hypernatremia. Exceptions to this guideline should be made for neonates, children undergoing neurosurgery, children with heart disease, liver diseases, acute kidney injury/chronic kidney disease, diabetes insipidus, severe watery diarrhea or burns and malignancies. IV fluid with osmolality lower than plasma osmolality can cause movement of free water from plasma to red blood cells leading to hemolysis. Therefore, infusing plain 5% dextrose in water or 0.2% or 0.45% saline (without dextrose) should be avoided in children.

Care must be taken in the special situation of diabetes insipidus, where administration of free water (directly or from hypotonic solutions) is the key to the resolution of the underlying metabolic disturbances resulting from the inability to excrete solutes in the urine. In children with diabetes insipidus, hypernatremia and significant hypovolemia, adequate free water administration is essential for correction of hypernatremia, after intravascular fluid repletion.

In children with weight 6–15 kg, body surface area (BSA)-based calculation for volume may be better than calculations using body weight. Weight-based formulae would deliver 20–50% more volume in children of this weight group

**Table 6.1:** Maintenance fluid requirement in healthy children*

| *Body weight* | *Per day* | *Per hour* |
|---|---|---|
| 0–10 kg | 100 mL/kg | 4 mL/kg |
| 10–20 kg | 1000 mL + 50 mL/kg for each kg above 10 kg | 40 mL + 2 mL/kg for each kg above 10 kg |
| >20 kg | 1500 mL + 20 mL/kg for each kg above 20 mg | 60 mL + 1 mL/kg for each kg above 20 kg |

*In smaller children (6–15 kg body weight), it is suggested to give fluid volumes at 1400–1500 mL/$m^2$ body surface area.

when compared to BSA-based calculation. Calculation using weight-based formulae also lead to overestimation of electrolyte-free water, leading to hyponatremia. It has been proposed that critically sick children receive 60–70% of calculated maintenance fluids to reduce the risk of fluid overload and hyponatremia. Patients with AKI and oligoanuria should receive fluids equivalent to 400 mL/$m^2$/day (insensible losses) plus urine output/other losses.

There is no single maintenance intravenous fluid (volume or composition) which is suitable for all clinical scenarios and maintenance fluid prescriptions should be individualized (Table 6.2). All children receiving IV maintenance fluid should be monitored with daily weight, fluid balance, clinical and biochemical parameters in order to maintain homeostasis. Additionally, maintenance IV fluids do not replace daily nutrient requirements and provide only about 20% of daily calories (enough to avoid starvation ketoacidosis and diminish protein degradation). Feasibility of transition to enteral fluids and nutrition should be actively considered.

## Deficit Therapy

The degree of volume depletion is assessed by physical examination (Table 6.3). The presence of hypernatremia or hypertonicity decreases the severity of physical signs of volume depletion. All fluid lost should be replaced to maintain euvolemia, within 24 hours. Steps for providing fluids and electrolytes to volume depleted patients are:

- If the patient shows signs of shock, compensated shock or features of severe dehydration (Table 6.3), rapidly infuse isotonic fluids to restore intravascular volume. This is done by infusing 1 to 3 fluid boluses of isotonic saline or Ringer's lactate, 20 mL/kg body weight, each over 10–30 minutes via a wide bore cannula or intraosseous needsle. Smaller volumes may be used for bolus therapy in case of pre-existing comorbidities like protein energy malnutrition, congestive cardiac failure, AKI or decompensated liver disease. In nephrotic syndrome with edema and clinical or biochemical hypovolemia, intravascular fluid repletion takes precedence over the presence of edema, so as to prevent significant end organ damage or vascular thrombosis.
- Provide fluids to replace calculated/observed volume deficit. This is calculated as volume at the rate of 10 mL/kg for each percentage weight loss. For example, in patients with moderate (some) dehydration, which is on an average 7.5% weight loss, the replacement volume is 75 mL/kg body weight. If the pre-dehydration weight is known, the volume of fluid needed is 1 liter for every kg of weight loss.

**Table 6.2:** Conditions requiring change in daily maintenance fluid volume

| *Decrease maintenance therapy volumes* | *Increase maintenance therapy volumes* |
|---|---|
| Postoperative children | Increased activity/fever |
| Children hospitalized with brain or lung disease (meningitis, encephalitis, bronchiolitis, pneumonia) | Increased skin loss: Burns/excessive sweating<br>Tachypnea/tachycardia<br>Dry environment |
| Coma | Hyperventilation |
| Hypothermia | Capillary leak, third spacing of fluid |
| Hypothyroidism | Extreme low birth weight |
| Oliguria/anuria (acute kidney injury) | Use of overhead heaters, phototherapy units |
| Highly humidified atmosphere | Polyuria |
| Humidified ventilator circuits | Surgical drains |

**Table 6.3:** Clinical assessment of dehydration

| | *No dehydration* | *Some dehydration* | *Severe dehydration* |
|---|---|---|---|
| Decrease in body weight | <5% in infants;<br><3% in older children | 5–10% in infants;<br>3–6% in older children | >10–15% in infants;<br>>6–9% in older children |
| Mental status | Normal | Irritable | Lethargic to comatose |
| Thirst | Normal | Increased | Unable to drink |
| Skin color and elasticity (turgor) | Normal | Cool, pale; mild delay | Cold, mottled; tenting |
| Sunken eyes | Normal | Sunken | Very sunken |
| Mucous membrane | Normal | Dry | Very dry |
| Fontanelle | Flat | Soft | Sunken |
| Pulse rate | Normal | Slightly increased | Tachycardia |
| Capillary refill | 2–3 seconds | 3–4 seconds | >4 seconds |
| Blood pressure | Normal | Normal | Normal or low |
| Urine output | Slightly decreased | Decreased | Oliguria, anuria |

**Table 6.4:** Electrolyte composition of body fluids and replacement choice

| *Losses* | *$Na^+$ (mEq/L)* | *$K^+$ (mEq/L)* | *$Cl^-$ (mEq/L)* | *$HCO_3^-$ (mEq/L)* | *Replacement fluid* |
|---|---|---|---|---|---|
| Gastric | 60–100 | 5–20 | 90–130 | 0 | ½ NS with potassium chloride |
| Small intestine | 80–140 | 5–15 | 90–140 | 40 | ½ NS or NS with sodium bicarbonate and potassium chloride |
| Colon | 60 | 30 | 40 | 15 | ½ NS with sodium bicarbonate |
| Pancreas | 135–145 | 5–10 | 70–90 | 95–120 | NS with sodium bicarbonate and potassium chloride; ORS |
| Diarrhea | 10–90 | 10–80 | 90–130 | 40 | ORS |
| Burns* | 135–140 | 5 | 105–110 | - | NS |

NS normal saline; ORS oral rehydration solution

*Fluid losses are usually estimated as 4 mL/kg per percentage body surface area involved; half the volume is administered over 8 hours and the remaining over the next 16 hours. Protein loss in burns may be estimated as 3–5 g/dL. This should be replaced by enteral or parenteral nutrition to avoid hypoalbuminemia/accelerated catabolism.

- Provide fluid and electrolytes to replace the amounts lost in normal daily metabolism (maintenance fluids; Table 6.1).
- Provide enough fluid to replace ongoing losses of various body fluids (Table 6.4). If losses cannot be measured appropriately, a rough calculation of 10 mL/kg for each large volume watery loose stool, and 2 mL/kg for every bout of emesis is appropriate.
- Enteral route is the safest and most preferred route for repletion therapy; if accessible and feasible.

Normal saline or balanced salt solutions (Ringer's lactate plasma-Lyte) can be used for replacement therapy. Infusion of large volumes of normal saline may be associated with hyperchloremic metabolic acidosis, and associated adverse effects. Balanced salt solutions are physiologically similar to human plasma and contain less chloride.

### Suggested Reading

1. Hasim N, Bakar MAA, Islam MA. Efficacy and safety of isotonic and hypotonic intravenous maintenance fluids in hospitalized children: A systematic review and meta-analysis of randomized controlled trials. Children 2021;8:785.
2. Feld LG, Neuspiel DR, Foster BA, et al. Clinical practice guideline: Maintenance intravenous fluids in children. Pediatrics. 2018; 142(6): e20183083.
3. Intravenous fluid therapy in children and young people in hospital. London: National Institute for Health and Care Excellence (NICE); 2020. Available from: https://www.ncbi.nlm.nih.gov/books/NBK563449/
4. Lehr AR, Rached-d' Astous S, Barrowman N, et al. Balanced versus unbalanced fluid in critically ill children. Pediatr Crit Care Med 2022;23(3):181–91.

*Competencies:* **PE15.2; PE15.3; PE15.4; PE15.5; PE24.13**

## SODIUM

### Physiology

Sodium is the most abundant ion of the extracellular fluid compartment and is critical in determining extracellular and intracellular osmolality. Normal serum $Na^+$ concentration varies between 135 and 145 mEq/L. Extracellular $Na^+$ balance is determined by its intake relative to its excretion. Daily $Na^+$ requirement is 2 to 3 mEq/kg body weight, although intakes are generally well in excess. The requirement varies with age. It is nearly two- to three-fold higher in term and very low birth weight preterm babies, a reflection of immaturity of renal tubular function and higher requirements for growth. Adult requirements decrease to 1.5 mEq/kg/d. Urinary $Na^+$ excretion represents the majority of the losses and approximately equals the daily intake of $Na^+$. Fractional excretion of $Na^+$ is generally less than 1% of filtered load. Extrarenal $Na^+$ losses can be significant during profuse sweating, burns, severe vomiting or diarrhea.

A fall in blood pressure, decrease in $Na^+$ delivery to the macula densa, or sympathetic stimulation activates the renin–angiotensin axis, generating angiotensin II. This enhances aldosterone secretion, which increases blood pressure and $Na^+$ retention (with $K^+$ excretion). Both these changes restore the effective circulating volume (the part of the ECF that effectively perfuses the tissues), providing renal or nonrenal losses are being effectively replaced. Extraneous $Na^+$ loading tends to produce volume expansion, whereas loss leads to volume depletion.

### Hyponatremia

Hyponatremia, defined as plasma $Na^+$ less than 135 mEq/L, can result from excessive loss of $Na^+$ from excessive sweating, vomiting, diarrhea, burns and the administration of diuretics (Table 6.5). The most common cause of hyponatremia, however, is not a deficiency of total body $Na^+$, but an excess of total body water, as in the syndrome of inappropriate antidiuresis (SIAD).

SIAD is seen in association with pulmonary and cranial disorders, postoperatively and can be drug induced. In SIAD, the osmostat is reset inappropriately, leading to high levels of vasopressin or antidiuretic hormone (ADH) being secreted at a lower threshold (lower plasma osmolality). This leads to euvolemic hyponatremia in the presence of low serum osmolality (<275 mOsm/kg $H_2O$) and inappropriately high urine osmolality (>100 mOsm/kg $H_2O$) and high urine $Na^+$ (>20–30 mEq/L). Adrenal, renal, hepatic and thyroid insufficiency should be ruled out before making the diagnosis. Low uric acid levels are also commonly observed in SIAD.

Another hyponatremic disorder associated with central nervous system disorders is termed as cerebral salt wasting (CSW). In CSW, there is hypovolemic hyponatremia with high urinary $Na^+$ (>80 mEq/L) due to increase in blood

**Table 6.5:** Causes of hyponatremia

| **Hypovolemic hyponatremia (sodium loss in excess of free water)** |
|---|
| • *Renal loss:* Diuretic use, osmotic diuresis, renal salt-wasting, adrenal insufficiency, pseudohypoaldosteronism<br>• *Extrarenal loss:* Diarrhea, vomiting, drains, fistula, sweat (cystic fibrosis), cerebral salt wasting, third-spacing effusions, ascites |
| **Normovolemic hyponatremia (conditions that predispose to SIAD)** |
| • Inflammatory central nervous system disease (meningitis, encephalitis), tumors<br>• Pulmonary diseases (severe asthma, pneumonia)<br>• Drugs (cyclophosphamide, vincristine)<br>• Nausea, postoperative |
| **Hypervolemic hyponatremia (excess free water retention)** |
| • Congestive heart failure, cirrhosis, nephrotic syndrome, acute or chronic kidney disease (CKD) |



levels of natriuretic factor(s). The treatments are different, as cerebral salt wasting requires replacement of urinary salt-water losses while SIAD is managed by fluid restriction.

Hyperosmolality resulting from non-$Na^+$ molecules (hyperglycemia, mannitol overdose) draw water from the intracellular space to dilute the extracellular $Na^+$ concentration. Factitious hyponatremia, reported in conditions of reduced plasma water (increased dissolved solids; hyperlipidemia, hypertriglyceridemia, hyperproteinemia) or otherwise, is currently uncommon with the use of ion-selective electrodes.

Patients are generally symptomatic when serum $Na^+$ <125 mEq/L or the decline is acute (<24 hours). Early features include headache, nausea, vomiting, lethargy and confusion. Advanced manifestations are seizures, coma, decorticate posturing, dilated pupils, anisocoria, papilledema, cardiac arrhythmias, myocardial ischemia and central diabetes insipidus. Cerebral edema occurs at levels of 125 mEq/L or less.

Hypo-osmolality causes influx of water into the intracellular space, which results in cytotoxic cerebral edema and increased intracranial pressure and can lead to brain ischemia, herniation and death. The brain's primary mechanism in adapting to hyponatremia is the extrusion of intracellular electrolytes and organic osmolytes (inositol, taurine, glutamine, aspartate). Some of these organic osmolytes are excitatory, such as glutamate and aspartate, that can produce seizures in the absence of detectable cerebral edema. Major risk factors for hyponatremic encephalopathy are young age, hypoxemia and neurological disease. Children are at significantly higher risk than are adults for developing hyponatremic encephalopathy due to their relatively larger brain to intracranial volume ratio compared with adults. Hyponatremia in association with increased intravascular volume can result in pulmonary edema, hypertension and heart failure. Asymptomatic hyponatremia in preterm neonates is associated with poor growth and development, and sensorineural hearing loss, and is a risk factor for mortality, if associated with perinatal asphyxia.

### *Treatment*

The first step is to determine whether hyponatremia is acute (<48 hours) or chronic (>48 hours), symptomatic or asymptomatic and evaluate the volume status. In hypovolemic hyponatremia with hypotension, volume resuscitation with normal saline takes precedence over treatment of hyponatremia even at the risk of sudden increase in serum $Na^+$. Symptomatic hyponatremia requires early recognition and prompt management with IV boluses of hypertonic saline irrespective of the chronicity of hyponatremia. In clinical practice, the distinction between acute and chronic hyponatremia is often unclear at initial evaluation. Therefore, hyponatremia should be assumed as chronic and corrected gradually (maximum 8–12 mEq/L/day). A diagnostic approach to hyponatremia is outlined in **Fig. 6.4**.

Management of acute symptomatic or asymptomatic hyponatremia (<120–125 mEq/L) is depicted in **Fig. 6.5**. Chronic asymptomatic hyponatremia should be managed as per steps outlined in **Box 6.1**. Chronic hyponatremia should be slowly corrected over 48–72 hours or even longer; depending on the severity. Aggressive therapy with hypertonic saline in patients with chronic hyponatremia (where brain adaptation to hypo-osmolality is set in by extrusion of intracellular electrolytes and organic osmoles) can lead to the osmotic demyelination syndrome **(Fig. 6.6)**. Patients who develop the demyelination syndrome show a biphasic course, with neurological improvement followed by deterioration 2–7 days later manifested by mutism, dysarthria, lethargy, spastic quadriparesis and pseudobulbar palsy.

In a volume expanded state, fluid restriction alone or in combination with diuretics is useful. Fluid restriction alone has no role in the management of symptomatic hyponatremia. Normal saline is also inappropriate for treating hyponatremic encephalopathy due to non-hemodynamic states of vasopressin excess, such as SIAD and postoperative hyponatremia, as it is not sufficiently hypertonic to induce reduction in cerebral edema. V2 receptor antagonists or vaptans that block the binding of ADH to its V2 receptor, are not yet recommended for treatment of hyponatremic encephalopathy in children. These agents may have a role in treating euvolemic hyponatremia from SIAD and hypervolemic hyponatremia in congestive heart failure.

**Box 6.1: Treatment of Chronic, Asymptomatic Hyponatremia**

- Treat underlying etiology
- Calculate $Na^+$ deficit (mEq) = (130–serum $Na^+$) × 0.6 × body weight (kg)
- Rise of serum $Na^+$ should not exceed 0.3–0.5 mEq/hour or 10 mEq/L in the first 24 hours and additional 8–12 mEq/L during every next 24 hours thereafter until the serum $Na^+$ reaches 130 mEq/L
- Hypovolemia: $Na^+$ deficit estimated is given as normal saline; WHO ORS rehydration solution is preferable for patients able to accept orally
- SIAD: Fluid restriction; furosemide and oral salt supplementation, if required
- Hypervolemia: $Na^+$ and fluid restriction, diuretics
- Cerebral salt wasting: Fludrocortisone

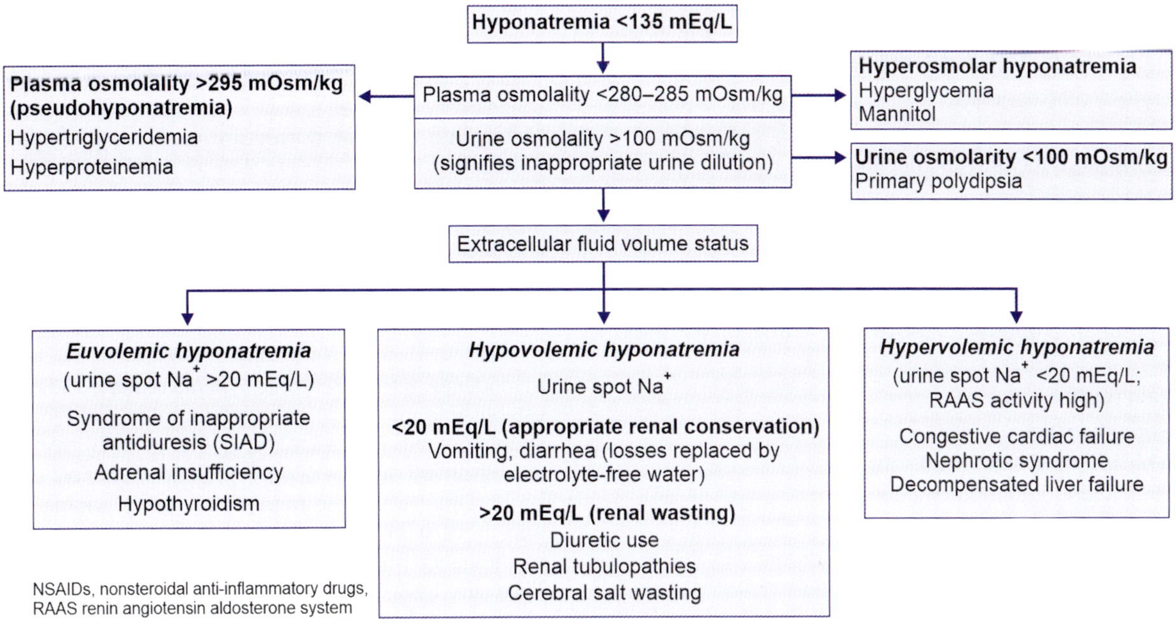


**Fig. 6.4:** Diagnostic approach to hyponatremia. Urine spot $Na^+$ should not be checked when the patient is being administered IV fluids. Syndrome of inappropriate antidiuresis can be observed in pain, nausea, vomiting, medications, pneumonia, bronchiolitis, meningitis and encephalitis. RAAS renin–angiotensin–aldosterone system

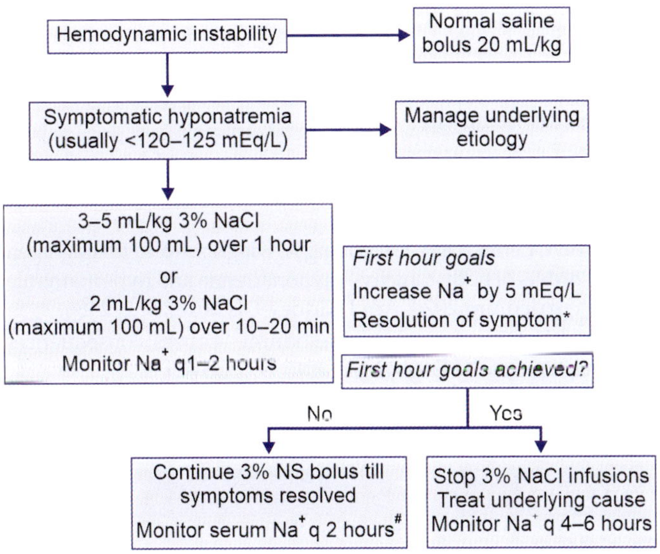


**Fig 6.5:** Management of acute symptomatic hyponatremia or asymptomatic hyponatremia <120–125 mEq/L.
*Symptom resolution is defined as patient being awake, alert, responding to commands with resolution of headache and nausea.
#Rise in serum $Na^+$ should not exceed 0.5 mEq/hr or 10 mEq/L in the first 24 hours and then 8 mEq/L every 24 hourly, till a serum level of 130 mEq/L

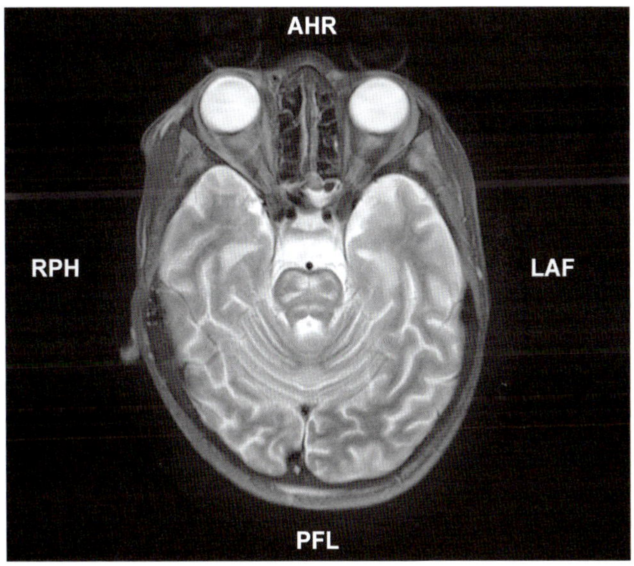


**Fig. 6.6:** MRI brain T2 axial image through the pons showing bilaterally symmetrical hyperintensities, consistent with osmotic demyelination syndrome. (*Courtesy:* Department of Radio-diagnosis, Christian Medical College Hospital, Vellore)

## Hypernatremia

Hypernatremia is defined as increase in serum $Na^+$ >145 mEq/L. It may be accompanied by the presence of low, normal or high total body $Na^+$ content. The major cause of hypernatremia is loss of body water, inadequate intake of water, a lack of antidiuretic hormone (ADH), or excessive intake of $Na^+$ (e.g. solutions with high $Na^+$ such as sodium bicarbonate) (Table 6.6). Diabetes insipidus may result from a deficiency of ADH or its end organ unresponsiveness.

In the presence of an intact thirst mechanism, a slight increase in serum $Na^+$ concentration (3 to 4 mEq/L) above the normal levels, elicits intense thirst. The lack of thirst in the presence of hypernatremia in a mentally alert child indicates a defect in either the osmoreceptors or the cortical thirst center. The most objective sign of hypernatremia is lethargy or mental status changes, which might progress to coma and convulsions. During acute and severe hypernatremia, the osmotic shift of water from neurons leads to shrinkage of the brain and tearing of the meningeal vessels and intracranial hemorrhage; slowly developing hypernatremia is generally well tolerated.

**Table 6.6:** Causes of hypernatremia

**Electrolyte-free water loss/deficient intake (common)**

*Pure water loss/deficient intake*
- Insensible losses
- Diabetes insipidus (central and nephrogenic)
- Inadequate breastfeeding

*Hypotonic fluid loss*
- Renal: Loop, osmotic diuretics; post obstructive diuresis; polyuric phase of acute tubular necrosis
- Gastrointestinal: Vomiting, nasogastric drainage, diarrhea; lactulose

**Sodium gain (rare)**
- Excess sodium intake
- Sodium bicarbonate, saline infusions
- Hypertonic feeds, boiled skimmed milk
- Ingestion of sodium chloride
- Primary hyperaldosteronism, Cushing syndrome



The latter adaptation occurs initially by movement of electrolytes into cells and later by intracellular generation of organic osmolytes, which counter plasma hyperosmolality. Thrombotic complications due to severe dehydration and possible hypercoagulability include stroke, cerebral venous sinus thrombosis, peripheral vein thrombosis and renal vein thrombosis. Associated hyperglycemia and mild hypocalcemia may also be observed.

### *Treatment*

Treatment involves restoring normal osmolality and volume. The speed of correction depends on the rate of development of hypernatremia and associated symptoms **(Box 6.2)**. Because chronic hypernatremia is well tolerated, rapid correction offers no advantage and may be harmful since it may result in brain edema. Usually, a maximum of 8–12 mEq/day or about 0.3–0.5 mEq/L per hour should be the rate of correction. Kidney replacement therapy using hemodialysis or peritoneal dialysis is indicated for concurrent acute kidney injury or chronic kidney disease and volume overload. As hypernatremia is commonly seen in infants, peritoneal dialysis, with dialysate $Na^+$ concentration 10–12 mEq/L below serum $Na^+$, can be used to manage hypernatremia and concomitant AKI.

Free water losses in hypernatremia are estimated to be: (i) 3 mL/kg per mEq/L increase in $Na^+$ above 145 mEq/kg if serum $Na^+$ >170 mEq/L, and (ii) 4 mL/kg per mEq/L increase in $Na^+$ above 145 mEq/L if serum $Na^+$ is between 145 and 170 mEq/L. This deficit needs to be corrected over the time periods mentioned below; along with maintenance fluids after initial resuscitation in hypernatremia.

Children with diabetes insipidus (DI) should have *ad libitum* access to free water. Management aims to reduce urine volume through use of vasopressin analogues (central DI), and low dietary sodium/osmolar load and hydrochlorthiazide (2–4 mg/kg/day) with or without amiloride (1–2 mg/kg/day) (nephrogenic DI). Volume resuscitation in DI should preferably be done with 5% dextrose water to reduce solute load and worsening hypernatremia.

**Box 6.2: Treatment of Hypernatremia**

- Restore intravascular volume with 1–2 boluses of 20 mL/kg normal saline over 20 min (till restoration of intravascular volume)
- Determine time for correction on basis of initial sodium concentration:

| *Serum sodium level* | *Target time to achieve ~145 mEq/L level* |
|---|---|
| 145–157 mEq/L | 24 hours |
| 158–170 mEq/L | 48 hours |
| 171–183 mEq/L | 72 hours |
| 184–196 mEq/L | 84 hours (may need kidney replacement therapy, if oliguric) |

- In moderate to severe chronic hypernatremia (>157 mEq/L), after establishing intravascular repletion, initial fluid for correction should contain 77–154 mEq/L of $Na^+$ (with 20 mEq/L KCl after establishment of urine output). Initially, higher Na content may be obtained in severe hypernatremia by adding 3% saline, and fluids with lower $Na^+$ content can be used later in the maintenance phase.
- *Fluid rate:* 1.25–1.5 times maintenance; institute oral rehydration early, if possible.
- Monitor serum $Na^+$ q4 hourly; should not fall by >0.5 mEq/L/hour or >8–12 mEq/day.
- Adjust fluid on basis of clinical status and serum $Na^+$ concentration; if child develops seizures (due to rapid correction) 3% NaCl (4–6 mL/kg over 30 min) is indicated.
- Replace ongoing losses as they occur; identify and treat the underlying cause.

### Suggested Reading


1. Hoorn EJ, Zietse R. Diagnosis and treatment of hyponatremia: Compilation of the guidelines. J Am Soc Nephrol 2017; 28:1340–49.
2. Seay NW, Lehrich RW, Greenberg A. Diagnosis and management of disorders of body tonicity—hyponatremia and hypernatremia: Core curriculum 2020. Am J Kidney Dis 2018;75: 272–86.
3. Sterns RH. Disorders of plasma sodium—causes, consequences, and correction. N Engl J Med 2015; 372: 55–65.


*Competencies:* **PE15.2; PE15.3; PE15.4; PE15.5; PE24.13**

## POTASSIUM

### Physiology

Blood levels of potassium (normal serum concentration 3.5 to 5 mEq/L) is not an indicator of total body stores as it is a predominantly intracellular cation (~98%). Common $K^+$-rich foods include meats, beans, fruits and potatoes. Gastrointestinal absorption is complete and $K^+$ homeostasis is maintained predominantly through the regulation of renal excretion. During normokalemia, the fractional excretion of $K^+$ ($FEK^+$) is about 10%, chiefly regulated by aldosterone at the collecting duct. In extrarenal and renal losses, $FEK^+$ is about 3% and >15%, respectively. Renal adaptive mechanisms maintain $K^+$ homeostasis until the glomerular filtration rate drops to less than 15–20 mL/min. In addition, splanchnic sensing of $K^+$ leads to dephosphorylation of sodium chloride cotransporters in the distal tubule, leading to increased $Na^+$ delivery, following a dietary load, to the aldosterone sensitive distal nephron. This results in increased aldosterone activity and subsequent $K^+$ excretion, independent of renal regulation. Another component independent of renal regulation is the circadian $K^+$ secretion (peak at noon and nadir at night). Both these mechanisms provide the ability to handle large $K^+$ loads in the diet, partially independent of renal regulation.

Excretion of $K^+$ is increased by aldosterone, high $Na^+$ delivery to the collecting duct (e.g. diuretics), urine flow (e.g. osmotic diuresis), blood $K^+$ level, glucocorticoids, acid–base status, vasopressin and delivery of negatively charged ions to the collecting duct (e.g. bicarbonate). In CKD, the proportion of $K^+$ excreted through the gut increases, chiefly by the colon in exchange for luminal $Na^+$.

Insulin stimulated by $K^+$ ingestion increases uptake of $K^+$ in muscle cells, through increased activity of the $Na^+$–$K^+$ ATPase pump. High $K^+$ levels stimulate its renal secretion via aldosterone-mediated enhancement of distal expression of secretory $K^+$ channels (renal outer medullary potassium channel; ROMK). Insulin, beta-adrenergic stimuli and alkalosis enhance $K^+$ entry into cells. The reverse happens with glucagon, α-adrenergic stimuli and acidosis.

The transtubular potassium gradient (TTKG) accounts for the confounding effect of urine concentration on interpretation of urine $K^+$ excretion. TTKG is the ratio of $K^+$ concentration in the lumen of the cortical collecting duct to that of the plasma; an indirect indicator of aldosterone activity. It is calculated as follows.

TTKG = (urine potassium × plasma osmolality)/(serum potassium × urine osmolality)

This test cannot be applied when the urine osmolality is less than the serum osmolality or in cases of poor distal tubular $Na^+$ delivery (urine $Na^+$ <25 mEq/L). Normal TTKG varies between 6 and 12. It should rise to >10 in patients with hyperkalemia. A value <5 signifies inappropriate aldosterone effect. An increase in TTKG >7 after administration of physiologic dose of fludrocortisone suggests mineralocorticoid deficiency; <7 suggests resistance.

The urinary $K^+$ to creatinine ratio can be used to assess $K^+$ handling by the kidneys; the near-constant rate of creatinine secretion in urine helps in correction for variation in urine concentration. A $K^+$: creatinine ratio <13 mEq/g creatinine (or <2.5 mEq/mmol creatinine) suggests an appropriate response to gastrointestinal $K^+$ loss, remote use of diuretics, decreased dietary intake, and $K^+$ shift into cells. Higher ratios imply an inappropriate response by the kidney. While cumbersome to collect, a 24-hour excretion of >25–30 mEq/day of $K^+$ in a hypokalemic patient also implies renal wasting.

### Hypokalemia

Hypokalemia is defined as a serum $K^+$ level below 3.5 mEq/L. The primary pathogenic mechanisms resulting in hypokalemia include increased losses, decreased intake or transcellular shift (Table 6.7). Vomiting, a common cause of hypokalemia, produces volume depletion and metabolic alkalosis. Volume depletion leads to secondary hyperaldosteronism, which enhances $Na^+$ resorption and $K^+$ secretion in the cortical collecting tubules. Metabolic alkalosis also increases $K^+$ secretion due to the decreased availability of $H^+$ for secretion in response to $Na^+$ reabsorption. Hypomagnesemia causes loss of inhibition of ROMK channels, leading to refractory hypokalemia which is corrected after magnesium repletion along with $K^+$ correction. Intracellular stores need to be corrected initially before changes in serum $K^+$ are noted (correction of serum $K^+$ from 2 to 3 mEq/L requires 400–600 mEq and correction from 3–4 mEq/L is achieved after 100–200 mEq $K^+$, for an adult).

**Table 6.7:** Causes of hypokalemia

**Increased losses**

*Renal*

- Renal tubular acidosis (proximal or distal)
- Medications (loop and thiazide diuretics, amphotericin B, aminoglycosides, corticosteroids)
- Cystic fibrosis
- Gitelman syndrome, Bartter syndrome, Liddle syndrome
- Ureterosigmoidostomy
- Mineralocorticoid excess (Cushing syndrome; hyperaldosteronism, congenital adrenal hyperplasia due to 11β-hydroxylase or 17α-hydroxylase deficiency)
- High renin conditions (renin-secreting tumors, renal artery stenosis)

*Extrarenal*

- Diarrhea, vomiting, nasogastric suction, sweating
- Potassium binding resins (sodium polystyrene sulfonate)

**Decreased intake or body stores**

- Malnutrition, anorexia nervosa
- Potassium-poor parenteral nutrition

**Intracellular shift**

Alkalosis, high insulin state, medications ($\beta_2$ adrenergic agonists, theophylline, hydroxychloroquine), refeeding syndrome, hypokalemic periodic paralysis, thyrotoxic periodic paralysis

Regardless of the cause, hypokalemia produces similar signs and symptoms, predominantly related to muscular or cardiac function. Severe hypokalemia (<2.5 mEq/L) may cause muscle weakness (neck flop, abdominal distension, ileus) and produce cardiac arrhythmias. Chronic hypokalemia is associated with interstitial renal disease of uncertain pathogenesis. Hypokalemia increases the risk of digoxin toxicity by promoting its binding to myocytes, potentiating its action and decreasing clearance.

#### Treatment

Patients should be evaluated to determine the underlying causes and determine whether it is associated with hypertension and acidosis or alkalosis (Fig. 6.7). Hypertension may be a clue to primary hyperaldosteronism, renal artery stenosis, or the rarer forms of genetically inherited hypertension such as, glucocorticoid remediable hypertension, apparent mineralocorticoid excess and Liddle syndrome. Relative hypotension and alkalosis suggest diuretic use, or a tubular disorder such as Bartter or Gitelman syndrome. Severe hypokalemia (<2.5 mEq/L) should be considered a medical emergency, since life-threatening arrhythmias may occur (Fig. 6.8).

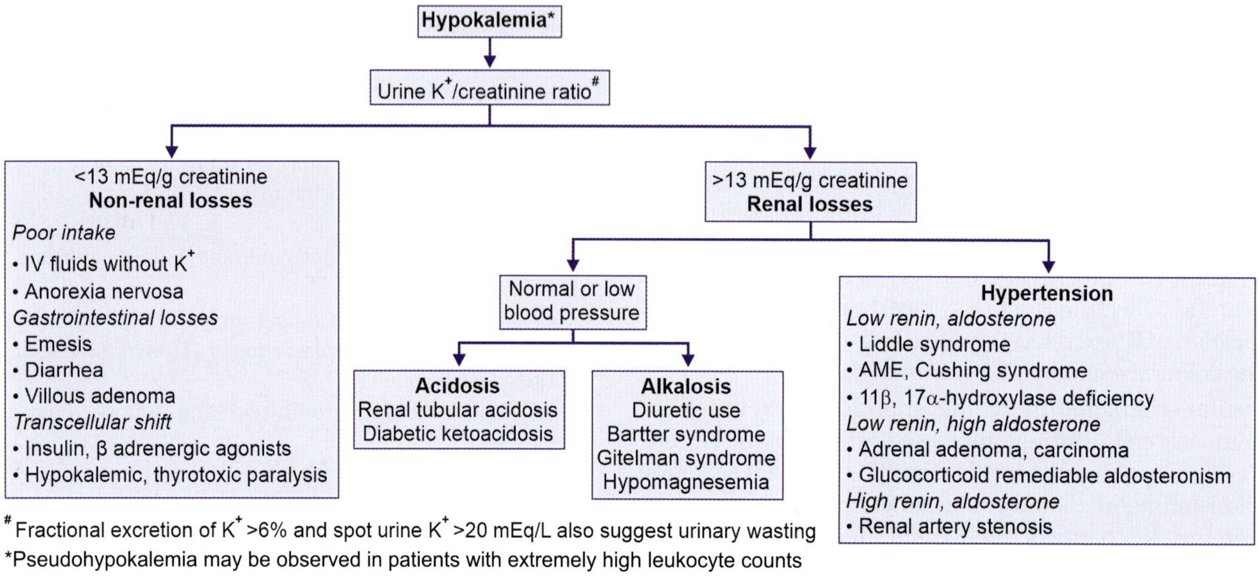


**Fig. 6.7:** Diagnostic approach to hypokalemia. AME apparent mineralocorticoid excess, CAH congenital adrenal hyperplasia

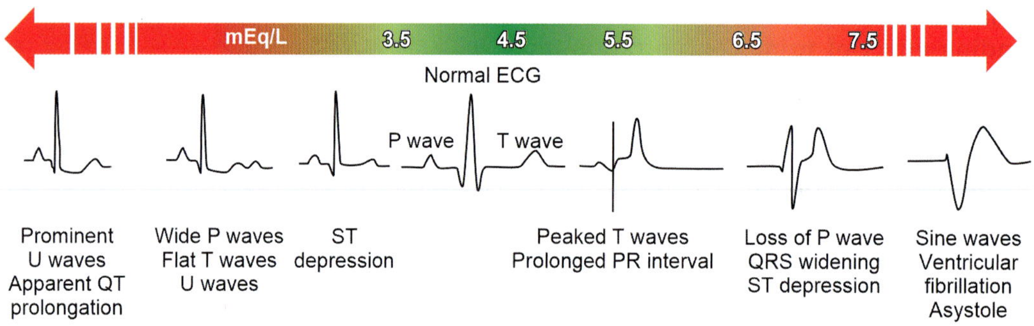


**Fig. 6.8:** Characteristic electrocardiographic changes with hypo- and hyperkalemia. While the changes in hyperkalemia correspond to serum potassium levels, those of hypokalemia do not always correlate with the serum levels (usually are seen with $K^+$ <2.5–2.7 mEq/L)

Therapy involves decreasing ongoing losses (e.g. discontinuation of diuretics, $\beta_2$-agonists), replenishing $K^+$ stores (oral or intravenous administration of potassium chloride) and disease-specific therapy for the conditions such as Bartter and Gitelman syndrome (e.g. indomethacin, angiotensin-converting enzyme inhibitors) **(Box 6.3)**.

**Box 6.3: Treatment of Hypokalemia**

- IV supplementation
  Indication: Symptomatic patients, severe hypokalemia (<2.5 mEq/L), ECG abnormalities
  - Potassium chloride (15%: 2 mEq/mL; 0.5–1 mEq/kg/dose) given as IV infusion over 1–2 hr. Infusion rate should not exceed 1 mEq/kg/hour; concentration of $K^+$ should not exceed 60 mEq/L (peripheral line) and 80 mEq/L (central line)
  - Avoid glucose containing fluids for hypokalemia correction, as insulin release will shift $K^+$ intracellularly
- Oral supplementation
  Dose: 2–4 mEq/kg/day in 3–4 divided doses
  - Potassium chloride (10%; 20 mEq/15 mL); potassium citrate used in renal tubular acidosis. Liquid preparations are bitter and may be diluted with juice or water
- Replace ongoing losses, volume resuscitation with normal saline, **correct hypomagnesemia**, treat underlying etiology (monogenic hypertension, Bartter and Gitelman syndromes)

## Hyperkalemia

Hyperkalemia, defined as serum potassium level exceeding 5.5 mEq/L, is most commonly associated with acute or chronic kidney disease, acidosis and diseases that involve defects in mineralocorticoid, aldosterone and insulin function. Sudden and rapid onset of hyperkalemia is one of the most serious electrolyte disturbances and result in severe cardiac arrhythmia.

Factitious or pseudohyperkalemia can occur because of the practice of squeezing of extremities during phlebotomy, blood sampled from a limb being infused with potassium-containing fluid or hemolysis of a standing sample. Thrombocytosis and leukocytosis can also lead to false elevation of serum $K^+$ levels. True hyperkalemia is caused by one or more of three mechanisms: Increased $K^+$ intake, extracellular potassium shifts and decreased excretion (Table 6.8). Increased $K^+$ intake may result from inappropriate intravenous or oral $K^+$ supplementation. Packed red blood cells have high concentrations of $K^+$ that can lead to hyperkalemia. Acidosis results in transcellular $K^+$ shift, but any cellular injury that disrupts the cell membrane (e.g. tumor lysis syndrome, rhabdomyolysis, crush injury, massive hemolysis) can cause hyperkalemia.

Patients may report nausea, vomiting and paresthesias or nonspecific findings of muscle weakness (skeletal,

**Table 6.8:** Causes of hyperkalemia

| **Decreased losses** |
|---|
| Acute kidney injury or chronic kidney disease |
| Renal tubular disorders: Pseudohypoaldosteronism, urinary tract obstruction |
| Medications: ACE inhibitors, angiotensin receptor blockers, potassium sparing diuretics, NSAIDs, heparin |
| Adrenal insufficiency: Congenital/acquired |
| **Increased intake** |
| Intravenous or oral $K^+$ intake, packed red cells transfusion |
| **Extracellular shift** |
| Acidosis, low insulin state, medications (β-adrenergic blockers, digitalis, succinylcholine, fluoride), hyperkalemic periodic paralysis, malignant hyperthermia |
| **Cellular breakdown** |
| Tumor lysis syndrome, rhabdomyolysis, crush injury, massive hemolysis |

respiratory), fatigue and ileus. Clinical manifestations are related to the effects of elevated $K^+$ levels on cardiac conduction since they interfere with repolarization of the cellular membrane. ECG changes **(Fig. 6.8)** appear progressively with rising serum $K^+$ and include tall, peaked T waves (5.5 to 6.5 mEq/L), prolonged PR interval, flat P waves, wide QRS complex (6.5 to 8.0 mEq/L), absent P waves, bundle branch blocks and eventually sine waves (>8.0 mEq/L).

### *Treatment*

Hyperkalemia is a medical emergency, requiring prompt discontinuation of $K^+$ containing fluids and administration of medications that ensure stability of myocardial membrane, intracellular shift of $K^+$ and enhance its elimination **(Box 6.4)**. Continuous ECG monitoring should be performed. Treatment should be individualized based upon the age, presentation, $K^+$ level, and ECG changes

**Box 6.4: Treatment of Hyperkalemia**

- Prompt discontinuation of $K^+$-containing fluids and medications that lead to hyperkalemia
- Stabilize myocardial cell membrane to prevent cardiac arrhythmia. Use IV 10% calcium gluconate at 0.5–1 mL/kg over 5–10 minutes under cardiac monitoring. Discontinue, if bradycardia develops
- *Enhance cellular uptake of potassium*

  Regular insulin and glucose IV: 0.3 U regular insulin/g glucose over 2 hr

  Sodium bicarbonate IV: 1–2 mEq/kg body weight over 20–30 minutes

  β-adrenergic agonists (salbutamol, terbutaline) nebulized or IV
- *Total body potassium elimination*

  Sodium polystyrene sulfonate (Kayexalate) oral/per rectal: 1 g/kg (max. 15 g/dose) oral or rectal enema in 20–30% sorbitol

  Loop or thiazide diuretics (if renal function is maintained)

  Kidney replacement therapy (hemodialysis or peritoneal dialysis): For severe symptomatic hyperkalemia, particularly in patients with impaired kidney function or tumor lysis syndrome

  Primary or secondary hypoaldosteronism: Maintenance steroids and fludrocortisone

(tall/peaked T waves: >5 mm in limb leads and >10 mm in chest leads).

If the hyperkalemia is severe ($K^+$ >7.0 mEq/L) or the patient is symptomatic with ECG changes, therapy should be initiated promptly with intravenous calcium gluconate, followed by sodium bicarbonate, insulin-glucose infusion and/or nebulized $\beta_2$-agonists. Hemodialysis may be needed in the more refractory patients. Milder elevations (5.5–6.5 mEq/L) are managed with elimination of $K^+$ intake, discontinuation of potassium sparing drugs and treatment of the underlying etiology. Children with primary or secondary hypoaldosteronism require stress-dose steroid supplements and mineralocorticoids.

### Suggested Reading


1. Bamgbola OF. Review of the pathophysiologic and clinical aspects of hypokalemia in children and young adults: An update. Curr Treat Options Pediatr. 2022. Doi.org/10.1007/s40746–022–00240–3.
2. Palmer BF, Clegg DJ. Physiology and pathophysiology of potassium homeostasis: Core curriculum 2019. Am J Kidney Dis 2019;74: 682–95.


*Competencies:* **PE13.11; PE13.12; PE20.14**

## CALCIUM

### Physiology

Ninety-eight percent of body calcium is found in the skeleton which is in equilibrium with the extracellular concentration of calcium. Approximately 1 to 2% of body calcium exists in the ECF for physiological functions like blood coagulation, cellular communication, exocytosis, endocytosis, muscle contraction and neuromuscular transmission. Calcium affects the intracellular processes, through its calcium-binding regulatory protein, calmodulin.

Most of the filtered calcium is reabsorbed in the proximal tubule (70%), ascending limb of Henle (20%), and the distal tubule and collecting duct (5–10%). Factors that promote calcium reabsorption include parathyroid hormone (PTH), calcitonin, vitamin D, thiazide diuretics and volume depletion. Volume expansion, increased $Na^+$ intake and diuretics such as mannitol and frusemide promote calcium excretion.

The intestine serves as a long-term homeostatic mechanism for calcium. Although the major source of calcium is dietary, less than 15% of dietary calcium is absorbed, primarily in the ileum and jejunum by means of active transport and facilitated diffusion via the TRPV6 channels. Calcium is controlled chiefly by PTH, calcitonin and vitamin D. Thyroid hormones, growth hormone, adrenal and gonadal steroids also influence calcium metabolism.

***Role of the calcium-sensing receptor:*** The calcium-sensing receptor (CaSR) is a G protein-coupled receptor, which allows the parathyroid chief cells, the thyroidal C cells and the ascending limb of Henle (renal tubular epithelial cells) to respond to changes in the extracellular calcium concentration. The ability of the CaSR to sense serum calcium is essential for the appropriate regulation of PTH secretion by the parathyroid glands and for the regulation of passive paracellular calcium absorption in the loop of Henle. Calcitonin secretion and renal tubular calcium reabsorption are directly regulated by the action of calcium ion on its receptor. Ionized calcium acts through calcitonin to inhibit its release from bones. Decrease in extracellular calcium concentration stimulates the CaSR in parathyroid glands, resulting in an increase in PTH secretion (Fig. 6.9). PTH increases distal renal tubular reabsorption of calcium within minutes and stimulates osteoclast activity with release of calcium from the skeleton within 1–2 hours. More prolonged PTH elevation stimulates 1α-hydroxylase activity in the proximal tubular cells, which leads to 1,25-dihydroxyvitamin D production. In the kidney, vitamin D and PTH stimulate the activity of the epithelial calcium channel and the calcium-binding protein (i.e. calbindin) to increase active transcellular calcium absorption in the distal convoluted tubule. These mechanisms help to maintain normal levels of serum calcium.

Plasma calcium exists in three forms: 50% as biologically active ionized form, 45% bound to plasma proteins (mainly albumin) and 5% complexed to phosphate and citrate. In the absence of alkalosis or acidosis, the proportion of albumin-bound calcium remains relatively constant. Metabolic acidosis leads to increased ionized calcium from reduced protein binding and alkalosis has the opposite effect. Plasma calcium is tightly regulated in the normal range of 9–11 mg/dL. As only the unbound (free or ionized) calcium is biologically active, the serum level must be adjusted for abnormal albumin levels. For every 1 g/dL drop in serum albumin below 4 g/dL, measured serum calcium decreases by 0.8 mg/dL. Corrected calcium can be calculated using the following formula:

$$\text{Corrected calcium} = [4 - \text{plasma albumin in g/dL}] \times 0.8 + \text{measured serum calcium}$$

Alternatively, serum free (ionized) calcium levels can be directly measured, negating the need for correction for albumin.

### Hypocalcemia

Hypocalcemia is defined as serum calcium less than 8 mg/dL or ionized calcium below 4 mg/dL. Its causes and a proposed algorithm for investigating the etiology are shown in Table 6.9 and Fig. 6.10. Hypocalcemia manifests as central nervous system irritability and poor muscular contractility. Newborns present with lethargy, poor feeding, jitteriness, vomiting, abdominal distension and seizures. Children may develop seizures, twitching, cramps and rarely laryngospasm. Tetany and signs of nerve irritability may manifest as muscular twitching, carpopedal spasm and stridor. Latent tetany can be diagnosed by maneuvers such as Chvostek sign (twitching of the orbicularis oculi and mouth elicited by tapping the facial nerve anterior to the external auditory meatus) and the Trousseau sign (carpopedal spasm elicited by inflating the arm blood pressure cuff above the systolic pressure for 3 min). ECG shows prolonged corrected QT interval (QTc) to more than 0.45 seconds. Cardiac function may be impaired because of poor muscle contractility. Prolonged hypocalcemia can present with features of rickets.

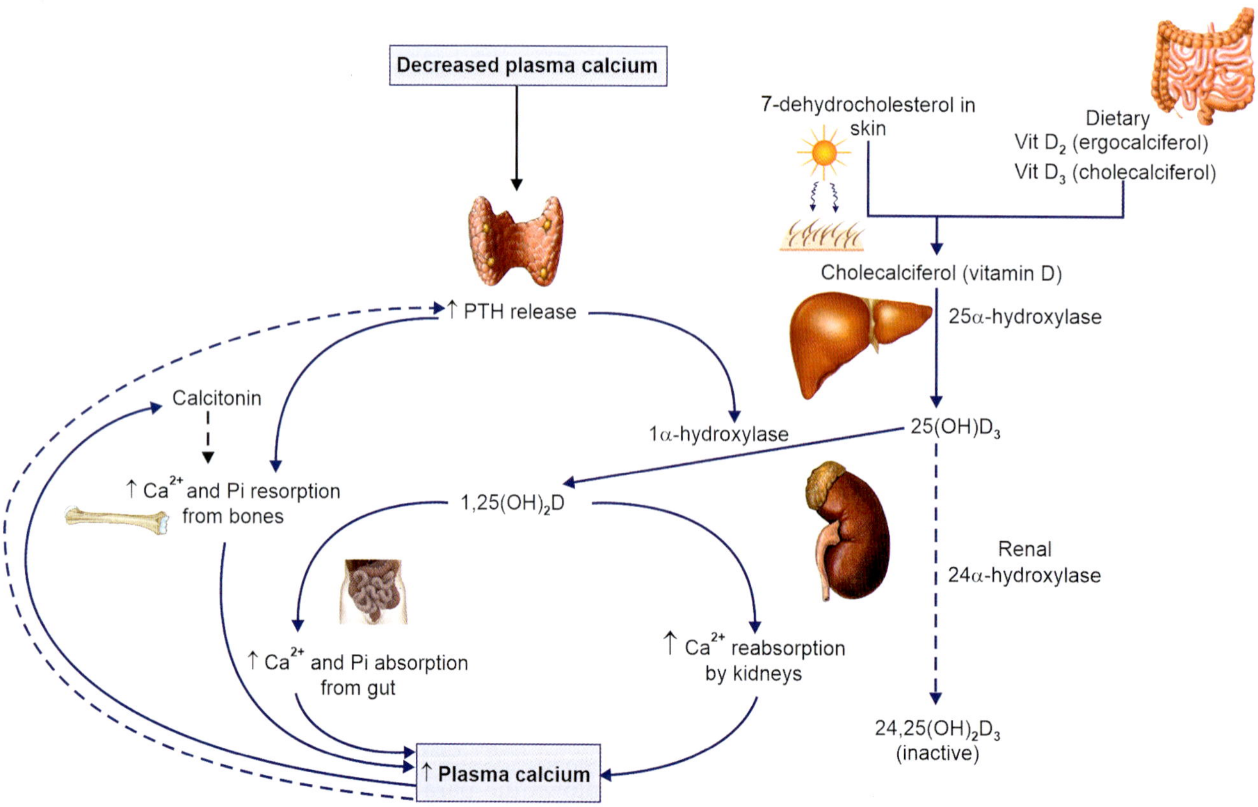


Fig. 6.9: Regulation of plasma calcium. Reduction in ionized calcium results in PTH secretion, which through direct and indirect actions on the bones, intestine and the kidneys results in positive calcium balance. Calcitonin results in accretion of bone mass. Discontinuous lines indicate inhibitory control

**Table 6.9:** Causes of hypocalcemia

| |
|---|
| **Neonatal:** Early (within 48–72 hours after birth) or late (3–7 days after birth) neonatal hypocalcemia; prematurity; infant of diabetic mother; neonates fed high phosphate milk |
| **Parathyroid:** Aplasia or hypoplasia of parathyroid glands, DiGeorge syndrome, idiopathic; pseudohypoparathyroidism; autoimmune parathyroiditis; activating mutations of calcium sensing receptor |
| **Vitamin D:** Deficiency; resistance to vitamin D action; acquired or inherited disorders of vitamin D metabolism |
| **Others:** Hypomagnesemia; hyperphosphatemia (excess intake, CKD); malabsorption; metabolic alkalosis; hypoproteinemia; acute pancreatitis |
| **Drugs:** Prolonged therapy with frusemide, corticosteroids or phenytoin |

### *Management*

Tetany, laryngospasm and seizures must be treated immediately with 2 mL/kg of 10% calcium gluconate, administered IV slowly under cardiac monitoring. Calcium gluconate 10% (100 mg/mL) IV solution contains 9.8 mg/mL (0.45 mEq/mL) elemental calcium; calcium chloride 10% (100 mg/mL) contains 27 mg/mL (1.4 mEq/mL). Initially, IV calcium boluses are given every 6 hours, followed by oral calcium supplementation at 40–80 mg/kg/day. Oral calcium therapy is used in asymptomatic patients and as follow-up to intravenous (IV) calcium therapy. Intravenous infusion with calcium-containing solutions can cause severe tissue necrosis; therefore, integrity of the IV site should be ascertained before administering calcium. Rapid infusion of calcium-containing solutions through arterial lines can cause arterial spasm and if administered via an umbilical artery catheter, intestinal necrosis. Magnesium administration is necessary to correct any hypomagnesemia because hypocalcemia does not respond until the low magnesium level is corrected. In patients with concurrent acidemia, hypocalcemia should be corrected first. Acidemia increases the ionized calcium levels by displacing calcium from albumin and hence, if acidemia is corrected first, ionized calcium levels decrease.

Calcium carbonate is an oral supplement providing 40% elemental calcium. Therapy with cholecalciferol is used in patients with vitamin D deficiency. Calcitriol, an active metabolic form of vitamin D (1,25-dihydroxycholecalciferol) is administered in liver or kidney disease.

## Hypercalcemia

Hypercalcemia is defined as a serum calcium level greater than 11 mg/dL. Even mild persistent elevations should be investigated as calcium metabolism is tightly regulated. Etiologies of hypercalcemia vary by age and other factors **(Table 6.10)**. Hypercalcemia is often asymptomatic, although it can cause symptoms at levels as low as 12 mg/dL and consistently at values above 15 mg/dL. Such high values are, however, rarely encountered and present as stupor and coma. Neonates may be asymptomatic or may have vomiting, hypotonia, hypertension or seizures. Clinical features in older children are summarized in **Box 6.5** and include irritability, malaise, headache, confusion, unsteady gait and proximal muscle weakness.

Levels of PTH are useful in assessment of hypercalcemia. Low PTH levels indicate 25-hydroxyvitamin D mediated hypercalcemia. High levels of 1,25-hydroxyvitamin D suggest extrarenal synthesis in granulomatous disease, malignancy, subcutaneous fat necrosis or increased renal

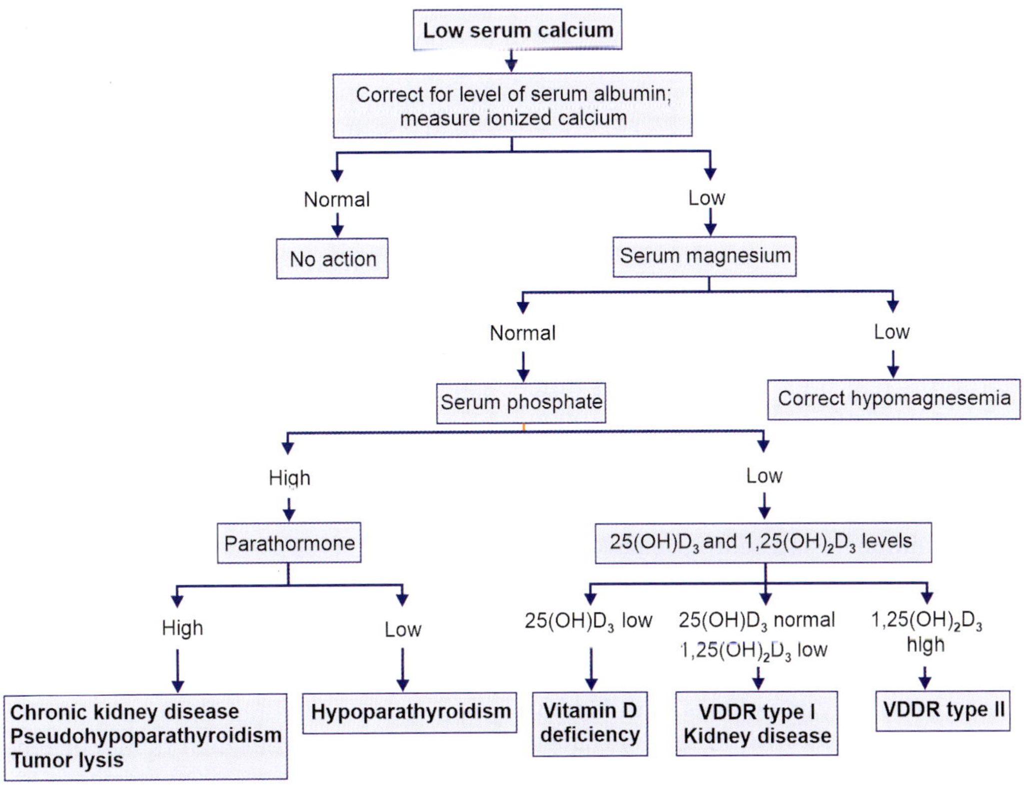


**Fig. 6.10:** Algorithm for evaluation of hypocalcemia. VDDR vitamin D dependent rickets

**Table 6.10:** Causes of hypercalcemia

**Neonates**

- Neonatal primary hyperparathyroidism (HPT; nonsyndromic or syndromic), secondary HPT
- Familial hypocalciuric hypercalcemia
- Excessive supplementation of calcium
- William syndrome, Down syndrome, hypophosphatasia, idiopathic infantile hypercalcemia

**Older children**

- HPT (parathyroid adenoma, autosomal dominant hereditary HPT, multiple endocrine neoplasia type 1; tertiary HPT in CKD or during therapy for hypophosphatemic rickets).
- *Malignancies:* Non-Hodgkin or Hodgkin lymphoma, Ewing sarcoma, neuroblastoma, Langerhans cell histiocytosis, rhabdomyosarcoma, acute leukemia.
- *Granulomatous disease:* Sarcoidosis, tuberculosis, polyangiitis with granulomatosis.

**Others:** Vitamin D or A intoxication; thiazide diuretics, milk-alkali syndrome; dietary phosphate deficiency; subcutaneous fat necrosis; thyrotoxicosis; retinoic acid therapy, prolonged immobilization, Jansen metaphyseal dysplasia.

**Box 6.5: Clinical Features of Hypercalcemia**

**Neurologic:** Lethargy, confusion, headache, depression, coma, hyporeflexia

**Cardiovascular:** Bradycardia, reduced QTc interval, systemic hypertension

**Renal:** Nephrocalcinosis, nephrolithiasis, polyuria, polydipsia

**Gastrointestinal:** Constipation, paralytic ileus, nausea, vomiting

**Ectopic calcification:** Pancreatitis, conjunctivitis, band keratopathy

synthesis/reduced degradation in idiopathic infantile hypercalcemia (*CYP24A1/SLC34A1* mutations). High levels of PTH and calcium are seen in patients with hyperparathyroidism.

#### *Treatment*

The initial treatment involves hydration to improve urinary calcium excretion. Rapid lowering of serum calcium can be expected with isotonic sodium chloride solution, because increasing $Na^+$ excretion enhances calcium excretion. Addition of a loop diuretic inhibits tubular reabsorption of calcium but attention should be paid to fluid status and other electrolytes (e.g. $Mg^{2+}$, $K^+$) during saline diuresis. Bisphosphonates serve to block bone resorption and decrease serum calcium within a couple of days. Pamidronate infusion is the drug of choice in children and a reduction in calcium is observed 12–24 hr, and might last for 2–4 weeks. Pamidronate and etidronate have been used in the treatment of hypercalcemia due to malignancy, immobilization and hyperparathyroidism. IV calcitonin may also be used with bisphosphonates.

Peritoneal dialysis or hemodialysis can be used in extreme situations, particularly in patients with kidney failure. Calcimimetics (cinacalcet hydrochloride) change the configuration of the CaSR in a manner that makes it more sensitive to serum calcium. Surgical intervention may be needed in patients with hyperparathyroidism, particularly with recurrent kidney stones or serum calcium levels higher than 12.5 mg/dL. Subtotal parathyroidectomy can be performed, or complete parathyroidectomy can be chosen with reimplantation of a small amount of tissue in the forearm.

### Suggested Reading

1. Davies JH, Shaw NJ. Investigation and management of hypercalcemia in children. Arch Dis Child 2012;97:533–38.
2. Kusumi K, Narla D, Mahan JD. Evaluation and treatment of pediatric calcium disorders. Curr Treat Options Pediatr. 2021;7(2):60–81.

*Competencies:* **PE13.13; PE13.14**

## MAGNESIUM

### Physiology

Magnesium is the third-most abundant intracellular cation predominantly located in muscle and liver cells. Most intracellular magnesium is bound to proteins; only approximately 25% is exchangeable. Magnesium plays a fundamental role in many functions of the cell, including energy transfer and storage and nerve conduction. Magnesium also plays important role in protein, carbohydrate, and fat metabolism, maintenance of normal cell membrane function and regulation of PTH secretion.

Dietary sources include green leafy vegetables, cereals, nuts and meats. Absorption of magnesium takes place primarily in the small intestine (major paracellular passive transport and minor transcellular active, saturable transport via transient receptor potential melastatin (TRPM) type 6 and 7 channels and is inversely related to the amount of magnesium, calcium, phosphate and fat. PTH, vitamin D and glucocorticoids increase magnesium absorption. Absorption is diminished in presence of substances that complex with magnesium (free fatty acids, fiber, phytate, phosphate, oxalate); increased intestinal motility and calcium also decreases magnesium absorption. Renal excretion is the principal regulator of magnesium balance. Reabsorption occurs chiefly in the thick ascending loop of Henle (70%) and to a smaller extent in the proximal (15%) and distal (5–10%) tubules. Reabsorption in the PCT and loop of Henle takes place predominantly via the paracellular pathways and transcellular pathway in the DCT. Claudin 10, 14, 16 and 19 channels mediate uptake in the loop of Henle, and TRPM6 channel in the DCT. Fractional excretion of magnesium exceeding 4% indicates renal magnesium wasting.

### Hypomagnesemia

Hypomagnesemia develops from decreased intake or more commonly increased losses which could be gastrointestinal (diarrhea, vomiting, nasogastric suction; upper gastrointestinal fluids contain less magnesium than lower gastrointestinal fluids) or renal (chronic use of thiazide diuretics, recovery phase of acute tubular necrosis, Gitelman syndrome, familial hypomagnesemia-hypercalciuria-nephrocalcinosis), drug induced (loop diuretics, aminoglycosides, proton pump inhibitors, epidermal growth factor receptor antagonists, calcineurin inhibitors and cisplatin/carboplatin).

Other genetic causes of hypomagnesemia include mutations in *CASR* (gain of function), *CLCKNB/BSND* or *KCNJ10* (Bartter syndrome), *FXYD2* (isolated autosomal dominant), *HNF1B* (autosomal dominant tubulointerstitial kidney disease), *TRPM6* (impaired dietary absorption), *CNNM2*, *EGF* and *EGFR*. Symptomatic magnesium depletion (occurs at levels below 1.2 mg/dL) is often associated with multiple biochemical abnormalities, including hypokalemia, hypocalcemia and metabolic acidosis. As a result, hypomagnesemia is sometimes difficult to attribute solely to specific clinical manifestations. Hypomagnesemia often leads to hypocalcemia, possibly by inhibition of PTH activity and also to hypokalemia, due to the removal of ROMK channel inhibition.

Neuromuscular manifestations of hypomagnesemia include muscle weakness, tremors, seizures, paresthesias, tetany, positive Chvostek or Trousseau sign, vertigo, ataxia, athetoid or choreiform movements and nystagmus. Cardiovascular manifestations include prolonged PR and QT intervals, U waves and "torsades de pointes" and arrhythmias (atrial tachycardia, fibrillation).

#### *Treatment*

Therapy can be oral for patients with mild symptoms or intravenous for patients with severe symptoms or those unable to tolerate oral administration. Severe hypomagnesemia is treated (in the presence of normal kidney functions) with slow intravenous infusion of magnesium sulfate (50% solution) at a dose of 25–50 mg/kg (2.5–5.0 mg/kg of elemental magnesium) [diluted to 5–10x volume in normal saline]. The dose is repeated every 6 hours, for a total of 2–3 doses; infusion of 100–200 mg/kg/day may be required in severe hypocalcemic states. Doses need to be reduced in children with CKD. Calcium gluconate should be available as an antidote during therapy.

Asymptomatic patients need to be administered oral replacement therapy for the short term; those requiring long-term replacement should preferably receive a sustained-release preparation, to avoid diarrhea. Oral magnesium preparation provides 5–7 mEq of magnesium per tablet. Two to four tablets may be sufficient for mild, asymptomatic disease while severe cases require up to six to eight tablets, to be taken daily in divided doses. Patients with renal magnesium wasting may benefit from diuretics with magnesium-sparing properties, such as spironolactone and amiloride. Concurrent hypokalemia and hypocalcemia warrant simultaneous correction.

### Hypermagnesemia

Serum magnesium >2.5 mg/dL is uncommon in children and may be seen in the setting of CKD, prolonged use of magnesium-containing antacids or in neonates born to mothers given magnesium sulfate as a treatment for eclampsia. Symptoms of hypermagnesemia are nonspecific at lower levels—nausea, vomiting, flushing, lethargy, weakness and dizziness. At higher levels, deep tendon reflexes are depressed which may progress to coma and respiratory depression. Cardiac effects include prolongation of intervals on ECG or arrhythmias, complete heart block and asystole.

#### *Treatment*

In patients with mildly increased levels, the source of magnesium may simply be removed. Intravenous calcium directly antagonizes the cardiac and neuromuscular effects of excess extracellular magnesium. Dialysis may be used for patients with severe hypermagnesemia and CKD, or those with serious cardiovascular or neuromuscular symptoms.

### Suggested Reading


1. Ahmed F, Mohammed A. Magnesium: The forgotten electrolyte—A review on hypomagnesemia. Med Sci (Basel). 2019; 7(4): 56.
2. Blaine J, Chonchol MB, Levi M. Renal control of calcium, phosphate, and magnesium homeostasis. Clin J Am Soc Nephrol. 2015;10(7): 1257–72.
3. Viering DHHM, de Baaij JHF, Walsh SB, et al. Genetic causes of hypomagnesemia, a clinical overview. Pediatr Nephrol 2017; 32: 1123–35.


## ACID–BASE DISORDERS

### Regulation of Acid–Base Equilibrium

The body is sensitive to changes in blood pH, as disturbances in acid–base homeostasis can result in denaturation of proteins and inactivation of enzymes that may be potentially fatal. Strong mechanisms exist to regulate acid–base balance and maintain arterial pH (7.35 to 7.45), $pCO_2$ (35 to 45 mm Hg) and $HCO_3^-$ (22 to 26 mEq/L) within a narrow range.

pH of body fluids is calculated using the Henderson-Hasselbach equation:

$$pH = pK + \log (HCO_3^-/pCO_2)$$

where pK is the dissociation constant of the acid.

Alteration in either serum bicarbonate concentration or the partial pressure of carbon dioxide causes acidosis (pH <7.35) or alkalosis (pH >7.45). Metabolic activity results in production of two types of acids—carbonic acid (a volatile acid, derived from carbon dioxide) and nonvolatile acids (including sulfuric acid, organic acids, uric acid and inorganic phosphates). Accumulation of $H^+$ ions of nonvolatile acids due to excess production or inadequate buffering, failure to excrete $H^+$ or loss of bicarbonate results in metabolic acidosis. If the reverse occurs, it results in metabolic alkalosis. The principal mechanism for carbon dioxide handling is by the lungs. Hyperventilation results in $CO_2$ washout and drop in arterial $pCO_2$ (respiratory alkalosis), hypoventilation has the opposite effect (respiratory acidosis). When only one primary acid–base abnormality occurs and its compensatory mechanisms are activated, the disorder is classified as simple acid–base disorder. A simple algorithm for defining simple acid–base disorders is shown in Fig. 6.11. When a combination of disturbances occurs, the disorder is classified as a mixed acid–base disorder. The latter are suspected when the compensation in a given patient differs from the predicted

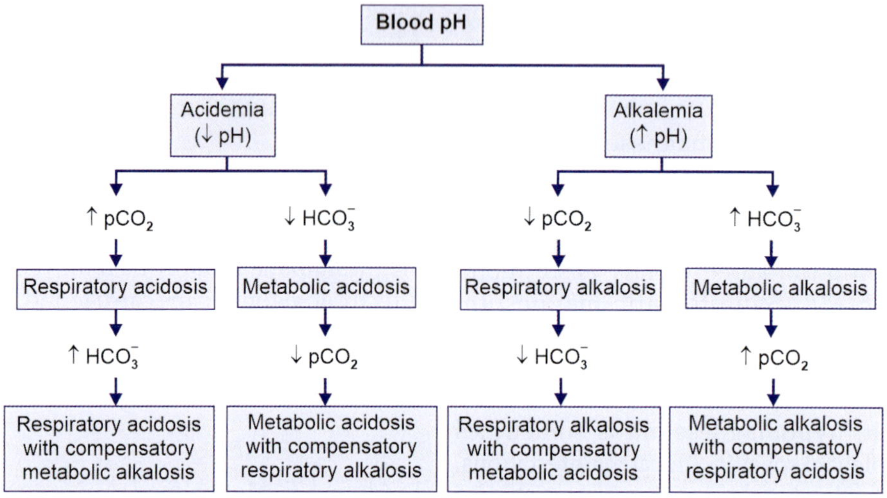


**Fig. 6.11:** Algorithm for simple acid–base disorders

values in **Table 6.11**. It should be kept in mind that overcompensation does not occur physiologically, and changes in same direction of metabolic and respiratory components should indicate a mixed acid–base disorder.

In order to maintain body homeostasis, changes in pH are resisted by a complex system of intracellular and extracellular buffers that reversibly bind hydrogen ions and reduce change in pH. In metabolic disorders, the extracellular buffers rapidly titrate the addition of strong acids or bases. Intracellular buffers chiefly accomplish the buffering of respiratory disorders. Secondary respiratory compensations to metabolic acid–base disorders occur within minutes and is completed by 12 to 24 hours. In contrast, secondary metabolic compensation of respiratory disorders begins more slowly and takes 2 to 5 days for completion. The compensatory mechanisms do not return the pH to normal until the underlying disease process has been appropriately treated. Extracellular buffers include bicarbonate and ammonia, whereas proteins and phosphate act as intracellular buffers. Hemoglobin is a powerful intracellular buffer because its negatively charged histidine moieties accept $H^+$, normalizing the pH. Other proteins also have negative charges that can accept $H^+$.

*Bicarbonate-carbonic acid buffer* in the extracellular fluid, is the key buffer as carbon dioxide ($CO_2$) can be shifted through carbonic acid ($H_2CO_3$) to hydrogen ions and bicarbonate ($HCO_3^-$):

$$H_2O + CO_2 \rightleftharpoons HCO_3^- \rightleftharpoons H^+ + HCO_3^-$$

Acid–base imbalances that overcome the buffer system can be compensated in the short-term by altering the rate of ventilation, which alters the $pCO_2$. While this is a relatively weak buffer, it accounts for 55% of the buffering capacity because of its sheer abundance. When $H^+$ concentration increases the above reaction shifts to the left, more $CO_2$ is generated and exhaled from the lungs, moderating the change in pH.

### Renal Regulation of Acid–Base Balance

The kidneys are slower to compensate, but renal physiology has several powerful mechanisms to control pH by the excretion of excess acid or base. Kidneys are the principal regulators of bicarbonate mainly by two methods: (i) Resorption of $HCO_3^-$ occurs mostly in proximal convoluted tubules, and (ii) excretion of $H^+$ and, therefore, generation of $HCO_3^-$, primarily by the distal tubules and collecting ducts. In response to acidosis, tubular cells reabsorb more bicarbonate from the tubular fluid, collecting duct cells secrete more hydrogen and generate more bicarbonate, and ammoniagenesis leads to increased formation of renal ammonia **(Fig. 6.12)**. In response to alkalosis, the kidneys excrete more bicarbonate by decreasing hydrogen ion secretion from the tubular epithelial cells, and lowering rates of glutamine metabolism and ammonia excretion.

***Bicarbonate-carbonic acid buffer in the renal tubules:*** $H^+$ ions secreted from the tubular cells combine with luminal $HCO_3^-$ to form water and $CO_2$. The $CO_2$ enters the tubular

**Table 6.11:** Compensation for primary acid–base disorders

| *Disorder* | *Primary event* | *Compensation* | *Expected compensation* |
|---|---|---|---|
| Metabolic acidosis | ↓ $[HCO_3^-]$ | ↓ $pCO_2$ | $pCO_2$ ↓ by 1–1.5 mm Hg for 1 mEq/L ↓$[HCO_3^-]$ |
| Metabolic alkalosis | ↑ $[HCO_3^-]$ | ↑ $pCO_2$ | $pCO_2$ ↑ by 0.5–1 mm Hg for 1 mEq/L ↑$[HCO_3^-]$ |
| Respiratory acidosis | | | |
| Acute (<24 hours) | ↑ $pCO_2$ | ↑ $[HCO_3^-]$ | $[HCO_3^-]$ ↑ by 1 mEq/L for 10 mm Hg ↑$pCO_2$ |
| Chronic (3–5 days) | ↑ $pCO_2$ | ↑↑ $[HCO_3^-]$ | $[HCO_3^-]$ ↑ by 4 mEq/L for 10 mm Hg ↑$pCO_2$ |
| Respiratory alkalosis | | | |
| Acute (<24 hours) | ↓ $pCO_2$ | ↓ $[HCO_3^-]$ | $[HCO_3^-]$ ↓ by 1–3 mEq/L for 10 mm Hg ↓$pCO_2$ |
| Chronic (3–5 days) | ↓ $pCO_2$ | ↓↓ $[HCO_3^-]$ | $[HCO_3^-]$ ↓ by 2–5 mEq/L for 10 mm Hg ↓$pCO_2$ |

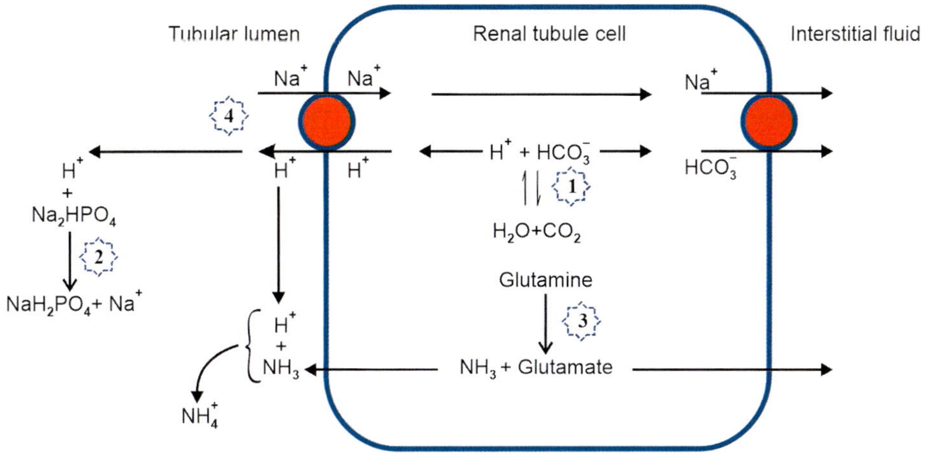


Fig. 6.12: Renal regulation of acid–base disorders. 1 = bicarbonate-carbonic acid buffer; 2 = monohydrogen phosphate-dihydrogen phosphate buffer; 3 = ammonia-ammonium buffer; 4 = sodium hydrogen exchanger



cell and combines with water, in presence of carbonic anhydrase, to regenerate $HCO_3^-$ that is reabsorbed into the bloodstream, thus conserving the filtered $HCO_3^-$.

*Monohydrogen phosphate-dihydrogen phosphate buffer:* This luminal buffer system buffers $H^+$ ions secreted from the tubular cells, as follows:

$$H^+ + Na_2HPO_4 \rightleftharpoons NaH_2PO_4 + Na^+$$

The weakly acidic sodium dihydrogen phosphate is excreted in the urine.

*Ammonia-ammonium buffer:* In tubular cells, glutamine is converted to glutamic acid and ammonia, the reaction catalyzed by glutaminase. Ammonia is secreted in the lumen and combines with $H^+$ to form ammonium ions, which are excreted in urine.

*Sodium-hydrogen exchange in the distal tubule:* Since the distal tubular cells actively reabsorb $Na^+$, to maintain electroneutrality, $H^+$ ions are exchanged. The latter combine with either monohydrogen phosphate or ammonia and are excreted.

### Anion Gap

To achieve electrochemical balance, the number of negatively charged ions (anions) should equal the positively charged ions (cations). Measured plasma anions are chloride and bicarbonate, and the unmeasured anions include phosphates, sulfates and proteins (e.g. albumin). Under typical conditions, unmeasured anions exceed unmeasured cations; this is referred to as the anion gap and can be represented by the following formula:

$$\text{Anion gap} = (Na^+) - (Cl^- + HCO_3^-)$$

The anion gap is normally 8 to 12 mEq/L. When a strong acid is added to or produced in the body, hydrogen ions are neutralized by bicarbonate, resulting in a fall in bicarbonate. These include inorganic (e.g. phosphate or sulfate), organic (e.g. ketoacids or lactate), or exogenous (e.g. salicylate) acids that are incompletely neutralized by bicarbonate. The accompanying unmeasured anion results in increased anion gap proportional to the fall in bicarbonate. In contrast, when the bicarbonate is lost from the body, no new anion is generated; therefore, there is a reciprocal increase in chloride ions (proportional to the fall in bicarbonate) resulting in normal anion gap. Hypoalbuminemia is the most common cause of a low anion gap. Albumin represents about half of the total unmeasured anion pool; for every decrease of 1 g/dL of plasma albumin, the plasma anion gap decreases by 2.5 mEq/L.

### Metabolic Acidosis

Metabolic acidosis is an acid–base disorder characterized by a decrease in serum pH that results from either a loss in plasma bicarbonate concentration or an increase in hydrogen ion concentration (Table 6.12). Primary metabolic

**Table 6.12:** Causes of metabolic acidosis

**Normal anion gap (hyperchloremic acidosis)**

*Renal loss of bicarbonate (urine anion gap positive)*

- Proximal (type 2) renal tubular acidosis, carbonic anhydrase inhibitors (e.g. acetazolamide), tubular damage due to drugs or toxins
- Chronic kidney disease stage 3–4

*Gastrointestinal bicarbonate loss (urine anion gap negative)*

- Diarrhea, ureteral sigmoidostomy, rectourethral fistula, fistula or drainage of small bowel or pancreas

*Decreased renal hydrogen ion excretion (urine anion gap positive)*

- Renal tubular acidosis type 1 and type 4 (aldosterone deficiency) potassium sparing diuretics

*Increased hydrogen chloride production*

- Parenteral alimentation, increased catabolism of lysine and arginine
- Ammonium chloride ingestion

**High anion gap (normochloremic acidosis)**

*Increased acid production/accumulation:* Sepsis, shock, poisonings (ethanol, methanol, ethylene glycol); inborn errors of metabolism

*Ketoacidosis:* Diabetic ketoacidosis, starvation

*Exogenous acids:* Salicylates, iron, isoniazid, paraldehyde

*Failure of acid excretion:* Acute or chronic kidney disease (eGFR <15 mL/min/1.73 m²)

acidosis is characterized by an arterial pH of less than 7.35 due to a decrease in plasma $HCO_3^-$ (<24 mEq/L; <20–22 mEq/L in neonates) in the absence of an elevated $PaCO_2$. Expected respiratory compensation for metabolic acidosis is then calculated as:

$$\text{Compensated } pCO_2 = (1.5 \times \text{serum } HCO_3^- + 8) \pm 2$$

If the measured $PaCO_2$ is higher than the expected $PaCO_2$, a concomitant respiratory acidosis is also present (caused by a depressed mental state, airway obstruction or fatigue). Acutely, medullary chemoreceptors compensate for metabolic acidosis through increase in alveolar ventilation, which results in tachypnea and hyperpnea that washes off $CO_2$ and corrects pH.

Calculation of plasma anion gap helps to classify metabolic acidosis into those with elevated anion gap (i.e. >12 mEq/L as in increased acid production or decreased losses) and those with normal anion gap (i.e. 8–12 mEq/L as in gastrointestinal or renal loss of bicarbonate or when hydrogen ions cannot be secreted because of AKI/CKD) (Table 6.12).

Another useful tool in the evaluation of metabolic acidosis with normal anion gap is the urinary anion gap.

$$\text{Urinary anion gap} = \text{urinary } [Na^+] + [K^+] - [Cl^-]$$

The urinary anion gap is negative in patients with diarrhea regardless of urinary pH, and is positive in renal tubular acidosis. The urinary anion gap is an indirect estimation of renal ammonium ($NH_4^+$) excretion. Appropriate response to systemic metabolic acidosis is an increase in urinary $NH_4^+$ and $Cl^-$ excretion. The increase in urinary chloride results in negative urine anion gap, if metabolic acidosis is secondary to extrarenal loss of $HCO_3^-$. A positive urinary anion gap in the presence of systemic acidosis implies impaired $NH_4^+$ excretion and a renal etiology. An elevated osmolal gap (>20 mOsm/kg) with metabolic acidosis suggests the presence of osmotically active agents such as methanol, ethylene glycol or ethanol.

### *Clinical Features*

Initially, patients with a metabolic acidosis develop a compensatory tachypnea and hyperpnea, which may progress if the acidemia is severe, and the child can present with significant work of breathing and distress (Kussmaul breathing). An increase in $H^+$ concentration results in pulmonary vasoconstriction, which raises pulmonary artery pressure and pulmonary vascular resistance. Tachycardia is the most common cardiovascular effect seen with mild metabolic acidosis. Cerebral vasodilation occurs as a result of metabolic acidosis and may contribute to an increase in intracranial pressure. Acidosis shifts the oxygen-hemoglobin dissociation curve to the right, decreasing hemoglobin's affinity for oxygen. During metabolic acidosis, excess hydrogen ions move toward the intracellular compartment and $K^+$ moves out of the cell into the extracellular space. Untreated severe metabolic acidosis may be associated with life-threatening arrhythmias, myocardial depression, respiratory muscle fatigue, seizures, shock and multiorgan failure. Chronic metabolic acidosis leads to demineralization of bones and growth retardation.

### *Treatment*

It is important to identify the cause of metabolic acidosis as most cases resolve with correction of the underlying disorder. The role of alkali therapy in acute metabolic acidosis is limited. It is definitely indicated in some situations, e.g. salicylate poisoning, inborn errors of metabolism, or in those with pH below or equal to 7.0 or $HCO_3^-$ less than 5 mEq/L, as severe acidosis can produce myocardial dysfunction. The amount of sodium bicarbonate (7.5%, 0.9 mEq/mL) required is = body weight (kg) base deficit × 0.3; usually diluted 1:1 and infused over 2–4 hours.

The recommendation is to replace only half of the total bicarbonate deficit during the first few hours of therapy. Rapid correction of acidosis with sodium bicarbonate can lead to extracellular volume expansion, exacerbating pulmonary edema in patients with cardiac failure. In the latter, the rate of infusion should be slower. If hypernatremia is a concern, sodium bicarbonate may be used as part of the maintenance intravenous solution. In newborns, frequent administration of hypertonic solutions such as sodium bicarbonate has led to intracranial hemorrhage resulting from hyperosmolality and resultant fluid shifts from the intracellular space.

During correction of acute metabolic acidosis, the effect of sodium bicarbonate in lowering serum $K^+$ and ionized calcium concentrations must also be considered and monitored. Since bicarbonate therapy generates large amount of $CO_2$, ventilation should increase proportionately otherwise this might worsen intracellular acidosis. The inability to compensate may be especially important in patients with diabetic ketoacidosis who are at risk for cerebral edema. In diabetic ketoacidosis, insulin therapy generally corrects the acidosis. Improving tissue perfusion should be the main therapeutic measure in patients with lactic acidosis (due to hypoperfusion) and sodium bicarbonate is not indicated. Children with inherited metabolic abnormalities, poisoning, or AKI/CKD may require hemodialysis. Mild to moderate acidosis in AKI or renal tubular acidosis improves on oral alkali therapy, the dose being 0.5 to 2 mEq/kg per day of bicarbonate in 3–4 divided doses. In cases of acidosis due to volume depletion, the volume deficit should be corrected.

## Metabolic Alkalosis

Metabolic alkalosis (pH >7.45, $HCO_3^-$ >26 mEq/L) is an acid–base disturbance caused by elevation in the plasma bicarbonate ($HCO_3^-$) concentration in the extracellular fluid that results from a net loss of acid, net gain of base or loss of fluid with more chloride than bicarbonate. The expected respiratory compensation for metabolic alkalosis is calculated by:

$$\text{Compensated } pCO_2 = 0.7 \times (\text{serum } HCO_3^- - 22)$$
$$\textit{or } \text{serum } HCO_3^- + 15$$

Consider mixed respiratory and metabolic disorder, if compensation is less than expected.

Common etiologies of metabolic alkalosis are listed in Table 6.13. When $H^+$ and $Cl^-$ are lost from any extrarenal site, the kidney avidly retains $Cl^-$ and $HCO_3^-$ forms the primary

**Table 6.13:** Causes of metabolic alkalosis

| **Chloride responsive** |
|---|
| • Gastric fluid loss (e.g. vomiting, nasogastric drainage)<br>• Volume contraction (e.g. loop or thiazide diuretics, metolazone)<br>• Congenital chloride diarrhea, villous adenoma<br>• Cystic fibrosis |
| **Chloride unresponsive** |
| *Normal blood pressure:* Bartter and Gitelman syndromes |
| *Elevated blood pressure*<br>• Primary aldosteronism (adenoma, hyperplasia)<br>• Renovascular hypertension, renin-secreting tumor<br>• Apparent mineralocorticoid excess<br>• Liddle syndrome<br>• Glucocorticoid remediable aldosteronism<br>• Congenital adrenal hyperplasia (11β- and 17α-hydroxylase deficiency)<br>• Adrenal adenoma, carcinoma<br>• Exogenous steroids |
| **Exogenous alkali load** |
| • Excess bicarbonate ingestion<br>• Milk alkali syndrome<br>• Blood transfusion (large volume citrate anticoagulants) |

anion in distal tubules ($HCO_3^-$ reabsorbed with simultaneous $H^+$ secretion). Volume depletion activates the renin-angiotensin-aldosterone axis, resulting in hypokalemia. This state of ECF volume depletion, hypochloremic metabolic alkalosis and hypokalemia is termed contraction alkalosis. Hypokalemia maintains metabolic alkalosis by increasing renal ammoniagenesis and renal $H^+$ secretion. Since alkalosis is driven by hypochloremia, it is responsive to administration (intravenous or oral). Usually urine $Cl^-$ levels are <10 mEq/L.

Retention of $HCO_3^-$ to accompany the major cation $Na^+$ can result in another scenario termed as chloride-unresponsive/resistant metabolic alkalosis, characterized by urine $Cl^-$ >20 mEq/L. This results from altered mineralocorticoid activity resulting in increased distal $Na^+$ reabsorption, increased $K^+$ secretion and increased intravascular volume. The resulting alkalosis is driven and compounded by hypokalemia. These patients do not respond to chloride administration.

The body compensates for metabolic alkalosis through buffering of excess bicarbonate and hypoventilation. Intracellular buffering occurs through sodium-hydrogen and potassium-hydrogen ion exchange, with eventual formation of $CO_2$ and water from $HCO_3^-$. Within several hours, elevated levels of $HCO_3^-$ and metabolic alkalosis inhibit the respiratory center, resulting in hypoventilation and increased $pCO_2$ levels. This mechanism produces a rise in $pCO_2$ of as much as 0.7 to 1 mm Hg for each 1 mEq/L increase in $HCO_3^-$.

### *Clinical Features*

Signs and symptoms observed with metabolic alkalosis usually relate to the specific disease process that caused the acid–base disorder. Though mild metabolic alkalosis is asymptomatic, severe alkalosis leads to reduced ionized calcium leading to increased neuromuscular excitability, paresthesias, muscle cramps, tetany, seizures, confusion, stupor and cardiac arrhythmias. Accompanying signs of dehydration may result from volume contraction. Difficulty in weaning from mechanical ventilation can be observed, as alkalosis shifts the oxygen hemoglobin dissociation curve to the left. Weight gain and hypertension may accompany metabolic alkalosis that results from hyperaldosteronism.

### *Treatment*

The overall prognosis in patients is good with prompt treatment and depends on the underlying etiology. Mild or moderate metabolic alkalosis or alkalemia rarely requires correction. Chloride responsive alkalosis is managed with normal saline with added potassium chloride. The initial target pH and bicarbonate level in correcting severe alkalemia are approximately 7.55 and 40 mEq/L, respectively.

Therapy with diuretics (e.g. furosemide, thiazides) should be discontinued. Chloride-resistant metabolic alkalosis may be more difficult to control. As with correction of any electrolyte or acid–base imbalance, the goal is to prevent life-threatening complications with the least amount of correction.

For persistent severe metabolic alkalosis in the setting of fluid overload, wherein saline cannot be given, cautious use of HCl or ammonium chloride may be considered. Acetazolamide may help patients with chloride-resistant metabolic alkalosis provided GFR is adequate. Correction of metabolic alkalosis in patients with AKI/ CKD may require hemodialysis or continuous renal replacement therapy with a dialysate that contains high levels of chloride and low $HCO_3^-$.

## Respiratory Acidosis

Respiratory acidosis occurs when the alveolar ventilation falls or when carbon dioxide production is increased, so that the arterial partial pressure of carbon dioxide ($PaCO_2$) is elevated above the normal range (>45 mm Hg) leading to a blood pH <7.35 (Table 6.14). $pCO_2$ is directly proportional to carbon dioxide production and inversely proportional to alveolar ventilation. The kidneys compensate for respiratory acidosis by increasing $HCO_3^-$ reabsorption, a process that begins in 6–12 hours but takes 3–5 days for maximal compensation.

**Table 6.14:** Causes of respiratory acidosis

| **Decrease in alveolar ventilation** |
|---|
| • Depressed central respiratory drive<br>• Acute paralysis of the respiratory muscles<br>• Acute or chronic parenchymal lung and airway diseases<br>• Progressive neuromuscular disease<br>• Worsening scoliosis (restrictive lung disease) |
| **High carbon dioxide production and inability to increase minute ventilation** |
| • Extensive burn injury<br>• Malignant hyperthermia<br>• Fever |

Fluid and Electrolyte Disturbances 6

The kidneys increase excretion of hydrogen ions (predominantly in the form of ammonium) that increases the plasma bicarbonate concentration by approximately 3.5–4 mEq/L for every 10 mm Hg increase in $CO_2$.

### Clinical Features

Patients with acute respiratory acidosis frequently demonstrate air-hunger with retractions and use of accessory muscles. Neurologic findings include anxiety, disorientation, confusion and lethargy followed by tremors, somnolence or coma at higher $pCO_2$. Hypercapnic neurologic changes are reversible with no residual effect. Cardiovascular findings include tachycardia, bounding arterial pulses and in severe cases hypotension.

### Treatment

The goal of therapy is to correct or compensate for the underlying pathologic process. Failure to consider a mixed acidosis can lead to missed therapies and diagnosis. Assisted ventilation is required in many cases.

## Respiratory Alkalosis

Respiratory alkalosis occurs in the setting of a primary decrease in $pCO_2$ as a consequence of hyperventilation (Table 6.15). In a child, this may result from high fever, sepsis, mild bronchial asthma, central nervous system disorders or overventilation of an intubated child in intensive care setting. In acute respiratory alkalosis, titration is done by intracellular buffers. Renal compensation begins within several hours and takes several days for the maximal response.

**Table 6.15:** Causes of respiratory alkalosis

| |
|---|
| **Hypoxia and hypoxemia** |
| High altitude or low fraction of inspired oxygen, anemia, hypotension, or lung disease |
| **Pulmonary disorders** |
| Pulmonary edema, embolism, airway obstruction, pneumonia, interstitial lung disease |
| Mechanical ventilation (ventilatory rate or tidal volume too high) |
| **Extrapulmonary disorders** |
| Stress, neurologic disease (stroke, infection, trauma, tumour) |
| *Medications:* Catecholamines, progesterone, methylxanthines, salicylates, doxapram, nicotine |
| Hyperthermia, hepatic encephalopathy, sepsis, recovery from metabolic acidosis |

### Clinical Features

Patients primarily have clinical manifestations of the underlying disorder. Alkalosis, by promoting the binding of calcium to albumin, can reduce the fraction of ionized calcium in blood which may manifest as feeling of tingling, paresthesias, dizziness, palpitations, tetany and seizures. Therapy is directed towards the causal process.

## Suggested Reading


1. Do C, Vasquez PC, Soleimani M. Metabolic alkalosis: Core curriculum 2022. Am J Kidney Dis 2022. doi: 10.1053/j.ajkd.2021.12.016.
2. Emmett M. Metabolic alkalosis. Clin J Am Soc Nephrol 2020; 15(12):1848–56.
3. Fenves AZ, Emmett M. Approach to patients with high anion gap metabolic acidosis: Core curriculum 2021. Am J Kidney Dis 2021;78(4):590–600.
4. Jung B, Martinez M, Claessens YE, et al. Diagnosis and management of metabolic acidosis: Guidelines from a French expert panel. Ann Intensive Care 2019; 9: 92.

Chapter 7

# Nutrition

Rakesh Lodha, Anuja Agarwala

## Introduction

Children need adequate nutrition to grow and develop to their full potential. The 1,000-day period from pregnancy until a child's second birthday is the most critical period for good nutrition.

The importance of breastfeeding in the first 2 years of life in saving lives, protecting children from diseases and boosting development of brain is well known. Beyond 6 months, children need to begin eating their first foods. The meals have to be frequent and of adequate quantity throughout the day; the meals should also be nutrient-dense. The child has to be fed a variety of foods. Food hygiene needs adequate attention.

Undernutrition is an important contributor to under-5 mortality. Despite the knowledge about the importance of nutrition in growth and development of a child, there are significant gaps. While undernutrition is a major challenge, the country also faces another one in form of overnutrition-overweight and obesity.

Given the burden of problem, the healthcare professionals should use every opportunity—every contact with a child and family to assess nutritional status, dietary intake and offer appropriate counseling. For sick children, specific measures are required, as will be for children with moderate and severe malnutrition.

*Competency:* **PE9.1**

## FOOD

Our food is made up of essential, natural substances called nutrients. Human body needs over 50 nutrients on a daily basis to stay healthy. Nutrients are categorized as macronutrients including carbohydrates, proteins, fat; and micronutrients such as vitamins, minerals and trace elements.

***Macronutrients*** are needed in large quantities and are the energy yielding components of diet, i.e., they breakdown into simpler compounds to provide energy (Table 7.1).

***Micronutrients*** are needed in small quantities, but are very essential to keep us healthy. They do not yield energy but have a protective role and are needed to enhance immunity. Micronutrients are discussed in detail in Chapter 8.

All nutrients work together to maintain overall health. Each of these nutrients is required in a specific amount by the body. The deficiency and excess of nutrients can be harmful, leading to a variety of complex diseases.

## Carbohydrates

Carbohydrates are the main source of energy in the Indian diet. Carbohydrates contribute to taste, texture and bulk to the diet. They are essential for digestion and assimilation of other foods. Lack of carbohydrates (less than 30%) in the diet may produce ketosis, loss of weight, and breakdown of proteins.

Carbohydrates are divided into simple carbohydrates (monosaccharides and disaccharides such as glucose and fructose found in fruits, vegetables and honey, sucrose in sugar, and lactose in milk) and complex carbohydrates (oligosaccharides and polysaccharides such as starch in cereals, millets, pulses and root vegetables).

The main source of energy in the body is glucose derived from starch and sugars present in the diet. Glucose is used as a fuel by the cells and is converted to glycogen by liver and muscles. Excess carbohydrates are converted to fat.

**Table 7.1:** Energy content of macronutrients

| *Nutrient* | *Energy (kcal) per gram* |
|---|---|
| Carbohydrate | 4 kcal |
| Protein | 4 kcal |
| Fat | 9 kcal |
| Dietary fiber | 2 kcal |
| Water | 0 kcal |

*Requirements:* As much as 55–60% of total energy intake should come from carbohydrates.

### Fiber

Fiber determines the quality of carbohydrates. Dietary fibers are also called "non-digestible or unavailable carbohydrates" as they are not digested by the enzymes in the gut. They are essential for the normal functioning of gut, elimination of waste, bile acid binding capacity and for maintaining the growth of normal intestinal microflora.

Polysaccharides such as cellulose, hemicelluloses, pectin, gums, mucilage and lignin are some examples of fiber, mainly provided by cereals, millets, vegetables and fruits.

Soluble fiber undergoing fermentation in the colon provides 2 kcal/g.

*Requirements:* Fiber intake is based on energy intake and 40 g/2000 kcal is recommended as safe level.

### Proteins

Protein is the second most abundant substance in the body after water. They are required for the growth and synthesis of tissues in the body; formation of digestive juices, hormones, plasma proteins, enzymes, vitamins, hemoglobin; as buffers to maintain acid–base equilibrium in the body; and as an alternate source of energy for the body.

Proteins are made of amino acids. Amino acids that can be synthesized in the body are called non-essential amino acids, while essential amino acids require to be supplied in the diet. Essential amino acids include leucine, isoleucine, lysine, methionine, phenylalanine, threonine, tryptophan and valine. Importantly, histidine and arginine are essential during infancy because the rate of their synthesis is inadequate for sustaining growth.

*Protein quality:* Food proteins differ in their nutritional quality depending on their amino acid profile and digestibility. Egg protein has the highest nutritive value and is, therefore, taken as the reference protein, and the value of others is expressed as relative to the biological value of egg protein (taken as 100%). Generally, animal proteins have a higher biological value than the plant proteins.

The nutritive value of a mixture of two proteins may be higher than the mean of the two because of mutual complementary effects. Cereal grains (wheat, rice) are deficient in lysine, threonine or tryptophan, whereas pulses are rich in lysine but are limited in sulfur-containing amino acids, mainly methionine. When cereals are taken in combination with the pulses, the deficiency in one is made good by an excess in other; thereby optimizing the overall quality of proteins in food.

*Requirements:* Nearly 10–12% of the total energy should be provided from protein sources. An intake of 8% proteins may be sufficient for food having a higher content of animal proteins or high value proteins in the diet.

### Fats

Fats are a major source of energy in diet. Fats function as structural elements of the cell membranes, act as vehicle for absorption and transport of fat-soluble vitamins (A, D, E and K) and are precursors of prostaglandins and hormones.

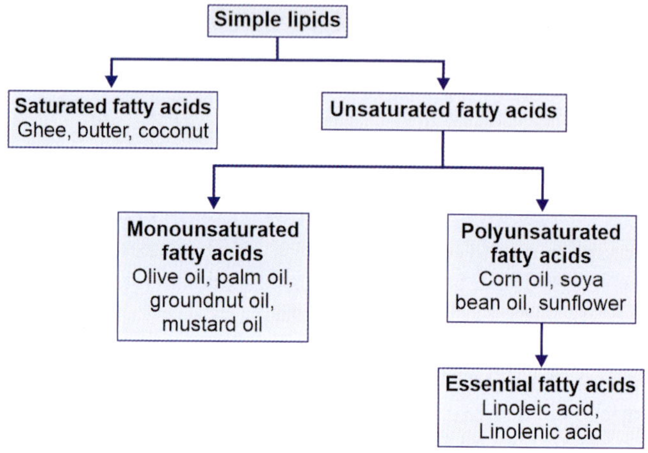


**Fig. 7.1:** Classification of fats

Fats are made of fatty acids. Dietary fats are mixture of largely triglycerides, phospholipids and cholesterol.

*Fatty acids are classified into 3 groups:* Saturated fatty acids (SFAs), monounsaturated fatty acids (MUFAs) and polyunsaturated fatty acids (PUFAs) (Fig. 7.1). Humans can synthesize SFAs and MUFAs besides obtaining them from diet, but PUFAs cannot be synthesized in the body and have to be provided through diet.

*Saturated fatty acids (SFA)* consisting of straight, even numbered chains of 4–24 carbon atoms. They are classified as short (C<10), medium (C12:0 and C12:0) or long (C16:0–C24:0) chain fatty acids based on carbon chain length. The degree of saturation determines whether the fat is solid or liquid at room temperature— more the saturation, harder and more solid is the fat.

*Unsaturated fatty acids (MUFAs and PUFAs)* have double bonds in *cis* or *trans* configuration. Double bonds in *cis* configuration are nutritionally good, while in *trans* configuration (*trans* fatty acids) are bad for health. Thus, *trans* fats are a type of unsaturated fats. These occur naturally in small quantity. Artificial *trans* fats are created when hydrogen is passed through liquid vegetable oils to make them more solid ('vanaspati'). Such fats are used in household cooking as well as in snack foods (packaged baked food, samosas, mathris, kachoris, pizzas, burgers, French fries, etc.). *Trans* fats increase the risk of coronary artery disease due, in part, by increasing levels of low density lipoproteins (LDL) and lowering high density lipoprotein (HDL). Hence, *trans* fat intake is best avoided.

*Polyunsaturated fatty acids (PUFAs)* are grouped into two series, namely, linoleic acid (LA) and alpha-linolenic acid (ALA) depending on the position of double bond. LA and ALA are long chain dietary essential fatty acids. LA gets metabolized to arachidonic acid (AA), while ALA to eicosapentaenoic acid (EPA), docosapentaenoic acid (DPA) and docosahexaenoic acid (DHA).

Medium chain triglycerides (MCT) are an immediate source of energy as they are transported directly from the small intestine to liver by portal vein and metabolized immediately to produce energy. MCT improves endurance performance, promote fat metabolism, spare muscle glycogen, increase metabolic rate, maintain muscle mass and lower blood cholesterol level. Supplementation with MCT is used in the dietary management of cystic fibrosis, obesity, pancreatic insufficiency, and fat malabsorption. Sources of MCTs are coconut oil, palm kernel oil, butter (15% of MCT). Prolonged use of MCTs in excess leads to essential fatty acid (EFA) deficiency.

Long chain triglycerides (LCT) provide essential fatty acids (EFAs) and require carnitine to produce energy. MCT and LCT should be ideally used in combination to prevent EFA deficiency.

Essential fatty acids (EFAs) cannot be synthesized in the body and have to be supplied through dietary fat. EPA and DHA are important components of gray matter of the brain. Deficiency of EFA leads to cessation of growth, alopecia, diarrhea, impaired wound healing, decreased calcium absorption, decreased calcium deposits in bones and decreased bone strength. It is recommended that ALA content of the diet should be about 0.5% of the total calories or 1.0–1.5 g/day.

Cholesterol is a component of cell membrane, and enables the body produce steroid hormones and bile acids.

*Invisible fat:* Fat presents naturally in our food but cannot be seen and separated from food. Milk and milk products, egg and meat, nuts contain good amount of invisible fat. Cereals, pulses, vegetables and fruits contain negligible amount.

*Visible fat:* Fat which is used for cooking or added while cooking such as edible vegetable oils and ghee.

*Requirements:* In normal children, about 25–30% of energy intake should be derived from fat which includes 10–15% invisible fat. In malnourished children, up to 45% of energy can be safely provided from fat.

To provide a healthy balance of visible fat, daily diet should provide <7% saturated fat, 10% polyunsaturated fat, and rest 13% should be derived from monounsaturated fats. A minimum of 3% energy should be derived from linoleic acid and 0.3% from linolenic acid.

There is no single edible oil/fat with the ideal composition. It is, therefore, recommended to use a blend of two or more vegetable oils/fat source.

### Energy

Energy requirements vary through childhood because of variations in growth rate, metabolic rate and physical activity. Although after infancy, the growth rate slows in toddlers, their activity levels are high. During adolescence, energy needs increase due to rapid growth and development.

There are three critical periods in early life of a child with regards to energy requirements: First, at 6 months when complementary feeding is to be initiated. Second, between 1 and 2 years when physical activity increases. Third, between 10 and 12 years for girls and 15–18 years for boys when pubertal growth spurt triggers increased nutrition requirement.

Calculation of energy requirement should account for the level of physical activity and the growth. For children with normal body weights, the energy requirements are calculated roughly as shown in Table 7.2.

**Table 7.2:** Simple calculation of daily energy requirements for children

| *Weight (Kg)* | *Energy requirement (kcal)* |
|---|---|
| At 10 kg body weight | 1000 kcal |
| Weight >10–20 kg | 1000 kcal + 50 kcal for each kg above 10 kg, e.g. for a 15 kg child, requirement will be 1250 kcal |
| Weight >20 kg | 1500 kcal +20 kcal for each kg above 10 kg, e.g. for a 30 kg child, requirement will be approximately 1700 kcal |

*Competencies:* **PE9.2; PE9.3; PE9.4; PE9.5; PE12.1; PE12.6; PE12.11; PE12.13; PE12.15; PE12.19; PE13.1; PE13.7; PE13.11, PE13.13**

## DIETARY STANDARDS

Infants and children have relatively higher requirements of nutrients than adults. While adults need nutrients for maintaining constant body weight and functions, infants and children require nutrients not only for maintenance, but also for promoting and supporting their growth and development.

The 2020 report of the ICMR—National Institute of Nutrition has brought in the concept of Estimated Average Requirements (EAR) for evaluating population level nutrient intake. Recommended Dietary Allowance (RDA) is to be considered for planning the diet of an individual child.

The EAR is the median daily intake value that is estimated to meet the requirement of half the healthy individuals in a life-stage and gender group. At this level of intake, the other half of the individuals in the specified group would not have their needs met. It is used to assess the nutrient intake of groups/populations.

The RDA is the average daily dietary intake level that is sufficient to meet the nutrient requirement of nearly all (97 to 98%) healthy individuals in a particular life-stage and gender group. The RDA is the goal for usual intake by an individual. The 2020 report provides RDA values for all macronutrients as well as micronutrients. However, RDA values for energy intake are not provided. Since RDA pertains to individuals, we will mainly be referring to RDA in this chapter.

### Recommended Dietary Allowances

RDA are nutrient specific, and technical in nature. These are formulated based on the current knowledge of nutritional requirements of different age and sex groups depending on anthropometry (weight, height), body composition, climate and environment, physical activity, physiological status, and body demands. These factors lead to variations in the required food intake and nutrient requirements.

Summary of RDA for protein and other nutrients revised in 2020, is shown in Table 7.3.

Table 7.4 shows the energy requirements for Indian infants. Table 7.5 shows the energy requirements of Indian children and adolescents assuming a moderate level of activity for boys and girls.

Table 7.6 portrays energy, protein, carbohydrates and fat composition of common Indian food items and portions.

**Table 7.3:** Summary of daily RDA for Indian children and adolescents 2020

| *Age group* | *Wt (kg)* | *Prot (g)*[a] | *CHO (g)*[b] | *Visible fat (g)*[c] | *Ca (mg)* | *Mg (mg)* | *Fe (mg)* | *Zn (mg)* | *I (µg)* | *Vit $B_1$ (mg)* | *Vit $B_2$ (mg)* | *Vit $B_3$ (mg)* | *Vit $B_6$ (mg)* | *Folate (µg)* | *Vit $B_{12}$ (µg)* | *Vit C (mg)* | *Vit A (µg)* | *Vit D (IU)* |
|---|---|---|---|---|---|---|---|---|---|---|---|---|---|---|---|---|---|---|
| **Infants** | | | | | | | | | | | | | | | | | | |
| 0–6 months | 5.8 | 8.1 | 55 | – | 300 | 30 | – | – | 100 | 0.2 | 0.4 | 2.0 | 0.1 | 25 | 1.2 | 20 | 350 | 400 |
| 6–12 months | 8.5 | 10.5 | 95 | 25 | 300 | 30 | 3.0 | 2.5 | 130 | 0.4 | 0.6 | 5.0 | 0.6 | 85 | 1.2 | 27 | 350 | 400 |
| **Children** | | | | | | | | | | | | | | | | | | |
| 1–3 yr | 11.7 | 11.3 | Min | 25 | 500 | 135 | 8.0 | 3.0 | 90 | 0.7 | 0.9 | 7.0 | 0.9 | 110 | 1.2 | 27 | 390 | |
| 4–6 yr | 18.3 | 15.9 | 130 | 25 | 550 | 155 | 11.0 | 4.5 | 120 | 0.9 | 1.3 | 9.0 | 1.2 | 135 | 1.2 | 32 | 510 | 600 |
| 7–9 yr | 25.3 | 23.3 | | 30 | 650 | 215 | 15.0 | 5.9 | 120 | 1.1 | 1.6 | 11.0 | 1.5 | 170 | 2.5 | 43 | 630 | |
| **Adolescents** | | | | | | | | | | | | | | | | | | |
| *Boys* | | | | | | | | | | | | | | | | | | |
| 10–12 yr | 34.9 | 31.8 | | 35 | 850 | 270 | 16.0 | 8.5 | 150 | 1.5 | 2.1 | 15.0 | 2.0 | 220 | 2.5 | 54 | 770 | |
| 13–15 yr | 50.5 | 44.9 | | 45 | 1000 | 355 | 22.0 | 14.3 | 150 | 1.9 | 2.7 | 19.0 | 2.6 | 285 | 2.5 | 72 | 930 | 600 |
| 16–18 yr | 64.4 | 55.4 | | 50 | 1050 | 405 | 26.0 | 17.6 | 150 | 2.2 | 3.1 | 22.0 | 3.0 | 340 | 2.5 | 82 | 1000 | |
| *Girls* | | | | | | | | | | | | | | | | | | |
| 10–12 yr | 36.4 | 32.8 | | 35 | 850 | 255 | 28.0 | 8.5 | 150 | 1.4 | 1.9 | 14.0 | 1.9 | 225 | 2.5 | 52 | 790 | |
| 13–15 yr | 49.6 | 43.2 | | 40 | 1000 | 325 | 30.0 | 12.8 | 150 | 1.6 | 2.2 | 16.0 | 2.2 | 245 | 2.5 | 66 | 890 | 600 |
| 16–18 yr | 55.7 | 46.2 | | 35 | 1050 | 335 | 32.0 | 14.2 | 150 | 1.7 | 2.3 | 17.0 | 2.3 | 270 | 2.5 | 68 | 860 | |

*Source:* ICMR-NIN Nutrient Requirements for Indians—2020 report. CHO carbohydrate; Ca calcium; Mg magnesium; Fe iron; Zn zinc; I iodine

a. Safe level of protein can be calculated up to 10% of the energy for an individual child.

b. Carbohydrate (CHO): Minimum carbohydrate for any individual over 1 year of age is set at 130 g/day based on basal brain glucose utilization. Below this level, energy need is met by breakdown of fat and endogenous protein. Carbohydrate intake varies from 50–60% of the energy requirement of an individual.

c. Visible fat (vegetable oil, ghee, butter) is used for cooking. Nearly 10–15% of energy is contributed by visible fat. Remaining 10–15% of the fat energy is contributed by invisible fat which is present in almost all food items.

**Table 7.4:** Daily energy requirement of normal infants during first year of life

| Age (months) | Boys | | | Girls | | |
|---|---|---|---|---|---|---|
| | *Weight (kg)* | *Daily energy requirement* | | *Weight (kg)* | *Daily energy requirement* | |
| | | *kcal/ d* | *kcal/kg/d* | | *kcal/d* | *kcal/kg/d* |
| 0–1 | 3.90 | 490 | 125 | 3.70 | 440 | 120 |
| 1–2 | 5.05 | 580 | 115 | 4.65 | 510 | 110 |
| 2–3 | 6.00 | 620 | 105 | 5.45 | 550 | 100 |
| 3–4 | 6.70 | 560 | 85 | 6.10 | 520 | 85 |
| 4–5 | 7.25 | 590 | 80 | 6.65 | 560 | 85 |
| 5–6 | 7.70 | 620 | 80 | 7.10 | 590 | 80 |
| 6–7 | 8.10 | 640 | 80 | 7.45 | 580 | 80 |
| 7–8 | 8.45 | 670 | 80 | 7.75 | 610 | 80 |
| 8–9 | 8.75 | 690 | 80 | 8.05 | 630 | 80 |
| 9–10 | 9.05 | 730 | 80 | 8.35 | 670 | 80 |
| 10–11 | 9.30 | 750 | 80 | 8.60 | 680 | 80 |
| 11–12 | 9.50 | 760 | 80 | 8.80 | 700 | 80 |

*Source:* ICMR-NIN Nutrient Requirements for Indians—2020 report.

*Note:* Total daily energy requirement (kcal/d) = total energy expenditure (TEE) on weight + allowance for energy deposition in tissues during growth.

**Table 7.5:** Energy requirement of normal moderately active Indian children and adolescents

| Age (yr) | Boys | | | Girls | | |
|---|---|---|---|---|---|---|
| | *Weight (kg)* | *Total energy requirement* | | *Weight (kg)* | *Total energy requirement* | |
| | | *kcal/d* | *kcal/kg/d* | | *kcal/d* | *kcal/kg/d* |
| 1–2 | 9.9 | 857 | 85 | 8.9 | 761 | 85 |
| 2–3 | 12.2 | 1056 | 87 | 11.5 | 969 | 84 |
| 3–4 | 14.3 | 1173 | 82 | 13.9 | 1097 | 79 |
| 4–5 | 16.3 | 1283 | 79 | 16.1 | 1209 | 75 |
| 5–6 | 18.5 | 1403 | 76 | 18.3 | 1318 | 72 |
| 6–7 | 20.5 | 1508 | 74 | 20.2 | 1408 | 70 |
| 7–8 | 22.9 | 1635 | 71 | 22.4 | 1510 | 67 |
| 8–9 | 25.4 | 1762 | 69 | 25.0 | 1626 | 65 |
| 9–10 | 28.1 | 1896 | 67 | 28.2 | 1761 | 62 |
| 10–11 | 31.2 | 2046 | 66 | 31.9 | 1905 | 60 |
| 11–12 | 34.6 | 2205 | 64 | 36.2 | 2054 | 57 |
| 12–13 | 38.9 | 2398 | 62 | 41.2 | 2209 | 54 |
| 13–14 | 44.3 | 2627 | 59 | 46.0 | 2333 | 51 |
| 14–15 | 50.6 | 2875 | 57 | 50.1 | 2417 | 48 |
| 15–16 | 56.6 | 3081 | 54 | 52.8 | 2461 | 47 |
| 16–17 | 61.3 | 3228 | 53 | 54.7 | 2486 | 45 |
| 17–18 | 64.8 | 3326 | 51 | 55.7 | 2498 | 45 |
| 18–19 | 67.3 | 3393 | 50 | 56.7 | 2511 | 44 |

*Source:* ICMR-NIN Nutrient Requirements for Indians—2020 report.

*Note:* This table reflects the gender specific energy requirement of healthy and moderately active children and adolescents. Requirement = TEE + energy cost of growth

Assessment of dietary intake as well as diet planning is done using nutritive value of foods.

### Dietary Intake Assessment by 24-hour Recall

There are many dietary assessment tools available but most widely used and recognized as gold standard is the "24-hour recall" method which captures the food eaten during the last 24 hours. However, "24-hour usual diet recall" is more appropriate and practical in most situations as it captures the food which an individual usually eats in 24 hours.

**Table 7.6:** Approximate nutritive value of some common foods

| *Food items* | *Household measures (cooked)* | *Raw edible amount (g or mL)* | *Calories (kcal)* | *Protein (g)* | *Carbohydrate (g)* | *Fat (g)* |
|---|---|---|---|---|---|---|
| **Milk and milk products** | | | | | | |
| Human milk | - | 100 mL | 65.0 | 1.1 | 7.4 | 3.4 |
| Milk (cow) | ½ glass | 100 mL | 73.0 | 3.2 | 4.9 | 4.4 |
| Milk (buffalo) | ½ glass | 100 mL | 107.0 | 3.6 | 8.3 | 6.5 |
| Paneer (homemade; cow milk) | 1 small piece | 30 g | 76.5 | 5.5 | 3.5 | 4.5 |
| Curd (homemade–cow milk) | 1 small cup | 100 mL | 62.0 | 3.2 | 3.2 | 4.0 |
| **Meat and poultry** | | | | | | |
| Chicken, thigh, boneless | 1 serving | 100 g | 200 | 18.0 | – | 14.0 |
| Egg whole (hen) | 1 no. | 45 g | 74.0 | 5.0 | – | 6.0 |
| Egg white (from 1 egg) | - | 25 g | 23.2 | 4.0 | – | 0.8 |
| Egg yolk (from 1 egg) | - | 20 g | 51.6 | 1.2 | – | 5.2 |
| **Cereals and millets** | | | | | | |
| Wheat daliya/ suji/ sevian | 1 katori boiled | 25 g raw | 80.0 | 2.5 | 16.0 | 0.3 |
| Wheat flour with choker | 1 medium roti | 25 g atta | 80.0 | 2.5 | 16.0 | 0.3 |
| Wheat flour refined (maida) | 2 small puris | 25 g | 90.0 | 2.5 | 18.5 | 0.2 |
| Rice | 1 katori cooked | 25 g raw | 90.0 | 2.0 | 19.5 | 0.1 |
| Bread (white) | 1 big slice | 30 g | 73.0 | 2.5 | 15.5 | 0.1 |
| Biscuits | 2 nos | 10 g | 50.0 | 1.0 | 7.0 | 2.0 |
| Cake | 1 small piece | 30 g | 129.0 | 1.8 | 18.0 | 5.5 |
| Sago/arrowroot/corn flour | 5 tsp | 25 g | 88.0 | – | 22.0 | – |
| Millet grains (includes bajra, jowar, jau, oats, kottu) | - | 25 g | 94.0 | 3.0 | 16.0 | 2.0 |
| Khichri - Raw rice 20 g, Raw dal 5 g (4:1) | 1 katori cooked (100 g) | 25 g raw | 85.0 | 3.0 | 18.0 | 0.1 |
| **Pulses** | | | | | | |
| Dhooli dals (moong/arhar, etc.) | 1 katori cooked | | 83.0 | 6.0 | 14.0 | 0.3 |
| Sabut dals (rajma/chana, etc.) | (100–125 g) | 25 g raw | 70.0 | 5.0 | 10.0 | 1.0 |
| Soyabean (white) | | | 95.0 | 10.0 | 2.5 | 5.0 |
| **Vegetables** | | | | | | |
| Green leafy and seasonal vegetables (spinach, bathua, bhindi, cauliflower, beans, etc.) | ½ katori cooked | 100 to 125 g | 24.0 | 2.0 | 2.5 | 0.6 |
| Root vegetables (includes arbi, potato, zimikand, etc.) | 1 small size | 100 g | 60.0 | 1.5 | 13.0 | 0.2 |
| Peas, fresh | 1 katori | 100 g | 80.0 | 7.0 | 13.0 | 0.1 |
| Low carb vegetables (lauki/ tori/ tinda/ kaddu/ cucumber) | ½ katori | 100 g | 11.0 | 0.53 | 1.68 | 0.13 |
| **Dried nuts** | | | | | | |
| Groundnuts | handful | 25 g | 130.0 | 6.0 | 4.0 | 10.0 |
| Almond/walnuts | | | 152.0 | 4.5 | 1.0 | 14.5 |
| Cashewnuts | | | 143.0 | 4.5 | 6.5 | 11.0 |
| **Fats and oils** | | | | | | |
| Refined oil/ghee | 1 tsp | 5 mL/g | 45.0 | – | – | 5.0 |
| Butter | 1 tsp | 5 g | 36.4 | – | – | 4.1 |
| Coconut oil | 1 tsp | 5 mL | 42.0 | – | – | 5.0 |
| **Sugars** | | | | | | |
| Table sugar/cornstarch | 1 levelled tsp | 5 g | 20.0 | – | 5.0 | – |
| Honey/jam | 1 levelled tsp | 5 g | 16.0 | – | 4.0 | – |
| Jaggery | 1 tsp | 5 g | 17.5 | – | 4.4 | – |
| **Drinks** | | | | | | |
| Sugarcane juice | ½ glass | 100 mL | 60.0 | - | 15.0 | - |
| Coconut water | ½ glass | 100 mL | 14.0 | 0.2 | 3.0 | 0.1 |
| Soft drinks | ½ glass | 100 mL | 37.0 | - | 9.2 | - |

*(Contd...)*

Table 7.6: Approximate nutritive value of some common foods (*Contd...*)

| *Food items* | *Household measures (cooked)* | *Raw edible amount (g or mL)* | *Calories (kcal)* | *Protein (g)* | *Carbohydrate (g)* | *Fat (g)* |
|---|---|---|---|---|---|---|
| **Processed dairy products** | | | | | | |
| Full cream milk | ½ glass | 100 mL | 90.0 | 3.5 | 5.0 | 6.2 |
| Toned milk | ½ glass | 100 mL | 58.0 | 3.2 | 4.5 | 3.0 |
| Double toned milk | ½ glass | 100 mL | 48.0 | 3.0 | 5.0 | 2.0 |
| Skimmed milk | ½ glass | 100 mL | 33.0 | 3.0 | 5.0 | - |
| Dahi (plain)/curd | 1 cup | 100 mL | 62.0 | 4.0 | 5.0 | 3.0 |
| Buttermilk (lassi–plain) | ½ glass | 100 mL | 32.0 | 2.0 | 2.0 | 2.0 |
| Sweet lassi | ½ glass | 100 mL | 95.0 | 2.5 | 15.5 | 2.5 |
| Salted lassi | ½ glass | 100 mL | 32.0 | 1.8 | 2.0 | 1.8 |
| Cottage cheese | 1 small piece | 30 g | 93.0 | 5.7 | 0.9 | 7.5 |
| Ice-cream | 1 small cup | 100 g | 180.0 | 4.0 | 23.0 | 8.0 |
| Ice-cream (sugar free) | 1 small cup | 100 g | 122.0 | 5.0 | 18.0 | 5.0 |

*Adapted from:*

1. Indian Food Composition tables, NIN, ICMR, 2017
2. Compilation of Food Exchange list (Technical series 6), Lady Irwin College, University of Delhi, 2017
3. For processed foods, nutritional facts are taken from the packets



A good dietary recall history elicited in terms of cooked foods using various household measures, food photographs and food models, is more accurate in terms of visual estimation of portion size and quantification. In the absence of visual aids, the respondent might refer to the size of the food item as small, medium, big and then, the interviewer quantifies based on his imagination. This may lead to false estimation of food and nutrient intake by the child.

## BALANCED DIET

Balanced diet is defined as nutritionally adequate and appropriate intake of food items that provide all the nutrients in required amounts and in proper proportions. A balanced diet ensures normal growth, development and optimum health. Wide variety and combination of foods are used to formulate balanced diet for various categories of people to meet their needs as per nutritional standards (RDA).

In order to plan nutritionally adequate balanced diet as per RDA, "food group system" is used that converts quantitative nutrient data into food-based information.

Based on major content of nutrients, foods are conventionally placed into 5 groups: (i) Cereals, millets, and cereal grains; (ii) pulses, legumes, and nuts; (iii) milk, egg, and flesh foods; (iv) vegetables and fruits; (v) fats and sugar. Food groups differ in their nutrient quality and quantity and hence while planning a diet, inclusion of one or more food items from each of these groups is essential to label a diet as 'balanced'.

The nutrient characteristics of common foods are depicted in Table 7.7.

Cereals, millets and pulses are the major source of most nutrients in Indian diet. Milk provides good quality protein and calcium and hence is an essential item of our diet. Eggs, flesh foods and fish enhance the quality of diet. Oils and nuts are calorie-rich foods and are useful in increasing the energy density. Vegetables and fruits provide protective substances such as vitamins, minerals, fiber and antioxidants.

**In a normal balanced Indian diet, recommended macronutrients as a proportion of total energy intake should be: Carbohydrates (55–60%), fats (25–30%) and proteins (10–12%).**

***Healthy plate concept:*** "My plate of the day" is an easy-to-understand visual guide representing regular consumption of foods using all food groups (designed by the NIN, ICMR) applicable for individuals without any specific medical condition. The proportion indicated in the plate represents healthy, balanced meal targeting prevention of hidden hunger and protection from diseases (Fig. 7.2).

A balanced diet is not just about eating the right foods, but also ensuring that the food on the plate is varied and in the appropriate proportion.

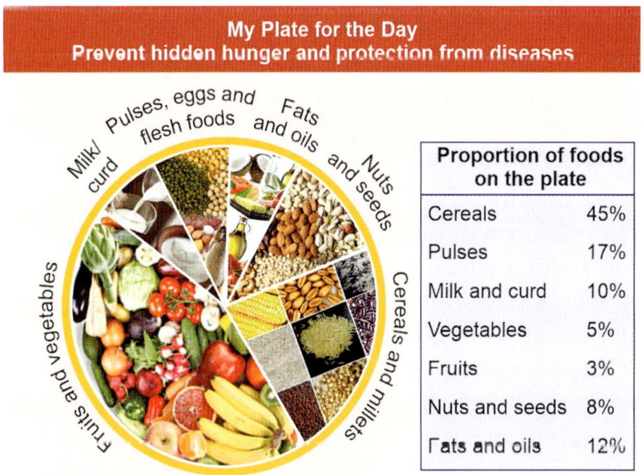


Fig. 7.2: Healthy plate

*Competencies:* **PE7.1; PE8.1; PE8.2; PE8.3; PE8.4; PE8.5; PE9.5**

## NORMAL BALANCED DIET FOR VARIOUS AGE GROUPS

### Exclusive Breastfeeding (0–6 months of age)

An infant should be exclusively breastfed till 6 months of age. During this phase, additional food or fluids are not

**Table 7.7:** Nutritional characteristics of common food items

| *Foods* | *Main nutrients* | *Other characteristics* |
|---|---|---|
| Milk and milk products | Protein, fat, calcium, phosphorus, vitamin $B_2$ | Provide high quality protein lactose and saturated fats; lack in iron and vitamin C |
| Egg (hen) | Protein, fat, phosphorus, riboflavin | Provide high quality protein and vitamin $B_{12}$; lacks in carbohydrates and vitamin C; contains saturated fats and is rich in cholesterol |
| Chicken | Protein, phosphorus | Provides high quality protein and all B vitamins; does not provide carbohydrate, fat and iron |
| Fish | Protein, fat, calcium, vitamin $B_{12}$ | Lacks in carbohydrates; good source of high quality protein and fat containing omega-3 fatty acids |
| Cereals grains and products | Carbohydrate, fiber, folic acid, vitamins $B_1$ and $B_2$, phytates, iron | Good source of energy; has poor quality protein that lacks in lysine; provides negligible amounts of unsaturated fat; phytates hinder the absorption of iron |
| Pulses, peas, beans | Carbohydrate, protein, folic acid, calcium, fiber, vitamins $B_1$ and $B_2$, iron, phosphorus | Good source of energy; contain proteins of lower quality that lack in methionine; provides negligible amount of unsaturated fat; absorption of iron is hindered by phytates |
| Soya bean | Protein (35%), fiber, fat (40%), calcium, iron, zinc, copper, magnesium, selenium, folic acid, potassium, all B vitamins, carotenoids, fiber, isoflavones | Source of high quality protein (twice of that in pulses) and fat (three times that in pulses); contains polyunsaturated, monounsaturated and saturated fats; vegetarian source of omega-3 fatty acids; deficient in sodium and vitamins C and $B_{12}$; phytates hinder the absorption of iron and calcium |
| Seasonal vegetables | Carotenoids, folic acid, calcium, fiber, vitamin C | Good source of carbohydrates in the form of roughage and fiber that provide bulk in diet; deficient in proteins and fat |
| Green leafy vegetables | Carotenoids, folic acid, calcium | Good source of soluble fiber; deficient in protein and fat fiber, vitamin C, iron, riboflavin |
| Root vegetables | Carbohydrate (chiefly starch) | Good source of energy; deficient in protein, fat and folic acid; carrots are a rich source of carotene; potatoes provide vitamin C; tapioca is rich in calcium |
| Fruits | Carbohydrate, potassium | Good source of fiber and roughage; deficient in proteins, fat and folic acid; juicy fruits have high potassium content; banana is a good source of energy but poor source of potassium |
| Nuts | Energy, protein, fat and B vitamins | Groundnuts are particularly rich in thiamine and nicotinic acid |

*Adapted from:* The 2010 recommendations of the National Institute of Nutrition (ICMR), Hyderabad on the Nutritive Value of Indian Foods

required as breast milk is nutritionally complete for the child's growth and development; it protects from infections and strengthens immune system.

### Complementary Feeding (6 months onwards)

After 6 months of age, breast milk alone is not enough for adequate growth of the infant. Complementary feeding refers to food which complements breast milk and ensures that the child continues to have enough energy, protein and other nutrients to grow normally.

*Complementary feeding is started at 6 months of age while continuing breastfeeding.* Breastfeeding is encouraged up to two years of age or more in addition with normal food. Key recommendations for breastfeeding and complementary feeding, based on recommendations on Infant and Young Child Feeding (IYCF) practices, are given in Table 7.8 and Fig. 7.3.

Between 6 and 12 months, child goes through a major food transition that depends on several cardinal factors, essential to be considered in feeding the child.

1. Consistency
   - Semisolid, thick liquid (does not flow out of spoon readily)
2. How much each time
   - 6 m–1 year: 1/2 to 1 katori
   - After 1 year: 1 to 1½ katori
3. How often
   - 6 m–1 year: 3 times
   - After 1 year: 5 times
4. How
   - *Pyar se, aaram se, bahla ke*

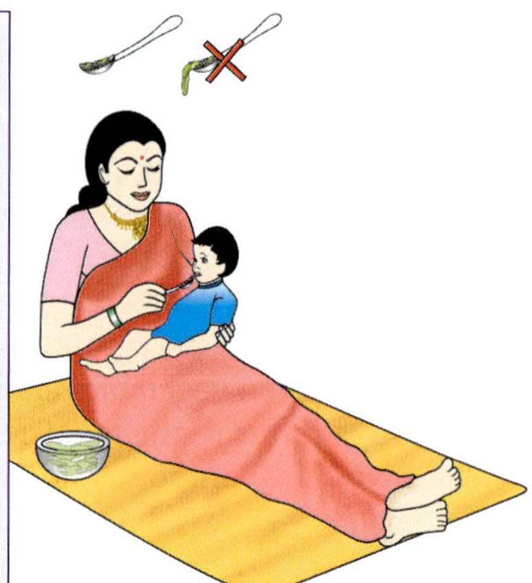

**Fig. 7.3:** Key messages for complementary feeding

### Factors to be Considered while Planning Food for Young Child

***Energy density:*** Most of our commonly consumed foods are bulky and a child cannot eat large quantities at a time.

**Table 7.8:** Counseling for optimal feeding of infants and children according to IYCF recommendations

| *Age (months)* | *Foods* |
|---|---|
| Up to 6 months | • Breastfeed as often as the child wants, day and night, at least 8 times in 24 hours<br>• Do not give any other foods or fluids, not even water<br>• Low birth weight babies to be fed expressed breast milk, if unable to suck directly from breast optimally<br>*Remember:* Continue breastfeeding, even if the child is sick |
| 6–12 months | • Breastfeed as often as the child wants<br>• Complementary feedings: Give at least 1 katori serving at a time of mashed roti/ bread/ biscuit/sattu mixed in sweetened undiluted milk; or mashed roti/rice/bread in thick dal with added ghee/oil; or khichri with added oil/ghee.<br>• Add cooked vegetables in these servings.<br>• Halwa/kheer/porridge—use sevain/dalia or any other cereal in milk<br>• Boiled mashed potato/fried potato/biscuits/banana/cheeku/mango/papaya as snacks in between the servings<br>• Feeds prepared using take home ration supplied by ICDS.<br>*Frequency:* 3 to 4 times/day, if breastfed; 5 times/day, if not breastfed.<br>*Remember:* Keep the child in your lap and feed with your own hands; wash your and child's hand with soap and water every time before feeding. Engage with the child actively while feeding; make feeding a lively and interactive affair. |
| 12 months–2 years | • Breastfeed as often as the child wants; offer food from the family pot.<br>• Give at least 1½ katori serving at a time of mashed roti/rice/bread mixed with thick dal or khichri or rice kanji with added ghee or oil<br>• Add cooked vegetables in the servings<br>• Mashed roti/rice/bread/biscuit mixed in sweetened undiluted milk<br>• Halwa/kheer/porridge—use sevian/dalia or any other cereal and cook in milk<br>• Mashed fried potato/biscuits/banana/cheeku/mango/papaya as snacks in between the servings<br>• Feeds prepared using take home ration supplied by ICDS<br>*Frequency:* 3 to 5 times/day<br>*Remember:* Sit by the side of the child and help him to finish the serving: Engage with the child actively while feeding; make feeding a lively and interactive affair. Wash your and child's hand with soap and water every time before feeding. |
| 2 years and older | • Give family food 3–4 times/day<br>• Feeds prepared using take home ration supplied by ICDS<br>• In addition, offer nutritious snack in-between meals at least twice daily, e.g. any fruit/ biscuits<br>*Remember:* Ensure that child finishes the servings. Teach your child to wash his hands with soap and water every time before eating. Engage with the child actively while feeding; make feeding a lively and interactive affair. |

NB: The food items mentioned above for complementary feeding are for some common examples. There are excellent suitable food items/recipes in every culture.

ICDS Integrated Child Development Services; IYCF Infant and Young Child Feeding

Children have low stomach capacity. Hence, it is important to give small and energy-dense feeds at frequent intervals to ensure adequate energy intake by the child.

Energy density of foods given to infants and young children can be increased without increasing the bulk by adding:

- *Oil or ghee, or sugar/jaggery:* Fat is a concentrated source of energy and increases energy content of food without increasing the bulk. The false belief that a young child cannot digest fat is not true. A young infant can digest fat present in breast milk as well as all other foods. Sugar and jaggery are also rich in energy though not as high in calories as fat but can also be added in infant foods to enhance energy content.
- *Thickening the gruel:* Thin gruels do not provide enough energy because of high water content. A young infant particularly during 6–9 months requires thick but smooth mixtures. For instance, advising *dal ka paani* as a complementary food recipe is absurd. Infant should be given medium thickness gruel of 'dal' with added oil instead.
- *Amylase-rich foods (ARF)* such as malted foods reduce the viscosity of the foods and, therefore, the child can eat more quantities at a time. Malting is germinating whole grain cereal or pulse, drying and then grinding; this process yields food rich in amylase which digests the carbohydrates. The ARF is added to the food item, e.g. Khichri.

**Often the energy needs of the child are underestimated by caregivers. A child between the age of 1 or 2 years needs as much as 50% the nutrition required by an adult.**

***Nutrient density*** of the feed can be ensured by including a variety of foods in order to meet all the nutrients. Even as early as 9 months, infants need small portions of food items from all food groups to be included in their diet to ensure intakes of all macronutrients and micronutrients.

*Amount of feed:* At 6 months of age, feed should be started with small amount as much as 1–2 teaspoons and the quantity is increased gradually as the child gets older and starts to accept food better. Child should be given time to adapt gradually to larger quantities from teaspoon to tablespoon and then to a katori.

*Consistency of feed:* Infants can eat pureed, mashed and semisolid foods beginning at 6 months. By 12 months, most children can eat the same types of foods as are consumed by rest of the family. As the child grows older, she should be shifted to more appropriate foods suitable for his age. The aim is to enable children accept the usual family food by second year of life.

*Frequency of feeding:* An average healthy breastfed infant needs complementary foods 3–4 times per day at 6–8 months of age, 3–4 times per day at 9–11 months and 4–5 times at 12–24 months of age. In addition, additional nutritious snacks such as a piece of fruit, should be offered 1–2 times per day or as desired. Snacks are defined as foods eaten between meals, usually convenient and easy to prepare. If energy density or amount of food per meal is low, or the child is no longer breastfed, more frequent meals may be required.

The water requirements of infants up to 6 months age is met with breastfeeding alone and no additional water needs to be given. Once semisolids and solids are started after 6 months of age, small amounts of water can be given; most of the requirements will still be met by milk.

*Hygiene:* Good hygiene and proper food handling should be practiced to prevent children from infections and malnutrition. Simple hygiene practices include: (a) Washing hands before food preparation and eating, (b) serving freshly cooked foods (cooked should not be kept for 2–3 hours), (c) using clean utensils and covered properly, (d) using clean cups and bowls when feeding children, and (e) avoiding use of feeding bottles.

### Make Feeding a Pleasant Experience for a Young Child

- The feeding time should be structured. Typical timings for 1–2-year-old child are: Morning (for breakfast), mid-morning (for snack), noon or early afternoon (for lunch), late afternoon (for snack), evening (for dinner).
- The caregiver should feed a young child with patience. The child eats slowly. Remember, it takes 30–40 min to feed a 9–18 months old child.
- The meal environment should be free from distractions; avoid viewing mobiles/television screens while feeding.
- The child should be comfortably seated.
- While feeding, the caregiver should interact with and talk to the child. *Bahlaa ke, manaa ke khilao* (Lure and persuade the child).

### Planning Diet for Individual Child

In clinical practice, it is imperative to plan diets for different conditions among children with various ages, both healthy and sick. In this exercise, it is important to ensure the right balance of macronutrients and food groups. A sample diet plan for 1000 kcal meant for a 12–18 months old child is shown in Table 7.9. This can serve as a template to plan diets of lower or higher energy content by varying amounts of ingredients.

#### Points to Remember

- Avoid adding extra salt in home-based foods given to children. Natural sodium in food is enough to take care

**Table 7.9:** Preparation of 1000 kcal diet—a sample balanced diet plan based on the food measures. The food portions are to be spread over 24 hours in multiple meals and snacks

***Step 1:*** Calculate carbohydrate, protein and fat energy distribution and convert in grams.
55 to 60% carbohydrate = 137 to 150 g; 10–12% protein = 25 to 30 g; 25–30% fat = 27 to 33 g

***Step 2:*** Plan the diet including all food groups, providing the amount of carbohydrates, protein and fat as calculated above and total energy adding up to 1000 kcal

| *Food Items* | *Amount (raw)* | *Household measures (cooked)* | *Energy (kcal)* | *Protein (g)* | *Carbohydrate (g)* | *Fat (g)* |
|---|---|---|---|---|---|---|
| Breast milk | | | | | | |
| Undiluted fresh cow's/toned milk | 300 ml | 2 small glasses | 174 | 9.6 | 13.5 | 9.0 |
| **Cereals** | **100 g** | **Variety of cereals** | | | | |
| Wheat flour | 50 g atta | 2 small rotis | 160 | 5.0 | 32 | 0.6 |
| Daliya/suji | 25 g | 1 small katori daliya | 80 | 2.5 | 16 | 0.3 |
| Rice | 25 g | 1 small katori cooked rice | 90 | 2.0 | 19.5 | 0.1 |
| Pulses | 15 g raw | 1 small katori cooked | 45 | 3.0 | 7.0 | 0.2 |
| Seasonal vegetables | 200 g | 2 small katori cooked | 48 | 4.0 | 5.0 | 1.2 |
| Potato | 100 g | 1 medium size | 60 | 1.5 | 13.0 | 0.2 |
| Fruits | 100 g | 1 Banana | 110 | 1.5 | 25 | 0.5 |
| Fat | 20 mL | 4 levelled tsp Refined oil/ ghee | 180 | - | - | 20.0 |
| Sugar | 15 g | 3 levelled tsp | 60 | - | 15.0 | - |
| **Total** | | | **1007 kcal** | **29.1 g** | **146 g** | **32.1 g** |

100 g cereal = 4 small rotis (1 roti = 25 g atta) OR
100 g cereal = 2 small rotis + 2 small katoris cooked rice

of their salt needs. Avoid canned/tinned commercial baby foods—they have high sodium content.

- Avoid excess sugar due to growing incidence of childhood obesity. Avoid getting children addicted to commercial canned/tinned baby foods, sugary drinks, squashes, juices, sweetened curd, etc.
- Avoid junk foods such as confectionaries, chocolate, mushrooms, ketchups, soft drinks
- Avoid chilies and strong spices
- Avoid foods such as whole nuts, seeds, corn chips, hard lollies, raw carrot, and chunks of fruits and vegetables, which can choke small children.
- Commercial ultra-processed foods are high in salt, sugar and trans fats, excess saturated fats should be strictly avoided.
- Prefer bland natural taste from a variety of foods by inclusion of all food groups.
- The eating environment is an important factor for the development of healthy eating behaviors.
- Child should be allowed to experiment/play with food items.

**Avoid honey, added sugar and salt, and hard foods tough to swallow till 1 year of age. By age 2 years, child eats almost everything.**

*Competencies:* **PE9.6; PE9.7**

## UNDERNUTRITION

Undernutrition is a set of conditions that result from inadequate consumption, poor accretion or excessive loss of nutrients. Overnutrition includes overweight and obesity and is caused by overindulgence or excessive intake of nutrients, or pathological conditions.

Malnutrition refers to deficiencies, excesses or imbalances in intake of energy and/or nutrients. Thus, malnutrition connotes both undernutrition as well as overnutrition. In practice, however, often the terms malnutrition and protein energy malnutrition (PEM) are used interchangeably with undernutrition.

In this chapter, we will focus on undernutrition among children less than 5 years of age.

### Consequences of Undernutrition

Undernourished children have higher risk of infections and mortality. Undernutrition is strongly associated with shorter adult height, poor lean weight, less schooling, low cognition, reduced economic productivity and, for women, lower offspring birth weight. Low birth weight and undernutrition in childhood are important risk factors for diabetes mellitus, hypertension and dyslipidemias in adulthood.

### Underweight, Stunting and Wasting

Undernutrition has three subgroups: *Underweight*, *wasting* and *stunting* (Table 7.10 and Fig. 7.4)

An *underweight* child has *low-weight-for-age*. It means that the weight of this child is less than minus 2 standard deviation scores (–2 SDS) on the WHO Growth Standard for her/his age. An underweight child could be wasted or stunted, or both.

*Stunting* denotes *low-height-for-age*. The height (or length) of a stunted child is below minus 2 standard deviation scores (<–2 SDS) at her/his age. A stunted child is short for her/his age. Stunting indicates chronic undernutrition.

*Wasting* implies *low-weight-for-height*. A child whose weight for her/his actual height is less than minus 2 standard deviation scores (<–2 SDS) at her/his age on the WHO Growth Standard has wasting. A wasted child has a thin appearance. Wasting indicates acute undernutrition as result of recent food deficit or an acute illness such as diarrhea.

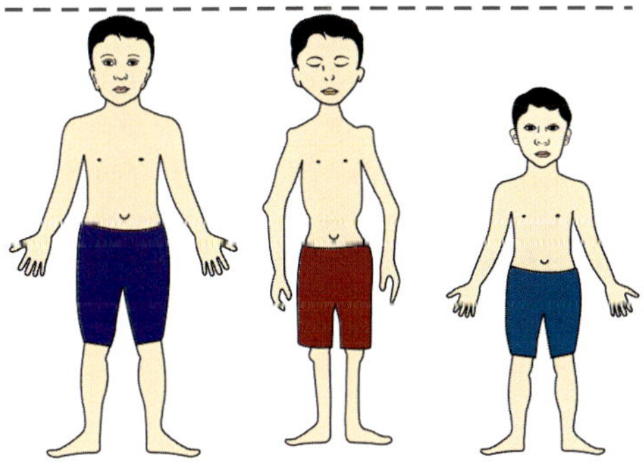


Fig. 7.4: Appearance of undernourished children

Table 7.10: Classification of undernutrition

| *Classification* | *Criteria* | *As per WHO growth standards* | *Subclassification* | *As per WHO reference standards* |
|---|---|---|---|---|
| Underweight | Low-weight-for-age | Weight-for-age <–2 SDS | Underweight<br>Severe underweight | Weight-for-age <–2 SDS and up to –3 SDS<br>Weight-for-age <–3 SDS |
| Stunting | Low-height*-for-age | Height-for-age <–2 SDS | Stunting<br>Severe stunting | Height-for-age <–2 SDS and up to –3 SDS<br>Height-for-age <–3 SDS |
| Wasting | Low-weight-for-height | Weight-for-height <–2 SDS | Wasting<br>Severe wasting | Weight-for-height <–2 SDS and up to –3 SDS<br>Weight-for-height <–3 SDS |

*Length is measured in the first two years of life
SDS standard deviation score

7 Nutrition

Growth charts based on WHO Growth Reference Standards are given in Chapter 2 and Annexures.

The term 'edematous malnutrition' is used, if edema is also present in an underweight child. Clinical classification of undernutrition as marasmus, kwashiorkor and marasmic kwashiorkor is also helpful (discussed below).

## Epidemiology

Childhood undernutrition is an underlying cause in an estimated 45% of all deaths among under-5 children. According to the National Family Health Survey (NFHS) 5, carried out in 2019–21, 32% of India's children under the age of five are underweight, 36% are stunted and 19% are wasted **(Fig. 7.5)**. Comparable figures for 2005–06 were 43%, 48% and 20%, respectively. There has been a slow reduction in undernutrition in the country over the years, especially stunting. Yet we continue to have the highest burden of childhood undernutrition in the world.

Undernutrition rates are highest among the scheduled tribes and scheduled caste families. Proportion of underweight children in rural areas (34%) is higher than urban areas (27%).

During the first 6 months of life, 20–30% of children already undernourished, often because they were born low birth weight **(Fig. 7.6)**. Breastfeeding coverage is far from satisfactory. Breastfeeding is initiated within one hour in 42% neonates and exclusive breastfeeding in 6 months is achieved in 64% infants. It is important that all mothers and their families are counselled and supported regarding breastfeeding. Special focus is required on feeding of low birth weight babies (Chapter 9).

Stunting rate climbs rapidly after 6 months of age due to 2 reasons **(Fig. 7.6)**.

- First, after 6 months of age, breast milk alone is not enough to meet the energy requirement of the child, and, therefore, solid food (complementary feeding) must be introduced, in addition to continuing breastfeeding. This often does not happen. Complementary feeding is introduced between 6–9 months only in 46% infants. In addition, it is estimated that only 11% of children between the age of 6–24 months receive minimal acceptable diet (NFHS-5). Minimal acceptable diet criteria: Breastfed children receiving 4 or more food groups and a minimum meal frequency, non-breastfed children fed with a minimum of 3 Infant and Young Child Feeding Practices (fed with other milk or milk products at least twice a day, a minimum meal frequency that is, receiving solid or semisolid food at least twice a day for breastfed infants 6–8 months and at least three times a day for breastfed children 9–23 months, and solid or semi-solid foods from at least four food groups not including the milk or milk products food group). Most children in the country are thus 'nutrition hungry' in this critical phase of life. Late introduction of complementary feeding and inadequate food intake leads to increasing predisposition to undernutrition.

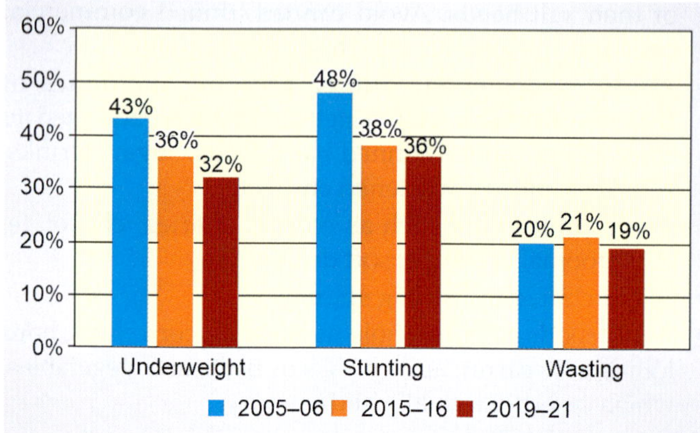


**Fig. 7.5:** Trends in undernutrition in India: Proportion of under-5 children with underweight, stunting and wasting. [*Source:* National Family Health Surveys-3 (2005–06), 4 (2015–16), and 5 (2019-21)]

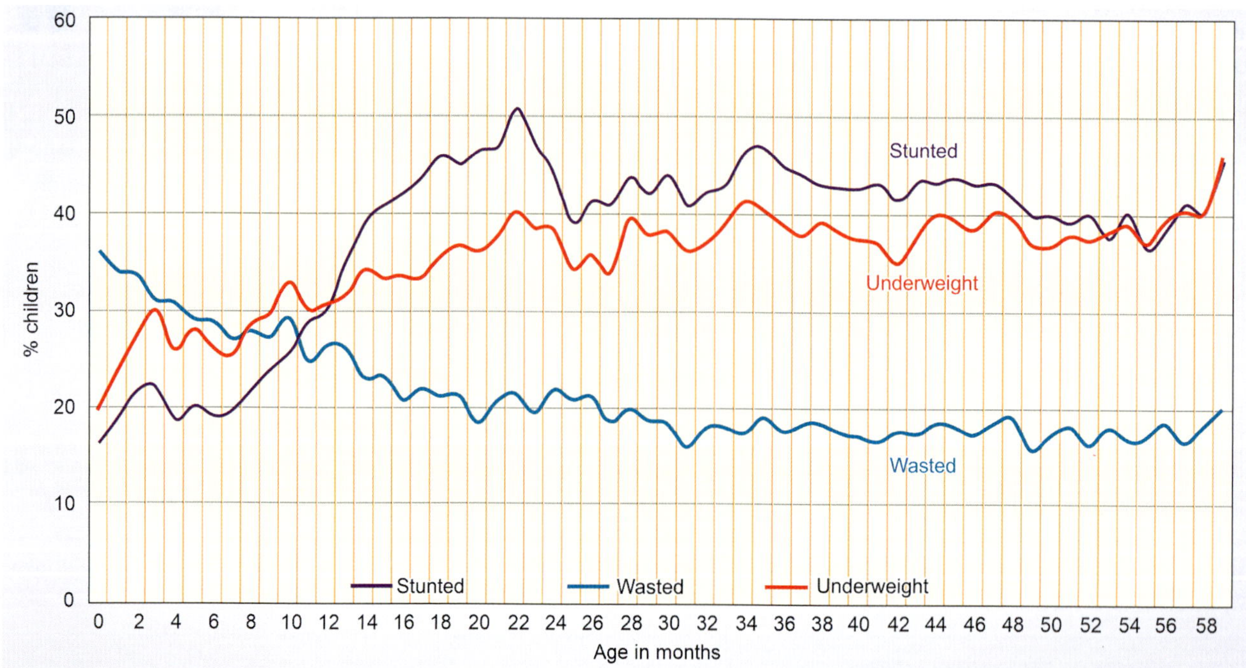


**Fig. 7.6:** Proportion of malnourished children according to age (National Family Health Survey 4, 2015–16)

- Second, after 6 months of age, the child becomes more prone of infections, particularly diarrhea, as she becomes mobile and puts unhygienic objects into mouth.

The proportion of children who are stunted or underweight increases rapidly with the child's age until about 18–24 months (Fig. 7.6).

*Importance of fetal life and the first two years of life (the first 1000 days 'window') for linear and brain growth.*

Length at 2 years is the predictor of adult height and productivity. Brain achieves a near adult size by two years of age. Nutrition during the first 1000 days since conception, encompassing pregnancy and the first 2 two years of life, is important for realizing the physical and intellectual potential. Ensuring optimum nutrition of the mother before and during pregnancy, and optimum feeding of children in the first 2 years of life is crucial.

### Determinants

The causes of malnutrition could be viewed as immediate, underlying and basic as depicted in Fig. 7.7.

The immediate determinants of a child's nutritional status work at the individual level. These include low birth weight, illnesses (particularly infections such as diarrhea and pneumonia) and inadequate dietary intake.

Finally, the underlying determinants are influenced by the basic determinants. These include the socioeconomic status and education level of the families, women's empowerment, cultural taboos regarding food and health, and access to water and sanitation.

**Three cardinal determinants of undernutrition**

1. ***Low birth weight:*** Infants born small often remain undernourished. About 20% childhood undernutrition is attributable to fetal growth restriction.
2. ***Infections:*** Diarrhea, pneumonia and other infections increase energy expenditure and hamper growth. Diarrhea causes nutrient loss in stools. About 25% of childhood undernutrition is attributable to diarrhea, pneumonia and other infections.
3. ***Low food intake:*** Inadequate breastfeeding, delayed complementary feeding and insufficient food intake means less energy and protein available for growth. This underlies about 55% of childhood undernutrition.

## Clinical Syndromes of Undernutrition

Moderate and severe malnutrition is associated with one of classical syndromes, namely, marasmus, kwashiorkor, or with manifestations of both. Classification as moderate and severe acute malnutrition (MAM, SAM) are discussed later.

### Marasmus

Marasmus is characterized by severe form of wasting. There is marked wasting of fat and muscle as these tissues are consumed to make energy. Acute starvation or acute illness over a borderline nutritional status precipitates this form of undernutrition. Severe marasmus is a typical form of severe acute malnutrition (SAM).

- The main sign is severe wasting. The child appears very thin (skin and bones) and has no fat. There is wasting of the shoulders, arms, buttocks and thighs (Fig. 7.8).
- The loss of buccal pad of fat creates the aged or wrinkled appearance, referred to as monkey facies (Fig. 7.8a). Baggy pants appearance refers to loose skin of the buttocks hanging down (Fig. 7.8b). Axillary pad of fat may also be diminished.
- Affected children may appear to be alert in spite of their condition.
- There is no edema

### Kwashiorkor

Uncommon in India now, it usually affects children aged 1–4 years. The main sign is pitting edema, usually starting in the legs and feet and spreading, in more advanced cases, to the hands and face. Because of edema, children with kwashiorkor may look healthy so that their parents view them as well fed.

- *General appearance:* Child may have a fat, sugar baby appearance.
- *Edema:* It ranges from mild to gross and may represent up to 5–20% of the body weight.
- *Muscle wasting:* It is always present. The child is often weak, hypotonic and unable to stand or walk.
- *Skin changes:* The skin lesions consist of increased pigmentation, desquamation and dyspigmentation. Pigmentation may be confluent resembling flaky paint or

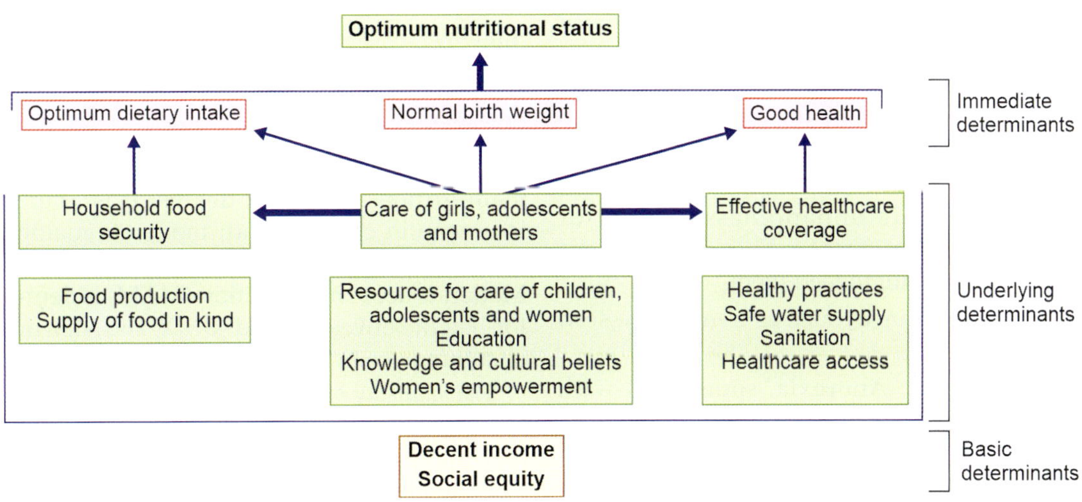


**Fig. 7.7:** Determinants of a child's nutrition status (*Adapted from:* Smith LC, Haddad L. World Develop 2015)

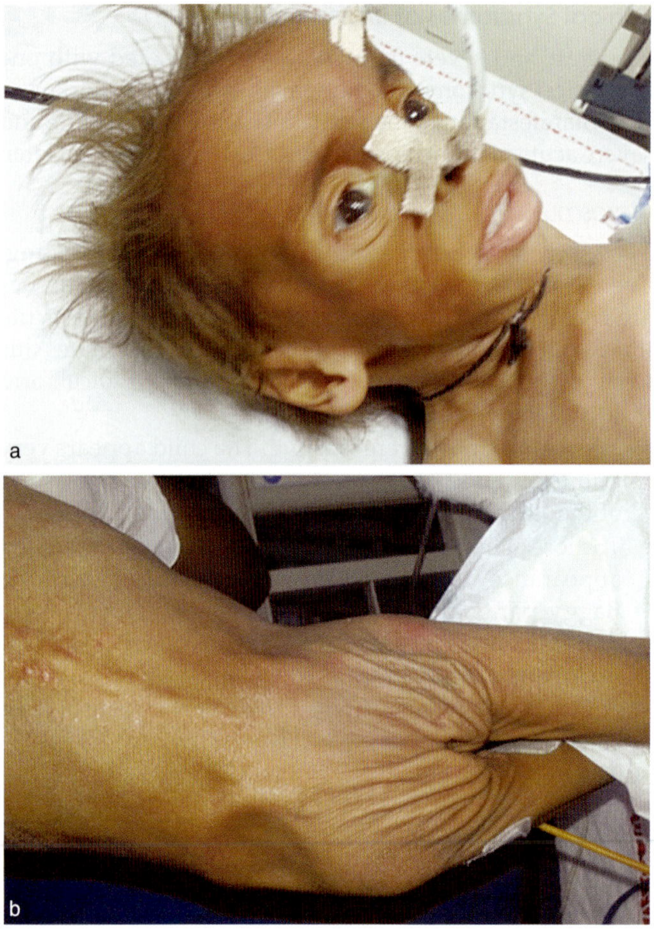

Fig. 7.8: A child with severe acute malnutrition. Note the: (a) Dull, lusterless, sparse hair; temporal hollowing; loss of buccal pad of fat; anxious look; (b) Loose folds of skin in the gluteal region giving a 'baggy pant' appearance



in individual enamel spots. The distribution is typically on buttocks, perineum and upper thigh. Petechiae may be seen over abdomen. Outer layers of skin may peel off and ulceration may occur. The lesions may sometimes resemble burns.

- *Mucous membrane lesions:* Smooth tongue, cheilosis and angular stomatitis are common. Herpes simplex stomatitis may also be seen.
- *Hair:* Changes include dyspigmentation, loss of characteristic curls and sparseness over temple and occipital regions. Hairs lose their luster and are easily pluckable. A flag sign which is the alternate bands of hypopigmented and normally pigmented hair pattern is seen when the growth of child occurs in spurts.
- *Mental changes:* Include unhappiness, apathy or irritability with sad, intermittent cry. They show no signs of hunger and it is difficult to feed them.
- *Neurological changes:* Changes such as tremors are seen during recovery.
- *Gastrointestinal system:* Anorexia, sometimes with vomiting, is the rule. Abdominal distension is characteristic. Stools may be watery or semisolid, bulky with a low pH and may contain unabsorbed sugars.
- *Anemia:* Nutritional anemia is almost always associated.
- *Cardiovascular system:* The findings include cold, pale extremities due to circulatory insufficiency and are associated with prolonged circulation time, bradycardia, diminished cardiac output and hypotension.
- *Renal function:* Glomerular filtration and renal plasma flow are diminished. There is aminoaciduria and inefficient excretion of acid load.

### Marasmic Kwashiorkor

It is a mixed form of undernutrition and manifests as edema occurring in children who may or may not have other signs of kwashiorkor and have varied manifestations of marasmus.

### Severe Acute Malnutrition (SAM)

This special classification is recommended by the WHO for identifying and managing children with life-threatening undernutrition in public health programme settings. Children with SAM have a mix of features of marasmus and kwashiorkor.

Severe acute malnutrition (SAM) among children 6–59 months of age is defined by WHO and UNICEF as any of the following three criteria:

i. Weight-for-height below –3 standard deviation score (<3 SDS) on the WHO Growth Standard; or
ii. Presence of bipedal edema; or
iii. Mid-upper arm circumference (MUAC) below 11.5 cm.

In a child below 6 months of age, the MUAC is not used as a criterion.

Children with SAM have a high risk of death in near future. In addition to debilitating undernutrition, they often have serious infections such as diarrhea, pneumonia, sepsis, malaria and skin infections. They require urgent attention.

*Competencies:* **PE9.7; PE10.1; PE10.2; PE10.3; PE10.4; PE10.5; PE10.6**

## MANAGEMENT OF MALNUTRITION

The management of malnutrition depends on its severity. While moderate malnutrition can be managed on ambulatory basis, severe malnutrition is preferably managed in hospital. The management of low birth weight infants is discussed in Chapter 9.

### Moderate Acute Malnutrition (MAM)

Moderate malnutrition makes up the greatest portion of malnourished children and accounts for >80% of malnutrition associated deaths. It is, therefore, vital to intervene in children with moderate malnutrition at the community level before they develop complications. Moderate acute malnutrition (MAM) is defined as weight-for-height between –2 and –3 SDS and/or a mid-upper arm circumference (MUAC) between 115 and 125 mm.

*The mainstay of treatment is provision of adequate amounts of protein and energy; at least 150 kcal/kg/day* or additional 25 kcal/kg/day should be given. Nutritious home food is recommended. The ICDS programme provides extra ration for such children.

In order to achieve these high energy intakes, frequent feeding (up to seven times a day) is often necessary. Because energy is so important and carbohydrate energy sources are bulky, fat is usually used to increase the energy in therapeutic diets. Nutrient-dense foods enable children to consume and maximize the absorption of nutrients in order to fulfil their requirements of energy and all essential nutrients.

According to the WHO, animal-source foods are more likely to meet the amino acid and other nutrient needs of recovering children. Milk and eggs are excellent animal origin foods for children. Plant-source foods, in particular legumes or a combination of cereals and legumes, also have high-quality proteins, although they may also contain some anti-nutrients such as phytates, tannins or inhibitors of digestive enzymes, which may limit the absorption of some micronutrients, particularly minerals.

It is recognized increasingly that a relatively small increase over normal protein requirements is sufficient for rapid catchup growth, provided energy intake is high. *A protein intake of 3 g/kg/day is sufficient*. Milk is the most frequent source of the protein used in therapeutic diets, though other sources, including vegetable protein mixtures, have been used successfully. Adequate minerals and vitamins should be provided for the appropriate duration. *The best measure of the efficacy of treatment of mild and moderate malnutrition is weight gain.*

## Severe Acute Malnutrition (SAM): Children 6 to 59 Months

The World Health Organization has developed guidelines for the management of severe acute malnutrition (SAM) and these have been updated in 2013. Guidelines are mainly for children of more than 6 months of age.

Once a child, 6 months or older, is diagnosed as SAM, she/he should be assessed by a physician for complications by looking for severe edema (+++), lack of appetite, medical complications (e.g. severe anemia, pneumonia, diarrhea, dehydration, cerebral palsy, tuberculosis, HIV, heart disease) and danger signs according to IMNCI algorithm (**Fig. 7.9**, also *see* Chapter 32). If any of these are present, it is classified as complicated SAM, and the child is referred for inpatient management.

If the above-mentioned signs are absent, the child has uncomplicated SAM and can be managed in the outpatient setting with care at home (**Fig. 7.9**). Good appetite is critically important in the home care of the child with SAM because oral intake of adequate energy dense food is the fundamental requirement for recovery.

## Supervised Home Management of Uncomplicated SAM

Children with uncomplicated SAM can be managed at home provided:

- Family is counseled and fully engaged
- Community health worker(s) and peer counselors are involved to support the family
- There is supply of adequate home food
- Periodic monitoring for growth and medical condition can be ensured.

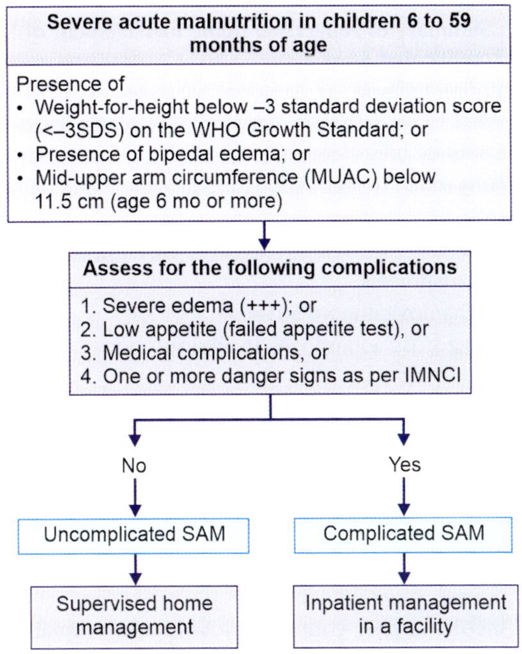


**Fig. 7.9:** Approach to child with severe acute malnutrition

Mainstay of home management is nutritional rehabilitation with high energy food. This could be adequate home foods prepared from locally available cereals and pulses, sugar, oil, milk and/or eggs, etc. ensuring 175 kcal/kg body weight/day. Initially, the catch-up diets (100 kcal/100 mL) may be used and, thereafter, home foods could be fed.

Caregiver should wash hands and utensils used for feeding. Breastfeeding should be continued, if the child is breastfed. The caregiver should lovingly engage the child, talk to her, play with her and make feeding exercise an interactive affair. In addition, the child should be provided sensory stimulation (play, physical activity, laughter, exposure to colors and shapes, storytelling, massage, etc.).

Optimum home management of a child with SAM is not possible without effective support by the health worker. Families will invariably need close facilitation and guidance by the health worker (ASHA, ANM or AWW). A home contact every day initially, and then twice a week is essential **(Panel 1)**.

The child should be monitored by health workers for signs of undernutrition (weight, height, MUAC, edema, anemia, etc.) every week.

In addition to nutrition, every child on SAM treatment should receive the following interventions: An antibiotic course (amoxicillin for 5 days), mega dose of vitamin (100,000 units) in the presence of clinical deficiency (xerophthalmia, Bitot's spots or keratomalacia), and albendazole single dose (for children over 1 years of age). The child should be provided all the due vaccines as per national immunization schedule.

Nutritional rehabilitation of a child with SAM would require 3–5 months. Hence, home contacts are extremely important. After completion of treatment, the child should be followed up in the Anganwadi regularly.

**Panel 1: Summary of supervised home management of a child with uncomplicated SAM**

I. Nutrition therapy
- *What to feed*: Initially catch-up diets; later home foods. Continue breastfeeding
- *How much to feed:* Enough to provide 175 kcal/kg/day
- *How often to feed:* 6–8 times a day
- *How to feed:* Lovingly, actively; ensuring hygiene

II. Other treatments
- Oral amoxicillin for 5 days
- Mega dose vitamin A, if obvious signs of vitamin A deficiency
- Albendazole single dose
- Age appropriate vaccines

III. Sensory stimulation
- Play, physical activity, interaction

IV. Supervision and support
- Home visits by health workers, initially daily, later twice a week; more if necessary
- Involve a peer counselor, a volunteer woman friend/ neighbor to support the family

V. Monitoring by health workers (ASHA/AWW/ANM)
- Assess intake, solve feeding issues
- Evaluate for medical problems; treat/refer
- Assess growth weekly

## Management of Complicated SAM in Hospital

All children with complicated SAM should be hospitalized. The government has established nutrition rehabilitation centres (NRCs) in all states.

The child with severe malnutrition has a complex backdrop with dietary, infective, social and economic factors underlying the malnutrition. A history of events leading to the child's admission should be obtained. Socioeconomic history and family circumstances should be explored to understand the underlying and basic causes.

Physical features of malnutrition as described above should be looked for. Following clinical features should be particularly looked for: Fever, hypothermia (temperature <35.5°C), signs of dehydration, shock (cold hands, slow capillary refill, weak and rapid pulse), anemia, eye signs of vitamin A deficiency, localizing signs of infections (pneumonia, skin infections, diarrhea, tuberculosis), signs of HIV infection, mouth ulcers and skin changes of kwashiorkor.

Median case fatality rate in children with SAM is approximately 23.5%, which may reach 50% in edematous malnutrition. The high case fatality has been attributed to various factors related to the management and includes:

1. Inability to distinguish between acute and rehabilitation phases
2. Excessive use of intravenous (IV) fluids
3. Fluid overload due to lack of monitoring during rehydration
4. Use of diuretics (for edema) and albumin
5. Not keeping the child warm and euglycemic (normal blood glucose levels)
6. Low index of suspicion for infection
7. Early use of diets with high protein, sodium, energy
8. Failure to monitor food intake
9. Early treatment of anemia with oral iron

The case fatality can be brought down to approximately 7–10% by standard case management protocol.

*The general treatment involves 10 steps in two phases:*
- The initial *stabilization phase* focuses on restoring homeostasis and treating medical complications and usually takes 2–7 days of inpatient treatment.
- The *rehabilitation phase* focuses on rebuilding wasted tissues and may take several weeks.

The 10 essential steps and the time frame are shown in Fig. 7.10 and Table 7.11.

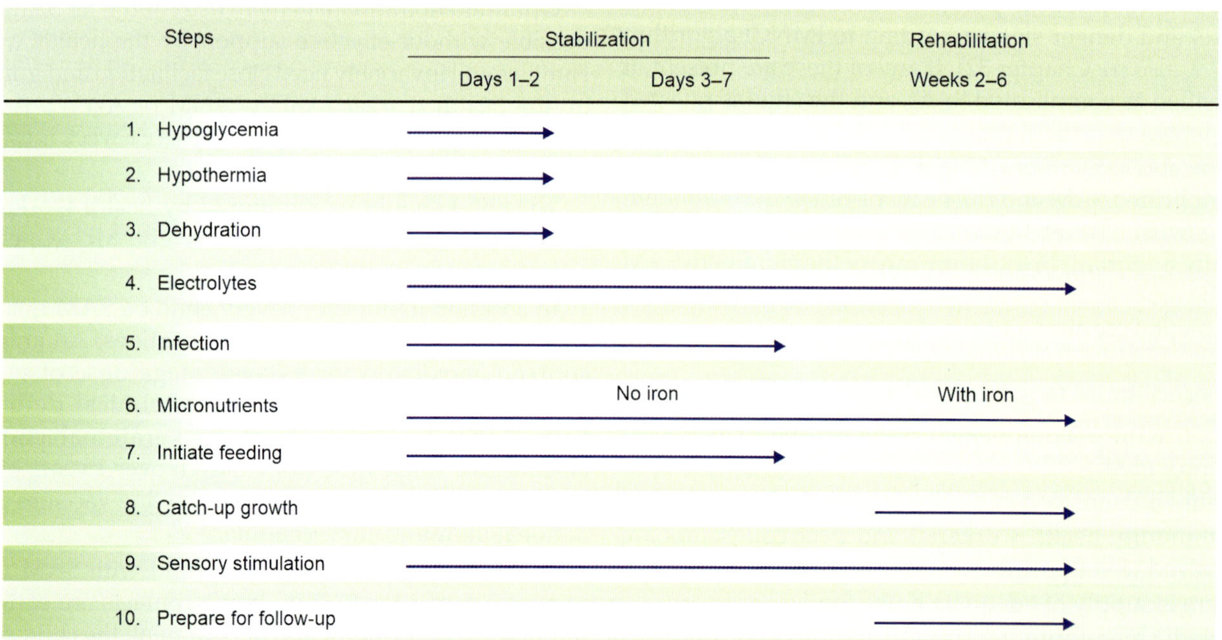


**Fig. 7.10:** The time frame for initiating and achieving 10 steps

**Table 7.11:** Summary of the management of severe acute malnutrition

| | |
|---|---|
| Hypoglycemia | Blood glucose level <54 mg/dL or 3 mmol/L<br>If blood glucose cannot be measured, assume hypoglycemia<br>Hypoglycemia, hypothermia and infection generally occur as a triad<br>**Treatment**<br>Asymptomatic hypoglycemia<br>Give 50 mL of 10% glucose or sucrose solution orally or by nasogastric tube followed by first feed<br>Feed with starter F-75 every 2 hourly day and night<br>Symptomatic hypoglycemia<br>Give 10% dextrose IV 5 mL/kg<br>Follow with 50 mL of 10% dextrose or sucrose solution by nasogastric tube<br>Feed with starter diet every 2 hours day and night<br>Start appropriate antibiotics<br>**Prevention**<br>Feed 2 hourly starting immediately<br>Prevent hypothermia |
| Hypothermia | Rectal temperature less than <35.5°C or 95.5°F or axillary temperature less than 35°C or 95°F<br>Always measure blood glucose and screen for infections in the presence of hypothermia<br>**Treatment**<br>Clothe the child with warm clothes; ensure that the head is also covered with a scarf or cap<br>Provide heat using overhead warmer, skin contact or heat convector<br>Avoid rapid rewarming as this may lead to disequilibrium<br>Feed the child immediately<br>Give appropriate antibiotics<br>**Prevention**<br>Place the child's bed in a draught-free area<br>Always keep the child well covered; ensure that head is also covered well<br>May place the child in contact with the mother's bare chest or abdomen (skin-to-skin)<br>Feed the child 2 hourly starting immediately after admission |
| Dehydration | Difficult to estimate dehydration status accurately in the severely malnourished child<br>Assume that all severely malnourished children with watery diarrhea have some dehydration<br>Low blood volume (hypovolemia) can coexist with edema<br>**Treatment**<br>Use reduced osmolarity ORS with potassium supplements for rehydration and maintenance<br>Amount depends upon how much the child wants, volume of stool loss, and whether the child is vomiting<br>Initiate feeding within two to three hours of starting rehydration; use F-75 formula on alternate hours along with reduced osmolarity ORS<br>Be alert for signs of overhydration<br>**Prevention**<br>Give reduced osmolarity ORS at 5–10 mL/kg after each watery stool, to replace stool losses<br>If breastfed, continue breastfeeding<br>Initiate refeeding with starter formula |
| Electrolytes | Give supplemental potassium at 3–4 mEq/kg/day for at least 2 weeks<br>On day 1, give 50% magnesium sulfate (equivalent to 4 mEq/mL) IM once (0.3 ml/kg; maximum of 2 mL). Thereafter, give extra magnesium (0.8–1.2 mEq/kg daily)<br>Excess body sodium exists even though the plasma sodium may be low; decrease salt in diet |
| Infection | Multiple infections are common; assume serious infection and treat<br>Usual signs of infection such as fever are often absent<br>Majority of bloodstream infections are due to gram-negative bacteria<br>Hypoglycemia and hypothermia are markers of severe infection<br>**Treatment**<br>Treat with parenteral ampicillin 50 mg/kg/dose 6 hourly for at least 2 days followed by oral amoxicillin 15 mg/kg 8 hourly for 5 days; and gentamicin 7.5 mg/kg or amikacin 15–20 mg/kg IM or IV once daily for 7 days<br>If no improvement occurs within 48 hours, change to IV cefotaxime (100–150 mg/kg/day 8 hourly) or ceftriaxone (50–75 mg/kg/day 12 hourly)<br>If other specific infections are identified, give appropriate antibiotics |

*(Contd...)*

**Table 7.11:** Summary of the management of severe acute malnutrition *(Contd...)*

| | |
|---|---|
| | **Prevention**<br>Follow standard precautions like hand hygiene<br>Give measles (MR) vaccine, if the child is >6 months and not immunized, or if the child is >9 months and had been vaccinated before the age of 9 months |
| Micronutrients | Use up to twice the recommended daily allowance of various vitamins and minerals<br>On day 1, give vitamin A orally (if age >1 year, give 2 lakh IU; age 6–12 months, give 1 lakh IU; age 0–5 months, give 50,000 IU)<br>Folic acid 1 mg/day (give 5 mg on day 1)<br>Zinc 2 mg/kg/day<br>Copper 0.2–0.3 mg/kg/day<br>Iron 3 mg/kg/day, once child starts gaining weight; after the stabilization phase |
| Initiate feeding | Start feeding as soon as possible as frequent small feeds<br>If unable to take orally, initiate nasogastric feeds<br>Total fluid recommended is 130 mL/kg/day; reduce to 100 mL/kg/day, if there is severe edema<br>Continue breastfeeding *ad libitum*<br>Start with starter feeds every 2 hourly<br>If persistent diarrhea, give a cereal based low lactose starter diet<br>If diarrhea continues on low lactose diets, give lactose free diets (rarely needed) |
| Catch-up growth | Once appetite returns in 2–3 days, encourage higher intakes<br>Increase volume offered at each feed and decrease the frequency of feeds to 6 feeds per day<br>Continue breastfeeding ad libitum<br>Make a gradual transition from starter to catch-up diet<br>Increase calories to 150–200 kcal/kg/day, and proteins to 4–6 g/kg/day<br>Add complementary foods as soon as possible to prepare the child for home foods at discharge |
| Sensory stimulation | A cheerful, stimulating environment<br>Age appropriate structured play therapy for at least 15–30 min/day<br>Age appropriate physical activity as soon as the child is well enough<br>Tender loving care |
| Prepare for follow-up | **Primary failure to respond** is indicated by:<br>Failure to regain appetite by day 4<br>Failure to start losing edema by day 4<br>Presence of edema on day 10<br>Failure to gain at least 5 g/kg/day by day 10<br>**Secondary failure to respond** is indicated by:<br>Failure to gain at least 5 g/kg/day for consecutive days during the rehabilitation phase |

### *Step 1: Treat/Prevent Hypoglycemia*

All severely malnourished children are at risk of hypoglycemia (blood glucose level <54 mg/dL or 3 mmol/L), hence blood glucose should be measured immediately at admission. If blood glucose cannot be measured, one must assume hypoglycemia and treat.

Hypoglycemia may be asymptomatic or symptomatic. Symptomatic hypoglycemia manifesting as lethargy, unconsciousness, seizures, peripheral circulatory failure or hypothermia is more common in marasmus, where energy stores are depleted or when feeding is infrequent.

For correction of asymptomatic hypoglycemia, 50 mL of 10% glucose or sucrose solution (1 rounded teaspoon of sugar in 3½ tablespoons of water) should be given orally or by nasogastric tube followed by the first feed. For correction of symptomatic hypoglycemia, 5 mL/kg of 10% dextrose should be given intravenously. This should be followed with 50 mL of 10% dextrose or sucrose solution by nasogastric tube. Blood glucose levels must be estimated every 30 min till the glucose level becomes normal and stabilizes. Once stable, the 2 hourly feeding regimens should be started.

Feeding should be started with starter diet (containing 75 kcal/100 mL and 0.9 g protein/100 mL) as quickly as possible and then continued 2–3 hourly day and night (initially a quarter of the 2 hourly feed should be given every 30 min till the blood glucose stabilizes). Most episodes of symptomatic hypoglycemia can be prevented by frequent, regular feeds and the child should be fed regularly throughout the night. Hypoglycemia, hypothermia and infection often occur as a triad.

### *Step 2: Treat/Prevent Hypothermia*

All severely malnourished children are at risk of hypothermia due to impairment of thermoregulatory control, lowered metabolic rate and decreased thermal insulation from body fat. Children with marasmus, concurrent infections, denuded skin and infants are at a greater risk. Hypothermia is diagnosed, if the axillary temperature is less than 35°C or 95°F. It can occur in summers as well. The child should be rewarmed providing heat using radiation (overhead warmer) or conduction (skin contact) or convection (heat convector). Rapid rewarming may lead to disequilibrium and should be avoided.

In case of severe hypothermia (temperature <32°C), warm humidified oxygen should be given followed immediately by 5 mL/kg of 10% dextrose IV or 50 mL of 10% dextrose by nasogastric route (if IV access is difficult). If clinical condition allows the child to take orally, warm feeds should be given immediately or else the feeds should be administered through a nasogastric tube. If there is feed intolerance or another contraindication for nasogastric feeding, maintenance IV fluids (prewarmed) should be started.

In a hypothermic child, hypoglycemia must be looked for and managed. The child's temperature should be monitored every 2 hours till it rises to more than 37.5°C. Temperature monitoring must be ensured especially at night when the ambient temperature falls.

In most cases, hypothermia may be prevented by frequent feeding. Therefore, the child should be fed immediately and subsequently, every 2 hourly. All children should be nursed in a warm environment, clothed with warm clothes and covered using a warm blanket. The head should also be covered well with a scarf or a cap. The child could also be put in contact with the mother's bare chest or abdomen (skin-to-skin) as in kangaroo mother care to provide warmth. Besides these measures, hypothermia can also be prevented by placing the child's bed in a draught-free area away from doors and windows, minimizing exposure after bathing or during clinical examination and keeping the child dry always.

#### *Step 3: Treat/Prevent Dehydration*

Dehydration tends to be over-diagnosed and its severity overestimated in severely malnourished children. Loss of elasticity of skin may either be due to loss of the subcutaneous fat in marasmus or loss of extracellular fluid in dehydration. In dehydration, the oral mucosa feels dry to the palpating finger gently rolled on the inner side of the cheek. Presence of thirst, hypothermia, weak pulses and oliguria are other signs of dehydration in severely malnourished children. It is important to recognize that low blood volume (hypovolemia) can coexist with edema. Since estimation of dehydration may be difficult in severely malnourished children, it is safe to assume that all patients with watery diarrhea have some dehydration.

WHO lays down following guidelines for treating dehydration with ORS in children with SAM:

- Children with severe acute malnutrition who present with some dehydration or severe dehydration but who are not in shock should be rehydrated slowly using ORS for malnourished children.
- WHO recommended ORS for SAM children (ReSoMal) is not commercially available in India.
- We can prepare modified ORS for SAM by dissolving one sachet (meant for 1 liter) of low-osmolarity oral rehydration salt, adding and dissolving 50 g of glucose/ sugar and 45 mL of potassium chloride syrup or 30 mL of potassium chloride injection containing (total 40 mEq/L of potassium) in water to make a total volume of 2 liters in place of 1 liter.
- In case preparation of modified ORS is not possible, start rehydration with low osmolarity ORS.
- If the child has profuse watery diarrhea or cholera is suspected, use low osmolarity ORS without any modification for rehydration.

ORS is given orally or by nasogastric tube at 5–10 mL/ kg/h up to a maximum of 12 hours. Thus, dehydration should be corrected slowly over a period of 12 hours.

Intravenous therapy should be given only for severe dehydration and shock or if the enteral route cannot be used. The exact amount actually depends on how much the child wants, volume of stool loss and whether child is vomiting. Ongoing stool losses should be replaced with approximately 5–10 mL/kg of the ORS after each watery stool. The frequent passage of small unformed stools should not be confused with profuse watery diarrhea as it does not require fluid replacement.

Breastfeeding should be continued during the rehydration phase. Refeeding must be initiated with starter diet within 2–3 hours of starting rehydration. The feeds must be given on alternate hr (e.g. 2, 4, 6 hours) with reduced osmolarity ORS (composition as described above) (hr 1, 3, 5). Once rehydration is complete, feeding must be continued, and ongoing losses replaced with ORS.

The progress of rehydration should be monitored every half hourly for first 2 hours and then hourly for the next 4–10 hours. Pulse rate, respiratory rate, oral mucosa, urine frequency or volume and frequency of stools and vomiting should be monitored.

One must be alert for signs of overhydration (increase in respiratory rate by 5/minute and pulse rate by 15/minute, increasing edema and periorbital puffiness), which can be dangerous and may lead to heart failure. In case of signs of overhydration, ORS should be stopped immediately and child reassessed after one hour. On the other hand, a decrease in the heart rate and respiratory rate (if increased initially) and increase in the urine output indicate that rehydration is proceeding. The return of tears, a moist oral mucosa, less sunken eyes and fontanelle and improved skin turgor are also indicators of rehydration. Once any four signs of hydration (child less thirsty, passing urine, tears, moist oral mucosa, eyes less sunken, faster skin pinch) are present, ORS for rehydration must be stopped and continued to replace the ongoing losses.

*Severe dehydration with shock:* It is important to recognize severe dehydration in malnourished children. Severe dehydration with shock is treated with intravenous fluids. Ideally, Ringer lactate with 5% dextrose should be used as rehydrating fluid. If not available, half normal saline (N/2) with 5% dextrose or Ringer lactate alone can be used. After providing supplemental oxygen, the rehydrating fluid should be given at a slow infusion rate of 15 mL/kg over the first hour with continuous monitoring of pulse rate, volume, respiratory rate, capillary refill time and urine output.

If there is improvement (pulse slows, faster capillary refill) at the end of the first hour of IV fluid infusion, a diagnosis of severe dehydration with shock is made, and IV fluid infusion repeated at the same rate of 15 mL/kg over the next hour. This should be followed by administration of reduced osmolarity ORS at 5–10 mL/kg/hr, either orally or by nasogastric tube. Patients should be monitored for features of overhydration and cardiac decompensation.

*Septic shock:* If at the end of the first hour of IV rehydration, there is no improvement or worsening, septic shock must be considered and appropriate treatment started.

### Step 4: Correct Electrolyte Imbalance

In severely malnourished children, excess body sodium exists even though the plasma sodium may be low. Sodium intake should be restricted to prevent sodium overload and water retention during the initial phase of treatment. Excess sodium in the diet may precipitate congestive cardiac failure.

All severely malnourished children have deficiencies of potassium and magnesium, which may take two weeks or more to correct. Severely malnourished children may develop severe hypokalemia and clinically manifest with weakness of abdominal, skeletal and even respiratory muscles. This may mimic flaccid paralysis. Electrocardiography may show ST depression, T waves inversion and presence of U waves. If serum potassium is <2 mEq/L or <3.5 mEq/L with ECG changes, correction should be started at 0.3–0.5 mEq/kg/hr infusion of potassium chloride in intravenous fluids, preferably with continuous monitoring of the ECG.

Once severe hypokalemia is corrected, all severely malnourished children need supplemental potassium at 3–4 mEq/kg/day for at least 2 weeks. Potassium can be given as syrup potassium chloride; the common preparation available has 20 mEq of potassium/15 mL.

On day 1, 50% magnesium sulfate (equivalent to 4 mEq/mL) should be given at 0.3 mL/kg to a maximum of 2 mL intramuscularly. Thereafter, 0.8–1.2 mEq/kg magnesium should be given orally as a supplement mixed with feeds.

### Step 5: Treat/Prevent Infection

Infection may not produce the classical signs of fever and tachycardia in severely malnourished children. Instead, severe infection may be associated with hypothermia. Localizing signs of infection are often absent. The most common sites for infection are the skin, the alimentary tract, the respiratory tract (including the ears, nose and throat) and the urinary tract. Majority of the infections and septicemia are caused by gram-negative organisms. Therefore, all severely malnourished children should be assumed to have a serious infection on their arrival in hospital. In addition, hypoglycemia and hypothermia are considered markers of severe infection in children.

The following investigations are done for identifying infections: (i) Hb, TLC, DLC, peripheral smear, (ii) urinalysis and culture, (iii) blood culture, (iv) chest X-ray, (v) Mantoux test, (vi) gastric aspirate for AFB, (vii) peripheral smear for malaria (in endemic areas), and (viii) CSF examination (if meningitis is suspected).

All children with suspected infection should be treated with broad spectrum parenteral antibiotics; ampicillin and gentamicin or amikacin (Table 7.12). Antimalarial and antituberculous treatment should only be given when the particular conditions are diagnosed.

Response to treatment will be indicated by resolution of initial symptoms and signs of infection, if any. The child's activity, interaction with parents and appetite should improve. If there is no improvement or deterioration of the symptoms/signs of infection, the child should be screened for infection with resistant bacterial pathogens, tuberculosis, HIV and unusual pathogens.

***Prevention of hospital acquired infection:*** The health care personnel should follow standard precautions. The effectiveness of hand hygiene should be emphasized to all healthcare providers, attendants and patients. It is essential that adequate safety measures are taken to prevent the spread of hospital-acquired infections, since these children are at higher risk of acquiring infections due to their compromised immune status.

### Step 6: Correct Micronutrient Deficiencies

All severely malnourished children have vitamin and mineral deficiencies. Micronutrients should be used as an adjunct to treatment in safe and effective doses. Up to twice the recommended daily allowance of various vitamins and minerals should be used. Although anemia is common, iron should not be given initially due to risk of promoting free radical generation and bacterial proliferation. It should be added only after a week of therapy when the child has a good appetite and starts gaining weight.

**Table 7.12:** Recommended antibiotics for infections in severely malnourished children

| *Type of infection* | *Recommended antibiotics* |
|---|---|
| No obvious infections or complications | Oral cotrimoxazole (5 mg/kg /dose 12 hourly of trimethoprim) or oral amoxicillin 10 mg/kg /dose 8 hourly for 5 days |
| Infected child or complications | IV ampicillin 50 mg/kg/dose 6 hourly and IV gentamicin 5–7 mg/kg/day in 1–2 divided doses; add IV cloxacillin 100 mg/kg/day 6 hourly, if staphylococcal infection is suspected; revise therapy based on the culture sensitivity report |
| Septic shock; no improvement or worsening | Add third generation cephalosporin, i.e. IV cefotaxime 100 mg/kg/day 8 hourly |
| Meningitis | IV cefotaxime 200 mg/kg/day in 4 divided doses with IV amikacin 15 mg/kg/day as a single dose (slow infusion) |
| Dysentery | Ciprofloxacin 20 mg/kg/day in 2 divided doses; IV ceftriaxone 50 mg/kg/day in 2 divided doses, if child is sick or has already received nalidixic acid |

Vitamin A deficiency is not an infrequent association and is an important cause of blindness caused by keratomalacia. Vitamin A should, therefore, be given to all severely malnourished children on day 1 at 50,000 IU, 100,000 IU and 200,000 IU for infants 0–5 months, 6–12 months and children >1 year of age unless there is definite evidence that a dose has been given in the last month. In presence of xerophthalmia, the same dose should be repeated on the next day and 2 weeks later. Children >1 year but weighing <8 kg should receive half the age related dose. In presence of clinical evidence of xerophthalmia, the administration of vitamin A should be considered an emergency as the changes may progress to keratomalacia within hours.

Vitamin K should be administered in a single dose of 2.5 mg intramuscularly at the time of admission. Daily multivitamin supplements containing thiamine 0.5 mg/1000 kcal, riboflavin 0.6 mg/1000 kcal and nicotinic acid (niacin equivalents) 6.6 mg/1000 kcal should be given. It is better to give a formulation that is truly multivitamin (e.g. one that has vitamin A, C, D, E and $B_{12}$). Folic acid 1 mg/day (5 mg on day 1), zinc 2 mg/kg/day and copper 0.2–0.3 mg/kg/day should be given daily. Iron 3 mg/kg/day should be added once child starts gaining weight, after the stabilization phase.

***Emergency treatment of severe anemia:*** If a severely malnourished child has severe anemia with a hemoglobin less than 4 g/dL or between 4 and 6 g/dL but with respiratory distress, a blood transfusion should be given with whole blood 10 mL/kg bodyweight slowly over 3 hours. Furosemide should be given at the start of the transfusion. If the severely anemic child has signs of cardiac failure, packed cells rather than whole blood should be transfused.

The hemoglobin concentration may fall during the first week of treatment. This is normal and no transfusion should be given. In mild to moderate anemia, iron should be given for two months to replete iron stores but this should not be started until after the initial stabilization phase has been completed.

### *Step 7: Initiate Refeeding*

Feeding should be started as soon as possible with a diet which has osmolarity less than 350 mOsm/L; lactose not more than 2–3 g/kg/day; appropriate renal solute load (urinary osmolarity <600 mOsm/L); initial percentage of calories from protein of 5%; adequate bioavailability of micronutrients and low viscosity. The preparation should be easy to prepare and socially acceptable and there should be facilities for adequate storage, cooking and refrigeration.

***Start cautious feeding:*** The suggested starter formulae are usually milk based, such as starter F-75 diet (containing with the starter diet containing 75 kcal/100 mL). The protein content is 0.9 g of protein/100 mL. Feeding should be started with starter diet as soon as possible as frequent small feeds. If child is unable to take orally with a cup and spoon or takes <80% of the target intake, nasogastric feeds should be initiated. Breastfeeding should be continued *ad libitum*. Older children could be started on cereal based diets **(Table 7.13)**.

One should begin with 80 kcal/kg/day and gradually increase to 100 kcal/kg/day. To fulfill this, one should start with 2 hourly feeds of 11 mL/kg/feed. Night feeds are essential. The volume of feeds are increased gradually while decreasing the frequency of administration. The calories are increased only after the child can accept the increased volume of feeds.

### *Step 8: Achieve Catch-up Growth with Catch-up Diet*

For catch-up growth, energy and protein intake has to be enhanced further; starter diet (75 kcal/100 mL) would not be enough. Starter feeds should be gradually replaced with

**Table 7.13:** Starter diets

| *Diet contents (per 100 ml)* | *Starter* | *Starter (cereal based) Example: 1* | *Starter (cereal based) Example: 2* |
|---|---|---|---|
| Cow milk or equivalent (mL) (approximate measure of one katori) | 30 (1/3) | 30 (1/3) | 25 (1/4) |
| Sugar (g) (approximate measure of one level teaspoon) | 9 (1½) | 6 (1) | 3 (1/2) |
| Cereal: Powdered puffed rice* (g) (approximate measure of one level teaspoon) | – | 2.5 (3/4) | 6 (2) |
| Vegetable oil (g) (approximate measure of one level teaspoon) | 2 (1/2) | 2.5 (1/2) | 3 (3/4) |
| Water: Make up to (mL) | 100 | 100 | 100 |
| Energy (kcal) | 75 | 75 | 75 |
| Protein (g) | 0.9 | 1.1 | 1.2 |
| Lactose (g) | 1.2 | 1.2 | 1.0 |

*Powdered puffed rice may be replaced by commercial precooked rice preparations (in same amounts).

Wherever feasible, actual weighing of the constituents should be carried out. Household measure should be used only as an alternative, as they may not be standardized.

The above charts give the composition for 100 mL diet. Wherever, there is a facility for refrigeration, 1 liter diet could be prepared by multiplying the quantity of each constituent by 10.

**Table 7.14:** Catch-up diets

| *Diet contents (per 100 mL)* | *Catch-up* | *Catch-up (cereal based)* |
|---|---|---|
| Cow milk/toned dairy milk (mL) (approximate one katori) | 95 (3/4) | 75 (1/2) |
| Sugar (g) (approximate one level teaspoon) | 5 (1) | 2.5 (1/2) |
| Cereal: Puffed rice (g) (approximate one level teaspoon) | – | 7 (2) |
| Vegetable oil (g) (approximate one level teaspoon) | 2 (1/2) | 2 (1/2) |
| Water to make (mL) | 100 | 100 |
| Energy (kcal) | 101 | 100 |
| Protein (g) | 2.9 | 2.9 |
| Lactose (g) | 3.8 | 3 |

feeds which have a higher calorie density (100 kcal/100 mL) and have at least 2.5–3.0 g protein/100 mL. These feeds are called catch-up diets (Table 7.14).

Once appetite returns, increasing intakes of catch-up diet should be encouraged. It is recommended that each successive feed is increased by 10 mL until some is left uneaten. The frequency of feeds gradually decreased to 6 feeds/day and the volume increased till the child is being offered 200 mL/kg/day of catch-up diet. Breastfeeding should be continued *ad libitum*.

Once the child achieves rapid weight gain, catch-up diet should be changed to energy dense home food.

Home foods should be added as soon as possible to prepare the child for home foods at discharge. They should have comparable energy and protein concentrations once the catch-up diets are well tolerated. Khichri, dalia, banana, curd-rice and other culturally acceptable and locally available diets can also be offered liberally.

***Special diets for diarrhea:*** For children with persistent diarrhea, who do not tolerate low lactose diets, lactose-free diet can be started. In these diets, carbohydrates (rice, sugar and glucose) can be given in varying proportions according to the patients' individual tolerance to achieve optimal balance between osmolarity and digestibility.

***Monitoring progress during treatment:*** If there is a good weight gain of >10 g/kg/day, the same treatment should be continued till recovery. If there is a moderate weight gain of 5–10 g/kg/day, food intake should be checked and the children should be screened for systemic infection. In case of poor weight gain of <5 g/kg/day, possible causes like inadequate feeding, untreated infection, psychological problems and coexisting infections like tuberculosis and HIV should be looked for and managed appropriately.

#### *Step 9: Provide Sensory Stimulation and Emotional Support*

Delayed mental and behavioral development often occurs in severe malnutrition. It is important to encourage a cheerful, stimulating environment; structured play therapy for at least 15–30 min/day; and physical activity as soon as the child is well enough.

#### *Step 10: Prepare for Follow-up*

Ideally, 6–8 weeks of hospitalization is required for optimum recovery. SAM children admitted to hospital can be transferred to outpatient care when their medical complications have settled, edema is resolving and they have a good appetite, they are consuming adequate diet and are clinically well and alert.

The decision to transfer children from inpatient to outpatient care should be determined by their clinical condition and not on the basis of specific anthropometric outcomes such as a specific mid-upper arm circumference or weight-for-height/length.

National guidelines recommend treatment for helminthic infections should be given to all children with SAM before discharge. Give a single oral dose of albendazole 200 mg for children aged 12–23 months, 400 mg for children aged 24 months or older.

### Post-Discharge Care at Home

A child with SAM may be considered to have completed treatment when:

- There is no edema for at least 2 weeks, plus
- Weight-for-height (or length) reaches –2 SDS or higher on WHO growth standard or mid-upper-arm circumference is more than 12.5 cm

After discharge, the principles of care are the same for supervised home care of uncomplicated SAM (as above). This is a very important phase and full support needs to be extended to the family by involving the frontline workers and community. The treatment of the child is not complete till the weight-for-height and MUAC reaches normal range (*see* below).

The caregiver should be advised to bring child back for regular follow-up checks, ensure booster immunizations, make sure that vitamin A is given every 6 months, feed frequently with energy and nutrient dense foods and give structured play therapy.

Until the above is reached, the child must be under constant care at hospital and/or home by a frontline health team. Support to the family must be continued during this phase and after discharge from treatment.

### Severe Acute Malnutrition (SAM): Under 6 Months of Age

Infants less than 6 months of age with SAM and any of the following complications should be admitted for inpatient care:

a. Any serious clinical condition or complication outlined for infants who are 6 months of age or older with SAM
b. Recent weight loss or failure to gain weight
c. Ineffective feeding (attachment, positioning and suckling) directly observed for 15–20 min, ideally in a supervised separated area
d. Pitting edema
e. Medical or social issue needing detailed assessment or support (e.g. disability, depression of the caregiver, or adverse social circumstances)

Infants less than 6 months of age with SAM should receive the same general medical care as infants with severe acute malnutrition who are 6 months of age or older:

a. Infants with SAM who are admitted for inpatient care should be given parenteral antibiotics to treat possible sepsis and appropriate treatment for other medical complications such as tuberculosis, HIV, surgical conditions or disability
b. Infants with SAM who are not admitted should receive a course of broad-spectrum oral antibiotic, such as amoxicillin.

Feeding approaches for infants who are less than 6 months of age should prioritize establishing, or re-establishing, effective exclusive breastfeeding by the mother.

*Infants who are admitted:*

a. Should be breastfed where possible and the mothers should be supported to breastfeed the infants. If an infant is not breastfed, support should be given to the mother to re-lactate.
b. Should also be provided a supplementary feed: Supplementary suckling approaches should, where feasible, be prioritized; for infants with severe acute malnutrition but no edema, expressed breast milk should be given, and, where this is not possible, commercial (generic) infant formula or starter diet or diluted catch-up diet may be given (prepared catch-up should be further diluted by adding 30% water), either alone or as the supplementary feed together with breast milk.
c. Should not be given undiluted catch-up at any time (owing to the high renal solute load and risk of hypernatremic dehydration); prepared catch-up should be further diluted by adding 30% water.
d. If there is no realistic prospect of being breastfed, the infant should be given appropriate and adequate replacement feeds such as commercial (generic) infant formula, with relevant support to enable safe preparation and use, including at home when discharged.
e. Assessment of the physical and mental health status of mothers or caregivers should be promoted and relevant treatment or support provided

Infants less than 6 months of age with SAM and have been admitted to inpatient care can be transferred to outpatient care when:

a. All clinical conditions or medical complications, including edema, are resolved
b. The infant has good appetite, is clinically well and alert
c. Weight gain on either exclusive breastfeeding or replacement feeding is satisfactory, e.g. above the median of the WHO growth velocity standards or more than 5 g/kg/day for at least 3 successive days
d. The infant has been checked for immunizations and other routine interventions, and
e. The mother or caregiver is linked with needed community-based follow-up and support.

## Preventing Undernutrition

Since undernutrition is multifactorial, it can only be prevented through interventions across sectors. Action is required at the individual and societal level **(Panel 2)**.

**Panel 2: Preventing undernutrition in children**

**Individual Level Action**

*Mother*

- Care of the adolescent girl
- Childbirth after 20 years
- Spacing between pregnancies
- No more than 2 children
- Iron and folic acid to ensure good hemoglobin
- Antenatal checks as per national program
- Additional food and micronutrients (especially iron and folic acid) in pregnancy

*Child*

- Initiation of breastfeeding within one hour of birth
- Exclusive breastfeeding for first 6 months, continuing till 2 years or more
- Special support to low birth weight babies for breastfeeding and kangaroo mother care
- Complementary feeding introduction at 6 months
- Optimum intake of food that is balanced, energy-dense and of good quality
- Hygiene, handwashing
- Full immunization especially, measles, BCG, rotavirus, *H. influenzae* and pneumococcal
- Prompt treatment of diarrhea with ORS and zinc
- Prompt treatment of pneumonia and other illnesses
- Growth monitoring and periodic checks

*Adolescent girls*

- Optimum nutrition
- Education in parenting and mothercraft
- Marriage after 18 years of age

**Society Level Action**

- Safe water and sanitation
- Ensuring appropriate nutrition
- Maternity and child care leave to enable women to breastfeed and to take care of infants and children
- Crèches for children of working women
- Promoting breastfeeding at workplace
- Cash support to pregnant and lactating women
- Socioeconomic development, high income, equity
- Education of women and men
- Women empowerment
- Food security at the household level
- Nutrition promoting agriculture

### *Integrated Child Development Services (ICDS)*

The ICDS program seeks to directly reach out to children, below 6 years, especially from vulnerable groups and remote areas. The Scheme provides an integrated approach for converging basic services through community-based workers and helpers. The services are provided at a center called the 'Anganwadi'. A package of six services is provided under the ICDS scheme:

a. Supplementary nutrition for mother and the child. The norms are given in Table 7.15.
b. Immunization of pregnant women and infants.

**Table 7.15:** Norms for supplementary nutrition in ICDS

| *Beneficiaries* | *Energy (kcal)* | *Protein (g)* |
|---|---|---|
| Children (6 to 72 months) | 500 | 12–15 |
| Severely malnourished children (SAM) (6 to 72 months) | 800 | 20–25 |
| Pregnant women and lactating mothers | 600 | 18–20 |

*Source:* http://icds-wcd.nic.in/icds/icds.aspx

c. Nonformal preschool education; stimulating learning.
d. Health check-up. This includes healthcare of children less than 6 years of age, antenatal care of expectant mothers and postnatal care of nursing mothers. These services are provided by the ANM and medical officers under the RCH programme. The various health services include regular health check-ups, immunization, management of malnutrition, treatment of diarrhea, deworming and distribution of simple medicines.
e. Referral services. During health check-ups and growth monitoring, sick or malnourished children are referred to the primary health center or its subcenter.
f. Nutrition and health education. Healthy behaviors and detection and treatment of sickness.

### Suggested Reading


1. Bhandari N, Mohan SB, Bose A, et al. Efficacy of three feeding regimens for home-based management of children with uncomplicated severe acute malnutrition: a randomized trial in India. BMJ Global Health 2016;1:e000144.
2. Dalwai S, Choudhury P, Bavdekar SB, et al. Indian Academy of Pediatrics. Consensus statement of the Indian Academy of Pediatrics on integrated management of severe acute malnutrition. Indian Pediatr 2013;50:399–404.
3. ICMR-National Institute of Nutrition. Nutrient Requirements for Indians. A report of the Expert Group, 2020.
4. National Family Health Survey 5. http://rchiips.org/nfhs/factsheet_NFHS-5.shtml
5. WHO. Guideline updates on the management of severe acute malnutrition in infants and children, 2013.
6. World Health Organization. Technical note Supplementary foods for the management of moderate acute malnutrition in infants and children 6–59 months of age, 2012.


*Competencies:* **PE9.6; PE11.1**

## OVERNUTRITION AND OBESITY

Obesity is defined as the condition of abnormal or excess fat deposition in the body leading to impaired health. In the last 2–3 decades, there has been a steep increase in the incidence of overweight and obesity, not only in adults but also in children and adolescents. Even among the 5–9 years old children, approximately 4% are overweight or obese. In the age group of 10–19 years, the prevalence of overweight or obesity is 5%. Nearly 50–80% of obese children become obese adults, who are at higher risk of diabetes mellitus, hypertension and heart disease.

Prevention of adult obesity and consequential diseases, therefore, rests in averting excessive weight gain in childhood.

### Measuring Overnutrition

The term overnutrition is used loosely to connote higher than normal weight of an individual. Two levels namely, overweight and obesity define a borderline overnutrition state (overnutrition) and overtly abnormal state (obesity). In children below 5 years of age, weight-for-height above +2 SDS deferes overweight and that above +3 SDS is considered as obesity (Table 2.4).

The commonly used measure of overweight and obesity in adults is the body mass index (BMI). Formula for BMI = weight (kg) ÷ height $(m)^2$. The cut off points for overweight and obesity for Indian adults are BMIs of 23 $kg/m^2$ and 27 $kg/m^2$, respectively. In children older than 5 years, threshold for overweight and obesity are defined as BMI SDS or centiles that correspond to adult BMI of 23 $kg/m^2$ and 27 $kg/m^2$, respectively. The approximate corresponding SDS values, in girls and boys, are shown in Table 2.4.

Other measures applicable to overnutrition are: Mid-upper arm circumference (MUAC), skin fold thickness and waist circumference.

### Reasons for Rising Overnutrition in Children

A variety of social, behavior, economic and lifestyle changes combine together to unbalance the intake and expenditure of energy.

i. ***Sedentary habits:*** Children are increasingly leading a sedentary life, more so in urban areas, and particularly among the middle and upper classes. School-going children are preoccupied with studies. Children and adolescents spend significant period of time watching TV, using computer or on the mobile. Outdoor activities and play are diminishing. Playgrounds in schools and open spaces in urban areas have shrunk.
ii. ***Obesogenic food:*** With affluence and commercial promotion, there has been a shift towards consumption of high energy, high fat, sugar and salted foods and beverages which are highly energy dense but usually low in vitamins, minerals and other micronutrients. Examples of such foods are chips, namkeens, French fries, pakoras, samosas, pizzas, burgers and sweets like cake, pastries, burfi, gulab-jamun and rasgulla. These foods , popularly called "fast foods" and "junk foods" are preferred by children and adolescents. Eating large portion sizes and mindless snacking are other contributing factors.

Apart form the above, obesity could be uncommonly caused by endocrine and other disorders. Infants with intrauterine growth retardation are particularly prone to obesity and associated metabolic disturbances in the face of high calorie food intake and lack of physical activity. Discussion of causes, differential diagnosis and management of obesity is covered in Chapter 18.

### Preventing Childhood Overnutrition

#### *Healthy Food*

Children must be encouraged to consume healthy wholesome food. Calorific values of some of the unhealthy food items along with suggestions of healthy meals and snacks are given in Table 7.16.

**Table 7.16:** Food items high in fat and refined carbohydrate and suggested healthy options

| *Food items high in energy* | *Calorie content (kcal)* | *Healthy meal and snack alternatives* |
|---|---|---|
| Samosa (1 medium) | 160 | Fresh whole fruits |
| Vegetable pakora (5 small pieces) | 200 | Steamed idli |
| Kachori (1 small) | 200 | Vegetable uttapam |
| Vegetable patty (1 piece) | 250 | Plain dosa |
| Aloo tikki (1 piece) | 300 | Besan cheela |
| Chicken burger (1 medium) | 500 | Grilled paneer |
| Cheese burger | 330 | Vegetable sandwich |
| Pizza (1 medium slice – big size) | 150–250 | Sprouts with vegetables |
| Cake (1 piece) | 225 | Dhokla |
| Pastry (medium size) | 300 | Salads |
| French fries | 220 (small); 300 (medium); 500 (large) | Fruit yogurt, curd |
| Chocolate (40 g) | 225 | Steamed corn, popcorn without salt and butter |
| Barfi (1 pc) | 100 | Bhelpuri with sprouts |
| Rasgulla (1 pc) | 150 | Fruit chaat |
| Jalebi (1 pc) | 200 | Nuts |
| Rasmalai (40 g) | 250 | Roasted papad |
| Laddo (40 g) | 250 | Roasted cereals |
| Packed juice (200 mL)–mixed fruit juice | 120 | Coconut water, lemonade, lassi, chhach, lime juice, milk, rasam |
| Cola (250 mL) | 105 | |
| Soft drinks (250 mL) | 94 | |
| Maida noodles, white bread<br>Processed cheese, butter chicken, meat in gravy, etc. | Variable | Multigrain bread instead of white bread, grilled cheese, soya nuggets, grilled fish or chicken |
| Junk meal–medium coke, medium French fries and medium cheese burger | 700 kcal | |

Introduce the healthy plate concept (Fig 7.3). Teach healthy food choices to parents and children. Mindful eating with proper chewing without distraction should be encouraged. Follow proper regular mealtimes; skipping meals is harmful. Equally harmful is frequent and excessive snacks. Breakfast should not be skipped.

### *Physical Activity*

Physical activity in children is important for maintaining weight, good bones and overall good health. Promotion of physical activity during childhood years should be considered as the top public health priority. It is recommended (NIN, 2020) that children should engage in moderately intense physical activity at least one hour per day. This need not be carried out at a stretch and can be accumulated in bouts of 10–20 minutes.

Participation in games, yoga and sports activities should be encouraged. Excessive TV viewing, video games, social media habits and use of computers should be restricted by parents and teachers. Physical education should be compulsory in schools and college curricula. Children may be encouraged to participate in household chores. Healthy and optimum sleep is also crucial.

Approximate energy expenditure in various physical activities are sumarized in Table 7.17.

**Table 7.17:** Approximate energy expenditure in various physical activities

| *Physical activity* | *Approximate energy expenditure* |
|---|---|
| Playing badminton for 1 hour | 250 kcal |
| Swimming for 1 hour | 330 kcal |
| Dancing for 1 hour | 200 kcal |
| Football for 1 hour | 350 kcal |
| Basketball for 1 hour | 350 kcal |
| Jogging for ½ hour (3 km) | 300 kcal |
| Lawn tennis (singles) for 1 hour | 300 kcal |
| Brisk walking for 2 km | 160 kcal |
| Bicycling for 1½ hours | 250 kcal |

## Calorie Restricted Diets in Obese Children

Unlike management of obesity in adults, calorie restriction is not usually recommended in younger children (<7 years). Focus should be on promoting healthy eating pattern and enforcing learned behaviour.

Older children and adolescents may benefit from calorie-restricted diet if BMI >95th centile or in presence of co-morbid conditions. Calorie-restricted diet (between 1200–1800 kcal/day) based on age and activity can be used. Reduction of calories below 1200 kcal/day is not recommended. It is necessary to involve all family members in supporting the child, and be consistent regarding counseling.

Chapter

8

# Micronutrients in Health and Disease

Rajni Sharma

In Chapter 7, we learnt about 'macronutrients' the major components of diet such as carbohydrates, protein and fat that are essential for energy provision and body structure. Micronutrients (vitamins and minerals) are also essential dietary components required for maintenance of health but in smaller amounts. Vitamins are organic compounds required for normal physiological processes. With few exceptions, they are not synthesized in the body and must be obtained from the diet. Vitamins can be categorized into fat-soluble (A, D, E, K) and water-soluble forms (B complex vitamins, C and folate). The former control protein synthesis at either transcriptional or post-transcriptional level and perform diverse biochemical functions, as hormones (e.g. vitamin D), antioxidants (e.g. vitamin E) and regulators of tissue growth and differentiation (e.g. vitamin A). Several vitamins (e.g. B complex vitamins) are precursors for cofactors of enzyme activity (coenzymes) in various metabolic pathways.

Certain minerals are essential to support biochemical processes involved in cell structure and function. The amount of mineral required varies from >100 mg/day (major minerals including calcium, magnesium, sodium, potassium, chloride, and phosphorus) to <100 mg/day (trace minerals including iron, copper, zinc). Ultra-trace minerals are required in miniscule amounts (<1 mg/day) and include iodine, chromium, selenium, cobalt, manganese, molybdenum, fluorine, boron and nickel. Deficiencies of micronutrients are common in specific high-risk groups and result in various deficiency diseases.

Dietary requirements and recommended intakes of various micronutrients for Indians have been published by the Indian Council of Medical Research-National Institute of Nutrition in 2020 (available at www.nin.res.in).

**Box 8.1: Breast-milk and Vitamins**

Breast-milk is the complete food for infants. However, it is deficient in vitamins D and K. Breast-milk contains only 30–40 IU/L of vitamin D whereas the RDA is much higher in infants predisposing exclusively breastfed children to its deficiency. Exclusively breastfed babies require vitamin D supplementation at the dose of 400 IU per day. As vitamin K is produced by the gut microflora, it may take sometime for a newborn gut to be colonized by bacteria and start producing vitamin K of its own. Thus, all babies should receive vitamin K at birth to prevent hemorrhagic disease of the newborn.

## FAT-SOLUBLE VITAMINS

*Competencies:* **PE12.1; PE12.2; PE12.3; PE12.4; PE12.5**

### Vitamin A

Vitamin A (retinol) is derived from natural plant pigments called carotenoids (provitamin A) that are converted to retinol in the body and stored as retinol palmitate in the liver. Retinol is further converted to the active forms of vitamin A: Retinal and retinoic acid. Being a fat-soluble vitamin, vitamin A is absorbed in the intestine as a part of chylomicrons.

#### Physiological Functions

***Night vision:*** Retinol is converted to retinal which plays an important role in vision especially night vision. Within the eye, 11-*cis*-retinal (an isomer of retinal) is bound to the visual proteins called opsins to form rhodopsin. As light enters the eye, 11-*cis*-retinal is isomerized to the all-*trans* form. The all-*trans*-retinal dissociates from the opsins in a series of steps called bleaching. This isomerization induces a nervous signal along the optic nerve to the visual center of the brain. Subsequently, the all-*trans*-retinal is recycled and converted to 11-*cis*-retinal form via a series of enzymatic reactions. Deficiency in vitamin A inhibits the reformation of rhodopsin and leads to night blindness.

***Growth:*** Retinal and its derivative retinoic acid bind to their intracellular receptor, regulate gene expression and induce the synthesis of proteins involved in growth and cell differentiation.

***Maintenance of epithelial tissue:*** Retinol is also required for production of glycoproteins and mucus and down-regulation of keratin synthesis. Vitamin A deficiency leads to drying of epithelial surfaces and excessive keratin formation of the surface. A break in the epithelial integrity of the cornea predisposes to infections.

### Sources

Carotenoids (provitamin A) are found in green and yellow plants including carrots, dark-green leafy vegetables, squash, oranges and tomatoes. β-carotene is the major carotenoid found in plants. Animal sources such as liver, shark/cod liver oil, egg yolk, whole milk and butter are good sources of preformed vitamin A (retinol). Many processed foods and infant formulas are fortified with preformed vitamin A.

### Recommended Daily Allowance

The recommended daily allowance of vitamin A is as follows: (i) Infants 300–400 μg; (ii) children 400–600 μg; (iii) adolescents 750 μg; (iv) pregnant women 800 μg. 1 μg retinol equivalent (RE) = 3.3 international units (IU) of vitamin A. Hence, 30 mg retinol = 100,000 IU vitamin A.

### Vitamin A Deficiency

Mild vitamin A deficiency manifests with follicular hyperkeratosis of the skin that consists of rough skin with raised hyperkeratotic patches resembling toad skin **(Fig. 8.1a)**. Defective dark adaptation is a characteristic early clinical feature, resulting in night blindness. The ocular epithelium becomes dry (xerophthalmia) **(Table 8.1)** and hyperkeratinized with the appearance of small foam-like silvery lesions on the conjunctiva (Bitot's spots) **(Fig. 8.1b)**. More severe deficiency leads to hyperkeratinization of the cornea with the appearance of corneal opacity, which can progress to ulceration and infection (keratomalacia) **(Fig. 8.2)**. In developing countries, vitamin A deficiency is the leading cause of blindness in preschool children. Due to loss of mucosal integrity of the respiratory, gastrointestinal tracts and impaired immunity, children with vitamin A deficiency are at high risk of contracting severe systemic infections especially measles with higher risk of mortality.

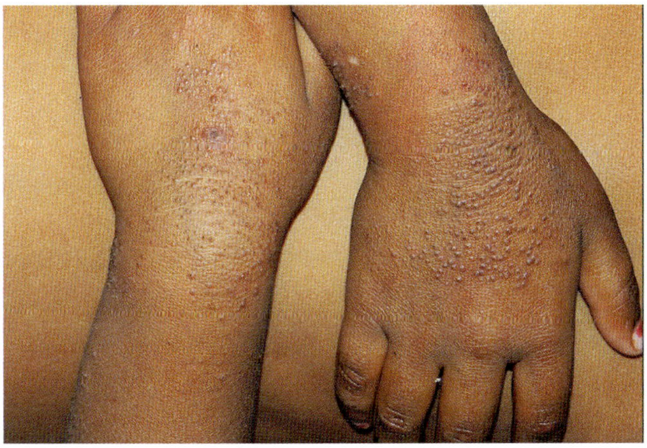

**Fig. 8.1a:** Follicular hyperkeratosis due to vitamin A deficiency (*Courtesy:* Prof M Ramam, AIIMS, New Delhi)

**Table 8.1:** WHO classification of xerophthalmia

| *Primary signs* | *Secondary signs* |
|---|---|
| X1A Conjunctival xerosis | XN Night blindness |
| X1B Bitot's spots | XF Fundal changes |
| X2 Corneal xerosis | XS Corneal scarring |
| X3A Corneal ulceration (<1/3 of cornea) | |
| X3B Corneal ulceration (>1/3 of cornea) | |

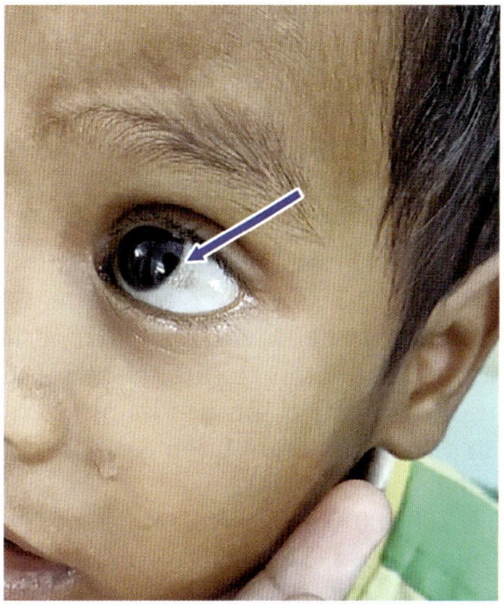

**Fig. 8.1b:** Bitot's spot showing foamy, frothy, sharply demarcated whitish spot on the temporal side of bulbar conjunctiva (blue arrow). It is formed by keratinization of the epithelium and accumulation of mucus, bacteria, and debris on the surface (*Courtesy:* Prof Praveen Kumar, KSCH, New Delhi)

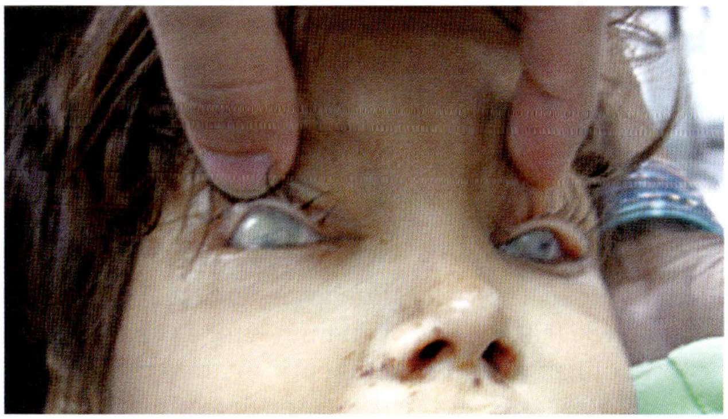

**Fig. 8.2:** Bilateral keratomalacia in a child with severe vitamin A deficiency precipitated by an episode of pneumonia. Note the bilateral corneal opacification and corneal perforation in the left eye

***High-risk groups:*** Malnourished children and those with fat malabsorption (celiac disease and liver disease) are predisposed to vitamin A deficiency. Laboratory tests may show low serum retinol level of 15 μg/dL or less (normal 20 to 80 μg/dL) but are not essential for diagnosis.

***Treatment of vitamin A deficiency:*** Specific treatment consists of oral vitamin A at a dose of 50,000 IU, 100,000 IU and 200,000 IU in children aged <6 months, 6–12 months and >1 year, respectively. The same dose is repeated the next day and 4 weeks later. Alternatively, parenteral water-soluble preparations are administered in children with persistent vomiting or severe malabsorption (parenteral dose is half the oral dose for children above 6–12 months and 75% in <6 months old). Clouding of the cornea in a child with vitamin A deficiency is an emergency and requires parenteral administration of 50,000 to 100,000 IU (15 to 30 mg retinol). In cases of keratomalacia, local treatment with antibiotic drops and ointment and padding of the eye enhances healing.

***Prevention:*** Vitamin A deficiency is a public health problem in India (Bitot's spots in preschool children ≥0.5%) with reported prevalence of xerophthalmia of 5–20% in school-going children. The Ministry of Health and Family Welfare initiated the 'National Prophylaxis Program against Nutritional Blindness' in 1970. According to this scheme, children between 9 months and 3 years were given oral doses of vitamin A every six months. It was later expanded to cover children of ages 6–59 months. Under this program, a dose of vitamin A 100,000 IU is given with measles vaccine at 9 months and 200,000 IU with the DPT booster at 15–18 months and then 6 monthly till the age of 5 years. Dietary diversification with inclusion of vitamin A rich food is necessary to prevent vitamin A deficiency in the long run. Children with measles or severe malnutrition should receive vitamin A at 100,000 IU, if <1-year-old and 200,000 IU, if older. Vitamin A supplementation significantly decreases the risk of mortality in children with measles.

### *Carotenemia*

Beta-carotene is an important precursor of vitamin A in vegetable-based diets; 10 µg β-carotene has the biological potency of 1 µg retinol. Excessive dietary intake of carotene containing foods, most commonly carrots, can lead to deposition of carotenoids in keratin and subcutaneous fat. At high plasma levels, yellow pigmentation (carotenemia) shows in superficial skin (face, palms and soles), but not in sclerae. The color returns to normal within 2–6 weeks of discontinuing intake of carrots.

### *Hypervitaminosis A and Teratogenicity*

Vitamin A toxicity may occur with ingestion of large doses more than 50,000 IU/day of vitamin A for several weeks in the form of fish liver oil, therapeutic vitamin preparations or, in adolescents, topical retinol or retinoic acid for acne. Acute manifestations include pseudotumor cerebri (vomiting, irritability, bulging fontanel, diplopia, headache). Patients with chronic hypervitaminosis may have anorexia, dry skin, alopecia, painful joints and hepatosplenomegaly. Vitamin A is teratogenic, if taken in high doses in early gestation. The WHO recommends that vitamin A intake during pregnancy for treating deficiency should not exceed a daily dose of 10,000 IU (3000 µg RE) per day or weekly 25,000 IU (7500 µg RE).

*Competencies:* **PE12.6; PE12.7; PE12.8; PE12.9; PE12.10**

## Vitamin D

Vitamin $D_3$ is produced in the skin on exposure to sunlight, or available through ingestion of vitamin D-rich food like fatty fish, fish oils and vitamin-D fortified milk/milk products. Under normal conditions, endogenous synthesis of vitamin D is sufficient to meet the body's requirement.

### *Metabolism and Mechanism of Action*

There are two forms of vitamin D: Cholecalciferol (vitamin $D_3$, made in animals) and ergocalciferol (vitamin $D_2$, made in fungi/plants). Vitamin $D_3$ is synthesized from 7-dehydrocholesterol in the skin upon exposure to ultraviolet B (UVB) radiation of wavelength 290–315 nm. It is bound to vitamin D-binding protein and transported to the liver where it is converted to 25-hydroxyvitamin D (25-OHD, 25-α calcidiol) by the enzyme 25-α hydroxylase. Vitamins $D_2$ and $D_3$, that are derived from diet are similarly transported to the liver and converted to the 25-hydroxy form. Being a fat-soluble vitamin, vitamin D absorption is decreased in conditions of fat malabsorption such as chronic pancreatitis, cystic fibrosis, etc.

25-OHD is stored in the liver and released into the bloodstream. It is the major circulatory form of vitamin D, with a long biological half-life of approximately 3 weeks. Due to this, 25-OHD is taken as the biochemical marker for vitamin D levels in the body. It undergoes further hydroxylation in the kidneys by the enzyme 1-hydroxylase to form 1,25-dihydroxyvitamin D [1,25$(OH)_2$D, calcitriol], the active form of vitamin D which mediates its actions via the vitamin D receptor. The activity of 1-α hydroxylase enzyme is increased by high parathyroid hormone or low phosphate levels. On th other hand, its activity is decreased by FGF-23 (Fig. 8.3).

The main physiological role of calcitriol is the maintenance of calcium homeostasis through its action on the intestine and bones. In the intestine, it increases absorption of dietary calcium and phosphate by the enterocytes. In the bone, it stimulates osteoclastic reabsorption of bone (release of calcium) and its proper mineralization. Thus, the overall effect of calcitriol is to increase the serum levels of calcium.

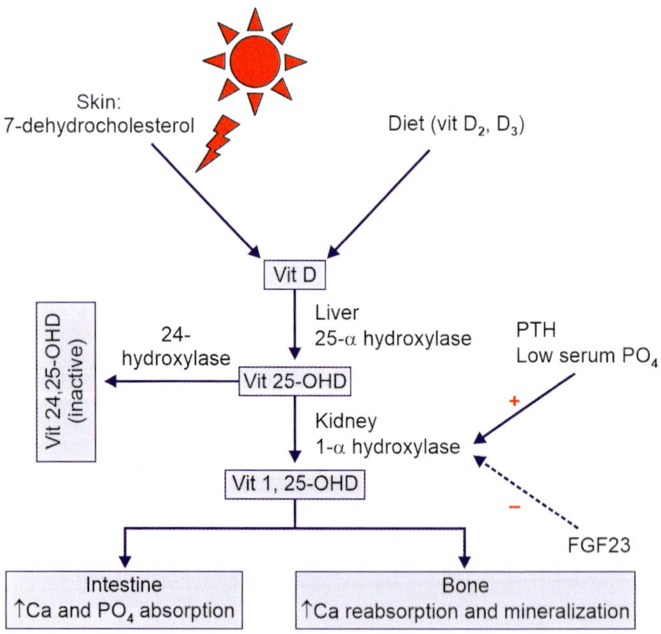


**Fig. 8.3:** Vitamin D metabolism

### Recommended Daily Allowance

The daily requirement of vitamin D is 10 μg (400 IU) per day in infants and 15 μg (600 IU) per day in children >1 year age.

### Sources

Endogenous production of vitamin D generally suffices to fulfill the nutritional requirements of vitamin D. Dietary sources include fish and fish oils, liver, egg yolk, mushrooms and vitamin D fortified milk/milk products. Natural diet contains very little vitamin D and dietary supplementation is essential to prevent deficiency when endogenous production is inadequate.

### Vitamin D Deficiency

Adequate vitamin D synthesis in the skin depends on various extrinsic factors that affect the amount of UVB radiation reaching the skin such as the time of the day, latitude, season, cloud cover and presence of air pollutants, as well as intrinsic factors such as area of skin exposed (amount of clothing), use of sunscreens and time spent outdoors **(Box 8.2)**. The dermal pigment melanin decreases the amount of UVB rays that reach the epidermal layers containing the substrate, 7-dehydrocholesterol. Hence, individuals with dark skin require more duration of sun exposure to make the same amount of vitamin D. Daily sunlight exposure of 17–30 minutes in infants and 30–45 minutes in older children over 15–40% body surface area at least five times a week during noon (11 AM to 3 PM) is recommended to prevent vitamin D deficiency.

### High-Risk Groups for Vitamin D Deficiency

The risk factors that predispose to vitamin D deficiency include limited exposure to sunlight, predominant indoor living due to any reason including debilitation or disability or full body clothing due to cultural or religious beliefs. Certain groups are at high risk of vitamin D deficiency. These include patients on anticonvulsant drugs (phenytoin, phenobarbitone, carbamazepine) or antitubercular therapy (isoniazid, rifampicin). These medications are hepatic p450 enzyme inducers and increase the metabolism of 25-OHD in the liver into inactive metabolites leading to low serum levels.

Breast milk is a poor source of vitamin D containing only 30–40 IU per liter and exclusively breastfed infants can develop vitamin D deficiency, unless adequately supplemented. Exclusively breastfed babies should receive 400 IU of supplemental vitamin D per day. Formula milk has 400 IU of vitamin D per litre; infants getting less than 1 litre formula per day also require supplementation.

### Pathophysiology of Vitamin D Deficiency

Vitamin D deficiency leads to decreased absorption of calcium in the gut and low serum calcium. The hormone PTH, secreted by the parathyroid glands, is the main regulator of serum calcium in the body. The parathyroid gland and kidneys have calcium-sensing receptors (CaSR), which are activated by serum calcium. When serum calcium is low, the CaSR stimulates the parathyroid glands to release increased amounts of PTH. PTH helps to restore serum calcium levels back to normal through its action on bones and kidney. Serum alkaline phosphatase levels are raised due to increased bone turnover. In the kidney, PTH activates renal 1α-hydroxylase and increases calcitriol synthesis. However, high PTH also increases phosphate excretion from kidney leading to urinary losses and low serum phosphate levels. Low phosphate levels are characteristic of vitamin D deficiency and lead to various manifestations of vitamin D deficiency including metabolic bone disease (see below) and muscle weakness. When vitamin D levels are very low or there is a simultaneous dietary calcium deficiency, even high PTH fails to compensate and restore serum calcium levels leading to hypocalcemia that can manifest with tetany or seizures.

### Assessment of Vitamin D Status

Serum levels of 25-OHD are used to assess vitamin D status **(Box 8.3)**. There is controversy regarding the cutoff values that should be used to define vitamin D sufficiency in adults. In children, the consensus guidelines defined vitamin D sufficiency as that level which is optimal to prevent rickets (serum 25-OHD >20 ng/mL). Vitamin D deficiency is defined by the level below which there is a compensatory increase in serum PTH and bone health is likely to be affected (serum 25-OHD <12 ng/mL), whereas insufficiency (serum 25-OHD 12–20 ng/mL) may affect bone health in the presence of other risk factors, such as low calcium intake.

### Hypervitaminosis D

Excessive vitamin D due to overdosage can result in hypervitaminosis D (serum levels >100 ng/mL). This can result in hypercalcemia and hypercalciuria increasing the risk of renal stones and nephrocalcinosis. Other manifestations of hypercalcemia include anorexia, vomiting, constipation, renal insufficiency, polyuria and hypertension. Such an "epidemic of hypercalcemia" was reported in England in the 1950s due to high dose vitamin D supplementation (between 2,000 and 3,000 IU/day) given for several months.

**Box 8.2 Factors Affecting Cutaneous Vitamin D Synthesis**

| *Extrinsic* | *Intrinsic* |
|---|---|
| Time of day | Time spent outdoors |
| Season | Skin area exposed (clothing) |
| Latitude | Skin pigmentation |
| Air pollutants | Use of sunscreens |

**Box 8.3 Serum Vitamin D Levels**

| | | |
|---|---|---|
| Deficient | <12 ng/mL | <25 nmol/L |
| Insufficient | 12–20 ng/mL | 25–50 nmol/L |
| Sufficient | >20 ng/mL | >50 nmol/L |
| Toxic | >100 ng/mL | >250 nmol/L |

Competencies: **PE12.7; PE12.8; PE12.9**

## RICKETS

Rickets is a metabolic disease of growing bones, hence seen only in children. It is derived from the word 'wrickets' meaning 'twisted' referring to the characteristic bony deformities or 'bow legs' of rickets. The most common cause of rickets is nutritional deficiency of vitamin D and/or calcium. Osteomalacia (soft bones) refers to undermineralization of the organic content of bone (osteoid), and is a feature of rickets as well as adult vitamin D deficiency. It should be distinguished from the term 'osteoporosis' used for overall decrease in bone mass (both mineral and organic content), most commonly seen in patients on prolonged corticosteroid therapy.

### Pathophysiology

In growing children, the metaphyseal ends of long bones are separated from the bony epiphyses by the cartilaginous growth plate. The cartilage cells (chondrocytes) of the growth plate undergo progressive maturation from the epiphyses to the metaphyses. The chondrocytes in the resting zone proliferate and undergo hypertrophy. Hypertrophied chondrocytes then undergo apoptosis followed by angiogenesis, invasion of bone forming cells (zone of provisional calcification) and replacement with mineralized bone. An adequate amount of phosphate is essential for the apoptosis of the chondrocytes. In the absence of adequate phosphate, the chondrocytes continue to hypertrophy and this leads to the characteristic hypertrophic swellings at the growth plates seen in rickets. Low levels of serum phosphate and calcium also lead to undermineralization of the bones leading to osteomalacia and tendency of weight-bearing bones to get bent.

### Etiology of Rickets (Table 8.2)

Rickets is broadly classified as calcipenic or phosphopenic forms. The unifying mechanism of all forms of rickets is an underlying phosphate deficiency. Calcipenic rickets is associated with low-normal calcium, high PTH levels (and secondary phosphate deficiency), whereas in phosphopenic rickets, there is primary defect in phosphate metabolism and normal PTH levels.

### Nutritional Rickets

Nutritional rickets due to vitamin D deficiency is the leading cause of rickets. Though nutritional rickets had once been virtually eradicated in developed nations by fortification of milk or direct administration of vitamin D, recent reports indicate its resurgence in exclusively breastfed infants especially immigrants and those who not get vitamin D supplements. Apart from insufficient exposure to sunlight and poor dietary intake, vitamin D deficiency may result from various malabsorption syndromes, chronic liver disease and use of anticonvulsant or antitubercular drugs.

Nutritional rickets may also occur secondary to severe dietary deficiency of calcium that can occur with or without concomitant vitamin D deficiency. Calcium deficiency rickets is commonly encountered in African countries where there is a high consumption of starchy food with low dairy intakes. Children with vitamin D deficiency are more likely to develop rickets, if they also have low dietary calcium intake.

#### *Clinical Features* (Box 8.4)

Children generally persent with knee deformities, motor delay and waddling gait. The classical features of rickets include swellings of the wrist and ankles and leg deformities in the form of bow-legs (genu varum) or knock-knees (genu valgum) (Fig. 8.4). The lateral malleolus of the ankles has two bony prominences instead of one (called the double-malleoli sign). From head to toe, the following signs may be seen: frontal bossing, delayed closure of anterior fontanelle, craniotabes (soft skull bones with ping-pong ball consistency), delayed dentition and enamel hypoplasia. The anterior chest wall may have a beaded appearance due to swelling of costochondral cartilage junctions (rachitic

**Table 8.2:** Etiological classification of rickets

| *Calcipenic rickets* | *Phosphopenic rickets* |
|---|---|
| **Nutritional vitamin D deficiency**<br>• Reduced cutaneous synthesis<br>• Exclusively breastfed infants<br>• Malabsorption, chronic liver disease; use of anticonvulsants | **Dietary phosphate deficiency**<br>• Prematurity<br>• Total parenteral nutrition<br>• Aluminum-containing antacids |
| **Nutritional calcium deficiency**<br>• Restricted intake of dairy products<br>• Prematurity | **Renal phosphate wasting (FGF23 dependent)**<br>• Familial hypophosphatemic rickets (X-linked/autosomal recessive/ autosomal dominant)<br>• Tumor-induced osteomalacia<br>• Linear nevus sebaceous syndrome<br>• McCune-Albright syndrome |
| **Non-nutritional**<br>• Vitamin D dependent rickets type 1 (1α-hydroxylase deficiency)<br>• Vitamin D dependent rickets type 2 (end-organ resistance) | **Renal phosphate wasting (non-FGF23 dependent)**<br>• Hereditary hypophosphatemic rickets with hypercalciuria<br>• Fanconi syndrome (proximal renal tubular acidosis) |
| **Others**<br>• Chronic kidney disease<br>• Distal renal tubular acidosis | |

**Box 8.4: Clinical Features Requiring Assessment in Rickets**

***History***

- Onset and progress of bony deformities
- Symptoms of hypocalcemia: Tetany, seizures; motor delay
- Sunlight exposure
- Malabsorption: Chronic diarrhea; liver disease
- Kidney disease: Polyuria, undernutrition
- Medications: Anticonvulsants, antitubercular, antacids
- Family history of similar disease
- Intake of calcium (dairy products); vitamin D supplements

***Examination***

- Craniotabes, open anterior fontanelle in infants
- Frontal bossing
- Delayed dentition
- Enamel hypoplasia; dental abscesses
- Rachitic rosary, Harrison sulcus
- Wrist widening
- Lower limb deformities; double malleoli
- Jaundice, other features of liver disease
- Anemia, hypertension
- Eye examination (intraocular pressure; lens; fundus exam)

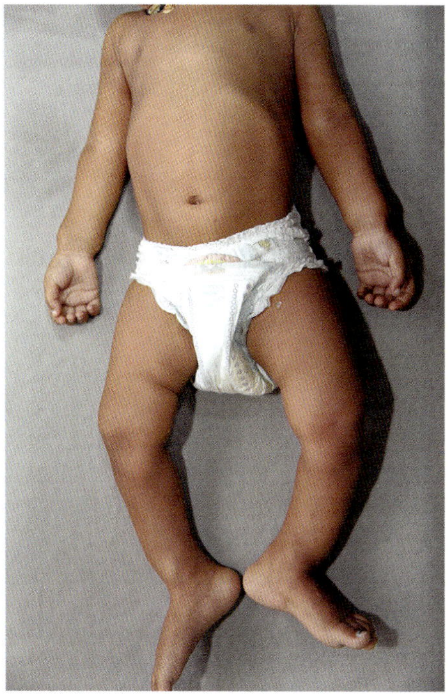

**Fig. 8.4:** A 15-month-old boy with nutritional rickets. Note the wrist widening, rachitic rosary, anterolateral blowing of legs and prominent malleoli

rosary). A depression may be evident along the lower border of the chest at the site of insertion of the diaphragm (Harrison sulcus) which appears due to the pull of the diaphragm on the weakened chest wall. The abdomen is protuberant due to lax abdominal muscles. Other features of rickets include tetany, failure to thrive and irritability. Rarely, severe vitamin deficiency and hypocalcemia can affect cardiac muscle function resulting in cardiomyopathy and congestive heart failure. There is an increased risk of fracture even with minimal trauma. Pelvic deformities lead to outlet narrowing, which can be troublesome in females at a later age due to the risk of obstructed labor.

### Evaluation

The initial evaluation includes blood biochemistry (calcium, phosphate, alkaline phosphatase, creatinine and albumin) and radiographs of the wrists and knee joints. The measurement of vitamin D and PTH is optional in a suspected case of nutritional rickets. Serum calcium may be normal or low, with low serum phosphate and high alkaline phosphatase. 25-OHD levels are low, and PTH levels are high (Table 8.3).

Radiologic changes are characteristically seen at the metaphysis. The first change is loss of normal zone of provisional calcification adjacent to the metaphysis seen as a blurring or a frayed appearance of the metaphyseal margin. Cartilage hypertrophy leads to widening of the growth plate giving the appearance of cupping and widening of metaphyseal ends (splaying) (Fig. 8.5a, b). Weight-bearing and stress on uncalcified bone gives rise to bowing of limbs. Eventually, a generalized reduction in bone density is seen (osteopenia on radiographs).

**Table 8.3:** Biochemical findings in rickets

| *Etiology of rickets* | *Calcium* | *Phosphate* | *Alkaline phosphatase* | *25-OHD* | *PTH* | *1,25(OH)₂D* | *Urine calcium* |
|---|---|---|---|---|---|---|---|
| Nutritional vitamin D deficiency | N or ↓ | ↓ | ↑ | ↓↓ | ↑ | ↓ /N/↓ | ↓ |
| Nutritional calcium deficiency | N or ↓ | ↓ | ↑ | N | ↑ | ↑ | ↓ |
| Vitamin D dependent rickets* | N or ↓ | ↓ | ↑ | N | ↑ | ↓; ↑↑ | N or ↓ |
| Familial hypophosphatemic rickets | N | ↓ | ↑ | N | N | ↓ | N |
| Hypophosphatemic rickets with hypercalciuria | N | ↓ | ↑ | N | N | ↑ | ↑ |
| Fanconi syndrome | N | ↓ | ↑ | N | N | N | N or ↑ |
| Distal renal tubular acidosis | N or ↓ | N or ↓ | ↑ | N | N or ↓ | N | N or ↑ |
| Chronic kidney disease–mineral bone disease | N or ↓ | ↑ | ↑ | N | ↑ | ↓ | ↓ or N |

*Patients with type 1 or type 2 disease are distinguished by elevated levels of $1,25(OH)_2D$ in the latter

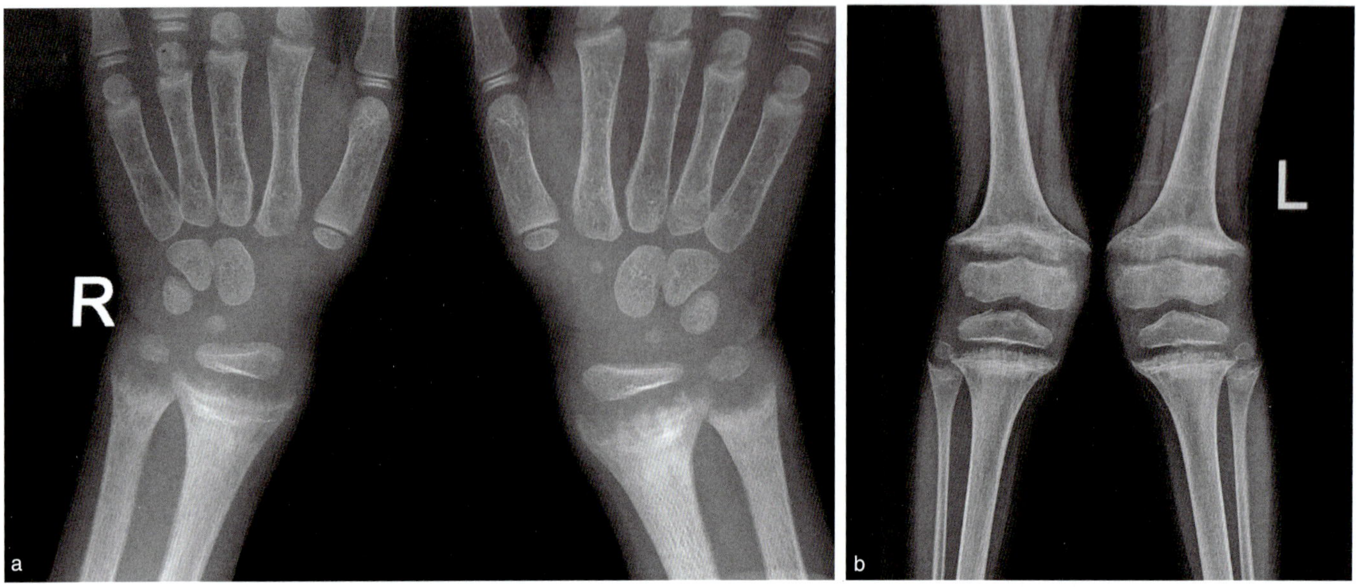


**Fig. 8.5:** (a) Radiograph of wrists in a 4-yr-old boy showing widening, cupping and fraying of metaphysis of both forearm bones. There is wide unossified cartilage (physis); (b) Similar lower limb findings as above in an older girl with hypophosphatemic rickets. Note the wide and frayed metaphyseal ends of both femora and tibia

### *Management*

Treatment of nutritional rickets requires administration of high doses of vitamin D. Previously rickets was treated by mega-doses of vitamin D (also called Stoss therapy), which consisted of a single oral or intramuscular bolus dose of 600000 units or 60,000 IU daily for 10 days. However, such a therapy was observed to lead to high serum calcium levels, hypercalciuria and the risk of nephrocalcinosis. According to current guidelines, lower daily doses of cholecalciferol $D_3$ taken over a period of 12 weeks is a safer and more effective way to treat rickets **(Table 8.4)**. Alternatively, higher doses (60,000 IU) can be given as fortnightly therapy in patients with suspected noncompliance to daily therapy. Oral calcium supplements (30–75 mg/kg/day, maximum 500 mg) should be given to all patients for 2 months. Following adequate therapy, most patients with vitamin D deficiency rickets show radiological evidence of healing within 4 weeks. This consists of a white dense line of calcification (white line of healing) in the metaphyses of wrist bones **(Fig. 8.6)**. Reduction in blood levels of alkaline phosphatase and resolution of clinical signs occur slowly. The X-ray and blood biochemistry should be rechecked after completion of therapy. If radiologic healing or biochemical improvement is not demonstrated, despite adequate therapy, patients should be evaluated for refractory rickets **(Fig. 8.7)**.

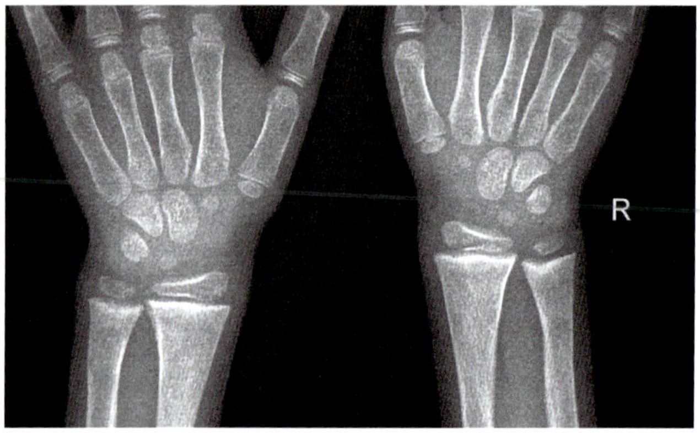


**Fig. 8.6:** Healing of the growth plate following vitamin D therapy

### *Prevention*

For prevention of rickets, all breastfed infants (or those taking less than 1 liter formula milk) should get

**Table 8.4:** Treatment guidelines for nutritional rickets

| *Age* | *Daily dose of vitamin $D_3$ for 12 wks*[a] | *Alternative intermittent dose regimen*[b] | *Daily calcium supplementation*[c] | *Daily maintenance dose*[d] |
|---|---|---|---|---|
| <6 months | 2000 IU | Not recommended | 30–75 mg/kg/day | 400 IU |
| 6–12 months | 2000 IU | Equivalent of 2000 IU/ day may be given on a weekly or monthly basis | 30–75 mg/kg/day | 400 IU |
| >12 months | 3000 IU | 60,000 IU every 2 weeks for 5 doses | 30–75 mg/kg/day (up to 500 mg) | 600 IU |

[a]Reassess after 12 weeks
[b]In certain situations where compliance to daily therapy is doubtful, alternative regimen can be given (only above 6 months of age)
[c]Maximum 500 mg per day
[d]Ensure daily intake of maintenance dose after completion of therapy through diet or supplementation.
Indian Academy of Pediatrics. Indian Pediatrics 2022;5:142.

400 IU/day, from birth to 12 months of age. High-risk groups for vitamin D deficiency (malabsorption, chronic liver disease or anticonvulsant therapy) should be supplemented with 600–800 IU cholecalciferol to prevent development of rickets.

### Refractory Rickets

Rickets that does not respond to the usual treatment of nutritional rickets is called refractory rickets **(Box 8.5)**. The diagnosis is made in patients with no radiological healing after vitamin D therapy. It can be broadly classified into two categories: Defects in vitamin D metabolism (calcipenic) and low phosphate disorders (phosphopenic). **Figure 8.7** outlines the approach to a case of refractory rickets.

#### *Vitamin D Dependent Rickets (VDDR)*

These are rare autosomal recessive forms of rickets due to inherited defects in vitamin D metabolism with early onset of disease in infants between 3 and 6 months of age.

***VDDR type I:*** This condition arises due to a deficiency of the enzyme, 1α-hydroxylase. Blood levels of 25-$OHD_3$ are normal but those of 1,25$(OH)_2$D are markedly decreased. It is characterized by low to normal serum calcium, low phosphate, elevated alkaline phosphatase and high PTH. The clinical features are similar to vitamin D deficiency rickets and include hypotonia, growth failure, motor retardation (poor head control, delayed standing and walking) and convulsions due to hypocalcemia. Physical examination shows frontal bossing, widely open anterior fontanelle, rachitic rosary, thickening of wrists and ankles, bony deformities and positive Trousseau and Chvostek signs. Dentition is delayed and development of tooth enamel is impaired.

The initial treatment of VDDR type I consists of supplementation of supraphysiological doses of 1-α OHD (1-alphacalcidiol) or 1,25$(OH)_2$D (1–2 μg daily) with oral calcium (30–50 mg/kg). Serum calcium levels rise and radiological healing occurs within 6 to 8 weeks. Thereafter, supplementation with physiological doses of 1α-hydroxy $D_3$ (1-alphacalcidiol) or 1,25$(OH)_2$D (0.25 μg daily) is continued lifelong.

***VDDR type II:*** It arises due to vitamin D receptor mutation and end organ resistance to 1,25$(OH)_2$D. Serum levels of 1,25$(OH)_2$D are markedly raised. Clinical features of rickets appear in early infancy and are characterized by hypocalcemia, secondary hyperparathyroidism, and an absence of response to vitamin D or its analogs. Other features of VDDR type II include alopecia and ectodermal defects (oligodontia, milia and epidermal cysts). The response to treatment in these patients is not satisfactory. An occasional patient may get clinical, biochemical improvement and radiological healing following long-term administration of large amounts of intravenous or oral calcium.

**Box 8.5: Pointers to Non-nutritional Rickets**

- History of polyuria; polydipsia; preference for savory foods
- Marked stunting; undernutrition
- Onset in early infancy
- Alopecia, epidermal cyst, milia
- History of tetany, seizures
- Family history of rickets
- Non-response to standard treatment of rickets
- Normal levels of 25-hydroxycholecalciferol (25-OHD)

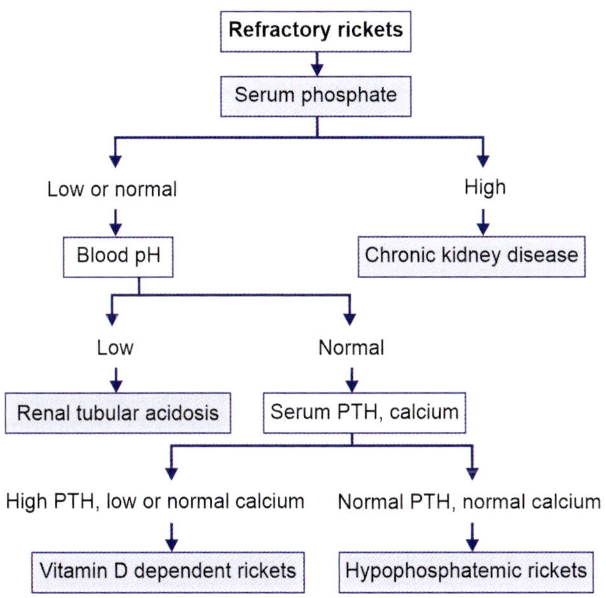


**Fig. 8.7:** Biochemical evaluation of a child with refractory rickets

#### *Phosphopenic Rickets*

Phosphopenic rickets arises mostly due to a defect in renal phosphate retention and high urinary losses of phosphate. Unlike vitamin D and calcium deficiency, dietary deficiency of phosphate is rare due to the sufficient availability of phosphate in normal diet. Nonetheless, it may occur certain situations as in preterm babies who have high calcium and phosphate requirements for growth and can have a combined dietary deficiency of both. Other high-risk patients include those on total parenteral nutrition with deficient phosphate content or those consuming aluminum-containing antacids that bind dietary phosphate.

#### *Familial Hypophosphatemic Rickets*

Some inherited clinical disorders lead to excessive loss of phosphate in the urine with very low serum phosphate levels and can present as refractory rickets that does not respond to standard treatment.

***Pathogenesis:*** Fibroblast growth factor 23 (FGF23), a bone-derived hormone, plays a major role in phosphate homeostasis and development of phosphopenic rickets. FGF23 is a phosphatonin and leads to increased urinary losses of phosphate by downregulating the sodium-phosphate ($Na^+$/Pi) co-transporter in the proximal renal tubules. High FGF23 levels lead to increased renal phosphate losses and low serum phosphate. FGF23 also inhibits the enzyme 1-α hydroxylase and PTH secretion. Therefore, the blood levels of 1,25$(OH)_2$D are low despite hypophosphatemia (which normally activates 1α-hydroxylase activity).

*Familial X-linked dominant hypophosphatemic rickets:* The most common inherited cause of hypophosphatemic rickets is the X-linked dominant form due to a mutation in *PHEX* (**PH**osphate-regulating gene with homology to endopeptidases on the chromosome Xp22.1). The endopeptidase produced by the normal gene inactivates FGF23, and mutations in this gene lead to increased levels of FGF23. In addition, autosomal dominant and recessive hypophosphatemic rickets are associated with mutations in FGF23, which make it resistant to enzymatic breakdown.

*Clinical features:* Lower limb deformities, such as coxa vara, genu valgum, genu varum and short stature, are more prominent in hypophosphatemic rickets. Abnormalities of maxillofacial region and premature fusion of cranial sutures may lead to deformities of skull. Dental abnormalities are commonly seen including pulp deformities with intraglobular dentin, and frequent dental abscesses. Symptoms of hypocalcemia including tetany and seizures (generally seen in disorders of vitamin D metabolism) are absent in hypophosphatemic forms. The mother of affected patient may have bowing of legs and short stature or fasting hypophosphatemia.

*Evaluation:* The level of serum calcium is normal or slightly low, that of phosphate decreased and serum alkaline phosphatase level is raised. PTH levels are normal. Blood levels of $1,25(OH)_2D$ are inappropriately low for the level of serum phosphate. Urinary phosphate excretion is increased. This can be quantified by measuring the tubular reabsorption of phosphate on timed urine samples.

*Management:* Oral phosphate and vitamin D supplements are the mainstay of therapy. Phosphates are provided at a dosage of 40–70 mg/kg (total 1–3 g elemental phosphorus) divided into 4 or more equal parts and can be given in the form of Joulie solution (30.4 mg phosphate/mL) or as neutral phosphate effervescent tablets. Diarrhea is a frequent problem with high doses of phosphate.

Since the levels of calcitriol are relatively low, therapy with 1α-hydroxyvitamin $D_3$ (1-alphacalcidiol) or calcitriol is necessary. Treatment is started at a dose of 20–40 ng/kg/day (maximum 2 μg/day) until there is biochemical and radiological evidence of healing of rickets. Periodic monitoring of serum calcium, phosphate and PTH is necessary. High phosphate doses may lead to hypocalcemia and secondary hyperparathyroidism, which can impair healing of rickets.

Anti-FGF23 monoclonal antibodies, burosumab, reverse the metabolic and biochemical changes associated with hypophosphatemic rickets. The agent which is currently not widely available, is being accepted as the standard of care of the disease.

### *Other forms of hypophosphatemic rickets*

***Hereditary hypophosphatemic rickets with hypercalciuria (HHRH):*** HHRH is a result of mutations in the renal sodium-phosphate (Na+/Pi) co-transporter gene, which leads to excessive phosphate loss in the urine. FGF23 levels are normal. Hypophosphatemia stimulates 1α-hydroxylase enzyme and $1,25(OH)_2D$ production leading to hypercalcemia and hypercalciuria. This distinguishes HHRH from other forms of familial hypophosphatemic rickets where $1,25(OH)_2D$ levels are low (due to high FGF23 levels).

*Fanconi syndrome:* It is an inherited or acquired condition of generalized proximal renal tubular dysfunction leading to urinary losses of bicarbonate, phosphate, glucose and amino acids. Urinary phosphate losses lead to a form of phosphopenic rickets. The presence of normal anion gap metabolic acidosis and hypokalemia is characteristic. Treatment consists of phosphate, potassium and bicarbonate supplementation.

*Tumor-induced osteomalacia (oncogenous rickets):* Benign mesenchymal tumors may secrete large amounts of FGF23 that results in phosphaturia, hypophosphatemia and refractory rickets. Removal of the tumor reverses the biochemical abnormalities and heals the rickets. Patients with fibrous dysplasia (McCune-Albright syndrome) may produce excessive FGF23 from bony lesions and develop phosphopenic rickets.

## Other Causes of Rickets

*Renal tubular acidosis* (*see* Chapter 17)*:* Renal tubular (proximal or distal) acidosis (RTA) is important cause of refractory rickets in children. The conditions are characterized by presence of polyuria, rachitic deformities, short stature, and failure to thrive. Investigations reveal hyperchloremic (normal anion gap) metabolic acidosis with normal blood levels of urea and creatinine. Patients with Fanconi syndrome have a proximal renal tubular defect and urinary phosphate wasting. Patients with distal RTA develop rickets due to severe metabolic acidosis, which leads to leaching and defective mineralization of bone and growth cartilage.

*Chronic kidney disease:* Patients with chronic kidney disease and low GFR have impaired excretion of urinary phosphate. High serum phosphate chelates calcium, leading to hypocalcemia and secondary hyperparathyroidism. High PTH levels are responsible for osteoclastic bone resorption. Chronic kidney disease also leads to impaired 1α-hydroxylase activity in the kidney and low $1,25(OH)_2D$ levels. Serum levels of calcium are low and those of urea, creatinine, phosphate and PTH are increased. Therapy consists of restricting dietary phosphate intake, oral phosphate binders and providing supplements of calcium and active calcitriol or 1-alphacalcidiol.

## Evaluation of Refractory Rickets

In children not responding to standard therapy of nutritional rickets or in cases with suspected non-nutritional cause of rickets, the following investigations are indicated: Serum PTH, 25-OHD and 1, $25(OH)_2D$, pH, bicarbonate, electrolytes; and urine dipstick analysis for glucosuria and protein (Fanconi syndrome). If PTH is normal, estimation of timed urinary phosphate reabsorption is indicated to diagnose a defect in urinary phosphate excretion. FGF23 levels are not routinely available. Genetic studies (where feasible) help confirm the clinical diagnosis.

### Differential Diagnosis of Bony Deformities in Children

Certain diseases are associated with bony deformities that resemble rickets but do not have the typical biochemical or radiological features of rickets.

***Metaphyseal dysplasia:*** Patients with metaphyseal dysplasia show bony deformities and radiological findings that mimic rickets. Short stature with bowing of legs and waddling gait are prominent. The classic biochemical findings of rickets, including low calcium, low phosphate or high alkaline phosphatase are usually absent. Hypercalcemia has occasionally been reported in the Jansen metaphyseal chondrodysplasia.

***Fluorosis:*** Endemic fluorosis may present with bony deformities and radiological features mimicking rickets in school-going children. It results from high levels of fluoride in the community drinking water source. There may be a history of similar cases in the community. It may be associated with mottling of teeth and pain in limbs, joints and spine. Radiographs of long bones show osteosclerosis and calcification of ligaments; levels of alkaline phosphatase and PTH may be raised.

*Competencies:* **PE12.11; PE12.12**

## Vitamin E

Vitamin E refers to a group of compounds called tocopherols (α, β, and δ), which play a major role in protecting of cell membranes and cellular components from free radical injury and peroxidation. Tocopherols are absorbed in the small intestine and being fat-soluble, their absorption is enhanced in the presence of dietary fat. It is incorporated into chylomicrons and stored in the liver from where it is released with low density lipoproteins (LDL) for delivery to peripheral tissues. Red blood cell membranes contain about 20% of blood vitamin E content.

***Nutritional requirements:*** Ages 0 to 6 months: 3 mg tocopherol, 6 to 12 months: 4 mg, 1 to 3 years: 6 mg, 4 to 10 years: 7 mg, 11 to 14 years: 10 mg, 14 years or more: 15 mg. Preterm babies require higher amounts 15 to 20 µg/day. One mg of tocopherol provides 1.5 IU activity of vitamin E.

***Sources:*** The common sources of vitamin E are leafy vegetables, whole grains, nuts, seeds and vegetable oils (corn, cottonseed, safflower).

### Vitamin E Deficiency

Vitamin E deficiency is rare except in few high-risk groups. Preterm babies (<34 weeks) are born in a state of relative tocopherol deficiency. This is attributed to limited placental transfer of vitamin E. Hemolytic anemia is a common presentation in these babies generally manifesting after 4–6 weeks of age. Investigations show levels of hemoglobin between 7 and 9 g/dL, reticulocytosis, hyperbilirubinemia and low serum levels of vitamin E (<0.5 mg/dL). Administration of iron can exacerbate the hemolysis unless vitamin E is co-administered. Treatment consists of parenteral vitamin E 20–50 IU/day for 1 week. All preterm babies (<34 weeks or birth weight <1500 g) should receive vitamin E to prevent hemolytic anemia. Vitamin E supplementation also protects them against oxygen free radical injury and development of chronic lung disease and retinopathy of prematurity.

The other high-risk groups for vitamin E deficiency include children with fat malabsorption, pancreatic insufficiency (cystic fibrosis), cholestatic liver disease, Crohn's disease or short bowel syndrome. Deficiency can result in muscle weakness, peripheral neuropathy and hemolytic anemia. Abetalipoproteinemia, caused by the genetic absence of apolipoprotein B, is associated with fat malabsorption, steatorrhea, and undetectable plasma levels of vitamin E. These patients present with progressive neuropathy and pigmented retinopathy in the first two decades of life. Other manifestations include spinocerebellar ataxia with loss of deep tendon reflexes, loss of vibration and position sense, ophthalmoplegia, muscle weakness, ptosis and dysarthria.

Most malabsorption syndromes respond to large doses of oral vitamin E (15–20 mg/kg/day or 20–30 IU/kg/day) with amelioration of deficiency and improvement in neurological symptoms.

### Hypervitaminosis E

Vitamin E is relatively non-toxic compared to other fat-soluble vitamins and side-effects are rare. The upper limit of intake is 1000 mg/day. High levels of vitamin E may cause antagonism to vitamin K action and increase the risk of bleeding. Occasionally, muscle weakness, fatigue, nausea and diarrhea are reported in persons ingesting >1000 mg/day for several months.

*Competencies:* **PE12.13; PE12.14; PE20.10**

## Vitamin K

Vitamin K exists in two forms: Vitamin $K_1$ (phylloquinone) derived from plants and vitamin $K_2$ (menaquinone) synthesized by intestinal bacteria.

***Nutritional requirements:*** Newborns and infants: 3 to 5 µg/day, >2 years: 10 µg/day, older children: 10 to 30 µg/day, adult women: 90 µg/day, adult men: 120 µg/day.

***Sources:*** Green leafy vegetables and liver are rich dietary sources of vitamin K. Endogenous synthesis by intestinal flora is usually sufficient to meet daily requirements.

***Absorption and metabolism:*** Like all fat-soluble vitamins, absorption of dietary vitamin K requires bile and pancreatic juice. Dietary vitamin K is absorbed in the jejunum, incorporated into chylomicrons and delivered to the circulation via the lymph. The liver is the primary site of storage and action of vitamin K.

***Physiological function:*** Vitamin K is a cofactor for post-translational hepatic carboxylation of glutamic acid to form gamma-carboxyglutamic acid. Several proteins involved in blood coagulation require vitamin K dependent carboxylation including factors II (prothrombin), VII, IX and X. This facilitates the chelation of calcium ions to glutamate and platelet phosphatide, which is essential for the coagulation cascade.

*Vitamin K Deficiency*

Vitamin K deficiency can occur in patients on chronic antibiotics due to the elimination of intestinal bacterial flora. Malabsorption syndromes such as biliary obstruction, cystic fibrosis, short bowel syndrome and celiac disease are other causes of deficiency. Manifestations include bleeding from various sites and presence of ecchymosis. Treatment includes intravenous injection of vitamin K 5–10 mg per day till bleeding stops. Severe bleeding is treated with infusion of fresh frozen plasma. Patients with malabsorption or chronic liver disease should receive high dose oral or intramuscular vitamin K for prevention of deficiency.

Newborn babies are particularly prone to vitamin K deficiency due to a combination of factors; vitamin K does not cross the placenta and they do not have adequate intestinal bacterial flora to synthesize it endogenously. Moreover, breast milk is a poor source of vitamin K.

*Hemorrhagic disease of the newborn* (HDN) is a syndrome of severe systemic bleeding due to vitamin K deficiency manifesting in the newborn period. Life-threatening bleeding occurs from various sites including skin (ecchymosis), gastrointestinal tract, nasal cavity or umbilical stump. Intracranial hemorrhage is a complication manifesting with seizures. HDN is characterized by undetectable plasma vitamin K levels and high concentrations of 'protein induced by vitamin K absence' (PIVKA), an uncarboxylated form of prothrombin. The prothrombin time and activated partial thromboplastin time are prolonged with normal platelet counts. HDN can be classified into three categories based on age of onset: Early onset manifests at <24 hours of age; classic HDN manifests in the first week of life, and late-onset manifests from 1 to 12 weeks of age. Maternal use of drugs such as primidone, warfarin and phenytoin that antagonize the action of vitamin K is usually responsible for early onset HDN, whereas normal breastfed babies who have not received vitamin K at birth show classic HDN. Late onset HDN is usually seen in infants with underlying liver disease or defects in vitamin K metabolism. Treatment includes IV vitamin K and fresh frozen plasma. Routine administration of prophylactic vitamin K is recommended at birth to all healthy newborns at a dose of 0.5–1 mg IM to prevent HDN.

*Competencies:* **PE12.15; PE12.16; PE12.17; PE12.18; PE12.19, PE12.20, PE12.21**

## WATER-SOLUBLE VITAMINS

Unlike fat-soluble vitamins, water-soluble vitamins are not stored in the body (except vitamin $B_{12}$) and their deficiency can develop in a short period of time on deficient diets. Toxicity is very rare even with very high doses. They mostly act as co-enzymes in various energy-releasing pathways. Table 8.5 outlines the function, sources and clinical features of deficiency of essential B vitamins.

### Thiamine (Vitamin $B_1$)

*Biologic action:* Thiamine pyrophosphate, the active form of thiamine, is an important cofactor for the key enzymes transketolase and pyruvate dehydrogenase involved in glycolysis. It is also important for energy generation in the citric acid cycle that is highly active in the heart and brain.

*Requirements:* Recommended daily allowance is 0.4 mg/1000 calories of carbohydrate intake.

*Dietary sources:* These include human milk, cow milk, unpolished grains, eggs, organ meats (liver, kidney) and legumes. Thiamine is sensitive to heat, sulfites, pasteurization and sterilization.

*Deficiency:* Thiamine deficiency results in beriberi that affects people who consume diets based on exclusive intake of polished rice. Three forms of beriberi are described: Dry, wet and infantile. Dry beriberi manifests as a peripheral neuritis with irritability, paralysis of lower limbs, loss of deep tendon jerks, muscle wasting and loss of position sense. Wet beriberi is characterized by congestive heart failure and peripheral edema. Infantile beriberi has a more subtle onset occurring in breastfed infants of thiamine-deficient mothers (who may not have signs of beriberi), or with very low thiamine intake. The clinical picture is dominated by cardiomegaly, cyanosis, dyspnea and aphonia. Severe thiamine deficiency causes Wernicke-Korsakoff syndrome most commonly seen in adults with chronic alcoholism. It consists of a triad of mental confusion, ataxia and ocular abnormalities (ophthalmoplegia and nystagmus), and may also occur in thiamine deficient children.

*Diagnosis:* Thiamine deficiency may be suspected in all cases of malnutrition. The diagnosis is confirmed by measuring 24 hours urinary thiamine excretion or red blood cell transketolase activity.

*Treatment:* Treatment with thiamine leads to resolution of neurologic and cardiac symptoms within 24–48 hours. Treatment of patients with mild beriberi with thiamine (5 mg/day) is satisfactory. Severely ill children should receive 10 mg IV twice daily.

### Riboflavin (Vitamin $B_2$)

Riboflavin is a constituent of two coenzymes involved in oxidation-reduction reactions of cellular respiration: Flavin adenine dinucleotide (FAD) and flavin mononucleotide (FMN). A number of redox enzymes, including glutathione reductase and xanthine oxidase, require flavin coenzymes.

*Riboflavin requirements:* The recommended daily intake is 0.4 mg/1000 calories for infants and 0.8–1.2 mg/1000 calories for children.

*Dietary sources:* Meat, milk, eggs and cereals are good sources of riboflavin. It is resistant to oxidation and heat and is not destroyed by pasteurization.

*Deficiency:* Riboflavin deficiency occurs from inadequate intake or malabsorption. It takes 1–2 months to develop and is associated with other vitamin deficiencies. Features include photophobia, glossitis, cheilosis, angular stomatitis (Fig. 8.8), seborrheic dermatitis (especially around the nasolabial folds) and corneal vascularization. Activity of the enzyme glutathione reductase in erythrocytes is a good indicator of riboflavin status in the body.

**Table 8.5:** Essential B vitamins: Function, sources, deficiencies and at-risk groups

| *Vitamin* | *Function* | *Sources* | *Daily requirement* | *Deficiency* | *At-risk groups* |
|---|---|---|---|---|---|
| $B_1$ (thiamine) | Coenzyme in glycolysis and citric acid cycle | Human milk, cow milk, unpolished grains, eggs, organ meats (liver, kidney), legumes | <6 mo: 0.2 mg<br>6–12 mo: 0.3 mg<br>1–3 yr: 0.5 mg<br>4–8 yr: 0.6 mg<br>9–13 yr: 0.9 mg<br>>14 yr: 1.2 mg | *Beriberi:* Peripheral neuritis, irritability, paralysis, heart failure<br>*Wernicke encephalopathy* | Diets based on polished rice, malnutrition, malabsorption, alcoholics |
| $B_2$ (riboflavin) | Part of flavoproteins FMN, FAD involved in redox reactions | Meat, milk, eggs, cereals, vegetables | <1 yr: 0.3 mg<br>1–3 yr: 0.5 mg<br>4–8 yr: 0.6 mg<br>9–13 yr: 0.9 mg<br>>14 yr: 1.2 mg | Photophobia, glossitis, cheilosis, angular stomatitis, seborrhea, corneal vascularization | Malnutrtion, malabsorption states, deficient diets |
| $B_3$ (niacin) | Cofactors (NAD, NADP) in redox reactions and cellular respiration | Meat, eggs, milk, legumes, peanuts | <1 yr: 2–4 mg<br>1–3 yr: 6 mg<br>4–8 yr: 8 mg<br>9–13 yr: 12 mg<br>>13 yr: 16 mg | Pellagra | Groups on predominant maize-based diet |
| $B_6$ (pyridoxine) | Synthesis of amino acids, myelin, neurotransmitters, hemoglobin | Meat, whole-grain cereals, vegetables, egg yolk, soya beans, walnuts | <6 mo: 0.1 mg<br>6–12 mo: 0.3 mg<br>1–3 yr: 0.5 mg<br>4–8 yr: 0.6 mg<br>9–13 yr: 1 mg<br>>13 yr: 1.3 mg | Peripheral neuropathy, refractory seizures, dermatitis, microcytic anemia | Malabsorption states, isoniazid use |
| $B_{12}$ (cobalamin) | Regeneration of folate; myelin synthesis | Dairy products, eggs and meat | <6 mo: 0.4 µg<br>6–12 mo: 0.5 µg<br>1–3 yr: 0.9 µg<br>4–8 yr: 1.2 µg<br>9–13 yr: 1.8 µg<br>>13 yr: 2.4 µg | Megaloblastic anemia, subacute combined degeneration of cord, infantile tremor syndrome | Exclusively breastfed infants of vegan mothers, vegan diets, intrinsic factor deficiency, ileal resection |
| Folate | DNA synthesis, cell growth | Green leafy peas, fruits, sunflower seeds | < 6 mo: 65 µg<br>6–12 mo: 80 µg<br>1–3 yr: 150 µg<br>4–8 yr: 200 µg<br>9–13 yr: 300 µg<br>>13 yr: 100 µg | Megaloblastic anemia | Preterm babies, pregnancy, malnutrition, malabsorption, hemolytic anemia, anticonvulsant therapy |

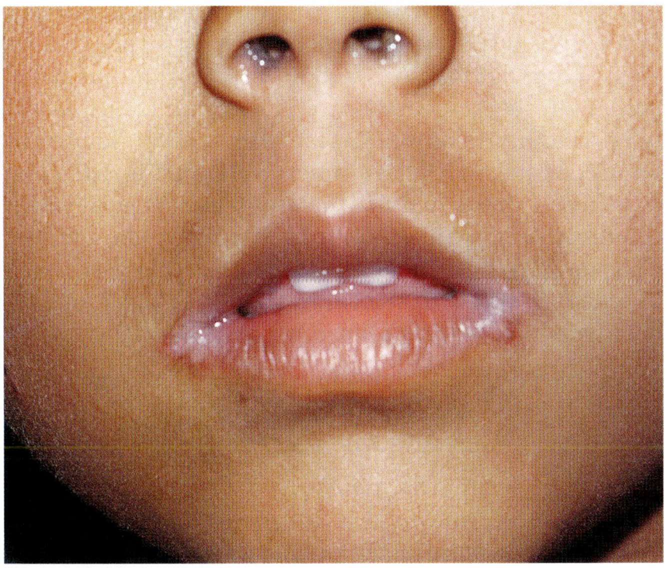

Fig. 8.8 Angular stomatitis due to vitamin $B_2$ (riboflavin) deficiency (*Courtesy:* Prof M Ramam, AIIMS, New Delhi)

*Treatment:* Children are treated with 3–10 mg of oral riboflavin daily for several weeks; infants respond to 1 mg daily. Therapeutic doses of vitamin help in improving corneal lesions rapidly.

### Niacin (Vitamin $B_3$)

Nicotinic acid and nicotinamide, biologically equivalent vitamins, are both referred to as niacin. Niacin is a part of NAD and NADP, coenzymes in oxidation-reduction reactions and cellular respiration.

*Sources:* Milk, eggs, meat, legumes and peanuts are good sources of niacin. Deficiency occurs in areas where maize is the staple food, as the niacin in maize is present in bound form and not easily absorbed. The vitamin is resistant to heating. Niacin can be synthesized in the body from tryptophan, however, the conversion ratio is 60:1, requiring large amounts of tryptophan to meet niacin needs.

*Niacin requirements:* Requirements are expressed in terms of niacin equivalents (NE). One NE equals 1 mg of niacin or 60 mg of tryptophan. RDA for niacin is related to dietary energy intake; the recommended intake is 6.4 to 8 NE/1000 calories.

*Niacin deficiency:* Niacin deficiency leads to pellagra which is characterized by three Ds: **d**ermatitis, **d**iarrhea and **d**ementia. The cutaneous lesions consist of a symmetrical pigmented rash in body parts exposed to sunlight especially the neck (Casal necklace) or back (**Fig. 8.9a**). The diagnosis is suspected on history of inadequate diet or chronic alcohol ingestion with typical clinical features.

*Treatment of pellagra:* The daily dose for treatment is about 10 times the recommended dietary intake (50–300 mg/day).

### Pyridoxine (Vitamin $B_6$)

Pyridoxine is converted to the coenzyme pyridoxal phosphate, which is involved in the metabolism of amino acids and synthesis of sphingolipids (myelin), neurotransmitters (GABA and serotonin) and hemoglobin. Rich sources of vitamin $B_6$ include meat, whole-grain cereals, vegetables, egg yolk, soya beans and walnuts. Primary dietary deficiency is rare but secondary deficiency can occur in malabsorptive states. The antitubercular drug isoniazid inhibits the activation of pyridoxine and may lead to its deficiency.

Pyridoxine deficiency may cause peripheral neuropathy, refractory seizures, dermatitis and microcytic (sideroblastic) anemia. Pyridoxine is given 10–50 mg/day to patients on INH (isoniazid) to prevent peripheral neuropathy. For refractory seizures 100 mg of pyridoxine is injected IM.

### Pantothenic Acid (Vitamin $B_5$)

Pantothenic acid is a part of coenzyme A (CoA), which is essential for metabolism of fatty acid, proteins and carbohydrates in the citric acid cycle and fatty acid synthesis. Pantothenic acid is present in virtually all naturally occurring foods. Isolated pantothenic acid deficiency is rare and includes burning feet, insomnia and gastrointestinal symptoms. The suggested daily intake is 2–3 mg for infants and 3–5 mg for children.

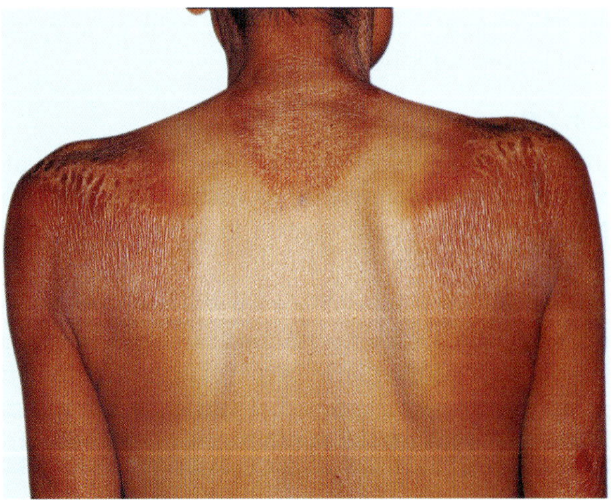

**Fig. 8.9a:** Pellagra: Note the symmetric hyperpigmented rashes on sun-exposed parts of back due to niacin deficiency (*Courtesy:* Prof M Ramam, AIIMS, New Delhi)

### Biotin (Vitamin $B_7$)

Biotin is a coenzyme for many carboxylase enzymes in the body, which are involved in multiple metabolic pathways like gluconeogenesis, amino acid metabolism and fatty acid synthesis. Dietary sources of biotin include liver, egg yolk, milk, yeast extracts and meat. Biotin deficiency has been observed in individuals who consume a large number of raw eggs (rich in avidin). Avidin is not hydrolyzed by gastrointestinal enzymes and binds to biotin preventing its absorption. Cooking of eggs destroys avidin.

Clinical features of biotin deficiency include anorexia, vomiting, dry scaly dermatitis, glossitis, developmental delay and seizures. Multiple carboxylase deficiency is a genetic disorder affecting the activity of carboxylase synthetase. This condition responds to large doses of biotin. Another genetic defect affects the activity of biotinidase, an enzyme involved in the recycling of biotin. Treatment of biotin deficiency consists of oral administration of 5–10 mg daily for 2 to 3 weeks.

### Cobalamin (Vitamin $B_{12}$)

Vitamin $B_{12}$ plays two major roles in the body. The methyl derivative of vitamin $B_{12}$ is required for conversion of homocysteine to methionine, a process that helps in folate regeneration (homocysteine + $N^5$methyltetrahydrofolate $\rightarrow$ methionine + folate). In the absence of cobalamin, folate gets trapped and cannot be utilized for DNA/RNA synthesis. In the second reaction, the 5-deoxyadenosyl derivative of vitamin $B_{12}$ is required to convert methylmalonyl CoA to succinyl CoA. Excessive accumulation of methylmalonyl CoA leads to defect in fatty acid synthesis and neural myelin sheath degeneration.

*Sources:* Vitamin $B_{12}$ is produced in the gut of certain species of animals by the intestinal bacteria. However, humans do not produce vitamin $B_{12}$ in their gut and have to depend on animal sources like meat, milk, eggs and fish to fulfill vitamin $B_{12}$ requirements. Animal meats such as liver, kidney, heart and muscle are rich sources of vitamin $B_{12}$.

*Absorption and metabolism:* Vitamin $B_{12}$ binds to intrinsic factor, a glycoprotein produced by the gastric parietal cells, and the complex is absorbed by specific receptor-mediated process in the ileum. Absence of intrinsic factor results in an inability to absorb ingested vitamin $B_{12}$ known as pernicious anemia. Passive diffusion accounts for a fraction of total absorption, but may be useful in the management of pernicious anemia with mega-doses of the vitamin. Cobalamin is stored in the liver and has a long half-life. The average total body pool in an adult is enough to sustain daily vitamin $B_{12}$ needs for several years.

*Requirements:* The recommended intake of vitamin $B_{12}$ for infants is 0.3 μg/day. Older children should receive 0.5–1.5 μg/day and adolescents 2.0 μg/day.

*Deficiency:* Vitamin $B_{12}$ deficiency can occur in patients with impaired intestinal absorption due to defects in intrinsic factor, or distal ileal disease. True dietary vitamin $B_{12}$ deficiency occurs in persons who follow vegan diets containing no animal or meat products. Content of vitamin

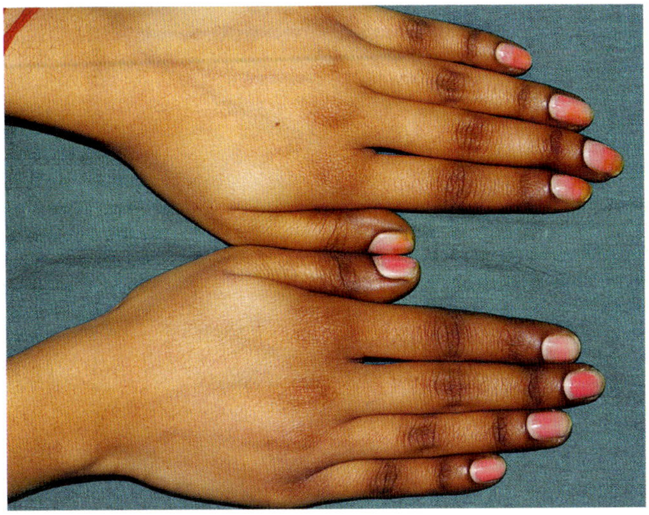

Fig. 8.9b: Knuckle pigmentation in vitamin $B_{12}$ deficiency (*Courtesy:* Prof M Raman, AIIMS, New Delhi)

$B_{12}$ in breast milk is determined by maternal intake. Hence, exclusively breastfed infants of strict vegan mothers can become vitamin $B_{12}$ deficient over a period of time especially if weaning is delayed.

Vitamin $B_{12}$ deficiency results in megaloblastic anemia due to secondary folate deficiency. Apart from pallor, there is hyperpigmentation of the knuckles and nail beds of the hands as well as skin (Fig. 8.9b). Neurological manifestations consist of progressive demyelination of the posterior and lateral columns of the spinal cord and peripheral nerves (subacute combined degeneration). In exclusively breastfed infants of deficient mothers, there is delayed neurodevelopment, seizures and a movement disorder characterized by fine tremor, called 'infantile tremor syndrome'.

*Diagnosis of deficiency:* The peripheral smear shows macrocytes (red cell volume >100 fL), immature neutrophils with hypersegmented nuclei (5 lobes in at least 5% neutrophils or ≥6 lobes in single neutrophil) and thrombocytopenia. Serum cobalamin levels are below 200 pg/mL and plasma homocysteine and methylmalonic acid levels are increased.

*Treatment:* The commercially available preparations of vitamin $B_{12}$ are cyanocobalamin and hydroxocobalamin. Deficiency associated with neurological manifestations is treated with IM administration of vitamin $B_{12}$ 1000 µg/day or thrice weekly for 2 weeks followed by weekly doses for 6 weeks. In case of thrombocytopenia, intravenous route may be used. In the absence of malabsorption, oral route is equally efficacious and can be given to patients with megaloblastic anemia at a dose of 500–1000 µg/day for 4–6 weeks followed by monthly doses. Reticulocytosis is seen within 2–4 days and hemoglobin levels return to normal in 4–8 weeks. Patients with intrinsic factor defect require lifelong parenteral therapy.

### Folic Acid (Pteroylmonoglutamic Acid, Vitamin $B_9$)

Folic acid is essential for normal growth and maintenance of cells, since it acts as a coenzyme for normal DNA and RNA synthesis.

*Sources:* Green leafy vegetables, peas, fruits and sunflower seeds.

*Requirements:* The recommended daily allowance of folic acid varies from 25 µg in infancy to 200 µg by adolescence. Requirements of folic acid are high in tissues with active cell division or regeneration such as intestinal cells or bone marrow.

*Deficiency:* Folate is absorbed in the small intestine. Deficiency is common in malabsorption states such as chronic gastrointestinal infections, short bowel syndrome and celiac disease. Preterm babies are at risk of folate deficiency due to increased tissue demands and lack of maternal placental transfer that generally occurs in the last trimester of pregnancy. Children with hemolytic anemia are also predisposed to deficiency due to increased bone marrow erythropoiesis and high folate requirements. Anticonvulsant drugs (phenytoin) increase the hepatic catabolism of folate leading to secondary deficiency. Deficiency of folate impairs DNA synthesis, limits cell division and affects normal growth and repair of tissues. The tissues that have the fastest rate of cell replacement are affected first. Erythropoiesis is hindered, resulting in megaloblastic anemia, which manifests with macrocytic peripheral smear.

Maternal deficiency of folate during the phase of embryogenesis in early pregnancy increases the risk of fetal neural tube defects. Periconceptional folate supplements begun 1-month before conception and continued for 3-month after, is recommended in all women for protection against these defects.

*Diagnosis:* Serum folate levels may be low (<3 µg/L) but may not be reliable due to fluctuating levels. RBC folate levels are more indicative of folate deficiency. Levels of homocysteine are high but methylmalonic acid are normal.

*Treatment:* Folate deficiency is corrected using folic acid at a dose of 0.5–1 mg/day orally for 3–4 weeks.

In patients with megaloblastic anemia, it is imperative to rule out and treat vitamin $B_{12}$ deficiency before empirically treating with folate. High doses of folate may reverse the megaloblastic anemia due to vitamin $B_{12}$ deficiency, but not the neurological signs which may progress irreversibly in the absence of correct treatment.

### Vitamin C (Ascorbic Acid)

Vitamin C plays many important roles in the body; it is a co-factor for oxidation–reduction reactions needed for hydroxylation of lysine and proline an important component of collagen. It is required for the maintenance of normal connective tissue, wound healing and bone (osteoid) formation, all of which contain collagen. Also, vitamin C reduces ferric to ferrous state and helps in iron absorption in the gut. Due to its antioxidant properties, it stabilizes a number of other compounds, including vitamin E and folic acid. Humans, unlike other animals, lack the enzyme (gulonolactone oxidase) required for conversion of glucose to ascorbic acid, hence vitamin C must be obtained from the diet.

***Sources:*** Rich sources of vitamin C include fresh citrus fruits (oranges, grapefruit, lime and gooseberry) and vegetables (cabbage, cauliflower, spinach, cucumber). Much of the vitamin is lost in cooking and storage, but is stable in canned and frozen foods. Human milk contains 5 to 15 mg/100 cal and cow milk 0.2–2.0 mg/100 cal of vitamin C. Daily requirements are 30–40 mg for infants and 40–70 mg for children.

***Absorption and metabolism:*** Ascorbic acid is absorbed by an active, sodium-dependent process in the upper small intestine. The vitamin circulates in plasma in its free, anionic form, reaching high concentrations in adrenal gland where it acts as a cofactor in catecholamine and glucocorticoid synthesis. It is not stored in the body and excreted freely in the urine.

***Deficiency:*** Vitamin C deficiency is associated with increased capillary fragility, appearance of petechiae on the skin, delayed wound healing and bleeding gums. Other features include irritability, anorexia and anemia. Scurvy is a severe form of vitamin C deficiency with bleeding into joints (hemarthrosis) and subperiosteal spaces resulting in painful joint swellings and generalized tenderness of the limbs. The child may present with inability to move limbs (pseudoparalysis) due to pain and assume a frog-like posture, with semiflexion at hips and knees. Characteristic angular swellings at the costochondral junction arising due to subperisoteal bleed (scorbutic rosary) are often apparent. Unlike rachitic rosary due to vitamin D deficiency, scorbutic rosary is tender and more angular. Scurvy can result in cerebral hemorrhage or hemopericardium and is potentially fatal, if left untreated. Children at risk for vitamin C deficiency include those who are fed boiled or evaporated milk and those with severe dietary restrictions with lack of fresh fruits and vegetables.

***Diagnosis of scurvy:*** The diagnosis is made by presence of characteristic physical findings and history of inadequate dietary intake of vitamin C. X-rays of long bones show a ground glass appearance with thinning of cortex (pencil thin cortex). An irregular thickened white line appears at the metaphysis (white line of Frankel), representing the zone of well-calcified cartilage. There is a zone of rarefaction proximal to this line, which represents poorly formed trabeculae (Trümmerfeld zone). The lateral part of the rarefaction appears as a triangular peaked defect called Pelken spurs. The epiphyses are rarefied and surrounded by a thin white calcified line (Wimberger ring sign) (Fig. 8.10).

***Therapy for scurvy:*** Therapy with 100–200 mg of vitamin C orally or parenterally prompts rapid improvement in symptoms and resolution of the radiological signs. Daily intake of 100 mL of orange juice or tomato pulp has the same effect.

*Competencies:* **PE13.11; PE13.12**

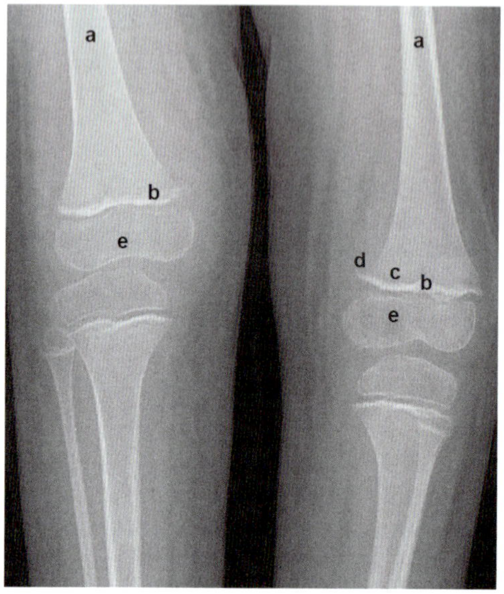


**Fig. 8.10:** Scurvy. X-ray of lower limbs showing: (a) Ground glass appearance with thinned cortex (pencil thin cortex); (b) Thickened metaphyseal white line (white line of Frankel); (c) Zone of rarefaction (Trümmerfeld zone); (d) Triangular peaked defect called Pelken spurs; (e) Rarefied epiphyses surrounded by thin white calcified line (Wimberger ring sign)

## MINERALS AND TRACE ELEMENTS

### Calcium

Calcium is the most abundant mineral in the body and is located primarily (98%) in bone. It is essential for the coagulation cascade, hormone action, neuromuscular function and muscle contractility. Intestinal absorption of calcium varies inversely with intake and is regulated by $1,25(OH)_2D$, which controls the synthesis of calcium-binding protein at the brush border. In the presence of vitamin D, calcium absorption can adapt to a wide range of dietary calcium intakes, varying from 10 to 80% of available calcium. Calcium absorption also depends on the interaction of calcium with other dietary constituents, including fiber, phytate, oxalates, fat and lactose.

The main sources of calcium for infants are milk and dairy products, with smaller amounts derived from grains and fruits once solid foods are introduced. Children consuming strict vegan diets develop calcium deficiency, either alone or with vitamin D deficiency. Strict vegan diets may provide as little as 250 mg of calcium per day, and include agents that inhibit calcium absorption, such as fiber and phytates. Secondary calcium deficiency may develop in association with steatorrhea, malabsorption syndromes, liver disease, or renal abnormalities of calcium metabolism.

The adequate intake of calcium is 200 mg and 260 mg/day for infants aged 0–6 and 6–12 months, respectively. Children aged 1 to 10 years require an intake of 500 to 800 mg per day. During the pubertal growth spurt, calcium requirements are as high as 1000 to 1200 mg per day. Pregnant and lactating women require 400 mg per day. Calcium deficiency may cause tetany characterized by muscle cramps, numbness and tingling in limbs. Rickets and osteoporosis may occur with chronic deficiency.

*Competencies:* **PE13.13; PE13.14**

### Magnesium

Magnesium is essential for reactions controlling carbohydrate metabolism, membrane transport and signal transmission. Over 80% of the total body magnesium is in bone and skeletal muscle. Rich sources of magnesium include legumes, nuts, bananas and whole grains. Magnesium is efficiently absorbed in the intestine and regulation of its balance depends on renal tubular reabsorption. Primary deficiency is common in children with protein energy malnutrition. Magnesium is eliminated during food processing and diets based on processed or junk food can lead to magnesium deficiency. Deficiency may also develop secondary to intestinal malabsorption, excessive gastrointestinal losses (through fistulae or continuous suction) or renal losses (due to tubular disease or diuretics). Manifestations of its deficiency include irritability, hypocalcemic tetany, hypo- or hyper-reflexia and arrhythmias. Magnesium requirements in the first 6 months range between 40 and 50 mg/day; 60 mg/day for 6–12 months, and ~200 mg/day for older children.

## Trace Elements

Eleven 'major' elements constitute 99% of human body weight. These essential-for-life elements are carbon, hydrogen, oxygen, nitrogen, sodium, potassium, chlorine, calcium, phosphorus, sulfur and magnesium. In addition, the body is composed of numerous "trace" elements. The term trace elements comprise minerals with proven or putative essentiality for human nutrition. Their major functions are related to enzyme systems where they act either as cofactor for metal-ion-activated enzymes or as specific constituents of metalloenzymes.

*Competencies:* **PE13.1**

### Iron

Iron deficiency remains a major nutritional problem among infants and young children. The National Family Health Survey (NFHS)-V (2019–21) showed that 67% children between the ages of 6 months and 5 years were anemic. Iron deficiency anemia is associated with impaired performance in mental and physical functions, including physical coordination and capacity, cognitive abilities, and social and emotional development (Chapter 13). The Anemia-Mukt Bharat intensified Iron-plus Initiative aims to strengthen the existing mechanisms and foster newer strategies for tackling anemia (*anemiamuktbharat.info*).

### Zinc

***Functions:*** Zinc is the second most common trace element in the body after iron. It is an essential micronutrient with diverse but critical physiological role, being part of more than 200 enzymatic reactions. As a component of zinc finger proteins, zinc regulates gene transcription and participates in nucleic acid metabolism, protein synthesis and cellular growth. Thymidine kinase, DNA polymerase and RNA polymerase are zinc dependent enzymes. Zinc is a major antioxidant being part of the enzyme superoxide dismutase. Due to its ubiquitous nature, zinc is required for normal functioning of almost all organ systems including immune, gastrointestinal, central nervous, skeletal, epidermal and reproductive system.

***Dietary sources:*** Zinc is derived mainly from animal protein. Liver, meat, fish, nuts and eggs are a rich source. Diets based on cereals/starch, plants and legumes with low content of animal protein are associated with zinc deficiency. This is due to the presence of increased dietary phytates that decrease the bioavailability or the capacity to absorb zinc.

***Absorption and metabolism:*** Zinc is absorbed throughout the small intestine by a process of facilitated diffusion. Most absorbed zinc is taken up temporarily by the liver, which plays a central role in zinc metabolism. In the systemic circulation, the major fraction of plasma zinc is loosely bound to albumin. Almost 90% of total body zinc is localized in bone and skeletal muscle. Zinc status is regulated both at the absorptive step and by intestinal re-excretion. The major excretory route for endogenous zinc is via the intestinal tract and fecal losses may be significantly increased in children with intestinal diseases or diarrhea.

***Deficiency:*** Infants, children, adolescents, pregnant and lactating women have increased demand of zinc due to active growth and tissue synthesis. Deficiency is also seen as a part of malnutrition and malabsorption syndromes, caused by low dietary intake or poor absorption. Excessive loss of zinc in stools can occur in children with recurrent or chronic diarrhea. Severe zinc deficiency syndromes can occur in patients on prolonged intravenous feeding without adequate trace element supplements.

Poor physical growth is an important feature of zinc depletion in preschool and school-age children. Delayed sexual maturation (hypogonadism) is also a prominent feature of zinc deficiency in adolescents. Other features include anemia, anorexia, diarrhea, alopecia, dermatitis, impaired immune function, poor wound healing and skeletal abnormalities.

Acrodermatitis enteropathica is an autosomal recessive disorder of severe zinc deficiency, caused by impaired intestinal absorption due to defect in intestinal zinc transporter protein, ZIP4. It presents in early infancy, with vesicobullous, dry, scaly or eczematous skin lesions chiefly in the periorificial (around the mouth and perineum), buttocks and acral areas (Fig. 8.11). Alopecia

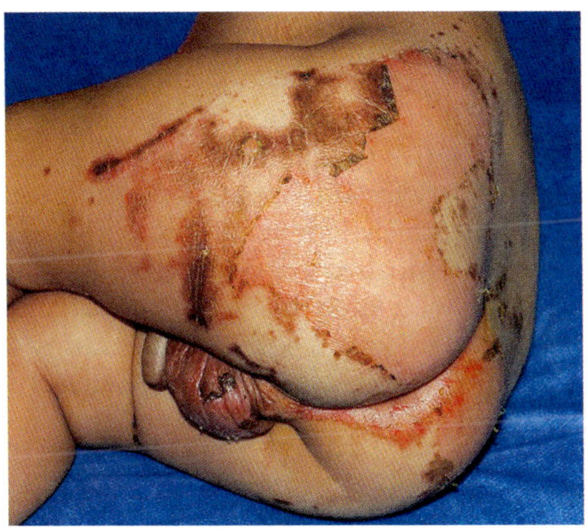

**Fig. 8.11** Acrodermatitis enteropathica in an infant. Erythematous and eczematous skin lesions chiefly in the periorificial area and buttocks (*Courtesy:* Prof. M Ramam, AIIMS, New Delhi)

and eye changes, such as conjunctivitis, blepharitis and photophobia, may be present. Chronic diarrhea, growth retardation, stomatitis, loss of taste sense, irritability and delayed wound healing are other findings. Resolution of symptoms with catch-up growth is noted following long-term oral zinc therapy, at a dose of 2–3 mg/kg/day.

The diagnosis of zinc deficiency is often derived from the combination of dietary history of chronic low zinc intake or excessive intestinal losses, presence of clinical features compatible with deficiency and low levels of zinc in plasma or hair.

***Requirement and treatment of deficiency:*** The normal requirements for children range between 3.5 and 5.0 mg per day. Acquired zinc deficiency states can be treated with 0.5 to 1.0 mg elemental zinc/kg/day for several weeks or months. Malnourished children have much higher requirements of 2–4 mg/kg/day due to zinc depletion and intestinal disease. One mg of elemental zinc is available from 4.5 mg zinc sulfate or 3 mg zinc acetate.

### Copper

Copper is a component of several metalloenzymes required for oxidative metabolism.

***Absorption and metabolism:*** Most of the ingested copper is absorbed in stomach and small intestine, from where it is transported to the liver and released into the systemic circulation bound to ceruloplasmin, the main transport protein for copper. Copper is mainly stored in the liver and muscle. It is excreted mainly through biliary secretions in the feces and urinary excretion is minimal.

***Sources:*** The richest sources are meats, liver, seafood, nuts and seeds. Additional copper may enter the food chain through pesticides and contamination of water by pipes and cooking utensils.

***Deficiency:*** Primary dietary deficiency is infrequent. Secondary deficiency may develop in malabsorption syndromes, liver disease, peritoneal dialysis and other conditions causing excessive copper losses. Copper deficiency decreases the lifespan of the erythrocyte and impairs mobilization of stored iron from liver and bone marrow. Features of deficiency are microcytic, hypochromic anemia unresponsive to iron therapy, depigmentation of hair, neutropenia, neurological problems and osteoporosis.

Copper transport is disrupted in two human diseases: Wilson's disease (*see* Chapters 12 and 19) and Menkes disease. Both have defects in copper transporting membrane proteins. Menkes steely-hair syndrome is a rare X-linked fatal disorder of impaired copper absorption presenting in early infancy with kinky hair, skin hypopigmentation, neurological regression and seizures. Laboratory findings include hypocupremia, low plasma ceruloplasmin, neutropenia and anemia.

### Selenium

Selenium is a constituent of glutathione peroxidase, an antioxidant in red blood cells and other tissues. Selenium also helps maintain normal immune function and is a part of the enzyme type 1 deiodinase which converts thyroxine to triiodothyronine. Dietary sources include whole grain, meat, egg, seafood, garlic and mushrooms. Endemic selenium deficiency results in Keshan disease, a form of cardiomyopathy in young children seen in some regions of China. In combination with iodine deficiency, lack of selenium can result in myxoedematous endemic cretinism, seen in certain parts of Africa. Selenium deficiency may be seen in patients on total parenteral nutrition who are not supplemented and manifests with brown hair, whitening of nails and macrocytosis.

### Chromium

Glucose intolerance, which complicates malnutrition in young children, has been attributed in part to chromium deficiency. Symptoms of chromium deficiency are usually in the setting of total parenteral alimentation and include glucose intolerance and peripheral neuropathy.

*Competencies:* **PE13.7; PE13.8; PE13.9**

### Iodine

Iodine, a micronutrient present in small quantities in the thyroid gland, is essential for the formation of thyroid hormones thyroxine ($T_4$) and triiodothyronine ($T_3$), the main determinants of basal metabolic rate. Thyroid hormones play a key role in body growth and brain development, especially in the fetus and first three years of postnatal life, periods of rapid brain growth. Iodine deficiency and consequent hypothyroidism in early life leads to lifelong mental retardation.

Iodine is most commonly found in sea water and sea food/plants are rich sources. Iodine is relatively deficient in soil especially in mountainous regions due to leaching and erosion. The Himalayan belt and Ganges valley are areas of severe iodine deficiency in India.

***Recommended daily intake:*** The recommended iodine intake is around 90 µg/day from birth to 5 years of age increasing to 120 µg/day at ages 6–12 years, and 150 µg/day in adolescents and adults. Pregnant and lactating women require higher amounts (200 µg/day). Iodine is excreted in urine and 24-hour urinary iodine excretion is a useful measurement of iodine sufficiency in a community. Urinary iodine <100 µg/L indicates iodine insufficiency, with values <20 µg/L pointing to severe deficiency.

***Iodine deficiency disorders:*** Nearly 1.5 billion people in 130 countries around the world live in areas of iodine deficiency and are at risk of developing iodine deficiency disorders (IDDs). IDDs are the commonest cause of mental retardation in these populations and are responsible for an average lowering of IQ scores by 13.5 points compared to populations living in iodine-sufficient areas. Goiter is the earliest manifestation of iodine deficiency and is an adaptive response to increase thyroid hormone production under the influence of increased TSH levels, but can eventually lead to decompensation in the form of hypothyroidism. Goiter rates are as high as 10–30% in endemic populations suffering from iodine deficiency (**Table 8.6**).

**Table 8.6:** Spectrum of iodine deficiency disorders (IDD)

| | |
|---|---|
| Fetus | Abortions, stillbirths<br>Endemic cretinism<br>Congenital anomalies<br>Increased perinatal mortality |
| Neonate | Neonatal goiter<br>Endemic mental retardation<br>Neonatal hypothyroidism |
| Child, adolescent | Goiter<br>Impaired mental function<br>Subclinical hypothyroidism<br>Retarded physical development |

*Iodine deficiency in the fetus:* Maternal hypothyroidism due to iodine deficiency leads to an increased risk of abortions and stillbirths. The fetal thyroid gland begins to function from the second half of gestation. Inadequate availability of $T_4$ due to maternal hypothyroidism adversely affects early brain development in the fetus leading to permanent manifestations of endemic cretinism including mental retardation, hearing impairment (deaf-mutism), spastic diplegia and squint.

*Iodine deficiency in the neonate:* Iodine deficiency affects functioning of the thyroid gland leading to neonatal goiter and hypothyroidism The brain of the human infant at birth has only reached about one-third of its full size and continues to grow rapidly until the end of the second year. The thyroid hormone, dependent on an adequate supply of iodine, is essential for normal brain development at this critical time. Neonatal hypothyroidism persists into infancy and childhood, if the deficiency is not corrected and results in retardation of physical and mental development.

*Iodine deficiency in children:* Moderate iodine deficiency is associated with abnormalities in psychoneuromotor and intellectual development of children who are clinically euthyroid, but who do not exhibit other features of endemic cretinism (Table 8.6). Some patients may show goiter (Fig. 8.12) (*see* Chapter 18). Studies in moderately iodine-deficient areas indicate that fine motor skills and visual problem solving improved in school children after iodine repletion.

*Therapy:* Universal iodization of salt is a successful public health intervention to prevent IDD in populations at risk of deficiency throughout the world. In India, the National Iodine Deficiency Disorders Control Program (formerly known as National Goitre Program) was started by establishment of salt iodination plants to ensure an adequate supply of iodized salt in the country. The target iodine content of salt as per the program is 30 and 15 parts per million (ppm) at the manufacturing and distribution levels, respectively.

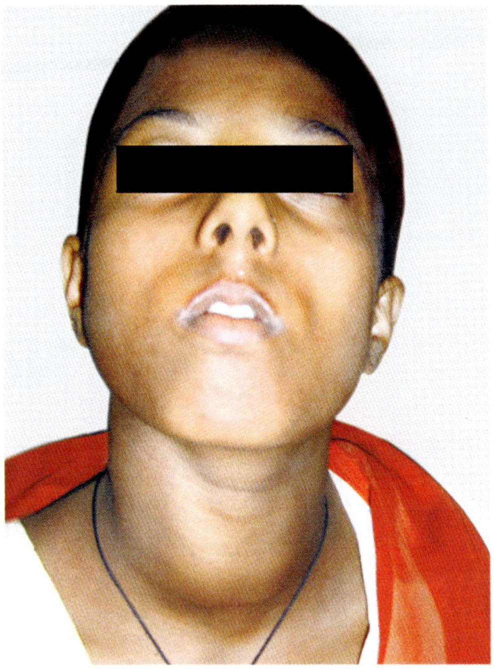

**Fig. 8.12** A 14-year-old girl with goiter

## Suggested Reading


1. Carpenter TO, Shaw NJ, Portale AA, et al. Rickets. Nature Rev Dis Primers 2017;3(1):1–20.
2. Gupta P, Dabas A, Seth A, et al. Indian Academy of Pediatrics Revised (2021) Guidelines on Prevention and Treatment of Vitamin D Deficiency and Rickets. Indian Pediatrics 2022 Feb; 59(2):142–58.
3. Kapil U, Kapil R, Gupta A. National Iron Plus Initiative" Current status and strategy. Indian J Med Res 2019;150:239–47.
4. Yadav K, Pandav CS. National Iodine Deficiency Disorders Control Program. Indian J Med Res 2018;48 (5):503–10.
5. Suskind DL. Nutritional deficiencies during normal growth. Pediatr Clin North Am 2009;56(5):1035–53.

Chapter

9

# Newborn Care

❍ Ramesh Agarwal ❍ Amanpreet Sethi

Newborn infants are unique in their physiology and health problems. The neonatal period is characterized by the transition to extrauterine life and rapid growth and development. Comprising just the first 28 days of life, this period carries the highest mortality risk during childhood. Despite being less than 2% of the under-5 childhood, the newborn period accounts for over half of U-5 child mortality. Therefore, optimum care improves children's survival and lays the foundation for optimal long-term physical and neurocognitive development.

Newborn health is the key to child health and survival. The current neonatal mortality rate (NMR) in India is 20 per thousand live births (SRS 2020). India has about five lakh neonatal deaths each year. Neonatal deaths account for 63% of U-5 and 71% of infant deaths. First-week deaths (<7 days; early neonatal deaths) at 15 per thousand live births alone account for 47% of total under-5 deaths at 32 per thousand live births (SRS 2020). Of all the neonatal deaths, about 40% occur within the first 24 hours, half within 72 hr, and three-fourths within one week of birth.

Preterm birth complications account for 44% of all neonatal deaths and constitute the most important cause of neonatal mortality (Fig. 9.1). Bacterial infections (sepsis and pneumonia) contribute to 20% of neonatal deaths. Birth asphyxia (19%) and congenital malformations (11%) are other important causes of neonatal deaths. Newborns with low birth weight (LBW) constitute nearly one-third of the neonatal population but account for three-fourths of neonatal deaths. The mother's health and care during pregnancy and childbirth profoundly influence neonatal outcomes.

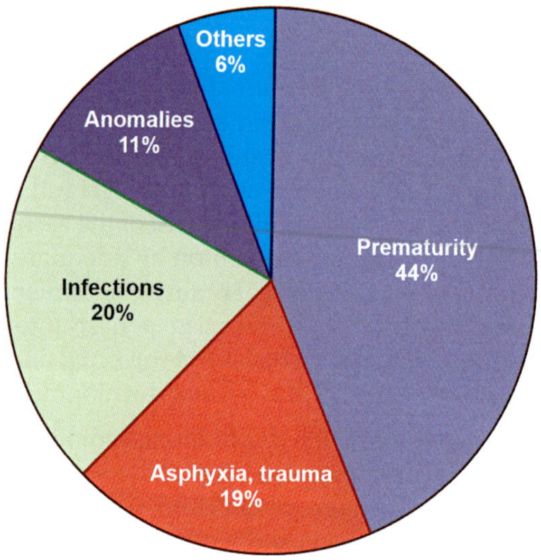


**Fig. 9.1:** The leading causes of neonatal deaths in India (WHO 2020) (*Courtesy:* Dr M Jeeva Sankar)

*Competency:* **PE20.1**

## DEFINITIONS (Fig. 9.2)

*Neonatal period:* From birth to under four weeks (0 to 27 days or 1 to 28 days, depending on whether the first day has been taken as day 0 or day 1 of life) of age. The early neonatal period is the first week of life (<7 days or <168 hr). The late neonatal period extends from the 7 to the 28 days.

*Post neonatal period:* Period of infancy from 28 days to <365 days (<1 year) of life.

*Perinatal period:* The perinatal period extends from the 22nd week of gestation (≥154 days or fetus weighing 500 g or more) to less than 7 days of life.

*Live birth:* A product of conception, irrespective of weight or gestational age, that, after separation from the mother, shows *any evidence of life* such as breathing, heartbeat, pulsation of the umbilical cord, or definite movement of voluntary muscles.

*Fetal death:* A fetal death is a product of conception that does not show any evidence of life after separation from the mother.

*Stillbirth (WHO):* Fetal death at a gestational age of ≥28 weeks or weight  1000 g before or during the birth

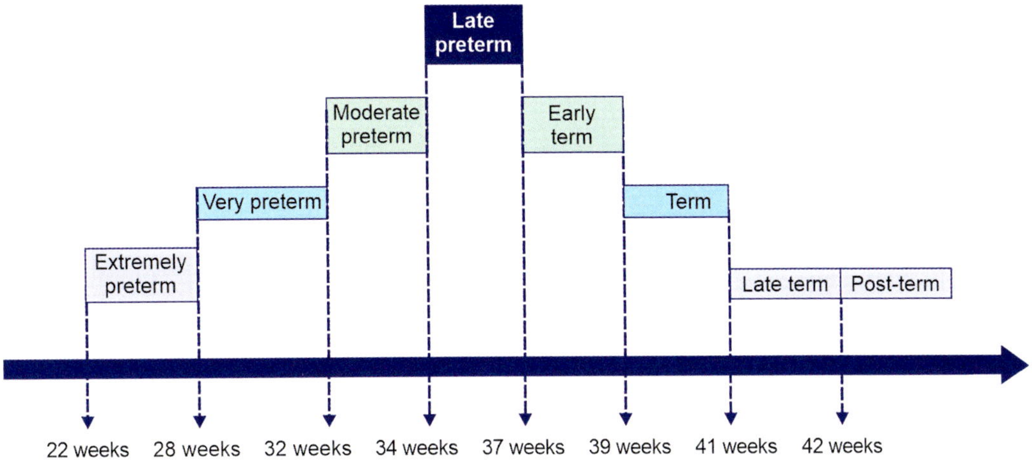


**Fig. 9.2:** Gestation-based definitions in newborns

process. Many developed nations, such as the USA and the UK, define stillbirths at 20 weeks of gestation.

***Term neonate:*** A neonate is born between 37 and <42 weeks (259–293 days) of gestation.

***Preterm neonate:*** A neonate born before 37 weeks (<259 days) of gestation, irrespective of the birth weight.

***Post-term neonate:*** A neonate is born at a gestation age of 42 weeks or more (294 days or more).

***Late preterm neonate:*** A neonate born between 34 and 36 weeks and 6 days of gestation.

***Moderate preterm neonate:*** A neonate born between 32 and 33 weeks and 6 days of gestation.

***Very preterm neonate:*** A neonate born between 28 and 31 weeks and 6 days of gestation.

***Extreme preterm neonate:*** A neonate born less than 28 of gestation.

***Low birth weight (LBW) neonate:*** A neonate weighs less than 2500 g at birth, irrespective of the gestational age.

***Very low birth weight (VLBW) neonate:*** A neonate weighs less than 1500 g at birth, irrespective of the gestational age.

***Extremely low birth weight (ELBW) neonate:*** A neonate weighs less than 1000 g at birth, irrespective of the gestational age.

***Neonatal mortality rate (NMR):*** Deaths of infants during the first 28 days of life per 1000 live births per year.

***Perinatal mortality ratio (PNMR):*** The number of perinatal deaths (stillbirths plus neonatal deaths before 7 days of life) per 1000 live births. It is designated as a ratio since the numerator is not the part of the denominator (for a rate, like in NMR, numerator must be part of the denominator).

*Competency:* **PE20.3**

## RESUSCITATION

Around 6 lakh newborns die every year in India. Approximately 19% of these deaths are attributed to birth asphyxia.

The term birth asphyxia connotes the inability of a newly born baby to establish optimum respiration after birth. Birth asphyxia leads to progressive hypoxia, hypercapnia, hypoperfusion and acidosis. It affects all major organ systems, including CNS, heart, GIT, and lungs. It may lead to multiorgan dysfunction. Hypoxic ischemic encephalopathy (HIE) resulting from asphyxia may lead to long-term neuromotor sequelae.

Approximately 85% of all neonates born at term gestation do not require resuscitation. The American Heart Association (AHA) and the American Academy of Pediatrics (AAP) have recently updated the resuscitation guidelines (2020). Around 10% of neonates require initial steps of drying and stimulation, and approximately 5% require positive pressure ventilation at birth.

### Pathophysiology of Asphyxia

When a fetus does not receive enough oxygen, a brief period of rapid breathing occurs. If the asphyxia continues, the respiratory movements cease, and the infant enters a period of apnea known as primary apnea. During primary apnea, the heart rate begins to fall, the neuromuscular tone gradually diminishes, but the blood pressure is preserved. In most instances, tactile stimulation during this period will reinitiate respiration.

If the asphyxia continues, the infant develops deep gasping respiration, the heart rate continues to fall, the blood pressure also begins to fall, and the infant becomes flaccid. The breathing becomes weaker until the infant takes the last gasp and enters a period of secondary apnea. The infant is now unresponsive to stimulation and does not spontaneously resume respiratory efforts unless resuscitation in the form of positive pressure ventilation (PPV) is initiated.

As a result of fetal hypoxia, the infant may go through primary and secondary apnea phases before birth. Hence, apnea at birth may be either primary or secondary apnea. These two are clinically indistinguishable; the infant is not breathing in both instances, and the heart rate may be below 100 beats per minute. Hence, when faced with an apneic infant at birth, assume that the infant is experiencing secondary apnea and, therefore, institute full resuscitation without wasting too much time in tactile stimulation.

*Lung Inflation*

During intrauterine life, the lungs do not participate in gas exchange, which is taken care of by the placenta. The lung alveoli in the fetus are filled with fluid secreted by type II alveolar cells. The process of fluid removal starts with the onset of labor. The fluid gets reabsorbed from the alveoli into the perivascular space and blood and lymphatic channels. The labor process may facilitate the removal of lung fluid, whereas removal is slowed when labor is absent (as in elective cesarean section).

Removal of lung fluid from the alveoli is facilitated by respiration soon after birth. The first few breaths after birth effectively expand the alveoli and replace the lung fluid with air. Problems in clearing lung fluid may occur in infants whose lungs have not inflated well with the first few breaths, such as those who are apneic at birth or have a weak initial respiratory effort as with prematurity or sedation.

*Pulmonary Circulation*

Oxygenation depends not only on air reaching the alveoli but also on pulmonary circulation. After birth, pulmonary vessels dilate, resulting in a fall in pulmonary vascular resistance and increased blood flow. As the pulmonary vessels remain constricted, there is hardly any blood flow in the lungs during fetal life.

The asphyxiated infant has hypoxemia and acidosis (low pH), failing pulmonary vasodilation, and closure of ductus arteriosus (persistence of fetal circulation). Due to poor pulmonary blood flow, proper oxygenation of the body's tissues does not occur as there is inadequate oxygen uptake in the lungs, even if the infant is adequately ventilated.

In mildly asphyxiated neonates, the oxygen and pH are slightly lower; it may be possible to increase pulmonary blood flow by quickly restoring ventilation. However, pulmonary perfusion in severely asphyxiated infants may not improve with ventilation alone. The combination of oxygenation and correction of metabolic acidosis would be necessary to improve pulmonary blood flow.

*Circulation*

Asphyxia redistributes the blood flow from nonvital to vital organs. There is reduced blood supply to the bowel, kidney, muscles, and skin, while the blood flow to the heart and brain is relatively preserved (diving-in reflex). As asphyxia is prolonged, myocardial function and cardiac output deteriorate, and the blood flow to all the organs is further reduced. This sets in the stage for progressive organ damage.

*Preparing for Resuscitation*

Even with knowledge of risk factors, we can predict asphyxia only in half of the cases. In the remaining half, asphyxia and the need for resuscitation would come as a surprise. Therefore, the team must view each delivery as an emergency and be ready to provide resuscitation and manage asphyxia in the neonate.

*Preparation for Delivery*

There should be at least one person available who is solely responsible for the neonate and is capable of undertaking full resuscitation. In an anticipated need for resuscitation, more than one person may be needed. A coordinated team effort is required to ensure adequate resuscitation:

a. Inquire about antepartum and intrapartum risk factors
b. Anticipate emergencies and plan accordingly
c. Assemble a team and choose a team leader
d. Team leader delegates roles and responsibilities as per the competence of the team members
e. Use effective closed-loop communication (the listener repeats what has been said to him)
f. Check the equipment and supplies (Table 9.1)
g. Ask for additional help, if required.

*Role of Apgar Scores in Resuscitation*

The Apgar score is an objective method of evaluating the newborn's condition (Table 9.2). It is generally performed at 1 minute and again at 5 minutes after birth. However, resuscitation must be initiated before the 1-minute score is assigned. *Therefore, the Apgar score is not used to guide the resuscitation.*

While the Apgar score does not help decide the need for resuscitation, the serial scores help in knowing how well the neonate responds to resuscitative efforts. Extended Apgar scores should be obtained every 5 minutes for up to 20 minutes, if the 5-minute Apgar score is less than 7.

## TABC of Resuscitation

The components of neonatal resuscitation can be summarized as TABC:

***T-Temperature:*** Provide warmth, dry the neonate and remove the wet linen.

**Table 9.1:** Neonatal resuscitation supplies and equipment

| |
|---|
| **Suction equipment** |
| Mechanical suction |
| Suction catheters 10, 12 or 14 F |
| Meconium aspirator |
| **Bag and mask equipment** |
| Neonatal resuscitation bags (self-inflating) |
| Face-masks (for both term and preterm babies) |
| Oxygen with flow meter and tubing |
| **Intubation equipment** |
| Laryngoscope with straight blades no. 0 (preterm) and no. 1 (term) |
| Extra bulbs and batteries (for laryngoscope) |
| Endotracheal tubes (internal diameter of 2.5, 3.0, 3.5 and 4.0 mm) |
| **Medications** |
| Epinephrine |
| Normal saline or Ringer lactate |
| Naloxone hydrochloride |
| **Miscellaneous** |
| Linen, shoulder roll, gauze |
| Radiant warmer |
| Stethoscope |
| Syringes 1, 2, 5, 10, 20, 50 mL |
| Feeding tube 6 F |
| Umbilical catheters 3.5, 5 F |
| Three way stopcocks |
| Gloves |

**Table 9.2:** Apgar score

| *Sign* | *Score* | | |
|---|---|---|---|
| | *0* | *1* | *2* |
| Color | Blue or pale | Body pink, extremities blue | Body and extremities both pink |
| Heart rate | Absent | Slow (<100 beat/min) | Normal (>100 beat/min) |
| Reflex irritability | No response | Grimace | Cough or sneeze |
| Muscle tone | Limp | Some flexion | Active movements |
| Respiration | Absent | Irregular/gasping | Good strong cry |

*A-Airway:* Position the infant; clear the airway if required (by wiping or suctioning of baby's mouth and nose). If necessary, insert an endotracheal (ET) tube to ensure an open airway.

*B-Breathing:* Tactile stimulation to initiate breathing, positive-pressure breaths using either bag and mask or bag and ET tube as necessary.

*C-Circulation:* Stimulate and maintain blood circulation with chest compressions and medications as indicated.

The resuscitation team must reach the birthing room well in time and interact with the obstetric and anesthesia team to elicit relevant information. Review the risk factors that can predispose the neonate to asphyxia. Ask these four pre-birth questions: (i) What is the gestation? (ii) if the amniotic fluid clear or stained with meconium, (iii) If there are additional risk factors as discussed before, and (iv) what is the plan for umbilical cord management?

### Resuscitation Algorithm

Figure 9.3 presents the algorithm of neonatal resuscitation. At the time of birth, one should ask three questions about the newborn:

1. Term gestation?
2. Good muscle tone? (Flexed posture and active movements of the neonate denotes good tone)
3. Breathing or actively crying?

If the answers to all three questions are 'Yes', the infant stays with the mother and receives "routine care."

Routine care consists of four steps:

i. *Warmth:* Provided by putting the neonate directly on the mother's abdomen and chest in skin-to-skin contact.
ii. *Clearing of airway if required:* Position the neonate and wipe the baby's mouth and nose using a clean cloth—no need to suction routinely.
iii. *Dry the neonate using a dry and warm cloth. Remove wet linen and cover the baby.*
iv. *Ongoing evaluation* for vital parameters. Helping mothers in breastfeeding will facilitate an easy transition to an extrauterine environment.

#### *Delayed Cord Clamping (DCC)*

*In all* neonates, *preterm and term, that do not require resuscitation, cord clamping must be delayed for 30 to 60 seconds—delayed cord clamping (DCC). There is not enough evidence to recommend DCC in* neonates *needing resuscitation. In such* neonates, *clamp and cut the cord immediately and initiate resuscitation without delay.*

If the answer to *any* of the three questions is "No", the neonate requires at least some resuscitation. After cutting the cord, perform what is known as the "*Initial steps*."

### Initial Steps

#### *Warmth*

Place the neonate under the heat source, preferably a radiant warmer. Do not cover the neonate with blankets or towels to ensure visualization and allow the radiant heat to reach the baby.

#### *Dry and Stimulate*

Dry the neonate adequately using pre-warmed linen to prevent heat loss. Remove the wet linen. Suctioning and drying themselves provide enough stimulation to initiate breathing. If the newborn continues to have poor breathing, additional tactile stimulation can be provided by gently rubbing the trunk, back, and extremities. However, one should not waste too much time providing tactile stimulation.

#### *Positioning*

Place the neonate on her back or side with the neck slightly extended (sniffing position). That keeps the airway open and facilitates breathing. Avoid hyperextension or flexion of the neck since either may interfere with respiration.

To help maintain the correct position, one may place a rolled blanket or towel under the shoulders of the infant, elevating her by ¾ or 1 inch off the mattress. This *shoulder roll* is particularly helpful, if the infant has a prominent occiput resulting from molding, edema, IUGR, or prematurity (Fig. 9.4).

#### *Clear Airway, if Necessary*

If present, remove secretion from the airway by wiping the nose and mouth with a clean cloth or suctioning with a bulb syringe or a suction catheter. Suction mouth before nose ('M' before 'N') to prevent aspiration in case the infant makes a breathing effort when the nose is suctioned. If the infant has copious secretions from the mouth, turn the head to one side to allow secretions to collect in the side of the mouth, where they can be easily removed.

For suctioning, the catheter size should be 12 or 14 Fr. Keep the suction pressure around 80 mm Hg (100 cm $H_2O$) and no more than 100 mm Hg (130 cm $H_2O$). Do not insert the catheter too deep in the mouth or nose as the stimulation of the posterior pharynx can cause vagal response resulting in bradycardia or apnea.

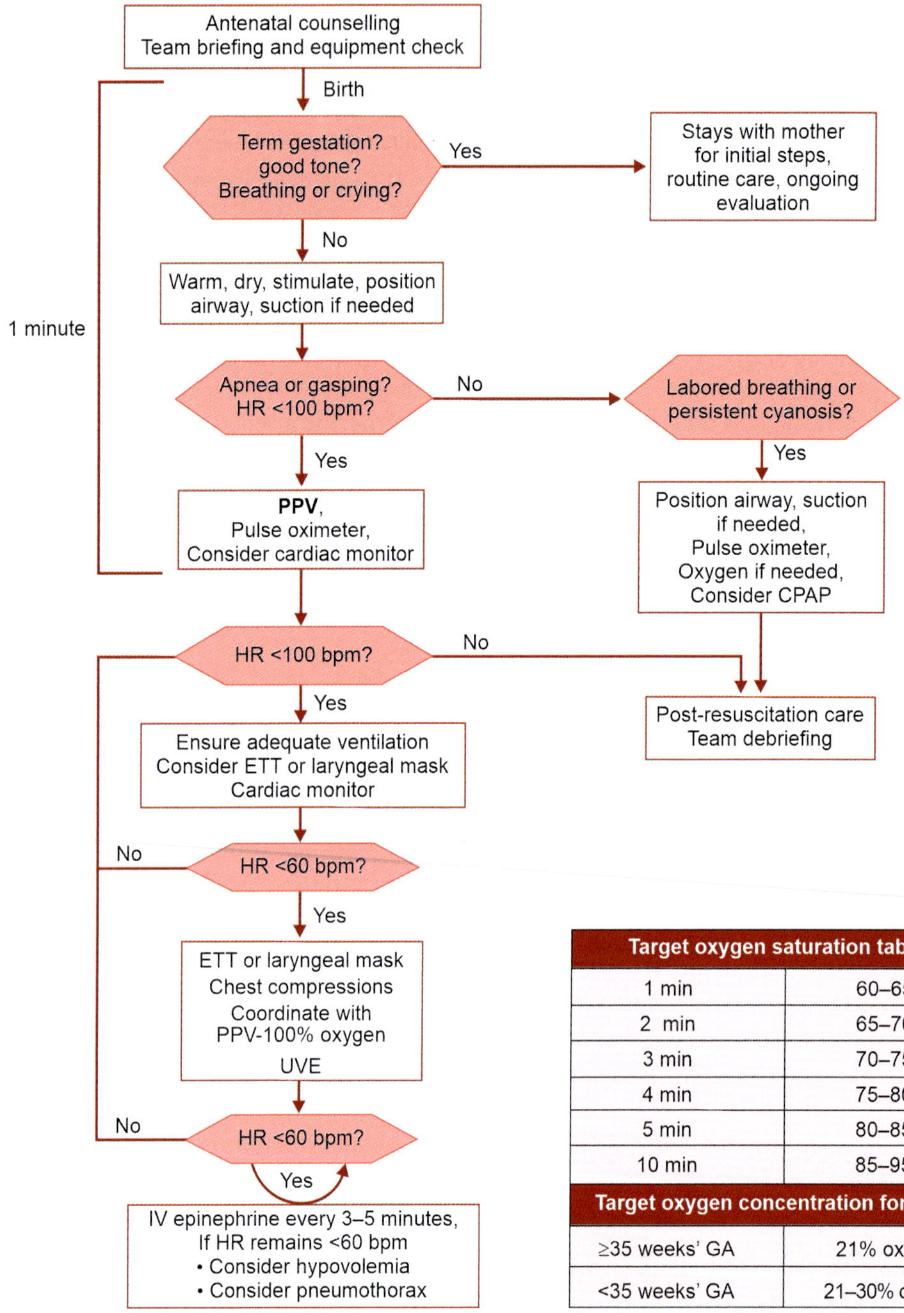


| Target oxygen saturation table | |
|---|---|
| 1 min | 60–65% |
| 2 min | 65–70% |
| 3 min | 70–75% |
| 4 min | 75–80% |
| 5 min | 80–85% |
| 10 min | 85–95% |
| **Target oxygen concentration for PPV** | |
| ≥35 weeks' GA | 21% oxygen |
| <35 weeks' GA | 21–30% oxygen |

**Fig. 9.3:** The resuscitation algorithm. CPAP continuous positive airway pressure; PPV positive pressure ventilation; $SpO_2$ saturation of oxygen; ETT endotracheal tube (Adapted with permission from American Academy of Pediatrics 2020)

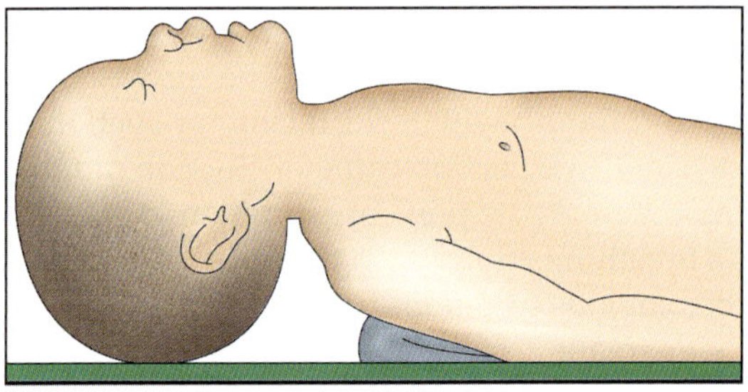

**Fig. 9.4:** Rolled towel under the shoulders

### Infant Born through Meconium-Stained Liquor (MSL)

A neonate born through meconium-stained liquor (MSL) may aspirate the meconium into the trachea and lungs. Recent evidence has demonstrated that procedures of intrapartum suctioning of the mouth and nose before delivery of the shoulders and postnatal tracheal suctioning of non-vigorous neonates (feeble breathing or low tone) are not beneficial. The new guideline does not recommend these procedures anymore.

### Evaluation

After providing initial steps, the neonate should be evaluated by assessing respiration, heart rate (HR), and color (or oxygen saturation by pulse oximetry).

Observe chest movements for evaluation of respiration. Auscultate the heart or palpate the umbilical cord pulsation for 6 seconds. Multiply the number of heart beats or pulsations in 6 seconds by 10 to get the HR per minute (e.g. a count of 14 in 6 seconds is an HR of 140 per minute). Look at the tongue, mucous membranes, and trunk to evaluate the color. A blue hue to the lips, tongue, and central trunk indicates central cyanosis. The presence of cyanosis in extremities (acrocyanosis) does not have any significance.

- *Good breathing efforts, HR 100/min or more, and no cyanosis:* No additional intervention is needed; monitor the neonate frequently.
- *Labored breathing or persistent central cyanosis:* Provide CPAP in preterm neonates and supplemental oxygen in term neonates. Monitor oxygen saturation and titrate supplemental oxygen to achieve the targeted saturations (Fig. 9.6).
- *Apnea, gasping breathing, or HR below 100 min:* Provide positive pressure ventilation (PPV)

### Supplemental Oxygen

Provide supplemental oxygen by an oxygen mask or oxygen tube held in a cupped hand over the baby's face or by a flow-inflating bag and mask. Do not attempt giving supplemental oxygen using a self-inflating bag. The flow of oxygen should be at least 5 L/minute.

### Positive Pressure Ventilation (PPV)

Provide PPV with a self-inflating bag and face mask (bag and mask ventilation or BMV). The self-inflating bag is easy to use as it reinflates entirely without any external compressed gas source.

The resuscitation bag (Fig. 9.5) should have a capacity of 240 to 750 mL. Connect the bag to a source of oxygen and air and a blender that provides the desired concentration of supplemental oxygen.

#### *Indications of PPV*

PPV is indicated, if:

i. The infant is apneic or gasping.
ii. HR is less than 100 beats per minute.

*In suspected or confirmed diaphragmatic hernia, bag and mask ventilation is contraindicated.*

Treat oxygen as a drug—too little or too much; both are bad for the baby. Even a brief exposure to a high oxygen concentration can have a detrimental effect on the baby. Studies have shown that term neonates resuscitated with room air compared to 100% oxygen have better survival and long-term outcomes. The recent evidence indicates that most preterm neonates needed supplemental oxygen during resuscitation. In preterm neonates, less than 35 weeks of gestation, start resuscitation with 21–30% oxygen followed by up- or downward titration based upon pulse oximetry. Starting with a lower oxygen concentration prevents the harms of hyperoxia like bronchopulmonary dysplasia and retinopathy of prematurity in this vulnerable population.

Use room air in neonates of 35 weeks or more and 21 to 30% oxygen in preterm neonates of 34 weeks or lower to initiate resuscitation. Monitor oxygen saturation using pulse oximetry and titrate oxygen concentration to maintain oxygen saturation in the targeted range (Fig. 9.3). Without pulse oximetry, room air should be substituted by 100% oxygen, if the neonate fails to improve (improvement in HR and breathing) by 90 seconds.

#### *Procedure*

Stand at the head end or on the side of the neonate to get a clear view of the neonate's chest and abdomen. Keep the infant's neck neutral or slight extension. Select an appropriate size face mask that covers the mouth and nose but not the eyes of the infant (Fig. 9.6). Hold the face mask firmly on the face to obtain a good seal. Compress the bag using your fingers and not your hands.

The *PPV is the single most effective step in neonates who fail to breathe* at birth. Ensuring adequacy of PPV is, therefore, critical for the successful resuscitation of neonates not breathing at birth.

Usually, neonates respond to PPV after birth with an immediate increase in their HR. If a neonate is not responding by a rapid increase in HR after 15 seconds of PPV, assess if the baby's chest is moving with PPV and auscultate for breath sounds. If the chest is not rising and there are no audible breath sounds, take ventilation corrective steps (MR SOPA; Table 9.3).

Once the effective chest rise is observed, perform PPV at a rate of 40 to 60 breaths per minute, following a 'squeeze, two, three' sequence (Fig. 9.7). Ensure the chest is rising as if the neonate is taking easy breaths. Avoid giving too deep breaths (too much tidal volume). Avoid delivering PPV at a high rate.

After the infant has received 30 seconds of PPV, evaluate the HR and take follow-up action as in Fig. 9.3.

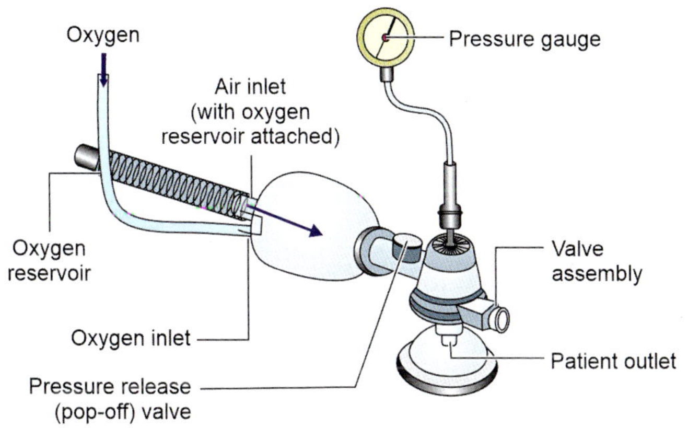


**Fig. 9.5:** Self-inflating bag (Adapted with permission from AAP 2005)

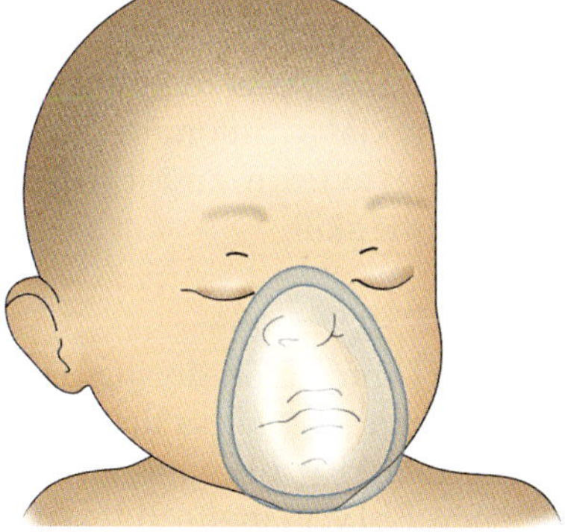

**Fig. 9.6:** Properly fitting mask

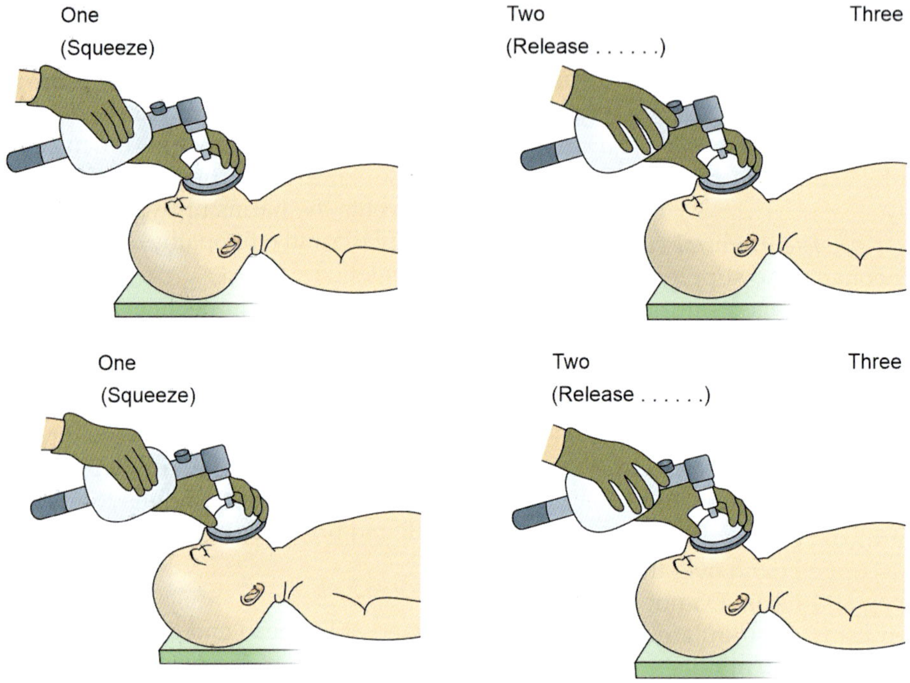


**Fig. 9.7:** Correct rhythm of providing positive pressure ventilation (Adapted with permission from American Academy of Pediatrics 2005)

**Table 9.3:** Ventilation corrective steps (MR SOPA)

| *Action* | *Condition* |
|---|---|
| Inadequate seal | Re-apply **m**ask |
| Blocked airway | **R**eposition the infant's head |
| Blocked airway | Clear **s**ecretions by suction |
| Blocked airway | Ventilate with mouth slightly **o**pen |
| Inadequate pressure | Increase **p**ressure slightly |
| Consider **al**ternate airway | Blocked **a**irway (endotracheal tube) |

Improving the infant's condition is judged by increasing HR, spontaneous respiration, and improving color. If the infant fails to improve, check for chest rise. If chest rise is inadequate, take ventilation corrective steps as outlined earlier.

PPV may cause abdominal distension as the gas escapes into the stomach via the esophagus. Distended stomach presses on the diaphragm and compromises ventilation. Therefore, if ventilation is continued for more than two minutes, an orogastric tube (feeding tube size 6–8 Fr) should be inserted and left open to decompress the abdomen.

## Endotracheal Intubation

Endotracheal (ET) intubation is required only in a small proportion of asphyxiated neonates. Intubation is a relatively difficult skill to learn, and it requires consistent practice to maintain the skill.

### *Indications*

The indications of ET intubation during resuscitation are: (i) If the neonate's heart rate is less than 100 bpm despite 30 seconds of effective PPV, (ii) when prolonged BMV is required, (iii) when BMV is ineffective, (iv) when chest compression is needed, and (v) when a diaphragmatic hernia is suspected, or the airway is blocked with thick secretions. ET intubation may be considered for administering epinephrine.

### *Endotracheal Tube (ET)*

ET should be of uniform diameter throughout the tube length (not tapered near the tip) and have a vocal cord guide at the tip and centimeter markings. ET tube size depends on the weight or gestation of the neonate (Table 9.4). The ET tube's insertion depth is now determined by a formula: Nasotragal length (NTL)+ 1 cm, as shown in Fig. 9.8.

Most ET currently manufactured for neonates have a black line near the tube's tip called a vocal cord guide. Such tubes are meant to be inserted so that the vocal cord guide is placed at the level of the vocal cords. This helps position the tip of ET above the bifurcation of the trachea.

A neonatal laryngoscope with straight blades of sizes 0' (for preterm neonates) and '1' (for term neonates) is required for intubation. Before intubating, the appropriate blade is attached to the laryngoscope handle, and the light is turned on.

### *Procedure*

The infant's head should be in the midline and the slightly extended neck. The laryngoscope is held in the left hand

**Table 9.4:** Appropriate endotracheal tube size

| *Inner diameter of tube (mm)* | *Weight (g)* | *Gestational age (weeks)* |
|---|---|---|
| 2.5 | <1000 | <28 |
| 3.0 | 1000–2000 | 28–34 |
| 3.5 | 2000–3000 | 34–38 |
| 4.0 | >3000 | >38 |

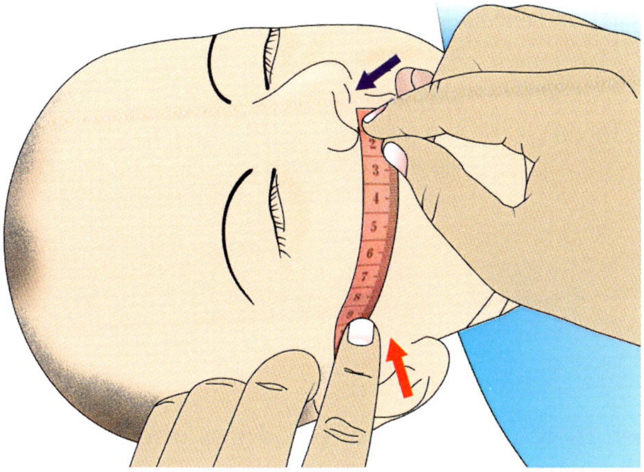

Fig. 9.8: Procedure to measure nasotragal length: Blue arrow indicates the bridge of the nose and red arrow indicates the tragus (*Courtesy:* Dr Sakshi Jindal, Faridkot)

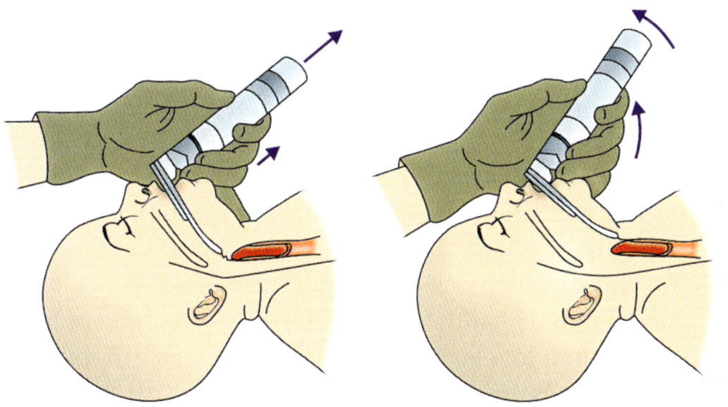


Fig. 9.9: Direction of pull on the laryngoscope (Adapted with permission from AAP 2005)

between the thumb and the first three fingers, with the blade pointing away from oneself. Standing at the head end of the infant, the blade is introduced in the mouth and advanced to just beyond the base of the tongue so that its tip rests in the vallecula. The blade is lifted as shown in Fig. 9.9, and landmarks looked for: The epiglottis and glottis should come into view. Vocal cords on the sides surround the glottic opening. Once the glottis is visible, the ET is introduced from the right side of the mouth, and its tip is inserted into the glottis until the vocal cord guide is at the glottis level. Thus, it positions it halfway between the vocal cords and the carina.

## Chest Compressions (CC)

The heart circulates blood throughout the body delivering oxygen to vital organs. When an infant becomes hypoxic, the HR slows, and myocardial contractility decreases. As a result, blood and oxygen flow to the vital organs is diminished.

CC helps mechanically pump blood to vital organs of the body. CC consists of rhythmic sternum compression that compresses the heart against the spine, increases intrathoracic pressure, and circulates blood to the body's vital organs. BMV must always accompany CC so only oxygenated blood is circulated during CC.

CC are indicated if HR is below 60/min, even after 30 seconds of PPV. Once the HR is 60/min or more, chest compressions should be discontinued.

### Procedure

The CC is delivered by the 2-thumb technique (Fig. 9.10). With the thumb technique, the two thumbs are used to depress the sternum, with the hands encircling the torso and the fingers supporting the back. *The earlier used two-finger technique for CC is no more recommended.*

When CC is performed on a neonate, pressure is applied to the lower third of the sternum (Fig. 9.10). Avoid using force on the xiphoid. To locate the area, slide the fingers on the lower edge of the thoracic cage to find the xiphisternum. The lower third of the sternum is just above it. Thumbs should remain in contact with the chest during compression and release. Complications of CC include broken ribs, lacerations of the liver, and pneumothorax.

### Rate

Ventilate between CC. A positive breath should follow every third CC: 90 CC and 30 PPV in one minute (totaling 120 events). The chest should be compressed three times over 1½ seconds, leaving out ½ second for ventilation in a 2-minute cycle. Check femoral or carotid pulsation periodically to determine the efficacy of CC.

### Evaluation

After 60 seconds of CC, the heart rate is checked:

***HR below 60:*** Continue CC along with PPV. In addition, medications (epinephrine) may have to be administered.

***HR 60 or above:*** Discontinue CC. PPV should be continued until the HR is above 100 beats per minute and the infant breathes spontaneously.

## Medications

Medications used in resuscitation include epinephrine and volume expanders (Table 9.5). There is no role of atropine, dexamethasone, calcium, mannitol, dextrose, and naloxone for newborn resuscitation in the delivery room.

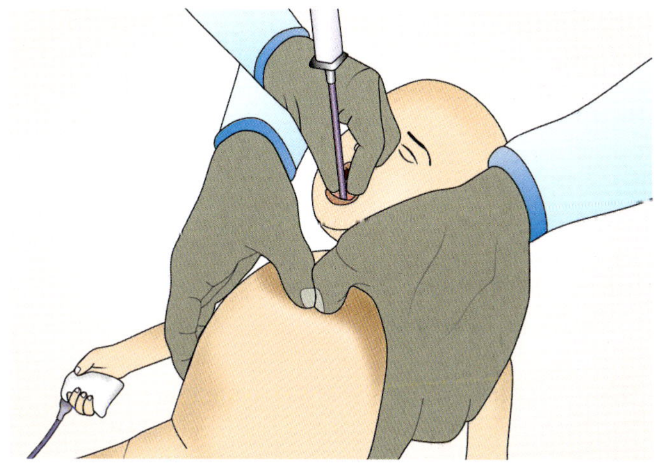

Fig. 9.10: Technique for chest compression using two thumbs placed side by side on the lower part of the sternum (Adapted with permission from AAP 2020)

Table 9.5: Medications to be used in the delivery room: Indications, dosage, and effects

| *Medication (concentration)* | *Indication* | *Effects* | *Concentration administered* | *Dose of the prepared solution* | *Route* |
|---|---|---|---|---|---|
| Epinephrine (1:1000) | HR <60/min after 60 seconds of effective PPV and chest compressions | Inotropic; chronotropic; peripheral vasoconstrictor | 1:10000 | 0.2 mL/kg (a repeat dose can be given every 3–5 minutes) | IV; through umbilical vein (endotracheal route, if no IV access) |
| Normal saline, Ringer lactate | Acute bleeding with hypovolemia (especially in the setting of antepartum hemorrhage) | Increased intravascular volume improves perfusion | | 10 mL/kg (over 5–10 minutes) | Umbilical vein |

Medications are preferably delivered through the umbilical vein. There is no role for intracardiac injection. For umbilical vein access, insert a 3.5 Fr or 5 Fr umbilical catheter into the umbilical vein just deep enough to get a free blood flow. In an emergency, epinephrine can be delivered through the trachea, if the newborn is intubated. Absorption is erratic in the tracheobronchial tree, and this method is to be used only if venous access cannot be obtained. The drug is injected by a syringe or a feeding tube (5 Fr) into the endotracheal tube and dispersed into the lungs by PPV.

### *Indications*

Use of adrenaline is indicated, if HR remains below 60 despite adequate ventilation of 30 seconds and 60 seconds of effective ventilation and chest compressions. The dose of epinephrine is 0.2 mL/kg (range 0.1 to 0.3 mL/kg) of 1:10 000 dilution (1 mg in 10 mL of saline). Follow the IV bolus with a saline bolus of 3 mL to flush the drug into the central circulation. Volume expander in the form of normal saline or Ringer's lactate is indicated when there is a history of blood loss or signs of shock in the neonate.

### Suggested Reading


1. Textbook of Neonatal Resuscitation, 8th edn. American Academy of Pediatrics and American Heart Association, 2020.


## LEVEL OF NEWBORN CARE

The newborn care has been planned at different levels to meet the needs of neonates that may be normal to extremely sick, requiring complex care. American Academy of Pediatrics specifies four levels: Normal newborn care at all birthing places (level 1) to subspecialty level care to meet the needs of highly sick neonates (Table 9.6 and Fig. 9.11).

The National Health Mission of the Government of India specifies three levels of care: Newborn care corners at all birthing places to meet the basic needs of all neonates, newborn stabilization units at the first referral level, and special newborn care units (SNCUs) at district hospitals and medical colleges to cater to need of sick neonates. Currently, India has nearly 1000 SNCUs.

Table 9.6: Level of newborn care

| *Level of newborn care* | *Target neonates/capabilities* |
|---|---|
| Level 1 | Normal term newborns<br>Stable newborns of 35 to 36 weeks' gestation<br>These units stabilize small and sick neonates and transfer them to a higher level |
| Level 2 | Neonates of 32 weeks or more of gestation or 1500 g or more at birth<br>Neonate with moderate sickness.<br>CPAP and brief ventilation<br>Serves as step-down units for level-3 and level-4 care. |
| Level 3 | Neonates of less than 32 weeks or less than 1500 g<br>Critical illnesses<br>Offer a full range of respiratory support. |
| Level 4 | Provide a full range of advanced subspeciality care, including options of cardiac surgery, pediatric surgery, extracorporeal membrane oxygenator (ECMO) |
| **National Health Mission (NHM), India** | |
| Newborn care corner (NBCC) | Present in all birthing facilities<br>Identify and refer at-risk and sick neonates to higher facilities |
| Newborn stabilization units (NBSU) | NBCC in all birthing facilities<br>Provide sick newborn care to neonates above 1800 g<br>Present in CHCs and first referral units |
| Special newborn care unit (SNCU) | In addition to the availability of NBCC and NBSU<br>Provides care to neonates <1800 g and limited ventilation facilities |

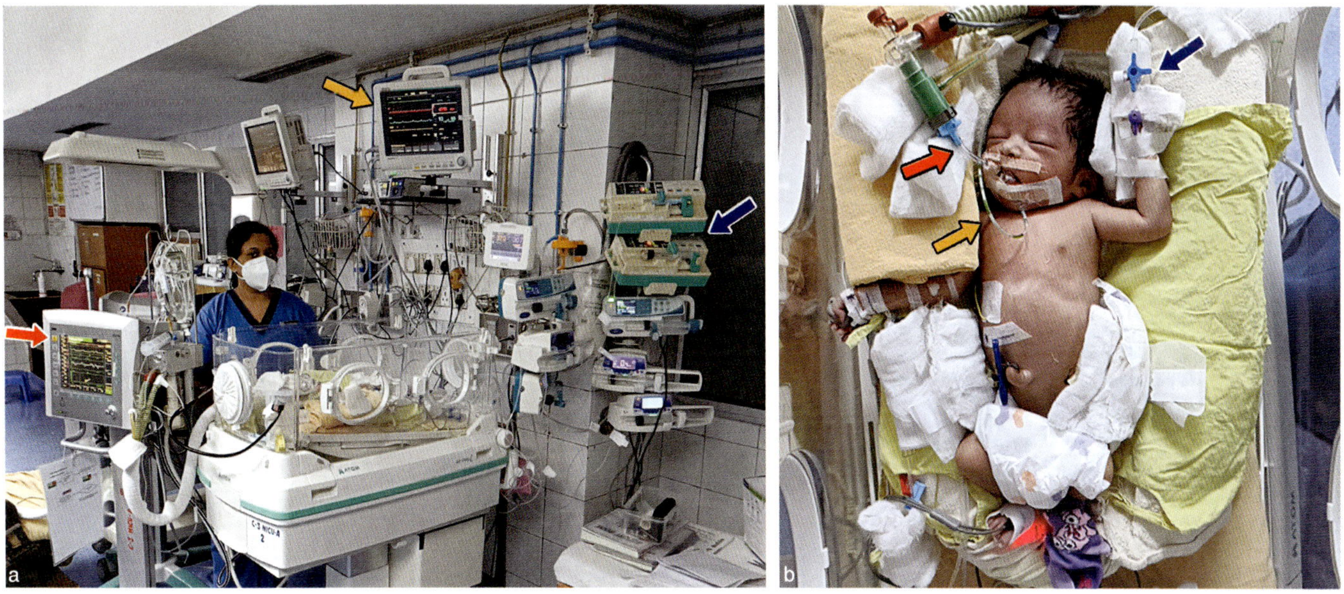

Fig. 9.11: (a) A sick baby being cared for in the neonatal intensive care unit (NICU). Note the ventilator (red arrow), multiple infusion pumps (blue arrow), and multipara monitor (yellow arrow); (b) The baby: Note the endotracheal tube connected to the ventilator tubing (red arrow), an arterial line (blue arrow), a pulse oximeter probe on the right foot, and a temperature probe on the abdomen. The abdomen of the baby appears distended. The feeding tube has a bilious discharge (yellow arrow). The baby is kept in a cloth boundary around him for developmentally supportive care



### Family Participatory Care

Family participatory care (FPC) involves family members caring for their sick and small neonates admitted to SNCU as caregivers and decision makers. The providers' team encourages, empowers, trains, and supports the family members to assist in caring for their sick and small neonate. FPC has been shown to improve exclusive breastfeeding rates, parent–infant bonding, infant weight gain, less hospital-acquired infections, thus leading to early discharge and fewer readmission rates. It lowers stress and anxiety among parents' workload of the nursing staff.

### Mother-Neonatal Intensive Care Unit (M-NICU)

Mother-neonatal intensive care unit (M-NICU) is a novel concept wherein the mothers and their sick and small neonate are kept together after delivery. In M-NICU, the mother's bed is kept side by side with the newborn's radiant warmer. Therefore, the mother becomes an active caregiver and can provide immediate KMC to her sick and small neonates. She can easily be trained about asepsis routine, danger signs, feeding, and recognizing danger signs. Such units can provide routine postpartum care and management of common postpartum morbidities of the mothers.

Care in M-NICU has improved neonatal survival, bonding, exclusive breastfeeding rates, weight gain, less hospital stay, and maternal stress. A recent multicountry study demonstrated that immediate KMC provided by the mother or other caregiver in the M NICU setting reduces mortality by 25% in infants 1.0 to 1.79 kg that were moderately sick. For M-NICU to be successful, proper coordination and collaboration is required with obstetrics and gynecology team.

*Competencies:* **PE20.2; PE20.5; PE20.6**

## CARE OF NORMAL NEONATES

### Care at Birth

*Standard precautions and asepsis at birth:* The personnel attending the delivery must exercise all the universal/ standard precautions in all cases. All fluid from the baby/ mother should be treated as potentially infectious. Gloves, masks, and gowns should be worn when resuscitating the newborn. Protective eyewear or face shields should be worn during procedures likely to generate droplets of blood or other body fluids.

'Five cleans' to prevent sepsis at birth:

i. ***Clean hands:*** Hand-hygiene and wear sterile gloves
ii. ***Clean surface:*** Use a clean and sterile towel to dry and cover the neonate
iii. ***Clean blade:*** The umbilical cord is to be cut with a clean and sterile blade/scissor
iv. ***Clean tie:*** The cord should be clamped with a clean and sterile clamp or tie
v. ***Nothing to be applied on the cord.*** Keep it dry.

*Prevention and management of hypothermia:* Immediately after birth, the newborn is at high risk of hypothermia. This early hypothermia may have a detrimental effect on the infant's health. Special care should be taken to prevent and manage hypothermia. The temperature of the delivery room should be 25°C, and the space should be free from the air draft. The neonate should be received in a prewarmed sterile linen sheet at birth. The infant should be dried thoroughly, including the head and face, and any wet linen should not remain in contact with the infant. The infant may be placed on the mother's abdomen immediately after the birth for early skin-to-skin (STS) contact (Fig. 9.12). This maintains the newborn's temperature, promotes early breastfeeding,

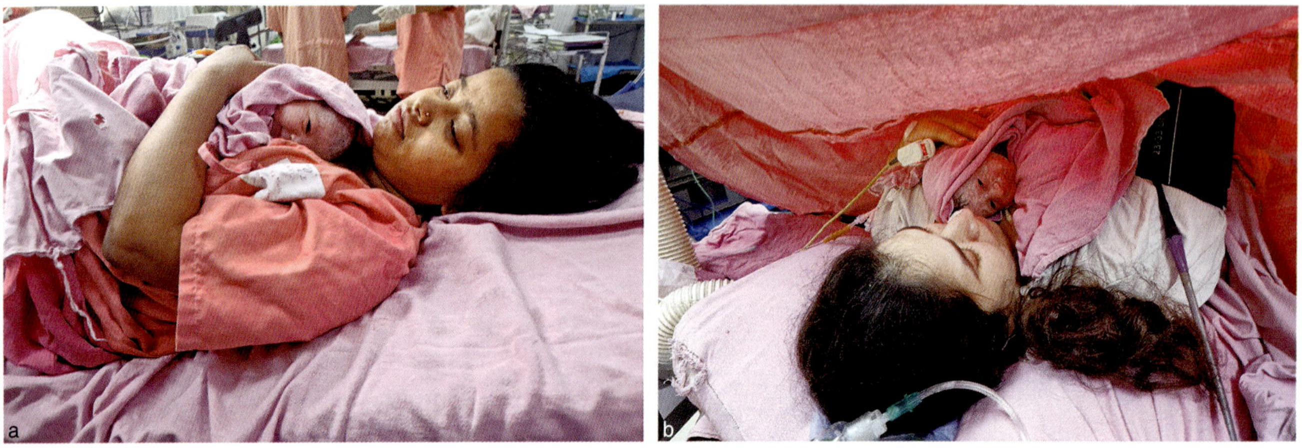

Fig. 9.12: Early skin-to-skin contact with mother after vaginal delivery (a) and cesarean section (b) (*Courtesy:* Dr Nidhi Jain)

and decreases the mother's pain and bleeding. The neonate should be observed during the transition.

***Early skin-to-skin contact:*** According to new Navjat Shishu Suraksha Karyakram-2020 (NSSK) guidelines provided by National Health Mission, all healthy neonates should be delivered on the mother's abdomen, and early skin-to-skin contact should be promoted for at least 1 hour. This enables the neonate to breast crawl and establishes early exclusive breastfeeding. This simple intervention has also been shown to prevent hypothermia in newborns.

***Delayed clamping of the umbilical cord:*** Clamp the umbilical cord 2–3 cm away from the abdomen with a clamp, a clean thread, or a sterile rubber band (Fig. 9.13). Umbilical cord clamping must be delayed for at least 30 to 60 seconds (in term and preterm neonates) to allow additional blood from the placenta to the infant.

The delayed cord clamping (DCC) in term neonates improves the infants' hemoglobin and iron stores and reduces clinical anemia at 2 to 6 months. In preterm infants, DCC is associated with reduced IVH and other morbidities. However, if the neonate is asphyxiated at birth, the cord should be clamped immediately after birth, and resuscitation should be initiated without delay.

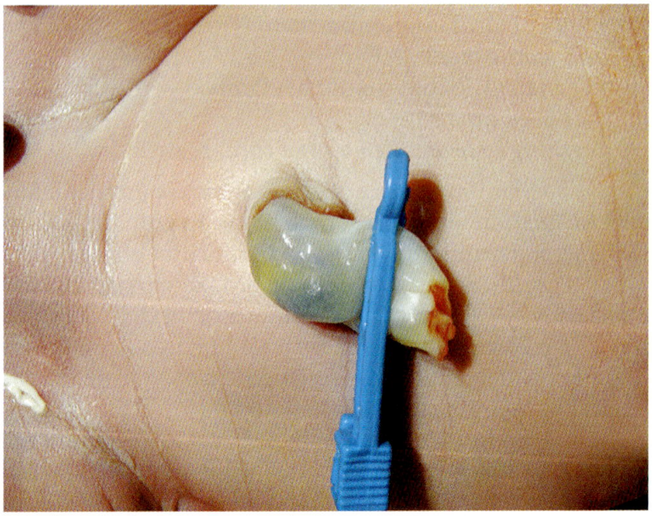

Fig. 9.13: Correct application of the umbilical clamp. Note the clamp should leave 1.2 cm of the cord length on each side of it

The cut umbilical stump should be kept away from the genitals to avoid fecal and urine contamination. The cord should be inspected every 15–30 minutes during the initial few hours after birth for early detection of any oozing.

***Cleaning of the baby:*** The neonate should be dried and cleaned at birth with a clean and sterile cloth. The cleaning should be gentle and only wipe out the blood and the meconium and not be vigorous enough to remove the vernix caseosa (whitish greasy material on the skin). The vernix protects the skin of the infant and helps maintain temperature. This gets absorbed on its own in a few days.

***Placement of identity band:*** Each infant must have an identity band containing the mother's name, hospital registration number, gender, and birth weight.

### Care of Neonate in Initial Few Hours after Birth

***Recording of weight:*** The neonate should be weighed after stabilization and early skin-to-skin contact for 1 hour after birth. A sterile pre-heated sheet (or a single-use paper towel) should be placed on a weighing machine with 10 g sensitivity. Electronic weighing scales are ideal. Zeroing of the device should be performed. The neonate is then gently placed on the weighing machine, and the weight is recorded.

***First examination:*** Examine the neonate thoroughly at birth from head to toe and record the findings in the neonatal sheet. Examine midline structures for malformations (e.g. cleft lip, neck masses, chest abnormality, omphalocele (Fig. 9.14), meningocele, cloacal abnormality). Examine if the anal opening is patent. There is no need for routine catheter passage in the stomach, nostrils, and rectum to detect esophageal atresia, choanal atresia, and anorectal malformation, respectively. The neonate should be examined for the presence of birth injuries. The axillary temperature of the neonate should be recorded before the neonate is shifted out from the birthing place.

***Initiation of breastfeeding:*** Initiate breastfeeding within one hour of birth. Assist the mother in putting the neonate to the breast, irrespective of the mode of delivery—proactive support of breastfeeding results in high rates of successful breastfeeding. Extra-help is needed in primipara mothers, small neonates, and multiple births.

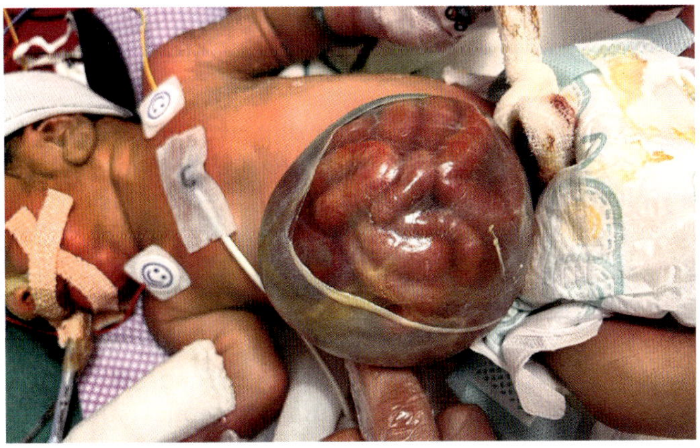

Fig. 9.14: Omphalocele major. Note loops of intestine lying outside the abdomen enclosed in a sac. In contrast to omphalocele, gastroschisis does not have an overlying sac and the intestinal loops lie outside the intestine uncovered. (*Courtesy:* Dr Aparna Chandrasekaran, Hyderabad)

*Vitamin K:* Give vitamin $K_1$ to all the neonates (0.5 mg in less than 1000 g and 1 mg in those more than 1000 g). Vitamin $K_3$ can cause hemolysis in G6PD-deficient neonates.

*Communication with the family:* Counsel the mother and the family members at birth: (i) Gender of the baby, (ii) birth weight, (iii) well-being of the baby, (iv) need for initiation of breastfeeding within one hour and need for continued observation.

*Rooming in:* A normal newborn should not be separated from the mother. In the initial few hours of life, the neonate is very active, and co-bedding the neonate with the mother facilitates early breastfeeding and bonding. Studies have shown that separation during initial hours may have a detrimental effect on successful breastfeeding.

### Care of Neonate Beyond a Few Hours after Birth

*Care of the cord:* The umbilical stump should be kept dry and devoid of any application. The nappy of the neonate should be folded well below the stump to avoid contamination. The cord falls off in 7 to 10 days in healthy-term neonates.

*Exclusive breastfeeding:* Follow a proactive approach to initiate and maintain breastfeeding. Inform the family of the benefits of breastfeeding.

*Position of sleep:* All healthy-term newborn should sleep in the supine position. Evidence has linked prone position to sudden infant death syndrome (SIDS).

*Traditional practices should be discouraged:* Applying kajal or surma in the eyes, putting oil in the ear, or applying cow dung on the cord must be strongly discouraged.

*When to discharge:* A normal neonate should stay in the health facility for at least 24 hr and preferably for 48 hours. Smaller neonates or those with feeding problems or sickness should remain in the hospital as required.

### Discharge Criteria

- The newborn has a normal examination.
- No breastfeeding problems and the mother can breastfeed the neonate well. The adequacy of feeds can be determined by:
  - Passage of urine 6 to 8 times every 24-hour
  - Neonate sleeping well for 2–3 hours after feeds.
- The newborn has received the immunization as per the schedule.
- The mother is confident in taking care of the neonate. She has been counseled regarding routine newborn care
- No significant jaundice or other illness requiring closer observation.
- 'Danger signs' explained (Fig. 9.15).
- Advice regarding the mother's health: The nursing mother's nutrition and health is important. She should take adequate healthy foods above the recommended dietary allowance to meet energy and protein needs while breastfeeding. Mothers should also drink enough water and other liquids to remain hydrated. Iron and folic acid supplementation should continue till three months of postnatal age. The family should be able to identify signs and symptoms of postpartum hemorrhage, infection, thromboembolism, and hypertension following the birth of a baby. Mental health issues are common in the postpartum period, and adequate care must be taken.
- A date for follow-up has been assigned. In the presence of any high-risk factor (e.g. low birth weight, prematurity, significant jaundice, or feeding not established), the neonates should be seen within 2–3 days of discharge. A normal newborn with the adequacy of breastfeeding and no significant jaundice by 72 hours can be seen at 6 weeks of age.

### Common Parental Concerns

*Weight loss in the first week:* Term neonates lose 7 to 10% of birth weight in the first week of life and regain their birth weight by 7–10 days. Subsequently, they gain 20 to 40 g of weight per day. The initial weight loss happens due to the loss of extracellular fluid, and subsequent weight gain is due to a gain in intracellular water and solids content leading to cellular growth. Preterm neonates tend to lose more weight (10 to 15%) owing to immaturity of the tubular function of the kidneys and skin; they tend to regain

- Difficulty in feeding or poor feeding
- Convulsions
- Lethargy (movement only when stimulated)
- Fast breathing (RR >60/min)
- Severe chest indrawing
- Temperature of more than 37.5°C or below 35.5°C
- Yellow soles (severe hyperbilirubinemia)

Fig. 9.15: Danger signs in newborns

9 Newborn Care

birth weight by 10 to 14 days. Small gestational-age infants have less weight loss than their appropriate counterparts.

***Crying during micturition:*** The sensation of a full bladder is uncomfortable to many neonates who may cry *before* passing urine, and they quieten as soon as the act of micturition starts—crying *during micturition* as opposed to *before* the act may indicate urinary tract infection.

***Bathing:*** Only sponging is recommended during the first week until the cord falls off, which can be given after the first 24 hr of life. Later, bathing every 2–3 days is enough. A draught-free warm room, warm water, and quick bath ensure that the neonate does not get cold during bathing. The head has a large surface area; therefore, it should be washed and dried immediately. Inspect the baby's cord, eyes, and skin for any discharge, rash, or redness during bathing.

***Cosmetics:*** Neonates have sensitive skin. Minimize the use of cosmetics. Advise parents to use a mild soap that is non-perfumed-non-medicated. They can use any oil except mustard for skin application or massage. Avoid sprinkling talcum powder, as that can be inhaled. Avoid boric acid-containing products (present in prickly heat preparations).

***Regurgitation (posseting):*** Neonates commonly regurgitate small amounts of curdled milk soon after feeding. This is normal, if the neonate gains weight and passes urine 6–8 times daily.

***Frequent stools:*** During the first few days of life, the stool color in breastfed neonates changes from black-green to yellow by the end of the first week. In between, the stools appear loose ('transitional stools'). The stool frequency may increase at this time. The transition of stools from black meconium to yellow-green stools by the end of the first week is an important indicator of the adequacy of breastfeeding. A neonate may pass a small stool after feeding (gastrocolic reflex). If the neonate remains hydrated, has no signs of sepsis, feeds well, passes urine 6–8 times per day, and gains weight, there is no cause for concern.

***Breast engorgement:*** The breasts in boys and girls may get hypertrophied and secrete milk-like fluid (witch milk; Fig. 9.16) because of transplacentally transmitted hormones. It resolves spontaneously in a few days. Do not squeeze or massage the engorged breasts, as it could lead to soreness and infection.

***Erythema toxicum:*** It starts on day two or three of life. These maculopapular lesions have an erythematous base distributed over the trunk and face. These are eosinophil-laden sterile lesions and resolve spontaneously **(Fig. 9.17a)**.

***Pyoderma (boil)*** is pus-filled lesions due to local skin infection commonly occurring in creases where dirt accumulates, such as the thigh fold and back of the neck **(Fig. 9.17b)**. If the boils are less than ten and there are no signs of sepsis, local cleaning with an antiseptic solution and

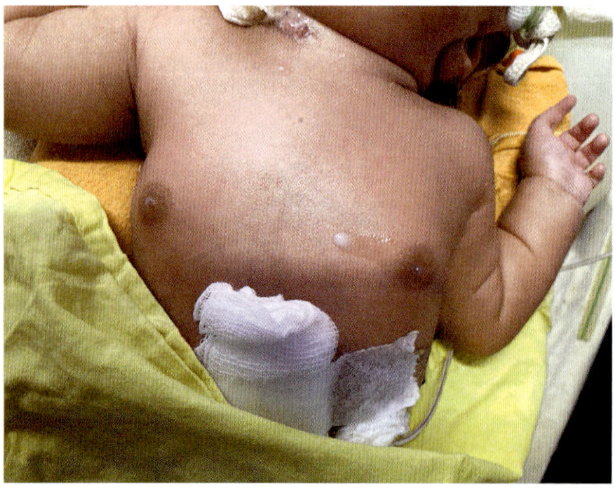

Fig. 9.16: Breast enlargement. Rarely, milk-like fluid may come out of these enlarged breasts (witch milk). (*Photo courtesy:* Dr Soumya Devarapalli)

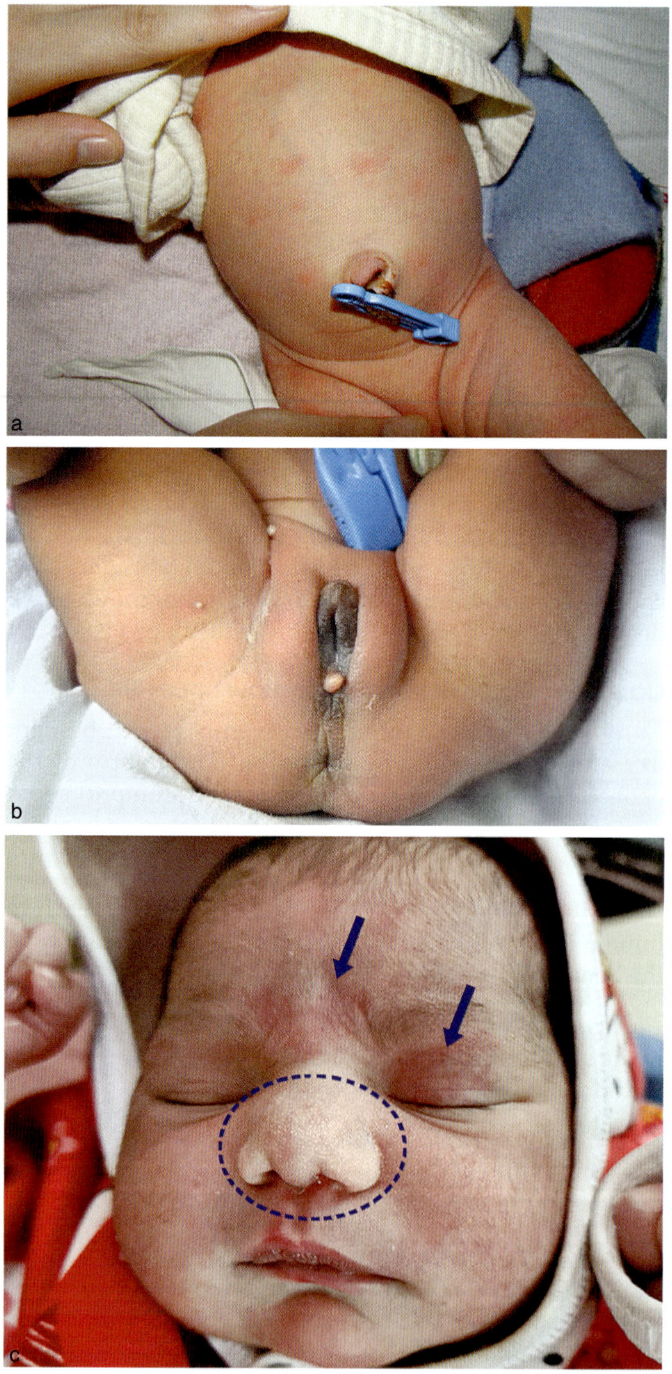


Fig. 9.17: (a) Erythema toxicum; (b) Hymenal tag and pustule; (c) Stork bite over eyelids and forehead (blue arrows) and milia on the nose (circle)

applying 1.0% gentian violet is sufficient. If the number is greater than 10, investigate for sepsis.

*Stork bite:* Sometimes, benign capillary malformation with flat red patches over the forehead and upper eyelids can be present in the newborn period (stork bites; **Fig. 9.17c**). Another common benign skin condition is milia, which consists of tiny white papular cystic lesions, especially over the face and nose **(Fig. 9.17c)**.

*Pink diapers:* Sometimes, male neonates pass pink-colored urine, usually on the 2nd or 3rd day of life, which stains diapers **(Fig. 9.18)**. This results from the passage of urate crystals and often occurs when there is feeding inadequacy causing dehydration. The other causes, like hematuria, hemoglobinuria, myoglobinuria, and porphyria, are infrequent in an otherwise normal neonate. The condition resolves spontaneously in a couple of days and does not require any treatment. Ensure breastfeeding adequacy.

Skin peeling is normal, especially in post-term and IUGR neonates. Oil massaging can decrease flaking, and no other intervention is required.

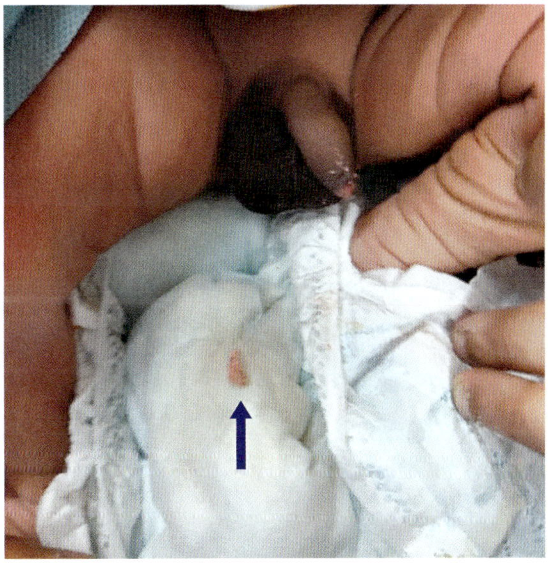

**Fig. 9.18:** Pink diaper in a neonate due to urate crystals (blue arrow)

*Diaper rash:* The diaper area is red and inflamed, and there is an excoriation of the skin due to maceration by stools and urine **(Fig. 9.19)**. The problem is more frequent with commercial than domestic cotton diapers. The treatment consists of keeping the area dry, avoiding skin rubbing for cleaning, and applying a soothing cream.

*Competency:* **PE20.4**

## EVALUATION OF NEWBORN

Most neonates are born healthy. Some 10% are sick and small and need admission to the neonatal unit for observation or treatment.

Newborns may have different physical findings at other time points. Hence, do the physical examination: (i) soon after birth, (ii) at 24 hr of age, (iii) before discharge, and (iv) at the follow-up visit **(Table 9.7)**.

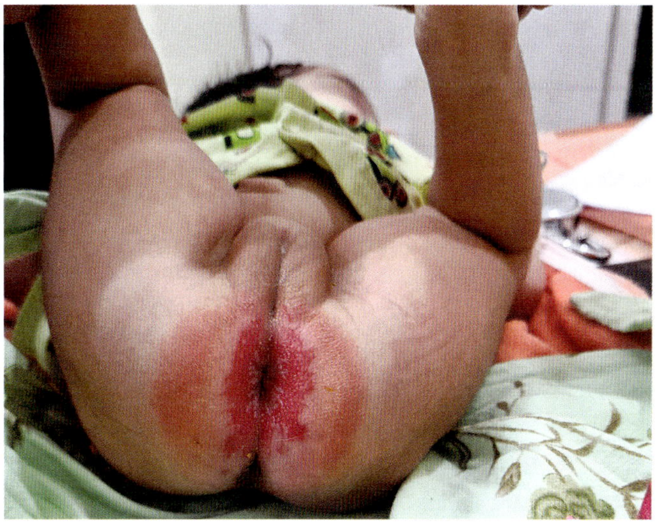

**Fig. 9.19:** Diaper rash

Assign Apgar scores at 1 and 5 minutes **(Table 9.2)**. If the score is less than 7, do it every 5 minutes until 20 minutes. Apgar score provides information regarding cardiopulmonary status at birth and adaptation to the postnatal environment. Apgar score of 0 to 3 at 5 minutes correlates well with mortality. However, low Apgar scores do not predict long-term neurodevelopmental outcomes.

### General Observation

Carefully observing a newborn provides important information at any time and should never be missed. Assess the state of alertness, behavior, response to handling, posture, spontaneous activity, color, breathing difficulty, or obvious malformation in the baby. Ideally, observe when the neonate is in light sleep or awake but quiet—typically 1 to 1.5 hour following feeding.

### Vital Signs

In a sick baby, assess the vital parameters at the outset to assess hemodynamic stability and find out if the neonate needs emergency treatment **(Table 9.8)**.

### Assessment of Size and Growth

Low birth weight (LBW) implies birth weight below 2500 g, very low birth weight (VLBW) less than 1500 g, and extremely low birth weight (ELBW) less than 1000 g. Plotting the weight against the gestational age on the intrauterine growth curve **(Fig. 9.20)** provides information regarding the status of intrauterine growth.

- Between 10th and <90th percentile—appropriate for gestational age (AGA)
- Below the 10th percentile—small for gestational age (SGA)
- At or above the 90th percentile—large for gestational age (LGA)

The SGA neonates have suboptimal growth during the intrauterine period (intrauterine growth restriction, IUGR). These neonates look thin and slender, have loose folds of wrinkled skin **(Fig. 9.21)**, and have monkey-like faces. Intrauterine growth charts are different from postnatal growth charts. The latter assesses growth after birth.

**Table 9.7:** Newborn history and examination: Format for case presentation

| | |
|---|---|
| **History** | |
| General | Mother's name and age, parity, last menstrual period, expected date of delivery |
| Past obstetric | Past pregnancies: When, gestation, fetal or neonatal problems, current status of children |
| Antenatal | Number of antenatal visits, tests (hemoglobin; urine albumin, sugar; ultrasound; blood group, VDRL, HIV), tetanus toxoid immunization, supplements (iron, folic acid, calcium, iodine) |
| Obstetric or medical complications | Obstetric complications (toxemia, urinary tract infections, twins/triplets, placenta previa, accidental hemorrhage); fetal problems (IUGR, hydrops, Rh isoimmunization); medical problems (diabetes, hypertension); investigations, medications, course |
| Labor | Presentation, onset of labor (spontaneous/induced), rupture of membranes (spontaneous/artificial), liquor (clear/meconium stained); duration of first and second stage of labor; fetal heart rate (tachycardia, bradycardia, irregular) |
| Delivery | Place of delivery, vaginal (spontaneous/forceps/vacuum), cesarean (indication, elective/emergency); local/general anesthesia; duration of third stage; postpartum hemorrhage |
| Immediate care at birth | Resuscitation; time of first breath and cry; Apgar score; cord care; passage of urine/stool |
| Feeding | Breastfeeding (when initiated, frequency, adequacy); other feeds |
| Postnatal problems | Feeding problems, jaundice, eye discharge, fever; current problems |
| Family | History of perinatal illness in other siblings |
| Past medical problems | History of past medical problems, if any |
| Personal/social | Socioeconomic status, family support |
| **General examination** | |
| Immediately after birth | Weight, gestation, congenital anomalies, sex assigning, Apgar scores, examination of umbilical vessel, and placenta |
| Appearance | Overall appearance: Well or sick looking; alert/unconscious |
| Vital signs | Temperature, cold stress; respiratory rate, retractions, grunt/stridor; heart rate, palpable femoral arteries; blood pressure, capillary refill time; cry; apneic spells |
| Anthropometry | Weight, length, head circumference, chest circumference |
| Gestation | Assessment by physical criteria; more detailed assessment by expanded New Ballard examination |
| Classification by intrauterine growth | Appropriate/small/large for gestational age; symmetric or asymmetric small for gestational age; signs of IUGR |
| Congenital anomalies | Head to toe examination for malformations |
| Birth trauma | Signs of trauma; cephalohematoma |
| Common signs | Cyanosis, jaundice, pallor, bleed, pustules, edema, depressed fontanel |
| Special signs | Caput; eye discharge; umbilical stump; discharge or redness; jitteriness; eye discharge; oral thrush; development peculiarities (toxic erythema, Epstein pearls, breast engorgement, vaginal bleeding, capillary hemangioma, mongolian spot) |
| Feeding | Observe feeding on breast (check positioning and attachment) |
| Reflexes | Moro, grasp, rooting |
| **Systemic examination** | |
| Chest | Shape; respiratory rate; retractions; air entry; adventitious sounds |
| Cardiovascular system | Apical impulse, heart sounds, murmur |
| Abdomen | Distension, wall edema, tenderness, palpable liver/spleen/kidneys, any other lump, ascites, hernial sites, gonads, genitalia |
| Musculoskeletal system | Deformities; tests for developmental dysplasia of hip; club foot |
| Central nervous system | State of consciousness; vision, pupils, eye movements; facial sensation; hearing; sucking and swallowing; muscle tone and posture; power; tendon reflexes |

IUGR intrauterine growth retardation

## Anthropometry

Weight is measured on a weighing scale with 10 g sensitivity, length by infantometer, and head circumference (HC) by a soft non-stretchable tape circling the head just above the eyebrows and the occiput. Measure chest circumference (CC) at the level of the nipples. Ponderal index (PI) is calculated by multiplying the weight in grams by a hundred and then dividing by a cube of length in cm.

The mean birth weight of Indian neonates at term gestation is approximately 2900 g. Their birth lengths and head circumferences are about 50 cm and 33 to 37 cm.

**Table 9.8:** Normal vital parameters in neonates

| *Vital parameter* | *Normal range* | *Remarks* |
|---|---|---|
| Heart rate (beats/minute) | Term neonates: 100–160 bpm | Relative bradycardia with HR as low as 80 bpm is normal in term neonates during sleep |
| | Preterm neonates: 120–180 bpm | Tachycardia suggests sepsis, anemia, fever, or congestive cardiac failure |
| Axillary temperature | 36.5°C to 37.4°C | Axillary temperature is a good proxy for the core temperature of the baby; no need to measure rectal temperature |
| Capillary refill time (CRT) | ≤3 seconds | Prolonged CRT (>3 seconds) suggests poor circulation as in shock or hypothermia. Assess CRT on the sternum by pressing the skin with the ball of your finger/thumb for five seconds and then noting the time taken to refill |
| Respiratory rate | 40 to 60 breaths per minute | Periodic breathing with short apneic pauses of 5–10 seconds is normal<br>A borderline count nearing 60 needs to be repeated<br>Apnea associated with cyanosis or bradycardia is abnormal. |

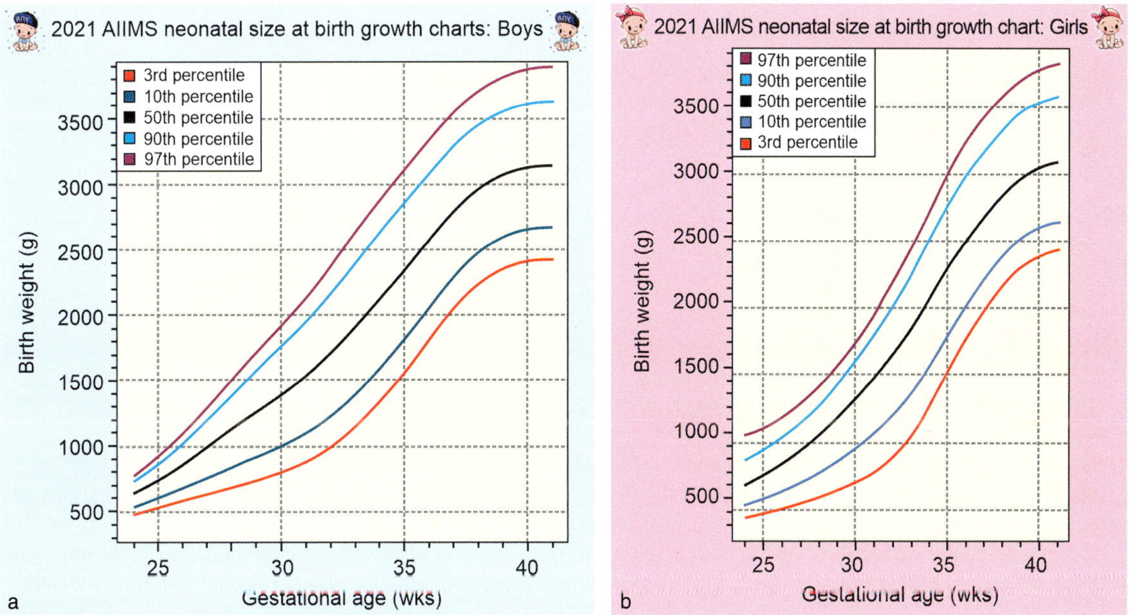


**Fig. 9.20:** New AIIMS intrauterine growth curve: (a) Boys; (b) Girls

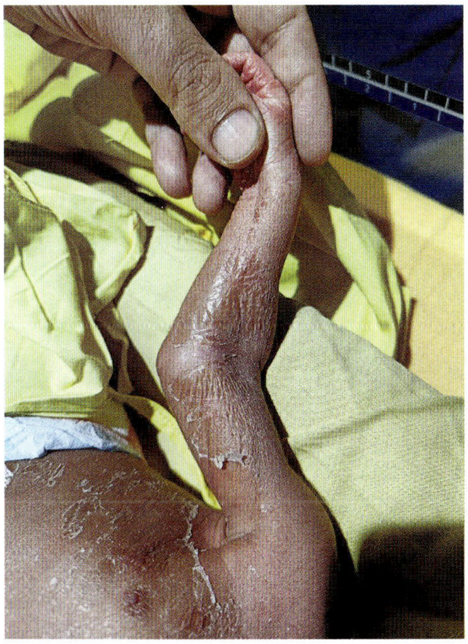

**Fig. 9.21:** An IUGR neonate showing wrinkled skin with peeling

The difference between HC and CC is usually less than 3 cm. An HC-CC difference of more than 3 cm may indicate IUGR in a term baby. PI is usually less than 2 in IUGR neonates and two or more in AGA neonates.

A large head is known as macrocephaly. Its causes include hydrocephalus (enlarged ventricles) and overgrowth of bone or brain tissues.

### Assessment of Gestational Age

Based on the gestation, neonates can be classified as preterm (<37 weeks), post-term (≥42 weeks), and term (37–41 weeks). The gestational age of a neonate can be assessed by the last menstrual period, if the periods have been regular and reliably known by first-trimester ultrasound or newborn examination.

The newborn examination for assessing gestation requires an assessment of physical features and neurological maturity (Fig. 9.22a to l). Expanded New Ballard Scores (ENBS), a commonly used scoring system, can provide gestation with an accuracy of 1 week.

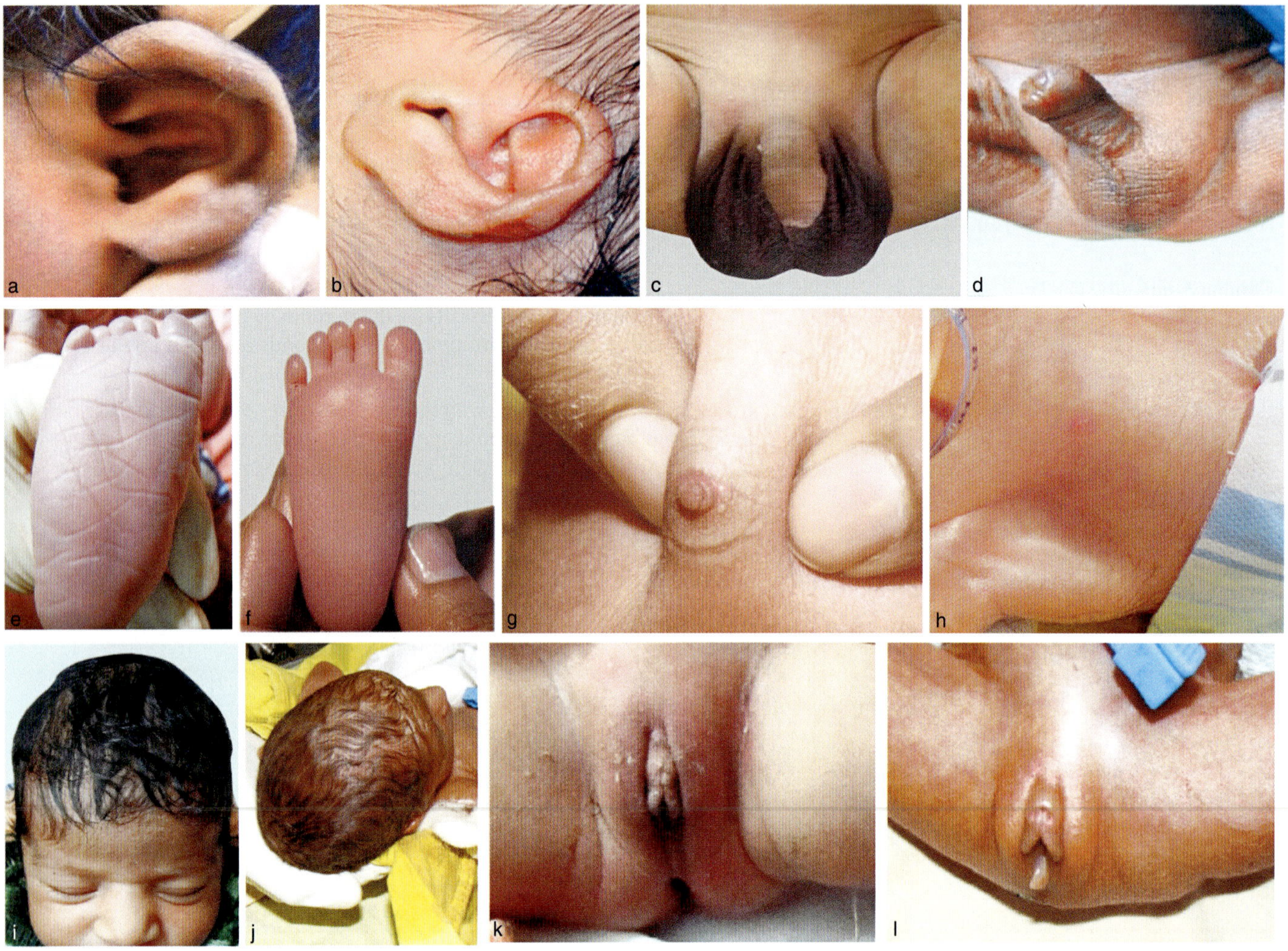

Fig. 9.22: Salient difference in physical characteristics of preterm and term neonates: (a) Well-curved pinna, cartilage reaching up to periphery; (b) Flat and soft pinna, cartilage not reaching up to periphery; (c) Well pigmented and pendulous scrotal sacs, with fully descended testes; (d) Light pigmentation and not yet descended testes; (e) Deep, transverse creases on the soles; (f) Faint marks on the sole, no deep creases; (g) Well-formed breast bud (>5 mm); (h) Poorly developed breast bud; (i) Silky hair, where individual strands can be made out; (j) Fuzzy hair; (k) Labia majora covering clitoris and labia minora; (l) Prominent labia minora

## General Examination

***Skin and hair:*** Examine skin for its thickness, color, transparency, and presence of edema, rashes, and lesions like hemangioma. The skin may exhibit minor features that are self-limiting. Assess the presence of jaundice by pressing the skin to reveal the yellow color of subcutaneous tissue. Ecchymoses or petechiae may relate to birth trauma. Examine the presence and texture of lanugo—the fine hair of the fetal period that is shed later (Fig. 9.23a).

Neonates can have significant seborrheic dermatitis in the initial few months that do not require any treatment (Fig. 9.23b).

***Head and fontanel:*** Examine the size and shape of the head, sutures, and fontanels. A small head indicates microcephaly. Caput succedaneum and cephalohematoma are common findings in normal neonates (Table 9.9). The ventouse application can cause the formation of chignon in the neonate (Fig. 9.24). A full and tense fontanel in a quiet neonate is abnormal and may indicate meningitis, hydrocephalus, or intracranial hemorrhage.

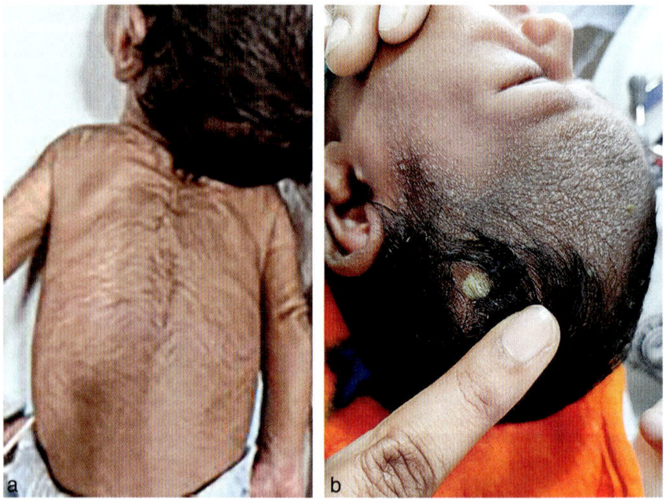

Fig. 9.23: (a) Lanugo hair in a preterm neonate; (b) Seborrheic dermatitis (cradle cap). A large yellow pustule is also seen

In vertex presentation, the shape of the head may change, and the skull bones may override (sutural override) during the process of vaginal birth. Large fontanels and wide

**Table 9.9:** Differences between caput succedaneum and cephalohematoma

| *Characteristic* | *Caput succedaneum* | *Cephalohematoma* |
|---|---|---|
| Incidence | Common | Less common |
| Location | Subcutaneous plane | Over parietal bones, between skull and periosteum |
| Time of presentation | Maximum size and firmness at birth | Increasing size for 12–24 hours and then stable |
| Time course | Softens progressively from birth | Takes 3–6 weeks to resolve and resolves within 2–3 days |
| Characteristic findings | Diffuse; crosses suture line | Does not cross suture line; has distinct margins |
| Association | None | Linear skull fracture (5–25%); hyperbilirubinemia |

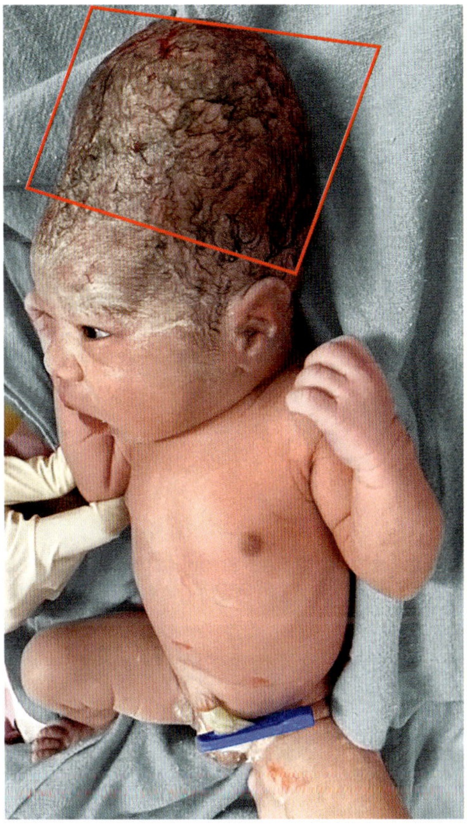

**Fig. 9.24:** Chignon in a neonate following ventouse delivery (box). It resolves without treatment in a few days

sutures are common in IUGR neonates. However, their presence can indicate increased intracranial pressure, trisomy 21, hypothyroidism, and osteogenesis imperfecta. Some neonates have delayed ossification of the skull bones that may feel like a ping pong ball (*craniotabes*). It is benign and resolves spontaneously.

***Neck, face, eyes, and ears:*** Examine the neck for masses such as enlarged thyroid gland and sternomastoid tumor. Newborns have short necks.

A birth injury can cause facial nerve paresis causing asymmetry of the face while the neonate is crying—the affected side having an open eye, absent nasolabial fold, and deviation of angle of mouth to the normal side. The absence of depressor anguli oris (DAOM) can mimic facial nerve palsy; however, in this condition, the eyes remain tightly shut while crying, and the nasolabial fold is intact (Fig. 9.25a and b). Examine the nose for its shape, secretions, and patency. The flaring of the nostrils indicates an increase in respiratory distress.

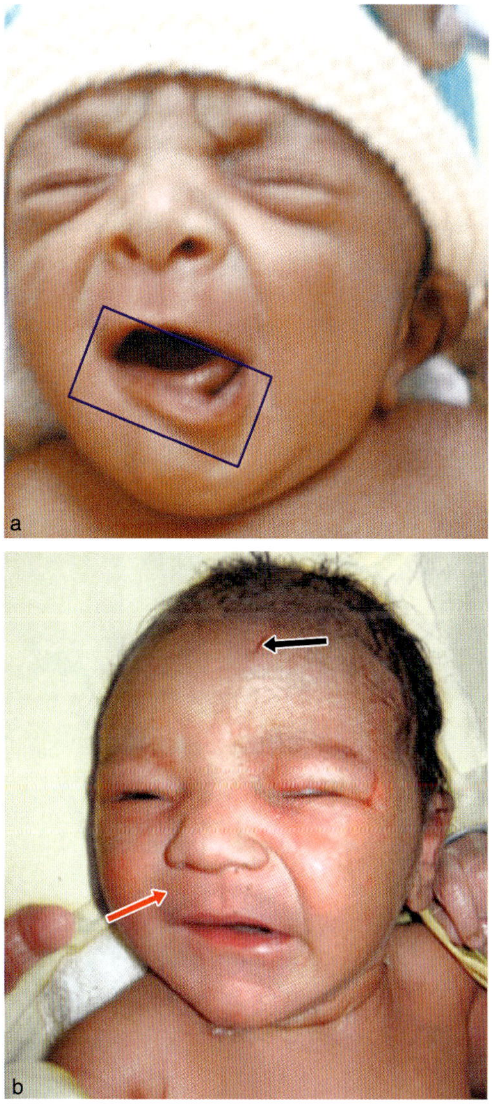

**Fig. 9.25:** (a) Absent depressor anguli oris muscle. Note the asymmetry of the face on crying and the presence of nasolabial folds and closed eyes. The uptick of the lower lip is typical of the condition (box); (b) Newborn with right-sided lower motor nerve facial palsy secondary to forceps application (red arrow) and forceps marks (black arrow). The upper lids of the baby looks puffy, which is often normal at birth

The alveolar ridge may have natal teeth. A white papule at the apex of the hard palate is a retention cyst (Epstein pearl) that disappears in a few weeks.

Subconjunctival hemorrhages are common after vaginal delivery and resolve spontaneously. The cornea should be clear; pupils should be equal in size, reactive to light, and symmetrical. Accessory auricles and preauricular tags are common.

***Umbilicus, anus, and spine:*** Inspect the number of vessels in the umbilical cord (Fig. 9.26). A single umbilical artery is found in 0.7% of live births; this may be associated with renal and gastrointestinal tract anomalies.

Palpate the base of the umbilical cord for a hernia (Fig. 9.27). Palpate the spine with a finger to exclude spina bifida, masses, and abnormal curvature. Check if the anal opening is intact. A sinus (Fig. 9.28a) or tuft of hair (Fig. 9.28b) in the lumbosacral area may mark an underlying neural tube defect.

***Genitalia (male and female):*** Examine the genital area for the urethral opening and clitoris. The presence of a hymenal tag is an innocuous finding). Examine the size and curvature of the penis. Hypospadias implies more ventral location of the urethra (normally, it is located on the tip) and the presence of ventral incurvation (chordee) and deficient foreskin (Fig. 9.29). Circumcision should be postponed in newborns with hypospadias.

***Extremities:*** Examine if arms and limbs are fully movable with no evidence of dislocation or asymmetry of movements.

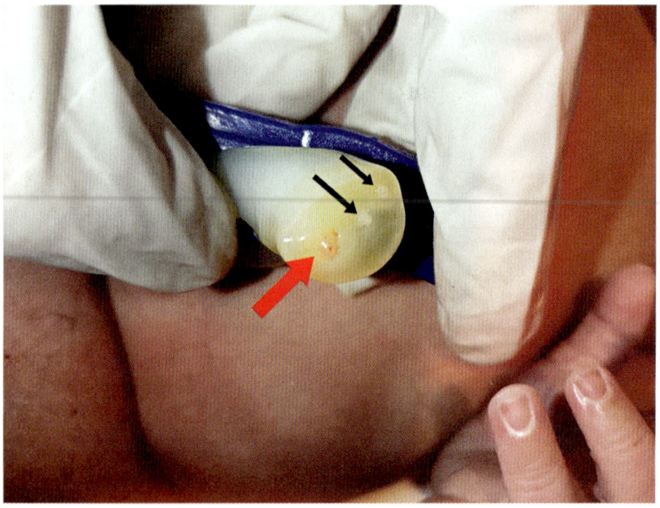

**Fig. 9.26:** The base of a freshly cut umbilical cord shows two arteries (2 black arrows) and a vein (red arrow)

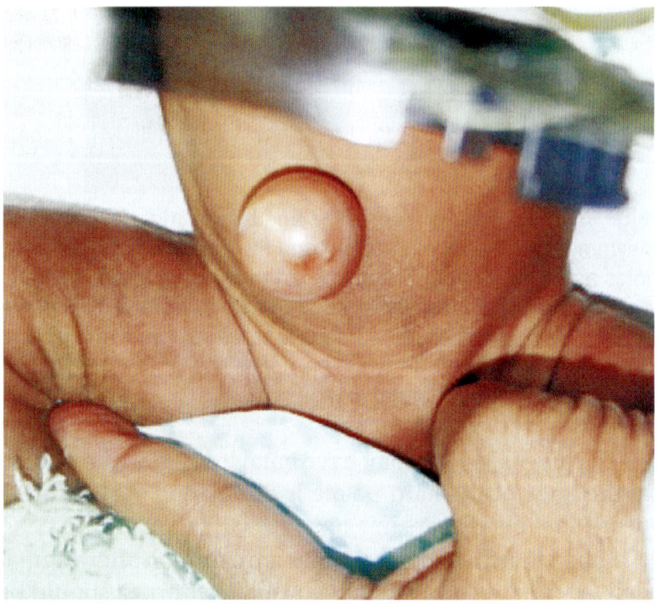

**Fig. 9.27:** Umbilical hernia

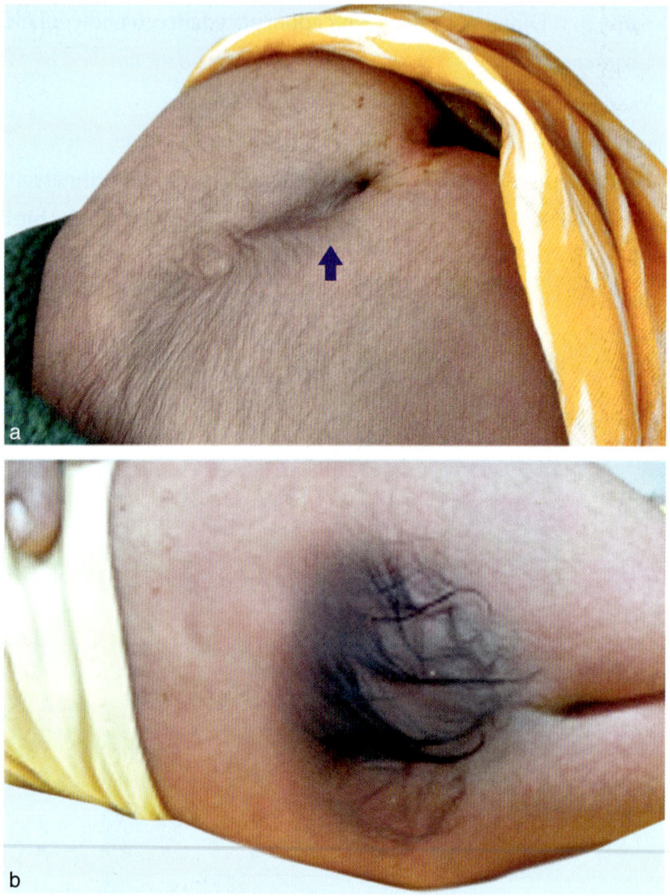


**Fig. 9.28:** Sinus shown by an arrow (a) or tuft of hair (b) in the lower back may signify an underlying neural tube defect

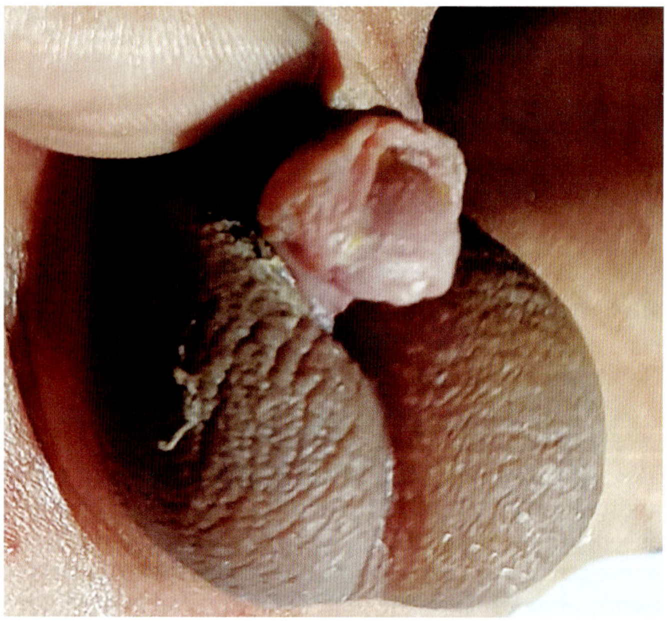

**Fig. 9.29:** A newborn male with hypospadias. Note the presence of chordee (ventral curvature of the penis) (*Courtesy:* Dr Parminder Singh)

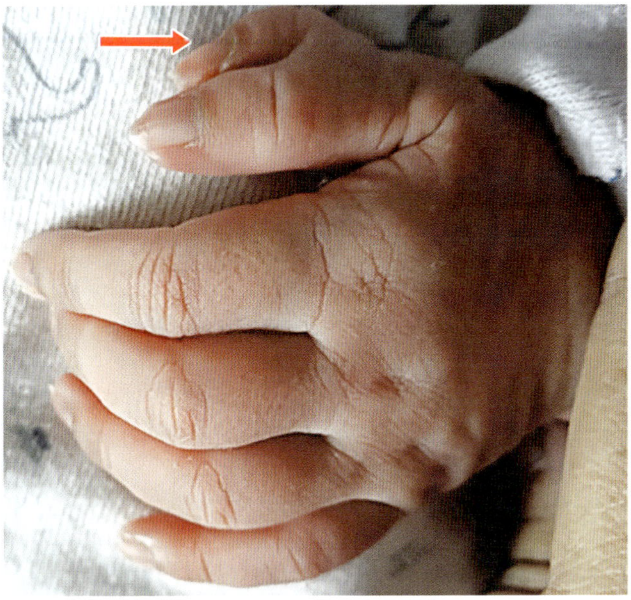

Fig. 9.30: Pre-axial polydactyly

Examine the fingers and toes for abnormality in the shape, size, or number: Syndactyly or polydactyly (Fig. 9.30). A calcaneovalgus deformity is usually self-correcting within the next few months, but equinovarus requires orthopedic consultation (Fig. 9.31a and b).

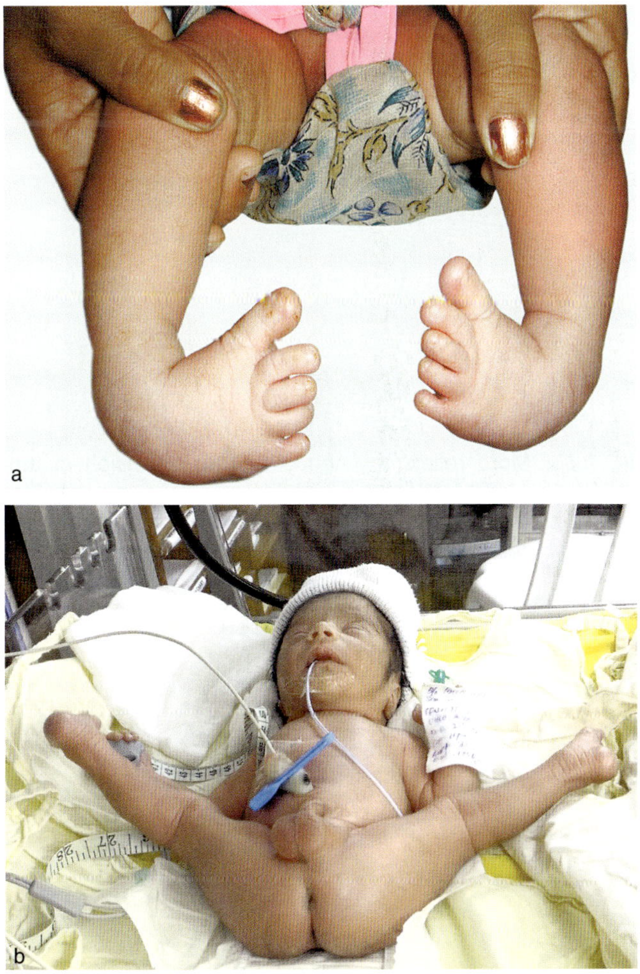

Fig. 9.31: (a) Congenital talipes equinovarus deformity; (b) A newborn delivered by the extended breech. Note lower limbs with extended knees and flexed hips

### Systemic Examination

*Chest:* The anteroposterior diameter of the neonate's chest is roughly equal to the transverse diameter. Nasal flare, grunting, fast breathing, and intercostal and subcostal retractions indicate respiratory distress. Such distress may reveal the presence of underlying pneumonia, respiratory distress syndrome (RDS), delayed reabsorption of lung fluid (transient tachypnea), or any other cardiorespiratory cause. Stridor indicates larger airway obstruction. Wheezing denotes small airway obstruction. The presence of bowel sounds in the chest may mean a congenital diaphragmatic hernia.

*Cardiovascular system:* The presence of abnormal heart sounds or murmurs may indicate congenital heart disease. Such neonates can have tachypnea, cyanosis, or both. Bilateral femoral artery pulsation may be absent in the coarctation of the aorta.

*Abdomen:* An unusual flatness or scaphoid shape may be associated with congenital diaphragmatic hernia. Visible gastric or bowel patterns may indicate ileus or intestinal obstruction (Fig. 9.32a and b). Normal neonates can have liver palpable below the costal margin, spleen tip, and left kidney lower pole may also be normally palpable.

*Musculoskeletal system:* The common alterations are deformations caused by adverse mechanical factors *in utero*. Most positional deformities are mild and resolve in time.

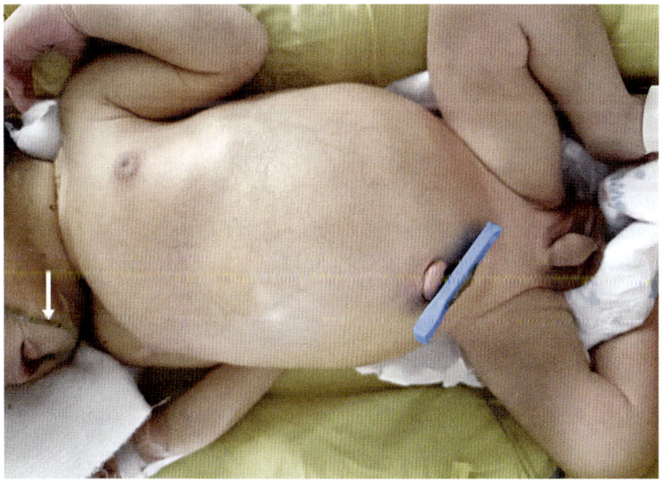

Fig. 9.32a: Abdominal distension in a term neonate suggestive of intestinal obstruction. The gastric tube (arrow) shows drainage of bile (green color fluid)

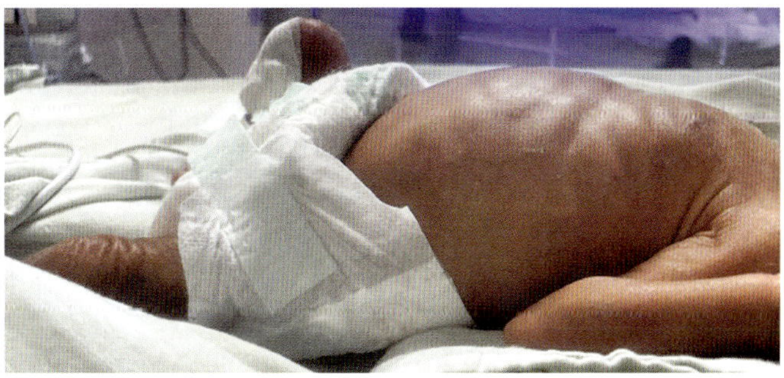

Fig. 9.32b: A preterm newborn showing abdominal distension with visible bowel loops. The differential diagnosis includes sepsis, feed intolerance, necrotizing enterocolitis, and intestinal obstruction

Developmental dysplasia of the hip occurs in 1 of 800 live births, more commonly in girls, those with family history, and delivered by the breech. This is examined by:

i. ***Barlow maneuver:*** Barlow test is done to dislocate the unstable hip joint. Test both hips separately. Stabilize the pelvis with one hand, with the thumb on the medial side of the thigh and fingers on the greater trochanter. With the other hand, flex and adduct the hip while applying posterior pressure to dislocate the hip.

ii. ***Ortolani sign:*** This sign is present, if the hip is already dislocated. The neonate is placed on its back with the knees fully flexed, and the hips flexed to a right angle. Test both hips separately. Stabilize the pelvis with one hand, with the thumb on the medial side of the thigh and fingers on the greater trochanter. Abduct the thigh and push the femoral head anteriorly with your fingers. In the dislocated hip, the femoral head suddenly slips into the acetabulum with a distinctly palpable "clunk."

*Neurological examination* consists of assessing the level of alertness, cranial nerves, motor and sensory system, and neonatal reflexes.

***Cranial nerves:*** Neonates respond to cotton soaked in peppermint by 32 weeks of gestation. By 26 weeks, the infant consistently blinks in response to light, and by term gestation, fixation and following (tested using fluffy red yarn ball) are well established. By 28 weeks, the infant startles or blinks at a loud noise. Normal sucking and swallowing denote proper functioning of the V, VII, IX, X, and XII cranial nerves.

Feeding requires the coordinated action of sucking, swallowing, and breathing. Suck-swallow coordination to accept paladai feeding is present by 32 weeks. Suck-swallow and breathing coordination for breastfeeding occurs by 34 weeks. However, perfect coordination of suck-swallow and breathing develops only by 38 weeks of gestation.

***Motor examination:*** By 28 weeks, there is minimal resistance to passive manipulation of all the limbs, and a distinct flexor tone is appreciated in the lower extremities by 32 weeks. By 36 weeks, flexor tone is palpable in both the lower and upper extremities.

***Primary neonatal reflexes:*** To elicit the Moro reflex, raise the baby's head slightly and drop it suddenly while the hand still supports the neonate. The response consists of the opening of the hands and extension and abduction of the upper extremities, followed by anterior flexion (embracing) of the upper extremities with an audible cry (Fig. 9.33a and b). The hand opening is present by 28 weeks, extension and abduction by 32 weeks, and anterior flexion by 37 weeks. Moro reflex disappears by 3–6 months in normal infants. The most common cause of depressed or absent Moro reflex is a generalized disturbance of the central nervous system. An asymmetrical Moro reflex indicates root plexus injury (Fig. 9.33c).

The palmar grasp is present at 28 weeks of gestation and is strong by 32 weeks. Palmar grasp is strong enough to allow the lifting of the neonate at 37 weeks of gestation (Fig. 9.34); it becomes less consistent and allows the appearance of a voluntary grasp at four months. The

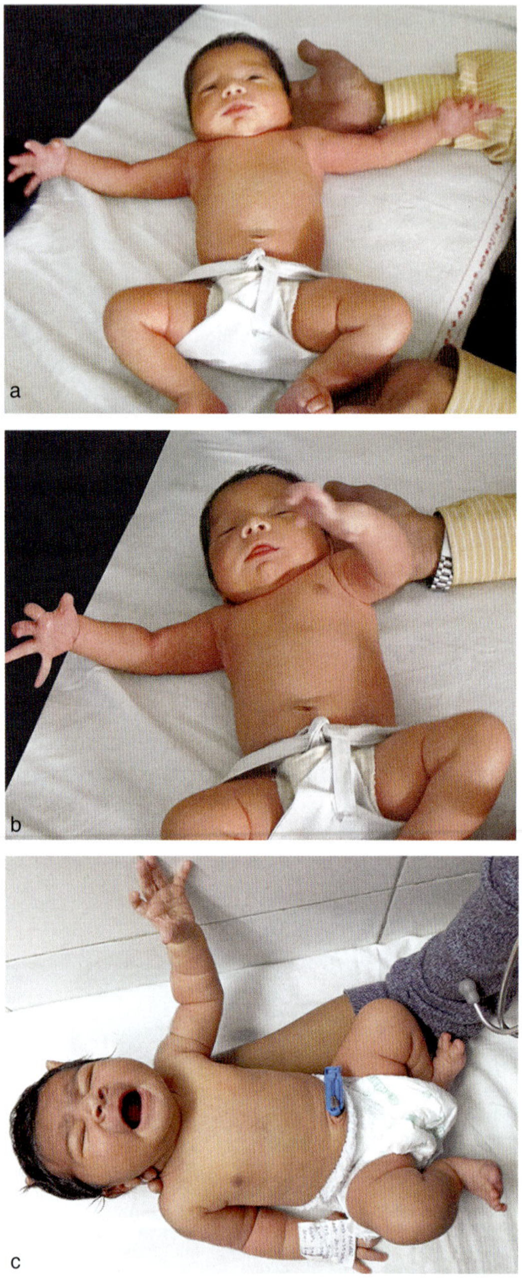

**Fig. 9.33:** Moro reflex: (a) Abduction and extension of arms are followed by (b) Adduction and flexion; (c) Asymmetric Moro reflex in brachial plexus injury (Erb's palsy on the right side—the upper limb does not move)

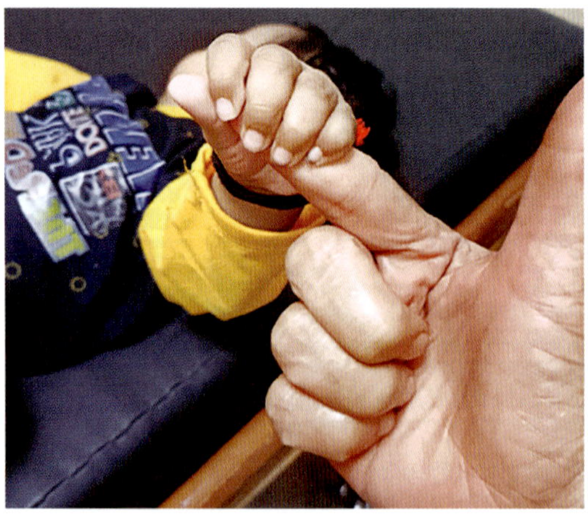

**Fig. 9.34:** Palmar grasp

asymmetric tonic neck response is an important response elicited by head rotation that causes extension of the upper extremity on the side to the face and flexion of the upper extremity on the opposite side. This reflex disappears by four months.

### Suggested Viewing

1. Video link for assessing respiratory distress in preterm infants: https://youtu.be/Hd8qH43HyVE

*Competencies:* **PE20.12; PE27.24; PE27.25; PE27.26; PE27.27**

## THERMAL PROTECTION

Newborn neonates are prone to hypothermia as they have immature heat-regulating mechanisms. The neonates have a limited capacity to generate heat, including brown fat. A larger surface area to body weight, thin and permeable skin, and lower subcutaneous fat put neonates at risk of hypothermia. The head constitutes a significant portion of the newborn's body surface area and can contribute significantly to overall heat loss. The low environmental temperature also contributes to the occurrence of hypothermia.

### Sources of Heat Loss

Heat loss in a newborn occurs in four ways:

i. *Radiation* to the surrounding environment not in direct contact with baby
ii. *Convection* to the air flowing in surrounding
iii. *Conduction* to substances in direct contact with baby
iv. *Evaporation* of fluid and moisture from baby's skin

### Sources of Heat Production

When exposed to a cold environment, the neonate tries to generate heat by increasing physical activity (crying, increased body movements). A cold environment stimulates the baby's sympathetic system causing cutaneous vasoconstriction and generation of heat by *non-shivering thermogenesis* in the brown fat. Brown fat, located in the axillae, groin, and nape of the neck, interscapular, and perirenal areas, has a rich vascular supply and sympathetic innervation. The release of norepinephrine uncouples beta-oxidation in fat, resulting in heat production. Blood passing through brown fat gets heated up and keeps the neonate warm. Preterm and small for gestational age infants have scanty brown fat stores.

*Response to hypothermia:* Hypothermia-induced peripheral vasoconstriction leads to increased metabolism with excess utilization of oxygen and glucose. When body temperature drops below 32°C, hemoglobin cannot release oxygen resulting in tissue hypoxia. The consequent anaerobic metabolism results in metabolic acidosis (Fig. 9.35), resulting in pulmonary vasoconstriction and further hypoxemia. Severe hypothermia, hypoxemia, bradycardia, hypoglycemia, and metabolic acidosis increase mortality in hypothermic neonates.

*Hyperthermia:* An immature thermoregulating mechanism and reduced ability to sweat predispose newborns to hyperthermia. Factors like over-clothing, the high environmental temperature in summer, poor feeding, and dehydration are common factors that can lead to hyperthermia.

### Definitions

*Thermoneutral environment:* The thermoneutral zone (TNZ) denotes a narrow environmental temperature range in which a neonate can maintain his normal body temperature with the least basal metabolic rate and oxygen utilization. The TNZ varies with gestation and postnatal age. It is higher at lower than higher gestation, naked than clothed, and early than later postnatal ages. The disorders can be categorized based on axillary temperature, as shown in Fig. 9.36.

### Temperature Measurement

Ideally, the axillary temperature should be measured as it is safer than the rectal temperature. Currently, we use digital thermometers as mercury thermometers have been phased out. To record axillary temperature, place the bulb of the thermometer on the roof of the dry axilla parallel to the trunk. Hold the baby's arm close to the body until the thermometer gives a beep.

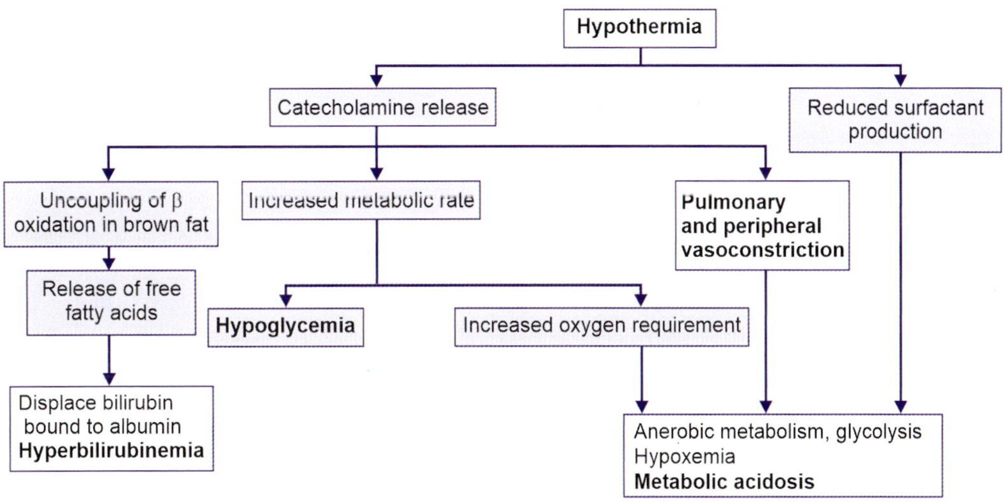


**Fig. 9.35:** Response to cold stress in the sick neonate

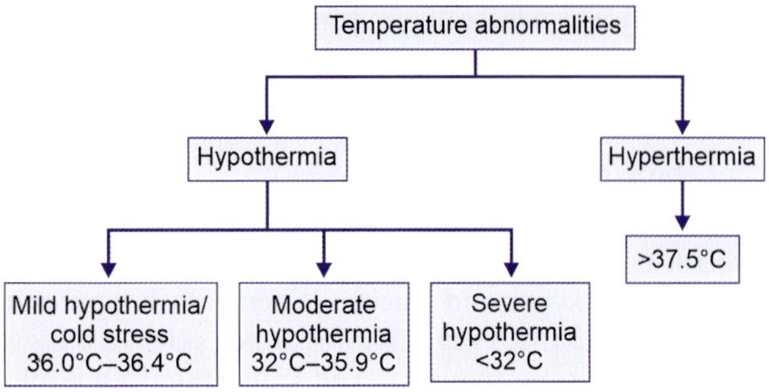


**Fig. 9.36:** Classification of temperature abnormalities (based on axillary temperature). The normal body temperature is between 36.5°C and 37.5°C

*One can get a reasonable idea about a baby's body temperature by touching the baby's hands and feet and the abdomen with the back of the examiner's hand. The baby's body temperature is normal if the hands, feet, and abdomen feel warm. Warm abdomen but cold feet and hands indicate mild to moderate hypothermia. Cold feet, hands, and abdomen would suggest that the* neonate *has severe hypothermia.*

#### *Frequency of Measurement*

WHO guidelines recommend the following schedule for temperature measurement:

- Once daily, preferably in the early morning hours, for healthy-term neonates who are otherwise well
- Three times daily for healthy small neonates (2 to 2.5 kg)
- Four times daily for very small neonates (<2 kg)
- Every two hours for sick neonates.

The mother should be encouraged to assess the neonate's body temperature by touching the baby.

### Disorders of Body Temperature

Hypothermia, as well as hyperthermia, can also indicate a severe underlying illness. Hypothermia may happen due to exposure to a cold environment, such as low ambient temperature, cold surface, or cold air, or if the neonate is wet or not clothed adequately. Hyperthermia may result from exposure to a warm environment, such as in summer, direct sun exposure, or overheating in the incubator or radiant warmer.

### Hypothermia

Hypothermia correlates well with an increased risk of mortality in neonates. Hypothermia is common in neonates in hospital as well as community settings. It also occurs in the tropical environment. The conditions, such as prematurity, hypoglycemia, and asphyxia, have a higher risk of mortality when associated with hypothermia.

#### *Prevention*

- Keep birthing rooms' ambient temperature at least 25°C, and they should be free from air drafts (keep windows and doors closed).
- After delivery, dry the neonate immediately, put in skin-to-skin contact on the mother's abdomen, and cover with warm and dry linen. Discard the wet towel. Dress the neonate in proper clothing, including a cap and socks **(Fig. 9.37a and b)**. Dressing the neonate in multiple layers of warm and light clothes provides better thermal protection than a single layer of heavy woolen clothing.
- Kangaroo mother care (KMC) keeps LBW neonates warm.
- Frequent breastfeeding allows the neonate to remain in touch with the mother's warm body and provides energy to keep the neonate warm.
- Postpone bathing and weighing. Provide sponge bathing to healthy term neonates after hospital discharge during summer months. Delay bathing during winters and in sick and small neonates until the umbilical cord falls off (end of the first week). Give bathing to small neonates once they weigh two kilograms.
- Keep the mother and the neonate on the same bed (co-bedding/rooming in).
- Warm transportation: This is the weakest link in the warm chain with a significant risk of severe hypothermia.
- Training/awareness of healthcare providers

***Incubators and radiant warmers:*** Radiant warmers and incubators help sick and small neonates maintain their

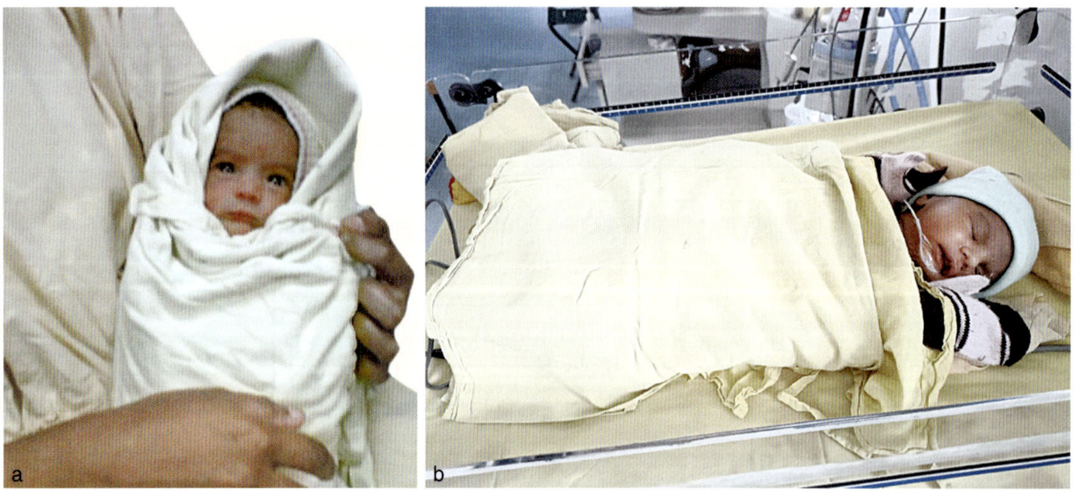


**Fig. 9.37:** (a) Well-clothed premature baby in mother's lap; (b) A well-covered baby in radiant warmer; clothing of baby under radiant warmer improves thermal protection and provides developmental supportive care

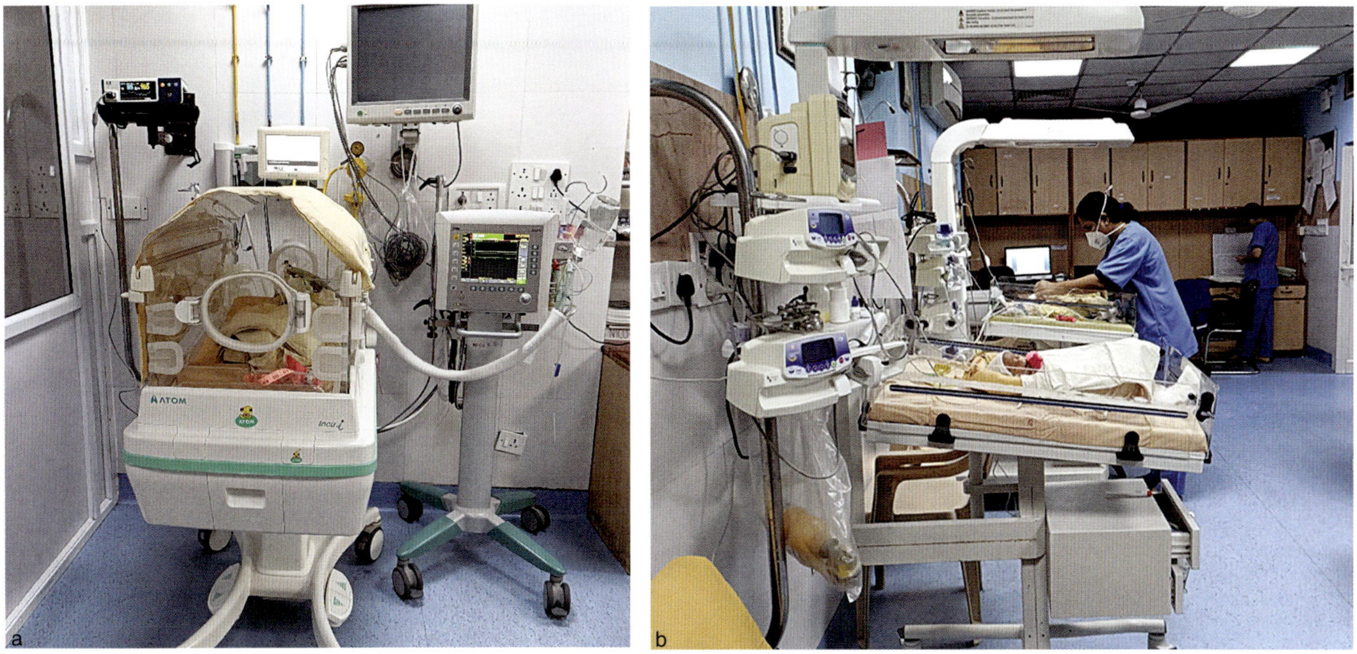

**Fig. 9.38:** (a) An incubator; (b) A radiant warmer. Note that the incubator has port holes on the sides to assess the baby (*Courtesy:* Dr Satya Prakash)

normal body temperature (Fig. 9.38a and b). An incubator is a transparent acrylic cabin (closed system) with a fan in its base that keeps circulating warm air around the neonate to keep him warm (convection). Often the incubators have a double wall for better thermal protection of the neonate. A radiant warmer is an open system with a radiant heater installed over a bassinet (Table 9.10). Both types of equipment have an inbuilt feedback system (servo-control) that controls the ambient temperature by altering heater output based on the baby's temperature, thereby maintaining the baby's temperature in the normal range (Fig. 9.39). Radiant warmer also has a 'manual' mode of operation, which allows manual adjustment of the heater output. That helps in the initial warming of the bed before the neonate occupies it.

Use radiant warmers and incubators in servo-control mode with the skin temperature probe attached to the baby. Set the skin temperature at 36.5°C to 37°C, which helps maintain the baby's temperature in the desired range.

*Signs and Symptoms*

Hypothermia affects all the body systems adversely. Peripheral vasoconstriction results in acrocyanosis, cool extremities, and delayed capillary refill time. The neonate becomes restless and lethargic. Bradycardia, hypotension, and raised pulmonary artery pressure can cause respiratory distress and hypoxemia. There may be apnea, lethargy, poor reflexes, and decreased oral acceptance. Abdomen distension and vomiting can make enteral feeding difficult. Significant metabolic disturbances such as acidosis, hypoglycemia, oliguria, azotemia, and generalized bleeding can occur in severe cases. Neonates experiencing hypothermia over more extended periods may not gain adequate weight.

*Management*

Methods for temperature maintenance include skin-to-skin contact, warm room, radiant warmers, incubators, and increasing ambient temperature using heaters.

**Table 9.10:** Differences between a radiant warmer and an incubator

| *Feature* | *Radiant warmer* | *Incubator* |
|---|---|---|
| Design | A radiant heater installed over a bassinet provides heat (radiation)<br>Open care system | Circulation of warm air by an inbuilt heater and fan (convection) into a canopy<br>Closed system |
| Access to the baby | Easy | Restricted |
| Insensible water loss | Greater (can result in dehydration in small neonates) | Lesser (suitable for neonates below 1500 g) |
| Option to add humidification | Not available | Available in advanced machines<br>Higher humidity reduces insensible water losses from the skin. That helps in maintaining fluid balance in neonates below 1500 g |
| Maintenance and disinfection | Easy | Difficult to maintain and disinfect |
| Cost | Low | High |

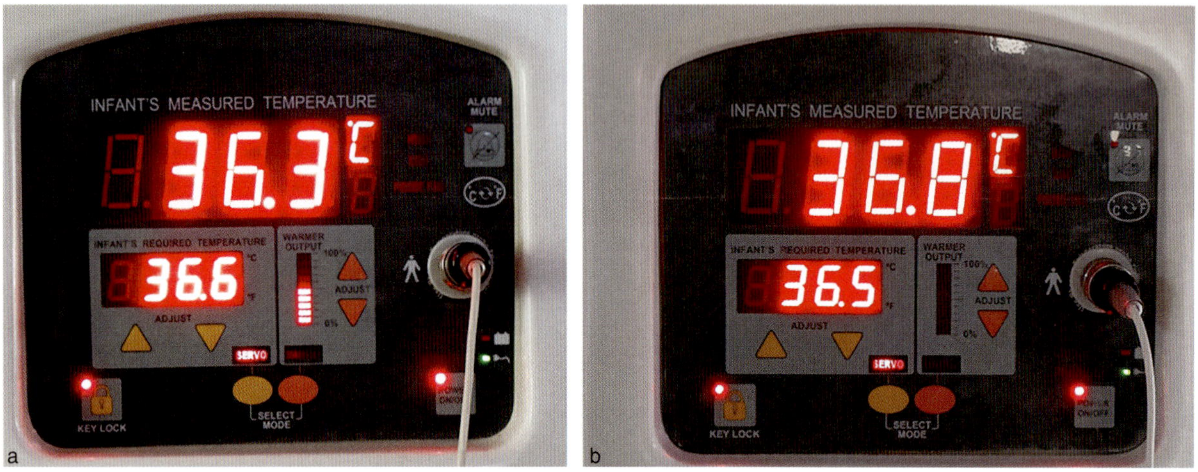


Fig. 9.39: The skin servo-control mode of the radiant warmer and incubator helps maintain the infant's desired temperature: (a) The infant temperature is 36.3°C as against the set temperature of 36.6°C. Accordingly, the heater output is nearly 50%; (b) The infant temperature is higher than the set temperature, and the heater output is zero



*Cold stress or moderate hypothermia*

- Remove the neonate from the source, such as a cold environment, cold clothes, or wet clothing.
- Initiate skin-to-skin contact or provide warm clothing. Keep the neonate in close contact with the mother in a warm room. Alternatively, nurse the neonate in a radiant warmer or incubator.
- Monitor temperature frequently. If the neonate does not get warm, ensure adequate warmth.
- Ensure frequent feeding to prevent hypoglycemia.
- Monitor vitals. Rule out sepsis, if the neonate continues to remain cold.

*Severe hypothermia:* Severe hypothermia is a life-threatening condition and requires treatment on an urgent basis.

- Remove the neonate from the source, such as a cold environment, cold clothes, or wet clothing.
- Nurse the neonate in an incubator or a preheated radiant warmer. Alternatively, use a room heater.
- Monitor oxygen saturation with a pulse oximeter. Provide oxygen, if required.
- The neonate requires a saline bolus, if in shock.
- Give IV dextrose infusion
- Give vitamin K (1 mg)
- Fast rewarming until the baby's temperature reaches 34°C. Slow the rewarming process after that.
- Measure body temperature and other vital signs frequently.
- Take blood culture and give empiric IV antibiotics.

### Suggested Reading

1. Lunze K, Bloom DE, Jamison DT, Hamer DH. The global burden of neonatal hypothermia: a systematic review of a major challenge for newborn survival. BMC Med. 2013 Jan 31;11:24.
2. Thermal protection of the newborn: A practical guide. WHO/FHW/MSM/97.2

*Competencies:* **PE7.1; PE7.2; PE7.3; PE7.4; PE7.5; PE7.7; PE7.8; PE7.9; PE7.10**

## BREASTFEEDING

*Breast milk* is the ideal nutrition containing all the nutrients for optimum growth and development of a neonate from birth to six months. Exclusive breastfeeding for 6 months is the most effective public health intervention that can reduce neonatal death by 20% and under-5 deaths by 13%. Exclusive breastfeeding reduces hospital admissions due to diarrhea and pneumonia by 72% and 57%, respectively.

Exclusive breastfeeding means giving only breast milk. It permits vitamin drops or any medication, if indicated. Initiate breastfeeding within one hour of the birth, and continue exclusively for 6 months. After 6 months, start complementary feeding and continue breastfeeding for 2 years or as long as the mother wants.

As per the latest NFHS-5 data (2019-20), the breastfeeding initiation within one hour was 41.8%. Exclusive breastfeeding for 6 months was 64%.

### Benefits of Breast Milk

*Nutritional superiority:* Breast milk contains all the nutrients in the proportions that a neonate needs for optimum growth and development. The neonate can digest breast milk easily.

*Carbohydrates:* Lactose helps absorb calcium and enhances the growth of lactobacilli, the good bacteria, in the intestine. Galactose is necessary for the formation of galactocerebrosides.

*Proteins:* The breast milk has a low protein concentration (0.9–1.1 g/dL); most of it is lactalbumin and lactoglobulin (60%), which neonates can easily digest. It contains taurine and cysteine, which are necessary for brain growth. These are lacking in cow milk and formula.

*Fats:* Breast milk is rich in polyunsaturated fatty acids (PUFA), necessary for the myelination of the neural tissue. It also contains omega-2 and omega-6 fatty acids for synthesizing prostaglandins and cholesterol for steroid hormones.

*Human milk oligosaccharides (HMO):* HMOs, the most abundant solid in breast milk, are non-digestible carbohydrates that reach the large intestine. They act as prebiotics, support the growth of friendly bacteria, and help develop a healthy microbiome in the large intestine. A healthy microbiome helps in preventing diarrhea and diseases like necrotizing enterocolitis.

*Vitamins and minerals:* The quantity and bioavailability of vitamins and minerals are sufficient for the baby's needs in the first 6 months.

*Water and electrolytes:* Breast milk has a water content of 88%; hence, a breastfed neonate does not require additional water in the first few months of life, even during summer. Breast milk has a low solute load and poses less burden to the kidneys.

*Immunological superiority:* A breastfed neonate is 14 times less likely to die of diarrhea and almost four times less likely to die of pneumonia. Breast milk contains many protective elements: Secretory IgA, macrophages, lymphocytes, lactoferrin, lysozyme, Bifidus factor, and interferon.

*Other benefits:* Breast milk contains several growth factors, enzymes, and hormones. Epidermal growth factor enhances the maturation of the intestinal cells and reduces the risk of allergy in later life. Enzymes like lipases increase the digestion of fats in the milk.

*Other illnesses:* Breastfed neonates have a lower risk of diabetes, heart disease, cancer, allergy, ear infections, and orthodontic problems in later life.

*Mental growth:* Breastfed neonates have a better bonding with their mothers. They have a higher IQ.

*Benefits to mother:* Breastfeeding helps in uterine involution and reduces the risk of postpartum hemorrhage. Lactation amenorrhea provides effective contraception for initial 6 months. Breastfeeding is convenient and time-saving. It reduces the risk of breast cancer and helps the mother shed the extra weight gained during pregnancy. It prevents type-2 diabetes in mothers.

### Breast Anatomy

The breast contains milk glands embedded in supporting tissues and fat (Fig. 9.40). Breast glands are clusters of tiny sacs that produce milk. These glands have a layer of myoepithelial cells outside of them that propel the milk into lactiferous ducts toward the nipple. Before opening at the nipple, the ducts widen to form lactiferous sinuses, which store milk. The lactiferous sinuses lie beneath the junction of the areola and the rest of the breast. Tiny oil-producing glands on the areola keep the nipple skin soft. The areola and nipples have a rich nerve supply making them extremely sensitive to the baby's suckling efforts.

For efficient milk transfer, the neonate's gumline must overlie at the junction of the areola and the rest of the breast.

### Physiology

Milk production (lactogenesis) involves the interaction of many hormones and reflexes. Two hormones, in particular, play a critical role: Prolactin and oxytocin.

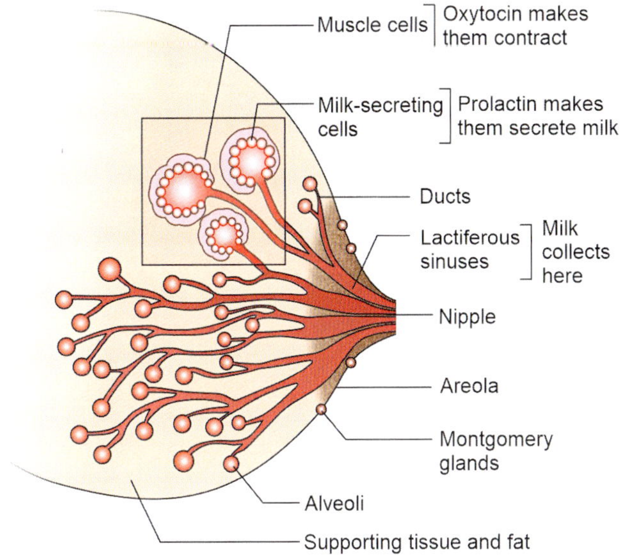


**Fig. 9.40:** Anatomy of breast

*Prolactin reflex (milk secretion reflex):* Prolactin acts on the alveolar glands of the breast to produce milk: The prolactin reflex or the milk secretion reflex. The anterior pituitary produces prolactin, which mediates milk production by the alveolar epithelial cells (Fig. 9.41a). When the neonate sucks, the nerve ending in the nipple carries the impulse to the anterior pituitary, which releases prolactin. The more the neonate sucks at the breast, the greater the milk production. Earlier the initiation, the sooner the reflex. The greater the demand more is the production. Therefore, mothers should initiate feeding early, do it frequently, and allow complete emptying of the breasts at each session. There is a higher production of prolactin during the night; therefore, night feeding helps maintain this reflex.

*Oxytocin reflex (milk ejection reflex):* The posterior pituitary produces oxytocin, which is responsible for *ejection of milk* from the milk glands into the lactiferous sinuses. A baby's thought, sight, or sound stimulates this reflex (Fig. 9.41b and c). The mother's positive emotions and relaxed and confident attitude help the milk ejection reflex. On the contrary, tension, lack of confidence, pain, and lack of sleep hinders the milk flow.

The factors reducing milk production include:

- Using dummies, pacifiers, and bottles. Not only does it interfere with breastfeeding, but it also predisposes neonates to diarrhea.
- Giving anything additional to breastfeeding, such as sugar water, tonic, honey, breast milk substitutes, or formula, either as *prelacteal* (before the first initiation of breastfeeding after birth) or supplemental (alongside breastfeeding) feeds. Studies have reported that even a single such feed may reduce the chances of successful breastfeeding.
- Painful conditions like sore or cracked nipples and engorged breasts.
- Lack of night feeding
- Inadequate emptying of the breasts (sick or small neonate and mother not expressing milk; less frequent feeding)

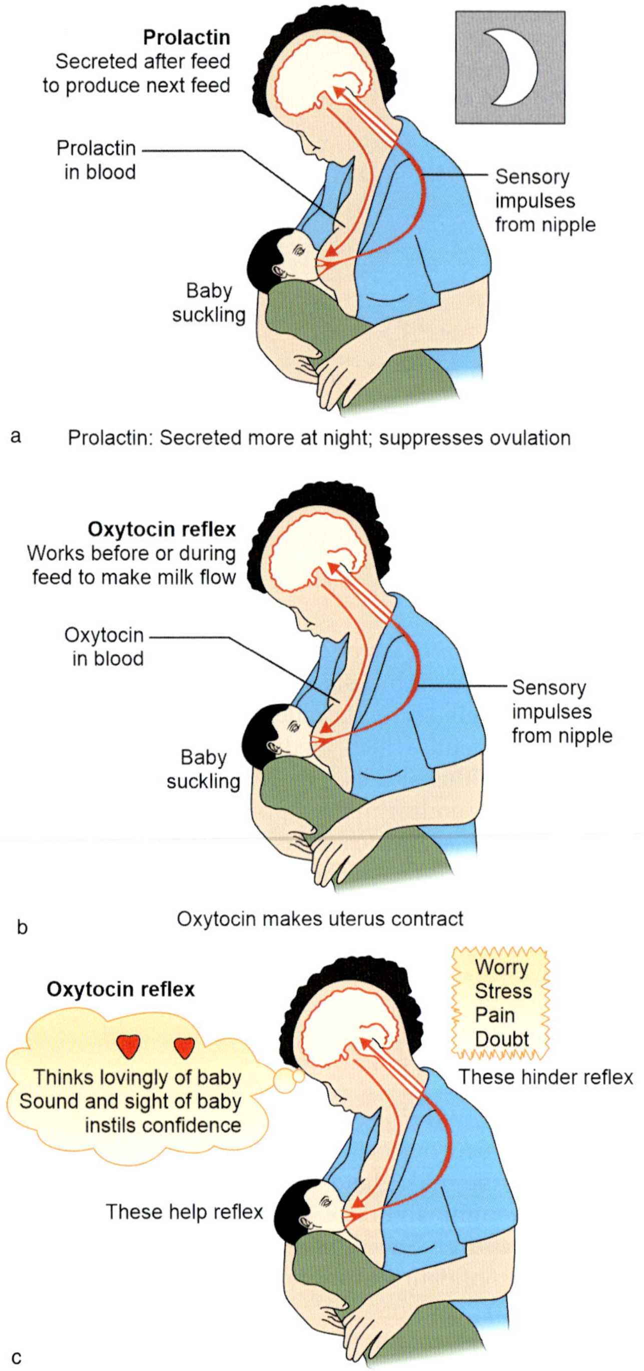


**Fig. 9.41:** (a) Prolactin and (b) oxytocin reflex; (c) Factors which help and hinder oxytocin reflex

## Reflexes in the Baby

A neonate has reflexes that help him in attachment and breastfeeding.

*The rooting reflex:* The neonate turns his head, opens his mouth, and searches the nipple when something touches his cheek or the side of the mouth.

*The suckling reflex:* Effective suckling requires correct attachment. The neonate starts sucking when the nipple touches his palate. Using rooting and sucking reflexes, the neonate grasps the nipple and areola in the mouth and elongates them into a teat. He compresses the teat between the tongue and the palate and draws milk from the lactiferous sinuses.

*The swallowing reflex:* The neonate suckles a few times to get enough milk, which triggers the swallowing reflex. When milk is in the mouth, the neonate reflexly swallows it.

Effective suckling and swallowing require coordination with breathing. The suckle-swallow-breathe cycle lasts for about one second. Reflexes mature fully for efficient breastfeeding by term gestation (Table 9.11).

Advise mothers not to bottle-feed the neonates as it interferes with successful breastfeeding. Suckling at the breast is entirely different from sucking at the bottle. Suckling on a milk-filled bottle is a passive process; the neonate has to control the free flow of milk with her tongue. While breastfeeding requires the baby's active efforts. Bottle-fed neonates develop *nipple confusion*, and that interferes with successful breastfeeding. Even a bottle-feeding session considerably lessens the chances of successful breastfeeding. Also, bottle feeding is associated with severe infections and malnutrition risk.

## Composition of Breast Milk

The breast milk composition varies with time and gestation and within a feeding session to meet the baby's requirements.

i. *Colostrum* is secreted during the initial 3–4 days of delivery. It is small in quantity, yellow and thick, and contains large amounts of antibodies, immune-competent cells, and vitamins A, D, E, and K.
ii. *Transitional milk* is secreted from 3–4 days until two weeks. The immunoglobulin and protein content decreases while the fat and sugar content increases.
iii. *Mature milk* follows transitional milk. It is thinner and watery but contains all the nutrients essential for optimal neonates' growth.
iv. *Preterm milk* contains more proteins, sodium, iron, immunoglobulins, and calories to meet a preterm baby's requirements. However, the milk may require fortification with additional nutrients to meet high calorie, protein, and mineral requirements for very preterm neonates.

**Table 9.11:** Maturation of breastfeeding reflexes

| *Reflexes* | *Gestation age in weeks* | | | |
|---|---|---|---|---|
| | *28 weeks* | *32 weeks* | *34 weeks* | *38 weeks* |
| Rooting | Absent | Weak and slow | Present | Strong |
| Sucking | Absent | Weak | Weak | Vigorous |
| Swallowing | Absent | Associated with a pause in respiration | Less frequently interruption of respiration | Well-coordinated with respiration |

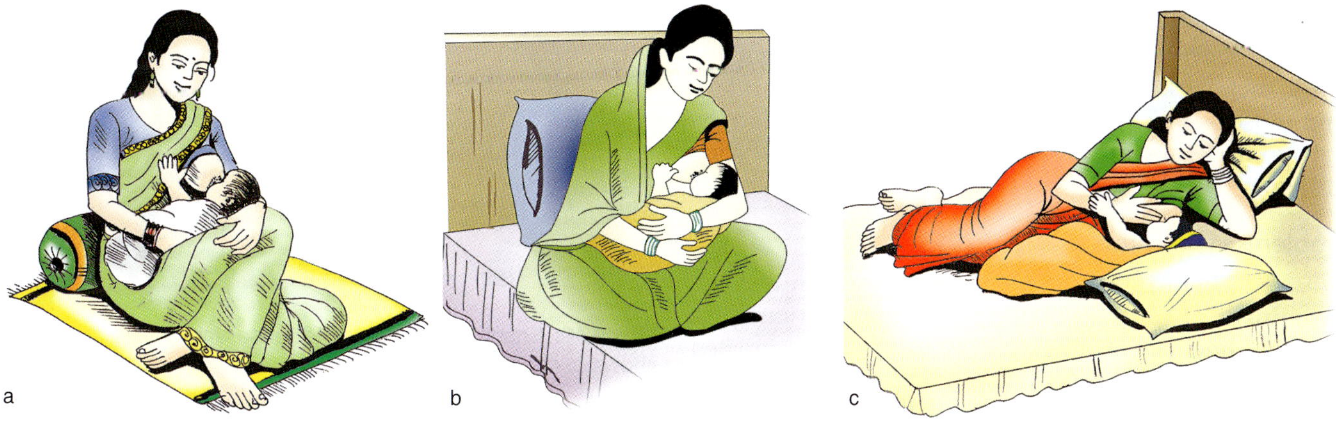


**Fig. 9.42a to c:** Different postures of a mother during breastfeeding. The mother can feed the baby in any position that is comfortable for her. If sitting, her back should be amply supported, and she should not lean on the baby

v. *Foremilk* is the milk secreted at the start of a feed. Watery and high in proteins, sugar, vitamins, and minerals, it quenches the baby's thirst.

vi. *Hindmilk* comes later and is richer in fat, providing more energy and a sense of satiety. For optimum growth, the neonate needs fore- and hindmilk. Therefore, the neonate should empty the breast before switching to the other.

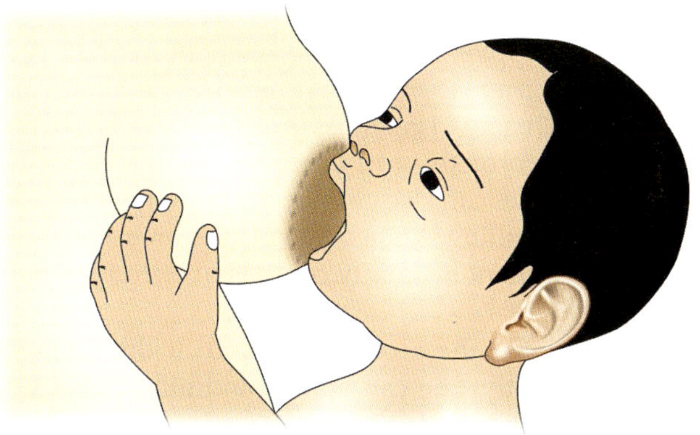

**Fig. 9.43:** Good attachment

### Technique of Breastfeeding

Breastfeeding is a natural and pleasurable experience for the mother. However, the mothers require assistance and support in learning the breastfeeding technique. Many mothers face breastfeeding problems that need support from health providers. A systematic approach to lactation support involving families, mothers, and providers greatly enhances breastfeeding success.

#### *Positioning*

***Position of the mother:*** The mother can assume any position of comfort—she can sit or lie down. Her back should be well supported, and she should not lean on her neonate **(Fig. 9.42a to c)**.

***Position of the baby***

i. Baby's *whole body is supported*, not just the neck or shoulders
ii. Baby's *head and body are in one line* without any twist in the neck
iii. Baby's *body turned towards the mother* (abdomens of the neonate and the mother touching each other)
iv. Baby's *nose is at the level of the nipple.*

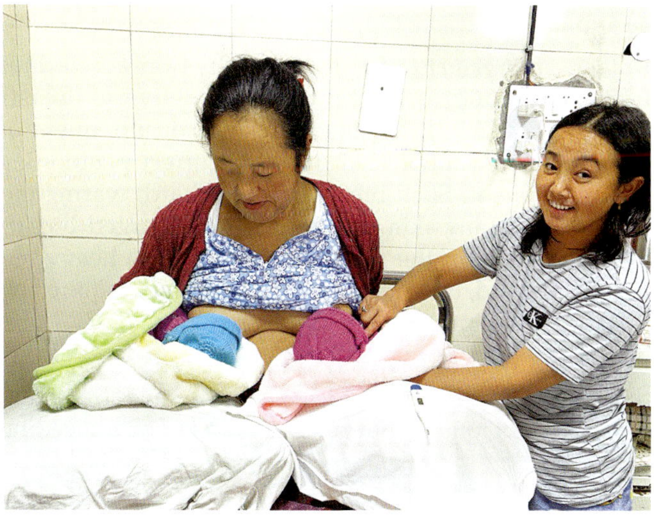

**Fig. 9.44:** The mother feeding both the twin neonates using football hold positions. Note a relative helping the mother. Supporting the babies with pillow reduces the exertion by the mother. Feeding of both the babies simultaneously saves time that mother can use for self-care

#### *Attachment (Latching)*

Ensure proper positioning of the mother and the baby. The mother touches the baby's upper lip with her breast. Wait until the neonate opens his mouth widely. Bring the neonate closer to the breast and put the nipple and most of the areola into the baby's mouth **(Fig. 9.43)**. The mother should not lean on the baby.

#### *Signs of Good Attachment*

i. The baby's mouth is *wide open.*
ii. *Most of the nipple and areola in the mouth*, only the upper areola visible, not the lower one.
iii. The baby's *chin touches the breast.*
iv. The baby's *lower lip is everted.*

The mother can feed twin neonates simultaneously, saving time, and she can rest adequately between feeding sessions **(Fig. 9.44)**.

### Effective Suckling

Neonate *slowly suckles a couple of times and pauses* to swallow (suck, suck, suck, and swallow). One can see throat cartilage and muscles moving and hear the gulping sounds. The baby's cheeks are full and not hollow or retracting during suckling.

## Problems in Breastfeeding

***Inverted nipples:*** Flat or small nipples, which become prominent on pulling out, do not pose difficulty in breastfeeding. However, genuinely inverted or retracted nipples can make latching difficult. As the neonate cannot fully take the nipple and areola in the mouth properly, the nipple becomes sore as the neonate sucks on the nipple. Treatment involves pulling out the nipple and rolling it between the finger and thumb several times daily. Alternatively, a cut plastic syringe can also be used **(Fig. 9.45)**.

***Sore nipple:*** Nipples become sore when the neonate *suckles on them rather than the areola and nipple* because of incorrect attachment. Unable to get milk, the neonate gets frustrated and sucks vigorously, and bites on the nipple, causing soreness. Nipples can also get sore due to frequent washing with soap or pulling the neonate off the breast while still sucking. Treatment primarily consists of *correct positioning and latching*.

In most cases, the mother can feed, if the neonate is attached correctly. She can apply hindmilk after feeding and keep the nipple dry between feeds. Cleaning of the breast and nipples can happen when the mother takes a bath without frequent washing. No cream or ointment should be applied to the sore nipples.

***Breast engorgement:*** *The* milk production accelerates from the second to the third day of delivery. Breasts can get engorged, if feeding is delayed or infrequent or if the neonate cannot feed due to incorrect positioning and attachment. Such breast becomes hard, warm, and tender with shiny skin **(Fig. 9.46)**. The engorged breasts are different from the full breasts, which are heavy but not warm, hard, or tender. Full breasts do not require any specific treatment.

***Early and frequent feeding and correct breastfeeding technique prevent engorgement of the breast:*** Treatment consists of hot fomentation, massage, and frequent feeding or expression of milk. Analgesics can be given to relieve the pain.

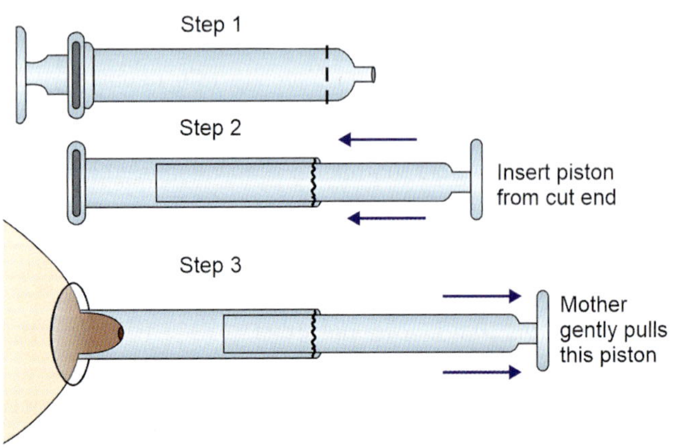


**Fig. 9.45:** Syringe treatment for inverted/flat nipple

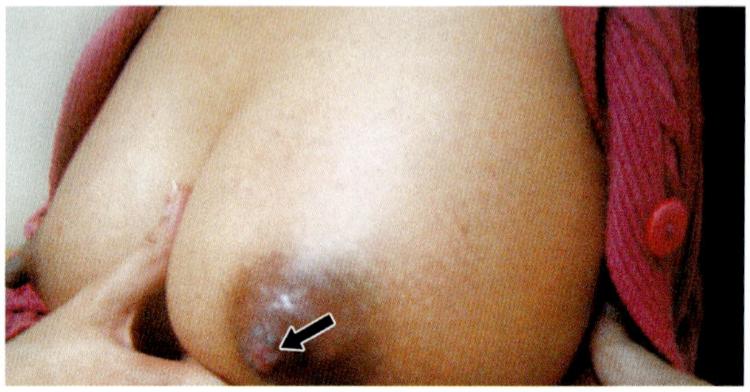

**Fig. 9.46:** Engorged breast. Note tense and shiny skin; nipple shows excoriation (arrow)

***Breast abscess:*** Breast abscess formation can occur, if an engorged breast, cracked nipple, blocked duct, or mastitis is not treated in the early stages. There are systemic signs such as high-grade fever and malaise and profound signs of breast inflammation. Management involves giving analgesics and if required, incision and drainage. Often mothers can continue breastfeeding.

***Not enough milk:*** First, ensure that the perception of "not enough milk" is correct. If the neonate is satisfied and sleeps for 2–3 hr after breastfeeding, passing urine at least 6–8 times in 24 hr, and gaining weight, the mother produces enough milk.

There could be several reasons for insufficient milk: Incorrect method of breastfeeding, supplementary or bottle feeding, no night breastfeeding, engorgement of the breast, maternal illness, stress, or tiredness.

Identify the possible cause and take appropriate action **(Table 9.12)**. Keeping the mother and the neonate in the same bed allows on-demand and frequent breastfeeding. The mother needs sufficient rest and fluids.

## Expressed Breast Milk (EBM)

A mother can express milk if she cannot feed her neonate (sick or working mother, sick or small baby). The neonate can receive expressed breast milk (EBM) or own mother's milk (OMM) by an alternate feeding method such as a paladai or gastric tube. EBM can be stored for 6–8 hours at room temperature, 24 hours in a refrigerator, and 3 to 6 months in a freezer at –20°C.

### Method of Milk Expression

After washing her hands thoroughly, the mother sits comfortably and massages the breast **(Fig. 9.47)**. She squeezes the breast at the areola and collects milk in a wide-mouth container. The proper hand position involves placing the thumb 4 cm away from the nipple and the index finger on the undersurface of the breast. She must first pull the grip towards her chest and then compress it. The milk generally starts flowing after a few compress-and-release cycles. Being at the baby's bedside or keeping the baby's picture can help stimulate the oxytocin reflex.

If there is no milk flow, change the position of the thumb and finger closer to the nipple and express as before. Compress and release all around the breast.

**Table 9.12:** Insufficient breast milk: Causes and remedial actions

| *Causes* | *Remedial action* |
|---|---|
| Delayed initiation of breastfeeding after birth | Start breastfeeding immediately after vaginal delivery and within 30 minutes after cesarean section<br>Early skin-to-skin contact |
| Cracked or sore nipple | Correct positioning and attachment<br>Apply hindmilk<br>Oral analgesics |
| Supplementary feeding | Avoid any supplementary feeding |
| Infrequent night feeding | Frequent night feeding |
| Breast engorgement | Correct positioning and attachment<br>Hot fomentation<br>Massage<br>Frequent breastfeeding of expression of milk<br>Oral analgesics |
| Maternal stress | Counseling |
| Maternal illness or painful condition in the mother | Specific treatment<br>Pain alleviation |
| Less sleep | Ensure proper sleep and rest<br>Keep neonate and mother together |

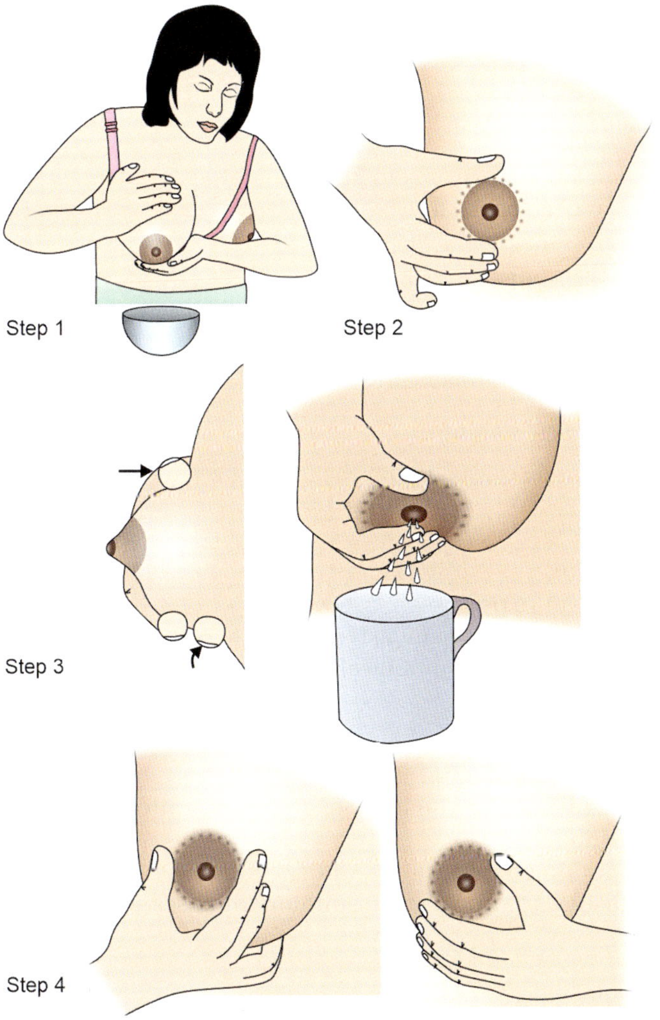


**Fig. 9.47:** Steps of breast milk expression: (1) Massage the breasts gently toward the nipples; (2) Place the thumb and index finger opposite each other just outside the areola; (3) Press back toward the chest, then gently squeeze to release milk; (4) Repeat step 3 in different positions around the areola

A mother should express milk from both breasts 6 to 8 times in 24 hr to maintain optimum lactation.

### Human Breast Milk Banking

Human milk banking (HMB) involves the supply of human donor milk for feeding sick and small neonates whose mothers cannot provide their milk. The first milk bank ("Sneha") was established in Mumbai in 1989. Following national guidelines on establishing "Lactational Management Centers", many centers now have human milk banks in India.

The banks accept voluntary milk donations from lactation women after screening them for a penal of infections. The milk is further cultured to detect bacterial contamination and pasteurized by the Holder method. However, pasteurized donor human milk (PDHM) is inferior to the fresh mother's own milk (MOM); infants tolerate it better than formula milk. The PDHM retains most macronutrients and micronutrients but lacks many immunocompetent substances of fresh human milk. Compared to formula milk, PDHM use reduces late-onset sepsis, necrotizing enterocolitis, feeding intolerance, retinopathy of prematurity, and length and cost of hospital stay. Long-term studies have also shown benefits in better motor and behavior scores and lower metabolic syndrome risk.

*Competency:* **PE20.11**

## CARE OF LOW BIRTH WEIGHT NEONATES

Low birth weight (LBW; birth weight less than 2500 g) neonates have higher morbidity and mortality. LBW results from either preterm birth (before 37 completed weeks of gestation), intrauterine growth restriction (IUGR), or both.

IUGR is like malnutrition and may present in term and preterm infants. Neonates affected by IUGR are usually undernourished and have loose skin folds on the face and

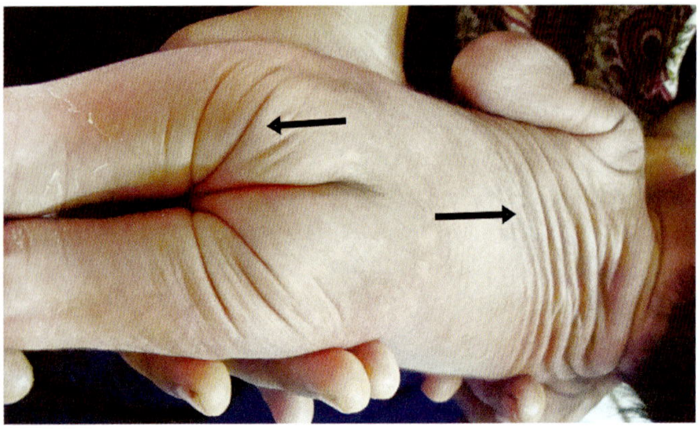

Fig. 9.48: Neonate with intrauterine growth retardation showing many loose folds of skin (arrows)



in the gluteal region (Fig. 9.48), absence of subcutaneous fat, and peeling of skin (Fig. 9.21). Problems faced by a preterm and IUGR neonate are different, although the management principles are common (Table 9.13).

IUGR results when fetal growth falters due to adverse factors affecting normal growth patterns that prevent the fetus's normal growth potential.

There are two types of IUGR:

- *Symmetric:* When insult occurs early in gestation, that reduces the head size, body weight, and length proportionately. The causes of such IUGR include genetic and chromosomal disorders or intrauterine infections (TORCH).
- *Asymmetric:* The insult occurs during late gestation, thereby sparing brain growth. Head size is relatively preserved compared to length and weight. Causes include placental insufficiency, pregnancy-induced hypertension, and maternal medical diseases.

Small for gestational age (SGA) denotes the weight of an infant less than two standard deviations or less than the tenth percentile of the population norms (intrauterine growth chart). For practical purposes, SGA and IUGR are synonymous.

**Table 9.13:** Major problems in preterm babies and those with intrauterine growth retardation (IUGR)

| |
|---|
| **Preterm babies** |
| Hypothermia |
| Perinatal asphyxia |
| Respiratory (hyaline membrane disease, pulmonary hemorrhage, pneumothorax, bronchopulmonary dysplasia, pneumonia) |
| Bacterial sepsis |
| Apnea of prematurity |
| Metabolic (hypoglycemia, hypocalcemia) |
| Hematologic (anemia, hyperbilirubinemia) |
| Feeding problems and poor weight gain |
| **Babies with IUGR** |
| Perinatal asphyxia |
| Meconium aspiration |
| Hypothermia |
| Hypoglycemia |
| Feed intolerance |
| Polycythemia |
| Poor weight gain |

## Issues in LBW Care

Besides common problems, LBW neonates may have additional problems requiring special care.

### Resuscitation

**_Problems_**

- Compromised intrauterine environment with higher chances of perinatal asphyxia
- Preterm neonates have immature lungs that may be more difficult to ventilate
- Immature blood vessels in the brain are prone to bleeding
- Thin skin and a large surface area, which contribute to rapid heat loss
- Increased risk of hypovolemic shock caused by small blood volume

**_Management_**

- Adequate preparation for a higher level of resuscitation
- Appropriate size of equipment such as resuscitation bags, face masks, and endotracheal tubes.
- CPAP device
- Take extra care to avoid hypothermia

### Temperature Control

**_Problems_**

- Higher surface area to body weight
- Low glycogen stores
- Low subcutaneous fat

**_Management_**

- Frequent monitoring and education of parents
- Special attention to the maintenance of the warm chain
- Kangaroo mother care

### Fluids and Feeding

They are discussed under the feeding section.

### Infection

**_Problems_**

- Immature defenses
- Higher need for invasive support such as mechanical ventilation and umbilical vessel catheterization.

**_Management_**

- Strict asepsis, hand hygiene
- Minimal handling
- High index of suspicion of sepsis, rationale use of antibiotics
- Limiting exposure to adults/children with infectious diseases, particularly respiratory illnesses.

### Metabolic Derangements

**_Problems_**

- High risk of hypoglycemia due to low hepatic glycogen stores and higher demands
- Early onset *hypocalcemia:* Presents within three days of life. It is especially seen in premature neonates, infants of diabetic mothers, and those with birth asphyxia.

It is usually asymptomatic and detected during the investigation.

- Late onset hypocalcemia presents as classical neonatal tetany, jitteriness, and seizures. The pathogenesis includes feeding the infant with animal milk that has high phosphate content. That result in hyperphosphatemia with subsequent hypocalcemia.

*Management:* They are discussed in appropriate sections.

*Competency:* **PE20.11; PE27.25**

## KANGAROO MOTHER CARE

Drs Edgar Rey and Hector Martinez conceptualized KMC for the care of LBW infants in Bogotá, Colombia, in 1978. Initially conceived as an alternative to conventional warmer care, KMC has become the standard of care as an alternative or adjunct to technology-based care **(Table 9.16)**. It refers to placing a preterm or LBW infant in skin-to-skin contact with the mother or another caregiver. KMC has three components:

1. Kangaroo position—skin-to-skin contact for prolonged periods.
2. Kangaroo feeding—infants receive breastfeeding.
3. Kangaroo discharge—early discharge as soon as the infant is stable enough.

### Benefits of KMC

KMC benefits the mothers and the babies. It reduces neonatal mortality, infection, and hypothermia and improves breastfeeding, growth, neurodevelopment outcomes, and bonding between the mother and the baby.

### Technique

Infants receive KMC once they have achieved cardio-respiratory stability, often on the second-third day or later. Recently, a large multicentric study undertaken in India, Ghana, Malawi, Nigeria, and Tanzania, reported a 25% improved survival in LBW neonates between 1.0 and 1.79 kg who received KMC starting immediately after birth. After birth, the neonates were transported in KMC position with a caregiver to the specially created mother-neonatal intensive care unit (M-NICU), which had the facility to provide care to the infants and their mothers. The infants received KMC continuously from their mothers or other caregivers. India is implementing the modality of immediate KMC in district and medical college hospitals. Another study demonstrated that KMC could be provided in homes, also.

### Eligibility

*Baby*

Stable LBW neonates below 2000 g are eligible for KMC **(Fig. 9.49)**. The LBW infants weighing 2000 to 2499 g can also receive KMC, depending upon the willingness of the family. Sick neonates need care under radiant warmers or incubators and should receive KMC once hemodynamically stable. Short KMC sessions can be performed during recovery while the infant receives IV fluids, oxygen therapy, and CPAP.

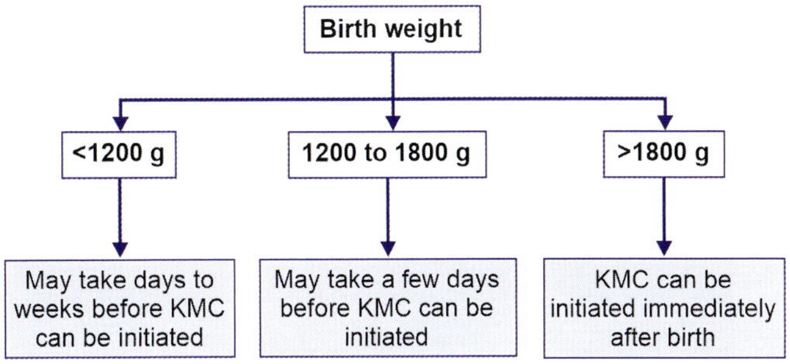


**Fig. 9.49:** Kangaroo mother care (KMC) protocol

*Mother*

All mothers, irrespective of age, parity, education, culture, and religion, can provide KMC. They should be free from significant illness and maintain good hygiene.

### Initiation of KMC

*Counselling:* When a neonate is ready for KMC, arrange a convenient time for the mother and her baby. The first few sessions are essential and require extended interactions. Demonstrate the KMC procedure in a caring and patient manner. Encourage her to bring her mother/mother-in-law, husband, or any other family member. It helps build a positive attitude and ensures the family supports the mother, which is crucial for maintaining KMC at home. Peer interaction between the mothers with someone already practicing KMC also helps.

*Mother's clothing:* KMC can be performed in any front-open dress acceptable to the mother. The garment should be able to retain the neonate for an extended period. KMC works well with a blouse, sari, gown, or shawl **(Fig. 9.50)**.

### Procedure

*Kangaroo positioning:* Place the neonate between the mother's breasts in an upright position **(Fig. 9.51)**. The head should be slightly extended and turned to one side. This head position keeps the airway open and allows the eye-to-eye contact between the mother and her baby. The hips of the neonate should be flexed and abducted in a 'frog' position with flexed arms. The baby's abdomen should be at the level of the mother's epigastrium. The mother's breathing stimulates the baby, thus reducing the occurrence of apnea. Support the baby's bottom with a sling or binder.

*Monitoring:* Neonates receiving KMC should be monitored carefully, especially during the initial stages. The nursing staff should ensure that baby's neck is neither too flexed nor too extended, the airway is clear, breathing is regular, the color is pink, and the neonate is maintaining temperature. The mother should observe the neonate during KMC so that she learns to monitor it.

*Feeding:* Explain to the mother how to breastfeed the neonate and express milk while the neonate is in the KMC position. Holding the neonate near the breast stimulates milk production. The expressed milk can be fed with *a paladai*, spoon, or tube.

*Privacy:* The staff must respect the mother's sensitivities and ensure culturally acceptable privacy.

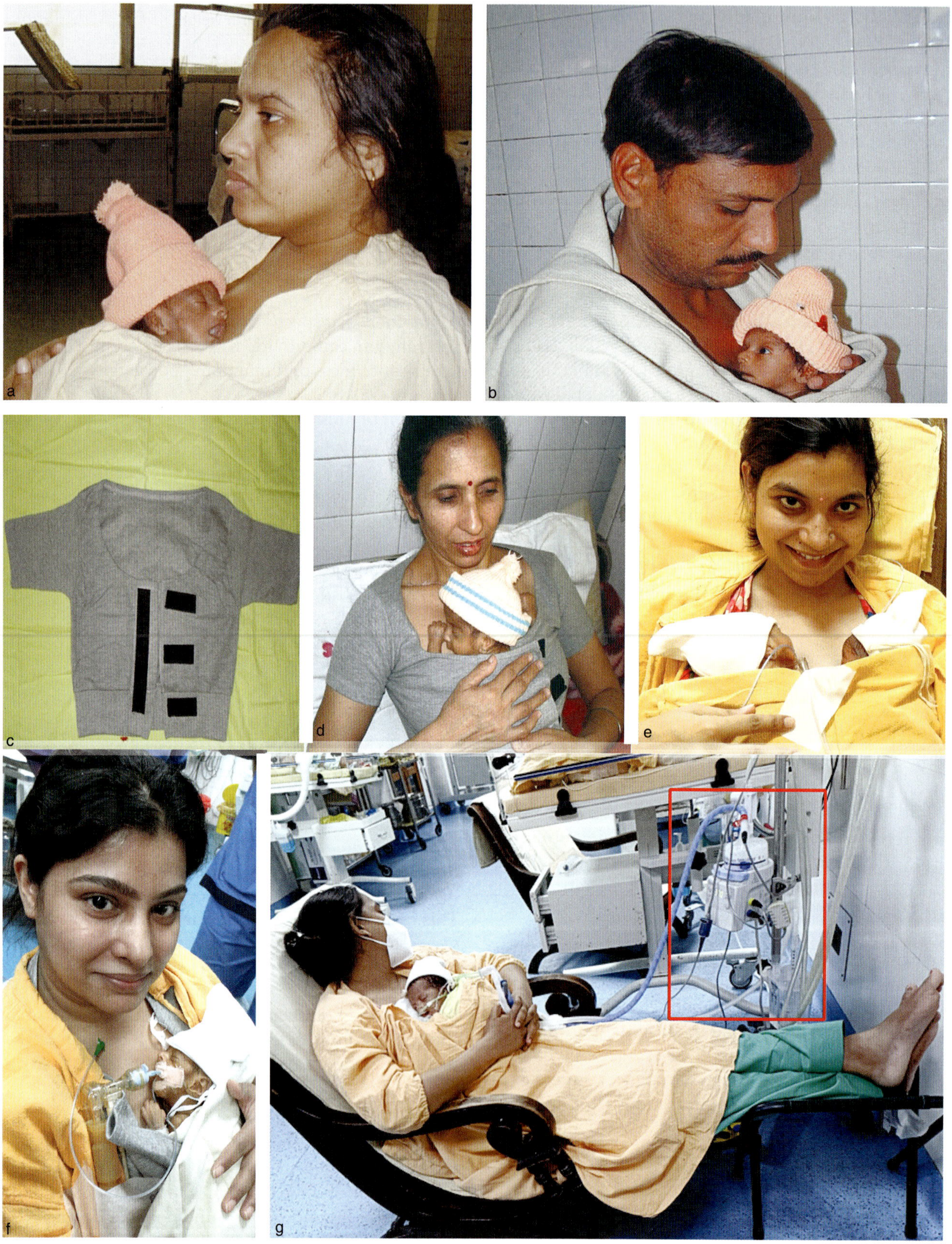


**Fig. 9.50:** (a) Mother and (b) father practicing KMC in front-open gown and shawl; (c) AIIMS KMC jacket; (d) Mother performing KMC using AIIMS KMC jacket; (e) Twins are receiving KMC; one of them receiving oxygen by open tube; (f) KMC in a ventilated baby; (g) A mother provinding KMC to a baby receiving CPAP support. Note both the mother and the baby are sleeping well

***Duration:*** Skin-to-skin contact should start gradually in the nursery, with a smooth transition from conventional care to continuous KMC. The length of skin-to-skin contact should be gradually increased up to 24 hr a day, interrupted for changing diapers. Sessions that last less than one hour should be avoided because frequent handling may be stressful for the baby. The neonate can receive KMC in the postnatal ward after transfer from the NICU.

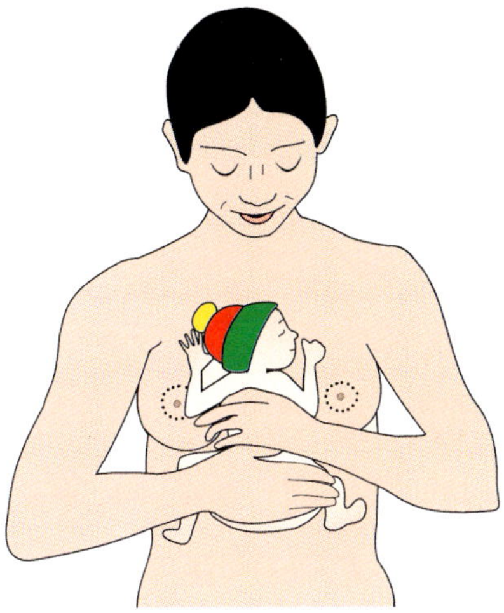

Fig. 9.51: Kangaroo positioning. Note the baby is placed between breasts in frog-legged position with face turned to one side

The mother can sleep with the neonate in a semi-recumbent position with the head end elevated to about 30° using an adjustable bed or pillows. A comfortable chair can also work.

### When to Stop KMC

KMC should be continued until the neonate likes it. When the neonate wriggles out and becomes uncomfortable, KMC is no longer needed. Generally, neonates do not tolerate KMC once they attain a weight of 2500 g and a gestation of 37 weeks.

### Suggested Reading

1. Ministry of Health and Family Welfare, Government of India. Kangaroo mother care and optimal feeding of low-birth-weight infants. Operational guidelines September 2014.

## FLUID AND ELECTROLYTE MANAGEMENT

Changes in body fluid composition happen during the transition from fetal to extrauterine life. Neonates are born with an excess of total body water (TBW), primarily in the extracellular fluid (ECF) compartment. The diuresis during the first week of life results in the loss of ECF and, thus, TBW. Term neonates lose about 7 to 10% of body weight during the first 3 to 5 days of life. Preterm neonates have proportionately higher TBW and may lose up to 10 to 15% of birth weight during the first week of life. SGA neonates have lesser TBW and lose less weight than their AGA counterparts.

The heart, kidneys, skin, and neuroendocrine system regulate fluid and electrolyte balance. In neonates, kidneys have a limited capacity to concentrate or dilute urine due to a lower glomerular filtration rate and reduced proximal and distal tubular sodium reabsorption. In addition to the kidneys and gastrointestinal system, water losses occur due to evaporation from the skin and respiratory tract (insensible water loss; IWL). IWL is higher in preterm infants owing to thin skin. Fever, increased respiratory rate, radiant warmers, and phototherapy increase IWL.

### Guidelines for Fluid Therapy

The neonates of 1000 g or more or 28 weeks or more, otherwise not sick, can be fed enterally with breast milk. The neonates between 1000 and 1800 g or 28 to 33 weeks require alternate feeding methods using a gastric tube or paladai, while the neonates 1800 g or more or 34 weeks or more can accept breastfeeding directly.

***Intravenous (IV) fluid:*** Small or sick neonates need IV fluids initially. Neonates less than 28 weeks should receive IV fluids routinely. Sick neonates, irrespective of weight or gestation, such as those with respiratory distress, significant asphyxia, feed intolerance, or hemodynamic instability, are also candidates for IV fluids. A peripheral intravenous line is the most common route used to provide fluids.

The amount of fluids required depends on the birth weight, day of life, and clinical assessment of fluid balance (well-hydrated versus over- or under-hydrated).

***Neonates with birth weight ≥1500 g:*** Infants receiving IV fluids must excrete a solute load of about 15 mOsm/kg/day in the urine. To excrete this solute load at a urine osmolarity of 300 mOsm/L, the infant would have to pass a minimum of 50 mL/kg/day of urine. The initial fluids should be 10% dextrose with no electrolytes to provide a glucose infusion rate of 4 to 6 mg/kg/min. With an IWL of 20 mL/kg, the initial fluids should amount to 60–80 mL/kg/day (Table 9.14).

As the infant grows and receives enteral feeds, the solute load increases, requiring more fluid to excrete the solute load. Fecal losses and growth also need extra water. Therefore, the fluid requirements increase by 15–20 mL/kg/day to a maximum of 150 mL/kg/day by the seventh day. The neonates need sodium and potassium after 48 hr.

***Neonates with a birth weight less than 1500 g:*** The urine output in these neonates is similar to neonates of 1500 g or more. Due to higher IWL, these neonates need 80 mL/kg/day of 10% dextrose on day 1 (Table 9.14).

Proper dressing of the neonates by providing frocks, caps, and socks reduces IWL under the radiant warmer. As the skin matures, the IWL decreases, and the fluid requirement becomes similar to bigger neonates. These neonates, therefore, need fluid increments of 10–15 mL/kg/day up to a maximum of 150 mL/kg/day by the fifth to the seventh day. Sodium and potassium should be added to IV fluids after 48 hr.

The complications of IV fluid therapy include extravasation, local phlebitis, and fluid overload. Because IV fluid therapy is a significant risk factor for healthcare-associated infections

Table 9.14: Daily fluid requirements during first week of life (mL/kg/day)

| *Birth weight* | *Day 1* | *Day 2* | *Day 3* | *Day 4* | *Day 5* | *Day 6* | *Day 7 and onwards* |
|---|---|---|---|---|---|---|---|
| <1500 g | 80 | 95 | 110 | 120 | 130 | 140 | 150 |
| ≥1500 g | 60 | 75 | 90 | 105 | 120 | 135 | 150 |

(HAIs), all asepsis precautions must be followed during the insertion of an IV cannula and administering fluids. To reduce the risk of HAI, neonates should receive oral feeding once stable. The IV fluid can be stopped once oral feeds constitute about two-thirds of the daily fluid requirement. IV sites should be inspected frequently.

### Monitoring of Fluid and Electrolyte Status

Monitor fluid therapy every 12 to 24 hr in a neonate on IV fluids.

***Body weight:*** Serial weight measurements can help in knowing the adequacy of fluids. Usually, term neonates lose 1–3% of their birth weight daily, with a cumulative loss of 7 to 10% in the first week. Preterm neonates lose 2 to 3% of their birth weight daily, with a cumulative loss of 10–15% in the first week of life. Failure to lose weight in the first week of life may indicate excessive fluid administration. Excessive weight loss during the initial few days, failure to regain birth weight by stipulated age, or failure to gain weight afterward would indicate fluid deficit.

***Clinical examination:*** The usual physical signs of dehydration are unreliable in neonates. Infants with 10% (100 mL/kg) dehydration may have sunken eyes and fontanel, cold and clammy skin, poor skin turgor, and oliguria. Infants with 15% (150 mL/kg) or more dehydration would have signs of shock (hypotension, tachycardia, and weak pulses).

***Urine output:*** A well-hydrated neonate would pass urine at 1 to 3 mL/kg/hr.

### Suggested Reading


1. Chawla D, Agarwal R, Deorari AK, Paul VK. Fluid and electrolyte management in term and preterm neonates. Indian J Pediatr 2008;75:255–9.
2. Segar L. A physiological approach to fluid and electrolyte management of preterm infant. J Neonatal Perinatal Med 2020;13(1):11–19.


*Competency:* **PE20.11**

## FEEDING OF LBW NEONATES

Good nutrition is key to the survival and optimum growth and development of LBW infants. Early nutrition influences long-term neurodevelopmental outcomes.

Healthy-term neonates can directly breastfeed with some assistance in the early postnatal period. In contrast, feeding LBW infants have the following limitations.

i. Over one-third of LBW infants are born preterm with inadequate feeding skills. They may not be able to breastfeed efficiently and require feeding by alternate methods such as paladai or gastric tube.
ii. Many LBW neonates are sick during the first few days of life, interfering with enteral feeding.
iii. Preterm infants have higher fluid requirements in the first few days due to higher IWL.
iv. Since intrauterine accretion of many nutrients occurs in the third trimester, preterm infants, particularly those born before 32 weeks of gestation, have lower body stores, necessitating supplementation.
v. *Because of gut immaturity, they frequently have feed intolerance.*

Direct and exclusive breastfeeding is the goal of feeding all LBW infants. However, many LBW infants may not be able to accept breastfeeding during the initial few days. These infants need spoon/*paladai or* gastric tube (gavage) feeding. Some neonates requiring intravenous (IV) fluids may not receive enteral feeding.

The appropriate method of feeding depends on the following factors:

- Whether the infant is sick or not; and
- Feeding ability of the infant (determined by the gestation and birth weight)

### Level of Sickness

***Sick infants:*** This group includes infants having significant illnesses such as respiratory distress requiring mechanical ventilation, shock, or seizures. These infants require IV fluids initially. These infants should receive enteral feeding at the earliest once reasonably stable. The choice of feeding method depends on the infants' gestation and clinical condition (*see* below).

Enteral feeding is vital for sick neonates. Many sick infants can receive enteral feeding once hemodynamically stable before complete recovery. Infants with respiratory distress receiving mechanical ventilation can be fed enterally once the acute phase is over. Similarly, sepsis or asphyxia in the absence of shock or NEC are not contraindications for enteral feeding.

***Healthy LBW infants:*** Enteral feeding should be initiated immediately after birth in healthy LBW infants with the appropriate feeding method.

### Ability to Feed

Breastfeeding requires effective sucking, swallowing, and proper coordination between sucking, swallowing and breathing. These skills mature with gestation (Table 9.15). A robust sucking may not present until 32–34 weeks gestation. Coordination between sucking, swallowing, and breathing may not mature until 34 weeks, and it fully matures by 37 to 38 weeks.

The initial feeding method is individualized based on the infant's gestation or birth weight and feeding skills (Fig. 9.52).

Stable LBW infants should be offered direct breastfeeding, irrespective of their initial feeding method. This helps faster maturation of smaller infants' feeding skills and improves lactation in their mothers (*non-nutritive sucking*). Figure 9.53a and b shows the method of *paladai* and gastric tube (gavage) feeding.

### Progression of Oral Feeds

The progression of feeding methods is summarized in Fig. 9.54.

Term LBW infants started on IV fluids (because of their sickness) can be put on the breast once they are hemodynamically stable.

**Table 9.15:** Maturation of oral feeding skills and the choice of initial feeding method in LBW infants

| *Gestational age, weeks* | *Maturation of feeding skills* | *Initial feeding method* |
|---|---|---|
| <28 weeks | Inadequate sucking efforts<br>Lack of propulsive gut motility | Intravenous fluids |
| 28–31 weeks | Sucking bursts develop<br>Lack of coordination between suck/ swallow and breathing | Orogastric or nasogastric tube feeding with occasional spoon or paladai feeding |
| 32–34 weeks | Slightly mature sucking pattern<br>Coordination between breathing and swallowing begins | Feeding by spoon or paladai |
| >34 weeks | Mature sucking pattern<br>Coordination between breathing and swallowing | Breastfeeding |

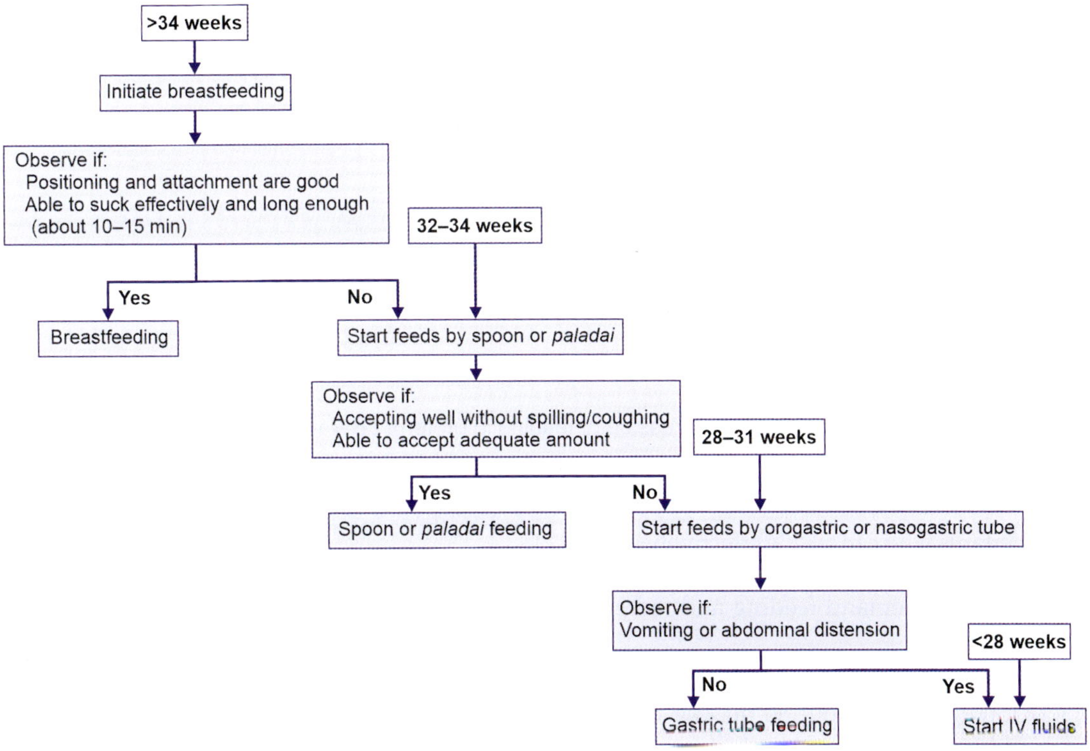


**Fig. 9.52:** Choosing initial methods of feeding

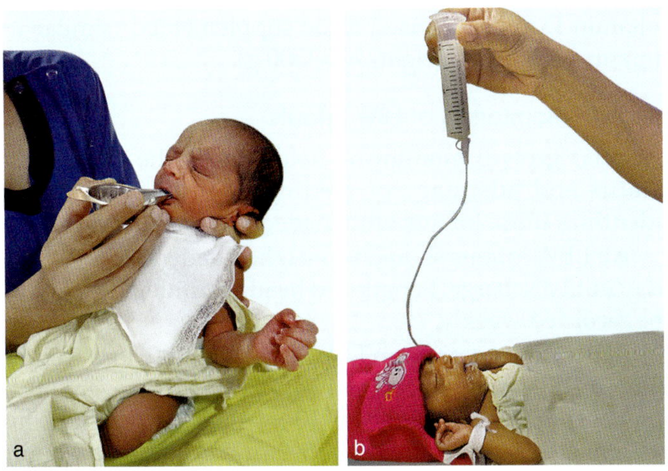


**Fig. 9.53:** (a) Paladai feeding; (b) Gavage feeding (*Courtesy:* Dr Deena Thomas, Akash Sharma)

## Choice of Milk

The choice for milk in LBW infants is the following:

1. Mothers' own milk (MOM)
2. Pasteurized donor human milk
3. Preterm formula
4. Term formula

***Expressed breast milk (EBM):*** All mothers should be counseled and supported in expressing breast milk for feeding their preterm infants (Fig. 9.47). The expression should ideally be initiated within hours of delivery so that the infant gets colostrum. After that, it should be done every 2 to 4 hours to maintain good lactation. Expressed breast milk can be stored for about 6 hours at room temperature and 24 hours in the domestic refrigerator (2 to 8°C).

***Sick mothers/contraindication to breastfeeding:*** In these rare circumstances, the options are:

a. Pasteurized donor human milk
b. Preterm formula in VLBW infants, and
c. Term formula in infants weighing 1500 g or more at birth

Once the mother becomes stable (or does not have the contraindication), these infants should be started on exclusive breastfeeding.

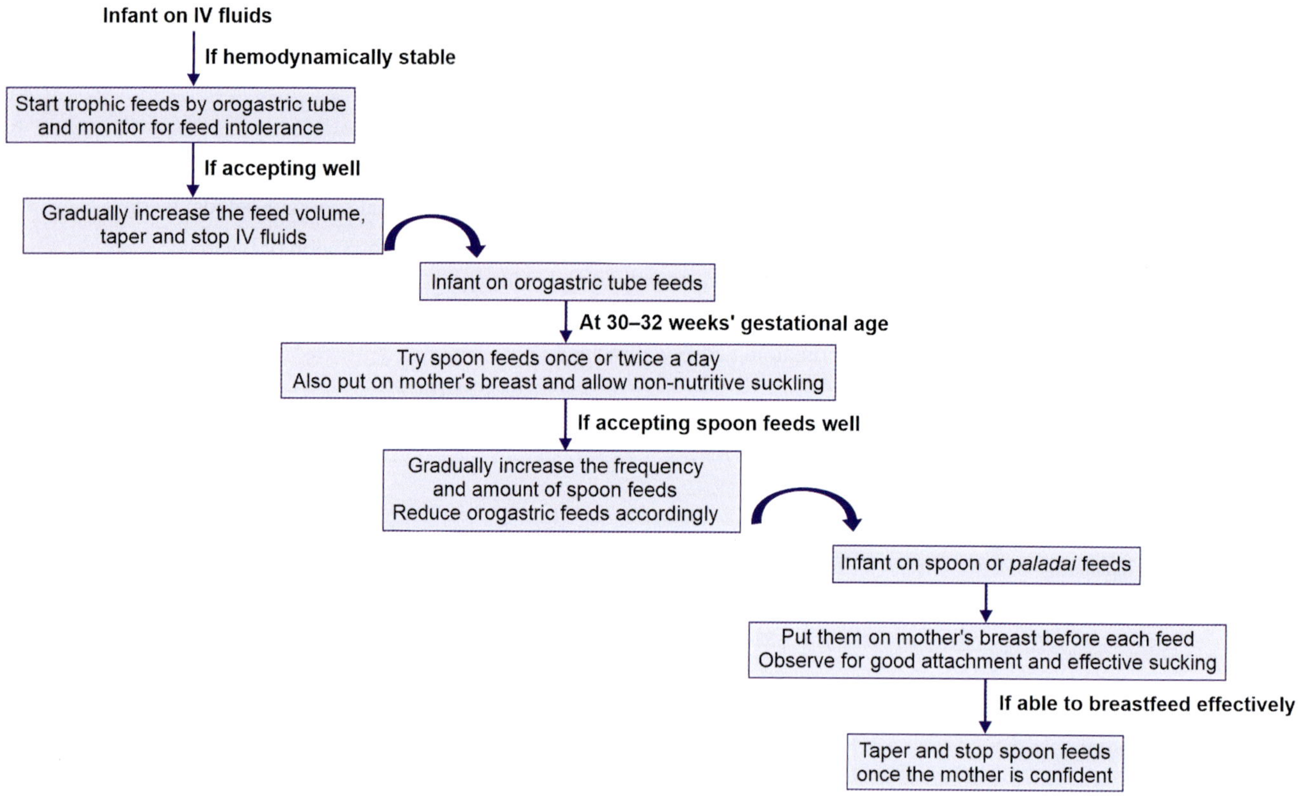


**Fig. 9.54:** Progression of feeding in preterm LBW infants

### How Much to Feed?

*Breastfed infants:* Infants who can suckle effectively should be breastfed on demand. Small neonates (<2000 g) may not be relied upon for on-demand feeding and fed every 2–3 hours.

*Infants who are fed by spoon/paladai or by gastric tube:* VLBW infants (<1500 g) need about 80 mL/kg of fluids on the first day of life (discussed earlier). It needs to be increased by 10–15 mL/kg/day to 150 mL/kg/day by the end of the first week of life. LBW infants ≥1500 g are usually given about 60 mL/kg fluids on the first day of life, and fluid intake is increased by about 15–20 mL/kg/day to a maximum of 150 mL/kg/day by the end of the first week of life. The volume of one feed can be calculated by dividing the total fluid given by the number of feeds planned in 24 hours.

### Nutritional Supplementation

*Birth weight of 1500–2499 g:* These infants are likelier to be born at or near-term gestation (≥34 weeks). They need vitamin D and iron (Table 9.16).

*Birth weight <1500 g:* These infants, usually born before 32–34 weeks gestation, have inadequate body stores of most nutrients. Since EBM has insufficient protein, energy, calcium, phosphorus, trace elements (iron, zinc), and vitamins D, E, and K, these infants need multi-nutrient supplementation until term gestation (40 weeks, i.e. until the expected date of delivery). These additional nutrients can be provided by fortification of expressed breast milk with human milk fortifiers (HMF). Fortification increases the nutrient content of the milk without compromising its other beneficial effects. As HMF does not provide adequate iron, the same has to be provided separately. Fortification or supplementation of minerals and vitamins should be continued till term gestation (40 weeks) in VLBW infants. After 40 weeks, only vitamin D and iron need to be supplemented (similar to infants with birth weights of ≥1500 g).

### Growth Monitoring of LBW Infants

Regular growth monitoring helps assess the nutritional status and adequacy of feeding in LBW infants and identifies those infants with inadequate weight gain.

All LBW infants should be weighed daily or every other day until discharge. Length and head circumference should be recorded weekly.

Both term and preterm LBW infants tend to lose weight (about 10% and 15%, respectively) in the first seven days; they regain birth weight by 10–14 days. After that, the weight gain should be at least 15–20 g/kg/day till a weight

**Table 9.16:** Nutritional supplements for infants with birth weight between 1500 g and 2499 g

| *Nutrients* | *Method of supplementation* | *Dose* | *Duration* |
|---|---|---|---|
| Vitamin D | Multivitamin drops or syrup | 400 IU/day | 2 weeks to 1 year of age |
| Iron | Iron drops or syrup | 2 mg/kg/day (maximum 15 mg) | 6–8 weeks to 1 year of age |

of 2–2.5 kg is reached. After this, a gain of 20 to 40 g/day is considered appropriate.

*Growth charts:* A growth chart (Fenton chart) is a simple way to monitor growth. Serial plotting of weight and other anthropometric indicators in the growth chart allows for tracking an infant's growth with respect to a reference. It helps in the early identification of growth faltering.

### Inadequate Weight Gain

Inadequate weight gain is a common problem (Table 9.17). It may result in failure to thrive and wasting in the first year of life.

Management consists of the following:

i. Ensuring adequate breastfeeding support. Mothers should use proper technique and the right feeding frequency, including night feeding.
ii. Ensuring optimum feeding frequency and quantity of milk for spoon or *paladai* feeds. Ensuring night feeds.
iii. Supplementing breastfeeding with a spoon or *paladai* feeds, if the infant tires out while sucking from the breast.
iv. Ensuring the correct technique of milk expression and *paladai* feeding.
v. Ensuring optimum thermal protection

### Suggested Reading


1. Nutrition. In: Edmond K, Bahl R (Eds). Optimal feeding of low-birth-weight infants—Technical Review. World Health Organization 2006; 1–131.
2. Sankar MJ, Agarwal R, et al. Feeding of low birth weight infants. Indian J Pediatr 2008;75:459–69.
3. Dutta S, Singh D, Chessell L, et al. Guidelines for feeding very low weight infants. Nutrients 2015;7(1):423–42.


### Jaundice

*Problems*

- Larger RBC volume for body weight
- Immaturity of hepatic enzymes and hepatic excretory capacity
- Immature blood–brain barrier—increased risk for bilirubin encephalopathy

*Management:* This has been discussed in the section on jaundice.

**Table 9.17:** Causes of inadequate weight gain

| |
|---|
| **Inadequate intake** |
| *Breastfed infants* |
| Incorrect feeding (improper positioning or attachment)* |
| Less frequent breastfeeding, not feeding in the night hours* |
| *Infants on spoon or paladai feeds* |
| Incorrect method of feeding* (e.g. excess spilling) |
| Incorrect measurement or calculation |
| Infrequent feeding* |
| Not fortifying the milk in VLBW infants |
| **Increased demands** |
| Hypothermia or cold stress* |
| Chronic illnesses, bronchopulmonary dysplasia |
| Medications such as corticosteroids |

*Common causes

### Hematological Abnormality

*Problems*

***Polycythemia:*** Placental insufficiency stimulates erythropoiesis, which results in polycythemia, especially in IUGR neonates. Polycythemia (>65% hematocrit) produces hyperviscosity with decreased organ perfusion. Manifestations include jitteriness, respiratory distress, cardiac failure, feeding intolerance, hypoglycemia, hypocalcemia, and hyperbilirubinemia.

***Anemia:*** The accelerated destruction of fetal RBCs, low reticulocyte count, and inadequate response of the bone marrow to erythropoietin cause anemia of prematurity. The need for frequent blood sampling can predispose LBW to the risk of severe anemia.

*Management*

- ***Treatment of polycythemia:*** Symptomatic infants or asymptomatic infants with hematocrit >75% require partial exchange transfusion, which involves removal of 25 to 50 mL per kg of blood and replacement with normal saline. For others, management includes increasing fluid intake.
- ***Anemia:***
  - All LBW neonates should receive iron supplementation with a dose of 2–3 mg/kg from 2 months until 2 yr of age.
  - Blood sampling should be minimized
  - Transfusions are given as per institution protocol.

### Immature Organ Systems in Preterm Infants

*Respiratory distress syndrome:* This is described in detail later.

*Intraventricular hemorrhage (IVH):* Preterm infants have a fragile and highly vascular germinal matrix near the brain's lateral ventricles. Respiratory distress, mechanical ventilation, or vigorous resuscitation can cause rupture of these vessels leading to adverse neurological sequelae. Preventive measures include giving antenatal steroids, minimal and gentle handling, avoiding rapid fluid boluses or infusion of hyperosmolar solutions, and avoiding high pressures during ventilation.

*Retinopathy of prematurity (ROP):* Retinal vessels grow from the optic disc to the periphery from 18 to 44 weeks of gestation. A host of postnatal factors, such as high or low oxygen saturations, sepsis, blood transfusions, sickness, and poor postnatal nutrition support, may injure the vascular growth of the retina. The retinal vascular injury can induce pathological proliferation of retinal vessels resulting in ROP. While in most neonates, ROP would regress in time, it can progress to retinal detachment and blindness if left untreated in some neonates. This complication can be reduced with rational use of oxygen, maintaining a $SpO_2$ between 91 and 95%, avoiding unnecessary transfusions, and regular screening of the eyes for early detection. Advanced stages of ROP require peripheral retinal ablation by laser.

*Hearing impairment:* Preterm infants are at higher risk of hearing loss. Rational usage of ototoxic drugs, preventing hypoxia, optimally treating jaundice, and routine early detection screenings can minimize this complication.

### Prolonged Hospital Stay

LBW neonates often need extended stay in the hospital, which could be substantial in very small or sick neonates. It is an emotionally and financially trying time for all families. It results in their long separation from their parents and usually incurs high expenses. Keeping parents involved in the decision-making and providing emotional support can help the families greatly.

### Criteria for Discharge

- The clothed neonate can maintain normal body temperature outside the radiant warmer or incubator.
- The neonate has been gaining weight consistently for a few days. Tracking weight, length, and head circumference using a growth chart can help determine whether growth is adequate. There are separate growth charts for the term and preterm infants (Table 9.18).
- Neonate should be breastfeeding well or accepting feeds using *paladai* or spoon. The mother is adequately trained in feeding the baby.
- Absence of significant morbidity, and the neonate not needing any treatment such as IV antibiotics. The parents have well understood how to give medicines or supplements after discharge.
- All screenings (ROP, hearing, metabolic) have been performed before discharge. Some infants may need ROP screening after discharge.
- Ensure the neonate receives all nutritional supplements, including multivitamins, iron, calcium, and vitamin D.
- Immunization with BCG, hepatitis B, and OPV is given (Fig. 9.55a and b).
- Parents have understood how to recognize danger signs (Fig. 9.15) and when to come back.
- Follow-up within 3–7 days of discharge to ensure the neonate has adapted well to the home environment.

### Suggested Reading

1. Fenton TR, Kim JH. A systematic review and meta-analysis to revise the Fenton growth chart for preterm infants. BMC Pediatr 2013;13:59.

**Table 9.18:** Growth charts

| *Gestation* | *Charts used for growth monitoring* |
|---|---|
| Preterm infants | Fenton's chart up to 50 weeks postmenstrual age (PMA), and WHO chart after that |
| Term infants | WHO growth chart |

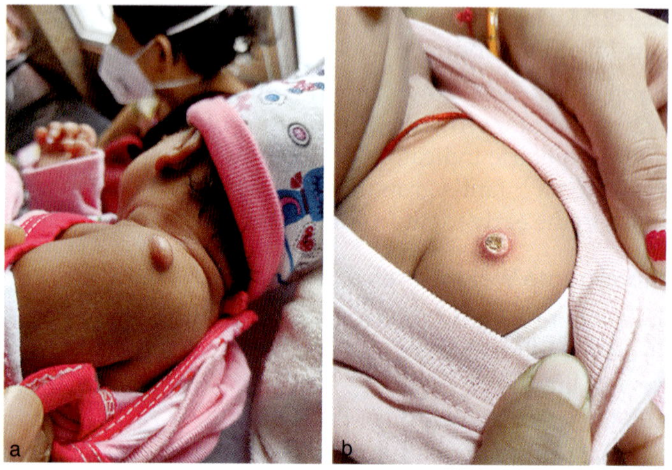


**Fig. 9.55:** Reaction to BCG vaccine: (a) Papule formation in 2 to 3 weeks; (b) The papule ulcerates, and later heals, leaving a scar, 4 to 8 mm in diameter. (*Courtesy:* Dr Md Tousifullah)

*Competency:* **PE20.8**

## RESPIRATORY DISTRESS

Respiratory distress is defined as the presence of tachypnea (RR >60 per min), with lower chest retractions, grunting, and cyanosis. It can be due to non-respiratory (Table 9.19) or respiratory causes (Table 9.20).

### Approach

The gestation of the neonate, age at onset and severity of distress, and presence of associated clinical features assist in the diagnosis. The chest retractions are mild or absent in respiratory distress due to non-respiratory causes. Downe's Score can objectively assess respiratory distress (Table 9.21).

**Table 9.19:** Non-pulmonary causes of rapid breathing

| | |
|---|---|
| Cardiac | Congestive heart failure; congenital heart disease |
| Metabolic | Hypothermia, hypoglycemia, metabolic acidosis |
| Central nervous system | Asphyxia, cerebral edema, hemorrhage |
| Chest wall | Asphyxiating thoracic dystrophy, Werdnig-Hoffman disease |

**Table 9.20:** Pulmonary causes of respiratory distress

| *Cause* | *Time of onset* | *Remarks* |
|---|---|---|
| Respiratory distress syndrome | First 6 hours of life | Common in preterm neonates |
| Meconium aspiration syndrome | First few hours of life | Common in term, post-term and small for date babies; history of meconium-stained liquor |
| Pneumonia | Any age | Often bacterial |
| Transient tachypnea of newborn | First 6 hours after birth | Tachypnea with minimal distress; lasts for 48–72 hours |
| Pneumothorax | Any age | Sudden deterioration; usually during assisted ventilation |
| Tracheoesophageal fistula, diaphragmatic hernia | Any age | May show associated malformations; polyhydramnios in esophageal atresia |

**Table 9.21:** Downe score

| *Parameters* | *Score** | | |
|---|---|---|---|
| | *0* | *1* | *2* |
| Respiratory rate/minute | <60 | 60–80 | >80 |
| Cyanosis | Absent | At room air (21% $O_2$) | At ≥40% $O_2$ |
| Grunting | Absent | Audible with stethoscope | Even audible without a stethoscope |
| Retractions | Absent | Mild | Marked |
| Air entry | Bilateral equal | Mildly decreased | Markedly decreased |

*A score >6 is suggestive of impending respiratory failure

***Respiratory causes:*** Conditions in Tables 9.19 and 9.20 can occur in preterm and term neonates. The respiratory distress in a preterm neonate soon after birth is likely to be respiratory distress syndrome (RDS) or delayed adaptation (transient tachypnea). Meconium aspiration syndrome is expected in a term neonate born through meconium-stained liquor and developing respiratory distress soon after birth. Respiratory distress soon after birth in a term neonate born by elective cesarean section is likely to have transient tachypnea of the newborn. The presence of suprasternal recessions with or without stridor indicates upper airway obstruction.

***Cardiac causes:*** The presence of respiratory distress with hepatomegaly or cyanosis may indicate heart disease. Transposition of great vessels (TGV) usually presents on day one with progressive distress. Most other cardiac conditions present after the first week of life. A preterm neonate having a systolic murmur, tachypnea and hepatomegaly are likely to have patent ductus arteriosus (PDA).

***Neurological causes:*** Neonates with birth asphyxia, cerebral hemorrhage, or meningitis can present with tachypnea and respiratory distress. These neonates are usually lethargic with poor neonatal reflexes.

### Transient Tachypnea of Newborn (TTN)

Transient tachypnea of the newborn (TTN) is a benign self-limiting disease usually occurring in term neonates. TTN is due to delayed lung fluid clearance, leading to impaired gas exchange and hypoxia at birth. Elective cesarean section before 39 weeks of gestation and prematurity are major risk factors. These neonates have tachypnea, which is often silent without much respiratory distress. TTN is a diagnosis of exclusion after ruling out serious disorders such as RDS and pneumonia. Chest X-ray may show high-volume lung fields, prominent vascular marking, and prominent interlobar fissure (Fig. 9.56a). Supportive treatment with oxygen therapy is often adequate, but some may need CPAP therapy. The prognosis is excellent.

### Respiratory Distress Syndrome (RDS)

RDS is common in neonates of less than 34 weeks of gestation. The overall incidence is 10–15% but can be as high as 80% in neonates <28 weeks. In addition to prematurity, asphyxia, acidosis, maternal diabetes, and cesarean section can increase the risk of RDS.

#### *Etiopathogenesis*

Surfactant production starts around 20 weeks of life and peaks at 35 weeks gestation. Therefore, any neonate less than 35 weeks is prone to develop RDS. The primary abnormality is surfactant deficiency. Surfactant, produced by type II alveolar cells, comprises lipoprotein containing phospholipids and proteins. The surfactant prevents the alveoli from deflating at the end of expiration by lowering surface tension within them. In the absence of surfactant, the alveoli tend to collapse during expiration, and the neonate has to exert additional to open the collapsed alveoli again. Increased work of breathing and hypoxemia causes acidosis, which results in pulmonary vasoconstriction, right-to-left shunting across the foramen ovale, and consequent hypoxemia. Ischemic damage to the alveoli causes the transudation of proteins forming a hyaline membrane.

#### *Clinical Features*

The onset of respiratory distress usually occurs within the first 6 hr of life. Clinical features include tachypnea, retractions, grunting, cyanosis, and decreased air entry. A chest X-ray depicts low-volume lungs, reticulogranular pattern, ground glass opacity, and air bronchogram (Fig. 9.56b). The lungs become white out in severe disease.

#### *Management*

Such neonates need admission to the neonatal intensive care unit, IV fluids, and appropriate respiratory support. Continuous positive airway pressure (CPAP) is generally enough for mild to moderate disease. CPAP is a noninvasive modality of support where a continuous distending pressure (5–7 cm $H_2O$) is applied at the nostril level to keep the alveoli open in a spontaneously breathing neonate (Figs 9.57 and 9.58; Box 9.1). CPAP is an excellent respiratory support modality that minimizes lung injury, air leaks, and sepsis. Preterm neonates developing severe RDS often require mechanical ventilation. Preterm neonates are at risk of lung injury by excessive pressure and high oxygen. High oxygen saturations (above 95%) can contribute to the development of retinopathy of prematurity (ROP) which can lead to blindness as discussed before.

Exogenous surfactant replacement therapy (SRT) is recommended as the treatment of choice for moderate to severe RDS. Though lung surfactants were initially manufactured synthetically, current surfactants are extracted from animal lungs (natural surfactant) such as bovine calves (beractant) or pigs (poractant). As opposed to

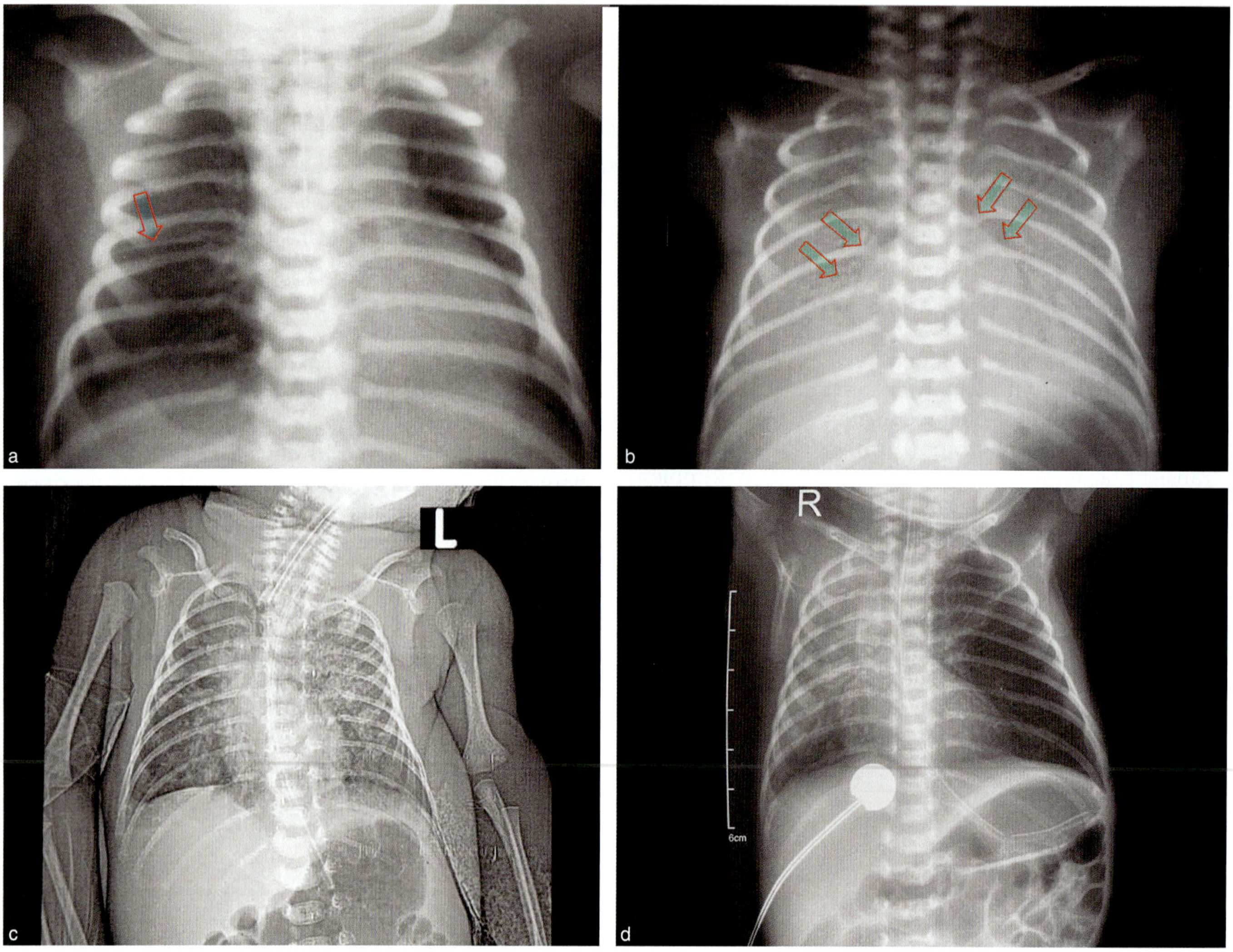


Fig. 9.56: (a) Transient tachypnea of the newborn. Note hyperinflated lungs, prominent bronchovascular markings, and horizontal fissure (arrow); (b) Moderate to severe respiratory distress syndrome. Note homogenous opacification of lungs obscuring heart borders and presence of air bronchogram (arrows); (c) Asymmetric patchy Infiltrates with hyperinflation suggesting meconium aspiration syndrome (MAS); (d) Pneumonia-involving one lung

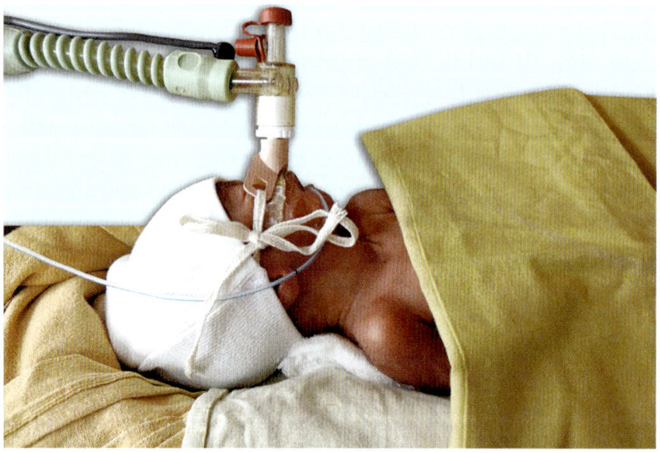

Fig. 9.57: Continuous positive airway pressure being provided to a preterm baby

artificial surfactants, which lack surfactant proteins, natural surfactants have surfactant proteins B and A, making the latter more effective. New synthetic surfactants with recombinant surfactant protein B are more effective than the previous synthetic surfactants.

SRT is indicated in preterm neonates with moderate to severe RDS. SRT can be given as rescue therapy to treat established RDS or prophylactic therapy in neonates less than 28 weeks. SRT has a synergistic action with CPAP. A preterm neonate with respiratory distress is treated initially with CPAP. The SRT is administered, if the RDS is severe enough to require $FiO_2$ of 40% or greater while on CPAP.

SRT decreases the duration and level of respiratory support in neonates and improves outcomes. Traditionally, the neonates were intubated, given surfactant in four or five boluses through an endotracheal tube, and later extubated after a few hours to days. Many neonates can now be INtubated, given SURfactant, and rapidly Extubated (InSurE approach) to CPAP, avoiding mechanical ventilation. Lately, giving surfactant using a thin catheter inserted in the trachea under vision has obviated the need for intubation, thus avoiding complications of intubation.

### Prevention of RDS

Antenatal steroids reduce RDS, intraventricular hemorrhage, and mortality in preterm neonates.

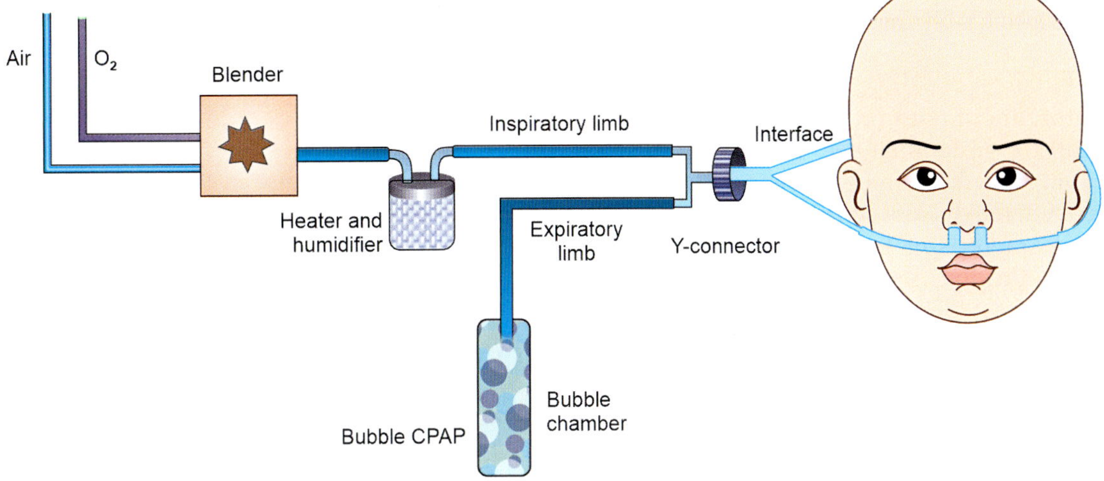


**Fig. 9.58:** Continuous positive airway pressure (CPAP) device. It blends air and oxygen in the desired concentration, heats to the body temperature and humidifies, and circulates it in the circuit to generate the desired pressure (3 to 10 cm $H_2O$) at the nostril level for a spontaneously breathing baby

### Box 9.1 CPAP in Newborns

Continuous positive airway pressure (CPAP) provides respiratory support to preterm neonates breathing spontaneously with respiratory distress. CPAP generates a positive pressure of 5 to 8 cm $H_2O$ at the nostril level, and it is delivered through an interphase of either a binasal prong or nasal mask.

Preterm neonates do not have adequate functional residual capacity (FRC) due to a compliant chest wall. The lung alveoli tend to collapse at the end of expiration, making breathing difficult and impairing the gas exchange. CPAP prevents the collapse of the alveoli and helps in better recruitment of alveoli resulting in optimal FRC.

**Components of CPAP system**

The CPAP system has the following elements:

- *Gas source* provides a continuous supply of warm, humidified, and blended gases, i.e. air and oxygen. The blender can provide desired oxygen concentration varying from 21 to 100%.
- *Pressure generator* creates a positive pressure in the circuit. In the most commonly used bubble CPAP machine, the expiratory limb of the circuit is dipped in a water column to generate the desired pressure.
- *Patient interface* connects the CPAP circuit to the infant's airway

**Common indications**

1. Respiratory distress in preterm neonates due to respiratory distress syndrome (RDS), transient tachypnea, and pneumonia
2. Apnea of prematurity despite methylxanthine therapy
3. Following extubation in preterm VLBW infants
4. Airway instability such as laryngomalacia, tracheomalacia and bronchomalacia

**Contraindications to CPAP**

- Severe cardiovascular instability
- Poor respiratory drive
- Progressive respiratory failure ($PaCO_2$ levels >60 mm Hg and/ or $PaO_2$ <50 mm Hg)
- Congenital malformations, e.g. tracheoesophageal fistula
- Congenital diaphragmatic hernia

**How to set up**

- *Initiation:* CPAP 5 cm $H_2O$, $FiO_2$ titrate to maintain $SpO_2$ 90–95%
- *Escalation:* Increase CPAP in steps of 1–2 cm to a maximum of 7–8 cm $H_2O$, increase $FiO_2$ in steps of 5% till 80%
- *Failure of CPAP:* Worsening respiratory distress, $PaO_2$ <50 mm Hg, $PaCO_2$ >60 mm Hg, despite CPAP of 7–8 cm and $FiO_2$ of 80%
- *Weaning from CPAP:* Reduce $FiO_2$ in steps of 5 to 40%, then decrease pressure in steps of 1–2 cm $H_2O$ until 4 cm $H_2O$

**Complications**

- Nasal injury
- Pulmonary air leaks
- Decreased cardiac output
- Increased pulmonary vascular resistance (with excessive CPAP)
- Gastric distension (CPAP belly syndrome)

*Compiled:* Dr Md Tousifullah

## Meconium Aspiration Syndrome (MAS)

Neonates born through MSAF can aspirate meconium into the lungs and develop respiratory distress (meconium aspiration syndrome; MAS). Aspirated meconium can block the large and small airways causing areas of atelectasis and emphysema, which can result in air leaks like pneumothorax (Fig. 9.59). Atelectasis and emphysema cause ventilation-

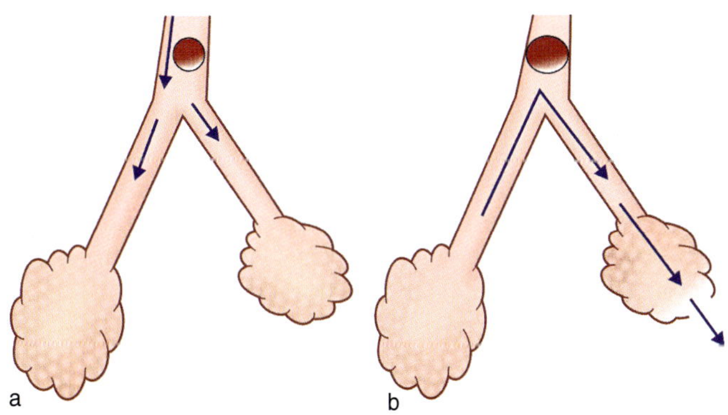


**Fig. 9.59:** Ball valve effect due to meconium plug: (a) During inspiration, air enters the alveoli; (b) During expiration, air cannot pass through the main airway leading to the rupture of small alveoli

perfusion mismatch that can progress to respiratory failure. Meconium also induces chemical pneumonitis.

#### Clinical Features and Course

MAS usually occurs in term or post-term neonates that are often small for gestational age. Respiratory distress develops within a few hours and worsens in the next 24–48 hr. If untreated, the distress can progress to respiratory failure. The characteristic X-ray picture is shown in Fig. 9.56c. Complications include pneumothorax, other air leak syndromes (pneumopericardium, pneumomediastinum), and hypoxia leading to persistent pulmonary hypertension.

#### Management

Unnecessary disturbance to the neonate can cause worsening of PPHN. Such neonates need supportive care by providing thermal protection, IV fluids, and monitoring. Judicious use of oxygen, CPAP, and mechanical ventilation helps maintain oxygenation and ventilation. Some neonates may need inhaled nitric oxide to reduce pulmonary artery hypertension. With improved NICU care and ventilatory support, the mortality has reduced to 18–20% in severe MAS. The survivors have a high risk of developing asthma in childhood.

### Pneumonia

Pneumonia is a common cause of respiratory distress in term and preterm neonates. It is a form of sepsis with a pathogen profile such as *E. coli*, *S. aureus*, and *K. pneumoniae*. It can be due to aspiration or viral or fungal infection. Though common in the Western world, group B Streptococcus is a rare cause of sepsis/pneumonia in India.

The affected neonate has features of sepsis in addition to respiratory distress. Chest X-ray shows assymmetric patchy parenchymal opacities (Fig. 9.56d), and the sepsis screen and blood culture may be positive.

Treatment includes supportive care and specific antibiotic therapy for sepsis.

### Surgical Problems

Excessive frothing in a neonate may indicate the presence of a tracheoesophageal fistula (TEF). A plain X-ray confirms the diagnosis with a red rubber catheter inserted in the esophagus; the catheter stops at the 10th thoracic vertebrae in the presence of esophageal atresia. The presence of the gastric bubble suggests concomitant TEF. Avoid the use of infant feeding tube since it may be coiled up in the esophagus (Fig. 9.73).

A neonate with respiratory distress and a scaphoid abdomen may have a diaphragmatic hernia. The antenatal ultrasound can make the diagnosis. Chest X-ray shows the presence of bowel loops in the thoracic cavity.

### Pneumothorax

Pneumothorax can occur in neonates with meconium aspiration syndrome and those receiving positive pressure ventilation (Fig. 9.60). Transillumination of the chest can help in diagnosis. Needle aspiration or chest tube drainage is a life-saving procedure in this situation.

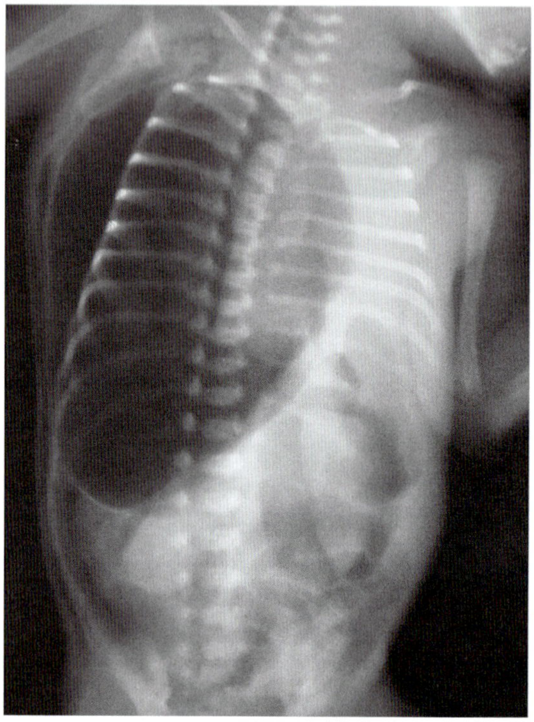

**Fig. 9.60:** Tension pneumothorax on the right side displacing the mediastinum and pushing down the diaphragm

### Apnea

Apnea denotes cessation of breathing for 20 seconds or shorter periods, if it is associated with cyanosis or bradycardia.

There are three types of apnea:

1. Central apnea resulting from the decreased central drive
2. Obstructive apnea resulting due to neck flexion or airway secretions
3. Mixed apnea, involving both mechanisms, is the most common.

Apnea of prematurity, the most common cause of apnea in preterm neonates, occurs between the second to fifth days of life. It is due to the immaturity of the respiratory center. Treatment is supportive, and the use of caffeine or aminophylline is advised. The prognosis is good.

Apnea within the first 24 hours or after seven days of birth is more likely to be secondary (Table 9.22). The treatment and prognosis depend on the underlying cause.

### Suggested Reading


1. Mishra S, Agarwal R, Jeevasankar M, et al. Apnea in the newborn. Indian J Pediatr. 2008;75:57–61.
2. Lemyre B, Davis PG, De Paoli AG. Nasal intermittent positive pressure ventilation (NIPPV) versus nasal continuous positive airway pressure (NCPAP) for apnea of prematurity. Cochrane Database of Systematic Reviews 2002.


## CYANOSIS IN NEWBORN

Central cyanosis in newborns always signifies an underlying pathological condition. Most of the time, cardiac and respiratory conditions lead to cyanosis. A stepwise clinical and radiological approach can facilitate early diagnosis and management (Fig. 9.61).

**Table 9.22:** Secondary causes of apnea

| *Conditions* | *Features* |
|---|---|
| Temperature instability | Hypothermia or hyperthermia (less frequently) |
| Hematological | Polycythemia; anemia |
| Neurological | Meningitis; intraventricular hemorrhage; perinatal asphyxia, maternal drugs like opiates |
| Metabolic | Hypoglycemia; hyponatremia; hypocalcemia |
| Respiratory | Any severe respiratory morbidity |
| Cardiac | Patent ductus arteriosus; shock; congestive cardiac failure |
| Gastrointestinal | Necrotizing enterocolitis; gastroesophageal reflux |
| Infections | Sepsis |

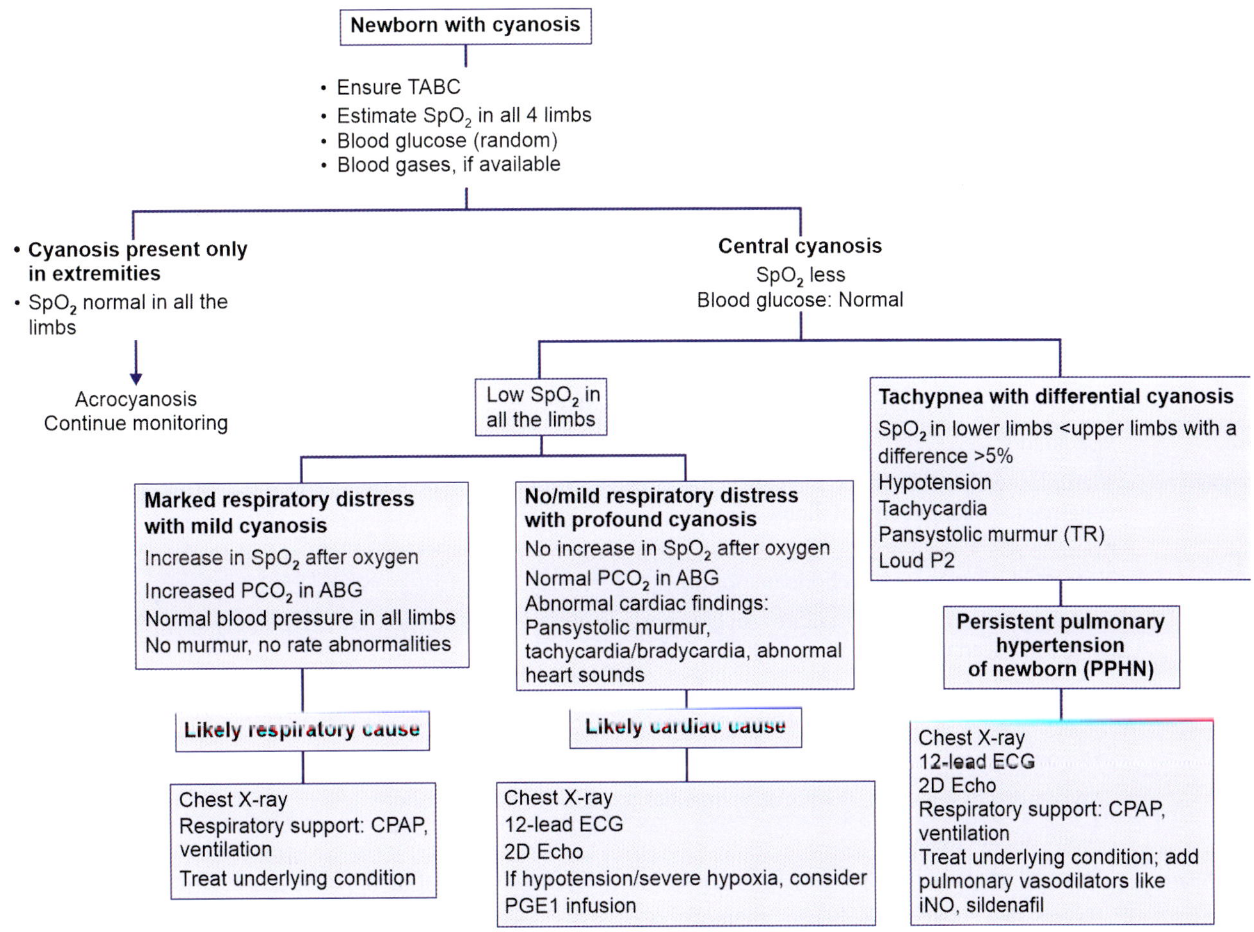


**Fig. 9.61:** Approach to a newborn with cyanosis (TABC temperature, airway breathing circulation; $SpO_2$ saturation pulse oximetry; RBS random blood sugar; ABG arterial blood gas $pCO_2$ partial pressure of carbon dioxide in mm Hg; CPAP continuous positive airway pressure; ECG electrocardiogram; PGE1 prostaglandin E1; PPHN persistent pulmonary hypertension of newborn; TR tricuspid regurgitation; iNO inhaled nitric oxide

## Suggested Reading


1. Gupta SK. Clinical approach to a neonate with cyanosis. Indian J Pediatr. 2015;82:1050–60.


*Competency:* **PE20.7**

## PERINATAL ASPHYXIA

Perinatal or birth asphyxia is an injury to the fetus or newborn occurring due to a lack of oxygen (hypoxia) or a lack of perfusion (ischemia) to various organs. It is often associated with tissue lactic acidosis and hypercarbia. Asphyxia accounts for an estimated 900,000 deaths each year globally and is one of the primary causes of early neonatal mortality. The most common cause of perinatal asphyxia is complications during childbirth.

There is no universally-accepted definition of perinatal asphyxia. The American Academy of Pediatrics has suggested essential criteria (Table 9.23) for defining perinatal asphyxia.

National Neonatology Forum of India (NNF) uses Apgar scores of 0–3 and 4–7 at 1 minute to define severe and moderate birth asphyxia, respectively. The risk factors for HIE are discussed in Table 9.24.

| Table 9.23: Essential criteria for perinatal asphyxia |
|---|
| Prolonged metabolic or mixed acidemia (pH <7.0) on an umbilical arterial blood sample |
| Persistence of Apgar score of 0–3 for >5 minutes |
| Neurological manifestations, e.g. seizures, coma, hypotonia or hypoxic ischemic encephalopathy (HIE) in the immediate neonatal period |
| Evidence of multiorgan dysfunction in the immediate neonatal period |

### Consequences of Asphyxia

PA is a multiorgan system disorder affecting virtually every organ system in the body, including the brain, heart, lungs, kidneys, and intestine (Table 9.25). The severity of organ system dysfunction determines an asphyxiated neonate's early and long-term outcomes.

Hypoxic ischemic encephalopathy (HIE) is the CNS dysfunction associated with asphyxia. It is often the prime concern while managing asphyxiated neonates because it is not only associated with a high risk of mortality but also carries a significant risk of long-term severe neuromotor sequelae among survivors.

### Neuropathology

These differ according to gestation and result in variable clinical sequelae (Table 9.26).

### Management

Hypoxia is an evolving process that starts at the onset of the insult, continues after resuscitation, and after that manifests as sequelae in childhood. The common differential diagnosis of encephalopathy masquerading as HIE is shown in Table 9.27.

A broad spectrum of clinical manifestations is seen depending on injury severity. The HIE manifestation in term neonates has been classified in different staging systems, including Sarnat, Sarnat, and Levene stages (Table 9.28). The HIE in preterm neonates also manifests as abnormalities of consciousness, tone, and seizures, but there is no distinct classification system.

HIE staging helps predict the evolution of the disease and long-term outcomes. Neonates with stage one have a uniformly good prognosis. Adverse neurological outcomes are present in 20% of neonates with stage 2 HIE. In stage 3 HIE, half of the neonates die, and the remaining half have poor neurodevelopment outcomes.

Table 9.24: Risk factors leading to hypoxic ischemic encephalopathy (HIE)

| *Phase* | *Risk factors* |
|---|---|
| Antenatal | Uteroplacental insufficiency manifesting as pregnancy-induced hypertension and intrauterine growth retardation; maternal medical or surgical illness |
| Natal | Abruptio placentae; cord prolapse; maternal hypotension due to acute blood loss, spinal anesthesia, use of oxytocin; obstructed labor; maternal chorioamnionitis |
| Postnatal | Severe hypoxic respiratory failure; severe sepsis leading to hypotension and respiratory failure; critical cyanotic congenital heart disease |

Table 9.25: Organ system dysfunction in perinatal asphyxia

| | |
|---|---|
| CNS | Hypoxic ischemic encephalopathy, intracranial hemorrhage, seizures, long-term neurological sequelae |
| Cardiac | Myocardial dysfunction, rhythm abnormalities, congestive cardiac failure |
| Renal | Acute tubular necrosis |
| Pulmonary | Delayed adaptation, respiratory failure, meconium aspiration, primary pulmonary hypertension |
| GI tract | Necrotizing enterocolitis, hepatic dysfunction |
| Hematological | Thrombocytopenia, coagulation abnormalities |
| Metabolic | Acidosis, hypoglycemia, hypocalcemia, hyponatremia |

Table 9.26: The hypoxic-ischemic insult and its neuropathological lesions and long-term consequences in term and preterm

| *Gestation predilection* | *Pattern of injury* | *Consequences* |
|---|---|---|
| Term neonates | Selective neuronal necrosis involving the cerebral cortex and deeper nuclei | Dystonic cerebral palsy<br>Seizures<br>Cognitive delay |
| | Parasagittal cerebral (watershed) injury | Spastic quadriplegic cerebral palsy<br>Delayed cognition |
| | Focal and multifocal ischemic necrosis (stroke) | Hemiplegia<br>Seizures<br>Delayed cognition |
| Preterm neonates | Periventricular leukomalacia (PVL) | Spastic diplegia<br>Cognition relatively preserved |

**Table 9.27:** Conditions causing encephalopathy other than HIE

| |
|---|
| Infections: Sepsis, meningoencephalitis |
| Metabolic: Hypoglycemia, inborn errors of metabolism |
| Neonatal onset epileptic encephalopathy |
| Brain malformations like holoprosencephaly |
| Maternal drug exposure like opiates |

## Post-Resuscitation Management of an Asphyxiated Neonate (Fig. 9.62)

***Temperature:*** Maintain the normal temperature of the neonate and avoid hyperthermia. In a resourceful setting, moderate induced hypothermia (core temperature of 33° to 34°C) reduces the death or severe neurodevelopmental handicap. A multicenter trial from 3 countries (India, Bangladesh, and Sri Lanka) showed that therapeutic hypothermia (TH) had no beneficial effect on neonatal mortality and disability at 18–24 months. Moreover, they also noticed an increased risk of death at discharge in neonates receiving TH. The results of this trial have raised doubts about the efficacy and safety of this novel treatment modality in our country, which is the standard of care in high-income countries. Following this, the National Neonatology Forum (NNF) India has given a position statement on the use of TH for treating HIE in India and recommended TH only in a tertiary care setting with a trained team for a select group of neonates with a precise diagnosis of asphyxia.

***Oxygen:*** Both hypoxia and hyperoxia can damage neurons. Oxygen saturations are maintained between 90 and 95%. $CO_2$ concentration in ventilated neonates should be maintained between 40 and 50 mm Hg as hypocarbia and hypercarbia are detrimental to the brain.

***Perfusion:*** Cerebral perfusion in asphyxiated neonates is in a 'pressure passive' state, which means there is loss of autoregulation, and blood supply to the brain is entirely dependent on BPs; it decreases when BP falls and increases when BP rises. Therefore, to maintain normal perfusion pressure, a systemic mean arterial pressure of 45–50 mm Hg (term), 35–40 (1–2 kg weight), and 30–35 mm Hg (<1 kg weight) is required. Judicious use of fluid boluses and use of vasopressors help maintain BP. Hyperviscosity due to polycythemia should be corrected by the partial exchange.

***Glucose:*** Levels between 75 and 100 mg/dL are recommended. Hyperglycemia enhances cerebral edema and compromises perfusion, while hypoglycemia potentiates excitotoxic damage. Hypoglycemia is commonly seen in asphyxiated infants and must be regularly monitored.

***Metabolic profile:*** Hypocalcemia and electrolyte disturbances should be regularly looked for until stabilization of neonate and corrected as indicated.

***Seizures:*** 20–50% of infants with HIE develop seizures during day 1 or 2. Seizures are commonly subtle or focal, or multifocal. Metabolic disturbances such as hypoglycemia, hypocalcemia, and hyponatremia must be ruled out. Seizures should be treated with anti-epileptic drugs (AEDs)



**Table 9.28:** Levene classification for hypoxic-ischemic encephalopathy

| *Feature* | *Mild* | *Moderate* | *Severe* |
|---|---|---|---|
| Consciousness | Irritability | Lethargy | Comatose |
| Tone | Hypotonia | Marked hypotonia | Severe hypotonia |
| Seizures | No | Yes | Prolonged |
| Sucking/respiration | Poor suck | Unable to suck | Unable to sustain spontaneous respiration |

*Modified from:* Levene MI. The asphyxiated newborn infant. In: Levene MI, Lilford RJ, eds. Fetal and Neonatal Neurology and Neurosurgery. Churchill Livingstone, Edinburgh 1995;405–26.

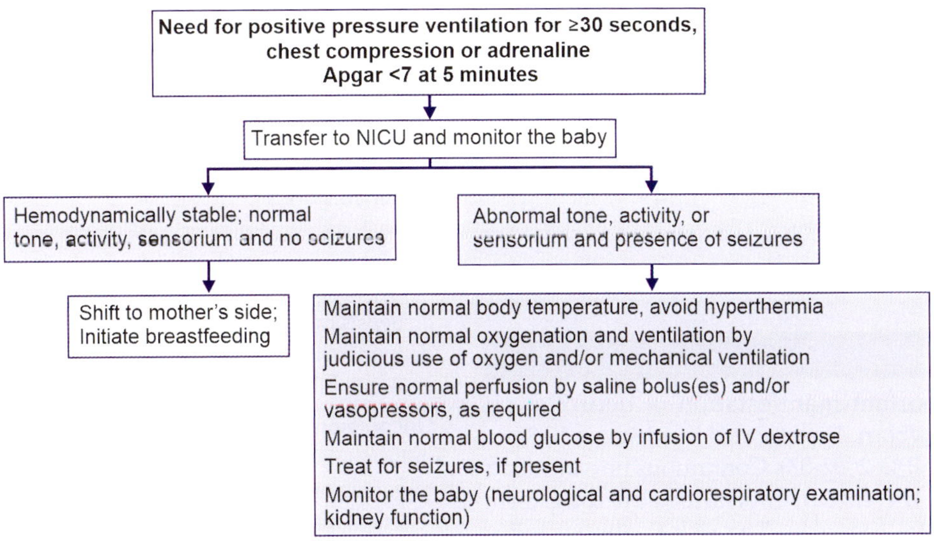


**Fig. 9.62:** Post-resuscitation management of an asphyxiated baby

**Table 9.29:** Types of clinical neonatal seizures and their presentation

| *Clinical type* | *Presentation* | *Prognosis* |
|---|---|---|
| Subtle seizures | Most common type (50%). Includes tonic deviation of eyes, repetitive lip or tongue movements, repetitive cycling-pedaling or boxing, and apnea | Subtle seizures secondary to HIE have a poor prognosis |
| Clonic seizures | Repetitive rhythmic movements/jerks of muscles with both fast and slow components (1–3/second). | Depends upon the etiology. |
| Tonic seizures | Sustained extension or flexion of appendicular or axial muscle groups often resembling decorticate or decerebrate posturing, respectively | Poor; often secondary to severe intraventricular hemorrhage of preterm infants |
| Myoclonic seizures | Lightning-fast jerks (multiple or single) of the lower or upper extremity with an absence of slow component | Worst prognosis |



such as phenobarbitone and phenytoin. The seizures may be intractable initially but usually tend to burn out by 48 hr. Subtle seizures lasting for a brief duration need not be treated.

Once the neonate is seizure free for 3–4 days, AEDs are stopped in the same order as they were started, except for phenobarbitone. Phenobarbitone is stopped at discharge, if the neurological examination is normal and the neonate feeds well on the breast. If the neurological examination is abnormal, phenobarbitone is continued until one month. If the neonate is normal neurologically at one month, phenobarbitone is stopped. If the neurological function is abnormal, continue phenobarbitone. The infant is assessed again at three months: If normal neurologically, phenobarbitone is stopped; if the neurological examination is abnormal, EEG is performed. Phenobarbitone can be stopped, if EEG does not show any seizure activity.

### Prognosis

The following features predict a poor outcome:

- Lack of spontaneous respiratory effort within 20–30 minutes of birth is associated with almost uniform mortality
- HIE stage 3
- Abnormal neurological findings persisting beyond the first 7–10 days of life

Thus, all these neonates should have regular follow-up and monitoring of neurodevelopmental milestones to detect any deficits early and intervene effectively.

### Suggested Reading

1. Agarwal R, Jain A, Deorari AK, Paul VK.Post-resuscitation management asphyxiated neonates. Indian J Pediatr 2008;75: 175–80.
2. Clinical Protocols in Neonatatology. www.newbornwhocc.org

*Competency:* **PE20.15**

## NEONATAL SEIZURES

Seizure is an important manifestation of neurological dysfunction in a newborn. The reported incidence is 10.3 per 1000 live births (NNPD-2002-03). Continuous uncontrolled seizures increase the risk of mortality and long-term neurodevelopmental sequelae. The risk is almost twice in preterm-low birth weight neonates. Neonatal seizures, unlike in older children and adults, have a distinct clinical presentation, etiopathogenesis, and management approach.

### Types and Definition

Three types of seizures are recognized:

1. *Electro-clinical seizures:* An abrupt change in neurological function (motor, autonomic, or behavior) in a neonate associated with corresponding EEG changes.
2. *Clinical-only seizures:* An abrupt change in neurological function (motor, autonomic behavior) in a neonate associated without corresponding EEG changes.
3. *Electric seizures:* Recognized seizure activity only on EEG without any clinical attribute.

### Classification

Neonatal seizures are classically differentiated into four major types, as shown in Table 9.29.

### Etiology

The common underlying causes of neonatal seizures are HIE (40–50% cases), and ischemic stroke in term neonates and, intraventricular bleeding in preterm neonates (Table 9.30).

**Table 9.30:** Etiology of neonatal seizures

**Common causes**

a. Hypoxic ischemic encephalopathy
b. Metabolic disorders like hypocalcemia, hypoglycemia, hyponatremia, hypomagnesemia
c. Sepsis/meningitis
d. Intracranial bleed
e. Acute bilirubin encephalopathy

**Uncommon causes**

- Inborn error of metabolism (galactosemia, urea cycle defects, organic acidemias)
- Cortical malformations (lissencephaly, cortical dysplasia)
- Epileptic syndromes

### Seizure Mimics

Seizure mimics may be challenging to differentiate from seizures unless carefully examined. Their recognition helps avoid unnecessary investigations and treatment.

The common seizure mimics include:

a. *Jitteriness:* It is sudden onset and characterized by rapid tremors or shaking activity. The common causes are mild

HIE, hypocalcemia, hypoglycemia, and drug withdrawal. A hungry neonate can have jitteriness that subsides after feeding.

The following features differentiate jitteriness from seizures are:

1. Absence of eye deviation or fixed gaze, heart rate changes.
2. Rhythmic tremors with equal to and fro movements. The frequency is 7 to 10 per second—no fast and slow components. In contrast, a clonic seizure is slower (1–2 per second), and the to and fro movements have rapid and slow components.
3. The tremors are usually stimulus sensitive, precipitated by hunger, crying, or loud noise, and stopped by gentle restraint.

b. ***Benign neonatal sleep myoclonus:*** It typically presents in quiet sleep and continues for several minutes. Benign neonatal sleep myoclonus is different from actual seizures as it is present only in sleep and disappears on waking the neonate. The neonate is normal otherwise. This condition does not require any treatment and subsides in 2 to 3 months. The neurodevelopmental outcome is normal.

## Investigations

The following investigations are required in all neonates with seizures:

- Random blood sugar
- Serum electrolytes (sodium and calcium)
- Serum bilirubin level, if the infant has significant jaundice
- Cerebrospinal fluid examination. This can be omitted if seizures occur in a typical setting of severe perinatal asphyxia.
- Cranial ultrasound in preterm neonates
- Electroencephalography (EEG)
- Neuroimaging (MRI brain)

## Management

A neonatal seizure is a medical emergency. The first step is correctly identifying and characterizing the seizure and then ensuring normal temperature, open airway, breathing, and circulation. After ruling out hypoglycemia, the initial medication for neonatal seizures is phenobarbitone. The algorithm for the management is shown in Fig. 9.63.

### *Long-term Anticonvulsant Therapy (ACT)*

Most of the drugs used in the ACT have the potential to damage long-term brain development, especially in the first two years of age. Therefore, World Health Organization guidelines suggest discontinuing ACT as soon as possible. We discontinue maintenance phenobarbitone therapy, if the neonate is breastfeeding well and the neurological examination is normal at discharge.

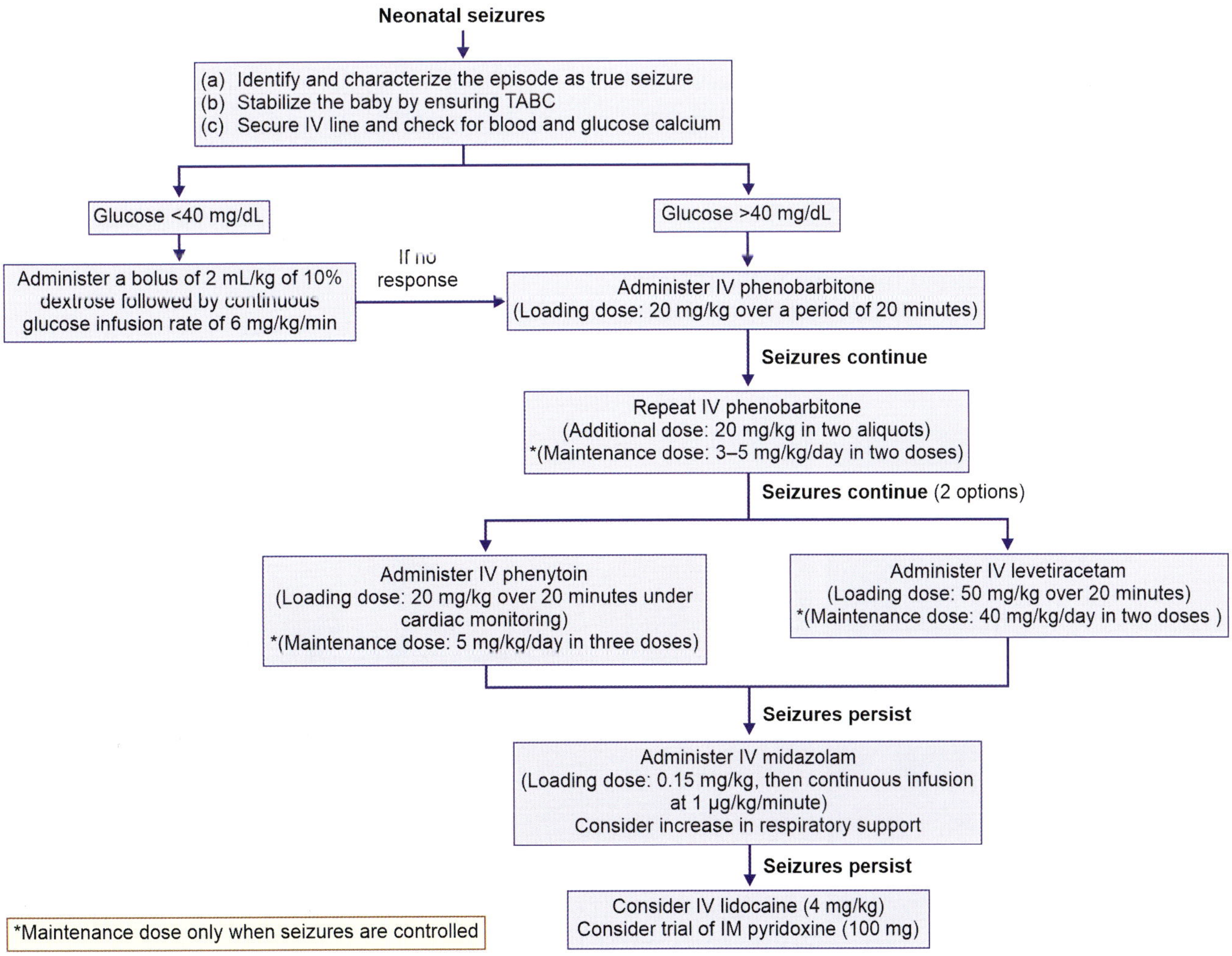


**Fig. 9.63:** Management of neonatal seizures. TABC temperature, airway, breathing, ciculation; IV intravenous

## Suggested Reading

1. Neonatal seizures. In: Volpe JJ, Inder TE (eds). Volpe's Neurology of the Newborn, 6th edition, Elsevier, 2018;275–321.
2. WHO. Guidelines on neonatal seizures. Geneva: World Health Organization, 2012.

*Competencies:* **PE20.16; PE20.17**

# INFECTIONS IN NEONATES

Various pathogens can infect neonates, including bacteria, viruses, and protozoa. Infections can be superficial or systemic.

## Superficial Infections

***Omphalitis:*** Omphalitis indicates redness or induration around the umbilicus or pus draining from it. Omphalitis starts as a local infection, usually from unclean handling or the application of unclean substances to the cord. It can spread to cause life-threatening systemic sepsis.

- *Local infection.* When the redness extends to less than one cm of the surrounding skin, there is no sign of sepsis. Local cleaning with an antiseptic solution, followed by application of 0.5% gentian violet four times a day till redness subsides, would suffice.
- *Severe infection.* When the area of redness extends beyond one cm of surrounding tissue, or there are signs of sepsis. It needs local treatment, as above, plus systemic antibiotics.

***Oral thrush:*** White patchy oral mucosa and tongue lesions can occur in healthy newborns. Actual oral thrush lesions are difficult to remove and leave hemorrhagic points when removed. Local nystatin or clotrimazole application is recommended four times a day after the feed.

***Conjunctivitis:*** It is from the common condition of sticky eyes. Sticky eyes have mucoid discharge without signs of inflammation and require cleaning with warm water. Conjunctivitis has a purulent discharge, and the eye has signs of inflammation (**Fig. 9.64a and b**). Treatment involves the instillation of antibiotics. Severe inflammation (pus or lid inflammation) may occur due to a gonococcal infection that can result in blindness and requires systemic antibiotics therapy.

***Pustules:*** Cutaneous infections (bacterial origin) in neonates usually present with pustules (**Fig. 9.64c**) or sometimes as bullous impetigo or peri-follicular lesions like folliculitis. *Staphylococcus aureus* and β-hemolytic streptococci are the most implicated bacteria. Treatment consists of local application of mupirocin and fusidic acid. If the number of pustules is extensive (more than 10), then a course of oral antibiotics can be given.

## Systemic Infections (Neonatal Sepsis)

When a pathogenic organism gains access to the bloodstream, it can result in neonatal sepsis, which may be generalized or localized to the lungs (pneumonia), the meninges (meningitis), or the bones and joints (osteomyelitis/arthritis). Neonatal sepsis encompasses generalized sepsis, pneumonia, meningitis, and bone-joint infections.

Neonatal sepsis is commoner in infants with lower birth weight and gestational age. It is ten times more common in infants with a weight less than 1,500 g than infants with a birth weight greater than or equal to 1,500 g. In developing countries, sepsis rates range from 20 to 41%.

Infections in neonates kill nearly 9% of under-5 children around the world, with around 69% (0.4 million) of them occurring in India alone; ~42% of these die within the first week of life. Recent estimates suggest around 50,000 neonatal deaths in India are attributable to resistance to first-line antibiotics and this figure is expected to rise by tenfold by 2050. Almost 40% of septic infants have long-term sequelae such as cognitive/learning difficulties or developmental delay, cerebral palsy, and visual and hearing impairment.

### *Early Versus Late Sepsis*

Early-onset sepsis (EOS) (up to 72 hr after birth) infections are caused by organisms prevalent in the maternal genital

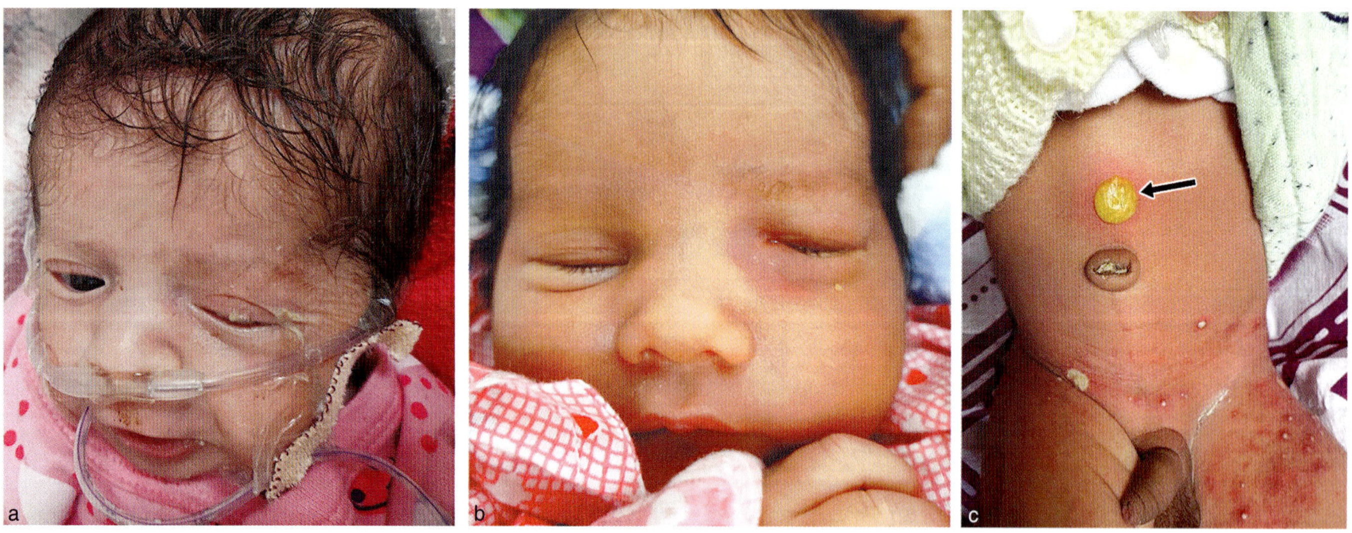

**Fig. 9.64:** (a) Conjunctivitis (left eye) with purulent discharge; (b) Conjunctivitis (right eye) with lid inflammation; (c) Multiple pustules with impetigo (arrow). (*Courtesy:* Dr Nikhil Arora, Faridkot)

**Table 9.31:** Key differences between early and late-onset sepsis

| *Parameter* | *Early-onset sepsis* | *Late-onset sepsis* |
|---|---|---|
| Timing | Up to 72 hours | After 72 hours |
| Risk factors | Perinatal risk factors like the spontaneous onset of preterm labor, prolonged rupture of membranes (>18 hours), foul-smelling liquor, multiple per vaginal examinations, maternal fever, and difficult or prolonged labor | Poor hand hygiene compliance, LBW, lack of breastfeeding, poor cord care, superficial infections (pyoderma, umbilical sepsis), aspiration of feeds, disruption of skin integrity with needle pricks, and use of intravenous fluids. |
| Presentation | Pneumonia and less commonly as septicemia and meningitis | Generalized sepsis, pneumonia, or meningitis |
| Organisms | In developed nations, the causative pathogens include those colonizing the maternal genital tract, such as group B streptococci, *E. coli*, and listeria.<br>In developing countries, there is not much difference in EOS pathogens resembling those of LOS. | *Klebsiella pneumoniae*, *Acinetobacter* spp, and *Staphylococcus aureus* are the predominant pathogens. Other organisms include coagulase-negative staphylococci, *Enterobacter*, *Pseudomonas*, and *E. coli*. |
| Case fatality rate | High | Relatively lower |



tract or the delivery area. EOS occurs in the presence of perinatal risk factors such as the spontaneous onset of preterm labor, prolonged rupture of membranes, foul-smelling liquor, and prolonged labor. EOS frequently manifests as pneumonia. The neonates with early onset sepsis born may be initially asymptomatic and suspected based on maternal risk factors.

Late-onset sepsis (LOS; onset after 72 hr of age) infections are caused by the organisms thriving in the external environment of the home or the hospital. The infection is often transmitted through the hands of the care providers. The presentation is that of generalized sepsis, pneumonia, or meningitis. The predisposing factors include LBW, lack of breastfeeding, poor cord care, superficial infections (pyoderma, umbilical sepsis), aspiration of feeds, disruption of skin integrity with needle pricks, and use of intravenous fluids.

The clinical manifestations of sepsis include tachypnea and chest retractions, hypoxemia, feeding difficulty, temperature instability (low or high body temperature), lethargy or drowsiness, abdominal distension, shock, and apnea. Table 9.31 highlights key differences between early and late-onset sepsis.

### Clinical Features

Neonatal sepsis often manifests with vague and ill-defined symptoms and, therefore, requires a high index of suspicion for early diagnosis. An early but non-specific manifestation is the alteration in the established feeding behavior. The neonate, who had been active and sucking normally, refuses to suck and becomes lethargic or unresponsive—poor cry, hypothermia, abdominal distension, vomiting, apneic spells, and other common manifestations. Diarrhea is uncommon. Fast breathing, chest retractions, and grunt indicate pneumonia. Most cases of meningitis do not have any distinct clinical picture per se, making it mandatory to suspect meningitis in all patients suspected of sepsis. Shock, bleeding, sclerema, and renal failure are indicators of overwhelming sepsis.

Diagnosis of sepsis is fraught with poor specificity. A host of conditions like hypothermia, hypoglycemia, hypoxia, late metabolic acidosis, congestive heart failure, and even simple conditions like nasal block may mimic sepsis. A careful clinical examination and relevant investigations are necessary to differentiate these conditions from NNS and avoid unnecessary antibiotic therapy. Clinically stable neonates can be observed, without admission and intravenous antibodies, while providing good supportive care (Fig. 9.65).

### Investigations

No investigation is required to start treatment in a sick neonate with a high probability of sepsis (Fig. 9.65). Blood culture provides a definitive diagnosis of NNS and should be taken before starting antimicrobial therapy. After cleaning the skin (with alcohol, povidone-iodine, and again alcohol), a specimen of 0.5 to 1.0 mL of blood can be taken in a small culture media bottle containing 5 to 10 mL of the liquid broth.

A panel of tests (sepsis screen) consisting of total leukocyte count (TLC), absolute neutrophil count (ANC), immature to the total neutrophil ratio (I/T ratio), CRP, and micro-ESR constitutes a useful sepsis screen for clinically doubtful cases. The sepsis screen is considered positive, if two of these parameters are positive. The cut-off of the parameters mentioned above is shown in Table 9.32.

Lumbar puncture should be performed in all cases suspected of neonatal sepsis except in asymptomatic neonates being investigated for maternal risk factors. Table 9.33 provides gestation-specific cut-offs for values of various parameters in cerebrospinal fluid.

**Table 9.32:** Sepsis screen parameters

| *Parameter* | *Cut-off* |
|---|---|
| Total leukocyte count | $<5000/mm^3$ |
| Absolute neutrophil count | $<1800/mm^3$ |
| Immature/total neutrophil (I/T) ratio | >20% |
| C-reactive protein | >1 mg/dL or 10 mg/L |
| Micro-ESR | ≥15 mm in the first hour |

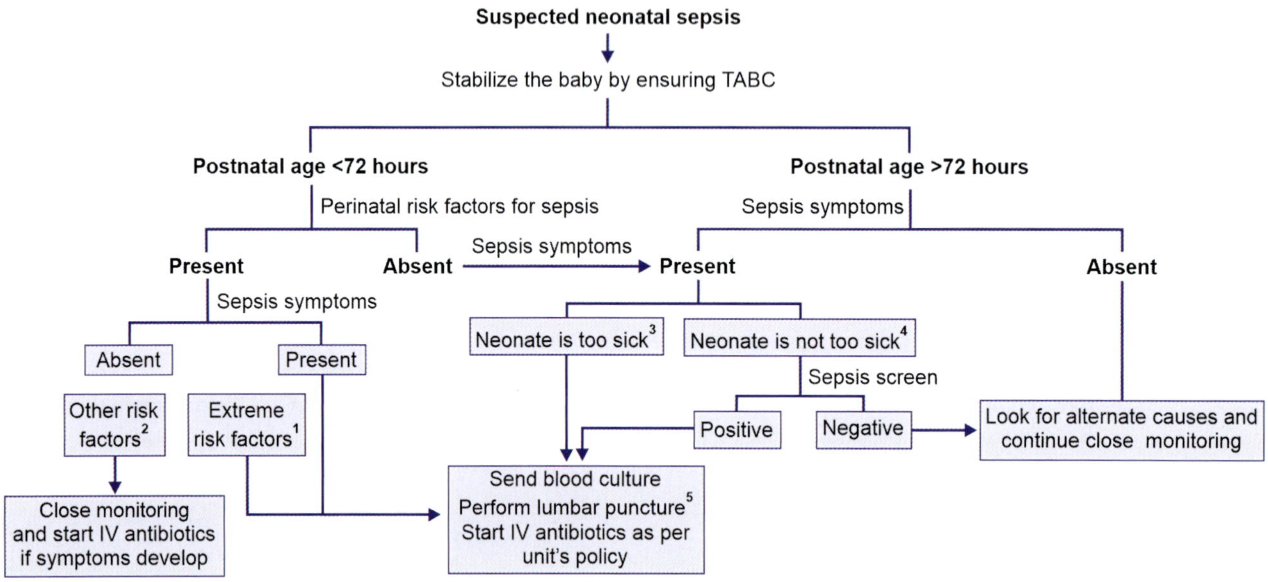


[1] Extreme risk factors: Chorioamnionitis, foul smelling liqor, or rupture of membrane >72 h
[2] Other risk factors: Spontaneous preterm labor, rupture of membranes (24 to 71 hr), or unclean PV examination
[3] Too sick: Presence of shock, bleeding tendency, respiratory failure requiring ventilation, seizures in absence of asphyxia, severe hypothermia, cellulitis, etc.
[4] Not too sick: Single episode of apnea, occasional vomiting, transient temperature instability, some reduced activity, mild tachypnea
[5] Perform LP: Before starting antibiotics in symptomatic neonates or If culture comes positive in asymptomatic neonates

**Fig. 9.65:** Approach to neonate suspected of sepsis. TABC temperature, airway, breathing, circulation; IV intravenous

**Table 9.33:** Normal CSF examination in neonates, mean (range)

| *Test* | *Term* | *Preterm* |
|---|---|---|
| Cells | | |
| Leukocytes | 7 (0–32) | 9 (0–29) |
| Polymorphonuclear cells | 61% | 57% |
| Protein (mg/dL) | 90 (20–170) | 115 (65–150) |
| Glucose (mg/dL) | 52 (34–119) | 50 (24–63) |

### New Screening and Diagnostic Tests

***Procalcitonin (PCT):*** It is a precursor of calcitonin, produced by C cells of the thyroid gland, and is an acute phase reactant. Serum PCT is not helpful in the diagnosis of neonatal sepsis. Recently, molecular diagnostic tests based on the amplification of bacterial DNA (e.g. polymerase chain reaction) have been used as an 'add-on' test for improving accuracy.

### Treatment

Institution of prompt treatment is essential in neonates with sepsis who often reach the healthcare facilities late and in critical condition. Supportive care and antibiotics are the two *equally important* components of treatment. Antibiotics take at least 12 to 24 hr to show any effect; optimum supportive care improves the outcomes in sick septic neonates.

***Supportive care:*** Good supportive care requires meticulous attention to various aspects:

- Provide warmth; ensure normal temperature (36.5–37.5°C).
- Start oxygen by hood or mask, if the neonate is cyanosed or grunting. Provide bag and mask ventilation, if breathing is inadequate. Instilling normal saline drops in the nostrils may help clear the nasal block.
- Assess peripheral perfusion by palpating peripheral pulses, capillary refill time (normally <2–3 seconds), and skin color. Serial measurement of urine output is helpful for this purpose. Infuse normal saline or Ringer lactate 10 mL/kg over 5–10 minutes, if perfusion is poor. Repeat the same 1–2 times over the next 30–45 minutes, if perfusion continues to be poor. Dopamine and dobutamine may be required to maintain normal perfusion.
- Insert intravenous line. If hypoglycemia is suspected, infuse glucose (10%) 2 mL/kg stat. Do not use glucose boluses routinely. Provide maintenance fluid, electrolytes, and glucose (4–6 mg/kg/min). Add potassium to IV fluids once the normal flow of urine is documented.
- Ensuring optimal nutrition is extremely helpful in sick neonates. Enteral feeds should be initiated early, if there is no abdominal distension and the neonate is hemodynamically stable. Feed mother's milk.

***Specific care:*** *Antimicrobial therapy* constitutes the mainstay of treatment of sepsis. In a seriously sick neonate suspected of sepsis, appropriate antibiotic therapy should be initiated without delay after obtaining blood samples for culture.

***Empiric therapy when the etiologic agent is not known:*** The empiric treatment of NNS should cover the significant causative pathogens while awaiting reports of culture studies.

Since the antimicrobial spectrum and susceptibility profile is different in different settings, there cannot be a universal policy of empiric regimen. Antibiotics are often used in neonates on the slightest suspicion of sepsis because of its grave and fulminant nature. However, rampant overuse of antibiotics is associated with the risk of developing resistant strains of pathogens. Most newborn units in the country are facing the problem of overwhelming antimicrobial resistance to practically all antibiotics. Rational use of antibiotics is the responsibility of every physician.

Each treating unit should adopt a suitable policy. Based on changes in the spectrum of etiologic agents and the antibiotics sensitivity pattern, the choice of antibiotics must be periodically reviewed and modified. Table 9.34 provides a possible regimen of empiric antibiotics.

***Therapy after an etiologic agent is known:*** Antimicrobial treatment can be specific once a positive culture and sensitivity report are available (2–3 days). BACTEC automated blood culture system utilizing fluorescence principle ($CO_2$ released by microorganisms) is increasingly being used in many centers for early detection of sepsis-causing microorganisms. Even in the best institutions, only approximately one-fourth of neonates suspected of sepsis have positive blood cultures.

***Mode of administration and dosage:*** Antibiotics should preferably be administered parenterally. In a neonate with septicemia or pneumonia (but not meningitis), who has received intravenous ampicillin and gentamicin initially and is clinically well after three days, the physician may consider an individual basis switching over to oral amoxicillin along with single-dose intramuscular gentamicin therapy for the rest of the course.

### Monitoring

Intensive care and monitoring are the key determinants of improved survival of neonates. The elements of monitoring in sepsis are not different from those in other life-threatening conditions. Proper monitoring of sick neonates enables care providers detection of complications at the earliest. The periodicity of documenting the various parameters should be individualized.

**Table 9.34:** Choice of initial antibiotic therapy

- Low resistance to common antibiotics
  - Ampicillin/cloxacillin + gentamicin/amikacin
  - Meningitis: Ampicillin + cefotaxime
- High resistance
  - Ciprofloxacin/piperacillin-tazobactam + amikacin

### Antibiotics Stewardship Program (ASP)

ASP aims to optimize antibiotics use and ensures each patient gets the "**R**ight antibiotic at the **R**ight time and dose for the **R**ight duration through the **R**ight route".

### Prevention of Sepsis

- Six cleans at the time of delivery: Clean hands, clean delivery surface, clean perineum, clean and dry cord care, clean cutting instruments, clean towels
- Exclusive breastfeeding or mother's own milk feeding
- Hand hygiene among healthcare staff **(Fig. 9.66)**
- Avoid unnecessary invasive interventions like IV fluids, IV cannula, and unnecessary medicines
- Kangaroo mother care for stable low birth weight neonates

## Suggested Reading


1. Antimicrobial Stewardship Program in health care facilities in low and middle-income countries. A WHO Practical Toolkit. 2019.
2. Investigators of the Delhi Neonatal Infection Study (DeNIS) collaboration. Characterization and antimicrobial resistance of sepsis pathogens in neonates born in tertiary care centers in Delhi, India: A Cohort study. Lancet Glob Health 2016 Oct;4(10):e752–60.
3. Jefferies AL, Candian Pediatric Society. Management of term infants at increased risk of bacterial sepsis. Pediatr Child Health 2017;22:223–28.
4. Puopolo KM, Benitz WE, Zaoutis TE, et al. Management of neonates with suspected or proven bacterial sepsis. Pediatrics 2018;142(6):e20182894.


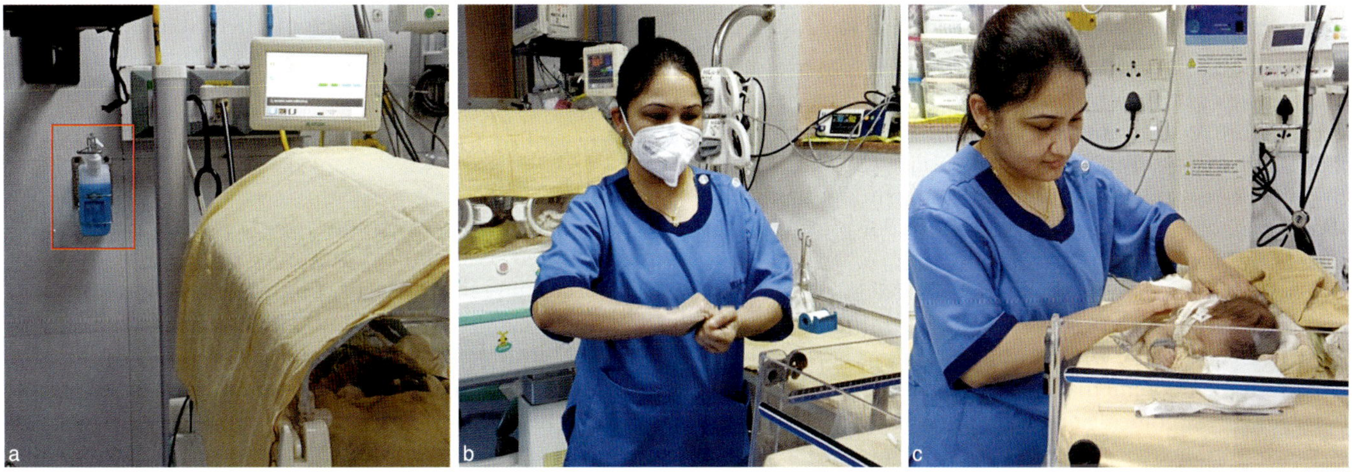

Fig. 9.66: Hand hygiene (HH) before and after touching the baby and her surroundings is the most critical factor in preventing healthcare-associated infections (HAI). Note: (a) The provision of an HH dispenser at the bedside (red box); (b) The physician doing proper HH using isopropyl alcohol; (c) Examining the baby after adequate HH. The provider wears half-sleeve scrub and keeps short nails; hands do not have any jewelry or cell phone

## NECROTIZING ENTEROCOLITIS

Necrotizing enterocolitis (NEC) often occurs in preterm infants born before 32 weeks of gestation. It mimics neonatal sepsis because of abdominal distension, apnea, bradycardia, temperature instability, cyanosis, and lethargy.

### Staging (Modified Bell's Staging)

*Stage I:* Mild abdominal distension and pre-feed residuals, apnea, temperature instability, and occult or frank blood in stools

*Stage II:* Gross abdominal distension and tenderness. X-ray shows the presence of gas in intestinal walls (pneumatosis intestinalis)

*Stage III:* Signs mentioned above, along with shock and ascites. X-ray shows features of ascites and pneumoperitoneum.

### Management

Oral feeding should be withheld. A nasogastric tube is inserted to relieve distension and to aspirate stomach contents. Fluids and electrolytes in adequate quantities should be administered. Parenteral nutrition may be administered. The neonate is given antibiotics after taking suitable cultures. Shock is managed by the replacement of fluids and the use of vasopressor agents. Plasma and platelet transfusion may be necessary to prevent bleeding tendencies.

*Competency:* **PE20.19**

## JAUNDICE

Nearly 60% of term newborns and preterm neonates become visibly jaundiced in the first week of life. High bilirubin levels may harm the developing central nervous system and cause neurological impairment even in term newborns. In most cases, jaundice is a self-limiting condition and does not require any treatment. Approximately 5–10% of neonates have significant jaundice that requires phototherapy or exchange transfusion.

### Physiological Versus Pathological Jaundice

Physiological jaundice results from the physiological immaturity of the neonates to handle increased bilirubin production. Visible jaundice usually appears between 24 and 72 hr of age. Total serum bilirubin (TSB) level peaks by three days of age and then falls in term neonates. TSB levels are below the designated cut-offs for phototherapy. It does not require any treatment.

There is no clear-cut distinction between pathological and physiological jaundice. Pathological jaundice refers to elevated TSB levels, wherein the treatment is more likely to benefit the neonate than cause harm. The differentiation between physiological and pathological jaundice is difficult in preterm neonates.

The presence of any of the following criteria generally indicates pathological jaundice in term neonates:

- Clinical jaundice detected before 24 hours of age
- TSB rises more than 5 mg/dL/day
- TSB more than 15 mg/dL
- Significant jaundice persisting beyond 3 or 4 weeks of life
- Clay/white colored stool or dark urine
- Direct bilirubin >1 mg/dL at any time

Breastfed infants have a different pattern of physiological jaundice than formula-fed neonates. Jaundice in breastfed neonates appears between 24 and 48 hours of age, peaks by 3 to 4 days, and disappears by the 10 to 14 days of life. In one-third of breastfed neonates, mild jaundice may persist in the third or fourth week. The formula-fed neonates have a lower peak of TSB, and jaundice disappears earlier.

### Breastfeeding Jaundice (BFJ)

Many neonates have higher TSB values due to inadequate breastfeeding. Such neonates have excess weight loss, and jaundice appears in the later part of the first week and can persist into the third and fourth week of life. This excess jaundice results from inadequate breast milk intake that promotes enterohepatic circulation. The BFJ is, therefore, more aptly termed "suboptimal intake hyperbilirubinemia." Maternal conditions, such as improper breastfeeding technique, breast engorgement, cracked or sore nipples, illness or fatigue, and neonatal factors, such as late preterm gestation (34 to 36 weeks), and ineffective sucking, can cause ineffective breastfeeding and, consequently, BFJ. Ensuring optimum breastfeeding would help decrease this kind of jaundice.

### Breast Milk Jaundice (BMJ)

Approximately 2–4% of exclusively-breastfed term neonates have TSB over 10 mg/dL beyond the third-fourth week of life. Breast milk jaundice (BMJ) is possible in neonates if the jaundice is unconjugated type (not staining nappies); and other causes for prolongation hyperbilirubinemia such as inadequate feeding, continuing hemolysis, extravasated blood, G6PD deficiency, and hypothyroidism have been ruled out.

Breast milk contains high concentrations of beta-glucuronidase, which deconjugates bilirubin excreted in the intestine after conjugation by the liver. Most such neonates would not have a dangerous level of TSB and do not require any treatment. The mothers would be able to continue breastfeeding their neonates. There is no need to stop breastfeeding for diagnosis or treatment of BMJ.

### Assessment of Jaundice

#### *Visual Assessment*

Originally described by Kramer, dermal staining of bilirubin may be used as a clinical guide to the level of jaundice. Dermal staining in newborns progresses in a cephalocaudal direction. Every newborn should be examined for jaundice every 12 hours **(Fig. 9.67)**.

Examine the neonate in natural light or bright white fluorescent light. Make sure there is no yellow or off-white background. You may have to move the neonate to a brightly lit area. Note the extent of jaundice. Blanch the skin of the forehead, chest, abdomen, thighs, legs, palms, and soles with digital pressure. Note the underlying color of skin and subcutaneous tissue. Look for the degree of

Visual assessment of jaundice (Modified Kramer Rule)

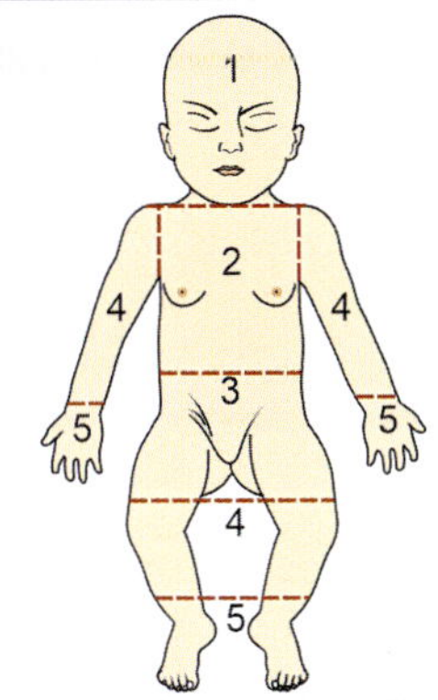

| Kramer zones | Approximate TSB level |
|---|---|
| 1. Face and neck | 5–7 mg/dL |
| 2. Chest and upper abdomen | 7–9 mg/dL |
| 3. Lower abdomen and thighs | 9–11 mg/dL |
| 4. Legs and arms/forearms | 11–13 mg/dL |
| 5. Palms and soles | 13–15 mg/dL |

**Fig. 9.67:** Dermal zones for estimation of total serum bilirubin levels

yellowness of the tissue and estimate the level of total serum bilirubin (TSB) as per modified Kramer's rule (Fig. 9.67).

### *Transcutaneous Bilirubin Level (TcB)*

This hand-held equipment can quantify the yellowness of the subcutaneous tissues and give TcB levels that approximate the TSB level (Fig. 9.68). TcB provides objective measurements and is reliable clinical tool and obviates the subjective nature and wide interobserver and intraobserver variations of visual assessment. Routine TcB measurements reduce the need for blood sampling to confirm TSB.

TcB and visual assessment are unreliable when the TSB levels are high during and after phototherapy and in preterm neonates.

### *Measurement of Serum Bilirubin Levels*

Measure TSB levels, if the jaundice is present in the legs or beyond or when visually-estimated TSB levels or TcB approach phototherapy range. TSB assessment has a marked interlaboratory variability. Treatment decisions should always be made on TSB levels.

## Causes of Jaundice

Important causes of jaundice in neonates include:

i. *Hemolytic:* Rh incompatibility, ABO incompatibility, G6PD deficiency, thalassemia, hereditary spherocytosis

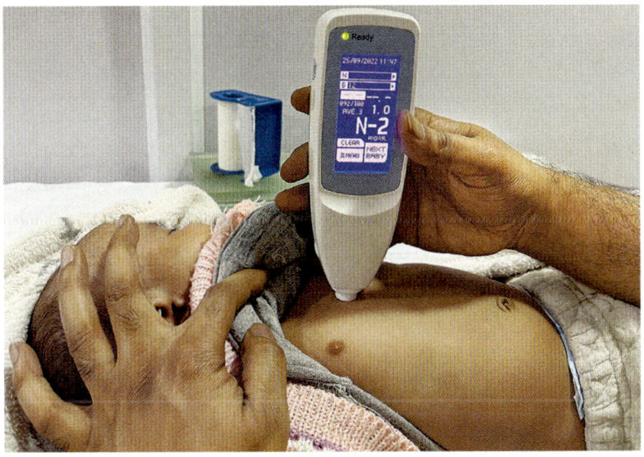

**Fig. 9.68:** Transcutaneous bilirubinometer. It gives a fair approximation of serum total bilirubin (TSB) when TSB levels are below 13 to 15 mg/dL (*Photo courtesy:* Dr Md Tousifullah)

ii. *Non-hemolytic:* Prematurity, extravasated blood, inadequate feeding, polycythemia, idiopathic, breast milk jaundice

## Risk Factors for the Development of Hyperbilirubinemia

i. Jaundice observed in the first 24 hr.
ii. Predischarge TcB or TSB concentration close to phototherapy cut-offs or need for phototherapy before discharge
iii. Blood group incompatibility with positive direct antiglobulin (Coombs) test and other known hemolytic diseases (e.g. G6PD deficiency). The rapid rise of TcB or TSB (0.3 mg/dL/hour in the first 24 hours and 0.2 mg/dL/hour after 24 hours of age indicates the presence of hemolysis.
iv. Lower gestation age (risk increases with each week decrease from 40 wk)
v. Previous sibling or parent received phototherapy
vi. Cephalohematoma or significant bruising
vii. If breastfeeding is inadequate with excessive weight loss
viii. East Asian race
ix. Macrosomic infant of a diabetic mother

## Risk Factors for Neurotoxicity

i. Gestation below 38 weeks
ii. A hemolytic condition such as blood group incompatibilities, G6PD deficiency
iii. Sepsis
iv. Low albumin level (less than 3 g/dL)
v. Significant clinical instability in the previous 24 hours

## Approach to a Jaundiced Neonate

All the neonates should be visually inspected for jaundice every 12 hr during the initial 3 to 5 days of life (Fig. 9.67). The simplified approach is shown in Fig. 9.69. For screening, TcB is preferable to visual assessment, if available. Visual assessment, if performed correctly, and TcB provides a reasonable estimation of TSB when the TSB level is below 15 mg/dL.

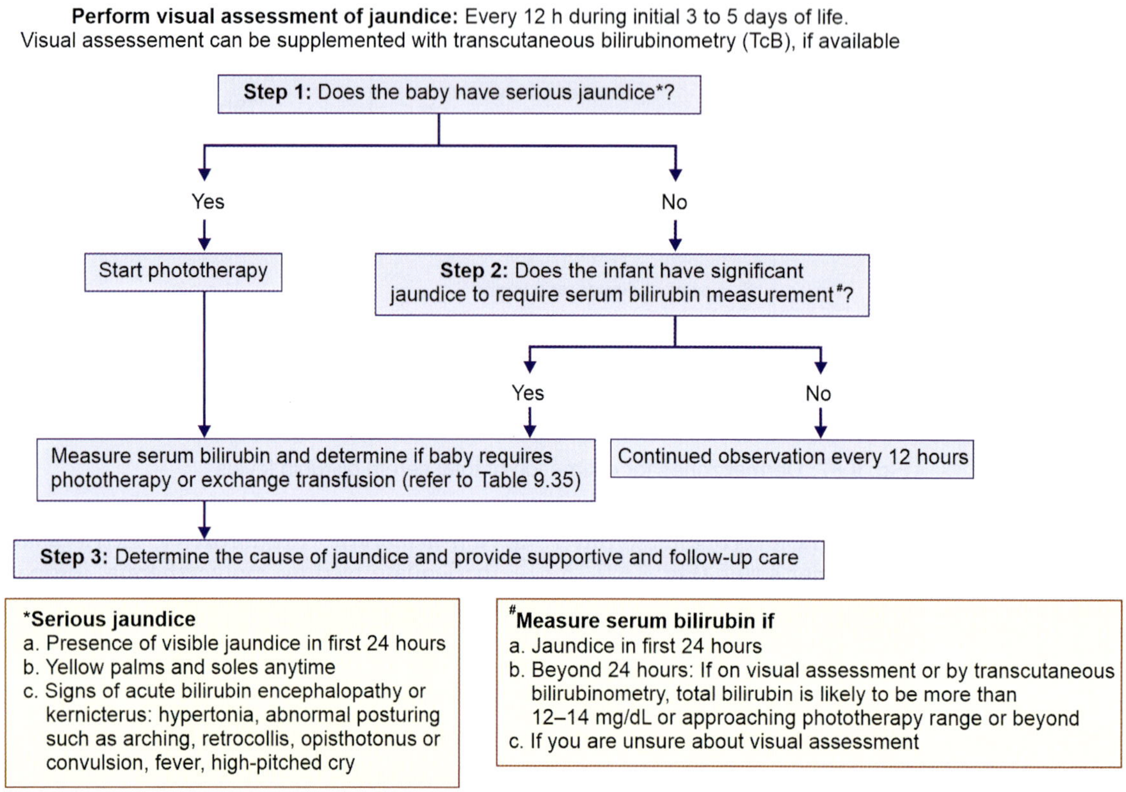


**Fig. 9.69:** Approach to an infant with jaundice

## Management

### Prevention of Hyperbilirubinemia

Pregnant women with Rh negative blood group need screening for anti-Rh antibodies. These women require prophylaxis with Rh immunoglobulin after delivery of an Rh-positive baby.

Ensuring adequate breastfeeding through best practices is critical for the prevention of hyperbilirubinemia. There must be a systematic approach to initiating and supporting breastfeeding, including promptly addressing breastfeeding problems.

### Investigations

The aim of performing investigations is to confirm the level of jaundice, identify the cause and follow the response to treatment.

#### First line

- Total serum bilirubin (and its fractions, if jaundice is prolonged or there is the yellow staining of nappies): All cases with suspected pathological levels either clinically or by transcutaneous measurements need confirmation by a blood test.
- Blood groups of mother and neonate (if the mother is 'O' or Rh negative): Detects any incompatibility
- Peripheral smear: Evidence of hemolysis

#### Second line

- Direct Coombs test: Detects the presence of antibody coating on fetal RBC
- Hematocrit: Decreased in hemolysis
- Reticulocyte count: Increased in hemolysis
- G6PD levels
- Others: Sepsis screen; thyroid function test; urine for reducing substances to rule out galactosemia; specific enzyme/genetic studies for Crigler-Najjar, Gilbert, and other genetic enzyme deficiencies.

### Physiological Jaundice

Counsel the parents regarding the benign nature of jaundice. Encourage the mother to breastfeed exclusively and return to the hospital, if the neonate looks deep yellow or if palms and soles have yellow staining. Direct exposure to sunlight is ineffective in reducing hyperbilirubinemia and may harm the baby, and it is best avoided.

*Call the infant again for re-evaluation of jaundice, if discharged before 72 hr of life, or if there is a high risk of developing hyperbilirubinemia such as suboptimal feeding, cephalhematoma, or late preterm gestation.*

### Pathological Jaundice

***Neonates of 35 weeks or more of gestation:*** American Academy of Pediatrics (AAP; 2022) has provided guidelines for managing hyperbilirubinemia in neonates of 35 weeks or more (**Figs 9.70a and b** for phototherapy and **9.71a and b** for exchange transfusion). The charts are separate for those without and with risk factors for neurotoxicity. The X-axis of the charts gives age in hours, and the y-axis shows TSB. Each line represents a different gestation.

***Neonates less than 35 weeks of gestation:*** We use cut-offs provided by the National Institute of Health and Care Excellence (NICE), UK, for managing jaundice in these neonates **(Table 9.35)**. The consensus is to use a lower

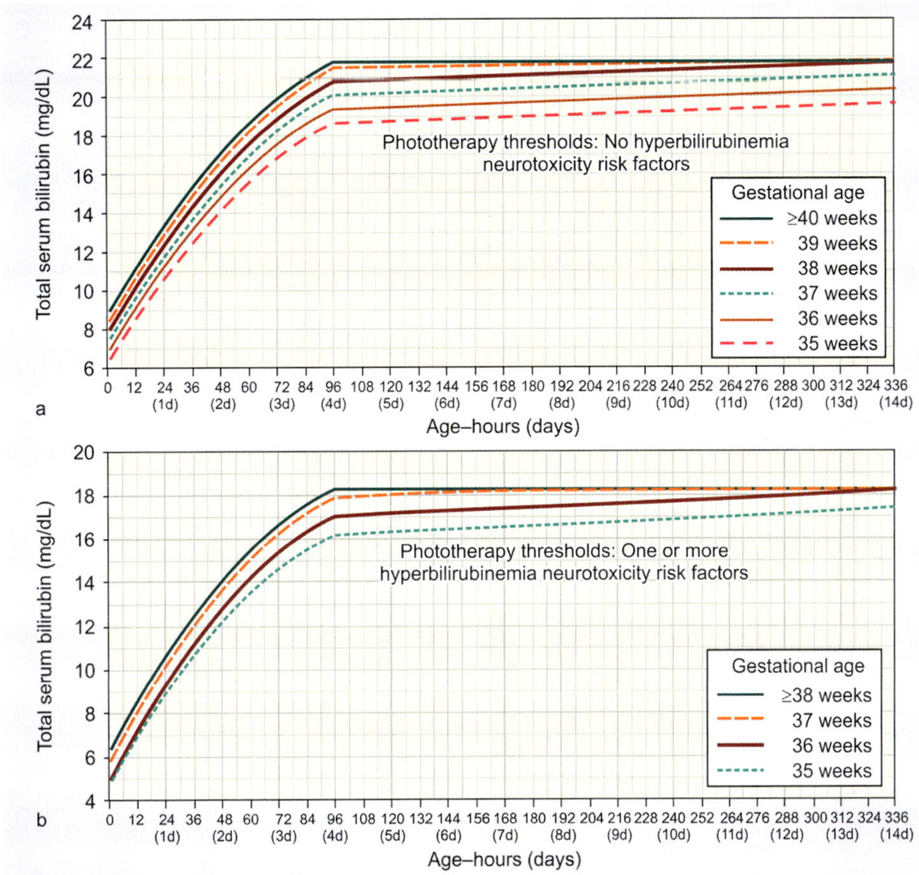


**Fig. 9.70:** Guidelines for phototherapy in infants of 35 or more weeks gestation: (a) Without neurotoxicity risk factors; (b) With neurotoxicity risk factors (Reproduced with permission from AAP 2022)

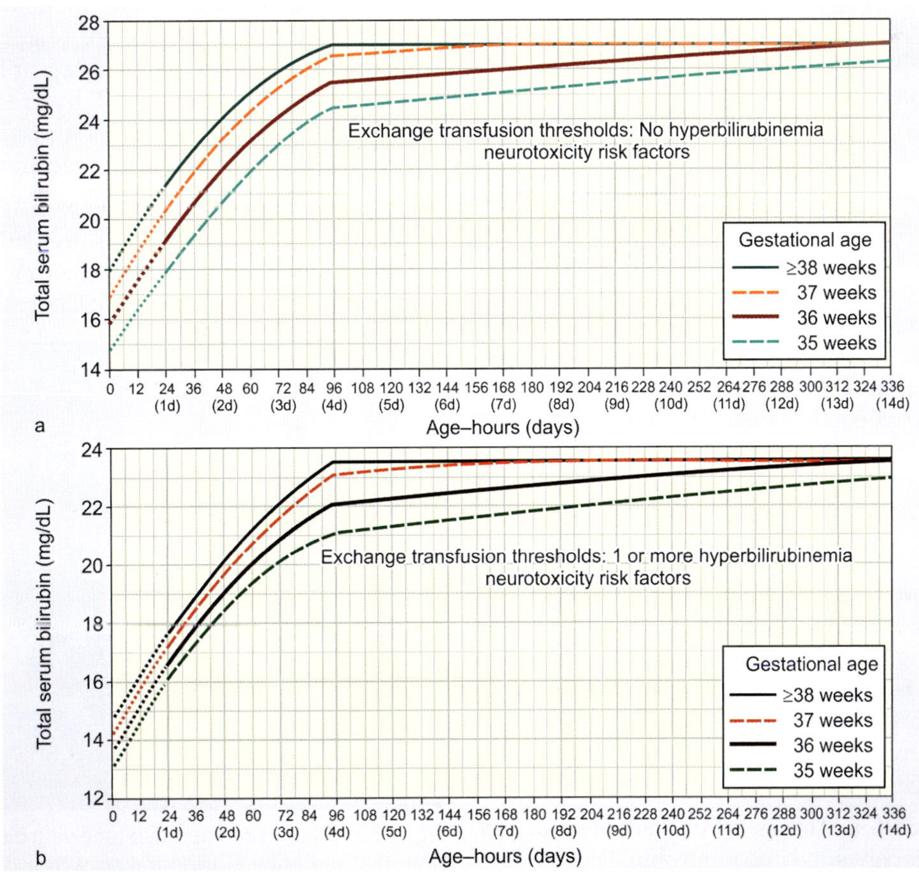


**Fig. 9.71:** Guidelines for exchange transfusion in infants of 35 or more weeks gestation: (a) Without neurotoxicity risk factors; (b) With neurotoxicity risk factors (Reproduced with permission from AAP 2022)

**Table 9.35:** Suggested total serum bilirubin (mg/dL) cut-offs for phototherapy and exchange transfusion in preterm neonates <35 weeks gestational age (NICE 2010)

| *Gestational age* | *24 hours* | | *48 hours* | | *72 hours or more* | |
|---|---|---|---|---|---|---|
| | *Phototherapy* | *Exchange transfusion* | *Phototherapy* | *Exchange transfusion* | *Phototherapy* | *Exchange transfusion* |
| <28 weeks | 4–5 | 7–8 | 6–8 | 10–12 | 7–10 | 13–16 |
| 28–31 weeks | 5–6 | 8–9 | 8–9 | 12–13 | 10–12 | 16–18 |
| 32 weeks or more | 5–6 | 9–10 | 9–10 | 14–15 | 12–14 | 18–20 |

These are broad levels of TSB for a given gestation. In general, lower the gestation, lower the TSB level, lower the postnatal age, and lower the cut-off. The user is advised to refer to these charts rather than trying to memorize these cut-offs.

(*Compiled by:* Dr Satya Prakash)

threshold for phototherapy and exchange transfusion as preterm neonates are more prone to develop bilirubin-induced neurological dysfunction than neonates with more than 35 weeks of gestation.

### Prolonged Jaundice Beyond 3 Weeks

This is defined as the persistence of significant jaundice (~10 mg/dL) beyond three weeks in a term baby. The common causes include inadequate feeding, breast milk jaundice, extravasated blood (cephalohematoma), ongoing hemolytic disease, G6PD deficiency, and hypothyroidism. Rule out cholestasis by noting the urine and stool color and checking the direct bilirubin level. If the neonate has dark urine or significant jaundice, investigations should be initiated to rule out the following:

i. Cholestasis (stool color, urine color, direct and indirect bilirubin levels)
ii. Ongoing hemolysis, G6PD screen
iii. Hypothyroidism
iv. Urinary tract infection

### Phototherapy

Phototherapy remains the mainstay of treating hyperbilirubinemia in neonates. Phototherapy is highly effective and has an excellent safety track record of over 50 years. It converts insoluble bilirubin (unconjugated) into soluble isomers that can be excreted in urine and feces. The bilirubin molecule isomerizes to harmless forms under blue-green light (460–490 nm), and the light sources having high irradiance in this particular wavelength range are more effective than the others.

For phototherapy to be effective, bilirubin needs to be present in the skin, so there is no role for prophylactic phototherapy. Phototherapy acts in several ways:

***Configurational isomerization:*** Here, bilirubin's Z-isomers are converted into E-isomers. The reaction is instantaneous upon exposure to light but reversible as bilirubin reaches the bile duct. After 8–12 hr exposure to phototherapy, this constitutes about 25% of TSB, which is non-toxic. Since this is excreted slowly from the body, this is not a significant mechanism for a decrease in TSB.

***Structural isomerization:*** This is an irreversible reaction where the bilirubin is converted into lumirubin. This product forms 2–6% of TSB, which is rapidly excreted from the body and thus is mainly responsible for phototherapy-induced decline in TSB. The response is directly proportional to the dose of phototherapy.

***Photo oxidation:*** This is a minor reaction where photo-products are excreted in the urine.

***Types of phototherapy lights:*** Most phototherapy units have blue LED lamps these days. LED lamps have the advantage of long life (up to 50,000 hr), use less electricity, and deliver high irradiance resulting in a faster decline in TSB levels.

***Maximizing the efficacy of phototherapy:*** The irradiance of phototherapy lights should be periodically measured and ensure a minimum level of 30 microwatt/cm$^2$/nm in the wavelength range of 460 to 490 nm. The lamps should be changed, if the irradiance falls below the specified level or per the manufacturers' recommendation.

Expose the maximal surface area of the neonate (Fig. 9.72). The light should fall on the neonate perpendicularly, if the neonate is in an incubator. Avoid blocking the lights with any equipment (e.g. radiant warmer), a large diaper or an eye patch, a cap or hat, tape, dressing, or electrode. Ensure good hydration by frequent breastfeeding. Minimize interruption of phototherapy during feeding sessions or procedures.

***Administering phototherapy:*** Ensure the ambient temperature is 25° to 28°C to prevent the neonate from becoming hypothermic or hyperthermic. Remove all clothes of the neonate except the diaper. Cover the baby's eyes with

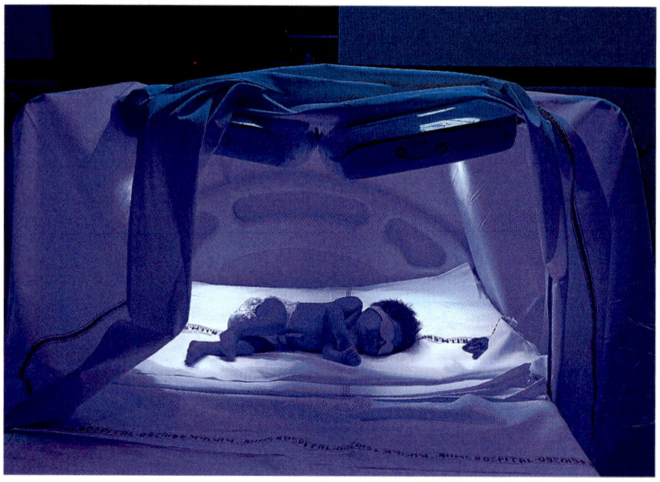

**Fig. 9.72:** A jaundiced neonate receiving blue light phototherapy. Note that the baby is lying naked with a diaper and eye cover. The bed cover and the curtains are white to reflect the light (*Courtesy:* Dr Richie Dalai)

an eye patch, ensuring that it does not block the baby's nostrils. Place the naked neonate under the lights in a cot or bassinet if the neonate weighs more than 2 kg or in an incubator or radiant warmer if the neonate is <2 kg. Keep the distance between neonate and light 30 to 45 cm (or as per manufacturer recommendation).

***Ensure optimum breastfeeding:*** The mother can remove the neonate from the bassinet for breastfeeding sessions. Removal of the eye patch can help improve mother–infant interaction. There is no need to supplement, if breastfeeding is adequate.

***Monitoring and stopping phototherapy:*** Monitor the temperature of the neonate every 2 to 4 hr. Measure TSB level every 12 to 24 hr. Discontinue phototherapy once two TSB values 12 hr apart fall below current age-specific cut-offs. The infant should be monitored clinically for rebound bilirubin rise within 24 hr after stopping phototherapy for neonates with hemolytic disorders.

#### Exchange Transfusion

Double volume exchange transfusion should be performed, if the TSB levels reach the age-specific cut-off for exchange transfusion or the infant shows signs of bilirubin encephalopathy, irrespective of TSB levels.

Indications for exchange transfusion at birth in infants with Rh isoimmunization include:

i. Cord bilirubin is 5 mg/dL or more
ii. Cord Hb is 10 g/dL or less

At birth, if a neonate shows signs of hydrops or cardiac decompensation in the presence of low PCV (<35%), partial exchange transfusion with 50 mL/kg of packed red blood cells should be done to restore oxygen carrying capacity of blood quickly.

### Follow-up

Neonates with serum bilirubin ≥20 mg/dL and those who require exchange transfusion should be kept under follow-up for neurodevelopmental surveillance. Some of these neonates develop anemia in first 6 to 12 weeks and require transfusion. A hearing assessment (BERA) should be done at three months of age.

### Suggested Reading


1. Clinical Practice Guideline Revision: Management of Hyperbilirubinemia in the Newborn Infant 35 or More Weeks of Gestation. Pediatrics. 2022 Sep 1;150(3):e2022058859.
2. Jaundice in newborn neonates under 28 days. National Institute of Health and Care Excellence, United Kingdom, 2010.
3. Kumar P, Chawla D, Deorari A. Light-emitting diode phototherapy for unconjugated hyperbilirubinemia in neonates. Cochrane Database Syst Rev. 2011 Dec 7;2011(12):CD007969.


## NEONATAL CHOLESTASIS

Neonatal cholestasis is an abnormal accumulation of conjugated bilirubin (CB) due to impaired formation or flow of bile. Cholestasis should be ruled out in case of prolonged hyperbilirubinemia. The history of deep yellow urine or clay-colored stools also suggests cholestasis. Conjugated bilirubin level exceeding 1 mg/dL is strongly suggestive.

The evaluation and management of neonatal cholestasis is discussed in Chapter 12.

*Competency:* **PE20.9**

## BIRTH INJURY

Birth injury includes impairments of the body's structure or function during birth (Table 9.36). It does not include therapeutic and diagnostic procedures like amniocentesis or intrauterine transfusion complications. Any neonate with birth injury should be examined for additional complications. Most birth injuries are temporary and self-limiting.

*Competency:* **PE20.20**

## CONGENITAL MALFORMATIONS

### Tracheoesophageal Fistula (TEF)

TEF occurs in 1 in 4000 live births. In the most common variety (type C; over 80% of cases), the upper part of the esophagus ends blindly, and the lower part is connected to the trachea by a fistula.

#### Clinical Features

Maternal polyhydramnios and single umbilical artery should alert to the possibility of atresia of the upper digestive tract. Congenital anomalies of vertebrae, anorectal region, heart, kidneys, or limbs should also make one suspect (VACTERL association). The affected neonate has excessive drooling soon after birth with frothing. There is choking and cyanosis during feeding. Overflow of milk and saliva from the esophagus and regurgitation of secretion through the fistulous tract (when present) into the lungs result in aspiration pneumonia.

#### Diagnosis

A nasogastric tube cannot be passed into the stomach as it gets arrested at a distance of 7–10 cm from the mouth (Fig. 9.73). After instilling 1–2 mL of air through the catheter, the skiagram may be obtained. It is not advisable to use barium as a contrast material since it may be aspirated in the lungs.

On X-ray, an air bubble is seen in the abdomen, if there is communication between the lower part of the esophagus and trachea, which occurs in the commonest variety of tracheoesophageal fistula. In other types, there is no communication between the esophagus and trachea, and there will be no gas in the stomach.

#### Management

The neonate should be nursed supine or upright, and the esophageal pouch should be gently suctioned every five minutes or continuously using a slow suction device. The neonate needs to be kept nil orally and requires intravenous fluids. Infection, if any, should be treated. The lesion needs surgical repair as early as possible.

**Table 9.36:** Common birth injuries, risk factors, and associated complications

| *Birth injury* | *Risk factors* | *Complications* | *Prognosis* |
|---|---|---|---|
| **Head and neck injury** | | | |
| Cephalohematoma/subgaleal hemorrhage | Instrumental delivery; macrosomia; precipitous delivery | Hypovolemia, prolonged jaundice, anemia, infection | Usually resolves within 4–6 weeks. Monitor for hypovolemia in subgaleal bleed. |
| Skull fracture (linear and depressed) | Instrumental delivery; breech delivery | Associated intracranial bleeds | Self-limiting; depressed fracture may require neurosurgical intervention |
| Sternocleidomastoid injury (sternocleidomastoid tumor) | Abnormal intrauterine positioning leads to rupture of muscle fibers leading to hematoma and fibrosis | Torticollis with a head tilt toward the injury site | Stretching exercises; recovers in 3 months in the majority. Some may require surgery |
| **Nerve injury** | | | |
| Facial nerve injury | Forceps application; Uterine fibroids | Lower motor neuron type injury | Most recover in 2–3 weeks |
| Brachial plexus injury<br>a. Duchene-Erb palsy (C5, C6 nerve root injury with occasional C7 involvement): 90% cases<br>b. Total brachial plexus injury (C5, C6, C7, C8, T1 nerve root injury): 10% cases<br>c. Klumpke palsy (C7, C8, T1 nerve root injury): Very rare | Macrosomia; malpresentation; shoulder dystocia; forceps or vacuum application | a. Weakness in shoulder abduction, elbow flexion, and external rotation ("waiter's tip" posture with intact grasp)<br>b. Flaccid paralysis of the entire arm with absent grasp reflex<br>c. Weakness of hand and wrist muscles with Horner syndrome | An intact grasp reflex suggests 80% chance of spontaneous recovery.<br>Complete injury has a poor outcome, with 30–50% chance of recovery. |
| **Bone injury** | | | |
| Clavicle fracture: Most common bone injury | Macrosomia; shoulder dystocia; breech presentation | Pseudoparalysis of affected arm with asymmetric Moro reflex **(Fig. 9.33c)** | Complete healing occurs after proper splinting |
| Long bone fractures: Such as humerus or femur | Difficult delivery | Swelling and pseudoparalysis of the affected limb | Closed reduction and casting for two weeks |

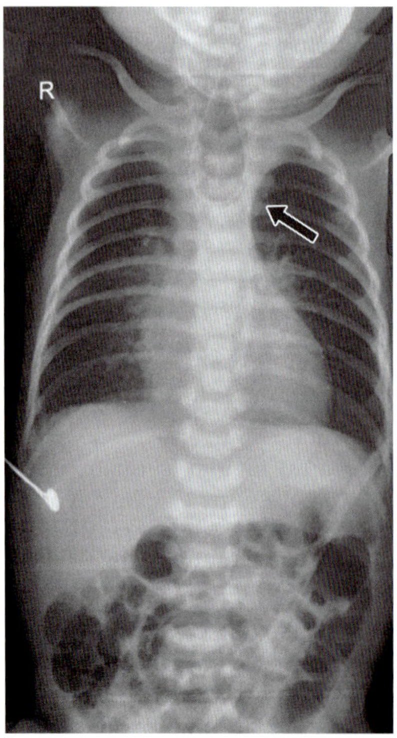


**Fig. 9.73:** Esophageal atresia with tracheoesophageal fistula with a coiled nasogastric tube (as shown by red arrow)

## Intestinal Obstruction

Neonatal intestinal obstruction is a common surgical emergency that occurs in 1 in 2000 live births. The diagnosis is usually based on the clinical presentation of abdominal distension or bilious vomiting and a plain X-ray abdomen. Early diagnosis and management are the keys to good outcomes.

Any newborn presenting with bilious vomiting with or without abdominal distension should be investigated for possible obstruction **(Fig. 9.74)**. **Table 9.37** shows the

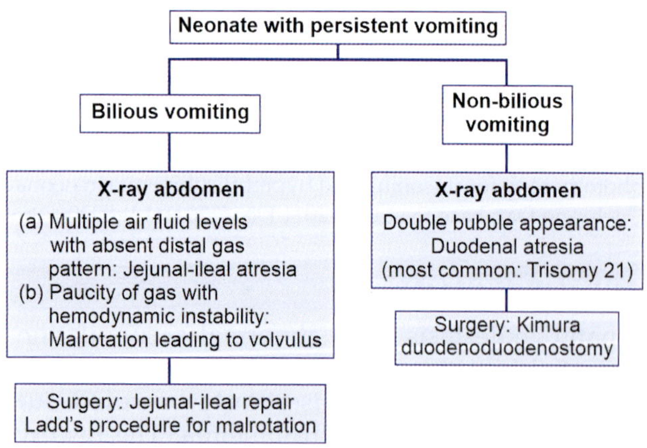


**Fig. 9.74:** Approach to a neonate with persistent vomiting

Table 9.37: Classification of neonatal intestinal obstruction and its common causes

| *Site of obstruction* | *Common causes* |
|---|---|
| Upper (up to second part of duodenum) | Malrotation of gut<br>Hypertrophic pyloric stenosis or atresia<br>Duodenal atresia or stenosis |
| Mid (up to middle transverse colon) | Ileal atresia<br>Jejunal atresia<br>Meconium ileus<br>Hirschsprung disease |
| Lower (up to anal aperture) | Anorectal malformation<br>Hirschsprung disease<br>Colonic atresia |

three main forms of intestinal obstruction. Sepsis causing paralytic ileus and necrotizing enterocolitis are close differential diagnoses.

### Anorectal Malformation

Anorectal malformation (ARM) is a common neonatal surgical emergency with an incidence of 1 in 5000 live births. ARM is an isolated anomaly in one-third of cases. The remaining two-thirds, especially the high types, have associated urogenital, vertebral, cardiac, or gastrointestinal anomalies.

The currently used 'Krickenbeck classification' of ARM has simplified and standardized the various anomalies into groups based on their treatment strategies. The most common ARM seen in males is the rectourethral fistula, while that in females is a rectovestibular fistula. The conventional terms, high and low type ARM, used in common parlance, were derived from the Wingspread classification. The ARMs were divided into high and low based on the level of the terminal bowel with respect to the levator ani muscle of the pelvic floor. Low ARM can be managed with perineal surgery in the neonatal period. In contrast, a high ARM requires an initial colostomy followed by a definitive procedure after 3–6 months.

Neonates with ARM usually present with an absent normal anal opening detected on routine neonatal assessment at birth. When missed, they are brought to attention after 24–48 hours once abdominal distension develops, in addition to the failure to pass meconium. An exception to this rule is rectal atresia, an ARM with a normal anal opening but atresia high up in the rectum that can only be diagnosed by probing with a stiff catheter. A decompressing vestibular or perineal fistula may be present in females, delaying the diagnosis.

History suggestive of pneumaturia or meconuria (suggesting a genitourinary communication) should be enquired about. Presence or absence of anal, vaginal, and urethral openings, site of any fistula in the perineum (low anomaly), site of the anal dimple, gluteal cleft (poorly developed in high anomaly), and scrotum (bifid or associated with hypospadias in high anomaly) should be examined. Any meconium-staining or meconium pearls (Fig. 9.75) in the perineum or perineal skin tags (low anomaly) should be noted. In the cloaca, the urinary tract, the vagina, and the terminal bowel communicate with a common channel of variable length with a single opening in the perineum.

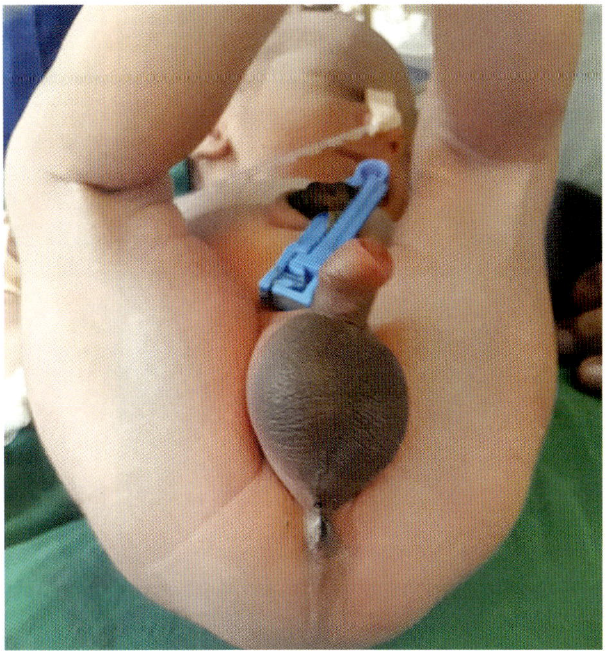

Fig. 9.75: Absence of normal anal opening. Note meconium trickling to the scrotum (meconium pearl; low ARM) (*Courtesy:* Dr Ashish Chhabra, Faridkot)

In ARM, once the level of the terminal pouch is established (clinically or radiologically), the decision regarding a diverting colostomy or a primary definite procedure is made. A diverting colostomy is performed in the neonatal period for male ARMs (high-type) and females with persistent cloacae. Later after 3–4 months, accurate anatomic information is obtained by a contrast colostogram or genitoscopy (for persistent cloacae); posterior sagittal anorectoplasty (PSARP) or a posterior sagittal anorecto-urethrovaginoplasty (for persistent cloacae) is undertaken. Stoma reversal is done after 3–4 months after the definitive reconstruction. For boys with a "low type" of malformation, a single-stage perineal procedure like anoplasty is usually sufficient. Females with ano-/recto-vestibular fistulas can be observed, if they can decompress the bowel and pass stools normally. An elective single-stage limited PSARP can be performed around 3–4 months of age.

### Neural Tube Defects

*Anencephaly:* Anencephaly is due to a defect in neural axis development and is incompatible with life.

*Encephalocele:* In encephalocele, the brain and its coverings herniate through a defect in the skull.

*Congenital hydrocephalus* (Fig. 9.76a): Congenital hydrocephalus results from impaired CSF circulation or absorption in basal cisterns. This usually follows intrauterine infections such as toxoplasmosis, rubella, cytomegalovirus, and syphilis but may also be the result of a congenital malformation of the aqueduct, Dandy-Walker syndrome (posterior fossa cyst and a defect of cerebellar

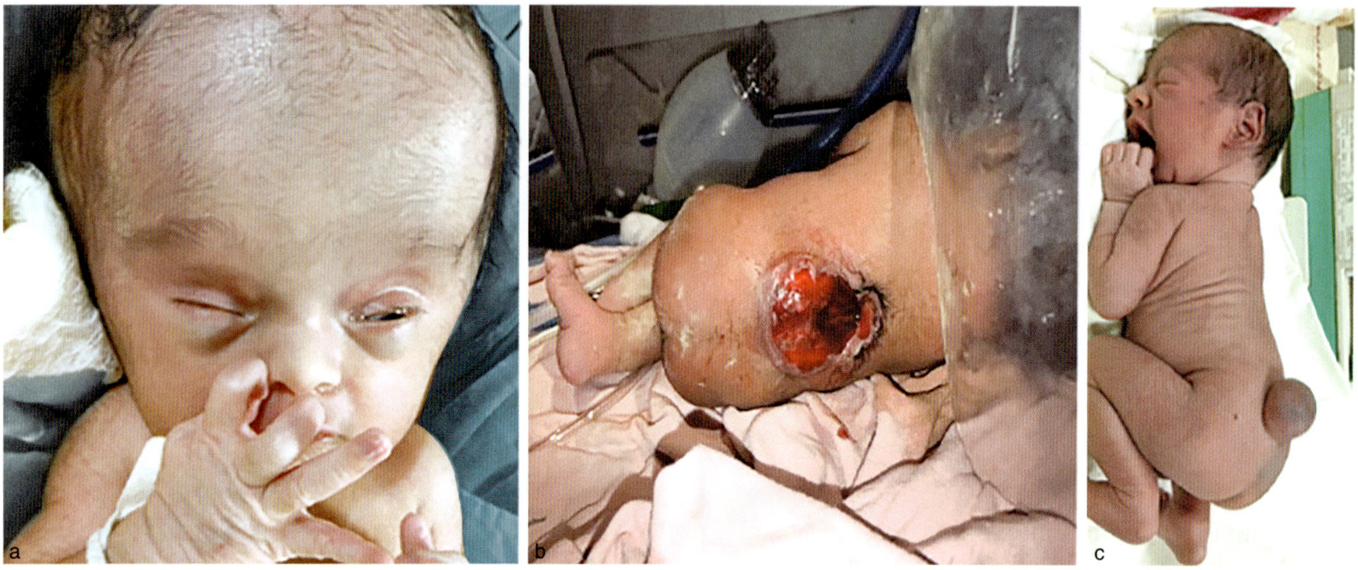


Fig. 9.76: Various congenital malformations: (a) Congenital hydrocephalus; (b) Open neural tube defect in the lumbar region; (c) Meningocele (*Courtesy:* Dr Neerja Gupta)



vermis), Arnold-Chiari malformation (displacement of brainstem and cerebellum in the spinal canal) or multiple congenital malformations of the nervous system.

Diagnosis should be suspected, if the head is too large, sutures and fontanels are wide open, or if the head circumference increases rapidly (more than 1 cm in a fortnight during the first three months). CT or MRI scan should be done to confirm the diagnosis. The type of dilatation of the ventricles indicates the site of obstruction. Isolated aqueductal stenosis has a better prognosis.

Treatment should be directed to find a specific cause, and surgical intervention such as ventriculocaval or ventriculoperitoneal shunt to decompress the brain.

***Myelomeningocele*** **(Fig. 9.76b and c)**: It presents as a membranous protrusion at the lumbosacral region and contains meninges, cerebrospinal fluid, nerve roots, and a dysplastic spinal cord. The defect is open and not covered by skin.

In contrast, the meningocele is covered with skin. There may be no associated neurological deficit, but Arnold-Chiari malformation and congenital hydrocephalus are often associated. Severe motor and sensory deficits are common, and urinary and fecal incontinence are usually present. Meningomyelocele is operated on, only if there is no paralysis of the lower limbs and if there is no bladder/bowel involvement.

Folic acid, at a dose of 4 mg/day, is advised to women in the periconceptional period to prevent a recurrence.

### Cleft Lip and Cleft Palate

An oral cleft is the most common craniofacial malformation in newborns. Oral clefts include cleft lip alone, cleft lip with cleft palate, or cleft palate alone. Cleft lip and palate can be unilateral or bilateral (Fig. 9.77a and b). The cleft palate may involve the anterior portion, posterior soft palate, or the entire palate. A cleft lip is recognized readily, but a careful inspection of the oral cavity is necessary to identify the cleft palate. A soft palate cleft can be easily missed unless the neonate is examined carefully. Associated malformations can be present in one-third of cases. A ventricular septal defect is a commonly associated anomaly with a cleft palate.

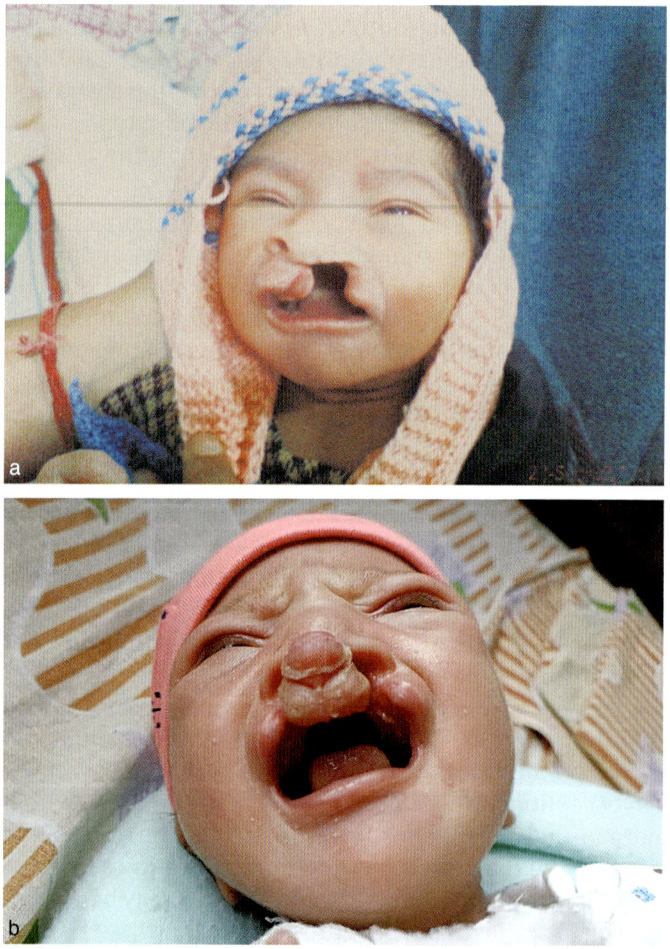


Fig. 9.77: (a) Unilateral cleft lip and cleft palate; (b) Bilateral cleft lip and palate

Feeding is problematic in cases of cleft palate. For the first few days, gavage feeding or spoon-feeding may be done. Bottle feeding may be tried with a long soft nipple.

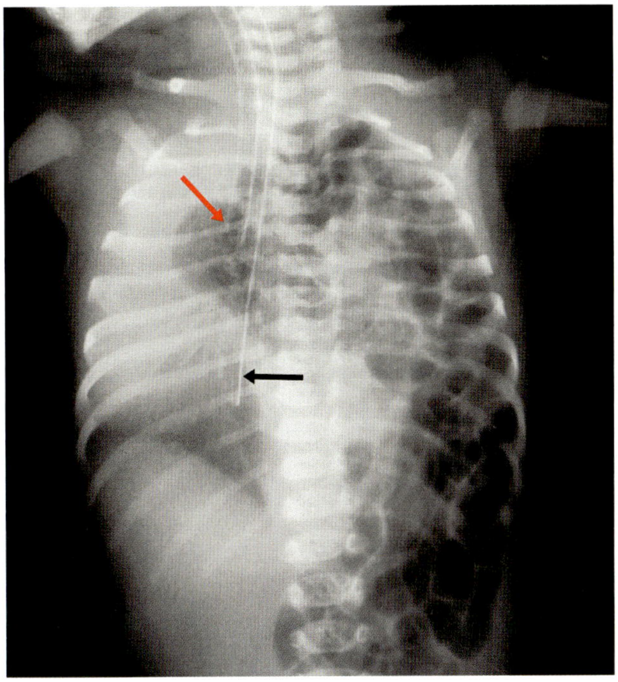

Fig. 9.78: Diaphragmatic hernia. Chest X-ray showing multiple air-filled cysts in the left hemithorax, the shift of the mediastinum to the right, and the absence of outline of the left diaphragm. Note endotracheal tube displaced to right side (red arrow) and feeding tube (black arrow)

*Management:* The cleft lip is repaired in the neonatal period. Operation for cleft palate is generally deferred until the second year. Management of cleft palate requires a team effort involving a pediatrician, a plastic surgeon, an orthodontist, an ENT specialist, and a speech therapist.

### Diaphragmatic Hernia

A diaphragmatic hernia occurs because of the failure to close the pleuroperitoneal membrane. This allows intestinal loops to ascend to the thorax, compress the developing lung, and can result in pulmonary hypoplasia (Fig. 9.78). At birth, a neonate may be suspected to have diaphragmatic hernia, if there is respiratory distress and a scaphoid abdomen. These neonates can present at any time after birth. Bag and mask ventilation should be avoided in these neonates. Surgical repair after stabilization is the treatment of choice.

## TRANSPORT OF NEONATES

Transport of a sick neonate to a higher facility requires careful attention to vital parameters, temperature, and blood glucose levels, as well as coordination with the receiving hospital (Fig. 9.79). Indication of the transport would depend on the level of referring facility and the sickness level of the infant:

- A small or sick neonate may need transportation from the birthing facility to a level 2 facility, if the neonate is <1800 g or <34 weeks of gestation or if there is sickness such as apnea, respiratory distress requiring level 2 care
- A level-2 unit may have to transfer a sick and small neonate to level-3 care, if the neonate is too small (e.g. <1000 g or needing prolonged ventilation or surgical care)

**Determine the indication* to transport the baby to higher health facility**

Birth weight <1200 g or gestation <30 weeks

Sickness: Severe respiratory distress, shock, severe jaundice, major malformations requiring surgery, refractory seizures

↓

**Prepare for transport**

*Baby*

Stabilize (temperature, airway, breathing, circulation and blood sugar)

Secure IV line and give necessary treatment before transfer

*Logistics*

Counsel the parents and family before transport

Communicate with referral facility. Provide a brief note

Arrange supplies, equipment and transport vehicle

↓

**Care during transport**

Monitor frequently (temperature, airway and breathing, circulation, IV cannula and infusions)

Ensure that the baby receives feeds or fluid

Stop the vehicle, if necessary, to manage problems

↓

**Feedback after transport**

Communicate with referral team for condition at arrival and outcome

*Indications may vary as per the facility

Fig. 9.79: Transport of sick neonates

- Sometimes, a sick neonate managed at a higher-level facility may need reverse transfer to a lower-level facility once reasonably stable.

In the anticipated birth of an at-risk neonate, the mother should be transported (*in utero* transport) to an equipped facility for optimum care of the mother and the baby.

If a neonate requires referral after birth, follow these principles:

1. Transfer the neonate for a genuine indication only. Explain the condition of the neonate and the need for transport to the family.
2. Stabilize the neonate as much as possible. It may worsen along the way. Correct hypothermia or provide initial shock treatment or first dose of antibiotics, if indicated before transport.
3. Provide a referral note giving adequate details about the baby, the need for referral, and the treatment given.
4. The mother should be encouraged to accompany the neonate or reach the facility soon.
5. A health provider must accompany the neonate to provide care en route.
6. Take the neonate to the nearest referral facility (inform them in advance) by the shortest route, using the fastest and most affordable mode of transport.

## FOLLOW-UP OF HIGH-RISK NEONATES

Improved perinatal and neonatal care has resulted in improved survival of many sick and small neonates who are at risk for long-term morbidities such as growth failure, developmental delay, and visual/hearing problems (Table 9.38).

A structured follow-up program helps in the prevention, early detection, and appropriate management of these problems, thereby maximizing the probability of disability- and morbidity-free survival.

**Table 9.38:** Growth and developmental outcomes of common neonatal morbidities

| *Condition* | *Outcomes* |
|---|---|
| Very preterm (gestation <32 weeks) | Very preterm neonates are at high risk of growth failure. Many of these babies remain stunted and wasted.<br>There is a higher need for repeat hospitalization during the first year for pneumonia, diarrhea, and other illnesses. There is a higher risk of respiratory syncytial virus infection. There is a higher risk of retinopathy of prematurity, and if not detected and treated timely, it can lead to blindness.<br>~10 to 15% of neonates are at risk of significant neurodevelopmental disabilities, including cerebral palsy (most commonly spastic diplegia), low cognition, blindness and deafness. |
| Hypoxic-ischemic encephalopathy | High risk of major neurodevelopmental disabilities (30–50% in moderate to severe encephalopathy), minor neuro-morbidities (10–20%), including cerebral palsy (dystonic, quadriplegia), low cognition, blindness, deafness, and seizures |
| Significant hyperbilirubinemia (total serum bilirubin >25 mg/dL) | High risk of intellectual disability (25%), choreoathetosis cerebral palsy, sensorineural hearing loss, and gaze abnormalities |
| Term small-for-gestational age | Poor catch-up growth (13–20%), low cognitive scores, increased risk of cardiovascular disease, and type II diabetes |

(*Contributed by:* Satya Prakash)



### Who Needs Follow-up Care?

Table 9.39 discusses the indications for high-risk follow-up.

### When to Follow-up?

The infant should have the following visits:

- Two weeks after discharge
- At 6, 10, and 14 weeks of postnatal age
- At 3, 6, 9, 12, and 18 months of corrected age and then six monthly until at least 5 yr.

The follow-up clinic follows a multidisciplinary approach, with a pediatrician being the nodal person. The team should include a nutritionist, psychologist, occupational therapist, and social worker.

The following parameters are assessed at each visit, and appropriate remedial action are taken.

i. *Nutrition:* Inquire about infants' diet, including frequency and adequacy of breastfeeding and details of supplementary and complementary feedings. Record the duration of exclusive breastfeeding. Measures are taken to improve breastfeeding, if there is inadequate weight gain. Complementary feeding should be started at 6 months of corrected age.

**Table 9.39:** Common newborn conditions requiring high-risk follow-up care

| *Newborn conditions requiring high-risk follow-up care* |
|---|
| Birth weight <1800 g or gestation <34 weeks |
| Newborns requiring respiratory support |
| Perinatal asphyxia: Apgar score 3 or less at 5 min and/or hypoxic ischemic encephalopathy (HIE) stage II and III |
| Small for date (<3rd centile) and large for date (>97th centile) |
| Hypoglycemia |
| Neonatal seizures |
| Meningitis, or culture-positive sepsis |
| Shock requiring inotropes |
| Total serum bilirubin nearing exchange transfusion cut-off |

ii. *Growth:* Measure weight, head circumference, mid-arm circumference, and length and plot them on an appropriate growth chart at each visit. If there is any deviation in growth, appropriate actions are taken.

iii. *Developmental assessment:* Assess developmental milestones according to the corrected age in four domains (Chapter 3). Infants who lag in any domain should undergo a formal developmental evaluation. Age-appropriate stimulation should be provided to these neonates. The family is encouraged to interact with the child appropriately.

iv. *Immunization:* Immunization should be ensured according to chronological age.

v. *Ongoing problems:* Ongoing morbidities such as diarrhea and pneumonia occur more frequently in these neonates and require appropriate treatment.

vi. *Neurological assessment:* Inquire about the history of seizures or involuntary movements. Perform neurological examination, including muscle tone assessment. Any asymmetry between the extremities should also be recorded.

vii. *Vision and hearing evaluation:* An ophthalmologist should evaluate the neonate for vision, squint, cataract, and optic atrophy. Subjective visual assessment can be made from clinical clues such as the inability to fixate eyes, roving eye movements, and nystagmus. An objective visual assessment should be done with the Teller Acuity Card. Preterm infants need screening for retinopathy of prematurity starting from 28 days of age.

Since clinical screening is often unreliable, brainstem auditory evoked responses (BAER/BERA) should be performed to determine any hearing impairment at discharge.

*Competencies:* **PE20.13; PE20.14**

## METABOLIC DISORDERS

### Hypoglycemia

Hypoglycemia is a blood glucose value of less than 45 mg/dL. Screening for hypoglycemia is recommended in high-

**Table 9.40:** Common causes of hypoglycemia

| |
|---|
| *Inadequate substrate:* Small for gestational age (weight for gestation <3rd percentile), gestation <35 weeks, birth weight <2000 g |
| *Relative hyperinsulinemia:* Infants of diabetic mother, large for date baby (weight for gestation >97th percentile). |
| *Sickness:* Hypothermia, sepsis, asphyxia |

risk situations (Table 9.40). Appropriate for gestational-age neonates who are breastfeeding adequately do not require screening for hypoglycemia.

Neonates should be screened for hypoglycemia at 2, 6, 12, 24, 48, and 72 hr after birth with reagent strips. Neonates showing a blood sugar value of less than 45 mg/dL should be treated for hypoglycemia, but have confirmation by a lab test as reagent strips have high false positive rates.

#### Clinical Features

Clinically, the neonate with hypoglycemia may be asymptomatic or have features like stupor, tremors, apathy, cyanosis, convulsions, apneic spells, tachypnea, weak and high-pitched cry, lethargy, difficulty in feeding, eye-rolling, episodes of sweating, sudden pallor, hypothermia and rarely, cardiac arrest.

#### Management of Hypoglycemia

***Prevention of hypoglycemia:*** Ensure the adequacy of breastfeeding. All high-risk neonates should receive breastfeeding counseling and support. Small neonates unable to breastfeed effectively should receive expressed breast milk by alternate methods.

***Asymptomatic neonates:*** If the blood sugar is more than 20 mg/dL in an asymptomatic baby, a trial of oral feeds is given, and blood sugar is tested after 30–45 minutes. If repeat blood sugar values are above 40 mg/dL, frequent feeding is ensured with six-hourly monitoring of blood sugar for 48 hr. However, if blood sugar values persist below 40 mg/dL, the neonate should receive an IV glucose infusion.

If the initial blood sugar value is less than 20 mg/dL, then intravenous glucose infusion is started.

***Symptomatic neonates:*** A bolus of 2 mL/kg of 10% dextrose should be given, followed immediately by glucose infusion at an initial rate of 6 mg/kg/min. Blood sugar is checked after 30–45 minutes and then 6 hours. Repeat hypoglycemic episodes may be treated by increasing the glucose infusion rate by 2 mg/kg/min until a maximum of 12 mg/kg/min. If two or more consecutive values are >50 mg/dL after 24 hr of parenteral therapy, the infusion can be tapered off at 2 mg/kg/min every 6 hr, with glucose monitoring. Tapering has to be accompanied by a concomitant increase in oral feeds.

### Hypocalcemia

Hypocalcemia is a common metabolic condition in the neonatal period characterized by total serum calcium less than 7 mg/dL in preterm (ionized calcium <4 mg/dL) and less than 8 mg/dL in term neonates (ionized calcium <4.8 mg/dL). According to the age of onset, hypocalcemia is classified into two main categories, as shown in Table 9.41.

### Key Maternal Interventions to Improve Fetal and Neonatal Health

Several interventions can improve the health of fetuses and neonates (Table 9.42). They should be appropriately included in the mother's care during pregnancy, childbirth, and postnatal care.

### Suggested Reading


1. Journey of the First 1000 Days. Foundation for a Brighter Future. RBSK, Ministry of Health and Family Welfare 2018.
2. WHO recommendations on antenatal care for a positive pregnancy experience, Geneva, WHO, 2016.


## EFFECT OF MATERNAL CONDITIONS ON FETUS AND NEONATES

### Diabetes Mellitus

The following complications are likely to occur during the pregnancy of a diabetic mother.

i. Fetus may die suddenly during the last trimester of pregnancy
ii. Macrosomia or large size of the neonate (Fig. 9.80a, b) increases the chances of birth trauma, asphyxia, and cesarean section
iii. Neonatal respiratory distress
iv. Metabolic problems such as hypoglycemia and hypocalcemia
v. Polycythemia, increased viscosity of blood, and hyperbilirubinemia
vi. Higher risk of congenital anomalies

**Table 9.41:** Types of hypocalcemia, their risk factors, and management

| | *Onset* | *Main risk factors* | *Clinical features* | *Management* |
|---|---|---|---|---|
| Early onset | First 3 days | Prematurity<br>Perinatal asphyxia<br>Infant of diabetic mother | Usually, asymptomatic | IV and PO calcium |
| Late onset | After seven days | Increased phosphate load: Cow milk feeds, renal insufficiency<br>Vitamin D deficiency in mother and neonate<br>Hypomagnesemia<br>Hypoparathyroidism | Tetany, seizures, tachycardia, prolonged QTc interval, apnea, tachypnea, cyanosis | Same as above<br>Etiological diagnosis is vital to treat the cause |

Table 9.42: Key maternal interventions to improve fetal and neonatal health

| For general fetal well-being | |
|---|---|
| Dietary interventions | Balanced energy and protein intake during pregnancy, especially in malnourished populations, can reduce the risk of preterm births and the chances of low birth weight. Mothers should be educated about healthy eating habits and remain physically active during pregnancy. |
| Iron and folic acid supplementation | The supplementation of oral iron (30 to 60 mg of elemental iron daily) and folic acid: 0.4 mg daily can reduce maternal anemia, LBW, and prematurity rates. Pre-conception folic acid supplementation (400 µg daily) prevents neural tube defects. |
| Calcium supplementation | Oral elemental calcium supplementation at a dose of 1.5 to 2 g daily, especially in mothers with low dietary intake of calcium, can reduce the risk of pre-eclampsia and preterm births |
| Vitamin A or multiple micronutrient supplementation | Routine supplementation is not recommended for improving fetal and neonatal outcomes |
| **For improving preterm birth outcomes** | |
| Antenatal corticosteroids | Dexamethasone, 6 mg IM 12 hourly for four doses<br>Gestation: 24 to 34 weeks of pregnancy presenting with preterm labor<br>Benefits<br>1. 30% reduction in respiratory distress syndrome<br>2. 40% reduction in intraventricular hemorrhage,<br>3. 40% reduction in sepsis in the first 48 hours<br>4. 50% reduction in necrotizing enterocolitis<br>5. 22% reduction in neonatal mortality<br>Contraindication: Frank chorioamnionitis |
| Magnesium sulfate | In preterm labor with gestation less than 32 weeks, magnesium sulfate at a dose of 4 g/kg IV loading over 30 minutes, followed by 1 g/hour for 24 hours reduces cerebral palsy and motor delay |
| Prophylactic antibiotics | Recommended only in pregnant women with preterm premature rupture of membranes (PPROM). It reduces neonatal sepsis and respiratory distress syndrome |

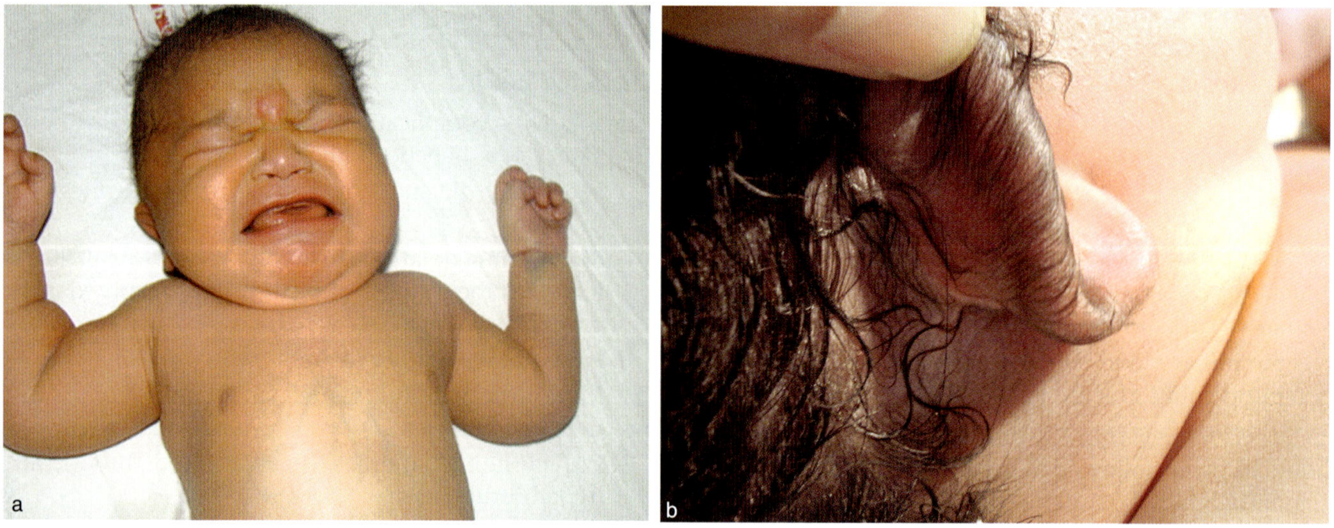

Fig. 9.80: (a) Infant of diabetic mother: Large size with broad shoulders and torso and a relatively smaller head; (b) Hairy pinna of the baby

### *Pathogenesis*

Maternal hyperglycemia leads to fetal hyperglycemia and fetal hyperinsulinemia (Pederson hypothesis). Insulin being an anabolic hormone promotes growth. Excess maternal glucose and amino acids provide the substrate for increased fetal protein, lipids, and glycogen synthesis. Large fetal size is due mainly to the accumulation of fat.

After birth, hyperinsulinemia causes respiratory distress, hypoglycemia, hypocalcemia, polycythemia, and hyperbilirubinemia. Hypocalcemia results from diminished production of parathormone. The increased red cell mass results in polycythemia and hyperbilirubinemia. As insulin retards the production of surfactant, that explains the higher risk of respiratory distress syndrome in these neonates.

### *Management*

Examine the infant at birth for malformations and injuries. Frequent breastfeeding prevents hypoglycemia. Monitor blood glucose levels periodically during the initial 48 to 72 hours. Other morbidities, such as respiratory distress and hyperbilirubinemia, require appropriate treatment.

*Competency:* **PE33.3**

### Hypothyroidism

Thyroid hormone is required for the fetus's and neonate's normal neural development.

Hypothyroidism is a common disorder during pregnancy. It can be overt or subclinical. Both types are associated with increased chances of miscarriage, pregnancy-induced hypertension, pre-eclampsia, placental abruption, postpartum hemorrhage, and stillbirths. The adverse neonatal outcomes include preterm birth, low birth weight, and increased perinatal mortality.

All pregnant women require TSH measurement during the first trimester. TSH level greater than 2.5 mIU/L in the first trimester and greater than 3.0 mIU/L in the second and third trimesters indicates hypothyroidism. Patients with overt hypothyroidism need treatment with levothyroxine. Certain patients with subclinical hypothyroidism and those with thyroid autoantibody also need treatment. Patients with pre-existing hypothyroidism often require dose escalation of levothyroxine during pregnancy.

### Tuberculosis

A neonate is at risk of tuberculosis infection, if the mother has active pulmonary tuberculosis that has been treated for less than two months before birth or if the diagnosis of tuberculosis was made after birth. However, such neonates should not be separated from their mothers. BCG vaccine is given at birth. Exclusive breastfeeding is encouraged.

The infant should be given isoniazid prophylaxis (10 mg/kg/day) and evaluated at 6 weeks:

- If there is evidence of tubercular infection, give anti-tubercular therapy
- If there is no evidence, continue isoniazid therapy for 6 months

### Hepatitis B Infection

Women who have hepatitis B infection (active or carrier stage) can transmit the infection to their neonates. Such neonates should receive the hepatitis B vaccine within 12 hr of birth, decreasing the risk of perinatal transmission by 70–90%. Additionally, hepatitis B immunoglobulins (HBIG; 100 IU, IM) can be given to enhance the protection by another 10–30%, but is costly and there are availability issues.

### Vitamin K Deficiency Bleeding

The incidence of the disorder, previously known as hemorrhagic disease of the newborn, has considerably reduced due to routine vitamin K prophylaxis at birth.

Neonates have low vitamin K levels due to the following reasons: (i) Poor transplacental transfer; (ii) low vitamin K content in the breast milk; and (iii) lack of gut colonization of bacteria synthesizing vitamin K.

There are three types of vitamin K deficiency bleeding during infancy (Table 9.43).

### Suggested Reading

1. Operational guidelines for injection of vitamin K prophylaxis at birth (in facilities). National Health Mission 2014.

## SPECIALIZED NEWBORN SCREENING BEFORE DISCHARGE

In most developed countries, all healthy neonates are screened for disorders like inborn error of metabolism (IEM), congenital hypothyroidism, congenital adrenal hyperplasia, critical cyanotic heart disease, and congenital hearing loss. These neonates are well in the initial few days of life. Timely screening helps in the early detection and treatment of these conditions and prevents serious complications.

### Pulse Oximeter Screening

Pulse oximetry screening at discharge or after 24 hours of birth helps detect critical congenital heart disease (CCHD). The CCHDs identified include hypoplastic left heart syndrome, pulmonary atresia, tetralogy of Fallot, total anomalous pulmonary venous return, D-transposition of the great arteries, tricuspid atresia, and truncus arteriosus.

**Table 9.43:** Types of vitamin K deficiency bleeding (VKDB)

| *Types* | *Risk factors* | *Clinical presentation* | *Prevention* |
|---|---|---|---|
| Early | Maternal intake of anticoagulants such as warfarin, anti-tubercular (rifampicin), and anticonvulsants (phenytoin, phenobarbitone) | Dangerous bleeding within 24 hours of birth. Intracranial bleeds are common | Mother should receive prophylactic vitamin K at least 24 hours before birth. Substitute the offending drugs, if possible<br>Neonatal vitamin K administration will not prevent early VKDB |
| Classic (most common) | No vitamin K prophylaxis at birth | Bleeding occurs after 24 hours of birth. The maximum incidence is in the first week of life.<br>Bleeding sites: Umbilical cord stump; GI tract; surgical wound<br>Intracranial bleed is rare | Vitamin K prophylaxis at birth prevents this complication<br>>1000 g: 1 mg IM<br><1000 g: 0.5 mg IM |
| Late | No vitamin K prophylaxis at birth; prolonged broad-spectrum antibiotic therapy; cholestasis and other malabsorption syndromes | Incidence: 2–12 weeks of age<br>Bleeding site: intracranial bleed (most common); GI tract | Vitamin K prophylaxis at birth prevents this complication |

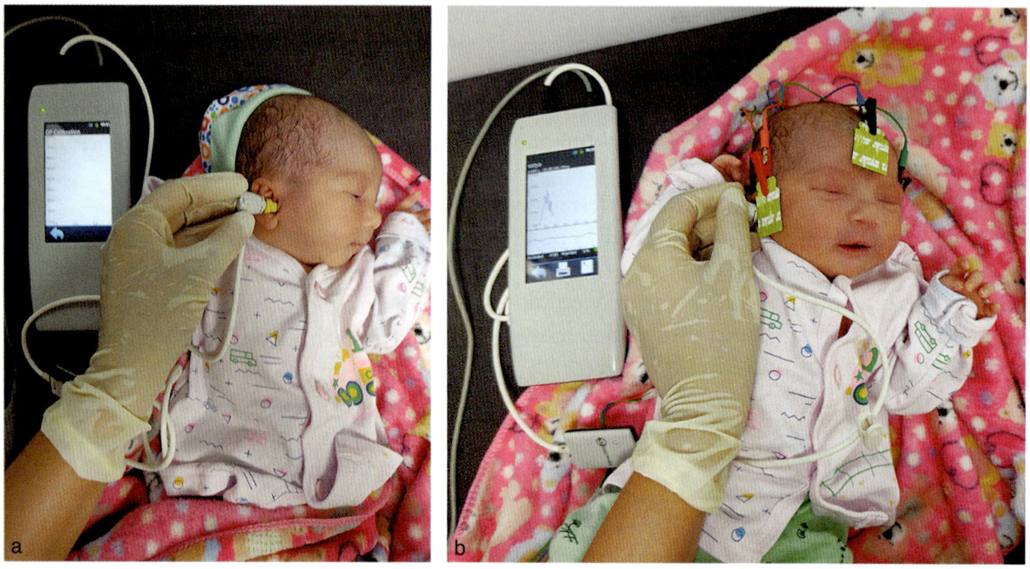

Fig. 9.81: (a) Hearing screening using otoacoustic emissions (a single probe emits the sound and receives the response); (b) Hearing screening with automated auditory brainstem response (the ear probe emits the sound, and scalp electrodes record the response) (*Photo courtesy:* Pragya Tyagi)

The screen has an excellent negative predictive value for ruling out CCHD.

### Hearing Screen

Normal hearing is critical for normal speech development. Routine screening can help early detection of hearing loss and facilitate the timely provision of hearing aid.

Hearing screening is performed at discharge/after 24 hours in neonates of 34 weeks or greater gestation. Perform screening in neonates lesser than 34 weeks once they complete 34 weeks of gestation. The screening tool could be either otoacoustic emissions (OAE) or automated auditory brainstem responses (AABR) for normal neonates. However, both OAE and AABR should be used for high-risk neonates **(Fig. 9.81)**. For those who fail the first screening, a repeat after 48 to 72 hours reduces the false positivity rate (two-step screening). Finally, a diagnostic auditory brainstem response (ABR) is performed to confirm the hearing loss. Such neonates need a hearing aid or cochlear implant by 6 months of age and speech rehabilitation. Any neonate with a normal hearing screen should be re-screened, if they develop any illness that can impair hearing, such as meningitis, if there is any parental concern for hearing, or if there is any red flag sign of normal speech development.

Chapter 10

# Immunization

Aditi Sinha

Immunization is a global health success story, ranking high among the most cost-effective strategies to prevent disease and save lives in all age groups. Globally, immunization is estimated to annually prevent 3.5–5 million deaths from common diseases. Important milestones achieved through immunization include the eradication of small-pox, widespread elimination (and near-eradication) of poliomyelitis. Currently licensed vaccines are designed to protect against 35 pathogens. Most recently, the development and rollout of vaccines against SARS-CoV-2 represent the fastest bench-to-bedside implementation in the history of vaccines, and the first large-scale implementation of vaccines based on mRNA and viral vectors.

## Definitions and Principles

A vaccine consists of killed or live-attenuated organisms or specific components of a pathogen that when administered to previously unexposed individuals, will elicit an immune response but not cause disease.

*Active immunity* is the protective response mounted by the immune system after a clinical or subclinical infection or vaccination. It comprises of humoral and/or cellular immune responses. Following first exposure (or first dose of a vaccine), the *primary* immune response develops slowly over 3–14 days and may not be sufficient to counteract the infection. The response involves formation of low titer IgM antibodies, followed by a smaller amount of IgG antibodies, activation of macrophages, induction of mononuclear inflammatory response, and delayed type hypersensitivity. Non-live vaccines usually require multiple doses to elicit satisfactory primary response. Host response to re-exposure to the infectious agent (or a booster dose of vaccine), termed *secondary* or *anamnestic* response, involves rapid (less than 3–4 days) production of high titers of high affinity IgG antibodies, which is usually sufficient to prevent disease, and provides protection for several years.

*Passive immunity* refers to protection from disease provided by introduction of preformed animal or human antibodies into the body. Examples include the passage of IgG from the mother across the placenta to the fetus, transmission of secretory IgA in breast milk, and administration of immunoglobulin or antisera to prevent disease. *Immunoglobulins* are glycoproteins produced by plasma cells that function as antibodies *in vivo*. *Antiserum* is blood-derived serum that contains polyclonal antibodies, e.g. against tetanus or diphtheria.

*Immunization* is the process of inducing immunity by administering a vaccine prior to natural exposure to infectious agent (active immunization), or preformed antibodies soon after exposure, in order to suppress disease (passive immunization).

*Vaccination* is the process of administering a vaccine. This elicits predominantly humoral immune response (*H. influenzae* vaccine), cellular immunity (BCG), or both responses (most vaccines).

*Adjuvants* are substances unrelated to the organism that, when added to a vaccine, enhance its immunogenicity, by stimulating lymphocytes nonspecifically or enabling slow release of antigen. Examples include aluminum hydroxide and lipids.

*Seroconversion* is the change from antibody negative to antibody positive state, due to induction of antibodies in response to infection or vaccination. In a person with detectable antibodies before vaccination, it is defined as at least a fourfold rise from the pre-vaccination titer.

*Seroprotection* is the state of protection from disease, due to the presence of detectable serum levels of antibody in protective titers.

*Immunogenicity* is the ability of a vaccine to induce antibodies to achieve seroprotective titers, and/or the desired level of cell-mediated immune response, as measured by specific tests.

*Protective efficacy* of a vaccine is its ability to protect against disease, assessed as follows:

$$\text{Efficacy} = \frac{\text{Rate of disease in unvaccinated} - \text{Rate of disease in vaccinated persons}}{\text{Rate of disease in unvaccinated persons}} \times 100$$

Live viral vaccines (measles, rubella) and toxoids are more efficacious than BCG and killed bacterial vaccines.

*Vaccine effectiveness* is the ability of a vaccine to protect the population from disease. It is usually assessed in the context of an immunization program. It depends on vaccine efficacy as well as various aspects of program implementation (e.g. coverage, cold chain maintenance, injection technique, age of recipients, and dosing frequency and interval). Vaccine effectiveness is usually lower than its efficacy, but may be increased by herd effect. Effectiveness is measured using disease rates, odds ratio of disease in vaccinated and unvaccinated population, and studies of seroprevalence.

*Vaccine failure* is the occurrence of disease in an individual despite vaccination. *Primary* vaccine failure is the inability of the recommended dose(s) to induce an immune response, while *secondary* failure refers to occurrence of disease despite an immune response. Vaccine failure is rare with measles, diphtheria and tetanus vaccines. Primary vaccine failure may occur with oral poliovirus vaccine (OPV); secondary failure is seen with BCG, pertussis and typhoid vaccines.

### Epidemiological Terms

*Disease control:* Reduction of disease incidence, prevalence, transmission, duration, morbidity or mortality to a level where the public health burden is significantly reduced; e.g. the control of infections causing acute watery diarrhea. However, continued intervention is required to maintain control.

*Disease elimination:* Reduction of the incidence of a specific infectious disease to zero in a defined geographical area, with no endemic transmission persisting; e.g. neonatal tetanus, measles, rubella, poliomyelitis. Continued measures are required to prevent re-establishment of transmission.

*Disease eradication:* Permanent reduction of the worldwide incidence of infection caused by a specific agent to zero; e.g. smallpox. This is usually achieved through prolonged containment and surveillance; intervention measures are no longer required.

*Disease extinction:* The specific infectious agent no longer exists in nature or in laboratories. This has not been achieved for any known human infection.

*Herd effect:* If a large proportion of susceptible individuals are protected from infection with an organism by simultaneous vaccination, the transmission chain is broken by reduced carriage of the microorganism by vaccinated individuals, thus decreasing the risk of disease even among the unimmunized. This phenomenon is less marked for vaccines: (i) that protect only against disease (diphtheria) than those that prevent infection (measles or OPV); (ii) with low protective efficacy (pertussis and typhoid); and (iii) against diseases where humans are not the chief reservoir (tetanus). Herd effect is a strategy for eradication of poliovirus, and measles epidemics. *Herd immunity* refers to the proportion of immune individuals in a population. The minimum proportion of population that must be immunized to eliminate disease is called the *herd immunity threshold.*

*Epidemiological shift* refers to a significant change in the pattern of disease in a population following immunization. Immunization with trivalent OPV caused selective extinction of type 2 poliovirus, due to higher efficacy against that subtype. Following partial immunization coverage, some diseases (hepatitis A, varicella, rubella) affect older individuals with more severe disease.

*Surveillance:* This refers to the collection, collation, analysis and dissemination of information regarding the epidemiology and burden of disease. Apart from monitoring progress towards disease control, elimination or eradication, it helps detect outbreaks, monitor the effectiveness of vaccines, and plan public health strategies. Examples of surveillance strategies for vaccine-preventable diseases include those used for poliomyelitis eradication, measles control, acute encephalitis syndrome or bacterial meningitis (sentinel surveillance), and understanding seroprevalence of SARS-CoV-2, HIV or hepatitis B infection (periodic population-based seroprevalence survey).

## Types of Vaccines

A good vaccine is easy to administer, induces permanent immunity, is free of toxic substances, has minimal side effects and is stable for prolonged time (Table 10.1).

Table 10.1: Types of vaccines

| *Description* | *Example* |
|---|---|
| Live attenuated | Bacillus Calmette–Guérin, oral typhoid (Ty21a), oral poliovirus, measles, mumps, rubella, varicella, rotavirus, yellow fever, influenza (intranasal), hepatitis A |
| Killed or inactivated | Whole cell pertussis, inactivated poliovirus, rabies, hepatitis A, influenza, SARS-CoV-2 |
| Toxoid | Diphtheria, tetanus |
| **Subunit vaccines** | |
| Capsular polysaccharide | Typhoid (Vi), *Hemophilus influenzae* b, meningococcal, pneumococcal |
| Conjugated | *Hemophilus influenzae* b, meningococcal, pneumococcal |
| Recombinant | Acellular pertussis, hepatitis B, papillomavirus |
| Viral vector-borne | SARS-CoV-2 |

Timing of administration depends on the ability to mount immune response, age at which the disease is anticipated and feasibility.

*Live attenuated vaccines* infect the recipient and replicate to elicit cellular and humoral immune responses. They mimic natural infection but do not cause disease, except rarely in immunocompromised hosts. While a single dose is usually sufficient to induce immunity, OPV may need multiple doses to infect the intestinal mucosa. Residual maternal antibody in infant blood may neutralize the organism before infection occurs, interrupting immune response. Hence, vaccines like measles and measles, mumps and rubella (MMR) are given after 9 months of age. Maternally derived antibodies do not interfere with vaccine response to BCG that induces cell-mediated immunity, and OPV that infects gut mucosa. Live vaccines may confer herd immunity.

*Killed vaccines,* prepared by growing organisms in media followed by heat or chemical inactivation, do not cause infection but elicit protective immune response. Interference by maternal antibodies is less significant. However, multiple doses are required since the organism cannot replicate in the vaccinee. The immunity is not permanent; booster doses are necessary to ensure prolonged protection.

*Toxoids* are modified and purified toxins that are not injurious to recipients. Primary immunization is provided as multiple divided doses in order to decrease adverse effects at each administration and to elicit high antibody titers. Booster doses are required to sustain the protection.

*Subunit vaccines,* including viral or bacterial antigens, are produced using recombinant DNA technology or genetic engineering **(Table 10.1)**. Conjugated vaccines are often preferred over polysaccharide vaccines **(Table 10.2)**.

### Vaccination Route

Locations for intramuscular (IM) administration (22–25 gauge needle) include the anterolateral aspect of the thigh in infants and deltoid in upper arm in older children and adults **(Fig. 10.1)**. Gluteal administration is avoided to reduce risk of injuring the sciatic nerve. Hepatitis B vaccine is particularly not given in the gluteal region as this has reduced efficacy. If required, two vaccines may be given in the same thigh, but separated by 1 inch. Separate sites are used when administering a vaccine and an immunoglobulin. Preferred locations for subcutaneous vaccines (25–27 gauge needle) include the anterolateral thigh in infants and upper outer aspect of triceps in older children. Intradermal injection (25–27 gauge needle) is given in skin overlying the deltoid.

### Principles of Immunization

Compliance with the recommended dose and route of vaccination is essential to retain efficacy and limit adverse events. Important considerations are shown in **Box 10.1**.

Vaccines available as lyophilized powder are reconstituted in: (i) Sterile or distilled water, e.g. vaccines against measles, mumps, rubella, meningococcus (MPSV4), rabies and varicella; (ii) normal saline, e.g. Hib vaccine; or (iii) another vaccine, e.g. combined vaccination with separately available DTaP, inactivated polio and Hib vaccines. The maximum time allowed between reconstitution and use varies from 30 minutes (DTaP-IPV-Hib, MMRV, Hib with MenCY, rabies, varicella and zoster), to 8 hours (MMR, meningococcal) or 24 hours (Hib, rotavirus vaccines). Reconstituted vaccines are not used, if there is discoloration, particulate matter and inability to suspend the lyophilized powder.

### Suggested Reading


1. Miller E, Wodi AP. General best practice guidance for immunization. In: Hall E, Wodi AP, Hamborsky J (eds). Centers for Disease Control and Prevention. Epidemiology and prevention of vaccine-preventable diseases. 14th edn. Washington DC, Public Health Foundation, 2021; pp: 9–28.


*Competencies:* **PE19.1; PE19.6**

## VACCINATION SCHEDULES AND IMMUNIZATION PROGRAMS

The *Expanded Programme on Immunization (EPI)*, introduced by the World Health Organization (1974), was the first global immunization initiative. Adopted by India in 1978, the EPI focused on vaccinating young children with BCG, diphtheria and tetanus toxoids and whole cell pertussis

**Table 10.2:** Comparison of subunit polysaccharide and conjugate vaccines

| *Characteristic* | *Polysaccharide vaccine* | *Conjugated vaccine* |
|---|---|---|
| Component | Carbohydrate present in bacterial cell surface (capsule) | Polysaccharide attached to carrier protein that is recognized by host as foreign antigen |
| Immune cells stimulated; response elicited | B cells; humoral immunity, thymic independent | B and T cells; humoral and cellular immunity; thymic dependent |
| Antibodies type and titer | Chiefly IgM; low titer (low immunogenicity) | Both IgM and IgG; high titer (high immunogenicity) |
| Duration of protection | Brief | Longer and consistent |
| Age at which effective | Poor immunogenicity and efficacy <2 years of age | Immunogenic and effective in infancy or older age |
| Response elicited by booster/repeated dose | Poor | Satisfactory |
| Examples | Pneumococcal (PPSV23), meningococcal (A, C, W135, Y) and typhoid polysaccharide vaccines | Pneumococcal (PCV7, PCV13), *Hemophilus influenzae* type b, typhoid and meningococcal conjugate vaccines |

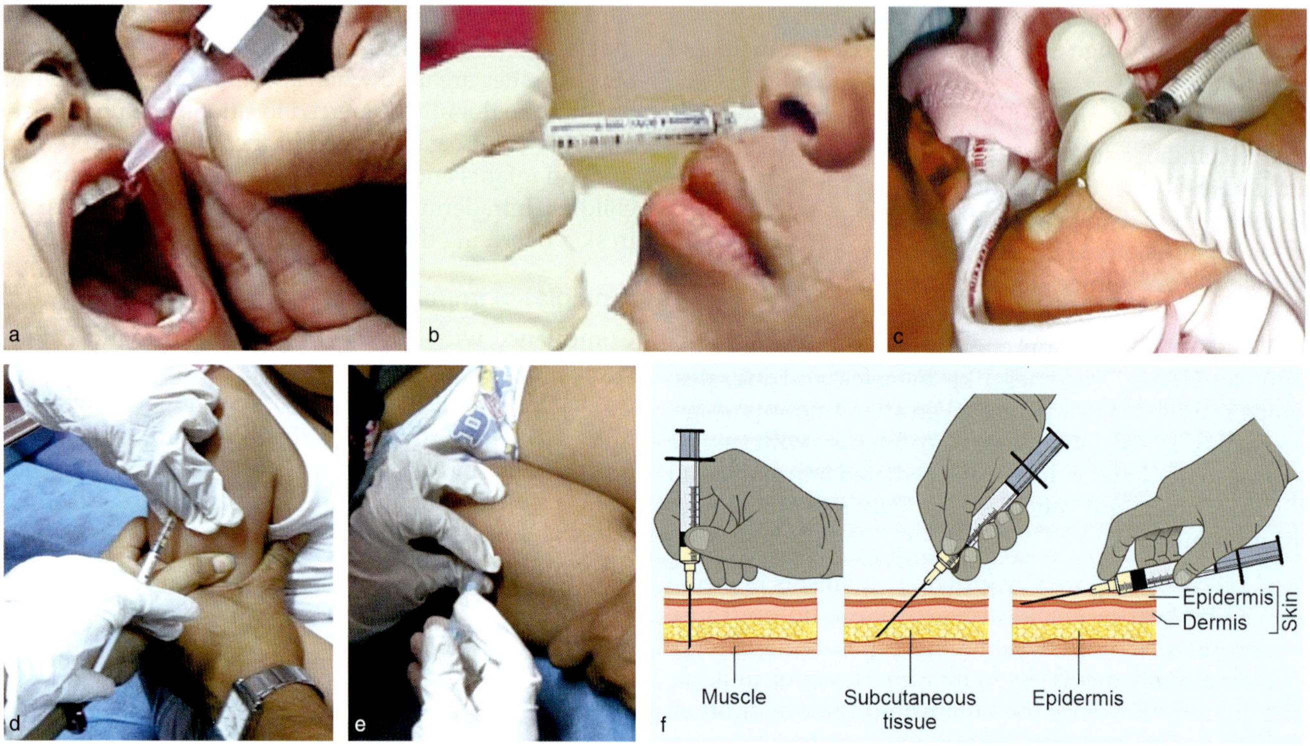


**Fig. 10.1:** Routes of vaccination: (a) Oral: Poliovirus, rotavirus; (b) Intranasal: Influenza virus; (c) Intradermal: BCG, inactivated poliovirus (fractionated dose) and (sometimes) rabies; (d) Subcutaneous: Measles, mumps, rubella, varicella, yellow fever, and pneumococcal polysaccharide; (e) Intramuscular: Most vaccines, including hepatitis A and B; diphtheria, tetanus and pertussis, *H. influenzae* b, pneumococcal polysaccharide, inactivated polio and influenza; (f) Note the variations in the angle of insertion of the needle through the skin when administering the vaccine by the intramuscular (90°), subcutaneous (45°), and intradermal (10–15°) routes

### Box 10.1: Principles of Immunization

- Different live (oral, parenteral, intranasal) vaccines may be given simultaneously, or 4 weeks apart.
- Different types of inactivated or subunit vaccines may be administered simultaneously or at any interval between their doses.
- Exceptions to these rules are as follows: (i) Pneumococcal conjugate and polysaccharide vaccines (to improve immunogenicity, the former should precede the latter by at least 8 weeks); (ii) varicella and smallpox vaccines; and (iii) in patients with functional or anatomic asplenia or HIV, pneumococcal conjugate and MenACWY-D (Menactra) vaccine (when both are indicated, the former should precede the latter, by at least 4 weeks)
- A minimum interval of 4 weeks between two doses of the same vaccine is necessary to ensure adequate immune responses. An exception is the rabies vaccine.
- There is no minimum recommended time interval between two types of vaccines. Hence, a live and an inactivated vaccine can be administered simultaneously or at any interval of time.
- When necessary, two vaccines can be given in the same limb at a single visit, preferring the anterolateral thigh for simultaneous IM injections; vaccines are administered at least 1-inch apart.
- Vaccines should not be given earlier than indicated or with shorter interval between doses than indicated in the routine immunization schedule. However, it is permissible to administer a dose up to 4 days before the minimum age or interval to avoid missing an opportunity to vaccinate.
- A delay or lapse in the administration of a dose does not require the schedule to be repeated; the missed dose is administered and the course resumed at the point it was interrupted. Delaying the dose does not affect adversely the rates of seroconversion or titers.
- Vaccines should not be mixed in a syringe, unless approved by the manufacturer.
- Patients should be observed for allergic reactions for 15–20 minutes after receiving immunization.
- Immunization is not contraindicated in minor illness, prematurity, allergies, malnutrition or during infection and antibiotic therapy.
- Live vaccines are contraindicated in inherited or acquired immunodeficiency and during therapy with immunosuppressive drugs, but may be given after a short (<2 weeks) course of low dose steroids.
- Immunoglobulins interfere with the immune response to certain live vaccines like mumps, measles and rubella, but not OPV, yellow fever, oral typhoid vaccine, and/or inactivated vaccines.
- Hepatitis B, tetanus toxoid and rabies vaccine may be given concurrently with corresponding immunoglobulin. However, the vaccine should be administered at a site distant from where the immunoglobulin is injected.
- Active, with or without passive, immunization should follow exposure to rabies, measles, varicella, tetanus and hepatitis B

(DTP or DTwP) and OPV vaccines, and chiefly covered urban areas. The *Universal Immunization Programme* (UIP, 1985) improved nationwide coverage of immunization and also included measles vaccine. The *Pulse Polio Immunization Programme* (1995) enabled polio control. UIP has remained a key component of the Child Survival and Safe Motherhood Programme (1992), the Reproductive and Child Health Programme (1997) and National Rural Health Mission (NHRM, 2005).

**Figure 10.2** depicts milestones in the national immunization program and current national schedule. Recent initiatives under the UIP include the introduction of inactivated poliovirus (2015), rotavirus vaccine (introduced in 2016 to reach all states in 2019), and the measles-rubella campaign (since 2019). Currently, the UIP provides free-of-cost immunization against 11 vaccine-preventable diseases in all states, including diphtheria, pertussis, tetanus, polio, measles, rubella, tuberculosis, rotavirus diarrhea, hepatitis B, meningitis and pneumonia caused by *Hemophilus influenzae* type B and pneumococcal pneumonia. Vaccination against Japanese encephalitis is provided in endemic districts and against human papillomavirus in selected states (**Table 10.3** and **Fig. 10.3**).

***Mission Indradhanush:*** Despite the UIP being operational for three decades, surveys had indicated that only 65% of infants received full immunization coverage. In 2014, the Government of India launched 'Mission Indradhanush' to strengthen UIP and achieve full immunization coverage rapidly **(Box 10.2)**. The mission derives its name from the seven diseases prevented through the vaccines (BCG, OPV, pentavalent and TT vaccines) initially included in the program, and focuses on complete immunization of all children less than 2-year-old and on pregnant women. Five additional vaccines that were subsequently included during various phases of the Intensified Mission Indradhanush

| Year | Vaccination policy change | Diseases, n |
|---|---|---|
| 1978 | Expanded Programme on Immunization (EPI) | 6 |
| | BCG, OPV, typhoid and DPT | |
| 1983 | TT vaccine | |
| 1985 | Universal Immunization Programme (UIP) | 6 |
| | Measles vaccine one dose introduced | |
| | Typhoid discontinued | |
| | Cold chain implemented nationwide | |
| 1995 | Pulse polio immunization campaign | |
| 2002 | Hepatitis B immunization (in some states) | 7 |
| 2006 | Japanese encephalitis (JE) vaccine (in endemic districts) | 8 |
| 2010 | Hepatitis B vaccine scaled up to entire country | |
| | Measles vaccine second dose | |
| 2011 | Pentavalent (DPT+HBV+HiB) vaccine (in some states) | 9 |
| 2013 | JE vaccine second dose (in endemic districts) | |
| 2014 | JE vaccine for adults (in endemic districts) | |
| 2015 | Inactivated poliovirus vaccine (IPV, in some states) | |
| | Mission Indradhanush | |
| 2016 | Rotavirus vaccine (in some states) | 11 |
| | Human papillomavirus vaccine (in some states) | |
| | Switch from trivalent to bivalent OPV, in entire country | |
| | IPV scaled up to entire country | |
| 2017 | Measles-rubella vaccination campaign | 13 |
| | Intensified Mission Indradhanush | |
| 2019 | Pneumococcal conjugate vaccine (PCV, in some states) | |
| | Td instead of TT at 10 yr, at 16 yr and in pregnant women | |
| 2021–22 | Rotavirus vaccine scaled up to entire country | 14 |
| | PCV scaled up to entire country | |
| | Measles rubella vaccine scaled up to entire country | |
| | SARS-CoV-2 vaccine in adults and adolescents | |

**Fig. 10.2:** Milestones in the National Immunization Program. The program that started with four vaccines against six infectious illnesses now provides coverage against 13 childhood infections

**Table 10.3:** Comparison of the national immunization schedule with the schedule recommended by the Indian Academy of Pediatrics

| *Age* | *National Immunization Schedule* | *Indian Academy of Pediatrics schedule*[1] |
|---|---|---|
| At birth | BCG, bOPV-0, HBV-0 | BCG, bOPV-0[#], HBV-1 |
| 6 weeks | bOPV-1, Pentavalent-1, Rota-1, fIPV-1, PCV-1 | DTP-1, Hib-1, HBV-2, IPV-1, Rota-1, PCV-1 |
| 10 weeks | bOPV-2, Pentavalent-2, Rota-2 | DTP-2, Hib-2, HBV-3, IPV-2, Rota-2, PCV-2 |
| 14 weeks | bOPV-3, Pentavalent-3, Rota-3, fIPV-2, PCV-2 | DTP-3, Hib-3, HBV-4, IPV-3, Rota-3, PCV-3 |
| 6–9 months | | Inactivated influenza-1 and -2[2]; typhoid conjugate vaccine |
| 9 months | MR-1, JE-1[3], PCV-3, fIPV-3 | MMR-1 |
| 12–15 months | | HAV-1, MMR-2, Varicella-1, PCV-B1, JE-1[3] |
| 16–18 months | DTwP-B1, bOPV-B, JE-2[3], MR-2 | DTP-B1, Hib-B1, IPV-B1, JE-2[3] |
| 18–24 months | | HAV-2, Varicella-2 |
| 5–6 years | DTwP-B2 | DTP-B2, MMR-3, IPV-B2 |
| 10–12 years | Td | Tdap[4] |
| 9–14 years | HPV-1, HPV-2[5] | HPV-1 and -2 (6 months apart)[6] |
| 16 years | Td | |

B booster; BCG Bacillus Calmette–Guerin; bOPV bivalent oral poliovirus; DTP diphtheria, pertussis, tetanus either whole cell (DTwP) or acellular (DTaP); fIPV fractionated inactivated poliovirus; HAV hepatitis A virus; HBV hepatitis B virus; Hib *Hemophilus (H.) influenzae b*; HPV human papillomavirus; IPV inactivated poliovirus; JE Japanese encephalitis; MMR mumps, measles, rubella; MR measles, rubella; PCV pneumococcal conjugate vaccine; Pentavalent DTwP + HBV + *H. influenzae* b; Rota rotavirus;

[1]Preferred schedule detailed under respective vaccines; vaccination in high-risk groups not shown; [2]Doses given one month apart, then annually till 5-yr-old; [3]Only in endemic areas; [4]Subsequently, a dose of Td every ten years; [5]Where implemented; [6]If >15-yr-old, give three doses at 0, 1 and 6 months

| Age | At birth | 6 weeks | 10 weeks | 14 weeks | 6–9 months | 9–12 months | 12–15 months | 16–18 months | 18–24 months | 4–6 years | 10–12 years | 9–14 years | 16 years |
|---|---|---|---|---|---|---|---|---|---|---|---|---|---|
| BCG | 1 | | | | | | | | | | | | |
| Hepatitis $B_1$ | 1 | 2 | 3 | 4 | | | | | | | | | |
| Poliovirus[1] | bOPV 0 | bOPV 1 | bOPV 2 | bOPV 3 | | | | bOPV B | | | | | |
| | | IPV-1 | IPV-2 | IPV-2 or -3 | | IPV-3 | | | IPV-B1 | | IPV-B1 | | |
| DTwP/DTaP | | 1 | 2 | 3 | | | | B1 | | B2 | | | |
| Hib | | 1 | 2 | 3 | | | | B1 | | | | | |
| PCV | | 1 | 2 | 2 or 3 | | 3 | B1 | | | | | | |
| Rotavirus | | 1 | 2 | 3 | | | | | | | | | |
| Measles-containing vaccine | | | | | | MR-1 or MMR-1 | | MR-2 or MMR-2 | | | MMR-3 | | |
| Tdap/Td | | | | | | | | | | | 1 | | 2 |
| Japanese encephalitis[2] | | | | | | 1 | 1 | 2 | | | | | |
| Human papillomavirus[2] | | | | | | | | | | | | 1 and 2 | 1, 2 and 3 |
| Typhoid conjugate | | | | | 1 | | | | | | | | |
| Influenza | | | | | 1 | | | | 2 | 3, 4 and 5 | | | |
| Hepatitis A | | | | | | | 1 | | 2 | | | | |
| Varicella | | | | | | | 1 | | 2 | | | | |

| KEY | Recommended age | Catch up immunization |
|---|---|---|
| Universal Immunization Programme only | | |
| Indian Academy of Pediatrics only | | |
| Both Schedules | | |

**Fig. 10.3:** Vaccination schedules of the Universal Immunization Programme and Indian Academy of Pediatrics (2022). Details are under respective vaccines. [1]Bivalent oral poliovirus (bOPV) or injectable inactivated poliovirus (IPV); [2]Only in selected areas. B booster; BCG Bacillus Calmette–Guerin; bOPV bivalent oral poliovirus; DTP diphtheria, pertussis, tetanus, either whole cell (w) or acellular (a) pertussis; HAV hepatitis A virus; HBV hepatitis B virus; Hib *Hemophilus influenzae* b; HPV human papillomavirus; IPV inactivated poliovirus; JE Japanese encephalitis; MMR mumps, measles, rubella; MR measles, rubella; PCV pneumococcal conjugate vaccine; Td tetanus toxioid, reduced dose diphtheria toxoid; Tdap Td with reduced dose acellular pertussis vaccine

are those that protect against measles-rubella (MR), and in selected states or districts, rotavirus diarrhea, Japanese encephalitis, and pneumococcal conjugate vaccine. The most recent phase of the Intensified Mission Indradhanush (4.0) is ongoing in 2022 and has focused on ensuring routine immunization coverage that was disrupted by the restrictions imposed during the COVID-19 pandemic **(Box 10.2)**. Data from the National Family Health Survey-5 (2019-21) suggests that three-fourth (76.4%) of Indian children have completed primary immunization, with similar coverage for urban and rural areas (75.5% versus 76.8%).

### *Immunization Schedule of the Indian Academy of Pediatrics (IAP)*

The IAP Advisory Committee on Vaccines and Immunization Practices (ACVIP) endorses the National Immunization Program, but recommends certain additional vaccines based on regional burden of vaccine preventable diseases and the availability, safety and efficacy of various vaccines. **Figure 10.3** and **Table 10.3** compare the national program and recommendations of the IAP.

### Suggested Reading

1. Kasi SG, Shivananda S, Marathe S, et al. IAP Advisory Committee on Vaccines and Immunization Practices (ACVIP): Recommended immunization schedule (2020-21) and update on immunization for children aged 0 through 18 years. Indian Pediatr 2021;58:44–53.
2. Ministry of Health and Family Welfare, GOI. Universal Immunization Programme (UIP). Available at www.mohfw.gov.in; last accessed 15 June 2022.

*Competencies:* **PE19.2; PE19.3; PE19.16**

## COMMONLY USED VACCINES

The following section describes vaccines recommended in the national immunization program or Indian Academy of Pediatrics for normal children and certain high-risk groups.

### BCG Vaccine

Bacillus Calmette–Guérin (BCG) vaccine contains bacilli derived from subcultures of live attenuated *M. bovis* Calmette–Guérin strain. The vaccine used in India is the Copenhagen (Danish 1331) strain produced at Guindy (Tamil Nadu) and is available as lyophilized powder in vacuum-sealed dark multidose vials. When reconstituted with sterile normal saline, each dose (0.1 mL) contains 0.1–0.4 million live viable bacilli. This heat and light sensitive vaccine is stable in lyophilized form at 2–8°C for one year, but loses potency rapidly when reconstituted.

BCG vaccine primarily induces cell-mediated immunity. The response to BCG vaccine ('take') is reduced by exposure to environmental non-tuberculosis mycobacteria, considered inversely proportional to the latitude; i.e. individuals living in the areas away from the equator have higher response to the vaccine. Meta-analyses estimate that

## Box 10.2: Mission Indradhanush

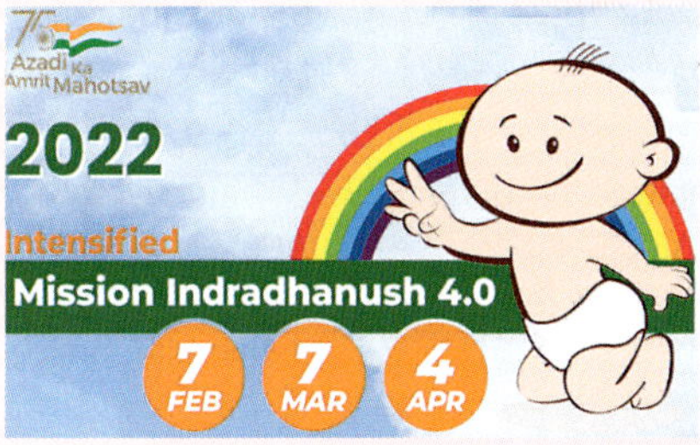


**Mission Indradhanush**

*Launched:* December 2014

*Objective:* Fully immunize >90% of infants by 2020

*Strategy:* Special immunization drives; intense efforts in focus areas

*Achievements:* By August 2017, annual increment in immunization coverage increased from 1% in 2014 to 6.7% in 2015

**Intensified Mission Indradhanush (IMI)**

*Launched:* October 2017

*Objectives:* Fully immunize >90% newborns by December 2018

*Additional aspects:* (i) Need based interventions; (ii) strengthen involvement of relevant non-health departments; (iii) enhanced accountability; (iv) vaccination on demand to children ≥5 years

*Implementation:* Week-long immunization drives from 7th of each month

**IMI 2.0**

*Launched:* December 2019

*Objectives:* Reach the unreached; accelerate coverage in identified areas

*Additional aspects:* Commemorated the 25th anniversary of Pulse Polio Campaign

*Focus areas for coverage:* 272 districts in 27 states

**IMI 3.0**

*Launched:* February 2021

*Objectives:* Reach the unreached with all available vaccines; accelerate the coverage in the identified districts and blocks

*Focus areas for coverage:* 250 high-risk districts; migrant populations and hard to reach areas

**IMI 4.0**

*Launched:* February 2022

*Objectives:* Reach the unvaccinated and partially vaccinated children <2-yr and pregnant women, especially those who missed vaccination during the pandemic

*Focus areas for coverage:* 416 districts, including 378 districts prioritized for immunization, and 75 districts selected for the 'Azadi ka Amrit Mahotsav', with focus on: (i) Areas with immunization services disrupted due to pandemic; (ii) areas with high burden of COVID cases (e.g. containment areas); (iii) high-risk areas, as defined for polio eradication activities including non-migratory/settled and migrant high-risk areas; (iv) newborns delivered at home; (iv) villages/areas with vacant subcenters, ≥2 consecutive missed routine immunization sessions; (v) hard-to-reach areas, areas with vaccine hesitancy; (vi) urban areas, especially slums; (vii) areas with high incidence of measles and other vaccine-preventable diseases; (viii) orphanage, prisons, red-light areas, riverine areas, agricultural migrants; (ix) tribal areas; (x) areas hit by natural calamities, geopolitical or other conflicts

**Outcomes**

- 701 districts covered in the first ten phases
- Increase in 'full immunization coverage' by 6.7% in the first two phases
- Increase in 'full immunization coverage' among 12–23-month-old from 62% (NFHS-4) to 76.4% (NFHS-5)

the vaccine has low protective efficacy against primary infection (~40%), pulmonary infection (8–79%), all forms (~50%) of tuberculosis, and re-infection. However, it enables satisfactory (72–100%) protection against severe forms of tuberculosis (miliary tuberculosis, tubercular meningitis) and reduces the risk of mortality. As childhood tuberculosis accounts for 15–20% cases and is often disseminated, vaccine administration in infancy prevents serious morbidity. Since maternal antibodies do not interfere with cellular immune responses, BCG is given at birth to ensure both compliance and early protection. While immunity typically wanes over 10–15 years, repeating vaccination in adolescence or adulthood does not extend protection.

BCG vaccine is now part of routine immunization at birth in many countries. While vaccination in newborn period is routine in east Europe, a few countries in Europe practice vaccinating chiefly in adolescence, and countries with low endemicity (e.g. United States, Canada) vaccinate only the high-risk groups (immigrants, healthcare professionals, children exposed to patients with tuberculosis). The BCG vaccine has also been examined for its role in protecting against leprosy and COVID-19, and as an immunomodulator in atopy or certain malignancies (e.g. bladder cancer).

Conventionally, BCG vaccine is administered at insertion of the deltoid on the left shoulder to allow easy identification of its scar **(Box 10.3)**. Intradermal injection using a 26 G needle raises a 5–7 mm wheal. Bacilli multiply to form a papule about 4–8 mm wide by one week, ulcerates by 3–6 weeks, and heals by scarring by 6–12 weeks. Alternative methods of intradermal injection, e.g. jet or multiple puncture, are not recommended.

Inadvertent subcutaneous injection causes persistent ulceration and ipsilateral axillary or cervical lymphadenopathy. Children with severe immunodeficiency may develop disseminated BCG disease 6–12 months after vaccination. Hence, vaccination is contraindicated in severe congenital and acquired immunodeficiency syndrome

**Box 10.3: Bacillus Calmette-Guérin (BCG) Vaccine**

| | |
|---|---|
| *Dose, route* | 0.1 mL; intradermal |
| *Site* | Left upper arm at insertion of deltoid |
| *Schedule* | |
| National program | At birth; catch up till 1-yr (if missed) |
| IAP 2021 | At birth; catch up till 5-yr |
| *Adverse reactions* | Local ulceration; discharging sinus; axillary lymphadenitis<br>If immunodeficient, disseminated infection, osteomyelitis; scrofuloderma |
| *Contraindications* | Cellular immunodeficiency; symptomatic HIV |
| *Storage* | 2–8°C; sensitive to heat and light<br>Discard reconstituted vaccine after 4 hr |



(SCID, AIDS). Given the benefits of vaccination, the WHO recommends vaccinating all HIV-positive infants, including patients stable on antiretroviral therapy, except in countries with low endemicity where the vaccine is not included in the routine immunization schedules.

Certain inactivated, protein subunit and viral-vector vaccines are being examined as safer candidates for immunosuppressed individuals. Proposed tuberculosis vaccines under evaluation for prevention of infection and/or disease include naturally attenuated mycobacteria (e.g. *M. vaccae*, *M. microti*), *M. tuberculosis* attenuated by deletion of virulent genes (e.g. MTBVAC); recombinant vaccines carrying *M. tuberculosis* antigen (e.g. 85A antigen) in living viral or bacterial vector (e.g. attenuated adenovirus, *Vaccinia*, influenza A, or *Salmonella*); and subunit vaccines, manufactured using natural, synthetic or recombinant technology, to carry one or more tubercular antigens (e.g. 85A, 85B, ESAT-6, Mtb32, Mtb39, CFP10,) as protein, DNA or DNA motifs, with or without adjuvants.

### Suggested Reading

1. Weerasuriya CK, Clark RA, White RG, Harris RC. New tuberculosis vaccines: Advances in clinical development and modelling. J Intern Med 2020; 288: 661–81.
2. Yadav J, Verma S, Chaudhary D, et al. Tuberculosis: Current status, diagnosis, treatment and development of novel vaccines. Curr Pharm Biotechnol 2019; 20: 446–58.

## Poliomyelitis Vaccines

Vaccination is an important strategy for preventing paralytic poliomyelitis, caused by poliovirus serotypes 1– 3, chiefly in young children. Two types of vaccines are available: live attenuated oral poliovirus vaccine (OPV) and inactivated poliovirus vaccine (IPV). Figure 10.4 depicts the currently used and proposed poliovirus vaccines.

### *Oral Polio Vaccine (OPV)*

OPV contains the live strain of Sabin polioviruses, which has been attenuated by repeated passage in monkey kidney cell cultures and stabilized with magnesium chloride. When administered orally, the vaccine viruses infect the intestinal mucosa and multiply in mucosal cells. Mucosal immunity protects from paralytic poliomyelitis by reducing

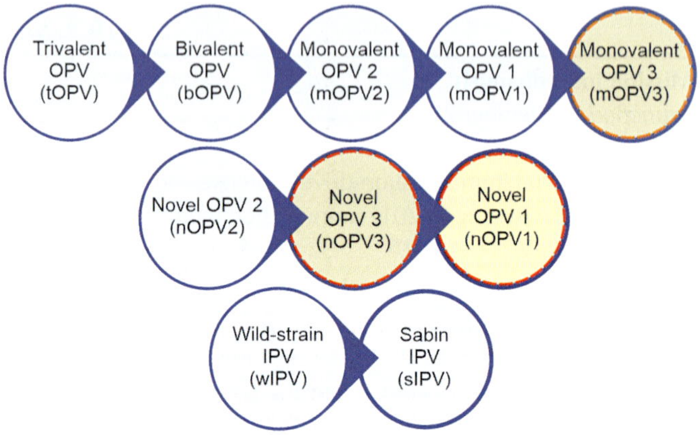


**Fig. 10.4:** Current and future vaccines against poliomyelitis: Those in development and yet to be deployed are shown in orange circles. The trivalent oral poliovirus vaccine (tOPV) has been replaced globally by the bivalent OPV (bOPV) to improve the vaccine's immunogenicity and reduce the risk of circulating vaccine-derived poliomyelitis viruses (cVPDV), by removing OPV serotype 2. Monovalent OPV types 1 (mOPV1) and 3 (mOPV3) are similarly more immunogenic than tOPV are used in supplemental immunization campaigns. The novel oral poliomyelitis vaccine type 2 (nOPV2) was developed from mOPV2 by genetically stabilizing it, making it less likely to revert to forms that cause cVPDV2 in settings of low population immunity. Similarly, novel genetically stable strains for serotypes 1 and 3 (nOPV1, nOPV3) are likely to replace mOPV1, mOPV3 and bOPV. The Sabin-inactivated poliovirus (sIPV) has lower biosafety risk than the conventional Salk-IPV, and can be produced at lower costs in developing countries

the chances of infection when wild-type poliovirus is encountered. Following vaccination, wild virus is excreted for shorter periods and in fewer numbers, reducing feco-oral transmission and interrupting wild virus circulation. However, multiple OPV doses are essential to ensure appropriate response. Compared to IPV, OPV induces better mucosal immunity, and hence, rapid protection and 'herd' immunity; however, mucosal responses are relatively short-lived as compared to systemic immunity generated by IPV. To decrease chances of vaccine failure, at least three doses are required 4–8 weeks apart. The administration of 'zero' dose at birth enhances seroconversion.

Each dose (2 drops) of trivalent OPV contained $10^5$–$10^6$ median cell culture infectious doses of each serotype 1, 2 and 3. There is no cross-protection between viral subtypes. Seroconversion rates following administration of trivalent OPV are overall lower in developing regions as compared to developed countries. Vaccine 'take' in the former setting is affected by competition by other enteroviruses, concomitant diarrhea, interference by maternal antibodies, and interruptions in the vaccine cold chain.

Serotype 2 is the most immunogenic of the three serotypes, and interferes with the immunogenicity of serotypes 1 and 3. It is estimated that 13–15 doses of trivalent OPV are required to achieve the population immunity threshold necessary to stop virus circulation for types 1 and 3, while 100% seroconversion against serotype 2 requires only 4–6 doses. Hence, the number of viral particles in trivalent OPV was lowest for type 2, such that the ratio of viral subtypes

1:2:3 is 10:1:6. Given its higher immunogenicity, OPV type 2 was the first serotype to be eliminated from India, in 1999.

OPV is very sensitive to temperature. Hence, its potency is monitored using vaccine vial monitor (VVM), a heat sensitive patch on the vial label (see section on 'Cold Chain'). Breastfeeding and mild diarrhea are not contraindications for OPV administration. Children with immunodeficiency and pregnant women should not receive the vaccine; its use is also avoided in household contacts of these patients.

In the past, OPV vaccine was given simultaneously with DPT vaccines at 6, 10 and 14 weeks, followed by two booster doses with DTP boosters at 15–18 months and 5 years. Since 1995, children below 5 years also received the vaccine during the (sub-) national immunization days and supplementary immunization activities in the Pulse Polio campaign, wherein simultaneous administration of OPV to all young children in the community interfered with feco-oral transmission of the circulating wild poliovirus. Together with surveillance and targeting of migrant populations and high-risk areas, wild poliovirus was eradicated from India; the last wild polio case (serotype 1) reported from Howrah in January 2011.

The attenuated OPV may rarely and sporadically be neurovirulent in a particular host, resulting in vaccine-associated paralytic poliomyelitis (VAPP). VAPP is observed in 1 of 1.5 million OPV recipients, chiefly due to OPV type 3 (in recipients) and OPV type 2 (in contacts).

Sabin OPV strains are genetically unstable, such that the attenuated virus can regain virulence during replication in the human gut through reversion of key attenuating mutations. Particularly in areas of low-vaccine coverage, where OPV strains have the opportunity to replicate unchecked and transmit for longer durations, this genetic instability may lead to emergence of *circulating vaccine-derived polioviruses (cVDPVs)* that cause paralytic poliomyelitis. Both wildtype and cVDPV transmit rapidly in areas of persistently low or declining immunization coverage to cause outbreaks. Approximately 90% of all cVDPV outbreaks are caused by the type 2 strain.

#### Inactivated Polio Vaccine (IPV)

IPV is a suspension of formaldehyde killed (Salk) poliovirus grown in monkey kidney, human diploid or Vero cell culture. The vaccine primarily induces humoral immune response, but pharyngeal and, possibly, intestinal mucosal antibodies are also induced. Vaccine potency is measured by its 'D' antigen content. Each dose of currently used third generation or enhanced potency IPV (eIPV) vaccines contains 40D, 8D and 32D units of types 1, 2 and 3 polioviruses, respectively, grown in Vero cell culture and purified before inactivation.

IPV is highly immunogenic; with seroconversion in 90–99% of infants over 8 weeks old administered 2–3 doses 4–8 weeks apart. Vaccination beginning at 6 weeks carries risk of interference with maternal antibodies. Despite low titers of secretory IgA and weak induction of herd immunity, IPV has excellent efficacy in preventing poliomyelitis. IPV administration has the theoretical advantage of not causing VAPP. However, inadequate inactivation of the polioviruses during the manufacturing process is know to have resulted in cases of VAPP.

***Newer poliovirus vaccines:*** In order to increase the immunogenicity of OPV types 1 and 3 and reduce the risk of cVPDV associated with type 2 OPV, a bivalent OPV containing only serotypes 1 and 3 (bOPV), and monovalent OPV types 1 (mOPV1) and 3 (mOPV3), were introduced for supplemental immunization campaigns following elimination of poliovirus type 2 **(Fig. 10.4)**. As part of Polio Eradication and Endgame Strategic Plan 2013–18, there was a global coordinated withdrawal of trivalent Sabin OPV and switch to bivalent OPV, and the use of OPV2 was discontinued globally in 2016.

Despite the withdrawal of Sabin OPV2, cVDPV outbreaks have continued to emerge in high-risk areas. To address the risk of cVPDV2, a novel oral poliomyelitis (polio) vaccine type 2 (nOPV2) was developed by modifying mOPV2 (Fig. 10.4). nOPV2 is a genetically stabilized variant that is as safe and effective in protecting against polio as the currently used mOPV2, but is significantly less likely to revert into forms that cause cVPDV2 in low immunity settings. Following emergency use listing by the WHO prequalification (PQ) program in November 2020, the nOPV2 is being rolled out for outbreak response in countries affected by cVDPV2 outbreaks. Achieving complete eradication of polioviruses (wildtype and cVPDV) requires that OPV be replaced with strains with less inherent risk of cVPDV. Hence, it is plausible that novel genetically stable strains for serotypes 1 and 3 (nOPV1, nOPV3) will later replace mOPV1, mOPV3 and bOPV **(Fig. 10.4)**.

The Sabin-inactivated poliovirus (sIPV) is another outcome of global efforts to develop poliovirus vaccines from less virulent strains. Compared to the conventional Salk-IPV, the manufacture of which carries strict containment requirements met only in developed countries, production of the sIPV carries lower biosafety risk, making it suited for mass production in developing countries, and therefore, more affordable and accessible than conventional (Salk) IPV.

#### Recommendations on Vaccination Against Poliovirus in India

Since February 2014, WHO no longer recommends an OPV only schedule. Apart from protecting from wildtype poliovirus, IPV also protects against poliomyelitis caused by cVDPV. Most countries practice a sequential IPV-OPV schedule, which has the advantage that the risk of OPV-induced VAPP is minimized by prior administration of IPV, while ensuring adequate mucosal immunity to interrupt wild poliovirus circulation. Following a phase of sequential or combined OPV- IPV use, most countries with sustained eradication of circulating wild poliovirus have switched to exclusive use of IPV. *WHO recommends that all countries using only OPV should add at least one dose of IPV to the national schedule*, and this was a major objective of the Polio Eradication and Endgame Strategic Plan 2013–2018 **(Fig. 10.5)**. The primary series, consisting of three bOPV doses and 1–2 IPV doses, is initiated at the age of 6 weeks, with at least 4 weeks interval between bOPV doses.

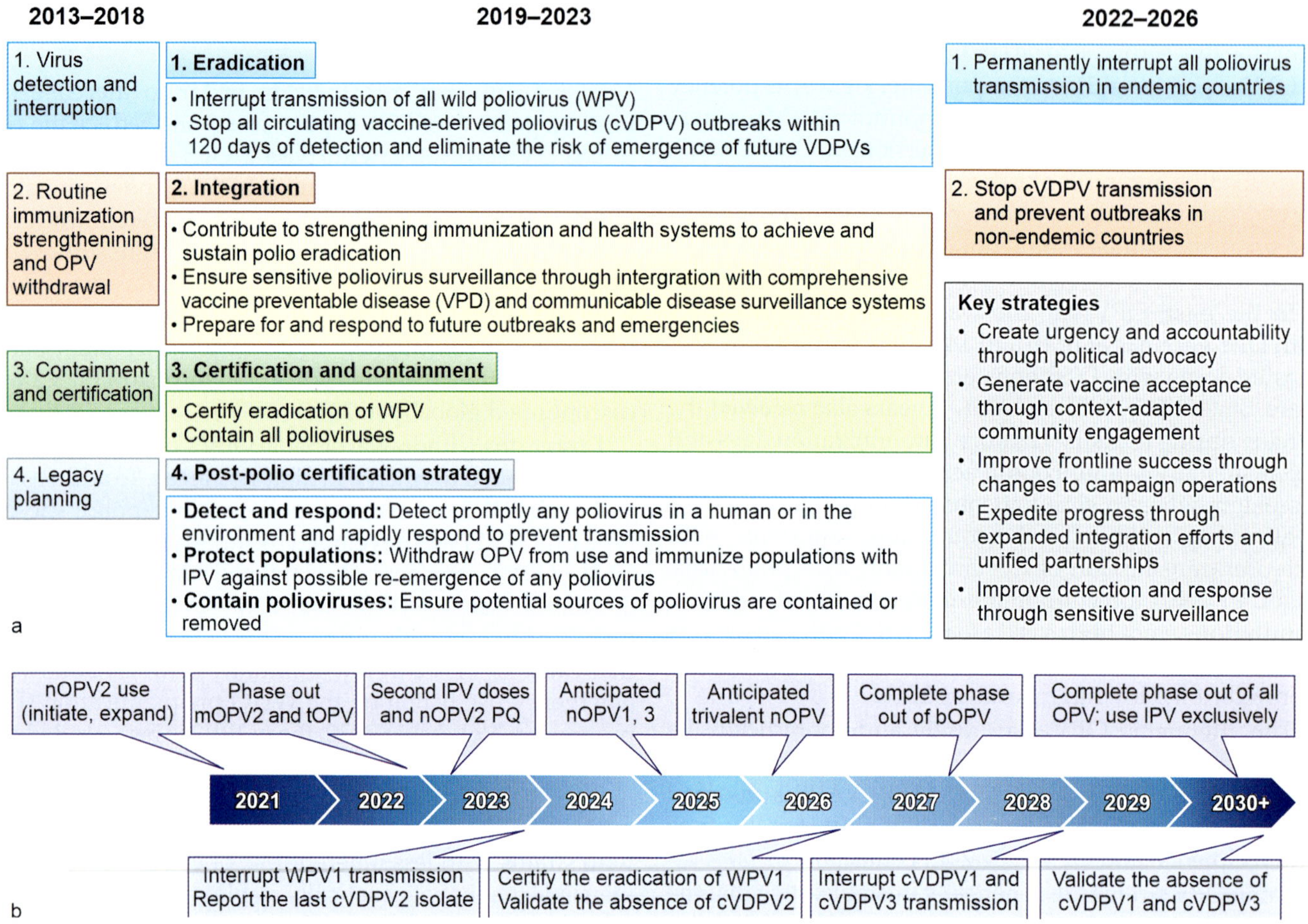


**Fig. 10.5:** Polio Endgame Strategy of the Global Polio Eradication Initiative (GPEI): (a) Goals of successive strategic plans; (b) Targeted global timeline of implementation and achievement of milestones. bOPV bivalent oral poliovirus; IPV inactivated poliovirus; OPV oral poliovirus; mOPV monovalent OPV; nOPV novel OPV; PQ pre-qualification

Evidence suggests that VDPV and wild type OPV may surface 4–10 years after global cessation of OPV. Even after global OPV withdrawal, national schedules should continue to provide at least two doses of IPV in their immunization schedule, administered either as full or fractional doses, for at least 10 years after OPV withdrawal. Until IPV supply is sufficient for use of 2–3 IM doses, a 2-dose fractional (fIPV) dose schedule would ensure that all eligible infants receive IPV. This strategy is dose sparing (one-fifth the IM dose) and results in better immunogenicity than a single

**Box 10.4: Bivalent Oral Poliovirus (bOPV) and Inactivated Poliovirus (IPV) Vaccines**

| | Bivalent oral poliovirus vaccine | Inactivated poliovirus vaccine |
|---|---|---|
| *Dose, route* | Two drops; oral | 0.5 mL, IM or SC<br>0.1 mL, intradermal |
| *Schedule*[1] | | |
| National program (OPV and IPV) | Dose at birth or <2 weeks (zero dose); 3 doses at 6, 10 and 14 weeks (primary); one booster dose at 15–18 months | Three intradermal fractionated doses at 6 weeks, 14 weeks and 9–12 months |
| IAP 2021 (OPV and IPV) | At birth | Three IM doses of IPV at 6, 10 and 14 weeks, or two IM doses at 8 and 16 weeks (primary); and two booster doses at 15–18 months and 4–6 years |
| Catch up | Up to 5 years: Three doses 4 weeks apart | Up to 5 years: 3 doses at 0, 2 and 6 months |
| *Adverse reactions* | Vaccine-derived poliovirus; vaccine-associated paralytic poliomyelitis | Local pain, swelling |
| *Contraindications* | Inherited or acquired immunodeficiency; symptomatic HIV | Known allergy |
| *Storage* | 2–8°C; sensitive to heat; use vaccine vial monitor | 2–8°C; sensitive to light and heat; use vaccine vial monitor |

[1]Additional doses of bivalent or monovalent OPV should be given on all supplementary immunization activities, regardless of receipt of scheduled vaccines

intramuscular dose of IPV. Administering fIPV during routine immunization visits at 6–14 weeks achieves high vaccine coverage and acceptability. IPV was, therefore, introduced in India in 2015–16 with two fractional (fIPV) intradermal doses at 6 and 14 weeks **(Box 10.4)**. From 1 January 2023, all infants should receive an additional fractionated IPVdose at 9–12 months. Children continue to receive bOPV at birth, at 6, 10 and 14 weeks, and on all supplementary immunization activities.

IPV is less immunogenic in the national immunization schedule (6 and 14 weeks) or when given at 6, 10 and 14 weeks, compared with vaccinating infants at older age in a three-dose schedule (2, 4 and 6 months), or two intramuscular doses beginning at 8 weeks and given 8 weeks apart **(Box 10.4)**. Hence, the IAP recommends an IPV-based schedule for primary immunization at 6, 10 and 14 weeks. Long-term studies show that antibodies wane over time, persisting usually only up to the school-entry age, with the highest titers observed in children who received a booster at 15–18 months. Following a second booster at 4–6 years, 100% seroprotection is achieved against all three serotypes, which persists for at least another 5 years. Hence, the IAP recommends three doses of IPV in infancy, and a booster each in the second and fifth years of life **(Box 10.4)**.

Both the national and IAP schedules continue to recommend the birth dose of OPV; this dose is necessary in areas with continued risk of wild virus transmission, and is unlikely to cause VAPP in presence of maternally transmitted antibodies. The risk of importing poliovirus (wild and cVDPV) from neighboring countries justifies the continued use of OPV during national and subnational pulse polio days for all children. Such additional OPV doses in IPV primed children should help augment mucosal immunity, which could interrupt circulation of poliovirus.

IPV is the vaccine of choice in patients with immunodeficiency including symptomatic HIV, and in siblings and close contacts of such patients. These children should not receive OPV, and should receive booster doses of IPV at 4–6 years.

### *Polio Eradication and Endgame Strategic Plan*

The Global Polio Eradication Initiative (GPEI), which was launched in 1988 with anticipated completion by 2000, has not yet reached its goal or eradicating poliovirus. The initial strategy was based on stopping transmission of wild polioviruses by global coordinated use of the trivalent OPV (OPV), followed by the destruction or containment of all its stocks and discontinuation of immunization in order to prevent the rare occurrence of VAPP. However, this plan was rendered ineffective by the emergence of cVDPV, which is now the cause of the majority of paralytic polio cases globally. Another obstacle to eradication was the persistence of wild poliovirus circulation in some regions, for geopolitical and cultural reasons and prejudices leading to vaccine hesitancy.

The last decade has seen steady progress on the path to eradication of poliovirus, with over 90% reduction in the incidence of cases of WPV type 1 since 2014. India reported its last case of wild poliovirus more than a decade ago in January 2011. Worldwide, the last case of wildtype poliovirus type 2 was reported in 1999 and that of WPV type 3 in 2012, leading to eradication of WPV types 2 and 3 in 2015 and 2019, respectively. However, WPV transmission continues in Afghanistan and Pakistan, and circulating vaccine-derived poliovirus (cVDPV) outbreaks have been reported from countries across Africa and Asia.

**Figure 10.5** summarizes key aspects and recent modifications in the eradication and endgame strategic plan of the GPEI, to overcome the final hurdles towards polio eradication and sustain a polio-free future. The chief objectives of the GPEI plan 2013–18 were to introduce at least one dose of IPV in national immunization programs, strengthen routine immunization and withdraw OPV in a phased manner, starting with OPV2. The strategic plan of 2019–2023 was built on the lessons and optimizes use of the tools of the 2013–2018 plan. The GPEI strategy has been further strengthened for 2022–2026, aiming for: (i) permanent interruption of all poliovirus transmission in the remaining WPV-endemic countries (Afghanistan and Pakistan), and (ii) stopping cVDPV transmission to prevent outbreaks in non-endemic countries.

### Suggested Reading


1. Chumakov K, Ehrenfeld E, Agol VI, Wimmer E. Polio eradication at the crossroads. Lancet Glob Health 2021; 9: e1172-e1175.
2. Martin J, Burns CC, Jorba J, et al. Genetic characterization of novel oral polio vaccine type 2 viruses during initial use phase under emergency use listing: Worldwide, March–October 2021. MMWR Morb Mortal Wkly Rep 2022; 71: 786–90.
3. World Health Organization. Global Polio Eradication Initiative (GPEI). Polio Endgame Strategy 2019–2023: Eradication, integration, certification and containment. Geneva, 2019. Available at https://polioeradication.org/who-we-are/polio-endgame-strategy-2019-2023, accessed 10 April 2021).
4. World Health Organization. Global Polio Eradication Initiative (GPEI). Polio Eradication Strategy 2022–2026: Executive summary. 2021; ISBN 978-92-4-002483-0 (electronic version)


## Diphtheria, Pertussis and Tetanus Vaccine

Diphtheria vaccine contains diphtheria toxin (DT) inactivated by formalin and adsorbed on aluminum hydroxide, the adjuvant. This is the most commonly used vaccine. The quantity of toxoid in the vaccine, expressed as limit of flocculation (Lf) content is 20–30 Lf of DT, 5–25 Lf of tetanus toxoid (TT) and >4 IU of whole cell killed pertussis.

Maternal antibodies protect the infant against disease and interfere with immune responses to DPT vaccination, particularly against pertussis. Protection in endemic regions requires that vaccination is begun within a few weeks of life and multiple doses are given. Primary immunization with 3 doses of the vaccine, given 4–8 weeks apart, induces satisfactory immune response to DT and TT in 95–100% infants. Protective efficacy against pertussis is lower, at ~70–90%, and wanes over 6–12 years. Immunization does not eliminate *C. diphtheriae* from the skin or nasopharynx. Booster doses are required to sustain a protective antibody titer of 0.1 IU/mL and protect from disease in the first decade of life. Natural infections and immunization against pertussis induce immunity lasting 4–12 years, making boosters necessary to prevent infection in adolescence.

### Box 10.5: Combinations of Diphtheria Toxoid, Tetanus Toxoid and Pertussis Vaccines

| | |
|---|---|
| *Dose, route* | 0.5 mL; intramuscular |
| *Schedule* | Anterolateral aspect of mid-thigh (gluteal region: sciatic nerve injury; inadequate response) |
| National program | DTwP at 6, 10 and 14 weeks (primary), and at 15–18 months and 5 years (boosters); Td at 10 years and 16 years, and during pregnancy |
| IAP 2021 | DTwP or DTaP for primary immunization and booster in schedule as above; Tdap or Td at 10–12 years, and then Td every 10 years |
| Catch up (IAP 2021) | <7 years: DTwP or DTaP at 0, 1 and 6 months<br>≥7 years: Tdap at 0 month; Td at 1 and 6 months, and then Td every 10 years |
| *Adverse reactions* | *Common:* Local pain, swelling, fever (DTwP>DTaP)<br>*Rare:* Hypotonic hyporesponsive episodes, inconsolable cry; fever >40.5°C; seizures; encephalopathy (DTwP=DTaP) |
| *Contraindications* | (i) Anaphylaxis after previous dose; (ii) encephalopathy within 7 days of previous dose; (iii) (relative contraindication) progressive neurological disease (administer DT or Td instead) |
| *Precautions* | Previous dose associated with (i) fever >40.5°C within 48 hours; (ii) hypotonic-hyporesponsive episode <48 hours; (iii) persistent inconsolable crying for >3 hours, <48 hours; (iv) seizures <72 hours |
| *Storage* | 2–8°C; sensitive to light |

DT diphtheria toxoid and tetanus toxoid; DTwP diphtheria toxoid, tetanus toxoid and whole cell killed pertussis vaccine; DTaP diphtheria toxoid, tetanus toxoid, and acellular pertussis vaccine; Td reduced dose diphtheria with tetanus toxoid; Tdap reduced dose diphtheria and pertussis with tetanus toxoid; TT tetanus toxoid



**Box 10.5** indicates the schedule for administration of DTwP or DTaP, containing DT, TT and acellular pertussis. DTwP vaccine is commonly associated with local (pain and redness) and systemic (fever) reactions, chiefly attributed to the pertussis component. The incidence of these adverse effects increases with the number of doses administered; hence the vaccine should not be used beyond 5 doses or beyond 7 years of age. DTP is rarely incriminated in serious neurological complications, though conclusive evidence is lacking. Hence, the vaccine is contraindicated in children with progressive neurological disease. Children with stable neurological diseases (e.g. developmental delay, cerebral palsy and idiopathic epilepsy) may receive the vaccine. Absolute contraindications to administration of the vaccine and adverse events that require precaution are listed. If an event listed as precaution recurs with a subsequent dose, further doses are contraindicated.

Individuals in which DTP is contraindicated should complete the immunization schedule with DT, which contains the same doses of DT and TT as DTP, but is devoid of the pertussis component. Beyond 7 years of age, Td is recommended.

#### *Acellular Pertussis Vaccine (DTaP)*

Since active pertussis toxin and endotoxin were implicated in causing the adverse events associated with DTwP, various types of purified acellular pertussis vaccines have been developed, termed DTaP. These vaccines contain inactivated pertussis toxin and one or more additional pertussis antigens, like filamentous hemagglutinin (FHA), pertactin, fimbrial protein and a nonfimbrial protein. Approved vaccines have at least 4 IU of inactivated pertussis toxin and 6.7–25 Lf of DT. The most common DTaP vaccine, Pentaxim®, is a two-component DTaP (containing pertussis toxin and FHA) combined with Hib and IPV vaccines; the availability of the three-component Infanrix® and five-component Tripacel® is not consistent. A DTaP/IPV combination vaccine (Tetraxim, Sanofi Pasteur), containing ≥30 IU of diphtheria toxoid, ≥40 IU of tetanus toxoid, two antigens of *Bordetella pertussis* (pertussis toxoid and filamentous hemagglutinin, 25 µg each), and IPV (40 DU, 8 DU and 32 DU of serotypes 1, 2 and 3, respectively), is highly immunogenic against all included antigens and can be administered as a booster dose, 0.5 mL intramuscularly, at 4–6 years (school entry).

Since the DTaP vaccines were reported to have efficacy similar to DTwP, but lower risk of systemic and local side effects, they gained popularity in developed countries where adverse effects form a major reason for vaccine hesitancy. Later studies indicated that the DTwP vaccine has superior immunogenicity (61–89% versus 46–92%), particularly so for pertussis, and provides longer lasting protection as compared to DTaP vaccines. However, *recent studies indicate that the duration of protection for all three components of both DTaP and DTwP vaccines, following three primary doses and one booster dose given at least after a year, is similar, at 6–12 years.*

The DTaP vaccine is not included in the National Program due to its prohibitive cost. Primary immunization comprises three doses of DTwP in the first year, and two booster doses are administered at 15–24 months and at five years **(Box 10.5)**.

Given the balance of benefit of low reactogenicity leading to improved vaccine acceptance, over harm through reduced efficacy, and knowing that the efficacy of DTaP improves with booster administration, the IAP recommends that primary vaccination should be completed with three doses of either DTwP or DTaP vaccines. The chief aim is to increase the vaccination coverage with either of the vaccines. Hence, the IAP recommends using either the DTwP or DTaP vaccine for primary immunization as well as booster doses **(Box 10.5)**. Further, the IAP recommends switching to DTaP in patients who show an adverse effect with DTwP.

Contraindications for DTaP vaccine are similar to that for DTwP. Hence, the vaccine should not be given, if a previous dose of DTwP or DTaP was associated with a contraindication (**Box 10.5**); these children should complete immunization with DT instead of DTwP or DTaP.

### *Tetanus Vaccine*

Extensive routine immunization of pregnant women has led to decline in the incidence of neonatal tetanus. Two doses administered during pregnancy, with the second dose given at least 4 weeks before delivery, provides passive immunity to the newborn due to the transplacental passage of IgG antibodies.

Tetanus toxin is inactivated by formalin and adsorbed onto aluminum salts to enhance immunogenicity. Each dose of the vaccine contains 5 Lf of toxoid. The vaccine is heat stable and remains potent for a few weeks even at 37°C. The efficacy of TT vaccine varies between 80 and 100%. While antitoxin level of 0.01 IU/mL is considered protective, the level of protection available also depends on the toxin load.

Since tetanus may occur at any age, primary immunization should begin in early infancy. Td (see below) or TT may be used as boosters at 10 and 16 years of age and for wound prophylaxis (**Table 10.4**). Children who have not received primary immunization should receive three doses of tetanus containing vaccine 1 month apart.

### *Reduced Antigen Acellular Pertussis Vaccine (Tdap), Reduced Antigen Diphtheria Toxoid Vaccine (Td) and Diphtheria Toxoid (DT)*

Natural immunity to diphtheria and pertussis is acquired through apparent or inapparent infections. Hence, a large proportion of adults in non-endemic regions are susceptible through lack of natural boosting and waning of immunity, and hence require revaccination every 10 years. Even in endemic regions, the increase in immunization coverage in children has led to shift in age-group of diphtheria cases to school-going children and adults. Healthcare workers are particularly susceptible to exposure to diphtheria. Vaccines useful in such situations include diphtheria and tetanus toxoids (DT) and combinations containing reduced toxoid content (Td, Tdap).

While standard dose DT is more immunogenic and less reactogenic than the conventional DTP combination vaccines, the reactogenicity of DT increases with age. Hence, beyond 7 years of age, primary immunization or booster doses against diphtheria should be provided as Tdap or Td, which contain smaller amount of diphtheria toxoid (2 Lf) and acellular pertussis vaccine compared to DTaP, which is adequately immunogenic. Td is available in India as Td-Vac® and BE-Td®, while DT is marketed by several vaccine manufacturers as Dual Antigen®.

Tdap reduces the incidence of pertussis in adults and adolescents, and decreases the risk of disease transmission to young children. Its reduced antigen content causes less severe adverse effects while being sufficient to induce protective response in previously immunized (booster effect). The available Tdap vaccines in India (e.g. Boostrix®, Adacel®) contain 5 Lf of tetanus toxoid, 2 Lf of diphtheria toxoid and three acellular pertussis components (pertussis toxoid 8 µg, filamentous hemagglutinin 8 µg and pertactin 2.5 µg). Contraindications to Tdap are the same as those listed for DTaP or DTwP.

In the national immunization schedule, TT was replaced by Td at 10 years, 16 years and during pregnancy. The Td vaccine may be used whenever TT is indicated in children above 7 years of age. The Tdap vaccine may be used instead of Td or TT above 10 years of age in children and adults who have not received Tdap in the past, and 5 years have elapsed since the receipt of previous TT or Td vaccine. The IAP recommends the administration of Tdap at 10 years and Td every 10 years thereafter.

### *Newer Approaches*

A vaccine, BPZEI, has been developed that is based on a live *B. pertussis* strain that has been attenuated by genetically removing, reducing or inactivating three major pertussis toxins. One dose of the intranasal vaccine induces protection lasting one year or longer, and through nasal colonization, provides nonspecific cross-protection against other respiratory pathogens. A Tdap vaccine, licensed in Thailand, containing a genetically inactivated pertussis toxin, FHA, tetanus toxoid and reduced dose diphtheria toxoid is more immunogenic than conventional Tdap.

## Measles-Containing Vaccines

Measles vaccine, derived from the Edmonston-Zagreb strain, is available as a monovalent preparation, or in combination with rubella (MR), mumps (MMR) and varicella (MMR-V). Both cellular and humoral responses are elicited. Since infants are protected by maternal antibodies till 6–9 months of age, administering the vaccine at 9 months in endemic countries balances the need for early protection with the ability to ensure seroconversion.

**Table 10.4:** Tetanus prophylaxis following wound

| *Doses of tetanus toxoid received previously* | *Clean minor wound* | | *All other wounds* | |
|---|---|---|---|---|
| | *Tetanus toxoid*[1] | *Tetanus immunoglobulin* | *Tetanus toxoid*[1] | *Tetanus immunoglobulin* |
| <3 doses or uncertain, or immunodeficient | Yes[2] | No | Yes[2] | Yes |
| ≥3 doses, >10 years back | Yes | No | Yes | No[3] |
| ≥3 doses, 5–10 years back | No | No | Yes | No[3] |
| ≥3 doses, <5 years back | No | No | No | No[3] |

[1]Administer any tetanus toxoid containing vaccine (DT or DTaP if <7-yr-old, Tdap, Td or TT if older) based on age-appropriateness and ease of availability

[2]The vaccination course should be completed with three doses of an age-appropriate vaccine containing tetanus toxoid, given 1 month apart

[3]Yes, if immunodeficient

**Box 10.6: Measles-containing Vaccines**

| | |
|---|---|
| *Dose, route* | 0.5 mL; subcutaneous |
| *Site* | Right upper arm (at insertion of deltoid) or anterolateral thigh |
| *Schedule* | |
| National program | At 9–12 and 15–24 months, as measles or measles rubella vaccine |
| IAP 2021 | At 9–12 months, 15–18 months and 4–6 years; preferably as MMR; avoid MMR-V <2 years |
| *Adverse reactions* | Local pain, tenderness; febrile seizures (especially with MMR-V in <2-yr-old)<br>Measles vaccine: Fever or transient macular rash (after 7–12 days)<br>MMR vaccine: Transient rash, arthralgia, aseptic meningitis, lymphadenopathy |
| *Contraindications* | Immunosuppression; malignancy; immunodeficiency (e.g. symptomatic HIV); recent infusion of immunoglobulin-containing blood product |
| *Storage* | 2–8°C; sensitive to heat and light; use within 4–6 hours of reconstitution |

MMR-V measles, mumps, rubella, varicella

However, interference by maternal antibodies causes primary vaccine failure in 15%, making a second dose necessary at 15 months. During outbreaks, the vaccine may be given even earlier (~6 months) with a repeat dose at 12–15 months. Each vaccine dose contains at least 1000 infective units of the attenuated virus. Measles vaccine loses potency rapidly after reconstitution; unused vaccine should be discarded after 4–6 hours since contamination may lead to staphylococcal sepsis and toxic shock syndrome.

As part of the commitment of the southeast Asia region's goal to eliminate measles and rubella by 2023, the measles rubella (MR) vaccine was introduced in February 2017 through a nationwide campaign targeting children aged between 9 months and 15 years. Additional doses continued to be given during routine immunization at 9–12 months and 16–24 months in the national immunization program are given in **Box 10.6**. The nationwide 'measles rubella' program involved administering one dose of the vaccine to all children 9 months to 15 years of age, irrespective of their immunization status.

Recognizing the significant morbidity associated with mumps infections, the IAP recommends MMR instead of MR at 9 and 16–24 months. IAP also recommends a third dose of MMR at 4–6 years, chiefly in order to boost anamnestic response.

Post-exposure prophylaxis with immunoglobulin is considered for immunocompromised contacts and 6–12-month-old infants within 6 days of exposure (*see* Passive Immunization). Unimmunized immunocompetent contacts older than 12 months should receive measles or MMR vaccine within 72 hours of exposure.

### Hepatitis B Vaccine

Hepatitis B virus (HBV) vaccine contains the surface antigen HBsAg, produced by recombinant DNA technology in yeast, adsorbed on aluminum salt as adjuvant. The dose of the vaccine differs between children and adults **(Box 10.7)**. The vaccine is available as monovalent vaccine in single-dose or multidose vials, and in combination with hepatitis A (Twinrix®), DTwP and Hib (pentavalent vaccine), and DTaP (Easyfour®) with or without Hib (Easyfive®).

If the mother's HBsAg status is not known, vaccination must begin at birth, since immunization at birth prevents horizontal transmission. The national immunization schedule recommends a zero dose at birth followed by three doses at 6, 10 and 14 weeks **(Box 10.7)**. Immunization at birth, 1 and 6 months has better immunological efficacy than the regime advised in the National Program **(Box 10.7)**. However, the latter integrates HBV vaccination into the existing schedule without increasing visits, and ensures compliance.

Seroconversion rates exceed 95% after three HBV doses. An antibody titer >10 mIU/mL is considered protective. Vaccination usually induces long-term immunity, and booster doses are not routinely recommended. Patients with immunodeficiency, malignancy, chronic liver disease,

**Box 10.7: Hepatitis B Vaccine**

| | |
|---|---|
| *Dose, route* | 0.5 mL (10 μg); 1 mL (20 μg) in adults[1]; intramuscular |
| *Site* | Anterolateral thigh or deltoid; avoid gluteal region |
| *Schedule* | |
| National program | At birth, 6 weeks, 10 weeks and 14 weeks |
| IAP 2021 | As above; ideally, a gap of ≥4 weeks between the first two doses; ≥8 weeks between doses 2 and 3; and ≥16 weeks between the first and final doses, with the final dose given at ≥6 months of age[2] |
| Catch up | Three doses at 0, 1 and 6 months; preferred gaps as detailed above |
| *Adverse reactions* | Local soreness; fever; fatigue |
| *Contraindication* | Anaphylaxis after previous dose |
| *Storage* | 2–8°C; do not freeze |

[1]The adult dose is also preferred in certain high-risk categories (see text)

[2]The following schedules are also acceptable: Birth, 1 and 6 months; birth, 6 weeks and 6 months; and birth, 6 weeks and 14 weeks; if mother HBsAg negative: 6, 10 and 14 weeks

chronic kidney disease (including those on hemodialysis) and diabetes may not mount seroprotective titers or titers may wane over time. In such cases, higher dose of the vaccine and periodic monitoring for seroprotective titers is useful to guide need for booster doses.

If the mother is known to be HBsAg positive, the child should receive the vaccine within a few hours of birth, and hepatitis B immunoglobulin (HBIG) within the first 24 hours at separate sites (*see* Passive Immunization). Subsequently, any of the schedules incorporating a birth dose of the vaccine can be used. If HBIG is not administered, the baby should be immunized in an accelerated schedule at 0, 1 and 2 months, with an additional dose at 9–12 months. Combined passive and active immunization with use of HBIG and HBV vaccine results in 90% reduced risk of HBV transmission in patients with needle stick injuries, sexual exposure, or transfusion of blood product that has not been screened for HBV.

### Hemophilus Vaccine

*Hemophilus influenzae* b (Hib) causes invasive infections such as pneumonia, meningitis and bacteremia, especially in children <2-year-old. Vaccination prevents 33% of pneumonia and 90% meningitis related to Hib. The chief antigen is Hib capsular polysaccharide, polyribosyl-ribitol- phosphate (PRP), which is conjugated to tetanus toxoid (PRP-T), diphtheria toxoid (PRP-D), a mutant nontoxic diphtheria toxin CRM-197 (Hib-OC), or meningococcal outer membrane protein (PRP-OMP). While PRP-OMP provides early protection with even 1–2 doses, three doses of PRP-T and PRP-OC, the vaccines currently available in India as monovalent and combination (with DTP and hepatitis B, and/or IPV) vaccines, have 88–95% efficacy. Adequate immunization coverage is also associated with herd immunity for unimmunized children through reduced nasopharyngeal carriage of the organism in immunized children.

The vaccination schedule depends on age of the child at immunization **(Box 10.8)**. As Hib infections chiefly affect preschool children, the vaccine is administered during the first year of life. The vaccine is part of the pentavalent vaccine (DTP, HBV and HibPRP-T vaccines) in the Universal Immunization Program since 2015. A booster in the second year of life is recommended to sustain protection; however, this is not yet included in the national schedule. IAP recommends the vaccine in all children under the age of 5 years, and older children in certain high-risk categories, including: (i) Immunosuppressed children; (ii) those planned for splenectomy or ear surgery; and (iii) those with chronic cardiac or pulmonary disease or sickle cell disease).

#### Suggested Reading


1. Das S, Ramakrishnan K, Behera SK, et al. Hepatitis B vaccine and immunoglobulin: Key concepts. J Clin Transl Hepatol 2019;7:165–71.
2. Drugs and Lactation Database (LactMed) [Internet]. Bethesda (MD): National Library of Medicine (US); 2006. Haemophilus vaccines. 2020. PMID: 29999947
3. Hall E, Wodi AP, Hamborsky J, et al (eds). Centers for Disease Control and Prevention. Epidemiology and Prevention of Vaccine-Preventable Diseases. 14th edn. Washington, DC Public Health Foundation, 2021.
4. Mother To Baby | Fact Sheets [Internet]. Brentwood: Organization of Teratology Information Specialists (OTIS); 1994. Measles, mumps, rubella and the MMR vaccine. 2020. PMID: 35951800.
5. Prygiel M, Mosiej E, Górska P, Zasada AA. Diphtheria-tetanus-pertussis vaccine: past, current & future. Future Microbiol 2022; 17:185–97.


### Pneumococcal Vaccine

*S. pneumoniae* causes 15–50% of community-acquired pneumonia, 30–50% of acute otitis media and 50% of deaths due to pneumonia. Pneumococcal pneumonia is the leading single cause of vaccine-preventable deaths, globally and in India. Twenty of 90 known serotypes account for 80% of invasive pneumococcal disease, and 13 serotypes cause 75% of invasive disease in young children. Children below two years of age are particularly susceptible to invasive pneumococcal disease. Children at high risk of disease, regardless of age, include: (i) Primary immunodeficiency, HIV, immunosuppressive therapy and organ transplant recipients; (ii) sickle cell disease, anatomical or functional asplenia or hyposplenia; (iii) chronic cardiac, liver or pulmonary disease; (iv) chronic kidney disease and nephrotic syndrome; (v) diabetes mellitus; (vi) cerebrospinal fistula or cochlear implants, and (vii) therapy with complement inhibitors (e.g. eculizumab).

**Box 10.8: Hemophilus Influenzae b Vaccine**

| | |
|---|---|
| *Dose, route* | 0.5 mL, intramuscular |
| *Site* | Anterolateral thigh |
| *Schedule* | |
| National program | Pentavalent vaccine with DTP and hepatitis B; three doses given at 6, 10 and 14 weeks |
| IAP 2021 | <6 months old: 3 doses at ≥6 weeks given ≥4 weeks apart; one booster at 12–18 months |
| Catch up | At 7–12 months: Two doses ≥8 weeks apart; one booster at 12–18 months[1] |
| | At 12–14 months: One dose and one booster at 15–18 months[1] |
| | At 15–59 months: One dose |
| | At ≥5-years: Not recommended, except if high risk[2] |
| *Adverse reactions* | Local pain or redness; fever, rash |
| *Contraindication* | Hypersensitivity to previous dose |
| *Storage* | 2–8°C |

[1]Ensure that the booster is given ≥8 weeks after the last dose of primary immunization schedule
[2]See text

10 Immunization

## Box 10.9: Pneumococcal Vaccines

| Type | Pneumococcal conjugate (PCV13: Prevenar 13®; PCV10: Synflorix®, Pneumosil®) | Pneumococcal polysaccharide (PPSV23: Pneumovax®) |
|---|---|---|
| *Dose, route* | 0.5 mL; intramuscular | 0.5 mL; intramuscular or subcutaneous |
| *Site* | Anterolateral thigh or deltoid | Deltoid |
| *Schedule* | | |
| National program | Three doses at 6 weeks, 14 weeks and 9 months | Not recommended |
| IAP 2021 | Three doses at ≥6 weeks age; given ≥4 weeks apart; one booster at 15–18 months[1] | Only in high-risk category[2]: One dose ≥8 weeks after primary course with conjugate vaccine; repeat once after 5 years, if risk persists[3] |
| Catch up (IAP) | At 7–11 months: Two doses ≥4 weeks apart; one booster at 15–18 months[1]<br>At 12–23 months: Two doses ≥8 weeks apart[1]<br>At 24–59 months: One dose[4]<br>≥60 months: One dose[4], if high risk[2] | Use only if high risk[2] and ≥2 years old |
| *Adverse reactions* | Fever, local pain, soreness, malaise | Local pain, redness, soreness (30–50%) |
| *Contraindication* | Anaphylaxis after previous dose | Anaphylaxis after previous dose |
| *Storage* | 2–8°C; do not freeze | 2–8°C |

[1]Pneumosil® is approved only for use at 6 weeks to 23 months, as 3 doses given ≥4 weeks apart and no booster
[2]See text for details
[3]No more than two doses are given in the entire lifetime
[4]Give two doses ≥8 weeks apart if receiving Synflorix® (not licensed at >5 years of age in India) or if high-risk and previously unimmunized (either Prevenar 13® or Synflorix®); Pneumosil® is not approved at this age

Two kinds of vaccines are available **(Box 10.9)**. The unconjugated polysaccharide vaccine has 25 µg capsular polysaccharide of each of the 23 serotypes, termed PPSV23 (Pneumovax). Since polysaccharides stimulate B cells independent of T cells, the vaccine is poorly immunogenic below 2 years of age and induces poor immunological memory. This vaccine does not reduce nasopharyngeal pneumococcal carriage or provide herd immunity. Its efficacy in preventing invasive pneumococcal disease in high-risk categories is <70%. The vaccine is recommended for use in children only in high-risk categories (see above) and should follow primary immunization using the conjugate vaccine. A gap of at least 8 weeks is necessary between the last dose of the conjugate vaccine and the PPSV23. No more than two doses of PPSV23 are administered throughout the lifetime because of lack of booster response and risk of hyporesponsiveness and adverse reactions.

The pneumococcal conjugate vaccines available currently in India have the capsular polysaccharide of either 13 most commonly pathogenic serotypes linked to a non-toxic diphtheria carrier protein CRM197 (PCV13, Prevenar 13®) or 10 serotypes combined with either the outer membrane protein (protein D) of non-typeable *H. influenzae* vaccine (Synflorix®) or diphtheria CRM197 (Pneumosil®). Two vaccines marketed internationally are 15-valent (Vaxneuvance®) or 20-valent (Prevnar 20®). Conjugated vaccines induce robust immune responses and immunological memory. They also reduce nasopharyngeal bacterial carriage by almost 50%, resulting in significant herd effect. The protective efficacy of current PCVs is estimated at 80% for invasive pneumococcal disease covered by the included serotypes, and 58% overall. The rates of protection against pneumonia and otitis media are lower. While there is concern regarding emergence of 'replacement' disease caused by non-vaccine serotypes, the rise in such cases is reported to be lower than the decline in invasive pneumococcal disease caused by vaccine serotypes.

Since pneumococcal infections cause significant morbidity and mortality in children <2 years of age, vaccination with the 13-valent PCV (Prevenar 13®) was launched in the national program in three states in May 2017. Vaccination has later been extended to the entire country in a phased manner, chiefly using the 10-valent PCV (Pneumosil®). However, the national schedule differs from that recommended by the IAP, with fewer doses (two primary and one booster, within 1 year of life) to reduce program costs and improve its implementation, as recommended by the WHO for low resource settings **(Box 10.9)**. Since the risk of invasive infections decreases with age, vaccination beyond 5 years is not necessary except in high-risk categories; the latter should additionally receive the polysaccharide vaccine in view of its broad-based protection. An additional dose of PPSV23 may be given in high-risk categories 3–5 years later.

### Rotavirus Vaccine

Rotavirus is the chief cause of diarrhea in infants and toddlers, accounting for 6–45% of diarrhea-related hospitalization in Indian children. Natural infection does not protect against reinfection or severe disease. Four live attenuated, oral vaccines are currently in use globally **(Box 10.10)**.

The first vaccine to be licensed was Rotashield, a live oral tetravalent vaccine which was withdrawn subsequently following an association with intussusception. Rotarix is a monovalent vaccine containing at least $10^6$ median cell culture infective doses of rotavirus strain G1P8 attenuated in Vero cell culture. RotaTeq is a pentavalent vaccine

**Box 10.10: Rotavirus Vaccines**

| Vaccine name | Rotavac | RotaTeq | Rotarix | Rotasiil |
|---|---|---|---|---|
| *Name by type* | Indian neonatal (116E); human bovine monovalent | Human bovine pentavalent (RV5) | Human monovalent (RV1) | Bovine pentavalent; thermostable |
| *Number of strains* | 1 | 5 | 1 | 5 |
| *Schedule*[1] | | | | |
| National program | 3 doses at 6, 10 and 14 weeks | Not included | Not included | Not included |
| IAP 2021 | 3 doses at 6, 10 and 14 weeks | 3 doses at 6, 10 and 14 weeks | 2 doses at 6 and 10, or 10 and 14, weeks[2] | 3 doses at 6, 10 and 14 weeks |
| *Dose, route* | 5 drops, oral | 2 mL (liquid), oral | 1 mL (lyophilized); 1.5 mL (liquid), oral | 2.5 mL, oral |
| *Catch up* | National program: Up to 1 year of age<br>IAP 2021: Give the first dose before 16 weeks of age and complete the schedule by 32 weeks of age | | | |
| *Adverse reactions* | Fever, diarrhea, vomiting, cough, rhinitis, rash, irritability; intussusception is rare | | | |
| *Contraindication* | Past history of intussusception; severe immunodeficiency | | | |
| *Precaution* | Postpone vaccination during ongoing diarrhea or moderate illness | | | |
| *Storage* | 2–8°C (except Rotasiil, which can be stored at <25°C); protect from heat; use within 4 hours of reconstitution or opening | | | |

[1]Administer ≥4 weeks apart beginning at ≥6 weeks of age

[2]The IAP recommends vaccinating at 6 and 10 weeks in view of the risk of encountering natural infections at an earlier age in India; elsewhere the latter schedule is preferred for higher rates of longer lasting protection

with 2–116 million infectious units each of five strains (G1–4 and P8) reassorted between bovine and human WC3 rotaviruses, and attenuated by Vero cell culture. Rotasiil is an indigenous lyophilized pentavalent vaccine containing five human bovine reassortant strains (G1–4 and G9). It is a thermostable vaccine that can be stored without refrigeration at or below 25°C. Rotavac is an indigenous monovalent human-bovine recombinant live attenuated vaccine based on the 116E strain. This vaccine has 49–54% efficacy against rotaviral diarrhea in the first 2 years of life, and is safe with a low risk of intussusception. The vaccine was included in the national immunization program in 2016, and has been rolled out across India in a phased manner.

Early reports from developed countries had suggested that Rotarix and RotaTeq have efficacy of 85–98% in preventing severe rotaviral gastroenteritis, thus reducing rotavirus hospitalizations by 49–92%, and all-cause diarrhea hospitalizations by 17–55%. Routine immunization also protects unimmunized children by providing herd immunity. However, the reported efficacy of available vaccines is much lower (40–70%) in developing regions, likely due to reduced 'take' due to competition for intestinal infection by wildtype virus and other intestinal pathogens. Booster doses are not recommended as rotavirus diarrhea most commonly affects children less than 2 years old.

The available rotavirus vaccines may be given with OPV without compromising efficacy of either vaccine. Vaccination is avoided during acute gastroenteritis, as it might compromise vaccine take. The most common adverse events following vaccination are fever and mild, self-limiting diarrhea and vomiting. The risk of intussusception is insignificant with currently used vaccines, reported in one per 20,000 to 100,000 infants. However, caution is necessary in infants at risk of intussusception due to chronic gastrointestinal disease or gut malformations. To reduce the risk, immunization should be initiated by 6–14 weeks and completed by 8 months of age.

### Human Papillomavirus (HPV) Vaccine

Cervical cancer, with a cumulative lifetime risk of 1.4%, is the second most common cancer in women, and is almost always caused by infection with oncogenic HPV belonging to 20 of 100 known serotypes. Serotypes 16 and 18 cause 80–85% of invasive cervical cancers. Other oncogenic serotypes cause anal, vulvar, vaginal, penile and oropharyngeal cancer. Non-oncogenic serotypes 6 and 11 cause 90% of anogenital warts.

HPV vaccines contain self-assembling virus like particles containing recombinant L1, a major capsid protein. These vaccines protect against 90% of infections with included serotypes, but do not provide cross-protection against other strains. The quadrivalent vaccine Gardasil (HPV4) protects against strains 6, 11, 16 and 18, while the bivalent Cervarix (HPV2) targets HPV 16 and 18. The Gardasil 9 vaccine has 5 additional strains but is not widely available. While immunity is type-specific, there is reasonable cross-protection against related strains.

All available vaccines prevent cervical *in situ* neoplasia grade 2 and 3, and adenocarcinoma *in situ*. Gardasil also prevents serotype-related anogenital warts, vulval and vaginal cancers, and vulvar intraepithelial neoplasia. Gardasil 9 additionally protects against anal, oropharyngeal and head and neck cancers caused by HPV.

These vaccines are most immunogenic at 9–14 years of age, with protection persisting for at least 8–10 years. The ideal age at vaccination and need of booster doses, if any, is not determined. The WHO recommends HPV vaccination predominantly for young girls in developing countries. Gender-neutral vaccination (i.e. also in boys), while less cost-effective, is shown to be more beneficial in reducing risk of HPV infection and disease compared to vaccinating

**Box 10.11: Human Papillomavirus Vaccine**

| Vaccine name | Cervarix (HPV2) | Gardasil (HPV4) | Gardasil 9 (HPV9) |
|---|---|---|---|
| *Number of strains* | 2 | 4 | 9 |
| VLP types of L1 | 16, 18 | 6, 11, 16, 18 | 6, 11, 16, 18, 31, 35, 45, 52, 58 |
| Host | Baculovirus | *Saccharomyces cerevisiae* | *Saccharomyces cerevisiae* |
| *Target age, years* | | | |
| Girls | 9-45 | 9–45 | 9–45 |
| Boys[1] | Not available | 9–26 | 9–45 |
| *Number of doses* | | | |
| Age <15 years | 2 | 2 | 2 |
| Age ≥15 years[1] | 3 | 3 | 3 |
| *Schedule*[2,3] | | | |
| Age <15 years | 0, 6–12 months | 0, 6–12 months | 0, 6–12 months |
| Age ≥15 years | 0, 1, 6 months | 0, 2, 6 months | 0, 2, 6 months |
| *Dose, route* | 0.5 mL, intramuscular | | |
| *Site* | Upper arm (deltoid) | | |
| *Schedule* | | | |
| National program | In some states, in girls 11–13 years, as above | | |
| IAP 2021 | All young girls, as above[2] | | |
| Catch up | Up to 45 years (IAP); preferably before initiation of sexual activity | | |
| *Adverse reactions* | Local pain, swelling, erythema; fever<br>Syncope (due to injection, not vaccine) | | |
| *Contraindication* | Anaphylaxis after previous dose | | |
| *Storage* | 2–8°C; protect from light | | |

[1]Also, in younger immunodeficient or immunosuppressed children

[2]The recommended vaccines for boys (Gardasil) are not yet licensed for use in India in boys

[3]Ensure a minimum interval of 4 weeks between doses 1 and 2 and 12 weeks between doses 2 and 3 (in three dose schedule) and 5 months between first and last dose (in either schedule)

VLP virus like particles of L1 protein

girls alone. The IAP recommends that the vaccine should be offered to all girls prior to sexual debut **(Box 10.11)**. The available vaccines are not yet licensed for use in boys in India.

While HPV vaccine is not yet included in the national immunization program, the governments of Delhi, Sikkim and Punjab have initiated school- based programs for girls aged 11–13 years old since 2016. Immunization carries the risk of complacency regarding routine screening for cancer, which, together with incomplete immunization coverage, might paradoxically raise cervical cancer-related mortality.

There are no serious adverse effects with HPV vaccines. Safety information from large databases indicates no risk of Guillain-Barr syndrome, complex regional pain syndrome, postural orthostatic tachycardia syndrome, venous thromboembolism or premature ovarian insufficiency or failure. Adolescent immunization with any vaccine carries risk of syncope; hence, they must be advised to lie down for 15 minutes after vaccination.

### Japanese B Encephalitis Vaccine

Japanese encephalitis (JE) is an important cause of viral encephalitis in India, chiefly affecting children below 15 years of age. The condition is associated with fatality in 5–35% cases and severe neurological sequelae in almost half of the survivors. Vaccination as a control measure is recommended for all children and adults residing in, or travelling to (for >4 weeks), highly endemic areas, comprising of 268 districts in 23 states and union territories, chiefly in eastern Uttar Pradesh, Bihar, West Bengal, Assam, and North-East states. Previously available vaccines, discontinued in 2005, included inactivated mouse brain-derived vaccine (Nakayama or Beijing-1 strains) and primary hamster kidney cell culture vaccine (Beijing-3 strain). Three of the five second generation vaccines are licensed for use in India **(Box 10.12)**.

The live attenuated cell culture-derived vaccine is used in the national program in hyperendemic districts of Uttar Pradesh, West Bengal, Assam and Karnataka. It is based on SA-14-14-2, a genetically stable neuro-attenuated JE strain, which is unlikely to revert to neurovirulence **(Box 10.12)**. While a single dose has protective efficacy of 85–99%, two doses are recommended to provide complete and sustained protection. In endemic districts, a strategy of mass immunization followed by routine vaccination is practiced.

The purified formalin inactivated SA-14-14-2 (IC51, e.g. IXIARO®, JEEV®) is a whole virus vaccine derived from Vero cell culture with aluminum hydroxide as adjuvant. The vaccine is highly immunogenic in children, with seroconversion >90% with two doses. The risk of adverse effects is lower than with live attenuated vaccines. The inactivated purified Vero cell culture-derived vaccine, based

**Box 10.12: Japanese B Encephalitis Vaccine**

| | Live attenuated cell culture derived SA-14-14-2 | Inactivated cell culture derived SA-14-14-2 [IC51] | Inactivated Vero cell culture derived Kolar [82156XY] |
|---|---|---|---|
| *Dose, route* | 0.5 mL; subcutaneous | 1–3 yr: 0.25 mL; ≥3 yr: 0.5 mL; intramuscular | 0.5 mL; intramuscular |
| *Site* | Anterolateral thigh, upper arm | Anterolateral thigh, upper arm | Anterolateral thigh, upper arm |
| *Schedule* | | | |
| National program | Only endemic areas; two doses at 9 and 16–18 months; also adults | Not used | Not used |
| IAP 2021 | Recommended in endemic areas; not available in the private sector | Recommended in endemic areas; ≥1 yr-old; two doses ≥4 weeks apart | Recommended in endemic areas; ≥1 yr-old; two doses ≥4 weeks apart; timing of booster not determined |
| *Catch up* | Up to 15 years; adults | Any age | Any age |
| *Adverse reactions* | Fever, malaise; hypersensitivity (rare) | Less common: Fever, pain, malaise | Uncommon |

on the Kolar strain (821564XY; e.g., JenVac®) is similarly safe and effective, with seroconversion in 93–98%.

The inactivated Vero cell culture-derived vaccine based on the Beijing-1 strain is not available in India. A live attenuated recombinant SA-14-4-2 chimeric vaccine (JE-CV, e.g. IMOJEV®) comprises nucleic acid sequences of two envelope proteins of SA-14-2 strain (prM, E) inserted into the yellow fever 17D strain used as backbone. This vaccine, used in Australia and Thailand as two intramuscular doses given 4 weeks apart, is yet to be licensed in India.

## Suggested Reading


1. Briles DE, Paton JC, Mukerji R, Swiatlo E, Crain MJ. Pneumococcal vaccines. Microbiol Spectr 2019; 7. doi: 10.1128/microbiolspec.GPP3-0028-2018.
2. Carvalho MF, Gill D. Rotavirus vaccine efficacy: Current status and areas for improvement. Hum Vaccin Immunother 2019;15: 1237–50.
3. Jit M, Prem K, Benard E, et al. From cervical cancer elimination to eradication of vaccine-type human papillomavirus: Feasibility, public health strategies and cost-effectiveness. Prev Med 2021; 144:106354.
4. Satchidanandam V. Japanese encephalitis vaccines. Curr Treat Options Infect Dis 2020;12:375–86.


## Typhoid Vaccine

Global incidence estimates indicate that India is highly endemic for typhoid, with more than 100 cases per 100,000 population annually. While the typhoid vaccine is recommended by WHO and IAP, it is currently not part of the national program **(Box 10.13)**. Four types of vaccines have been available.

The whole cell-inactivated typhoid vaccine, containing heat-killed phenol-preserved or acetone-inactivated whole cell *S. typhi* and *S. paratyphi* A and B, was administered subcutaneously in two doses 4 weeks apart, and induced humoral antibodies that were protective in 50–80% cases. However, revaccination was required every 2–3 years. While used commonly in the past, the vaccine was discontinued due to the risk of adverse events, chiefly fever, local pain and headache, observed in 10–35% cases.

An oral live attenuated vaccine, not marketed in India, is supplied as enteric coated capsules containing 2–6

**Box 10.13: Typhoid Vaccines**

| | Typhoid conjugate (PedaTyph, Typbar-TCV, TyphiBEV) | Vi capsular polysaccharide (Typbar, Vactyph, Biovac) | Live attenuated Ty21a (no Indian brands) |
|---|---|---|---|
| *Dose; route* | 0.5 mL (25 μg[1]); IM | 0.5 mL (25 μg); SC or IM | Oral; capsule |
| *Site* | Anterolateral thigh or deltoid | Anterolateral thigh or deltoid | Oral |
| *Schedule* | | | |
| National program | Not included | Not included | Not included |
| IAP 2021 | (Preferred) One dose at ≥6 months of age | (If conjugate vaccine not available) One dose at ≥2 years | Not available; 3 doses at >5 years (based on ability to swallow) |
| Booster doses | No[2] | Every 3 years | Every 3 years |
| Catch up | One dose, up to 18 years | One dose at ≥2 years | Any age |
| *Adverse reactions* | Local pain, swelling, redness; fever | Local pain, swelling, redness; fever | Abdominal discomfort, fever |
| *Contraindication* | Anaphylaxis after previous dose | Anaphylaxis after previous dose | Immunodeficiency |
| *Storage* | 2–8°C | 2–8°C; do not freeze | 2–8°C |

IM intramuscular; SC subcutaneous
[1]Except in PedaTyph, which has only 5 μg of Vi polysaccharide
[2]Whether boosters are required and when they should be given, is not yet determined

million lyophilized bacteria of Ty21a, a genetically stable mutant of *S. typhi* that is unlikely to revert to a virulent form. The vaccine induces intestinal mucosal immunity that is protective in 50–60% cases within 7 days. Since the capsules must be swallowed intact to avoid inactivation by gastric acidity, the vaccine is unsuitable for young children. Antibiotics should be avoided for 3 days before to 7 days after vaccination to avoid interference with response. Revaccination is necessary every 3 years.

The virulence (Vi) capsular polysaccharide vaccine is an injectable subunit vaccine containing the purified Vi capsular antigen of *S. typhi* strain Ty2. Vaccination induces anti-Vi IgG antibodies, which are protective in 30–70% cases at 3 years, and do not interfere with the Widal test. However, polysaccharide vaccines do not protect against *S. paratyphi*, are not immunogenic below 2 years of age, and induce T cell independent responses that lack memory, making revaccination necessary every 3 years **(Box 10.13)**.

Typhoid conjugate vaccines (TCV) contain the Vi polysaccharide antigen coupled to a carrier protein, such as tetanus toxoid (PedaTyph® and Typbar-TCV®) or the mutant diphtheria toxoid CRM197 (TyphiBEV®). Conjugate vaccines are preferred to polysaccharide vaccines since they generate T cell dependent humoral responses that are elicited even in infancy, are sustained for longer, and show strong anamnestic responses, reducing the need for redosing. In highly endemic regions such as India, the WHO recommends the vaccine in infants as young as 6 months old. Since immunity lasts at least 5 years, and natural boosting is likely in endemic regions, currently no booster doses are recommended **(Box 10.13)**. If a child has already received the polysaccharide vaccine, a dose of TCV can be given after a minimum gap of 6 months. Unlike previously recommended, a gap of 4 weeks between TCV and measles containing vaccine(s) is not necessary, if the former is given beyond 9 months of age.

### Varicella Vaccine

Varicella is a benign self-limiting illness, except when it affects adults or immunocompromised children, in whom serious complications can occur including bacterial superinfection, pneumonia, laryngitis, cerebellar ataxia, encephalomyelitis, thrombocytopenia, myocarditis, and arthritis. Maternal infection during early pregnancy causes congenital varicella syndrome, while that in perinatal period (5 days before to two days after birth) carries high risk of neonatal mortality.

Varicella vaccine is not included in the National Immunization Program because the illness is not a public health priority, the vaccine is expensive, and the risk that inadequate immunization coverage can lead to an epidemiological shift to affect older individuals, causing severe disease. The IAP recommends the vaccine for all children **(Box 10.14)**. Vaccination is specifically necessary in the following high-risk groups: (i) Chronic cardiac or lung disease; (ii) asymptomatic HIV infection with CD4 >15%; (iii) leukemia in remission and off chemotherapy >3 months; (iv) anticipated prolonged immunosuppression (before transplantation; periods off immunosuppression in nephrotic syndrome); and (v) prolonged aspirin therapy.

Vaccination should also be considered for the following individual if they lack evidence of immunity against varicella: (i) Household contacts of immunocompromised patients, (ii) immunocompetent children and adults exposed to varicella, and (iii) adolescents and adults, particularly in institutional settings (school, hospital or army). Evidence of immunity against varicella includes any of the following: (i) Confirmed past history of varicella or zoster which was documented by a healthcare professional, (ii) documented receipt of two doses of varicella vaccine in an age-appropriate schedule, and (iii) seroprotective titers of varicella antibody. Exposure is defined as face-to-face contact exceeding five minutes, or being indoors for more than one hour, with an individual who has infectious varicella (from two days before rash till after all lesions have crusted).

Each dose of varicella vaccine has at least 1000 plaque-forming units of the live virus of Oka strain attenuated in human diploid cell culture. Both cellular and humoral immune responses are elicited, providing 95–99% protective efficacy. Following one dose, seroconversion is seen in 95% young children and 80% of those >12 years. Two doses of

**Box 10.14: Varicella Vaccine**

| | |
|---|---|
| *Dose, route* | 0.5 mL, subcutaneously |
| *Site* | Anterolateral thigh or upper arm |
| *Schedule* | |
| National program | Not included |
| IAP 2021 | All children, especially high-risk categories; following exposure to varicella; and adolescents/adults without evidence of immunity[1]: Two doses 3–6 months apart, with first given at 15–18 months (minimum 12 months)[2] |
| Catch up | Complete two doses ≥3 months apart (≥4 weeks apart, if ≥13-yr-old), if lacking evidence of immunity[1] |
| *Adverse reactions* | Fever, rash, local pain or redness; mild rash after 2–3 weeks (5%) |
| *Contraindications* | Anaphylaxis after previous dose; immunodeficiency; active leukemia or lymphoma; during immunosuppressive therapy |
| *Precautions* | Moderate to severe illness; thrombocytopenia; recent receipt of blood products or immunoglobulins; therapy with aspirin |
| *Storage* | Freeze dried, lyophilized; 2–8°C; protect from light; use within 30 minutes of reconstitution |

[1]See text; interval of ≥4 weeks is acceptable in high-risk setting, post-exposure and in adolescents (>12 years)
[2]Avoid MMR-V in children <2-yr-old

the vaccine lead to seroconversion in 90% of older children and adults. If breakthrough infection occurs, it is usually a mild afebrile illness with a few lesions and predominance of papules over vesicles. Two doses are recommended to reduce the risk of primary vaccine failure and provide sustained protection, since breakthrough infections can occur within 5 years following a single dose due to waning immunity. The second dose of varicella vaccine is preferably administered 3–6 months after the first dose, and is suggested to not be delayed to school entry age in countries like India with poor vaccine coverage, where the wildtype virus circulates predominantly.

When used for post-exposure prophylaxis (within 72 hours of contact), the protective efficacy of one dose of the vaccine is only ~70%.

Internationally available monovalent preparations (Varilrix® and Variped®) and its combination with MMR (MMR-V, Priorix-Tetra®) show similar immunogenicity and efficacy. While MMR-V is safe in children older than 2 years, in patients 12–23 months old, the vaccine is associated with a higher rate of adverse events (fever, rash, febrile seizures) compared to MMR and varicella administered separately. *Hence, the IAP cautions against the use of MMR-V below 2 years of age.*

Two forms of zoster vaccines are licensed for adults >50-yr-old. Zostavax®, containing a higher number of live attenuated viral particles than conventional varicella vaccines, is available in India. The FDA-approved Shingrix® is a subunit vaccine which is preferred over Zostavax for its superior efficacy and safety, permitting its use even in immunocompromised adults.

### Influenza Vaccine (Box 10.15)

Influenza virus has three antigenic types (A to C), and several subtypes based on its surface antigens hemagglutinin and neuraminidase. Mutations due to antigenic drifts and shifts result in frequent changes in circulating strains. Influenza viruses (A, B) cause global flu epidemics with severe disease in young children, the elderly and immunocompromised, and those with chronic illnesses. In south Asia, outbreaks of influenza are most common during June to November, have attack rates of 10–50%, and typically last 2–3 months. Available vaccines elicit a strain-specific humoral response with protective efficacy of 30–90%. Hence, vaccine composition is reviewed by the WHO annually for changes in component antigens.

***Inactivated influenza vaccines:*** These tri- or quadrivalent vaccines, containing two influenza A and one or two influenza B strains, are derived from viruses grown in chick embryos or cell culture. Whole virus vaccines, associated with significant adverse effects, are no longer used. Current vaccines are either split product, produced from detergent-treated purified viruses, or surface antigen subunit vaccines, containing purified hemagglutinin and neuraminidase. These are highly immunogenic, associated with minimal adverse events, and can be used safely above 6 months of age. The quadrivalent inactivated influenza vaccines (e.g., Influvac Tetra®, Fluarix Tetra®, Vaxiflu-4®, FluQuadri®) are preferred over the trivalent ones (e.g., Vaxigrip®, Vaxiflu®, Influvac®, Fluarix®). Protective efficacy for inactivated vaccines ranges from 30–90% and varies by subtype.

***Live attenuated intranasal vaccine:*** These trivalent or quadrivalent vaccines are developed by repeated passage of viruses at low temperature, to form a temperature sensitive variant that grows well at 25°C but does not replicate at 37–39°C. The vaccine (e.g. FluMist®, Nasovac-5®) is recommended for healthy children older than 2 years, and is more immunogenic than the inactivated vaccines. Efficacy varies from 25–90%, and is higher during outbreaks. Despite theoretical risk, reversion to virulent phenotype is not reported. Still, live vaccines are avoided in high-risk categories (*see* below). Children, 2–18 years old and

**Box 10.15: Influenza Vaccines**

| | **Inactivated vaccine** | **Live attenuated vaccine** |
|---|---|---|
| *Dose, route* | 0.5 mL (15 μg); intramuscular | 0.25 mL in each nostril |
| *Site* | Anterolateral thigh or upper arm | Intranasal using *accuspray* device |
| *Schedule* | | |
| National program | Not included | Not included |
| IAP 2021 | All children >6 months to 5-yr-old; children >5-yr-old with high-risk category[1]<br>First time vaccination:<br>6 months to 9-yr-old: Two doses ≥4 weeks apart[2]<br>≥9-yr-old: Single dose<br>Subsequently: Annual revaccination with one dose, preferably before rainy season[3] | All healthy children 2–18 years old<br>First time vaccination:<br>2–9 years old: Two doses ≥4 weeks apart[2]<br>≥9 years old: Single dose<br>Subsequently: Annual revaccination with one dose, preferably before rainy season[3] |
| *Adverse reactions* | Mild (10–35%): local pain, fever, nausea; severe (rare): anaphylaxis; Guillain-Barre syndrome[4] | Runny nose, headache, wheeze, myalgia, fever, sore throat, vomiting |
| *Contraindications, precautions* | Anaphylaxis after a previous dose, intake of egg or chicken, or thiomerosal; use cautiously in children with suspected chicken or egg allergy | Severe allergy after any influenza vaccine; high risk categories[1] |
| *Storage* | 2–8°C; do not freeze | 2–8°C; do not freeze |

[1]See text; [2]Also applicable to children <9 years old who have received fewer than two doses in the past; [3]Based on the latest (annual) WHO recommendation for the Southern hemisphere strain; if not available, use the latest vaccine available; [4]Unclear association, with 1 additional case per million adult recipients

otherwise healthy, may receive either the live or inactivated vaccine.

Routine vaccination is currently not part of the national immunization program. The IAP recommends the inactivated vaccine in all children 6 months to 5 years old, and in older children (5–18 years old) with certain high-risk settings, including: (i) Chronic cardiac, pulmonary, hematological, kidney or liver disease; (iii) asthma, or wheeze during the past one year; (iii) other chronic medical conditions, such as sickle cell disease, diabetes mellitus, systemic lupus erythematosus or morbid obesity; (iv) immunodeficiency; (v) prolonged therapy with aspirin; and (vi) laboratory personnel and healthcare workers **(Box 10.15)**. Due to a theoretical risk of reactivation of the attenuated strain, the live vaccine is avoided in patients with the above conditions, and in individuals who have received influenza antiviral therapy in the last 48 hours. Influenza vaccine should altogether be avoided in children who have experienced severe allergic reactions to a previous dose of either vaccine or any of its components **(Box 10.15)**.

The most optimal time to vaccinate against influenza would be before the onset of peak influenza activity which, in India, peaks during the rainy season, and in the extreme northern part of India, during the winter months. Hence, the optimum time to vaccinate is the pre-monsoon period (i.e., before June and October in north and south India, respectively). Vaccination should be performed using the latest available Southern hemisphere strain since the WHO classifies India under the 'South Asia' transmission zone of influenza circulation, which is more aligned with the Southern, rather than Northern, hemisphere strains.

### Rabies Vaccine

India is endemic for rabies, accounting for 50% of global deaths. Nerve tissue vaccines are not recommended due to poor efficacy and high incidence of adverse effects. Modern tissue or cell culture vaccines, available as lyophilized preparations that are reconstituted to provide at least 2.5 IU per intramuscular dose, include: (i) Purified duck embryo vaccine (Vaxirab®); (ii) purified chick embryo cell vaccine (Rabipur®, Vaxirab-N®); (iii) human diploid cell vaccine (Rabivax®); and (iv) purified vero-cell culture-derived vaccines (Indirab®, Verorab®, Verovax-R®, Abhayrab®, Verovax-R®). All these vaccines have comparable and high efficacy. Since they lack myelin basic protein, all modern vaccines are safer than the nerve tissue vaccines.

***Post-exposure prophylaxis:*** An animal bite/wound is characterized as follows: (i) Category I: Animal touch or lick on intact skin; (ii) Category II: Minor scratches or abrasions without bleeding, licks on broken skin or nibbling of uncovered skin; and (iii) Category III: Single or multiple transdermal bites, abrasions that bleed, scratches or contamination of mucous membranes with saliva/licks, and any bite from a wild animal. Individuals with category II or III wounds need wound management and rabies vaccine **(Box 10.16)**. Patients with wound category III, and immunocompromised patients with wound category II, should also receive rabies immunoglobulin. Individuals who have received pre- or post- exposure prophylaxis with rabies vaccine in the past do not require immunoglobulin.

Wound management includes immediate irrigation with running water for 10 minutes, thorough cleaning with soap and water, and application of povidone-iodine, 70% alcohol or tincture iodine. Tetanus toxoid and antibiotics are administered as indicated. Wound suturing is avoided; if necessary, it is performed after administering immunoglobulin.

Rabies immunoglobulin provides passive immunity by neutralizing rabies viruses (*see* Passive Immunization). Its dose is 20 U/kg for human immunoglobulin (ImogenRab®, KamRab®, BeriRab-P®; maximum 1500 U) and 40 U/kg for equine immunoglobulin (Equirab®, Vinrig®; maximum 3000 U) or equine anti-rabies serum. Human rabies immunoglobulin (HRIG) is preferred. This is infiltrated in and around the wound as soon as possible, not later than day 7 of injury. For large or multiple wounds, immunoglobulin is diluted with normal saline to infiltrate the entire wounded region. Any remaining immunoglobulin is administered intramuscularly at a site away from vaccination site, usually the deltoid or anterolateral thigh.

Recently, two monoclonal rabies antibodies have been licensed for use in India that are based on recombinant technology and are cell-culture derived, offering a potent

**Box 10.16: Rabies Vaccine**

| | |
|---|---|
| *Type* | Modern tissue culture vaccine |
| *Dose, route* | Intramuscular (IM): 0.5 mL (1 mL for non-Vero cell vaccine) |
| | Intradermal (ID)[1]: 0.1 mL (0.2 mL for non-Vero cell vaccine; 0.25 IU) |
| *Site* | Deltoid (≥2 years old) or anterolateral thigh (<2-year-old); never gluteal region |
| *Schedule* | |
| National program | Not recommended |
| IAP 2021 | *Pre-exposure:* Specific indications[2]; three IM doses on days 0, 7 and 28 |
| | *Post-exposure:* After animal bites; usually 5 IM or ID doses[2] |
| | *Re-exposure*[3]: Two doses, on days 0 and 3 |
| *Adverse reactions* | Common: Local pain, swelling, induration (more with ID dose) |
| | Uncommon: Fever, malaise, abdominal pain, headache, dizziness; hypersensivity (seen with diploid cell vaccine) |
| *Storage* | 2–8°C; use within 6 hours of reconstitution |

[1]Licensed in India only for specific purified chick embryo or vero cell-derived vaccines, in centers with adequate training and frequent use of the vaccine; not licensed in India for pre-exposure prophylaxis; [2]See text; [3]With documentation of having completed pre-exposure prophylaxis in the past

and preferred alternative to the current blood-derived rabies immunoglobulins. These include Rabishield®, a human monoclonal antibody against rabies virus glycoprotein (RAB1 or 17C7), and Twinrab®, a combination of two murine anti-rabies monoclonal antibodies, docaravimab (62-71-3) and miromavimab (M777-16-3). These antibodies are associated with minor and uncommon adverse effects, including injection site pain, swelling or redness, headache, myalgia, and upper respiratory tract infection. The IAP endorses the use of either monoclonal for post-exposure prophylaxis of category III wounds, in preference to rabies immunoglobulin, along with the vaccine.

Vaccination is usually planned using the Essen or WHO schedule, in which 5 intramuscular (IM) doses are given on days 0, 3, 7, 14 and 28; an additional dose on day 90 is advised in immunocompromised or severely malnourished individuals. The Updated Thai Red Cross schedule (2-2-2-0-2-0) involves administering two intradermal (ID) doses each on days 0, 3, 7 and 30. Abbreviated and effective alternate schedules include: (i) Zagreb (2-1-1: two IM doses on day 0; one dose each on days 7 and 21; not used in India); (ii) Thai Red Cross (2-2-2-0-1-1: two ID doses on days 0, 3 and 7, and one ID dose each on days 30 and 90); (iii) abbreviated multisite (similar to Zagreb, except that last dose is on day 14; not used in India), and (iv) eight site (8-0-4-0-1-1: eight ID doses on day 0, four doses on day 7, and one each on days 30 and 90; not used in India). A reduced four-dose (IM doses on 0, 3, 7 and 14 days) is not endorsed by the IAP. Following re-exposure, patients who have previously completed pre-exposure prophylaxis should receive two doses on days 0 and 3. For all schedules, the same product should be used for all the doses.

*Pre-exposure prophylaxis:* This is offered to individuals at high risk of rabies, such as laboratory staff handling virus or infected material, care providers to patients with rabies, veterinarians, animal handlers and catchers, taxidermists, wildlife workers, wardens, quarantine officers, municipal workers, postmen and travelers to endemic areas. The IAP recommends its use in certain high-risk categories of children, chiefly (i) children having pets in home, and (ii) children perceived with higher threat of being bitten by dogs such as hostellers, risk of stray dog menace while going outdoor. Three IM doses are given on days 0, 7 and 28; the third dose may be given on day 21, if risk is imminent. In high-risk settings and in immunocompromised individuals, the antibody titer is monitored 6–12 monthly and boosters given in order to maintain protective titers (>0.5 U/mL).

### Hepatitis A Vaccine

India is hyperendemic for hepatitis A, with 50% children acquiring seropositivity by 5 years of age, usually following asymptomatic or mildly symptomatic infection. Disease severity, complications and mortality are higher in adolescents, adults and children with underlying chronic liver disease. While hepatitis A vaccination is not a public health priority, improving hygiene has resulted in a later age at infection, leading to serious complications. Further, almost half the cases of fulminant hepatic failure in childhood are still caused by hepatitis A vaccine. Hence, the IAP recommends vaccinating all children against hepatitis A. High-risk categories in which vaccination must be considered, in view of higher risk of exposure or unfavorable outcomes, include: (i) Patients with chronic liver disease; (ii) seronegative travelers to endemic areas; (iii) children attending crèches and daycare; (iv) seronegative adolescents; and (v) liver and kidney transplant recipients.

Two types of vaccines are available. Formalin-inactivated viral vaccines usually have aluminum hydroxide or a virosome adjuvant, and are available either singly or in combination with hepatitis B. Two doses, when administered 6–12 months apart at >1 year age, provide protective efficacy of 95% which lasts for 40–50 years **(Box 10.17)**. Two live vaccines are available which are based on H2 and L-A-1 strains of hepatitis A virus, attenuated through repeated cell culture and grown on human diploid lung fibroblasts. A single dose of live vaccine is immunogenic and safe, with protection lasting at least 10 years **(Box 10.17)**. Since maternal antibodies interfere with immune responses, both vaccines are avoided in infancy.

The vaccine is effective as pre- and post-exposure prophylaxis. Pre-exposure prophylaxis with vaccine alone

**Box 10.17: Hepatitis A Vaccine**

| | Inactivated vaccine | Live attenuated vaccine |
|---|---|---|
| *Dose, route* | 0.5 mL (720 U); intramuscular | 0.5 mL; intramuscular |
| *Site* | Deltoid | Deltoid |
| *Schedule* | | |
| National program | Not included | Not included |
| IAP 2021 | >1 year: Two doses 6 months apart | >1 year: One dose |
| Catch up | 1–10 years: As above<br>>10 years: After confirming seronegativity, give two doses 6–12 months apart; use higher dose (1440 U; 1 mL) if >18-yr-old | As for inactivated vaccine |
| *Adverse reactions* | Local pain, headache, malaise | Soreness, erythema, fever, malaise |
| *Contraindications* | Anaphylaxis after previous dose | Hypersensitivity to egg protein; immunodeficiency, chemotherapy or radiotherapy |
| *Storage* | 2–8°C; protect from light<br>Use within 30 minutes of reconstitution | 2–8°C; do not freeze<br>Use within 30 minutes of reconstitution |

is sufficient for most international travelers to endemic areas; however, young infants (<6-month-old) and immunocompromised individuals additionally require passive immunization with specific immunoglobulin (see later). Similarly, vaccine alone is sufficient for post-exposure prophylaxis, if administered within 14 days of exposure to unimmunized household or institutional contacts of symptomatic patients, if they are otherwise healthy and 1–40 years old. Specific immunoglobulin is additionally administered, if the exposed individual is an infant (<1-yr-old), immunocompromised or has chronic liver disease.

### Meningococcal Vaccine

*Neisseria meningitidis* accounts for 30–40% cases of bacterial meningitis in children, with high case fatality. Invasive infections are caused by serogroups A, B, C, Y, W135 and X are reported chiefly in either pre-school children or adolescents. Outbreaks of meningitis due to serogroup A (and sometimes C) are frequently reported in north India. However, the overall burden of endemic meningococcal disease is low in India, hence vaccination is not indicated routinely.

Two types of vaccines are available. Like other polysaccharide vaccines, the unconjugated polysaccharide vaccines contain serogroup-specific capsular polysaccharides, which induce T cell independent humoral responses, do not provide immunological memory, and are poorly immunogenic below 2 years of age. These are available as bivalent (containing groups A and C) and tetravalent (groups A, C, Y and W135) vaccines. Conjugate vaccines are preferred over polysaccharide vaccines due to higher immunogenicity, prolonged efficacy and potential for herd effect, especially in childhood. Two types of polysaccharide-protein conjugate vaccines are available in India **(Box 10.18)**. The quadrivalent conjugate vaccine (groups A, C, Y and W135; Menactra® and Menveo®) use diphtheria toxin or its protein CRM197 as carriers, while the monovalent (serogroup A or C) vaccine uses tetanus toxoid (MenA) or CRM197 (MenC) as carrier protein. The former is preferred in India, and the latter is used predominantly in Africa (MenA) or Europe (MenC).

The quadrivalent conjugate vaccine is recommended for use in India in certain high-risk situations, including: (i) Immunocompromised patients, including HIV and complement component deficiency; (ii) functional or anatomical asplenia, hyposplenia, or splenectomy (ideally given 2 weeks prior); (iii) before therapy with complement inhibitors (e.g. eculizumab, ideally given 2 weeks prior); (iv) chronic cardiac, pulmonary, or severe systemic disease (including renal or hepatic disease, diabetes mellitus); (v) adolescents and adults residing in crowded institutions, e.g. boarding school; (vi) before cochlear implant; (vii) before travel to endemic regions, e.g. the African meningococcal belt; and (viii) after close contact with patients with meningococcal disease.

### Yellow Fever Vaccine

The yellow fever vaccine is a live attenuated vaccine of either 17D-204 or 17DD strain that is effective against all known strains of yellow fever. Neutralizing antibodies develop in 90% vaccinees by 10 days and in 100% by 3 weeks, and persist for three decades. A single dose is administered at least 10 days before planned travel to endemic areas in Africa and South or Central America **(Box 10.19)**. Adverse effects are common; administration in young infants and pregnant women is avoided.

### Suggested Reading


1. Centers for Disease Control and Prevention. Yellow fever vaccine recommendations. Available at: https://www.cdc.gov/yellowfever/vaccine/vaccine-recommendations.html; last accessed 10 September 2022.
2. Ertl HCJ. New rabies vaccines for use in humans. Vaccines (Basel) 2019; 7: 54.
3. Gershon AA, Gershon MD, Shapiro ED. Live attenuated varicella vaccine: Prevention of varicella and of zoster. J Infect Dis. 2021; 224 (12 Suppl 2): S387–S397.
4. Masuet-Aumatell C, Atouguia J. Typhoid fever infection - Antibiotic resistance and vaccination strategies: A narrative review. Travel Med Infect Dis 2021; 40: 101946.


**Box 10.18: Meningococcal Vaccine**

| | Polysaccharide vaccine | Quadrivalent conjugate vaccine |
|---|---|---|
| *Dose, route* | 0.5 mL, SC or IM | 0.5 mL, IM |
| *Site* | Anterolateral thigh or upper arm | Anterolateral thigh or upper arm |
| *Schedule* | | |
| National program | Not included | Not included |
| IAP 2021 | High-risk categories only (less preferred)[1] and at >2-year-old[2]: Two doses 8 weeks apart; one booster dose every 5 years, if risk persists | High-risk categories only (preferred)[1]: 9–23 months old: (Menactra, not Menveo) Two doses 3 months apart; >2 years old (Menactra, Menveo): Single dose; one booster dose every 5 years, if the risk persists |
| *Adverse reactions* | Fever, local pain or redness | Local pain, swelling or redness; rarely, Guillain-Barre syndrome |
| *Contraindications; precautions* | Anaphylaxis after previous dose | May interfere with pneumococcal conjugate vaccine; separate administration by ≥4 weeks |
| *Storage* | 2–8°C; protect from light; use within 30 minutes of reconstitution | 2–8°C; do not freeze |

[1]See text
[2]Except in outbreaks, when infants >3-month-old may be given the vaccine

**Box 10.19: Yellow Fever Vaccine**

| | |
|---|---|
| *Type* | Live attenuated (17D-204) |
| *Dose, route* | 0.5 mL, subcutaneous |
| *Site* | Anterolateral thigh or upper arm |
| *Schedule* | |
| National program | Not included |
| IAP 2021 | Single dose ≥10 days before travel to endemic areas; revaccinate after 10 years |
| *Indications* | Residence in, or travel to, endemic area; age >9 months |
| *Adverse reactions* | Mild (20–30%): Fever, headache and myalgia |
| *Contraindication* | Age <6 months; symptomatic HIV or CD4 <15% or <200/mm$^3$; primary or secondary immunodeficiency; radiation; malignancy; organ transplantation; chemotherapy; anaphylaxis after a previous dose; allergy to a vaccine component |
| *Precaution* | Age 6–9 months or >60 years; pregnancy and lactation; asymptomatic HIV or CD4 ≥15% or 200–499/mm$^3$; family history of vaccine-associated adverse effects |
| *Storage* | 2–8°C; use within 30 minutes of reconstitution |

5. Pizza M, Bekkat-Berkani R, Rappuoli R. Vaccines against meningococcal diseases. Microorganisms 2020;8:1521.
6. Sekiya T, Ohno M, Nomura N, et al. Selecting and using the appropriate influenza vaccine for each individual. Viruses 2021; 13: 971.
7. Song KR, Lim JK, Park SE, et al. Oral cholera vaccine efficacy and effectiveness. Vaccines (Basel). 2021; 9: 1482.
8. Zhang L. Hepatitis A vaccination. Hum Vaccin Immunother 2020; 16: 1565–73.

## SARS-CoV-2 Vaccines

The process of development of vaccines against SARS-CoV-2 represents an unprecedented global effort which culminated in rapid implementation of vaccination programs within a few months of the infection being labeled a pandemic.

### *Rationale for Vaccinating Children*

There has been considerable debate over the benefits versus potential harm of vaccinating children against SARS-CoV-2 infections, since the majority (~70%) of infections in children are asymptomatic, and most symptomatic children have mild disease, rarely requiring hospitalization. While children did not participate significantly in the transmission chain during the early phases of the pandemic when lockdowns were imposed, with reopening of schools and resumption of normal activities, it was necessary to vaccinate children to reduce the rates of symptomatic infections as well as reduce viral transmission. A cross-sectional study conducted across India in 2021 indicated serological evidence of infection in 57% of children aged 6–9 years, and 62% of those aged 10–17 years. Despite this, vaccinating children was considered necessary since antibody response declines with time, and unvaccinated individuals appear to have higher risk of reinfection and lower antibody titers than those who were fully vaccinated.

### *Available Vaccines*

The attributes of the most commonly used vaccines are compared in **Table 10.5**. The three vaccines that have been licensed for use in India's national program are Covishield (Serum Institute of India), Covaxin (Bharat Biotech) and CorBEvax (Biological E), sanctioned for use in patients ≥18-yr-old, ≥15-yr-old, and 12–14-yr-old, respectively **(Box 10.20)**. Other vaccines authorized in India for emergency use (EUA) in children ≥12-yr-old include ZyCov-D (Zydus Cadila) and Covovax (Serum Institute of India). Vaccines commonly used in children elsewhere, but not yet licensed or marketed in India, include BNT162b2 (Pfizer), mRNA-1273 (Moderna), and Gam-COVID-Vac (Sputnik). Recently, the intranasal vaccine iNCOVACC (Bharat Biotech) was approved in India for >18-yr-olds.

### *National Policy on COVID-19 Vaccination*

The national policy for vaccination against COVID-19 was implemented in a stepwise manner. Within a span of nine

**Box 10.20: SARS-CoV-2 Vaccine**

| | |
|---|---|
| *Dose, route* | 0.5 mL; intramuscular |
| *Site* | Upper arm |
| *Schedule (Post-pandemic)* | |
| National program; IAP 2021 | Covaxin, 2 doses ≥4 weeks apart; booster ≥9 months |
| *Indications* | Age ≥12 years |
| *Adverse reactions* | Mild fever, pain, headache; myocarditis (mRNA vaccines); thrombocytopenia |
| *Contraindication* | Anaphylaxis following previous dose |
| *Precaution* | Coagulopathy |
| | Avoid vaccination until 4–8 weeks later, in individuals with: (i) acute infection with SARS-CoV-2; (ii) past infection with SARS-CoV-2 and having received anti-SARS-CoV-2 monoclonal antibodies or convalescent plasma; and (iii) any acute illness requiring hospitalization |
| *Storage* | 2–8°C |

**Table 10.5:** Globally used SARS-CoV-2 vaccines

| | *Covaxin (BBV-152)* | *Covishield; Oxford-Astra Zeneca (AZD1222)* | *Corbevax* | *ZyCoV-D* | *Covovax (Novovax)* | *Moderna (mRNA-1273)* | *Sinopharm (BBIBP-CorV)* | *BNT162b2 (Pfizer)* | *Gam-COVID-Vac (Sputnik)* |
|---|---|---|---|---|---|---|---|---|---|
| Manufacturer, country | Bharat Biotech and ICMR, India | Oxford University, UK and Astra-Zeneca Inc; Serum Institute of India | Texas Children's Hospital, Baylor College of Medicine, Houston; Dynavax Technologies, California; Biological E, India | Zydus Cadila Healthcare, India | Serum Institute, India | Moderna Inc., NIAID and BARDA | Beijing Institute of Biologic Products, China | Pfizer, USA and BioNtech, Germany | Gamaleya Research Institute of Epidemiology and Microbiology, Russia |
| Age licensed[1] | ≥2 yr | ≥18 yr | ≥12 yr | ≥12 yr | ≥12 yr | 12–17 yr (EUA: >5 yr) | ≥18 yr (EUA: >3 yr) | ≥5 yr | ≥18 yr |
| Countries of use | India; ≥19 other countries | India; Brazil; Australia; ≥169 other countries | India | India | India | Switzerland, USA, ≥79 other countries (EUA in India) | China, Bahrain, UAE, ≥75 other countries | USA, Switzerland, ≥114 other countries | Russia, Pakistan, ≥58 other countries |
| Vaccine type | Inactivated virus[2-1] | Spike protein in chimpanzee adenovirus vector ChAdOx[1] | Receptor binding domain of the spike protein adjuvanted to aluminum hydroxide gel and CpG1018 | DNA plasmid carrying the spike protein gene | Recombinant[2-2] SARS-CoV-2 spike proteins in a nanoparticle | Modified mRNA encoding nucleoside-stabilized prefusion protein in nanoparticle | Inactivated virus[2-1] | Modified mRNA encoding nucleoside-stabilized prefusion protein | Full-length spike protein in recombinant adenovirus vector |
| Dose, route | 0.5 mL, IM | 0.5 mL, IM | 0.5 mL, IM | Two ID injections, 0.1 mL each | 0.5 mL; IM | 100 μg; IM | 0.5 mL; IM | <5-yr: 10 μg ≥5-yr: 3 μg; IM | 0.5 mL; IM |
| Doses; interval | 2 doses 4 weeks apart | 2 doses 8–12 weeks apart | 2 doses 4 weeks apart | 3 doses 4 weeks apart | 2 doses 3 weeks apart | 2 doses 4 weeks apart | 2 doses 3–4 weeks apart | <5-yr-old: 1 dose ≥5-yr-old: 2 doses 3 weeks apart | Two doses 3 weeks apart[3] |
| Interval between doses | 4 weeks | 8–12 weeks | 4 weeks | 4 weeks | 3 weeks | 4 weeks | 3–4 weeks | 3 weeks | 3 weeks |
| Vaccine efficacy, % | 63.4 to 93.4% | 55 to 80% | ~90% | 66.7 | 89.7% | 94.5% | 78.1% | 80 to 100% | 50 to 81% |

BARDA Biomedical Advanced Research and Development Authority; ICMR Indian Council of Medical Research; ID intradermal; IM intramuscular; NIAID United States National Institute of Allergy and Infectious Diseases

All vaccines are stored at temperature of +2°C to +8°C except Moderna (–25°C to –15°C), BNT162b2 or Pfizer (–70°C), and the freeze-dried powder of Gam-COVID-Vac or Sputnik (<-18°C)

[1]Use in children has often been based on emergency use authorization (EUA)

[2]Produced by [2-1]replication in Vero cell lines, followed by inactivation by β-propriolactone and adjuvanted to alhydroxyquim-II or aluminum hydroxide alum; and [2-2]recombination in a baculovirus expression system in an insect cell line derived from Sf9 cells of *Spodoptera frugiperda* and adjuvanted to *Quillaja saponaria* molina extract

[3]The two doses differ in the serotype of the replication-defective adenovirus vector, with Ad26 used for delivering dose 1 and Ad5 for dose 2

months, one billion Indians were immunized with at least one dose of the COVID-19 vaccine. Phase 1 focused on vaccinating the healthcare workers (since 16 January 2021) and other frontline workers (1 February 2021). In phase II, beginning on 1 March 2021, vaccination was initiated for the elderly (≥60-yr-old) and unwell older adults (≥45-yr-old with comorbidities), following which vaccination was opened to all older adults (≥45-yr-old). Phases III and IV enabled vaccination of all adult patients (≥18-yr-old) through private and public sector hospitals and later, free of cost. In phase V, initiated since January 2022, precaution/booster doses were administered to persons included in phases I and II, and vaccination was extended to include children ≥15-yr-old, and later, ≥12-yr-old.

Currently available COVID-19 vaccines can be administered alongside other scheduled childhood vaccines, either simultaneously or at any interval between them. Nationwide reporting of all vaccinations, using the COWIN portal and app, has been mandatory. Real-time remote temperature monitoring of cold-chain points is done through COVID Vaccine Intelligence Network (Co-WIN) vaccine delivery and E-VIN.

#### Suggested Reading


1. Creech CB, Walker SC, Samuels RJ. SARS-CoV-2 vaccines. JAMA. 2021;325:1318–20.
2. Kasi SG, Dhir SK, Shah A, et al; For Advisory Committee on Vaccines and Immunization Practices (ACVIP), Indian Academy of Pediatrics. Coronavirus Disease 2019 (COVID-19) vaccination for children: Indian Pediatr 2022; 59:51–57.
3. Kouhpayeh H, Ansari H. Adverse events following COVID-19 vaccination: A systematic review and meta-analysis. Int Immunopharmacol 2022;109:108906.


*Competency:* **PE19.16**

## Vaccines not Yet in Use

### *Dengue Vaccine*

Dengue infection, a common mosquito-borne disease in the tropical regions, most commonly affecting adolescents and young adults. Efforts to develop safe and effective vaccines to prevent dengue virus infections have been thwarted by challenges related to vaccine immunogenicity, limited efficacy, and the risks of vaccine-induced dengue hemorrhagic syndrome or shock. Of seven vaccines currently in stages of testing of safety and efficacy, three are considered most promising.

Dengvaxia is the only dengue vaccine which has been licensed globally. This chimeric vaccine has a yellow fever virus backbone from which two genes have been removed and replaced by one gene each from the four dengue virus serotypes. When used in individuals 9–45 years old, the vaccine had modest efficacy (25–59%), with particularly low protection against type 2 dengue virus strain, thus leading to need for multiple doses. A worrisome and widely criticized drawback has been the vaccine's association with risk of severe dengue infection in individuals who were seronegative at vaccination. The WHO has approved the use of Dengvaxia in highly endemic countries where the majority (~90%) of eligible individuals would be seropositive at vaccination. Children of age 9–16 years living in dengue endemic areas and with laboratory confirmation of previous dengue infection are administered three doses at 0, 6, and 12 months. However, the risk of severe dengue makes it unsuitable for large-scale implementation in India's immunization program.

Two dengue vaccines, namely LATV and DenVax, are currently in phase III clinical trials. The former vaccine has a dengue virus 4 backbone into which recombinant genes from the other three dengue virus types have been inserted. The latter vaccine is based on a live-attenuated dengue virus type 2 strain in which two genes are replaced by one homologous gene each from the other three dengue virus serotypes.

### *Malaria Vaccine*

The RTS, S vaccine is the first malaria vaccine to be licensed. The vaccine is based on the fact that immunization with attenuated *Plasmodium* sporozoites induces protective immune responses that protect against parasitic infection. The vaccine comprises a hepatitis B virus-like particle containing genetically recombined portions of the repeat domain and the C-terminal region of the circumsporozoite protein (CSP) of *P. falciparum*. CSP is expressed on the surface of sporozoites of different *Plasmodium* species and contains a central domain of tandem repeats. Antibodies binding to the CSP immobilize the sporozoites, thus preventing infection of hepatocytes, an obligatory stage in infection with malaria.

Multiple phase 2 and 3 clinical trials in malaria endemic areas show that immunizing children 6–12 weeks and 5–7 months old induces protective immunity that neutralizes sporozoite infection and attenuates the severity of malaria. Based on these studies, the World Health Organization (WHO) has recommended this vaccine for widespread use among children living in malaria endemic areas. However, efficacy wanes with time, from 63–74% a few weeks after immunization, to 11–28% at 1 year and 3–9% at 5 years. Further, the vaccine-induced immune responses do not inhibit gametocytes; hence, transmission of *Plasmodium* and, therefore, endemicity remains unchanged.

A new vaccine candidate, termed R21, comprising of an antigenic domain similar to RTS, S expressed in a nanoparticle, may offer 77% protection from severe malaria.

#### Suggested Reading


1. Torres-Flores JM, Reyes-Sandoval A, Salazar MI. Dengue vaccines: An update. BioDrugs. 2022; 36: 325–36.
2. Zavala F. RTS,S: The first malaria vaccine. J Clin Invest 2022; 132: e156588.


## Combination Vaccines

A combination vaccine consists of multiple immunogens physically combined in a single preparation, including antigens or serotypes of the same pathogen (e.g. trivalent polio vaccine) or different pathogens (e.g. pentavalent or DTP vaccines). This is distinct from simultaneous administration of multiple separate vaccines at the same time at separate sites. The immune system of an infant can respond to a large number of antigens simultaneously, and the efficacy of most vaccines is not altered by concurrent administration. With the requirement of vaccination against several infections, a child needs to be administered more than 20 antigens in the first 2 years. Combining vaccines offers several benefits. Fewer injections at each visit and fewer visits increases compliance. The immunization program also benefits from decreased expenditure on packaging, storage and transportation and enhanced immunization coverage. The uptake of a new vaccine is improved by replacing a previously used vaccine with a vaccine combining the new and existing vaccines, e.g. the immunization coverage for Hib was ensured by replacing DPT with the pentavalent vaccine.

Development of combination vaccines is challenging. The antigens should be compatible and not interfere with each other's immunological 'take' (relevant for live viral vaccines) and be indicated at the same time. Some antigens may require an adjuvant to be present in the combination. The total volume of the vaccine should not be excessive and the product should be stable for at least a year. The efficacy of the combination must be evaluated and cost benefit analyses done before licensing. Common combination vaccines include pentavalent, DTwP, DTaP, DT, dT, OPV, IPV, MMR, MR and influenza (Table 10.6).

**Table 10.6:** Combination vaccines used in children and infants

| *Vaccine* | *Examples* |
|---|---|
| DTwP-HB-Hib | Pentavalent vaccine; Pentavac PFS®, Comvac-5®, ComBE Five®, Shan-5® May combine in same syringe, e.g. Qvac® + HibPro®, Hiberix® + Tritanrix® |
| DTwP | Tripvac®, Triple antigen®, Comvac3® |
| DTaP-HB-Hib | Easy-5® |
| DTaP-Hib-IPV | Pentaxim® |
| DTaP-IPV | Tetraxim® |
| DTaP | Infanrix®, Boostrix®, Tripacel® |
| Tdap | Boostrix®, Adacel® |
| Td | Td-Vac®, BE-Td® |
| DTwP-HB | Shantetra®, Q-VAC®, Tritanrix-HB®, Tripvac-HB®, Comvac-4-HB® |
| DTaP–Hib | Easy-4® may combine Tripacel® + ActHib®, Infanrix® + Hiberix® |
| DTwP–Hib | Quadrovax®, Shan-4®, Tetract Hib®; Triple antigen® + HibPro® |
| HepA-HepB | Twinrix® |
| MMR-V | Priorix tetra®, Proquad® |
| Meningococcal | A, C, Y and 135 (Mencevax ACWY®); A, C, Y and 135 DT conjugate (Menactra®); quadrivalent conjugate (Menveo®) |
| Pneumococcal | 10 or 13-valent conjugate vaccine (Prevenar®), 10-valent conjugate vaccine (Pneumosil®), 23-valent conjugate vaccine (Pneumo23®), polyvalent polysaccharide vaccine (Pneumovax®) |

aP acellular pertussis; ap acellular pertussis reduced dose; D/DT diphtheria toxoid; d/Td diphtheria toxoid reduced dose; HB hepatitis B; HepA hepatitis A; Hib *Hemophilus influenzae* b; MMR measles, mumps, rubella; T/TT tetanus toxoid; V varicella; wP whole cell pertussis

## ADVERSE EVENTS FOLLOWING IMMUNIZATION (AEFI)

An adverse event following immunization (AEFI) is defined as any untoward medical event that follows immunization. Not all events have a causal relationship with the vaccine, and can be categorized as follows: (i) *Vaccine induced:* Event caused or precipitated by an active component of vaccine, e.g. anaphylaxis after measles vaccine, vaccine associated paralytic poliomyelitis, BCG related adenitis, pertussis encephalopathy; (ii) *Vaccine potentiated:* Event precipitated by vaccination but may have occurred without vaccination, e.g. first febrile seizure; (iii) *Injection reaction:* Event from anxiety, pain due to the injection (rather than the vaccine), e.g. syncope after vaccination; (iv) *Program or immunization errors:* Event due to error in vaccine preparation, handling or administration, e.g. toxic shock syndrome due to contaminated measles vaccine, abscess at injection site; (v) *Coincidental:* Temporally linked, by chance or due to unrelated illness, e.g. gastroenteritis after MMR injection.

Each AEFI must be assessed for its severity and causality. An AEFI is considered serious, if it results in recipient's death, hospitalization or persistent or significant disability, or occurs in clusters, i.e. two or more cases are reported within a geographical area. These events should be reported immediately, and investigated appropriately. Overall, immunization error-related reactions (also called program errors) are the most cause of serious AEFI.

The assessment of causality should follow guidance provided by the World Health Organization in 2013, which relies chiefly on: (i) Whether there is a known causal association with the vaccine; (ii) timing of the event in relation to the vaccination and anticipated period of risk; and (iii) presence of evidence against a causal relationship.

Minor reactions are common, and include fever, irritability, malaise and pain, and swelling or redness at the injection site. These are self-limiting or settle following cold compresses and paracetamol. Severe local reactions, termed 'arthus' reaction, may follow administration of excessive doses of a toxoid vaccine.

Live vaccines that have been reconstituted (e.g. measles, BCG, JE, rotavirus) carry risk of bacterial contamination since they usually lack preservatives. These vaccines should be kept in contact with ice packs during the immunization session, and be discarded beyond 4 hours of reconstitution in order to decrease the risk of infections such as bacterial abscess and toxic shock syndrome, which is most commonly by caused by *Staphylococcus aureus*.

Immediate allergic reactions are rare and difficult to predict. Severe reactions (anaphylaxis) are usually caused by vaccine constituents, rather than by microbial contamination. *Anaphylaxis might need to be differentiated from vasovagal reaction*. While anaphylaxis is rare (1 per million doses) and may follow any vaccination, yellow fever, MMR and tetanus vaccines are most commonly implicated. *Each patient must be observed for at least 15 minutes after vaccination*. All providers who administer vaccines must be trained in management of emergencies, and have necessary supplies to treat anaphylaxis. Components implicated in allergic reactions include: (i) *Egg protein:* Yellow fever, measles, MMR, rabies PCEV, influenza (killed injectable and live-attenuated) vaccines; (ii) *Gelatin:* Influenza, measles, MMR, rabies, varicella, yellow fever and zoster vaccines; (iii) *Latex in the vaccine vial stopper or syringe plunger;* (iv) *Casein:* DTaP vaccine; (v) *Saccharomyces cerevisiae:* hepatitis B and HPV vaccines; (vi) *Neomycin* which, if present even in trace amounts, may cause allergic reactions.

Thiomersal (50% ethyl mercury), aluminum and phenoxyethanol, added as preservatives in multidose vials, may cause delayed type hypersensitivity or contact dermatitis. The use of thiomersal, an organomercury compound with bacteriostatic properties, is being minimized due to risks of mercury toxicity. A causal relationship between thiomersal exposure through vaccination and neurodevelopmental disorders has not been confirmed.

There is no causal relationship between MMR vaccine and autism or inflammatory bowel disease. Similarly, there is no relationship between vaccines and asthma, sudden infant death syndrome, or chronic fatigue syndrome.

Systemic adverse reactions, such as fever or rash, may follow live attenuated vaccines, mimicking a mild form of the natural infection, usually occur 3 through 21 days after vaccination.

Specific events associated with individual vaccines and serious AEFI are listed in Table 10.7.

Table 10.7: Reportable or serious adverse events following immunization

| |
|---|
| **Serious adverse events following any vaccine** |
| Anaphylaxis or anaphylactic shock ≤7 days of immunization |
| Adverse effects listed as contraindications to vaccination |
| Any serious or unusual event; and |
| Any sequelae of reportable events |
| **Vaccine-specific serious adverse events, considered reportable and/or 'precautions' for subsequent doses** |
| *Oral polio:* Paralytic polio or vaccine strain polio within 1–6 months of vaccine administration |
| *Measles:* Thrombocytopenic purpura within 7–30 days; measles infection in an immunodeficient recipient ≤6 months |
| *Measles, mumps and/or rubella:* Encephalopathy or encephalitis <15 days |
| *Tetanus:* Brachial neuritis ≤28 days |
| *Pertussis:* Encephalopathy or encephalitis ≤7 days |
| *Rotavirus:* Intussusception ≤30 days |
| *Rubella:* Chronic arthritis <6 weeks |
| **Vaccine-specific serious adverse events, not considered reportable** |
| *Diphtheria, pertussis, tetanus:* Hypotensive hyporesponsive episode (acute pallor, loss of muscle tone or consciousness) |
| *Diphtheria, pertussis, tetanus:* Inconsolable cry (<72 hr) |
| *Diphtheria, pertussis, tetanus:* Generalized seizure with fever |
| *Measles:* Toxic shock syndrome (usually due to contamination with *Staphylococcus aureus*) |
| *BCG:* Axillary lymphadenitis (1–6 months) |
| *Yellow fever:* Yellow fever vaccine-associated neurotoxin disease (post-vaccinal encephalitis) |

### Suggested Reading


1. Miller E, Wodi AP. General best practice guidance for immunization. In: Centers for Disease Control and Prevention. Epidemiology and prevention of vaccine-preventable diseases. Hall E, Wodi AP, Hamborsky J, et al. (eds) 14th edn. Washington, DC. Public Health Foundation, 2021; pp: 9–28.


*Competency:* **PE19.4**

## Vaccine Storage and Cold Chain

Maintenance of temperature is critical to the viability and potency of a vaccine. Vaccines such as OPV, measles and BCG (especially after reconstitution) are sensitive to heat but may be frozen without harm (Fig. 10.6). In contrast, vaccines like hepatitis B, DTP, penatavalent vaccine and tetanus toxoid are less sensitive to heat and are damaged by freezing. Certain vaccines lose their potency, if exposed to bright light, and are, therefore, packaged in dark brown glass (BCG, MMR, measles and rubella vaccine). Within the refrigerator, OPV vials are stored in the freezer compartment (0 to –4°C). BCG, measles and MMR vaccines are kept in the top racks of the main compartment (4–10°C) (just below the freezer); DTP, DT, TT, hepatitis A and typhoid are stored in the middle racks; and hepatitis B, varicella and diluents are stored in the lower racks.

Table 10.8 lists specific equipment used at various sites in the cold chain system. Temperatures are monitored to ensure that the cold chain system is maintained. Vaccine vial monitors comprise a tag, present on the label of liquid vaccines or cap of freeze-dried vaccines. The tag contains a heat sensitive material, which changes color in response to cumulative heat exposure (Fig. 10.7a).

Freeze-sensitive vaccines must never be frozen since they may lose their potency, and the agglutination of aluminum containing excipients on freezing of 'adsorbed' vaccines increases the risk of sterile abscesses. A 'shake test' is often used to determine if an adsorbed vaccine (e.g. DTP, DT, TT, pentavalent vaccine and hepatitis B) has been erroneously frozen anytime in the past. As shown in Fig. 10.7b, the suspected freeze damaged vial is labeled as 'test'. Another vaccine vial of the same batch and manufacturer, labelled as 'control', is deliberately frozen (≥10 hours at –10°C) and then thawed completely at room temperature. Both vials are shaken vigorously for 10–15 seconds and then placed side by side on a flat surface against a source of light to compare the sedimentation in the two vials. If the rate of sedimentation is similar in the two vials or the 'test' vial sediments faster than the 'control', the 'test' vial is discarded. If the 'test' vial shows no sediment or sediments slower than the 'control', it can be used (Fig. 10.7b).

### Suggested Reading


1. Effective vaccine management (EVM). Available from: https://www.who.int/teams/immunization-vaccines-and-biologicals/essential-programme-on-immunization/supply-chain/effective-vaccine-management-(evm). Accessed 20 September 2022.

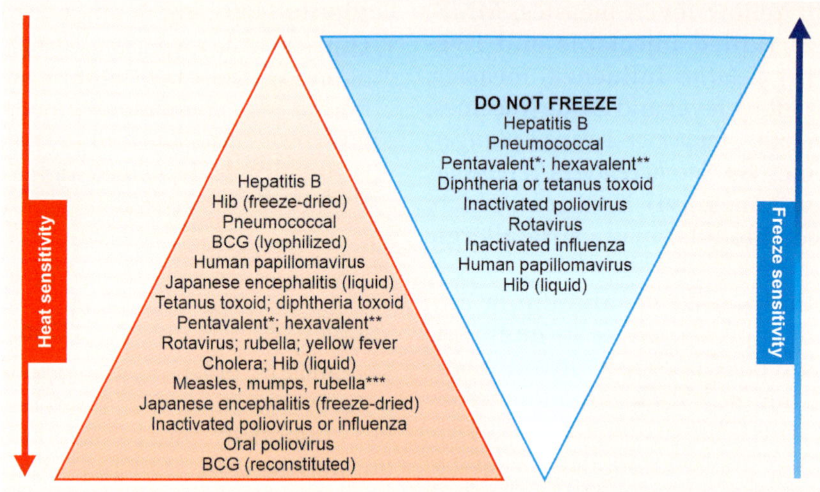


**Fig. 10.6:** Heat and freeze sensitivity of various vaccines. *Pentavalent: diphtheria, (whole cell) pertussis, tetanus, hepatitis B and *Hemophilus (H.) influenzae* b; **Hexavalent: diphtheria, (acellular) pertussis, tetanus, hepatitis B, *H. influenzae b*, inactivated poliovirus; ***Together, or as measles alone or measles rubella combination; BCG Bacillus Calmette–Guerin; Hib *H. influenzae* type b

**Table 10.8:** Implementation of cold chain

| *Center* | *Storage* | *Temperature* | *Duration of storage; comments* | *Transport to next level* |
|---|---|---|---|---|
| Manufacturer; national store; subnational stores | Walk in cooler<br>Walk in freezer | –25°C to –15°C<br>+2°C to +8°C | ≥3 months; bulk storage<br>≥3 months; bulk storage | Air transport<br>Refrigerated or insulated vans |
| District vaccine store | Deep freezer<br>Ice lined refrigerator | –25°C to –15°C<br>+2°C to +8°C | Chiefly for OPV and ice packs<br>1–3 months; useful in power failure | Vaccine vans<br>Vaccine vans |
| Sub-district vaccine store; primary health center | Ice lined refrigerator<br>Cold boxes<br>Vaccine carriers | +2°C to +8°C<br>+2°C to +8°C | 1–3 months; useful in power failure<br><5 days; useful in power failure<br>Useful for transport to vaccination site | Vaccine vans<br>Vaccine carriers<br>None |

OPV oral poliovirus vaccine

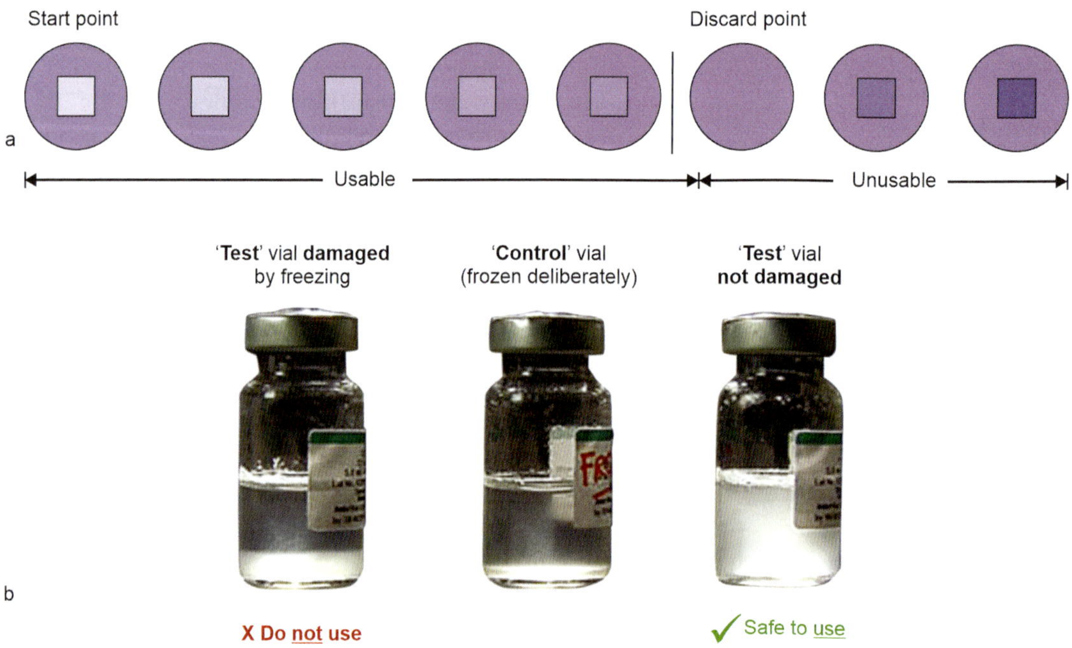


**Fig. 10.7:** Practical check of heat and freeze sensitivity of vaccine vials: (a) Vaccine vial monitor (VVM): This comprises an inner lighter square within an outer dark circle. The inner square darkens gradually and irreversibly following exposure to heat in a time dependent manner. The vaccine is usable as long as the inner square is lighter than the outer circle, and should be discarded if the color of the square matches to or is darker than the circle. Time to color change varies with the vaccine type; e.g. two days for OPV (VVM2) and 14 days for the DTP-hepatitis B combination (VVM14); (b) Shake test: Three vials of liquid freeze-sensitive vaccine are shown with light behind them. From left to right, are shown a frozen 'test' vial in which a sediment has settled to the bottom after vigorous shaking; a frozen 'control' vial in which the sedimentation rate is compared with the rate in suspected frozen 'test' vials; and a non-frozen 'test' vial showing the uniformly cloudy appearance of a vaccine that has not been damaged by freezing.

Competency: **PE19.5**

## IMMUNIZATION IN SPECIAL CIRCUMSTANCES

In addition to routine immunization, certain high-risk categories need additional vaccines, which are detailed below (Table 10.9). Table 10.10 details recommendations for immunization in specific circumstances beyond childhood.

*Primary or secondary immunodeficiency:* Immunodeficiency may be primary, or secondary to malignancy, HIV infection, corticosteroids and immunosuppressive therapy (*see* Chapter 25: Inborn Errors of Immunity). The risk of certain infections and severity of most vaccine-preventable diseases is increased compared to immunocompetent children. On the other hand, the immune response to vaccination may be inadequate and live vaccines are considered unsafe since they may cause disease in an immunocompromised host.

In general, all inactivated, killed or subunit vaccines (e.g. pneumococcal and inactivated influenza vaccines) can be administered safely. However, their efficacy may be compromised; hence, additional or higher doses may be required, and antibody titers should be monitored to ensure seroprotection (e.g., hepatitis B). Live vaccines (BCG, OPV, measles, MMR, varicella) are usually contraindicated, except in milder immunodeficiency states (e.g. isolated deficiency of IgA, IgG subclass, or a complement component) where benefits outweigh risk of harm. Live viral (but not live bacterial) vaccines can be administered to patients with neutrophil or phagocyte defects. Vaccines not routinely administered in healthy children beyond a certain age may be necessary in immunocompromised children, such as the *Hemophilus influenzae* and pneumococcal vaccines. Where feasible, such patients should receive additional vaccines, such as inactivated influenza, meningococcal and hepatitis A vaccines.

***Children infected with HIV*** are susceptible to severe and/or recurrent infections with usual or unusual pathogens. Efficacy and safety of vaccines in such children depends on the degree of immunodeficiency. Most vaccines are safe and effective in early infancy when immune functions are relatively intact, but efficacy declines and immune responses wane as disease advances. Live vaccines (BCG, OPV, measles, MMR, varicella) may be given in early stage of HIV infection (CD4 count 15% for 6 months at age ≤5-yr, or >200/mm$^3$ for ≥6 months at age ≤5-yr) after counseling regarding anticipated benefits versus risks, but are considered unsafe in advanced HIV disease. Where feasible, IPV is preferred over OPV. Symptomatic infants should not receive BCG. The neonate of an HIV positive mother with indeterminate HIV status should receive initial vaccination as per schedule. Where feasible, serological response should be documented, and additional doses administered, as necessary.

***Patients on immunosuppression*** are considered significantly immunosuppressed, if the dose of prednisolone (or its equivalent) is ≥2 mg/kg/day or 20 mg/day for 14 days or more. These children should not receive live vaccines until after 4 weeks of stopping corticosteroid therapy. Live vaccines may be given, if corticosteroids are given for <14 days, in lower doses, on alternate days, or by inhaled, topical or intra-articular routes. Wherever possible, vaccination should be completed prior to initiation of chemotherapy, immunosuppressive drugs or radiation. Live vaccines are not given for 3 months after such treatment; inactivated vaccines during therapy might need to be repeated.

***Following chemotherapy***, live vaccines are contraindicated, at least up to 6 months after the end of chemotherapy. Non-live vaccines are also best deferred until that time point, to provide sustained protection. All children should receive the inactivated influenza vaccine annually and complete immunization with hepatitis B vaccine, even during chemotherapy. Post-treatment immunization depends on the pre-chemotherapy immunization status.

***Household contacts*** may transmit infection to immunocompromised children. Hence, they should be immunized with live vaccines against common or serious pathogens in order to provide indirect protection to the index patient, e.g. varicella and MMR vaccines. However, household contacts should not receive those live vaccines in which the organism may be transmitted to the patient (e.g. oral poliovirus vaccine); they should instead receive an alternative killed vaccine, if feasible (e.g. IPV).

### Other High-Risk Categories

*Splenectomy:* Children with splenectomy or anatomical or functional asplenia (sickle cell disease) are at an increased risk of infections with encapsulated organisms (pneumococci, meningococci, *H. influenzae*). Where feasible, vaccines against these organisms should be administered at least two weeks before elective splenectomy.

*Chronic diseases:* Patients with chronic illnesses (Table 10.9) are at risk of serious infections and should preferably receive pneumococcal, inactivated influenza, varicella, hepatitis A and rotavirus vaccines. Pneumococcal and inactivated influenza vaccines are particularly important in patients with cardiac or pulmonary disease and hepatitis A and B vaccines in liver disease.

*Prematurity:* Most preterm and low birth weight babies mount adequate immune responses, with seroconversion rates comparable to term newborns. They should receive immunization at the same chronological age, at the same doses, and according to the same schedule as for full term infants. Since seroconversion rates for hepatitis B vaccine are lower for preterm neonates weighing <2 kg, the initial may be postponed by 1-month, if the mother is known to be HBsAg negative. Preterm or low birth weight newborns of HBsAg positive mothers or mothers with unknown status should receive the vaccine and hepatitis B immunoglobulin within 12 hours of birth.

### Miscellaneous

*Immunization during illness:* Minor illnesses are not a contraindication to immunization. Immunization is deferred during moderate to severe sickness, since it might inhibit immune response. If permitted, children with

Table 10.9: Vaccination in specific risk subgroups

| *Type of vaccine* | *Inborn error of immunity* | | *Asplenia or splenectomy* | *Acquired: HIV infection* | | *Acquired: Immune dysfunction* | | | *Specific risk groups*[4] |
|---|---|---|---|---|---|---|---|---|---|
| | *Severe*[1] | *Limited*[2] | | *Asymptomatic, and CD4+ >15%*[3] | *Symptomatic, or CD4+ ≥15%*[3] | *Chemotherapy* | *After HSCT* | *Post-solid organ transplantation; on immunosuppression* | |
| ***Live vaccines:*** *Principle* | *Avoid* | *Consider* | *Consider* | *Consider* | *Avoid* | *Avoid until >3–6 months after close of therapy* | *Avoid live vaccines; re-administer other vaccines 6–24 months after transplant* | *Avoid until >4 weeks after stopping intense immunosuppression; administer before, if feasible* | *Administer* |
| BCG | No | Consider | Consider | Yes | No | No | No | No | Yes |
| OPV | No | Consider | Consider | If IPV not afforded | No | No | No | No | Yes |
| Measles | No | Consider | Consider | Yes | No | No | No | No | Yes |
| MMR | No | Consider | Consider | Yes | No | No | No | No | Yes |
| Varicella | No | Consider | Consider | Yes | No | No | No | No | Yes; ensure given |
| Rotavirus | No | Consider | Consider | Yes | No | No | No | No | Yes |
| **Killed/inactivated/subunit vaccines:** Can give in most cases, efficacy often reduced; where feasible administer before risk ensues (e.g. before chemotherapy, transplant or immunosuppression) | | | | | | | | | |
| DPT/Tdap/Td | Yes | Yes | Yes | Yes | Yes | Yes | Yes | Yes | Yes |
| Hepatitis B | Yes[5] | Yes[5] | Yes[5] | Yes; ensure | Yes[5]; ensure | Yes[5]; ensure | Yes5; ensure | Yes[5]; ensure | Yes[5]; ensure |
| Hib | Yes | Yes | Yes | Yes; ensure | Yes; ensure | Yes; ensure | Yes | Yes; ensure | Yes; ensure |
| Pneumococcal | Yes[6] | Yes[6] | Yes[6] | Yes[6]; ensure | Yes[6]; ensure | Yes[6]; ensure | Yes6; ensure | Yes[6]; ensure | Yes[6]; ensure |
| Meningococcal | Yes | Yes | Yes | No specific advice | No advice | No advice | No advice | No advice | Yes; ensure |
| Influenza | Yes[7] | Yes[7] | Yes[7] | Yes[7]; ensure | Yes[7] | Yes[7] | Yes[7] | Yes[7] | Yes; ensure |
| Hepatitis A | Yes[5] | Yes[5] | Yes[5] | Yes | Yes[5] | Yes[5] | Yes[5] | Yes[5] | Yes |
| Typhoid | Yes | Yes | Yes | Yes; ensure | Yes | Yes | Yes | Yes | Yes |
| HPV | Yes | Yes | Yes | Yes | Yes | Yes | Yes | Yes | Yes |

[1]Examples: Severe combined immunodeficiency disorder, combined variable immunodeficiency disorder, X-linked (Bruton) agammaglobulinemia, complete DiGeorgie syndrome, Chediak-Higashi syndrome, leukocyte adhesion defects and myeloperoxide deficiency

[2]Examples: Selective IgA or IgG subclass deficiency, partial DiGeorgie syndrome, Wiskott-Aldrich syndrome, ataxia telangiectasia; phagocyte, neutrophil & complement defects without T and NK cell dysfunction or deficiency

[3]CD4+ cells should have been at this level for ≥6 months, if ≤5-yr-old, or >200/μL for ≥6 months, if >5-yr-old

[4]Include: Congenital or acquired heart disease, chronic pulmonary disease (including asthma treated with prolonged high-dose oral corticosteroids), chronic kidney disease (including nephrotic syndrome), hematological or liver disease, diabetes mellitus; patients with cerebrospinal fluid leaks or cochlear implants must receive vaccines against encapsulated organisms

[5]Check for seroconversion; give boosters as necessary; for hepatitis B, an anti-HBs antibody titer of ≥10 mIU/mL is considered seroprotective

[6]Primary immunization with PCV is given as per schedule, followed by a dose of PPSV23 at ≥2-yr-old and another ≥5 years after the first PPSV23 dose

[7]One dose of the inactivated influenza vaccine is given annually

DPT diphtheria, pertussis and/or tetanus; Hib *Hemophilus influenzae* type b; HPV human papillomavirus; HSCT hematopoietic stem cell transplantation; IPV inactivated poliovirus vaccine; MMR measles mumps rubella; OPV oral poliovirus vaccine

**Table 10.10:** Vaccination beyond early childhood

| *Other at-risk groups* | *Adolescents* | *Healthcare workers* | *Pregnant women* | *Elderly (>50 years)* | *Comment* |
|---|---|---|---|---|---|
| Diphtheria | Yes | Yes | Yes | Yes | *If previously unimmunized:* One dose of Tdap, followed ≥4 weeks later by two doses of Td given 6–12 months apart; then one dose of Td every 10 years (and one dose of Td during each pregnancy) |
| Tetanus | Yes | Yes | Yes | Yes | *If previously immunized:* One dose of Tdap, followed by Td every 10 years (and a dose of Td during each pregnancy) |
| Hepatitis B | Consider | Yes | Yes | No | *If previously unimmunized or lacking seroprotection*[1]: Three doses (20 µg or 1 mL each) at 0, 1 and 6 months; confirm seroprotection after 1–2 months |
| Pneumococcal | No | Yes | No | Yes | One dose of PCV13, followed ≥8 weeks later by one dose of PPSV23; repeat PPSV23 once after ≥5 years if first dose of PPSV23 was given at <65-yr-old |
| Influenza | No | Yes | Yes | Yes | One dose of the inactivated vaccine annually (only once in pregnant women) |
| MMR | Consider | Yes | Postpartum | No | *If previously unimmunized or lacking seroprotection:* Two doses ≥4 weeks apart |
| Varicella | Consider | Yes | No | No | *If previously unimmunized:* Two doses of varicella vaccine ≥4 weeks apart |
| Shingles/zoster | No | No | No | Yes | Two doses of zoster vaccine 2–6 months apart |
| SARS-CoV-2 | Yes | Yes | Yes | Yes | Two doses, followed by booster, as per national schedule for the specific vaccine |
| HPV | Yes | No | No | No | As per schedule |
| **Specific risks (children or adults, including healthcare workers)** | | | | | |
| Travel to endemic areas | | | | | Cholera, yellow fever, Japanese encephalitis and rabies |
| High risk of exposure to specific pathogens | | | | | Typhoid, polio, rabies and/or meningococcal vaccines |

[1]An anti-HBs antibody titer of ≥10 mIU/mL is considered seroprotective

HPV human papillomavirus vaccine; MMR measles, mumps and rubella vaccine; PCV pneumococcal conjugate vaccine; PPSV23 pneumococcal polysaccharide vaccine; SARS-CoV-2 severe acute respiratory syndrome coronavirus 2; Tdap tetanus toxoid with reduced content of diphtheria and pertussis

**Table 10.11:** Vaccination of previously unimmunized child

| *Visit* | *At evaluation* | *After 1 month* | *After 2 months* | *After 6 months* |
|---|---|---|---|---|
| Age ≤7 years | BCG<br>Oral poliovirus<br>DTwP/DTaP<br>Hepatitis B | Oral poliovirus<br>DTwP/DTaP<br>Hepatitis B | Oral poliovirus<br>Measles-containing vaccine<br>Typhoid | DTwP/DTaP<br>Hepatitis B |
| Age >7 years | Tdap<br>Hepatitis B | Td<br>Hepatitis B | Measles-containing vaccine<br>Typhoid | Td<br>Hepatitis B |

Td diphtheria pertussis with reduced content of diphtheria; DTaP diphtheria tetanus acellular pertussis; DTwP diphtheria tetanus whole cell pertussis; Tdap tetanus toxoid with reduced content of diphtheria and pertussis; BCG Bacillus Calmette-Guérin

bleeding or coagulation defects should receive vaccine by subcutaneous rather than IM route. Live vaccines (except OPV, yellow fever) should be avoided for 3 months after administration of blood product(s); blood products are preferably not given for 2 weeks following live vaccination.

***Lapsed immunization:*** Table 10.11 suggests schedules for children who have missed routine immunization. For vaccines with multiple doses, the entire schedule need not be repeated and only limited doses are given. The vaccination schedule for adolescents is discussed in Chapter 5.

### Passive Immunization

Table 10.12 lists indications for passive immunization for vaccine-preventable diseases, usually required in the setting of an unimmunized host.

Human immunoglobulin is a concentrated antibody-containing solution prepared from plasma from normal donors, which consists primarily of IgG, but may contain trace amounts of IgA, IgM, and other serum proteins. This is given intravenously (IVIG) as soon after exposure as possible, in settings where specific immunoglobulin is not

**Table 10.12:** Passive immunization for vaccine-preventable diseases

| *Infection* | *Target population* | *Dose* |
|---|---|---|
| **Normal human immunoglobulin**[1] | | |
| Hepatitis A | Unimmunized contact of infected individual, if <1-yr-old[2], immunocompromised, or with chronic liver disease; newborn whose mother was symptomatic <2 weeks before to <1 week after delivery | 0.1 mL/kg once, within 14 days of exposure |
| | Travel to endemic area and immunocompromised or <6 months old[2] | 0.1 mL/kg, if travel for <1 month; 0.2 mL/kg, if travel for 1–2 months; repeat every 2 months if travelling for longer |
| Measles | Immunocompromised person; unimmunized pregnant woman; infant exposed to infection <6 days back | 0.5 mg/kg (immunocompromised; pregnant woman); 0.25 mg/kg (infant) |
| **Specific (hyperimmune globulin)** | | |
| Hepatitis B (HBIG) | Newborn of HBsAg positive mother; percutaneous (e.g. needlestick) or mucosal exposure; sexual contact | Newborn: 100–200 IU <5 days (preferably <48 hr) of birth<br>Others: 0.06 mL/kg (32–48 IU/kg; maximum 2000 IU) <7 days (preferably <48 hr) of exposure<br>Give another dose after 1 month if the source is HBsAg positive and/or seroprotection is lacking |
| Varicella (VARIZIG)[2] | Newborn of infected mother with lesions noted ≤5 days before to ≥2 days after birth; preterm or very low birth weight neonates; and immunocompromised unimmunized children exposed to varicella <6 days back | 12.5 (5–25) U/kg (maximum 625 units)[3] |
| Rabies immunoglobulin (human, equine RIG); monoclonal antibody (Rabishield, Twinrab) | Category III bite by rabid animal | Human RIG: 20 units/kg (maximum 1500 IU)<br>Equine RIG: 40 units/kg (maximum 3000 IU)<br>Rabishield: 3.33 IU/kg<br>Twinrab: 40 IU/kg |
| Tetanus immunoglobulin (Human, equine TIG) | Wound/exposure in unimmunized or incompletely immunized individual; treatment of tetanus | *Prevention (wound prophylaxis)*<br>Human TIG: 250 units<br>Equine TIG: 3,000–5,000 units<br>*Treatment of tetanus*<br>Human TIG: 3000–6000 units<br>Equine TIG: 50,000–100,000 units |
| **Antisera, antitoxin** | | |
| Diphtheria antitoxin (equine) | Susceptible contact | Severe diphtheria (extensive membrane, severe edema, bull neck); laryngeal, pharyngeal or nasopharyngeal disease of >48 hours: 100,000 IU (10 ampoules)<br>Laryngeal, pharyngeal or nasopharyngeal disease of <48 hours: 70,000 IU (7 ampoules)<br>Skin lesions, >2 cm$^2$: 40,000 IU (4 ampoules) |
| Anti-tetanus serum (horse) | Wound/exposure in unimmunized or incompletely immunized individual | 1,500 U, subcutaneous or IM |
| Rabies antiserum (equine) | Category III bite by potentially rabid animal | 40 IU/kg (maximum 3000 IU) |

[1]An interval of at least 2 weeks is necessary between live vaccines and immunoglobulin containing products; hepatitis A vaccine can be administered simultaneously with immunoglobulin at a different site

[2]Immunoglobulin may be administered to persons aged >40 years or 6–12 months old depending on the provider's risk assessment

[3]If VARIZIG is not available, administer oral acyclovir (80 mg/kg in 4 divided doses daily, maximum 3.2 g daily) or valacyclovir (if ≥3-mo-old, 60 mg/kg in 3 divided doses daily, maximum 3 g daily) for 7 days, beginning 6–10 days from first exposure; also vaccinate after >4 months, if varicella vaccine is not contraindicated

available, e.g. to protect from hepatitis A or measles. The half-life of IVIG is about 3 weeks.

Hyperimmune globulin, prepared from the plasma of individuals with high titers of antibody against a specific organism or antigen, following natural infection or immunization. Hyperimmune globulins are available against rabies, tetanus and varicella. Antisera are purified and concentrated preparations of serum of horses which have been actively immunized against a specific antigen. While antisera and hyperimmune globulin carry higher risks of reactions and anaphylaxis, monoclonal antibodies against specific infectious agents, where available, are safer and usually more effective.

## Suggested Reading


1. Kasi SG, Shivananda S, Marathe S, et al. Indian Academy of Pediatrics (IAP) Advisory Committee on Vaccines and Immunization Practices (ACVIP): Recommended Immunization schedule (2020-21) and update on immunization for children aged 0 through 18 years. Indian Pediatr 2021; 58: 44–53.
2. Miller E, Wodi AP. General best practice guidance for immunization. In: Centers for Disease Control and Prevention. Epidemiology and Prevention of Vaccine-Preventable Diseases. Hall E, Wodi AP, Hamborsky J, et al., eds. 14th edn. Washington, DC. Public Health Foundation, 2021; pp: 9–28.
3. Moulik NR, Mandal P, Chandra J, et al. Immunization of children with cancer in India treated with chemotherapy: Consensus Guideline from the Pediatric Hematology-Oncology Chapter and the Advisory Committee on Vaccination and Immunization Practices of the Indian Academy of Pediatrics. Indian Pediatr 2019; 56: 1041–48.
4. Slifka MK, Amanna IJ. Passive immunization. Plotkin's Vaccines. 2018:84–95.e10. doi: 10.1016/B978-0-323-35761-6.00008-0.

Chapter 11

# Infections and Infestations

Tanu Singhal ❍ Rakesh Lodha ❍ Sushil K Kabra

*Competencies:* **PE34.14; PE34.15; PE34.16; PE34.17**

## FEVER

Fever is a controlled increase in body temperature over the normal values for an individual. The normal body temperature in children is higher as compared to adults, exhibits a normal circadian diurnal variation and varies between 36.1°C and 37.8°C (97°F and 100°F) on rectal measurement. There is a normal diurnal variation in the body temperature; it is lowest between 0 and 6.00 hours and maximum between 17.00 and 19.00 hours.

### Definition

The core body temperature can be measured at several sites including the oral cavity, axilla, rectum, ear canal and over the temporal artery. The rectal method is the most reliable site for measurement of temperature with fever defined as rectal temperature of more than 38°C or 100.4°F. However, measurement of rectal temperature is not always possible in clinical practice. In children below the age of 4–5 years, axillary temperature may be used. The axillary temperature is on an average 0.5–1°C or 1–2°F lower than the rectal temperature. Fever, if measured in the axilla, is defined as temperature more than 37.2°C or 99°F. In children above the age of 4–5 years, the oral method is suitable. The oral temperature is on an average 0.5–1°F or 0.25–0.5°C lower than rectal temperature. Fever as measured in the oral cavity is defined as temperature more than 37.5°C or 99.5°F.

### Types of Thermometers

*Digital thermometers:* They can be used to measure temperature in the mouth, armpit or rectum. They are the most commonly used devices, but are subject to calibration errors.

*Digital ear thermometers:* They are quick and give an estimate of the core temperature. However, they are expensive.

*Forehead infrared thermometers:* The temperature is same as armpit temperature. They have to be keep at a 2-inch distance from the forehead for reliable estimate. They are expensive and used for mass screening in airports, etc. and were widely used during the COVID pandemic.

*Mercury thermometers:* These are no longer recommended due to risk of breakage and contamination of environment.

*Forehead strip thermometer:* This is not accurate and not recommended.

### Etiopathogenesis

Fever may be caused by multiple causes including infection, vaccines, biologic agents, tissue injury, malignancy, drugs, autoimmune diseases, granulomatous diseases, metabolic disorders (gout) and genetic disorders such as familial Mediterranean fever. All these insults result in the production of endogenous pyrogens, such as interleukin (IL)-1, IL-6, tumor necrosis factor (TNF)-$\alpha$, interferon-$\beta$, interferon-$\gamma$ and lipid mediators such as prostaglandin $E_2$, which alter the temperature set point in the anterior hypothalamus leading to elevation in body temperature. In contrast to fever, the high body temperature in heat illness is due to increased heat production or reduced heat loss, with the hypothalamic set point being normal. Here, the core temperatures can rise to beyond 106°F. Common causes of heat illness are hyperthyroidism, anhidrotic ectodermal dysplasia, drugs such as anticholinergics and phenothiazines, heat stroke and malignant hyperthermia.

### Evaluation of a Febrile Patient

Fever is a symptom and not a disease; hence, evaluation for cause is important. If temperatures are very high, heat illness should be suspected. It is useful to classify fevers as short duration fevers and prolonged fevers as etiology and management strategies differ. The pattern of fever is rarely useful in arriving at a diagnosis and is altered by use of antipyretics. Intermittent fevers are characteristic of malaria (but may not always be present); biphasic fevers are seen in illnesses such as dengue, influenza and leptospirosis; and periodic fevers (fever syndromes with regular periodicity) are seen in cyclic neutropenia, PFAPA syndrome (periodic fever, adenopathy, pharyngitis, aphthous ulcers) and hyperimmunoglobulin (Ig) D syndromes.

## Management

Fever is a symptom and, therefore, treatment of the underlying cause is important. Treatment of fever per se may not always be needed. Fever has been shown to improve the immunologic response to certain infections in experimental models; whether this is clinically significant is unknown. However, fever may be associated with adverse effects such as discomfort, paradoxical suppression of immune response, increased insensible water losses, cardiopulmonary stress and triggering febrile seizures in predisposed patients.

Reduction of fever should be a priority in patients with past/family history of febrile seizures, those critically ill, those with cardiorespiratory failure, those with disturbed fluid and electrolyte balance, or with temperature exceeding 40°C (104°F). For the rest, treatment should be individualized; parental counseling is important. This counseling should include ensuring adequate fluid intake, watching for danger signs and safe usage of antipyretics.

The two commonly used drugs for fever control in children are paracetamol and ibuprofen. Other agents such as aspirin, nimesulide and mefenamic acid are associated with high incidence of adverse effects and are better avoided. Ibuprofen decreases fever at the same rate as paracetamol, the nadir with ibuprofen is slightly lower and duration of action is longer (6 hr) as compared to paracetamol (4 hr). However, the risk of side effects, such as acute kidney injury and gastrointestinal bleeding, is theoretically higher with ibuprofen (not substantiated by observational studies). Conversely, the consequences of paracetamol overdose (hepatic failure) are more sinister than those with ibuprofen (kidney failure, neurological depression). Considering all factors, it is reasonable to use paracetamol at a dose of 10–15 mg/kg every 4 hours (5–6 doses/day; maximum daily dose 90 mg/kg; 4 g) as the first-line medication. It is reasonable to shift to ibuprofen in those patients who have not adequately responded to paracetamol and administer at a dose of 10 mg/kg every 6 hr (maximum daily dose 40 mg/kg; 2.4 g). There is evidence to suggest that combining paracetamol and ibuprofen or alternating between paracetamol and ibuprofen is more efficacious in reducing fever as compared to a single drug. This strategy may be used in recalcitrant fevers. The oral route is the preferred route. Rectal and intravenous route may be used in presence of vomiting or when oral medications cannot be given. Tepid water sponging or showering may be complementary to medications, in bringing down fever quickly in children.

Heat illness is a medical emergency. The high temperatures can cause irreversible organ damage and should be brought down quickly. Since the hypothalamic set point is not altered, non-steroidal anti-inflammatory drugs, which act by reducing prostaglandin production, are ineffective. External cooling is needed with ice water sponging, cooling blankets, cold water enemas, gastric washes and infusion of cold saline. At the same time, measures should be taken to correct the underlying condition.

### Suggested Reading

1. Chiappini E, Bortone B, Galli L, et al. Guidelines for the symptomatic management of fever in children. BMJ Open 2017; 7:e015404.
2. Section on Clinical Pharmacology and Therapeutics; Committee on Drugs, Sullivan JE, Farrar HC. Fever and antipyretic use in children. Pediatrics. 2011;127(3):580–87.

## Short Duration Fevers

Short duration fevers lasting for less than 5–7 days are one of the most common reasons for pediatric outpatient visits. Most of these are due to self-limiting viral infections. Fever without localizing signs is of concern since it may be due to serious bacterial infections. The concern in the past was pneumococcal and Hib bacteremia but with increasing immunization coverage, these infections have declined. Urinary tract infections (UTI), pneumonia, tropical infections (dengue, enteric fever) are currently the most common causes of fever without localizing signs in the Indian setting. Since 2020, COVID-19 has emerged as an important cause of fever at all ages.

### *Fever without Focus in Less Than 1 Month*

Fever in a neonate (<1 month of age) is generally a medical emergency. This is because of (i) 5–15% risk of serious bacterial infection such as sepsis, bacteremia, urinary tract infections, pneumonia, enteritis and bacterial meningitis, (ii) neonates may look well and still have serious bacterial infection, and (iii) the implications of missing or delaying diagnosis of sepsis are serious. Sometimes neonates get fever due to over clothing and warm weather ('dehydration fever') in which the baby looks well and active. This only warrants frequent feeding and nursing in less warm environment. The infant is kept under observation for other signs of sepsis and investigated, if in doubt.

Since fever in neonate has important implications it should ideally be confirmed by rectal temperature measurement. Fever is defined as rectal temperature more than 100.4°F.

A detailed clinical assessment should be performed for a febrile neonate (Fig. 11.1). Investigations recommended include a complete blood count with differential, C-reactive protein (CRP), one set of blood cultures, urinalysis and urine culture, chest radiograph and lumbar puncture with CSF analysis. The urine specimen should be obtained by suprapubic aspiration/catheterization/clean catch specimen and not as a bag collection. If the CSF is abnormal, HSV PCR should also be sent. If diarrhea is present, then stool should be examined for leukocytes.

Empiric antibiotics should be started after sending cultures and CSF examination. The usual choice of antibiotics includes a third generation cephalosporin (cefotaxime) with aminoglycoside (amikacin/gentamicin). However, with

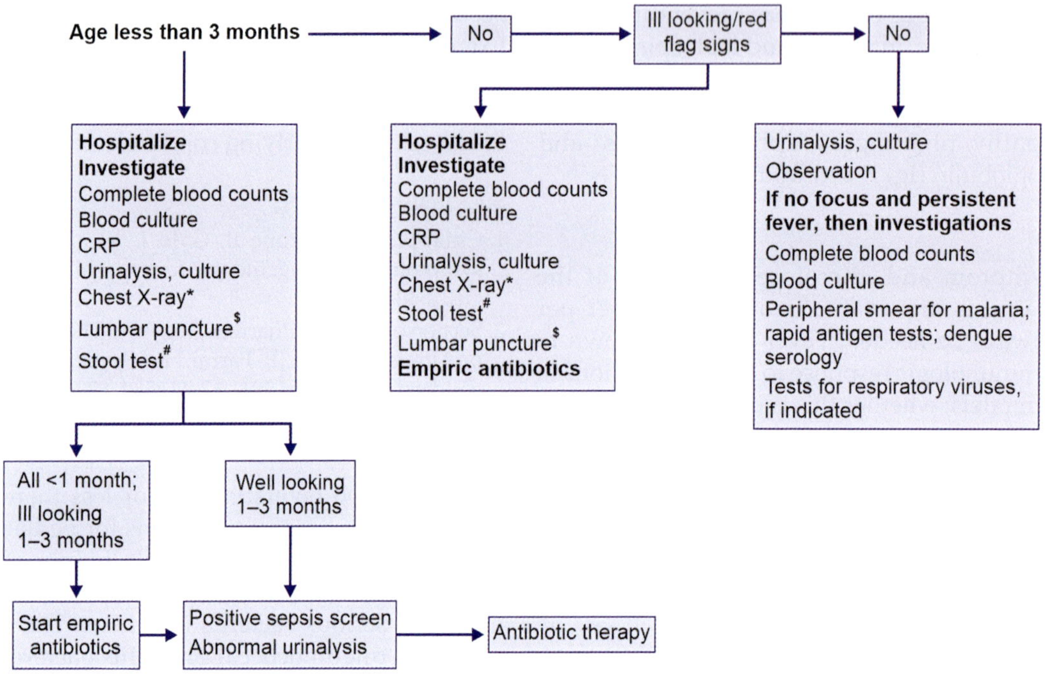


**Fig. 11.1:** Management of fever without focus in children 0–36 months of age

*Chest X-ray is done in all neonates, if high fever >102°F, leukocyte counts >20000/cu mm or if respiratory signs

$Stool examination if diarrhea

#Lumbar puncture in all neonates and all 1–3 months who are sick, or >3 months with neurologic signs

increasing prevalence of extended spectrum beta-lactamase (ESBL) producing gram-negative infections, one may choose either piperacillin tazobactam and amikacin, or meropenem and amikacin in sick/toxic neonates.

If the sepsis screen is positive (leukocytes <5000 or >15,000/cu mm and CRP more than 1 mg/dL), then antibiotics are continued and modified as per cultures and results of other investigations. Duration of therapy is 7 days for culture negative sepsis, 14 days for culture positive sepsis and 3 weeks for meningitis. If the screen is negative, then antibiotics may be stopped after 48 hours, if cultures are negative and fever resolves, or an alternative diagnosis is made.

### *Fever without Focus in an Infant 1–3 Months of Age*

Infants in this age group like those aged less than 1 month are at high risk of serious bacterial disease. They may look well and still have bacterial disease. The algorithm for management of these babies is fairly similar to those less than 1 month (Fig. 11.1). The red flags for serious illness in infants more than 1 month are listed below and presence of any of these signs has a positive likelihood ratio of 5 for serious illness:

#### *Red flag signs for serious illness*

- ***Child behavior:*** Changes in crying pattern, drowsiness, inconsolability, moaning
- ***Circulatory, respiratory:*** Crackles, cyanosis, decreased breath sounds, poor peripheral circulation, rapid breathing, shortness of breath
- ***Other factors:*** Decreased skin elasticity, hypotension, meningeal irritation, petechial rash, seizures, unconsciousness

All babies should ideally be hospitalized for evaluation and treatment. The investigative approach is same as an infant less than 1 month except that lumbar puncture is only recommended if the baby appears ill, and chest X-ray done only if there is high fever/ high WBC count or presence of respiratory signs.

### *Fever without Focus in Children Aged 3–36 Months*

The risk of serious bacterial infections decreases with advancing age and in this age group it is less than 5%. Detailed history is taken about vaccination, history of sick contacts in family and the condition of the child when fever is down.

Ill-appearing babies should be hospitalized and undergo complete blood counts with differential, CRP, blood culture, urinalysis and urine culture. Testing for malaria and dengue should be included, if suspected. Lumbar puncture is recommended, only if the baby has neurologic signs, and chest X-ray, if the fever is high/WBC count is >20,000/cu mm or if there are respiratory signs. Stool should be examined, if there is diarrhea.

Well-looking babies can be subjected to urinalysis and culture (if below 24 months) and observed as outpatients for the next 48-hour. Molecular tests for viruses including influenza/other respiratory viruses/COVID-19 may be done depending on epidemiology and availability. If no focus develops and the fever persists, then investigations as listed above should be done.

## Suggested Reading

1. Cioffredi LA, Jhaveri R. Evaluation and management of febrile children: A Review. JAMA Pediatr. 2016;170:794–800.
2. Hamilton JL, John SP. Evaluation of fever in infants and young children. Am Fam Physician. 2013;87:254–60.

## Fever of Unknown Origin

### Definition

The definition of fever of unknown origin (FUO) is fever >101°F lasting for 3 weeks or more for which no cause is apparent after 1 week of outpatient investigation. A practical definition of FUO is fever >101°F lasting for more than 7 days where preliminary clinical assessment, investigations (blood counts, peripheral smear, urinalysis, blood culture, chest X-ray and ultrasound abdomen) do not yield a diagnosis.

### Causes

The principal causes of FUO are listed in Table 11.1 and depend greatly on regional epidemiology. Infections account for most of the cases of FUO in children (60–70%). Common among infectious causes are enteric fever, malaria, pulmonary or extrapulmonary tuberculosis and urinary tract infections. Malignancies including leukemia/lymphoma and autoimmune diseases account for the remaining cases. Following the COVID-19 pandemic, multisystem inflammatory syndrome (MIS-C) has emerged as a novel cause of prolonged fever in children. Relatively rare causes include drug fever, temperature dysregulation, diabetes insipidus, sarcoidosis, ectodermal dysplasia, sensory autonomic neuropathies, etc. Even with extensive investigations, the cause of FUO may remain undiagnosed in 10–20% of the cases.

### Approach to FUO

The first step is to identify sick patients who need stabilization and urgent referral to a tertiary care centre. Subsequently all attempts should be made to reach an etiologic diagnosis. A detailed history is crucial. History should include:

- Whether and how fever was documented (it is not uncommon to find children with history of prolonged fever not to have fever documented by a thermometer)
- Duration and pattern of fever (in order to distinguish from recurrent fever)
- Symptoms referable to all organ systems and weight loss
- History of recurrent infections, oral thrush (HIV infection and primary immunodeficiency disorders)
- History of joint pain, rash, photosensitivity, oral ulcers, hair loss (autoimmune disease)

**Table 11.1:** Causes of fever of unknown origin (FUO)

| |
|---|
| **Infectious causes:** Enteric fever, malaria, urinary tract infections, tuberculosis, chronic hepatitis, human immunodeficiency virus infection, hidden abscesses (liver, pelvic), mastoiditis, sinusitis, osteomyelitis, meningitis, infectious mononucleosis, infective endocarditis, brucellosis, CMV disease, kala-azar, rickettsial infections |
| **Autoimmune causes:** Systemic onset juvenile idiopathic arthritis, Kawasaki disease, MIS-C, systemic lupus erythematosus, inflammatory bowel disease, vasculitis including polyarteritis nodosa, Kikuchi disease |
| **Neoplastic causes:** Leukemia, lymphoma, Langerhans cell histiocytosis, hemophagocytic lymphohistiocytosis |

- History of contact with infectious tuberculosis in past two years and animals (brucellosis)
- Travel to endemic zones (kala-azar, rickettsial infections)
- Drug history particularly anticonvulsants and anticholinergics (drug fever)

History should be followed by a complete physical examination. Documentation of fever is necessary, followed by assessment of general activity, nutritional status and vitals. A head to toe examination, after removing all clothes, is vital. The physical examination should be repeated on daily basis as new findings may emerge that provide a clue to the etiology. Results of previous investigations should be carefully reviewed. One must keep Kawasaki disease in mind, since early diagnosis is crucial to prevent coronary complications (Fig. 11.2). Patients who are sick and Kawasaki disease suspects should be identified and fast tracked for appropriate management.

Investigative work-up for a patient with FUO is guided by the clinical differential diagnosis. First-line investigations are detailed in Table 11.2 and may be repeated even is

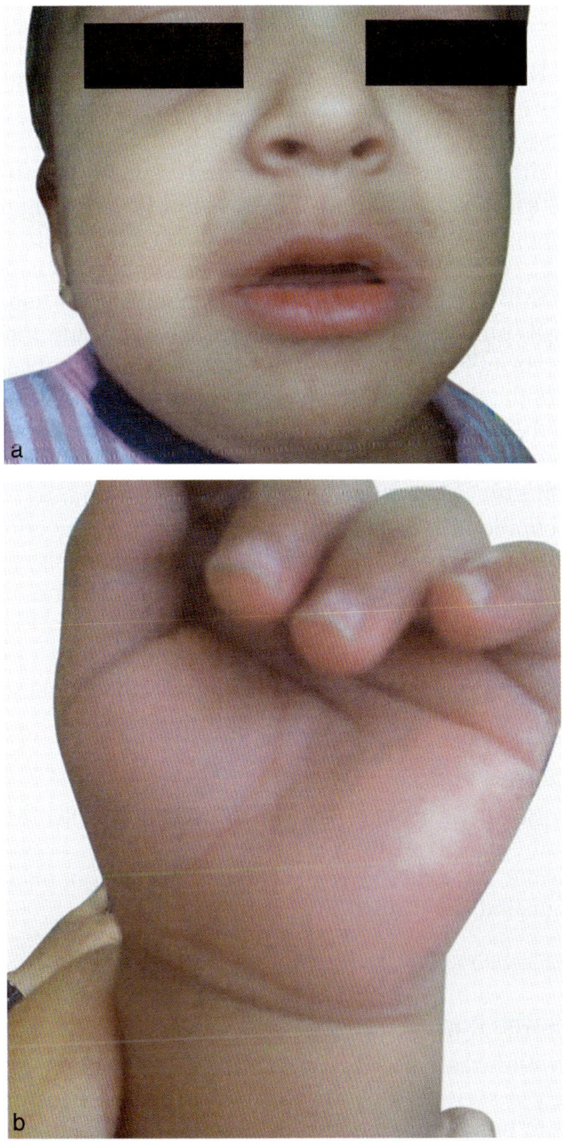


**Fig. 11.2:** Kawasaki disease: (a) Red and cracked lips; (b) Palmar rash and swelling

| Table 11.2: Investigative evaluation of fever of unknown origin (FUO) |
|---|
| **First-line investigations** |
| Complete blood counts with platelet count and peripheral smear |
| C-reactive protein, ESR, liver and kidney function tests |
| Urinalysis; at least 1 and preferably two sets of blood cultures (aerobic and anaerobic), urine culture |
| Chest radiograph; ultrasound abdomen and pelvis |
| HIV serology |
| **Second-line investigations** |
| Repeat blood counts, ESR, C-RP |
| Contrast enhanced CT scan of chest and abdomen |
| 2D echocardiography |
| Serology for: Brucella, infectious mononucleosis, kala-azar |
| Bone marrow aspiration and biopsy; bone marrow aspirate cultures |
| ANA, ANCA, complement C3, hepatitis B serology |
| Lumbar puncture and cerebrospinal fluid analysis |
| Tissue biopsies, fluid analysis, cultures, molecular tests (as relevant) |
| Positron emission tomography-CT scan |
| **Investigations of limited value** |
| Tuberculin skin test, interferon gamma release assays, serology for tuberculosis |

ANA antinuclear antibody; ANCA antineutrophil cytoplasmic antibody

performed earlier. Serology for enteric fever is commonly performed, but should be interpreted carefully. If a diagnosis is established, appropriate treatment is instituted. If no diagnosis is made, clinical reassessment and further investigations are merited. While second-line investigations are being planned (Table 11.2), treatment with IV ceftriaxone may be considered as enteric fever is an important cause of FUO in our country (especially in patients with negative clinical/preliminary investigations). Doxycycline may be added in areas endemic for rickettsia. Contrast enhanced CT scan of the chest and abdomen has emerged as a very useful second-line investigation, since it can detects pulmonary/extrapulmonary tuberculosis. An expert opinion is also a very useful 'second-line investigation'.

It should be possible to make a diagnosis of the etiology of FUO in most cases. In patients where a diagnosis cannot be made, periodic reassessments should be done as the disease may finally evolve (e.g. lymphoma, systemic onset juvenile idiopathic arthritis). Some cases of FUO may self-resolve over time. The use of empirical antitubercular therapy and steroids is not recommended.

### Suggested Reading


1. Chusid MJ. Fever of unknown origin in childhood. Pediatr Clin North Am. 2017;64:205–30.
2. Dayal R, Agarwal D. Fever in children and fever of unknown origin. Indian J Pediatr 2016;83:38–43.


*Competency:* **PE34.15**

## Fever with Rash

Fever with rash is a common and vexing problem. It may signify a serious disorder such as meningococcemia or dengue hemorrhagic fever or may be associated with a minor drug allergy. There are many infectious and non-infectious causes of fever with rash; the common causes are listed in Table 11.3. MIS-C has also emerged as an important cause of fever with rash in the post COVID-19 setting.

| Table 11.3: Common causes of exanthematous illnesses in India |
|---|
| ***Macular, maculopapular rash*** |
| **Measles, rubella, dengue, roseola infantum, erythema infectiosum, drug rash,** infectious mononucleosis, chikungunya, HIV, **adenoviral infections, enteroviral infections,** *Mycoplasma pneumoniae* infections, secondary syphilis, brucellosis, scrub typhus, chronic hepatitis B, cytomegalovirus infection, lupus, systemic onset idiopathic arthritis, **multisystem inflammatory syndrome in children (MIS-C)** |
| ***Diffuse erythema with peeling or desquamation*** |
| Scarlet fever, erythema multiforme, drug reaction with eosinophilia and systemic symptoms (DRESS), **Stevens-Johnson syndrome, toxic epidermolysis,** staphylococcal and streptococcal toxic shock syndrome, **Kawasaki disease, MIS-C** |
| ***Vesicular rash*** |
| Chicken pox, herpes simplex, herpes zoster, **enteroviral infections** (hand foot mouth disease), papulonecrotic TB |
| ***Petechial, purpuric rash*** |
| **Meningococcemia, dengue hemorrhagic fever, Indian spotted fever, scrub typhus,** gonococcemia, hemorrhagic measles, cutaneous vasculitis, **IgA vasculitis** |
| ***Urticarial rash*** |
| Scabies, cutaneous larva migrans (hookworm, strongyloides), **insect bites,** pediculosis |
| ***Nodular rash*** |
| **Molluscum contagiosum,** disseminated histoplasmosis, cryptococcosis, **erythema nodosum** |

*Common conditions are in bold

### Evaluation

The most important feature that helps to determine the etiology of an exanthematous febrile illness is the nature of rash. Rashes may be macular, maculopapular, vesicular, nodular, urticarial or purpuric (Fig. 11.3). These are not watertight compartments and considerable overlap may occur with one etiology having varying presentations. Other factors that enable diagnosis are local epidemiology, season, history of exposure, incubation period, age, vaccination status, previous exanthems, nature of prodromal symptoms and relation of rash with fever, distribution and progression

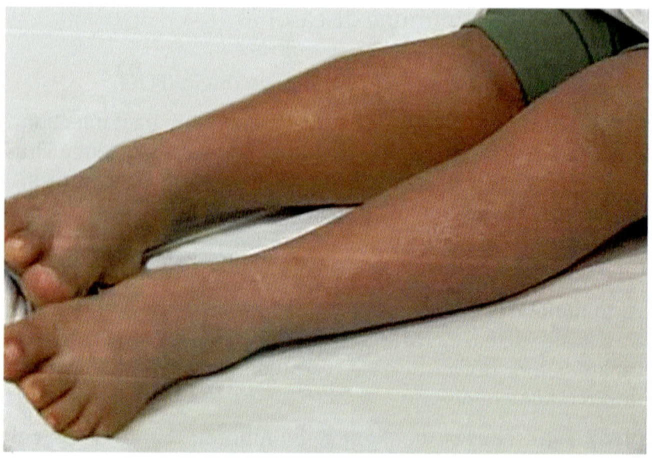

Fig. 11.3: The diffuse erythematous rash of dengue

of the rash, involvement of mucous membranes, history of drug intake, and associated symptoms.

Examination should include nature of the rash and distribution, involvement of palms and soles (seen in dengue, spotted fever, Kawasaki disease and Stevens-Johnson syndrome), involvement of mucous membranes, adenopathy, organomegaly and signs of meningeal irritation. Laboratory investigations that assist in diagnosis include complete blood counts, CRP, ESR, blood cultures, specific serology, and sometimes biopsy.

#### *Management*

All efforts should be made to diagnose the serious entities first and institute immediate treatment. For stable children a specific diagnosis may not always be possible. In this situation, symptomatic therapy, close observation, explanation of danger signs to parents and staying away from school until the rash resolves are recommended.

Often drugs and antibiotics are given to a child with fever who then breaks out into a rash. Distinguishing this rash as a viral exanthem from drug related rash is difficult. Intense itching is more commonly seen with a drug rash. The usual practice is withholding the drug, symptomatic therapy and observation. Rechallenge with the same drug later under observation is permitted, if the rash was mild.

#### Suggested Reading

1. Sarkar R, Mishra K, Garg VK. Fever with rash in a child in India. Indian J Dermatol Venereol Leprol 2012;78:251–62.

### Recurrent Fevers

The term 'recurrent fevers' refers to repeated episodes of fever and is a common phenomenon in children. Recurrent fevers are commonly seen with upper respiratory tract infections in children below 5-yr (especially those with allergic rhinitis, adenoid enlargement), urinary tract infections due to structural anomalies of the urinary tract, and malaria. Infective endocarditis and brucellosis may also present with recurrent fevers, if treatment is partial or incomplete. Primary and secondary immunodeficiency disorders are also associated with recurrent fevers referred to different organ systems.

There are a set of diseases termed as autoinflammatory diseases of genetic origin which present with recurrent or periodic fevers (Table 11.4). These disorders are characterized by recurrent episodes (3 more episodes over a 6-month period occurring more than 7 days apart) with constellation of symptoms referred to different organ systems. They may occur with a regular/ irregular periodicity. There is usually associated rise in inflammatory markers including white cell count, CRP and ESR. The attacks usually last from 3–7 days and resolve without any specific therapy. The patient is well between the episodes of fever. Diagnosis entails recognition of the clinical syndrome and sophisticated genetic tests. Some of the disorders are amenable to specific therapy, e.g. tonsillectomy for PFAPA, colchicine for FMF, etc.

| **Table 11.4:** Common autoinflammatory diseases |
|---|
| Periodic fever, aphthous stomatitis, pharyngitis and cervical adenopathy (PFAPA) |
| TNF receptor associated periodic syndrome (TRAPS) |
| Familial Mediterranean fever |
| Mevalonate kinase deficiency (hyper-IgD syndrome; hyper-immunoglobulinemia D and periodic fever) |
| Cryopyrin-associated periodic syndrome (Muckle-Wells syndrome, neonatal onset multi-inflammatory disease) |
| Familial cold autoinflammatory syndrome (rash, fever, joint pain triggered by exposure to cold temperature) |

#### Suggested Reading

1. Soon GS, Laxer RM. Approach to recurrent fever in childhood. Can Fam Physician 2017; 63:756–62.

## COMMON VIRAL INFECTIONS

### Coronavirus Disease (COVID-19)

The COVID-19 pandemic has been the biggest global public health crises since the 1918 influenza pandemic.

#### *Etiology and Epidemiology*

The coronaviruses are enveloped RNA viruses with spike-like projections on its surface giving it a crown-like appearance; hence the name coronavirus. Four corona viruses have been in circulation in humans, causing mild respiratory disease. There have been two outbreaks in the past two decades wherein crossover of bat coronaviruses to humans has resulted in severe respiratory disease. This was the SARS-CoV-1 outbreak in 2002–2003 and the Middle Eastern respiratory syndrome coronavirus virus (MERS-CoV) in 2012.

In December 2019, adults with severe pneumonia started presenting to hospitals in Wuhan city of China. The outbreak was notified to the WHO on 31 December 2019 and the virus was sequenced on 7 January 2020. It had more than 95% homology with the bat coronavirus and >70% with SARS-CoV-1. While the virus originated from bats, the intermediary animal through which it crossed over to humans is still not known. The virus was named as SARS-CoV-2 and the disease as COVID-19. The disease spread rapidly from China to other parts of the world and was unstoppable despite travel restrictions, closing of borders and lockdowns. The WHO declared SARS-CoV-2 disease as a pandemic on 11 March 2020. The last 30 months have seen infection and disease at an unprecedented scale globally. The reported 520 million cases and 6 million deaths worldwide till May 2022 (www.worldometers.info) and 43 million cases and 500,000 deaths in India may be an underestimate of the actual burden. Disease has occurred in the form of waves and some countries are experiencing the 4th or 5th wave at this time. The pandemic also witnessed the fastest development of vaccines in history of mankind. While these vaccines have impacted disease severity and mortality, they have not been really effective in preventing disease transmission. Another significant feature of the pandemic has been emergence of variants due to mutations in the viral genome. The variants of concern (alpha, beta, gamma, delta and omicron) have fueled the pandemic by escaping natural and vaccine-induced immunity. The delta variant which originated in India in 2021 was the most devastating. Apart from the direct effects, the virus has caused huge economic losses, social disruptions and mental health issues.

### Transmission, Pathogenesis, Clinical Features and Complications

Patients are infectious 1–2 days before and 5–7 days after symptom onset and even if they are asymptomatic. Infection occurs by inhalation of droplets generated during breathing, coughing and sneezing. The virus attaches itself to the ACE2 receptors in the respiratory epithelium followed by endocytosis. Since ACE2 receptors are widely distributed in the body, the disease affects many organ systems. The initial phase of viral replication is followed by development of the host immune response, which leads to recovery. However, in some individuals, this immune response is associated with hyperinflammation and cytokine storm leading to severe disease **(Fig. 11.4)**. Affection of the vascular endothelial cells by the virus, hyperinflammation and activation of the coagulation cascade leads to widespread thrombosis.

The incubation period varies from 2–14 days with a median of 5 days. With the original Wuhan strain of the virus, the rate of asymptomatic infection was 20%. In symptomatic individuals, the usual symptoms were fever, headache, body ache, fatigue, sore throat, cough and rhinorrhea and uniquely enough loss of sense of smell and taste. Recovery occurred by the end of the first week in 80% cases. In others, the development of complications was heralded by persistence or reappearance of fever, breathlessness, hypoxia and finally acute respiratory distress syndrome. Other complications included venous and arterial thrombosis and embolism, encephalitis, myocarditis and acute kidney injury. Risk factors for development of complications included advanced age, obesity, male sex, diabetes, family history of severe COVID-19, race, hypertension, underlying chronic diseases, pregnancy and immunocompromised state. Case fatality rate was around 3%. Another late complication seen was "long COVID" wherein adults with COVID-19 continued to have persistent symptoms of fatigue, low grade fever, chest pain, cough, breathlessness, insomnia even 4–12 weeks after the initial infection.

The disease manifestations have since changed with the appearance of variants and development of natural/vaccine-induced immunity. For example, with the Delta strain, complications occurred relatively early by day 4–5 and even in those with no risk factors. In contrast, with Omicron, the transmissibility was higher, incubation period shorter, asymptomatic infection higher, clinical features milder (with no loss of smell and taste) and complication rate and mortality were significantly lower.

### Epidemiology and Clinical Features in Children

Children below 18 years have contributed to ~12% of the total COVID-19 cases worldwide and in India, despite constituting 25–40% of the population. However, the seroprevalence rates in children are same as adults. This implies that while children are infected to the same extent as adults, they are tested less often. Besides, hospitalization rates in children are <5% as compared to 15–20% in adults. Mortality rates in children are <0.1% as compared to 2–3% in adults, with children contributing to only 0.3% of all COVID-19 deaths. This mild affection of children is attributed to immature ACE2 receptors, better innate immunity, higher circulating lymphocyte numbers, fewer comorbidities, and healthier lungs. It is the indirect effects of COVID-19 in children that overshadow the direct effects. These indirect effects include loss of parents/grandparents, learning crises, mental health issues, obesity, excess screen time, poverty, child abuse, missed immunization, and inattention to other diseases. The most dramatic manifestation of childhood COVID-19 is the multisystem inflammatory syndrome in children (MIS-C).

Symptoms in children are nonspecific and mimic other viral illnesses. Common symptoms include fever, sore throat, cough, runny nose, skin rash, vomiting, diarrhea, and abdominal pain. Headache, fatigue, loss of sense of smell and taste are less commonly reported as compared

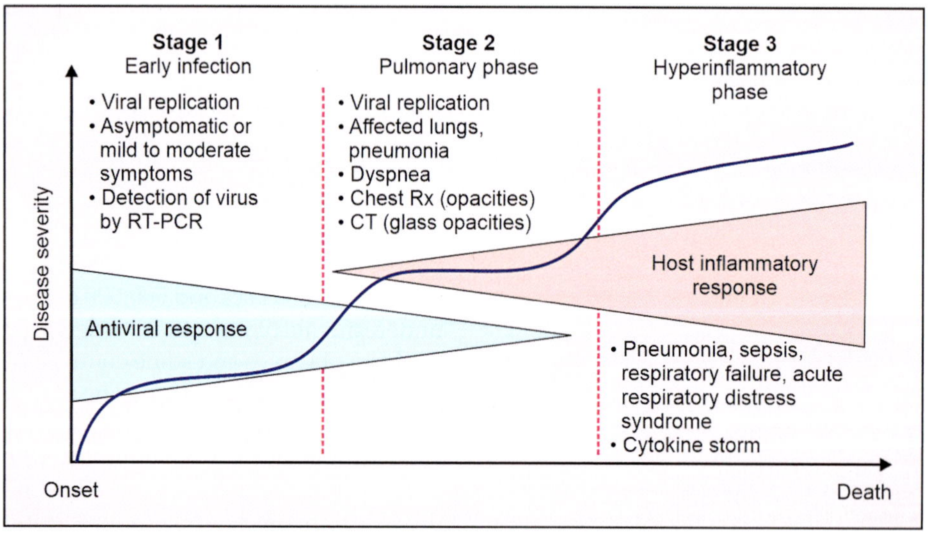


**Fig. 11.4:** Natural history of COVID-19

to adults. Most children recover in a few days. Febrile seizures and encephalitis like presentations have also been reported. Severe disease in children is usually seen in infants, adolescent children and those with comorbidities.

The ICMR criteria for classification of the disease are as follows:

- *Mild:* Symptoms of COVID-19 with no features of lower respiratory tract involvement
- *Moderate:* Fast breathing (as per age-related cutoffs) or hypoxemia (saturation 90–93%)
- *Severe disease:* Presence of retractions, saturation <90%, severe dehydration or drowsiness/seizures
- *Critical disease:* A subset of severe disease with either acute respiratory distress syndrome, shock, multiorgan dysfunction syndrome and acute thrombosis

### Diagnosis

Nucleic acid amplification tests (NAAT) are the gold standard for diagnosis in respiratory secretions (saliva, nasopharyngeal swab, oropharyngeal swab, sputum, bronchoalveolar lavage). The RT-PCR tests are the most commonly used NAAT tests and are based on detection of two genes of the SARS-CoV-2 genome. Different kits have different targets. The result is expressed as cycle threshold (Ct) value. The cycle threshold (Ct) is the number of cycles needed to amplify the RNA to make it detectable and a value below 35–40 is considered positive. A low Ct value implies a high viral load and vice versa. However, there is no correlation of Ct value with disease severity. A positive test is one where both the genes test positive while indeterminate is where only one gene tests positive. The sensitivity of test is higher in early illness and in lower respiratory specimens (sputum, bronchoalveolar lavage). The overall sensitivity is around 70%. The specificity of these tests is very high but since the tests detect RNA, they can continue to be positive for a long time after infection. Repeating tests to document negativity is not recommended. COVID-19 suspects who test negative should be retested and evaluated for other illnesses.

Rapid antigen tests (RAT) in the nasopharyngeal swab have emerged as cheap, point of care tests for diagnosis of COVID-19. These tests are based on the lateral flow principle and can also be done at home. The sensitivity is around 30–50% (lower than RT-PCR) but specificity in symptomatic individuals is high. Patients who test negative with RAT should be evaluated by NAAT tests. *Antibody detection tests* are not useful for detection of acute infection but are mainly used for diagnosis of MIS-C, epidemiologic surveys and immunogenicity of vaccines.

Complete blood count and C-reactive protein (CRP) are usually normal in mild COVID-19. Children with severe disease may demonstrate lymphopenia, thrombocytopenia, and high CRP. In patients with clinical evidence of lower respiratory tract involvement, the chest X-ray is abnormal with peripheral lower lobe infiltrates. The chest CT scan may show changes even in patients with mild symptoms. The characteristic features are ground glass opacities in subpleural locations of one/both lower lobes **(Fig. 11.5)**. The routine use of CT scan for diagnosis of COVID-19 in children is not recommended.

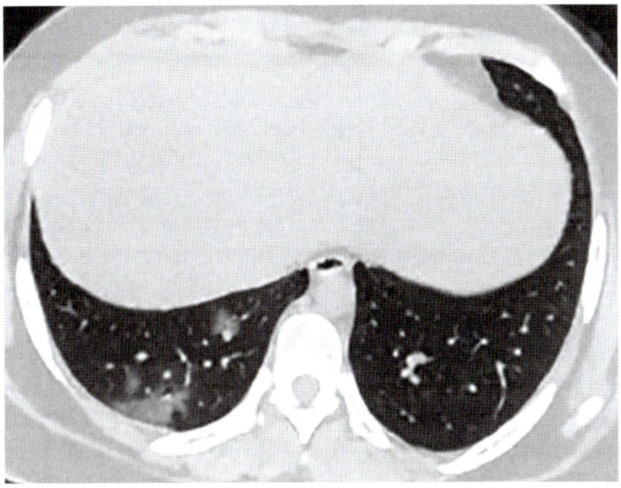

**Fig. 11.5:** CT scan showing the characteristic subpleural ground glass opacities of COVID-19

The differential diagnosis of COVID-19 in children includes other common causes of fever including respiratory viral and bacterial infections, gastrointestinal infections, tropical infections such as enteric fever, malaria and urinary tract infections.

### Treatment

Treatment of COVID-19 in children is largely symptomatic and supportive. Allaying parental anxiety is important. Polypharmacy should be avoided. There is currently no role of azithromycin, hydroxychloroquine, doxycycline, ivermectin, antibiotics, favipiravir, and convalescent plasma in the management. The parents should be asked to monitor for red flag signs such as persistent high fever, rapid breathing and in older children drop in oxygen saturation to below 94%. The IAP protocol for management of COVID-19 is depicted in **Fig. 11.6**. Children can be deisolated 7 days from onset of symptoms in mild disease and 14 days in severe disease.

### COVID-19 in the Newborn

Infection of the newborn usually occurs from an infected mother during delivery. Intrauterine transmission and transmission through breast milk is rare. The risk of perinatal transmission is around 10%. Most of the infected babies are asymptomatic or have mild symptoms. In around 20% of perinatally infected babies, there may be severe disease with fever, cough and respiratory distress. Neonatal MIS-C may be seen in babies born to mothers who were infected in pregnancy.

Babies born to infected mothers should be roomed in with the mother and breastfeeding continued. If sick, they should be admitted to an isolation intensive care unit. Babies should be tested at 24-48 hours for COVID-19. Vaccination with BCG, oral polio and hepatitis B should be given. Infected and uninfected babies can be discharged with the mother with instructions to return, if symptoms develop. Treatment of symptomatic babies is essentially supportive.

### Prevention of COVID-19

The prevention of COVID-19 is multipronged and can be considered at various levels including society, home,

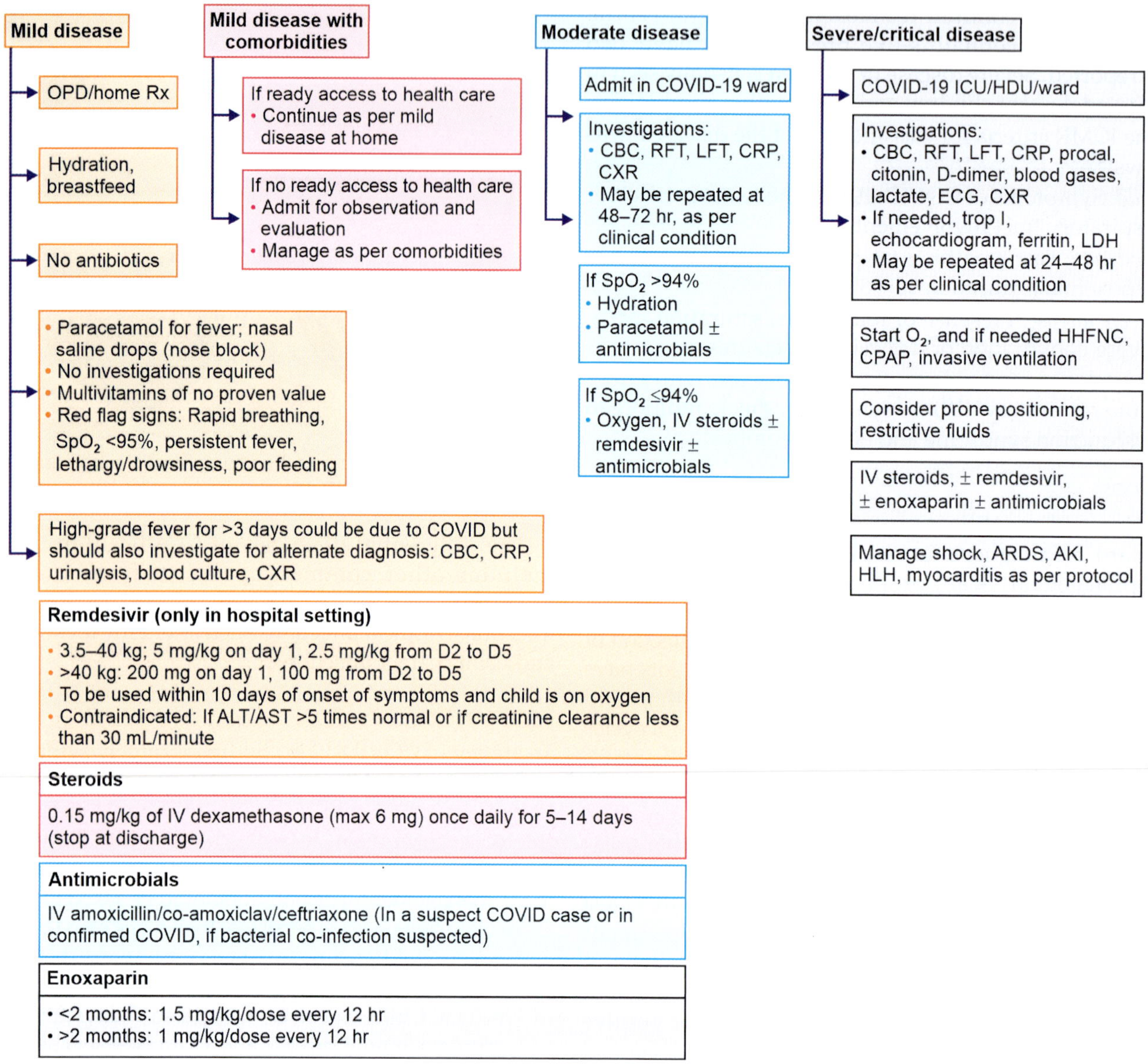


**Fig. 11.6:** IAP protocol for management of COVID-19 in children, June 2021. CBC complet blood counts; RFT renal function tests; LFT liver function tests; CRP c-reactive protein; HLH hemophagocytic lymphohistiocytosis; CPAP continuous positive airway pressure; CXR chest X-ray; HHFNC humidified high flow nasal cannula

work place, schools and hospitals. The rigor of preventive measures has changed in India over the past 2 years from a country-wide lockdown at the beginning of the pandemic to complete relaxation and return to normalcy in May 2022. The basic tenet of prevention has been universal masking, social distancing and hand hygiene. Masking is currently recommended for children above the age of 5 years. Indian children have endured one of the longest periods of school closure in the world. Vaccination has been a game changer in the pandemic and is discussed in Chapter 10.

### Suggested Reading

1. Borrelli M, Corcione A, Castellano F, Nastro FF, Santamaria F. Coronavirus disease 2019 in children. Front Pediatr 2021;9: 668484.
2. Chawla D, Chirla D, Dalwai S, et al. Perinatal-neonatal management of COVID-19 infection. Indian Pediatr 2020;57:536–48.
3. Indian Academy of Paediatrics. IAP COVID-19 management guidelines. Available at https://iapindia.org/news.php?news=49&title=IAP_Covid_19_Management_Guidelines_April_2021. Accessed on May 20, 2022.
4. Singhal T. A review of coronavirus disease-2019 (COVID-19). Indian J Pediatr 2020; 87:281–86.

## Multisystem Inflammatory Syndrome in Children (MIS-C)

### *Epidemiology and Pathogenesis*

In April 2020, 4–6 weeks after the peak of the first wave in the UK, cases of children presenting with a Kawasaki or toxic shock syndrome were first reported. These children had a history of COVID-19 or contact with a COVID-19 case 3–4 weeks earlier and were either COVID-19 PCR or COVID antibody positive. This entity was termed as pediatric inflammatory multisystem syndrome temporally related to SARS-CoV-2 (PIMS-TS). Similar cases were reported from Italy and USA. The syndrome was named as MIS-C by the US CDC and the WHO. Cases were reported from India in May 2020, and from all over the world.

MIS-C occurs in clusters usually after 4 weeks of the peak incidence of COVID-19 in the region. MIS-C is a rare complication of COVID-19 occurring in less than 1% of infected children. In one report from the US, while the incidence of lab confirmed COVID-19 in individuals less than 21 years of age was 322/100,000 the incidence of MIS-C was 2 per 100,000. The disease is more common in children of Black and Hispanic origin. Most of the cases occur in previously healthy children. The incidence of MIS-C has declined over the course of pandemic. Most cases of MIS-C were reported after the waves due to the Wuhan strain and Delta strain and very few cases after the Omicron wave.

MIS-C is due to a dysfunctional immune response to SARS-CoV-2 in a genetically susceptible child. This hyperimmune response occurs 3–4 weeks after the acute infection unlike adults where it happens a week after the infection.

### Clinical Features

Children with MIS-C present with persistent fever >3 days along with one or more of gastrointestinal symptoms (abdominal pain, vomiting, diarrhea), mucocutaneous symptoms (non-purulent conjunctivitis, cheilitis, rash) (Fig. 11.7), neurocognitive symptoms (headache, lethargy, confusion) and, in severe cases, hypotension and shock (Table 11.5). Respiratory symptoms are mild and this differentiates MIS-C from the cytokine storm of severe COVID-19. Other presentations seen during the acute phase of illness include encephalopathy, seizures, coma, or meningoencephalitis, acute kidney injury, serositis (small pleural, pericardial, and ascitic effusions) and hepatitis. Cardiac manifestations include ventricular dysfunction, coronary artery dilation or aneurysms, arrhythmia and conduction abnormalities, and rarely pericarditis and valvulitis.

MIS-C can be classified into the following three common phenotypes:

- *Kawasaki phenotype:* Usually seen in children below 5 years where mucocutaneous manifestations are prominent.

**Table 11.5:** WHO criteria for diagnosis of MIS-C

| 0–19-year-old child with fever >3 days |
|---|
| **AND** Two of the following<br>• Rash or bilateral non-purulent conjunctivitis or mucocutaneous inflammation signs (oral, hands or feet)<br>• Hypotension or shock<br>• Features of myocardial dysfunction, pericarditis, valvulitis, or coronary abnormalities (including ECHO findings or elevated troponin/NT-proBNP)<br>• Evidence of coagulopathy (PT, PTT, elevated d-dimers)<br>• Acute gastrointestinal problems (diarrhea, vomiting, or abdominal pain) |
| **AND**<br>• Elevated ESR, C-reactive protein, or procalcitonin |
| **AND**<br>• No other obvious microbial cause of inflammation, including bacterial sepsis, staphylococcal or streptococcal shock syndromes |
| **AND**<br>• Evidence of COVID-19 (RT-PCR, antigen test or serology positive) or likely contact with patients with COVID-19 |

NT-proBNP N-terminal prohormone brain natriuretic peptide; PT prothrombin time; PTT partial thromboplastin time; ESR erythrocyte sedimentation rate

- *Toxic shock phenotype:* Seen in older children where shock, myocarditis are seen.
- *Febrile inflammatory phenotype:* Here there is fever with no other organ affection. It may self-resolve or evolve into other phenotypes. This entity has to be differentiated from other illnesses.

  Incomplete and mixed phenotypes may also be seen.

### Diagnostic Criteria

In the Indian setting, diseases such as typhoid, malaria, dengue, rickettsial infections, chikungunya are closer differentials to MIS-C than streptococcal and staphylococcal toxic shock syndromes. While the WHO criteria are very

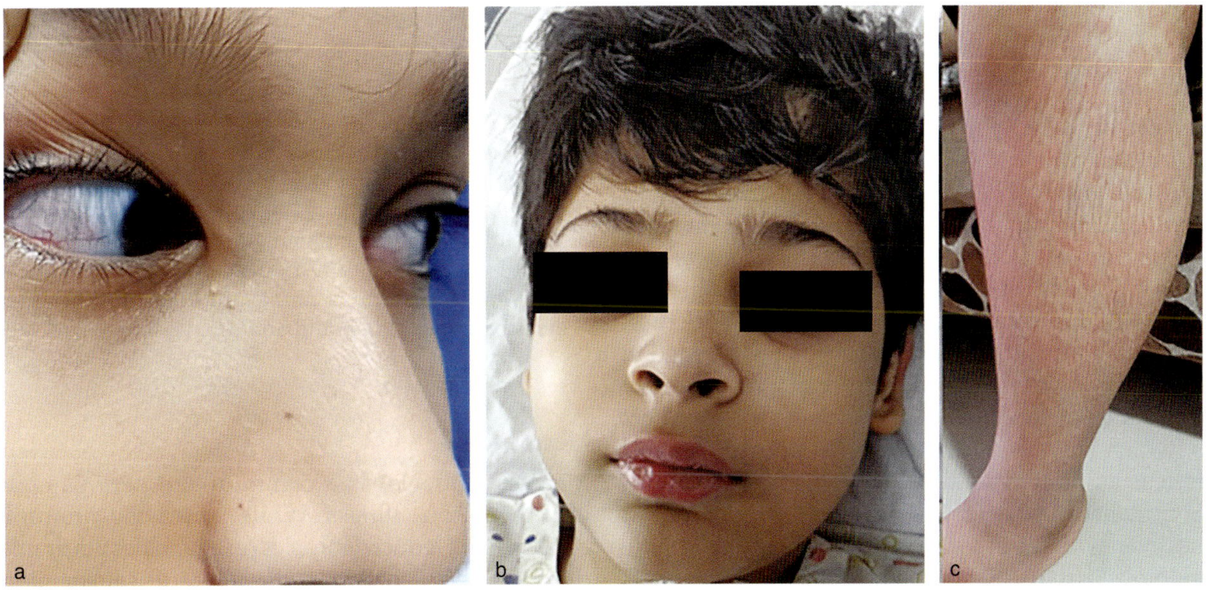

**Fig. 11.7:** Multisystem inflammatory syndrome in children (MIS-C) showing: (a) Conjunctival congestion; (b) Cracked erythematous lips; (c) Polymorphic rash on lower extremities

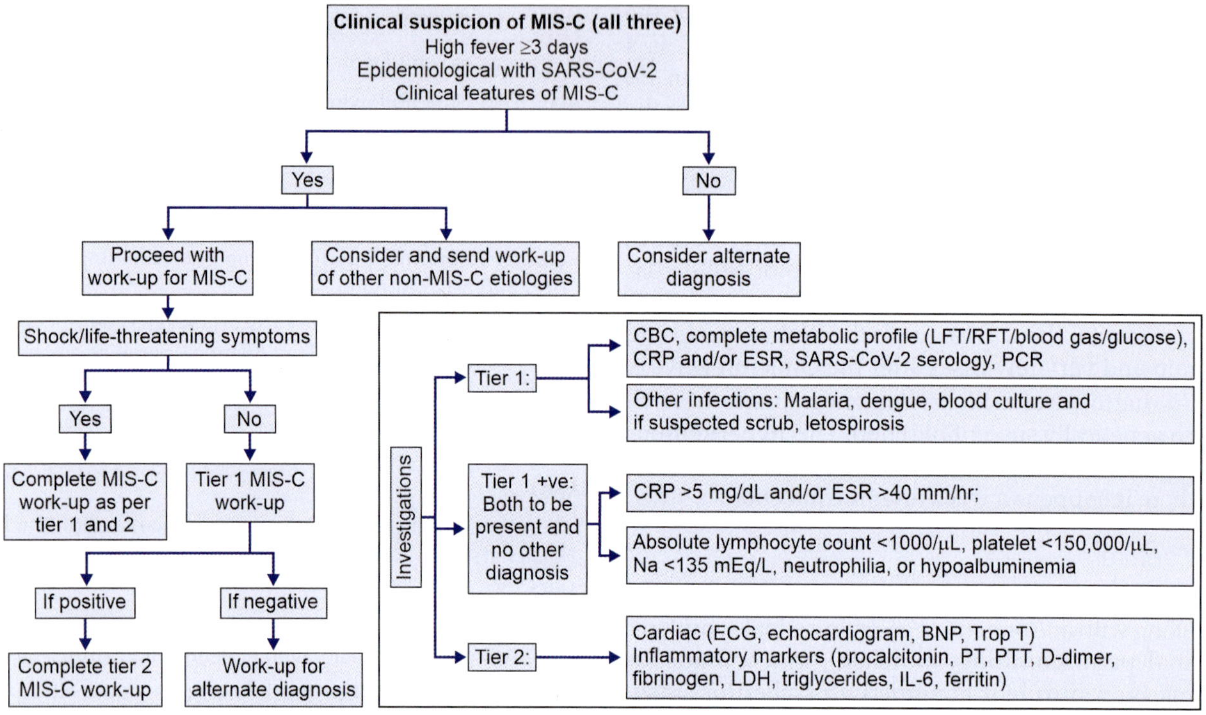


**Fig. 11.8:** India Academy of Pediatrics algorithm for diagnosis for MIS-C

sensitive, they are not specific. For instance, patients with acute appendicitis, shigellosis, enteric fever, rickettsial infections or leptospirosis will fulfill the clinical and lab criteria. Following a wave, most children will either have had COVID-19 like illness previously or contact with a COVID-19 patient. As the pandemic progressed, seroprevalence rates increased to more than 80%, thus lowering the specificity of the antibody criteria in diagnosis.

### *Lab Diagnosis*

The purpose of laboratory investigations is to confirm the diagnosis and exclude other mimics **(Fig. 11.8)**.

Antibodies to nucleocapsid protein should be tested and not the anti-spike protein, since the latter can be positive even in vaccinated children.

### *Management*

Management of MIS-C needs supportive care and multidisciplinary input from pediatricians, intensivists and cardiologists **(Fig. 11.9)**. The corner stone of treatment is use of immunomodulators. Immunomodulatory therapy includes intravenous immunoglobulin (IVIG), corticosteroids and other biologic agents such as infliximab, tocilizumab or anakinra. Since initial cases resembled Kawasaki disease, IVIG was the first-line drug; corticosteroids were added to therapy later. Biologics were used in children with refractory disease. Then came in evidence from retrospective cohort studies, which suggested that combination of IVIG and steroids was associated with better outcomes than IVIG alone. Simultaneously, several Indian centers reported good outcomes even with use of corticosteroids alone. While there is no randomized trial evidence comparing IVIG and steroids to steroids alone, recent WHO guideline recommends that steroids alone can be used in patients with non-Kawasaki phenotype of MIS-C. After initial intravenous therapy of 3–5 days, therapy should be switched to oral steroids, which are then tapered and stopped over 2–3 weeks.

Apart from use of immunomodulators, low dose aspirin in a dose of 3–5 mg/kg (max 75 mg) is recommended for 6 weeks. Anticoagulation is only recommended for those with low ejection fraction (<35%), documented thrombosis and giant coronary artery aneurysms (Z score of >10). Follow-up echocardiography is recommended at 2 and 6 weeks, and then as per need. The short-term prognosis of children MIS-C has been good with mortality rates between 0 and 5%. Long-term cardiac follow-up data is awaited.

## Suggested Reading

1. Indian Academy of Pediatrics. IAP COVID-19 guidelines. Available at https://iapindia.org/news.php?news=49&title=IAP_Covid_19_Management_Guidelines_April_2021.
2. McArdle AJ, Vito O, Patel H, et al. Treatment of multisystem inflammatory syndrome in children. N Engl J Med 2021;385:11–22.
3. WHO. Multisystem inflammatory syndrome in children and adolescents with COVID-19; 2020. Available at: https://www.who.int/publications-detail/multisystem-inflammatory-syndrome-in-children-and-adolescents-with-covid-19.

*Competency:* **PE34.15**

## Measles

Measles (rubeola) is a common and serious childhood exanthematous illness. While increasing immunization coverage has reduced measles cases and deaths dramatically over the past 2 decades, measles still causes more than 100,000 deaths per year. India contributes to around 25% of the global measles burden.

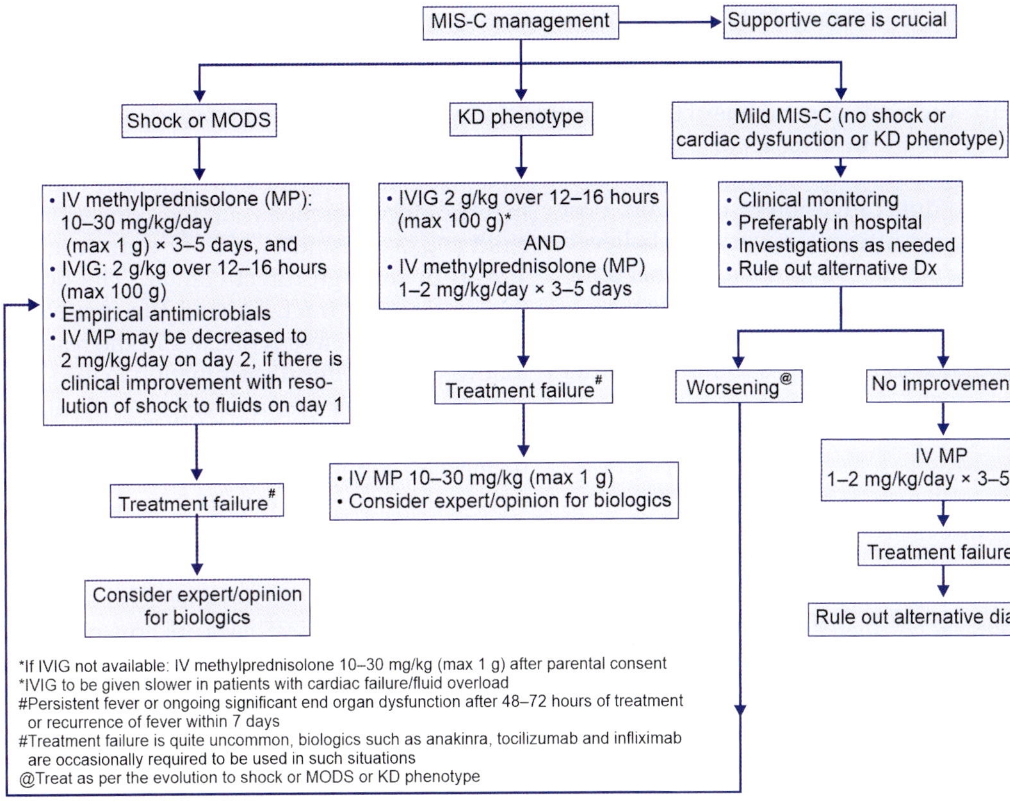


**Fig. 11.9:** Indian Academy of Pediatrics protocol for management of MIS-C. KD Kawasaki disease; MODS multiple organ dysfunction syndrome; MP methylprednisolone; IVIG intravenous immunoglobulin

### Etiopathogenesis

Measles is caused by an RNA virus belonging to the paramyxovirus family. The virus is transmitted by droplet nuclei spread from the secretions of the nose and throat usually 4 days before and 5 days after the rash. The disease is highly contagious with secondary attack rates in susceptible household contacts exceeding 90%. The portal of entry is the respiratory tract where the virus multiplies in the respiratory epithelium. Primary viremia occurs resulting in infection of the reticuloendothelial system followed by secondary viremia, which results in systemic symptoms. The incubation period is around 10 days.

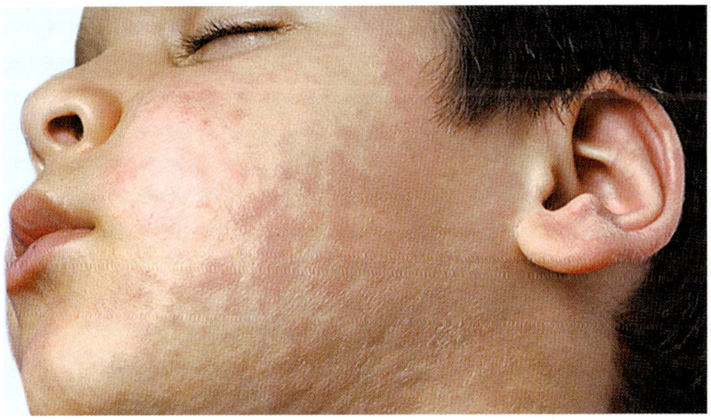

**Fig. 11.10:** The morbilliform rash of measles

### Clinical Features

The disease is most common in preschool children; infants are protected by transplacental antibodies, which generally decay by 6–9 months (hence the rationale for vaccination at this age). The prodromal phase is characterized by fever, rhinorrhea, conjunctival congestion and a dry hacking cough. Koplik spots appear on the second or third day of the illness as gray/white grains of sand-like lesions with surrounding erythema opposite the lower second molars on the buccal mucosa, and are pathognomonic for measles. The rash usually appears on the fourth day with rise in fever as faint reddish macules behind the ears, along the hairline and on the posterior aspects of the cheeks **(Fig. 11.10)**. The rash rapidly becomes maculopapular and spreads to the face, the neck, chest, arms, trunk, thighs and legs in that order over the next 2–3 days. It then starts fading in the same order that it appeared and leaves behind branny desquamation and brownish discoloration, which fades over the next 10 days.

Modified measles, seen in partially immune individuals, is a much milder and shorter illness. Hemorrhagic measles is characterized by a purpuric rash and bleeding from the nose, mouth or bowel.

### Complications

Widespread mucosal damage and significant immuno suppression induced by measles account for the frequent complications seen with this viral infection. Complications are more frequent in the very young, the malnourished and the immunocompromised. The most common complications are otitis media and bacterial bronchopneumonia. The usual bacterial pathogens are pneumococcus, *Staphylococcus aureus* and sometimes gram-negative bacteria. Other respiratory complications include laryngitis, tracheitis, bronchitis, giant cell pneumonia, bronchiectasis and flaring up of latent *M. tuberculosis* infection. Transient loss of tuberculin hypersensitivity reaction is common following measles. Gastrointestinal complications include persistent diarrhea, appendicitis, hepatitis and ileocolitis. Measles can precipitate malnutrition and can cause noma or gangrene of the cheeks.

Acute encephalitis occurs in measles at a frequency of 1–2/1000 cases most commonly during the period of the rash, consequent to direct invasion of the brain. Post measles encephalitis occurs after recovery and is believed to be due to an immune mechanism, similar to other para-infectious/demyelinating encephalomyelitis. Measles is also responsible for the almost uniformly fatal subacute sclerosing panencephalitis (SSPE) seen several years after infection at a frequency of 1/100,000 cases.

### Diagnosis

The diagnosis is clinical; it may be confirmed by estimating the levels of IgM antimeasles antibody that is present 3 days after the rash and persists for at least 1 month. Measles needs to be differentiated from other childhood exanthematous illnesses. The rash is milder and fever less prominent in rubella, enteroviral and adenoviral infections. In roseola infantum, the rash appears once fever disappears, while in measles the fever increases with rash. In rickettsial infections, the face is spared which is always involved in measles. In meningococcemia, the upper respiratory symptoms are absent and the rash rapidly becomes petechial. Drug rashes have history of antecedent drug intake. While Kawasaki disease closely mimics measles, glossitis, cervical adenopathy, fissuring of lips, extreme irritability, edema of hands and scaling in Kawasaki disease are distinguishing clinical features.

### Treatment

Treatment is mainly supportive and comprises antipyretics, maintenance of hygiene, ensuring adequate fluid and caloric intake, and humidification. Vitamin A reduces morbidity and mortality of measles and a single oral dose of 100,000 units below 1 year and 200,000 units over the age of 1 year is recommended. Complications should be managed appropriately.

### Prevention

Measles is a preventable and potentially eradicable disease through universal immunization, as discussed in Chapter 10. The MR campaign between 2017 and 2019 in which all children below age 15 years were immunized with the measles vaccine has helped improve vaccine coverage. Measles and measles-like illnesses are now reportable diseases, akin to acute flaccid paralysis surveillance.

### Suggested Reading

1. Strebel PM, Orenstein WA. Measles. N Engl J Med 2019; 381:349–57.
2. Moss WJ. Measles. Lancet 2017; 390:2490–2502.

*Competency:* **PE34.15**

## Varicella (Chickenpox)

Chickenpox usually a mild exanthematous illness in most healthy children can occasionally be a serious disease in neonates, immunocompromised, pregnant women and healthy adults.

### Etiopathogenesis

Chickenpox is caused by the varicella-zoster virus (VZV), a DNA virus of the herpes virus family. The virus is present in respiratory secretions and the skin lesions of an affected child and is transmitted either by air-borne droplet nuclei spread or through direct contact. The portal of entry is the respiratory tract. During the incubation period of 10–21 days, the virus replicates in the respiratory mucosa followed by viremic dissemination to the skin and various organs. The host immune response limits infection and promotes recovery. In immunocompromised children, unchecked replication and dissemination of virus leads to complications. During the latter part of the incubation period, the virus is transported to the respiratory mucosa and leads to infectivity even prior to appearance of the rash. The period of infectivity lasts from 24–48 hours before the rash until all the vesicles are crusted (the scabs are not infective unlike smallpox). The disease is highly contagious with secondary attack rates of 80% among susceptible household contacts. VZV establishes lifelong latent infection in the sensory ganglia. Reactivation, especially during periods of depressed immunity, leads to the dermatomal rash of herpes zoster.

### Clinical Features

Chickenpox is rarely subclinical; however, in some children only a few lesions may be present. The peak age of disease is 5–10 years. The prodromal period is short with mild to moderate fever, malaise, headache and anorexia. The rash appears 24–48 hours after the prodromal symptoms as intensely pruritic erythematous macules first on the trunk. The rash rapidly spreads to the face and extremities while it evolves into papules, clear fluid-filled vesicles, clouded vesicles and then crusted vesicles (Fig. 11.11). Several crops

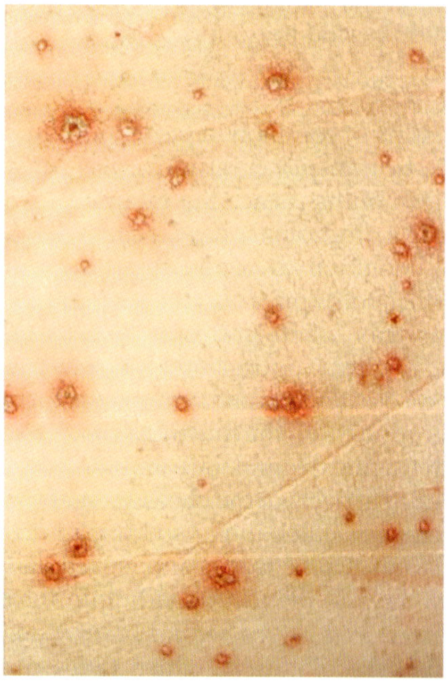

Fig. 11.11: The polymorphic rash of chickenpox

of lesions appear and simultaneous presence of skin lesions in varying stages of evolution is a characteristic of varicella. The median number of lesions is around 300 but may vary from 10–1500. Systemic symptoms persist for 2–4 days after appearance of the rash. The rash lasts 3–7 days and leaves behind hypopigmented or hyperpigmented macules that persist for days to weeks. Scarring is unusual unless lesions are secondarily infected.

### *Complications*

Secondary bacterial infections of the skin lesions may occur, occasionally resulting in necrotizing fasciitis. Commonly implicated organisms are *S. aureus* and *S. pyogenes*. Neurologic complications include meningoencephalitis, acute cerebellar ataxia, transverse myelitis, LGB syndrome and optic neuritis. Other complications include purpura fulminans due to antibodies against protein C, cold antibody mediated hemolytic anemia, CNS vasculitis leading to stroke, autoimmune thrombocytopenic purpura and Reye syndrome.

The progressive varicella syndrome is a dreaded complication of chickenpox in the immunocompromised, neonates, pregnant women and even healthy adults and adolescents. This syndrome is characterized by continued development of lesions, hemorrhagic lesions, coagulopathy and visceral organ involvement including hepatitis, pneumonia and encephalitis; mortality rates are high despite therapy.

Chickenpox in pregnancy is associated with an increased risk of severe disease in the mother. Congenital varicella syndrome may occur following infection in the first and second trimester at a frequency of 0.4–2% and is characterized by skin scarring, malformed extremities, cataracts and brain abnormalities (e.g. aplasia, calcifications). Finally, if the disease occurs in the mother 5 days before and 2 days after delivery, severe and often fatal neonatal disease may result.

Herpes zoster in children is characterized by a mild vesicular rash with dermatomal distribution; unlike adults, pain is less and post-herpetic neuralgia unusual. The risk of herpes zoster is more in children who acquire chickenpox in infancy, in those whose mothers developed varicella in the third trimester and in the immunocompromised.

### *Diagnosis*

The diagnosis is clinical and usually not difficult. Chickenpox should be differentiated from other vesicular exanthemata such as herpes simplex, enteroviral infections (hand foot mouth disease), insect bites and drug reactions. In atypical cases, the diagnosis is made on Tzanck smear of the lesions (showing multinucleated cells) and demonstration of anti-IgM antibodies to varicella.

### *Treatment*

Management is symptomatic and includes antipyretics (aspirin is contraindicated due to risk of Reye syndrome and ibuprofen due to risk of necrotizing fasciitis), antipruritic agents and good hygiene. The child should not attend school until no new lesions appear and all lesions have crusted. Administration of oral acyclovir (20 mg/kg/dose four times a day for 5 days) within 24 hours of onset of rash in healthy children reduces the duration of rash by one day and lesions by 25%. There may be some benefit, if started within 24–48 hrs of the rash but none beyond 48 hours. IV acyclovir (10 mg/kg every 8 hours or 500 mg/m$^2$ 8 hourly for 7–10 days) is given to patients with complicated varicella and illness of any severity in high-risk patients (neonates, immunocompromised children, pregnant women).

### *Prevention*

Prevention against varicella with the live attenuated varicella vaccine and use of varicella zoster immune globulin (VZIG) and oral acyclovir for post-exposure prophylaxis are detailed in Chapter 10.

### Suggested Reading


1. Arvin AM. Varicella-zoster virus. Clin Microbiol Rev 1996; 9:361–81.
2. Blumental S, Lepage P. Management of varicella in neonates and infants. BMK Pediatrics Open 2019;3:e000433.
3. Sauerbrei A. Diagnosis, antiviral therapy, and prophylaxis of varicella-zoster virus infections. Eur J Clin Microbiol Infect Dis 2016;35:723–34.


## Infectious Mononucleosis

Infectious mononucleosis, a syndrome characterized by fever, fatigue, sore throat and lymphadenopathy, is caused by the Epstein-Barr virus (EBV). A similar illness can be caused by toxoplasma, CMV, adenoviruses and primary HIV infection.

### *Etiopathogenesis*

The EBV, a DNA virus of the herpes virus family, is transmitted in oral secretions by close intimate contact like kissing or exchange of saliva from close child contact. The virus replicates in the oral epithelial cells then spreads to salivary glands with eventual viremia to the B lymphocytes in the blood and lymphoreticular system including liver and spleen. CD8 lymphocytes proliferate to check this replication of virus in the B lymphocytes and represent the atypical lymphocytes seen in EBV infection. Like other herpes viruses, EBV establishes lifelong latent infection after the primary infection, with frequent asymptomatic reactivations.

The symptoms of EBV are related to the age of primary acquisition of EBV infection. In developing countries, most of EBV infection occurs in infancy and early childhood when it is either asymptomatic or similar to other childhood infections. For this reason, infectious mononucleosis is uncommonly seen or reported in India. In developed countries, the age of acquisition of EBV infection shifts upwards and thus infectious mononucleosis is seen more commonly.

### *Clinical Features*

Symptomatic EBV infections in older children and adults are characterized by insidious onset with symptoms such as malaise, fatigue, fever, headache, nausea, sore throat, abdominal pain and myalgia. Examination shows pharyngeal inflammation with exudates and petechiae at the junction of soft and hard palate, generalized lymphadenopathy (cervical, less often axillary and inguinal), mild splenomegaly (50%) and hepatomegaly (10%). Maculopapular rashes are seen in 3–15%, and in 30–50% of those who have received ampicillin or amoxicillin.

Complications are rare and include splenic rupture following minor trauma, airway obstruction due to enlargement of oropharyngeal lymphoid tissue, meningitis, seizures, ataxia, myocarditis, hemolytic anemia, thrombocytopenia, neutropenia, aplastic anemia, interstitial pneumonitis and pancreatitis. Hemophago-lymphohistiocytosis (HLH) is another life-threatening complication.

#### *Diagnosis*

Most patients show leukocytosis and absolute lymphocytosis, with presence of atypical lymphocytes. The platelet counts may be low and hepatic transaminases mildly elevated in 50% patients. IgM antibody to viral capsid antigen (IgM VCA) is the confirmatory test to diagnose acute EBV infection. The Paul Bunnell test and monospot test are no longer recommended.

Infectious mononucleosis should be differentiated form other causes of mononucleosis enumerated earlier, and from streptococcal pharyngitis and acute leukemia.

#### *Treatment*

Rest and symptomatic therapy is the mainstay of management. Participation in strenuous activities and contact sports should be prohibited in the first 2–3 weeks of illness due to risk of splenic rupture. Treatment with prednisolone (1 mg/kg/day for 7 days) is advised for complications such as hemolytic anemia, airway obstruction, meningitis and thrombocytopenia with bleeding. Intranasal steroids may be used to relieve nasal obstruction caused by enlarged adenoids. There is no clear role of acyclovir in treatment of EBV in the immunocompetent.

#### *Other Manifestations of EBV Infections*

EBV has oncogenic potential and has been causally associated with aggressive proliferative disorders such as virus associated hemophagocytic syndrome, oral hairy leukoplakia and lymphoid interstitial pneumonitis in patients with AIDS, nasopharyngeal carcinoma, Burkitt lymphoma, Hodgkin disease and tumors in immunocompromised patients (X-linked lymphoproliferative disease, leiomyosarcoma, CNS lymphoma).

#### Suggested Reading

1. Luzuriaga K, Sullivan JL. Infectious mononucleosis . N Engl J Med 2010; 362:1993–2000.
2. Stanfield BA, Luftig MA. Recent advances in understanding EB virus. F 1000Res. 2017;6:386.
3. Womack J, Jimenez M. Common questions about infectious mononucleosis. Am Fam Physician 2015;91:372–76.

### Roseola Infantum

Roseola infantum or exanthem subitum or sixth disease is a common childhood exanthematous illness caused by primary infection mainly by a DNA virus, human herpes virus (HHV)-6 and less commonly by HHV-7 and echovirus 16. HHV-6 and HHV-7 target the CD4 T cells and like other herpes viruses can remain latent in the body for several years after acute infection.

The peak age for roseola is between 6 months and 3 years. The prodromal period is characterized by upper respiratory signs such as rhinorrhea, pharyngeal inflammation, conjunctival redness, mild cervical or occipital adenopathy, and sometimes, palpebral edema. The classic clinical illness is heralded by high fever ranging from 38°C to 40°C associated with febrile seizures in 5–10% and lasting for 3–4 days. Fever declines abruptly and is followed by development of a rash within 12–24 hrs. The rash is discrete erythematous and maculopapular which first appears on the trunk and then spreads to the face, neck and proximal extremities. It is non-pruritic, rarely becomes confluent and fades in 3–4 days. Infectiousness is low and outbreaks have not occurred. Roseola should be differentiated from childhood illnesses such as rubella, measles, enteroviruses and drug hypersensitivity. Treatment is symptomatic and prognosis excellent. HHV-6 may be associated with meningoencephalitis in immunocompromised patients, including stem cell transplant recipients.

#### Suggested Reading

1. Agut H, Bonnafous P, Gautheret-Dejean A. Laboratory and clinical aspects of human herpesvirus 6 infections. Clin Microbiol Rev 2015;28:313–35.

### Erythema Infectiosum

Erythema infectiosum or fifth disease is a common exanthematous illness of childhood caused by a small DNA virus, parvovirus B19. This virus has tropism for cells of the erythroid lineage at the pronormoblast stage.

The peak age for erythema infectiosum is between 5 and 15 years. Transmission of infection is by the respiratory route and the incubation period is 4–28 days (average, 16–17 days). The prodromal phase is mild and consists of low-grade fever, headache and symptoms of mild upper respiratory tract infection. The characteristic rash first appears as erythematous flushing on the face in what is a slapped cheek appearance (Fig. 11.12). It spreads rapidly to

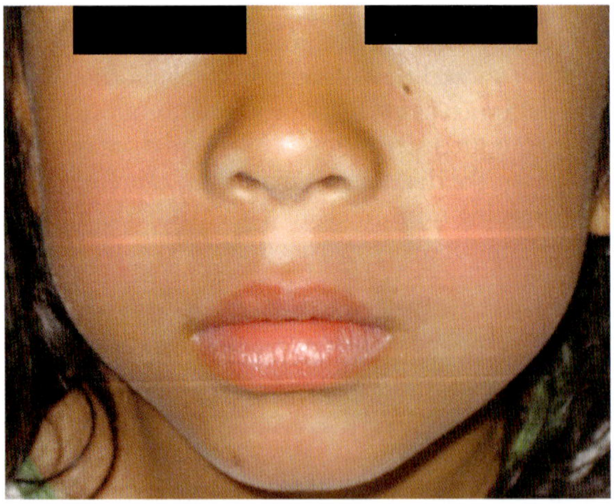

Fig. 11.12: The slapped cheek rash of erythema infectiosum

trunk and proximal extremities as a diffuse erythematous macular rash that rapidly undergoes central clearing to give it a lacy or reticulated pattern. The rash gradually fades over a 1–3-week period. Complications include arthropathy, idiopathic thrombocytopenic purpura and aseptic meningitis. Fifth disease should be differentiated from measles, roseola, rubella and drug rash. Treatment is symptomatic.

Other serious manifestations of parvovirus B19 infection include arthralgia and arthropathy in adolescents and adults; transient aplastic crises in patients with chronic hemolytic anemias; chronic anemia, pancytopenia and marrow suppression; virus associated hemophagocytic syndrome in the immunocompromised; hydrops fetalis in pregnant women; and rare episodes of myocarditis in healthy children and adults.

### Suggested Reading

1. Heegaard ED, Brown KE. Human parvovirus B19. Clin Microbiol Rev 2002;15:485–505.

*Competency:* **PE34.15**

## Mumps

Mumps is an acute viral infection characterized by painful enlargement of the salivary glands (most commonly the parotid glands). Mumps is caused by an RNA virus of genus Paramyxovirus in the family Paramyxoviridae; only one serotype is known.

### *Epidemiology and Etiopathogenesis*

Most cases occur between the ages of 5 and 15 years; infants are rarely affected due to presence of transplacentally acquired maternal antibodies. Man is the only reservoir of infection; carrier state does not exist. The incidence is higher in winter and spring.

The virus is spread from infected patient by direct contact, air-borne droplets and fomites contaminated by saliva and urine. The virus proliferates in the respiratory epithelium and enters the circulation; it then gets localized to the glandular and neural tissue. The virus has been isolated from saliva as long as 6 days before and 9 days after appearance of salivary gland swelling. The secondary infection rate is as high as 80%. Mumps infection or immunization is believed to confer lifelong immunity.

### *Clinical Features*

Following an incubation period of 2–4 weeks, the symptoms begin acutely with fever, malaise and headache. Mumps infection is characterized by unilateral or bilateral parotitis. This presents as earache, jaw tenderness while chewing, dryness of mouth and swelling at the angle of jaw. The ear lobe may appear to be pushed upwards and outwards. The defervescence and resolution takes about a week. Occasionally other salivary glands including the submaxillary and sublingual glands are affected.

The occurrence of epididymoorchitis is more common in adolescent boys or postpubertal men (unilateral in 85% cases) and occurs 1–2 weeks after parotitis. The testes are enlarged and tender. Some degree of atrophy develops in the testes affected by this viral infection but sterility is rare.

CNS involvement in the form of aseptic meningitis is seen in about 1–10% patients with parotitis. Recovery is generally uneventful. Mumps is perhaps the commonest cause of aseptic meningitis in children. The risk of encephalitis is 0.02–0.3%. Mumps encephalitis has a satisfactory prognosis with a mortality rate of less than 2%. Other CNS manifestations include auditory nerve damage leading to deafness, cerebellar ataxia, facial neuritis, transverse myelitis and Guillain-Barre syndrome. Uncommon presentations include pancreatitis (5% may trigger insulin dependent diabetes mellitus), mastitis, oophoritis, nephritis and myocarditis.

### *Diagnosis*

The diagnosis is based on clinical features. Serum amylase is elevated in almost 90% patients. The diagnosis may be confirmed by serum IgM ELISA. Mumps parotitis needs to be differentiated from suppurative parotitis, submandibular lymphadenitis, recurrent juvenile parotitis, calculus in Stensen duct and other viral infections causing parotitis, e.g. Coxsackie A and cytomegalovirus.

### *Treatment*

Symptomatic treatment is given in the form of antipyretics and warm saline mouthwashes. Orchitis is treated by bed rest and local support. Aseptic meningitis responds well to mannitol. Steroids may be used for symptomatic relief of orchitis and arthritis but do not alter the course of disease.

### *Prevention*

The affected patient should be isolated until the parotid swelling has subsided. Mumps can be prevented by timely immunization (Chapter 10).

### Suggested Reading

1. Hviid A, Rubin S, Mühlemann K. Mumps. Lancet. 2008;371:932–44.
2. Su SB, Chang HL, Chen AK. Current status of mumps virus infection: Epidemiology, pathogenesis, and vaccine. Int J Environ Res Public Health 2020;17:1686.

*Competency:* **PE30.13**

## Poliomyelitis

The polioviruses belong to the genus Enterovirus in the family Picornaviridae and comprise three related serotypes: Types 1, 2 and 3, all of which can cause paralysis. Type 1 is most frequently responsible, type 3 plays a lesser role and type 2 is only rarely involved. Wild polio virus infection has been eliminated in most parts of the world with only a handful of cases in a few countries.

### *Epidemiology*

The disease was seasonal, occurring more commonly in summer and early autumn in temperate climates. In tropical countries, seasonality was less clearly defined; some areas experience increase during the rainy season. While feco-oral route was the predominant mode of transmission in developing countries where sanitation is poor, oral-pharyngeal transmission predominated in industrialized countries and during outbreaks. The incubation period of the disease is 7–10 days (range, 4–35 days). The virus is shed in stools for six to eight weeks after infection. Humans are the only reservoir of poliovirus, and infection is spread from person-to-person. The virus spreads rapidly to non-immune persons; transmission is usually widespread in the community by the time of onset of paralysis in a child. It is estimated that for every one case of symptomatic infection there may be 1000 cases of asymptomatic disease.

The Global Polio Eradication initiative was launched in 1988 using oral polio vaccine (OPV) as the eradication tool and employing a four-pronged strategy comprising maintaining high routine immunization coverage, supplementary immunization activities (SIA) and pulse immunization, AFP surveillance and outbreak response immunization. The initiative was hugely successful with reduction of polio cases from 350,000 in 1988 to 650 in 2011 and only 17 cases in 2021. The last wild polio case was reported from India on 13 January 2011 and India has been removed from the endemic country list for more than a decade now. Only 2 countries, Afghanistan and Pakistan remain polio endemic as of today.

One of the biggest current challenges related to polio eradication is circulating vaccine-derived polio viruses (CVDPV). The term CVDPV is used for those oral polio vaccine strains that revert to neurovirulence and are capable of transmitting from person-to-person. CVPDV is most common with polio virus type 2. There have been more than 600 cases of CVDPV reported in the past 1 year (May 2021–May 2022) of which two-thirds are from Nigeria, and all but 10 are due to type 2.

The other issue is importation of wild polio into countries which were free of polio. Malawi has reported a case of wild polio virus in February 2022, which is same as the one circulating in Pakistan and another case was reported from Mozambique linked to the one in Malawi. This is the first time in 5 years when the wild virus was detected in the African continent.

All these events are a grim reminder that efforts need to be strengthened to achieve the goal of polio eradication.

### Pathogenesis

The mouth is the usual portal of entry. The virus is usually present in the pharynx and in the stool before the onset of paralytic illness. It invades local lymphoid tissue, enters the bloodstream and invades certain nerve cells. It may damage or destroy the nerve cells.

### Clinical Features

In 90–95% of infected individuals, poliovirus infection is in apparent. In the remaining 5–10% of individuals infected by poliovirus, one of the following syndromes may occur.

***Abortive polio:*** It occurs in 4–8% of infections and is characterized by a minor illness with low grade fever, sore throat, vomiting, abdominal pain, loss of appetite and malaise. Recovery is rapid and complete; there is no paralysis. It cannot be distinguished from other viral infections.

***Non-paralytic aseptic meningitis:*** It occurs in 1–2% of infections, with headache, neck, back, and leg stiffness several days after a prodrome similar to abortive polio. Recovery occurs within 2–10 days.

***Paralytic poliomyelitis:*** It occurs in 0.5–1% of infections. Symptoms occur in two phases, minor and major, separated by several days without symptoms. The minor phase consists of symptoms similar to those of abortive poliomyelitis. The major phase of illness begins with muscle pain, spasms and the return of fever. This is followed by rapid onset of flaccid paralysis that is usually complete within 72 hours.

***Spinal paralytic poliomyelitis:*** It is the most common form of paralytic poliomyelitis, accounting for approximately 80% cases. Severe cases may develop quadriplegia and paralysis of the trunk, abdominal and thoracic muscles. The affected muscles are floppy and reflexes are diminished. The senses of pain and touch are normal. Paralysis is often asymmetrical, affecting legs more often than arms. Paralytic manifestation in extremities begins proximally and progresses to involve distal muscle groups (i.e. descending paralysis). *Bulbar polio* accounts for 2% cases and results from a cranial nerve lesion, resulting in respiratory insufficiency and difficulty in swallowing, eating or speaking. *Bulbospinal polio* accounts for 20% cases and is a combination of spinal paralytic and bulbar polio.

Depending on the strain of poliovirus, the ratio between subclinical and clinical infections is estimated to range between 100:1 and 1000:1. Older children and adults run a greater risk of developing paralytic illness. The case fatality rate ranges between 2 and 20% among persons who do develop the paralytic form of the disease. However, if there is bulbar or respiratory involvement, the case fatality rate may be as high as 40%.

### Residual Paralysis

As the acute phase of illness (0–4 weeks) subsides, the recovery begins in paralyzed muscles. The extent of recovery is variable ranging from mild to severe residual paresis at 60 days, depending upon the extent of damage caused to the neurons by the virus. Maximum neurological recovery takes place in the first 6 months of the illness; slow recovery continues up to two years. After two years, no more recovery is expected and the child is said to have post polio residual paralysis, which persists throughout life.

### Diagnosis

The diagnosis is based on the history and the characteristic clinical manifestations of asymmetric flaccid paralysis. *Stool examination* is recommended in every case of acute flaccid paralysis (AFP). Virus can be detected from onset to 8 or more weeks after paralysis; the highest probability of detection is during the first 2 weeks after onset of paralysis. Examination of the *cerebrospinal fluid* (cell count, Gram stain, protein and glucose) is useful in eliminating other conditions that cause AFP. *Current serologic tests* cannot differentiate between wild and vaccine virus strains. Collection of blood specimens for culture or serology is not recommended.

### Differential Diagnosis

It is not possible to clinically differentiate between wild and vaccine associated paralytic polio (VAPP). The two diseases most commonly confused with polio are Guillain-Barré syndrome and transverse myelitis. Other conditions with a presentation similar to those of paralytic poliomyelitis include traumatic neuritis, rabies, meningitis/encephalitis, as well as illnesses produced by a variety of toxins (diphtheria, botulism).

### Treatment

Treatment should be early and appropriate to the stage and degree of paralysis. Children with bulbospinal polio and respiratory paralysis require hospitalization. In acute stage, children with isolated limb/limbs paralysis can be managed at home.

As the acute phase of illness subsides, recovery in muscle power is helped by giving physiotherapy, helping ambulation and prevention of deformities. Some children require orthosis at some stage for ambulation. Others with fixed deformities and contractures require orthopedic intervention.

### Prevention

The available vaccines and the recommended schedule along with principles of polio eradication are discussed in Chapter 10.

### Suggested Reading

1. Bahl S, Bhatnagar P, Sutter RW, Roesel S, Zaffran M. Global polio eradication – way ahead. Indian J Pediatr 2018;85:124–31.
2. Bao J, Thorley B, Isaacs D, et al. Polio - The old foe and new challenges: An update for clinicians. J Paediatr Child Health 2020;56:1527–32.

## Hand-Foot-and-Mouth Disease (HFMD)

Hand-foot-and-mouth disease is a common viral illness affecting primarily children below the age of 5 years.

### Etiology and Epidemiology

HFMD is caused by viruses of the enterovirus genus belonging to family Picornaviridae. The enterovirus genus has the polioviruses, ECHO viruses, Coxsackieviruses and enteroviruses. Though many viruses can cause HFMD, Coxsackievirus A16 and enterovirus 71 are the most common. The disease commonly presents as outbreaks often in preschools and transmission is by direct contact with an affected patient or with infected fomites.

### Clinical Features

The onset is with a prodrome characterized by low grade fever, feeling of being unwell, sore throat. This is followed by development of ulcers/blisters in the oral cavity mostly on the posterior aspect and then a papulovesicular skin rash on the palms and soles and less commonly on buttocks, knees, elbows and genital area (Fig. 11.13). All manifestations may not be present in all patients. The illness resolves quickly over the 4–5 days in most children.

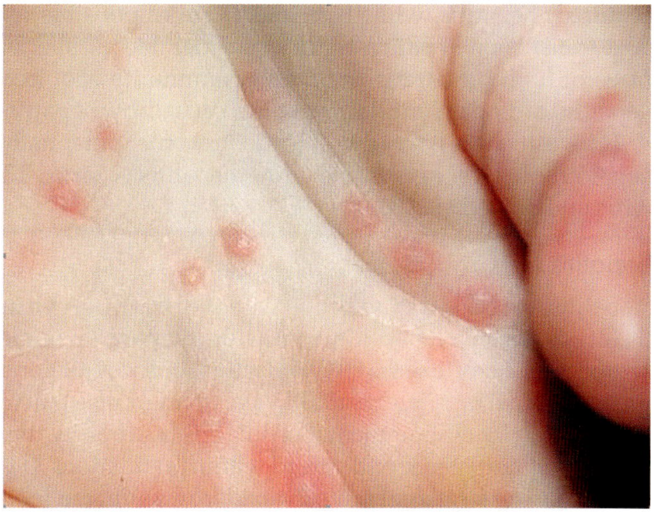

**Fig. 11.13:** The vesicular rash of hand foot mouth disease

Complications include loss of toe nails or finger nails 4 weeks after onset of disease which is temporary. Rare complications include aseptic meningitis, encephalitis, polio-like paralysis, myocarditis and respiratory distress syndrome. HFMD outbreaks due to enterovirus 71 with neurologic complications and deaths have been increasingly reported from China, Vietnam, Taiwan and Malaysia. Some experts believe that HFMD enteroviruses are occupying the ecologic niche created by eradication of polio viruses.

### Diagnosis

Diagnosis is clinical and the disease should be differentiated from other illnesses causing oral ulcers such as herpangina, herpetic gingivostomatitis and apthous ulcers, and also from chickenpox and insect bite allergy.

### Treatment and Prevention

Treatment is mainly symptomatic with analgesics and soft diet. Isolation of affected children at home and promotion of hand hygiene to prevent disease spread is important. Currently, there is no vaccine available against HFMD.

### Suggested Reading

1. Saguil A, Kane SF, Lauters R, Mercado MG. Hand-foot-and-mouth disease: Rapid evidence review. Am Fam Physician 2019;100:408–14.
2. Yi Z, Pei S, Suo W, et al. Epidemiological characteristics, routine lab diagnosis, chemical signs and risk factors for hand, foot and mouth disease: Systematic review and meta-analysis. PLoS One 2022;17:e0267716.

*Competency:* **PE26.1**

## Viral Hepatitis

Hepatitis is a general term meaning inflammation of the liver and can be caused by a variety of different hepatotropic viruses such as hepatitis A, B, C, D and E. Hepatitis A and E are responsible for most of the water-borne (community acquired) hepatitis, while B, C and D are responsible for post-transfusion hepatitis. Since a considerable number of cases of both post-transfusion and community-acquired hepatitis are not identified as being caused by hepatitis A–E, investigators have sought to identify other potentially hepatotropic viral agents, including hepatitis G virus, TT virus and SEN virus.

### Hepatitis A

Hepatitis A is caused by infection with the hepatitis A virus (HAV), a nonenveloped RNA virus. In humans, a single serotype of HAV exists. HAV infection induces lifelong protection against reinfection. HAV is extremely resistant to degradation by environmental conditions, a property that allows its maintenance and spread within populations. It is spread via the fecal–oral route through contaminated food and water, and person-to-person spread under poor sanitary conditions. The severity of the disease increases with age at time of infection. In children less than 5-year-old, infection is asymptomatic or presents as an acute undifferentiated febrile illness. Classic hepatitis is seen in older children, adolescents and adults. In developing countries with poor environmental hygienic conditions where most people are infected in childhood, symptomatic disease is less common and outbreaks rare. India is a country with intermediate endemicity. Hence, a subset of population, which is of good socioeconomic status escapes infection in childhood and gets symptomatic disease as adults.

#### Clinical Features

The *incubation period* ranging from 10 to 50 days (median 30 days), during which the patient remains asymptomatic despite active replication of the virus. Thereafter there is a short prodromal phase lasting for up to a week characterized by symptoms like loss of appetite, fatigue, abdominal pain, nausea and vomiting, fever, diarrhea, dark urine and pale stools. In older patients, this prodromal phase is followed by an *icteric phase*, during which jaundice develops at total bilirubin levels exceeding 2–4 mg/dL and liver enzymes in hundreds or thousands. The icteric phase generally begins within 10 days of the initial symptoms. Fever improves after the first few days of jaundice. During the next few weeks in the *convalescent period*, patient shows complete recovery.

In around 0.1–1% of patients, extensive necrosis of the liver occurs during the first 6–8 weeks of illness. In this case, high fever, marked abdominal pain, vomiting, jaundice and the development of hepatic encephalopathy associated with coma and seizures occur. These are the signs of fulminant hepatitis, which is more common as age advances and leads to death in 70–90% of the patients. In patients who survive, neither functional nor pathologic sequelae are common despite the widespread necrosis. Infection with HAV does not lead to chronic or persistent hepatitis.

In some patients, there is a prolonged febrile cholestatic phase and some patients have a relapsing pattern.

#### Diagnosis

The specific diagnosis of acute hepatitis A is made by finding anti-HAV IgM in the serum of patients. Anti-HAV IgM is detectable about 3 weeks after exposure, always by the time symptoms occur, its titer increases over 4 to 6 weeks, then declines to non-detectable levels within 6 months of infection. As IgG anti-HAV persists lifelong after acute infection, detection of IgG anti-HAV alone indicates past infection. Laboratory evaluation of liver function includes estimation of total and direct bilirubin, transaminases, alkaline phosphatase, prothrombin time, total protein and albumin.

Hepatitis A needs to be differentiated from other viral hepatitis chiefly E, sometimes also from Wilson disease and autoimmune hepatitis.

#### Treatment

Therapy is supportive and is aimed at maintaining adequate nutrition. There is no evidence to suggest that restriction of fats has any beneficial effect on the course of the disease. Eggs, milk and butter may actually help provide a correct caloric intake. Antiviral agents have no role because the hepatic injury appears to be immunopathologically mediated. Referral to a liver transplant centre is recommended for patients with fulminant hepatitis. Steroids are sometimes indicated in patients with cholestatic and relapsing hepatitis.

#### Prevention

The ideal preventive strategy is improvement in sanitation, hygiene and water supply. Immunization is very effective and discussed further in Chapter 10. Immunoglobulin G may be used for post exposure prophylaxis; if administered within 2 weeks of exposure, it either prevents or attenuates sevrity of disease.

### Suggested Reading


1. Abutaleb A, Kottilil S. Hepatitis A: Epidemiology, natural history, unusual clinical manifestations and prevention. Gastroenterol Clin North Am 2020;49:191–99.
2. Mathur P, Arora NK. Epidemiological transition of hepatitis A in India: Issues for vaccination in developing countries. Indian J Med Res 2008;128:699–704.


*Competency:* **PE26.12**

### Hepatitis B

Hepatitis B virus is a 3.2 kb, circular, partially double stranded DNA virus containing 3200 nucleotides coding for core protein (HBcAg), precore protein (HBeAg), envelope glycoprotein (HBsAg), a DNA polymerase with reverse transcriptase activity and the HBV-X protein that acts as a transcriptional activator for many host and viral genes and may have a role to play in hepatocellular carcinoma.

#### Epidemiology of HBV Infection

It is estimated that 400 million (5% of the world's population) people are living with hepatitis B infection worldwide and that hepatitis B resulted in an approximately 887,000 deaths in 2015 from cirrhosis and hepatocellular carcinoma. Global prevalence of HBV infection varies from 0.7% in the WHO Americas region, 2% in the Southeast Asian region to 6% in Africa. Carrier rates in India range from 2–5%. HBV is transmitted through contact with blood and body fluids of an infected person. In highly endemic areas, HBV infections occur mainly due to perinatal transmission from carrier mothers to their infants or less commonly through horizontal transmission resulting from casual contact with infected children during the first 5 years of life. It is estimated that in the absence of prophylaxis, 70–90% of HBsAg and HBeAg positive mothers will transmit infection as against only 10–40% of HBsAg positive but HBeAg negative mothers. HBV is not transmitted by breastfeeding. Other routes of transmission are unsafe injections, drug abuse, tattooing, medical procedures including dialysis and sexual transmission.

#### *Pathogenesis—Natural Course and Clinical Course*

It is estimated that 90% of perinatally infected children become chronic carriers as against 30–50% of those infected in early childhood and 5% of those infected in adulthood. Perinatally infected children are usually asymptomatic. Most of them have high levels of viral replication in the liver with high levels of HBV DNA and HBeAg but normal liver enzymes and no clinical symptoms. This is called the immunotolerant phase. However, in the second and third decade of life, the phase of immune tolerance converts to a phase of immune clearance, wherein there is immune-mediated destruction of the virus infected cells leading to abrupt increase in liver enzymes and less commonly symptoms of hepatitis and rarely hepatic decompensation. In some, this immune clearance is associated with loss of HBeAg and development of anti-HBe antibody, and later clearance of HBsAg (0.6% of infected children per year) **(Fig. 11.14)**. However, in most, this phase is associated with only temporary loss of HBeAg and clearance of HBV DNA with return of antigenemia. Several such episodes occur during the following years with development of chronic hepatitis, and later, cirrhosis and hepatocellular carcinoma. Treatment is discussed in Chapter 12.

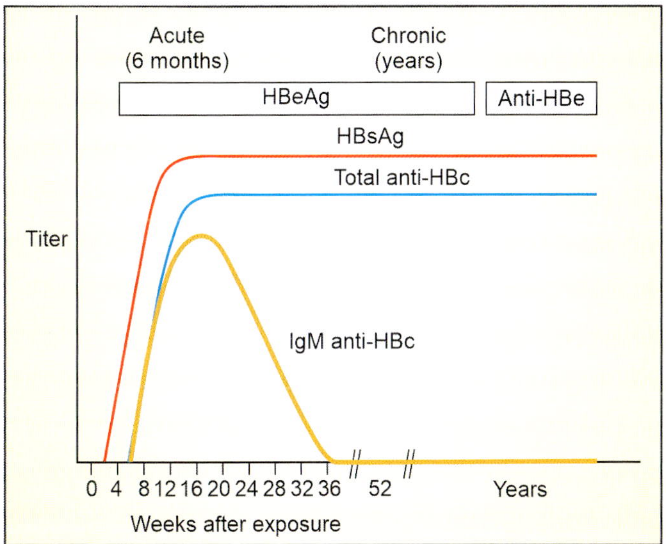


**Fig. 11.14:** Progression of hepatitis B virus infection

#### *Prevention and Immunoprophylaxis*

Hepatitis B immunoglobulin (HBIG) is used in the post-exposure prophylaxis of newborns of HBV-infected women. It is administered intramuscularly as soon as possible after birth and is given concurrently with HBV vaccine, at a different site. The dose for infants is 0.5 mL. Combination of HBIG and HBV vaccination in infants born to HBsAg positive mothers has around 95% efficacy in preventing transmission.

Vaccination is discussed in Chapter 10.

### Hepatitis D

Hepatitis delta virus (HDV) was first detected as a new nuclear antigen in the hepatocytes of patients infected with hepatitis B virus (HBV) and was frequently associated with severe acute or chronic hepatitis. Transmission of HDV requires either co-infection with HBV or superinfection in individuals who are HBV carriers. Although HDV infection is closely associated with HBV, HDV clearly belongs to a distinct virus group. Currently, HDV is assigned a floating genus, Deltavirus.

### Hepatitis C

Hepatitis C virus (HCV) was recognized in 1989 as a major cause of non-A, non-B hepatitis. HCV is an enveloped, single-stranded, positive-sense ribonucleic acid (RNA) virus, classified as an independent genus (*Hepacivirus*) within the Flavivirus family.

#### *Viral Variants*

The HCV RNA-dependent RNA polymerase lacks proof-reading ability, which results in HCV being genetically heterogeneous. Based on analysis of HCV sequences, six major HCV genotypes are recognized. HCV genotypes 1 and 2 are the most prevalent worldwide. HCV genotype 3 is most common in Australia and the Indian subcontinent. The viral genotypic distribution in children generally parallels that reported regionally in adults. HCV genotype 1 correlates with higher serum viral levels and a less favorable response to antiviral treatment.

#### *Epidemiology*

The worldwide prevalence of HCV infection is approximately 3%, which represents an estimated 170 million infected persons. Infection occurs due to contact with blood and body fluids of infected people. The primary modes of infection in children are vertical transmission from infected mothers (rates ranging from 2–10% depending on the level of maternal viremia and coinfection with HIV) and receipt of blood transfusions prior to the period when HCV testing became routine. HCV is not transmitted by breastfeeding. Transmission by unsafe injections, drug abuse, tattooing are other routes for disease transmission. Unlike HBV, HCV is not transmitted to household contacts and sexual transmission is infrequent.

#### *Natural Course and Clinical Features*

In adults, 85% of patients exposed to HCV will develop chronic infection, of which approximately 10 to 20% develop cirrhosis and some hepatocellular carcinoma. Chronic HCV is a common indication for liver transplant in the developed nations. However, the prognosis of childhood HCV infection is generally good. A significant percentage (up to 40%) of vertically infected children spontaneously clear HCV over a few years. The rate of spontaneous clearance reduces as age of acquisition of infection advances. Even chronically infected children remain asymptomatic. Most have normal liver enzymes and minimal changes on liver biopsy. Progression to chronic disease, hepatic decompensation and hepatocellular carcinoma are rare events in children.

#### *Diagnosis*

The diagnosis of HCV infection is based on detection of antibodies against recombinant HCV antigens by enzyme immunoassay or rapid immunoblot assays or by detection of HCV RNA using nucleic acid tests. Enzyme immunoassays are fairly sensitive but less specific and false positive results are seen in patients with elevated globulin levels such as those with autoimmune hepatitis. The rapid immunochromatographic tests are more specific and less sensitive. Hence, the EIAs are recommended as screening tests and the rapid immunochromatographic tests as confirmatory. Patients with positive EIA and negative rapid tests are labeled as indeterminate, and repeating tests after 4–6 weeks or conducting an HCV RNA PCR is recommended. Antibodies against HCV are non-protective and may last for life even if the patient has cleared HCV from the body. Diagnosis of perinatal infection, early infection (in the first 4–8 weeks) or active infection is made by performing the HCV RNA PCR

Therapy is discussed in Chapter 12.

#### Suggested Reading


1. Karnsakul W, Schwarz KB. Hepatitis B and C. Pediatr Clin North Am 2017; 64:641–58.
2. Sathiyasekaran M, Ramaswamy G. Diagnosis and management of hepatitis B and hepatitis C infections in children. Pediatr Infectious Dis 2020;2:12–18.


### Hepatitis E

Hepatitis E virus was first described in 1978 following a large epidemic in Kashmir. HEV is a single-stranded RNA virus, with four genotypes 1–4. Genotypes 1 and 2 are water borne and cause epidemics and acute hepatitis in the resource-limited nations, while genotypes 3 and 4 are zoonotic infections in industrialized nations and transmitted by close contact with animals (pigs) and eating undercooked pork.

#### *Clinical Features*

The incubation period following exposure to HEV ranges from 3 to 8 weeks, with a mean of 40 days. The usual clinical presentation is of acute hepatitis similar to that seen with hepatitis A. Fulminant hepatitis can occur especially in pregnant women with third trimester infections associated with mortality rates of 20%. Premature deliveries with high infant mortality up to 33% are observed. Chronic hepatitis E infection is a rare complication seen in severely immunocompromised hosts. Hepatitis E is also being implicated as a cause of many extrahepatic neurologic and hematologic manifestations.

#### *Diagnosis*

Laboratory evaluation of HEV is similar to that of HAV and is based on detection of HEV IgM. Antibodies to HEV (IgM and IgG) develop at the time symptoms occur, usually before the development of jaundice. IgM anti-HEV titer declines rapidly during early convalescence, while IgG anti-HEV persists and provides protection against subsequent infections.

#### *Treatment*

Treatment is supportive and symptomatic. There is some evidence of benefit of ribavirin therapy in patients with fulminant hepatitis and in chronic infection in immunocompromised hosts.

#### *Prevention*

The basic tenets of prevention include optimum food, water hygiene and personal hygiene. Boiling water inactivates HEV, but the effectiveness of chlorination is unknown. A recombinant genotype 1 vaccine has been commercially licensed in China since 2011 which has demonstrated good long-term protection and cross protection against genotypes 2 and 4.

#### Suggested Reading


1. Aslan AT, Balaban HY. Hepatitis E virus: Epidemiology, diagnosis, clinical manifestations, and treatment. World J Gastroenterol 2020;26:5543–60.


*Competency:* **PE34.18**

### Chikungunya

Chikungunya is an acute disease, which results in fever, arthritis and skin rash, caused by an enveloped flavivirus. Due to the severe arthritic symptoms, the disease is given the Swahili name of chikungunya (that which bends up). Since an outbreak of chikungunya in Tanzania in 1952, large epidemics were reported in South Africa, India (1971), South East Asia and Philippines. Re-emergence of chikungunya disease occurred in India during 2005–06, causing 1.3 million cases in 13 states, chiefly Andhra Pradesh and Karnataka.

#### *Epidemiology*

The rural cycle of chikungunya transmission involves *Aedes africans*, *A. fancifer*, and wild primates, while the urban cycle involves *A. aegypti* and humans. In urban areas, the outbreaks are sporadic and explosive with infection of a large population within weeks. In Asia, the virus may be maintained in urban cycle, with *A. aegypti*, or require reinoculation before onset of epidemic. Outbreaks typically occur during the rainy season, associated with the population density of the mosquito vector, which breeds in household containers and puddles with peak activity in mid-morning and late afternoon. After an epidemic, the disease typically vanishes for years, because a large proportion of the population is immune.

### Clinical Features

The disease has a sudden onset, with an incubation period of 2–12 days. Infection is characterized by fever, headache, fatigue, nausea, vomiting, muscle pain, rash and joint pain. Fever rises abruptly to 103–104°F and is accompanied by rigors. The acute phase lasts for 2–3 days. Joint pain appears suddenly and is often very severe in intensity; the arthralgia/arthritis is polyarticular, migratory, and predominantly affects the small joints of hands, wrist, ankle and feet, with less involvement of larger joints. Headache is present in 80% of cases. Photophobia and retro-orbital pain may also occur. An itchy, transient maculopapular rash appears 4–8 days later affecting the trunk and limbs. Inguinal lymph nodes may be enlarged. The joint pains may continue for many months after the illness. Acute complications include encephalitis, shock and bleeding. Disease can be transmitted vertically and presents in neonates as a febrile illness with rash and rarely neurological complications.

### Diagnosis

Chikungunya should be suspected in patients who presents with the characteristic triad of fever, rash and arthritis. The CBC may show leukopenia and thrombocytopenia ( though not as severe as dengue). Viremia is present in most patients during the initial 2–4 days of disease and can be detected commercially by PCR. Virus specific IgM antibodies may be detected by capture ELISA and hemagglutination inhibition assays after 5–7 days of illness.

The disease should be differentiated from dengue, zika and other tropical infections.

### Treatment

No specific treatment is available. Symptomatic treatment in the form of rest, fluids, and ibuprofen, naproxen, acetaminophen, or paracetamol may relieve symptoms. Chloroquine and steroids have been used to treat debilitating joint symptoms. Aspirin should be avoided during the acute phase of illness.

### Prevention and Control

Strategies for prevention and control include breaking the transmission cycle of *A. aegypti* and by holding the mosquito population at extremely low levels. A live attenuated vaccine, developed recently, which induces long-term production of neutralizing antibodies, is being examined.

## Suggested Reading


1. Ravi V. Reemergence of chikungunya virus in India. Indian J Med Microbiol 2006;24:83–84.
2. Vairo F, Haider N, Kock R, Ntoumi F, Ippolito G, Zumla A. Chikungunya: Epidemiology, pathogenesis, clinical features, management, and prevention. Infect Dis Clin North Am 2019; 33:1003–25.
3. Ward CE, Chapman JI. Chikungunya in children: A clinical review. Pediatr Emerg Care 2018;34:510–15.


*Competency:* **PE34.18**

## Dengue

Dengue fever is an acute febrile illness characterized by fever, myalgia, arthralgia and rash. Severe dengue infection is characterized by abnormalities in hemostasis and by leakage of plasma from the capillaries; the latter may lead to shock (dengue shock syndrome).

### Epidemiology

The global prevalence of dengue has increased, with the disease now being endemic in more than 100 countries in Africa, the Americas, the Eastern Mediterranean, southeast Asia and Western Pacific. Southeast Asia and the Western Pacific are most seriously affected. Modelling studies estimate more than 90 million annual symptomatic cases of dengue across the world. During epidemics, attack rates among susceptible are ~40–50%. An estimated 500,000 cases with severe dengue infection require hospitalization every year; 2.5% patients die. Without proper treatment, case fatality rates in severe dengue infection (earlier called dengue hemorrhagic fever, DHF) can exceed 20%. The spread of dengue is attributed to expanding geographic distribution of the four dengue viruses and their mosquito vectors, chiefly the pre-dominantly urban species *Aedes aegypti*. A rapid rise in urban populations is bringing ever greater numbers of people into contact with this vector, especially in areas that favor mosquito breeding, e.g. where household water storage is common and where solid waste disposal services are inadequate.

***Virus:*** Dengue fever is caused by any of the 4 dengue serotypes. Dengue virus is an arbovirus of the family Flaviviridae. These RNA viruses are spherical, approximately 50 nm in diameter with approximately 11000 nucleotides. The envelop protein bears epitopes that are unique to the serotypes. Antibodies to these epitopes neutralize the virus by interfering with entry of virus into the cells. There are other epitopes that are shared between dengue viruses (dengue subgroup antigens) and other flaviviruses (group antigens). Four well-defined dengue viruses are identified—DENV-1, DENV-2, DENV-3 and DENV-4. Genotyping is used to trace the movement of dengue viruses between different geographic regions.

***Transmission:*** Dengue viruses are transmitted to humans through the bites of infected female *Aedes* mosquitoes. Mosquitoes acquire the virus while feeding on blood of an infected person. After incubation for 3–7 days, an infected mosquito is capable, during probing and blood feeding of transmitting the virus to susceptible individuals for the rest of its life. Infected female mosquitoes may also transmit the virus to their offspring by transovarial (via the eggs); this transmission is not well studied. Humans are the main amplifying host, although monkeys may become infected and serve as a source of virus for uninfected mosquitoes. The virus circulates in the blood of infected humans for 2–7 days, at approximately the same time as fever. *Aedes* mosquitoes may acquire the virus when feeding on an infected individual.

### Pathophysiology

The major pathophysiology that differentiates severe dengue from dengue fever is plasma leakage and abnormal hemostasis leading to rising hematocrit values, moderate to marked thrombocytopenia and varying degrees of bleeding. The cause of abnormal leakage of plasma is not entirely understood. However, rapid recovery without residual abnormality in vessels suggests it to be the result of release and interaction of biological mediators, capable of producing severe illness with minimal structural injury.

The pathogenesis of dengue and severe dengue infection is not clear. It is observed that sequential infection with any two of the four serotypes of dengue virus results in DHF/DSS in an endemic area. It is suggested that antibodies produced during the first infection are able to neutralize a second viral infection with the same serotype. However, when no neutralizing antibodies are present (i.e. infection due to another serotype), the second infection is under the influence of enhancing antibodies and the resulting infection and disease are severe. It is proposed that serotype cross-reactive antibodies generated from previous infection with a particular dengue virus serotype are not specific for other serotypes. Hence, they bind to the virions but do not neutralize them, and instead increase their uptake by antigen presenting cells (tissue dendritic cells, monocytes, macrophages). Enhanced antigen presentation by these cells results in activation and proliferation of memory T cells, and release of cytokines that contribute to the pathogenesis of DHF/DSS.

Endothelial cell dysfunction manifests as increased capillary permeability with microvascular leak, hemoconcentration and circulatory insufficiency. The transient nature of plasma leakage suggests that this might be mediated by a soluble mediator. Dengue viral infection is commonly associated with thrombocytopenia, due to molecular mimicry between dengue virus proteins (especially NS1) and endogenous self-proteins. There is activation of blood clotting and fibrinolytic pathways. Mild disseminated intravascular coagulation, liver injury and thrombocytopenia contribute to hemorrhage. Liver may show diffuse hepatitis with focal necrosis and steatosis; viral antigen may be detected on immunohistochemistry. Central nervous system involvement is attributed to direct neurotropic effect of the virus.

Risk factors for DHF/DSS are:

- Virus strain: DENV-2 > DENV-3; DENV-4 > DENV-1
- Pre-existing antidengue antibody
- Age: Younger children are at increased risk
- Secondary infection
- Genetic predisposition
- Hyperendemicity: Two or more virus serotypes circulating simultaneously at high level.

### Clinical Manifestations

Dengue infection has varying clinical presentations and often with unpredictable clinical evolution and outcome. Incubation period varies between 3 and 7 days. Infants and young children may present with an undifferentiated febrile illness. The classic presentation of dengue fever is usually seen in older children, adolescents and adults and can be described under three phases—febrile, critical and recovery.

***Febrile phase:*** Characterized by sudden onset of high- grade fever that may last for 2–7 days, there is facial flushing, skin erythema, body aches, myalgia, arthralgia, headache, anorexia, nausea and vomiting. Occasionally the child may have sore throat, injected pharynx and conjunctival injection. A positive tourniquet test and minor hemorrhagic manifestations (petechiae, mucosal bleeding from nose and gums) may be seen in some patients. Liver may be enlarged and tender from 2 to 5 days and indicates risk for developing severe illness. There is progressive decrease in total white cell count and platelet count. Most children will recover from febrile phase without moving to critical phase.

***Critical phase:*** During defervescence, 3–7 days from onset of fever, some of the patients may develop bleeding and shock with fall in platelet count and increase in packed cell volume (PCV) (indicating capillary leak). Some children show organ dysfunction with severe hepatitis, encephalitis or myocarditis and/or severe bleeding, even in the absence of plasma leakage or shock.

***Recovery phase:*** After 24–48 hours in critical phase, a gradual reabsorption of extravascular compartment fluid takes place in next 48–72 hours. The general well-being improves, appetite returns, gastrointestinal symptoms abate, hemodynamic status stabilizes and diuresis ensues. Some patients may have a rash of 'isles of white in the sea of red.' Others exhibit pruritus, bradycardia and electrocardiographic changes; respiratory distress due to pulmonary edema is uncommon. PCV stabilizes or may be lower due to dilution. While leukocyte counts rise after defervescence, recovery of thrombocytopenia may take longer.

***Unusual features:*** A few patients may present with persistent thrombocytopenia mimicking idiopathic thrombocytopenia, hemophagocytic lymphohistiocytosis and an extended course of illness in form of multiorgan dysfunction (extended dengue syndrome). Dengue in immunocompromised children shows higher incidence of organ dysfunction and longer time for platelet recovery.

### Disease Classification

The current classification of dengue by WHO had been in use since 2009 and it identifies three categories based on the severity **(Fig. 11.15)**. The main purpose of the classification is to aid the physicians where and how intensively patient should be treated and monitored.

### Differential Diagnosis

Differential diagnosis includes other hemorrhagic fever, chikungunya infection, influenza, malaria, enteric fever, leptospirosis and less commonly meningococcemia and rickettsiosis. Malaria, leptospirosis, flu, enteric fever and chikungunya infections may be coinfected with dengue. The features of chikungunya infection are similar to dengue. However, fever is of shorter duration, and thrombocytopenia and bleeding are less frequent. Patients with chikungunya often have skin eruptions, mucosal lesions, polyarthralgia and encephalopathy.

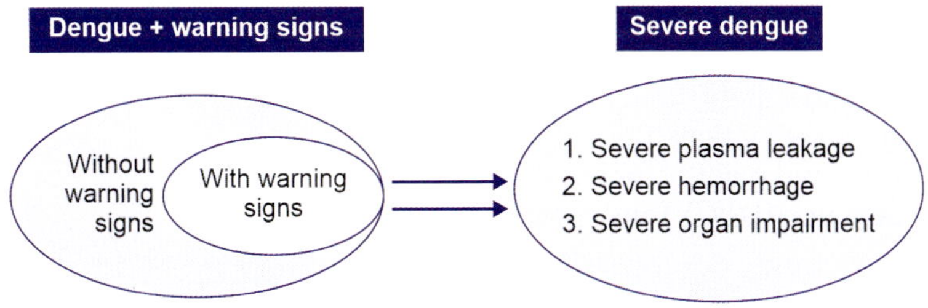


| Criteria for Dengue ± warning signs | | Criteria for severe dengue |
|---|---|---|
| **Probable dengue**<br>Live in/travel to dengue endemic area<br>Fever and 2 of the following<br>• Nausea, vomiting<br>• Rash<br>• Aches and pains<br>• Tourniquet test positive<br>• Leukopenia<br>• Any warning sign<br><br>**Laboratory confirmed dengue** | **Warning signs**<br>• Abdominal pain/tenderness<br>• Persistent vomiting<br>• Clinical fluid accumulation<br>• Mucosal bleed<br>• Lethargy, restlessness<br>• Liver enlargement >2 cm<br>• Laboratory increase in HCT concurrent with rapid decrease in platelet count | **Severe plasma leakage**<br>Leading to<br>• Shock (DSS)<br>• Fluid accumulation with respiratory distress<br>**Severe bleeding**<br>As evaluated by physician<br>**Severe organ impairment**<br>• Liver: AST/ALT ≥1000 u/L<br>• CNS: Impaired consciousness<br>• Heart and other organs |

HCT hematocrit, DSS dengue shock syndrome, AST aspartate aminotransferase, ALT alanine aminotransferase, CNS central nervous system

**Fig. 11.15:** Revised WHO classification of dengue infections. (Dengue Guidelines for Diagnosis, Treatment, Prevention and Control. Geneva, Switzerland: WHO; 2009)

Following clinical and laboratory features suggest presence of severe dengue infection.

*Clinical criteria:* Acute onset high-grade fever, hemorrhagic manifestations (positive tourniquet test), tender hepatomegaly, effusion in body cavities and/or shock.

*Laboratory criteria:* Thrombocytopenia (≤100 000 cells per mm$^3$; <1–2 platelets per oil immersion field), rising hematocrit.

*Tourniquet test:* This test is part of the WHO case definition for dengue, and a marker of capillary fragility. The test is performed by inflating the blood pressure cuff to a point midway between the systolic and diastolic blood pressure for 5 minutes. The cuff is deflated and removed. After waiting for 2 minutes, the number of petechiae is counted in the antecubital fossa. The presence of 10 or more petechiae per 1 square inch indicates a positive finding. This finding is present in more than 50% of cases.

### Laboratory Investigations

Children with severe dengue infection show increasing PCV and low platelet and leukocyte counts with lymphocyte predominance. A low leukocyte count in a child with febrile illness during the endemic season suggests possible dengue infection. While malaria and enteric fever may have low white cell counts, leukopenia is more severe in dengue.

Blood levels of total protein and albumin are reduced, more marked in patients with shock. Levels of transaminases are raised; higher increase in SGOT than SGPT suggests dengue rather than other virus infection.

Patients with severe dengue may show hyponatremia and acidosis, with increase in urea and creatinine. X-ray chest or ultrasound examination may show varying degrees of pleural effusion that is more common on the right, but occasionally bilateral. Ultrasound examination of abdomen may show ascites and enlarged gallbladder.

*Confirmation of diagnosis* of dengue is established by the following.

*Direct methods:* Virus isolation by culture; genome detection by PCR; NS1 antigen detection.

*Indirect methods:* IgM detection; IgG detection.

Virus isolation or detection by PCR requires the sample to be obtained within the first 5 days of fever, is technically demanding, not universally available and hence of limited practical use. NS1 antigen is a highly conserved glycoprotein of dengue virus and secreted during the initial phase of illness. It disappears as antibodies appear and hence declines as illness advances and in secondary dengue infections. The specificity is ~100% and sensitivity in the first 4 days of illness is 90% in primary dengue and 70% in secondary dengue infection.

Antibody determination needs careful interpretation. Following primary dengue infection, 80% patients show detectable IgM antibodies by day 5, 99% by day 10 that peak by day 14 and are undetectable by 2–3 months. IgG antibodies rise later, peak to levels lower than IgM, decline slowly and remain detectable at low levels for life. Diagnosis of primary dengue infection is thus based on elevated IgM antibodies.

### Management

*Undifferentiated fever:* Patients have non-specific symptoms. Treatment consists of paracetamol for fever and regular monitoring for development of any complications.

*Dengue infection without warning signs:* Patients with fever, body ache, rashes or minor bleeding may be treated symptomatically. Fever and body ache are best treated with paracetamol. Salicylates and other non-steroidal, anti-inflammatory drugs should be avoided as these may predispose to mucosal bleeds. Child should be encouraged to drink plenty of fluids. In epidemic situations, the primary care physician or health worker should monitor for warning signs (see below) along with hematocrit (PCV) and platelet count, if possible.

*Dengue with warning signs:* Children with suspected dengue infection who have any of the following need hospitalization:

i. Abdominal pain or tenderness
ii. Persistent vomiting
iii. Clinical fluid accumulation
iv. Mucosal bleeding
v. Lethargy, restlessness
vi. Liver enlarged >2 cm
vi. Increase in PCV with concurrent or rapid decrease in platelet count.

These patients should be admitted in hospital and need intravenous fluids. Crystalloids are the preferred fluids.

In the hospital, all children without hypotension should be given Ringer lactate or normal saline infusion at a rate of 7 mL/kg over one hour. After one hour, if PCV has decreased and vital parameters are improving; fluid infusion rate should be decreased to 5 mL/kg over next hour and to 3 mL/kg/hour for 24–48 hours with frequent monitoring of PCV and vital parameters. When the patient is stable as indicated by normal blood pressure, good oral intake and urine output, the child can be discharged (Fig. 11.16).

If at 1 hour, the PCV is rising and vital parameters do not show improvement, the infusion rate is increased to 10 mL/kg over next hour. In case of no improvement, fluid infusion rate may further be increased to 15 mL/kg in the 3rd hour. If no improvement is observed in vital parameters and PCV at end of 3 hours, colloids are given at 10 mL/kg. Once PCV and vital parameters are stable, the infusion rate is gradually reduced and stopped over 24–48 hours.

*Severe dengue:* Children having any of the following:

i. Severe plasma leakage leading to shock or fluid accumulation with respiratory distress
ii. Severe bleeding
iii. Severe organ involvement: high AST, ALT >1000 U/L, impaired consciousness or involvement of heart and other organs.

Children classified as severe dengue should be hospitalized (preferably in intensive care) and treated with normal saline or Ringer lactate; 10–20 mL/kg is infused over 1 hour or as bolus, if blood pressure is unrecordable (earlier known as dengue shock syndrome, DSS IV). In critically sick children, it is preferable to establish two IV lines, one for administration of normal saline and other for infusing 5% dextrose and potassium. If there is no improvement in vital parameters and PCV is rising, colloids 10 mL/kg are given rapidly. If PCV is falling without improvement in vital parameters, blood transfusion is recommended (Fig. 11.17). Once improvement begins, fluid infusion rate is gradually decreased.

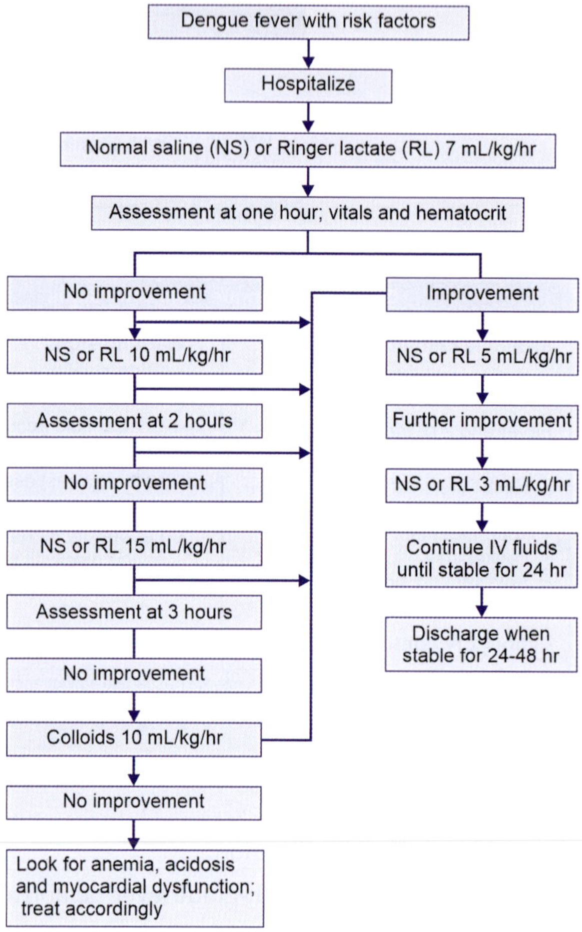

**Fig. 11.16:** Management of dengue fever with risk factors

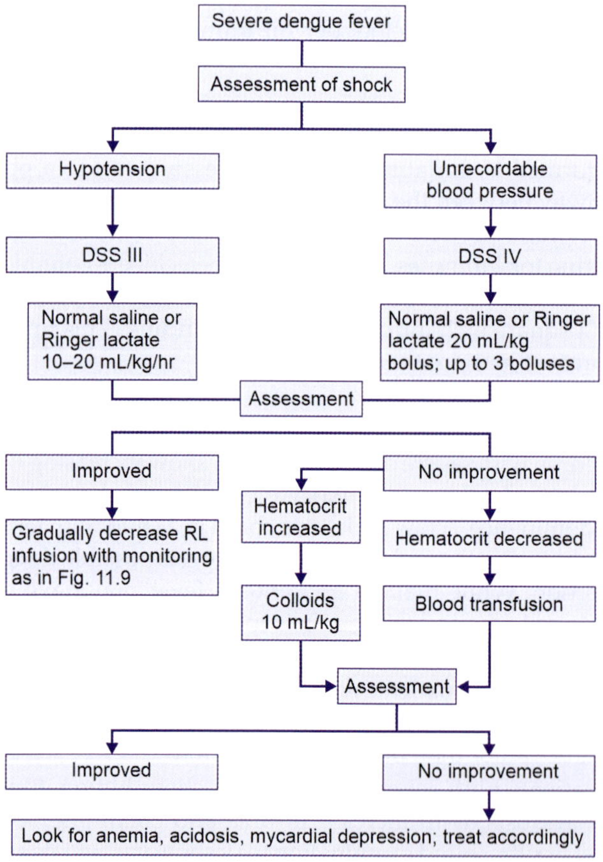

**Fig. 11.17:** Management of severe dengue fever

In addition to fluid management, oxygen should be administered to all patients with shock.

#### Management of Bleeding

***Petechial spots or mild mucosal bleed, hemodynamically stable:*** Such patients need supportive care including bed rest, maintenance of hydration and monitoring. There is no role for use of prophylactic platelet-rich plasma even with severe thrombocytopenia. Procedures predisposing to mucosal trauma and IM injections are avoided.

***Severe bleeding and hemodynamic instability, excessive mucosal bleed:*** These patients are treated with blood transfusions and monitoring. There is little evidence to support use of platelet concentrates and/or fresh-frozen plasma for severe bleeding. When massive bleeding cannot be managed with fresh whole blood/fresh-packed cells and there is possibility of DIC, combination of fresh frozen plasma and platelet concentrates should be considered.

#### Management of Fluid Overload

Stable hemodynamic status and out of critical phase (>24–48 hours of defervescence): Intravenous fluids are discontinued, but close monitoring should continue. Oral frusemide 0.1–0.5 mg/kg/dose once or twice daily or continuous infusion of furosemide 0.1 mg/kg/hour may be administered judiciously.

***Stable hemodynamic status but still within critical phase:*** The IV fluids are reduced. Diuretics are, however, avoided, to prevent intravascular volume depletion. Patients with fluid overload, shock and low PCV may have occult hemorrhage should receive careful fresh whole blood transfusion. Patients in shock and high PCV should receive repeated small boluses of colloids.

***Other supportive care:*** Organ dysfunction (liver, kidney) should be managed using standard guidelines. There is no role of therapy with corticosteroids, intravenous immunoglobulins or activated factor VII. Broad-spectrum antibiotics are indicated in case of superadded bacterial infection. Blood transfusion (20 mL/kg) is indicated when shock persists despite declining PCV (which indicates adequate fluid replacement). All children with hypotension should receive oxygen inhalation by nasal cannula/face mask or oxygen hood.

#### Monitoring

Monitoring of the patient is crucial in the first few hours of illness. Heart rate, respiratory rate, blood pressure and pulse pressure are monitored every 30 minutes till the patient is stable, then every 2–4 hours as long as the child is in the hospital. Critically ill children should preferably be monitored in ICU; central venous pressure and accurate urine output with an indwelling urinary catheter should be monitored. Absolute platelet counts should be checked once a day till there is a rising trend.

#### Prognosis

Dengue fever is a self-limited disease but mortality in severe dengue may be as high as 20%, if untreated. Early recognition of illness, careful monitoring and appropriate fluid therapy has resulted in considerable reduction of case fatality rate to <1%. Early recognition of shock is of paramount importance as the outcome of a patient with DSS depends on the duration of shock. If shock is identified when pulse pressure starts getting narrow and IV fluids are administered at this stage, the outcome is excellent.

#### Prevention

Preventive measures are directed towards elimination of adult mosquitoes and their larvae. During epidemics, aerial spraying/fogging with malathion is recommended for adult mosquitoes. Larval control measures by source reduction and use of larvicides are even more crucial. Mesocyclops and the shellfish are credited to eat and effectively eliminate larvae of *Aedes*. The strategy has been used with success by Australian scientists working in Vietnam by growing shellfish in ponds and water traps. *A. aegypti* breed in and around human dwellings and flourish in fresh water. Special drives must be launched during and soon after the rainy season to interrupt their breeding. There should be no stagnation of water in the bathroom, kitchen, terrace, lawn and other open places; stored water should be covered. Cooperation from every house owner, public establishment and the government and its employees is crucial for the success of control program. A live-attenuated quadruple vaccine has been approved for use in some countries between 9 and 45 years of age.

### Suggested Reading


1. National guidelines dengue case management during COVID-19 Pandemic. Government of India, 2020. nvbdcp.gov.in
2. Lodha R, Kabra SK. Dengue infection: Challenges and way forward. Indian J Pediatr 2015; 82:1077–79.
3. Royal College Physician of Thailand. Practical guideline for management of Dengue in adults. Southeast Asian J Trop Med Public Health 2015;46 Suppl 1:169–85.
4. World Health Organization (2009). Dengue guidelines for diagnosis, treatment, prevention and control. WHO; ISBN: 9789241547871.


## HIV Infection, Acquired Immunodeficiency Syndrome

HIV infection has become an important contributor to childhood morbidity and mortality, especially in developing countries and has undone many of the major gains in child health.

#### Epidemiology

It is estimated that in 2020, nearly 38 million persons worldwide were living with HIV infection; 2.78 million of these were children under 20 years of age. In 2020 alone, 680,000 people were estimated to have died due to AIDS, including 120,000 children. In 2020, an estimated 310,000 children were newly infected with HIV. More than 90% of HIV-infected individuals live in developing nations. Sub-Saharan Africa accounts for nearly 68% of the world's total population of HIV-infected children. India and Thailand dominate the epidemic in Southeast Asia, with more recent expansion into Vietnam, China, and Cambodia.

There has been considerable progress in improving access to antiretroviral therapy. Without access to such therapy, 20% of vertically infected children will progress to AIDS or death in their first year of life and more than half of HIV-infected children will die before their fifth birthday.

### HIV-1, HIV-2

HIV-1 and HIV-2 are members of the Retroviridae family and belong to the Lentivirus genus. The HIV-1 genome is single-stranded RNA that is 9.2 kb in size. The genome has three major sections: The gag region, which encodes the viral core proteins (p24, p17, p9, p6; these are derived from the precursor p55), the pol region, which encodes the viral enzymes (reverse transcriptase [p51], protease [p10], and integrase [p32]); and the env region, which encodes the viral envelope proteins (gp120 and gp41). The major external viral protein of HIV-1 is a heavily glycosylated gp120 protein which contains the binding site for the CD4 molecule, the most common T lymphocyte surface receptor for HIV.

Following viral attachment, gp120 and the CD4 molecules undergo conformational changes, allowing gp41 to interact with the fusion receptor on the cell surface. Viral fusion with the cell membrane allows entry of viral RNA into the cell cytoplasm. Viral DNA copies are then transcribed from the virion RNA through viral reverse transcriptase enzyme activity, and duplication of the DNA copies produces double-stranded circular DNA. Because the HIV-1 reverse transcriptase is error-prone, many mutations arise, creating wide genetic variation in HIV-1 isolates even within an individual patient. The circular DNA is transported into the cell nucleus where it is integrated into chromosomal DNA; this is called the provirus. The provirus can remain dormant for extended periods. HIV-1 transcription is followed by translation. A capsid polyprotein is cleaved to produce, among other products, the virus-specific protease (p10). This enzyme is critical for HIV-1 assembly. The RNA genome is then incorporated into the newly formed viral capsid. As the new virus is formed, it buds through the cell membrane and is released.

HIV-2 is a rare cause of infection in children, more prevalent in western and southern Africa. If HIV-2 is suspected, a specific test that detects antibody to HIV-2 peptides should be used.

### Transmission

Transmission of HIV-1 occurs via sexual contact, parenteral exposure to blood, or vertical transmission from mother to child. The primary route of infection in the pediatric population is vertical transmission. Most large studies in the United States and Europe have documented mother-to-child transmission rates in untreated women between 12 and 30%; in contrast, transmission rates in Africa and Asia are higher, up to 50%.

Vertical transmission of HIV can occur during the intrauterine or intrapartum periods, or through breastfeeding. Up to 30% of infected newborns are infected *in utero*. The highest percentages of HIV-infected children acquire the virus intrapartum. Breastfeeding is an important route of transmission, especially in the developing countries. The risk factors for vertical transmission include preterm delivery (<34 weeks gestation), a low maternal antenatal CD4 count, use of illicit drugs during pregnancy, >4 hours duration of ruptured membranes and birth weight <2500 g.

Transfusions of infected blood or blood products have accounted for a proportion of pediatric AIDS cases. Heat treatment of factor VIII concentrate and HIV antibody screening of donors have virtually eliminated HIV transmission to children with hemophilia. Blood donor screening has dramatically reduced, but not eliminated, the risk of transfusion-associated HIV infection. Sexual contact is a major route of transmission in adolescents.

### Natural History

Before highly active antiretroviral therapy (HAART) was available, three distinct patterns of disease were described in children. Approximately 10–20% of HIV-infected newborns in developed countries presented with a rapid disease course, with onset of AIDS and symptoms during the first few months of life; if untreated, these patients died from complications by 4 years of age. In resource-poor countries, >85% of the HIV-infected newborns may have such a rapidly progressing disease.

It has been suggested that if intrauterine infection coincides with the period of rapid expansion of CD4 cells in the fetus, it could effectively infect the majority of the body's immunocompetent cells. Most children in this group have a positive HIV-1 culture and/or detectable virus in the plasma in the first 48 hours of life. This early evidence of viral presence suggests that the newborn was infected *in utero*. In contrast to the viral load in adults, the viral load in infants stays high for at least the first 2 years of life.

Majority of perinatally infected newborns (60–80%) present with the second pattern: Slower progression of disease with a median survival of 6 years. Many patients in this group have a negative viral culture or PCR in the first week of life and are, therefore, considered to be infected intrapartum. In a typical patient, the viral load rapidly increases by 2–3 months of age, and then slowly over 24 months. The third pattern (i.e. long-term survivors) occurs in a small percentage (<5%) of perinatally infected children who have minimal or no progression of disease with relatively normal CD4 counts and very low viral loads for longer than 8 years.

HIV-infected children have changes in the immune system that are similar to those in HIV-infected adults. CD4 cell depletion may be less dramatic because infants normally have a relative lymphocytosis. Therefore, a value of 1500 CD4 cells/$mm^3$ in children <1 year of age is indicative of severe CD4 depletion and is comparable to <200 CD4 cells/$mm^3$ in adults. Lymphopenia is relatively rare in perinatally infected children and is usually only seen in older children or those with end-stage disease.

B cell activation occurs in most children, as evidenced by hypergammaglobulinemia with high levels of anti-HIV-1 antibody. This response may reflect both dysregulation of T cell suppression of B cell antibody synthesis and active CD4 enhancement of B lymphocyte humoral responses.

CD4 depletion and inadequate antibody responses lead to increased susceptibility to various infections and clinical features vary with the severity of immunodeficiency.

### Clinical Features

The clinical manifestations of HIV infection vary widely among infants, children and adolescents. In most infants, physical examination at birth is normal. Initial signs and symptoms may be subtle and non-specific, such as lymphadenopathy, hepatosplenomegaly, failure to thrive, chronic or recurrent diarrhea, interstitial pneumonia or oral thrush and may be distinguishable from other causes only by their persistence. While systemic and pulmonary findings are common in the United States and Europe, chronic diarrhea, wasting, and severe malnutrition predominate in Africa. Symptoms more common in children than adults include recurrent bacterial infections, chronic parotid swelling, lymphocytic interstitial pneumonitis (LIP), and early onset of progressive neurologic deterioration.

Pediatric HIV disease is staged using two parameters: Clinical status (Table 11.6) and degree of immunologic impairment (Table 11.7). However, the classification of the degree of immunologic impairment is less relevant now with expansion of indication of initiation of antiretroviral therapy for all HIV-infected children.

### Opportunistic Infections

Children with HIV infection and advanced or severe immunosuppression are susceptible to develop various opportunistic infections. The important pathogens include: *Pneumocystis jirovecii*, *Cryptosporidium*, *Cryptococcus*, *Isospora* and CMV.

### Respiratory Diseases Complicating HIV Infection

*P. jirovecii* (previously *P. carinii*) pneumonia is the opportunistic infection that led to the initial description of AIDS. This is one of the commonest AIDS defining illnesses in children in the US and Europe; most cases occur between 3rd and 6th months of life. Even if a child develops the illness while on prophylaxis, therapy may be started with cotrimoxazole. With the use of appropriate therapy, the mortality decreases to less than 10%. Risk factors for mortality are severity of the episode and severity of the immunosuppression.

***Recurrent bacterial pneumonia*** may be present in up to 90% HIV-infected children. Initial episodes often occur before the development of significant immunosuppression. As the immunosuppression increases, the frequency increases. The common pathogens for community-acquired pneumonia are *S. pneumoniae*, *H. influenzae* and *S. aureus*. In children with severe immunosuppression and hospital-acquired infections, gram-negative organisms, such as *Pseudomonas aeruginosa*, gain importance. Clinical features in HIV-infected children are similar to those in other children. However, in severely immunocompromised children, the signs may be subtle. Often, the response to therapy is slow and the relapse rates are high. Bacteremia may be more common, seen in up to 50%.

Choice of antibiotics is based on local patterns of etiologies and susceptibilities. An appropriate choice

**Table 11.6:** WHO clinical staging of HIV/AIDS for children with confirmed HIV infection

**Clinical stage 1**
- Asymptomatic
- Persistent generalized lymphadenopathy

**Clinical stage 2**
- Unexplained[a] persistent hepatosplenomegaly
- Papular pruritic eruptions
- Fungal nail infection
- Angular cheilitis
- Lineal gingival erythema
- Extensive wart virus infection
- Extensive molluscum contagiosum
- Recurrent oral ulceration
- Unexplained[a] persistent parotid enlargement
- Herpes zoster
- Recurrent or chronic upper respiratory tract infections (otitis media, otorrhea, sinusitis, tonsillitis)

**Clinical stage 3**
- Unexplained[a] moderate malnutrition or wasting not adequately responding to standard therapy
- Unexplained[a] persistent diarrhea (14 days or more)
- Unexplained[a] persistent fever (above 37.5°C intermittent or constant, for longer than one month)
- Persistent oral candidiasis (after the first 6–8 weeks of life)
- Oral hairy leukoplakia
- Acute necrotizing ulcerative gingivitis/periodontitis
- Lymph node TB
- Pulmonary TB
- Severe recurrent bacterial pneumonia
- Symptomatic lymphoid interstitial pneumonitis
- Chronic HIV-associated lung disease including bronchiectasis
- Unexplained anemia (<8 g/dL), neutropenia (<$0.5 \times 10^9$/L) or chronic thrombocytopenia (<$50 \times 10^9$/L)

**Clinical stage 4[b]**
- Unexplained severe wasting, stunting or severe malnutrition not responding to standard therapy
- Pneumocystis pneumonia
- Recurrent severe bacterial infections (empyema, pyomyositis, bone, joint infection, meningitis; excluding pneumonia)
- Chronic herpes simplex infection (orolabial or cutaneous for >1 month duration; visceral at any site)
- Esophageal candidiasis (or candidiasis of trachea, bronchi or lungs)
- Extrapulmonary/disseminated TB
- Kaposi sarcoma
- Cytomegalovirus infection (retinitis or CMV infection affecting another organ, with onset at age >1 month)
- Central nervous system toxoplasmosis (after one month of life)
- Extrapulmonary cryptococcosis (including meningitis)
- HIV encephalopathy
- Disseminated endemic mycosis (extrapulmonary histoplasmosis, coccidioidomycosis)
- Disseminated non-tuberculous mycobacterial infection
- Chronic cryptosporidiosis (with diarrhea)
- Chronic isosporiasis
- Cerebral or B cell non-Hodgkin lymphoma
- Progressive multifocal leukoencephalopathy
- Symptomatic HIV (associated nephropathy or cardiomyopathy)

[a]Unexplained refers to where the condition is not explained by other causes
[b]Additional specific conditions may be included in the regional classifications (e.g. reactivation of American trypanosomiasis, meningoencephalitis and/or myocarditis in Americas region, penicilliosis in Asia and HIV-associated rectovaginal fistula in Africa)

**Table 11.7:** Classification of immune suppression in children (CD4 levels in relation to severity of immune suppression)

| *HIV-associated immunodeficiency* | *Age-related CD4 cell values* | | | |
|---|---|---|---|---|
| | *<11 months* | *12–35 months* | *36–59 months* | *≥5 years* |
| Not significant (normal CD4 cells) | >35% | >30% | >25% | >500 cells/mm$^3$ |
| Mild | 30–35% | 25–30% | 20–25% | 350–499 cells/mm$^3$ |
| Advanced | 25–30% | 20–25% | 15–20% | 200–349 cells/mm$^3$ |
| Severe | <25% | <20% | <15% | <15% |
| | <1500 cells/mm$^3$ | <750 cells/mm$^3$ | <350 cells/mm$^3$ | 200 cells/mm$^3$ |

is the combination of a broad-spectrum cephalosporin and an aminoglycoside. In areas with large proportion of MRSA, vancomycin, clindamycin, linezolid or other drugs may be used. Children with non-severe pneumonia can be managed as out-patients using a second or a third generation cephalosporin or coamoxiclav. Since *P. jirovecii* pneumonia cannot be excluded in most children with severe respiratory symptoms, cotrimoxazole is also used unless another diagnosis has been made.

***Tuberculosis*** is a common medical concern. Co-existent TB and HIV infections accelerate the progression of both diseases. HIV-infected children are more likely to have extrapulmonary and disseminated tuberculosis; the course is also likely to be more rapid. The overall risk of active TB in children infected with HIV is at least 5- to 10-fold higher than in children not infected with HIV. The duration of antitubercular therapy in patients is same as that for not-HIV infected; a few children may need prolongation of treatment to 9–12 months. Close follow-up is essential to diagnose non-response or drug resistance. Rifampicin may show drug interactions with some antiretroviral agents (nevirapine, protease inhibitors).

***Viral infections,*** chiefly respiratory syncytial virus, influenza and parainfluenza viruses, often result in symptomatic disease. Infections with adenovirus and measles virus might result in serious sequelae. Disseminated CMV is a known opportunistic infection, but pneumonia caused by the virus is rare.

***Fungal infections*** present as a part of disseminated disease in immunocompromised children. Primary pulmonary fungal infections are uncommon.

***Lymphoid interstitial pneumonitis (LIP)*** has been recognized as a distinctive marker for pediatric HIV infection and is considered in the criteria for AIDS in children. In absence of antiretroviral therapy, nearly 20% of HIV-infected children developed LIP. The etiology and pathogenesis of LIP are not well understood, but include: Exaggerated immune response to inhaled or circulating antigens, and/or primary infection of the lung with HIV, Epstein-Barr virus (EBV), or both. LIP is characterized by nodule formation and diffuse infiltration of the alveolar septa by lymphocytes, plasmacytoid lymphocytes, plasma cells and immunoblasts. There is no involvement of the blood vessels or destruction of the lung tissue. Children with LIP have a relatively good prognosis.

LIP is usually diagnosed in children with perinatally acquired HIV infection when they are older than 1 year of age. Most children with LIP are asymptomatic. Children with severe disease show tachypnea, cough, wheezing and hypoxemia; crepitations are uncommon. Clubbing is present in advanced disease. These patients can progress to chronic respiratory failure. Long-standing LIP may be associated with bronchiectasis. The presence of a reticulonodular pattern, with or without hilar lymphadenopathy, that persists on chest radiograph for 2 months or greater and that is unresponsive to antimicrobial therapy is considered presumptive evidence of LIP. A definitive diagnosis is made by histopathology. Early disease is managed conservatively. The effect of antiretroviral agents is limited. Steroids are indicated, if children with LIP have symptoms and signs of chronic pulmonary disease, clubbing and/or hypoxemia. Treatment includes an initial 4- to 12-week course of prednisolone (2 mg/kg/d) followed by tapering to low dose medication, using oxygen saturation and clinical state as guide to improvement.

### Gastrointestinal Diseases

Multiple microbes can cause gastrointestinal disease, including bacteria (*Salmonella*, *Campylobacter*, *Mycobacterium avium intracellulare* complex), protozoa (*Giardia, Isospora, Cryptosporidium*, microsporidia), viruses (CMV, HSV, rotavirus) and fungi (*Candida*). Protozoal infections are severe and can be protracted in children. Children with *Cryptosporidium* infestation can have severe diarrhea leading to hypovolemic shock. AIDS enteropathy, a syndrome of malabsorption with partial villous atrophy not associated with specific pathogens, is the result of direct HIV infection of the gut.

Chronic liver inflammation is relatively common in HIV-infected children. In some children, hepatitis caused by CMV, hepatitis B or C viruses, or MAC may lead to liver failure and portal hypertension. It is important to recognize that several of the antiretroviral drugs such as didanosine, and protease inhibitors may also cause reversible elevation of transaminases.

Pancreatitis is uncommon in HIV-infected children. This may be the result of drug therapy, e.g. didanosine, lamivudine, nevirapine, or pentamidine. Rarely, opportunistic infections, such as MAC or CMV, may be responsible for acute pancreatitis.

### Neurologic Diseases

The incidence of central nervous system (CNS) involvement in perinatally infected children may be more than 50% in developing countries but lower in developed countries, with a median onset at about 1½ years of age. The most common presentation is progressive encephalopathy with loss or plateau of developmental milestones, cognitive deterioration, impaired brain growth resulting in acquired microcephaly, and symmetric motor dysfunction. CNS infections: Meningitis due to bacterial pathogens, fungi such as *Cryptococcus* and a number of viruses may be responsible for the clinical features. CNS toxoplasmosis is exceedingly rare in young infants, but may occur in HIV-infected adolescents; the overwhelming majority have serum IgG antitoxoplasma antibodies.

#### *Cardiovascular Involvement*

Cardiac abnormalities in HIV-infected children are common, persistent, and often progressive; the majority is subclinical. Left ventricular structure and function progressively may deteriorate in the first 3 years of life, resulting in subsequent persistent cardiac dysfunction and increased left ventricular mass. Children with encephalopathy or other AIDS-defining conditions have the highest rate of adverse cardiac outcomes. Resting sinus tachycardia has been reported in up to nearly two-thirds and marked sinus arrhythmia in one-fifth of HIV-infected children. Gallop rhythm with tachypnea and hepatosplenomegaly appear to be the best clinical indicators of congestive heart failure; anticongestive therapy is generally very effective, especially when initiated early.

#### *Renal Involvement*

Nephropathy is an unusual presenting symptom of HIV infection, more commonly occurring in older symptomatic children. Nephrotic syndrome is the most common manifestation; polyuria, oliguria, and hematuria have also been observed. Hypertension is unusual.

#### *Diagnosis*

All infants born to HIV-infected mothers test antibody-positive at birth because of passive transfer of maternal HIV antibody across the placenta. Most uninfected infants lose maternal antibody between 6 and 12 months of age. As a small proportion of uninfected infants continue to have maternal HIV antibody in the blood up to 18 months of age, positive IgG antibody tests cannot be used to make a diagnosis of HIV infection in infants up to this age. In children >18 months old, demonstration of IgG antibody to HIV by a two or three reactive enzyme immunoassay (EIA) can establish the diagnosis of HIV infection.

Specific diagnostic assays, such as HIV proviral DNA or RNA PCR, HIV culture, or HIV p24 antigen, are useful for diagnosis of young infants born to HIV-infected mothers. By 6 months of age, the HIV culture and/or PCR identifies all infected infants, who are not having continued exposure due to breastfeeding. HIV RNA PCR is the preferred virological assay in developed countries. HIV culture has similar sensitivity to HIV RNA PCR; however, it is more technically complex and expensive, and results are often not available for 2–4 weeks; the test is not routinely available. The p24 antigen assay is less sensitive than the other virological tests. Figure 11.18 shows the algorithm for diagnosis of HIV infection in infants. The national program (Early Infant Diagnosis) now uses HIV total nucleic acid

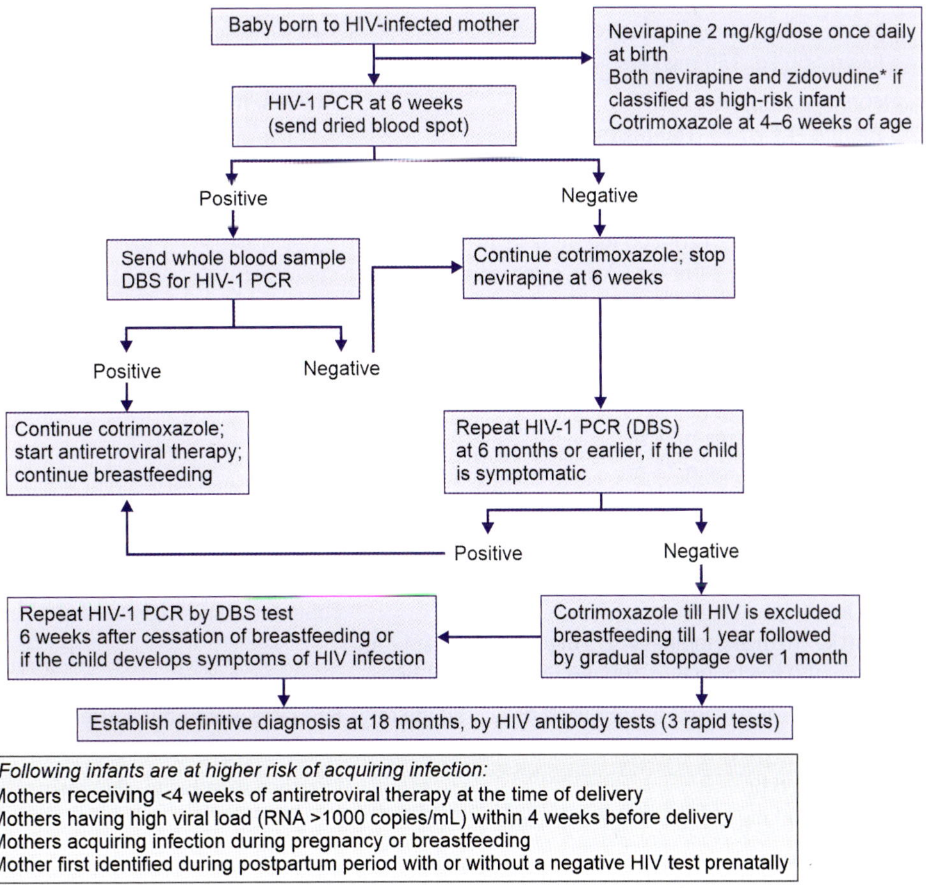


**Fig. 11.18:** HIV diagnosis in children <18 months with HIV-total nucleic acid-PCR. DBS dried blood spot

(RNA + proviral DNA) PCR test on dried blood spot samples; positive tests need confirmation with HIV PCR test on another sample.

### Management

The management of HIV-infected child includes antiretroviral therapy, prophylaxis and treatment of opportunistic and common infections, adequate nutrition and immunization. Decisions about antiretroviral therapy (ART) for HIV-infected patients were earlier based on the magnitude of viral replication (i.e. viral load), CD4 lymphocyte count or percentage and clinical condition. The current World Health Organization and the Indian guidelines recommend ART for all children irrespective of the immunologic or clinical stage.

Availability of antiretroviral therapy has transformed HIV infection from a uniformly fatal condition to a chronic infection, where children can lead a near normal life. Current therapy does not eradicate the virus and cure the child; it rather suppresses the virus replication for extended periods of time. The main groups of drugs are nucleoside reverse transcriptase inhibitors (NRTI), non-nucleoside reverse transcriptase inhibitors (NNRTI), protease inhibitors (PI), and integrase strand transfer inhibitors (Table 11.8). Highly active antiretroviral therapy (HAART) is a combination of 2 NRTI with a PI or an integrase strand transfer inhibitor or an NNRTI. The national program for management of HIV-infected children recommends combination of zidovudine or abacavir + lamivudine + PI/integrase inhibitor as first-line therapy (Table 11.9). Pediatric fixed dose combinations (FDC) have also been developed.

***Cotrimoxazole prophylaxis:*** In resource-limited settings, cotrimoxazole prophylaxis is recommended for all HIV-exposed infants starting at 4–6 weeks of age (or at first encounter with the health care system) and continued until HIV infection can be excluded. Cotrimoxazole is recommended for HIV-exposed breastfeeding children of all ages; prophylaxis should be continued until HIV infection is excluded by antibody testing (beyond 18 months of age) or virological testing (before 18 months of age), at least 6 weeks after cessation of breastfeeding. Infants documented to be living with HIV should receive cotrimoxazole prophylaxis regardless of symptoms or CD4 percentage. After one year of age, cotrimoxazole prophylaxis is given to symptomatic children (WHO clinical stages 2, 3 or 4 for HIV disease) or children with CD4 <25%. All children

**Table 11.8:** Commonly used antiretroviral drugs

| *Drug* | *Dose* | *Side effects* |
|---|---|---|
| **Nucleoside reverse transcriptase inhibitors** | | |
| Abacavir | 3 months–13 yr: 8 mg/kg/ dose q 12 hr<br>>13 yr: 300 mg/dose q12 hr (max: 300 mg/dose) | Hypersensitivity |
| Lamivudine (3TC) | 1 month–13 yr: 4 mg/kg q 12 hr<br>>13 yr; <50 kg: 4 mg/kg/dose q 12 hr<br>>13 yr; >50 kg: 150 mg/kg/dose q 12 hr | Pancreatitis, neuropathy, neutropenia |
| Zidovudine | Neonates: 2 mg/kg q 6 hr<br>3 months–13 yr: 90–180 mg/m² q 6–8 hr | Anemia, myopathy |
| **Non-nucleoside reverse transcriptase inhibitors** | | |
| Nevirapine (NVP) | 2 months–13 yr: 120 mg/m² (max: 200 mg) q 24 hr for 14 days; follow by 120–200 mg/m² q 12 hr<br>>13 yr: 200 mg q 24 hr for 14 days; increase to 200 mg q 12 hr, if no rash or other side effects | Skin rash, Steven Johnson syndrome |
| Efavirenz | >3 yr: 10–15 kg: 200 mg q 24 hr<br>15–20 kg: 250 mg q 24 hr<br>20–25 kg: 300 mg q 24 hr<br>25–32.5 kg: 350 mg q 24 hr<br>32.5–40 kg: 400 mg q 24 hr<br>>40 kg: 600 mg q 24 hr | Skin rash, CNS symptoms, increased transaminase levels |
| **Protease inhibitors** | | |
| Lopinavir/ ritonavir | 7–15 kg: 12 mg/kg lopinavir; 3 mg/kg ritonavir q 12 hr with food<br>15–40 kg: 10 mg/kg lopinavir; 2.5 mg/kg ritonavir q 12 hr<br>>12 yr: 400 mg lopinavir; 100 mg ritonavir q 12 hr | Diarrhea, fatigue, headache, nausea; increased cholesterol and triglycerides |
| Ritonavir | <13 yr: 350–400 mg/m² q 12 hr (start dose: 250 mg/m²)<br>>13 yr: 600 mg q 12 hr (start dose: 300 mg) | Bad taste, vomiting, nausea, diarrhea, rarely, hepatitis |
| Saquinavir | 50 mg/kg q 8 hr<br>>13 yr: 1200 mg q 8 hr soft gel capsules | Diarrhea, headache, skin rash |
| **Integrase strand transfer inhibitor** | | |
| Dolutegravir (DTG) | Age >6 yr and weight >20 kg: 50 mg once a day | Increased serum lipase, hyperglycemia, GI symptoms |

**Table 11.9:** First-line antiretroviral regimens for infants and children with HIV infection

| | *Regimen* |
|---|---|
| Age less than 6 years, and body weight less than 20 kg | Abacavir + Lamivudine + Lopinavir/ritonavir (AL+LPV/r) |
| Age between 6 and 10 years, and body weight between 20 kg and 30 kg | Abacavir + Lamivudine + Dolutegravir (ALD) |
| Age more than 10 years, and body weight more than 30 kg | Tenofovir + Lamivudine + Dolutegravir (TLD) |

Note:

- Any infant or child initiated on any regimen must be based on body weight; refer to NACO guidelines for weight-band dosage charts to determine the appropriate doses.
- On every visit, check body weight of the infant/child before writing the prescription. Even though the drug regimen remains the same, drug dosages have to be modified according to change in body weight.

*Source:* National AIDS Control Organization. National Guidelines for HIV Care and Treatment, 2021. New Delhi: NACO, Ministry of Health and Family Welfare, Government of India.

who begin cotrimoxazole prophylaxis (irrespective of age) should continue until the age of 5 years, when they can be reassessed.

*Isoniazid prophylaxis:* Current NACO guidelines recommend administration of isoniazid prophylaxis to all HIV-infected children who do not have evidence of active tuberculosis.

*Nutrition:* HIV-infected children often show failure to thrive and require nutritional rehabilitation.

*Immunization:* Vaccines recommended in the national schedule can be administered to HIV-infected children, except that symptomatic HIV-infected children should not be given OPV and BCG.

*Prevention of mother-to-child transmission (MTCT):* The risk of MTCT can be reduced to under 2% by interventions that include antiretroviral therapy given to women during pregnancy and labor and antiretroviral prophylaxis to the infant in the first week of life, obstetrical interventions including elective cesarean delivery (prior to the onset of labor and rupture of membranes), and complete avoidance of breastfeeding.

***Antiretroviral drug regimens for pregnant women:*** For all HIV infected pregnant women, antiretroviral therapy is indicated. The recommended regimen is a combination of Tenofovir + Lamivudine + Dolutegravir (TLD).

***Antiretroviral regimens for infants born to HIV-infected mothers:*** If mother received triple drug ART during pregnancy and entire breastfeeding, the infant should receive daily AZT or NVP from birth until 6 weeks of age (irrespective of feeding).

***Intrapartum interventions:*** Artificial rupture of membranes should be avoided, unless medically indicated. Delivery should be by elective cesarean section at 38 weeks before onset of labor and rupture of membranes. Procedures increasing exposure of child to maternal blood should be avoided.

***Breastfeeding:*** The risk of HIV infection via breastfeeding is highest in the early months of breastfeeding. Factors that increase likelihood of transmission include detectable levels of HIV in breast milk, presence of mastitis and low maternal CD4+ T cell count. Exclusive breastfeeding has been reported to carry a lower risk of HIV transmission than mixed feeding and risk of mortality in non-breastfed infants in resource-limited settings is increased. Currently, exclusive breastfeeding is recommended during the first months of life. WHO recommends that the transition between exclusive breastfeeding and early cessation of breastfeeding should be gradual and not an "early and abrupt cessation".

### Suggested Reading


1. National AIDS Control Organization. National Guidelines for HIV Care and Treatment, 2021. New Delhi: NACO, Ministry of Health and Family Welfare, Government of India. Available at: http://naco.gov.in/sites/default/files/National_Guidelines_for_HIV_Care_and_Treatment_2021.pdf
2. World Health Organization. Consolidated guidelines on HIV prevention, testing, treatment, service delivery and monitoring: recommendations for a public health approach. Geneva: World Health Organization; 2021.
3. WHO/UNAIDS. AIDS epidemic update Dec 2021.


## Influenza

The influenza virus is capable of causing disease in humans, birds and animals. Interestingly, the burden of influenza has reduced considerably during the COVID-19 pandemic.

### *Etiology and Epidemiology*

The influenza virus is an RNA virus of the Orthomyxoviridae family. Influenza A and B are the two types that cause human disease. Influenza A is further classified into subtypes based on the two surface proteins hemagglutinin (H) and neuraminidase (N). Influenza B is classified into two distinct lineages—Yamagata and Victoria, but not into subtypes. Influenza has a highly segmented genome that is prone to frequent mutations and reassortment. This leads to frequent antigenic "drifts" (seen in both A and B) when there is minor change in antigenicity, and "shifts" (seen only in A) where there is major change in antigenicity. These phenomena of antigenic change lead to evolution of new viruses with little population immunity, causing annual outbreaks and occasionally pandemics. The novel H1N1 pandemic of 2009 occurred due to emergence of a new swine origin influenza virus H1N1 which was pathogenic to humans and capable of rapid human-to-human transmission, and with no pre-existing immunity. It has been estimated that the novel H1N1 pandemic caused 18,000 deaths globally with case fatality rates ranging from 0.0004 to 1.5% (0.83% in India). Avian H5N1, commonly referred as bird flu, is a highly pathogenic strain of influenza virus that infects and kills humans in close contact with diseased birds but has not acquired pandemic potential due to limited human-to-human transmissibility.

Influenza is transmitted from person-to-person through airborne droplet spread or through contact. The portal of entry is the respiratory tract and the virus attaches itself to the respiratory epithelium through the hemagglutinin, which is the main virulence factor. The incubation period is 1–3 days and the period of infectivity is usually 7 days after illness onset and sometimes longer in those with severe disease. The attack rates are the highest in children and young adults. In temperate climates, there is a clear defined influenza season in fall and winters but in tropical countries like India, it occurs throughout the year with a peak during the monsoons.

### Clinical Features

In most individuals, influenza is a minor illness characterized by a combination of fever, runny nose, sore throat, cough, body ache, headache, abdominal pain, diarrhea and vomiting. The illness may have a biphasic course. Recovery usually occurs within a week. Asymptomatic and subclinical infections are also very common.

A small proportion of individuals (less than 1%) can have complications and severe disease. The risk of complications is higher at extremes of age (children below 2-yr and the elderly), pregnant women and those who have just delivered, those with underlying comorbidities such as any chronic neurologic, metabolic, cardiac, pulmonary or renal disease, those who are immunocompromised and those with severe asthma. In the novel H1N1 epidemic, morbid obesity was an important risk factor.

The most dreaded complication of influenza is pneumonia with acute respiratory distress syndrome, respiratory failure and sometimes shock and kidney failure.

Approximately 30% of these patients have bacterial coinfection with *S. pneumoniae* and *S. aureus*. Progression is very rapid and most patients require ventilator support over the next 24 hours. Occasionally other complications such as encephalitis, seizures, quadriparesis and myocarditis have been reported. Transplacental transmission to newborn and neonatal complications have also been reported. Complications usually set in by day 4 or 5 of illness. The red flag symptoms are persistent high fever of more than 3 days duration, reappearance of fever after initial defervescence, breathlessness, dyspnea, tachypnea, hemoptysis in older children and adolescents, extreme weakness, poor oral intake and altered sensorium.

### Diagnosis

Influenza is primarily a clinical diagnosis. Complete blood count may show leukopenia and thrombocytopenia; liver enzymes and CPK may be mildly elevated. Diagnosis is confirmed by antigen detection tests (sensitivity of 20%), or PCR on throat or nasopharyngeal swabs. PCR tests for influenza may be standalone, or as part of multiplex PCR panels. These tests are expensive and have a turnaround time varying from 2 to 24 hours. The sensitivity is around 70–80% and higher in lower respiratory secretions such as sputum and bronchoalveolar lavage.

Since the symptoms and lab findings of severe flu overlap those of other infections such as COVID-19, malaria, dengue, enteric fever, viral hepatitis and leptospirosis, it is important to conduct appropriate laboratory tests to exclude these illnesses.

### Treatment

Definitive treatment is with a neuraminidase inhibitor (oseltamivir, zanamivir, peramivir). These drugs reduce duration of symptoms, risk of complications, death and infectiousness. Though they are most effective, if given within the first 48 hours of illness, they should be given in severe illness even if the patient presents late. The therapeutic dose of oseltamivir is 30 mg twice daily in those with weight less than 15 kg, 45 mg twice daily for 15–24 kg, 60 mg twice daily for 25–34 kg, and 75 mg twice daily for those 35 kg and above. Oseltamivir, though formally not approved for infants, may be used at a dose of 2–3 mg/kg twice daily. The duration of therapy is 5 days. In patients with very severe disease, double the recommended dose for 10 days may be used. Oseltamivir is well tolerated with occasional GI and neurological side effects. Baloxavir is a novel anti-influenza drug recently approved in the USA.

For any patient presenting with influenza-like illness (ILI), the treatment strategy depends on two factors: The severity of illness and the likelihood of complications. In patients with mild disease who are not at risk for complications, only symptomatic treatment is indicated. Antibiotics and antivirals should not be prescribed. Patients should be counseled about the red flag signs and asked to seek medical care in the event these occur. These patients should be asked to stay at home till they are afebrile to prevent disease transmission to others.

Patients with ILI who are at high risk for complications should be started on antiviral therapy irrespective of the severity of disease.

For patients who present with symptoms of severe illness or who have complications, antiviral treatment with oseltamivir should be started without delay. An effort should be made to rule out other illnesses with similar symptomatology. In patients with signs of lower respiratory involvement, antibiotics like coamoxiclav or cephalosporins (cefuroxime, ceftriaxone) should also be used, if bacterial coinfections are suspected. Supportive and intensive care is as for pneumonia or ARDS.

### Prevention

Vaccination is the most effective preventive strategy and is discussed in Chapter 10.

Chemoprophylaxis with oseltamivir is also effective in preventing influenza. The dose is 30–75 mg of oseltamivir (as per weight) to be taken once daily for 10 days. Since chemoprophylaxis is associated with side effects and risk of development of drug resistance, it must be reserved only for very high-risk household contacts.

Household transmission can be reduced by good ventilation in the room, proper hand hygiene and adherence to cough etiquettes by the index case. Nosocomial transmission to other patients and health care workers is a concern. Vaccination for all health care workers and placing all patients with suspected ILI on droplet precautions is recommended.

School children show one of the highest infection rates and outbreaks are common in school. For reducing transmission in schools, the classrooms should be kept well ventilated, children should be trained in hand hygiene and cough etiquettes and sick children should be prohibited from attending school till they are afebrile. Temporary school closure may be considered during a massive pandemic.

### Suggested Reading


1. Committee on Infectious Disease. American Academy of Pediatrics. Recommendations for Prevention and Control of Influenza in Children 2021–22. Pediatrics 2021;148:e2021053744.
2. Dharmapalan D. Influenza. Indian J Pediatr. 2020; 87:828–32.
3. Writing Committee of the WHO Consultation on Clinical Aspects of Pandemic (H1N1) 2009 Influenza. Clinical aspects of pandemic 2009 influenza A (H1N1) virus infection. NEJM 2010; 362: 1708–19.


## Zika Virus

Zika is an RNA flavivirus closely related to the dengue and chikungunya viruses, which has recently assumed prominence due to its association with newborn microcephaly.

### Epidemiology

The virus was first identified in a rhesus monkey in the Zika forest of Uganda in 1947 with only 13 human cases diagnosed till 2007. Since then large outbreaks have happened in the Pacific islands of Micronesia, French Polynesia and New Caledonia. A very large outbreak was reported in Brazil in 2015 with almost a million cases. The virus has since spread worldwide including Asia. The WHO has declared it as a public health emergency of international concern. Cases of zika virus infection have also been reported sporadically from India.

The virus is transmitted primarily by the bite of *Aedes aegypti*. Other routes of transmission include vertical transmission from mother to child, sexual and possibly through blood transfusion.

### Clinical Features and Complications

Many infections are asymptomatic. Clinical disease is characterized by low grade fever with arthralgia, myalgia, rash, conjunctivitis and lymphadenopathy. Symptomatology resembles dengue and chikungunya except that rash and conjunctivitis is more prominent than the other two illnesses.

There are two major complications of zika infection. The first is acute neurologic syndromes such as Guillain-Barre syndrome, myelitis and meningoencephalitis. However, more important are the teratogenic effects. Infections in the first trimester and less commonly in the second trimester are associated with abortions, intrauterine deaths and stillbirths, microcephaly (13%) and ocular abnormalities.

### Diagnosis

Diagnosis in the first seven days is by performing a RT- PCR in blood and after seven days is by IgM antibody capture (MAC), ELISA. The ELISA can demonstrate cross-reactivity with the other flaviviruses.

### Treatment and Prevention

There is no specific treatment and care is symptomatic and supportive. Prevention revolves around avoiding travel to zika afflicted areas especially by pregnant women, vector control. Candidate vaccines are in development.

### Suggested Reading


1. Marban-Castro E, Gonce A, Fumado V, et al. Zika virus infection in preganant woman and their children. Gynecol Reprod Biol 2021;265:162–68.
2. Peterson, et al. Zika virus. NEJM 2016; 374:1552–63.


## Ebola Virus

The ebola virus is an RNA virus belonging to the family Filoviridae first described in 1976 near the Ebola river in the Democratic Republic of Congo. It causes hemorrhagic fever with very high mortality. Several outbreaks have been reported in Africa. The most recent outbreak in 2014 in West Africa caught international attention due to likelihood of spread to distant countries and nosocomial transmission.

### Epidemiology

The Old World fruit bat is the natural reservoir of ebola virus. Infection is transmitted to wild or farm animals (chimpanzees, pigs, monkeys) and humans through direct contact with bats or consumption of plants or their products contaminated with bat feces or body fluids. Humans can also be infected by direct contact with infected animals or handling or consuming meat of infected animals. Human-to-human transmission to family members, caretakers and health care workers can occur through close contact or handling the fluids of infected patients.

### Clinical Features

The incubation period varies from 2–21 days and initial symptoms are nonspecific and consist of fever, headache, weakness, nausea, vomiting, abdominal pain and joint and muscle aches. This is followed by bleeding from multiple sites and multiorgan failure. The average case fatality rate is 60%.

### Diagnosis and Treatment

Investigations show leukopenia and thrombocytopenia. Definitive diagnosis is by antigen detection, IgM ELISA, RT-PCR and viral isolation. Treatment is supportive and symptomatic. However, several novel therapies including serum of infected patients who have recovered from disease, and nucleic acid based therapies are under evaluation.

### Prevention

Prevention centers around strict isolation of infected cases, safe burial practices and avoidance of consumption of bush meat. Vaccines against ebola virus are now available and have been used to control the outbreaks in African nations.

### Suggested Reading

1. Malvy D, McElroy AK, de Clerck H, Günther S, van Griensven J. Ebola virus disease. Lancet 2019; 393:936–48.

## Emerging Viruses

This section deals briefly with some of the new emerging viral diseases seen in India.

### *Crimean Congo Hemorrhagic Fever Virus (CCHF)*

Crimean Congo hemorrhagic fever virus is an RNA virus of the Bunyaviridae family normally infecting cattle and occasionally transmitted to humans by infected ticks. The virus is highly contagious and human-to-human transmission in household and hospital setting is not uncommon. Outbreaks of CCHF have been reported from various countries including Pakistan. It was first reported from India in 2011 from Gujarat. The presentation is that of a viral hemorrhagic fever with fever, body pain, headache, profuse bleeding, leukopenia, thrombocytopenia, altered liver functions, deranged coagulation parameters, rhabdomyolysis and renal failure. The disease mimics dengue with salient differences being early and more rapid platelet fall and rhabdomyolysis. Diagnosis is by specific PCR. Treatment is supportive; early administration of ribavirin is beneficial. Strict isolation of affected patients is crucial to prevent nosocomial transmission.

### *Hantaviruses*

Hantaviruses, which are rodent borne causes two important clinical syndromes: Hemorrhagic fever and renal syndrome (HFRS) in Europe and Asia including India and hantavirus cardiopulmonary syndrome in America. Rodents are natural hosts and humans acquire infection by inhalation of aerosols contaminated by rodent excreta or saliva. In India, HFRS and asymptomatic hantavirus infection has been reported from Tamil Nadu. The disease presents as a febrile illness with body pain, headache, thrombocytopenia, elevated liver enzymes, bleeding and renal failure. Leukocytosis with shift to left differentiates it from dengue. Diagnosis is by specific IgM antibodies. Treatment includes ribavarin and supportive care.

### *Nipah Virus*

Nipah virus, a Hendra virus from the genus Henipavirus, is an important cause of encephalitis, has been reported from West Bengal, India. The latest outbreak was from Kerala in 2018 which caused 17 deaths. The natural asymptomatic hosts are fruit bats who can transmit infection and disease to pigs and humans. Human-to-human transmission is also reported. Clinical features in humans are fever followed by features of encephalitis and sometimes pneumonia and respiratory distress. Mortality can be as high as 70% and there are sequelae in survivors. Treatment is symptomatic; prevention centers around limiting human exposure to raw date palm juice contaminated by fruit bat excreta and infected pigs.

### *Chandipura Virus*

Chandipura virus, a rhabdovirus is implicated as a cause of epidemic viral encephalitis in children in several states in India. It is transmitted by bite of infected sandflies and is associated with high mortality and neurologic sequelae.

### Suggested Reading

1. Aditi, Shariff M. Nipah virus infection: A review. Epidemiol Infect. 2019;147:e95.
2. Chandy S, Abraham S, Sridharan G. Hantaviruses: An emerging public health threat in India? A review. J Biosci 2008;33: 495–504.
3. Mourya DT, Pragya YD, Patil DY, et al. Experience of ICMR with tick-borne zoonotic infection. Indian J Med Res 2021;153:339–47.
4. Sudeep AB, Gaurav YK, Bondre VP. Changing clinical scenario in Chandipura virus infection. Indian J Med Res 2016;143:712–21.

*Competencies:* **PE34.1; PE34.2; PE34.3; PE34.4; PE34.5; PE34.7; PE34.8; PE34.9; PE34.10; PE34.13**

# COMMON BACTERIAL INFECTIONS

## Tuberculosis

Tuberculosis, caused by *Mycobacterium tuberculosis*, killed nearly 1.4 million people in year 2019. More than 90% cases occur in the developing countries, where resources for optimal treatment are limited.

### *Magnitude*

Since most children acquire the organism from adults, the epidemiology of childhood tuberculosis follows that in adults. While the global burden of the illness is unclear, it is estimated that 10–12% cases occur in childhood. Tuberculosis infection and disease among children are much more prevalent in developing countries, where resources for control are scarce. It is estimated that in developing countries, the annual risk of tuberculosis infection in children is 2–5%. In India, childhood tuberculosis remains a significant problem, contributing to approximately 31% of the global burden. Over the last decade, consistently, children constitute 6–7% of all the patients treated under National Tuberculosis Elimination Program (NTEP) annually, pointing to a gap of 4–5% in total notification against the estimated incidence.

The estimated lifetime risk of developing tuberculosis for a young child infected with *M. tuberculosis*, as indicated by positive tuberculin test, is about 10%. About 5% of those infected are likely to develop disease in the first year after infection and the remaining 5% later. These rates increase about sixfold in HIV-infected individuals.

Reasons for an increase in childhood tuberculosis include inadequate facilities for diagnosis, prevention and therapy, the HIV pandemic, and emergence of drug resistance. Due to improved standards of living, the incidence of tuberculosis has declined in affluent and highly developed countries. However, it continues to be a public health problem in underprivileged countries of Asia, Africa and South America.

### Epidemiology

*Agent:* All patients of pulmonary tuberculosis and most cases of extrapulmonary disease are caused by human type strain of *M. tuberculosis*. A few cases of extrapulmonary illness particularly the tubercular lymphadenitis may be due to the bovine strain.

*Reservoir of infection:* Infection is spread by patients suffering from pulmonary tuberculosis, who discharge tubercle bacilli in sputum or nasopharyngeal secretions during bouts of coughing or sneezing. Such patients are called open or infective cases. In children, a few infections may occur transplacentally (congenital tuberculosis).

*Mode of infection:* The usual mode of infection is through inhalation of droplets of infected secretions. Infected sputum from open cases of tuberculosis dries up, and tubercle bacilli are resuspended in dust and air that might be inhaled. Infection through ingestion of infected material is rare. Rarely infection is transmitted through skin, mucous membrane or transplacentally.

### Host Factors

No age is exempt from tuberculosis. Tubercle bacilli are not transferred across the healthy placenta but the fetus may be infected from an infected placenta. The frequency of infection increases with age. An infant is more likely to develop disease after an infection compared to an older child.

Adolescents, especially girls, are prone to develop active tuberculosis disease during puberty. Undernourished children are more susceptible to develop tuberculosis, probably due to depressed immune defense. Tuberculosis may precipitate severe malnutrition in infants with undernutrition. A malnourished patient who does not respond to dietary therapy should be investigated for tuberculosis.

Children with primary or secondary immune deficiencies develop disseminated disease. Illnesses that affect cell-mediated immunity (including measles) increase the susceptibility of disease. The risk of infection is associated with the extent of contact and burden of organisms in the sputum. Patients with smear positive pulmonary tuberculosis are more likely to transmit infection. An increased risk of infection is seen in institutional settings (nursing homes, correctional centers and homeless shelters).

### Pathology

The inhaled tubercle bacilli lodge in pulmonary alveoli and cause inflammation with hyperemia and congestion. Initially, polymorphonuclear leukocytes infiltrate the site, but their phagocytic ability is low and they are soon eliminated. The further course depends on the immune response of the host. If host resistance is good, the inflammatory exudate around the primary focus is absorbed and the caseous area inspissated. Healing occurs by fibrosis and calcification. When the cell-mediated immune response is weak, the bacilli continue to multiply and the inflammatory process extends to the contiguous areas.

Progressive primary disease (PPD) is a serious complication of the pulmonary primary complex (PPC) in which the PPC, instead of resolving/calcifying, enlarges steadily and develops a large caseous center. The center liquefies and may empty into an adjacent bronchus leading to formation of a cavity, which characteristically is associated with a large number of tubercle bacilli. Next, the bacilli may spread to other parts of the lobe or the entire lung, resulting in lobar consolidation or bronchopneumonia. The enlarged lymph nodes may compress the neighboring airway. Ball-valve effect due to incomplete obstruction may lead to trapping of air distal to obstruction (emphysema). Enlarged paratracheal nodes may cause stridor and respiratory distress, and subcarinal nodes impinge on the esophagus and cause dysphagia. If obstruction of the bronchus is complete, atelectasis may occur. The whole spectrum is labelled as progressive primary disease.

*Outcome of bronchial obstruction*

i. Complete expansion and resolution of chest X-ray findings
ii. Disappearance of the segmental lesions
iii. Scarring and progressive compression of the lobe or segment leading to bronchiectasis

A caseated lymph node may erode through the wall of the bronchus, leading to tuberculous bronchitis or endobronchial tuberculosis. Fibrosis and bronchiectatic changes may supervene. Discharge of bacteria into the lumen may lead to their bronchial dissemination.

Hematogenous dissemination from infected lymph nodes occurs early in course, resulting in foci of infection in various organs (e.g. Simon focus in apex of the lungs). If the host immunity is good, these foci are contained and disease does not occur. Lowered host immunity, as in infants, severely malnourished children, and immunodeficiency may lead to activation of these metastatic foci and occurrence of disease. Massive hematogenous seeding with *M. tuberculosis*, usually within 3–6 months after initial infection, leads to miliary tuberculosis where all lesions are of similar size.

Pulmonary tuberculosis resulting from endogenous reactivation of foci of infection is uncommon in children; but may be seen in adolescents. The commonest site for this type of disease is the apex of the lung (Puhl lesion), because blood flow is sluggish at apex. Regional lymph nodes are usually not involved. Miliary and meningeal tuberculosis usually occur within 1 year of the primary lesion.

### Clinical Features

The incubation period varies between 4 and 8 weeks. The onset of symptoms is insidious, but may be acute in miliary tuberculosis. Primary infection usually passes off unrecognized. Asymptomatic infection is defined as infection associated with tuberculin hypersensitivity and a positive tuberculin test, without significant clinical or radiological findings.

Symptoms in children with PPC include mild fever, anorexia and weight loss; occasionally PPC are detected during evaluation of intercurrent infection. Cough is inconsistent and may be absent even in advanced disease. Irritating dry cough can be a symptom of bronchial and tracheal compression due to enlarged lymph nodes. Lymph nodes may continue to enlarge even after resolution of parenchymal infiltrates, and lead to compression of neighboring bronchi.

Children with PPD present with high-grade fever and cough. Expectoration of sputum and hemoptysis are associated with advanced disease and development of cavity or ulceration of bronchi. Cavitating pulmonary tuberculosis is uncommon in childhood. Children with endobronchial tuberculosis usually present with fever, troublesome cough (with or without expectoration). Dyspnea, wheezing and cyanosis may be present. Partial compression of the airway can lead to emphysema; features of collapse are seen with large airway compression.

Miliary tuberculosis, characterized by hematogenous spread and multiple systemic foci, is common in infants and young children. The onset of illness is sudden and clinical features depend on the number of disseminated organisms and involved organs. Unlike other forms of tuberculosis, the child shows high-grade fever; dyspnea, cyanosis and altered sensorium. There are hardly any pulmonary findings, but fine crepitations and rhonchi may be present. Patients often show lymphadenopathy and hepatosplenomegaly. Choroid tubercles may be seen in ~50% and meningitis in 20–30%.

Pleural effusion follows the rupture of a subpleural focus into pleural cavity, but may also occur following hematogenous spread from the primary focus. The effusion occurs because of hypersensitivity to tubercular proteins. Minor effusions are usually asymptomatic. Tuberculous effusion is uncommon in children younger than 5 years of age, and is rarely associated with segmental lesion and miliary tuberculosis. The onset may be insidious or acute with fever, cough, dyspnea, pain and a pleural rub. Increase in effusion may make breathing shallow and difficult. Early signs include decreased chest wall movement, impaired percussion note and reduced air entry on affected side. As fluid collection increases, signs of pleural effusion are more definite.

### Extrathoracic Tuberculosis

The most common forms of extrathoracic disease in children include tuberculosis of the superficial lymph nodes (scrofula) and the central nervous system. Other rare forms of extrathoracic disease include osteoarticular, abdominal, gastrointestinal, genitourinary, cutaneous and congenital disease.

Tuberculosis of superficial lymph nodes may be associated with drinking unpasteurized cow milk or extension of primary lesions of upper lung or abdomen leading to involvement of the supraclavicular, anterior cervical, tonsillar and submandibular nodes. Although lymph nodes may become fixed to surrounding tissues, low grade fever may be the only systemic symptom. A primary focus is visible radiologically in 30 to 70% patients; tuberculin test is usually reactive. Although spontaneous resolution may occur, untreated lymphadenitis frequently progresses to caseating necrosis, capsular rupture, and spread to adjacent nodes and overlying skin, resulting in a draining sinus tract.

Central nervous system disease is the most serious complication of tuberculosis and arises from formation of a caseous lesion in the cerebral cortex or meninges, due to occult lymphohematogenous spread. Infants and young children are likely to experience rapid progression to hydrocephalus, seizures and raised intracranial pressure. In older children, signs and symptoms progress over several weeks, beginning with fever, headache, irritability and drowsiness. The disease advances with lethargy, vomiting, nuchal rigidity, seizures, hypertonia and focal signs. The final stage of disease is marked by coma, hypertension, decerebrate and decorticate posturing and death. Rapid confirmation of the diagnosis can be difficult because of variable cerebrospinal characteristics, nonreactive tuberculin tests (40%) and normal chest radiographs (50%). Since better outcomes are associated with early institution of therapy, the diagnosis should be considered in any child with basilar meningitis, hydrocephalus or cranial nerve involvement.

Tuberculosis of abdomen is due to hematogenous spread from the lungs. It may, however, be secondary to swallowing of the infected sputum by a patient with pulmonary lesions. Patients with abdominal tuberculosis may remain asymptomatic initially. Symptomatic patients show toxemia and have colicky abdominal pain, vomiting and constipation. The abdomen feels characteristically doughy; abdominal wall is not rigid but tense. The rolled up omentum and enlarged lymph nodes appear as irregular nodular masses with ascites; liver and spleen are often enlarged.

Children may rarely present with hemophagocytic lymphohistiocytosis (HLH), immune hemolytic anemia, superior mediastinal syndrome, pneumothorax and immune reconstitution inflammatory syndrome (IRIS) in form of paradoxical worsening of symptoms after starting antituberculous drugs, especially in children with immune deficiency.

### Diagnosis

The diagnosis of tuberculosis in children is based on clinical features, chest roentgenogram, tuberculin testing and history of contact with adult patients. Clinical features may be nonspecific and chest radiograph and tuberculin test are difficult to interpret. In addition, these do not give conclusive evidence for the disease. While demonstration of *Mycobacterium* in various clinical specimens is the gold standard, this is often not possible in children due to the paucibacillary nature of the illness.

***History of contact:*** A contact is defined as a child who lives in a household with an adult taking antitubercular therapy or having taken such therapy in the past 2 years. A history of contact is available in less than one-third of the patients. Contacts can often be traced to a maid servant, cook, domestic aid or gardener in case of patients from well-to-do families with healthy parents. Tracing of contact is useful for confirming the diagnosis, as well as protection of other susceptible children from the disease.

Children with persistent fever and/or cough greater than two weeks, loss of weight (>5% weight loss) and/or no weight gain, and/ or gradually enlarging painless lymph node, especially in the neck, swelling in the back—Gibbus deformity and/or history of contact are considered to having presumptive childhood TB and must be evaluated for the disease.

Any child displaying the presence of organ-specific symptoms and signs such as swelling of lymph nodes, pain and swelling in joints, neck stiffness, disorientation, etc. and/or constitutional symptoms like significant weight loss, persistent fever for 2 weeks or more and night sweats must be considered to have presumptive extrapulmonary TB and should be evaluated.

In all children with presumptive intrathoracic TB, microbiological confirmation should be sought through examination of clinical specimens (e.g. sputum by expectoration, nasopharyngeal aspirate, gastric aspirate, gastric lavage, induced sputum, bronchoalveolar lavage, or other appropriate specimens) with rapid molecular diagnostic tests, preferably CB-NAAT/TrueNat, culture or smear microscopy.

For children with presumptive extrapulmonary TB, appropriate specimens from the presumed sites of involvement should be obtained for rapid molecular diagnostic tests, microscopy, culture and drug susceptibility testing, and histopathological examination.

### Laboratory Tests

Diagnostic tests for pulmonary tuberculosis can be divided into two categories based on demonstration of: (i) *M. tuberculosis* or one of its components; (ii) host response to *M. tuberculosis*.

Tubercle bacteria can be demonstrated by (i) Ziehl-Neelsen (acid-fast) staining, (ii) special stains, (iii) cultures, and (iv) cartridge-based nucleic acid amplification test. The above methods can be used on sputum, induced sputum, gastric or bronchoscopic lavage fluid, or pleural fluid. The best specimen for demonstration of *M. tuberculosis* in children is the early morning gastric aspirate obtained by using a nasogastric tube. For better results, at least two specimens of gastric aspirates are recommended. Fluorescence microscopy (using auramine-rhodamine stains) may improve yield further. In children who are not able to provide sputum, expectoration can be induced by nebulized hypertonic saline (3–5%). Older children may provide sputum at end of the procedure. In young children, a nasopharyngeal aspirate is collected and processed like sputum for smear and culture.

***Culture:*** Lowenstein-Jensen (LJ) medium is the most widely used medium for determination of characteristic features of colonial morphology, growth rate and pigment production. Though the culture technique is simple, 7–10 weeks of incubation is necessary for detection of organisms. Microscopic examination of thin layer culture plate may lead to detection of microcolonies of *M. tuberculosis* as early as after 7 days. The yield of culture of gastric aspirate varies from 30–50% in children with tuberculosis. In view of the excessively long period for isolation of *M. tuberculosis* by conventional culture, LJ medium has been replaced by mycobacterial growth indicator tube (MGIT) system. In this system, culture is positive in majority by end of 2 weeks, though final result is available by the end of 6 weeks.

***Cartridge-based nucleic acid amplification test (CBNAAT):*** The test, based on real-time polymerase chain reaction, is preferred for diagnosis of pulmonary tuberculosis; results are available in less than 2 hours. CBNAAT identifies presence of *M. tuberculosis* and provides information on rifampicin resistance. The sensitivity and specificity of two gastric aspirates for diagnosing pulmonary tuberculosis in children ranges between 60 and 70% and 90 and 100%, respectively. Its utility in extrapulmonary tuberculosis is lower. The commercially available tests include GeneXpert, GeneXpert Ultra, TrueNAT.

***Serodiagnosis:*** ELISA has been used to detect antibodies to various antigens of the bacillus. Despite a number of studies, current techniques have no role for the diagnosis of tuberculosis in children.

***Methods to diagnose latent infection:*** Till date, tuberculin skin test was the only method to diagnose latent tuberculosis infection. Recently, a new test based on interferon gamma release assay (IGRA) has been developed. This *in vitro* test estimates a component of cell-mediated immunity to *M. tuberculosis*, based on quantitation of interferon-gamma (IFN-$\gamma$) released from sensitized lymphocytes in whole blood incubated overnight with antigens specific for the bacterial species. Two tests are available: QuantiFERON® gold TB test (QFT) and ELISPOT. In countries with high prevalence of tuberculosis, it is recommended to continue using tuberculin skin test that is considerably less expensive than IGRA.

***Tuberculin skin test:*** The tuberculin or Mantoux test is commonly used to make the diagnosis of tuberculosis in children. Although currently available test antigens are not 100% sensitive or specific, no better diagnostic test is widely available. Infection with *M. tuberculosis* produces a delayed hypersensitivity reaction to its specific antigenic components. All purified protein derivative (PPD) lots are bioassayed to demonstrate equal potency. The standard test dose of a preparation is defined as dose of that product that is biologically equivalent to 5 TU of PPD-S or 2 TU of tuberculin PPD RT23. The reaction to tuberculin typically begins 5–6 hours after the intradermal injection and reaches maximal induration at 48–72 hours; vesiculation and necrosis are rare.

Variability of the tuberculin test may be reduced by attention to administration and reading. A 26-gauge needle and tuberculin syringe are used to inject 0.1 mL of PPD intradermally into the volar aspect of the forearm. Forty-eight to 72 hours later, the diameter of induration is measured transversely to the long axis of forearm and recorded in millimeters. A non-reactive tuberculin test does not exclude latent or active tuberculosis. Numerous factors can diminish tuberculin reactivity, resulting in a false negative reaction (Table 11.10). Because some antigens in PPD are shared with other mycobacteria and Bacillus Calmette–Guerin (BCG), false-positive reactions can occur in those infected with other mycobacteria or following vaccination. Although BCG vaccination of older children

**Table 11.10:** Causes of false positive and false negative tuberculin skin test (Mantoux test)

**False negative results**

*Infections*

- Viral (measles, mumps, chickenpox, HIV)
- Bacterial (enteric fever, typhus, leprosy, pertussis, severe TB)
- Live vaccines (measles, mumps, polio, varicella)
- Chronic renal failure, liver failure
- Hodgkin disease, lymphoma, chronic leukemia, sarcoidosis
- Corticosteroids, immunosuppressive agents
- Newborn, elderly patients

*Factors related to tuberculin*

- Exposure to light, heat, chemicals; contamination
- Improper dilution; adsorption

*Factors related to technique*

- Injection of too little antigen
- Subcutaneous injection
- Delayed administration after drawing into syringe
- Injection close to other skin tests
- Inexperienced reader; errors in recording

**False positive results**

- Infections due to atypical mycobacteria
- BCG vaccination
- Infection at the site of test

**Table 11.11:** Interpretation of Mantoux test

| *Size of induration* | *Interpretation* |
|---|---|
| <10 mm | Negative; no active disease |
| 5–10 mm | Borderline; consider positive in immunocompromised host; contact with adult patient with sputum AFB positive tuberculosis |
| >10 mm | Positive; suggests disease in presence of clinical features |

or adults results in greater initial and more persistent cross-reactivity, most individuals lose cross-reactivity within 10 years of vaccination. Interpretation of the skin test is based on risk of infection and progression to disease (Table 11.11).

***BCG test:*** An accelerated response after injection of the vaccine is observed in individuals suffering from tuberculosis. Induration of more than 5–6 mm after 3 days of BCG vaccine is considered a positive reaction. However, due to high antigen load, there are higher chances of false positive results and this test is not recommended. Certain newer skin tests are being evaluated which use recombinant antigens (e.g. C-TB).

***Radiology:*** Chest radiograph has an important role in diagnosis of pulmonary tuberculosis. In extrapulmonary tuberculosis, presence of lesions on chest radiograph supports diagnosis. The typical chest X-ray appearance of a pulmonary primary complex (PPC) is that of a consolidation of variable size, usually unifocal and homogenous (Fig. 11.19). Enlarged lymph nodes are seen in the hila and right paratracheal region. Adenopathy alone may be the sole feature of primary tuberculosis.

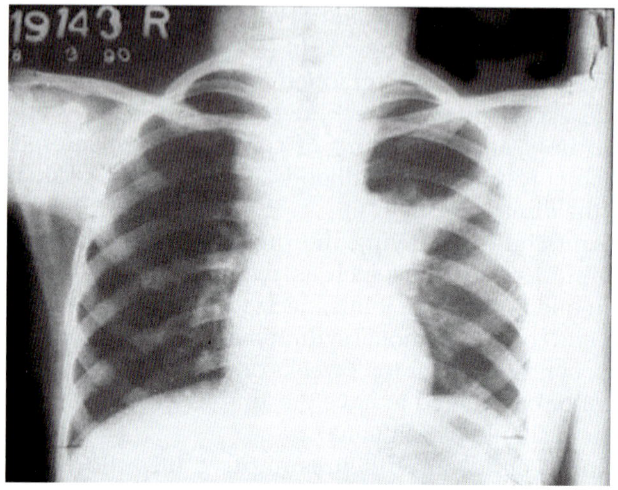


**Fig. 11.19:** Pulmonary primary complex (PPC) showing left hilar adenopathy with ill-defined parenchymal lesion

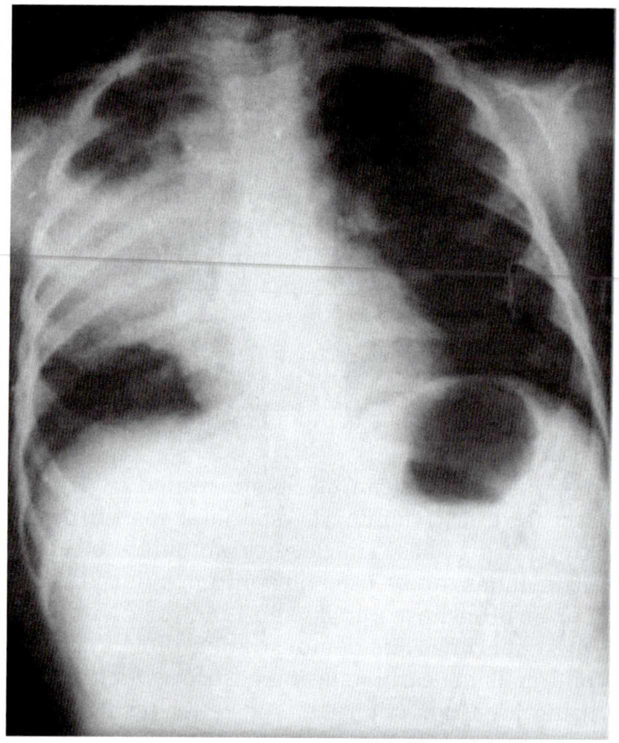

**Fig. 11.20:** Progressive pulmonary disease showing consolidation

Consolidation in progressive primary disease (PPD) is usually heterogeneous, with poorly marginated predilection for apical or posterior segments of upper lobe or superior segment of lower lobe (Fig. 11.20). There may be features of collapse (Fig. 11.21). Bronchiectasis may occur because of (i) destruction and fibrosis of lung parenchyma resulting in retraction and irreversible bronchial dilatation, and (ii) cicatricial bronchostenosis secondary to localized endobronchial infection resulting in obstructive pneumonitis and distal bronchiectasis. In children, cavitary disease is uncommon.

Pleural effusion may occur with or without lung lesions (Fig. 11.22). In miliary tuberculosis, there are multiple lesions of size 2–5 mm (Fig. 11.23). Occasionally, the chest radiograph may be normal and lymphadenopathy is

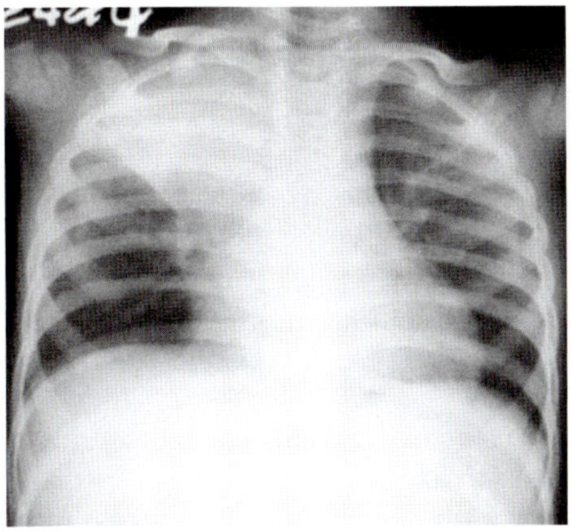

Fig. 11.21: Collapse with consolidation of right upper lobe

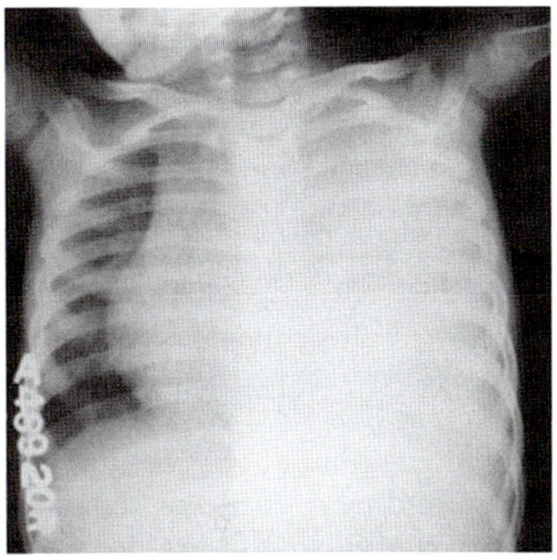

Fig. 11.22: Massive pleural effusion on left side, with mediastinal shift

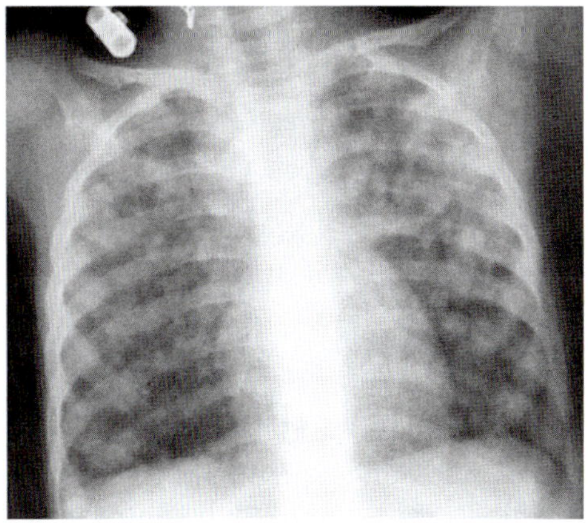

Fig. 11.23: Miliary shadows with right paratracheal adenopathy

detected on computed tomography. CT features such as low attenuation lymph nodes with peripheral enhancement, lymph node calcification, branching centrilobular nodules and miliary nodules are helpful in suggesting the diagnosis where the radiograph is normal or equivocal. Contrast MRI is useful for CNS tuberculosis, since it demonstrates localized lesions, meningeal enhancement, brainstem lesions and ventricular dilatation.

*Histopathology:* Lymph nodes, liver and other tissues may be examined for histological evidence of tuberculosis by fine needle aspiration cytology.

*Diagnostic algorithm for tuberculosis:* The diagnosis of tuberculosis disease in children is challenging. Even in advanced nations, the diagnosis is made by combination of a positive tuberculin test, chest radiograph, physical examination and history of contact with a patient (Fig. 11.24). Newer diagnostic methods, such as CBNAAT, have improved the yield of microbiologically confirmed tuberculosis.

### Treatment

The principles of therapy in children with tuberculosis are similar to that of adults. Medications used for treatment of tuberculosis in children are given in Table 11.12.

*Drug regimens:* Changes have occurred in the therapeutic approach to childhood tuberculosis. Short course therapy with treatment duration of 6 months is now standard practice. This includes 2 months of 4-drug therapy (HRZE) followed by 4 months of 3-drug therapy (HRE).

Three drugs (HRE) are used instead of two drugs (HR) in the continuation phase, in view of increasing resistance to INH.

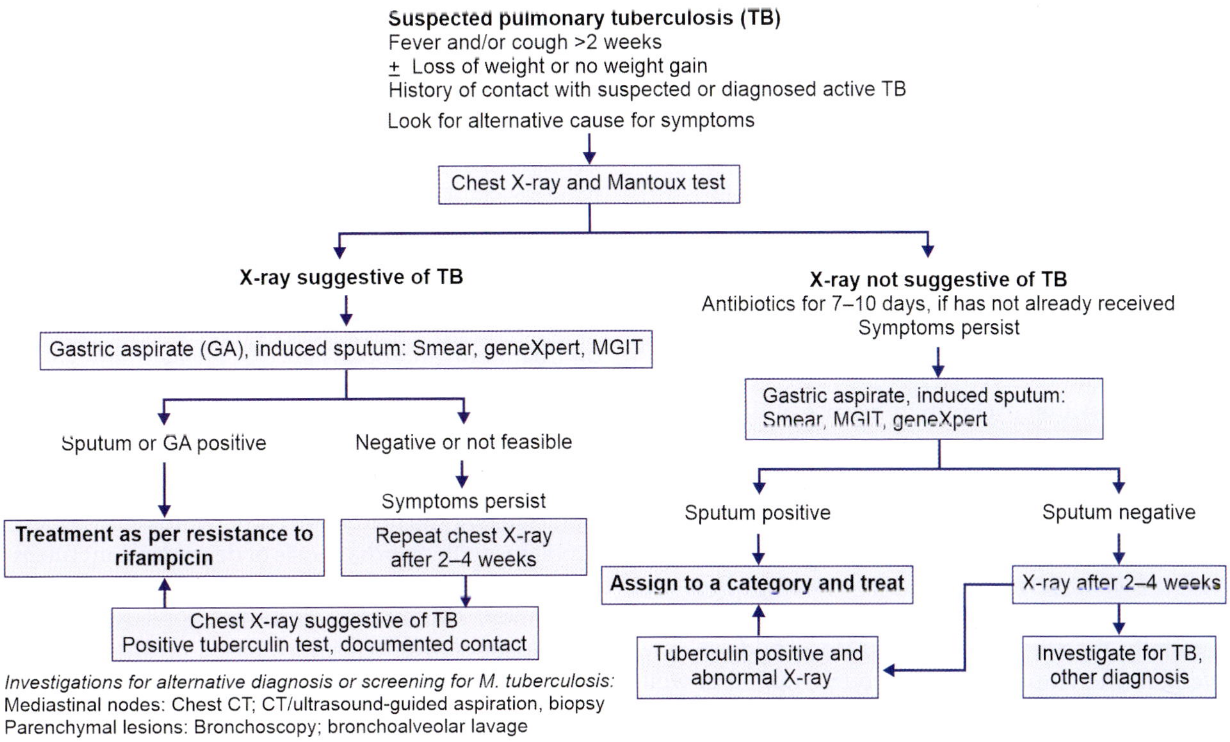


Fig. 11.24: Diagnostic algorithm for pediatric tuberculosis

**Table 11.12:** Doses and side effects of first-line antitubercular drugs

| *Medication* | *Dose (mg/kg/ day; frequency)* | *Side effects* |
|---|---|---|
| Isoniazid | 7–15; q 24 h | Hepatotoxicity, hypersensitivity rash, fever, peripheral or optic neuritis, psychosis, seizures |
| Rifampicin | 10–20; q 24 h | Nausea, vomiting, hepatotoxicity, flu-like syndrome, blood dyscrasia, arthralgia, wheezing |
| Ethambutol | 15–25; q 24 h | Hypersensitivity reaction: Rash, fever, joint pain; optic neuritis, GI upset, confusion, dizziness |
| Pyrazinamide | 25–35; q 24 h | GI upset, hepatotoxicity, hyperuricemia, photosensitivity, dysuria, malaise, arthralgia, fever, thrombocytopenia |

***Corticosteroids:*** Additional therapy with these agents is useful in treating patients with CNS and rarely pulmonary tuberculosis, especially when host inflammatory reaction contributes to tissue damage. Short courses of corticosteroids are indicated in children with endobronchial tuberculosis (with localized emphysema, segmental pulmonary lesions or respiratory distress) and severe miliary tuberculosis (if alveolocapillary block is suspected). Significant improvement in symptoms is seen in children with tuberculous pericardial effusion, but not pleural effusion. The medication used is prednisolone, at doses of 1–2 mg/kg/day for 4–6 weeks.

***Infant born to mother with tuberculosis:*** Congenital tuberculosis is rare, the fetus infected either hematogenously (through umbilical vessels) or by ingestion of infected amniotic fluid. In the former, the primary focus is in the liver and in latter, the lungs. It is often difficult to differentiate between congenital and postnatally acquired tuberculosis. Infants born to mothers with active tuberculosis should be screened for disease by examination, tuberculin test and X-ray chest. If examination and investigations are negative for the disease, the infant should receive INH prophylaxis (10 mg/kg/day for 6 months). The infant is examined regularly for features suggestive of tuberculosis. Infants with congenital tuberculosis are treated with 4 medications (INH, rifampicin, pyrazinamide, ethambutol) in intensive phase for 2 months, followed by 3 drugs (isoniazid, rifampicin, ethambutol) during maintenance for 4 months.

***Management of a child in contact with an adult with tuberculosis:*** One-third of children with adult contacts with active tuberculosis show features of infection. Infection is more common in younger children, and those with severe mal- nutrition, absence of BCG vaccination, sputum positive contacts and exposure to tobacco smoke. Children <5-year-old who are in contact with adult patients with pulmonary tuberculosis should receive INH prophylaxis (10 mg/kg/day for 6 months) after excluding presence of disease.

### Monitoring of Therapy

Response to treatment is judged by clinical, radiological, bacteriological and laboratory assessment.

***Clinical criteria:*** Clinical improvement judges the response of therapy. The child should be seen every 2–4 weeks initially, then every 4–8 weeks. Most children show improvement in symptoms (fever, cough, appetite, well-being) within a few weeks. The child is examined for weight gain and improvement in chest findings. Compliance to therapy should be ensured.

In presence of unsatisfactory response or worsening of features, the initial basis of diagnosis is reviewed, especially if there are no issues with compliance. The possibility of drug resistant tuberculosis should be considered. Following completion of therapy, patients are reviewed every 3–6 months for 2 years.

***Radiological criteria:*** Clinical improvement precedes radiological clearance. The first chest X-ray is done after 8 weeks' therapy, i.e. at the end of intensive phase. In patients who show increase or little change in radiological features coupled with delayed clinical response, prolongation of intensive phase by one-month is suggested. Further films are taken after 4 weeks and child, if better, should be shifted to continuation phase; else the patient is investigated for failure of treatment and drug resistance. The degree of radiological clearance is graded as: (i) complete, (ii) moderate (½–⅓ clearance), (iii) mild (⅓ decrease in size), or (iv) no clearance or appearance of new lesion(s). One need not treat till complete radiological clearance, since improvement may continue even after stoppage of therapy.

***Microbiological criteria:*** Childhood tuberculosis is paucibacillary. In children, where isolation of *M. tuberculosis* was possible at the time of diagnosis, efforts are made to document disappearance of bacilli during therapy. If smear was positive initially, repeat sampling is done at 2 and 6 months.

### Suspecting Drug-Resistant Tuberculosis

Children in the following categories are at risk of developing drug resistant tuberculosis: Contact with adult patients with proven drug resistance; irregular treatment or recent death due to tuberculosis; children not responding to standard antitubercular therapy; children who respond initially but later show deterioration. Appearance of new lymph nodes on treatment, and persistence or isolated non-clearance of radiologic shadows are not considered indicators of drug resistant tuberculosis.

### Drug-Resistant Tuberculosis

Clinicians should neither miss nor overdiagnose the disease. Problems with overdiagnosis of drug-resistant tuberculosis are multiple: Second-line drugs are less effective; they have more side effects; and are expensive. A physician may suspect drug resistance based on the above criteria, but before making a diagnosis, all attempts are made to demonstrate AFB from appropriate samples and obtain culture and sensitivity. If the diagnosis is confirmed or not established, these patients must be referred to centers treating patients with drug resistance. The National Tuberculosis Eradication Program currently offers shorter duration regimen for drug resistant tuberculosis; the use of drugs such as bedaquiline and delaminid have made this possible.


### Suggested Reading

1. MoHFW, GoI. India TB Report 2022. Available at: https://tbcindia.gov.in/WriteReadData/IndiaTBReport2022/TBAnnaulReport2022.pdf
2. Mukherjee A, Singh S, Lodha R, et al; Delhi Pediatric TB Study Group. Ambulatory gastric lavages provide better yields of *Mycobacterium tuberculosis* than induced sputum in children with intrathoracic tuberculosis. Pediatr Infect Dis J 2013; 32:1313–17.
3. Lodha R, Kabra SK, Seth V (Eds). Essentials of tuberculosis in children, 5th edn. New Delhi, Jaypee Publishers; 2023.
4. WHO consolidated guidelines on tuberculosis. Module 5: management of tuberculosis in children and adolescents. Geneva: World Health Organization; 2022


## Nontuberculous Mycobacteria (NTM)

Atypical mycobacteria or nontuberculous mycobacteria or mycobacteria other than tuberculosis (MOTT) are environmental pathogens that are being increasingly recognized as cause of human disease. More than 200 NTM species have been recognized till date and new species are being identified constantly. NTM are classified depending on the rapidity of growth in media as rapid growers, which grow within 7 days and slow growers that take longer to grow. Acquisition of NTM is through contact with the environment and human-to-human or animal-to-human transmission almost never occurs. NTM infections may occur in previously healthy or those with underlying immunodeficiencies, like HIV. The main clinical syndromes recognized with NTM infection are pulmonary, disseminated, lymph node disease, and skin and soft tissue infections. The smear reveals acid-fast bacilli, which are short and fat (unlike MTB) but is negative for NAAT tests used for detection of MTB. The organism can be identified with biochemical and molecular tests after it grows on culture. Treatment of NTM disease depends on the causative organism and its sensitivity. MOTT are frequently confused with tuberculosis with consequent delay in diagnosis and treatment.

Lymphatic disease is the most common manifestation of NTM disease in children. Unlike the West where NTM lymphadenopathy is very common; in India, NTM account for 10% of mycobacterial lymphadenitis (rest being MTB). It usually presents as painless cervical adenitis in children aged 1–5 years with no systemic symptoms. Histopathology reveals granulomatous inflammation. The main differential is tuberculous lymphadenitis. The definitive diagnosis is by culture, the causative organisms being *Mycobacterium avium-intracellulare* (MAC), *M. scrofulaceum* and *M. hemophilium*. Treatment of choice is complete excision of the lymph nodes. This may not always be possible and is associated with risk of facial nerve injury. Medical treatment is with clarithromycin, rifabutin and ethambutol.

Pulmonary disease due to NTM usually occurs in adults with underlying pulmonary problems and is usually due to MAC, *M. kansasii* and *M. abscessus*. In children, it is seen in cystic fibrosis and bronchiectasis. Presentation is with fever, cough and hemoptysis. Diagnosis is by cultures in sputum or bronchoalveolar lavage. Treatment depends on the species and usually includes rifampicin, ethambutol, clarithromycin and isoniazid.

Disseminated NTM disease is usually due to MAC and seen mainly in adults and less commonly children with advanced HIV infection and presents as fever, weight loss, night sweats, abdominal pain, diarrhea and anemia. Blood cultures are often positive. MAC is usually treated with combination therapy consisting of a macrolide (clarithromycin/azithromycin), rifampicin/rifabutin, ethambutol and in some cases quinolones or aminoglycoside for around 12–18 months. Primary prophylaxis is indicated in patients with CD4 counts below 50/μL with daily clarithromycin or weekly azithromycin.

Skin and soft tissue infections are usually a consequence of trauma (*M. ulcerans* and *M. marinum*) or health care procedures (*M. abscessus*, *M. chelonae*, *M. fortuitum*). Health care associated procedures have been seen following injections, central lines, peritoneal dialysis catheters, laparoscopic procedures, liposuction, cosmetic procedures, implants and prosthesis, and ocular and other surgeries. These mycobacteria species are usually hardy, resist the commonly used disinfectants and hence occur when endoscopic equipment is rinsed with tap water or inadequately cleaned and disinfected. These infections usually present as indolent infections that do not respond to the usual antibiotics. Treatment of these depends on sensitivity, but usually includes combination therapy with clarithromycin, linezolid, clofazimine and amikacin.


### Suggested Reading

1. López-Varela E, García-Basteiro AL, Santiago B, Wagner D, van Ingen J, Kampmann B. Non-tuberculous mycobacteria in children: Muddying the waters of tuberculosis diagnosis. Lancet Respir Med 2015; 3:244–56.


# OTHER BACTERIAL INFECTIONS

## Brucellosis

Brucellosis is a chronic infection that is often misdiagnosed and underdiagnosed. It occurs worldwide especially in the Mediterranean region, Middle Eastern Countries, Central Asia and India.

### *Etiopathogenesis*

Brucella species are intracellular gram-negative coccobacilli. The classification of brucella species is based on its preferred hosts namely *B. melitensis* (sheep and goats), *B. abortus* (cattle), *B. suis* (pigs), and *B. canis* (dogs). Brucellosis is a zoonosis and transmission to humans can occur through the consumption of infected unpasteurized milk and animal products, through direct contact with infected animal parts such as placenta by inoculation of skin and mucous membranes, and by inhalation of infected aerosolized particles. The vast majority of cases worldwide are attributed to *B. melitensis*.

#### Clinical Features

Human brucellosis is an illness with protean manifestations and can be an acute (<2 months), subacute (2–12 months), or chronic (>1 year). The incubation period is usually between 7 days and 3 months. A history of exposure to animals especially drinking unpasteurized milk without boiling is present. Fever is the cardinal feature, which can be continuous or intermittent and go on for several months especially due to partial response to antibiotics. Fever is usually accompanied by profuse sweating, joint pains (particularly knee), back pain, hepatosplenomegaly and less common lymphadenopathy. In untreated cases, complications such as spondylitis, osteoarthritis, meningoencephalitis, brain abscesses, pneumonia and endocarditis can occur.

#### Diagnosis

Blood count usually reveals anemia, leukopenia and thrombocytopenia. The liver enzymes are mildly elevated (SAP and GGT, more than transaminases).

The gold standard for diagnosis is blood culture, which has good sensitivity if done prior to antibiotic therapy and specimen incubated for 4 weeks. In today's automated systems, most cultures are positive by the 10th day. The sensitivity of bone marrow cultures is even higher than blood cultures as organisms are present in large amounts in the reticuloendothelial system. Serologic tests for diagnosis include ELISA (IgG and IgM) and serum agglutination tests (SAT). IgG ELISA should be used for screening as it has high sensitivity, while agglutination tests have high specificity. False positive results with IgM antibodies to brucella are common and should be interpreted carefully.

Important differential diagnoses include tuberculosis, enteric fever, chronic malaria, HIV, sarcoidosis and lymphoproliferative disorders.

#### Treatment

Treatment of human brucellosis (adult or pediatric) is with a combination of antibiotics for 6 weeks, as monotherapies and short treatments are characterized by unacceptably high relapse rates. Brucella is sensitive *in vitro* to multiple antibiotics, but the medications should penetrate macrophages and act in an acidic intracellular environment. The standard regime is a combination of doxycycline and rifampicin for 6 weeks. For children less than 8 years old, combinations containing rifampicin and cotrimoxazole with or without aminoglycosides are recommended. Brucella spondylodiscitis should be treated for 3 months with combination therapy along with streptomycin or gentamicin for the first 1–2 weeks. Treatment needs to be modified and prolonged for endocarditis and neurobrucellosis.

#### Prevention

Preventive strategies include control of disease in livestock and preventing human exposure particularly boiling milk before use.

### Suggested Reading


1. Bukhari EE. Pediatric brucellosis. An update review for the new millennium. Saudi Med J. 2018; 39:336–41.
2. Pappas G, Akritidis N, Bosilkovski M, Tsianos E. Brucellosis: Review. N Engl J Med 2005; 352:2325–36.


## Staphylococcal Infections

*Staphylococcus*, a gram-positive coccus, is a common cause of both community acquired and nosocomial disease in children.

#### Etiopathogenesis

Staphylococci are functionally classified on basis of production of an enzyme and virulence factor coagulase. Coagulase positive staphylococcus is termed as *S. aureus* while *S. saprophyticus* and *S. epidermidis* are important coagulase negative staphylococci (CONS). CONS usually colonize the skin of all people and *S. aureus* the nares, axilla and perineum of around 20–25% of the population. Staphylococci can survive for days in the environment, and infection is acquired by direct contact with an infected patient or carrier, and sometimes contaminated objects. Airborne spread is less common. Predisposing factors for staphylococcal infections include breach in the mucocutaneous barrier, previous viral infections such as measles, depressed immunity and prosthetic material such as shunts, central venous catheters and prosthetic joints.

#### Clinical Features

*S. aureus* can cause a myriad of infections involving almost all organs of the body. Infections are associated with suppuration, and often require drainage and prolonged antibiotic therapy.

The commonest are infections of skin and soft tissues like furuncles, impetigo, carbuncles, abscesses and cellulitis. In some situations, *S. aureus* can invade the fascia and muscle causing necrotizing fasciitis, an infection that is associated with very high morbidity and mortality. Staphylococcal scalded skin syndrome is another bullous infection commonly seen in infants produced by 'exfoliatin' toxin producing *S. aureus* that can lead to massive desquamation and denudation.

*S. aureus* is an important cause of respiratory infections such as sinusitis, otitis media, pneumonia, lung abscess and empyema. Staphylococcal pneumonia commonly occurs after antecedent viral infections, is rapidly progressive and associated with a high rate of complications such as pneumatocoeles, abscess and empyema (Fig. 11.25). *S. aureus* is the commonest cause of acute infective endocarditis in both patients with native and prosthetic valves and sometimes with no risk factors. It is rapidly progressive, locally destructive and is associated with significant complications. It is also the commonest cause of pyopericardium, an illness with high rates of constrictive pericarditis that often requires pericardiectomy.

*S. aureus* is the commonest cause of musculoskeletal infections such as osteomyelitis, septic arthritis and pyomyositis. CNS infections such as meningitis usually occur following trauma or neurosurgery. *S. aureus* is also a common etiologic agent of subdural empyema, brain abscess and shunt infections. Enterotoxin producing *S. aureus* is a common cause of food poisoning that is characterized by fever and profuse vomiting.

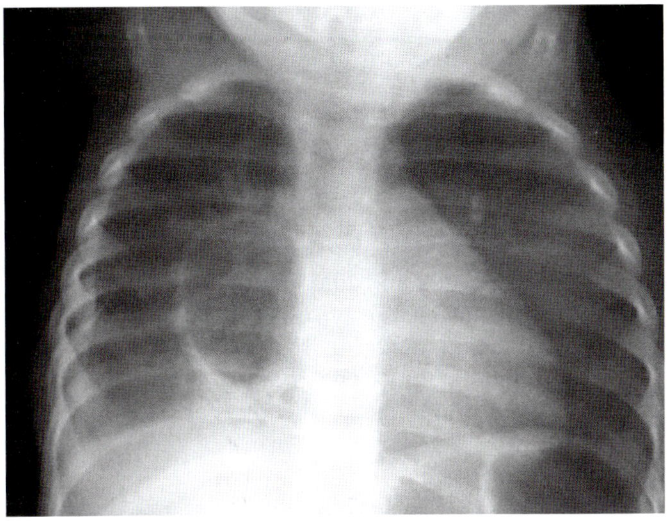

**Fig. 11.25:** Staphylococcal pneumonia with pneumatocele

Toxic shock syndrome (TSS) results from a locally non-invasive toxigenic strain of *S. aureus*, characterized by fever, shock, erythematous skin rash, hepatic derangement, sensorial changes and high mortality. Disseminated staphylococcal disease is another illness usually seen in previously healthy children. It is characterized by suppurative staphylococcal infections at multiple sites, either together or serially and a prolonged course.

CONS are usually pathogens of lower virulence than *S. aureus*. Since they colonize the skin, they are often cultured as contaminants, if blood cultures are not collected by aseptic techniques. They are commonly implicated in bacteremia in low birth weight babies or in those with central venous catheters, subacute infective endocarditis, CNS shunt infections, infections associated with peritoneal dialysis catheters and prosthetic joints, urinary tract infections and postoperative surgical site infections.

### *Treatment*

The most important treatment strategies are surgical drainage and antibiotics.

Antibiotic therapy of staphylococcal infections has become complicated due to evolving resistance. More than 90% staphylococci are resistant to penicillin due to production of a beta-lactamase/penicillinase. Those isolates sensitive to penicillinase-resistant penicillins such as cloxacillin/methicillin and cephalosporins are termed as MSSA. There is an increased incidence of methicillin-resistant *S. aureus* (MRSA) in both hospital and community acquired infections. There are sporadic reports of vancomycin intermediate and resistant *S. aureus* (VISA and VRSA) and linezolid resistance.

The drug of choice for treating MSSA infections is cloxacillin. Other alternatives are first generation cephalosporins (cephalexin, cefadroxil or cefazolin), second generation cephalosporins (cefuroxime), coamoxiclav and clindamycin. If MRSA infections are proven or suspected, medications like vancomycin, linezolid and teicoplanin are preferred. Daptomycin works well for both MSSA and MRSA organisms.

Most *S. aureus* infections need removal of any prosthetic material to ensure cure and prolonged therapy ranging from 2 weeks for bacteremia and 4–6 weeks for osteomyelitis, septic arthritis and endocarditis.

### Suggested Reading


1. Kalu IC, Kao CM, Fritz SA. Management and prevention of *Staphylococcus aureus* infections in children. Infect Dis Clin North Am 2022;36:73–100.
2. Tong SYC, Davis JS, Eichenberger E, et al. *S. aureus* infections: Epidemiology, pathophysiology, clinical manifestations and management. Clin Microbiol Rev 2015;28:603–61.


## Pneumococcal Infections

Pneumococcus is one of the most common bacterial causes of pediatric infections particularly pneumonia. It is currently estimated that 50% of deaths due to severe pneumonia are caused by pneumococcus. Of the 4,00,000 deaths in children below the age of 5-yr in India due to acute respiratory infections, 2,00,000 are due to pneumococcus.

### *Etiopathogenesis*

Pneumococcus is a gram-positive diplococcus with a thick polysaccharide capsule. This capsule is the most important virulence factor and determines the various serotypes of the pneumococcus. Almost 90 serotypes of pneumococcus exist but only a handful cause disease. Serotypes 1, 4, 5, 6A and 6B, 9V, 14, 18C, 19A, 19F and 23 are those that commonly cause human disease and are the incorporated in the vaccines (further discussed in Chapter 10). Pneumococci colonize the nasopharynx; colonization rates are highest in young children. Colonization can lead to infection in some individuals. Risk factors for pneumococcal disease include extremes of age (age less than two years), splenic dysfunction, immunodeficiency especially HIV, any chronic disease and CSF leaks.

### *Clinical Features*

Pneumococcal infections are distributed like a pyramid, the base of the pyramid being non-invasive disease like otitis media, sinusitis and pneumonia and the apex comprising invasive disease like bacteremic pneumonia, bacteremia and meningitis. It is estimated that for every 1000 cases of otitis media, there is one case of meningitis. Other less common invasive diseases due to pneumococci are osteomyelitis, septic arthritis, cellulitis and peritonitis.

Pneumococcus is responsible for most of the cases of acute bacterial meningitis and is associated with high rate of complications like subdural empyema, morbidity and mortality. Pneumococcal bacteremia presents usually as fever without focus in infants and children below 3 years, and needs aggressive therapy. It is estimated that pneumococcus causes 30–50% of severe pneumonia. Pneumococcal pneumonia classically has a lobar distribution with necrosis and empyema being common complications.

### *Diagnosis*

The gold standard for diagnosis of pneumococcal disease is culture. However, culture yields are poor because of several reasons. Pneumococcus, unlike *Salmonella*, is difficult to culture, especially if antibiotics have been administered.

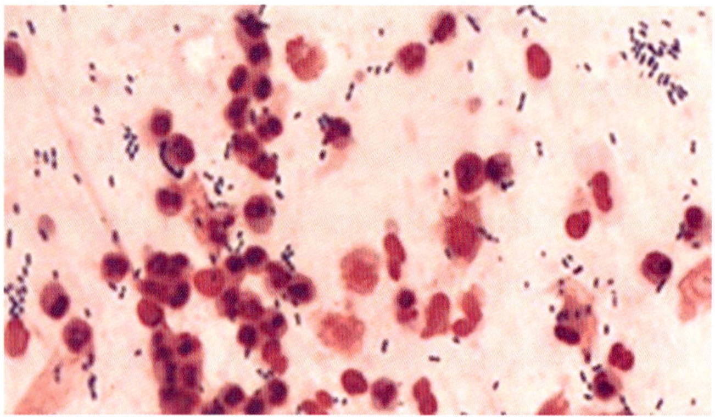

**Fig. 11.26:** Gram stain of pus showing abundant gram-positive diplococci, suggestive of pneumococci

Special media containing sheep blood are required and delays in transportation and improper storage further reduce recovery. Moreover, in pneumonia, isolation rates from blood are low and the ideal sample of lung aspirate cannot be obtained in routine clinical practice. Low culture yields are responsible for under recognition of pneumococcus as a common pathogen.

Other tests useful for diagnosis are Gram stain **(Fig. 11.26)**, latex agglutination tests in CSF and pleural fluids, and now PCR in CSF.

### *Treatment*

Penicillin and its derivatives such as ampicillin and amoxicillin are the drugs of choice for treatment of pneumococcal infections. The cephalosporins especially ceftriaxone are also satisfactory alternatives. Like many other bacteria, resistance in pneumococcus is being increasingly reported (more from the West and relatively less from India). There is high prevalence of resistance to macrolides and cotrimoxazole in India. Resistance to beta lactams is due to altered penicillin binding protein and may be of intermediate or high level. Intermediate resistance can be overcome by using higher doses of penicillin or amoxicillin, but high level resistance requires use of alternative drugs like fluoroquinolones or vancomycin. The current rates of penicillin and ceftriaxone resistance in meningeal isolates of pneumococcus in India have risen, mandating the use of ceftriaxone with vancomycin for treatment of bacterial/pneumococcal meningitis.

### Suggested Reading


1. Maraqa NF. Pneumococcal infections. Pediatr Rev. 2014;35:299–310.


*Competency:* **PE34.16**

## Diphtheria

Diphtheria is an acute bacterial infection caused by gram-positive bacillus, *Corynebacterium diphtheriae*. The incidence of diphtheria has dramatically declined over the years with only 3500 cases reported in 2020 in India. However, cases in unvaccinated/partially vaccinated children continue to be reported.

### *Etiopathogenesis*

The secretions and discharges from infected person or carrier are the main source of infection. The infection is transmitted by contact or via droplets of secretion. The portal of entry is commonly the respiratory tract. The incubation period of the disease is 2–5 days. *C. diphtheriae* proliferate and liberate a powerful exotoxin which is the principal cause of systemic and local lesions. The exotoxin causes necrosis of the epithelial cells and liberates serous and fibrinous material which forms a grayish white pseudomembrane that bleeds on being dislodged. The surrounding tissue is inflamed and edematous. The organs principally affected by the exotoxin include the heart, kidney and myocardium.

### *Clinical Features*

The onset is generally acute with fever, malaise and headache. The child has a toxic look. The clinical features depend on the site of involvement. The commonest form is faucial or tonsillopharyngeal diphtheria in which there is redness and swelling over the fauces. The exudates coalesce to form a grayish white pseudomembrane, which extends to surrounding areas. The cervical lymph nodes are enlarged leading to a bull neck appearance. Sore throat, dysphagia and muffled voice are frequently present. In nasal diphtheria, there is unilateral or bilateral serosanguinous discharge from the nose and excoriation of upper lip. In laryngotracheal diphtheria, the membrane over the larynx leads to brassy cough, stridor and respiratory distress. Diphtheritic lesions may occasionally also be found in skin and conjunctiva.

The commonest complication is respiratory failure due to occlusion of the airways by the membrane. Myocarditis generally occurs by second week of illness and can lead to symptoms of congestive cardiac failure, arhythmias and sudden death. Neurological complications include: (i) Palatal palsy, which occurs in second week and is clinically manifested by nasal twang and nasal regurgitation; (ii) ocular palsy in third week; (iii) loss of accommodation, manifested by visual blurring and inability to read; and (iv) generalized polyneuritis by 3–6 weeks of illness. Renal complications include oliguria and proteinuria.

### *Diagnosis*

There should be a high index of suspicion in patients presenting with exudative pharyngitis. Rapid diagnosis is enabled by Albert stain of a swab from the oropharynx or larynx. Culture, however, takes 8-hr to become available. Faucial diphtheria should be differentiated from acute streptococcal membranous tonsillitis (patients have high fever, but are less toxic and the membrane is confined to the tonsils), viral (adenovirus) membranous tonsillitis (high fever, sore throat, membranous tonsillitis with normal leukocyte count, self-limited course of 4–8 days), herpetic tonsillitis, aphthous stomatitis, thrush, infectious mononucleosis (generalized rash, lymphadenopathy, abnormal lymphocytosis, positive Paul Bunnell test), agranulocytosis and leukemia.

### *Management*

The most important component of therapy is neutralization of bacterial toxin by administration of antitoxin. Diphtheria antitoxin (10000–30000 IU/IM) should be administered as soon as possible before the bacteria have fixed to the tissues. The degree of protection offered by the diphtheria antitoxin is inversely proportional to the duration of clinical illness. Repeat doses of antitoxin may be given, if clinical improvement is not satisfactory.

Antibiotics, such as penicillin or erythromycin, should be used to terminate toxin production, limit proliferation of bacteria, to prevent spread of organism to contacts and to prevent the development of carriers. This should be followed by active immunization as clinical disease does not confer active immunity.

Bed rest is advocated for two to three weeks. Children should be monitored for airway obstruction and managed; tracheostomy may be required in some cases. Sudden exertion should be avoided and changes in rate and rhythm of heart should be looked for. Children with palatal palsy should be fed by nasogastric feeding. Generalized weakness due to polyneuritis is treated as for poliomyelitis or Guillain-Barre syndrome.

### Prevention and Control

The patient should be isolated until two successive cultures of throat and nose are negative for diphtheria bacillus. All contaminated articles from discharges should be disinfected. All household and other contacts should be observed carefully for development of active lesions, cultured for *C. diphtheriae* and given chemoprophylaxis with oral erythromycin for 7 days or single dose benzathine penicillin. Previously immunized asymptomatic patients should receive a booster dose of diphtheria toxoid. Those not fully immunized should receive immunization for their age. Immunization is discussed in Chapter 10.

### Suggested Reading


1. Nicholson L, Adkins E, Karyanti MR, et al. What is the true burden of diphtheria, tetanus, pertussis and poliovirus in children aged 3–18 years in Asia? A systematic literature review. Int J Infect Dis 2022;117:116–29.
2. Zibners L. Diphtheria, pertussis, and tetanus: Evidence-based management of pediatric patients in the emergency department. Pediatr Emerg Med Pract 2017;14:1–24.


Competency: **PE34.16**

## Pertussis (Whooping Cough)

Pertussis is an acute highly contagious respiratory tract infection, caused by *Bordetella pertussis*. It may affect any susceptible host but is more common and serious in infancy and early childhood. The disease is characterized by intense spasmodic cough. Similar illness is also caused by *B. parapertussis*, *B. bronchoseptica* and adenoviral infections. The worldwide prevalence of the illness has declined following widespread vaccination. However, since protection offered by both vaccination and natural infection is of limited duration, the disease continues to remain endemic. India reported 12000 cases of pertussis in 2020. There is gross underreporting due to lack of awareness and lack of diagnostic facilities.

### Epidemiology

Pertussis is extremely contagious with attack rates as high as 100% in susceptible individuals exposed to aerosol droplets. *B. pertussis* does not survive for prolonged periods in the environment. Chronic carriage in humans is not known. After intense exposure as in households, the rate of subclinical infection is as high as 80% in fully immunized and naturally immune individuals. Protection against typical disease wanes 3–5 years after vaccination, and is unmeasurable after 12 years. Coughing adolescents and adults are the major reservoir of *B. pertussis* and are the usual sources for index cases in infants and children.

### Features

The incubation period of the disease is 7–14 days. The clinical presentation is divided into three stages.

The *catarrhal phase* lasts for 1–2 weeks and is the most infectious period. The initial manifestations are indistinguishable from upper respiratory tract infections. The child has cough, coryza with little nasopharyngeal secretions. Unlike the upper respiratory infections, the cough does not improve in a few days but becomes more severe and frequent with the passage of time. Though the cough may not be typically paroxysmal in early stages, it tends to be annoying and frequent at night. The paroxysmal nature of the cough is suspected towards the latter part of this phase.

The *paroxysmal stage* lasts for 2–6 weeks in which cough progresses to episodic paroxysms of increasing intensity ending with high-pitched inspiratory whoop. The whoop is produced by the air rushing in during inspiration through the half-open glottis. The whoop may not always be present in infants who present with apneic or cyanotic spells. The child coughs up thick tenacious mucus. The paroxysms of cough may occur frequently and terminate by vomiting. Repeated thrusting of tongue over the teeth causes ulceration of the frenulum of the tongue. Paroxysms of cough are precipitated by food, cold air and cold liquids. In infants <3 months, this stage may be considerably prolonged.

In the *convalescent phase*, the intensity and paroxysms of cough decrease gradually over 1–4 weeks. The vomiting becomes less frequent. Appetite, general condition and health gradually improve.

### Complications

- *Respiratory:* Otitis media, pneumonia, atelectasis, emphysema, bronchiectasis, pneumothorax and pneumomediastinum.
- Young infants may present with recurrent apnea, extreme leukocytosis and pulmonary hypertension and have high mortality.
- *Neurological:* Seizures and encephalopathy (2–7%)
- *Bleeding episodes:* Epistaxis, retinal or subconjunctival bleeds, intracranial hemorrhage
- Inguinal hernia, rectal prolapse
- Malnutrition due to persistent vomiting and disinclination to eat (fear of paroxysms of cough with attempts at feeding)
- Flare up of tuberculosis

Older children and adolescents may have non-classical presentation with prolonged, paroxysmal cough without the whoop or post-tussive vomiting.

### Diagnosis

The diagnosis of whooping cough is based on clinical features. There may be a lymphocytic leukocytosis and low ESR. Specific diagnosis depends on isolation of the organism from nasopharyngeal swab or cough plate cultured on Bordet-Gengou medium, which is often positive in the catarrhal and paroxysmal stage. Other tests include serology and PCR on the throat swab. PCR for pertussis is now available as part of multiplex PCR respiratory panels.

Other differentials for pertussis include adenoviral infection, endobronchial tuberculosis, inhaled foreign body, extrinsic compression of airway by lymph nodes, and reactive airway disease.

### Management

General measures include providing adequate nutrition and hydration and avoiding factors aggravating cough. Macrolides including erythromycin, azithromycin or clarithromycin are the drugs of choice. Antibiotics terminate the respiratory tract carriage of *B. pertussis*, reduce the period of communicability but do not shorten the course of illness. Nebulization with salbutamol is sometimes effective in reducing bronchospasm and controlling bouts of cough. Cough suppressants and antihistaminic agents should be used carefully.

### Prevention

Chemoprophylaxis with erythromycin is recommended for close family contacts especially children <2-yr-old. Unvaccinated and partially vaccinated contacts should be given booster dose of vaccination. Vaccination is discussed separately.

### Suggested Reading


1. Kilgore PE, Salim AM, Zervos MJ, Schmitt HJ. Pertussis: Microbiology, disease, treatment, and prevention. Clin Microbiol Rev 2016;29:449–86.
2. Pertussis Guidelines Group. Guidelines for the public health management of pertussis in England, 2018, 1–48.www.gov.uk/phe.


Competency: **PE34.17**

## Enteric Fever

The term enteric fever includes typhoid fever caused by *Salmonella enterica* var *typhi* and paratyphoid fever caused by *S. enterica* var *paratyphi* A, B or C. Paratyphoid infections constitute about 20% of all cases of enteric fever worldwide. As enteric fever is a disease transmitted by the feco-oral route, its greatest burden is in resource-limited countries where water supply and sanitary conditions are poor. It is estimated that there are 2–3 million cases of enteric fever in India annually. Enteric fever contributes to 10% of all fevers in hospitalized children.

### Etiopathogenesis

*S. enterica* serotype *typhi/paratyphi* is a gram-negative, non-lactose fermenting, flagellate bacterium. The somatic or O antigen is shared among various salmonellae; the flagellar or H antigen is specific to the serovar. *S. enterica* var *typhi* also possesses a Vi polysaccharide capsule.

The infective dose of typhoid/paratyphoid bacillus varies from $10^3$ to $10^6$ organisms. The organism must survive the gastric barrier to reach the small intestine; hence, conditions which reduce gastric acidity, such as antacids, H2 receptor blockers and proton pump inhibitors reduce the infective dose. On reaching the small intestine, the organism penetrates the mucosa and infects the lymphoid follicles and subsequently the draining mesenteric lymph nodes and the liver and spleen. It multiplies in the reticuloendothelial system and after incubation period varying from 7–14 days spills into the bloodstream and is widely disseminated, especially to liver, spleen, bone marrow, gallbladder and the Peyer's patches of the terminal ileum. This spill marks the onset of clinical manifestations of enteric fever. Infection leads to both local and systemic immune responses, which are, however, inadequate to prevent relapse or reinfection.

### Clinical Features

There is no appreciable difference between the manifestations of typhoid and paratyphoid fever. The hallmark of enteric fever is fever which starts as a low grade fever and then shows stepwise increase peaking to as high as 103–104°C by the end of the first week. This pattern differentiates it from viral fever where the peak is usually at the onset of fever. With fever, there is associated malaise, dull headache, anorexia, nausea, poorly localized abdominal discomfort, mild cough and malaise. There may be diarrhea; constipation in children is rare. Physical findings are unremarkable with the exception of a coated tongue, tumid abdomen and sometimes hepatosplenomegaly. The rash described in Western textbooks is seldom or never seen in Indian subjects. Infants and young children with enteric fever may have diarrhea as a predominant manifestation or a short-lasting undifferentiated febrile illness. In the absence of treatment, fever may continue for 3–4 weeks followed by natural remission or by development of complications.

### Complications

The commonest intestinal complications are bleeding or perforation seen in the 2nd or 3rd week of illness in 10–15% adult patients, but less frequently in children. Bleeding is due to erosion of a necrotic Peyer's patch through the wall of a vessel and is usually mild but can, sometimes, be life-threatening. Perforation is a dreaded complication manifesting as acute abdomen, with high mortality unless appropriately treated.

The term severe or complicated enteric fever is used for patients presenting with neurological complications such as delirium, coma, obtundation or stupor, and/or shock and is associated with mortality rates as high as 50%. Other complications of enteric fever include splenic abscesses, hepatitis, cholecystitis, osteomyelitis, pneumonia, disseminated intravascular coagulation and other manifestations such as psychosis, ataxia or meningitis. Hemophagocytic lymphohistiocytosis is a rare complication. The case fatality rate is less than 1% in appropriately treated cases, but may be 10–20% in inadequately treated or complicated cases.

### Relapse

Relapse may occur in 5–15% of treated cases, usually due to the organism with the same susceptibility as the original attack and is relatively a milder illness. Rate of relapse is dependent on choice of drug therapy. It is higher with beta lactams such as cefixime or ceftriaxone as compared to quinolones and azithromycin.

### Carrier State

Although 5–10% adult patients may shed *Salmonella* in stool following an acute attack for up to 3 months, only 1–4% excrete bacilli for more than 1 year. These individuals are potential sources of infection for family members and contacts, and for the community if they are in occupations that involve food-processing. There is no data on carrier prevalence in children and routine examination of stool following recovery from enteric fever is not recommended.

### Diagnosis

Leukocyte counts may be normal to low with absolute eosinopenia and neutrophilic predominance. Anemia and thrombocytopenia may occur in advanced illness. There may be mild elevation of transaminases to 2–3 times normal (SGOT being higher than SGPT). A high C reactive protein (CRP) helps differentiate enteric from viral fevers, especially dengue. USG abdomen may show terminal ileal thickening, mesenteric adenitis and splenomegaly.

The gold standard for diagnosis is blood culture, which continues to be the most important investigation for diagnosis of enteric fever. The sensitivity is greatest in the first week at around 90%, but drops to 40% in the 4th week. Its overall sensitivity is 60%, which reduces to 20–40% after antibiotics; its specificity is 100%. *Salmonella* is an easy organism to culture and use of bile broth media and automated culture systems such as BACTEC improve recovery. Sufficient blood should be collected (10 mL in adults and 5 mL in children) and a blood: media ratio of 1:5 should be maintained. The use of clot culture methods does not significantly improve recovery rates. Bone marrow cultures have higher yield as compared to peripheral blood cultures as *Salmonella* is a pathogen of the reticuloendothelial system. Owing to very low recovery rates, stool cultures and urine cultures are not recommended. Antimicrobial susceptibility testing of the isolate is important in the era of multidrug resistance.

The Widal test has been in use for around 100 years for the serological diagnosis of typhoid. It detects presence of IgG and IgM antibodies to H (flagellar antigen) of *S. enterica* var *typhi* and *paratyphi* A and B, and O (somatic antigen) common to typhi and paratyphi A and B. Anti-O titers are both IgG and IgM that rise and decline early, while anti-H are primarily IgG that rise and decline late in course of the disease. The conventional method of interpretation of the Widal test has been to demonstrate fourfold rise in antibody titers in two samples. Since this is often not practical, a single titer of at least 1:160 for both O and H is considered positive. Even with this compromise, the Widal test has several limitations. Sensitivity is low in the first week of illness and in patients treated with prior antibiotics. Specificity is low owing to anamnestic reactions, prior vaccination, cross reactivity with other Enterobacteriaceae and subclinical infections in endemic areas. Other tests such as Tubex and Typhidot that detect IgM antibodies against typhoid have not proven to be superior to the Widal test.

### Treatment

***Indications for inpatient treatment:*** Most cases of enteric fever can be managed at home with oral antibiotics and advice to seek medical follow up in case of failure to respond to therapy or development of complications. Children with persistent vomiting, inability to take orally, severe diarrhea or abdominal distension usually require intravenous antibiotic therapy and intravenous fluids, necessitating admission to hospital.

***Antimicrobial susceptibility:*** The antimicrobial sensitivity of *S. typhi/paratyphi* has shown changes over the decades. Though resistance to chloramphenicol was first noted soon after its first use in the 1940s, it was not until 1972 that chloramphenicol-resistant typhoid fever became a major problem. Multidrug-resistant typhoid fever (MDRTF) became a common occurrence by the end of 1990s, with emergence of *S. typhi* simultaneously resistant to all the drugs that were used as first-line treatment (chloramphenicol, trimethoprim, sulfamethoxazole and ampicillin). Fluoroquinolones were introduced in the late 1980s and early 1990s and produced very good results initially, but the past decade has seen a progressive increase in the minimum inhibitory concentrations (MIC) of ciprofloxacin in *S. typhi* and *S. paratyphi*. Alongside the recent rise in resistance to quinolones, there has been some return in sensitivity to first-line antibiotics such as chloramphenicol, cotrimoxazole and ampicillin. However, concerns of toxicity preclude their widespread use.

Currently, third-generation cephalosporins such as ceftriaxone and cefixime are the first-line agents for therapy of enteric fever. Azithromycin is another drug that is being used as an alternative agent. However, there are recent reports of emergence of plasmid borne ceftriaxone resistance in *S. enterica* that is of serious concern.

***Choice for empirical therapy:*** Where enteric fever is clinically suspected but cultures are awaited or are sterile, empirical therapy may be started. Choice for empirical therapy is guided by various factors including the severity of the illness, inpatient/outpatient therapy, presence of complications and local sensitivity patterns.

Current choice of empiric therapy is summarized in Table 11.13.

Once culture results are available, therapy can be modified. Cefixime should be continued for a period of 14 days; lesser duration of therapy is associated with relapse.

**Table 11.13:** Choice of antimicrobial therapy for enteric fever

| | *First line* | *Alternative* |
|---|---|---|
| Uncomplicated illness | Cefixime @ 20 mg/kg/day q 12 hourly (max 1200 mg) | Azithromycin 20 mg/kg/day q 24 hourly (max 1000 mg) |
| Severe illness | Ceftriaxone 100 mg/kg/day q 12 hourly (max 4 g) | Aztreonam 150 mg/kg/day q 8 hourly (max 6 g/day) |

Azithromycin should be continued for 7–10 days. In a patient on ceftriaxone, treatment can be switched to oral cefixime to complete 14 days of therapy. There is no data at present to support use of combination therapy in enteric fever. Recently extensively drug resistant *S. typhi* infections have been reported from Pakistan and Iraq. The use of carbapenems or azithromycin may be indicated in these cases.

Some patients with culture proven enteric fever do not defervesce by day 7 of treatment despite being on a susceptible drug. In such situations, drug fever, thrombophlebitis, coinfections, and complications should be suspected. If all are excluded, it implies clinical failure and treatment can be switched to an alternative agent. If cultures are negative and defervescence has not occurred by day 7, a thorough search for alternative etiology for fever should be made.

***Therapy of relapses:*** Relapse rates vary with the type of drug and are most common with beta lactams (ceftriaxone, cefixime) especially if shorter duration of therapy is used. Relapses may be satisfactorily treated with the same drug as used for primary therapy but for at appropriate dose and duration. Alternatively azithromycin may be used, if not used earlier.

### Prevention

The most effective and desirable method for preventing enteric fever is by improving hygiene and sanitation. This will yield additional dividends of reduction in the burden of other water-borne illnesses as well. Since this is unlikely in the near future in developing countries, vaccination is a major preventive strategy, as detailed in Chapter 10.

### Suggested Reading


1. Appiah CD, Hughes MJ, Chatham-Stephens K. Typhoid and paratyphoid fever. www.cdc.gov/typhoid-fever.
2. Basnyat B, Qamar FN, Rupali P, et al. Enteric fever. British Med J 2021;372:n437.
3. Kumar P, Kumar R. Enteric Fever. Indian J Pediatr. 2017;84(3):227–30.


## Leptospirosis

Leptospirosis is an emerging zoonotic disease of worldwide distribution, caused by spirochetes of the genus *Leptospira*. Most cases of leptospirosis occur in tropical and subtropical countries. While rats are the principal source of human infection, dogs, cats, livestock and wild animals are other important animal reservoirs. Infected animals may excrete spirochete in urine for several weeks. The survival of excreted organisms depends on the moisture content and temperature of the soil. Humans acquire infection after getting exposure to water or soil contaminated with rat urine. Agricultural workers, veterinarians, meat handlers, sewage workers, rodent control workers and laboratory personnel are at higher risk of getting infected because of occupational exposure. Infection is also common in the monsoons and during flooding.

### Pathogenesis

*Leptospira* enter the body through abrasions and cuts in skin or through mucous membranes, and spread to all organs hematogenously. The organisms damage the endothelial lining of small blood vessels, with leakage and extravasation of blood cells, hemorrhage, and ischemic damage to various organs including liver, kidneys, meninges and muscles.

### Clinical Features

Human infection with *Leptospira* may range from asymptomatic infection to a severe multiorgan involvement, which is often fatal. Symptomatic infection is relatively mild as an anicteric febrile illness in over 70% of patients; about 20% present as aseptic meningitis, while severe leptospirosis with hepatorenal dysfunction (Weil's disease) develops in 5–10% of individuals. The incubation period is usually 1–2 weeks.

The illness was earlier thought to be biphasic with an initial febrile phase characterized by high grade fever with rigors and chills, lethargy, severe myalgia, headache, nausea, vomiting. This is followed by a brief period of remission of symptoms followed by the development of complications. In clinical practice, however, most complicated cases of Weil's disease are uniphasic. Here along with high fever, there is jaundice, myositis and non-oliguric renal failure. There may be associated myocarditis, shock and acute respiratory distress syndrome, with high rates of mortality.

### Diagnosis

The complete blood count shows anemia, leukocytosis with polymorph predominance and thrombocytopenia. CRP is high, and liver enzymes are elevated with SGOT more than SGPT. The creatinine kinase level is high. In Weil's disease, there is elevated serum creatinine, deranged coagulation parameters and direct hyperbilirubinemia with elevated transaminases, but less than in viral hepatitis.

Specific diagnosis is established by serologic testing, microscopic demonstration of the organism or culture. The gold standard for serologic diagnosis is the microscopic agglutination test, which is only available in reference centres. Commercial kits for serologic diagnosis include rapid tests and IgM ELISA. These tests are positive after 5 days of illness. Cross reactivity and false positivity is seen with other infections like enteric fever and malaria. Demonstration of organism in tissues or urine by dark field microscopy or immunofluorescence, and cultures are not routinely available. *Leptospira* PCR is now commercially available with satisfactory sensitivity and specificity.

Leptospirosis should be differentiated from other febrile illnesses commonly seen in the monsoon season like malaria, dengue, enteric fever, acute viral hepatitis, rickettsial infections and hantavirus infections.

### Treatment

Treatment should be initiated as early as possible. For a severe case of leptospirosis, parenteral penicillin G (6–8 million U/m²/day IV; in 4 divided doses) for 7 days is the drug of choice. Ceftriaxone and IV tetracycline are also acceptable alternatives. For oral treatment, amoxicillin and doxycycline (in children above 8 years) are used.

### Prevention

Prevention entails avoidance of exposure to contaminated water. Doxycycline (200 mg orally, once weekly) is sometimes employed following short-term exposure to flood water; in children below 8 years azithromycin @10 mg/kg single dose may be used.

### Suggested Reading


1. Karpagam KB, Ganesh B. Leptospirosis: A neglected tropical zoonotic infection of public health importance. Eur J Clin Microbiol Infect Dis 2020;39:835–46.
2. Ministry of Health and Family Welfare. Program for prevention and control of leptospirosis, www.ncdc.gov.in
3. Tullu MS, Karande S. Leptospirosis in children: A review for family physicians. Indian J Med Sci 2009;63:368–78.


*Competency:* **PE34.16**

## Tetanus

Tetanus is caused by the bacterium *Clostridium tetani*, a spore forming, anerobic, gram-positive motile bacillus, found in human and animal feces. Its spores are widespread in the environment. The bacterium predominates in areas where soil is cultivated, in rural areas, in warm climates, and during summer months. Neonatal tetanus has been eliminated in India due to high rates of antenatal vaccination and clean delivery practices.

### Pathogenesis

*C. tetani* is a noninvasive organism. The spores of the organism remain nonpathogenic in soil or contaminated tissues until conditions are favorable for transformation into vegetative form. Transformation occurs in the presence of locally decreased oxygen reduction potential, typically in devitalized tissue, in the presence of a foreign body, trauma and crush injury and suppurative infections. Two types of toxins are produced by the organism—*tetanolysin* and *tetanospasmin*. *Tetanospasmin* is the main toxin responsible for manifestations of the disease. It binds to the neuromuscular junction at the site of injury, and undergoes retrograde axonal transport to reach the presynaptic nerve terminal where it prevents the release of inhibitory neurotransmitters, glycine and GABA leading to uncontrolled contraction of muscles.

### Clinical Features

Tetanus mainly affects the unimmunized and partly immunized individuals. The disease may occur in various forms: Neonatal, generalized, localized, and cephalic. The most common forms are generalized and neonatal tetanus.

***Generalized tetanus:*** It has an incubation period of approximately 8 days (range 2–14 days). Characteristically, there is descending paralysis, with initial involvement of the jaw muscles. There is spasm of the masseters leading to trismus or lockjaw. Subsequent involvement of the neck, back and abdominal muscles occurs, soon involving the whole body. As the disease progresses, minimal stimuli may lead to generalized spasms, which are the hallmark of the disease, and contribute to serious complications and eventually death. Typically, the sensorium of the patient is preserved. There is difficulty in swallowing. Autonomic instability may occur, with blood pressure fluctuations in the form of hypertension or hypotension, diaphoresis and arrhythmias. Recovery usually begins after 3 weeks and approximately takes four weeks. Recovery from tetanus occurs by sprouting new nerve terminals in the spinal cord leading to relaxation of the contracted muscles.

***Neonatal tetanus:*** In neonatal tetanus, symptoms appear by the third day after birth; symptoms are not seen in the first two days of life and rarely after the age of two weeks. Excessive unexplained crying followed by refusal of feeds and apathy are the common initial symptoms. The baby develops progressive feeding difficulty, becomes rigid, develops paralysis, and may develop opisthotonic posturing and experience painful spasms. The mouth is kept slightly open due to pull and spasm of the neck (Fig. 11.27). Reflex spasm of the masseter makes feeding painful. Pharyngeal muscles go into spasm and cause dysphagia and choking, lockjaw or reflex trismus followed by spasms of limbs. There is generalized rigidity and opisthotonus in extension. Spasm of larynx and respiratory muscles are characteristically induced by stimuli such as touch, noise and bright light, resulting in episodes of apnea and cyanosis. Constipation persists until the spasms are relieved. Intercurrent infections, dehydration and acidosis may complicate the clinical picture. It has a very high case fatality rate of 70 to 100%.

***Localized tetanus:*** It is less severe in comparison, and is characterized by rigidity and pain confined to the muscles adjacent to the wound. It may lead to generalized tetanus later. In patients with isolated localized tetanus, the mortality is less than 1%. Cephalic tetanus is a form of local

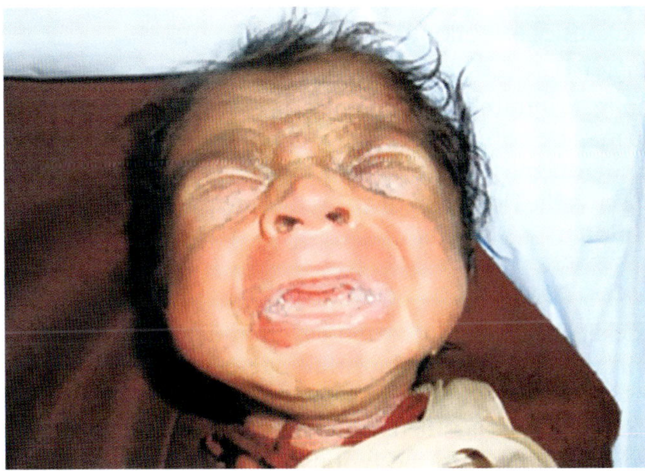

**Fig. 11.27:** Neonatal tetanus (*Courtesy:* Dr Amarjeet Mehta, Jaipur)

tetanus, which occurs due to injury of the bulbar muscles. It has a poor prognosis.

### *Treatment*

Most patients require intensive care management and good supportive care. The aims of treatment are airway maintenance, prevention of further toxin absorption, relieving clinical features, e.g. spasms, controlling autonomic instability and antibiotics. Airway management may require intubation and mechanical ventilation, especially in severe cases and if the infant gets frequent episodes of largyngeal spasms, apneic attacks with cyanosis or central respiratory failure. Neutralization of free toxin is done by administering human tetanus immunoglobulin (TIG); however, antitoxin cannot dislodge the toxin already fixed to the nerve roots. The usual dose is 3000 IU administered IM or intrathecally. Antibiotic therapy is needed to abolish the bacteria from the wound site. The commonly used antibiotics are crystalline penicillin or metronidazole.

Management of spasms is accomplished with diazepam and paralytic agents. Supportive care includes maintaining adequate hydration, early detection of myoglobinuria, prevention of renal shutdown and prevention of infections. All patients should receive a complete course of immunization with tetanus toxoid once recovered, as the disease does not induce protective antibodies.

### *Prevention*

Immunization with tetanus toxoid leads to induction of protective antibodies, and is discussed in Chapter 10. Maternal and neonatal tetanus can be effectively prevented by immunizing the mother during pregnancy, and ensuring clean delivery and cord care.

### Suggested Reading


1. Okoromah CN, Lesi FE. Diazepam for treating tetanus. Cochrane Database Syst Rev 2004; CD003954.
2. Rodrigo C, Fernando D, Rajapakase S. Pharmacological management of tetanus: An evidence based review. Critical Care 2014;18:217.
3. Yen LM, Thwaites CL. Tetanus. Lancet 2019; 393:1657–68.


*Competency:* **PE34.20**

## Rickettsial Infections

Rickettsial diseases are a group of febrile illnesses caused by obligate intracellular gram-negative bacilli and transmitted to man by arthropod vectors. Rickettsial diseases are often underdiagnosed due to poor awareness. Here we briefly discuss the rickettsial diseases that are prevalent in Indian children.

### *Etiopathogenesis and Epidemiology*

Rickettsia are a group of motile, gram-negative, non-spore forming highly pleomorphic bacteria that present as cocci, rods or thread-like obligate intracellular parasites. Rickettsia are classified on the basis of clinical features and epidemiology into the typhus group (epidemic typhus, endemic typhus and scrub typhus), the spotted fever group (Rocky mountain spotted fever, Indian spotted fever), Q fever, trench fever and ehlirichiosis. Scrub typhus caused by *R. tsutsugamushi*, Indian spotted fever caused by *R. conorii*, and Q fever caused by *C. burnetti* are prevalent in India. Cases have been reported from all states chiefly from rural and forested areas and occasionally also from urban areas.

Scrub typhus is transmitted by bite of the trombiculid mite, and Indian spotted fever by ticks. Rickettsial disease is due to invasion of the endothelial region of the vasculature and subsequent microvasculitis. This process especially affects the brain, cardiac and skeletal muscle, skin, liver, lungs and kidneys.

### *Clinical Manifestations*

Incubation period in children varies from 2 to 14 days. A history of exposure to tick, history of origin from an endemic area or a similar illness in family members may be forthcoming. Severity of manifestations varies from a mild, self-limiting illness to a life-threatening disease.

Initially, patients present with headache, very high fever, anorexia, myalgias, restlessness, calf muscle pain and tenderness. Gastrointestinal symptoms include abdominal pain, nausea, vomiting, and diarrhea. Skin rash is usually not present until after 2–4 days of illness. The typical triad of fever, headache and rash is observed in only half of the patients. In spotted fever, rash is initially discrete pale rose red blanching macules or maculopapules on the extremities including the ankles, wrist, or lower limbs. Later, the rash spreads rapidly to involve the entire body including palms and soles and becomes more petechial sometimes with palpable purpura **(Fig. 11.28a)**. In severe form of the disease, petechiae may enlarge into ecchymosis, which can become necrotic **(Fig. 11.28b)**. Severe vaso-occlusive disease secondary to rickettsial vasculitis and thrombosis is infrequent but can result in gangrene of the digits, toes, earlobes, scrotum, nose or entire limbs. In scrub typhus, rash is seen initially on trunk or may not be present at all. Scrub typhus is characterized by presence of a painless eschar, the *tache noire*, at the initial site of tick attachment in 25–50% of cases. It is often present in the genital area, under breasts, axilla and may be missed, if the patient is not examined carefully.

Complications may involve any organ systems and include encephalopathy, pulmonary edema, myocarditis, acute kidney injury and vascular collapse.

### *Laboratory Diagnosis*

Laboratory findings are usually non-specific. Total leukocyte count may be initially normal or low but leukocytosis develops as the disease progresses. Anemia, thrombocytopenia, hyponatremia and elevated serum aminotransferases are some other features. CSF findings are usually normal.

Specific diagnosis of a rickettsial illness is most often confirmed by serological testing. Serological evidence of infection occurs not earlier than the second week of illness in any of the rickettsial diseases and hence a specific diagnosis may not be available until after the patient has fully

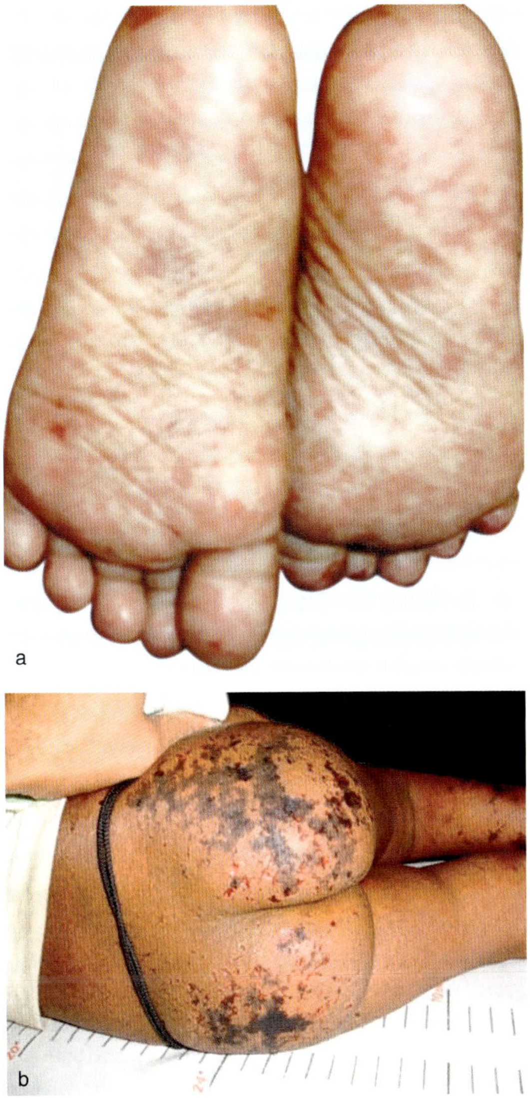

Fig. 11.28: Rash in rickettsial infection; (a) Maculopapular rash on the soles, (b) Necrotic rash on the buttocks, in a patient with spotted fever (*Courtesy:* Dr Atul Kulkarni, Sholapur)

recovered or worsened. The gold standard for serodiagnosis of rickettsial disease is the immunofluorescence assay for detection of IgG and IgM. However, it is expensive and not widely available. ELISA is specific and sensitive allowing detection of IgG and IgM antibodies. Detection of IgM antibodies to scrub typhus and Indian spotted fever, now available in India, is the preferred test for diagnosis. The Weil-Felix test depends on detection of antibodies to various *Proteus* species containing OX antigens, with cross reacting epitopes to antigens from members of the genus *Rickettsia*. It is widely available, but has only 50% sensitivity and specificity. PCR on tissues for rickettsia is available in research labs.

If clinical suspicion for rickettsia is high, then empirical therapy should begin without waiting for any confirmatory test.

#### *Differential Diagnosis*

Spotted fever can mimic a number of febrile illnesses. These include meningococcemia, malaria, dengue, measles, typhoid fever, secondary syphilis, leptospirosis, toxic shock syndrome, scarlet fever, rubella, Kawasaki disease, parvovirus B19 infection, idiopathic thrombocytopenic purpura, thrombotic thrombocytopenic purpura, hemolytic uremic syndrome, Henoch-Schonlein purpura (IgA vasculitis), hepatitis, and infectious mononucleosis.

#### *Treatment*

Since no reliable diagnostic test is available to confirm rickettsial infection in the early stage, initial diagnosis and suitable treatment should be based on a high index of suspicion and appropriate clinical, epidemiological and laboratory findings.

Doxycycline is the drug of choice for all age groups. The therapy should be continued for a minimum of 5–7 days and for at least 3 days until the patient is a febrile in order to avoid relapse. Patients usually become afebrile within 48 hours and thus the entire therapy lasts for less than 10 days. In patients with severe disease, admission to an intensive care unit and appropriate supportive therapy is required. Alternative drugs for mild disease include azithromycin and rifampicin.

#### *Prevention*

No vaccines are available. Known tick infested areas should be avoided. Daily inspection of body for ticks is particularly important. Disinfection of dogs will minimize the tick population. Health education of people about mode of transmission by ticks and means of personal protection is equally important. Prophylactic antimicrobial therapy is not recommended.

### Suggested Reading


1. Rahi M, Gupte MD, Bhargava A, Varghese GM. DMR-ICMR Guidelines for diagnosis and management of rickettsial diseases in India. Indian J Med Res 2015;141:417–22.
2. Rathi N, Kulkarni A, Yewale V; for Indian Academy of Pediatrics. IAP guidelines on rickettsial diseases in children. Indian Pediatr 2017;54:223–29.
3. Sood AK, Sachdeva A. Rickettsioses in children—a review. Indian J Pediatr 2020;87:930–36.


## Mycoplasma Infections

#### *Etiology*

Mycoplasma are the smallest of free living life forms with characteristics somewhere between bacteria and viruses. The most important species causing human disease is *M. pneumoniae*. The genital mycoplasmas (*M. hominis* and *Ureaplasma urealyticum*) are associated with genital tract disease in adults and sometimes neonatal disease.

#### *Epidemiology*

Newborns can get infected by genital mycoplasmas during delivery. Some studies show *U. urealyticum* as only second to respiratory syncytial virus as a cause of neonatal sepsis. *M. pneumoniae* can infect children of any age but disease is uncommon below 3–5 years. In school-aged children and adolescents, it causes up to 30–40% of all community acquired pneumonias; almost 20% of such pneumonias requre hospitalization.

### Clinical Manifestations

The chief manifestations of mycoplasma disease are low grade fever, cough, headache, malaise, pharyngitis, rhinorrhea and sometimes otitis media. Pneumonia is associated with few clinical signs and is of varying severity. Patients rarely appear ill and hence the term "walking pneumonia". There is marked disparity between the clinical symptoms and signs and the radiographic picture. The radiographic picture is variable; the most common finding is thickened bronchial shadow, streaks of interstitial infiltration, and areas of atelectasis primarily in lower lobes. One-third children have hilar adenopathy. Pleural effusions occur in 5–20% of the cases. In some children, fulminant pneumonia and respiratory failure may occur.

Extrapulmonary manifestations can coexist, follow or occur independently of respiratory disease and include dermatologic manifestations (morbilliform rash, papulovesicular exanthem, erythema nodosum, erythema multiforme, or Stevens-Johnson syndrome), and neurologic manifestations (encephalitis, aseptic meningitis, transverse myelitis, peripheral neuropathies, and radiculopathies). Cold-antibody mediated immune hemolytic anemia may have variable severity. Rarely the gastrointestinal tract, heart, kidneys and joints may be involved.

Neonates with genital mycoplasma infection may present with cough, wheezing or sepsis, meningitis and brain abscess.

### Diagnosis

Complete blood count shows anemia, leukocytosis with neutrophilia and elevated ESR. Liver transaminases can be mildly elevated. Cold agglutinins may be present and a high titer is considered significant. Specific diagnosis is most commonly done by demonstration of anti-*Mycoplasma* IgM by ELISA. IgM antibodies appear usually 7 days after infection and may be negative in early disease. They remain elevated for a long time and hence have low specificity. Most multiplex PCR kits for diagnosis of respiratory infections include *Mycoplasma*.

### Treatment

Since mycoplasma lack cell walls, all cell wall active antibiotics including beta lactams are inactive. The role of anti-*Mycoplasma* therapy in improving the outcome of pneumonia is controversial. However, empiric treatment for *Mycoplasma* should be initiated in children above age 5 years presenting with:

- Clinical features of pneumonia
- Pneumonia not responding to standard beta lactam therapy
- Severe or very severe pneumonia.

Macrolides are the drugs of choice for *Mycoplasma*. Recommended regimens include azithromycin 10 mg/kg in one dose on the first day and 5 mg/kg in one dose for four days, clarithromycin 15 mg/kg per day in two divided doses for 10 days, or erythromycin 30 to 40 mg/kg per day in four divided doses for 10 days. In children older than 8 years, tetracycline 20 to 50 mg/kg per day in four divided doses (maximum daily dose 1 to 2 g) and doxycycline 2 to 4 mg/kg per day in one or two divided doses (maximum daily dose 100 to 200 mg) for 10 days also are effective.

Extrapulmonary mycoplasma infection is often immune-mediated and may need other therapeutic modalities including steroids, plasmapheresis apart from antimicrobial therapy.

### Suggested Reading


1. Colin AA, Yousef S, Forno E, Korppi M. Treatment of mycoplasma pneumoniae in pediatric lower respiratory infection. Pediatrics. 2014; 133:1124–25.
2. Krafft C, Christy C. Mycoplasma pneumonia in children and adolescents. Pediatr Rev 2020;41:12–19.


## FUNGAL INFECTIONS

Fungi have become increasingly common cause of disease in humans. Superficial fungal infections are discussed in Chapter 27. Here, we discuss some of the common and serious invasive fungal infections, viz. invasive candidiasis, aspergillosis, mucormycosis, cryptococcosis and endemic fungal infections. Invasive fungal infections are assuming increasing importance, due to increase in the critically ill and immunocompromised population.

### Invasive Candidiasis

Candida is a yeast with major species being *C. albicans*, *C. tropicalis*, *C. parapsilosis*, *C. krusei*, *C. glabrata*, and others. *C. auris* is emerging as an important cause of candidiasis in ICUs. Invasive infections with *Candida* happen usually as nosocomial infections in individuals with impaired defenses. Children at risk for invasive candidiasis include neonates, children in PICU and children with cancer.

While neonatal candidiasis is usually seen in preterm and extremely or very low birth weight babies, it is also being reported in term babies in India. The presenting features are those of neonatal sepsis. The disease tends to disseminate widely to the brain and kidneys. Diagnosis is established by blood cultures, examination of urine for budding yeasts, and ultrasonography kidneys for fungal balls. Lumbar puncture and CSF examination are mandatory to rule out meningitis. The drug of choice is amphotericin B deoxycholate and treatment for 2 weeks, after last negative culture is recommended; longer therapy is needed if there is meningitis. Prevention against neonatal candidiasis entails good infection control practices. Use of fluconazole twice or thrice weekly in extremely low birth weight babies in NICU with high rates of candidiasis is recommended.

Candida is among the top pathogens causing bloodstream infections in the PICU and in neutropenic children. Risk factors for *Candida* bloodstream infection include central lines, neutropenia, mucositis, prolonged ICU stay, use of antimicrobials, immunosuppressive therapy, gut surgery, total parenteral nutrition, mechanical ventilation and multifocal colonization with *Candida*. Clinical presentation is indistinguishable from bacterial sepsis. Since the sensitivity of blood cultures is around 50%, high index of suspicion and early empiric therapy is important. Choice of empiric therapy depends on local epidemiology and local prevalence of azole-resistant fungi and may include fluconazole, liposomal amphotericin B, or echinocandins (caspofungin, micafungin). Source control and removal of the central line especially in the non-neutropenic population is crucial.

### Aspergillosis

*Aspergillus* is a ubiquitously distributed filamented fungus; the two common species causing human infection are *A. fumigatus* and *A. flavus*. Invasive aspergillosis occurs usually in the immunocompromised. Common predisposing factors include children on cancer undergoing chemotherapy and resultant neutropenia, stem cell or solid organ transplant recipients, patients on other immunosuppressive drugs and children with primary immunodeficiency disorders such as chronic granulomatous disease. Common sites of involvement are the lungs and sinuses. Clinical symptoms and signs depend on the site of involvement. Diagnosis is primarily by radiology (CT chest which shows nodular lesions with surrounding halo; Fig. 11.29) and histopathologic demonstration of the invasive hyphae in samples and culture. Galactomannan estimation in serum and bronchoalveolar lavage samples has emerged as a useful diagnostic test. The medication of choice is voriconazole. Other options are isavuconazole, amphotericin B and echinocandins. Fluconazole has no activity against *Aspergillus*.

### Mucormycosis

Mucormycosis refers to infection with the filamented fungi of the family Mucorales. The hyphae are broad and aseptate unlike those of Aspergillus that are narrow and septate. Mucormycosis is an invasive infection that primarily occurs in patients with risk factors such as diabetic ketoacidosis, cancer chemotherapy, transplant recipients, iron overload and receipt of immunosuppressive drugs. Recently, India witnessed a surge of mucormycosis cases in patients with COVID-19. The sites of involvement are mainly the nasal sinuses with orbit and less commonly pulmonary, gastrointestinal and skin/soft tissue. Infection can sometimes occur due to direct inoculation in traumatic or surgical wounds, and injection sites. Clinical features depend on the site involved; in the rhinoorbital form pain, swelling, bloody nasal discharge, tooth/jaw pain and presence of blackish eschars on palate are the usual presenting features (Fig. 11.30). Diagnosis is established by imaging of the affected area and nasal endoscopy. Confirmation of diagnosis is by demonstration of the characteristic hyphae on histopathology and cultures. Treatment includes radical surgical debridement, antifungal therapy with amphotericin B and correction of underlying predisposing factors. Other effective medications include posoconazole and isavuconazole. The disease is associated with mortality rates averaging around 50%.

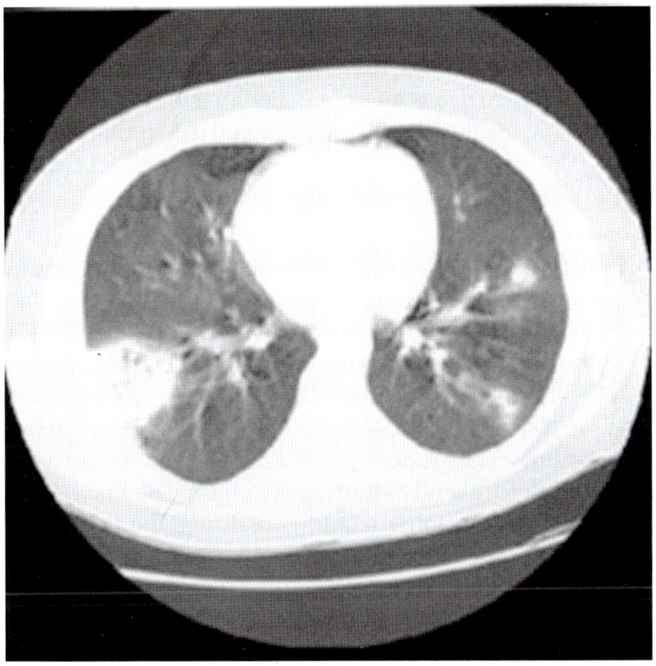

Fig. 11.29: CT scan showing multiple nodules with irregular borders, internal cavitation and surrounding halo suggestive of invasive aspergillosis

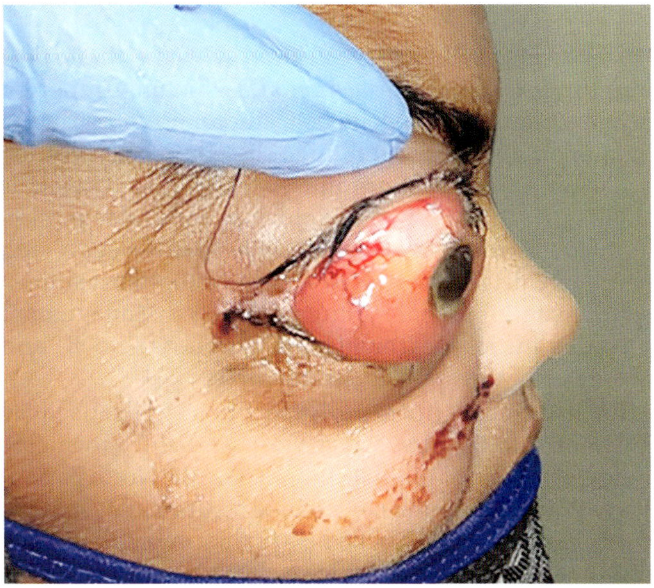

Fig. 11.30: Proptosis due to rhinoorbital mucormycosis in a 14-year-old girl following COVID-19 (*Courtesy:* Department of Ophthalmology, Dr RN Cooper Hospital, Mumbai)

### Cryptococcosis

Infection with *Cryptococcus neoformans* is most commonly seen in HIV-infected individuals with advanced immunosuppression. It can also occur in other immunocompromised states and rarely in immunocompetent individuals. The disease most often affects the central nervous system; pulmonary and disseminated forms are less common. Clinical symptoms include headache, vomiting, altered sensorium, signs of meningism and less commonly neurologic deficits. The diagnosis is confirmed by demonstrating cryptococci in the CSF by India ink, cryptococcal antigen testing and fungal culture. CSF is usually under increased pressure and has high protein with pleocytosis. Treatment includes antifungal therapy with amphotericin B and flucytosine for 2–6 weeks, followed by fluconazole for prolonged periods. Reduction of elevated pressure by serial lumbar punctures is also crucial.

## Endemic Fungal Infections

Histoplasmosis is due to infection with the dimorphic fungus *Histoplasma capsulatum* and is mainly reported in India from the Gangetic belt. Infection occurs due to inhalation and is self-limiting. Disseminated infection occurs in immunocompromised hosts and disease is characterized by fever, weight loss, oral ulcers, skin lesions, gastrointestinal symptoms, splenomegaly and pancytopenia. Diagnosis is by a urine histoplasma antigen test, tissue biopsy and fungal cultures. Management includes initial treatment with amphotericin B, and maintenance therapy with itraconazole.

Talaromycosis (formerly penicilliosis) is caused by a dimorphic fungus *Talaromyces marneffei* (formerly *Penicillium marneffei*) and is reported from the North Eastern states in India. Disseminated disease occurs mainly in those with advanced HIV infection and rarely in other severely immunocompromised states. Clinical manifestations include fever, weight loss, respiratory symptoms, hepatosplenomegaly, lymphadenopathy, diarrhea and skin lesions. Diagnosis is by culture and treatment includes antifungals such as amphotericin B, itraconazole and fluconazole for prolonged periods.

### Suggested Reading

1. Downes KJ, Fisher BT, Zane NR. Administration and dosing of systemic antifungal agents in pediatric patients. Pediatr Drugs 2020; 22:165–88.
2. Otto WR, Green AM. Fungal infections in children with haematologic malignancies and stem cell transplant recipients. Br J Haematol 2020; 189:607–24.
3. Weimer KED, Smith PB, Puia-Dumitrescu M, Aleem S. Invasive fungal infections in neonates: A review. Pediatr Res 2022;91: 404–12.

*Competency:* **PE34.19**

# PROTOZOAL INFECTIONS

## Malaria

Malaria the most important protozoal disease of man is caused by the genus *Plasmodium*. There are four species pathogenic to man, *P. vivax*, *P. falciparum*, *P. malariae* and *P. ovale* of which the first two occur in India. *P. knowlesi*, a primate pathogen, has been infrequently reported to cause human disease.

### *Epidemiology*

Malaria is currently endemic in 87 countries. While the global burden of malaria is declining due to vector control measures, it still causes more than 200 million cases and 400,000 deaths annually. Sub-Saharan Africa is responsible for 93% of the global burden and deaths. Most of the deaths happen in children below age 5 and in pregnant women. The COVID-19 pandemic has caused substantial disruption and setback to malaria control measures across the world, including Africa.

In India, as per WHO estimates, there are 6 million cases and 10,000 deaths annually. Seventy percent of the cases are due to *P. falciparum* and 30% due to *P. vivax*. The states with the highest burden of malaria are Orissa (25%), Chhattisgarh (13%), West Bengal (11%), Jharkhand (7%) and Karnataka (7%). About 10% cases are reported from the urban areas, due to construction activities, population migration, and inappropriate water storage and disposal. The National Vector Borne Disease Control Program (NVBDCP) aims to eliminate malaria in India by 2030.

### *Transmission*

The infectious stage of the parasite, the sporozoite, is transmitted to the host by the bite of the female anopheline mosquito. Six species of anopheline mosquitoes are important in the transmission of the disease in India, namely *Anopheles culicifacies* (rural), *A. fluvitalis*, *A. stephensi* (urban), *A. minimus*, *A. philippinesis* and *A. sundaicus*. *Anopheles* bites mainly in evening, night or early morning unlike *Aedes* which bites mainly during the day. To enable development of parasites in the vector's body and make it capable of transmitting the disease, the vector must be susceptible, feed on human blood and live at least for 10–12 days after an infective blood meal. The vector should be present in large number or sufficient density to be of importance. Resting habits of the mosquito are important for planning control measures. Mosquitoes usually breed in edges of streams, water tanks, pits, cisterns and overhead tanks. *A. stephensi* breed in wells, cisterns, fountains and overhead tanks, *A. fluviatilis* in moving water and *A. sundaicus* in brackish water. Breeding sites such as burrowed pits, pools, ponds, marshy areas and unregulated irrigation channels are conducive to mosquito breeding and spread of malaria. Mosquitoes thrive best in temperature between 20 and 30°C, relative humidity 60% and in areas with good rainfall. The peak transmission season of malaria is between July and November. Malaria is uncommon at altitudes over 2000 m above sea level.

Efficient vectors are those that have bite humans in preference to cattle, have high biting rates and where the duration of sporogony is shorter and who are long lived (hence they outlive sporogony). More efficient the vector, greater the burden of malaria; *A. gambiae* the vector in Sub-Saharan Africa is a very efficient vector and is largely responsible for the huge burden of malaria in that area.

### *Life Cycle of the Parasite*

#### ***Humans***

- *Hepatic or tissue phase:* When an infectious mosquito bites a human, it injects sporozoites, which circulate and invade hepatocytes and reticuloendothelial tissues within 30 minutes of the bite. During hepatic infection, *P. vivax* produces 2000–15000 merozoites and *P. falciparum* produces 40000 merozoites by repeated divisions. These merozoites are released and invade erythrocytes at end of the hepatic phase. The first hepatic phase is asymptomatic and constitutes the incubation period. This cycle lasts at least 10 days (1–2 weeks for falciparum infection).
- *Erythrocytic phase:* After replication in the liver (exoerythrocytic schizogony), the parasites undergo asexual multiplication in the erythrocytes (erythrocytic schizogony). In erythrocytes, parasites develop into ring forms, mature trophozoites and then multinucleated

schizonts, which rupture and release more merozoites. Repeated cycles of erythrocyte invasion and rupture lead to chills, fever, headache, fatigue, nonspecific symptoms and, with severe malaria, signs of organ dysfunction.

A key feature of the life cycle of *P. falciparum* is cytoadherence, whereby erythrocytes infected with mature parasites adhere to endothelial cells in the microvasculature. This process is presumably advantageous to the parasite, since it prevents the passage of abnormal erythrocytes through the spleen. High concentrations of *P. falciparum* infected erythrocytes in the microvasculature and a complex interplay of host and parasite factors lead to the manifestations of severe malaria, including cerebral malaria, noncardiogenic pulmonary edema and acute kidney injury. Because of the ability of mature *P. falciparum* organisms in the erythrocytic stage to adhere to endothelial cells, only ring forms circulate (except in very severe infections), and levels of peripheral parasitemia may be low despite substantial infection.

- *Gametocytic phase:* After several stages of schizogony, some merozoites are converted to gametocytes which are taken up by the mosquitoes. They do not cause symptoms but are responsible for transmission of malaria.
- *Exoerythrocytic phase:* Termination of the erythrocytic schizogony does not necessarily terminate the infection with malaria because merozoites of *P. vivax/P. ovale/P. malariae*, but not those of *P. falciparum*, may go into, a dormant stage (hypnozoite) in the liver and cause relapses by invading the bloodstream weeks or even years later. This intermittent release of schizonts in case of *P. vivax* and *P. ovale* may last for 2–3 years and for *P. malariae* for 10–20 years.

***Mosquito:*** The gametocytes are ingested by an *Anopheles* mosquito during a blood meal. Only the gametocyte forms survive in the stomach of the mosquito; all other stages are destroyed. The parasites' multiplication in the mosquito is known as the sporogonic cycle. While in the mosquito's stomach, fertilization of female gametes generates motile and elongated zygotes (ookinetes) that invade the midgut wall and develop into oocysts (resting stage). These oocysts grow, rupture and release sporozoites, which make their way to the salivary glands. Inoculation of the sporozoites into a new human host perpetuates the malaria life cycle.

### Immunity Against Malaria

Innate resistance in malaria may be due to differences in the surface receptor, intraerythrocytic factors or yet unknown causes. Epidemiologic observations suggest that patients with sickle cell trait, thalassemia and glucose-6-phosphate dehydrogenase deficiency are relatively immune to malaria. Homozygotes of sickle cell disease are not protected from malaria but heterozygotes are immune. Variations in HLA frequency may also determine the prevalence of malaria.

Acquired immunity against malaria is both cell mediated and humoral. The first response to malarial infection is *phagocytosis* in the spleen or the hyperplastic reticuloendothelial cells of the parasitized erythrocytes. IgM antibodies against the merozoites help in opsonophagocytosis of the RBC in spleen. Malarial immunity in endemic areas increases with age and disappears when the individual leaves the endemic area, a phenomenon known as premunition.

### Clinical Features

The clinical manifestations and severity of malaria depend largely on the species of the parasite and endemicity of disease. Most cases of severe or complicated malaria are due to *P. falciparum*; recently there is an increasing number of reports due to severe disease by *P. vivax*. In highly endemic areas with "stable malaria" such as Sub-Saharan Africa, children below 5 years are most affected with severe anemia and cerebral malaria being prominent manifestations. In areas of lower endemicity, all ages including children and young adults are affected.

The incubation period of malaria varies between 9 and 30 days, being the least for *P. falciparum* and the longest for *P. malariae* infections. The onset of the disease is not as characteristic as is believed, especially in infections with *P. falciparum*. The onset of the disease is sudden with fever, headache, loss of appetite, lassitude and pain in the limbs. The fever may be continuous or remittent for several days before it becomes classically intermittent. The illness, then, is characterized by a *cold stage* (chills and rigors with headache, nausea, malaise and anorexia); *hot stage* (dry flushed skin, rapid respiration and marked thirst); and *sweating stage* (temperature falls by crisis). In most cases, however, the classic intermittent fever is not seen in children.

On basis of severity, malaria is classified as "complicated or severe" and uncomplicated malaria which has treatment and prognostic implication. Severe malaria can affect virtually every organ system (Table 11.14) and has a mortality rate of approximately 20%. Any of the criteria, if present with asexual parasitemia with *P. falciparum* or *P. vivax*, classifies malaria as severe and should be treated as such.

### Diagnosis

***Specific diagnosis:*** The gold standard for diagnosis is careful examination of a properly prepared thick film. Thick smears have sensitivity of detecting 5–10 parasites/μL. Thin smears have a lower sensitivity of 200 parasites/μL, but enable species identification (Fig. 11.31). Microscopy also provides information about the parasite load (infected RBC/total RBC), prognosis (mature schizonts and pigmented neutrophils indicate a poor prognosis) and tracks response to therapy. Additionally, peripheral smears are inexpensive and readily available. The main drawback is need for expertise and that they are time consuming (a careful examination of 100 fields needs 20 minutes). Sometimes peripheral smears may be negative due to partial antimalarial treatment or sequestration of parasitized cells in deep vascular beds. Repeating smears every 6–8 hourly at least three times is recommended if the clinical suspicion for malaria is high and the initial smear is negative.

*Rapid diagnostic tests* detect malaria antigens (PfHRP2/pLDH/aldolase) from asexual and/or sexual forms of

**Table 11.14:** Manifestations of severe malaria

| |
|---|
| *Impaired consciousness:* Glasgow Coma Score <11 in adults; Blantyre Coma Score <3 in children |
| *Prostration:* Generalized weakness so that the person is unable to sit, stand or walk without assistance |
| *Multiple convulsions:* More than two episodes within 24 hours |
| *Acidosis:* Base deficit >8 mEq/L, bicarbonate <15 mEq/L, or venous plasma lactate ≥5 mmol/L. Severe acidosis manifests clinically as respiratory distress (rapid, deep, labored breathing) |
| *Hypoglycemia:* Blood or plasma glucose <2.2 mmol/L (<40 mg/dL) |
| *Severe anemia:* Hemoglobin concentration ≤5 g/dL, or hematocrit ≤15% in children <12 years old (<7 g/dL and <20%, respectively, in adults) with a parasite count >10 000/µL |
| *Kidney impairment:* Plasma or serum creatinine >265 µmol/L (3 mg/dL) or blood urea >20 mmol/L (120 mg/dL) |
| *Jaundice:* Plasma or serum bilirubin >50 µmol/L (3 mg/dL) with a parasite count >100 000/µL |
| *Pulmonary edema:* Radiologically confirmed, or oxygen saturation <92% on room air with a respiratory rate >30/min, often with chest indrawing and crepitations on auscultation |
| *Significant bleeding:* Including recurrent or prolonged bleeding from the nose, gums or venepuncture sites; hematemesis or melena |
| *Shock:* Compensated shock is defined as capillary refill ≥3 s, or temperature gradient on leg (mid to proximal limb), but no hypotension |
| *Decompensated shock* is defined as systolic blood pressure <70 mm Hg in children or <80 mm Hg in adults, with evidence of impaired perfusion (cool peripheries or prolonged capillary refill) |
| *Hyperparasitemia: P. falciparum* parasitemia >10% |

the parasite as color changes on antibody coated lines on the strips. In general, these are quick and simple to use, distinguish between the major forms of human malaria, and are useful when reliable microscopy is not available. Disadvantages include cost, lower sensitivity than microscopy (detect 100–200 parasites/µL), variation in quality from batch to batch and need for rigorous storage conditions. In addition, they do not give information about the parasite load and cannot be used to monitor response to therapy.

*Polymerase chain reaction* (PCR) is highly sensitive and specific for detecting all species of malaria, particularly in cases of low level parasitemia. The limit of detection is 5 parasites/µL. It is, however, expensive and can be positive for some time after treatment. It is now available commercially and may be used when disease suspicion is high, and smears and rapid antigen tests are negative.

***Investigations that are useful for management:*** These include complete hemogram, and blood levels of glucose, electrolytes, pH, bicarbonate, anion gap, lactate PT and PTT, bilirubin, transaminases and creatinine. Urinalysis is done in patients with acute kidney injury. Blood cultures should be sent in patients presenting with shock. Repeated assessments of blood glucose are very important. CNS imaging is indicated in children presenting with suspected cerebral malaria, and shows significant brain swelling patients. The WHO recommends that a lumbar puncture should be done in patients presenting with acute febrile encephalopathy, even if asexual parasitemia is demonstrated in the peripheral smear. This is true in the African context where asymptomatic parasitemia with *P. falciparum* is fairly common and hence it is difficult to establish a cause effect relationship. In Indian, a lumbar puncture is not required, if the smear diagnosis of falciparum malaria is unequivocal.

### Differential Diagnosis

Common differential diagnoses include other tropical and monsoon infections such as typhoid fever, leptospirosis, dengue, viral hepatitis, rickettsial infections and chikungunya. Cerebral malaria should be differentiated from other causes of acute febrile encephalopathy, such as meningitis and encephalitis. Patients with algid malaria (those in shock) mimic meningococcemia and gram-negative shock.

### Treatment of Uncomplicated Malaria

In a setting of suspected uncomplicated malaria, establishing a lab diagnosis is a must before giving empirical therapy. This is to prevent irrational therapy and consequent drug resistance and also to avoid missing other causes of fever.

***Vivax malaria:*** The drug of choice for managing vivax malaria is still chloroquine (Table 11.15). Resistance to

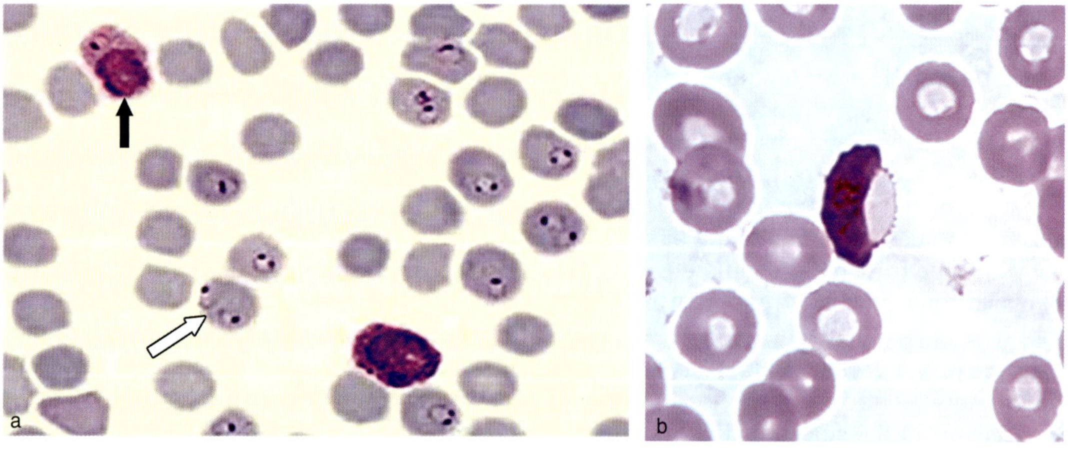


**Fig. 11.31:** Peripheral smear in diagnosis of malaria: (a) Trophozoites of *P. vivax* (black arrow) and *P. falciparum* (white arrow) indicating mixed infection; (b) Gametocyte of *P. falciparum*

**Table 11.15:** Drug doses for oral antimalarial drugs

| *Drug* | *Oral dose* |
|---|---|
| Chloroquine (Tablets 250 mg salt with 150 mg of base; syrup 50 mg of base/ 5 mL) | 10 mg/kg of base loading and then 10 mg/kg after 24 hr and then 5 mg/kg at 48 hr |
| Primaquine (7.5/15 mg tablets) | 0.25–0.75 mg/kg |
| Artemether lumefantrine (Tablets having 20 mg artemether and 120 mg lumefantrine; syrup having similar constituents per 5 mL) | 5–14 kg, 15–24 kg, 25–34 kg and >34 kg: 1, 2, 3 and 4 tablets, respectively at 0, 8, 24, 36, 48 and 60 hours<br>1.7 mg/kg of the artemether component twice daily for 3 days |
| Artemether (50 mg tablets) | 4 mg/kg/day single dose |
| Mefloquine (250 mg tablets) | 25 mg/kg given as two doses, of 15 mg/kg and 10 mg/kg 8 hours apart |
| Pyrimethamine sulfadoxine (25 mg pyrimethamine and 500 mg sulfadoxine tablet) | 1.25 mg/kg of pyrimethamine (maximum 75 mg) single dose |
| Doxycycline (100, 200 mg tablets) | 3.5 mg/kg/day |
| Clindamycin (300 mg capsule) | 10 mg/kg/day twice daily |
| Quinine (Tablets having 300 mg of salt) | 10 mg/kg of salt thrice daily |

chloroquine has been rarely reported in India. The total dose is 25 mg/kg; first dose given as 10 mg/kg and then 10 mg/kg at 24 hours and 5 mg/kg at 48 hours. Fever should be brought down before giving chloroquine to reduce the risk of vomiting. Radical therapy with primaquine is indicated for vivax malaria to eliminate the exoerythrocytic stages in liver and reduce risk of relapses. Primaquine also has schizonticidal effect and due to this effect functions as combination therapy for vivax malaria along with chloroquine; G6PD level should be checked prior to administering primaquine. The dose of primaquine is 0.25–0.3 mg/kg/day for 14 days. The risk of relapse is reduced significantly following therapy with primaquine. For patients who relapse despite primaquine, higher doses of 0.5 or 0.75 mg/kg may be used. Primaquine is contraindicated in infants, pregnant and breastfeeding women and those with G6PD deficiency. For patients with mild G6PD deficiency, primaquine may be given at a lower dose (0.75 mg/kg) once weekly for 8 weeks. In patients who cannot be given primaquine, relapses may be prevented by administering chloroquine as suppressive therapy at a dose of 10 mg/kg weekly for 3–6 months. Tafenoquine, an 8-aminoquinoline agent related to primaquine, is approved in the USA as a single dose radical treatment for vivax malaria; it cannot be used in patients with G6PD deficiency. Artemisinin based combination therapy may be used as an alternative to chloroquine for treatment of vivax malaria.

Quinine and pyrimethamine sulfadoxine do not have adequate activity against vivax malaria and should not be used for its treatment.

***Uncomplicated falciparum malaria:*** The WHO recommends that falciparum malaria should always be treated with combination therapy. This is because combination therapy is more effective and reduces the risk of emergence of resistance. Both the partner drugs should have independent mode of action and both partner drugs should be effective in the area where they are used. Hence pyrimethamine–sulfadoxine is not combination therapy as both partner drugs have similar mechanism of action. Similarly, if an area has resistance to pyrimethamine–sulfadoxine and mefloquine, then these should not be used as part of combination therapy.

Artemisinin based combination therapy (ACT) is at present the treatment of choice for falciparum malaria (Table 11.15). Artemisinin (qinghaosu) is the antimalarial extract isolated from *Artemisia annua*. Artemisinin and its derivatives (artemether, artesunate, arteether, dihydroartemisinin, arterolane) are the most rapidly acting of all antimalarials; they also have a broad time window of antimalarial effect from ring forms to mature trophozoites (like chloroquine and unlike quinine that acts only on mature forms). Artemether and lumefantrine combination is the most commonly used oral ACT at this time in India (Table 11.15). Other drugs such as mefloquine and pyrimethamine–sulfadoxine, amodiaquine, piperaquine may be used in combination with artemisinin derivatives. The combination of atovaquone with proguanil is also efficacious for treatment of uncomplicated falciparum malaria but is not available in India.

Oral quinine for 3 days, with clindamycin or doxycycline or tetracycline (in children aged more than 8 years) for 7 days is alternative effective treatment, but may be associated with poor tolerability of oral quinine and prolonged therapy.

At the end of therapy, a single gametocidal dose of primaquine at a dose of 0.75 mg/kg is recommended to reduce community transmission of malaria.

***Uncomplicated mixed malaria:*** Uncomplicated mixed malaria should be treated as *P. falciparum* malaria with ACT. Primaquine should also be used as mentioned earlier for vivax malaria.

### Treatment of Complicated/Severe Malaria

The treatment of severe malaria is a medical emergency as it is associated with high mortality rates of up to 20%. If the suspicion of malaria is strong, then treatment should be initiated without waiting for confirmation of diagnosis. Severe malaria whether due to falciparum or vivax should be treated similarly. Supportive care and treatment of complications are as important as antimalarial therapy.

***Antimalarial therapy:*** Treatment should be parenteral as most patients are not able to take orally and the bioavailability of oral drugs is unpredictable. Artemisinins are associated with a 25% lower mortality as compared to quinine and are the current drugs of choice.

***Artemisinin-based therapy:*** Parenteral formulations of artesunate, artemether and arteether are commercially available. Artesunate is the preferred agent and is available as a dry powder which is reconstituted with sodium bicarbonate and given as a bolus injection. The drugs of second choice are artemether and arteether, given by the

IM route. The dose of artesunate is 2.4 mg/kg (3 mg/kg in children below 20 kg), and that of artemether 3.2 mg/kg given stat and then repeated after 12 and 24 hours and then daily. Parasite counts start declining 5–6 hours after institution of therapy with artemisinin derivatives, unlike quinine. Asexual parasitemia generally disappears after a mean time of 72 hours. Once the patient is better, treatment can be shifted to oral and a full course of oral ACT and single dose primaquine should be given as detailed earlier. Since there are issues with drug quality, care should be taken to use drugs from standard companies.

Artemisinin derivatives have a good safety profile. Local reactions after IM administration are rare and much less frequent as compared to IM quinine. Cardiotoxic effects in the form of prolongation of the QT interval in patients being administered high dose artemether have been reported. No clinical significance of this has been noted except that artemisinins should not be combined with other cardiotoxic drugs such as quinine or halofantrine. Neurotoxic side effects and neuropathologic changes have been consistently reported in animal studies with dogs and rats. In two human trials, use of artemether was associated with frequent convulsions and longer recovery time from coma as compared to quinine, long-term sequelae being comparable in both the groups. Since use of artesunate is associated with delayed hemolytic anemia, patients should be monitored with weekly hemoglobin levels after discharge.

***Quinine-based therapy:*** Quinine acts principally on the mature trophozoite stage of parasite development; it does not prevent sequestration or further development of formed meronts and does not kill the pre-erythrocytic or sexual stage of *P. falciparum*.

It should be used, only if artemisinins are not available or if resistance is suspected. It is dosed initially as 20 mg/kg of salt given either as intramuscular injection or as an infusion in 5% dextrose over 4-hr. After the loading dose, quinine should be continued at a dose of 10 mg salt/kg as infusion over 2-hr, every 8 hr. Therapy should be converted to oral after 48 hours. If parenteral quinine has to be continued beyond 48 hours or if renal failure supervenes, the maintenance dose should be reduced to 5–7 mg salt/kg, 8 hourly to avoid quinine toxicity. Total duration of therapy is 7 days. A second drug such as sulfadoxine-pyrimethamine, doxycycline or clindamycin should be added. A single dose of primaquine 0.75 mg/kg is recommended on completion of quinine therapy to eradicate gametocytes and hence prevent transmission. Quinine is associated with significant side effects including QT prolongation, arrhythmias, hypoglycemia and cinchonism. It is also known to cause intravascular hemolysis, hemoglobinuria and acute kidney injury (black water fever).

There is no benefit of combining quinine with artesunate for treatment of malaria.

***Supportive therapy:*** Supportive care is crucial in managing severe malaria. The child should be admitted to intensive care, if possible. Rapid clinical assessment should be done with respect to level of consciousness, blood pressure, pallor, rate and depth of respiration and hydration status. Fundus should be examined, and the patient weighed. The relevant investigations should be sent as detailed earlier. Parenteral antimalarial therapy is started empirically awaiting confirmation of diagnosis. Doses should be calculated as mg/kg body weight. Good nursing care is needed, especially if patient is unconscious; oxygen therapy, respiratory support, fluids and inotropes are used, if required. Broad-spectrum antibiotics (third generation cephalosporins and aminoglycoside, beta-lactam–beta-lactamase inhibitor combinations) are given in: (a) Any child with localized signs suggesting bacterial infection, (b) any child in shock, (c) any child with severe respiratory distress in whom deep breathing does not rapidly improve with correction of dehydration or anemia. Complications such as raised intracranial pressure, hyperpyrexia, seizures, shock, anemia, hemolysis, hypoglycemia, ARDS, metabolic acidosis, acute kidney injury, and bleeding should be managed appropriately.

Cerebral malaria is associated with mortality rates of 20% despite appropriate treatment and neurologic morbidity in survivors. There have been trials with several adjuvant drugs including mannitol, dexamethasone, anti-TNF, IVIG, heparin, aspirin, levamisole, UDCA, nitric oxide, prophylactic phenobarbitone, pentoxifyline, deferoxamine, deferiprone and IV albumin with no benefit. Similarly, red blood cell exchange transfusion (erythrocytapheresis) is currently not recommended, as a form of therapy.

#### *Response to Therapy, Treatment Failures, Recrudescence and Relapse*

Treatment of malaria is plagued by development of resistance. In India, there is resistance in falciparum malaria to chloroquine and sulfadoxine-pyrimethamine. Artemisinin resistance is anecdotally reported from East India, which is associated with prolonged parasite clearance times.

An optimal response to therapy is defined as a count which on day 1 is less than day 0, a count on day 3 which is less than 25% of count on day 0, no parasites in peripheral blood 72-hr after starting therapy and up to 28 days, and no fever after 72-hr.

Patients with parasitologically confirmed malaria who continue to have fever 72-hr after starting antimalarials are occasionally encountered in clinical practice. If they are smear negative, causes could be IV line associated thrombophlebitis, secondary bacterial infections, coinfections such as typhoid or rarely immune phenomena. If the smear is positive, then this is early treatment failure; causes are choice of wrong drug, sub-standard drug, wrong dose, poor compliance or drug resistance. If drug resistance is suspected, then treatment should be changed to an alternative ACT combination or quinine.

Reappearance of asexual parasites within 28 days of treatment is defined as recrudescence or late treatment failure. Causes again are choice of wrong drug, wrong dose, poor compliance or drug resistance. Treatment of recrudescence includes optimizing drug therapy or change to an alternative regime.

Appearance of parasites after 28 days in *P. vivax* could be due to relapse or reinfections. Accurate distinction is possible only by genomic analysis. Management includes use of either ACT or chloroquine, followed by primaquine in higher doses.

### Control and Prevention of Malaria

Control and prevention of malaria is based on elimination of the vector by strategies like use of insecticide treated bed nets (most important), indoor insecticide spraying, and elimination of breeding places. In holoendemic areas like sub-Saharan Africa, the WHO recommends chemoprophylaxis with pyrimethamine sulfadoxine to pregnant women, infants and children below 5 years. A vaccine against falciparum malaria (Mosquirix) is now licensed for use and has been deployed in sub-Saharan Africa. The vaccine (RTS, S/AS01) based on the circumsporozoite protein is given as 3 doses IM at 1 month interval in children aged from 17–25 months and provides 30% protection against severe malaria for 4 years.

Chemoprophylaxis against malaria is recommended for travelers from non-endemic areas to endemic areas. The indication and medication depends on the risk of malaria at the destination, patient risk profile and drug resistance. Drugs commonly used are weekly chloroquine (for areas known to be fully chloroquine sensitive) and weekly mefloquine, weekly tafenoquine, daily doxycycline or daily atovaquone-proguanil (for chloroquine resistant areas). Prophylaxis is generally started at least 1–2 weeks before departure and continued for 4 weeks after return except for atovaquone-proguanil where it can be started on the day of departure and stopped 7 days after return.

### National Vector-Borne Disease Control Program (NVBDCP)

The NVBDCP strategies are twofold: Early case detection and prompt treatment and vector control. It has laid out guidelines for detection and management of malaria and are more or less similar to what has been discussed earlier. NVBDCP recommends treatment of uncomplicated vivax malaria with chloroquine and falciparum malaria with ACT. Lumefantrine is recommended as the partner drug in Northeast India. Artemisinin monotherapy is banned in India and artemisinin derivatives are marketed only as combinations. Strategies for vector control include source control, elimination of breeding places, biologic control with use of larvivorous fish in water bodies and finally chemical vector control by indoor residual spray, space fogging and use of chemical larvicides like abate in water bodies.

## Suggested Reading


1. Guidelines for Diagnosis and Treatment of Malaria in India, 2014. Available at https://nvbdcp.gov.in/WriteReadData/l892s/20627628441542176662.pdf.
2. Venkatesan P. The future of malaria control in light of RTS,S. Lancet Microbe 2022;3:E251.
3. World Health Organization, 2022. WHO guidelines on malaria, 3 June 2022. Available at https://www.who.int/publications/i/item/guidelines-for-malaria.


## Leishmaniasis

Leishmaniasis is a disease caused by parasites of the genus *Leishmania*, which are transmitted by the bites of female sandflies. There are three major clinical forms of leishmaniasis: Visceral leishmaniasis (VL), cutaneous leishmaniasis, and mucocutaneous leishmaniasis (espundia). The visceral and cutaneous forms of the disease seen in India are caused by *Leishmania donovani*. Kala-azar, the Indian term for the visceral form of leishmaniasis, denotes hyperpigmentation in these patients (*kala*–black; *azar*–sickness). In India, annually about 1–3 lakh cases of kala-azar are reported, most often from Bihar and eastern UP.

### Transmission and Etiopathogenesis

The parasite exists in the human or animal reservoir as amastigotes, which are non-flagellated, round or oval in shape (Leishman-Donovan bodies), and in the sandfly and culture medium as flagellated promastigotes. In countries such as India and Sudan, humans are the chief reservoir (anthroponotic cycle). The female sandfly of the genus *Phlebotomus* ingests amastigotes into its digestive tract when feeding on an infected animal/human. The amastigote develops into a promastigote in the digestive tract, migrates to the salivary glands and is injected into the susceptible host when the sandfly takes its next feed. Within the host, promastigotes infect macrophages where they develop into amastigotes. These amastigotes multiply in the cells of the mononuclear phagocyte system including blood monocytes, macrophages, histiocytes, Kupffer cells and reticuloendothelial cells in spleen and lymphoid tissue.

Although disease occurs irrespective of age, children aged 1–4 years appear to be more susceptible. The protective immune response in VL is primarily cell-mediated immunity which results in subclinical infection and spontaneous cure in majority of cases. Failure of immunity leads to the clinical syndrome of VL. For every case of VL, there are about 30 subclinical infections. Malnutrition and HIV predispose to clinical disease.

### Clinical Features

***Visceral leishmaniasis:*** The incubation period is generally 3 to 8 months (range 10 days–34 months). Features include high grade fever, weight loss, hepatosplenomegaly, abdominal discomfort, lymphadenopathy, and pallor. Fever may be high or low grade, remittent, intermittent or continuous; the '*double-rise*' of temperature in a day (*double quotidian*), although characteristic is uncommon. There are no rigors and the patient does not appear 'toxic'. Splenohepatomegaly, with the spleen much larger than the liver, is usual. Spleen is usually huge, firm, smooth and non-tender and is palpable by the end of first month of illness. Moderate hepatomegaly is seen in over 80% of cases. Unlike African VL, lymphadenopathy is infrequent in Indian VL (<5%). Hyperpigmentation of skin is characteristically a feature of Indian VL and occurs in about two-thirds of patients in late stages of disease, affecting the face, hands and upper trunk. Progressive emaciation occurs in all cases of VL, though appetite is well preserved. Cough and diarrhea are common. Bleeding manifestations in the form of petechial hemorrhages, epistaxis and gum bleeding may be seen. Pedal edema may occur due to hypoalbuminemia. Jaundice is uncommon. Diminished cell-mediated immunity in VL may account for the high incidence of secondary infections. Pancytopenia and hypergammaglobulinemia are characteristic.

The disease may begin insidiously and be asymptomatic initially, but usually runs a chronic course that may be fatal without or despite treatment. Death usually occurs within 2 years in 75–95% cases, because of severe secondary bacterial infections or gastrointestinal bleeding in advanced disease.

***Post kala-azar dermal leishmaniasis (PKDL):*** PKDL develops after resolution of VL and is seen in a small percentage of patients in Africa and India. This is usually due to infection by the *L. donovani* cluster. The time interval to development of PKDL is variable; it usually occurs 1–10 years after successful treatment of VL. Hypopigmented macular, maculopapular or nodular skin lesions are seen first in the perioral area, chin and lips, and later appear over the neck, extensor surfaces of the arms, trunk, and legs. Lesions spare the scalp, palms, soles, axillae and perineum. Lepromatous leprosy is a close differential, but peripheral nerves are spared. Skin lesions may persist for up to 20 years. These patients may act as chronic reservoir of infection.

### Diagnosis

VL should be suspected in a patient from an endemic area presenting with prolonged pyrexia and splenomegaly. Cases in non-endemic areas have also been reported but are very rare. Clinical differentials include chronic malaria, storage disorders, leukemia, lymphoma, chronic liver disease with portal hypertension, and HIV. Preliminary tests show pancytopenia, mild elevation of liver enzymes and hypergammaglobulinemia with reversal of albumin globulin ratio. The aldehyde test has poor sensitivity and specificity and is no longer used.

Diagnosis in VL is usually based on microscopic detection of amastigotes in smears of tissue aspirates or biopsy samples. Bone marrow aspirate or biopsy is frequently the tissue of choice with sensitivity between 55 and 97%. Lymph node aspirate smears or biopsy (sensitivity 60%), liver biopsy (sensitivity 85%), and splenic aspirates (sensitivity 97%) may also be used for diagnosis. Though splenic aspirate has the highest sensitivity, the procedure may result in life-threatening hemorrhage. Recently PCR methods on tissue samples and peripheral blood with very high sensitivities have been developed.

Immunochromatographic strip (dipstick) testing of blood from a finger prick for leishmanial anti-K39 antibody has been used successfully in field serodiagnosis with a sensitivity of 90–100% (~93%) in symptomatic patients, and high specificity (90.6%). Titers to K39 decrease following successful therapy and tend to rise in cases of relapse, thus making it useful to recognize treatment failures. This test is useful in clinical management in resource-poor areas. Newer methods with high sensitivity and specificity include the detection of leishmania antigen and antibody in the urine.

### Treatment of Visceral Leishmaniasis

Options for drug therapy are discussed in **Table 11.16**

Other agents including sitamaquine are under evaluation. Since lipid formulations of amphotericin B are expensive, the simple mixing of amphotericin B with a commercially available fat emulsion has been proposed (at 2 mg/kg on alternate days for a duration of 10 days).

The NVBDCP in its 2015 guidelines has made the following recommendations for treatment of kala-azar in India:

- The first-line agent is single dose liposomal amphotericin B at a dose of 10 mg/kg
- If liposomal amphotericin B cannot be given, then options include:
  - Oral miltefosine for 28 days (contraindicated below 2-yr, in pregnant and lactating women and women of childbearing age who refuse contraception, and HIV infected patients)
  - Oral miltefosine and IM paramomycin for 10 days
  - Amphotericin B deoxycholate (1 mg/kg alternate day for 30 days, or 15 doses)
- Amphotericin B lipid emulsion (Amphomul) at a dose of 15 mg/kg single dose has been introduced on a pilot basis in some districts.

**Table 11.16:** Treatment options for VL

| *Drug* | *Dose* | *Side effects* | *Comments* |
|---|---|---|---|
| Pentavalent antimonials | 20 mg/kg IV or IM for 28 days | QT prolongation, arrythmias | High rates of resistance in Bihar; no longer used |
| Pentamidine | 4 mg/kg IM or IV thrice weekly for 6 weeks | Pancreatitis, diabetes, bone marrow suppression | Limited availability, risk of toxicity; response rates ~75% |
| Paromomycin (aminosidine) | 16–20 mg/kg/day IV or IM for 21 days | Gastrointestinal side effects, malabsorption | Usually used in combination |
| Miltefosine | 2.5 mg/kg/day oral for 28 days | GI side effects, teratogenicity | Cure rates of 95-100%; can be given as outpatient |
| Amphotericin B deoxycholate | 1 mg/kg daily for 2 weeks or alternate day for 30 days | Nephorotoxicity, infusion related side effects | Cumbersome to give, side effects |
| Lipid formulations of amphotericin B | 3 mg/kg on day 1–5<br>10 mg/kg single dose | Nephrotoxicity; infusion related reactions | Treatment of choice, but expensive |

Supportive care is crucial. Severe anemia and thrombocytopenia may necessitate packed cell and platelet transfusion. The child should receive a nutritious diet, and nutritional deficiencies should be corrected. Concurrent infections should be treated appropriately.

Fever, spleen size, hemoglobin, blood cell counts, serum albumin, and body weight are monitored for response to therapy. In most patients, the fever subsides within 7 days, blood counts and hemoglobin levels rise, the patient feels better, and spleen becomes smaller within 2 weeks. Parasitological cure should be documented at the end of therapy by splenic or bone marrow aspiration. As relapses are common in this disease, patient should be followed for at least 6 months before a long-term definite cure is pronounced. The spleen may take 6 months to 1 year to regress completely. Relapse is suggested by an increase of spleen size, a fall in hemoglobin levels and should be confirmed by the demonstration of parasites.

#### Treatment of PKDL

Treatment of PKDL is important to reduce the community reservoir and transmission, and is more aggressive as compared to VL. The recommended treatment options are:

- *Miltefosine:* 100 mg orally per day for 12 weeks
- *Amphotericin B deoxycholate:* 1 mg/kg/day over 4 months (60–80 doses)
- *Liposomal amphotericin B:* 5 mg/kg/day by infusion two times per week for 3 weeks, for a total dose of 30 mg/kg.

#### Prevention and Control

Control of leishmaniasis involves controlling the source of infection and eradicating the vector, and depends on local epidemiology. Where sandflies are mostly endophilic (rest mostly indoors after feeding), spraying houses with insecticide is effective, while use of treated and untreated bed nets is effective where sandflies are endophagic (feed mainly indoors). Insecticide treatment of dogs and dog collars is useful where canines are important reservoirs. In India, where anthroponotic transmission is important, effective treatment of patients, especially those with PKDL (who may act as long-term reservoirs), has been found to be effective in controlling transmission when combined with vector control. There is no effective vaccine for prevention of leishmaniasis at present.

### Suggested Reading


1. Bhattacharya SK, Sur D, Karbwang J. Childhood visceral leishmaniasis. Indian J Med Res 2006; 123:353–56.
2. Burza S, Croft SL, Boelaert M. Leishmaniasis. Lancet 2018;392:951–70.
3. NVBDCP. Operational guidelines on kala-azar elimination in India 2015. Available at www.nvbdcp.gov.in. Accessed on 16 May 2022.
4. Sundar S, Singh OP, Chakravarty J. Visceral leishmaniasis elimination targets in India, strategies for preventing resurgence. Expert Rev Anti Infect Ther 2018;16:805–12.


## Amebiasis

Amebiasis is defined as infection with *Entamoeba histolytica*. Clinical features of amebiasis due to *E. histolytica* range from asymptomatic colonization to amebic dysentery and invasive extraintestinal amebiasis.

#### Epidemiology

*E. histolytica* is thought to infect 10% of the population in developing countries, and perhaps 30–40% in India. However, these may be overestimates, because three morphologically identical, genetically distinct but apparently nonpathogenic Entamoeba species, namely *E. dispar*, *E. moshkovskii*, *E. bangladeshi* are now being recognized in asymptomatic cases. In a study from Northeast India in adults, the average prevalence of Entamoeba was 30%, of which one-third were *E. histolytica* and the rest were the nonpathogenic species. Amebic dysentery and extraintestinal amebiasis are associated with a high morbidity and mortality in the resource-limited settings causing 50,000 deaths annually each. Amebiasis is less common in children and some estimates suggest that it is responsible for less than 3% of diarrhea in children below 2 years.

#### Etiopathogenesis

The organism exists in nature as a cyst and a trophozoite. The cysts are resistant to gastric acidity and chlorination but are destroyed by boiling. Each ingested cyst excysts in the small intestine to produce eight trophozoites that colonize the mucosa of the large intestine and produce more cysts. Trophozoites may cause tissue invasion, inflammation and destruction through several virulence factors resulting in characteristic flask-shaped ulcers, seen commonly in cecum, transverse colon and sigmoid colon. Extraintestinal complications occur when trophozoites invade the bloodstream and migrate through the portal circulation, to lodge usually in the liver. Rare extraintestinal complications include amebic involvement of peritoneum, pericardium, pleura, lungs, brain, genitourinary system and skin.

#### Clinical Features

Asymptomatic cyst passage is the most common manifestation of *E. histolytica*, in most cases, the infection resolves spontaneously, but uncommonly, these individuals may later present with amebic dysentery and other invasive manifestations.

After a variable incubaton period of weeks to months, about 10% individuals colonized with *E. histolytica* develop symptomatic disease, in form of colitis or extraintestinal disease. Amebic colitis presents as abdominal pain or tenderness (seen in 80%), with watery, bloody or mucous diarrhea. Some may have only intermittent diarrhea alternating with constipation. Fever is unusual. Occasionally fulminant amebic colitis may occur, with profuse bloody diarrhea, fever, widespread abdominal pain, diffuse tenderness and pronounced leukocytosis. Risk factors for fulminant colitis include use of corticosteroids and anti-motility agents. Toxic megacolon (mortality rate of 40–80%), ameboma (mimics colon cancer), cutaneous amebiasis and rectovaginal fistulae can occur as complications of intestinal amebiasis.

Amebic liver abscess (ALA), seen in about 1% of infected individuals, may occur months to years after infection. It is usually single (95%) and more frequently involves the right lobe of the liver (posterosuperior part). The abscess may regress, rupture or disseminate; transdiaphragmatic rupture may cause amebic empyema and pulmonary amebiasis. While some individuals may have concurrent amebic colitis, more commonly there are no bowel symptoms. The patient usually presents with fever with chills and rigors and right upper quadrant pain of acute onset (<10 days). Examination reveals toxic appearance, right upper quadrant tenderness and hepatomegaly; jaundice is unusual (10–15%). Cough, along with dullness or crepitations in the right lung base may be present. Complications include rupture into the pleura, which has a relatively good prognosis, and rupture into the pericardium and superinfection with bacteria, which are more serious.



*Diagnosis*



Amoebic colitis has to be differentiated from other causes of colitis and dysentery (*Shigella, E. coli, Campylobacter*). Diagnosis of amoebic colitis can be established by demonstration of motile trophozoites by direct microscopic examination of fresh fecal sample. At least 3 stool specimens taken on consecutive days should be examined because the test has poor sensitivity (<60% with 1 sample; ~90% with 3 fresh samples). Stool contains plenty of erythrocytes but few leukocytes, unlike bacillary dysentery where leukocytes are plentiful. Presence of ingested erythrocytes within trophozoites is pathognomonic for *E. histolytica*. Multiplex PCR-based gastrointestinal diagnostic panels also detect *E. histolytica* with satisfactory sensitivity and specificity, but are expensive. Presence of cysts of *E. histolytica* in stool samples is of no clinical significance and should not be treated.

ALA has to be differentiated from pyogenic liver abscess (more common in children than ALA) and hydatid disease. In case of a liver abscess, chest radiograph shows elevated diaphragm and pleural reaction on the right side. Ultrasound, CT, MRI or isotope scan can localize the abscess in most cases. Leukocytosis without eosinophilia, mild anemia, raised alkaline phosphatase, and a high erythrocyte sedimentation rate (ESR) are common laboratory findings. Serological tests (ELISA, IHA and IFA) are routinely employed for diagnosis of extraintestinal disease with *E. histolytica* and especially for differentiating amebic from pyogenic liver abscess. They are positive in 70–80% patients with invasive disease at presentation, and in >90% cases beyond first week of symptoms. However, the specificity is poor as they may be positive due to previous infection. Aspiration of the abscess reveals the characteristic "anchovy sauce" (dark chocolate color) pus. Microscopy of the pus can reveal the motile trophozoites. PCR for *E. histolytica* in pus is also now available.

*Treatment*

The practice of giving empiric anti-amebic drugs for all children presenting with diarrhea should be strongly discouraged since amebiasis is relatively uncommon in young children.

Metronidazole is the drug of choice for treating amebic colitis or ALA. It is given at a dose of 35–50 mg/kg/day in 3 divided doses (adult dose 750 mg 8 hourly) for 7–10 days. Alternatives include tinidazole (50 mg/kg/day, adult dose 2 g) for 3 days. Ornidazole, secnidazole and nitazoxanide are alternative, but less effective agents. Since metronidazole does not destroy the cysts, a luminal agent (paromomycin, iodoquinol, or diloxanide furoate) should be used to in all cases of amebic colitis/ALA to eradicate colonization. Diloxanide furoate is dosed as 20 mg/kg/day in 3 divided doses (adult dose 500 mg thrice daily) for 10 days.

When possible, fulminant amebic colitis, even with perforation, is managed conservatively, with the addition of antibiotics to deal with bowel flora. Radiographic monitoring of the abdomen by CT scan, coupled with the judicious use of percutaneous catheter drainage to obtain suspect fluid, might aid in management.

Most ALA, even large ones, can be cured without drainage. Most patients show a response to treatment (reduced fever and abdominal pain) within 72–96 hours. Therapeutic image-guided aspiration is not indicated in the treatment of uncomplicated ALA. Aspiration is usually reserved for individuals in whom diagnosis is uncertain (where pyogenic abscess or bacterial superinfection is a concern), those who have not responded to metronidazole therapy (persistent fever or abdominal pain after 4 days of treatment), individuals with large left lobe abscesses (because of the risk of rupture into the pericardium), size more than 8–10 cm (suggesting impending rupture) and severely ill patients with an accelerated clinical course and large abscesses suggesting imminent rupture. Aspiration or percutaneous catheter drainage, or both improve outcomes in the treatment of amebic empyema after liver abscess rupture, and percutaneous catheter (or, if necessary, surgical) drainage is mandatory in the treatment of amebic pericarditis. ALA rupture into the peritoneum is managed conservatively, along with percutaneous catheter drainage for localized collections of fluid.

### Suggested Reading


1. Kumanan T, Sujanitha V, Sreeharan N. Amebic liver abscess: A neglected tropical disease. Lancet Infect Dis 2020;20:160–62.
2. Shirley DT, Farr L, Watanabe K, Moonah S. A review of the global burden, new diagnostics, and current therapeutics for amebiasis. Open Forum Infect Dis 2018; 5:ofy161.
3. Stanley SL. Amoebiasis. Lancet 2003; 361:1025–34.


## Giardiasis

Giardiasis, caused by *Giardia lamblia* (also known as *G. intestinalis* or *G. duodenalis*), is a major cause of diarrhea in children and in travelers.

*Epidemiology*

Based on the latest figures provided by WHO, *G. lamblia* is the third most common agent of diarrheal disease worldwide with over 300 million reported cases per annum, preceded only by rotavirus and *Cryptosporidium parvum* in children under five years of age. The prevalence of giardiasis in humans ranges from 2–3% in industrialized countries, and up to 30% in low-income and developing countries. Giardiasis was formerly included in the WHO

Neglected Diseases Initiative and is directly associated with poverty and poor quality of drinking water. Individuals with malnutrition, humoral immunodeficiencies and cystic fibrosis are particularly susceptible. Children appear to be more severely affected than adults.

### *Etiopathogenesis*

Giardia exists in two stages—cysts and trophozoites. Outside the human body, it exists in the form of cysts. Cysts are hardy, capable of surviving in cool, moist environments for up to 2 months and in water that has been routinely chlorinated, but are destroyed by boiling for 10 minutes. Transmission of infection is through cysts, which may be ingested in contaminated water or food or spread by direct person-to-person contact. Ingestion of 10–100 cysts is sufficient for causing infection. Low pH of the duodenum facilitates excystation and release of trophozoites. Trophozoites colonize the duodenum and proximal jejunum of the host, where they attach to the intestinal brush border. Unlike amebiasis, there are no invasive or locally destructive lesions. It is believed that the infection causes diarrhea via a combination of intestinal malabsorption and hypersecretion. These effects cause malabsorption and maldigestion and, in addition, may facilitate the development of chronic enteric disorders, including inflammatory bowel disease, irritable bowel syndrome, and allergies, via mechanisms that remain poorly understood. Steatorrhea that is often seen may occur due to pancreatic involvement, or due to bacterial overgrowth in the duodenum and upper jejunum, and bile salt deconjugation liberating free bile acids.

### *Clinical Features*

The incubation period after ingestion of cysts is 1–2 weeks. Most infections in both children and adults are *asymptomatic*. *Symptomatic* infections are more common in children than in adults, and usually take the form of acute diarrhea with sudden onset of explosive, watery, foul smelling stools, along with nausea and anorexia; others may also have abdominal distension, flatulence, epigastric cramps and mild fever. There is no blood or mucus in stools. The illness may last 3–4 days and is usually self-limiting in normal immunocompetent children. Variable degree of malabsorption may occur. Some patients may have a protracted course, with persistent or recurrent mild to moderate symptoms such as brief episodes of loose foul smelling stools alternating with constipation. Persistent diarrhea may be seen in 30–50% cases. A few children may develop chronic diarrhea, lactose and fat malabsorption and failure to thrive.

### *Diagnosis*

Diagnosis of giardiasis is traditionally established by microscopic examination of stools. At least three fresh specimens of stools collected on alternate days should be examined to achieve sensitivity of 90%, because the multiplication and passage of the giardial cysts is often intermittent. There is no blood or leukocytes in stools. Enzyme immunoassay (EIA) and direct fluorescent antibody test for *Giardia* antigens in stools have been reported to have better sensitivity and require less expertise than traditional microscopy. *Giardia* is also a part of currently available multiplex PCR panels for diagnosis of GI pathogens. Where diagnosis is strongly suspected but stool testing is negative, duodenal aspirate or biopsy may yield high concentration of *Giardia* when fresh wet mount is examined for trophozoites. Where duodenal aspirate is negative, intestinal biopsy may be considered in presence of any suggestive feature like lactose malabsorption or abnormal radiographic findings (edema or segmentation in small intestine), or a suggestive setting like absent secretory IgA or hypogammaglobulinemia.

### *Treatment*

All symptomatic cases acute and persistent diarrhea, failure to thrive and malabsorption syndrome—require drug treatment. Unlike amebiasis, asymptomatic carriers of cysts should also be treated. At present, treatment options include the nitroimidazoles derivatives (metronidazole and tinidazole), benzimidazoles (albendazole and mebendazole) and nitazoxanide. Metronidazole is given at a dose of 15 mg/kg/day for 5–7 days; it has 80–90% efficacy and is inexpensive, but has frequent adverse effects and has to be given three times a day. Tinidazole has the advantage of high efficacy (>90%) and single dose treatment (50 mg/kg once). Albendazole given as single dose of 400 mg once daily for 5 to 10 days has similar efficacy as compared to metronidazole, but is better tolerated. Nitazoxanide also has high efficacy (80–90%), low incidence of adverse effects and is available in suspension form. Nitazoxanide is given for 3 days, in two doses, with the dose depending on age (100 mg bid for 1–4 years, 200 mg bid for 4–12 years, 500 mg bid for >12 years). There is an increase in incidence of refractory giardiasis and these patients are best treated with a combination of metronidazole/tinidazole with albendazole.

### Suggested Reading


1. Desai AN. Giardiasis. JAMA 2021;325:1356.
2. Mmbaga BT, Houpt ER. Cryptosporidium and giardia infections in children: A review. Pediatr Clin North Am 2017;64:837–50.


## Amebic Meningoencephalitis

Amebic meningoencephalitis is the infection of the central nervous system by free-living amebae. The disease occurs in two clinical forms: Primary amebic meningoencephalitis (PAM) caused by *Naegleria fowleri* and granulomatous amebic encephalitis (GAE) induced by *Acanthamoeba* and *Balamuthia*.

### *Primary Amebic Meningoencephalitis (PAM)*

*Naegleria fowleri* causes fulminant meningoencephalitis, mostly in children and healthy young adults who have a recent history of swimming in fresh water lakes, pools and ponds, usually during hot summer months. The amebae enter the nose through contaminated water (or air), penetrate the nasal mucosa and the cribriform plate and travel along the olfactory nerves to the brain leading to a diffuse hemorrhagic necrotizing meningoencephalitis. Around 300 cases have been reported worldwide.

Signs and symptoms are suggestive of acute pyogenic meningitis including severe headache, photophobia, irritability. Microscopic demonstration of motile amebae in fresh cerebrospinal fluid is required for diagnosis. Intracranial pressures can be very high and lumbar puncture should be done carefully. CSF evaluation is otherwise similar to that seen with acute pyogenic meningitis with a high laukocyte count (usually in thousands) with polymorphonuclear predominance, and elevated proteins. Disease progression is usually rapid and death occurs within 5–10 days. Mortality rates are around 99%. Survivors have been reported occasionally. Infection with *Naegleria* must be considered in differential diagnosis of a patient with pyogenic meningitis presenting with history of swimming in fresh water, non-specific cerebral edema on CT, and no evidence of bacteria on Gram stain, antigen detection assays and culture. The drug of choice is intravenous and intrathecal amphotericin B. Other drugs which have been used include fluconazole, azithromycin and rifampicin. There are recent anecdotal reports of successful outcome with miltefosine.

#### *Granulomatous Amebic Encephalitis (GAE)*

This is an infection with the free living amoeba *Acanthamoeba* species and *Balamuthia* species that are ubiquitous in the environment including soil and water. *Acanthamoeba* is more commonly recognized as a cause of sight-threatening keratitis often seen in contact lens users. Systemic infection is acquired through inhalation or skin contact and then spreads hematogenously. The CNS disease is usually seen in immunocompromised children such as those with AIDS, SLE or post-transplant. Immunocompetent individuals may also be affected. Only a few hundred cases have been reported. Clinically, GAE runs a subacute or chronic course similar to tubercular or other chronic meningitis and is fatal in more than 95% of the cases. CT/MRI scan of brain may reveal ring enhancing lesions and ventricular dilatation. CSF examination may show elevated proteins and lymphocytic leukocytosis. Trophozoites are rarely found in the CSF, unlike *Naegleria*. Brain biopsy is needed to demonstrate the protozoan. A triplex real time TaqMan PCR assay for simultaneous identification of *Acanthamoeba* spp., *Balamuthia mandriallaris*, and *N. fowleri* has been developed and may be used for rapid laboratory diagnosis. Treatment has been attempted with combination therapy with fluconazole, ketoconazole, sulfonamides, pentamidine, cotrimoxazole and miltefosine.

### Suggested Reading


1. Bhosale NK, Parija SC. Balamuthia mandrillaris: An opportunistic, free-living ameba—an updated review. Trop Parasitol. 2021;11:78–88.
2. Bunsuwansakul C, Mahboob T, Hounkong K, et al. Acanthamoeba in Southeast Asia—Overview and challenges. Korean J Parasitol 2019;57:341–57.
3. Gharpure R, Bliton J, Goodman A, et al. Epidemiology and clinical characteristics of primary amebic meningoencephalitis. Clin Infect Dis 2021;73:e19–27.
4. Parija Sc, Dinoop KP, Venugopal H. Management of granulomatous amebic encephalitis. Trop Parasitol 2015;5:23–28.


## CONGENITAL AND PERINATAL INFECTIONS

Congenital and perinatal infections are often referred to by the acronym "TORCH". This refers to toxoplasmosis (T), rubella (R), cytomegalovirus (C) and herpes simplex (H). The others' group (O) is ever expanding and includes several other infections like syphilis, malaria, tuberculosis, HIV, HCV, HBV, varicella, enterovirus, parvovirus, zika virus infections among many others. This section is restricted to postnatal aspects of toxoplasmosis, rubella, cytomegalovirus, herpes simplex and syphilis.

### General Principles

- These infections are mild/asymptomatic in the pregnant women but can be disastrous for the fetus and newborn.
- Fetal and neonatal infection and affection due to TORCH usually occurs with primary infection in the mother. Latent infection or reactivation affects the baby infrequently (exception CMV, syphilis) unless the woman is immunocompromised.
- Not all infection in the mothers is transmitted to the baby due to the placental barrier and not all infected babies are affected. The transmissibility and severity of fetal affection depends on the timing of gestation. As a general rule, infection during the first trimester have the most devastating consequences.
- Congenital and perinatal infections can manifest during pregnancy as ultrasonographic findings, soon after birth or later in life. The common manifestations of intrauterine infections are abortions (recurrent only with syphilis, not with others), intrauterine growth retardation, intrauterine death, stillbirth, prematurity, deafness, chorioretinitis, aseptic meningitis, microcephaly, mental retardation, lymphadenopathy, hepatosplenomegaly, neonatal hepatitis, anemia, thrombocytopenia and skeletal abnormalities. Certain features are classical for each infection.
- Tests that are useful in diagnosis in the newborn include a complete blood count, liver and renal functions, skeletal survey, fundus examination, hearing evaluation and imaging of the central nervous system. Specific diagnosis is generally by serology and the "TORCH" screen is often ordered for. However, it must be remembered that serologic diagnosis by IgM and IgG estimation is tricky, should be done in both baby and mother and interpreted with caution. Molecular tests in urine, blood, CSF and tissues are also available.
- Treatment is possible and rewarding for toxoplasmosis, syphilis, herpes simplex, only partly successful for CMV and not available for rubella.
- Prenatal screening for syphilis, HIV and HBV, and preconceptional immunization with rubella and varicella vaccines is important to reduce the burden of the "TORCH" infections.

### Congenital Toxoplasmosis

It is only maternal primary infection (which is generally subclinical) that leads to fetal infection and disease. In HIV-infected or immunocompromised women, reactivation of latent infection may also affect the fetus. The transmissibility increases but the risk of fetal disease decreases with advancing pregnancy. The classic clinical triad of congenital toxoplasmosis includes intracranial calcification, hydrocephalus and chorioretinitis (Fig. 11.32). Infants asymptomatic at birth may later present with mental retardation and deafness. Diagnosis is confirmed by demonstrating a positive toxoplasma IgM in the serum of the affected child or by toxoplasma PCR in CSF/tissues. Treatment is recommended for all affected babies even if they are asymptomatic, and includes pyrimethamine, sulfadiazine and folinic acid for a period of 1 year. Since maternal infection results from ingestion of food/water contaminated with oocysts or infected meat containing tachyzoites, prevention revolves around advising pregnant women to wash fruits and vegetables carefully, limit contact with soil and refrain from eating undercooked meat.

### Congenital Rubella

Transmissibility is highest in the first trimester, and so is the rate of fetal disease (90% at <11 weeks). The fetus is completely spared, if infection occurs beyond 16 weeks. The classical triad of congenital rubella syndrome consists of deafness, cataract and congenital heart disease (commonly patent ductus arteriosus). Expanded rubella syndrome comprises delayed manifestations such as diabetes mellitus and renal disease have also been described. Diagnosis is by demonstration of positive rubella IgM in cord or neonatal blood. No treatment exists. A unequivocal diagnosis of rubella in the first trimester of pregnancy is an indication for maternal termination of pregnancy. Preconceptual counselling should include testing women for rubella IgG and vaccinating them with MR or MMR if IgG is negative. Vaccinating all children including adolescent girls against rubella is strongly recommended to reduce the burden of congenital rubella. The universal immunization program of India substituted measles vaccine, with the MR vaccine, and carried out a country wide pulse MR campaign in 2017 to achieve this objective.

### Congenital/Perinatal CMV

Congenital CMV is reported to be the commonest congenital infection in developed countries. The rate of transmission of CMV from mother to baby depends on whether it is primary maternal infection or reactivation/reinfection in the mother. The overall transmission rate with primary infection is 30% and 10% of all babies infected are symptomatic. The transmission risk with reactivation or reinfection is only 1% and only 5–10% of infected babies are symptomatic. But since the total numbers of reactivations and reinfections are higher than primary infections, these contribute to half the burden of congenital CMV. In India where 99% of the mothers are CMV IgG positive, congenital infections are due to reactivations/reinfections. CMV transmission and fetal disease occur throughout pregnancy. Congenital CMV can affect all organ systems; periventricular calcification is characteristic of CMV (Fig. 11.33). Babies who are asymptomatic at birth can manifest later with sensorineural deafness. The diagnosis of congenital CMV can be confirmed by a positive IgM or urine CMV PCR in the first 2 to 3 weeks of life. The sensitivity of IgM is low and a negative IgM does not rule out CMV. A positive CMV IgM/urine CMV PCR after the first 2–3 weeks of life can also occur due to postnatal transmission and is not specific for diagnosis. Antiviral treatment with ganciclovir is indicated in patients with neurologic involvement, progressive disease and deafness. The treatment duration is 6 weeks and should be followed with oral valganciclovir for up to 6 months.

CMV transmission can also occur during delivery and breastfeeding and is of consequence mainly in the preterm and very low birth weight babies. In this setting, it presents as a sepsis-like illness with pneumonia and respiratory distress. CMV transmission due to blood and blood products can also cause anemia, thrombocytopenia and hepatosplenomegaly in preterm infants. Here, treatment is symptomatic and antiviral therapy is usually not indicated.

### Perinatal HSV

The transmission of HSV to babies usually occurs during delivery in mothers who develop primary genital herpes

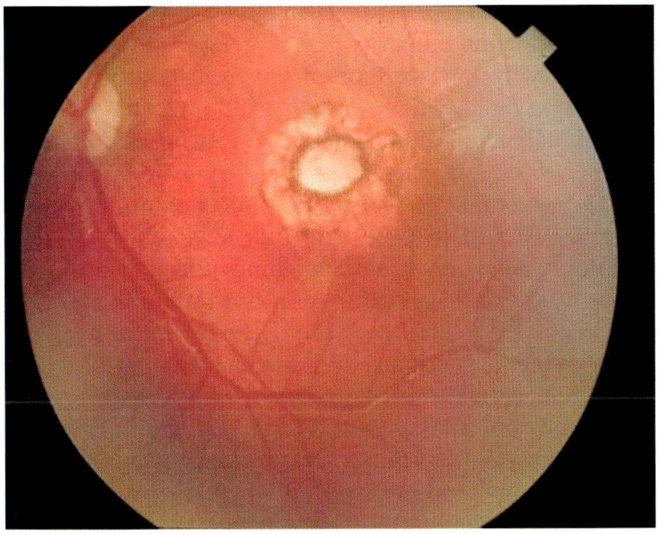

Fig. 11.32: Retinitis in congenital toxoplasmosis

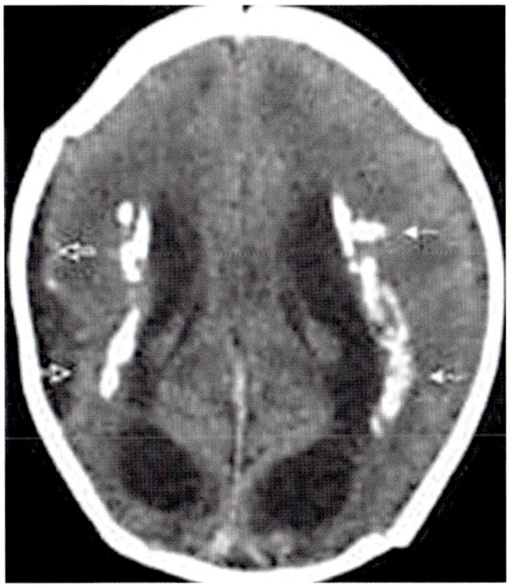

Fig. 11.33: Classical periventricular calcification of CMV

before or at the time of delivery. Reactivation of genital herpes is associated with very low rates of transmission and disease. Infected babies may be asymptomatic or have fulminant disease. Three forms of disease have been described—that limited to skin, eyes and mouth (SEM) with a vesicular eruption, CNS disease that presents with seizures and altered sensorium, and disseminated disease that presents as sepsis-like illness with high mortality. The latter two may not have associated skin eruption which further complicates diagnosis. Diagnosis is by Tzanck smear of the skin lesions, culture/PCR of lesions or the CSF for the virus. HSV serology plays no role in diagnosis. Treatment of neonates with suspected or confirmed infection with intravenous acyclovir 20 mg/kg 8 hourly should be started promptly. Duration of therapy is intravenous for 2–3 weeks, followed by 6 months of oral acyclovir to prevent reactivation of the disease. Babies born to mothers with active herpetic lesions during delivery should have cultures sent from skin and mucosa and started on empiric acyclovir pending results and should be watched carefully for disease. Elective cesarean section should be considered in mothers with active primary genital herpes and unruptured membranes.

### Congenital Syphilis

There has been a resurgence of syphilis in many countries including the USA. Syphilis is the only maternal infection that is associated with recurrent abortions; hence requesting the TORCH screen (that does not include VDRL/RPR) for recurrent abortions is of no use. All mothers should be screened for syphilis by VDRL/RPR at least once in pregnancy. If the quantitative VDRL/RPR titer is 1:8 or more, a specific treponemal test such as TPHA or TPPA should be used to confirm the diagnosis. Infected mothers should be treated with benzathine penicillin. Maternal syphilis can be transmitted throughout pregnancy, more commonly during later pregnancy as the placenta thins down. Apart from the usual clinical features mentioned earlier, infected babies have other pathognomonic features like skeletal lesions, snuffles, pneumonia and bullous skin lesions. Some babies manifest with delayed features like depressed nasal bridge, notched central incisors, keratitis, saber shins, and frontal bossing. Diagnosis is by quantitative VDRL estimation in serum. A VDRL titer four times that of the mother is defined as significant. All babies suspected to have congenital syphilis should undergo CSF evaluation and VDRL estimation. Apart from symptomatic babies and those who have significant VDRL titers, asymptomatic babies born to mothers who were untreated/inadequately treated/treated with non-penicillin based regimes/treated less than 4 weeks before delivery should also be treated irrespective of VDRL titers. Treatment is recommended with crystalline penicillin or procaine penicillin with probenecid. Benzathine penicillin may be used, if there is no CNS or long bone abnormalities and normal complete blood count. In case penicillin is not available, ceftriaxone may be used. Infected babies should be followed up with serial VDRL titers till these become non-reactive.

#### *Summary*

Congenital and perinatal infections are illnesses that result in significant morbidity and mortality. Diagnosis is complicated, expensive and not readily available. The results of the laboratory tests, chiefly TORCH serology, should be interpreted carefully. In India, illnesses like malaria and tuberculosis which mimic the classical "TORCH" infections should not be forgotten as they are commoner and readily treatable.

### Suggested Reading

1. Khalil A, Sotiriadis A. Chaoui R, et al. JSUOG practice guidelines: role of ultrasound in congenital infection. Ultrasound Obstet Gynaecol 2020;56:128–51.
2. Moodley A, Payton KSE. The term newborn: Congenital infections. Clin Perinatol 2021;48:485–511.
3. Neu N, Duchon J, Zachariah P. TORCH infections. Clin Perinatol. 2015;42:77–viii.

## HELMINTHIC INFECTIONS

Helminthic infestations contribute to significant disease burden in children particularly in the underprivileged and in developing countries. Helminthiasis is caused by three groups of worms, nematodes (roundworms), cestodes (tapeworms) and trematodes (flukes). Nematodes may be further classified as intestinal nematodes and tissue nematodes. Trematode infections are uncommon in India and will not be considered further.

### Intestinal Nematodes

Intestinal nematodes are the commonest type of helminthic infestations. This group includes *Ascaris lumbricoides* (roundworm), *Enterobius vermicularis* (pinworm, threadworm), *Ankylostoma duodenale* (Old world hookworm) *Necator americanus* (New world hookworm), *Trichuris trichura* (whipworm) and *Strongyloides stercoralis*. These infections are common in areas with unsatisfactory hygiene and sanitation, open air defecation and improper disposal of sewage.

#### *Life Cycle*

*Ascaris*, *Strongyloides*, *Necator* and *Ankylostoma* inhabit the small intestine, *Enterobius* is lodged in the cecum and *Trichuris* inhabits the large intestine. Eggs are released in the feces with the exception of *Enterobius* where they are released on the perianal skin. The eggs embryonate in the environment and become infective. In *Ascaris* and *Trichura*, infection occurs by ingestion of embryonated eggs from the enviroment. In *Enterobius*, autoinfection occurs due to ingestion of embryonated eggs lodged on hands or from contaminated bedlinen, etc. Sometimes infection may occur through inhalation and ingestion or rarely retroinfection may occur by release of larvae which migrate back in the intestine. It is because of these reasons that pinworm infections are recurrent and recalcitrant. The larvae are released in the intestines and mature into adult worms locally in case of trichuriasis and enterobiasis, while in case of ascariasis they migrate through the intestinal wall, into the portal circulation, the liver, heart, lungs, trachea, are swallowed into the pharynx and finally mature into adult worms in the small intestine. In case of *Necator*, *Ankylostoma* and *Strongyloides*, infection occurs by penetration of the skin by filariform larvae through the systemic circulation reach the heart, the lungs, trachea, pharynx and finally mature into adult worms in the intestines. *Strongyloides* is unique among the intestinal nematodes in several respects; larvae divide parthenogenetically in the small intestine, development of the eggs into infective larvae occurs within the intestine leading to autoinfections, retroinfections and hyperinfections.

### Clinical Manifestations

Clinical manifestations depend on the worm burden and vary from asymptomatic infection to severe morbidity. Penetration of the skin by the larvae of *Ancylostoma*, *Necator* and *Strongyloides* may cause a maculopapular itchy rash. Migration of the larvae through the lungs in case of ascariasis and hookworm may cause Loeffler's (Loffler) syndrome characterized by fever, cough, dyspnea, wheeze, urticaria, eosinophilia and lung infiltrates. Other causes of this syndrome include tropical pulmonary eosinophilia, visceral larva migrans, schistosomiasis and allergic bronchopulmonary aspergillosis. Visceral larva migrans refers to infection by dog or cat ascaris where the larvae have an aberrant life cycle and cause prominent visceral manifestations such as fever, eosinophilia, bronchospasm and hepatosplenomegaly. Cutaneous larva migrans characterized by an erythematous, serpiginous, pruritic eruption refers to infection by non-human hookworms where the larvae migrate through the epidermis and are unable to mature.

Ascaris being the largest worm has the most prominent intestinal manifestations. Heavy infestation can lead to vague abdominal discomfort, abdominal distension, vomiting, irritability, poor growth and nutritional deficiencies. A large mass of worms may cause bowel obstruction and migration of the worms can result in cholecystitis, cholangitis, pancreatitis and rarely intrahepatic abscess.

Hookworms (*Ankylostoma, Necator*) suck blood from the intestine and lead to iron deficiency anemia, hypoalbuminemia and edema. The severity of anemia varies and with heavy infestations, transfusion may be needed. Heavy infestation with *Trichuris* may cause dysentery, anemia, rectal prolapse, abdominal pain, distension, hypoproteinemia and growth retardation. Manifestations of enterobiasis include perianal or vulval itching caused by migration of the gravid females to the perianal skin to lay eggs. *Strongyloides* is associated with abdominal pain, vomiting, diarrhea, bleeding, steatorrhea and weight loss. Ulceration and strictures of the duodenum may occur. Hyperinfection syndrome occurs in the immunocompromised (high dose steroids, chemotherapy, transplant, HIV) and is characterized by dissemination of massive numbers of larvae into various body organs, concurrent gram-negative sepsis and high mortality.

Contrary to popular belief, symptoms including night teeth grinding, craving for sweets, poor weight gain are not due to worm infestation.

### Diagnosis

The diagnosis of most intestinal nematodes is by examination of feces for the characteristic eggs. In enterobiasis, the eggs are present on the perianal skin from which they can be lifted using the scotch tape method. In strongyloidiasis, fresh stool should be examined for larvae as eggs are rarely present; wet mount examination of centrifuged CSF and bronchoalveolar lavage may also help. Serology may also be used to diagnose *Stronglyloides* but is not readily available. Peripheral blood examination may reveal eosinophilia (striking in *Strongyloides*, visceral larva migrans). In ascariasis, the worms may be incidentally observed in the biliary and pancreatic ducts by ultrasound, or in the intestines during contrast studies of the gastrointestinal tract.

### Treatment

As a rule, all family members should be treated. Antiparasitic drugs available for nematode infections including albendazole (200 mg for children aged 1–2 years; 400 mg for those aged 2 years and above, taken with a fatty meal), mebendazole (100 mg twice daily for 3 days or 500 mg single dose), pyrantel pamoate (11 mg/kg, max dose 500 mg), or ivermectin in a daily dose of 150–200 μg/kg. Therapy with nitazoxanide is also effective (100 mg for children aged 1–3 years; 200 mg for children aged 4–11 years; 500 mg for older children and adolescents dosed twice daily for 3 days) **(Table 11.17)**. Since, in pinworm, autoinfections are common, it is essential to stress on personal hygiene, keep nails clipped short, clean bed linen thoroughly and ensure hand washing before meals.

### Prevention

Eradication of intestinal nematodes is possible only with improvement of hygiene and sanitation and appropriate disposal of sewage. Periodic deworming is of no benefit in individual children and should be discouraged. A systematic review of mass deworming programs for soil transmitted helminths has shown no benefit of mass deworming on childhood growth, cognition, school attendance and mortality. Hence, mass deworming is also not currently recommended.

### Suggested Reading


1. Jourdan PM, Lamberton PHL, Fenwick A, Addiss DG. Soil-transmitted helminth infections. Lancet 2018;391:252–65.
2. Welch VA, Ghogomu E, Hossain A, et al. Mass deworming to improve developmental health and wellbeing of children in low-income and middle-income countries: A systematic review and network meta-analysis. Lancet Glob Health 2017; 5:e40–e50.


## Tissue Nematodes

The tissue nematodes of significance in India include *Wuchereria bancrofti*, *Brugia malayi* (causes of lymphatic filariasis) and *Dracunculus medinensis* (guinea worm). Guinea worm disease has been eradicated and India was declared as disease free by WHO in 2000. Further discussion is limited to lymphatic filariasis, an infection acquired in

Table 11.17: Treatment of intestinal nematode infections

| *Helminth* | *Primary drug* | *Alternative(s)* | *Comment* |
|---|---|---|---|
| Round worm (*Ascaris*) | Single dose albendazole | Mebendazole, pyrantel pamoate, ivermectin, nitazoxanide | |
| Hookworm (*Ankylostoma, Necator*) | Albendazole | Mebendazole, pyrantel pamoate | Daily for 3 days<br>Ivermectin ineffective<br>Iron supplements |
| Pinworm (*Enterobius*) | Single dose albendazole | Single dose pyrantel, mebendazole | Repeat in 2 weeks<br>Treat all family members<br>Reinfection common<br>Hand hygiene, keeping nails clipped short, bed linen hygiene |
| Whipworm (*Trichuris*) | Mebendazole 100 mg twice daily | Albendazole 200–400 mg daily or ivermectin 0.2 mg/kg daily | Treat for 3 days |
| Strongyloides | Ivermectin for 2 days | Albendazole twice daily for 7 days (not as effective) | For hyperinfection repeated or prolonged treatment may be needed |
| Cutaneous larva migrans | Ivermectin for 1–2 days | Albendazole twice daily for 3 days | |
| Visceral larva migrans | Antihistaminics and steroids<br>Albendazole or mebendazole twice daily for 5 days | | Ocular toxocariasis may threaten vision |



childhood but usually manifesting in adulthood. Lymphatic filariasis is endemic in several Indian states the most affected being Bihar and Kerala.

### *Life Cycle*

Humans are infected by bite of the vector which in most instances in India is the *Culex* mosquito. The bite releases the infective larvae which migrate to the lymphatics and grow into adult males and females in about a year's time. They mate and release thousands of larvae termed as microfilaria which stay in the lung arterioles during the day and emerge in the systemic circulation at night. They are then taken up the insect vector where they develop further and become infective to humans. The lifespan of the adult worms is usually 5–10 years but can occasionally be up to 40 years.

### *Clinical Features*

The acute symptoms of filarial disease are fever, lymphangitis, epididymoorchitis and adenolymphangitis (Fig. 11.34). In around 0.5% of infected patients, a distinct immunologic reaction to the microfilaria results in an entity called tropical pulmonary eosinophilia (TPE). Features of TPE include cough that worsens at night, wheezing, low grade fever, enlarged neck nodes, interstitial infiltrates on CXR, marked peripheral blood eosinophilia (more than 3000/cu mm) and very high serum IgE levels. This syndrome can also result from the pulmonary phase of ascariasis and hookworms, visceral larvae migrans due to zoonotic *Ascaris* and *Strongyloides* infections. The chronic manifestations of lymphatic filiariasis seen usually in adults include hydrocele, lymphedema and elephantiasis.

### *Diagnosis*

This is largely clinical and confirmed by demonstrating the microfilaria in Geimsa stained thin and thick blood smears obtained from finger pricks. The time of collection depends on the feeding habits of vector, in case of *W. bancrofti*, night time collection is preferred. Diethylcarbamazine (DEC)

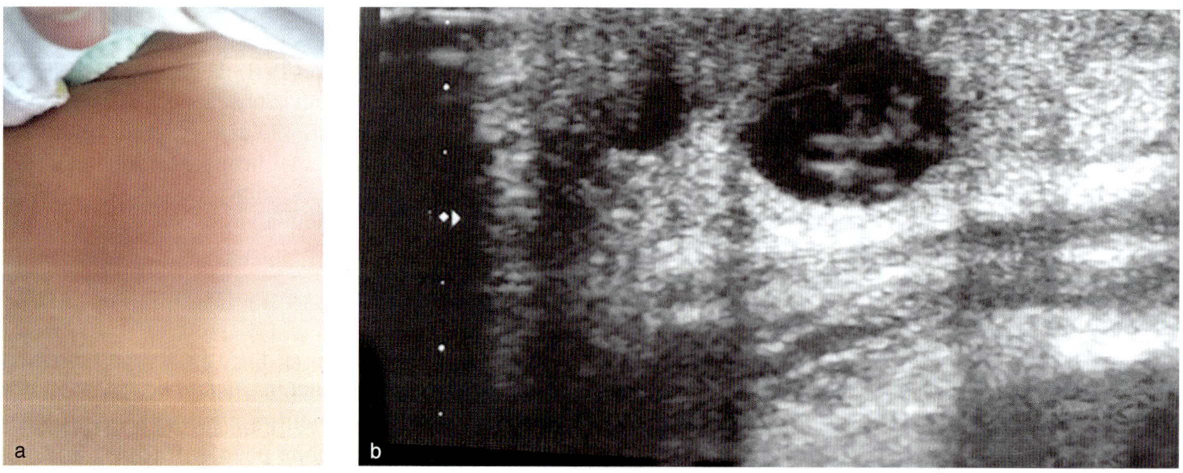


Fig. 11.34: Filariasis manifesting as: (a) An erythematous swelling on the chest of a 2-year-old child; (b) Ultrasonography showing the convoluted worm in the soft tissue

can be used as a provocative agent to facilitate daytime collections. Filarial antigen test in blood is also available.

### Treatment

Most of the symptoms are due to the adult worms, but treatment suppresses or reduces microfilaria but does not affect the adult worms. Adult worms cannot be eradicated. The treatment of choice for lymphatic filariasis is diethylcarbamazine (DEC) dosed at 6 mg/kg/day given either as single dose or in 2–3 divided doses for a period of 12 days. Addition of doxycycline 3 mg/kg/day for a maximum daily dose of 200 mg for 6 weeks improves the lymphedema. Corticosteroids may need to be used to manage allergic reactions of dying microfilaria. Treatment may need to be repeated every 6–12 months for the reappearing microfilaria till the adult worms spontaneously die. Chronic complications need surgical treatment.

Patients with tropical pulmonary eosinophilia (TPE) due to *W. bancrofti* infection should be treated with 14 to 21 days of DEC (6 mg/kg/day).

### Prevention

Since lymphatic filariasis causes considerable morbidity, the National Vector-Borne Disease Control Program (NVBDCP) had proposed elimination of lymphatic filariasis by 2021. The strategy employed is mass drug administration of single dose of DEC with or without albendazole annually to all residents of an endemic district for 5 years. A recent trial demonstrated superior efficacy of three-drug combination with albendazole 400 mg with DEC 6 mg/kg/ dose and ivermectin 150 µg/kg/dose in eradication of microfilaria as compared to single or dual therapy. Vector control is also important.

### Suggested Reading


1. King CL, Suamani J, Sanuku N, et al. A trial of a triple-drug treatment for lymphatic filariasis. N Engl J Med 2018; 379:1801–10.
2. Raju K, Jambulingam P, Sabesan S, Vanamail P. Lymphatic filariasis in India: Epidemiology and control measures. J Postgrad Med 2010; 56:232–38.


## Cestodes

The cestodes that infect humans include giant tapeworms like *Taenia saginata*, *T. solium* and *Diphyllobothrium latum*, dwarf tapeworms like *Hymenolepis nana* and zoonotic cestodes like *Echinococcus granulosus* and *E. multilocularis*. Infection with *T. saginata* and *T. solium* is acquired through ingestion of cysticerca in contaminated food, while *Echinococcus* infection is through ingestion of eggs, and *D. latum* infection is carried to man by ingestion of cysts in freshwater fish.

### Taeniasis and Cysticercosis

Two species of tapeworms infest humans, *Taenia solium* or the pork tapeworm and *T. saginata* or beef tapeworm, the names reflecting the principal intermediate hosts for each of them. Man is the only definitive host for both the parasites. While the pork tapeworm has a scolex with suckers and hooks that aid its attachment to the intestinal wall, hooks are absent in *T. saginata*. Taeniasis refers to intestinal infection by the adult tapeworm, and cysticercosis results from larval lodging in various sites.

**Epidemiology:** Cysticercosis is the most common parasitic disease worldwide, with an estimated prevalence of more than 50 million persons. It is endemic in Mexico, Central and South America, and parts of Africa, Asia, and India. Neurocysticercosis, the neurologic manifestation of cysticercosis, is the most prevalent infection of the brain worldwide and may be responsible for up to 20–50% of all seizures.

**Pathogenesis:** The life cycle of *Taenia solium* and *Taenia saginata* begins as a larva in pigs/cattle, and human infection is acquired by ingestion of these larvae in undercooked pork or beef. The larvae attach to the human gut and grow into adult tapeworms. The adult tapeworm sheds proglottids containing hundreds of tapeworm eggs into human feces. When ingested by pigs or cattle, these eggs develop into larvae that invade the intestinal wall, enter the bloodstream and lodge in various tissues to develop into cysts.

The eggs of beef tapeworm are not infectious to humans. Humans may ingest *T. solium* eggs, usually by feco-oral transmission (via contamination of food by food handlers with poor hand hygiene, or by ingestion of raw fruits or vegetables fertilized with contaminated human waste), or sometimes through autoinfection (by reflux of eggs from intestine into the stomach by reverse peristalsis). Thus humans become dead-end hosts of the larval stage of the parasite, and develop cysticercosis in various body tissues. Ingestion of encysted pork does not directly cause cysticercosis; rather, it causes an intestinal infection with the adult tapeworm and a human reservoir for *T. solium* eggs. Cysticercosis can, therefore, occur in persons who do not eat pork.

Initially the larvae become encysted, which helps viable cysts avoid initial host reaction and destruction by the host. This phase, which may last for 5–10 years, is often clinically silent except when cyst location or size causes signs or symptoms. Degenerating cysts release larval antigens that produce a vigorous host response with release of inflammatory mediators and surrounding edema. After this phase, the encysted larvae degenerate entirely, die and often calcify. Calcified cysts can produce symptoms by unclear mechanisms.

**Clinical features:** Infection with adult worm is mostly symptomatic, but some children may have non-specific symptoms like nausea, abdominal pain and diarrhea. These patients may also develop cysticercosis through autoinfection.

The clinical features of cysticercosis depend on the location of the cysts and overall cyst burden. In about 2 months, the larvae mature into cysticerci of about 2 mm to 2 cm size. Cysts can lodge in the brain, skeletal muscle, subcutaneous tissues, spinal column and eyes. The two sites associated with high morbidity are the brain—the most common (60–90%) location for cysts, and the eye—the least common site (1–3%). Cysts in the brain parenchyma (parenchymal neurocysticercosis) cause focal or generalized seizures and, less commonly, headache, focal neurologic deficits, or behavioral abnormality. Heavy cyst burden can cause encephalopathy with fever, headache, nausea, vomiting, altered mental status and seizures. Cysts in the subarachnoid or ventricular spaces may cause meningeal signs and symptoms, obstructive hydrocephalus or cranial nerve palsies; those located in the spinal column can cause radicular pain or paresthesias. Ocular cysts in the subretinal space or vitreous humor can impair vision by inflammation or through retinal detachment, while those in the extraocular muscles may limit the range of eye movements and those in the subconjunctival tissue present as a nodular swelling. Skeletal muscle or subcutaneous cysticercosis may be either asymptomatic or cause localized pain and nodules.

*Diagnosis:* The diagnosis of taeniasis is made by demonstration of eggs or proglottids in the stools. Patients may pass motile segments of worms through anus.

Diagnosis of neurocysticercosis is based on CT, with or without contrast, or MRI of brain. Demonstration (by CT/MRI) of a solitary contrast-enhancing lesion less than 20 mm in diameter and producing no midline shift is suggestive of neurocysticercosis; if the scolex is visible, it is pathognomonic. Cystic, nonenhancing lesions suggest viable, nondegenerating cysts; cystic, enhancing lesions indicate degenerating cysts with some surrounding inflammation; and calcified cysts suggest old cysts that have already died. MRI is superior to CT in demonstrating spinal, brainstem, or intraventricular lesions (Fig. 11.35). Ocular or extraocular muscle cysticercosis can be picked up on CT or ultrasound, or by dilated ophthalmologic examination.

Detection of antibodies by enzyme-linked immunoblot assay or enzyme-linked immunosorbent assay of the serum or cerebrospinal fluid has sensitivity of 65–98% and specificity of 67–100%, varying with the cyst burden,

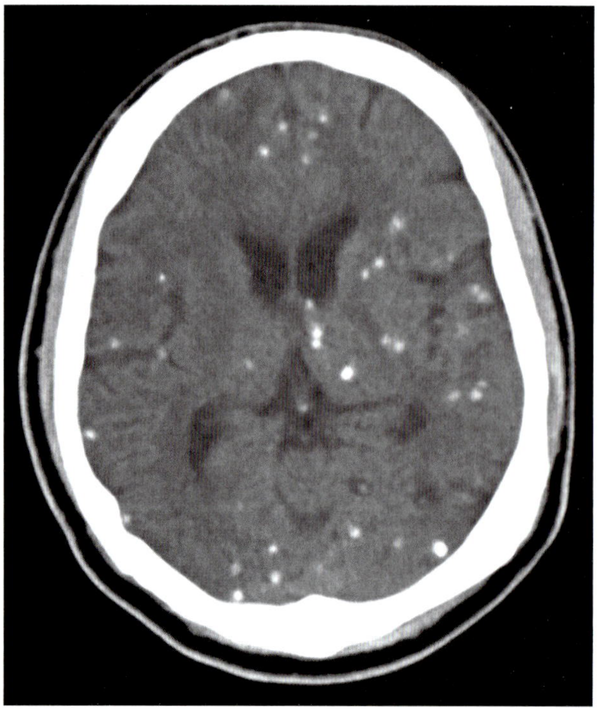

Fig. 11.35: Multiple lesions of neurocysticercosis on computed tomography of the brain

location, and phase of the infection; the immunoblot assay is preferred. Biopsy of the skin or muscle provides a definitive diagnosis in ambiguous situations, and may be the diagnostic method of choice for ocular, extraocular muscle, or painful muscular or subcutaneous cysts.

*Treatment:* Infestation with the adult tapeworm (taeniasis) is treated with praziquantel (5–10 mg/kg once) or niclosamide (50 mg/kg once).

Therapeutic modalities in neurocysticercosis include antiparasitic drugs, surgery, anti-inflammatory drugs and antiseizure medications. The decision depends upon multiple factors, including symptoms and the location, number, stage, and size of cysts. Prior to initiation of therapy, all patients should have an ophthalmologic examination to exclude ocular cysticercosis as inflammation around degenerating cysticerci in the eye due to antiparasitic therapy can threaten vision. Antiparasitic therapy is also generally contraindicated in patients with signs or symptoms of elevated intracranial pressure, regardless of the cause. Such patients should be assessed regarding the need for antiparasitic therapy only after appropriate intervention to reduce intracranial pressure.

***Parenchymal neurocysticercosis:*** Although active parenchymal lesions usually resolve spontaneously and thus may not require anticysticercal drugs, a meta-analysis showed that cysticidal drug therapy is associated with reduced seizures and increased resolution of lesions in the brain parenchyma. Two effective anticysticercal drugs are available—albendazole and praziquantel. Current evidence suggests combination therapy is associated with better outcomes than single therapy. The preferred drug regime is albendazole 15 mg/kg/day in two divided doses (maximum 800 mg/day) with praziquental 50 mg/kg/day in three divided doses for 10 days. Therapy is also combined with dexamethasone 0.1 mg/kg starting 1 day prior to cysticidal therapy and continued for 10 days, with slow taper. If there are multiple cysts, then the duration of therapy may be extended to >30 days. If there are only 1–2 cysts on MRI, only albendazole 15 mg/kg (maximum 1200 mg) with dexamethasone may be used for 10 days. Retreatment after 6 months is indicated, if viable cysts remain. Antiseizure medications are also given, the duration of which may vary. If only calcified cysts are present, only antiseizure medications are used.

***Subarachnoid neurocysticercosis:*** A ventriculoperitoneal shunt and control of raised intracranial pressure with corticosteroids is needed before starting opticidal therapy. Recommended treatment is albendazole 15 mg/kg/day (maximum 1200 mg) for30 days, and dexamethasone 0.1 mg/kg/day for 30 days, with slow taper. This regime may need to be repeated based on clinical and MRI evaluation. If albendazole is used for prolonged periods, blood counts and liver functions should be monitored every 2 weeks. Long courses of albendazole and praziquental may be tried for refractory disease.

***Intraventricular neurocysticercosis:*** This usually necessitates neuroendoscopic removal of the cyst. If the cyst is not accessible then one may place a VP shunt followed by use of albendazole and dexamethasone for prolonged periods.

***Cysticerci elsewhere:*** No treatment generally needed, if asymptomatic. If symptomatic, surgical excision is preferred.

***Prevention:*** Prevention of cysticercosis requires provision of safe water and sanitation to the population.

### Suggested Reading


1. Guideline for preventive chemotherapy for the control of Taenia solium taeniasis. Washinton DC. PAHO; 2021.
2. Sankhyan N, Kadwa RA, Kamate M, et al. Management of neurocysticercosis in children: Consensus guidelines. Indian Pediatr 2021;58:871–80.
3. White AC, Coyle CM, Rajshekhar V, et al. Diagnosis and Treatment of Neurocysticercosis: 2017 Clinical Practice Guidelines by the Infectious Diseases Society of America and the American Society of Tropical Medicine and Hygiene. Am J Trop Med Hyg 2018;98(4):945–66.


#### *Hymenolepiasis*

Infection with *Hymenolepis nana*, also known as the dwarf tapeworm, is very common in developing countries. Man acts as both definitive and intermediate host because the entire life cycle may be completed in human host; however, rodents, ticks and fleas may serve as the intermediate host. The infestation usually results from poor hygiene. The adult worm lives in the jejunum. Transmission is mainly feco-oral, but autoinfection may also occur, such that one host may harbor up to thousands of adult worms. Symptoms are usually non-specific, including mild abdominal discomfort and poor appetite; some have linked growth retardation to *H. nana* infection. The infection is a major cause of eosinophilia. The diagnosis is based on the demonstration of characteristic eggs in stools. Treatment is with praziquantel (25 mg/kg once) or niclosamide (50 mg/kg once, maximum 2 g).

#### *Echinococcosis (Hydatid Disease)*

Human echinococcosis is an infestation caused by larval stages of members of the genus *Echinococcus*, and is characterized by production of unilocular or multilocular cysts in the lung and liver. Echinococcosis is endemic in most contintents of the world, with hyperendemic areas in Western China, North Africa, West Asia and areas of South America.

***Pathogenesis:*** Hydatidosis is a zoonosis caused by two *Echinococcus* species, *E. granulosus* and *E. mulilocularis*. The parasite eggs are transmitted from members of the canine family like dogs and wolves, to various wild and domestic animals like sheep, cattle and goats, which act as intermediate hosts. Humans are accidental hosts. Eggs from the adult worm are passed in the stools that may contaminate the water and soil, and also the fur coats of dogs. Ingestion of food or water contaminated with eggs or direct contact with infected dogs may result in humans being infected accidentally. Eggs hatch in the intestines to release larvae that penetrate the intestinal mucosa, and traverse the venous or lymphatic system to reach the liver, lungs and, less commonly, other target organs.

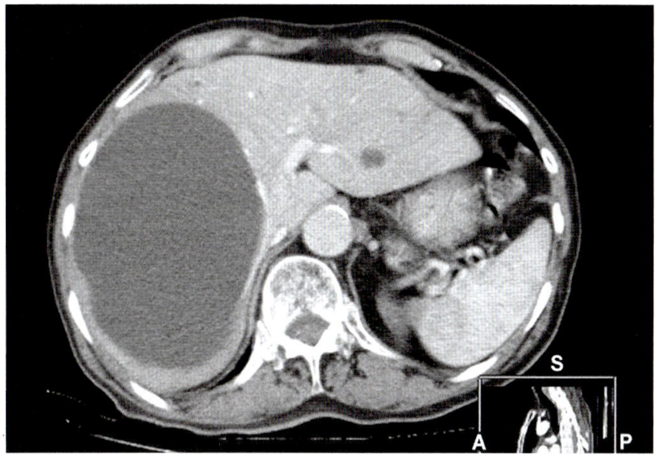


**Fig. 11.36:** Large hydatid cyst of the liver

In the target organs, larvae develop into characteristic multiloculated fluid-filled cysts, called *hydatid cysts*. In children, lung cysts are common, whereas in adults cysts are more commonly seen in the right lobe of the liver (Fig. 11.36). Other tissues that may be involved include bone, brain, genitourinary tract, intestines and subcutaneous tissue. The cyst may keep on expanding over several years.

Life cycle of *E. multilocularis* is the same except that rodents and mice serve as intermediate hosts and the cysts are multilocular that proliferate exogenously and also metastasize. The infection often mimics a malignancy.

***Clinical features:*** Symptoms depend on the target organ involved. Very often, liver cysts may regress spontaneously without becoming symptomatic. Otherwise, cysts may become symptomatic after several years when significant mass effect results in abdominal pain, vomiting, increase in abdominal girth and a palpable mass; jaundice is rare. Alveolar cysts have a more malignant course. Direct spread of infected tissue may result in cysts in the peritoneal cavity, kidneys, adrenal gland or bones. Lung cyst may present with chest pain, cough, hemoptysis and breathlessness. Involvement of the genitourinary tract may manifest as passage of cysts in the urine (hydatiduria) and hematuria. Rupture or leakage from a hydatid cyst may cause anaphylaxis, manifest as fever, itching and rash, and results in dissemination of infectious scolices. Rare but potentially serious complications include compression of important structures in the central nervous system, bone, heart, eyes or genitourinary tract.

***Diagnosis:*** Physical examination may reveal a palpable mass, hepatomegaly or subcutaneous nodules. Ultrasonography is the most valuable tool in diagnosing echinococcal cysts. Lung hydatids may be visible on plain X-ray. MRI and CT may be used for further delineation. Diagnostic aspiration is generally contraindicated because of risk of infection and anaphylaxis. Antibody detection by ELISA is more sensitive but less specific. The test uses partially purified antigens that cross-reacts with other parasites such as cysticercosis and schistosomiasis.

***Management:*** The available options of treatment are: (i) Percutaneous intervention, (ii) surgery, (iii) drug therapy; and (iv) observation alone (for dead calcified cysts). The appropriate approach depends on the size, location and clinical features.

***Liver cysts:*** Percutaneous-aspiration-injection-reaspiration (PAIR) is recommended for uncomplicated larval cysts in the liver. Adjunctive drug therapy with albendazole for 28 days should be administered to minimize risk of secondary echinococcosis from spillage. Surgery and albendazole therapy is the treatment of choice for management of complicated cysts (e.g. ruptured cyst, cysts with biliary fistulae, cysts compressing vital structures, cysts with secondary infection, or hemorrhage) and for management of cysts with many daughter vesicles that are not suitable for percutaneous treatment.

The optimal duration of medical treatment is uncertain. Treatment should be initiated at least 4 days prior to surgery (WHO suggests 4–30 days preoperatively) and should be continued for at least 1-month (albendazole) or 3 months (mebendazole) following surgery. For circumstances in which intact removal of the cyst is not feasible, a protoscolicidal agent such as 20% hypertonic saline should be injected into the cyst prior to removing the contents. Drug therapy alone may be indicated for cysts smaller than 5–10 cm. The dose is 15 mg/kg/day, divided into two doses, to maximum 400 mg orally twice daily with food given for 30 days, for a total of 3 times with a 2-week gap between each course. Watchful waiting is recommended for asymptomatic and calcifying cysts.

***Pulmonary cyst:*** Surgical resection is the treatment of choice. Preoperative albendazole should be avoided. It may, however, be given postoperatively 400 mg twice daily for 28–30 days. Ruptured and complicated cysts may require longer therapy.

***Disseminated disease:*** Patients are administered albendazole 400 mg twice daily till clinical response, with periodic debulking surgery, if possible.

### Suggested Reading


1. Brunetti E, White AC Jr. Cestode infestations: Hydatid disease and cysticercosis. Infect Dis Clin North Am 2012; 26:421–35.
2. Mihmanli M, Idiz UO, Kaya C, et al. Current status of diagnosis and treatment of hepatic echinococcosis. World J Hepatol 2016;8:1169–81.
3. World Health Organization. Echinococcosis, 2021. www.who.int/home/healthtopics/echinococcosis


## HEALTH CARE-ASSOCIATED INFECTIONS

### Introduction

Health care-associated infections (HAI) are termed as those infections that occur in hospitalized patients and were neither present nor incubating at the time of admission. They include those infections that occur as a result of hospital visit (e.g. varicella following exposure in the emergency room or outpatient visit), or in hospitalized children (e.g. diarrhea), or in health care personnel.

### Types of HAI

These may range from minor infections such as viral upper respiratory tract infections to serious infections. Immunocompromised children, children in the neonatal and pediatric intensive care units, and post-surgical patients are at the highest risk for serious infections. Serious HAI include central line-associated bloodstream infections (CLABSI), health care-associated pneumonia (HAP), catheter-associated urinary tract infections (CAUTI), surgical site infections (SSI) and *C. difficile*-associated diarrhea.

### Etiology of HAI

HAI in India are predominantly due to infection with resistant gram-negative bacilli, including ESBL (extended spectrum beta-lactamase), AmpC beta-lactamase and carbapenamase producing *E. coli*, *Klebsiella*, *Pseudomonas* and *Acinetobacter*. Gram-positive pathogens including *S. aureus* and *Enterococcus* are less common. *Candida* is an emerging pathogen.

### Clinical Features

The clinical features include new onset fever, hemodynamic compromise, respiratory deterioration and diarrhea depending on the site of HAI. Some of the HAI can be rapidly progressive and lead to septic shock and multiorgan dysfunction in a few hours. HAI need to be differentiated from non-infectious causes of fever such as drug fever, thrombophlebitis, pulmonary embolism and atelectasis. Mere isolation of bacteria from non-sterile site cultures, such as trachea, urine, stool and drains, is not indicative of HAI and should be interpreted carefully.

### Consequences of HAI

HAI can lead to significant morbidity and mortality, and lengthen duration and cost of hospital stay. More importantly they lead to increased use of high end antimicrobials that further amplify the problem of antimicrobial resistance.

### Treatment

Management entails early recognition and sending appropriate cultures including blood, endotracheal aspirates, urine, pus and starting broad-spectrum antibiotics pending reports. The choice of antibiotics varies with the severity and site of infection, prior antibiotic exposure, local antimicrobial resistance patterns and host comorbidities such as kidney or liver dysfunction. Usually this regime comprises beta-lactam–beta-lactamase inhibitor combinations such as piperacillin–tazobactam, cefoperazone–sulbactam, or carbapenems with or without amikacin and antifungals. In settings with high prevalence of carbapenem resistance, therapy with colistin, fosfomycin and tigecycline may be needed. Source control such as removal of infected lines and drainage of pus is crucial. In the interests of antimicrobial stewardship, de-escalation and optimization of therapy, once culture results are available, is important. Treatment for 7–10 days is sufficient in most cases.

### Prevention

Infection prevention and control is the cardinal strategy to prevent HAI. The most important is hand hygiene with antimicrobial soap and water or alcohol-based hand rub before and after each patient contact, before sterile procedures and after contact with patient surroundings. Implementing prevention bundles for CLABSI/HAP/CAUTI and SSI are integral to any infection control program. Maintaining a clean hospital environment with attention to air and water quality, and following standard and transmission-based precautions are other components of preventive strategy.

### Suggested Reading


1. Foster CB, Sabella C. Health care associated infections in children. JAMA 2011; 305:1480–81.
2. Indian Council for Medical Research. Antimicrobial Resistance Research and Surveillance Network, 2020. Available at: https://main.icmr.nic.in/sites/default/files/guidelines/AMRSN_annual_report_2020.pdf


## RATIONAL ANTIMICROBIAL THERAPY

Rational antimicrobial therapy refers to using antimicrobials only when indicated; the right drug for the right duration through the right route and in the right dose. Irrational use of antibiotics compromises treatment outcomes, increases adverse effects and cost of therapy. Irrational use of antimicrobials is the biggest driver for antimicrobial resistance. Rising antimicrobial resistance is responsible for increasing morbidity, mortality and treatment cost of infections.

### Antimicrobial Resistance

The most important antimicrobial resistance challenges facing us at the current time in India are antimicrobial resistance in gram-negative bacilli due to production of extended spectrum beta-lactamases (ESBL) and carbapenemases, and emergence of multidrug resistant and extremely drug resistant (XDR) tuberculosis.

### Irrational Antimicrobial Therapy

**Examples of irrational therapy** include:

- Prescribing antimicrobials when not indicated. For example, using antibiotics to treat viral upper respiratory tract infections and viral gastroenteritis.
- Prescribing multiple antimicrobials at the same time, using irrational combinations, and changing them frequently.
- Using high-end antimicrobials such as carbapenems to treat community-acquired infections, and using drugs for MRSA such as vancomycin when not indicated.
- Using fewer drugs than indicated for diseases where combination therapy is indicated such as tuberculosis, HIV, malaria.

**Reasons for irrational therapy** include:

- Practitioner errors owing to inadequate knowledge about microbial etiology and resistance patterns. Other reasons for irrational prescriptions are fear of missing a diagnosis, in order to circumvent investigations and sometimes due to pressure from parents. The belief that the newer the drug and more the number of drugs the better it is also drives practitioners to over use antibiotics.
- Self-medication by parents and as per pharmacist recommendations.
- Aggressive marketing of antimicrobials by representatives of pharmaceutical companies.
- Ready availability of antimicrobials over-the-counter and licensing of irrational fixed drug combinations such as cefixime–ofloxacin.

#### *Management*

The following measures are proposed as strategies to reduce antimicrobial resistance:

- Education of medical practitioners about rational antimicrobial practices right from the undergraduate level through postgraduation and for practicing doctors.
- Development of evidence-based guidelines to treat common infections and ensuring that they are implemented.
- Educating the public and parents about the hazards of overuse of antibiotics.
- Legislation to prevent over-the-counter availability of antimicrobials and licensing of irrational fixed drug combinations.
- Preventing overuse of antimicrobials in the veterinary industry.
- Establishing antimicrobial stewardship programs in hospitals targeting use of antimicrobials in inpatients especially intensive care units.

#### *Conclusions*

We are facing an antimicrobial resistance crises. We are running out of treatment options and not many new drugs are in the pipeline. If we do not use our existing antmicrobials wisely, we are destined to return to the pre-antibiotic era and era of untreatable infections.

### Suggested Reading


1. Ghafur A, Mathai D, Muruganathan A, et al. The Chennai Declaration: A roadmap to tackle the challenge of antimicrobial resistance. Indian J Cancer 2013;50:71–73.
2. Marston HD, Dixon DM, Knisely JM. Antimicrobial resistance. JAMA 2016; 316:1193–1204.

Chapter 12

# Diseases of Gastrointestinal System and Liver

❍ Anshu Srivastava ❍ Barath Jagadisan ❍ Surender Kumar Yachha

*Competencies:* **PE26.5; PE26.8**

Most diseases of the gastrointestinal (GI) tract present with a few symptoms, such as vomiting, dysphagia, abdominal pain, distension, diarrhea, constipation, gastrointestinal bleeding and failure to thrive. Appropriate evaluation involves assessment of symptoms and signs, listing differential diagnosis and planning investigations so as to arrive to the correct diagnosis and initiate treatment.

*Competencies:* **PE26.5; PE26.6**

## VOMITING

Vomiting refers to expulsion of gastric contents through the mouth. Vomiting should be differentiated from regurgitation, especially in infants. Regurgitation is the involuntary and effortless expulsion of small amounts of gastric contents that is not accompanied by nausea. Recurrent or persistent vomiting requires thorough evaluation. Persistent vomiting may be complicated by dehydration, hypokalemic hypochloremic metabolic alkalosis, malnutrition and constipation. Vigorous vomiting can uncommonly result in mucosal tear (Mallory-Weiss syndrome) or esophageal rupture (Boerhaave syndrome).

Vomiting is a common, but often nonspecific, symptom that may be acute, chronic or recurrent (Table 12.1). Acute onset, short duration vomiting is the most common and is often caused by viral infections. Chronic vomiting may be (i) cyclic, characterized by stereotype episodes occurring infrequently with complete normalcy in between, or

**Table 12.1:** Causes of vomiting

| *Gastrointestinal* | *Nongastrointestinal* |
|---|---|
| **Acute** | |
| Gastroenteritis | Infections, e.g. urinary tract infection, meningitis, encephalitis, pertussis |
| Hepatitis | Raised intracranial tension |
| Appendicitis | Diabetic ketoacidosis |
| Small intestinal obstruction (malrotation, volvulus, intussusception) | Defects in fatty acid oxidation or respiratory chain |
| Cholecystitis | Drug or toxin induced |
| Pancreatitis | |
| **Chronic** | |
| Gastroesophageal reflux | Raised intracranial tension |
| Gastritis | Chronic sinusitis |
| Gastric outlet obstruction (hypertrophic pyloric stenosis, peptic ulcer) | Uremia |
| Small bowel obstruction (duodenal stenosis, annular pancreas, superior mesenteric artery syndrome) | Overfeeding |
| Food allergy | |
| Achalasia cardia; gastroparesis; eosinophilic esophagitis | |
| **Recurrent** | |
| Cyclic vomiting | Urea cycle defects |
| Abdominal migraine | Diabetic ketoacidosis |
| Malrotation with volvulus | Addison disease |

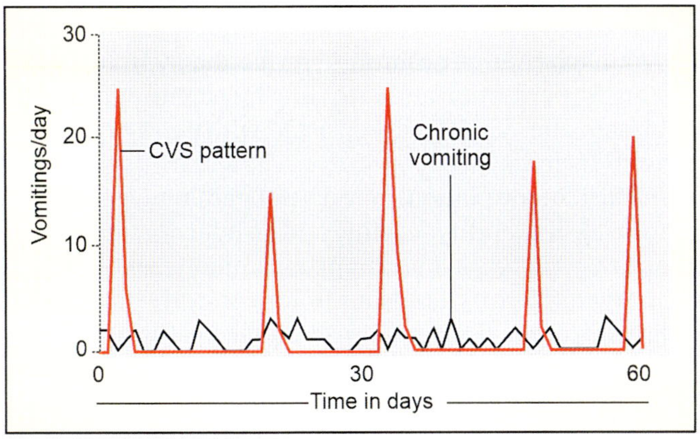


Fig. 12.1: Chronic and cyclic (cyclic vomiting syndrome, CVS) pattern of vomiting

(ii) chronic, characterized by ongoing low frequency vomiting for weeks (Fig. 12.1).

## Evaluation

A detailed history and examination often gives clue to the diagnosis. The etiology of vomiting varies according to age; while infectious causes occur across all ages, most congenital anomalies, e.g. atresia and metabolic disorders, present in the neonatal period or infancy. The first step is to determine whether the vomitus is bilious or non-bilious. Lesions beyond the ampulla of Vater cause bilious vomiting and those proximal to it lead to non-bilious vomiting. Associated features may indicate etiology, e.g. vomitus containing stale food ingested on the previous day (gastric outlet obstruction), visible peristalsis (obstruction), vomiting in early morning (intracranial neoplasm or cyclic vomiting syndrome), vertigo (middle ear disorder) and hypotonia (mitochondrial disorders). The 'red flags' in a child with vomiting include presence of blood or bile in the vomitus, severe abdominal pain with abdominal distension or tenderness, projectile vomiting, persistent tachycardia or hypotension, neck stiffness and/or photophobia. These patients need admission and urgent evaluation.

Workup for chronic vomiting depends upon the suspected diagnosis. It includes blood chemistry (sugar, electrolytes, creatinine, amylase, lipase and transaminases); abdominal imaging (ultrasound abdomen, CT or MRI abdomen with small bowel enterography), upper gastrointestinal endoscopy, gastric emptying scan, CT or MRI brain, metabolic testing or urinalysis. It is important to remember that children with cyclic vomiting should be evaluated during symptomatic phase before starting intravenous fluids since investigations may be non-contributory during asymptomatic periods.

Evaluation of a child with acute vomiting should include assessment of hydration, electrolytes, creatinine and plain X-ray abdomen (in suspected surgical causes). Promethazine and ondansetron are useful in postoperative vomiting and to abort episodes of cyclical vomiting. Ondansetron given alone or with dexamethasone is preferred for chemotherapy-related vomiting. Domperidone and metoclopramide are useful in patients with gastroparesis. Antihistaminics like diphenhydramine, help in motion sickness. Management of the underlying condition is essential.

Some common disorders presenting with vomiting are described below.

## Idiopathic Hypertrophic Pyloric Stenosis

Hypertrophic pyloric stenosis is the most common surgical disorder of the gastrointestinal tract in infants. The pylorus is thickened and elongated with narrowing of its lumen due to hypertrophy of the circular muscle fibers.

### *Clinical Presentation*

Patients present with non-bilious vomiting that gradually increases in frequency and severity to become projectile in nature. The disorder is 4–6 times more common in boys than girls. Most patients are symptomatic beyond 3 weeks of age, however, about 20% are symptomatic since birth. Constipation is common. Recurrent and persistent vomiting causes dehydration, malnutrition and hypochloremic alkalosis. As the stomach muscles contract forcibly to overcome the obstruction, a vigorous peristaltic wave can be seen to move from left hypochondrium to umbilicus, particularly on examination after feeding. A firm olive-shaped mass is palpable in the mid-epigastrium in 75–80% infants, especially after feeds.

### *Evaluation*

Ultrasound abdomen is diagnostic (100% sensitive and ~90% specific). It shows thickened (muscle thickness ≥4 mm) and elongated pylorus (length ≥16 mm. However, in case of doubt, an upper GI barium study (Fig. 12.2) or an upper GI endoscopy should be performed.

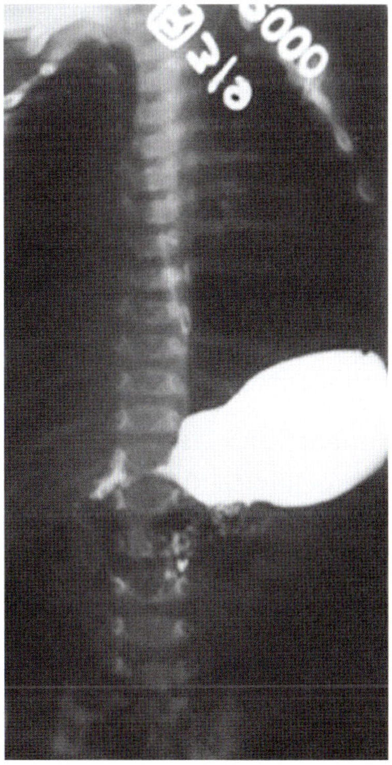

Fig. 12.2: Upper gastrointestinal barium study showing narrowing and elongation of pyloric channel in idiopathic hypertrophic pyloric stenosis

### Management

The treatment includes correction of dehydration and electrolyte abnormalities, followed by surgery (Ramstedt pyloromyotomy).

## Cyclic Vomiting

This is defined as occurrence of stereotypic episodes of intense nausea and vomiting satisfying the following criteria:

- Minimum 5 episodes, or 3 attacks in 6 months time
- Episodic intense nausea and vomiting, lasts 1-hr to 10 days, separated by ≥1 week
- Stereotypical
- Vomiting >4 times/hr, for ≥1 hr
- Return to baseline health between episodes
- Not attributed to other metabolic, neurologic or gastrointestinal disorders

Typically, the attacks begin in early morning with symptoms of autonomic surge, e.g. lethargy, pallor, mild fever, headache, tachycardia, hypertension, diarrhea and abdominal pain. Most subjects have onset in preschool or school age. Family history of migraine and/or motion sickness is noted in 30–40% cases. Symptoms may overlap with abdominal migraine. Age <2 years at onset or presence of alarm features like attacks precipitated by fasting/high protein meal, presence of abdominal distension/bilious vomiting/severe pain, or altered mentation (confusion/severe irritability) needs exclusion of other causes by appropriate investigations.

### Management

Known precipitants (like fasting, lack of sleep, stress, specific dietary components, etc.) of the episodes should be avoided. Management of an attack includes providing a quiet environment, administration of intravenous fluids, use of serotonin 5-$HT_3$ antagonists such as ondansetron (0.3–0.4 mg/kg/dose IV q 4–6 hr up to 20 mg) and sedation with lorazepam (0.05–0.1 mg/kg/dose IV every 6 hr). Prophylaxis against future attacks is recommended in patients with severe and frequent episodes of vomiting. They include cyproheptadine (0.25–0.5 mg/kg/day in two or three divided doses) or propranolol in younger children (<5 years), and amitriptyline (initiate at 0.2–0.3 mg/kg/day at bedtime; may increase up to maximum of 1.0–1.5 mg/kg/day) or propranolol (0.25–1 mg/kg/day; upto 10 mg q 8–12 hr) in older children.

## Gastroesophageal Reflux Disease (GERD)

Gastroesophageal reflux (GER) is passage of gastric contents into the esophagus with or without regurgitation and vomiting. GER is a normal physiologic process that occurs several times a day in healthy infants, children and adults. When this reflux of gastric contents causes troublesome symptoms and/or complications, it is known as GERD. About 50% of healthy 3–4-month-old infants regurgitate at least once per day and most of them outgrow this by 1 year of age. Children with obesity, repaired esophageal atresia, cystic fibrosis, hiatal hernia, neurological impairment (cerebral palsy), preterm babies and a family history of GERD are at an increased risk of developing GERD.

### Clinical Features

As younger children cannot describe the symptoms, we rely on the perception and reporting by parents which may be biased. The symptoms associated with GERD vary with age and include:

- *Infants:* Regurgitation, emesis, not gaining weight, feed refusal, irritability, crying and grimace, anemia and apnea. *Sandifer syndrome* is an uncommon manifestation, characterized by spasmodic torsional dystonia with arching of the back and opisthotonic posturing.
- *Young child:* Regurgitation, abdominal pain, anorexia, feeding refusal, and poor weight gain.
- *Older children and adolescents:* Heartburn, epigastric/retrosternal pain, regurgitation. Hematemesis and dysphagia indicate presence of esophagitis or stricture esophagus.

Extraesophageal symptoms (like asthma, pneumonia, bronchiectasis, acute life-threatening events, laryngotracheitis, recurrent otitis media) have been associated with GERD, but a causal relationship with reflux is not well established.

### Evaluation

A detailed history and physical examination are generally sufficient to establish the diagnosis of GERD. Presence of symptoms like hematemesis, undernutrition, organomegaly and seizures in a suspected GERD patient requires investigations. Efforts should be made to differentiate GERD from rumination, eosinophilic esophagitis and achalasia cardia (especially in younger children). Rumination is defined as regurgitation of recently ingested food with rechewing or expulsion, which begins soon after ingestion of a meal, does not occur during sleep and does not respond to standard anti-GER therapy.

### Investigations

Useful investigations are as follows:

- *24 hours ambulatory esophageal pH monitoring* is a validated method for quantitative measurement of esophageal acid exposure (Fig. 12.3). It is also used to evaluate the efficacy of anti-secretory therapy and to correlate symptoms (e.g. cough, chest pain) with acid reflux episodes.
- *Combined 24 hours multichannel intraluminal impedance and pH monitoring (pH-MII)* detects acid, weakly acid and nonacid reflux episodes. It is superior to pH monitoring alone which detects episodes of acid reflux. Its main utility is to evaluate the temporal relationship between symptoms and GER episodes.
- *Upper GI endoscopy* may show erosions or mucosal breaks in the distal esophageal mucosa, the most reliable evidence of reflux esophagitis. Mucosal erythema and pallor are highly subjective and nonspecific findings. Complications like stricture esophagus (Fig. 12.4) and Barrett's esophagus can be picked up. Endoscopic biopsy is important to exclude other causes of esophagitis and to diagnose Barrett's esophagus. Elongated rete pegs, basal cell layer hyperplasia and dilated intercellular spaces, alone or in combination, are suggestive of reflux esophagitis on histology.

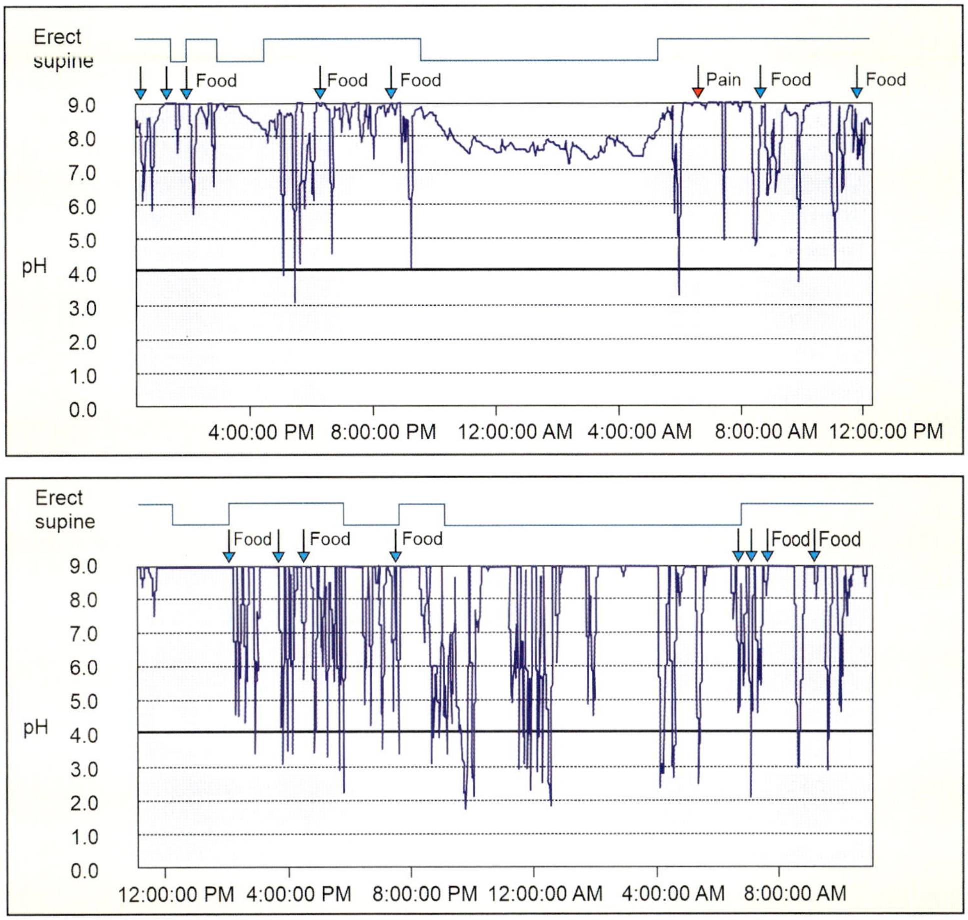


**Fig. 12.3:** 24 hours esophageal pH study. Upper panel shows a normal study and lower panel shows frequent episodes of acidic reflux with drop in pH to <4 suggestive of gastroesophageal reflux disease

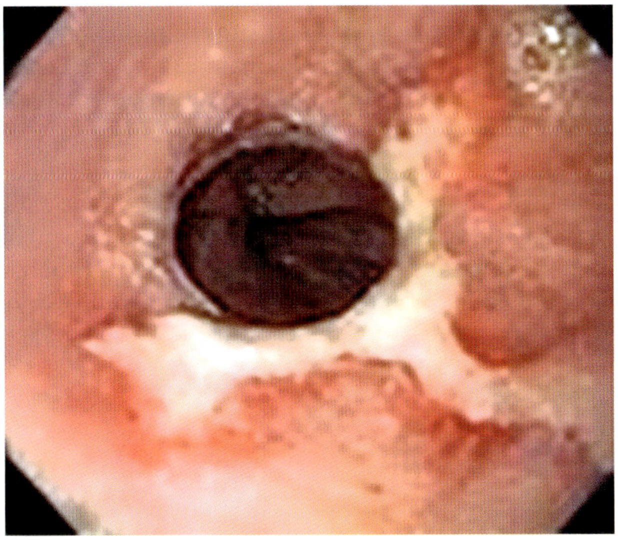

**Fig. 12.4:** Upper gastrointestinal endoscopy showing ulceration with stricture formation in reflux esophagitis

- *Barium contrast radiography* helps to rule out anatomic abnormalities of the upper gastrointestinal tract that may cause similar symptoms. It should be done in all infants with vomiting. However, it is not useful for the diagnosis of GERD.
- *Nuclear scintigraphy* has a role in the diagnosis of pulmonary aspiration in patients with chronic and refractory respiratory symptoms.
- *Empiric trial of acid suppression:* Using proton pump inhibitors for up to 4 weeks is justified in older children or adolescents with typical symptoms suggesting GERD.

The investigation of choice depends on the question being asked like 24 hours pH+MII for symptom correlation, gastroscopy for detecting erosions or excluding eosinophilic esophagitis. Approach to an older child with GERD is shown in Fig. 12.5.

### Management

It depends on patient's age, nature and severity of symptoms. Alarm systems include dysphagia (difficulty swallwing) and odynophagia (painful swallowing). Other alarm features include anemia, bleeding and weight loss. The main components are lifestyle changes, medications and surgery.

*Lifestyle changes:* Infants should be burped well and overfeeding should be avoided. Cow milk protein allergy is sometimes a cause of unexplained crying and vomiting in infants. Therefore, formula-fed infants may benefit from a 2–4 weeks trial of an extensively hydrolyzed protein formula. Thickening of feeds not only increases the calorie content but also reduces visible regurgitation. Careful follow-up with charting of caloric intake and weight gain is essential.

Children and adolescents with GERD, should avoid caffeine, chocolate and spicy foods. Weight loss if obese, sleeping in the left lateral position with elevation of the

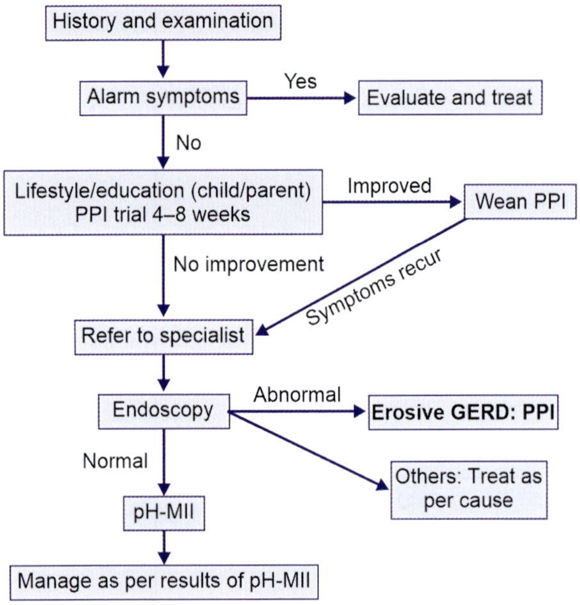


**Fig. 12.5:** Approach to an older child with suspected gastro-esophageal reflux disease (GERD). PPI proton pump inhibitor, pH-MII pH testing and multichannel intraluminal impedance monitoring

head-end of the bed, avoidance of alcohol and cessation of smoking are helpful.

*Histamine-2 receptor antagonists* like ranitidine [2–4 mg/kg/day, max 10 mg/kg/day (300 mg/d) in 2–3 divided doses] decrease acid secretion by inhibiting receptors on gastric parietal cells. They are less effective than PPI and tachyphylaxis occurs with chronic use.

*Proton pump inhibitors (PPI):* Inhibit acid secretion by blocking $Na^+$–$K^+$-ATPase, the final common pathway of parietal cell acid secretion. PPI are the agents of choice for GERD and maintain intragastric pH >4 for long periods and inhibit meal-induced acid secretion. They are mostly given once a day, 30 minutes before breakfast. PPI should not be given to all infants with suspected GERD due to lack of benefit. Only esomeprazole is approved in USA for infants with erosive esophagitis. Omeprazole, lansoprazole, pantoprazole and rabeprazole can be given to >1-yr-old. There is no data to support one PPI over another. In patients with reflux esophagitis or non-erosive reflux disease, PPI for 3 months constitute initial therapy. Important side effects include headache, diarrhea, community-acquired pneumonia, calcium malabsorption, hypomagnesemia, and acute interstitial nephritis; prolonged use should be avoided.

*Antacid therapy:* It is not recommended for most patients with GERD.

There is also insufficient evidence to justify the routine use of prokinetics (cisapride, metoclopramide, domperidone, erythromycin) or other agents like bethanechol or baclofen for GERD.

*Surgical therapy:* Fundoplication (open or laparoscopic) decreases reflux by increasing the lower esophageal sphincter (LES) pressure, decreasing the episodes of transient lower esophageal sphincter relaxation and increasing the nadir pressure during swallow-induced relaxation, increasing the length of intra-abdominal esophagus, accentuating the angle of His and reducing hiatal hernia, if present. Antireflux surgery may be of benefit in selected children with chronic GERD with intractable symptoms or risk of life-threatening complications.

### Suggested Reading

1. Li BUK, Lefevre F, Chelimsky GG, et al; North American Society for Pediatric Gastroenterology, Hepatology and Nutrition. Consensus statement on the diagnosis and management of cyclic vomiting syndrome. J Pediatr Gastroenterol Nutr 2008;47:379–93.
2. Rosen R, Vandenplas Y, Singendonk M, et al. Pediatric Gastroesophageal Reflux Clinical Practice Guidelines: Joint Recommendations of the North American Society for Pediatric Gastroenterology, Hepatology, and Nutrition (NASPGHAN) and the European Society for Pediatric Gastroenterology, Hepatology, and Nutrition (ESPGHAN). J Pediatr Gastroenterol Nutr. 2018; 66: 516–54.
3. Shields TM, Lightdale JR. Vomiting in children. Pediatr Rev. 2018;39:342–58.

*Competencies:* **PE26.5; PE26.6**

## DYSPHAGIA

Dysphagia refers to a sensation of food being hindered in its passage from the mouth to the stomach, i.e. difficulty in swallowing. *Odynophagia* is painful swallowing and *globus* is the sensation of a lump in the throat. Dysphagia can be divided into two distinct groups:

*Oropharyngeal or transfer dysphagia:* Presence of drooling, choking, coughing and nasal regurgitation suggests oropharyngeal dysphagia. The main causes are cerebral palsy, bulbar poliomyelitis, muscular dystrophy, brainstem tumors and neuropathy.

*Esophageal dysphagia:* Etiology of esophageal dysphagia can be broadly divided into two groups: Motor causes (e.g. achalasia cardia and diffuse esophageal spasm) and structural causes (e.g. strictures, foreign body, Schatzki's ring, esophageal web, eosinophilic esophagitis and extrinsic compression by aberrant vessel or mediastinal mass).

### Differential Diagnosis and Evaluation

The important causes of esophageal dysphagia and their evaluation is shown in Table 12.2.

*Congenital esophageal stenosis:* This may be of three types: Web or diaphragm, fibromuscular stenosis and stenosis due to cartilaginous tracheobronchial remnants. Symptoms of vomiting or chest infection due to aspiration typically develop around 6 months of age when weaning is started.

*Foreign bodies in esophagus:* Button battery and magnet ingestions have increased in last couple of years. Sharp foreign bodies and batteries can cause damage by perforation secondary to pressure or chemical necrosis and can present with dysphagia, mediastinitis and/or upper gastrointestinal bleeding. Multiple magnets, if ingested, attract each other across bowel loops and cause necrosis,

Table 12.2: Evaluation and management of esophageal lesions that cause dysphagia

| *Etiology* | *Investigation* | *Finding* | *Treatment* |
|---|---|---|---|
| Corrosive (acid or alkali) stricture | Barium swallow and meal; upper GI endoscopy | Narrowing in one or multiple, short or long, segments of esophagus; may show contracted stomach or pyloric stenosis | Endoscopic dilatation (Balloon or Savary-Gilliard dilators) |
| Stricture after repair of tracheoesophageal fistula | Barium swallow (**Fig. 12.6**) | Narrowing of a short segment of esophagus | Endoscopic dilatation |
| Congenital stricture | Barium swallow; CT chest | Stricture in middle or lower esophagus; cartilaginous tissue in stricture | Endoscopic dilatation or surgery |
| Post-sclerotherapy stricture | Barium swallow; upper GI endoscopy | Narrowing in lower end of esophagus | Endoscopic dilatation |
| Peptic stricture | Barium swallow; endoscopy; 24 hours pH study | Narrowing in lower esophagus; may show hiatus hernia or erosions | Endoscopic dilatation; proton pump inhibitor after dilatations |
| Foreign body | Plain X-ray; upper GI endoscopy (**Fig. 12.7**) | Type of foreign body and site of impaction | Endoscopic retrieval |
| Achalasia cardia | Barium swallow; endoscopy esophageal manometry | Beak-like narrowing in lower esophagus | Pneumatic dilatation; Heller's cardiomyotomy; POEM (peroral endoscopic myotomy) |
| Infectious esophagitis (in immunocompromised children) | Upper GI endoscopy; endoscopic biopsy | White curd-like deposits (*Candida*); ulcers (cyto-megalovirus, herpes) | Fluconazole (*Candida*); ganciclovir (cytomegalovirus) or acyclovir (herpes) |

GI gastrointestinal

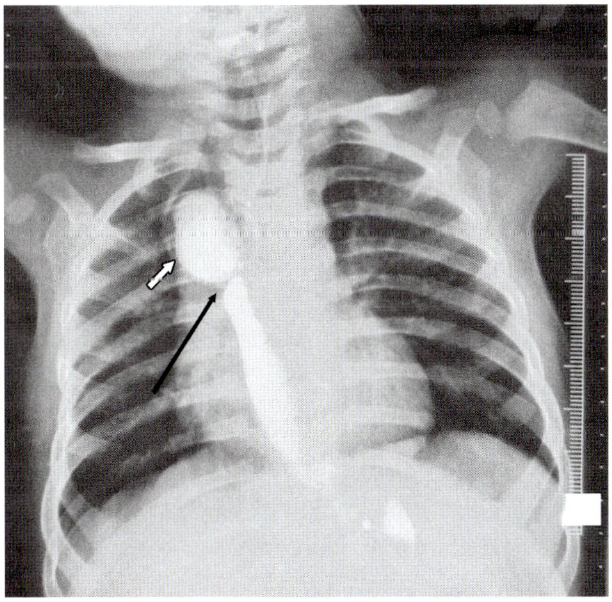

**Fig. 12.6:** Post-TEF stricture. Black arrow shows the short stricture and white arrow shows the dilated proximal esophagus

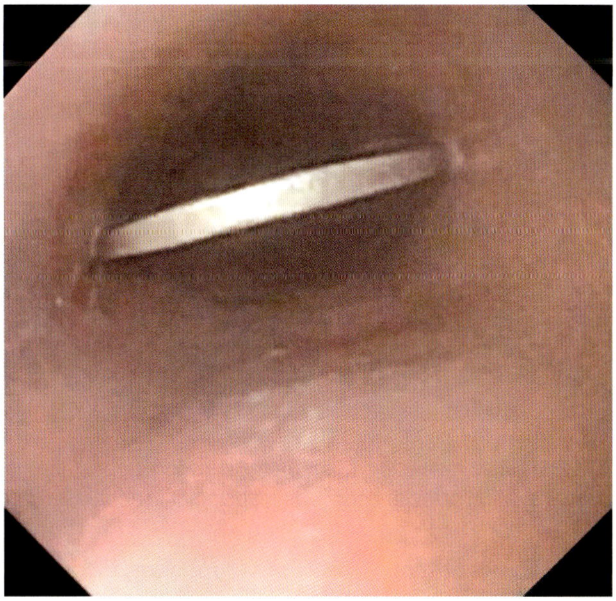

**Fig. 12.7:** Upper GI endoscopy showing foreign body (coin) in esophagus

fistula formation, and perforation. All patients with suspicion of foreign body ingestion should have an X-ray, even if asymptomatic. The vast majority of foreign bodies pass unimpeded through the GI tract. The most frequent sites of impaction are at the cricopharynx, mid-esophagus at tracheal bifurcation and just above the LES. Endoscopic removal by experts is the standard of therapy. The urgency of removal depends on the nature of the foreign body. No foreign body should be left in esophagus for >24 hours; however, button battery and sharps should be removed at the earliest possible.

*Achalasia cardia:* Children present with dysphagia, vomiting, weight loss, respiratory symptoms and slow eating whereas toddlers present with coughing and feeding aversion with failure to thrive. The average age at diagnosis is around 8–9 years. Barium swallow shows esophageal dilatation with beak-like narrowing at the LES (**Fig. 12.8**). Manometry is the most sensitive and specific

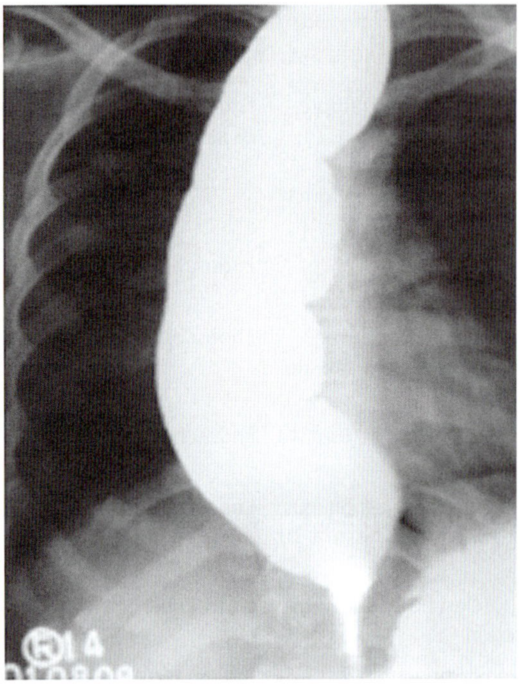

Fig. 12.8: Barium swallow showing achalasia cardia

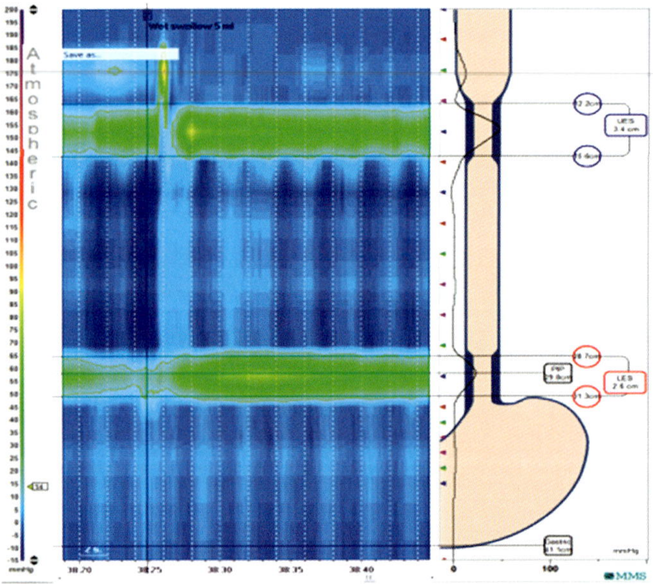

Fig. 12.9: High resolution manometry showing aperistalsis and lack of relaxation of lower esophageal sphincter in achalasia cardia

tool and shows absent peristalsis in esophagus; incomplete/absent LES relaxation and raised intraesophageal pressure (Fig. 12.9). Achalasia is classified as type I, II and III based on manometry. Endoscopy is useful to exclude other etiologies of dysphagia. Endoscopic pneumatic balloon dilatation, Heller's cardiomyotomy with fundoplication, and POEM (peroral endoscopic myotomy) are the main therapies.

## Suggested Reading

1. Mubarak A, Benninga MA, Broekaert I, et al. Diagnosis, Management, and prevention of button battery ingestion in childhood: A European Society for Paediatric Gastroenterology Hepatology and Nutrition Position Paper. J Pediatr Gastroenterol Nutr 2021;73:129–36.
2. van Lennep M, van Wijk MP, Omari TIM, et al. Clinical management of pediatric achalasia. Expert Rev Gastroenterol Hepatol 2018; 12: 391–404.

*Competency:* **PE26.5**

## CONSTIPATION

Constipation is defined as a delay or difficulty in defecation sufficient to cause significant distress to the patient. If the duration is >4 weeks, it is labeled as chronic constipation, and if less, it is acute. It is increasingly being recognized as a common problem in children and is associated with both physical and psychological morbidity and a poor quality of life. The normal stool frequency of Indian children decreases from 2–4 per day during infancy to once per day after 2 years of age. A stool frequency of ≤2/week is considered abnormal for all ages. The majority of patients have functional constipation; organic cause is found in ~10–15% (Table 12.3).

### Approach

Details about time of first passage of meconium, pattern of stooling, presence of blood in stools, diet, stressful life events, urinary symptoms, drug intake and previous surgeries should be known. A predominantly low fiber diet (milk based) and sedentary lifestyle contributes to constipation. A complete physical and neurological examination is essential. Examination should look for features of spina bifida (pigmentation or tuft of hair on lower back), power in lower limbs, perianal sensation, tone of anal sphincter, and fecoliths on abdominal/per rectal examination. '*Red flags*' like failure to thrive, blood in stools, recurrent fever with loose stools (enterocolitis), recurrent vomiting, lump in abdomen, and recurrent chest infections should alert the physician to suspect an organic etiology.

### Functional Constipation

Functional constipation (FC) is defined by the presence of at least two or more of the following criteria for >1 month: (i) Two or fewer defecations per week; (ii) at least 1 episode of fecal incontinence per week after the acquisition of toileting skills; (iii) history of retentive posturing; (iv) history of painful or hard bowel movements; (v) presence of a large fecal mass in the rectum or on per

| Table 12.3: Causes of constipation |
|---|
| *Intestinal nerve/muscle disorders:* Hirschsprung disease, intestinal neuronal dysplasia, pseudo-obstruction, spinal cord abnormalities (tethered cord, myelomeningocele) |
| *Anorectal:* Anteriorly placed anus, anal stenosis, rectal stricture, pelvic mass (sacral teratoma) |
| *Systemic disease:* Hypothyroidism, celiac disease, diabetes insipidus, diabetes mellitus, hypercalcemia, cystic fibrosis, myotonic dystrophy |
| *Developmental:* Mental retardation, autism |
| *Drugs:* Opiates, anticholinergic agents, phenobarbitone, vincristine, lead |

abdomen examination; and (vi) history of passage of large diameter stools that may obstruct the toilet (applicable only for children who use the Western type of toilet).

Children with FC pass large, hard stools and display stool withholding behavior, characterized by stiffening of whole body and screaming in infants, to walking on tiptoes or tightening of buttocks in older children. This is often misunderstood by parents as if the child is trying to defecate. Often an acute illness, change in diet, coercive toilet training or non-availability of clean toilet leads to delay or non-passage of stools. The stools become hard and cause pain on passage which leads to association of defecation with pain and further withholding. This further increases stool size and hardness with more pain on defecation. Children with FC often have abdominal pain (10–70%), anorexia (10–25%), enuresis or urinary tract infections (30%), and psychological problems (20%).

### Management

No investigations are required for diagnosis in the majority of children with FC. The management approach is shown in Fig. 12.10. It includes disimpaction and maintenance therapy.

***Disimpaction:*** It is required in patients who have a rectal impaction, i.e. presence of a large hard mass of feces on per rectal examination or abdominal fecoliths or retentive encopresis. Rectal impaction is responsible for progressive dilatation of the rectum over time and increased threshold volume for rectal sensation and defecation. This 'clean out' is essential for maintenance therapy to be effective. The oral route is preferred over rectal as it is less invasive. This can be done at home using polyethylene glycol (PEG) in a dose of 1.5 g/kg/day for 3–4 days. Alternatively, PEG electrolyte solution can be given in the dose of 15–40 mL/kg/hr till the rectal output is clear and devoid of solid fecal material. In young children, this should be done using a nasogastric tube and in hospital under supervision. Intravenous fluids may be required in small children to maintain adequate hydration. An alternative to oral administration of PEG is the use of phosphate enema (contraindicated in <1-year-old) or sodium dioctyl sulfosuccinate enema, 30–60 mL/10 kg body weight to a maximum of 120 mL, once or twice daily for 1–2 days. Repeated rectal enemas should be avoided.

***Maintenance therapy:*** The aim of maintenance therapy is to promote regular stooling and prevent reimpaction. Successful therapy is defined as passage of 1–2 soft stools per day and no soiling. It includes the following:

i. *Behavioral training* involves establishing a positive routine of sitting on toilet for passing stools after meals (2–3 times per day for 5–10 min) and documenting all stool passage. Embarrassment or punishment should be avoided.
ii. *Dietary changes:* A nutritious diet with fruit/vegetables and adequate fluids is given. A short trial of milk and milk product free diet may be done in refractory cases suspected to have bovine milk allergy.
iii. *Medication:* Regular and tailor-made (as per response) laxative use is the key to success. Osmotic laxatives, like lactulose (1–3 mL/kg/day), and PEG (0.8–1.0 g/kg/day) are the first-line agents. Stimulant laxatives like senna or bisacodyl are to be used intermittently as a rescue therapy to avoid impaction. Prokinetics like cisapride are not recommended. In infants, mineral oil and stimulant laxatives should not be used. Glycerin suppository is preferred over enema for impaction in infants. Premature withdrawal of medications is a very common cause of relapse.

### Prognosis

Most of the children need maintenance therapy for few months. Regular follow-up is essential to ensure continuation of toilet training and dietary advice and detect relapse. In nearly 25% patients, constipation persists even after puberty.

## Other Causes of Constipation

A subgroup of children with red flags or constipation that fails to respond to ≥3 months of optimal medical

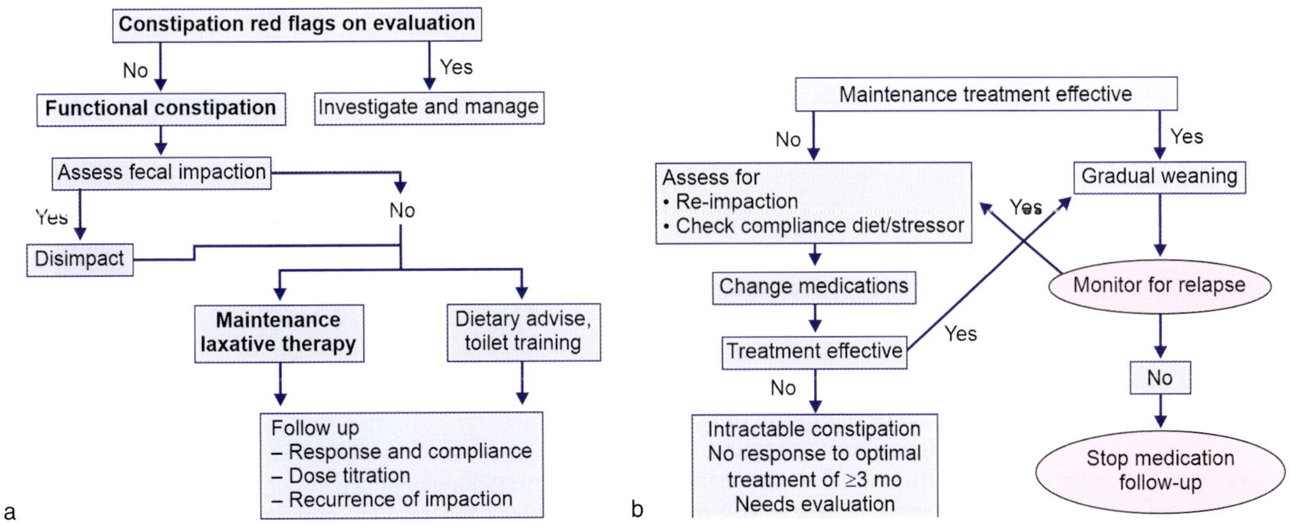


Fig. 12.10: Evaluation (a) and follow-up (b) of a child with constipation

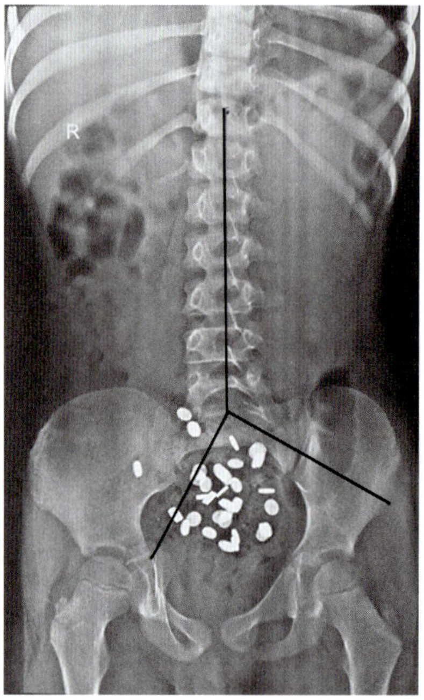

Fig. 12.11: Colonic transit study showing retained radiopaque markers in the left colon suggestive of outlet obstruction in a child with constipation

management despite compliance (refractory constipation) need evaluation. The main modalities of investigation are as follows:

*Rectal biopsy:* A full thickness rectal biopsy or suction biopsy is required to rule out Hirschsprung disease, neuronal intestinal dysplasia and hypoganglionosis.

*Anorectal manometry:* In normal persons, the internal anal sphincter shows relaxation on distension of rectum with a balloon. This is known as rectoanal inhibitory reflex and its presence excludes the diagnosis of Hirschsprung disease.

*MRI of lumbosacral spine:* It is useful for diagnosis of spina bifida occulta or tethered cord.

*Colonic transit study:* Assessment of total and segmental colonic transit time is done either by radiopaque markers or by scintigraphy. Based on transit studies, colonic motility is defined as: normal colonic transit, slow transit constipation (prolonged transit throughout the colon) and outlet obstruction (delayed transit through anorectum) (Fig. 12.11).

*Metabolic, endocrine and others:* It is useful to screen for hypothyroidism, cystic fibrosis, hypercalcemia, celiac disease and lead poisoning.

### Hirschsprung Disease (HD)

This is the commonest congenital gut motility disorder with an incidence of 1 in 5000 and is characterized by lack of ganglionic cells in the submucosal and myenteric plexuses of the distal intestine. The distal rectum is aganglionic and the aganglionosis extends proximally in a variable length of colon. The absence of enteric neurons leads to tonic contraction of the aganglionic segment and functional obstruction. This multigenic disorder can be familial or sporadic. Down syndrome is one of the most common associated malformations. HD is classified by the length of involved bowel, with ~75% cases having classic or short segment (rectosigmoid), ~15–20% having long segment (colon proximal to splenic flexure), ~5% having total colonic aganglionosis (entire colon with <50 cm distal ileum) and rarely total intestinal aganglionosis (involves longer segments of small bowel).

Affected infants present shortly after birth with constipation and signs of distal obstruction. About 60–90% children with HD fail to pass meconium in first 48 hours of life. Occasionally, the disease is missed and the child presents later with chronic constipation, failure to thrive and episodes of enterocolitis (loose stools with blood and mucus). Presence of empty rectum on per rectal examination with a gush of liquid stools on withdrawal of finger suggests the diagnosis.

In neonatal period, plain X-ray abdomen reveals bowel distension with multiple air-fluid levels and paucity of air in pelvis. A carefully performed barium enema without prior colonic preparation and slow injection of contrast clearly delineates the narrow aganglionic bowel, transition zone and proximal dilated colon in HD (Fig. 12.12). In contrast, in functional constipation, the rectum is grossly dilated, with a rectum to sigmoid ratio of >1 and absence of transition zone. However, a normal barium study does not exclude HD. Absence of rectoanal inhibitory reflex on anorectal manometry suggests HD. Rectal biopsy is the gold standard for diagnosis, with full thickness biopsy being ideal. Absence of ganglionic cells in the myenteric and submucosal plexus confirms the diagnosis. Hypertrophied nerves with increase in acetylcholinesterase activity in the parasympathetic nerve fibers are seen in the aganglionic segment. The main differences between functional constipation and HD are shown in Table 12.4.

Management depends on timing of diagnosis and is essentially surgical; medical management is restricted to stabilizing the general condition and treating episodes of enterocolitis. Definitive surgical treatment involves

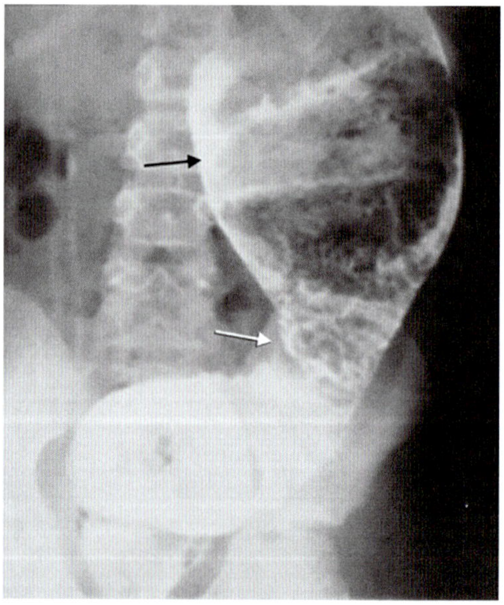

Fig. 12.12: Barium enema showing Hirschsprung disease. Black arrow shows the dilated proximal segment and white arrow shows the transition zone

Table 12.4: Differences between functional constipation and Hirschsprung disease

| Feature | Functional constipation | Hirschsprung disease |
|---|---|---|
| Passage of meconium | Normal | Delayed |
| Onset of symptoms | Beyond 1 year of age | Within infancy |
| Encopresis | Yes | No |
| Stool withholding behavior | Yes | No |
| Episodes of enterocolitis | No | Yes |
| Growth failure | No | Yes |
| Abdomen | Not distended; may have palpable fecoliths | Distended |
| Per rectal examination | Soft to hard stools present | Empty rectum with gush of stools on removing the finger |
| Barium enema | Rectum larger than sigmoid; ratio >1 | Rectosigmoid ratio <1; transition zone seen |
| Anorectal manometry | Rectoanal inhibitory reflex present | Rectoanal inhibitory reflex absent |
| Rectal biopsy | Ganglion present | Ganglion absent |

resection of the aganglionic bowel, pull through and anastomosis of normally innervated ganglionic bowel close to the anal margin. Effort is made to preserve the anal canal and sphincter mechanism, thus preserving continence. In patients with delayed presentation, a colostomy in the ganglionic bowel is performed initially to relieve the obstruction and allow the dilated hypertrophied proximal bowel to return to normal. Subsequently, definitive surgery is performed. Now less invasive, laparoscopic and single staged surgeries are performed, in comparison to previous 2–3-staged procedure. In the long-term, majority show improvement but nearly two-thirds of patients have some form of constipation or continence problem.

### Suggested Reading


1. Koppen IJN, Di Lorenzo C, Saps M, et al. Childhood constipation: finally something is moving! Expert Rev Gastroenterol Hepatol 2016; 10: 141–55.
2. Langer JC. Hirschsprung disease. Curr Opin Pediatr. 2013; 25: 368–74.
3. Poddar U, Singh S, Pawaria A, et al. Aetiological spectrum, clinical differentiation and efficacy of polyethylene glycol over lactulose in children with constipation: Experience of 316 cases. J Paediatr Child Health 2019; 55: 162–67.
4. Yachha SK, Srivastava A, Mohan N, et al. Management of childhood functional constipation: Consensus Practice Guidelines of Indian Society of Pediatric Gastroenterology, Hepatology and Nutrition and Pediatric Gastroenterology Chapter of Indian Academy of Pediatrics. Indian Pediatr 2018; 55: 885–92.


*Competencies:* **PE21.14; PE26.5**

## ABDOMINAL PAIN

Abdominal pain is a common manifestation of multiple pathologies which vary from benign to life-threatening conditions. The pain may be acute or chronic in nature. To be able to arrive at a diagnosis, careful history and examination and appropriate investigations are necessary. An understanding of pain perception and location of pain provides valuable information (Fig. 12.13). Stretching of the overlying visceral peritoneum or inflammation results in pain. The pain from the stomach and proximal intestine is sensed in the epigastrium; from the midgut to the periumbilical area; and from the hindgut to the suprapubic area. The inflammation in the parietal peritoneum causes pain in the overlying abdominal wall. Thus, the pain of appendicitis is referred to the periumbilical area when the inflammation is restricted to the visceral peritoneum, but is perceived in the right iliac fossa when the inflammation involves the parietal peritoneum. Referred pain is common in abdominal pathologies; a subdiaphragmatic collection may manifest as same side shoulder pain, ureteric pain is referred from loin to groin and pancreatic pain can radiate to the back.

Physicians must distinguish abdominal pain due to emergent diagnoses like appendicitis or intussusception from benign conditions like gastroenteritis or constipation. Details like site, duration, radiation, trend (improving or worsening), association with meals, nocturnal pain, associated features, and specific triggers that worsen the pain are essential for making a correct diagnosis. Examination should be meticulous including examination of genitalia as torsion of testes or incarcerated hernia can be easily overlooked. Acute onset, severe, localized pain, associated with bilious vomiting and/or distension, absent or increased bowel sounds, localized tenderness, or peritoneal signs (rebound tenderness, rigidity, guarding) suggest a surgical abdomen and needs immediate evaluation.

Differential diagnosis should be considered in terms of age as many diagnoses are more common in younger or older children (Table 12.5).

### Acute Appendicitis

Acute appendicitis is a surgical emergency and is more common in older children. Obstruction of the appendiceal lumen by either fecolith or lymphoid tissue (e.g. following viral infection) is the initiating event. The obstruction, distention and infection in the appendix causes progressive inflammation and, subsequently, perforation. The patient presents with fever and anorexia followed by pain in the periumbilical area. Vomiting follows the periumbilical pain, unlike in gastroenteritis. As the inflammatory fluid spreads, the pain is then felt in the right iliac fossa (McBurney point) towards which the child characteristically points with a

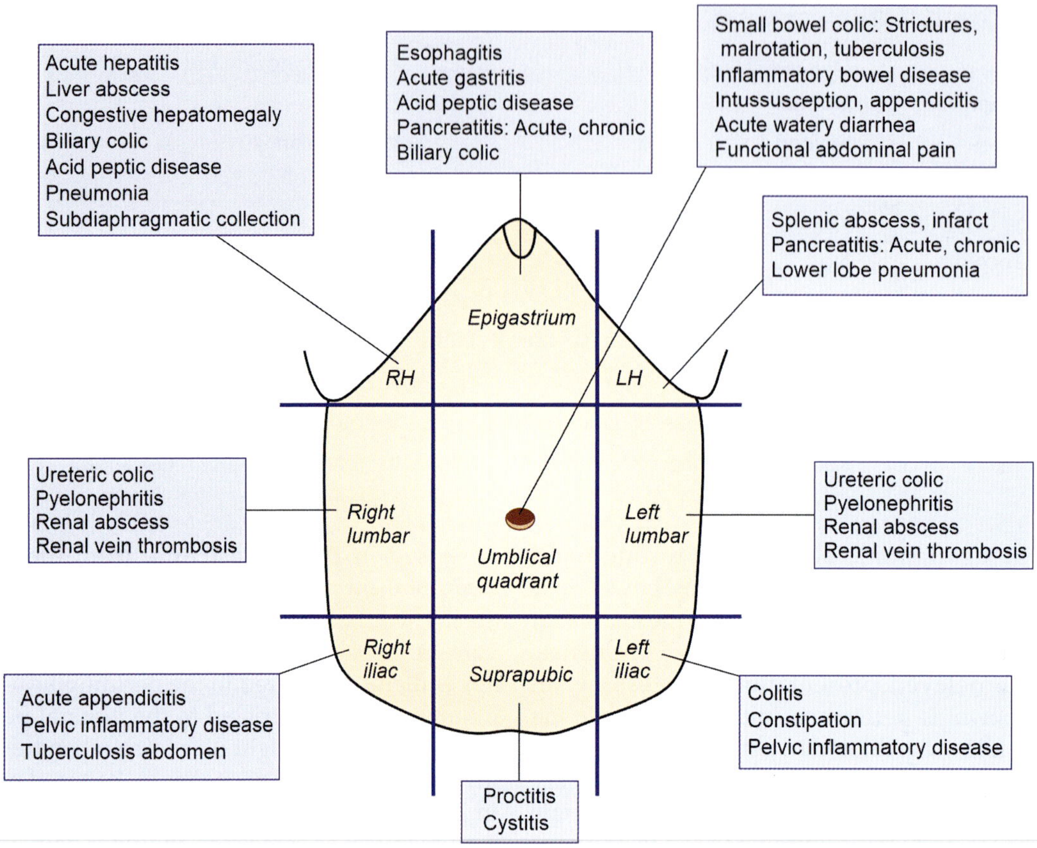


**Fig. 12.13:** Causes of abdominal pain as per site of pain. RH right hypochondrium; LH left hypochondrium

**Table 12.5:** Common causes of abdominal pain

| | |
|---|---|
| Infants and young children (<2 yr of age) | Colic, acute gastroenteritis, necrotizing enterocolitis, urinary tract infection (UTI), constipation, **intussusception, malrotation of gut with volvulus, incarcerated hernia, intestinal obstruction** |
| Preschool children (2–5 yr) | Acute gastroenteritis/colitis, UTI, constipation, lower lobe pneumonia, acute pancreatitis, ureteric colic, diabetic ketoacidosis, Henoch-Schönlein purpura, peptic ulcer disease, hepatitis, gallstone disease, **intussusception, acute appendicitis, malrotation of gut with volvulus, intestinal perforation with peritonitis, incarcerated hernia, torsion testis, Meckel's diverticulum, choledochal cyst** |
| Older children and adolescents | Acute gastroenteritis, gastritis, pancreatitis, cholecystitis, pneumonia, acute viral hepatitis, peptic ulcer disease, gallstone disease, Crohn's disease, constipation, UTI, tubo-ovarian disease, ovarian cyst menstrual pain, pelvic inflammatory disease, renal calculi, **acute appendicitis, complicated acute cholecystitis, choledochal cyst, testicular or ovarian torsion, intestinal obstruction, obstructed inguinal hernia, perforation or peritonitis, ectopic pregnancy** |

Causes highlighted in bold need surgical attention

finger. A retrocecal inflamed appendix may be difficult to diagnose and may manifest as spasm at the hip. The diagnosis is most often based on clinical suspicion after history and examination. Palpation reveals localized tenderness in the right lower abdomen, rebound tenderness or guarding or a mass.

#### *Diagnosis and Management*

Hemogram shows polymorphonuclear leukocytosis. Urine microscopy should be done to rule out urinary tract infection. Abdominal ultrasound detects a dilated (>6 mm) tubular, aperistaltic structure which is not compressible and is surrounded by fluid. Ultrasound has a sensitivity of 85–90% and specificity of 95–100% for diagnosing appendicitis. Computed tomography may be done occasionally, if the diagnosis is in doubt. In up to one-third of patients, the appendix ruptures before surgery. Intravenous fluids and antibiotics for gram-negative and anerobic coverage should be given in all cases. Early surgery (preferably laparoscopic appendectomy) is necessary to prevent complications like perforation, appendiceal abscess and sepsis.

### Intussusception

This is a common cause of intestinal obstruction in children between 3 months and 6 years. Intussusception refers to the telescoping of a proximal segment of intestine (intussusceptum) into a distal segment (intussuscipiens). This causes venous congestion, bowel edema leading to arterial obstruction, bowel ischemia, necrosis, perforation and shock. It may be ileocolic, colocolic or ileoileal. Ileocolic intussusception is most common (~75–80%), with the terminal ileum acting as the intussusceptum and the ascending colon as the intussuscipiens. Most cases occur in infants during the weaning period following upper respiratory tract infection or vaccination. An area of enlarged submucosal Peyer patch probably acts as a lead point. Beyond two years of age, the possibility of a submucosal lead point like lipoma and polyp that needs surgical resection should be considered as failure to resect them will lead to recurrence. Inflammatory conditions, like Henoch- Schönlein purpura, also result in intussusception. Iatrogenic intussusception occurs in patients with enteral feeding tubes, where the tip of the feeding tube acts as a lead point. The classic triad of abdominal pain, red currant jelly stools (blood and mucus) and palpable mass is seen only in a small percentage of children.

### *Diagnosis and Management*

X-ray abdomen shows paucity of air in right lower quadrant. Ultrasound is the investigation of choice that confirms the diagnosis ('doughnut' sign), provides information about presence of a mass as lead point and evaluates for other causes of abdominal pain. Vascularity of bowel is best assessed on color Doppler. Barium enema shows a characteristic 'claw' sign, if the intussusception involves colon. Early reduction either with saline (under ultrasound guidance), barium contrast (both diagnostic and therapeutic) or with air insufflation is advisable. Reduction with air is safer and preferred. Apart from fluoroscopy, USG is now used for monitoring the reduction of the intussusception, as it avoids radiation exposure. Failure of radiological reduction or suspected intestinal gangrene may necessitate surgery and resection.

## Gallstones (Cholelithiasis)

Gallstones are of three main types: Cholesterol stones with >50% cholesterol, pigment (black or brown) stones and mixed type. Pigment stones are common in children with hemolytic anemia. High-risk groups for gallstones include children with hemolytic anemia, obesity, ileal resection or disease, intake of drugs like ceftriaxone, progressive familial intrahepatic cholestasis type III and total parenteral nutrition. Overall, hemolytic anemia and other predisposing conditions account for 20–30% and 30–40% of gallstones, respectively, while 30–40% cases remain idiopathic.

Typical presentation is with acute or recurrent episodes of right upper quadrant or epigastric pain which may radiate to the right shoulder. Icterus and pain radiating to the back is suggestive of a stone in common bile duct or ampulla causing pancreatitis. Fever is uncommon; however, if present, it suggests cholecystitis or cholangitis.

### *Diagnosis and Management*

Serum bilirubin and alkaline phosphatase are elevated, if the stone is in the common bile duct. Raised amylase/lipase suggests pancreatitis. Ultrasonography is the investigation of choice for diagnosis of gallstones. MRCP and ERCP have a better accuracy than ultrasonography in diagnosing common bile duct stones. Hemoglobin, reticulocyte count, peripheral blood picture and other investigations should be done to look for hemolytic disease.

Symptomatic cholelithiasis is treated by open or laparoscopic cholecystectomy. Common bile duct calculi can be removed by ERCP or surgery. Children with asymptomatic gallstones without underlying predisposing factors can be safely followed up. Prophylactic cholecystectomy is preferred in patients with sickle cell disease and asymptomatic gallstones. Children with other hemolytic anemias undergoing splenectomy should be screened for gallstones. Cholecystectomy should be done along with splenectomy in those having gallstones.

## Choledochal Cyst

Choledochal cyst refers to abnormal cystic dilatation of biliary tree. Based on the site (intrahepatic or extrahepatic) and number (single vs multiple) of biliary dilatations, choledochal cyst is classified as type 1–5 (Todani classification). Type 5 is known as Caroli disease and has multiple fusiform or saccular dilatations of the intrahepatic ducts. Caroli syndrome is when congenital hepatic fibrosis occurs with Caroli disease.

Choledochal cyst has a variable presentation. In neonates, it mimics biliary atresia (~5% of all neonatal cholestasis), and in older children, it presents with recurrent episodes of pain, obstructive jaundice or mass in right upper quadrant. The disorder can cause pancreatitis either due to stone impaction at lower end of common bile duct, or due to anomalous pancreatobiliary junction. Biliary peritonitis secondary to spontaneous bile duct perforation is an important complication in younger children. If left untreated, patients can progress to secondary biliary cirrhosis.

### *Diagnosis and Management*

Ultrasonography is the first investigation for diagnosis. MRCP is done to define the anatomy of the pancreaticobiliary

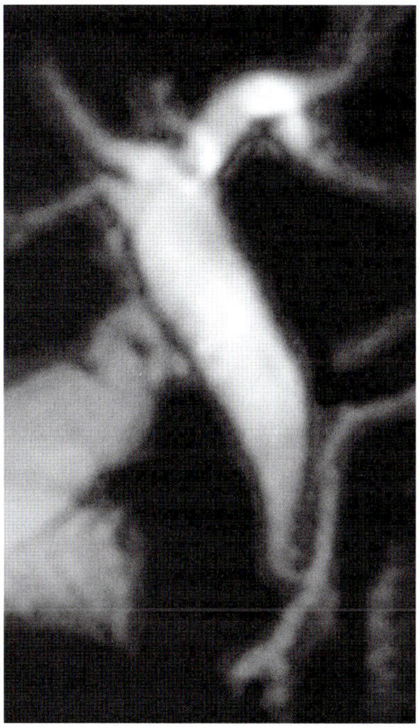

**Fig. 12.14:** Magnetic resonance cholangiopancreatography (MRCP) showing choledochal cyst

ductal system before surgical excision (Fig. 12.14). Antibiotics and supportive therapy are given to a child presenting with obstructive jaundice and cholangitis. Surgical resection of the cyst with hepaticojejunostomy is the definitive therapy as there is a risk of malignancy (cholangiocarcinoma).

### Intestinal Malrotation

Failure or interruption of the normal process of rotation, positioning and fixation of the gut during development results in malrotation. This causes recurrent obstruction, either due to congenital bands of fibrous tissue (Ladd's band) or volvulus of the gut over the narrow mesenteric pedicle. This can cause infarction and gangrene of long segments of gut and can be fatal, if not recognized. Majority (60–80%) of malrotation cases present in the first month of life. Recurrent episodes of abdominal pain with bilious vomiting suggest small bowel obstruction; abdominal distension may not be a prominent finding in proximal small bowel obstruction. Some children can have recurrent abdominal pain with failure to thrive secondary to chronic intermittent volvulus with malabsorption due to impaired lymphatic or venous drainage of the gut.

#### *Diagnosis and Management*

USG abdomen is a useful screening tool. It can detect volvulus (whirlpool sign) and an abnormal relation of superior mesenteric vein and artery in malrotation. Normally, the SMV lies to the right of the SMA. In malrotation, the SMV may be anterior or to the left of the SMA. Diagnosis of malrotation is confirmed on barium meal follow through (BMFT), which shows duodenojejunal junction on the right of the spine (rather than to the left of midline at the level of pylorus), an abnormally positioned cecum and small bowel loops on the right side of abdomen (Fig. 12.15). If volvulus is also present, the contrast abruptly tapers into a corkscrew appearance at the level of the second portion of duodenum.

The presence of bilious vomiting is an alarm sign and requires urgent evaluation. In patients with volvulus, resuscitation (correction of fluid and electrolyte balance) followed by emergency laparotomy and Ladd's procedure is done. This includes derotation of the volvulus, division of the Ladd's band, widening of the base of the mesentery, placement of bowel in a state of nonrotation and appendicectomy.

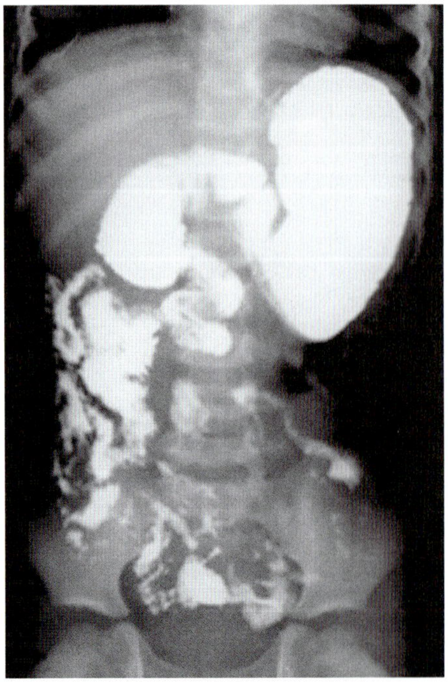

Fig. 12.15: Barium meal follow through showing malrotation of intestine

### Peptic Ulcer Disease

Ulcers may be primary, i.e. related to *Helicobacter pylori* or secondary to drugs (NSAIDs, steroids), stress (shock, sepsis and ischemia), corrosives, Ménétrier's disease, Crohn disease and Zollinger-Ellison syndrome. Both gastric and duodenal ulcers are uncommon in children as compared to adults. Clinical presentation depends on the age. Neonates typically present with bleeding and perforation from a gastric ulcer occurring in the setting of sepsis or respiratory distress. Older infants and toddlers have vomiting, feeding issues and upper GI bleeding. Older children may have epigastric pain similar to that seen in functional dyspepsia, which may be relieved by eating. Gastrointestinal bleeding, large volume vomiting due to gastric outlet obstruction and severe pain due to perforation suggest complicated ulcers. Ulcers associated with *Helicobacter pylori* infection usually affect older children. Nearly 20% patients have a positive family history and upper GI endoscopy shows antral nodularity.

#### *Diagnosis and Management*

Upper GI endoscopy confirms the diagnosis by direct visualization of location (gastric or duodenal), number and size of ulcer/s (Fig. 12.16). Endoscopic therapy with sclerosant or adrenaline injection, application of heater probe or bipolar electrocoagulation, or placement of hemoclip over bleeding vessel is indicated in ulcers with active bleeding, ooze or those with a visible vessel. Antral and corpus biopsies should be taken for diagnosis of

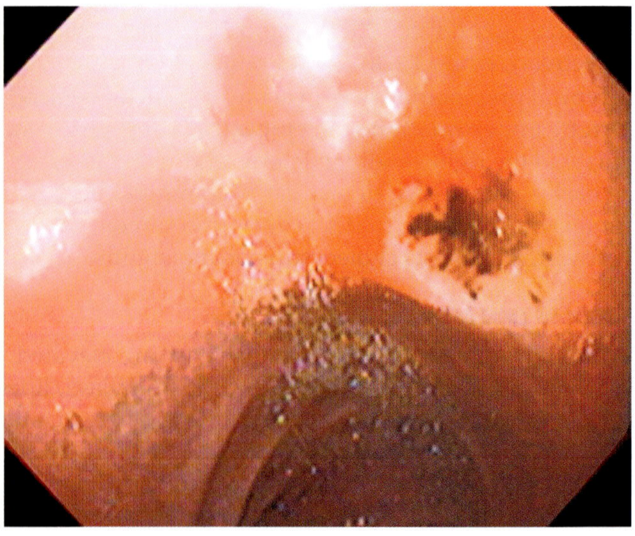

Fig. 12.16: Upper gastrointestinal endoscopy showing duodenal ulcer in the first part of duodenum

*H. pylori* using combination of rapid urease test, culture, Gram staining and histology.

Proton pump inhibitors are the mainstay of therapy. *H. pylori* eradication therapy (two of three antibiotics: Amoxicillin, metronidazole, clarithromycin and proton pump inhibitor) is essential to prevent recurrence of peptic ulcer. Predisposing factors, including NSAIDs, should be avoided. Prophylactic PPI in high-risk (respiratory failure, coagulopathy and high PRISM score) critically ill children in the PICU will reduce the risk of bleeding. Surgery is indicated in children presenting with gastric outlet obstruction or uncontrolled bleeding despite drug and endoscopic treatment.

## Acute Pancreatitis

Acute pancreatitis is increasingly being recognized in children. The main causes include trauma, drugs (valproate, L-asparaginase), viral infections (mumps), hemolytic uremic syndrome, congenital biliary anomalies (choledochal cyst), Henoch-Schönlein purpura, gallstones, hypercalcemia and hypertriglyceridemia. Abdominal pain is the main symptom, pain is mostly in epigastrium but ~20% may have diffuse pain. Pain radiating to the back is classical but uncommon. Infants and toddlers may present with vomiting, irritability and abdominal distension.

### *Diagnosis and Management*

Presence of at least two of the following three criteria is required for diagnosis:

- Abdominal pain compatible with pancreatic origin
- Amylase and/or lipase ≥3 × upper limit of normal, and
- Imaging (ultrasonography, CT scan) findings suggestive/compatible with pancreatic inflammation.

If the patient has organ failure for <48 hours, he has severe pancreatitis, if he has organ failure for <48 hours and/or local complications or exacerbation of comorbidity, he has moderately severe disease; and if there is no organ failure or local or systemic complications, then mild disease.

The management is supportive, with analgesia and hydration. Early fluid replacement corrects hypovolemia, increases the perfusion of pancreas, improves microcirculation and reduces necrosis. There is no role of antibiotics in mild pancreatitis. Antibiotics are given, if patient has infected necrosis or extrapancreatic infection (blood/urine/pneumonia/cholangitis). Early enteral feeding should be started; oral if child is accepting, otherwise nasogastric/nasojejunal tube feeding. Acute severe pancreatitis may result in acute respiratory distress syndrome, acute renal failure, shock, GI bleed, disseminated intravascular coagulation, hypoglycemia or hypocalcemia. Ascites, pleural effusion may develop apart from fluid collections (pseudocyst or walled off necrosis: Sterile/infected) (Fig. 12.17). Radiological, endoscopic or surgical interventions may be required for patients with pseudocyst, pancreatic abscess or infected necrosis. If a child has ≥2 episodes of acute pancreatitis plus complete resolution of pain (≥1 month pain-free interval between episodes), or complete normalization of amylase and lipase between the episodes, he is labelled as *acute recurrent pancreatitis* (ARP).

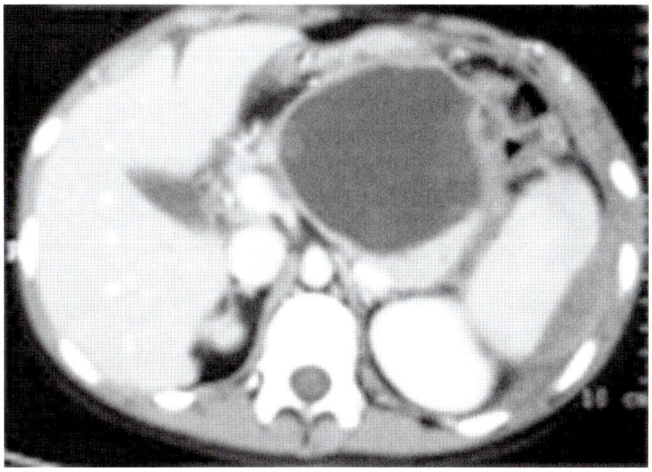

Fig. 12.17: Contrast-enhanced CT scan showing pseudocyst in a patient with acute pancreatitis

About 10–30% of patients with acute pancreatitis have ARP. Nearly one-third to one-half of children with idiopathic ARP progress to chronic pancreatitis.

## Chronic Pancreatitis (CP)

Children present with repeated episodes of pancreatic pain. Chronic diarrhea with fat malabsorption (exocrine insufficiency) and symptoms of diabetes mellitus develop later along with failure to thrive. CP may be idiopathic, hereditary, autoimmune, tropical or metabolic (hypercalcemia). Local complications include pseudocyst, pancreatic ascites, pancreatic duct stricture, biliary strictures and portal hypertension due to splenic vein thrombosis. There is an increased risk of pancreatic carcinoma, particularly in those with hereditary pancreatitis (mutations in PRSS1 encoding cationic trypsinogen).

### *Diagnosis and Management*

Diagnosis of CP needs one or more of the following three criteria:

i. Abdominal pain consistent with pancreatic origin and imaging findings of CP
ii. Evidence of exocrine pancreatic insufficiency and suggestive pancreatic imaging
iii. Evidence of endocrine pancreatic insufficiency and suggestive pancreatic imaging

X-ray abdomen may show pancreatic calcification. Ultrasound and CT scan demonstrate ductal dilatation (Fig. 12.18), strictures, calcification and altered size or echotexture of pancreas. ERCP and MRCP help in defining the pancreatic ductal anatomy (e.g. prominent stricture, intraductal calculi) and planning of endoscopic or surgical therapy. Exocrine pancreatic insufficiency is confirmed by demonstrating excess stool fat and reduced pancreatic fecal elastase or chymotrypsin. Elevated fasting and postprandial blood sugar suggest endocrine insufficiency.

Treatment includes supportive therapy during acute attacks, antioxidants, analgesics and dietary advice. Oral pancreatic enzymes for exocrine pancreatic insufficiency and management of diabetes mellitus is essential. Endoscopic or radiological treatment is done for pseudocyst, ductal

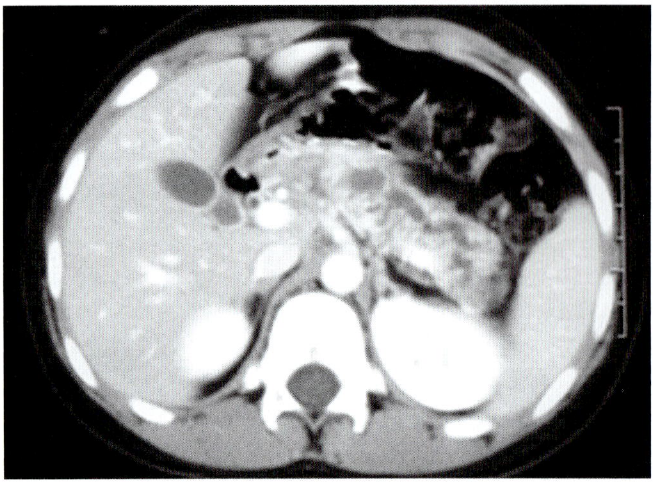

Fig. 12.18: CT scan showing dilated main pancreatic duct in chronic pancreatitis

stricture and calculi. Celiac ganglion block may be used for pain control. Surgical procedures like partial pancreatectomy or lateral pancreatojejunostomy are required in patients not responding to medical/endoscopic therapy.

### Chronic Abdominal Pain

Chronic abdominal pain refers to the pain that is either episodic or continuous and lasts for a period of at least 2 months. The prevalence of chronic abdominal pain in children varies from 0.5 to 19% and depends on the age group evaluated. In addition to organic causes, an important cause is nonorganic abdominal pain which is responsible for nearly 75% of all cases and is termed 'abdominal pain related to functional gastrointestinal disorders'.

#### *Abdominal Pain Related to Functional Gastrointestinal Disorders*

Functional gastrointestinal disorders (FGID) are a group of conditions characterized by a specific set of symptoms related to the gastrointestinal tract but without underlying structural or biochemical abnormalities. The exact pathophysiology of FGID is unknown. The diagnosis of FGID is based on the clinical history and physical examination, as per the Rome IV criteria. There are no objective tests which can be used to diagnose FGID. The absence of an organic cause of inflammatory, anatomic, metabolic and neoplastic nature is required for the diagnosis of FGID. The different types of FGID in children are shown in Table 12.6.

After extensive studies, the most accepted pathogenesis of childhood functional abdominal pain is of 'visceral hyperalgesia', referring to an altered excessive perception of normal gut motility that is interpreted by the child as pain. This perception is influenced by the psychosocial stressors in school and home which further impairs the child's coping. The focus on the pain is further heightened by the growing concern in the family and the frequent visits to the doctors. Children of parents with increased anxiety and functional GI problems have an increased risk of developing functional pain in abdomen.

*Functional dyspepsia:* It is defined as presence of ≥1 of the following symptoms—postprandial fullness, early satiety, epigastric pain or burning not associated with stooling for at least 4 times a month for ≥2 months. Based on the predominant symptoms, the condition is classified as postprandial distress syndrome or epigastric pain syndrome.

*Irritable bowel syndrome:* It is defined as abdominal pain for at least 4 days per month for ≥2 months, associated with 1 of the following: Pain related to defecation, onset of pain associated with a change in frequency of stool and onset of pain associated with a change in consistency of stool. Based on the main stool pattern, it is further subtyped as IBS with constipation, IBS with diarrhea, IBS with constipation and diarrhea, and unspecified IBS. In children with constipation and abdominal pain, we should first treat the constipation and if the pain persists despite successful therapy of constipation, we can put a label of IBS constipation.

*Abdominal migraine:* Paroxysmal episodes of intense, acute periumbilical/midline or diffuse pain, lasting for ≥1 hour during the last 6 months with normal health of weeks–months between the pain episodes. The pain is severe, interferes with normal activities and associated with ≥2 of the following: Anorexia, nausea, vomiting, headache, photophobia and pallor.

*Functional abdominal pain—not otherwise specified (FAP-NOS):* It is diagnosed if a child has episodic or continuous periumbilical pain (at least 4 times a month), for >2 months and it does not meet the criteria for IBS, abdominal migraine or functional dyspepsia.

Table 12.6: Types of functional gastrointestinal disorders (FGID) from infants to adolescents as per Rome IV criteria

| *Infants and toddlers* | *Children and adolescents (4–18 years)* |
|---|---|
| Infant regurgitation | Functional nausea/vomiting syndrome |
| Infant rumination syndrome | Rumination syndrome |
| Cyclic vomiting syndrome | Cyclic vomiting syndrome<br>Aerophagia |
| Infant colic | Functional dyspepsia |
| Functional diarrhea | Functional abdominal pain, not otherwise specified<br>Abdominal migraine |
| Infant dyschezia | Irritable bowel syndrome |
| Functional constipation | Functional constipation<br>Non-retentive fecal incontinence |

**Table 12.7:** 'Red flag' signs or features that indicate serious illness in a child with abdominal pain

| |
|---|
| Pain localized away from umbilicus in right/left upper or lower quadrant |
| Nocturnal pain |
| Failure to thrive; weight loss |
| Significant vomiting; bilious vomiting |
| Gastrointestinal blood loss |
| Chronic diarrhea |
| Persistent fever |
| Jaundice |
| Arthritis; rash |
| Dysphagia |
| Secondary amenorrhea |
| Family history of inflammatory bowel disease |
| Examination: Anemia, clubbing, edema, tenderness or mass; organomegaly, perianal fistulae/tags |
| Abnormal laboratory testing: Low hemoglobin, elevated CRP and ESR, occult blood in stool, raised fecal calprotectin |

Among the various types of functional pain mentioned above, FAP-NOS is the most common. When evaluating a child with abdominal pain, efforts should be made to differentiate functional from organic causes. The history should include not only details of pain but also family details, child's emotional environment in home and school, personality, coping skills, school performance and stress factors. The presence of 'red flag' signs (alarming symptoms and signs) (Table 12.7) increases the probability of an organic disorder and justifies further diagnostic testing as per the likely diagnosis. Only limited investigations like hemogram, inflammatory markers (ESR/CRP), urine examination and stool for ova/parasite are needed for patients with suspected functional pain disorders. Fecal calprotectin may be done in select cases; normal levels suggest functional pain. Abdominal ultrasonography is not helpful and the presence of small mesenteric lymph nodes (<10 mm in short axis) is not a cause of concern.

The aim of management of children with FAP-NOS is to make a positive diagnosis, normalize the lifestyle to not allow pain to curtail daily activities or school performance, and to rectify psychological factors. The crux of management is counseling the parents and the child, both jointly and separately. Parents need to be reassured about the benign nature of the ailment and emphasis is laid upon avoiding too much attention to the child. The concept of visceral hyperalgesia should be explained to parents. Provision of a nutritious diet with adequate fiber and avoiding intake of carbonated beverages and refined food helps in reducing bloating. The role of amitriptyline and hypnotherapy is restricted to refractory cases.

## Suggested Reading


1. Andrews ET, Beattie RM, Tighe MP. Functional abdominal pain: what clinicians need to know Arch Dis Child 2020; 105: 938–44.
2. Koppen IJN, Nurko S, Saps M, et al. The pediatric Rome IV criteria. Expert Rev Gastroenterol Hepatol 2017; 11:193–201.
3. Raymond M, Marsicovetere P, DeShaney K. Diagnosing and managing acute abdominal pain in children. JAAPA 2022;35:16–20.
4. Uc A, Husain SZ. Pancreatitis in children. Gastroenterology 2019;156:1969–1978.


*Competencies:* **PE24.1; PE24.2; PE24.3; PE24.4; PE24.5; PE24.8; PE24.9; PE24.10; PE24.14; PE27.23**

## ACUTE DIARRHEA

Diarrhea is defined as a change in consistency and frequency of stools, i.e. liquid or watery stools, that occur >3 times a day. In the vast majority of cases, these acute episodes subside within 7 days. If there is associated blood in stools, it is termed *dysentery*. Acute diarrhea may persist for >2 weeks in 5–15% cases, which is labeled as *persistent diarrhea*.

The global annual burden of diarrhea is huge, affecting 1.7 billion cases every year and accounting for ~11% of all childhood deaths world-wide. The two most important consequences of diarrhea in children are malnutrition and dehydration. Malnutrition and diarrhea form a vicious cycle, since malnutrition increases the risk and severity of diarrhea. Impaired absorption, loss of nutrients, increased catabolism and improper feeding in diarrhea aggravate the severity of malnutrition. A child may lose as much water and electrolytes from the body during an episode of diarrhea as an adult, which translates into a higher proportion of total body water loss in the child. Significant dehydration with abnormal electrolyte and acid-base status occurs in 2–5% of cases of diarrhea, which may be fatal.

### Etiology

Intestinal infections are the most common cause of acute diarrhea (AD). However, certain drugs, food allergy, systemic infections (e.g. urinary tract infection and otitis media) and surgical conditions (e.g. appendicitis or Hirschsprung disease) can also present as AD. Causative agents of AD (Table 12.8) can be identified in nearly

**Table 12.8:** Causes of acute diarrhea

| |
|---|
| **Bacterial**<br>• *Escherichia coli:* Enterotoxigenic, enteropathogenic, entero-invasive*, enterohemorrhagic* and enteroaggregative types<br>• *Shigella**: *S. sonnei*, *S. flexneri*, *S. boydii* and *S. dysenteriae*<br>• *Vibrio cholerae* serogroups O1 and O139<br>• *Salmonella**: Chiefly *S. typhi* and *S. paratyphi* A, B or C<br>• *Campylobacter* species* |
| **Viral**<br>• Rotavirus<br>• Human caliciviruses: *Norovirus* spp.; *Sapovirus* spp.<br>• Enteric adenoviruses serotypes 40 and 41<br>• Others: Astroviruses, coronaviruses, cytomegalovirus, picornavirus |
| **Parasitic**<br>• *Giardia lamblia*<br>• *Cryptosporidium parvum*<br>• *Entamoeba histolytica**<br>• *Cyclospora cayetanensis*<br>• *Isospora belli* |

*Cause diarrhea with or without dysentery

70–80% episodes. Rotavirus remains the leading cause of severe, dehydrating gastroenteritis worldwide. In India, rotavirus and enterotoxigenic *E. coli* account for nearly half of the diarrheal episodes among children. In rotavirus diarrhea, vomiting is an early feature and diarrhea is more severe. Cholera accounts for 5–10% cases; it is endemic in some parts and may occur in outbreaks. In cholera, stools are like rice water, vomiting is common and severe dehydration occurs rapidly within hours. Apart from enterotoxin producing *E. coli* (ETEC), which accounts for nearly 20% of childhood diarrhea, enteroinvasive *E. coli* (EIEC) and enterohemorrhagic *E. coli* (EHEC) can cause dysentery. EHEC may also cause hemolytic uremic syndrome. *Shigella* and *Salmonella* species are isolated in 3–7% of childhood diarrheas. Shigella accounts for majority of cases of dysentery whereas *Entamoeba histolytica* accounts for only 5% of dysentery. Giardia lamblia rarely causes AD. Infection with *Candida albicans* can cause AD in patients with malnutrition, immunocompromised state or after prolonged antibiotic treatment. *Clostridium difficile* should be suspected in patients who have received broad-spectrum antibiotics.

#### Risk Factors

Factors determining susceptibility to diarrhea include poor sanitation and personal hygiene, non-availability of safe drinking water, unsafe food preparation practices and low rates of breastfeeding and immunization. Young (<2 years) and malnourished children are more susceptible to AD, and tend to have severe and prolonged episodes. Other risk factors for prolonged and recurrent episodes of diarrhea include hypo- or achlorhydria (due to *Helicobacter pylori* infection or therapy with proton pump inhibitors) and immunodeficiency (selective IgA deficiency, HIV, etc.).

### Pathogenesis and Clinical Features

Approximately 60% of a child's body weight is water, present in two fluid compartments—extracellular fluid (ECF) and intracellular fluid (ICF). The ECF includes circulating blood, intestinal fluid and secretions. Diarrheal losses come from ECF, which is relatively rich in sodium and has low potassium. Loss of water from the body causes a reduction or shrinkage of ECF volume. In half of these cases, the concentration of sodium in the plasma remains nearly normal (about 140 mEq/L); in another 40–45% cases, excessive sodium is lost in the stools leading to a relative decline in serum sodium (hyponatremia) and a fall in ECF osmolality. This causes movement of water from the ECF to ICF compartment, causing further shrinkage of the already reduced extracellular compartment volume in hyponatremic dehydration. In about 5% cases of diarrhea, especially if the child has been given fluids with extra salt, serum sodium increases to >150 mEq/L and ECF osmolalilty is also increased.

Normally, skin turgor or elasticity is maintained by tissue water and fat. Shrinkage of extracellular water in both hypo- and isonatremic dehydration impairs skin elasticity. On pinching, it takes a few seconds for the skin fold to return to normal. In patients with hypernatremic dehydration, water moves from inside the cells to the ECF compartment due to the increased osmolality of ECF, and therefore, partially masks the loss of skin turgor. The skin appears soggy, doughy or leathery. Thus, a severe case of hypernatremic dehydration is likely to be erroneously underestimated as mild dehydration, unless severe sequelae of dehydration such as circulatory or renal impairment are noted.

As the ECF compartment is depleted, the blood volume is reduced. This results in a weak, thready pulse, low blood pressure and cold extremities. Because of low hydrostatic pressure, the filtration of urine is reduced. This is ominous because poorly functioning kidneys cannot regulate metabolic derangements. Urine flow is a good indicator of the severity of diarrhea. Severe cases are associated with acute kidney injury.

Diarrheal stools contain large amounts of potassium. Therefore, serum potassium invariably falls, if diarrhea persists for more than a few days. This is more pronounced in children with severe malnutrition with already depleted potassium stores. Affected children present with abdominal distension, paralytic ileus and muscle hypotonia. Electrocardiogram may show ST depression and flat T waves. Since intestinal secretions are alkaline, considerable bicarbonate is lost in diarrheal stools and acidosis usually accompanies dehydration. Patients remain asymptomatic till the base excess falls to 12 mEq/L. Below this level, breathing becomes deep and rapid (Kussmaul breathing).

The child is thirsty and slightly irritable in early and mild cases of diarrhea. As the diarrhea continues and dehydration worsens, the child becomes more irritable with depressed fontanelle (if open), sunken eyes and dry tongue and the inner side of cheeks. Abdomen may become distended in hypokalemia. As acidosis worsens, the breathing becomes deep and rapid. In extreme cases, the child appears moribund, with weak and thready pulses, low blood pressure and oliguria.

### Assessment of Child with Acute Diarrhea

*Goals of assessment:* These are to: (i) determine the type of diarrhea, i.e. acute watery diarrhea, dysentery or persistent diarrhea; (ii) look for dehydration and other complications; (iii) assess for malnutrition; (iv) rule out non-diarrheal illness especially systemic infection; and (v) assess feeding, both pre-illness and during illness.

*History:* This should include information on: (i) Onset of diarrhea—duration and number of stools per day; (ii) blood in stools; (iii) number of episodes of vomiting; (iv) presence of fever, cough, or other significant symptoms (e.g. convulsions, recent measles); (v) type and amount of fluids (including breast milk) and food taken during the illness and pre-illness feeding practices; (vi) drugs or other local remedies taken (including opioids or anti-motility drugs like loperamide that may cause abdominal distension); and (vii) immunization history.

*Examination:* The most important assessment is for dehydration. The degree of dehydration is assessed as per Table 12.9. One should look at the child's general condition and sensorium (alert, restless, irritable,

Table 12.9: Assessment of dehydration in patients with diarrhea

| Look at | | | |
|---|---|---|---|
| Condition[1] | Well alert | Restless, irritable | Lethargic or unconscious; floppy |
| Eyes[2] | Normal | Sunken | Very sunken and dry |
| Tears | Present | Absent | Absent |
| Mouth and tongue[3] | Moist | Dry | Very dry |
| Thirst | Drinks normally; not thirsty | Thirsty, drinks eagerly | 'Drinks poorly' or is not able to drink |
| **Feel** | | | |
| Skin pinch[4] | Goes back quickly | Goes back slowly | Goes back very slowly |
| **Decide** | The patient has *no signs* of *dehydration* | If the patient has two or more signs, there is *some dehydration* | If the patient has two or more signs, there is *severe dehydration* |
| **Treat** | Use treatment **Plan A** | Weigh the patient, if possible, and use treatment **Plan B** | Weigh the patient and use treatment **Plan C** urgently |

[1]A lethargic child is not simply asleep; the child cannot be fully awakened; has a dull mental state and the child may appear to be drifting into unconsciousness.

[2]In some infants and children, the eyes normally appear somewhat sunken. It is helpful to ask the mother, if the child's eyes are normal or more sunken than usual.

[3]Dryness of the mouth and tongue can also be palpated with a clean finger. The mouth may be dry in a child who habitually breathes through the mouth. The mouth may be wet in a dehydrated child owing to recent vomiting or drinking.

[4]The skin pinch is less useful in infants or children with marasmus (severe wasting), kwashiorkor (severe malnutrition with edema) and in obese children

lethargic or unconscious). Other assessments include appearance of eyes (normal or sunken) and the ability to drink water or ORS solution (normal, taken eagerly, refused or unable to drink due to lethargy or coma). Dehydration is assessed by feeling for skin turgor; following pinching, the abdominal skin may flatten immediately, go back slowly or return very slowly (more than 2 seconds). Based on the degree of dehydration after history and examination, the estimated fluid loss is calculated as follows:

| *Degree of dehydration* | *Assessment of fluid loss* |
|---|---|
| No dehydration | <50 mL/kg |
| Some dehydration | 50–100 mL/kg |
| Severe dehydration | >100 mL/kg |

In addition, we look for features of malnutrition and for for systemic infection.

***Laboratory investigations:*** Most episodes of acute diarrhea can be managed even in absence of laboratory investigations. Stool microscopy is not helpful except in selected situations, such as cholera (darting motion suggests *Vibrio cholerae*) and giardiasis (trophozoites). *Stool culture* is of little value in routine management. It helps decide on antibiotic therapy in patients with *Shigella* dysentery who do not respond to initial antibiotics. Tests for stool pH and reducing substances are not indicated routinely. Hemogram, pH, bicarbonate, electrolytes and renal function tests are performed, only if the child has pallor, labored breathing, altered sensorium, seizures, paralytic ileus or oliguria.

## Principles of Management

Management of acute diarrhea has four components: (i) Rehydration and maintaining hydration; (ii) ensuring feeding; (iii) oral supplementation of zinc; and (iv) early recognition of danger signs and treatment of complications.

The cornerstone of management is the use of oral rehydration solutions. The dehydration status is classified as no dehydration, some dehydration or severe dehydration and appropriate treatment is started.

### *Physiological Basis for Oral Rehydration Therapy*

In most cases of acute diarrhea, sodium and chloride are actively secreted from the gut mucosa due to pathogen-induced dysfunction of several actively functioning absorption pumps. However, glucose dependent sodium pump remains intact and functional, transporting one molecule of glucose and dragging along a molecule of sodium and of water across the intestinal mucosa resulting in repletion of sodium and water losses.

The glucose dependent sodium and water absorption is the principle behind replacing glucose and sodium in 1:1 molar ratio in the WHO oral rehydration solution (ORS). An important consideration in making ORT is that the osmolarity of the replacement fluid should not exceed that of blood (290 mOsm/L). Keeping the intestinal lumen at lower osmolarity as compared to blood allows for greater absorption of fluids into the bloodstream across concentration gradient, which also results in electrolyte absorption (by solvent drag). Since the concentration of glucose increases osmolarity, it is suggested that glucose concentration should not exceed 111 mmol/L. Meta-analyses have shown that use of low osmolarity ORS causes reduction of stool output, decrease in vomiting and reduced use of intravenous fluids, without increasing the risk of hyponatremia. For this reason, the recommendation for use of standard ORS (osmolarity of 311 mOsm/L) was changed to low osmolarity ORS (osmolarity of 245 mOsm/L).

Since 2004, based on the WHO/UNICEF and IAP recommendations, the Government of India has adopted the low osmolarity ORS as the single universal ORS to be used for all ages and all types of diarrhea. The composition of the low osmolarity ORS is given in Table 12.10. In the

**Table 12.10:** Composition of WHO recommended ORS

| Constituent | g/L | Osmole or ion | mmol/L |
|---|---|---|---|
| Sodium chloride | 2.6 | Sodium | 75 |
| Glucose, anhydrous | 13.5 | Chloride | 65 |
| Potassium chloride | 1.5 | Glucose, anhydrous | 75 |
| Trisodium citrate, dihydrate | 2.9 | Potassium<br>Citrate | 20<br>10 |
| Total osmolarity | | | 245 |

**Table 12.11:** Home available fluids for acute diarrhea

| **Acceptable home available fluids** | |
|---|---|
| Fluids that contain salt (preferred) | Salted drinks (e.g. salted rice water, yoghurt drink), vegetable or chicken soup with salt |
| Fluids that do not contain salt (acceptable) | Plain water, water in which a cereal has been cooked (e.g. unsalted rice water), unsalted soup, yoghurt drinks without salt, green coconut water, weak unsweetened tea, unsweetened fresh fruit juice |
| Unsuitable home available fluids | Commercial carbonated beverages, commercial fruit juices, sweetened tea |

absence of WHO ORS, one may administer culturally acceptable appropriate homemade fluids (Table 12.11). Oral solutions should be given by a spoon or *katori* and in sips or small volumes rather than a large volume at one time as this increases the retention of oral fluids.

### *Treatment Plan A: Treatment of "No Dehydration"*

Such children may be treated at home after explanation of feeding and the danger signs to the mother/caregiver. The mother may be given WHO ORS for use at home as per Table 12.12. Danger signs requiring medical attention are continuing diarrhea beyond 3 days, increased volume/frequency of stools, repeated vomiting, increasing thirst, decreased urine output, refusal to feed, fever or blood in stools.

### *Treatment Plan B: Treatment of "Some Dehydration"*

All cases with obvious signs of dehydration need to be treated in a health center or hospital. However, oral fluid therapy must be commenced promptly and continued during transport. Fluid requirement is calculated under the following three headings:

i. *Provision of normal daily fluid requirements:* Up to 10 kg = 100 mL/kg, 10–20 kg = 50 mL/kg, >20 kg = 20 mL/kg. As an example, the daily fluid requirement in a child weighing 15 kg will be 1250 mL (first 10 kg, 10 × 100 = 1000 mL; another 5 kg, 5 × 50 = 250 mL, total 1000 + 250 = 1250 mL).

ii. *Rehydration to correct the existing water or electrolyte deficits:* Calculated as 75 mL/kg of ORS, to be given over 4 hours. If ORS cannot be taken orally, then nasogastric tube can be used. If child's weight cannot be taken, then only age may be used to calculate fluid requirement as shown in Table 12.13. If, after 4 hours, the child still has some dehydration, then another treatment with ORS (as in rehydration therapy) is to be given. This therapy is effective in 95% cases. Oral rehydration therapy may be ineffective in children with a high stool purge rate of >5 mL/kg body weight/hr, persistent vomiting >3/hr, paralytic ileus and incorrect preparation of ORS (very dilute solution).

iii. *Maintenance to replace ongoing losses to prevent recurrence of dehydration:* This phase should begin when signs of dehydration disappear, usually within 4 hours. ORS should be administered in volumes equal to diarrheal losses, usually to a maximum of 10 mL/kg per stool. Breastfeeding and semisolid food are continued after replacement of deficit. Plain water can be offered in between.

**Table 12.12:** Oral rehydration therapy to prevent dehydration (Plan A)

| Age | ORS or other culturally appropriate ORT fluids after each loose stool | ORS to provide for use at home |
|---|---|---|
| <24 mo | 50–100 mL | 500 mL/day |
| 2–10 yr | 100–200 mL | 1000 mL/day |
| >10 yr | Ad lib | 2000 mL/day |

Explain use of ORS, i.e. the amount to be given, how to mix. Give a teaspoonful every 1–2 min for a child under 2 years. Give frequent sips from a cup for an older child

If the child vomits, wait for 10 min. Then give the solution more slowly (for example, a spoonful every 2–3 min)

If diarrhea continues after the ORS packets are used up, tell the mother to give other fluids as described above or return for more ORS

### *Treatment Plan C: Children with "Severe Dehydration"*

Intravenous fluids should be started immediately using Ringer lactate with 5% dextrose. Normal saline or plain Ringer solution may be used as an alternative, but 5% dextrose alone is not effective. A total of 100 mL/kg of fluid is given, over 6 hours in children <12 months and over 3 hours in children >12 months as shown on page 313.

**Table 12.13:** Guidelines for treating patients with some dehydration (Plan B)

| Age | <4 mo | 4–11 mo | 12–23 mo | 2–4 yr | 5–14 yr | >15 yr |
|---|---|---|---|---|---|---|
| Weight | <5 kg | 5–8 kg | 8–11 kg | 11–16 kg | 16–20 kg | >30 kg |
| ORS, mL | 200–400 | 400–600 | 600–800 | 800–1200 | 1200–2200 | >2200 |
| Number of glasses | 1–2 | 2–3 | 3–4 | 4–6 | 6–11 | 12–20 |

The approximate amount of ORS required in some dehydration is 75 ml/kg. When body weight is not known, the approximate amount of ORS solution to give in the first 4 hours is given according to age

For infants under-6 months who are not breastfed, also give 100–200 mL clean water during this period

Encourage breastfeeding

| Age | 30 mL/kg | 70 mL/kg |
|---|---|---|
| <12 mo | 1 hr* | 5 hr |
| >12 mo | 30 min* | 2½ hr |

*The above can be repeated, if child continues to have feeble/non-palpable radial pulse

ORS solution should be started simultaneously, if the child can take orally. If IV fluids cannot be given (for reasons of access, logistic availability or during transport), nasogastric feeding is given at 20 mL/kg/hr for 6 hours (total 120 mL/kg). The child should be reassessed every 1–2 hours; if there is repeated vomiting or abdominal distension, the oral or nasogastric fluids are given more slowly. If there is no improvement in hydration after 3 hours, IV fluids should be started as early as possible.

The child should be reassessed every 15–30 min for pulses and hydration status after the first bolus of IV fluid. Management following the first bolus of intravenous hydration is as follows:

i. *Persistence of severe dehydration:* Intravenous infusion is repeated.
ii. *Hydration is improved but some dehydration is present:* IV fluids are discontinued; ORS is administered over 4 hours according to Plan B.
iii. *There is no dehydration:* IV fluids are discontinued; treatment Plan A is followed.

The child should be observed for at least 6 hours before discharge, to confirm that the mother is able to maintain the child's hydration by ORS.

***Unique problems in infants below 2 months of age:*** Breastfeeding must continue during the rehydration process, whenever the infant is able to suck. Complications like septicemia, paralytic ileus and severe electrolyte disturbance are more likely in young infants with diarrhea than at later ages. Diarrhea in these infants should be ideally treated as inpatient by experienced physicians at treatment centers with appropriate facilities. This allows for careful assessment of need of systemic antibiotics and monitoring.

### Nutritional Management of Diarrhea

Children with severe malnutrition (marasmus or kwashiorkor) are at an increased risk of acute diarrhea and its complications, such as severe systemic infection, dehydration, heart failure, vitamin and mineral deficiencies. Feeding should not be restricted in such patients as this aggravates complications and increases morbidity and mortality. Early feeding during diarrhea not only decreases the stool volume by facilitating sodium and water absorption along with the nutrients, but also facilitates early gut epithelial recovery and prevents malnutrition. Once the child's status starts improving, a higher than recommended intake is given to facilitate complete catch-up growth. Following are the recommendations on dietary management:

i. In exclusively breastfed infants, breastfeeding should continue as it helps in better weight gain and decreases the risk of persistent diarrhea.
ii. Optimally energy dense foods with the least bulk, recommended for routine feeding in the household, should be offered in small quantities but frequently (every 2–3 hours).
iii. Staple foods do not provide optimal calories and should be enriched with fat or oil and sugar, e.g. *khichri* with oil, rice with milk or curd and sugar, mashed banana with milk or curd, mashed potatoes with oil and lentil.
iv. Foods with high fiber content, e.g. coarse fruits and vegetables should be avoided.
v. In non-breastfed infants, cow or buffalo milk can be given undiluted after correction of dehydration together with semisolid foods. Milk should not be diluted with water during any phase of diarrhea. Alternatively, milk cereal mixtures, e.g. dalia, sago or milk-rice mixture, are preferable.
vi. Routine lactose-free feeding, e.g. soy formula is not required, even when reducing substances are detected in the stools. Also, do not use cold drinks, fruit juices or glucose solutions as they have high osmolarity and can aggravate diarrhea, nausea and vomiting.
vii. During recovery, an intake of at least 125% of recommended dietary allowances should be attempted with nutrient dense foods; this should continue until the child reaches pre-illness weight and ideally until the child achieves a normal nutritional status.

#### Zinc Supplementation

Zinc deficiency is widespread among children in developing countries. Intestinal zinc losses during diarrhea aggravate pre-existing zinc deficiency. Zinc supplementation is now part of the standard care along with ORS. It is helpful in decreasing severity and duration of diarrhea and the risk of persistent diarrhea. Zinc is supplemented as sulfate, acetate or gluconate formulation, at a dose of 20 mg of elemental zinc per day for children >6 months for 14 days.

#### Symptomatic Treatment

An occasional vomit in a child with acute diarrhea does not need antiemetics. If vomiting is severe or recurrent and interferes with ORS intake, then a single dose of oral ondansetron (0.15 mg/kg/dose) should be given. Preferably wait for 45–60 minutes before restarting ORT. Children with refractory vomiting despite administration of ondansetron may require intravenous fluids.

Abdominal distension does not require specific treatment, if bowel sounds are present and the distension is mild. Paralytic ileus should be suspected, if bowel sounds are absent and abdomen is distended. Paralytic ileus can occur due to hypokalemia, intake of antimotility agents, necrotizing enterocolitis or septicemia. Subjects with paralytic ileus require IV fluids, nasogastric aspiration, correction of hypokalemia and no oral feeding. Potassium chloride (30–40 mEq/L) should be administered intravenously with parenteral fluids provided the child is passing urine.

Convulsions associated with diarrhea may be due to (i) hypo- or hypernatremia; (ii) hypoglycemia; (iii) hypocalcemia following bicarbonate therapy for acidosis; (iv) encephalitis; (v) meningitis; (vi) febrile seizures; or (vii) cerebral venous or sagittal sinus thrombosis. The management depends on the etiology.

#### Drug Therapy

Most episodes of diarrhea are self-limiting and do not require any drug therapy. Antibiotics are not recommended for routine treatment of acute diarrhea in children. Antimicrobials are indicated in bacillary dysentery, cholera, amebiasis and giardiasis. *Escherichia coli* are normal gut flora and their growth on stool culture is not an indication for antibiotics. Diarrhea may be the features of systemic infection especially in malnourished, prematurely born and young infants. Presence of (i) poor sucking; (ii) abdominal distension; (iii) fever or hypothermia; (iv) fast breathing; and (v) significant lethargy or inactivity in well-nourished, well-hydrated infants points towards sepsis.

***Antimotility agents*** such as synthetic analogues of opiates (diphenoxylate hydrochloride and loperamide) reduce peristalsis or gut motility and should not be used in children with diarrhea. Reduction of gut motility allows more time for the harmful bacteria to multiply. These drugs may cause paralytic ileus, bacterial overgrowth and sepsis, and can be dangerous in infants.

***Antisecretory agents*** have been used in AD. Racecadotril is an antisecretory drug that exerts its antidiarrheal effects by inhibiting intestinal enkephalinase. Recent studies reported some evidence in favour of racecadotril over placebo in reducing the stool output and duration of diarrhea. However, the overall quality of the evidence is limited.

***Probiotics***, defined as microorganisms that exert beneficial effects when they colonize the bowel, have been proposed as adjunctive therapy in the treatment of AD. *Lactobacillus rhamanosus* GG >$10^{10}$ CFU/day or *Saccharomyces boulardii* 250–750 mg/day for 5–7 days can be used as an adjuvant therapy. The quality of evidence is moderate-low for *L. rhamanosus* GG, and very low-low for *S. boulardii*. The marginal cost-benefit advantage must be carefully considered before prescribing these agents.

### Prevention of Diarrhea and Malnutrition

Chief measures to prevent diarrhea and its nutritional consequences are:

i. *Proper nutrition:* Since breast milk offers distinct advantages in promoting growth and development of the infant and protection from diarrheal illness, its continuation should be encouraged. Exclusive breast-feeding may not be adequate to sustain growth beyond the first 6-months of life. Supplementary feeding with energy-rich natural food mixtures containing adequate amounts of nutrients should be introduced by 6-month of age, without stopping breastfeeding.

ii. *Adequate sanitation:* Improvement of environment sanitation, clean water supply, adequate sewage disposal system and protection of food from exposure to bacterial contamination are effective long-term strategies for control of all infectious illnesses including diarrhea. Three 'Cs'—clean hands, clean container and clean environment are the key messages. Complementary foods should be protected from contamination during preparation, storage, and at administration.

iii. *Vaccination:* With improvement in sanitation and hygiene in developing countries, the burden of bacterial and parasitic infection has decreased. The use of rotavirus vaccine is an effective strategy for preventing acute diarrhea.

### Suggested Reading


1. Bhatnagar S, Lodha R, Choudhury P, et al. IAP Guidelines 2006 on management of acute diarrhea. Indian Pediatr 2007; 44: 380–89.
2. Kumar A, Basu S, Vashishtha V, Choudhury P. Burden of rotavirus diarrhea in under-five children. Indian Pediatr 2016; 53:607–17.
3. Piescik-Lech M, Shamir R, Guarino A, Szajewska H. Review article: The management of acute gastroenteritis in children. Aliment Pharmacol Ther. 2013; 37: 289–303.
4. Yachha SK, Sarma MS, Mohan N, et al. Indian Academy of Pediatrics: Consensus guidelines for probiotic use in childhood diarrhea. Indian Pediatr 2022; 59:543–51.


## Dysentery

Dysentery refers to the presence of grossly visible blood in the stools and is a consequence of infection of the colon by either bacteria or ameba. Bacillary dysentery is much more common in children than amebic dysentery. The bacteria causing bloody diarrhea are *Shigella* species (*S. dysenteriae*, *S. flexneri*, *S. boydii* and *S. sonnei*), enteroinvasive and enterohemorrhagic *E. coli*, *Salmonella* and *Campylobacter jejuni*. *S. flexneri* is the commonest organism reported in developing countries and *S. dysenteriae* is associated with epidemics of dysentery.

A child with bacillary dysentery presents with fever and diarrhea. Diarrhea may be watery to start with, but then shows mucus and blood mixed with stools. There is tenesmus, which refers to ineffectual defecation along with straining and suprapubic discomfort. The illness may be complicated by dehydration, dyselectrolytemia, hemolytic uremic syndrome, convulsions, toxic megacolon, intestinal perforation, rectal prolapse and, very rarely, Shigella encephalopathy.

Administration of ORS, continuation of oral diet, zinc supplementation and antibiotics are the components of treatment. Stool culture and sensitivity should be sent before starting empirical antibiotics. Antimicrobial agents are the mainstay of therapy of all cases of shigellosis. Based on safety, low cost and efficacy, ciprofloxacin (15 mg/kg/day in two divided doses for 3 days) has been recommended by World Health Organization (WHO) as the first-line antibiotic for shigellosis. However, antimicrobial resistance to fluoroquinolones had increased significantly from 2002 to 2011 and only ceftriaxone has been shown to be uniformly effective. Keeping this in mind, intravenous ceftriaxone (50–100 mg/kg/day for 3–5 days) should be the first line of treatment in a sick child. In a stable child, either ciprofloxacin or oral cefixime may be given, but the patient should be monitored for clinical improvement within

48 hours (decrease in fever, stool frequency and blood in stools). If no improvement is seen at 48 hours, antibiotics should be changed appropriately. Oral azithromycin (10 mg/kg/day for 3 days) can be used for shigellosis, but the experience is limited.

Amebic dysentery is less common among children. The onset is insidious. Tinidazole or metronidazole is the drug of choice. Any young child presenting with blood in stools and *persistent abdominal pain* should also be suspected to have intussusception and evaluated accordingly.

*Competency:* **PE24.6**

## PERSISTENT DIARRHEA

Persistent diarrhea is an episode of diarrhea, of presumed infectious etiology, which starts acutely but lasts for >14 days. It should not be confused with chronic diarrhea which has a prolonged duration but an insidious onset.

### Etiopathogenesis

Although persistent diarrhea starts as acute infectious diarrhea, the prolongation of diarrhea is not entirely due to infection. Various factors that are implicated in pathogenesis include:

i. The predominant problem is the worsening nutritional status that, in turn, impairs the reparative process in the gut. This worsens nutrient absorption and initiates a vicious cycle that can only be broken by proper therapy. Persistent diarrhea is more common in malnourished children. Apart from malabsorption, malnutrition also results from inadequate calorie intake due to anorexia, faulty feeding and improper counseling regarding feeding. One of the major obstacles to nutritional recovery is secondary lactose intolerance, and in some cases, impaired digestion of other complex carbohydrates due to decrease in brush border disaccharidases.
ii. Pathogenic *E. coli*, especially the enteroaggregative and enteroadherent types, result in malabsorption by causing persistent infection.
iii. Associated infections of the urinary tract or other sites contribute to failure to thrive and mortality.
iv. Prolongation of an acute diarrhea may rarely be a manifestation of cow milk protein allergy. The increased gut permeability in diarrhea predisposes to sensitization with oral food antigens.
v. The use of antibiotics in acute diarrhea suppresses normal gut flora. This may result in bacterial overgrowth with pathogenic bacteria and/or overgrowth of fungi, resulting in persistent diarrhea and malabsorption.
vi. *Cryptosporidium* infection is frequently implicated, even in immunocompetent children.

### Clinical Features

Majority of patients with persistent diarrhea pass several loose stools daily but remain hydrated. Dehydration develops only in some patients due to high stool output or when oral intake is reduced due to associated systemic infections. The major consequences of persistent diarrhea are growth faltering, worsening malnutrition and death due to diarrheal or non-diarrheal illness. The presence of secondary lactose intolerance should be considered when the stools are explosive (i.e. mixed with gas and passed with noise) and in presence of perianal excoriation. The stool pH is low and stool test for reducing substances is positive. Unabsorbed dietary lactose once delivered to colon is converted to hydrogen and lactic acid by colonic bacteria. Lactic acid results in decreased stool pH, explosive stools are due to hydrogen and unabsorbed lactose gives positive reducing substances. There is no need for laboratory testing for stool pH and reducing substances when the history is classical and excoriation is marked. Secondary fungal infection should be suspected, if the anal excoriation extends to groins with or without oral thrush.

### Management

The principles of management are: (i) Correction of dehydration, electrolytes and hypoglycemia; (ii) evaluation for infections using appropriate investigations (hemogram, blood culture and urine culture) and their management; and (iii) nutritional therapy. Two-thirds of patients with persistent diarrhea can be treated as outpatients. Patients in need of hospital admission are those with (i) age <4 months and not breastfed; (ii) presence of dehydration; (iii) severe malnutrition (weight for height <3 SD, mid-upper arm circumference <11.5 cm for children between 6 and 60 months of age, or bilateral pedal edema); or (iv) presence or suspicion of systemic infection.

#### Nutrition

Feeding should be started at the earliest. Initially 6–7 feeds are given per day and a total daily caloric intake of 100 kcal/kg/day is ensured. Caloric intake should be increased gradually over 1–2 weeks to 150 kcal/kg/day in order to achieve weight gain. Tube (nasogastric) feeding may be done initially in children with poor appetite. To ensure absorption and decreased stool output, one may attempt to overcome varying degrees of carbohydrate maldigestion by using diets with different degrees of carbohydrate exclusion in the form of diet A (lactose reduced), diet B (lactose free) and diet C (complex carbohydrate free) diets (Table 12.14).

***Initial diet A (reduced lactose diet; milk rice gruel, milk sooji gruel, rice with curds, dalia):*** This is based on the fact that secondary lactose intolerance exists in children with persistent diarrhea and malnutrition. Clinical trials have shown that reduced lactose diet is tolerated equally well as totally lactose-free diet, without significantly increasing stool output or risk of dehydration. If the patient is fed entirely on animal milk, the quantity should be reduced to 50–60 mL/kg providing not more than 2 g of lactose/kg/day. To reduce lactose concentration in animal milk, it should be mixed with cereals, but not diluted with water as that reduces the caloric content. Milk cereal mixtures, e.g. milk or curd mixed rice gruel, milk *sooji* gruel, or *dalia,* are palatable, provide good quality proteins and some micronutrients and result in faster weight gain than milk-free diets.

***Second diet B (lactose-free diet with reduced starch):*** About 65–70% of children improve on the initial diet A.

**Table 12.14:** Diets for persistent diarrhea

| *Diet A (reduced lactose)* | *Diet B (lactose free)* | *Diet C (monosaccharide based)* |
|---|---|---|
| **Constituents** | | |
| • Milk (1/3 katori/50 mL)<br>• Puffed rice powder/cooked rice or *Sooji* (2 tsp/6 g)<br>• Sugar (1½ tsp/7 g)<br>• Oil (1 tsp/4.5 g)<br>• Water (2/3 katori/100 mL) | • Egg white (3 tsp/half egg white)<br>• Puffed rice powder/cooked rice (3 tsp/9 g)<br>• Glucose (1½ tsp/7 g)<br>• Oil (1½ tsp/7 g)<br>• Water (3/4 katori/120 mL) | • Chicken puree (5 tsp/15 g) or egg white (3 tsp/half egg white)<br>• Glucose (1½ tsp/7 g)<br>• Oil (1½ tsp/7 g)<br>• Water (1 katori/150 mL) |
| **Preparation** | | |
| Mix milk, sugar and rice, add boiled water and mix well, add oil. | After whipping the egg white, add rice, glucose and oil and mix well. Add boiled water and mix rapidly to avoid clumping | Boil chicken and make puree after removing bones. Mix it with glucose and oil. Add boiled water to make a smooth flowing feed |
| **Nutrient content** | | |
| 85 kcal and 2.0 g protein per 100 g | 90 kcal and 2.4 g protein per 100 g | 67 kcal and 3.0 g protein per 100 g |



The remainder have impaired digestion of starch and disaccharides other than lactose. These children, if free of systemic infection, are advised diet B which is free of milk (lactose) and provides carbohydrates as a mixture of cereals and glucose. Milk protein is replaced by chicken, egg or protein hydrolysate. The starch content is reduced and partially substituted by glucose. Substituting only part of the cereal with glucose increases the digestibility but at the same time does not cause a very high osmolarity.

***Third diet C (monosaccharide-based diet):*** Overall, 80–85% of patients with severe, persistent diarrhea will recover with sustained weight gain with diet A or diet B. A small percentage may not tolerate a moderate intake of the cereal in diet B. These children are given diet C, which contains only glucose and a protein source as egg white or chicken or commercially available protein hydrolysates. Energy density is increased by adding oil to the diet.

The strategy of serial carbohydrate exclusion to varying degrees in plan A, B and C diets are meant to circumvent the problem of carbohydrate malabsorption. In addition, green (unripe) banana diet is gaining acceptance for treatment of persistent diarrhea. Fermentation of non-digestible soluble fibers in cooked green (unripe) banana by colonic bacteria generates short chain fatty acids that are absorbed along with sodium in the colon, thereby facilitating water absorption by solvent drag and also conserving dietary nutrients.

***Indications for change from the initial diet (diet A) to the next diet (diet B or diet C):*** The diet should be changed to the next level, if the child shows (i) marked increase in stool frequency (usually more than 10 watery stools/day) at any time after at least 48 hours of initiating the diet; (ii) features of dehydration any time after initiating treatment; or (iii) failure to gain weight gain by day 7 in the absence of initial or hospital acquired systemic infection. Unless signs of treatment failure occur earlier, each diet should be given for a minimum period of 7 days.

***Resumption of regular diet after discharge:*** Children discharged on totally milk-free diet should be given small quantities of milk as part of a mixed diet after 10 days. If they tolerate this and have no signs of lactose intolerance (abdominal pain, abdominal distension and excessive flatulence), then milk can be gradually increased over the next few days. Age appropriate normal diet can then be resumed over the next few weeks.

***Supplement vitamins and minerals:*** Supplemental multivitamins and minerals, at about twice the RDA, should be given daily to all children for at least 2–4 weeks. Iron supplements should be introduced only after the diarrhea has ceased. Vitamin A (as a single dose) and zinc are supplemented as both of them enhance the recovery from persistent diarrhea. A single oral dose of vitamin A should be given to those children with persistent diarrhea having severe acute malnutrition or with manifestation of vitamin A deficiency, at 2,00,000 IU for children >12 months or 100,000 IU for children 6–12 months of age. Children weighing <8 kg, irrespective of their age, should be given 100,000 IU of vitamin A. Zinc is given at a dose of 10–20 mg per day for at least 2 weeks to children between 6 months and 3 years of age.

***Additional supplements for severely malnourished infants and children:*** Magnesium and potassium supplementation is provided to these children. Magnesium is given by intramuscular route at 0.2 mL/kg/dose of 50% magnesium sulfate twice a day for 2–3 days. Potassium is supplemented at 5–6 mEq/kg/day orally or as part of intravenous infusion during the initial stabilization period.

***Role of antibiotics:*** The indiscriminate use of antibiotics in the treatment of acute diarrhea is one of the reasons for persistent diarrhea. Hence, the use of empirical antibiotics at admission is to be individualized and reserved for children with either severe malnutrition (majority of these children have associated systemic infections and clinical signs of infection may not be obvious) or those with evidence of systemic infection. A combination of cephalosporin and aminoglycoside can be started empirically and thereafter changed according to reports of culture/sensitivity. Urinary tract infection is common (seen in 10–15%) and should be treated appropriately.

### *Monitoring Response to Treatment*

Successful treatment is characterized by adequate food intake, reduced frequency of diarrheal stools (<2 liquid stools/day for 2 consecutive days) and weight gain. Most children will lose weight in the initial 1–2 days and then show steady weight gain as associated infections are treated and diarrhea subsides. All children should be followed regularly even after discharge to ensure continued weight gain and compliance with feeding advice.

### Prognosis

Most patients with persistent diarrhea recover with an approach of stepped-up dietary management as discussed above. A small subgroup (<5%) may be refractory and require parenteral nutrition and extensive workup. These patients generally have high purge rate, continue to lose weight, do not tolerate oral feeds and require referral to specialized pediatric gastroenterology centers.

### Suggested Reading


1. Bandasma RHJ, Sadiq K, Bhutta ZA. Persistent diarrhoea: Current knowledge and novel concepts. Paediatr Int Child Health 2019 Feb;39(1):41–47.
2. Gaffey MF, Wazny K, Bassani DG, Bhutta ZA. Dietary management of childhood diarrhea in low- and middle-income countries: A systematic review. BMC Public Health. 2013;13 Suppl 3:S3–S17.
3. Williams PCM, Berkley JA. Guidelines for the treatment of dysentery (shigellosis): A systematic review of the evidence. Paediatr Int Child Health 2018; 38:S50–S65.


*Competencies:* **PE24.7; PE25.1**

## CHRONIC DIARRHEA

Chronic diarrhea is a common problem in children. It is defined as an insidious onset diarrhea of >2 weeks duration in children and >4 weeks in adults. The term chronic diarrhea is not synonymous with persistent diarrhea. In children, diarrhea can be defined as a stool volume of >20 g/kg/d. Usually the parents can identify diarrhea by the increase in frequency and fluid content of the stool as compared to the normal for that child. The approach, etiology and management of chronic diarrhea along with a brief outline of some common causes is discussed as follows.

### Approach

Approach to chronic diarrhea must be considered with the following points in mind:

*Age of onset:* A list of common causes according to age of onset is shown in Table 12.15.

**Table 12.15:** Common causes of chronic diarrhea according to age of onset and nature of diarrhea

| *Age at onset <6 months* | *Age >6 months to 5 years* | *>5 years* |
|---|---|---|
| **Watery**<br>• Cow milk protein allergy[#]<br>• Lymphangiectasia<br>• Post enteritis syndrome<br>• Immunodeficiency[#]<br>• Anatomical defects<br>• Urinary tract infection*<br><br>**Rare causes*****<br>• Autoimmune enteropathy<br>• Microvillus inclusion disease<br>• Tufting enteropathy<br>• Glucose glactose malabsorption<br>• Congenital sodium/chloride diarrhea | **Small bowel**<br>• Cow milk protein allergy[#]<br>• Toddler diarrhea<br>• Celiac disease<br>• Lymphangiectasia<br>• Post enteritis syndrome<br>• Giardiasis<br>• Crohn's disease[#]<br>• Immunodeficiency[#]<br>• Autoimmune enteropathy<br>• Abetalipoproteinemia<br>• Drug induced<br>• Short bowel syndrome**<br>• Bacterial overgrowth | **Small bowel**<br>• Celiac disease<br>• Parasitic infections: Giardiasis, IBS (diarrhea), lactose intolerance<br>• Tropical sprue<br>• Drugs<br>• Lymphangiectasia<br>• Crohn's disease[#]<br>• Immunodeficiency[#]<br>• Drug induced<br>• Short bowel syndrome**<br>• Bacterial overgrowth<br>• Immunoproliferative small intestinal disease |
| **Bloody**<br>• Cow milk protein allergy<br>• Cytomegalovirus colitis<br>• Very early onset inflammatory bowel disease (VEOIBD)<br>• Hirschsprung enterocolitis<br>• Nectrotizing enterocolitis | **Large bowel**<br>• Cow milk protein allergy<br>• CMV colitis<br>• Hirschsprung enterocolitis<br>• Pseudomembranous colitis<br>• Ulcerative colitis<br>• Crohn's disease<br>• Tuberculosis | **Large bowel**<br>• Ulcerative colitis<br>• Crohn's disease<br>• Tuberculosis<br>• Pseudomembranous colitis<br>• CMV<br>• Radiation colitis<br>• Hirschsprung enterocolitis, etc. |
| **Fatty**<br>• Cystic fibrosis<br>• Cholestasis | **Fatty**<br>• Cystic fibrosis<br>• Chronic pancreatitis<br>• Cholestasis<br>• Shwachman-Diamond syndrome | **Fatty**<br>• Chronic pancreatitis<br>• Cystic fibrosis<br>• Cholestasis |

*Should be considered in young infants with chronic diarrhea, particularly if fever is noted.

**Consider if there is antecedent history of small bowel surgery.

***These rare conditions should only be considered, if the diarrhea is very early in its onset (neonate to 3 months) and common conditions have been ruled out.

[#]Some etiologies can present with watery and/or bloody diarrhea depending on the site of involvement

**Table 12.16:** Differentiating small bowel from large bowel diarrhea

| *Features* | *Small bowel diarrhea* | *Large bowel diarrhea* |
|---|---|---|
| Stool volume; color | Large; pale | Small; normal |
| Blood in stool | No | Usually present |
| Rectal symptoms, e.g. urgency, tenesmus | No | Yes |
| Steatorrhea (greasy stools); smell | Yes; offensive smell | No; normal |
| Carbohydrate malabsorption | Yes, explosive stools | No |
| Protein malabsorption | Yes | No |
| Pain (if any) | Periumbilical, no reduction after stool | Hypogastric, reduced after passage of stool |
| Nutrient deficiency | Frequent | Can occur due to blood loss |



*Nature of stools:* Stools can be broadly divided into three main categories—watery, fatty, and bloody. Watery stool has a high liquid content and can be mistaken for urine in infants. Fatty stools are bulky, foul smelling and pale with visible oil sometimes. Bloody stools contain gross blood mixed with stools and suggest a large bowel disease. Features that help in differentiating small bowel from large bowel diarrhea are shown in Table 12.16.

*Response to fasting:* Once the baseline stool output with normal feeding has been noted, the patient can be kept nil orally for 24 hours to assess the response. If the stool volume is same or minimally changed after fasting, it suggests the presence of secretory diarrhea. However, if there is significant reduction in the stool output, it suggests osmotic diarrhea.

*Site of disease:* Diarrhea is most commonly of intestinal origin (small, large or both) and sometimes pancreatic, or hepatobiliary in etiology. Cholestasis due to biliary obstruction or intrahepatic causes leads to fat malabsorption and diarrhea. Pruritus and malabsorption of fat-soluble vitamins (A, D, E and K) are commonly associated. Maldigestion due to deficiency of pancreatic enzymes leads to fatty stools. Diarrhea may be a systemic manifestation of other conditions like immunodeficiency states, diabetes, or collagen vascular disorders. Other uncommon causes include Zollinger-Ellison syndrome, VIPoma, carcinoid or mastocytosis.

The approach to a case with chronic diarrhea is shown in Fig. 12.19 and the important clues to some of the etiologies are given in Table 12.17. A brief description of the common causes of chronic diarrhea is given below.

## Celiac Disease

This is an enteropathy caused by permanent sensitivity to gluten in genetically susceptible subjects. Nearly 99% of patients are positive for the human leukocyte antigen-DQ2 or -DQ8. Celiac disease is the most common cause of chronic diarrhea in children over 2 years of age in North India. High-risk groups include type 1 diabetes mellitus, Down syndrome, selective IgA deficiency, autoimmune thyroid disease, Turner syndrome, Williams syndrome, autoimmune liver disease and first-degree relatives of patients with celiac disease.

**Approach to a child with chronic diarrhea**

↓

**Detailed history**

- Age at onset
- Stool characteristics: Nature, frequency, nocturnal, volume, relation with food, presence of blood, oil
- Dietary history: Relation with introduction of animal milk, gluten, intake of fruit juices, food aversions
- Previous abdominal surgery: Resection, adhesions
- History of repeated infections: Immunodeficiency, cystic fibrosis
- Drug intake: Causing diarrhea, immunosuppressive medications can increase risk of GI infections
- Associated illness: Diabetes mellitus, thyrotoxicosis, post-bone marrow transplant
- Family history: IBD, celiac disease, cystic fibrosis, immunodeficiency
- Previous history of acute gastroenteritis: Post infectious IBS, post enteritis syndrome
- Other manifestations: Extraintestinal in IBD, rash/aphthous stomatitis in celiac disease

↓

**Detailed examination**

- Anthropometry, signs of dehydration
- Anemia, edema—pitting/non-pitting (lymphedema), clubbing, oral thrush, skin infection/rash
- Vitamin (water or fat soluble)/mineral deficiency
- Perianal: Rash, tags, fissures, fistulae, blood on finger, features of Hirschsprung disease
- Abdomen: Distension, ascites, scars, organomegaly, visible peristalsis
- Systemic examination: Joint/eye—IBD; chest for cystic fibrosis, tuberculosis

↓

**Determine**

- Likely differential diagnosis as per nature of diarrhea, age of onset, associated findings
- Plan investigative work-up. Select from the list below

↓

**Investigations: No uniform protocol; case based**

- Hemogram including ESR and C-reactive protein
- Biochemistry: Liver functions, electrolytes, calcium, lipid profile
- Stool examination: Reducing substances, microscopy and antigen test for opportunistic infections, *Clostridium difficile* toxin, fecal fat/elastase
- Serology: Celiac disease, HIV, antienterocyte antibody
- Immune profile: Cellular and humoral immunity
- Endoscopy with biopsies: Upper GI/colon/enteroscopy
- Radiologic imaging: USG, CT enterography
- Others: D-xylose, glucose hydrogen/lactose breath tests, endocrine evaluation

**Fig. 12.19** Approach to a patient with chronic diarrhea. IBD inflammatory bowel disease, USG ultrasonography

### *Clinical Features*

The classical presentation is with small bowel diarrhea, growth failure and anemia. A temporal association of

**Table 12.17:** Clues to important causes of chronic diarrhea

| | |
|---|---|
| Cow milk protein allergy | • Onset of diarrhea after introduction of cow or buffalo milk or formula<br>• Rectal bleeding (due to colitis)<br>• Anemia; failure to thrive<br>• Family history of allergy or atopy<br>• Response to milk withdrawal |
| Lymphangiectasia | • Nonpitting pedal edema suggesting lymphedema<br>• Recurrent anasarca<br>• Hypoalbuminemia and hypoproteinemia<br>• Lymphopenia<br>• Hypocalcemia |
| Cystic fibrosis | • History of meconium ileus<br>• Predominant or associated lower respiratory tract infections<br>• Severe failure to thrive<br>• Clubbing<br>• History of sibling deaths<br>• High sweat chloride (>60 mEq/L) |
| Immunodeficiencies | • Predominant fever<br>• Recurrent infections involving other sites<br>• History of sibling deaths<br>• Organomegaly<br>• Opportunistic infections on stool examination |

diarrhea and introduction of wheat products at weaning may be present. Onset of diarrhea before introduction of wheat products in diet negates a diagnosis of CD. Other presentations include refractory iron deficiency (not responding to oral supplements) or dimorphic anemia, short stature, delayed puberty, rickets and osteopenia. Examination reveals failure to thrive, loss of subcutaneous fat, clubbing, anemia, rickets and signs of other vitamin deficiencies. A high index of suspicion for the disease is the key to diagnosis.

### *Diagnosis*

The main investigations required for making a diagnosis include:

***Serology:*** IgA antibody against tissue transglutaminase (tTG) is an ELISA-based test, with high sensitivity (92–100%) and specificity (91–100%) and is recommended for initial testing. IgA antiendomysial antibody is an equally accurate test (sensitivity 88–100%; specificity 91–100%), but is difficult to perform and not readily available. Serology helps in making a diagnosis of celiac disease and also in assessing compliance to dietary therapy.

***Upper GI endoscopy and histology:*** The endoscopy may be normal or show absence of folds or scalloped duodenal folds **(Fig. 12.20a)**. Multiple biopsies should be taken from the second/third part of duodenum and also from the duodenal bulb. The characteristic histological changes in celiac disease are increased intraepithelial lymphocytes (>30/100 enterocytes), increased crypt length, partial to total villous atrophy, decreased villous to crypt ratio and infiltration of plasma cells and lymphocytes in lamina propria **(Fig. 12.20b)**. Both serology and biopsy should be done when the subject is on a normal gluten-containing diet.

The diagnostic criteria have been changing in recent years with differences in recommendations between children and adults. Traditionally, the diagnosis of celiac disease required the following:

i. Clinical features compatible with diagnosis
ii. Positive intestinal biopsy
iii. Positive serology and
iv. Unequivocal response to gluten-free diet (GFD) within 12 weeks of its initiation.

The recent 2020 ESPGHAN guidelines suggest that in all suspected cases (symptomatic, asymptomatic, and at-risk group), the first test should be total serum IgA and IgA-tTG. In patients with IgA-tTG ≥10 times the upper limit of normal, the diagnosis of celiac disease may be made without a duodenal biopsy provided that the antiendomysial

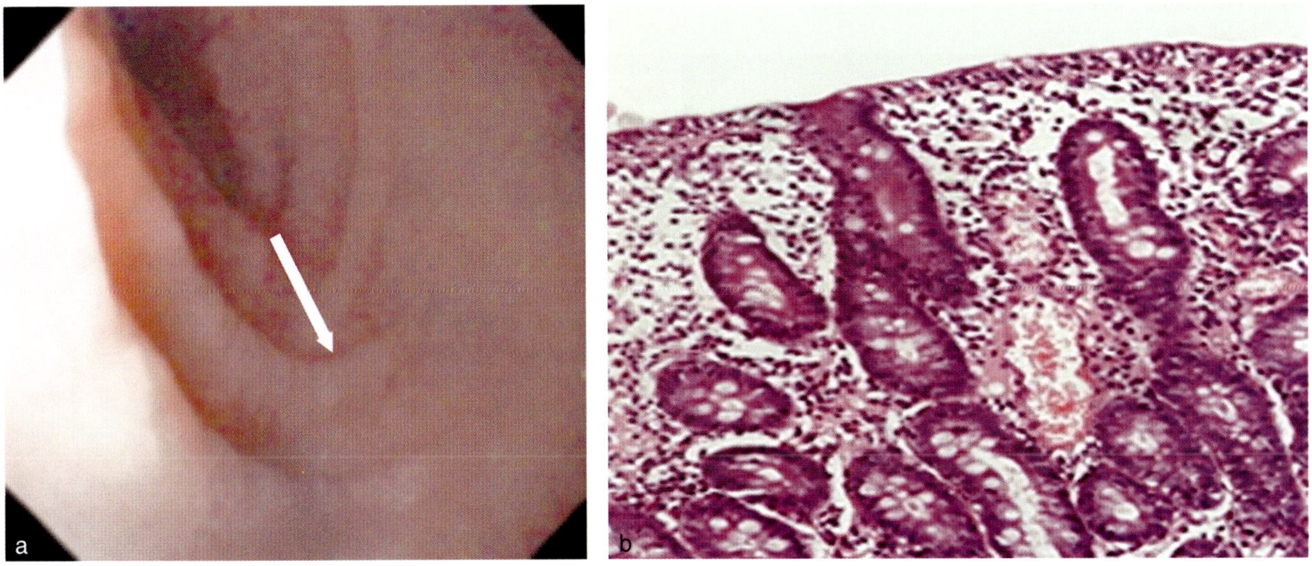


**Fig. 12.20:** Celiac disease: (a) Upper gastrointestinal endoscopy showing scalloping of duodenal folds (arrow); (b) Duodenal histology showing total villous atrophy

antibody (EMA, separately drawn blood sample) is also positive and there is a definite response to gluten-free diet. However, in view of restricted availability and cost of EMA and multiple labs reporting IgA-tTG only as positive (without actual titers), the non-biopsy approach is not yet preferred in our country. This is especially important as it is very difficult to confirm or refute the diagnosis of celiac disease after initiation of gluten-free diet. Thus, all efforts should be made to make a correct diagnosis with full work-up at onset prior to initiation of dietary therapy.

#### Treatment

Treatment involves lifelong gluten-free diet (no intake of wheat, rye and barley). Oats should also be avoided in the initial period due to the risk of gluten contamination. Nutritional deficiency of iron, folate and other vitamins and minerals should be corrected by supplementation. After initiation of gluten-free diet, the symptoms should subside (2–4 weeks) and there should be weight and height gain. Repeated explanation to patient and parents by doctors is essential for sustaining compliance after the child has become asymptomatic.

Celiac disease should be differentiated from nonceliac gluten sensitivity (NCGS) which is a condition in which gluten ingestion leads to GI and non-GI symptoms but the patients does not have celiac disease or wheat allergy (i.e. no enteropathy, negative serology). Gluten challenge is required to make a diagnosis of NCGS.

### Cow Milk Protein Allergy

Cow milk protein allergy (CMPA) affects 2 to 5% of all children in the West, with the highest prevalence during the first year of life. CMPA accounted for one-third of all children with chronic diarrhea of <5 years of age from a tertiary care centre in India. A family history of atopy is common. Nearly 50% children outgrow the allergy by 1 year and ~95% by 6 years. It is the most common food allergy in small children who are top-fed but can occasionally occur in exclusively breastfed babies, due to passage of cow milk antigen in breast milk.

There are two kinds of reactions to cow milk: (i) Immediate (IgE mediated). It occurs within minutes of milk intake and is characterized by vomiting, pallor, shock-like state, urticaria and swelling of lips. (ii) Delayed (cell mediated): It has an indolent course and presents mainly with GI symptoms.

#### Clinical Features

The chief presentation is with diarrhea with blood and mucus. Depending upon the site and extent of involvement, the child may have small bowel, large bowel or mixed type diarrhea. In an Indian study, 40% children presented with bloody diarrhea, 33% watery and 7% with a mixed type of diarrhea. Uncommonly reflux symptoms and hematemesis may be present. Respiratory symptoms (allergic rhinitis and asthma) and atopic manifestations (eczema, angioedema) may be seen in 20–30% and 50–60% cases, respectively. Iron deficiency anemia, hypoproteinemia and eosinophilia are commonly present.

#### Diagnosis

In patients with GI symptoms, non-IgE-mediated CMPA is more common. The gold standard for diagnosis is the elimination and challenge test. Typically, the symptoms subside after withdrawal of milk and milk products and recur after re-exposure to milk. Eosinophilia and family history of atopy are suggestive. Sigmoidoscopy (aphthous ulcers and nodular lymphoid hyperplasia, Fig. 12.21a) and rectal biopsy (plenty of eosinophils, Fig. 12.21b) can be used in patients with only gastrointestinal symptoms. Skin prick test and specific IgE levels are useful for IgE-mediated CMPA.

#### Treatment

All animal milk/milk products have to be removed from the diet. Soy or extensively hydrolyzed formula (EHF), both of which are equally effective in terms of growth and nutrient intake can be used as alternatives. Although soy is more palatable and cheap, it is not recommended in infants <6 months of age. 10–15% children of CMPA have

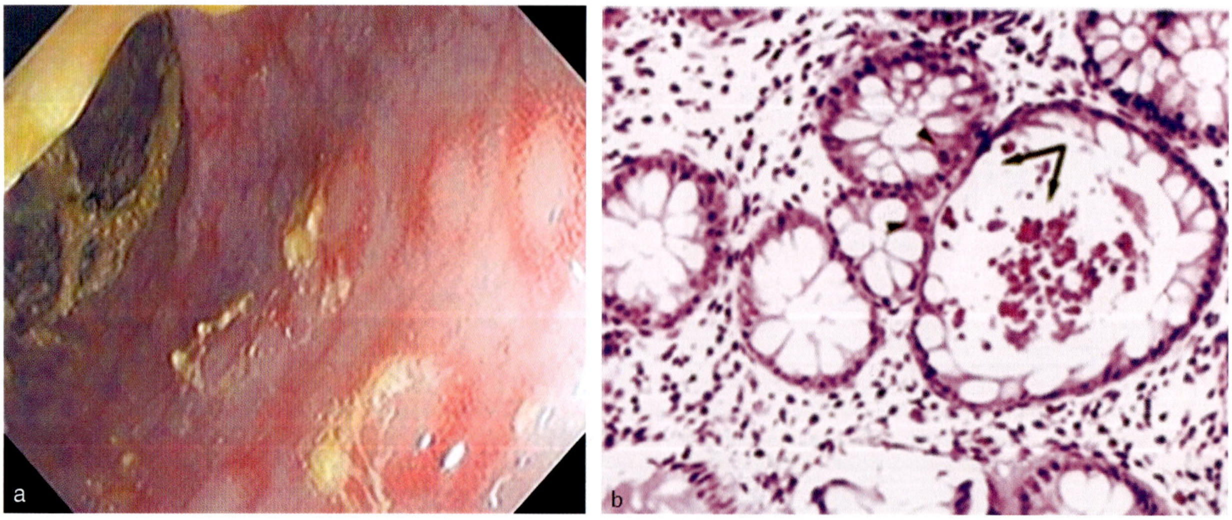

Fig. 12.21: Cow milk protein allergy: (a) Sigmoidoscopy showing aphthous ulcers; (b) Rectal biopsy showing eosinophilic infiltration with crypt abscess

concomitant soy allergy, and they need extensively hydrolyzed formulae for therapy. A minority of children with severe enteropathy or intolerant to hydrolyzed formulae need amino acid formulae.

CMPA is usually a mild disease in exclusively breastfed babies. A trial of continued breastfeeding till 6 months of age while the mother is placed on a milk/milk product free diet may be done in them. Parental education regarding diet and calcium supplementation is essential. Reevaluation should be done to determine development of tolerance and avoid prolonged restrictive diet.

*Toddler diarrhea* is a diagnosis of exclusion after common causes have been ruled out. The onset of diarrhea is between 6 and 36 months of age. The child passes 3–6 loose stools, mostly during waking hours. Diarrhea worsens with low residue, low fat or high carbohydrate diet. The child is well thriving, there is no anemia or vitamin deficiencies and the diarrhea resolves spontaneously by about 4 years of age. Treatment is with dietary modification; a high (>40%) fat, low carbohydrate diet (reduced intake of juices) and increase in dietary fiber is recommended.

### Intestinal Lymphangiectasia

Intestinal lymphangiectasia (IL) is an important cause of protein-losing enteropathy (PLE). It can either be primary or secondary to conditions causing obstruction of intestinal lymphatics. It is characterized by ectasia of the bowel lymphatic system, which on rupture causes leakage of protein-rich chyle into the intestinal lumen with resultant hypoproteinemia and hypoalbuminemia. Patients present with diarrhea, edema, ascites (chylous or non-chylous), pleural effusion, and failure to thrive. The edema can be bilateral and pitting due to hypoalbuminemia or asymmetrical and non-pitting due to lymphedema. Some children may present with steatorrhea and fat-soluble vitamin deficiencies. Presence of hypoalbuminemia, low immunoglobulins, hypocalcemia and lymphopenia is characteristic. The risk of recurrent and opportunistic infections is increased.

On UGI endoscopy (fat loading with 2 g/kg of butter at bedtime increases the yield), scattered white plaques or chyle-like substance covering the mucosa may be seen (Fig. 12.22a). Duodenal biopsy reveals dilated lacteals in villi and lamina propria (Fig. 12.22b) and confirms the diagnosis. However, in some patients, the UGI endoscopy may be normal and they need visualization and biopsy from jejunum by capsule endoscopy/enteroscopy for diagnosis. Treatment consists of a high protein, low fat diet with supplementation of MCT oil, calcium and fat-soluble vitamins. Intravenous albumin is required for symptomatic management. Total parenteral nutrition (TPN) and octreotide are used for management of chylous effusions. Bowel resection may be curative in patients with disease localized to a small segment of the intestine.

### Immunodeficiency

Both congenital and acquired immunodeficiency can cause chronic diarrhea. It should be suspected, if there is history of recurrent infections at multiple sites (chest/GI/skin) and wasting. The common immunodeficiency conditions presenting with diarrhea include IgA deficiency, severe combined immunodeficiency, common variable immunodeficiency and chronic granulomatous disease. There is increased risk of celiac disease (10–20-fold increase) and Crohn's disease in patients with IgA deficiency. Diagnosis is made by measuring serum immunoglobulins, T cell counts and functions, phagocytic function (nitroblue tetrazolium reduction test) depending upon the suspected etiology. Treatment depends on the cause of diarrhea and includes antimicrobials for bacterial overgrowth and opportunistic infections and therapy for underlying immunodeficiency (IV immunoglobulins, or bone marrow transplantation).

*Acquired immunodeficiency syndrome (AIDS):* Chronic diarrhea is a common feature in children with AIDS. The impaired mucosal immunity results in recurrent opportunistic infections and the altered maturation and function of enterocytes results in increased permeability and decreased functional absorptive surface with or

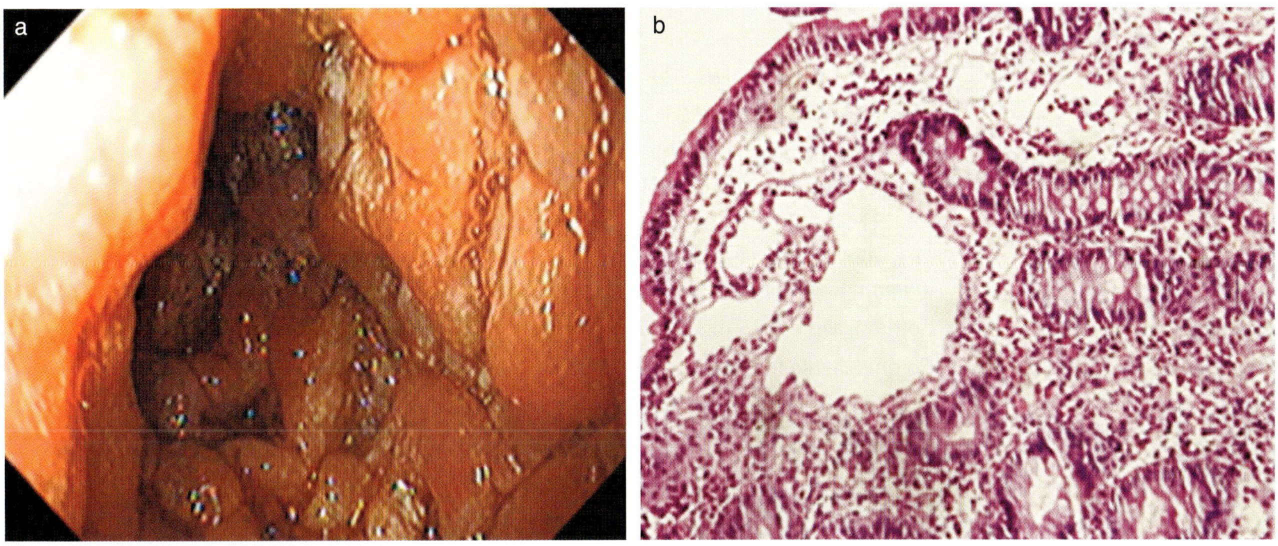

Fig. 12.22: Intestinal lymphangiectasia: (a) Upper gastrointestinal endoscopy showing snow-flake appearance; (b) Duodenal histology shows dilated lacteals

without bacterial overgrowth. AIDS enteropathy is characterized by chronic diarrhea and marked weight loss in absence of enteric pathogens. Presence of oral thrush, lymphadenopathy, hepatosplenomegaly and parotitis (10–20% cases) gives clue to the diagnosis. Common infections include:

i. *Viral:* Cytomegalovirus, herpes simplex, adenovirus, norovirus
ii. *Bacterial*: *Salmonella, Shigella, Mycobacterium avium* complex (MAC), *C. jejuni, C. difficile*
iii. *Fungi*: Candidiasis, histoplasmosis, cryptococcosis
iv. *Protozoa*: *Microsporidium, Isospora belli, Cryptosporidium, E. histolytica, G. lamblia, Cyclospora, Blastocystis hominis*

Multiple stool examinations are required to identify the etiology, using special stains and PCR techniques. Colonic/terminal ileum biopsy and duodenal fluid examination are useful for diagnosing some infections. Treatment is with specific antimicrobials **(Table 12.18)** along with HAART (highly active antiretroviral therapy).

## Drug-Induced Diarrhea

Diarrhea can be a side effect of many pharmacologic agents. Altered GI motility, mucosal injury and/or change in intestinal microflora are the main etiologic factors. Antibiotics can cause loose watery stools by altered bacterial flora or bloody stools secondary to *Clostridium difficile* overgrowth and pseudomembranous colitis. Stopping the offending agent is often enough. If suspicion of pseudomembranous colitis is present, then stool for toxin assay and sigmoidoscopy is required for confirmation. Metronidazole or oral vancomycin is the drug of choice.

## Inflammatory Bowel Disease (IBD)

IBD is a chronic inflammatory disease of the GI tract and is of two main types—Crohn's disease (CD) and ulcerative colitis (UC). In ~10% cases, with isolated colonic involvement, the subjects cannot be classified into UC or CD and they are labeled as indeterminate colitis. 15–25% of all IBD presents in children ≤17 years of age and they are labeled as pediatric IBD. The incidence of pediatric IBD is increasing all over the world including India. The average age of presentation in children is ~10–11 years. Very early onset IBD is used to define children with symptoms at <6 yr of age. The etiopathogenesis of IBD is multifactorial and includes genetic factors, environmental triggers, and altered gut microflora, the interaction of which initiates an abnormal mucosal immune response and intestinal inflammation.

### Clinical Features

Children with UC present with diarrhea and rectal bleeding which raises alarm and leads to early work-up and diagnosis. In CD, abdominal pain is the most common presenting symptom, followed by diarrhea, poor growth or weight loss, and anorexia. Patients with predominant colonic disease present as colitis. The classical triad of CD, i.e. pain, diarrhea and weight loss is seen in only 25% cases. Fever, fatigue and anorexia are present in 25–50% cases.

Extraintestinal manifestations (EIM) are seen in 25–30% children with IBD. Arthralgia/arthritis is the most common EIM seen in 15–17% cases. Uveitis, aphthous stomatitis, erythema nodosum, pyoderma gangrenosum, and sclerosing cholangitis are the other EIM. They can precede, follow or occur concurrently with the intestinal disease and may be related/unrelated to activity of the intestinal disease.

***Disease distribution:*** UC is classified as proctitis (E1: rectum only), left-sided (E2: distal to splenic flexure), extensive (E3: distal to hepatic flexure), and pancolitis (E4), with majority of children having pancolitis. CD is classified as—L1: Distal one-third ileal alone ± limited cecal involvement, L2: Colonic alone, L3: Ileocolonic, L4: Isolated upper GI based on disease extent and as inflammatory (B1), stricturing (B2) and penetrating (B3), based on disease behavior. Majority of patients with CD (50–70%) have ileocolonic disease. Upper GI involvement is present in 30–40% cases and perianal disease in ~15–20% cases. As the management and prognosis of CD and UC is different, so a correct diagnosis is

**Table 12.18:** Treatment recommendations for infectious diarrhea

| *Infection causing diarrhea* | *Drug of choice for treatment* |
|---|---|
| *Giardia lamblia* | Metronidazole 7.5 mg/kg/dose thrice daily for 5 days |
| *Entamoeba histolytica* | Metronidazole 7.5 mg/kg/dose thrice daily for 10 days |
| *Cryptosporidium* | Nitazoxanide: In immunocompetent children<br>• 1–3 years: 100 mg two times a day × 3 days<br>• 4–11 years: 200 mg two times a day × 3 days |
| *Microsporidium* | Oral albendazole (15 mg/kg/day twice a day) for 14 days in immunocompetent. Longer therapy in immunocompromised. |
| *Cyclospora* | Cotrimoxazole 5/25 mg/kg/day for 7 days |
| *Isospora belli* | Cotrimoxazole for 7 days |
| Cytomegalovirus | Ganciclovir or valganciclovir for 14–21 days |
| *Clostridium difficile* | Stop other antibiotics. Oral metronidazole (30 mg/kg/day in 4 divided doses) for 7–10 days for mild disease. Oral vancomycin (40 mg/kg/day in 4 divided doses; maximum, 2 g/day), with or without metronidazole for severe disease |
| Candidiasis | Fluconazole 6 mg/kg/day oral once a day |
| *Cryptococcus neoformans* | Fluconazole for 4 weeks |

**Table 12.19:** Differentiation between Crohn's disease and ulcerative colitis

| | *Crohn's disease* | *Ulcerative colitis* |
|---|---|---|
| Distribution | • Entire gastrointestinal tract<br>• Discontinuous lesions | • Colon only<br>• Continuous involvement |
| Bloody diarrhea | Less common | Common |
| Abdominal pain | Common | Less common |
| Growth failure | Common | Less common |
| Perianal disease | Abscess; fistulae | Absent |
| Serology | Anti-*Sacchromyces cerevisiae* antibody (ASCA) positive | Perinuclear anti-neutrophil cytoplasmic antibody (p-ANCA) positive |
| Endoscopy | Deep irregular serpigenous or aphthous ulcers with normal intervening mucosa (skip lesions) | Granularity, loss of vascular pattern, friability and diffuse ulceration |
| Histopathology | Transmural inflammation with non-caseating granuloma | Mucosal disease with cryptitis, crypt distortion, crypt abscess and goblet cell depletion |

essential. Table 12.19 lists the main differentiating features between UC and CD.

### Diagnosis

The initial evaluation of a child with suspected IBD includes a detailed clinical, family and treatment history. A complete examination with growth charting, perianal and rectal examination for fistulae, tags and fissures is essential. Simple lab tests like hemogram, ESR, C-reactive protein, total protein, serum albumin and fecal calprotectin help in screening for IBD and confirming presence of bowel inflammation. Raised fecal calprotectin is a reliable test for differentiating patients with functional abdominal pain from those with IBD.

According to the recommendations of the IBD working group, upper GI endoscopy with biopsy, colonoscopy with ileal intubation and biopsy is essential for all IBD cases (Fig. 12.23). Small bowel evaluation with CT or MR enterography is required for correct classification of IBD type (UC, CD) and to determine the disease extent. Capsule endoscopy may also be used for small bowel evaluation in patients who do not have any suggestion of small bowel obstruction. Multiple biopsies should be taken from all segments of bowel and the UGI tract for diagnosis. Children with infantile-onset IBD require genetic screening for monogenic IBD.

### Treatment

The goal of treatment is to control inflammation, improve growth and ensure a good quality of life with the least toxic therapeutic regimen. As IBD is a chronic disease with remissions and exacerbations, proper counseling of both patient and family at diagnosis is essential. The main drugs used for IBD are 5-aminosalicylates (5-ASA), steroids, immunomodulators (6-mercaptopurine, azathioprine, methotrexate) and biologicals (monoclonal antibodies against tumor necrosis factor: α-infliximab, adalimumab). The treatment can be divided into induction and maintenance therapy. For induction, we use 5-ASA, steroids, exclusive enteral nutrition, and biologicals as

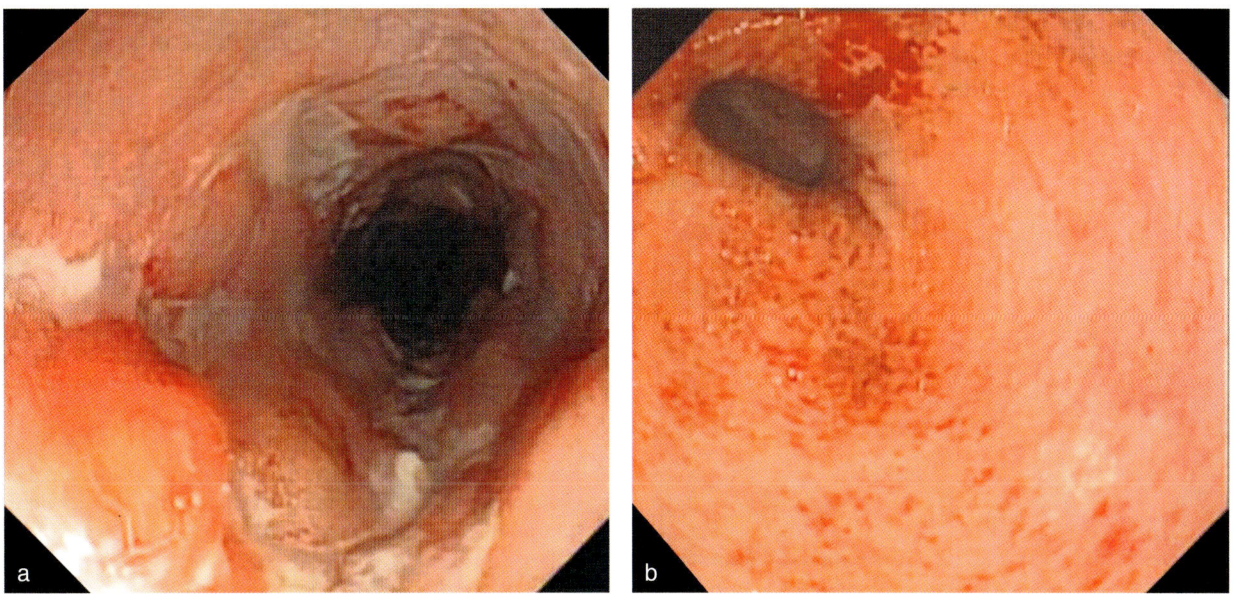


Fig. 12.23: Inflammatory bowel disease: (a) Deep, linear, serpigenous ulcers on colonoscopy in Crohn's disease; (b) Confluent superficial ulcerations with friability on colonoscopy in ulcerative colitis

per disease severity and for maintenance, we use 5-ASA, immunomodulators and biologics. Ensuring proper nutrition with caloric supplementation (~120% of RDA), adequate protein intake and correction of anemia is a necessity. Calcium and vitamin D supplementation should be given as these children are at an increased risk of osteoporosis.

Surgery (proctocolectomy with ileoanal pouch anastomosis) is curative in UC. Its indications include severe acute colitis refractory to medical disease, toxic megacolon, uncontrolled hemorrhage or colonic malignancy. In CD, surgery is not curative and is done in patients with bowel obstruction, abscesses, nonhealing fistulae, perforation, or GI bleeding.

## Abdominal Tuberculosis

The gastrointestinal tract, peritoneum, lymph nodes and/or solid viscera can be involved in abdominal tuberculosis. The peritoneal involvement is of two types: Wet (or ascitic) and dry (or plastic) type. On the other hand, the intestinal involvement may be ulcerative, hypertrophic or ulcero-hypertrophic type. Nearly 20% cases may have evidence of TB elsewhere in the body.

*Clinical features:* The clinical presentation is varied and depends upon the site of disease and type of pathology. Symptoms may include features of subacute intestinal obstruction (abdominal pain, distension, vomiting, obstipation), ascites, chronic diarrhea, lump in abdomen (ileocecal mass, loculated ascites, lymph nodes) and/or systemic manifestations (fever, malaise, anorexia and weight loss).

*Diagnosis:* A high index of suspicion followed by documenting presence of acid-fast bacilli (fine needle aspiration cytology from lymph nodes, ascitic fluid, endoscopic biopsies) on Ziehl-Neelsen staining, PCR or culture leads to a definitive diagnosis. Presence of tubercular granuloma with caseation in the biopsies (endoscopic, peritoneal or liver) also helps make the diagnosis. CT abdomen shows enlarged lymph nodes with central necrosis (Fig. 12.24). An exudative ascites (low serum ascites albumin gradient, SAAG <1.1) with lymphocyte predominance and high adenosine deaminase is typical of tubercular ascites. Colonoscopy classically shows transverse ulcers in ascending colon/cecum, deformed/ulcerated ileocecal valve and ulceration/stricture in terminal ileum (Fig. 12.25). Laparoscopy is required in select cases, it shows peritoneal tubercles and provides tissue for histopathological diagnosis. In absence of above features, a probable diagnosis of abdominal tuberculosis is made when suggestive clinical features and response to antitubercular therapy is present. It is important to differentiate intestinal TB from Crohn's disease as they mimic each other in clinical presentation but have very different treatments.

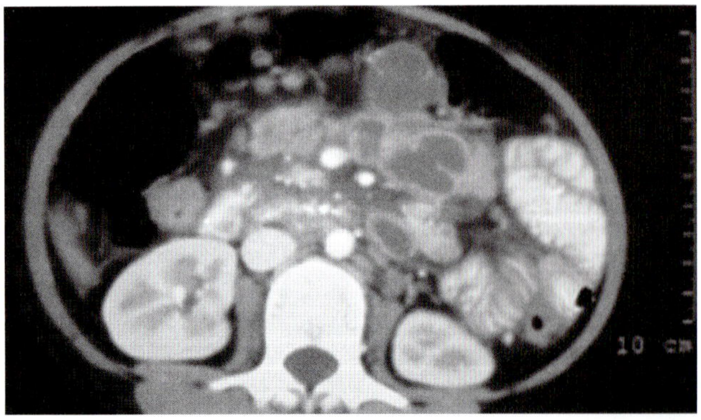


Fig. 12.24: CT scan showing multiple enlarged lymph nodes with central necrosis in para-aortic and mesenteric regions in abdominal tuberculosis

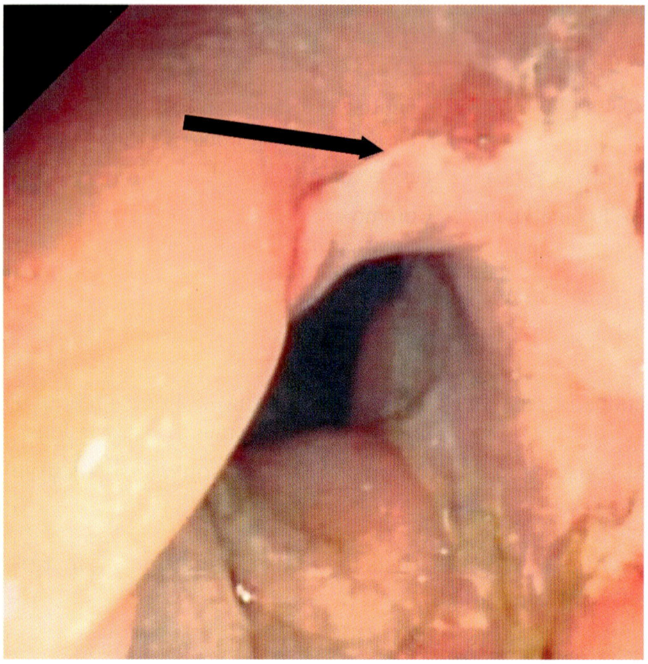

Fig. 12.25: Colonoscopy shows ulceration with gaping ileocecal valve in a patient with ileocecal tuberculosis

*Treatment:* Antitubercular drugs are the mainstay of treatment. Surgery is indicated, if there is bowel perforation, obstruction or massive hemorrhage. One should suspect multidrug resistant tuberculosis in patients with a definite diagnosis of abdominal tuberculosis but a poor response to standard antitubercular therapy despite good compliance. Nutritional support with high calorie and protein diet and correction of anemia and other deficiencies is required.

## Suggested Reading


1. Conrad MA, Rosh JR. Pediatric inflammatory bowel disease Pediatr Clin North Am 2017;64:577–91.
2. Husby S, Koletzko S, Korponay-Szabó I, et al. European Society Paediatric Gastroenterology, Hepatology and Nutrition Guidelines for Diagnosing Coeliac Disease 2020. J Pediatr Gastroenterol Nutr 2020;70:141–56.
3. Lal SB, Bolia R, Menon JV, et al. Abdominal tuberculosis in children: A real-world experience of 218 cases from an endemic region. JGH Open 2019;4:215–20.
4. Matthai J, Sathiasekharan M, Poddar U, et al; Indian Society of Pediatric Gastroenterology, Hepatology and Nutrition; Pediatric Gastroenterology Chapter of Indian Academy of Pediatrics. Guidelines on Diagnosis and Management of Cow Milk Protein Allergy. Indian Pediatr 2020;57:723–29.
5. Shankar S, Rosenbaum J. Chronic diarrhea in children: A practical algorithm-based approach. J Paediatr and Child Health 2020;56:1029–38.

Competencies: **PE26.5; PE26.11**

## GASTROINTESTINAL BLEEDING

Gastrointestinal bleeding is a commonly encountered problem in children. Upper gastrointestinal bleeding (UGIB) is defined as bleeding from a site proximal to the ligament of Treitz (at the level of duodenojejunal flexure). Lower gastrointestinal bleeding (LGIB) is defined as bleeding from a site distal to ligament of Treitz.

***Hematemesis*** is passage of blood in vomiting and suggests an upper GI site of bleeding. The vomitus may be bright red or coffee-ground in color depending upon the severity of hemorrhage and the duration it stayed in contact with gastric secretions. ***Melena*** is passage of black tarry stools and suggests an upper GI or small bowel source of bleed. ***Hematochezia*** is passage of bright red blood in stools. ***Hemobilia*** refers to bleeding from the biliary tree while ***hemosuccus pancreaticus*** is bleeding from the pancreas. Small bowel bleeding can be overt (presents with either melena or hematochezia) or occult (presents with iron-deficiency anemia and guaiac-positive stools). ***Obscure GI bleed*** is used to define patients where the source of bleeding is not identified after upper and lower endoscopy, small bowel evaluation with video capsule endoscopy and/or enteroscopy, and radiographic testing. It can be obscure-overt or obscure-occult.

### Upper GI Bleeding

UGIB is more common and often massive than LGIB in children. Most children with UGIB have hematemesis, however, a small proportion may also present with just melena or hematochezia. The causes of UGIB vary in different age groups as shown in Table 12.20. Varices, esophagitis and gastritis are the common causes in Indian children. NSAIDs are an important cause of UGIB and history of drug intake should always be taken.

Painless passage of large amount of blood in vomitus suggests variceal bleeding, especially in the presence of splenomegaly. However, the spleen may reduce in size after a bout of massive hematemesis and thus become non-palpable. In portal hypertension, esophageal varices are the most common cause of upper GI bleeding (Fig. 12.26a), others being gastric varices (Fig. 12.26b), portal hypertensive

**Table 12.20:** Common causes of upper gastrointestinal bleeding

| *Neonate or infant* | *Children >2 years* |
|---|---|
| Swallowed maternal blood | Esophagitis due to reflux, medications, infections |
| Esophagitis | Gastroduodenal erosions/ulceration |
| Gastroduodenal erosions/ulceration | Portal hypertension: Esophageal, gastric varices, portal hypertensive gastropathy |
| Sepsis/coagulopathy/stress | Sepsis/coagulopathy/stress |
| Hemorrhagic disease of newborn | Caustic ingestion, Mallory-Weiss tear |
| Esophageal varices (infants >3–4 months) | IgA vasculitis (Henoch-Schönlein purpura) |
| Vascular malformation | Vascular malformation; gastric antral vascular ectasia |
| Foreign body impaction | Foreign body impaction |
| Cow milk allergy | Gastrointestinal duplication |
| Gastrointestinal duplication | Hemobilia/hemosuccus pancreaticus |
| Tumors: Teratoma | Tumors: Leiomyoma, lymphoma, teratoma |

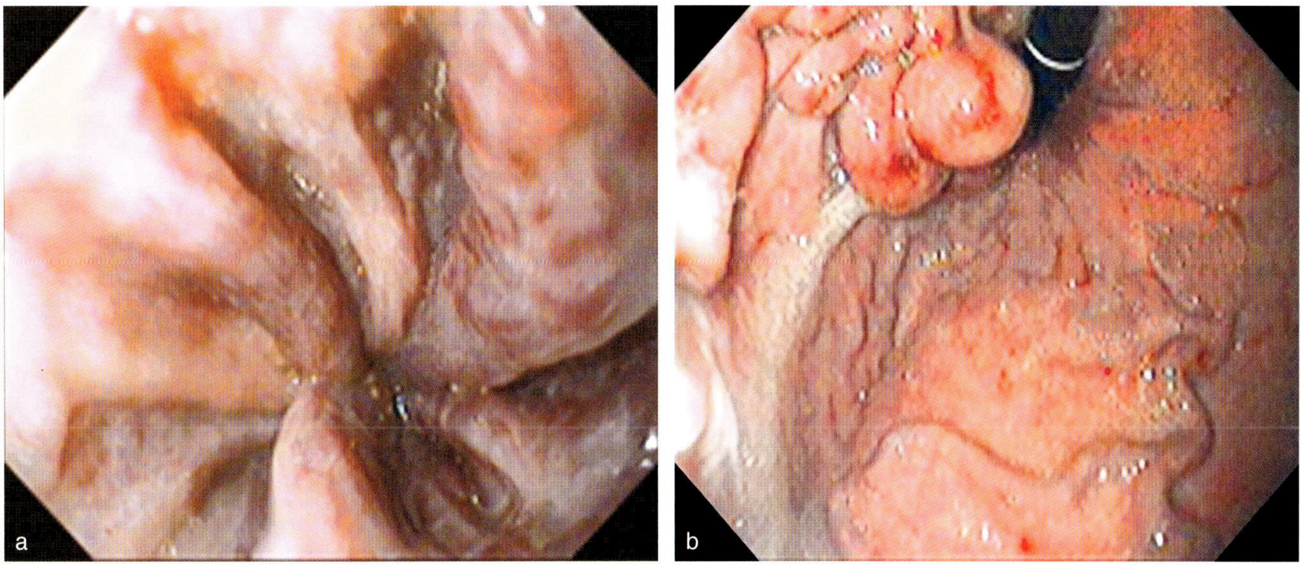


**Fig. 12.26:** Upper gastrointestinal endoscopy showing: (a) Esophageal varices; (b) Large gastric varices

gastropathy and gastric antral vascular ectasia. Children in the ICU requiring mechanical ventilation and those with coagulopathy have an increased risk of UGIB due to stress-related mucosal disease.

### Management

The management approach is shown in Fig. 12.27. General supportive measures include a good venous access, intake output monitoring, oxygen supplementation (if required) and vital charting. Presence of shock or orthostatic changes in heart rate and blood pressure (increase in pulse rate by 20 beats/min or a decrease in systolic blood pressure of 10 mm Hg upon changing the position from supine to sitting) suggest significant losses and need of urgent fluid replacement. Blood transfusion should be given to achieve hemoglobin of 7 g/dL. Short-term antibiotic prophylaxis (third generation cephalosporin for 7 days) should be given in children with cirrhosis and variceal bleeding as it reduces bacterial infection and mortality.

*Specific treatment* depends on the patient's condition, cause of bleed and expertise of the available personnel. UGI endoscopy is extremely useful for evaluating the cause and site of bleeding and offering therapy. UGIB is broadly classified as variceal and non-variceal for the purpose of management. A combination of pharmacologic and endoscopic therapy is preferred. Early administration of vasoactive drugs should be followed by endoscopic therapy within 12 hours of bleed.

*Variceal bleeding:* Administration of somatostatin or octreotide decreases the splanchnic and azygous blood flow, thus reducing portal pressures. Both agents are equally effective; limited studies in children have shown control of variceal bleeding in ~70% children. Infusion should be given for at least 24–48 hours after the bleeding has stopped and should not be discontinued abruptly.

*Endoscopic sclerotherapy (EST) and variceal ligation (EVL)* are the two main methods used to manage esophageal varices. In EST, 1–3 mL of sclerosant (1% ethoxysclerol) is injected into each variceal column. Variceal ligation is done with a device called multiple band ligator. The variceal column is sucked into a cylinder attached at the tip of the endoscope and the band is deployed by pulling the trip wire around the varix. Both procedures have 90–100% efficacy in controlling acute bleeding, but variceal ligation is preferred due to lesser side effects except in smaller children (<2 y). Following an episode of variceal bleeding, all patients should receive secondary prophylaxis till variceal eradication to prevent re-bleeding.

*Gastric varices* are managed with endoscopic injection of tissue adhesive glue, i.e. N-butyl-2-cyanoacrylate or isobutyl-2-cyanoacrylate. These agents harden within 20 seconds of contact with blood and result in rapid control of active bleeding.

*Tamponade of varices* is required only when the endoscopic and pharmacologic measures have failed which is very

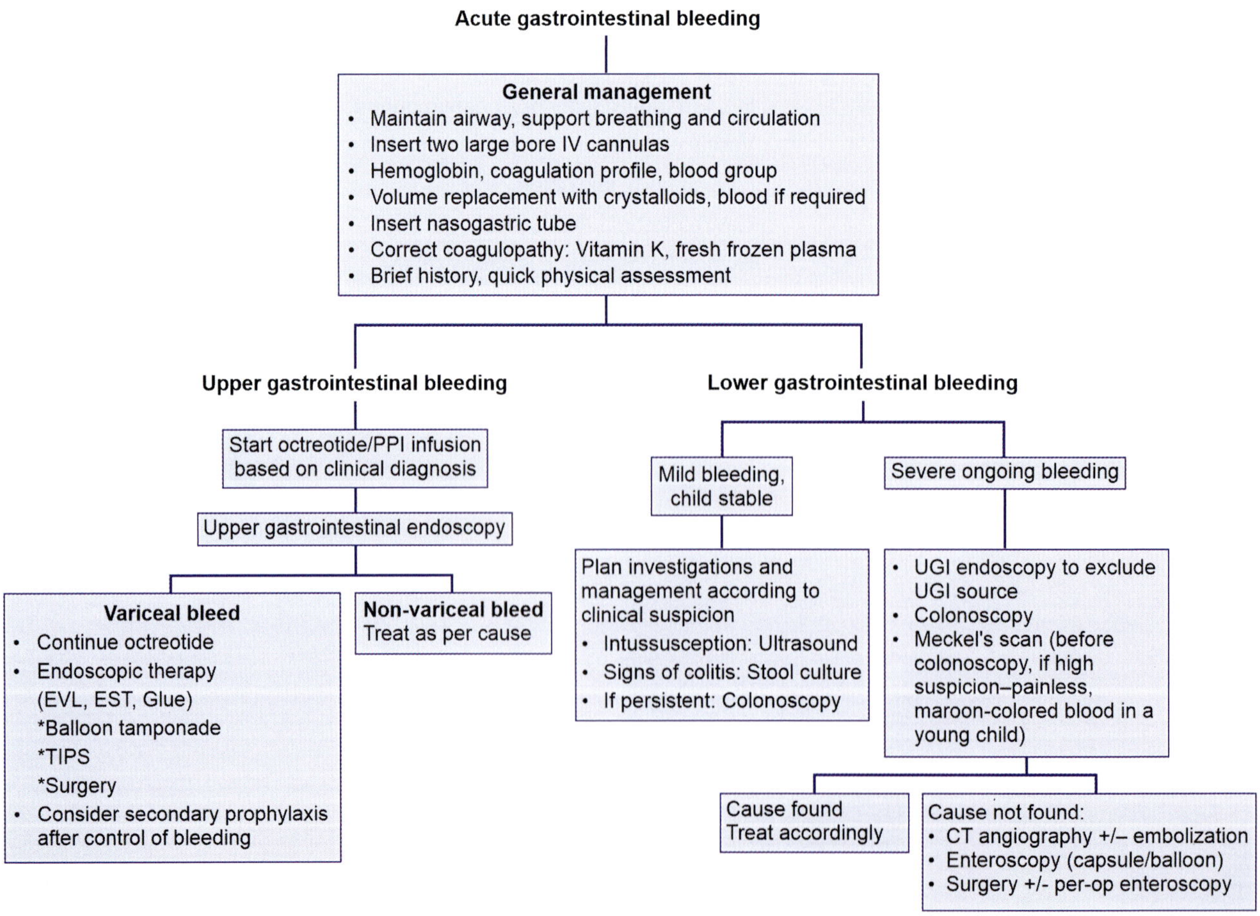


Fig. 12.27: Approach to a child with upper or lower GI bleeding

rare. Sengstaken-Blakemore tube is a triple lumen tube with connection to an esophageal balloon, a gastric balloon and one perforated distal end which helps in aspiration of the stomach contents.

*Transjugular intrahepatic portosystemic shunt (TIPS)* is an interventional radiology technique that establishes a communication between the portal vein and the hepatic vein by placing a metallic stent between them. This procedure results in bypassing liver resistance and consequently decreases the portal pressure. TIPS is indicated in refractory acute variceal hemorrhage or bleeding from ectopic varices. It is a less invasive alternative to surgical therapy. It requires skills and the experience in children is limited.

*Surgical management* is required when above measures have failed or when bleeding is from ectopic varices that cannot be effectively controlled by endoscopic procedures. Surgery can be done either in the form of portocaval shunt (selective or nonselective) or devascularization with esophageal staple transection.

***Non-variceal bleeding (NVB):*** Intravenous proton pump inhibitors should be started in children suspected to have non-variceal UGIB. High-dose infusion of intravenous pantoprazole 2 mg/kg (maximum 80 mg loading followed by 0.2 mg/kg/hr infusion, maximum 8 mg/hr) promotes clot stability and facilitates hemostasis by raising the intragastric pH. The infusion can be changed to oral medications after 72 hours provided there is no re-bleeding.

After stabilization, an UGI endoscopy is done for finding the cause and offering therapy.

### Lower Gastrointestinal Bleeding

The causes of LGIB as per the age is shown in Table 12.21. History and physical examination help narrow down the differential diagnosis.

Increased frequency of stools with blood and mucus, with crampy abdominal pain points towards a colitic illness and infectious colitis is by far the commonest cause in children across all ages. A sick preterm with abdominal distension, blood in stools, feed intolerance and systemic instability is likely to have necrotizing enterocolitis. Delayed passage of meconium followed by constipation, abdominal pain and distension is seen in Hirschsprung disease. Allergic colitis is mostly seen in infants who are top fed with cow milk and present with loose stools mixed with blood and anemia. Onset of bloody diarrhea after antibiotic use suggests pseudomembranous colitis. Presence of extra-intestinal manifestations, like aphthous ulcers, joint pains and iritis, gives clue to the diagnosis of inflammatory bowel disease (IBD). History of painful defecation and passage of hard stools with blood streaking of stools is seen in anal fissure. In a patient with history of constipation, straining at stools and digital evacuation, the most likely cause of bleeding is solitary rectal ulcer syndrome. Intussusception is characterized by episodes of abdominal pain, vomiting and red currant-jelly stools, i.e. mixture of blood, mucoid exudates and stool. Painless bleeding is seen commonly in polyps (Fig. 12.28), Meckel diverticulum (Fig. 12.29), rectal varices (Fig. 12.30), ulcer or vascular anomaly. Presence of typical cutaneous lesions as seen in blue rubber bleb nevus syndrome often suggests the diagnosis. Children with HIV infection or immunosuppression secondary to chemotherapy can develop CMV enterocolitis or polymicrobial inflammation of cecum (typhlitis), both of which can lead to significant rectal bleeding.

The aim of investigations in a child with LGIB is to localize the site of bleeding, i.e. small bowel or colon and to determine the etiology. The approach is as shown in Table 12.22 and Fig. 12.27. Supportive treatment is similar to that of UGIB and specific treatment depends upon the underlying cause.

**Table 12.21:** Causes of lower gastrointestinal bleeding

| *Neonate or infant* | *Children >2 years* |
|---|---|
| **Colitis** | |
| • Infectious colitis<br>• Cow milk protein allergy<br>• Necrotizing enterocolitis<br>• Hirschsprung disease<br>• Enterocolitis<br>• Cytomegalovirus | • Infectious colitis<br>• Inflammatory bowel disease<br>• Tuberculosis<br>• Pseudomembranous colitis<br>• Cow milk protein allergy<br>• Amebiasis, cytomegalovirus<br>• Neutropenic colitis<br>• Systemic vasculitis<br>• Immunodeficiency<br>• Radiation proctitis |
| **Others** | |
| • Anal fissure<br>• Intussusception<br>• Arteriovenous malformation<br>• Rectal prolapse<br>• Meckel's diverticulum<br>• Hemorrhagic disease of newborn<br>• Coagulopathy | • Anal fissure<br>• Polyp or polyposis syndrome<br>• Solitary rectal ulcer syndrome<br>• Meckel's diverticulum<br>• NSAID-induced ulcer<br>• Duplication cyst<br>• Hemorrhoids, rectal prolapse<br>• IgA vasculitis<br>• Rectal varices, portal colopathy<br>• Arteriovenous malformation<br>• Coagulopathy<br>• Leiomyoma, lymphoma |

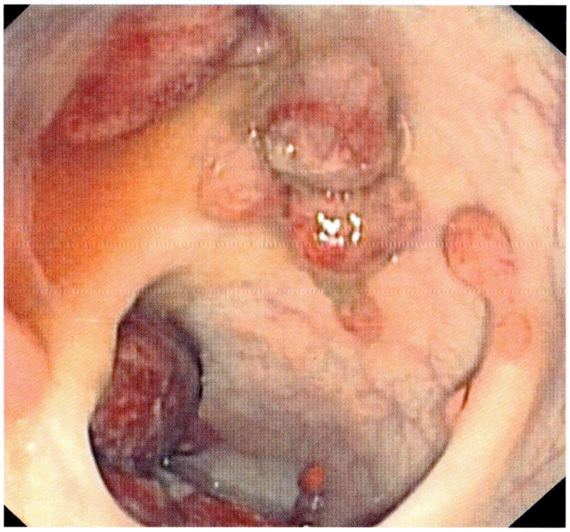

**Fig. 12.28:** Colonoscopy showing multiple sessile and pedunculated polyps in a child with polyposis coli

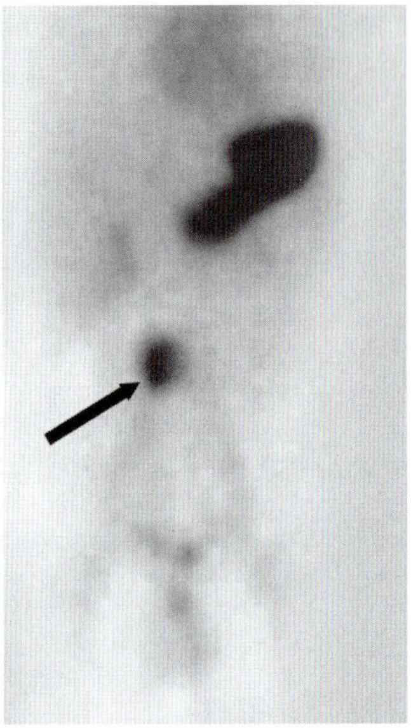

Fig. 12.29: Technetium-99m pertechnetate scan showing Meckel's diverticulum

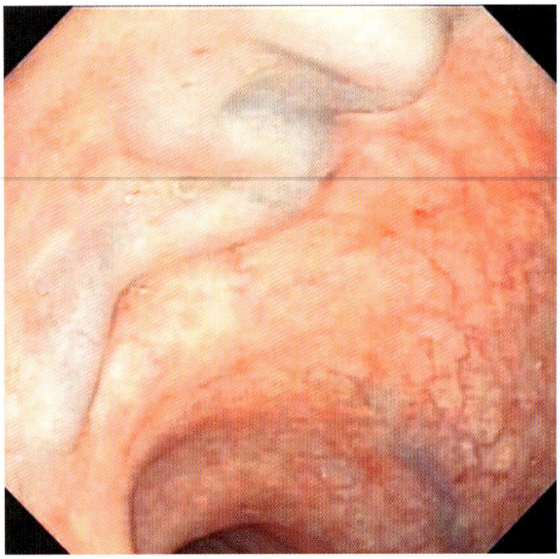

Fig. 12.30: Colonoscopy showing rectal varix in a patient with EHPVO and lower GI bleeding

**Table 12.22:** Evaluation for etiology of lower gastrointestinal tract bleeding

**Colitic presentation**
- Hemogram, ESR, CRP, albumin
- Stool examination for trophozoites, culture, *C. difficile* toxin
- Colonoscopy with biopsy for histology, culture, immunohistochemistry
- UGI endoscopy, enteroscopy (CT/MRI, capsule) for disease extent

**Noncolitic presentation**
- Hemogram, prothrombin time
- Colonoscopy and biopsy or polypectomy

*Based on presentation*
- Ultrasound abdomen (intussusception)
- $^{99m}$Tc pertechnate scan (Meckel's diverticulum, intestinal duplication)
- CT angiography (aneurysmal bleed)
- Capsule endoscopy, enteroscopy (small bowel source)

### Suggested Reading


1. AK, Fox VL. Gastrointestinal bleeding and management. Pediatr Clin North Am 2017; 64: 543–61.
2. Lal R, Yachha SK, Mandelia A, et al. Non-variceal gastrointestinal bleed in children: Surgical experience with emphasis on management challenges. Pediatr Surg Int 2019; 35: 1197–1210.
3. Nett A, Binmoeller KF. Endoscopic management of portal hypertension-related bleeding. Gastrointest Endoscopy Clin N Am. 2019; 29: 321–37.


*Competencies:* **PE26.5; PE26.8; PE26.9**

## DISORDERS OF THE HEPATOBILIARY SYSTEM

### Evaluation

The evaluation of disorders of hepatobiliary system begins with an accurate history and physical examination and involves a judicious selection of laboratory tests for a definitive diagnosis.

### Hepatomegaly

A palpable liver does not always indicate enlargement. It only reflects the relation of the liver to adjacent structures. In normal children, the liver is palpable one cm and in infants up to 2 cm below the costal margin. It is important to measure the liver span to determine the presence of hepatomegaly (Table 12.23). The liver span varies with age: Infants 5–6.5 cm; 1–5 years: 6–7 cm; 5–10 years: 7–9 cm; and 10–15 years: 8–10 cm. The liver is also examined for tenderness, consistency, surface characteristics, differential lobe enlargement and presence of bruit.

### Splenomegaly

Common causes of splenomegaly are listed in Table 12.24. The conditions in which the spleen is massively enlarged, >8 cm or crossing the umbilicus are underlined.

### Liver Function Tests

***Bilirubin:*** Total and fractionated (unconjugated and conjugated) bilirubin help to differentiate between elevation caused by hemolysis (leading to unconjugated

**Table 12.23:** Causes of hepatomegaly

| |
|---|
| *Infective:* Viral hepatitis, liver abscess (pyogenic or amebic), tuberculosis, salmonella, malaria, kala-azar, hydatid disease |
| *Chronic liver disease (cirrhosis or chronic hepatitis):* Wilson disease, chronic hepatitis B and C, autoimmune liver disease, Budd-Chiari syndrome, cryptogenic |
| *Metabolic or storage disorders:* Glycogen storage disease, Gaucher disease, Niemann-Pick disease, progressive familial intrahepatic cholestasis, nonalcoholic fatty liver disease |
| *Tumors:* Lymphoma, leukemia, histiocytosis, neuroblastoma, benign hemangioendothelioma, mesenchymal hamartoma, hepatoblastoma, hepatocellular carcinoma |
| *Biliary:* Caroli disease, choledochal cyst, congenital hepatic fibrosis, cystic disease of liver; extrahepatic biliary obstruction |
| *Miscellaneous:* Congestive heart failure, constrictive pericarditis, sarcoidosis |

| **Table 12.24:** Common causes of splenomegaly |
|---|
| *Portal hypertension:* Cirrhosis, **Extrahepatic Portal Venous Obstruction**; congenital hepatic fibrosis, **Noncirrhotic Portal Fibrosis**, Budd-Chiari syndrome |
| *Storage disorders:* Niemann-Pick disease, **Gaucher Disease**, mucopolysaccharidosis |
| *Hematological malignancies:* Acute leukemia, **Chronic Myeloid Leukemia**, **Myeloproliferative Disorders**, lymphoma, histiocytosis |
| *Increased splenic function:* Collagen vascular disorders, autoimmune hemolytic anemia, inherited hemolytic anemias (thalassemia major, hereditary spherocytosis) |
| *Infections:* **Malaria**, enteric fever, viral hepatitis, infectious mononucleosis, kala-azar, congenital infections |
| *Extramedullary hematopoiesis:* **Osteopetrosis** |

*Conditions that may cause massive splenomegaly are in bold

hyperbilirubinemia) versus hepatocellular or biliary diseases (causing conjugated hyperbilirubinemia). Deficiency of enzymes involved in bilirubin conjugation causes unconjugated bilirubinemia (Gilbert and Crigler-Najjar syndromes).

***Transaminases:*** Serum aspartate aminotransferase glutamate-oxaloacetate transferase (AST/SGOT) and alanine aminotransferase/serum glutamate pyruvate transferase (ALT/SGPT). ALT is present mainly in liver and in lower concentration in muscle while AST is derived from other sources as well (muscles, kidney, red blood cells). Disorders of muscle such as dystrophy and myositis can cause elevation of transaminases, and also elevation of creatinine phosphokinase (CPK). Raised ALT and AST indicate liver injury in the absence of an elevated CPK. Most marked increase in transaminases occurs with acute hepatocellular injury secondary to inflammation or ischemia, e.g acute viral hepatitis, drug- induced hepatitis, and shock. In chronic liver disease, transaminases are mildly or moderately elevated.

***Alkaline phosphatase (ALP) and gamma glutamyl transpeptidase (GGT):*** Normal ALP values are higher in growing children due to bone isoenzyme fraction. GGT is more specific for hepatobiliary disease. The values of GGT are higher in newborns and reach normal adult values by 6–9 months. Thus, elevation of ALP associated with increased GGT suggests a hepatic origin. Predominant elevation of ALP and GGT in comparison to the transaminases suggests a dominant biliary pathology, in contrast to hepatocellular disorders where transaminases are higher in comparison to ALP or GGT.

***Prothrombin time (PT) and international normalized ratio (INR):*** Deficiency of factor V and vitamin K dependent factors (II, VII, IX and X) occurs in liver disease. Thus, PT is a marker of synthetic function of liver. INR is a standardized way of reporting the prothrombin time. It is the ratio of a patient's prothrombin time to a normal sample, raised to the power of the international sensitivity index (ISI) value for the analytical system used. ISI ranges between 1.0 and 2.0 and shows how a batch of tissue factor compares to an internationally standardized sample.

$$\text{INR} = (\text{PT test}/\text{PT normal})^{\text{ISI}}$$

The reference range for prothrombin time is usually around 11–16 seconds; the normal range for INR is 0.8–1.2. A prolongation of PT by >3 seconds is abnormal.

***Serum proteins:*** The half-life of albumin is 20 days; albumin is a marker of liver synthetic function and is low in chronic liver disease. Gamma globulins are increased in autoimmune hepatitis; the ratio of albumin to globulin is reversed in cirrhosis. Low serum albumin and prolonged PT (unresponsive to vitamin K) indicates poor synthetic liver function.

***Serum ammonia:*** Levels are raised in significant liver dysfunction in acute liver failure or chronic liver disease. High levels are seen in hepatic encephalopathy even though the level may not necessarily correlate with the grade of encephalopathy. High ammonia levels are also seen in congenital portosystemic shunts that direct blood away from the liver.

### Liver Biopsy

Liver biopsy has been used to make a histological diagnosis, assessment of fibrosis, quantification of metal load such as copper in Wilson disease, immunohistochemical tests to diagnose infections and quantification of enzyme activity in metabolic disorders. Histological diagnosis plays a major role in the diagnosis of autoimmune liver disease and neonatal cholestasis. Genetic investigations have largely replaced liver biopsy in the diagnosis of some of the disorders causing neonatal cholestasis, such as Alagille syndrome and progressive familial intrahepatic cholestasis. Noninvasive measurement of fibrosis with transient elastography (TE) or acoustic radiation forced impulse (ARFI) have largely replaced the need for liver biopsy in assessing moderate to higher grades of fibrosis.

### Imaging Modalities

Ultrasound is the most common modality of imaging liver diseases. The information required in an individual case depends on the clinical context and may include liver size, echotexture, liver masses, nodularity, biliary dilatation, vascular structures and their patency, ascites, nodes and splenomegaly. Further delineation of the anatomy may be with MRI or CT scan. Ultrasound may also be used to guide liver biopsies.

*Nuclear scintigraphy* studies are used in the context of evaluating biliary drainage and connections.

## Liver Abscess

Pyogenic liver abscess is more common than amebic liver abscess in children. The infection reaches the liver by one of the following routes: (i) Portal vein, e.g. in intra-abdominal sepsis, umbilical infection in newborns; (ii) biliary tree obstruction and cholangitis, e.g. choledochal cyst; (iii) systemic sepsis, e.g. endocarditis, osteomyelitis; and (iv) direct inoculation, e.g. in trauma. In children on immunosuppressive medications or with defects of neutrophil function (e.g. chronic granulomatous disease), there is an increased risk of developing abscesses, especially due to *S. aureus*. In children with liver abscess without cholangitis or pyelophlebitis, gram-positive infections are the commonest. Invasive intestinal amebiasis can lead to amebic liver abscess although a history of amebic colitis in the preceding period is not common. Amebic abscess is usually solitary whereas pyogenic abscesses may be multiple (when secondary to portal pyemia or cholangitis) or single. The diagnosis of liver abscess in children should prompt a work-up for immunodeficiency disorders in the absence of an obvious predisposing pathology.

### Clinical Features

The child presents with fever and right upper quadrant abdominal pain. Jaundice is uncommon. Examination reveals tender hepatomegaly. Empyema, pneumonia, subphrenic abscess and cholecystitis can have a similar clinical presentation and should be differentiated.

Complications include spontaneous rupture into peritoneum, pericardium, pleura or bronchial tree and metastatic spread to lungs or brain.

### Diagnosis

Leukocytosis and elevated ESR are usually present. Transaminases and alkaline phosphatase are mildly elevated. X-ray abdomen may show an elevated right dome of diaphragm with or without pleural effusion. Diagnosis is confirmed by imaging; ultrasound provides good details about abscess size, number, rim and liquefaction. Contrast-enhanced CT scan may be required in patients with complications (Fig. 12.31). Amebic serology (indirect hemagglutination test) is positive in >95% children with amebic liver abscess, but does not help in differentiation from pyogenic abscess. In the developing world, amebic serology may be positive due to prior intestinal amebiasis, and thus a negative amebic serology helps exclude ALA.

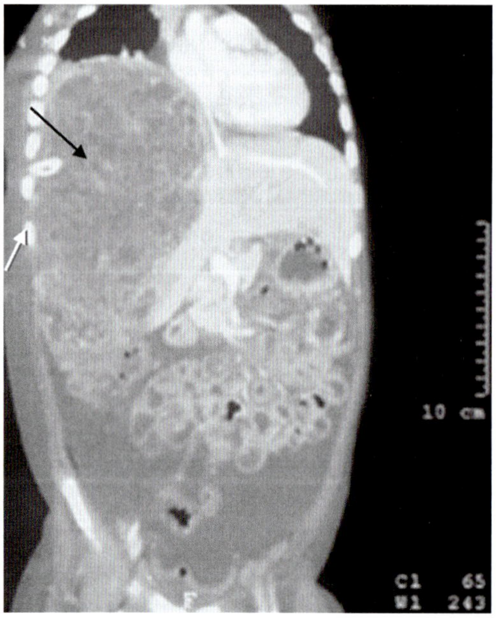


**Fig. 12.31:** Computed tomography scan shows a multi-loculated liver abscess in the right lobe (black arrow) with elevated right dome of diaphragm and ascites. Percutaneous drainage catheter is seen *in situ* (white arrow)

### Management

Patients with pyogenic abscess are treated with broad-spectrum antibiotics (against gram-positive, gram-negative aerobic and anerobic bacteria) for 4–6 weeks. Metronidazole is used for 10–14 days in patients with amebic liver abscess. Ultrasound-guided percutaneous needle aspiration and/or catheter drainage is required for abscesses that fail to clinically improve after 3–5 days of antibiotic therapy, large abscess in left lobe and those with impending rupture (narrow rim <1 cm). Surgery is required for abscesses complicated by frank intraperitoneal rupture or multiseptate abscesses not responding to percutaneous catheter drainage and antibiotics.

### Prognosis

The abscess cavity takes 3–6 months to resolve completely. Cure rate following management with antibiotics and percutaneous drainage is excellent.

## Liver Tumors

Liver tumors account for ~0.5–2% of all neoplasms in children. Hepatoblastoma, hemangioendothelioma and mesenchymal hamartoma are seen primarily in young children, whereas hepatocellular carcinoma, undifferentiated embryonal sarcoma and focal nodular hyperplasia present in the older child. The most common tumors are hepatoblastoma, hepatocellular carcinoma and infantile hemangioendothelioma.

Infantile hepatic hemangioendothelioma is a benign tumor and presents mostly in first 6 months of life with an abdominal mass. Jaundice, skin hemangiomas and congestive heart failure may be associated. The lesion may be single or multiple and is made of thin vascular channels. Observation is recommended for focal lesions. Treatment options for multifocal and diffuse lesions include propranolol, hepatic artery ligation, hepatic artery embolization, surgical resection or liver transplantation.

Hepatoblastoma is the most common malignant liver tumor in children. It may be epithelial (fetal or embryonal malignant cells) or mixed (epithelial and mesenchymal elements). It presents with an abdominal mass and anorexia. Weight loss and pain in abdomen usually appear late; metastasis occurs to lungs and lymph nodes and alpha-fetoprotein is raised in the majority of cases. Ultrasound helps to differentiate between malignant and vascular lesions. CT and MRI are used to define tumor extent and resectability (Fig. 12.32). The survival of patients with a hepatoblastoma has markedly improved in recent years by combining surgery with pre- and postoperative chemotherapeutic agents such as cisplatin and doxorubicin. Liver transplantation is an option for unresectable hepatoblastoma following chemotherapy in absence of visible extrahepatic disease.

Hepatocellular carcinoma is usually multicentric. The risk is increased in patients with chronic hepatitis B or C infection, tyrosinemia, glycogen storage disease or prior androgen therapy. The tumor presents as a liver mass with abdominal distension, anorexia and weight loss. Liver

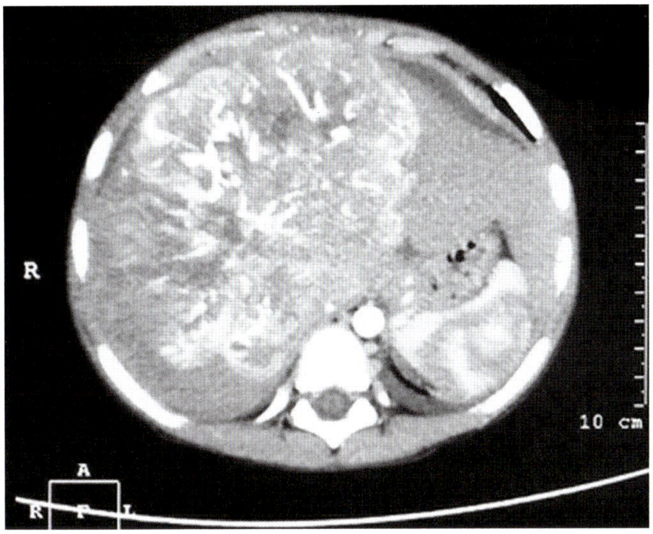


Fig. 12.32: CECT showing a large hepatoblastoma

functions are usually normal and anemia may be present; alpha-fetoprotein is raised. Imaging with CT/MRI helps in defining tumor extent, resectability and metastasis. Bone scan and CT chest should be done to screen for distant metastasis. Treatment options include surgical resection along with chemotherapy, chemoembolization and liver transplantation.

## Suggested Reading


1. Fuchs J, Warmann SW, Urla C, et al. Management of benign liver tumors. Semin Pediatr Surg 2020;29(4):150941.
2. Meyers R, Hiyama E, Czauderna P, Tiao GM. Liver tumors in pediatric patients. Surg Oncol Clin N Am 2021;30(2):253–74.
3. Srivastava A, Yachha SK, Arora V, et al. Identification of high-risk group and therapeutic options in children with liver abscess. Eur J Pediatr 2012; 171:33–41.


# JAUNDICE

The term jaundice means a yellow discoloration of skin, sclera and mucous membrane due to increase in the serum bilirubin levels. Nearly 250–300 mg of bilirubin is produced daily, approximately 70% from breakdown of old erythrocytes in reticuloendothelial system. Bilirubin is cleared by the liver in three steps. It is first transported into hepatocytes by specific carriers. Then it is conjugated to 1–2 molecules of glucoronide. Thereafter, the conjugated bilirubin moves to the canalicular membrane where it is excreted into the bile canaliculi by other carrier proteins. Most of the conjugated bilirubin is excreted in the stool and small amount is reabsorbed after deconjugation by colonic bacteria. Colonic bacteria also reduce bilirubin to urobilinogen, which is reabsorbed and excreted in urine.

Serum bilirubin should be >2.5–5 mg/dL for jaundice to be visible. Hyperbilirubinemia is classified as unconjugated (conjugated bilirubin fraction <15% of total bilirubin and normal colored urine) and conjugated hyperbilirubinemia (conjugated bilirubin fraction >20% with high colored urine). Any abnormality of the above steps can cause jaundice (Table 12.25).

Table 12.25: Causes of jaundice in children

**Unconjugated hyperbilirubinemia**
- *Hemolysis:* Blood group incompatibility (Rh, ABO), drugs, infection related, glucose-6-phosphate dehydrogenase deficiency, autoimmune hemolysis
- *Bilirubin overproduction:* Ineffective erythropoiesis, large hematoma
- *Specific conditions in neonates:* Physiologic jaundice, breast milk jaundice
- *Enzyme defects:* Gilbert syndrome, Crigler-Najjar syndrome
- *Miscellaneous:* Hypothyroidism, fasting

**Conjugated hyperbilirubinemia**
- Neonatal cholestasis
- *Infections:* Sepsis, acute viral hepatitis, enteric fever, malaria, leptospirosis
- Chronic liver disease
- *Liver tumor:* Primary, secondaries
- *Infiltration:* Histiocytosis, leukemia
- *Enzyme defects:* Dubin-Johnson syndrome, Rotor syndrome
- *Biliary:* Choledochal cyst, choledocholithiasis, ascariasis, sclerosing cholangitis
- *Miscellaneous:* Drug toxicity (hepatocellular, cholestatic), total parenteral nutrition, veno-occlusive disease

## Congenital Enzyme Deficiencies

Gilbert syndrome is the most common cause of unconjugated hyperbilirubinemia and affects 3–8% of the population. The condition may have an autosomal recessive as well as autosomal dominant transmission with variations in *UGT1A1* gene. It results from a partial deficiency of the enzyme uridine diphosphate glucuronyltransferase (UDP-GT) and thus, impaired conjugation. Most patients are asymptomatic and exhibit chronic or recurrent jaundice (up to 6 mg/dL) precipitated by intercurrent illness, fasting or stress. Mild fatigue, nausea, anorexia or abdominal pain may be present in some patients. Other liver functions remain normal. No specific treatment is necessary for this disorder.

*Crigler-Najjar syndrome (CN) type I:* It is an autosomal recessive disorder characterized by significant variations in *UGT1A1* and absence of UDP-GT activity. Patients develop severe unconjugated hyperbilirubinemia and die by 18–24 months of age, if untreated. Phototherapy, plasmapheresis and exchange transfusion are required for managing these cases in initial phases. Serum bilirubin levels should be kept below 20 mg/dL during first several months of life to prevent brain damage. Definitive treatment is possible by liver transplantation, preferably auxiliary, if available.

*Crigler-Najjar syndrome type II:* There is marked reduction of UDP-GT. In comparison to type I, jaundice is less severe and does not result in kernicterus. The condition responds to drugs, like phenobarbitone, that stimulate hyperplasia of the endoplasmic reticulum. The bilirubin level significantly decreases in type II CN following administration of phenobarbitone, while no change is seen in type I patients.

*Dubin-Johnson syndrome:* It is an autosomal recessive disorder resulting from impaired hepatic excretion of bilirubin from hepatocytes into bile canaliculi. Children present with conjugated hyperbilirubinemia (2–6 mg/dL). The transaminases and synthetic liver functions are normal. Most patients are asymptomatic apart from jaundice. Pregnancy and oral contraceptives may worsen jaundice. This disorder is diagnosed by genetic testing showing variation in *ABCC2*, which encodes the multidrug-resistance-associated protein 2 (MRP2). Liver biopsy, if done, shows brown-black pigmentation.

***Rotor syndrome:*** It is a rare, autosomal recessive disorder manifesting as mild conjugated hyperbilirubinemia. The primary defect appears to be a deficiency in the intracellular storage capacity of the liver for binding anions. The liver histology is normal.



Competency: **PE26.1**

## Acute Viral Hepatitis

Viruses can affect the liver, either primarily, e.g. hepatitis A, B, C, E or as part of a systemic involvement, e.g. cytomegalovirus (CMV), Epstein-Barr virus (EBV), herpes simplex virus (HSV). In Indian children, hepatitis A is the commonest cause (40–60%) of acute viral hepatitis, followed by hepatitis E (10–20%) and hepatitis B (7–17%). Nearly 8–20% patients have coinfection with more than one virus, HAV and HEV being most common. Hepatitis A and E are transmitted by feco-oral route whereas HBV and HCV are transmitted by parenteral or vertical (mother to baby) route **(Table 12.26)** (*see* also Chapter 11).



### Clinical Features

Following exposure, patients show a prodrome characterized by low grade fever, malaise, anorexia and vomiting, followed by appearance of jaundice. Examination shows icterus, hepatomegaly and splenomegaly (small, soft in 15–20%). Mild ascites may be present in 10–15% cases, which resolves completely on follow-up. Over the next few weeks, the appetite improves, jaundice resolves and the child gets better. In young children, asymptomatic and anicteric presentation of hepatitis A infection can occur.

### Differential Diagnosis

The conditions, which mimic the clinical features of viral hepatitis include enteric fever, falciparum malaria, leptospirosis and viral hemorrhagic fever. Unlike some of these disorders, the children usually become afebrile after appearance of jaundice in viral hepatitis. Other conditions that need to be differentiated include drug-induced hepatitis, acute presentation of autoimmune liver disease, or Wilson disease.

### Investigations

Liver function tests show a direct hyperbilirubinemia with markedly elevated ALT/AST, and normal albumin and prothrombin time. Mild leukopenia with relative lymphocytosis is seen. Ultrasound shows mildly enlarged liver with increased echogenicity and edema of gallbladder wall. Viral serologies help determine the etiology of acute viral hepatitis **(Table 12.26)**.

### Complications

- *Acute liver failure:* The appearance of irritability, altered sleep pattern, persistent anorexia and uncorrectable coagulopathy (despite administration of vitamin K) suggests the development of acute liver failure.
- *Aplastic anemia*
- *Pancreatitis*
- *Serum sickness*, vasculitis-like reaction may be seen in hepatitis B infection
- *Hemolysis* (cola-colored urine) with renal failure in subjects with glucose-6-phosphate dehydrogenase deficiency
- *Chronic liver disease:* In patients with acute viral hepatitis due to HBV, repeat testing for hepatitis B surface antigen should be done after 6 months to document clearance or persistence of infection. A majority (95%) clear hepatitis B infection after acute icteric infection.

### Management

Maintaining adequate oral intake is essential and intravenous fluids are given, if persistent vomiting and dehydration are present. There is no advantage of enforced bed rest, but vigorous activity may be avoided. No specific dietary modification is recommended. The child should be monitored for appearance of complications like encephalopathy.

**Table 12.26:** Epidemiological profile of different hepatitis viruses

| *Virus* | *A* | *B* | *C* | *E* |
|---|---|---|---|---|
| Type of virus | RNA | DNA | RNA | RNA |
| Incubation period, days | 15–40 | 50–150 | 30–150 | 15–45 |
| *Route of infection* | | | | |
| • Feco-oral | + | – | – | + |
| • Parenteral | Rare | Yes | Yes | – |
| • Others | | Perinatal by sexual contact | Perinatal sexual contact | – |
| Chronic liver disease | – | + | + | – |
| Vaccine | Available | Available | No | No (being developed) |
| Diagnostic test | IgM; anti-HAV | HBsAg; IgM anti-HBc | Anti-HCV antibody; HCV RNA | IgM anti-HEV |

### Prevention

Public health measures like sanitation, safe drinking water supply, handwashing and food hygiene are of utmost importance, especially in epidemics of hepatitis A or E. Effective vaccination is available for hepatitis A. Screening of blood and blood products and safe injection practices are essential. Universal immunization for hepatitis B is the most effective way of preventing hepatitis B related disease.

### Suggested Reading


1. Abutaleb A, Kottilil S. Hepatitis A: Epidemiology, natural history, unusual clinical manifestations, and prevention. Gastroenterol Clin North Am 2020;49:191–99.
2. Memon N, Weinberger BI, Hegyi T, Aleksunes LM. Inherited disorders of bilirubin clearance. Pediatr Res 2016;79:378–86.
3. Singh SK, Borkar V, Srivastava A, et al. Need for recognizing atypical manifestations of childhood sporadic acute viral hepatitis warranting differences in management. Eur J Pediatr 2019;178:61–67.


*Competency:* **PE26.2**

## LIVER FAILURE

Liver failure refers to a clinical state resulting from hepatocyte dysfunction or necrosis and not a specific disease etiology. It may be a result of chronic liver disease (CLD) or it may occur in normal children without any evidence of pre-existing liver disease where it is known as acute liver failure (ALF).

### Acute Liver Failure

An international normalized ratio (INR) of 1.5 with hepatic encephalopathy or INR of 2 with or without encephalopathy, along with biochemical evidence of liver injury in the absence of underlying chronic liver disease (CLD) is considered as ALF. The presence of encephalopathy is not essential for diagnosis of ALF in children unlike in adults. All INR values refer to that measured after 8-hr of parenteral vitamin K administration. This definition has evolved with the understanding that detection of mild grades of hepatic encephlopathy in small children is difficult, and any behavioral change or irritability in this age group may not be necessarily due to encephalopathy.

Patients with CLD may manifest with features of hepatocellular failure due to progressive worsening of liver function as part of the natural course of the disease or as a sudden dysfunction due to a superimposed hepatic insult resulting in acute on chronic liver failure. Superimposed insult can be due to hepatotropic virus (hepatitis A, E, B) infection, hepatotoxic drug intake or sepsis.

ALF is associated with high mortality and the etiology varies among different age groups (Table 12.27). Autoimmune liver disease and Wilson disease are two important causes of CLD in children which may have an acute presentation mimicking ALF. Drugs, especially antitubercular agents (isoniazid, rifampicin, pyrazinamide) and anticonvulsants are a major cause of ALF. In the West, paracetamol poisoning is a common cause of ALF. Herbal medicines and mushroom poisoning are also known to cause ALF. In the neonatal period, liver failure may be a result of metabolic conditions (neonatal hemochromatosis, galactosemia, hereditary fructose intolerance, tyrosinemia type 1, Niemann-Pick disease), infections and hematological conditions like hemophagocytic lymphohistiocytosis. A careful history and rapid investigations are necessary to identify the etiology, which has prognostic and therapeutic implications (Table 12.28). However, 30–40% cases are idiopathic.

**Table 12.27:** Causes of acute liver failure in children

| | |
|---|---|
| Infections | Common: Viral hepatitis (A, B, E)<br>Uncommon: Adenovirus, Epstein-Barr, parvovirus, cytomegalovirus, echovirus, varicella, dengue, herpes simplex virus I and II* |
| Others | Septicemia*, malaria, leptospirosis |
| Drugs | Isoniazid with rifampicin, pyrazinamide, acetaminophen, sodium valproate, carbamazepine, ketoconazole |
| Toxins | Herbal medicines, *Amanita phalloides* poisoning, carbon tetrachloride |
| Metabolic | Wilson disease, galactosemia*, tyrosinemia*, hereditary fructose intolerance*, hemochromatosis*, Niemann-Pick disease type C*, mitochondrial cytopathies*, congenital disorder of glycosylation |
| Autoimmune | Autoimmune liver disease |
| Vascular | Acute Budd-Chiari syndrome, acute circulatory failure |
| Infiltrative | Leukemia, lymphoma, histiocytosis* |
| Idiopathic | |

*More common in neonates and infants

### Clinical Features

The early clinical manifestations of ALF are nonspecific and characterized by lethargy, anorexia, malaise, nausea and vomiting. Central nervous system manifestations include encephalopathy and cerebral edema with raised intracranial tension. Hepatic encephalopathy is classified into four stages (Table 12.29). Its identification can be challenging as in the early stages they present with non-specific findings such as excessive somnolence, reversal of sleep-wake cycle or behavioral and personality changes. Coagulopathy due to impaired production of coagulation factors results in bleeding. Platelet counts are affected in the setting of infection. The patient may manifest with hypoglycemia, electrolyte imbalance and metabolic acidosis. Infections are common in ALF as the immune system is dysfunctional and invasive procedures are performed commonly. This results in gram-positive, gram-negative and fungal infections, which manifest as hypotension, disseminated intravascular coagulation, worsening metabolic acidosis, worsening encephalopathy, oliguria and azotemia.

Investigation for the causes is important as specific treatment is needed in some instances (Table 12.28).

### Management

The management of liver failure in children is based on: (i) Diagnosis of etiology as it influences the prognosis

**Table 12.28:** Disorders causing ALF that have etiology-specific treatment options

| *Etiology* | *Treatment* |
|---|---|
| Tyrosinemia type 1 | Nitisinone; dietary restriction of phenylalanine and tyrosine |
| Paracetamol toxicity | N-acetylcysteine |
| Hemophagocytic lymphohistiocytosis | Immunosuppression protocols |
| HSV infection | Acyclovir |
| Drug induced liver injury | Withdrawal of offending drug |
| Galactosemia | Galactose free formula |
| Fatty acid oxidation disorders | Dextrose infusion |
| *NBAS* mutations | Dextrose/lipid infusion |
| Gestational alloimmune liver disease | Double volume exchange transfusion and intravenous immunoglobulin administration |
| Acute HBV infection | Anti-HBV antivirals |
| Acute Budd-Chiari syndrome | Hepatic venoplasty and stenting |



**Table 12.29:** Stages of hepatic encephalopathy in children

| *Stage* | *Features* | *Reflexes* |
|---|---|---|
| I | Inconsolable crying, inattention to task, not acting like self, disturbed sleep-wake cycle | Normal or hyper-reflexic; asterixis absent |
| II | Same as in stage I | Normal or hyper-reflexic; asterixis easily elicited |
| III | Somnolence, stupor, combative | Hyper-reflexic; asterixis present |
| IV | Comatose, responsive to pain (IVA) or non-responsive to pain (IVB) | Decerebrate or decorticate; asterixis absent |

and management; (ii) assessment of severity of liver failure and timely liver transplantation, if indicated; and (iii) anticipation, prevention and treatment of complications. Patients should be treated and monitored closely in an intensive care unit (Table 12.30).

In spite of adequate supportive care, the mortality in ALF is as high as 60–70% without liver transplantation. Early identification of children who would benefit only from liver transplantation is essential. The King's College criteria are one of the commonly used criteria to identify patients requiring liver transplantation.

### Suggested Reading

1. Bhatia V, Bavdekar A, Yachha SK, et al. Management of acute liver failure in infants and children: Consensus statement of the Pediatric Gastroenterology chapter, Indian Academy of Pediatrics. Indian Pediatr 2013; 50:477–82.
2. Jagadisan B, Dhawan A. Emergencies in pediatric hepatology. J Hepatol 2022 Jan 3:S0168-8278(21)02304-7.
3. Lutfi R, Abulebda K, Nitu ME, et al. Intensive care management of pediatric acute liver failure. J Pediatr Gastroenterol Nutr. 2017;64:660–70.
4. Taylor SA, Whitington PF. Neonatal acute liver failure. Liver Transpl 2016;22:677–85.

*Competencies:* **PE26.3; PE26.4**

## CHRONIC LIVER DISEASE

Chronic liver disease (CLD) refers to a spectrum of disorders characterized by ongoing chronic liver damage and a potential to progress to cirrhosis or end stage liver disease. Although a 6-month duration cut off is used for defining chronicity related to hepatitis B and C, it does not apply to the other causes as irreversible chronic liver damage may have already taken place even before symptoms of liver disease are recognized.

Cirrhosis is a histopathological diagnosis. It is a diffuse liver process characterized by fibrosis in response to inflammation/injury and nodular regeneration. CLD with cirrhosis presenting with normal synthetic function without ascites or encephalopathy is termed as compensated cirrhosis. When the patient develops coagulopathy, jaundice, ascites and/or hepatic encephalopathy, it is known as decompensated cirrhosis.

### Etiology

The main causes of CLD in children are listed in Table 12.31. When there is no known etiology, it may be labeled cryptogenic.

### Clinical Features

The presentation depends on the etiology and pace of disease progression. Patients may present with insidious onset disease with failure to thrive, anorexia, muscle weakness and/or jaundice or abruptly with massive gastrointestinal bleed, acute onset jaundice, along with altered sensorium and ascites. Sometimes the patient may be asymptomatic and found to have hepatosplenomegaly or elevated transaminases on investigation for some unrelated illness. Clinical features that suggest presence of CLD are:

- *Characteristics of liver:* The liver is firm to hard, nodular or have irregular margins in cirrhosis. Differential left lobe enlargement is a feature of CLD. A small, non-palpable shrunken liver is a feature of post-necrotic cirrhosis.

**Table 12.30:** Management of a child with acute liver failure

| *Systems* | *Evaluation* | *Intervention, remarks* |
|---|---|---|
| Airway and respiratory support | • $SpO_2$, $pO_2$, $pCO_2$ and pH<br>• Pulse oximetry, pH, oxygen saturation | • Assisted ventilation in grade III/IV encephalopathy or agitation with lower encephalopathy grades<br>• Atracurium not dependent on hepatic elimination; useful when needing paralysis |
| Fluid, electrolyte and metabolic management | • Blood sodium, potassium, phosphate, urea creatinine; glucose, calcium, magnesium, lactate, pH<br>• Central venous pressure<br>• Urine ouput | • Start with 80% dextrose-based maintenance fluid for age and weight<br>• Target euvolemia to ensure cerebral perfusion<br>• Rapid fluid boluses can worsen cerebral edema<br>• No evidence to support use of lactulose, L-ornithine, L-asparate and rifaximin<br>• Consider kidney replacement therapy, if fluid overload, metabolic derangement |
| Cardiovascular support | • Heart rate, blood pressure, invasive arterial pressure, capillary refill time<br>• Mixed venous oxygen saturation in patients on inotropes, trend in CVP, stroke volume variations, pulse pressure variations and response to fluid administration in hypotension | • Noradrenaline is the inotrope of choice to treat hypotension<br>• Corticosteroids may alleviate adrenal insufficiency and treat refractory hypotension<br>• Plasmapheresis, if high inotrope requirement<br>• Consider emergency liver transplantation |
| Neurological monitoring and support | • Stage hepatic encephalopathy (Table 12.29)<br>• Glasgow coma/AVPU score<br>• Monitor for raised intracranial pressure, hypoglycemia, worsening of neurological signs, intracranial bleed | • Prevent raised intracranial pressure (ICP)/ neurological injury: Fever control, head end elevation to 30°, avoid fluid overload<br>• Maintain serum sodium between 145 and 150 mEq/L. Nurse with minimal stimulation in a quiet environment<br>• 3% saline, 20% mannitol (contraindicated in AKI) and transient hyperventilation may be used for increased ICP<br>• Sedate, agitated or ventilated patient; avoid benzodiazepines. Morphine/fentanyl preferred<br>• Early CRRT with renal impairment, HE grade III-IV with ammonia >150 µmol/L, or absolute ammonia >200 µmol/L<br>• Hepatectomy, if necrotic liver is believed to be causing raised intracranial hypertension, while awaiting emergency liver transplantation |
| Coagulation and hematological support | • Bleeding manifestations<br>• Prothrombin time (INR), fibrinogen level, platelet count<br>• INR does not predict bleeding risk | • Correction of INR by fresh frozen plasma, if bleeding manifestations and invasive procedures<br>• Platelet count >50,000/mm$^3$ reduces risk of bleeding<br>• Consider plasma exchange for life-threatening bleeds or increased requirement for coagulation factor support (>30 mL/kg FFP in 24 hr)<br>• Stress ulcer prevention using proton pump inhibitor |
| Secondary Infection | • Features of systemic inflammatory response syndrome are non-specific, and could be result of liver failure/necrosis<br>• Daily surveillance cultures<br>• Suspect infection, if sudden worsening/ hypotension/ unexplained AKI/encephalopathy/ SIRS | • Prophylactic broad-spectrum antibiotics and antifungals decrease frequency of infections.<br>• Selective gut decontamination not recommended<br>• CRP unreliable as a marker of sepsis |
| Nutrition | | Enteral feed when possible; ensure 1 g/kg/day of protein |
| Non-specific supportive medications | | • Role of N-acetylcysteine infusion in non-paracetamol-associated ALF is controversial |

AVPU alert, verbal, pain, unresponsive; INR International normalised ratio, CRRT continuous renal replacement therapy

- *Stigmata of CLD:* These include spider angiomata, palmar erythema, clubbing, leukonychia, muscle wasting, delayed puberty and gynecomastia. Testicular atrophy and parotid enlargement are present in adults with alcoholic liver disease, but not in children.
- *Portal hypertension:* Splenomegaly, ascites, tortuous veins over abdominal wall with flow away from umbilicus, i.e. caput medusae; esophageal or gastric varices.
- *Hepatic encephalopathy:* Asterixis, constructional apraxia or altered sensorium (Table 12.29) may be seen.

**Table 12.31**: Causes of chronic liver disease

| | |
|---|---|
| Viral hepatitis | Hepatitis B (common), hepatitis C (uncommon) |
| Autoimmune liver disease | Autoimmune hepatitis (common), autoimmune sclerosing cholangitis |
| Metabolic | Wilson disease, glycogen storage disease (IV)*, progressive familial intrahepatic cholestasis*, galactosemia*, NASH related, tyrosinemia*, Indian childhood cirrhosis*, cystic fibrosis, hereditary fructose intolerance*, alpha-1-antitrypsin deficiency, bile acid synthetic defects |
| Venous obstruction | Budd-Chiari syndrome, veno-occlusive disease, constrictive pericarditis, congestive heart failure |
| Biliary | Biliary atresia*, choledochal cyst*, primary sclerosing cholangitis, Caroli disease, Alagille syndrome |
| Rare causes | Niemann-Pick disease, Gaucher disease; drug induced (valproate, carbamazepine) |

NASH nonalcoholic steatohepatitis
*Causes in infants and young children >5 yr of age

## Evaluation

Evaluation of patients with suspected CLD is two-pronged: (i) Determine etiology of CLD, and (ii) assess degree of liver dysfunction and presence of complications. Based on clinical and laboratory features, liver damage is graded using scores like the CHILD Score and Pediatric End-Stage Liver Disease (PELD) Score.

Complications of CLD include: (i) Hepatic encephalopathy; (ii) portal hypertension with variceal bleeding, portopulmonary hypertension and hepatopulmonary syndrome; (iii) ascites and spontaneous bacterial peritonitis; (iv) hepatorenal syndrome; (v) coagulopathy; (vi) nutrition failure; (vii) increased risk of infections; and (viii) hepatocellular carcinoma.

### *Hepatic Encephalopathy*

Hepatic encephalopathy refers to neuropsychiatric abnormalities that result from liver dysfunction. It is a principal manifestations of both chronic and acute liver failure, and graded at least in older children (Table 12.29). Various factors like gastrointestinal bleed, infection, use of sedatives, dehydration due to aggressive diuresis, constipation and electrolyte imbalance can precipitate encephalopathy. Identification and reversal of the precipitating event is of importance. As ammonia is an important putative metabolite, efforts are targeted towards reducing its production and absorption and facilitating its excretion. Oral antibiotics and synthetic disaccharides have been shown to be effective in minimizing ammonia production in these patients. Neomycin was used in the past but it has serious side effects of deafness and renal toxicity. Rifaximin is a new drug with a better safety profile. Nonabsorbable disaccharides like lactulose and lactitol reach the colon intact and then are metabolized by bacteria into variety of small molecular weight organic acids, that act by acidifying fecal contents and trapping the diffusible ammonia as ammonium ion in the fecal stream along with alteration in colonic flora (loss of ammonia producing bacteria). In infants and children, protein intake should not be restricted to the point of causing growth failure or compromising overall nutritional status and a target range of 1–2 g/kg/day is recommended. Vegetable proteins, which are rich in branched chain amino acids, are preferred over animal proteins.

### *Nutrition Failure*

Children with end-stage liver disease are at risk for developing nutritional compromise, which increases the disease-related morbidity. Nutritional failure in the end-stage liver disease is multifactorial, due to a combination of decreased caloric intake, increased energy expenditure, malabsorption of macro- and micronutrients and altered physiologic anabolic signals. Children with CLD also have reduced levels of liver-derived insulin-like growth factor 1, and thus a growth hormone-resistant state.

Clinical recognition of malnutrition in infants and children with end-stage liver disease relies on monitoring for clinical features like growth failure, loss of muscle mass, delayed motor development or signs of fat-soluble vitamin or essential fatty acid deficiencies (skin rash, peripheral neuropathy, rickets/fractures or bruising). The presence of ascites, edema and organomegaly makes weight an unreliable indicator of nutrition. Therefore, height monitoring, along with other anthropometric markers of body fat and muscle mass (triceps skin fold, mid-arm circumference) should be used.

All patients need increased caloric intake ~120–150% of their estimated daily requirements. Formulae containing medium-chain triglycerides are used to maximize fat absorption in the setting of severe cholestasis. Daily supplements of vitamins and other nutrients like calcium and iron need to be given. For patients who cannot meet the needs by oral feeding, nasogastric tube feedings should be started. Patients with CLD are especially vulnerable to viral and bacterial infections. All infants and children with CLD should receive the recommended childhood vaccinations.

### *Hepatorenal Syndrome*

Hepatorenal syndrome is a functional renal impairment as changes are reversible after liver transplant. It is defined as severe acute kidney injury in absence of other known causes (prerenal, nephrotoxic drugs) in patients with severe liver disease. Acute management might requisre the use of renal replacement therapy. Terlipressin is effective in a few patients.

*Competencies:* **PE26.5; PE26.6**

## ASCITES

Ascites is the pathologic accumulation of fluid within the peritoneal cavity and it can occur at any age and also *in utero*. The main causes of ascites are given in Table 12.32. Sometimes a large intra-abdominal cyst, i.e. cystic lymphangioma, omental or ovarian cyst can masquerade as ascites and hence referred to as pseudoascites.

**Table 12.32:** Causes of ascites

| |
|---|
| **Common** |
| • Cirrhosis and portal hypertension |
| • Budd-Chiari syndrome |
| • Nephrotic syndrome |
| • Protein losing enteropathy |
| • Tubercular ascites |
| • Constrictive pericarditis |
| • Cardiac failure |
| • *Chylous:* Lymphatic obstruction, thoracic duct injury, intestinal lymphangiectasia |
| **Uncommon** |
| • *Pancreatic:* Pancreatitis, pancreatic duct injury |
| • *Urinary:* Obstructive uropathy, bladder rupture |
| • *Hepatobiliary:* Bile duct perforation, veno-occlusive disease |
| • *Serositis:* SLE, eosinophilic enteropathy |
| • *Infections:* Parvovirus, syphilis, cytomegalovirus |
| • *Others:* Intestinal perforation, peritoneal dialysis, ventriculo-peritoneal shunt, epidemic dropsy |

## Evaluation

A careful history, physical examination, imaging studies and paracentesis are required for ascertaining the etiology. Physical examination reveals abdominal distension, bulging flanks, shifting dullness, fluid thrill or puddle sign depending on the volume of ascites. The liver and spleen may be difficult to palpate in patients with tense ascites. Dilated abdominal collaterals and caput medusae may be seen in ascites due to liver disease, while collaterals in flanks and on the back suggest inferior vena cava block. Markedly elevated jugular venous pressure suggests a cardiac origin, e.g. constrictive pericarditis.

Ultrasound is a sensitive imaging technique for the detection of ascites. Abdominal paracentesis is a simple test for determining the etiology. Diagnostic paracentesis should be done when ascites is first detected, at the time of hospitalization, or when there is clinical deterioration with unexplained fever, abdominal pain or diarrhea. Ultrasound-guided tap is warranted in children with loculated ascites.

## Investigations

Ascitic fluid should be evaluated for total and differential cell count, SAAG (serum ascites albumin gradient, i.e. difference in concentration of albumin in serum and ascitic fluid) and culture.

High gradient ascites (SAAG 1.1 g/dL) suggests portal hypertension and is seen in cirrhosis, fulminant hepatic failure, Budd-Chiari syndrome and portal vein thrombosis.

Low gradient ascites (SAAG <1.1 g/dL) occurs in absence of portal hypertension in conditions such as peritoneal carcinomatosis, tuberculous peritonitis, pancreatic ascites, biliary leak ascites, nephrotic syndrome and serositis.

Elevated ascitic fluid level of amylase indicates pancreatitis or intestinal perforation. Polymicrobial infection is consistent with intestinal perforation, whereas monomicrobial infection suggests spontaneous bacterial peritonitis. Uroascites is present when the concentration of urea and creatinine are higher in the ascitic fluid than in serum. In biliary ascites, the ascitic fluid bilirubin is >6 mg/dL and in chylous ascites the ascitic fluid is milky in appearance and has a triglyceride concentration of >200 mg/dL.

## Treatment

Small amounts of ascitic fluid that do not produce symptoms require no treatment. Tense ascites causing respiratory compromise, severe pain, or other major clinical problems should be treated promptly. Treatment largely depends upon the cause, e.g. antitubercular therapy for tubercular ascites, diuretics for CLD and surgery for bile duct or bowel perforation.

### *Management*

For patients with ascites related to liver disease, mobilization of ascitic fluid is accomplished by creating a negative sodium balance until ascites has diminished or resolved; then the sodium balance is maintained so that ascites does not recur. Oral diuretic therapy consists of single morning dose of spironolactone (2–5 mg/kg/day) along with furosemide (0.5–2 mg/kg/day), that facilitates maintenance of normokalemia. If weight loss and decrease in abdominal girth are inadequate, the doses of both spironolactone and furosemide should be increased simultaneously.

Along with diuretic therapy, patients should be on a sodium restricted diet. One gram of table salt contains 17 mEq of sodium and one gram of sodium approximates 44 mEq of sodium. Restriction of sodium in diet is limited to 1–2 mEq/kg/day for infants and children and 1 to 2 g/day (44 to 88 mEq of sodium/day) in adolescents. Escalation of therapy involves albumin infusion along with intravenous furosemide. Rationalization of diuretic dosage may be necessary in those with electrolyte imbalances. Fluid restriction is recommended only in those with hyponatremia. Excessive fluid restriction may impair nutrition of the child.

If the ascites is massive or the patient is having respiratory discomfort, large volume paracentesis is done preferably under cover of albumin infusion. Patients resistant to the above therapy can be treated with transjugular intrahepatic portosystemic shunting (TIPS) as a temporary measure till orthotopic liver transplantation is done, of course with the risk of hepatic encephalopathy.

## Spontaneous Bacterial Peritonitis

This refers to bacterial peritonitis not associated with gut perforation or any other secondary cause. Presence of 250 polymorphonuclear cells/mm$^3$ with a positive culture of ascitic fluid is diagnostic. The other variants of ascitic fluid infection in patients with liver disease are culture negative neutracytic ascites (≥250 polymorphonuclear cells/mm$^3$ with negative culture), and monomicrobial non-neutracytic ascites (<250 polymorphonuclear cells/mm$^3$ with positive culture). Patients present with rapid onset abdominal distension, fever, malaise and abdominal pain with tenderness on abdominal examination. However, symptoms may be absent in 30–40% cases with SBP. Therefore, patients with new onset ascites and those with unexplained clinical deterioration should undergo diagnostic paracentesis to look for abnormalities. Third generation cephalosporins or piperacillin-tazobactum, for a total of 5 to 7 days, are recommended for treatment. Long-term administration of oral norfloxacin 5–7.5 mg/kg once a day in patients with cirrhosis and ascitic protein content of <1 g/dL, or prior episode of spontaneous bacterial peritonitis is recommended. Despite advances in supportive care, bacterial peritonitis is an indicator of poor prognosis.

### Suggested Reading


1. Biggins SW, Angeli P, Garcia-Tsao G, et al. Diagnosis, Evaluation, and management of ascites, spontaneous bacterial peritonitis and hepatorenal syndrome: 2021 Practice Guidance by the American Association for the Study of Liver Diseases Hepatology. 2021 Aug;74(2):1014–48.
2. Hadjihambi A, Arias N, Sheikh M, Jalan R. Hepatic encephalopathy: A critical current review. Hepatol Int 2018 Feb; 12(Suppl 1):135–47.
3. Mouzaki M, Bronsky J, Gupte G, et al. Nutrition Support of children with chronic liver diseases: A joint position paper of the North American Society and the European Society for pediatric gastroenterology, hepatology, and nutrition. J Pediatr Gastroenterol Nutr 2019 Oct;69(4):498–511.




## PORTAL HYPERTENSION

The portal vein is formed by the splenic and the superior mesenteric veins. Normal portal pressure is between 5 and 10 mm Hg and portal hypertension is an increase in portal pressure of >12 mm Hg. It occurs due to increased portal resistance. The causes of portal hypertension may be either intrahepatic or extrahepatic (prehepatic and posthepatic) (Table 12.33).

**Table 12.33:** Causes of portal hypertension

| | |
|---|---|
| Prehepatic | Portal venous thrombosis, extrahepatic portal venous obstruction (cavernous transformation of portal vein), isolated splenic vein thrombosis |
| Intrahepatic | Liver cirrhosis (common), congenital hepatic fibrosis, veno-occlusive disease, noncirrhotic portal fibrosis, schistosomiasis, nodular regenerative hyperplasia |
| Posthepatic | Budd-Chiari syndrome (hepatic vein or inferior vena cava obstruction), constrictive pericarditis |

The spectrum of portal hypertension in children from developed vs. developing world is different. Unlike in the West where cirrhosis is the commonest cause, in India, extrahepatic portal venous obstruction (EHPVO) is the commonest cause (50–75%) followed by cirrhosis (25–35%); uncommon causes are congenital hepatic fibrosis, non-cirrhotic portal fibrosis and Budd-Chiari syndrome. Portal hypertension results in development of portosystemic venous channels at different sites giving rise to esophageal, gastric or colonic varices. The main pointers which help in differentiating portal hypertension due to cirrhosis from that due to non-cirrhotic causes are shown in Table 12.34.

### Clinical Features

The age of presentation is dependent on the etiology and varies from infancy to teenage. A majority of patients with EHPVO present with upper gastrointestinal bleeding and splenomegaly. Hematemesis and melena occur due to esophageal or gastric variceal bleeding. The bleed may be recurrent and is well tolerated in EHPVO without development of post-bleed hepatic encephalopathy. Splenomegaly alone is the presentation in 10–20% cases of EHPVO.

Patients with portal hypertension due to cirrhosis have jaundice, ascites, hepatosplenomegaly and less often, upper gastrointestinal bleeding. In Budd-Chiari syndrome, patients present with ascites and hepatomegaly. Tortuous prominent back veins are seen in Budd-Chiari syndrome with inferior vena cava block.

### Investigations

The diagnosis of portal hypertension is made by the following investigations:

i. Ultrasound and Doppler study. The vascular anatomy is defined and any block in portal, splenic or hepatic veins can be detected. Increased size of portal vein is suggestive of intrahepatic portal hypertension. Presence of collaterals, ascites, splenomegaly and liver abnormalities (altered echotexture, size and space occupying lesions) are also seen.
ii. Endoscopy can reveal varices in esophagus, stomach and congestive gastropathy.
iii. Colonoscopy is useful in children with lower GI bleeding as it can show presence of rectal varices or colopathy.

**Table 12.34:** Differences between cirrhotic and non-cirrhotic portal hypertension

| *Features* | *Cirrhotic* | *Non-cirrhotic* |
|---|---|---|
| History of jaundice, edema and ascites | Common | Uncommon. Transient ascites may be seen after variceal bleed |
| Overt hepatic encephalopathy | Common | Not seen |
| Stigmata of liver disease, e.g. spider angioma, palmar erythema, gynecomastia, etc. | May be seen | Not seen |
| Splenomegaly | Mild-moderate | Mild-moderate-massive splenomegaly |
| Synthetic function of liver (prothrombin time/serum albumin) | Deranged | Well preserved |
| Transaminases (SGOT/SGPT) | Deranged frequently (except in burnt out liver disease) | Usually normal |

iv. Selective CT and MR portovenography is useful for delineation of vascular anatomy in Budd-Chiari syndrome or in preparation for shunt surgery in EHPVO.
v. Liver function tests are deranged in subjects with cirrhosis. Hemogram may show anemia, leukopenia and thrombocytopenia that suggests hypersplenism.

### Complications

The most common complication is GI bleeding secondary to esophageal varices. Hypersplenism usually is not symptomatic. The enlarged spleen is prone to splenic infarcts and accidental rupture with trauma. Other complications like ascites and hepatic encephalopathy occur in children with cirrhosis.

*Hepatopulmonary syndrome:* The triad of chronic liver disease or portal hypertension, alteration of arterial oxygenation (defined as widened age corrected alveolar arterial oxygen gradient with or without arterial hypoxemia) and evidence of intrapulmonary vascular dilatations defines hepatopulmonary syndrome. Patients with hepatopulmonary syndrome present with dyspnea, platypnea (dyspnea induced in upright position and relieved by recumbency) and orthodeoxia (arterial deoxygenation accentuated in upright position and relieved by recumbency). Examination shows clubbing and cyanosis. Contrast echocardiography is the most sensitive test to demonstrate intrapulmonary shunting. The only established effective therapy is liver transplantation.

*Portopulmonary syndrome:* This is defined as pulmonary arterial hypertension (pulmonary artery pressure >25 mm Hg) associated with severe portal hypertension. Most patients of portopulmonary syndrome have underlying cirrhosis but it can also develop in non-cirrhotic portal hypertension. Symptoms include dyspnea and syncope; echocardiography is required for diagnosis.

### Management

This is based on two goals: (i) Management of complications including upper gastrointestinal bleeding and ascites; and (ii) definitive management that depends on the etiology of portal hypertension. The prognosis is better for children with EHPVO than those with cirrhosis where liver transplantation is often necessary.

### Extrahepatic Portal Venous Obstruction (EHPVO)

It is the commonest cause of portal hypertension in children in India. It is characterized by obstruction of the main portal vein (PV) with or without involvement of the superior mesenteric vein and splenic vein and with variable involvement of the intrahepatic branches of the PV. The main PV is replaced by a cavernoma that shunts blood across the obstruction along with portosystemic collaterals. Umbilical catheterization/sepsis, pyelophlebitis, and procoagulant disorders have been implicated as etiology. However, in vast majority of cases, no cause is identified. These children present with splenomegaly or hematemesis due to variceal bleed. Caput medusae is characteristically absent in these patients as the PV is thrombosed. With improved endoscopic management, the survival of these children has improved and the long-term complications have become evident. These include effects on growth, hypersplenism, portal hypertensive gastropathy/colopathy/enteropathy, rectal varices, ectopic varices, portal biliopathy (compression of biliary system by collaterals) and minimal hepatic encephalopathy due to shunting of blood away from the liver. Meso-Rex bypass (shunt across the obstruction from superior mesenteric vein to the left branch of portal vein) can restore the portal flow and alleviate all complications of EHPVO.

#### *Congenital Hepatic Fibrosis (CHF) and Non-Cirrhotic Portal Fibrosis (NCPF)*

CHF and NCPF cause non-cirrhotic intrahepatic fibrosis leading to portal hypertension. The former often manifests early in childhood. It occurs in genetic disorders which are referred to as ciliopathies as they are inherited disorders of primary ciliary function. They may occur in combination with cystic disorders of the liver. NCPF manifests in teenage often in tropical countries. A definite etiology for this disorder is not known. It is characterized by obliterative portovenopathy (perivenular fibrosis of the small and medium branches of the portal vein) and fibrosis leading to portal hypertension.

#### *Budd-Chiari Syndrome*

Budd-Chiari syndrome is caused by the occlusion of the hepatic veins and/or the suprahepatic inferior vena cava. Right heart failure and sinusoidal obstruction syndrome (formerly known as veno-occlusive disease) impair hepatic venous outflow and share features with Budd-Chiari syndrome, but are grouped separately as its etiology and treatment is different. Budd-Chiari syndrome is considered primary when obstruction of the hepatic venous outflow tract is result of an endoluminal venous lesion (thrombosis or web). It is considered secondary when the obstruction originates from a lesion outside the venous system (tumor, abscess, cysts). The lesion can obstruct outflow by invading the lumen or by extrinsic compression.

The majority of patients with Budd-Chiari syndrome are primary and present with a chronic course; only a small number of patients present with acute or fulminant forms. Acute disorder presents clinically with abdominal pain, ascites, hepatomegaly and rapidly progressive hepatic failure. The chronic form is characterized by hepatomegaly, ascites and portal hypertension. In inferior vena cava block, the back veins become prominent, dilated and tortuous with flow from below upwards (Fig. 12.33).

Doppler ultrasound and venography confirm the diagnosis. Investigations should be done to look for presence of hypercoagulable states. Treatment is directed towards restoring the patency of hepatic vein/inferior vena cava by radiological means (angioplasty, stenting or transjugular intrahepatic portosystemic shunt). Surgery (mesoatrial shunt, mesocaval shunt) is used only in select cases. Orthotopic liver transplant is reserved for patients with end stage liver disease or fulminant failure.

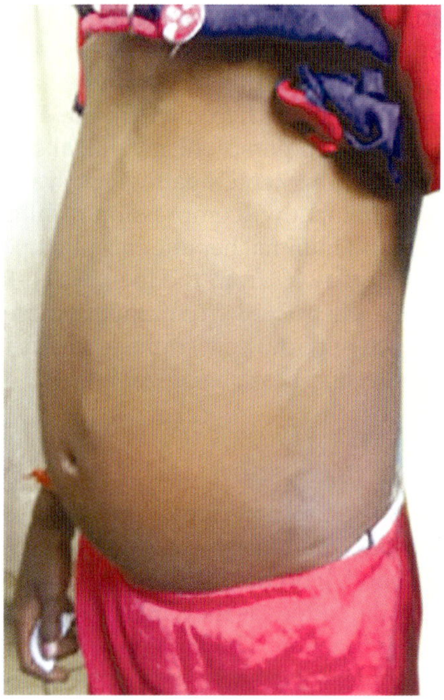

**Fig. 12.33:** Prominent and tortuous abdominal and flank veins in a child with Budd-Chiari syndrome

### Suggested Reading


1. Chapin CA, Bass LM. Cirrhosis and portal hypertension in the pediatric population. Clin Liver Dis 2018;22(4):735–52.
2. Kathuria A, Srivastava A, Yachha SK, et al. Budd-Chiari syndrome in children: Clinical features, percutaneous radiological intervention and outcome. Eur J Gastroenterol Hepatol 2014; 26:1030–38.
3. Khanna R, Sarin SK. Noncirrhotic portal hypertension: Current and emerging perspectives. Clin Liver Dis 2019;23(4):781–807.


## AUTOIMMUNE LIVER DISEASE

Autoimmune liver disease is characterized by hypergammaglobulinemia, presence of circulating autoantibodies, necroinflammatory histology (interface hepatitis, portal lymphoplasmacytic cell infiltration) on biopsy and response to immunosuppressive agents. The condition is common in girls. In children, autoimmune liver disease includes autoimmune hepatitis, autoimmune sclerosing cholangitis and *de novo* autoimmune hepatitis after liver transplantation. The following two types of autoimmune hepatitis are recognized:

- Type 1: Presence of antinuclear antibody and/or antismooth muscle antibody; constitutes 60–70% cases.
- Type 2: Presence of anti-liver kidney microsomal antibody (LKM-1); accounts for 20–30% cases.

### Clinical Presentation

Children can present in one of the following ways:

i. Acute viral hepatitis like presentation (40%) with malaise, nausea, vomiting and jaundice. It may progress to acute liver failure particularly in children with type II disease.
ii. Insidious onset liver disease (30–40%) with progressive fatigue, relapsing or prolonged jaundice lasting for months to years.
iii. Chronic liver disease and its complications (10–20%) with splenomegaly, ascites, variceal bleeding or hepatic encephalopathy.

### Diagnosis

The diagnosis of autoimmune liver disease should be made after exclusion of other known causes of liver diseases, based on the following criteria:

i. Positive autoantibodies
ii. Raised gammaglobulins and IgG levels
iii. Typical histology on liver biopsy
iv. Absence of known etiology, e.g. viral hepatitis, Wilson disease, drug hepatotoxicity or biliary disease
v. Response to immunosuppression confirms the diagnosis.

Seronegative autoimmune liver disease is similar to classical seropositive cases in all aspects.

### Management

Steroids and azathioprine are the primary immunosuppressive agents while mycophenolate mofetil may be a second line drug. Tacrolimus and rituximab are further options in non-responsive cases. The endpoint of therapy is normalization of transaminases and histological inflammatory activity with treatment. A majority of patients including those with cirrhosis respond to medical therapy. Liver transplantation is required for patients with end stage liver disease. Patients presenting with acute liver failure often need liver transplantation, as they often do not respond to medical treatment. A high index of suspicion and timely diagnosis of autoimmune liver disease is crucial.

### Suggested Reading


1. Mack CL, Adams D, Assis DN, et al. Diagnosis and Management of Autoimmune Hepatitis in Adults and Children: 2019. Practice Guidance and Guidelines From the American Association for the Study of Liver Disease. Hepatology 2020;72(2):671–722.
2. Mieli-Vergani G, Vergani D, Baumann U, et al. Diagnosis and Management of Pediatric Autoimmune Liver Disease: ESPGHAN Hepatology Committee Position Statement. J Pediatr Gastroenterol Nutr 2018;66(2):345–60.


## CHRONIC HEPATITIS B INFECTION

Hepatitis B virus (HBV) infection is a worldwide health problem and may result in acute viral hepatitis, acute liver failure, chronic hepatitis, cirrhosis and hepatocellular carcinoma (HCC). The age at time of HBV infection affects the outcome, with >90% of infected neonates becoming chronic carriers as compared to 20–25% of children infected in preschool age and only 5% of adults.

### Clinical Features

Chronic HBV infection is defined as persistence of HBsAg for >6 months. Three potentially successive phases have been described in the natural course of chronic HBV infection:

i. Immune tolerant phase is characterized by active viral replication and minimal liver damage. In this phase, serum HBsAg and HBeAg are positive, serum HBV

DNA levels are high (in millions), anti-HBe antibody is negative and serum ALT levels are normal.

ii. Immune clearance phase occurs years after immune-tolerant phase and is characterized by effort of clearing the chronic HBV infection by the host. In this serum, HBV DNA levels are reduced and ALT levels increase. Serum HBsAg and HBeAg are positive and anti-HBe is negative. The patient may become symptomatic in this phase with ALT flares.

iii. Inactive carrier phase or non-replicative phase follows HBeAg seroconversion, i.e. HBeAg is negative and anti-HBe is positive. It is characterized by very low serum HBV DNA levels (<2000 IU/mL), HBsAg positivity and normal ALT. It may lead to resolution of infection where serum HBsAg becomes undetectable and anti-HBs is present.

Most children with early acquired HBV infection spontaneously clear HBeAg by 15–30 years of age. Majority of the children with chronic HBV infection are asymptomatic during first two decades of life. Cirrhosis develops in 3–10% and hepatocellular carcinoma (HCC) in 1–4% of children with chronic HBV infection.

### Management

The recommendations for management of children with chronic HBV include: (i) Detailed examination and liver function tests; (ii) serology tests: HBeAg, anti-HBe, HBV DNA (quantitative by PCR). HCV RNA and HIV testing to rule out coinfection in high-risk groups (e.g. following multiple transfusions); (iii) consideration for liver biopsy for grading and staging of liver disease prior to initiation of treatment and (iv) identifying and treating patients that merit therapy for hepatitis B. The ideal drug for treatment of chronic HBV infection in children is one that is cheap, safe, orally administered, given at all ages for long duration without any risk of viral resistance and capable of interrupting viral replication to undetectable levels. Medications licensed for use in children include, interferon (>1 year of age), pegylated interferon (≥3 years) and oral antivirals (lamivudine and entecavir for >2 years, adefovir and tenofovir >12 years of age).

As per the recent guidelines, subjects are divided into chronic HBV infection (normal ALT and includes immune tolerant and inactive carrier groups) and chronic HBV hepatitis (raised ALT and can be HBeAg +ve [DNA >20,000 IU/mL] or HBeAg -ve [DNA>2000 IU/mL]). Treatment is indicated for patients with chronic hepatitis after liver biopsy. Follow-up, with elastography, for assessment of fibrosis is recommended for the HBV infection group.

Other aspects of managements include:

i. Follow-up of all infected children for disease flares and surveillance for hepatocellular carcinoma. Risk of cancer in HBV-infected subjects is 100-fold more than in HBV-negative patient. Alpha-fetoprotein and abdominal ultrasound are used to screen for hepatocellular cancer.

ii. Educating the child or adolescent regarding avoidance of other hepatotoxic factors, e.g. obesity, alcohol and intravenous drugs.

iii. Screen all family members of HBsAg positive patient for HBsAg. Vaccination of negative members against HBV and evaluating other HBsAg positive members for liver disease are required.

### Prevention of Chronic HBV Infection

Prevention is the most effective method of successfully controlling HBV infection and its complications. The hepatitis B vaccine is highly immunogenic with seroconversion rates of >90% after three doses. Antibody titers (anti-HBs) of >10 mIU/mL signify a response and are protective. The dose in children and adolescents (aged <18 years) is 0.5 mL (10 mg), given in 3 doses at 0, 1 and 6 months as an intramuscular injection in the deltoid/anterolateral thigh. For prevention of perinatal infection in HBsAg positive mother, the baby should be given hepatitis B immunoglobulin (0.5 mL IM) along with hepatitis B vaccine within 12 hours of birth, using two separate syringes and separate sites for injection. The other two doses of hepatitis B vaccine may be given at 1 and 6 months or at 6 and 14 weeks to piggy back it with the DPT vaccination. The efficacy of prophylaxis with both HBIG and hepatitis B vaccine is 90–95%. All infants born to HBsAg positive mothers should be tested for HBsAg and anti-HBs antibodies at 9–15 months of age to identify HBV-infected (HBsAg positive, anti-HBs antibody negative) and protected (HBsAg negative, anti-HBs antibody positive) children.

Universal infant vaccination, adequate screening of blood products and use of sterile syringes are necessary for preventing chronic HBV infection.

## HEPATITIS C INFECTION

HCV is an enveloped, single-stranded positive-sense RNA virus of the flavivirus family. Based on phylogenetic analysis of HCV sequences, 6 major HCV genotypes are recognized, designated 1 to 6, with multiple subtypes within each viral genotype. In India, genotype 3 is more prevalent.

### Epidemiology

Worldwide prevalence of chronic HCV infection is estimated at 3%, with 150 million chronically infected people. Routes of transmission of HCV are similar to HBV. Mother-to-infant transmission of HCV is the main mode of transmission in children. Hepatitis C affects 4–10% of children born to infected mothers, and 80% of them develop chronic infection.

### Clinical Presentation

Most children with chronic hepatitis C virus infection are asymptomatic or have mild nonspecific symptoms, with persistent or intermittently elevated or even normal serum transaminases. Hepatomegaly may be present. Severe liver disease may develop 10–20 years after onset of infection, with a less than 2% overall risk during the pediatric age group.

### Evaluation

All children of HCV-infected women need testing for HCV infection. Antibody-based testing is done at or after

18 months of age. HCV-RNA assay may be done in infancy as early as 2 months of age, but there is no consensus on the appropriate timing for the same. Children positive for anti-HCV antibody after the age of 18 months need to be tested by HCV-RNA assay after 3 years of age to confirm chronicity of hepatitis C infection. Extrahepatic manifestations of chronic hepatitis C infection include cryoglobulinemia and glomerulonephritis.

Siblings of such children should also be tested for HCV infection.

### Treatment

Children with hepatitis C infection are monitored for disease progression with liver function tests and physical examinations at diagnosis and annually thereafter. This may include noninvasive markers of fibrosis such as elastography in older children. Children with cirrhosis will need surveillance for hepatocellular carcinoma and surveillance for clinically significant portal hypertension. Vaccinations against hepatitis B and hepatitis A infection to prevent such infections.

Direct-acting antiviral (DAA) treatment has been approved for all children over 3-yr-old with chronic HCV infection. Extrahepatic manifestations and advanced fibrosis warrant early antiviral therapy. Combination of ledipasvir/sofosbuvir for 12 weeks may be used for children aged 3 years infected with HCV genotype 1, 4, 5, or 6. Combination of sofosbuvir/velpatasvir for 12 weeks, or combination of glecaprevir/pibrentasvir for 8 weeks may be used for children infected with any genotype. Choice of therapy is also influenced by prior exposure to DAA or the presence of cirrhosis and liver dysfunction.

### Suggested Reading


1. Clemente MG, Antonucci R, Sotgiu G, et al. Present and future management of viral hepatitis B and C in children. Clin Res Hepatol Gastroenterol 2020;44(6):801–09.
2. https://www.hcvguidelines.org/unique-populations/children.
3. Karnsakul W, Schwarz KB. Hepatitis B and C. Pediatr Clin North Am 2017;64(3):641–58.


## METABOLIC LIVER DISEASE

Metabolic diseases account for up to 15–20% of chronic liver disease in Indian children, with Wilson disease being the most frequent.

### Clinical Features

The clinical features are secondary to hepatocyte injury with development of cirrhosis, storage of lipids or glycogen, or metabolic effects secondary to hypoglycemia or hyperammonemia. Clinical signs and symptoms of most metabolic liver diseases are similar and indistinguishable from those seen in acquired hepatic disorders due to other causes. Presentations can be broadly subdivided into:

i. Isolated unconjugated hyperbilirubinemia, e.g. Gilbert syndrome, Crigler-Najjar syndrome types I and II
ii. Conjugated hyperbilirubinemia, e.g. progressive familial intrahepatic cholestasis, cystic fibrosis, bile acid synthesis defects
iii. Severe liver dysfunction with ascites and coagulopathy, e.g. galactosemia, neonatal hemochromatosis, tyrosinemia
iv. Hepatomegaly, hepatosplenomegaly, e.g. glycogen storage disease, lysosomal storage disorders
v. Reye like illness, e.g. mitochondrial hepatopathies, urea cycle defects
vi. Chronic liver disease or acute liver failure, e.g. Wilson disease

The settings in which metabolic liver disease should be suspected include: (i) Recurrent episodes of rapid deterioration with minor illnesses; (ii) recurrent unexplained encephalopathy, hypoglycemia, acidosis and hyperammonemia, as in mitochondrial hepatopathies, urea cycle defects, organic acidurias; (iii) consanguinity, sib deaths or positive family history, as in Wilson disease; (iv) food intolerance or aversions, e.g. sugars in hereditary fructose intolerance, protein in urea cycle defects; (v) rickets or unusual urine odors, e.g. tyrosinemia; (vi) developmental delay and multisystem involvement, e.g. mitochondrial hepatopathies; and (vii) fatty liver on ultrasonography or liver biopsy.

### Diagnosis

Apart from the high index of suspicion, investigations include complete blood count, arterial blood gases with lactate, electrolytes, glucose, ammonia; plasma and urine amino acids and organic acids; urine for ketones and sugars. Samples of urine and plasma, skin and liver biopsy are frozen for future evaluation. Liver biopsy provides information about the extent of damage and tissue for estimation of abnormal material (copper, iron or glycogen) and enzyme assay. Confirmation of the diagnosis requires specific tests like enzyme assay and genetic analysis depending on the suspected etiology.

### Management

Management is two pronged—specific treatment of underlying disease and therapy for liver damage. Supportive therapy includes measures like provision of optimal nutrition with vitamin supplementation, antioxidants, correction of hypoglycemia, coagulopathy and ascites, vaccination against infections like hepatitis B and monitoring for hepatocellular carcinoma in high-risk groups like tyrosinemia. Specific therapy is most important and should be given whenever available and affordable, e.g. chelation therapy for Wilson disease, and dietary modification for galactosemia. Liver transplantation might be offered for specific disorders.

### Wilson Disease

Wilson disease (WD) is an inborn error of metabolism due to toxic accumulation of copper in liver, brain, cornea and other tissues.

#### *Clinical Presentation*

The age of presentation can vary from 4 to 60 years. Manifestations are more likely to be hepatic in early childhood and neurological in adolescents or adults. The spectrum of hepatic manifestations includes all forms of chronic or acute liver disease, i.e. asymptomatic hepatomegaly, chronic hepatitis, portal hypertension, cirrhosis, 'viral hepatitis' like illness and sometimes acute liver failure. Neurological abnormalities are varied and include clumsiness, speech difficulties, scholastic deterioration, behavioral problems, convulsions and choreoathetoid/dystonic movements.

### *Investigations*

Serum ceruloplasmin is decreased (<20 mg/dL) in most patients. In symptomatic patients, the 24 hours urinary copper excretion is >100 µg/day. Kayser-Fleischer (KF) ring indicates long-standing disease and severe copper overload. KF rings are more common in children with neurological (96%) than hepatic (60%) and asymptomatic (10–20%) Wilson disease. Hepatic copper quantification on liver biopsy with ≥250 µg/g dry weight of liver may be useful in making a diagnosis where the diagnosis is ambiguous based on other tests. Genetic diagnosis is helpful in patients where diagnosis is difficult using usual biochemical parameters and in screening family members of an index patient with known mutation.

### *Diagnosis*

WD is strongly suggested by the presence of low ceruloplasmin, high urinary copper and KF ring. Leipzig scoring is used for diagnosis of WD, a score of 4 makes the diagnosis very likely. All siblings of patients with WD should be screened to detect asymptomatic WD.

### *Treatment*

Foods with high copper content like organ meats (liver), chocolates and nuts should be avoided especially in the early phase of chelation treatment, or while on zinc therapy. Long-term strict dietary restriction may not be necessary for stable patients on maintenance chelation therapy. Continuous life-long pharmacotherapy is essential for management.

Children diagnosed by genetic screening rarely become symptomatic before 2 years of age, and are kept under surveillance with periodic biochemical investigations. In the absence of any manifestations, zinc therapy used as acetate, sulfate or gluconate salts is commenced at 2 years of age.

***Chelators:*** D-penicillamine or trientine is often used as chelation therapy for manifest Wilson disease (asymptomatic liver biochemical abnormalities attributable to WD or symptomatic patients). Penicillamine is the first choice of medication and is started in slowly escalating doses while monitoring for allergic and non-allergic adverse events and emergence or worsening of neurological features. Adverse effects include skin rash, bone marrow depression and proteinuria. Trientine has been used as an alternative chelating agent especially for children intolerant to penicillamine. Neurological worsening on trientine is less than that on penicillamine as it is a less potent chelator. Ammonium tetrathiomolybdate though not widely available may be useful in neurological Wilson disease that show worsening on the above two chelators. The long-term target of 24-hour urine copper while on chelators is >200 µg/day, while avoiding over-chelation in the long term.

Zinc acts by reducing copper absorption, and it takes a longer time to achieve a negative copper balance. It is unsuitable as the first-line medication in patients with symptomatic WD. It has been used as monotherapy in patients showing neurological deterioration on chelators. The use of zinc monotherapy for long-term maintenance to replace chelators in stable patients is not routine practice, and requires close monitoring.

The role for routine use of combination therapy with chelators and zinc is not supported by evidence. If administered together, zinc might impair the action of chelators by binding to them.

Liver transplantation is indicated in patients with WD who present as acute liver failure or have decompensated cirrhosis unresponsive to medical therapy.

## Glycogen Storage Disorders

Glycogen storage disorders are important metabolic disorders manifesting in childhood with varied clinical picture ranging from asymptomatic hepatomegaly (type VI) to hypoglycemia (type I, III) and decompensated end-stage liver disease (type IV).

***Type I glycogen storage disease (von Gierke disease):*** Inability to convert glucose-6-phosphate to glucose in the liver results in inability to mobilize glycogen. Depending on whether this is due to glucose-6-phosphatase deficiency or translocase deficiency, it is classified as type 1A or 1B. Hepatomegaly, doll-like facies (Fig. 12.34), hypoglycemia, seizures, growth retardation, hyperuricemia, hypertriglyceridemia and lactic acidosis are main manifestations. Hypoglycemia is more marked after first few months of life when the frequency of feeding decreases.

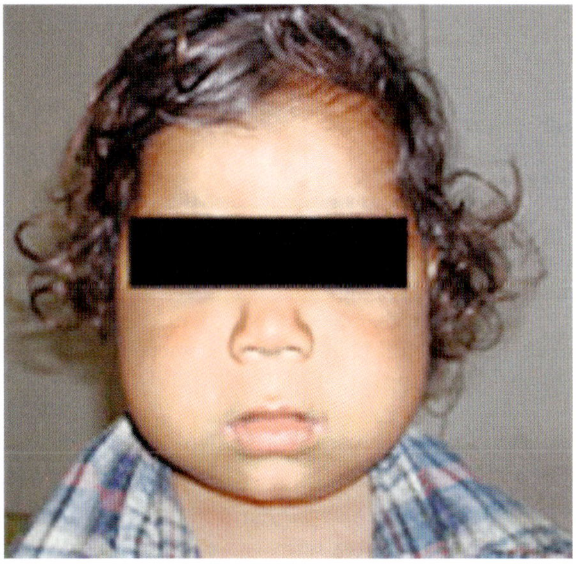

**Fig. 12.34:** Classical cherubic facies with prominent cheeks in a child with glycogen storage disease

Liver adenoma might develop with risk of bleeding and malignant transformation.

Hepatomegaly and nephromegaly is appreciated on imaging. Platelet dysfunction may be present. Neutropenia is specific to type 1B. There is mild transaminase elevation. Liver biopsy shows hepatocytes with vacuolated cytoplasm and glycogen accumulation (PAS stain positive, diastase sensitive); fibrosis is absent. Definite diagnosis depends on measuring enzyme activity in the liver or mutational analysis.

Management hinges on providing a constant source of glucose in the form of slowly digested complex carbohydrates. This is achieved by frequent daytime feeding, supplementation of uncooked corn starch both in day and specifically at night. As the child grows into adolescence, longer periods of fasting may be tolerated. Since the metabolism of other carbohydrates also yield glucose-6-phosphate, galactose and fructose also need to be restricted. Strict metabolic control with dietary therapy is the key to avoiding complications.

*Type III glycogen storage disorder:* There is a deficiency of debranching enzyme manifesting as hepatosplenomegaly, hypoglycemia, fibrosis in the liver and elevation in transaminases. While hypoglycemia and hepatosplenomegaly improve, 80–85% develop a myopathy in type IIIa disease while the other 15% (type IIIb) have only liver involvement. These cases are managed with diet similar to that in type I GSD, except that a high protein diet is preferred and there is no need to restrict galactose and fructose.

*Type IV glycogen storage disorder:* In type IV GSD, there is a deficiency of branching enzyme resulting in deposition of an amylopectin-like structure in the liver. The presentation is with chronic liver disease, portal hypertension and hepatic decompensation. Most children are symptomatic by 3 years of age. Treatment is largely supportive and liver transplantation is required for patients with advanced disease.

### Suggested Reading


1. Beyzaei Z, Geramizadeh B, Karimazadesh S. Diagnosis of hepatic glycogen storage disease patients with overlapping clinical symptoms by massively parallel seguencing. Orphanet J Rare Dis 2020;15:286.
2. Mayatepek E, Hoffmann B, Meissner T. Inborn errors of carbohydrate metabolism. Best Pract Res Clin Gastroenterol 2010; 24:607–18.
3. Nagral A, Sarma MS, Matthai J, et al. Wilson's Disease: Clinical Practice Guidelines of the Indian National Association for Study of the Liver, the Indian Society of Pediatric Gastroenterology, Hepatology and Nutrition, and the Movement Disorders Society of India. J Clin Exp Hepatol. 2019;9(1):74–98.


## Nonalcoholic Fatty Liver Disease (NAFLD)

This is a common cause of liver disease in children and is closely associated with obesity and insulin resistance. The prevalence is increasing with the expanding prevalence of childhood obesity. NAFLD is a clinicopathological diagnosis characterized by macrovesicular steatosis in hepatocytes, in absence of other causes of chronic liver disease. It ranges from simple steatosis (macrovesicular steatosis in hepatocytes without inflammation) to non-alcoholic steatohepatitis (NASH, macrovesicular steatosis in hepatocytes associated with inflammation and fibrosis) to cirrhosis of liver and hepatocellular carcinoma. Insulin resistance and hyperinsulinemia is regarded as essential to the disease mechanism.

### Clinical Presentation

Most children are asymptomatic. Some have vague abdominal pain; examination shows generalized obesity, cutaneous striae and hepatomegaly. Splenomegaly is uncommon. Acanthosis nigricans, a velvety brown-to-black pigment in skin folds and axillae, typically associated with hyperinsulinemia can be found in 30–50% patients.

### Investigations

The evidence of fatty liver is from radiological studies, usually an ultrasound. Typical biochemical abnormalities in NASH include moderately raised serum aminotransferases (with ALT more raised than AST). Metabolic abnormalities include hypertriglyceridemia, elevated fasting serum insulin and hyperglycemia. Apart from ruling out other causes of fatty liver, liver histology may be required to diagnose NASH and significant fibrosis in those with raised transaminases, splenomegaly, type 2 diabetes mellitus or panhypopituitarism.

### Treatment

The first step in treating NAFLD is to identify it. Besides height and weight, waist circumference provides highly informative data and is a surrogate for visceral obesity. The treatment has two goals—to reverse liver disease and to promote healthy growth. Lifestyle changes aimed at weight reduction are essential. Dietary changes and increased physical activity lead to diminished insulin resistance and are the main stay of therapy. Drugs, such as vitamin E, have been used. Children with significant liver fibrosis/inflammation and very high BMI may be referred to speciality obesity services. Prevention of over-weight and obesity in children is the best strategy to overcome the problem of NAFLD.

### Suggested Reading


1. Nobili V, Alisi A, Valenti L, et al. NAFLD in children: new genes, new diagnostic modalities and new drugs. Nat Rev Gastroenterol Hepatol 2019;16(9):517–30.
2. Vos MB, Abrams SH, Barlow SE, et al. NASPGHAN Clinical Practice Guideline for the Diagnosis and Treatment of Nonalcoholic Fatty Liver Disease in Children: Recommendations from the Expert Committee on NAFLD (ECON) and the North American Society of Pediatric Gastroenterology, Hepatology and Nutrition (NASPGHAN). J Pediatr Gastroenterol Nutr 2017;64(2):319–34.


## HEPATIC MANIFESTATIONS OF SYSTEMIC DISEASES

Apart from disorders that directly involve the liver, a number of disorders affecting other organ systems also have hepatic manifestations. While, in some disorders, these manifestations may be benign, in others the hepatic manifestations might significantly affect the outcome.

### Ischemic Hepatitis

Severe shock may lead to hypoperfusion of the liver. This shock may be the result of sepsis, acute cardiogenic shock or severe intraoperative hypoperfusion as in cardiac surgery. It usually manifests as an elevation of transaminases to high levels. The degree of hepatic injury depends on the duration and severity of shock. Thus, coagulopathy as evidenced by prolonged prothrombin time and encephalopathy may result. Jaundice is a late manifestation.

### Cardiac Disorders

Apart from an acute cardiogenic shock or intraoperative hypoperfusion in cardiac surgery, liver involvement may be seen as a result of congestion in right heart failure or as part of syndromes that involve both the liver and the heart. Chronic right heart failure may lead to hepatomegaly, splenomegaly and over long periods result in cardiac cirrhosis as seen in Fontan-associated liver disease. There may be an increased risk of hepatocellular carcinoma in children with Fontan-associated liver disease. Alagille syndrome, caused by syndromic paucity of intralobular bile ducts results in infantile cholestasis; patients also show peripheral pulmonary stenosis, tetralogy of Fallot and atrial or ventricular septal defects. In biliary atresia, splenic malformation syndrome anomaly, there may be vascular malformations and congenital heart disease.

### Sepsis and Systemic Infections

Gram-positive and gram-negative bacterial infections may result in jaundice. Up to one-third of neonatal jaundice has been attributed to sepsis. The mechanism may vary. It may be impaired canalicular bile transport due to defective transporter polarization in hepatocytes without hepatic necrosis as in gram-negative infections or elevated bilirubin load due to hemolysis as in clostridium infections or hepatocellular necrosis as in pneumococcal infections. Typhoid might result in elevated alkaline phosphatase, transaminases and lactate dehydrogenase. Transaminase elevation and liver dysfunction is also present in dengue hemorrhagic fever and malaria.

### Immunological Disorders

Juvenile idiopathic arthritis may be associated with hepatomegaly and elevated transaminases. Liver dysfunction due to macrophage activation syndrome is seen in systemic onset juvenile idiopathic arthritis. Systemic lupus erythematosus may be associated with hepatomegaly or autoimmune hepatitis. Transplacental transfer of autoantibodies might lead to neonatal SLE with transient cholestasis, congenital heart block, dermatitis and hematological abnormalities.

### Hemolytic Anemias

Repeated transfusions and the increased iron absorption due to ineffective erythropoiesis leads to chronic iron overload, fibrosis and cirrhosis. Recurrent transfusions increase the risk of acquiring hepatitis B and hepatitis C infections. These individuals are also at higher risk of pigment gallstones resulting in acute and chronic cholecystitis. Intrahepatic sickling of erythrocytes in sickle cell anemia leads to acute sickle cell hepatic crisis, acute hepatic sequestration, and acute intrahepatic cholestasis. Sickle cell anemia is also a cause of secondary sclerosing cholangitis.

### Malignancies

Leukemias and lymphomas might be associated with hepatic infiltration, presenting as jaundice, drug-induced liver disease or opportunistic liver infections and sepsis. Hemophagocytic lymphohistiocytosis, either familial or infection induced, presents with fever, jaundice, hepatosplenomegaly, liver dysfunction and cytopenia. It is an important differential diagnosis for liver failure in the first few months of life. Sclerosing cholangitis may be a complication of Langerhans cell histiocytosis.

### Bone Marrow Transplant

Conditioning chemotherapy and total body irradiation may lead to veno-occlusive disease manifesting as weight gain, hepatomegaly, ascites and jaundice. Other causes of liver dysfunction after bone marrow transplant include graft versus host disease (acute or chronic), sepsis, infectious hepatitis and drug toxicity.

### Endocrine Disorders

Uncontrolled diabetes mellitus presents with hepatomegaly due to glycogen hepatopathy. They may have associated autoimmune hepatitis or associated celiac disease leading to raised transaminases. Hypothyroidism manifests predominantly as unconjugated jaundice in the neonatal period due to impaired conjugation of bilirubin but may also result in conjugated jaundice due to decreased bile flow.

### Celiac Disease

Elevated transaminases may be observed, which normalize with gluten-free diet in the majority. Persistent rise of transaminases should lead to evaluation for co-existing autoimmune liver disease or other causes of liver disease.

## NEONATAL CHOLESTASIS

Jaundice is common in neonates as physiological jaundice is found in a majority. This jaundice usually resolves by two weeks of age. Also, most pathological causes of unconjugated jaundice are detected and treated by two weeks of age. Though breast milk jaundice can be a cause of unconjugated hyperbilirubinemia beyond two weeks of age, cholestatic jaundice is an important and potentially serious condition that needs evaluation and early treatment.

All bottle-fed newborns having jaundice beyond 2 weeks of postnatal age and breastfed infant with jaundice for longer than 3 weeks of postnatal age should have a fractionated bilirubin estimation. Conjugated hyperbilirubinemia is defined as direct bilirubin value greater than 1 mg/dL, if the total bilirubin is less than

5 mg/dL, or a value of direct bilirubin that represents more than 20% of the total bilirubin, if the total bilirubin is >5 mg/dL. Conjugated hyperbilirubinemia presents with high colored urine staining the diapers unlike unconjugated hyperbilirubinemia. Those with conjugated jaundice with or without acholic stools should be referred immediately to tertiary health facilities for further investigations and treatment. The need for time-bound early evaluation and treatment is manifold as mortality and poor outcomes are common in children with metabolic liver diseases and biliary atresia respectively when the referral is delayed. Often, valuable time is lost by work-up in less equipped primary health centres. Referral should be after a dose of vitamin K injection. This may be given intramuscular route but in those with bleeding this may be given by intravenous route. Vitamin K deficiency due to malabsorption resulting from cholestasis is not an uncommon cause of morbidity and mortality. This includes intracranial bleeds, exsanguinating gastrointestinal bleeds and intramuscular hematomas during vaccination.

### Clinical Features

Neonatal cholestasis is characterized by high colored urine along with jaundice. Referral of children with biliary atresia is often delayed as they are healthy looking and gaining weight. In contrast, failure to thrive is common in children with metabolic liver diseases. Stool color is best assessed by looking at the core of the stools as otherwise pale stools covered by bile pigment-stained intestinal epithelial cells may be mistaken for pigmented stools. The presence of pale stools does not necessarily reflect an extrahepatic obstructive cause as many metabolic liver diseases with significant liver dysfunction present with pale stools. Also, intrahepatic diseases with severe paucity of bile ductules or significant canalicular transporter dysfunction may present with pale stools. However, presence of persistently pigmented yellow stools is not seen in biliary atresia. A subset of patients present with signs of coagulopathy like skin or intracranial bleeds (seizures, irritability and bulging fontanel). Hepatomegaly or hepatosplenomegaly is common. Early decompensation of the liver synthetic function is a feature in patients with an underlying metabolic disorder. In a sick infant, one should consider the diagnosis of galactosemia, tyrosinemia, hemochromatosis, herpes and sepsis. Patients with biliary atresia and choledochal cyst are otherwise healthy looking. Bilateral cataract and *E. coli* sepsis is typical of galactosemia, whereas rash (maculopapular or petechial), fever, chorioretinitis, microcephaly and lethargy are suggestive of congenital infections. Triangular facies, pointed chin, prominent ears, cardiac murmurs and butterfly vertebrae are seen in Alagille syndrome. Splenohepatomegaly with cherry-red spot on fundus examination suggests storage disorder. Clinical clues to the diagnosis are shown in Table 12.35.

### Diagnosis

Neonatal cholestasis has a multifactorial etiology. The etiological spectrum in referral western centres is as follows—biliary atresia (25%), Alagille syndrome and bile acid synthetic disorders (25%), metabolic (20%), idiopathic neonatal hepatitis (INH, 15%), alpha-1-antitrypsin deficiency (10%), and viral (5%). This data is relevant as the

**Table 12.35:** Clinical clues to diagnosis in an infant with liver disease

| *Clinical features* | *Diagnosis* |
|---|---|
| Facial dysmorphism | Down syndrome, Zellweger syndrome, Arthrogryposis-renal dysfunction-cholestasis (ARC), Smith-Lemli-Opitz syndrome, Alagille syndrome |
| Eye examination | *Cataract:* Congenital rubella, galactosemia, Zellweger syndrome, Wolman disease<br>*Posterior embryotoxon and Drusen:* Alagille syndrome<br>*Cherry-red spot:* Gaucher and Niemann-Pick disease<br>*Septo-optic dysplasia:* Hypopituitarism |
| Skin changes | *Icthyosis, hypotrichosis:* Neonatal sclerosing cholangitis<br>*Cutaneous laxity:* ARC syndrome, transaldolase deficiency<br>*Lymphedema:* Aagenaes syndrome |
| Cardiovascular defects | *Pulmonary and peripheral pulmonary stenosis, tetrology of Fallot:* Alagille syndrome<br>*Atrial and ventricular septal defects, preduodenal portal vein, absent inferior vena cava:* Biliary atresia |
| Skeletal abnormalities | *Vertebral anomalies:* Alagille syndrome<br>*Patellar stippling on X-ray:* Zellweger syndrome |
| Neuromuscular involvement | *Hypotonia:* Down syndrome, Zellweger syndrome, Wolman syndrome, congenital disorders of glycosylation, mitochondrial disorders, Gaucher and Niemann-Pick disease<br>*Seizures:* Congenital intrauterine infections, disseminated herpes infection, hypoglycemia due to any cause of liver failure, galactosemia, fructosemia<br>*Arthrogryposis:* ARC syndrome |
| Ascites | *Ascites without liver failure:* Spontaneous rupture of bile duct<br>*Ascites with liver dysfunction:* Any cause of neonatal liver failure |
| Genital abnormalities | *Micropenis:* Septo-optic dysplasia<br>*Ambiguous genitalia:* Smith-Lemli-Opitz syndrome |
| Renal anomalies | *Cysts:* Ciliopathies; *Dysplasia:* ARC syndrome |

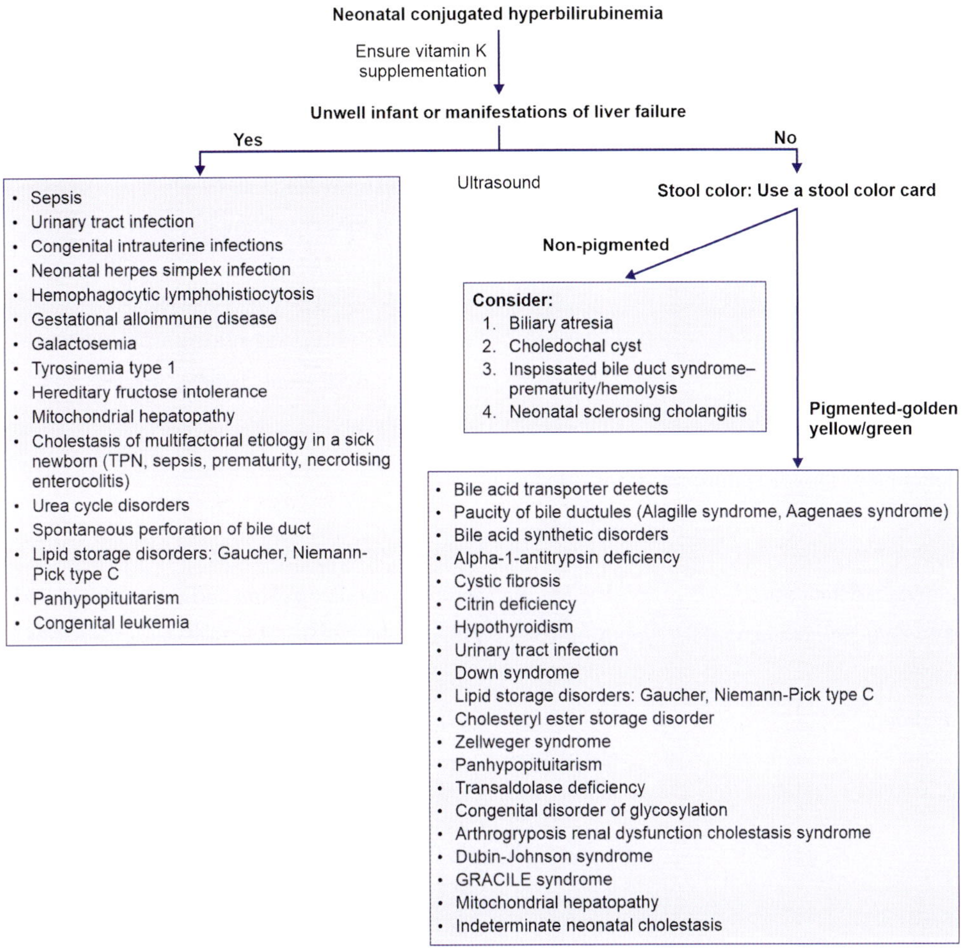


**Fig. 12.35:** Evaluation of an infant with cholestasis

proportion of cases with INH reduces when all necessary investigations especially metabolic tests are done. Alpha-1-antitrypsin is not as prevalent in India as in European countries. Liver dysfunction, general condition and stool color are important features in the differential diagnosis.

These infants need a detailed investigative work-up based on a rational approach so as to avoid unnecessary and costly investigations. The etiology and algorithm of evaluation is different in a 'sick' and 'not sick' infant with cholestasis as shown in the flowchart (Fig. 12.35). Table 12.36 mentions the etiology specific investigations in neonatal cholestasis.

In a non-sick infant with pale stools, the main objective is to quickly establish the diagnosis or rule out biliary atresia. Liver biopsy is an accurate (90–95%) test for differentiating biliary atresia from other causes of neonatal cholestasis. In biliary atresia, portal tract expansion, ductular proliferation and fibrosis are seen, whereas in neonatal hepatitis, there is alteration in lobular architecture, focal hepatocellular necrosis and giant cells formation. Hepatobiliary iminodiacetic acid (HIDA) scan is useful to see for excretion of bile in the gut. Priming with UDCA or phenobarbitone for 3 days before HIDA scan improves the diagnostic efficacy of HIDA. HIDA is more relevant for its negative predictive value (100%) as the presence of excretion into gut rules out biliary atresia. However, a non-excretory pattern, i.e. no activity in intestine at 24 hours in HIDA scan can be seen in both biliary atresia and severe intrahepatic cholestasis. Thus, the absence of excretion does not necessarily mean biliary atresia. Laparotomy and peroperative cholangiography may be required in an infant with equivocal biopsy, findings and no excretion on HIDA scan, to evaluate for biliary atresia. In experienced centres, with rapid reporting of liver biopsy, a histological diagnosis is possible much earlier than an HIDA report and helps in avoiding a negative laparotomy.

Ultrasound of abdomen is more relevant in determining the presence of dilated CBD/intrahepatic biliary radicle dilatation (seen in choledochal cyst), cysts at the porta (seen in cystic variants of biliary atresia and choledochal cyst), multiple intrahepatic cysts communicating with biliary tree (Caroli disease), hemangioma (relevant for liver biopsy) and looking for situs inversus (seen in some cases of biliary atresia—relevant for liver biopsy). Even though an absent, poorly contractile, small gallbladder, and triangular cord sign (echogenic density of more than 3 mm located immediately cranial to the portal vein bifurcation) are finding associated with biliary atresia, the condition should not be ruled out or diagnosed on the basis of an ultrasound alone. Dilatation of intrahepatic biliary radical is not seen in biliary atresia as it is a panductular fibrotic disease.

In an infant with frankly pigmented stools, intrahepatic causes need to be considered. There is no utility of HIDA in this situation as it will definitely be excretory. Liver biopsy

**Table 12.36:** Disease specific investigations for young infants with liver disease

| *Disorder* | *Investigations* |
|---|---|
| Sepsis, urinary tract infection | Blood culture, urine culture |
| Intrauterine infections | Review of maternal serology, history of infection during pregnancy Serological tests for infants; PCR for cytomegalovirus, Epstein-Barr virus |
| Neonatal herpes simplex infection | Blood PCR for herpes simplex virus |
| Gestational alloimmune disease | Buccal mucosal biopsy for salivary gland iron staining, MRI abdomen, serum ferritin, total iron binding capacity |
| Galactosemia | Galactose-1-phosphate uridyltransferase levels |
| Tyrosinemia type 1 | Urine succinylacetone; genetic studies |
| Hereditary fructose intolerance, arthrogryposis renal dysfunction cholestasis syndrome, Dubin-Johnson syndrome, GRACILE syndrome, citrin deficiency, Down syndrome, transaldolase deficiency, ciliopathies | Genetic testing |
| Mitochondrial hepatopathy | Serum lactate, pyruvate; genetic testing |
| Ornithine transcarbomylase deficiency | Serum ammonia, plasma and urine amino acids; genetic testing |
| Lipid storage disorders: Gaucher, Niemann-Pick type A, B, C | White cell enzymes, skin biopsy for fibroblast culture; genetics |
| Bile acid transporter defects | Genetics, liver immunohistochemistry |
| Bile acid synthetic disorders | GGT, serum and urine bile acid profile; genetic studies |
| Biliary atresia | *Ultrasound:* Cyst at the porta, triangular cord sign, small irregular gallbladder, polysplenia/asplenia, situs inversus<br>*Liver biopsy:* Expanded portal tract with fibrosis and inflammation, bile ductular reaction, bile plugs<br>Operative cholangiogram to confirm the diagnosis |
| Choledochal cyst, Caroli disease | Ultrasound, magnetic resonance cholangiopancreatography |
| Neonatal sclerosing cholangitis | Liver biopsy; genetic studies |
| Bile acid transporter defects | GGT, serum and urine bile acid profile; genetic studies |
| Syndromic paucity of bile ducts (Alagille syndrome) | Echocardiography, eye examination, vertebral radiography, liver biopsy; genetic studies |
| Cystic fibrosis | Immunoreactive trypsinogen, sweat chloride; genetic studies |
| Zellweger syndrome | Very long chain fatty acid; genetic studies |
| Congenital disorder of glycosylation | Transferrin electrophoresis; genetic studies |

(light microscopy and immunohistochemistry) is useful in making a specific diagnosis but is not of much use in most situations where a metabolic cause is suspected. A detailed metabolic workup is required for infants with conditions like progressive familial intrahepatic cholestasis, tyrosinemia, mitochondrial cytopathies, bile acid synthesis defects, etc.

## Management

Delayed diagnosis leads to problems of undernutrition, coagulopathy, pruritus (older infants), portal hypertension, ascites and hepatic encephalopathy.

*General management:* This includes the following:

i. Nutritional. Adequate caloric intake (125–150% of RDA based on ideal body weight) with medium chain triglyceride supplementation is necessary. Breastfeeding should be continued and supplementation with high MCT formulae should be done; 2–3% calories should come from long chain triglycerides to prevent deficiency of essential fatty acids. Nasogastric feed is offered to anorexic infants. Supplementation of fat-soluble and water-soluble vitamins is essential.
ii. For infants with pruritus, ursodeoxycholic acid (UDCA, 10–20 mg/kg/day), rifampicin (5–10 mg/kg/day) and cholestyramine (250 mg/kg/day, max 8 g/day) are used. UDCA is the first agent of choice and others are used in patients with persistent symptoms.
iii. Management of other complications like ascites, gastrointestinal bleeding and hepatic encephalopathy.

*Specific management* may be available, some of which have been listed below:

i. Biliary atresia is managed by Kasai procedure (hepatoportoenterostomy). The best results are obtained, if it is done early (<60 days of age) and at centers with expertise. Liver transplantation is indicated in children who progress to end stage cirrhosis either despite surgical treatment or due to late diagnosis.
ii. *Choledochal cyst:* Excision of cyst and hepaticojejunostomy

**Table 12.37:** Indications for liver transplantation

| **Indications** |
|---|
| • Decompensated chronic liver disease and its complications (ascites, encephalopathy, spontaneous bacterial peritonitis, hepatopulmonary syndrome, hepatorenal syndrome) |
| • Acute liver failure fulfilling liver transplant criteria |
| • Portal hypertension refractory to medical and endoscopic therapy |
| • Refractory pruritus |
| • Recurrent cholangitis in cholangiopathies |
| • Severe growth failure/sarcopenia in chronic liver disease in spite of optimal nutritional management |
| • Unresectable liver tumors |
| • Liver based non-cirrhotic metabolic defects |

iii. Herpes simplex: Intravenous acyclovir
iv. Bacterial sepsis: Intravenous antibiotics
v. Toxoplasmosis: Pyrimethamine and sulfadiazine with folinic acid
vi. Galactosemia: Galactose-free diet
vii. Hemochromatosis: IV immunoglobulins (IVIG) with exchange transfusion may be useful.
viii. Bile acid synthetic disorders: Cholic acid

There is considerable delay in referral of patients with neonatal cholestasis to higher centers in India. This results in delayed etiologic diagnosis, missed opportunity for corrective biliary atresia surgery in first 60 days and liver decompensation in patients with metabolic etiology. All efforts should be targeted towards early identification of neonates with conjugated hyperbilirubinemia and their referral to centres with expertise. The use of stool color cards to identify pale stools is a proven population screening strategy for biliary atresia.

### Suggested Reading


1. Feldman AG, Sokol RJ. Recent developments in diagnostics and treatment of neonatal cholestasis. Semin Pediatr Surg 2020;29(4):150945.
2. Jagadisan B, Dhawan A. Emergencies in pediatric hepatology. J Hepatol. 2022 Jan 3:S0168 8278(21)02301 7.
3. Lane E, Murray KF. Neonatal cholestasis. Pediatr Clin North Am. 2017;64(3):621–39.


## LIVER TRANSPLANTATION

Liver transplantation may be necessary in children with end stage liver disease, unresectable liver tumors, liver-based metabolic defects, and liver disorders leading to suboptimal quality of life. The graft is obtained either from the cadaver or can be from a living donor. The graft may be the whole liver from a cadaver or often part of the liver from a cadaveric or living donor. In auxiliary liver transplantation, a portion of the native liver is retained and a liver graft from the donor is transplanted in addition to the native liver. This is usually done for non-cirrhotic metabolic disorders of the liver where the graft provides the function of the deficient enzyme. It is also done in acute liver failure when it can be safely performed and there is potential for liver regeneration. This provides an opportunity to withdraw immunosuppression when there is regeneration of native liver.

The main indications for liver transplantation are biliary atresia, fulminant hepatic failure and other causes of chronic liver disease and hepatic tumors (Table 12.37).

### Suggested Reading


1. Mazariegos G, Shneider B, Burton B, et al. Liver transplantation for pediatric metabolic disease. Mol Genet Metab 2014:111:418–27.
2. Pham YH, Miloh T. Liver transplantation in children. Clin Liver Dis 2018;22(4):807–21.

Chapter

13

# Hematological Disorders

Tulika Seth

## Hematopoiesis

The hemangioblast is believed to be the stem cell from which endothelial and hematopoietic cells develop. These pluripotent stem cells give rise to two colony-forming units (CFU)—one is the common myeloid precursor (granulocytes, erythrocytes, monocytes and megakaryocytes) named CFU-GEMM; the second is the common lymphoid precursor called CFU-L. This complex and sequential development of hematopoietic cells is driven and regulated by local growth factors and cytokines.

*Competencies:* **PE29.1; PE29.10; PE29.11**

## APPROACH TO ANEMIA

Anemia is a sign. It is important to investigate the cause of anemia to ensure that it is not due to a serious underlying ailment and to decide the correct management approach.

### Definition

Anemia is present when the hemoglobin level in the blood is two standard deviations below the mean for the particular age and sex being evaluated (Tables 13.1 and 13.2). The physiologic definition of anemia is a condition in which tissue hypoxia occurs due to inadequate oxygen carrying capacity of blood. In the National Family Health Survey 2019–20 (NHFS-5), 67.1% children aged between 6–59 months had anemia.

### Physiological Adaptations

Anemia leads to decreased oxygen-carrying capacity of the blood and compensatory physiological adjustments. The maintenance of blood volume occurs by an increase in the volume of plasma and redistribution of blood flow. Cardiac output increases in anemia as a consequence of increased stroke volume, this high output state increases

**Table 13.1:** Hemoglobin and hematocrit in infancy and childhood

| | *Hemoglobin (g/dL)* | | *Hematocrit (%)* | |
|---|---|---|---|---|
| *Age* | *Mean* | *Mean –2SD* | *Mean* | *Mean –2SD* |
| Birth (cord blood) | 16.5 | 13.5 | 51 | 42 |
| 1–3 days (capillary) | 18.5 | 14.5 | 56 | 45 |
| 1 week | 17.5 | 13.5 | 54 | 42 |
| 2 weeks | 16.5 | 12.5 | 51 | 39 |
| 1 month | 14.0 | 10.0 | 43 | 31 |
| 2 months | 11.5 | 9.0 | 35 | 28 |
| 3–6 months | 11.5 | 9.5 | 35 | 29 |
| 0.5–2 years | 12.0 | 10.5 | 36 | 33 |
| 2–6 years | 12.5 | 11.5 | 37 | 34 |
| 6–12 years | 13.5 | 11.5 | 40 | 35 |
| Girls 12–18 years | 14.0 | 12.0 | 41 | 36 |
| Boys 12–18 years | 14.5 | 13.0 | 43 | 37 |

Values two standard deviations below the mean (–2 SD) indicate the lower limit of normal

Table 13.2: Cutoffs for hemoglobin and hematocrit proposed by the World Health Organization to define anemia

| Age group | Hemoglobin (g/dl) | Hematocrit % |
|---|---|---|
| Children, 6 mo to 5 years | <11.0 | <33 |
| Children, 5–11 years | <11.5 | <34 |
| Children, 12–13 years | <12.0 | <36 |
| Non-pregnant women | <12.0 | <36 |
| Men | <13.0 | <39 |

Source: WHO 1997

oxygen delivery to tissues by increasing the flow of blood. Diversion of blood flow occurs from tissues with lesser oxygen requirements to those with greater needs. Skin blood flow is reduced, while cerebral and muscle blood flow are increased. Tissue hypoxia develops when release of oxygen from hemoglobin and blood flow to the tissues is insufficient to meet requirements.

## Clinical Approach

The history can give important clues to the etiology; causes vary with age and in some cases the etiology may be multifactorial (Table 13.3).

## Clinical Features

The hemoglobin level at which symptoms of anemia develop depends on two main factors—the rate of development of the anemia and state of the cardiovascular system of the patient. In general, symptoms occur at a higher hemoglobin level with rapidly developing anemia, e.g. due to acute hemorrhage.

Tiredness, lassitude, easy fatigability and generalized muscular weakness are the most common and the earliest symptoms of anemia. In children, this can present as poor feeding, irritability and inadequate school performance. Pallor is the most prominent sign. Pallor of the nail beds, oral mucous membranes and palpebral conjunctivae are a reliable indication of anemia. Observing palmar creases and skin pallor is insufficient in children as the skin creases do not show pigmentation. Facial pallor varies with skin pigmentation and presence of facial edema. Dyspnea on exertion, tachycardia and palpitation are common symptoms. Murmurs become prominent as the degree of anemia increases. Hemic murmurs are mid-systolic 'flow' murmurs, reflecting the increased velocity of blood passing through the valves. They are best heard in the pulmonary area, but audible in all areas corresponding to the heart valves. Systolic bruits and postural hypotension can be demonstrated in patients with moderate to severe anemia. Very severe anemia can precipitate cardiac failure.

Severe anemia is characterized by a high output state with an elevated pulse pressure and a 'collapsing' pulse. Electrocardiographic changes may be found in approximately 30% of patients with hemoglobin of less than 6 g/dL. Findings on ECG are normal QRS waves, depression of the ST segments, and flattening or inversion of T waves.

Central nervous system symptoms such as dizziness, headache, humming in the ears, fainting, tinnitus, lack of

Table 13.3: Important age-related information on history in evaluation of anemia

| | |
|---|---|
| Infants | ***Obstetric history***<br>Maternal anemia, blood loss, collagen vascular diseases, infections, drugs<br>***Perinatal history***<br>• Prematurity<br>• Perinatal blood loss, phlebotomy<br>• Neonatal jaundice (ABO or Rh incompatibility; G6PD deficiency, sepsis)<br>• Hemangiomas<br>• Cephalhematoma<br>***Age of onset of anemia***<br>• *Physiological anemia:* Occurs at 2 months<br>• *Thalassemia major:* Occurs around 9 (6–12) months<br>• Diamond-Blackfan anemia: In newborn period/ infancy<br>***Dietary factors***<br>• Breast milk, formula or cow milk (iron deficiency), cow milk allergy; goat milk (folate deficiency)<br>• Diet, intake of vitamin and hematinics<br>• Adequacy of weaning<br>***Other leads***<br>• Fever, infections, infestations<br>• Jaundice, gallstones, persistent or intermittent jaundice<br>• Chronic illness or medication history<br>• Family history of problems in other siblings<br>• Inherited bone marrow failure syndromes: Dysmorphic features, growth retardation |
| Young children | • Diet, timing and nutritional quality of weaning foods<br>• Pica<br>• Blood loss: Worms, epistaxis, hematuria<br>• Acute illness<br>• Infections: Malaria, tuberculosis<br>• Transient erythroblastopenia of childhood<br>• Family history of thalassemia, sickle cell disease, other hemoglobinopathies<br>• Jaundice, early onset gallstones, leg ulcers: Sickle cell disease, enzyme disorders, or thalassemia intermedia<br>• Recurrent jaundice, blood transfusions: Hemolytic anemias, membranopathies, enzymopathies or congenital dyserythropoietic anemia<br>• Chronic illness, e.g. juvenile rheumatoid arthritis, chronic kidney disease<br>• Medications, e.g. anticonvulsants, ACE inhibitors anticancer drugs<br>• Lead toxicity by exposure to lead-based paints and chemicals |
| Adolescents | History of pica<br>Infections, infestations<br>Acute and chronic illnesses<br>Autoimmune disorders<br>Dietary fads: Vegan diets, ketogenic diet |

concentration and drowsiness, and with severe anemia, clouding of consciousness may occur.

Examination should be done to find etiological clues such as radial limb abnormalities seen in bone marrow failure syndromes; splenomegaly in infants with hemolytic anemia, infection or storage diseases; and lymphadenopathy and hepatosplenomegaly in malignancies or infections. Petechia, purpura, icterus, bossing or other phenotypic abnormalities may help in diagnosis.

## Laboratory Investigations

It is important to know the age of onset and detailed history; this information will provide direction to the laboratory investigation. The complete hemogram will reveal, if there is isolated anemia, or if other cell lines are affected. The red cell indices show the type of anemia, mean corpuscular volume (MCV) denotes the size of the red cells, the mean corpuscular hemoglobin (MCH) and mean corpuscular hemoglobin content (MCHC) provide information on red cell hemoglobinization (Table 13.4). Using the MCV, anemias can be classified into microcytic, normocytic or macrocytic anemia (Figs 13.1–13.3). Abnormal red cell indices can exist even when the underlying disorder is not sufficiently severe to cause anemia. In thalassemia minor or iron deficiency, the MCV, MCH and MCHC are low and in megaloblastic anemia, the MCV is elevated. The red cell distribution width (RDW) gives the size difference in the red blood cells, low RDW means all the red blood cells are



**Table 13.4:** Red cell indices and serum iron studies in normal children

| *Red cell indices* | *Birth* | *0.5–2 yr* | *6–12 yr* | *Girls, 12–18 yr* | *Boys, 12–18 yr* |
|---|---|---|---|---|---|
| Mean corpuscular volume (fl) | 108 | 78 | 86 | 90 | 88 |
| Mean corpuscular hemoglobin (pg) | 34 | 27 | 29 | 30 | 30 |
| Mean corpuscular hemoglobin concentration (g/dL) | 33 | 33 | 34 | 34 | 34 |
| Red cell distribution width (RDW)* | 12.8 ±1.2% | | | | |
| Serum iron | 60–170 µg/dL (10–30 µmol/L) | | | | |
| Serum ferritin, median (range) | 100 (15–300) ng/mL (boys); 40 (15–200) ng/mL (girls) | | | | |
| Total iron binding capacity | 250–400 µg/dL (47–70 µmol/L) | | | | |
| Transferrin saturation** | 20–50% | | | | |

*RDW = Standard deviation (SD) of red blood cell volume × 100/mean corpuscular volume

**Transferrin saturation = Serum iron × 100/total iron binding capacity

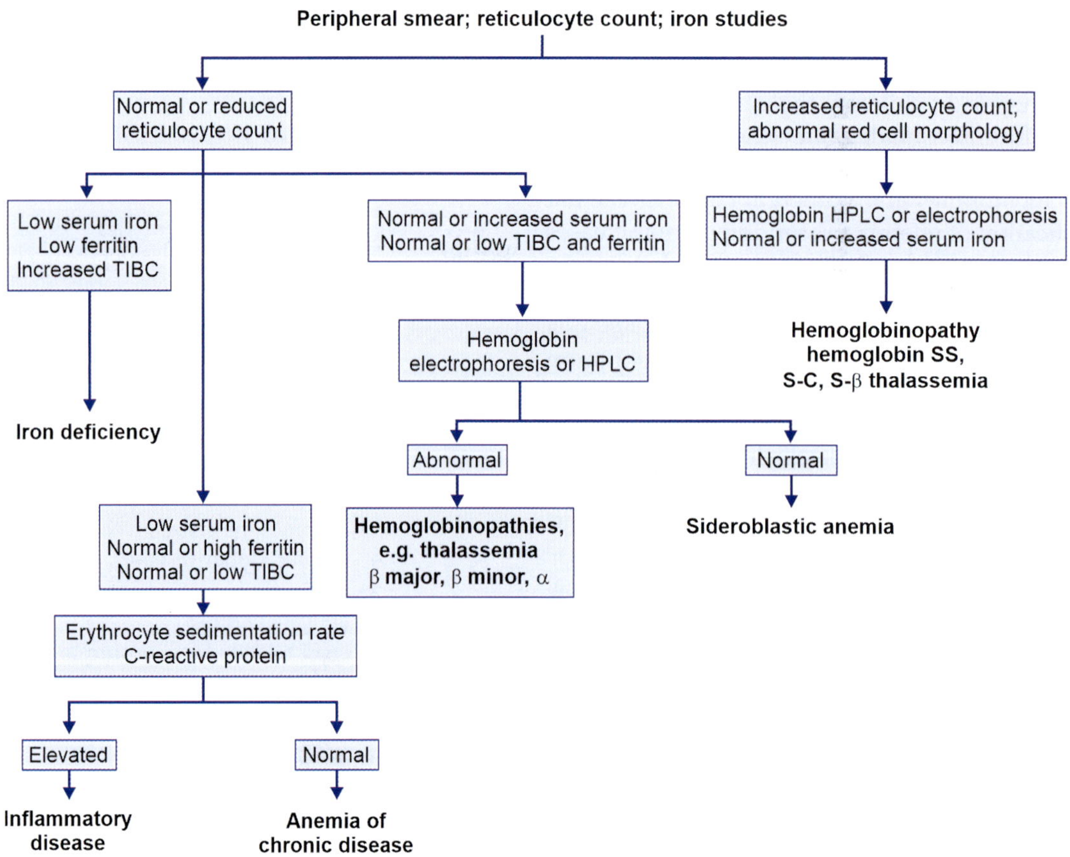


**Fig. 13.1:** Approach to microcytic anemia (mean corpuscular volume <80 fl). HPLC high performance liquid chromatography; TIBC total iron binding capacity

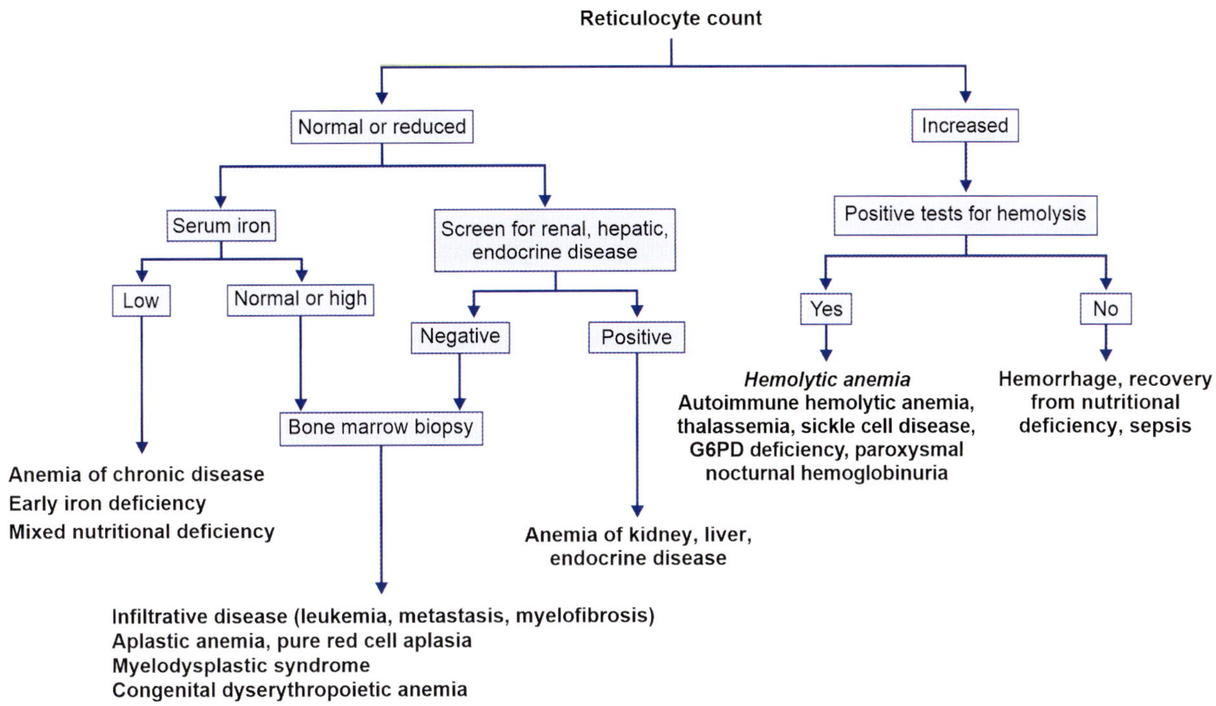


**Fig. 13.2:** Approach to normocytic anemia (mean corpuscular volume 80–100 fl)

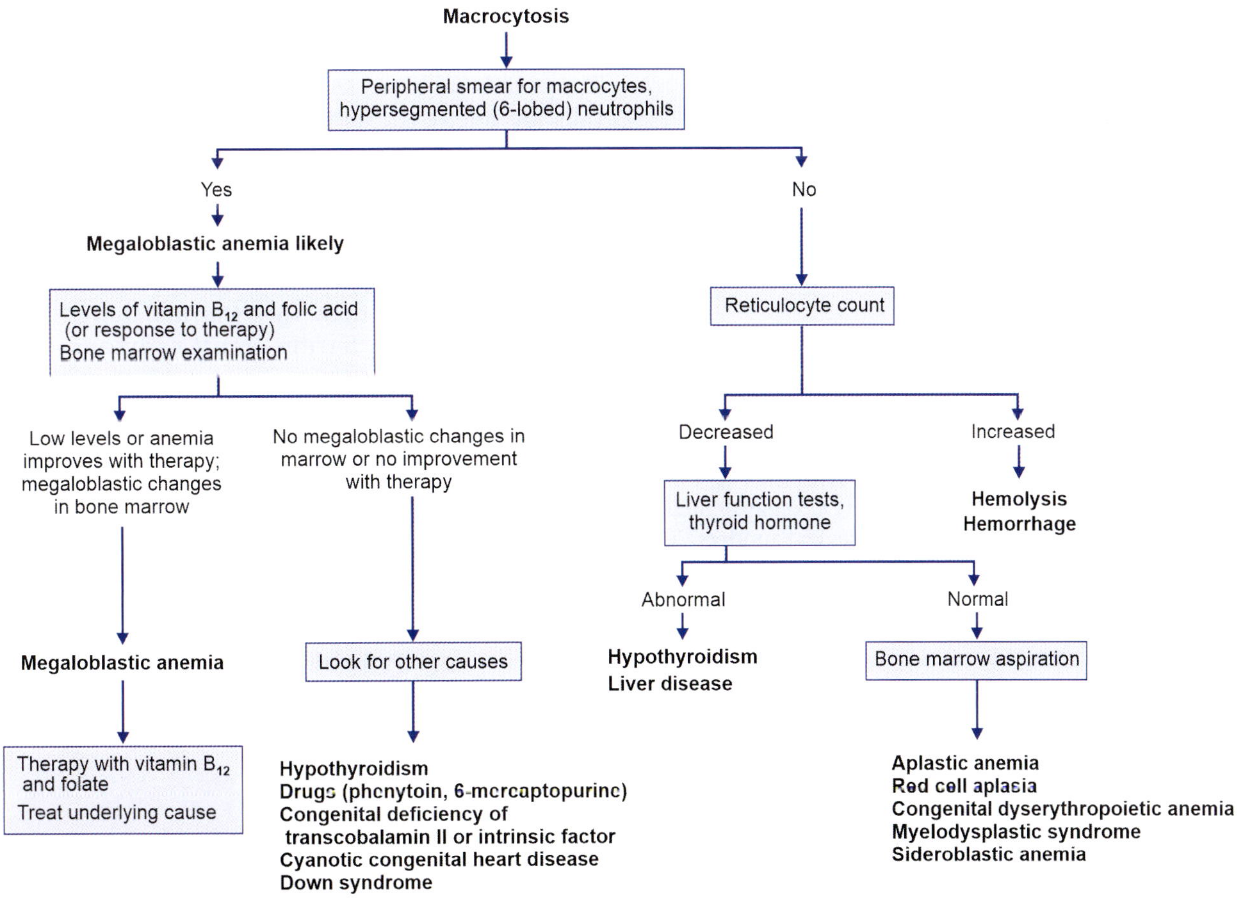


**Fig. 13.3:** Approach to macrocytic anemia (mean corpuscular volume >100 fl)

small and uniform in size, while a large RDW shows that the cells vary greatly in size.

Examination of the peripheral smear reveals the red cell morphology, presence of schistocytes, polychromasia, specific red cell morphology or parasites. When nutritional anemia is suspected, assessment of iron status, vitamin $B_{12}$ and folic acid levels is useful. The reticulocyte count differentiates, if anemia is caused by increased red cell

**Table 13.5:** Etiology of anemia based on the corrected reticulocyte count

*Low reticulocyte count*
- Congenital or acquired, aplastic or hypoplastic anemia
- Transient erythroblastopenia of childhood
- Pure red cell aplasia
- Parvovirus B19 infection
- Deficiency of vitamin B12, folic acid, iron
- Infiltration of bone marrow by malignancy, storage disorder
- Bone marrow suppression after serious infections, radiation or chemotherapy

*High reticulocyte count*
- Hemolytic anemia, including autoimmune and inherited causes (e.g. hereditary spherocytosis)
- Hemorrhage
- Splenic sequestration
- Recovery from deficiency of iron, vitamin $B_{12}$, or folic acid
- Systemic sepsis

destruction or decreased production from the bone marrow. When the hemoglobin is normal, the reticulocyte count is 1–2%. In some cases of anemia, the reticulocyte count may appear elevated, but is insufficient for the degree of anemia. The reticulocyte count corrected for hemoglobin or hematocrit, as follows, helps distinguish between etiologies of anemia (Table 13.5).

Corrected reticulocyte count

= Reticulocyte % × hemoglobin/15, *or*

= Reticulocyte % × patient hematocrit/normal hematocrit for age

In cases of anemia with increased reticulocyte count, a positive Coombs test suggests the diagnosis of immune hemolytic anemia.

## Suggested Reading

1. http://rchiips.org/nfhs/ National Family Health Survey 2019-21 (NFHS-5). India Fact Sheet. International Institute for Population Sciences
2. Orkin SH, Nathan D, Ginsburg D, Look AT, Fisher D, Lux S, (eds). Nathan and Oski's Hematology and Oncology of Infancy and Childhood. 8th edn. Philadelphia: Elsevier Saunders, 2015.

*Competencies:* **PE13.2; PE13.3; PE13.4; PE13.5; PE29.2**

## Iron Deficiency Anemia

Iron deficiency anemia (IDA) occurs when there is a decrease in total iron body content, severe enough to diminish erythropoiesis and cause anemia.

### *Pathophysiology*

Diminished dietary content or reduced iron absorption in the proximal small intestine or excessive loss of body iron can result in iron deficiency; intercurrent infections such as hookworm infestation and malaria compound the problem. Dietary constituents such as phytates, phosphates and tannates can interfere with non-heme iron absorption. Iron is essential for multiple metabolic processes, including oxygen transport, DNA synthesis, and electron transport. Iron deficiency anemia can result in diminished growth and learning and have serious consequences in children. In severe iron deficiency, other iron-containing enzymes are low and can even affect immune and tissue function.

Healthy newborn infants have a total body iron of 250 mg (approximately 80 parts per million, ppm); this decreases to ~60 ppm in the first 6 months of life. Breast milk iron content is more bioavailable than cow milk. Infants who consume cow milk have more iron deficiency because bovine milk has a higher concentration of calcium, which competes with iron for absorption and they may have gastrointestinal blood loss due to cow milk allergy.

### *Clinical Evaluation*

A careful dietary history is important; enquire about type of milk, weaning foods and supplements. Pica increases the risk of helminthic parasites and lead poisoning. The common features of anemia are present in proportion to the severity and rate of development. Behavioral symptoms such as irritability, anorexia usually precede weakness, fatigue, leg cramps, breathlessness and tachycardia. Congestive cardiac failure and splenomegaly may occur with severe, persistent, untreated iron deficiency anemia. Angular stomatitis, glossitis, koilonychia and platynychia are also seen in severe iron deficiency.

### *Laboratory Diagnosis*

The peripheral blood smear (Fig. 13.4) reveals that the red cells are microcytic and hypochromic, with anisocytosis, poikilocytosis, and increased red cell distribution width (RDW). The MCV and MCHC are reduced. Red cell number is reduced, unlike in thalassemias where it is increased.

In iron deficiency, serum iron is reduced while total iron binding capacity (TIBC) is increased; transferrin saturation is reduced to less than 16% (normal range 25–50%). Reduction in serum ferritin occurs early, and correlates well with the total body iron stores. However, ferritin is

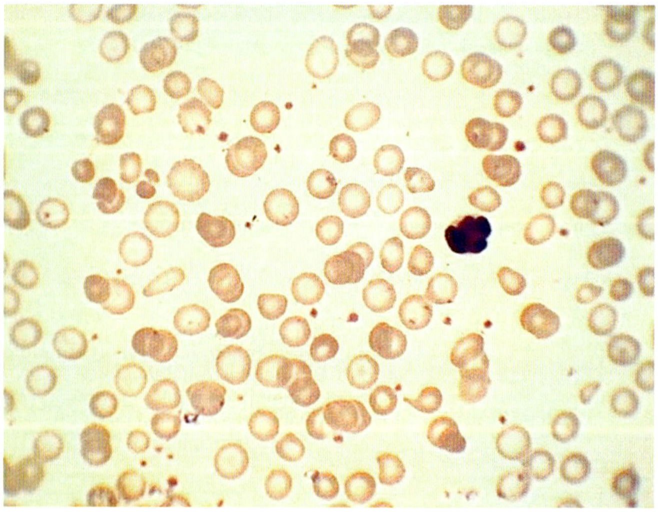

**Fig. 13.4:** Peripheral smear from a child with iron deficiency anemia, shows microcytosis (the red blood cells are smaller than the small lymphocyte in the field), hypochromia (central pallor >1/3rd of cell diameter), thrombocytosis, and a few ovalocytes and tear drop cells (moderate anisopoikilocytosis). Jenner-Giemsa ×1000

an acute phase reactant and is elevated in inflammatory conditions. High free erythroprotoporphyrin (FEP) is seen before anemia develops.

### Treatment

The cause of anemia should be identified and corrected. Hookworm infestation is the commonest cause of occult gastrointestinal blood loss at all ages. Dietary counseling and treatment of any other causative factors are required to prevent recurrence or failure of therapy (Table 13.6). Close follow-up is required to assess for adequate response and correction of anemia.

***Oral iron medications:*** Oral iron preparations should be taken on an empty stomach or in between meals for best absorption. The most effective and economical oral preparation is ferrous sulfate (20% elemental iron). About 10–20% patients will develop gastrointestinal side effects such as nausea, epigastric discomfort, vomiting, constipation and diarrhea. Enteric-coated preparations have fewer side effects, but are less efficacious and more expensive. In children, the dose for treatment of anemia is 3–6 mg/kg/day elemental iron. The reticulocyte count should increase within 72–96 hours after initiating therapy. After correction of anemia, oral iron should be continued for 4–6 months to replenish iron stores.

***Parenteral iron:*** The indications of parenteral iron therapy are limited to conditions such as: (i) Intolerance to oral iron; (ii) malabsorption states; and (iii) ongoing blood loss at a rate where the oral replacement cannot match iron loss. The use of intravenous preparations is increasing as these are safe and effective. Iron sucrose preparation is most commonly used in children with advanced chronic kidney disease on maintenance hemodialysis and in inflammatory bowel disease. Injection iron sucrose can be given as 1 mg/kg per session dialysis for correction of anemia, and subsequently at a dose of 1–2 mg/kg per week of dialysis as maintenance dose. The preparation is diluted in 150 mL of normal saline and administered as a slow intravenous infusion over 30–90 minutes. Injection ferric carboxymaltose is approved for children with malabsorption as a single dose of 15 mg/kg up to 1000 mg given over 15–20 minutes by intravenous route (Table 13.7).

**Table 13.6:** Reasons for non-response to hematinic therapy for iron deficiency anemia

| |
|---|
| Poor compliance with therapy, inadequate dosing |
| Poorly absorbed iron preparations, e.g. enteric coated |
| Use of antacids or H2 blockers causing achlorhydria |
| Ongoing blood loss at a rate greater than iron absorption |
| Associated vitamin $B_{12}$ or folic acid deficiency |
| Malabsorption states, e.g. celiac disease, giardiasis, *Helicobacter pylori* infection, inflammatory bowel disease, autoimmune gastritis |
| Underlying hemolytic anemia, inflammation or infection |
| Sideroblastic anemia |
| Congenital causes, e.g. *TMPRSS6* variations |

TMPRSS6 transmembrane protease, serine 6

**Table 13.7:** Dose calculation for parenteral iron

*Calculation of total iron deficit for initial repletion*

Total cumulative dose (mg) = [Target Hb* – actual Hb*] × weight (kg) × 2.4 + [15 × weight (kg)]

*Dosing*

- Divide cumulative dose; administer doses every 3–7 days until total dose is administered
- Recommended maximum single dose is 300 mg or 7 mg iron/kg, to prevent adverse effects

*Administration*

- Test dose is not necessary in children over 1 month of age
- Dilute doses ≤100 mg 1:1 with normal saline; infuse over 30 minutes
- Dilute doses of 100–200 mg 1:1 in normal saline; infuse over 60 minutes
- Dilute dose of 300 mg in 250 mL normal saline; infuse over at least 90 minutes

*Hemoglobin (Hb) in g/dL

### Blood Transfusions

As iron deficiency anemia is readily corrected with medication, blood transfusions should be avoided. Packed red cell transfusions are needed in emergencies where the rate of blood loss exceeds the expected rise of hemoglobin, for urgent surgery, hemorrhage or severe anemia with congestive cardiac failure. In very severe anemia with congestive cardiac failure, transfusions must be given very slowly (2–3 mL/kg) with monitoring and, if necessary, diuretic therapy.

### Suggested Reading


1. Crary SE, Hall K, Buchanan GR. Intravenous iron sucrose for children with iron deficiency failing to respond to oral iron therapy. Pediatr Blood Cancer 2011; 56: 615–19.
2. Kapil U, Kapil R, Gupta A. Prevention and control of anemia amongst children and adolescents: Theory and practice in India. Indian J Pediatr 2019; 86: 523–31.
3. Karelia BN, Buch JG. Analysis of hematinic formulations available in the Indian market. J Pharmacol Pharmacother 2012; 3: 35–38.


*Competency:* **PE29.3**

## Megaloblastic Anemia

Megaloblastic anemia is a distinct type of anemia characterized by red blood cells, which are macrocytic (MCV >100–120 fl; Fig 13.3). Concomitant iron deficiency can lead to less marked changes. The erythroid precursors show nuclear dysmaturity. The incidence varies with the dietary practices and socioeconomic patterns. A study in north Indian children showed folate deficiency in 6.8%, vitamin $B_{12}$ deficiency in 32%, and combined deficiency in 20%.

### Pathophysiology

Megaloblastic changes affect all hematopoietic cell lines with resultant anemia, thrombocytopenia and leukopenia. DNA synthesis is impaired because of lack of methyltetrahydrofolate (a folic acid derivative); vitamin $B_{12}$ plays an important role as cofactor in this reaction which is necessary for DNA base synthesis.

### Etiology

The two most common causes of megaloblastic anemia are vitamin $B_{12}$ deficiency (cobalamin) and folic acid deficiency (Table 13.8). Folate deficiency is caused by decreased ingestion, impaired absorption (e.g. celiac disease, malabsorption states) and impaired utilization. Vitamin $B_{12}$ deficiency is caused by its dietary deficiency due to vegan or other unsatisfactory diets. Maternal deficiency and prolonged exclusive breastfeeding may result in deficiency in infancy. Other important causes are infections, medications and rare inherited disorders.

### Clinical Manifestations

Anemia, anorexia, irritability and easy fatigability are common. Features characteristically found in megaloblastic anemia include glossitis, stomatitis and hyperpigmentation of the skin on knuckles and terminal phalanges; 30–40% have enlargement of liver and spleen. Neurologic signs may precede the onset of anemia. Petechiae and hemorrhagic manifestations have been reported in 25% cases. Pancytopenia and hepatosplenomegaly can make it difficult to differentiate from leukemia or aplastic anemia. The child should be evaluated for signs of malabsorption such as weight loss, abdominal distension, diarrhea, and steatorrhea.

Neurologic examination may reveal loss of position and vibratory sensation, which are the earliest neurologic signs. Later, other posterior and lateral column deficits may be found. Memory loss, confusion and neuropsychiatric symptoms can occur. Persistence of neurological sequelae can be found even after treatment of the deficiency.

**Table 13.8:** Causes of megaloblastic anemia

| |
|---|
| *Folate deficiency* |
| • Decreased ingestion or impaired absorption: Celiac disease, malabsorption states |
| • Increased requirements: Infancy, hyperthyroidism, chronic hemolytic disease |
| • Prolonged parenteral nutrition; losses during hemodialysis |
| *Vitamin $B_{12}$ (cobalamin) deficiency* |
| • Decreased ingestion: Vegetarian or vegan diet |
| • Impaired absorption: Intestinal microbes (*Giardia*, *H. pylori*, HIV); intrinsic intestinal disease; therapy with proton pump inhibitors |
| • Prolonged antibiotic use: Change in normal gastrointestinal flora |
| *Medications* |
| • Impaired folate absorption: Phenytoin, phenobarbital |
| • Interference with folate metabolism: Methotrexate, trimethoprim, pyrimethamine |
| • Purine analogs: 6-mercaptopurine, 6-thioguanine, azathioprine |
| • Ribonucleotide reductase inhibitors: Hydroxyurea, cytarabine arabinoside |
| • Pyrimidine analogs: Zidovudine, 5-fluorouracil |
| • Interference with cobalamin metabolism: Metformin, neomycin |
| *Inborn errors of folate metabolism* |
| • Dihydrofolate reductase deficiency |
| • N5-methyltetrahydrofolate homocysteine methyltransferase deficiency |
| *Inborn errors of cobalamin metabolism* |
| • Deficiency of transcobalamin I and II |
| • Defect in intestinal receptor (Imerslünd-Grasbeck syndrome) |
| • Methylmalonic aciduria |
| • Homocystinuria |
| • Congenital intrinsic factor deficiency |
| *Other inborn errors* |
| • Hereditary orotic aciduria |
| • Lesch-Nyhan syndrome |
| • Thiamine responsive megaloblastic anemia |

### Laboratory Evaluation

Red cell indices reveal macrocytic red cells (MCV >110 fl is highly suggestive of megaloblastic anemia), leukopenia and thrombocytopenia. Hypersegmented neutrophils (nucleus with >5 lobes) in more than 5% of neutrophils may be seen (Fig. 13.5). If available, blood $B_{12}$ and folate levels are assayed before starting supplementation. Serum level of homocysteine is increased in folate or vitamin $B_{12}$ deficiency and other conditions; however, high serum level of methylmalonic acid (MMA) is seen only in vitamin $B_{12}$ deficiency. Serum chemistry may show elevated lactate dehydrogenase and mild jaundice.

Bone marrow evaluation should be performed in any child with more than one abnormal hematological cell line. Bone marrow is indicated, if the history or labs are inconclusive, as it can help to rule out leukemia, myelodysplasia, and aplastic anemia. In megaloblastic anemia, the bone marrow is cellular, and red blood cell precursors show nuclear-cytoplasmic asynchrony. Erythroid and even granulocytic precursors may be dysplastic and confused with myelodysplastic syndrome. However, these changes get corrected following vitamin $B_{12}$ and folate supplementation.

### Differential Diagnosis

Other causes of macrocytosis should be considered in the differential diagnosis of megaloblastic anemia. These causes include aplastic anemia and other marrow

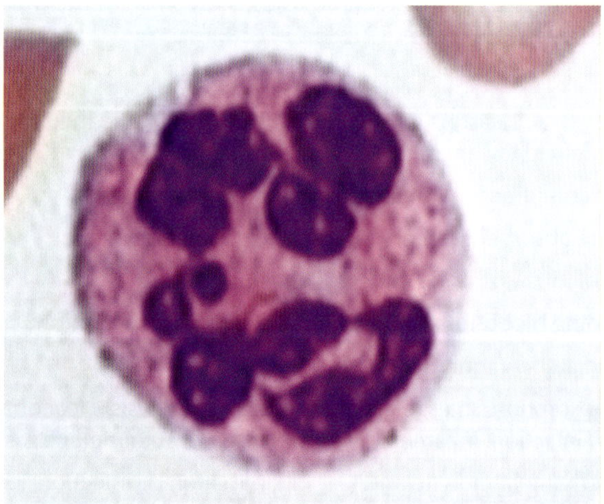

**Fig. 13.5:** Peripheral smear of a 12-year-old girl with megaloblastic anemia showing hypersegmented polymorphonuclear cell. Note that the nucleus has more than 5 lobes

failure syndromes (pure red cell aplasia, Fanconi anemia, transient erythroblastopenia of childhood), congenital dyserythropoietic anemia, chronic liver disease, hypothyroidism, cold agglutinin disease, myelodysplastic syndromes, and HIV.

### Treatment

The treatment depends on the underlying cause. If the cause cannot be determined, a therapeutic trial of folate (1–5 mg/day) and vitamin $B_{12}$ (1000 μg) can be given. Only folate therapy may correct the anemia, but can worsen the cobalamin-induced neurological problems, so both must be given together.

A parenteral dose of vitamin $B_{12}$ at a dose of 1 mg (1000 μg) is recommended in children older than 10 years, and administered intramuscularly or intravenously (check preparation). A decrease in MCV, increase in the reticulocyte count, and improvement in platelet and neutrophil counts are observed within a few days of therapy. Hemoglobin rise may take 1–2 weeks. Vitamin $B_{12}$ (1000 μg) should be given parenterally daily for 2 weeks, then weekly until the hematocrit value is normal. Therapy is continued monthly lifelong in patients with pernicious anemia and malabsorptive states. Patients with neurological complications should receive 1000 μg everyday for 2 weeks, then every 2 weeks for 6 months, and subsequently, monthly for life. Lower doses (250 μg) can be used in infants and young children.

Folate deficiency due to dietary insufficiency or increased demands is best treated with folate supplements. Folate deficiency caused by the use of anti-folate medications is best remedied by reducing or eliminating the implicating drug and supplementation. Patients with celiac disease require treatment of the underlying disorder and adequate supplementation. Folate is available as a 5 mg tablet and overdose is not associated with adverse effects; a dose of 1–5 mg/day is administered for 3–4 weeks.

### Suggested Reading


1. Chandra J. Megaloblastic anemia: Back in focus. Indian J Pediatr 2010;77:795–99.
2. Green R, Datta Mitra A. Megaloblastic anemias: Nutritional and other causes. Med Clin North Am 2017;101:297–317.
3. Seth T, Suri V, Balat D, Murthy S, Agarwal A, et al. Indian Academy of Pediatrics. Megaloblastic anemia: Standard treatment guidelines 2022.


*Competencies:* **PE29.4; PE29.10; PE29.11; PE29.15**

## APPROACH TO HEMOLYTIC ANEMIAS

The term 'hemolytic anemia' is limited to conditions in which the rate of red cell destruction is accelerated and the ability of the bone marrow to respond to anemia is unimpaired. Under maximal stimulation, the normal marrow is capable of increasing its production rate to 6 to 8 times its basal level. The reticulocyte count is useful in determining the rate of red cell destruction. The normal reticulocyte count value in the newborn is 3.2 ±1.4% and in children 1.2 ±0.7%.

### Etiology

Hemolytic disorders may be divided into inherited and acquired varieties (Table 13.9). This classification has a pathogenetic significance because the nature of hereditary lesions differs from that of acquired. Most intrinsic defects are inherited and the extrinsic are acquired. There are a few exceptions to this generalization; paroxysmal nocturnal hemoglobinuria, is an acquired disorder characterized by an intrinsic red cell defect.

### Clinical Signs

In acute hemolysis, the symptoms are related to the rate of fall of hemoglobin. If the hemolysis is rapid, the symptoms are more numerous and pronounced. Jaundice is a prominent finding in most hemolytic anemias. Increase in icterus, anemia, presence of fever, and red urine occurs in intravascular hemolysis. Splenomegaly is seen in autoimmune and many congenital types of hemolytic anemias. Other features include gallstones and icterus (hereditary spherocytosis), hemolytic or thalassemic facies (Fig. 13.6), splenomegaly (thalassemia major or intermedia, congenital dyserythropoietic anemia (CDA) and leg ulcers (sickle cell disease).

### Laboratory Manifestations

Laboratory test findings in hemolytic anemia can be divided into three groups: (i) Increase in erythrocyte destruction; (ii) compensatory increase in the rate of erythropoiesis; and (iii) specific features found only in a particular type of hemolytic anemia (Table 13.10).

An elevated corrected reticulocyte count may be the only manifestation of mild hemolytic anemia in a well-

**Table 13.9:** Causes of hemolytic anemia

| |
|---|
| ***Acquired*** |
| *Mechanical:* Macroangiopathic (artificial heart valves, march hemoglobinuria); microangiopathic (disseminated intravascular coagulation, hemolytic uremic syndrome, thrombotic thrombocytopenic purpura) |
| *Infections:* Malaria, kala-azar, *Clostridium welchii* |
| *Antibody mediated:* Autoimmune hemolytic anemia (warm and cold types) |
| *Transfusion reactions:* Immediate and delayed |
| Hemolytic disease of the newborn |
| *Drugs:* Cefotetan, ceftriaxone |
| Hypersplenism |
| Cryopathy, e.g. cold agglutinin disease, paroxysmal cold hemoglobinuria |
| Physical injury, e.g. burns |
| *Chemical injury:* Snake bite, lead and arsenic toxicity |
| ***Inherited*** |
| Hemoglobinopathies, e.g. thalassemia, sickle cell disease |
| Red cell enzyme defect, e.g. glucose-6-phosphate dehydrogenase deficiency |
| Disorders of the cytoskeletal membrane, e.g. hereditary spherocytosis |
| Unstable hemoglobins |
| Lipid membrane defects, e.g. abetalipoproteinemia |
| Porphyria |

**Table 13.10:** Investigations in patients with hemolytic anemia

| *Features of accelerated erythrocyte destruction* | *Features of accelerated erythropoiesis* |
|---|---|
| Fall in hemoglobin >1.0 g/dL per week<br>Increased serum unconjugated bilirubin<br>Increased urinary urobilinogen excretion<br>Increased lactate dehydrogenase<br>Reduced haptoglobin and hemopexin | *Peripheral blood:* Polychromasia, reticulocytosis, macrocytosis, increase in nucleated red cells<br>*Bone marrow:* Erythroid hyperplasia<br>*Iron kinetic studies:* Increased plasma iron turnover, increased erythrocyte iron turnover |

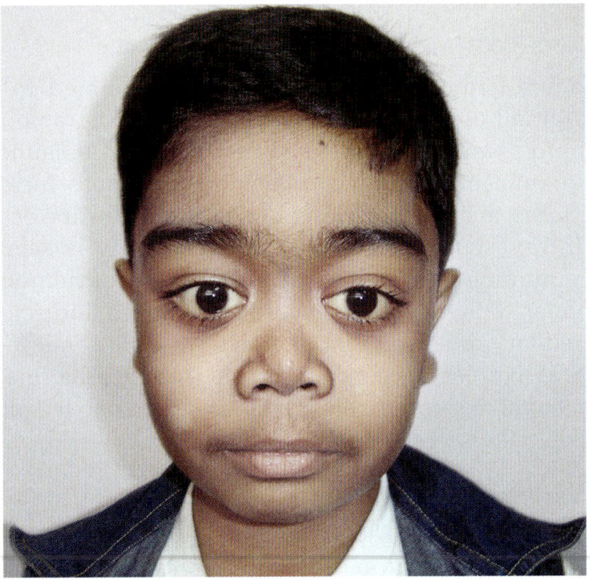

**Fig. 13.6:** Child with hemolytic anemia, showing hemolytic facies and icterus

compensated child. The Coombs test is the most important initial test for the etiology of hemolysis. A direct antiglobin (direct Coombs) test will be positive in most cases of immune hemolytic anemias. A positive test means that the erythrocyte is coated with IgG or C3 component of complement. The test may be rarely negative in about 2–5% of immune-mediated cases.

Haptoglobin and hemopexin are proteins that bind to hemoglobin and heme released from red cells following their destruction. The protein complexes formed after intravascular hemolysis are removed by circulation. As a consequence, haptoglobin and hemopexin levels are low in patients who have hemolytic anemia. When haptoglobin is saturated, free plasma hemoglobin can be detected. The indirect bilirubin level provides evidence for a hemolytic process; however, it is an insensitive measurement of hemolysis as it is only elevated when liver function is impaired or when hemolysis is extensive.

***Hallmarks of intravascular and extravascular hemolysis:*** Intravascular hemolysis occurs when the released hemoglobin is released into the plasma (hemoglobinemia). A part of the circulating free hemoglobin is converted to methemoglobin that binds with albumin to form methemalbumin that confers a brown color to the plasma. When the amount of hemoglobin exceeds the haptoglobin binding capacity it is excreted in the urine (hemoglobinuria), and to some extent reabsorbed in the proximal renal tubules. The loss of heme laden tubular cells is seen as hemosiderinuria. In extravascular hemolysis, hyperbilirubinemia is seen, but no free hemoglobin is seen in the plasma. Hence, no hemoglobinemia, hemoglobinuria or hemosiderinuria is found.

A peripheral smear is useful for evaluation. Increased spherocytes may be seen in hereditary spherocytosis and autoimmune hemolytic anemia, bite cells suggest glucose 6-phosphate dehydrogenase (G6PD) enzyme deficiency, microcytosis with many fragmented red cells suggests thalassemia, and thrombocytopenia with schistocytosis (fragmented red cells) is seen in microangiopathic hemolytic anemia or disseminated intravascular coagulopathy (DIC).

The Ham test, or sucrose hemolysis test, may be positive in a patient with underlying paroxysmal nocturnal hemoglobinuria (PNH) (red cells lysed by patient's acidified sera) and type II congenital dyserythropoietic anemia (in which the red cells lysed by other acidified sera but not patient's sera). A better test for PNH is the assay for deficiency of complement regulatory proteins on red blood cells such as CD55 (decay accelerating factor) and CD59 (membrane inhibitor of reactive lysis). Granulocyte and monocyte assays by flow cytometry are most specific for PNH. A bone marrow test is usually not required for diagnosis of hemolytic anemias, where it will show erythroid hyperplasia. The exception is dyserythropoietic anemia, where it can help make the diagnosis and identify the subtype.

### Management

In an acute attack of hemolysis, it is important to maintain fluid balance and urine output. Management of shock is by the usual measures, but blood transfusions, so useful in acute anemia of other types, must be used with caution in patients with acquired hemolytic anemia. Even with careful blood matching, rapid destruction of transfused packed red blood cells may lead to kidney dysfunction. Therapy varies according to the diagnosis.

## HEREDITARY SPHEROCYTOSIS

Hereditary spherocytosis is an autosomal dominant cause of chronic hemolytic anemia. Several mutations have been attributed to cause this disorder, the mutations lead to membrane protein defects on the red blood cell wall and result in instability of spectrin and ankyrin, the major skeletal membrane proteins. The degree of skeletal membrane protein deficiency correlates with the degree of hemolysis. The structural deficiency leads to membrane instability, loss of surface area, and abnormal membrane permeability, leading to the spherocytic red blood cell. The spleen is the site of destruction of these nondeformable erythrocytes. There is an increase in osmotic fragility after 18–24 hours incubation of blood at 37°C, which can be used for diagnosis. Special tests to characterize the defect by flow cytometry or next generation sequencing are available.

Patients with hereditary spherocytosis may have a mild to moderate chronic hemolytic anemia. The MCV is decreased and MCHC is increased due to cellular dehydration. The red cell distribution width (RDW) is increased due to the presence of spherocytes and there is marked increase in reticulocytes. Patients present with anemia and jaundice; the degree varies between other family members. Splenomegaly is found in over 75% patients. Pigment gallstones are frequently found, and the incidence increases with age.

Patients require lifelong folic acid supplementation of 1–5 mg/day. Splenectomy does not cure the hemolytic disorder, but may reduce the degree of hemolysis. It is the treatment of choice in patients who have severe hemolysis and high blood transfusion requirement. In pediatric patients who have an excessively large spleen, splenectomy diminishes the risk of traumatic splenic rupture. Splenectomy may be performed after 6-years of age with pre-surgical immunizations for *Hemophilus influenzae* type B, *Streptococcus pneumoniae* and *Neisseria meningitidis*. Prophylactic penicillin is required to prevent sepsis, this is usually given till early adulthood.

## ABNORMALITIES IN RED CELL GLYCOLYSIS

Glucose is the primary metabolic substrate for erythrocytes. Since the mature red cell does not contain mitochondria, glucose is metabolized by anerobic pathways; the two main metabolic pathways are Embden-Meyerhof pump (EMP) and the hexose monophosphate shunt (HMS). The EMP accounts for 90% of glucose utilization. The inability to maintain adenosine triphosphate required for cellular functions such as deformability, membrane lipid turnover and membrane permeability results in a shortened red blood cell lifespan. The HMS is responsible for the remaining 10% of glucose metabolism, and generates substrates which protect the red cells against oxidant injury. A defect in the HMS causes oxidized hemoglobin (Heinz bodies), lipids and membrane proteins to collect in the red cell and results in hemolysis. The reticulocyte count is raised, and bone marrow shows erythroid hyperplasia.

### Glucose-6-Phosphate Dehydrogenase Deficiency

Glucose-6-phosphate dehydrogenase (G6PD) deficiency is the most common red blood cell enzyme deficiency. It is an X-linked disorder with full expression in affected males. These children may present with jaundice in neonatal period or have bouts of jaundice precipitated by fever or medications. Many variants of G6PD deficiency have been identified by their biochemical and molecular differences. They vary in antioxidant reserve and enzyme levels. After oxidant exposure, hemoglobin is oxidized to methemoglobin and denatured to form intracellular inclusions also known as Heinz bodies. These Heinz bodies get attached to the red cell membrane and aggregate intrinsic membrane proteins such as band 3. Reticuloendothelial cells identify these changes as a new antigenic site on the red cell membrane and ingests a part of the RBC (resulting in bite cells), shortening the life of the cell.

The hallmarks of the intravascular hemolytic crises are pallor, icterus, hemoglobinemia (free hemoglobin in plasma), hemoglobinuria and increase in size of the spleen. Plasma haptoglobin and hemopexin are low. The peripheral blood smear shows fragmented bite cells and polychromasia. Special stains demonstrate Heinz bodies during the initial few days of hemolysis. The diagnosis of G6PD deficiency is based on family history, clinical findings, laboratory features and exposure to oxidants prior to the hemolytic event. Confirmation of the diagnosis is by quantitative enzyme assay or molecular gene analysis. Management consists of supportive care for the acute crisis (hydration, transfusions, if needed, and monitoring) along with folic acid supplementation. Counseling to avoid the intake of oxidant drugs is imperative **(Table 13.11)**.

### Pyruvate Kinase Deficiency

Pyruvate kinase deficiency is an EMP enzyme defect, inherited in an autosomal recessive manner. This changes metabolism in the RBC and causes deficiency in ATP. Homozygotes present with splenomegaly, icterus and hemolytic anemia and heterozygotes are asymptomatic. The clinical spectrum is variable. Splenectomy is a therapeutic option in these patients, though not curative. The reticulocyte count increases dramatically after splenectomy. Folic acid supplementation is required to prevent megaloblastic complications due to relative folate deficiency. Therapy with mitapivat, which upregulates erythrocyte pyruvate kinase, increases adenosine triphosphate (ATP) production and reduces levels of 2,3-diphosphoglycerate is approved for use in the patients.

## AUTOIMMUNE HEMOLYTIC ANEMIA

Autoimmune hemolytic anemia (AIHA) is caused by autoantibodies targeting the red blood cells. It may arise as an isolated problem (idiopathic) or as a complication of an infection (upper respiratory tract viral infections, mononucleosis, and cytomegalovirus infection); along with systemic lupus erythematosus or other autoimmune syndromes; immunodeficiency states; or even malignancies.

#### *Symptoms and Signs*

AIHA has an acute onset, is manifested by sudden onset of weakness, pallor, fatigue and dark urine. Jaundice is a prominent finding and splenomegaly is often present. Some cases may relapse after therapy or rarely become chronic. Clinical evidence of an underlying disease may be present.

**Table 13.11:** Drugs that cause oxidant stress and hemolysis in patients with glucose-6-phosphate dehydrogenase deficiency

| |
|---|
| *Sulfonamides:* Sulfamethoxazole |
| *Antimalarials:* Primaquine, quinine |
| *Analgesics:* Aspirin, non-steroidal anti-inflammatory drugs, phenazopyridine (pyridium) |
| *Others:* Nitrofurantoin, dapsone, methylene blue, rasburicase, toluidine blue, nalidixic acid, furazolidine, quinidine |

### Laboratory Findings

The anemia is normochromic and normocytic. It may vary from mild to severe (hemoglobin concentration <5 g/dL). The reticulocyte count is increased. Spherocytes and nucleated red cells may be seen on the peripheral blood smear. Other data consistent with hemolysis includes increased levels of lactate dehydrogenase, indirect and total bilirubin, aspartate aminotransferase, and urinary urobilinogen. Intravascular hemolysis is indicated by hemoglobinemia or hemoglobinuria. Examination of the bone marrow shows marked erythroid hyperplasia, but is seldom required.

Serologic studies are helpful in defining pathophysiology, planning therapeutic strategies, and assessing prognosis. In almost all cases, the direct Coombs test is positive. Further evaluation allows distinction into one of three syndromes: (a) The presence of IgG on the patient's red blood cells, maximal *in vitro* antibody activity at 37°C, specificity for Rh-like antigen constitute *warm AIHA* with extravascular destruction by the reticuloendothelial system. This can also be due to many drugs causing hapten or autoantibody type hemolysis. (b) In contrast, the detection of complement alone on red blood cells, optimal reactivity *in vitro* at 4°C and i or I antigen specificity is diagnostic of *cold AIHA* with intravascular hemolysis. This condition is usually found only in adults. In children, Donath-Landsteiner hemolytic anemia, usually associated with an acute viral syndrome is common and mediated by cold hemolysis. This paroxysmal cold hemoglobinuria is identical to cold AIHA, except for P antigen specificity and the exhibition of *in vitro* hemolysis. Paroxysmal cold hemoglobinuria is associated with infections, such as *Mycoplasma*, Epstein-Barr virus and cytomegalovirus. (c) Occasionally IgG and complement-associated AIHA due to warm antibody or, very rarely, due to drug-associated AIHA may occur.

### Complications

The anemia may be severe and result in cardiovascular collapse, requiring urgent management. The complications of the underlying disease, such as systemic lupus or an immunodeficiency state, may be present.

### Treatment

Patients with warm AIHA (in which hemolysis is extravascular) respond well to prednisone 1 mg/kg for 4–8 weeks or till the hemoglobin is stable. After the initial treatment, the dose of corticosteroids must be tapered very slowly over 4–6 months. Some patients respond to 1 g/kg per day of intravenous immunoglobulin (IVIG) for 2 days. Splenectomy does lead to sustained remission in ~50%, but should be limited to selected patients. In severe cases, unresponsive to steroids or dependent on steroids, other immunosuppressive agents such as cyclophosphamide, azathioprine, cyclosporine and rituximab may be considered. Work-up and treatment for primary immunodeficiency or autoimmune lymphoproliferative syndrome may be useful.

Patients with cold AIHA and paroxysmal cold hemoglobinuria are less likely to respond to corticosteroids or even intravenous immunoglobulin. These syndromes are associated with infections and have an acute, self-limited course; supportive care may be all that is necessary.

Transfusion may be necessary in patients with severe anemia but should be monitored closely. In most patients, crossmatch compatible blood will be difficult to arrange, and consultation with the transfusion medicine team is important. Transfusions must be conducted carefully, beginning with a test dose.

### Prognosis

In general, children with warm AIHA are at greater risk for more severe and chronic disease with higher morbidity and mortality rates. Hemolysis and the positive antiglobulin tests may continue for months or years. Patients with cold AIHA or paroxysmal cold hemoglobinuria usually have acute self-limited disease (<3 months).

## Suggested Reading


1. Choudhry VP, Seth T, Saxena R. Hemolytic anemias. deGruchy's Clinical Haematology in Medical Practice. Wiley India, 6th edn, 2013; pp146–83.
2. Go RS, Winters JL, Kay NE. How I treat autoimmune hemolytic anemia. Blood 2017; 129: 2971–79.
3. Michalak SS, Olewicz-Gawlik, et al. Autoimmune hemolytic anemia: Current knowledge and perspectives. Immunity and Ageing 2020;17; 38.


*Competencies:* **PE29.11; PE29.13; PE29.16**

## THALASSEMIAS

The major hemoglobin in children after 1-yr of age, called HbA, constitutes approximately 90% of all hemoglobin, while a minor component, HbA2, accounts for 2–3%. The main hemoglobin in fetal life is HbF, of which only traces remain after 1-yr of life.

The word thalassemia is a Greek term derived from *thalassa*, which means 'the sea', and *emia*, which means 'related to blood'. Thalassemias are hemoglobinopathies that occur due to mutations in the globin gene and over 200 mutations are described. β (beta) thalassemia carrier rates reported in Indians varies in different communities from 3–17%. Thalassemia major is inherited in an autosomal recessive manner. When a person carries a single mutation on only one of their alleles, they are called thalassemia trait or carriers. When two persons with thalassemia trait/carriers have a child, they may inherit the mutations from both parents, resulting in mutations on both their alleles, leading to thalassemia disease (intermedia or major).

## Pathophysiology

The homozygous β gene mutation leads to an alteration in the rate of globin chain production. A decrease in the rate of production of a globin (α, β, γ, δ) impedes hemoglobin synthesis and creates an imbalance with normally produced globin chains. Because two types of chains (α and non-α) pair with each other at a ratio close to 1:1 to form normal hemoglobin, the excess of the normally produced type is present and this accumulates in the cell as an unstable product, leading to early destruction of the red blood cells, before their usual 120-days lifespan. The type of thalassemia usually carries the name of the under produced chain or chains. The reduction may vary from a slight decrease to a complete absence. When β chains are produced at a lower rate, the thalassemia is termed β+, whereas $\beta^0$ thalassemia indicates a complete absence of production of β chains from the involved allele. The disease is inherited in a Mendelian recessive fashion. Carriers who are heterozygous for the mutation are easy to identify and screen, though they are asymptomatic. Homozygous thalassemia major occurs when two thalassemia carriers marry; there is 25% risk that they will have an affected child who inherits the mutation from both parents. The risk can be zero, if only one parent is a carrier or by doing prenatal testing of the baby at 10–12 weeks of gestation.

### Presentation

Infants with β thalassemia major usually demonstrate no symptoms until about six months of age (when β chains are needed to pair with α chains to form HbA, after γ chain production is turned off). However, the condition may not be recognized because of the delay in cessation of HbF production in some cases.

Symptoms of severe anemia as intolerance to exercise, irritability, heart murmur or even signs of frank heart failure may be present. Severe pallor and hepatosplenomegaly are almost always present. Bony abnormalities, such as frontal bossing, prominent facial bones and dental malocclusion are usually present (Fig. 13.6). Ineffective erythropoiesis creates a hypermetabolic state associated with fever and failure to thrive. Icterus is usually not present initially, but at a later age some patients have mild to moderate jaundice due to liver dysfunction from iron overload and chronic hepatitis. Hyperuricemia may be encountered.

#### Spectrum of β Thalassemia Disease

***Thalassemia major:*** This condition is characterized by transfusion-dependent anemia (onset 9–12 months), splenomegaly, bone deformities, growth retardation, and hemolytic facies in untreated or inadequately treated individuals. Examination of the peripheral blood smear shows severe hypochromia, microcytosis, marked anisocytosis, fragmented red blood cells, polychromasia, normoblasts and occasionally immature leukocytes. Organomegaly is mild in well-transfused patients, but is moderate in patients receiving irregular or inadequate transfusion support.

***Thalassemia intermedia:*** Also called non-transfusion dependent thalassemia, presents with anemia of varying severity, which may or may not require regular blood transfusions. Usually presents after 2 years or even later in life. Icterus and splenomegaly are present. This is primarily a clinical diagnosis and requires monitoring of the child over time to see the clinical spectrum of disease. Blood levels of iron and ferritin are raised. The condition may be found in compound heterozygous states, with inheritance of two different hemoglobinopathies.

***β thalassemia associated with β chain structural variants:*** The most frequent condition in this group is the HbE disease, these usually present with mild anemia and mild icterus. Patients with HbE/β thalassemia may present with symptoms of anemia and organomegaly. Variability is seen because of the different genotypes(i.e. $\beta^0$ or $\beta^+$), co-inheritance of an α thalassemia gene, level of HbF and the presence of other modifying genes.

***β thalassemia trait/minor:*** Patients have mild anemia, microcytosis and increased red blood cell number, the RDW is low. The peripheral blood film examination reveals marked hypochromia, microcytosis (without anisocytosis which is usually found with iron deficiency anemia) and presence of target cells. High-performance liquid chromatography (HPLC) or hemoglobin electrophoresis shows elevated levels of HbA2 or HbF, or increase of both. Table 13.12 contrasts iron deficiency and thalassemia trait. The diagnosis of thalassemia trait should be considered in any child with hypochromic, microcytic anemia that does not respond to iron supplementation (Table 13.6). While

**Table 13.12:** Differences between beta thalassemia trait and iron deficiency anemia

| | *Beta thalassemia trait (beta thalassemia carriers or thalassemia minor)* | *Iron deficiency anemia (IDA)* |
|---|---|---|
| Symptoms | None | Mild to severe depending on degree of iron deficiency |
| Hemoglobin | Usually 10–12 g/dL (unless additional iron deficiency is present) | Less than 10 g/dL |
| Mean corpuscular volume (MCV) and hemoglobin (MCH) | MCV <80 fl; MCH <27 pg | Very low MCV (<80 fl) |
| Red cell count | Elevated | Reduced |
| Red cell distribution width, % | Normal or mildly increased | 13–15 (high) |
| Serum iron and ferritin | Normal (unless concomitant iron deficiency) | Low |
| HbA2 levels (on HPLC) | Increased (may be borderline low and missed, especially with concomitant iron deficiency, which lowers HbA2 levels) | Normal |

HPLC high performance liquid chromatography

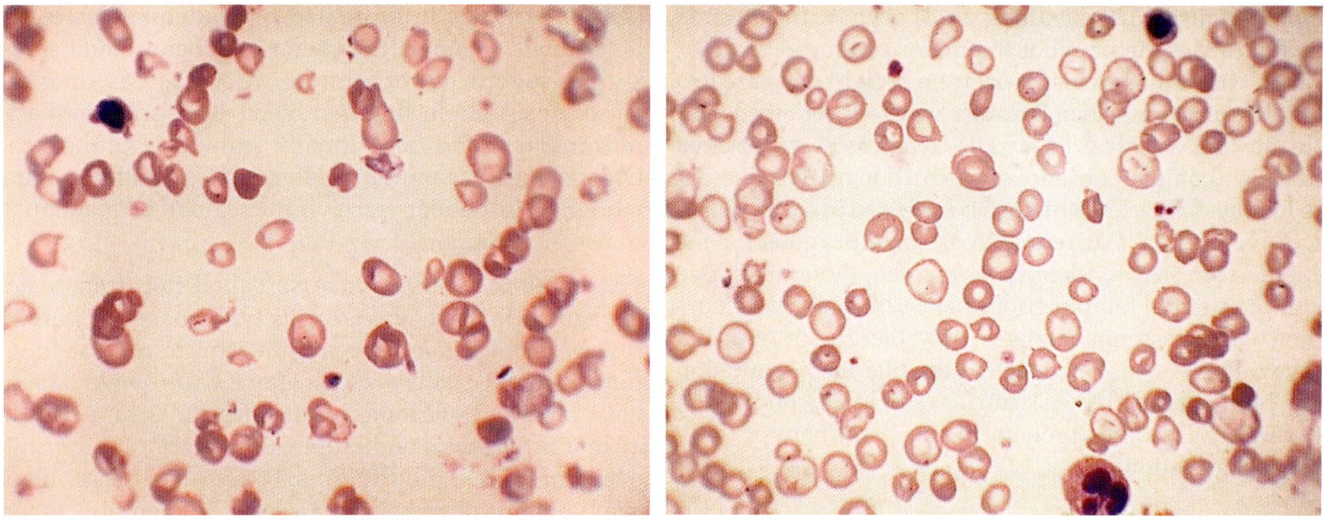

Fig. 13.7: Peripheral smears from a transfusion dependent patient with beta thalassemia major showing marked anisopoikilocytosis, microcytosis, hypochromia, polychromatophilia, nucleated red blood cells and a few fragmented erythrocytes. Jenner-Giemsa ×1000





this condition does not require treatment, patients and their families need to be counseled regarding risks in other family members and their progeny.

### Laboratory Studies

The complete blood count and peripheral blood film examination results are usually sufficient to suspect the diagnosis. In thalassemias major or intermedia, the hemoglobin level ranges from 2–8 g/dL. MCV and MCH are significantly low. Reticulocyte count is elevated to 5–8% and leukocytosis is usually present. A shift to the left is also encountered, reflecting the hemolytic process. The platelet count is usually normal, unless the spleen is markedly enlarged and causing hypersplenism.

Peripheral blood film examination reveals marked hypochromasia and microcytosis, polychromatophilic cells, nucleated red blood cells, basophilic stippling, and occasional immature leukocytes (Figs 13.7 and 13.8). A sample must be sent for high performance liquid chromatography (HPLC) prior to the first blood transfusion. This confirms the diagnosis in β thalassemia disease states. There is absence of HbA and elevation of HbF; the level of HbA2 is not needed for the diagnosis of thalassemia major or intermedia. The demonstration of elevated HbA2 fraction is important to identify patients with thalassemia trait.

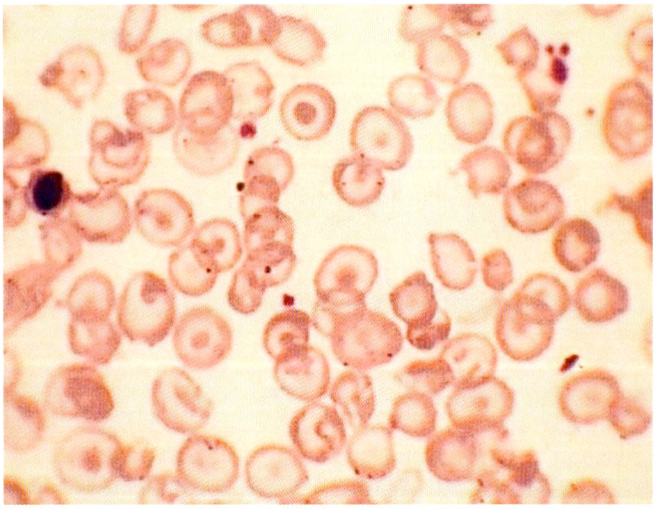

Fig. 13.8: Peripheral smear from an asymptomatic patient with hemoglobin E disease, showing microcytosis, hypochromia, target cells and nucleated red blood cells. Jenner-Giemsa ×1000

### Options for Management and Common Complications

Genetic counseling is needed for family to prevent the birth of other children with thalassemia major. Prenatal testing to see if the fetus is affected can be done by chorionic villus sampling (CVS) at 10–12 weeks.

Blood transfusion should be initiated at an early age, if hemoglobin persists below 7 g/dL; on regular transfusion therapy attempts to keep pretransfusion hemoglobin levels 9–10 g/dL (to promote growth and prevent deformity). Chelation therapy to deal with the accumulated iron is vital to prevent iron overload and organ dysfunction. Iron preparations should not be given to patients with thalassemia intermedia or major. A normal diet is recommended, with the following supplements: Folic acid, small doses of ascorbic acid (vitamin C), and alpha-tocopherol (vitamin E). Drinking tea with meals has been shown to decrease absorption of iron from the gut.

The introduction of hematopoietic stem cell transplantation offers the possibility of cure for thalassemia major patients; early transplant before the onset of complications has the best results. Therapy of non-transplanted children consists of regular blood transfusions and iron-chelating agents. If both are pursued vigorously, it will allow these children to survive into adulthood with fewer complications. Medications like hydroxyurea and luspatercept are effective in thalassemia intermedia and some patients with thalassemia major.

#### *Blood Transfusion Reactions and Infections*

After multiple transfusions, patients may develop transfusion reactions or alloimmunization to red cell antigens. These complications can be minimized by using leukocyte filters during transfusion or better still by having the blood bank preparing leukocyte depleted packed red blood cells. Administration of acetaminophen and diphenhydramine hydrochloride before each transfusion will minimize febrile or allergic reactions. The major complications of blood transfusions are those related to transmission of infections, hepatitis B, C and HIV. These can be reduced by good blood banking practices. Hepatitis B vaccination and regular assessment of hepatitis and HIV status are part of routine care.

Lactoferrin, a prominent component of the granules of polymorphonuclear leukocytes, is bacteriostatic for pathogens. The high transferrin saturation in patients with iron overload compromises the bacteriostatic properties of the protein. Infection with *Yersinia enterocolitica* can occur in iron overloaded patients, and presents with fever and diarrhea; these patients are treated with gentamicin and cotrimoxazole. Other important infections, which may occur are mucormycosis (*Rhizopus oryazae*), and *Listeria monocytogenes*.

#### Iron Overload

Iron overload is the major causes of morbidity and organ toxicity. Excessive iron is due to increased gastrointestinal iron absorption as well as repeated transfusions. Patients with iron overload demonstrate endocrinopathy caused by iron deposition in organs leading to hypothyroidism, decreased growth and lack of sexual maturation, diabetes mellitus, and hypoparathyroidism. Death is secondary to cardiac or hepatic iron overload. In older patients, bone and renal problems may occur.

Iron status is monitored by serum ferritin measurements. However, liver and cardiac iron may be underestimated by this test. A highly accurate and noninvasive tool to assess the iron status is the cardiac T2* magnetic resonance imaging. This can predict cardiomyopathy up to 2 years prior to its presentation and enabling effective iron chelation therapy.

#### Chelation Therapy

The introduction of chelating agents, capable of removing excess iron from the body, has dramatically increased life expectancy. Combination therapy may be needed in some children not controlled by appropriate use of a single iron chelator. The optimal time to initiate chelation therapy is dictated by the amount of accumulated iron. This usually occurs after 2–3 years of transfusions or when the serum ferritin level is above 1000 µg/L.

The gold standard was deferoxamine (DFO), but this has to be administered by a prolonged subcutaneous infusion due to its short half-life. DFO total dose of 40–60 mg/kg/day is infused over 8–12 hours for 5–6 days/week by a mechanical pump. Patients should be warned that their urine will become orange due to the iron-deferoxamine complex (ferrioxamine) being excreted. Eye examinations, hearing tests and kidney function tests are required to monitor the effects of deferoxamine (DFO) therapy.

Deferasirox is an oral chelating agent, the molecule is a tridentate ligand that binds iron with a high affinity, forming a 2:1 complex that is excreted in bile and eliminated in feces. It is highly selective for iron, chelating both intracellular and extracellular iron throughout the body: Liver, heart, reticuloendothelial system and circulation. It may cause skin rashes, nausea, vomiting, renal or hepatic toxicity. Monitoring of creatinine, liver function tests and urine for proteinuria is required. The recommended starting dose is 20–30 mg/kg/day.

Deferiprone, another oral agent, though effective for removing cardiac iron might cause cartilage problems, neutropenia and even agranulocytosis. It is administered at a dose of 50–75 mg/kg/day.

The spleen acts as a store for nontoxic iron, and its early removal may be harmful. Splenectomy is justified only in hypersplenism, leading to excessive destruction of erythrocytes and increased need for frequent blood transfusions, which results in further iron accumulation. Patients who require more than 200–250 mL/kg of packed red blood cells per year to maintain hemoglobin may benefit from this procedure. Pre-splenectomy immunizations and prophylactic antibiotics significantly decrease post splenectomy infections. The procedure is delayed until the child is aged 5-year or older.

### Complications

***Bone problems:*** The classic "hair on end" appearance of the skull results from widening of the diploic spaces. The maxilla may overgrow, resulting in maxillary overbite and prominence of the upper incisors. These changes contribute to the classic hemolytic facies (Fig. 13.6) observed in patients with thalassemia major. Bone density problems increase with age. The osteoporosis and osteopenia will require treatment with vitamin D and bisphosphonates.

***Extramedullary hematopoiesis:*** This usually occurs in patients with thalassemia intermedia, but can occur in thalassemia major in those who are not receiving adequate transfusion therapy. Compression fractures and paravertebral expansion of extramedullary masses, which behave clinically like tumors, may occur during the second decade of life.

***Psychosocial issues:*** As these children are surviving into adulthood, newer problems related to employment, marriage and having families, as well as the stress of chronic illness will need to be addressed. Patients with thalassemia, hemophilia and sickle cell disease are recognized as a disability under the Right of Persons with Disabilities (RPWD) Act, 2016.

### Curative Therapy

Hematopoietic stem cell transplant or allogeneic bone marrow transplant from an HLA-matched sibling is curative. A government program in partnership with Coal India (Thalassemia Bal Sewa Yojana) covers the cost of patients who are suitable and most likely to benefit from such procedures. Novel therapies like gene therapy and gene editing are being tried in clinical trials.

Thalassemia intermedia patients require monitoring to assess the need for transfusion as persistently low hemoglobin may retard growth. Hydroxyurea at a dose of

10–20 mg/kg/day may be used in an attempt to increase HbF production and reduce the need for transfusions. This therapy is most effective in those children with *XLM1* mutation. Iron overload is a problem due to its increased absorption; chelation is required if serum ferritin is more the 1000 μg/L.

### Prevention of Thalassemia Major

Persons with thalassemia trait do not require medical follow-up after the initial diagnosis, iron therapy should not be used unless a definite iron deficiency is confirmed. Genetic counseling is indicated to create awareness and prevent thalassemia major in subsequent offspring. Prevention program of the National Health Mission advocates awareness, and screening of adolescents to make them aware of their carrier state so they can choose their future partner. Antenatal testing of thalassemia carrier state of mothers is important. The option of prenatal testing should be given, if both partners are thalassemia carriers.

### Suggested Reading


1. Lal A, Bansal D. Thalassemia: Common clinical queries in management. Indian J Pediatr 2020; 87: 75–81
2. Prevention and control of hemoglobinopathies in India: Thalassemias, sickle cell disease and other variant hemoglobins. National Health Mission, Government of India, 2016 http://nhm.gov.in/images/pdf/programmes/RBSK/Resource_Documents/Guidelines_on_Hemoglobinopathies_in%20India
3. Sinha S, Seth T, Colah RB, Bittles AH. Hemoglobinopathies in India: estimates of blood requirements and treatment costs for the decade 2017-2026. J Community Genet 2020; 11: 39–45.


*Competencies:* **PE29.11; PE29.13; PE29.16; PE29.18**

## SICKLE CELL DISEASE

Sickle cell anemia occurs in India with a total gene frequency of 4.3%. It is present in a wide geographical distribution with very high incidence found in the tribal populations of Orissa, Maharashtra, Madhya Pradesh, Jharkhand, and Gujarat. These patients can present with serious and varied hematological manifestations.

### Pathophysiology

Sickle cell anemia is an autosomal recessive disease that results from the substitution of valine for glutamic acid at position 6 of the beta-globin gene. The sickle red blood cells are less deformable, and obstruct the microcirculation. This results in tissue hypoxia, which further promotes sickling. Deoxygenation of the heme moiety of sickle hemoglobin (HbS) leads to hydrophobic interactions between adjacent HbS molecules that aggregate into larger polymers. Sickle-shaped red blood cells are rapidly hemolyzed and have a lifespan of only 10–20 days. Patients who are homozygous for *HbS* have sickle cell disease. Patients who are heterozygous for *HbS* have sickle trait.

### Clinical Evaluation

Patients with sickle cell disease may have anemia and some require regular blood transfusion, but the most important symptom is vaso-occlusive crisis (**Table 13.13**). This is characterized by sudden onset of pain, following stress, fever or dehydration. The silent vaso-occlusion and crisis are associated with an increased risk of organ damage and death. Severe crises can last for 1–2 weeks. Icterus due to elevated unconjugated hyperbilirubinemia, pallor and mild splenomegaly in a young child are usual presentations. Patients are also at risk for infections and complications like pneumonia, acute chest syndrome, osteomyelitis and splenic sequestration. Every episode of fever needs to be investigated for focus of infection and promptly treated as patients have functional hyposplenism and are prone to infections from encapsulated organisms. Sudden increase in pallor, syncope or sudden pain, or hyposplenism a left-sided abdominal mass may indicate a splenic sequestration crisis.

Tachypnea suggests pneumonia, congestive heart failure, or acute chest syndrome. Hypoxia is commonly seen in patients with acute chest syndrome. Severe anemia may occur with aplastic crisis, and patients show signs of congestive heart failure. Hypotension and tachycardia may be signs of septic shock or sequestration crisis. Growth retardation and gallstones are common. The spleen undergoes auto-infarction and is usually not palpable beyond 6 years of age. Neurological symptoms such

**Table 13.13:** Types of crises in sickle cell disease

| | |
|---|---|
| Vaso-occlusive crisis | • Caused by obstruction of the microcirculation by sickled red blood cells, resulting in ischemic injury<br>• Presentation with pain in the femur, tibia and lower vertebrae; dactylitis; or as hand and foot syndrome (painful and swollen hands and/or feet) in children<br>• Kidneys, lungs, central nervous system and retina may be affected |
| Acute chest syndrome | • Caused by vaso-occlusive crisis involving the lungs<br>• Presentation with chest pain, cough, tachypnea, dyspnea, fever, hypoxemia, and/or new pulmonary infiltrates |
| Sequestration crisis (spleen or liver) | Results from obstruction of splenic veins by sickled cells, which causes sequestration of peripheral blood in an engorged spleen |
| Infectious crises | Caused by increased susceptibility to infection by encapsulated organisms (*Hemophilus influenzae*, *S. pneumoniae*), as well as common pathogens (*Salmonella*, *M. pneumoniae*, *S. aureus*, *E. coli*) |
| Aplastic crisis | • Results from cessation of erythropoiesis in the bone marrow, usually following infections (most commonly, parvovirus B19) or folate deficiency<br>• Usually self-limited; managed with supportive care; occasionally require packed red blood cells |

when peripheral stem cells are used instead of bone marrow cells. The advantage of autologous transplant is that there is no graft versus host disease, and once engraftment occurs then graft rejection is unlikely. However, there is a higher risk of tumor relapse as compared to allogeneic transplants.

### Complications

*Failure of engraftment:* Failure to engraft after HSCT (graft dysfunction) or inability to sustain graft (graft rejection) is a formidable complication. The causes include inadequate stem cell dose, infections, graft-versus-host disease (GVHD) and immunological mediated processes. The incidence is higher in unrelated donor and HLA mismatched transplant.

*Toxicity related to conditioning:* Conventional myeloablative therapy, given before HSCT, may be associated with complications such as: (a) veno-occlusive disease of the liver characterized by jaundice, hepatomegaly and ascites; (b) hemorrhagic cystitis; (c) seizures; (d) pulmonary complications, which can be infectious or non-infectious; (e) skin and mucosal changes including alopecia, nail changes and oral mucositis.

*Acute graft versus host disease:* This occurs within the first 3 months after transplant. It classically affects three tissues, namely the skin, gut and liver and may be accompanied by fever.

*Chronic graft versus host disease:* This develops later than 100 days after transplant and often follows acute GVHD but may also develop *de novo*. It is classified as limited or extensive chronic GVHD. Clinically it resembles autoimmune disorders like scleroderma with skin rash, sicca complex, sclerosing bronchiolitis and hepatic dysfunction. Management is with immunosuppressive agents.

*Tumor relapse:* A certain number of patients will relapse from the original malignancy, as the tumor cells survive the chemo/radiotherapy and graft versus tumor effect.

*Infections:* Bacterial and fungal infections are seen in the immediate post-transplant period; viral infections are important causes of morbidity and mortality later. The chief viral infections are cytomegalovirus, herpes simplex virus and varicella zoster. Bacterial infections with encapsulated organisms may occur after 3 to 6 months. The patient needs to be on immunosuppression after allogeneic HSCT for 6–12 months. Reimmunization with all childhood vaccines is required after stopping immunosuppression.

### Suggested Reading

1. Bazinet A, Popradi G. A general practitioner's guide to hematopoietic stem cell transplantation. Curr Oncol 2019; 26: 187–91.
2. Indian Council of Medical Research, Ministry of Health and Family Welfare. National guidelines for hematopoietic stem cell transplantation; January 2021, available at https://main.icmr.nic.in/sites/default/files/upload_documents/Nat-Guide-HCT.pdf.

*Competencies:* **PE29.6; PE29.10; PE29.11**

## APPROACH TO A BLEEDING CHILD

When a child with acute bleeding presents, the most important initial step is to stabilize the child. Assessment of the vitals will give an important clue to the severity of the disorder and magnitude of blood loss. Adequate administration of replacement fluids and blood is done. Following this, the child should be evaluated for the etiology of bleeding, which may be due to platelet factors (Tables 13.17 and 13.18), coagulation disorders (Table 13.19) or fibrinolytic dysfunction. The clinical assessment, type of bleeding, antecedent events and initial screening tests help identify the cause.

### Pathogenesis

The process of hemostasis is divided into cellular and fluid phases. The former involves platelets and the vascular wall,

| Table 13.17: Causes of thrombocytopenia |
|---|
| Immune thrombocytopenic purpura |
| *Infections:* Disseminated intravascular coagulation, malaria, kala-azar, dengue hemorrhagic fever, hepatitis B and C, HIV, congenital (TORCH) infections, infection associated hemophagocytosis syndrome |
| *Medications:* Valproate, penicillins, heparin, quinine, digoxin |
| *Thrombotic microangiopathy:* Thrombotic thrombocytopenic purpura; hemolytic uremic syndrome |
| *Malignancies:* Leukemia, lymphoma, neuroblastoma |
| *Autoimmune or related disorders:* Systemic lupus erythematosus, Evans syndrome, antiphospholipid syndrome, neonatal immune thrombocytopenia |
| *Immunodeficiency:* Wiskott-Aldrich syndrome, HIV/AIDS |
| *Bone marrow failure:* Thrombocytopenia with absent radii, Fanconi anemia, Shwachman-Diamond syndrome |
| *Marrow replacement:* Osteopetrosis, Gaucher disease |
| *Others:* Hypersplenism, Kasabach-Merritt syndrome |

| Table 13.18: Qualitative disorders of platelet function |
|---|
| **Inherited disorders**<br>Glanzmann thrombasthenia (GP IIb–IIIa deficiency)<br>Bernard-Soulier syndrome (GP Ib deficiency)<br>Gray platelet syndrome<br>Dense body deficiency |
| **Acquired disorders**<br>Medications, e.g. aspirin, clopidogrel<br>Chronic kidney disease<br>Cardiopulmonary bypass |

| Table 13.19: Common coagulation disorders |
|---|
| **Inherited disorders**<br>• Hemophilia A and B<br>• von Willebrand disease<br>• Other deficiencies<br>– Factor VII, X, XIII deficiency<br>– Afibrinogenemia |
| **Acquired disorders**<br>• Liver disease<br>• Vitamin K deficiency<br>• Warfarin overdose<br>• Disseminated intravascular coagulation |

while the latter involves plasma proteins. The physiology of hemostasis is complex and involves a fine balance between flow of blood (i.e. fluid) and local responses to vascular injury (i.e. clotting).

The fluid phase is divided into three processes: (i) The multiple-step zymogen pathway that leads to thrombin generation; (ii) thrombin-induced formation of fibrin clot; and (iii) complex fibrinolytic mechanisms which limit clot propagation.

The physiology of hemostasis includes the generation of insoluble fibrin and activation of platelets to form a hemostatic plug (Fig. 13.12). Pro- and anticoagulant pathways, platelet number, their function, vascular factors and other metabolic processes control this process. The coagulation cascade is depicted as involving two pathways—intrinsic and extrinsic. The extrinsic pathway is the primary initiating pathway for coagulation, it is measured by the prothrombin time (PT), and the intrinsic system works as a regulatory amplification loop, measured by the activated partial thromboplastin time (aPTT).



## Clinical Evaluation

It is important to know the age of onset of bleeding, site of bleeding (Table 13.20), spontaneous or after intervention, e.g. dental extraction, surgery or circumcision. In the case of new onset bleeding, history of antecedent infections, rash (IgA vasculitis, varicella), icterus (liver failure, hepatitis B and C), diarrhea (hemolytic uremic syndrome) and medication intake needs to be taken. Important medications that may cause bleeding include anticonvulsants, penicillins, warfarin, aspirin, non-steroidal anti-inflammatory medications and heparin. The family history is important, documentation of the sex of affected members and details of bleeding manifestations should be noted. Specific types of bleeding may give a clue, e.g. poor wound healing and prolonged bleeding from the umbilical stump suggests factor XIII deficiency.

Examination should assess the degree of anemia, fading and new ecchymoses (Fig. 13.13). The presence of petechia, vascular malformations and rashes should be documented. Presence of splenomegaly suggests infections, malignancy, collagen vascular disorders or hypersplenism, rather than a primary bleeding defect. Examination of the mouth and nose to rule out local causes of bleeding should be done. Hemangiomas and telangiectasias, may lead to mucocutaneous bleeding in Kasabach-Merritt syndrome and hereditary telangiectasia.

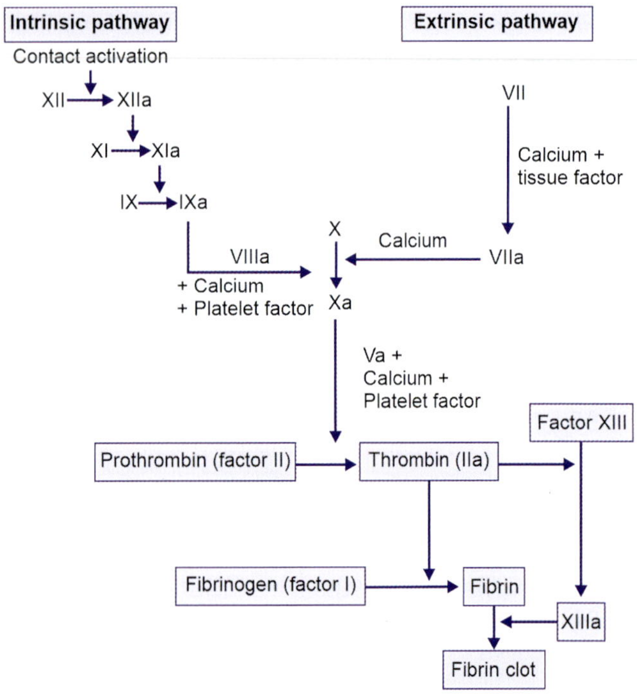


Fig. 13.12: *In vivo* coagulation cascade

## Investigations

A complete hemogram should be done to evaluate the platelet count, morphology of platelets and red cells, and for evidence of microangiopathic hemolysis. The optimal peripheral smear is made from a fresh finger stick. Initial

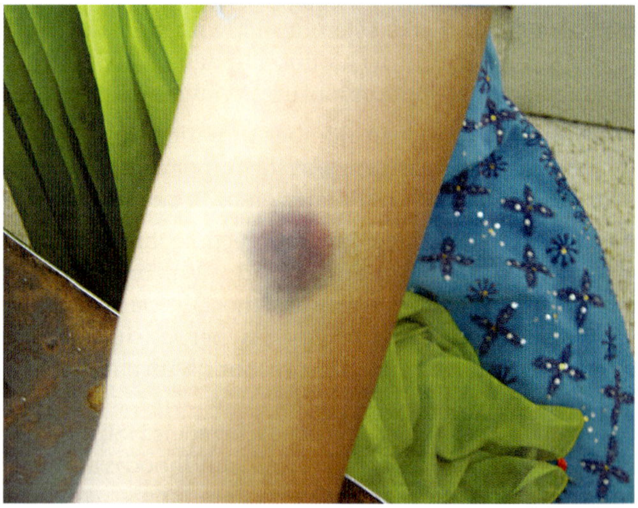

Fig. 13.13: Large ecchymotic patch on the upper limb of a young girl with von Willebrand disease

Table 13.20: Differences in bleeding patterns between platelet and coagulation disorders

| | *Platelet disorder* | *Coagulation disorder* |
|---|---|---|
| Site of bleeding | Skin, mucous membranes (mucosal bleeds: epistaxis, oral, gastrointestinal tract) | Soft tissues, joints, muscles (deep bleeds) |
| Petechiae | Yes | No |
| Ecchymoses | Small, superficial | Large, deep |
| Hemarthrosis, muscle bleeding | Extremely rare | Common |
| Bleeding after minor trauma | Yes | No |
| Bleeding after surgery | Immediate; usually mild | Delayed (1–2 days); often severe |

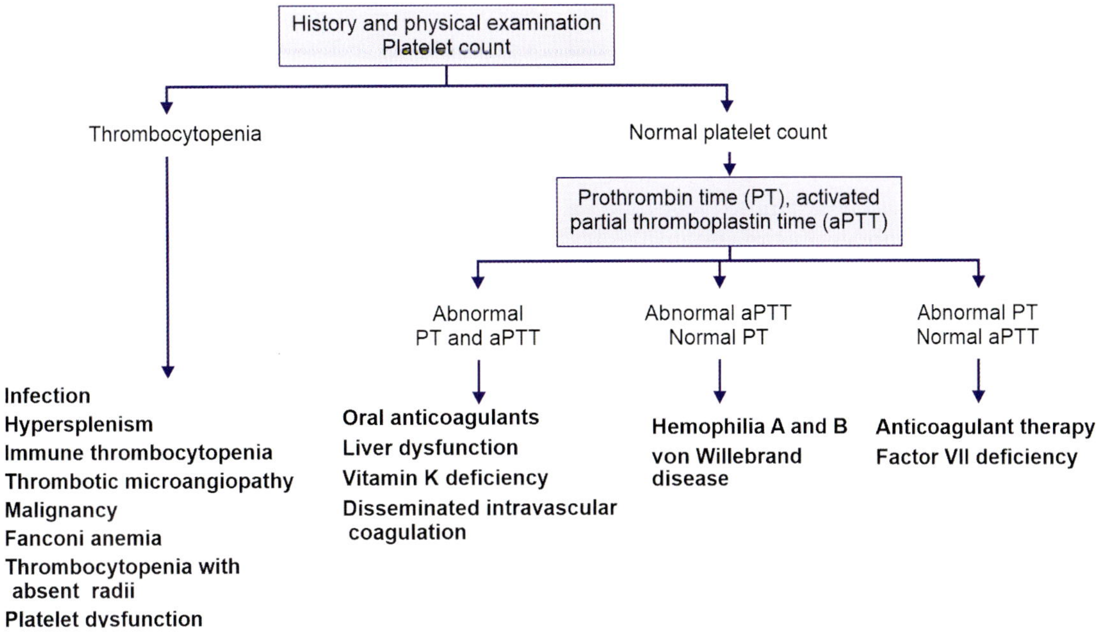


**Fig. 13.14:** Work-up of a child presenting with bleeding

screening tests for coagulation disorders include PT and aPTT (Fig. 13.14). Specific factor assays can be done to identify factor deficiencies; the degree of factor VIII and IX deficiency will dictate the management. The aPTT also is used for monitoring the efficacy of heparin; PT and the ratio of PT to an international normalized standard (INR) are used to assess therapeutic warfarin effect.

Bleeding time (BT) is now rarely used due to the problems of reproducibility and reliability. This test is also abnormal, if the platelet count is below 100,000/µL. In systemic vasculitic disorders, e.g. IgA vasculitis and connective tissue defects like Ehlers-Danlos syndrome, the bleeding time is also prolonged (Table 13.21). Bleeding time is largely being replaced by platelet aggregation studies for inherited and acquired platelet dysfunction. Evaluation for von Willebrand disease (vWD) includes the von Willebrand cofactor assay, quantitation of von Willebrand antigen, factor VIII assay, ABO blood group, and electrophoretic analysis of von Willebrand multimeric subtypes. In a sick child, evaluation for disseminated intravascular coagululopathy is performed.

*Competency:* **PE29.6**

## Immune Thrombocytopenic Purpura

In view of its immune pathology, this condition is now named immune thrombocytopenic purpura (ITP), in place of idiopathic thrombocytopenic purpura. This is the commonest bleeding disorder presenting in children between 1 and 7 years of age. It is important to correctly diagnose this entity and differentiate it from other more ominous conditions.

| Table 13.21: Vascular causes of bleeding |
|---|
| IgA vasculitis |
| Vasculitis in systemic lupus erythematosus |
| Ehlers-Danlos syndrome |
| Scurvy |
| Prolonged steroid use; Cushing disease |
| Hereditary hemorrhagic telangiectasia |

### *Pathogenesis*

ITP has an immune basis, due to antibodies against the platelet glycoprotein IIb/IIIa complex. Platelets with antibodies on their surface are trapped in the spleen, where they removed by splenic macrophages. Recent data describes a Th1 dominant proinflammatory cytokine state in these individuals. Increased megakaryocyte number in the bone marrow is the hallmark of immune-mediated platelet destruction. However, a relative decrease in megakaryocyte production due to specific anti-platelet autoantibodies has also been implicated in the pathogenesis.

Thrombocytopenia lasting less than 3 months is termed acute, persistent is up to 12 months and greater than 12 months is termed chronic. The majority of children (60–75%) are likely to have acute ITP, which usually resolves within 2–4 months of diagnosis, regardless of therapy.

### *Clinical Features*

Normal platelet counts are $150–400 \times 10^3/mm^3$ in all children above one week of age. In ITP, the bleeding mostly occurs when there is a sudden drop in the platelet counts or with prolonged bleeds with superficial trauma. Patients usually present with epistaxis, oral oozing, petechiae and purpura. The incidence of intracranial hemorrhage in children with ITP is <1%. There is often an antecedent febrile illness, but on presentation most patients are afebrile. There is a seasonal clustering, more frequent during the change in seasons.

It is important to estimate the duration of symptoms and confirm if this is the initial episode or there are prior events, as seen in the relapsing course of ITP. Symptoms and signs depend on the platelet count. Bleeding is usually mild unless the platelet count drops below 10,000/µL. With platelet counts from 20,000–50,000/µL, petechiae and ecchymoses are observed following mild trauma.

Oral mucosa bleeding or hematuria, menorrhagia may be present. The presence of lymphadenopathy or splenomegaly suggests other causes of thrombocytopenia rather than ITP. Patients should be examined for stigmata of bone marrow failure, e.g. Fanconi anemia (hypoplastic/absent thumb, short stature and hyperpigmentation), and thrombocytopenia with absent radii (radial bone abnormality, normal thumb). Infants should be examined for the presence of hemangiomas and ultrasound of abdomen may be useful. Hypersplenism, HIV and hepatitis C may also cause thrombocytopenia.

### *Laboratory Evaluation*

Complete blood count shows thrombocytopenia; other hematological parameters are normal. A peripheral smear screens for abnormal cells such as blasts, malarial parasites and importantly to know the precise platelet count, and exclude spurious thrombocytopenia. It also helps to assess platelet size; giant platelets are young and an indicator of platelet production.

If the child is febrile and ill, appropriate evaluation for infections is required, including chest X-ray, blood culture, tests for malaria, and dengue. Screening for disseminated intravascular coagulopathy should be done, if sepsis is suspected. Liver and kidney function tests, and lactate dehydrogenase (LDH) are done to rule out hepatitis, occult malignancy, hemolysis and hemolytic uremic syndrome. Bone marrow examination shows increased production of megakaryocytes, and exclude marrow infiltration or marrow failure.

### *Management*

Minimizing the risk of hemorrhage and decreasing the long-term side effects of treatment are the goals of therapy. Many children are stable with a platelet count (20–30000/µL), and have no symptoms or only few petechiae or occasional bruise. In acute ITP (symptoms lasting from 0–3 months), all children do not require therapy. Expectant watch-and-wait policy can be used, if there is no bleeding. If treatment is required, *intravenous immunoglobulin* (IVIG) is given as a single dose of 0.8 to 1.0 g/kg or over two days. *Prednisone* may be given at a dose of 4 mg/kg per day in 3 divided doses for 4–5 days with no taper, or at 1 to 2 mg/kg/day for 2–3 weeks. If serious life-threatening hemorrhage occurs, platelet transfusions may be necessary.

For persistent ITP (>3 months to one-year) or chronic ITP, many options of treatment are available. The goal of therapy is to keep platelets in a safe range to prevent serious bleeding; normal platelet count is not the treatment goal. Steroids can be used for bleeding episodes. For chronic treatment, the recommended medication is a thrombopoietin receptor agonist (TPO-RA). Two medications are available in India, *eltrombopag* and *romiplostim*. Injection romiplostim (dose 1–10 µg/kg once a week, subcutaneously) and eltrombopag (12.5–25 mg/day orally once daily) are both effective. Other options include alternate day low-dose steroids, splenectomy and various combinations of danazol, vincristine, cyclosporine, azathioprine, and rituximab.

The plethora of treatment for chronic ITP demonstrates the difficulty in managing this illness. The physician needs to take care of growth, bone density and psychosocial problems inherent in this and any chronic disease.

### Suggested Reading


1. Kim TO, Despotovic JM. Pediatric immune thrombocytopenia treatment. Ann Blood 2021;6:4 https://aob.amegroups.com
2. Provan D, Arnold DM, Bussel JB, et al. Updated international consensus report on the investigation and management of primary immune thrombocytopenia. Blood Adv 2019;3: 3780–3817.


*Competencies:* **PE29.7; PE29.10**

## Hemophilia

The hemophilias are the commonest hereditary clotting disorders. Both hemophilia A and B are inherited in an X-linked recessive manner. Hemophilia A is due to factor VIII deficiency and hemophilia B due to insufficient factor IX. Their clinical manifestations are indistinguishable, and presentation depends on the level of factor present. The patients have delayed bleeding after tooth extraction or minor surgery that is prolonged and severe, and is not controlled without giving clotting factor replacement. In severe cases where factor levels are less than 1%, repeated, spontaneous, debilitating joint bleeds (Fig. 13.15) lead to permanent disability and intracranial bleeds can be life-threatening.

### *Laboratory Investigation*

Different clotting disorders can have very similar symptoms. An accurate diagnosis can only be made with comprehensive and accurate laboratory tests. Screening tests such as prothrombin time (PT), and activated partial thromboplastin time (APTT) are necessary to identify the potential cause of bleeding.

In hemophilia A and B, the APTT is prolonged. The specific factor assay for factor VIII or IX reveals the deficient

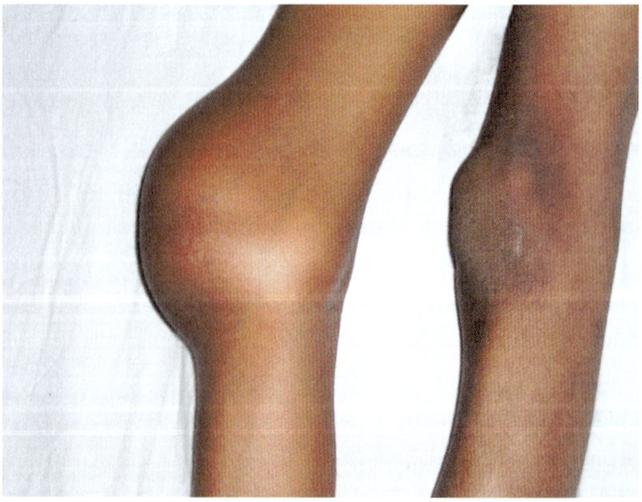

**Fig. 13.15:** Child with hemophilia with knee hemarthrosis with severe pain and signs of inflammation

clotting factor. Factor level <1% is severe hemophilia, 1–4% is moderate hemophilia and 5–40% is mild hemophilia.

### Complications

Patients suffer recurrent joint and muscle bleeds and can develop permanent disability. Treatment requires appropriate replacement therapy with judicious physiotherapy to prevent chronic joint disease, and counseling for injury prevention. Some sites of bleeding such as CNS and neck are life-threatening; iliopsoas muscle bleeding is also dangerous as large bleeds can occur.

The most serious complication of therapy is the development of inhibitors, which are alloantibodies to the clotting factor product. The presence of inhibitors makes the clotting factors ineffective. Use of recombinant and non-factor products, and double viral inactivated plasma derived products has reduced the risk of transfusion associated infections.

### Management

Children with hemophilia should be managed at centers equipped for their special needs. Replacement therapy with concentrates of factor VIII or IX are now available. Each unit of factor VIII/kg increases the level by 2%, and the half-life is 8–12 hours. To achieve a target of 40% factor VIII, which is required for management of most hemarthroses, a dose of 20 U/kg every 12–24 hours for 1–2 days is required. In a major bleed, e.g. intracranial hemorrhage, the target for factor level is 80–100% correction; the dose needed to achieve this is 50 U/kg every 12 hours for 7–10 days.

Cryoprecipitate and fresh frozen plasma (FFP) were used to control bleeding in the past but are not recommended except in an emergency or when diagnosis is unknown. Cryoprecipitate contains factor VIII, fibrinogen and von Willebrand factor, but not factor IX. As fresh frozen plasma is frozen, it retains all factors at their hemostatic levels including the labile factors V and VII. Epsilon-aminocaproic acid or tranexamic acid may be effective as adjunct therapy in mild cases of hemophilia. The non-factor product *emicizumab* is effective in patients with hemophilia A, with or without inhibitors.

The principles of therapy of hemophilia B are similar. One unit of factor IX per kg raises factor level by 1% and the half-life is 24 hours. In emergencies when factor IX is unavailable, only fresh frozen plasma, and not cryoprecipitate, is used.

***Management of hemophilia patients with inhibitors:*** These patients will not respond to clotting factor VIII or IX, or FFP or cryoprecipitate. They require bypassing agents, such as *recombinant activated factor VIIa* (Novoseven) or *activated prothrombin complex like factor VIII inhibitor bypass activity* (FEIBA). Both bypassing agents should be available at hemophilia treatment centers as some patients respond better to one agent compared to the other. The non-factor product emicizumab, is a monoclonal antibody that bypasses the function of factor VIII and can be used in patients of hemophilia A with or without inhibitors. The added benefit is that it can be used subcutaneously and can be given every 1–4 weeks. Newer non-factor therapies are being tested, including *concizumab* and *fitusiran*. Inhibitors may be eradicated by immune tolerance induction, which involves repeated and frequent administration of factor VIII that downregulates the antibody response and induces immune tolerance.

Prophylaxis is a better mode of management; children with severe hemophilia are given factor replacement two to three times a week to reduce the risk of bleeds. Doses of factor VIII at 15–20 IU/kg three times a week for hemophilia A are effective. Now extended half -life products are available and this can further reduce the frequency of therapies. Prophylaxis results in less deformity and allows the child to play normally, allowing satisfactory quality of life. All children should receive hepatitis B immunizations, vaccines are given by the subcutaneous route and the parents should be counseled regarding injury prevention. Genetic counseling is required and families should be informed of the availability of prenatal diagnosis.

### Suggested Reading


1. Sachdeva A, Gunasekaran V, Ramya HN, et al. Consensus statement of the IAP in diagnosis and management of hemophilia. Indian Pediatr 2018; 55: 582–90.
2. Seth T. Experience of immune tolerance induction therapy for hemophilia A patients with inhibitors from a single center in India. Indian J Hematol Blood Transfus 2020; 36: 458–63.
3. Srivastava A, Santagostino E, Dougall A, et al. WFH guidelines for the management of hemophilia. Hemophilia 2020; 26(S6): 1–158.


## Disseminated Intravascular Coagulopathy

Disseminated intravascular coagulopathy (DIC) is an acquired disorder characterized by systemic activation of coagulation. This dysregulated process leads to fibrin production and microvascular thrombi and consumption of the clotting factors and platelets, which can lead to bleeding. The fibrinolytic system also gets deranged and can cause either clotting or bleeding depending on the defect. The presentation ranges from an isolated derangement of laboratory parameters to severe bleeding from multiple sites, associated with high mortality. DIC is triggered by a variety of conditions all of which result in activation of the clotting cascade.

### Pathophysiology

There are three main pathologic processes involved.

***Initiation of fibrin deposition:*** Thrombin generation in DIC is mediated by the extrinsic pathway. The tissue factor accumulates on activated platelets by binding to platelet P-selectin, which results in thrombin generation.

***Amplification role of thrombin:*** Thrombin generated, as above, amplifies inflammation and clotting by activation of platelets, and activation of factors V, VIII and IX leading to more thrombin production. Activated factor XIII (XIIIa) cross-links with fibrin clots making them insoluble, while thrombin activatable fibrinolysis inhibitor (TAFI) makes fibrin clots resistant to fibrinolysis.

***Propagation of fibrin deposition:*** There is suppression of fibrinolysis secondary to sustained increase in plasma levels of plasminogen-activator inhibitor 1 (PAI-1).

Following injury, infection or other precipitating factors, there is release of cytokines (tumor necrosis factor, interleukin (IL)-1, and IL-6 which change the endothelium from an anticoagulant to a procoagulant surface and interferes with fibrinolysis. As DIC continues, fibrinogen, prothrombin, platelets and other clotting factors are consumed beyond the capacity of the body to compensate and bleeding ensues. Activated protein C has an anti-inflammatory effect and downregulates the tissue factor and decreases calcium ion flux. It is consumed in DIC and its supplementation may have an important role in sepsis, associated disease.

### Causes

The main groups of illnesses causing DIC are: Infections, malignancy, tissue necrosis, ABO incompatible blood transfusion and snakebites (Table 13.22).

Acute DIC is the most common form of DIC seen in clinical practice. Bleeding manifestations predominate and the patient is critically ill (Fig. 13.16). Chronic DIC occurs due to a weak or intermittent activating stimulus. The process of destruction and production of clotting factors and platelets is balanced, and the DIC is thus 'compensated'. Chronic DIC occurs in patients with giant hemangiomas, certain vasculitic disorders and in some solid tumors.

### Laboratory Features

***Screening tests:*** Peripheral blood film examination and hemogram reveal schistocytes and thrombocytopenia. Prothrombin time (PT), activated partial thromboplastin time (aPTT), and thrombin time (TT) are prolonged, and fibrinogen level is low.

**Table 13.22:** Disorders which cause disseminated intravascular coagulopathy (DIC)

| *Acute DIC* | *Chronic DIC* |
|---|---|
| **Medical conditions** | |
| Septicemia or infections* | Solid tumors |
| Fulminant hepatic failure | Kasabach-Merritt syndrome |
| Heat stroke, hyperpyrexia | Liver cirrhosis |
| Severe burns | |
| Acute promyelocytic leukemia, neuroblastoma | |
| Snakebite | |
| Collagen vascular disorders | |
| **Surgical conditions** | |
| Severe trauma—crush injury, multiple fractures with fat emboli | Vascular tumors<br>Aortic aneurysm |
| Major operations | |
| Severe renal allograft rejection | |
| **Iatrogenic** | |
| Hemolytic transfusion reaction; massive transfusion | Artificial surfaces |
| Heparin-induced thrombosis | |

*Include the following infections:
*Bacterial:* Meningococcus, gram-negative bacteria, group B streptococci
*Viral:* Arboviruses, varicella, variola, rubella, paramyxoviruses, HIV, Ebola
*Parasitic:* Malaria
*Mycotic:* Candida, Aspergillus
*Rickettsial:* Rocky Mountain spotted fever

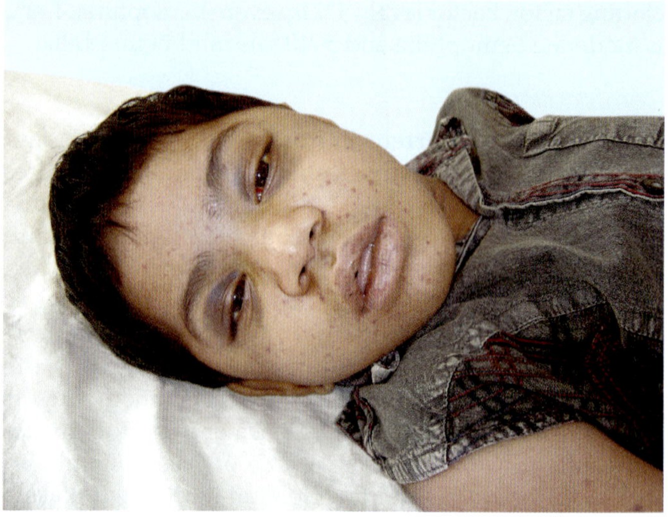

**Fig. 13.16:** An ill child with disseminated intravascular coagulation shows ecchymoses, purpura and subconjunctival hemorrhage

***Supportive tests:*** Increase in fibrin degradation products (FDP) or D-dimers is characteristic. Laboratory information of thrombocytopenia and hypofibrinogenemia (50% drop in either value) are the most sensitive in making a diagnosis.

A DIC scoring system has been proposed by the International Society on Thrombosis and Hemostasis (Table 13.23). An underlying disorder known to be

**Table 13.23:** Diagnosis of disseminated intravascular coagulation (DIC) using the DIC score

| | |
|---|---|
| *Risk assessment* | |
| Does the patient have an underlying disorder known to be associated with disseminated intravascular coagulopathy? (If Yes, proceed. If No, do not use this algorithm). | |
| *Order global coagulation tests* | |
| Platelet count; prothrombin time, fibrinogen, soluble fibrin monomers or fibrin degradation products | |
| *Score test results* | *Score* |
| (a) Platelet count >100,000/mm³ | 0 |
| 50,000–100,000/mm³ | 1 |
| <50,000/mm³ | 2 |
| (b) Elevated fibrin-related marker (soluble fibrin monomers or fibrin degradation products)* | |
| No increase | 0 |
| Moderate increase | 2 |
| Strong increase | 3 |
| (c) Prothrombin time | |
| <3 sec | 0 |
| >3 but <6 sec | 1 |
| >6 sec | 2 |
| (d) Fibrinogen level | |
| >1 g/L | 0 |
| <1 g/L | 1 |
| *Calculate score* | |
| Score ≥5: Compatible with overt DIC; repeat daily | |
| Score ≤5: Suggestive of non-overt DIC; repeat in 1–2 days | |

*Values of D-dimer above the upper limit of normal are moderately elevated; values above 5 times the upper limit of normal are strongly increased.

associated with DIC is a pre-requisite for the use of this algorithm; score of >5 is compatible with the diagnosis.

### Treatment

***Treatment of underlying cause and general care:*** The underlying disease must be managed appropriately. In cases of sepsis, antibiotics are the mainstay of treatment. In snakebites, anti-snake venom should be administered. Tissue perfusion and respiratory function must be maintained by intravenous fluids and provision of oxygen support to correct hypoxia. The coagulopathy may be compounded by vitamin K deficiency, which needs to be corrected.

***Hemostatic support (replacement therapy):*** Patients who have low levels of platelets, fibrinogen and other clotting factors, as demonstrated by prolonged PT, aPTT, TT, require replacement of deficient components. Monitoring is essential for guiding management and checking adequacy of replacement component support. Different blood components available (Table 13.24) for use in DIC are: Fresh frozen plasma (FFP), cryoprecipitate, platelet concentrates and packed red cells (also *see* Chapter 29). Replacement therapy can be halted when stabilization in platelet counts, fibrinogen levels and fall in fibrin degradation products (FDP) is observed.

***Heparin therapy:*** For a patient who is actively bleeding, heparin aggravates the bleeding. In most typical cases of acute DIC, heparin therapy has not proved to be useful and may be harmful. Heparin might be considered in patients with arterial, or large vessel venous thrombosis. Patients should be monitored by repeated platelet counts, fibrinogen levels and PT, APTT and TT.

## Suggested Reading


1. Papageorgiou C, Jourdi G, Adjambri E. Disseminated intravascular coagulation: An update on pathogenesis, diagnosis, and therapeutic strategies. Clin Appl Thromb Hemost 2018; 24 (9_suppl): 8S–28S.
2. Rajagopal R, Thachil J, Managle P. Disseminated intravascular coagulation in pediatrics. Arch Dis Child 2017; 102: 187–93.


*Competencies:* **PE29.10; PE29.11**

## APPROACH TO THROMBOSIS

The incidence of thrombosis is lower in children than in adults; however, thrombosis-related pediatric morbidity and mortality are significantly higher. Children till 6 months of age have lower levels of the vitamin K dependent coagulation factors II, IX, and X, compared to adults. Levels of thrombin inhibitors, chiefly protein C and S, antithrombin, heparin cofactor II and plasminogen are lower. Protein S levels approach adult values by the age of 3–6 months, but protein C levels remain low even into childhood. The incidence of thrombosis is maximum in infants younger than 1 year and during adolescence (Table 13.25).

### Clinical Evaluation

The patients are examined for features suggestive of congenital heart disease, collagen vascular diseases, and for fever, recent surgery, trauma, central venous catheter use, nephrotic syndrome, dehydration, varicella, or underlying malignancy. The age at which thrombosis occurred and the type of thrombosis (deep vein thrombosis, arterial thrombosis or stroke) should be documented. A family history suggests genetic predisposition to the disease.

**Table 13.24:** Types of blood component therapy, their constituents and guidelines for use

| *Component* | *Constituents* | *Indication* | *Dose* | *Precautions* |
|---|---|---|---|---|
| Fresh frozen plasma (FFP) | All coagulation factors as in normal plasma; contains 0.7–1.0 U/mL of factors II, V, VII, VIII, IX, X, XI, XII, XIII; and 2.5 mg/mL fibrinogen | Coagulation factor deficiencies with prolonged prothrombin time; thrombotic thrombocytopenic purpura | 15 mL/kg or 1 bag per 10 kg (constitutes 25–30% replacement therapy for coagulation factors) | Infuse soon after thawing; need ABO compatible units; may cause fluid overload |
| Cryoprecipitate | Fibrinogen 150 mg/bag; factor VIII 80–120 units/bag; factor XIII and vWD (does not contain factor IX) | Fibrinogen deficiency or consumption; factor VIII deficiency (hemophilia A), vWD disease; factor XIII deficiency | 1 bag per 5 kg will raise fibrinogen levels by 70 mg/dL | |
| Random donor platelets (RDP) | Platelets; ≥5.5 × $10^{10}$ platelets per bag | Thrombocytopenia | One unit raises platelet counts by 5000–10,000/$mm^3$; 1 unit every 10 kg raises counts by 30,000–50,000/$mm^3$ | Infuse rapidly; do NOT refrigerate prior to transfusion |
| Single donor platelets (SDP) | Platelets; contains at least 3 × $10^{11}$ platelets | Thrombocytopenia | One collection is equivalent to approximately 6 units of RDP | Precautions as above |
| Fresh blood | All components of blood | To replace acute and massive blood loss | Only to be used in severe trauma | Not a good source for platelets or coagulation factors |

**Table 13.25:** Factors which increase risk of thrombosis in children

**Acquired conditions**
- Infections: Viral, bacterial sepsis
- Disseminated intravascular coagulopathy
- Dehydration
- Central venous catheter
- Surgery, trauma
- Cyanotic congenital heart disease
- Antiphospholipid antibody syndrome
- Acute lymphoblastic leukemia; therapy (L-asparaginase and steroids)
- Nephrotic syndrome

**Inherited prothrombotic disorders**
- Factor V Leiden
- Protein C deficiency
- Protein S deficiency
- Antithrombin deficiency
- Prothrombin gene G20210A mutation
- Elevated lipoprotein (a) level
- Hyperhomocysteinemia

Symptoms vary according to site of thrombosis (Table 13.26). Symptoms of central nervous system thrombosis include vomiting, lethargy, seizures, or weakness in an extremity. Signs of pulmonary embolism are nonspecific and include diaphoresis, tachycardia and tachypnea. Signs of arterial thrombosis include diminished or absent peripheral pulses and coolness of extremity skin. Limb edema, erythema and tenderness on dorsiflexion of the foot (positive Homan sign) are present in deep vein thrombosis. Patients with renal vein thrombosis may present with flank pain and hematuria.

### Laboratory Evaluation

In acute thrombosis, there is consumption of clotting factors, resulting in low factor levels, hence assessment should be done only after 3 months. The diagnosis of disseminated intravascular coagulopathy should be excluded.

*Color Doppler* imaging signals are absent in thrombosed vessels and the lumen cannot be compressed with direct pressure. However, this may not be sufficiently sensitive to detect thrombosis in vessels such as subclavian veins, superior vena cava or brachiocephalic veins.

*Echocardiography* is useful for evaluation of thrombosis involving the vena cava and proximal subclavian vein.

*Computerized tomogram of the head* with intravenous contrast material is useful for detecting venous sinus thrombosis. However, both MRI and MRA are better at detecting early arterial ischemic strokes.

*Chest radiography* may reveal findings of pulmonary embolism which include small pleural effusions with wedge-shaped pleural-based opacity of pulmonary infarction; X-ray chest may be normal.

*Ventilation-perfusion (V/Q) scanning* is the procedure of choice in children with suspected pulmonary embolism. If D-dimer levels are elevated and V/Q scan indicates intermediate probability, then *spiral CT scan* may be useful.

### Management

Initial therapy requires heparin (unfractionated or low molecular weight) followed by oral warfarin therapy or direct acting anticoagulation (DOAC) medicines. IVC filters are only indicated in patients who are unable to receive anticoagulation medicines, and if placed must be removed as soon as possible. When doing therapeutic anticoagulation, close monitoring is required to prevent bleeding. The international normalized ratio (INR), which is PT of the patient compared to the international standard, is the most useful test for monitoring vitamin K antagonist medications. The INR therapeutic range is 2–3. The duration of therapy depends on the risk of recurrence. Detailed assessment of inherited thrombophilia is best done after 3 months of the event and after stopping anticoagulation medications, but the molecular tests can be done on treatment.

Initial treatment is usually with low molecular weight heparin (LMWH), which has primarily anti-Xa function (Table 13.27), and then the patient is switched to a vitamin K antagonist or a DOAC for 3–6 months or as long as the cause of thrombosis exists.

*Recurrent thrombosis:* Children with no adverse genetic factors have a 4.8% recurrence rate (RR), single genetic risk factor 17.6% RR and with two or more risk factors, almost 50% RR. Recurrent thrombosis can be due to inadequate anticoagulation therapy.

**Table 13.26:** Symptoms vary with the site of thrombosis

| *Site* | *Clinical features* |
|---|---|
| Cerebral sinuses | Headache, vomiting, lethargy, focal neurology deficit, seizures |
| Pulmonary thrombus | Chest pain, cough, dyspnea, respiratory failure |
| Mesenteric vein | Abdominal pain |
| Renal vein | Flank pain, hematuria |
| Hepatic vein | Pain in the right upper quadrant, hepatomegaly |
| Portal vein, splenic vein | Abdominal pain, splenomegaly |
| Inferior vena cava | Tenderness and edema in the lower limbs, abdominal pain |
| Superior vena cava | Headache, pain, edema neck and face |
| Limb | Pain, edema |

Table 13.27: Pediatric dosing of enoxaparin (LMWH), administered subcutaneously

| *Indication* | *Age <2 months* | *Age 2 months–18 years* |
|---|---|---|
| Therapy | 1.5 mg/kg/dose twice a day | 1 mg/kg/dose twice a day |
| Prophylaxis | 0.75 mg/kg/dose once daily | 0.5 mg/kg/dose once daily |

Avoid or use with caution, if kidney dysfunction, obesity or prematurity

### Suggested Reading


1. Seth T. Thrombosis in neonates and children. Eastern Med 2009; 14: 36–45.
2. Witmer C, Raffini L. Treatment of venous thromboembolism in pediatric patients. Blood 2020; 135: 335–43.


## WHITE BLOOD CELLS

Evaluation of quantitative and qualitative changes in the lymphocytes and myeloid series will help to diagnose many infectious, immunologic, malignant and even endocrine disorders.

Quantitative changes in counts are the most frequently found anomaly on the hemogram report. The differential count will help pinpoint the expanded population of cells. The percentage increase over normal range is important, very high counts are indicative of leukemoid reaction or leukemias. The absolute count is required in certain cases, e.g. absolute eosinophil count for diagnosis of hypereosinophilic syndromes and absolute neutrophil count for degree of immunodeficiency. The morphology of cells may reveal abnormal size, immaturity, change in nuclear-cytoplasmic ratio, inclusions and abnormal granules. Howell-Jolly bodies are found in cases of absent splenic function due to asplenia or post splenectomy, toxic granulations and left shift suggests sepsis, and Epstein-Barr virus infection results in large monocytoid cells.

### Leukocytosis

The onset and duration of illness may provide a clue to the diagnosis. History is taken for infections, inflammatory, malignant and metabolic disorders.

*Neutrophilia:* Increase in acute bacterial infections; other causes including acute blood loss, hemolysis and diabetic ketoacidosis (Table 13.28). Leukocyte alkaline phosphatase (LAP) is an enzyme present in mature neutrophils; this is increased in infections and leukemoid reaction and low in chronic myeloid leukemia.

*Monocytosis:* The circulating tissue macrophage precursors are called monocytes. These cells migrate to tissues and transform into macrophages, e.g. Kupffer cells in liver. These cells are important for ingestion and killing of many pathogenic bacteria and organisms like *Mycobacterium tuberculosis* and *Leishmania*. Monocytes are the first cells to recover in post chemotherapy states, when white blood cell counts recover. Abnormality of macrophage activation leads to disorders like hemophagocytic syndrome. Langerhans cell histiocytosis is a clonal proliferative disorder of histiocytes.

*Eosinophilia:* This occurs in many allergic disorders, e.g. atopic dermatitis and asthma, systemic inflammatory conditions, e.g. inflammatory bowel disease and rheumatoid arthritis, and malignancies, e.g. Hodgkin lymphoma.

Table 13.28: Common causes of neutrophilia

**Acute**

- Acute bacterial infections
- Epinephrine, corticosteroids, granulocyte colony-stimulating factor
- Hemorrhage; hemolysis
- Hypoxia
- Trauma, burns, exercise, heat stroke
- Acute kidney injury, diabetic ketoacidosis, hepatic failure
- Hodgkin lymphoma

**Chronic**

- Chronic myeloid leukemia
- Rheumatological and inflammatory diseases
- Hemolytic anemias; sickle cell anemia
- Post-splenectomy
- Chronic blood loss
- Thyrotoxicosis
- Chronic idiopathic neutrophilia

**Genetic causes or syndromes**

- Down syndrome
- Asplenia
- Leukocyte adhesion defects

Table 13.29: Common causes of eosinophilia

**Acute**

- *Allergic disorders:* Asthma, atopic dermatitis, urticaria, drug hypersensitivity, pemphigoid
- *Parasitic infestations:* Toxocara, ascaris, amebiasis, strongyloidiasis, filaria, toxoplasmosis, trichinosis, schistosomiasis, malaria, scabies
- *Fungal infections:* Bronchopulmonary aspergillosis, coccidiomycosis
- *Malignancy:* Hodgkin lymphoma, T cell lymphoma, acute myelogenous leukemia, myeloproliferative syndrome
- *Hypereosinophilic syndrome*

**Chronic**

- *Allergic disorders:* Pemphigus, dermatitis herpetiformis
- *Autoimmune disorders:* Inflammatory bowel disease, rheumatoid arthritis
- *Immunodeficiency syndromes:* Hyper-IgE, Wiskott-Aldrich syndrome; Omenn syndrome; graft versus host reaction
- *Miscellaneous:* Thrombocytopenia with absent radii; Addison disease

Parasites, which invade tissues, are more likely to cause eosinophilia, e.g. *Toxocara* that causes visceral larva migrans (Table 13.29). Elevated sustained eosinophil counts are associated with cardiac toxicity. Moderate elevated absolute eosinophil count are above 1500–5000 cell/μL, and severe eosinophilia is >5000 cells/μL.

**Table 13.30:** Common causes of lymphocytosis

| |
|---|
| *Infections:* Infectious mononucleosis, infectious hepatitis, cytomegalovirus, tuberculosis, pertussis |
| *Endocrine:* Thyrotoxicosis, Addison disease |
| *Malignancy:* Acute lymphoblastic leukemia, lymphoma |

***Lymphocytosis:*** Lymphocytosis is a common feature of many infections, particularly in children (**Table 13.30**). It is important to identify reactive from neoplastic lymphocytosis.

### Leukopenia

Important causes of leukopenia include viral infections (influenza, HIV, COVID-19), some medications (chemotherapy agents, anticonvulsants), megaloblastic anemia, aplastic anemia, bone marrow infiltration (malignancy, Gaucher disease, osteopetrosis) and hypersplenism.

***Neutropenia:*** The absolute neutrophil count is calculated by [WBC count/µL × percentage of neutrophils + band forms]. Severe neutropenia occurs when the absolute neutrophil count is below 500/µL. Neutropenia can be due to infections, inflammatory conditions, bone marrow failure syndromes, and due to malignancy or as a consequence of treatment for malignancy. It can also be due to rare metabolic disorders like glycogen storage disease type 1b, Shwachman-Diamond syndrome and Kostmann syndrome.

***Lymphopenia:*** Lymphopenia is found in patient with inherited immunodeficiency syndromes due to decreased production of B or T lymphocytes. It is also seen in patients with SARS-CoV-2 infection, acquired immunodeficiency syndrome, systemic lupus, rheumatoid arthritis, post antithymocyte globulin treatment for aplastic anemia, following use of corticosteroids, and in protein losing enteropathy.

### Suggested Readings


1. Orkin S, et al (eds). Nathan and Oski's Hematology and Oncology of Infancy and Childhood, 8th edn. Philadelphia, Pennsylvania: Elsevier Saunders, 2015.
2. Riley LK, Rupert J. Evaluation of patient with leukocytosis. Am Fam Physician 2015; 92: 1004–11.

Chapter 14

# Otorhinolaryngology

❍ Prem Sagar ❍ Alok Thakar ❍ Sandeep Samant

*Competency:* **PE28.4**

## DISEASES OF THE EAR

### Acute Otitis Media

Otitis media is a common early childhood morbidity that refers to viral or bacterial infection of the 'middle ear cleft'. The middle ear cleft is a term that includes the pneumatic spaces of the middle ear cavity medial to the tympanic membrane, the attic superiorly, the mastoid antrum posterior to the attic, and pneumatized air cells in temporal bone that surround the mastoid antrum and extend to the petrous apex. Anatomic features that predispose a young child to ear infections include a shorter, more horizontal and compliant eustachian tube, and bacterial carriage in the adenoids. Risk factors include bottle feeding, use of pacifier, day care center attendance, passive smoking, overcrowding, cleft palate, Down syndrome, allergy, immune dysfunction and gastroesophageal reflux.

*Incidence:* The peak incidence of acute otitis media in childhood is in infancy and decreases with advancing age. Acute otitis media is uncommon beyond the age of 7 years.

*Etiology:* The most common causative organisms are *Streptococcus pneumoniae*, *Hemophilus influenzae* and *Moraxella catarrhalis* in ~75% cases; less common pathogens include *S. pyogenes*, *S. aureus* and *Pseudomonas aeruginosa*; viruses may be the sole pathogen in 15% of cases.

*Diagnosis:* The condition is characterized by rapid onset of symptoms such as otalgia or ear tugging, fever, crying and irritability. Older children may report impaired hearing. History of recent upper respiratory tract infection is common. Otoscopy reveals a red and bulging tympanic membrane or perforated tympanic membrane with mucopurulent otorrhea (Fig. 14.1). The spontaneous perforation closes promptly following release of accumulated mucopus in the middle ear cleft. The diagnosis of otitis media is considered in the presence of the following criteria: Rapid onset of symptoms, signs of middle ear effusion and tympanic membrane inflammation.

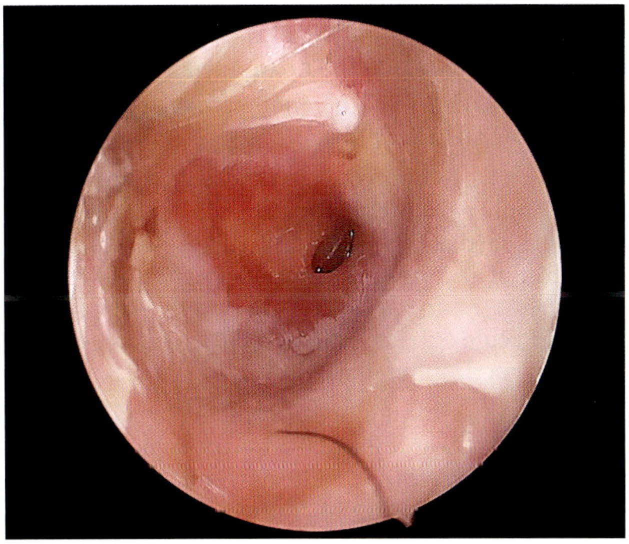

Fig. 14.1: Small perforation in congested tympanic membrane with otorrhea seen in acute otitis media

*Treatment:* Antimicrobial therapy is recommended in all patients except a few who may qualify for a trial of observation (Table 14.1). Amoxicillin is the first choice of therapy. Higher doses (75–90 mg/kg/day) are considered where streptococcal resistance is endemic. Coamoxiclav, cefaclor, cefuroxime and newer generation cephalosporins are useful second-line drugs. Macrolides are considered in patients allergic to penicillin and/or cephalosporins. Antibiotic therapy is continued for at least 7 days. Otoscopy should be repeated after 3–4 days and at 3 weeks to ensure resolution of infection and healing of tympanic membrane perforation. Adjuvant treatment with oral and topical decongestant agents is not necessary. Antihistaminic agents contribute little to resolution of otitis media and may precipitate sinus infections by drying mucosal secretions.

**Table 14.1:** Recommendations for initial management for uncomplicated acute otitis media

| *Age, months* | *Severe symptoms*, otorrhea or uncertain access to follow-up* | | *No severe symptoms* or otorrhea; follow-up assured* | |
|---|---|---|---|---|
| | *Unilateral* | *Bilateral* | *Unilateral* | *Bilateral* |
| 6–23 | Antibiotic therapy | Antibiotic therapy | Treat or observe** | Antibiotic therapy |
| ≥24 | Antibiotic therapy | Antibiotic therapy | Treat or observe** | Treat or observe** |

Clinical practice guideline: Diagnosis and management of acute otitis media. Pediatrics 2013; 131:e964–99

*Include toxic-appearance; otalgia persisting for >48 hours; temperature >39°C (102.2°F) in last 48 hours

**If observation is offered, follow up must be ensured and antibiotics are started if the child worsens or fails to improve within 48 to 72 hours of onset of symptoms

### Recurrent Acute Otitis Media

Recurrent acute otitis media refers to three or more episodes in any 6 months or four or more episodes in a year. Children experiencing recurrent otitis media are considered for tympanostomy tube insertion to reduce the frequency of the episodes. Adenoidectomy may be considered, if there is associated airway obstruction. Patients with recurrent acute otitis media do not benefit from concurrent tonsillectomy.

### Otitis Media with Effusion

Otitis media with effusion refers to serous or mucoid fluid occupying the normally air-filled spaces of the middle ear cleft. Inflammatory signs are absent and the prime symptom is hearing loss due to poor conduction of sound pressure from the external to inner ear.

*Etiology:* Otitis media with effusion occurs due to eustachian tube obstruction and may follow an episode of acute otitis media. Effusions are found in ~40% patients at 1 month after acute otitis media and in 10% after 3 months. Otitis media with effusion may occur *de novo* (without history of acute otitis media), particularly in patients with adenoid hypertrophy or nasal allergies.

*Diagnosis:* Most children are asymptomatic or complain of hearing loss and ear fullness; there is no otalgia. Otoscopy reveals dull gray, yellow or blue tympanic membrane with middle ear effusion (Fig. 14.2). Air fluid level or bubbles may be observed medial to the tympanic membrane. Diagnosis is confirmed by demonstrating reduced tympanic membrane mobility on pneumatic otoscopy (Seigel speculum examination) or type B pattern on tympanometry.

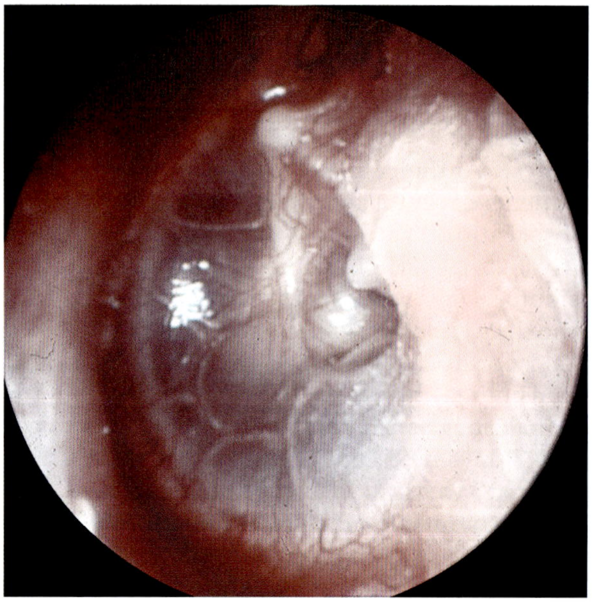

Fig. 14.2: Otitis media with effusion. Note the dull lusterless tympanic membrane (*Courtesy:* Textbook of ENT, Hazarika)

*Therapy and outcome:* About two-thirds of serous middle ear effusions in children (2–7 years old) resolve spontaneously within 3 months. Older children who are not at risk for speech and learning disabilities may be kept under observation without medical or surgical intervention. Children who can cooperate should be advised auto-inflation during the period of observation. Age appropriate hearing tests should be performed, if effusion persists beyond 3 months or if hearing loss, speech delay or learning difficulty is suspected. Use of antihistamines, decongestants, corticosteroids and antibiotics is not routinely required.

*Surgery is indicated in patients with:* (i) Otitis media with effusion lasting 3 months or longer along with persistent hearing loss, poor scholastic performance, behavioral problems, ear discomfort or difficulty in balance; (ii) recurrent or persistent otitis media with effusion in a child at increased risk of speech and learning disabilities (permanent hearing loss, speech and language disorder, autism spectrum disorder, Down syndrome, uncorrectable visual impairment or developmental delay); and (iii) otitis media with effusion associated with structural damage to the tympanic membrane or middle ear.

The initial surgical procedure consists of myringotomy and tympanostomy tube placement. The tympanic membrane is penetrated by a small radial myringotomy incision (approximately 1 mm) in the anteroinferior quadrant, the middle ear effusion is aspirated and a tympanostomy tube (grommet) is placed through the incision (Fig. 14.3). Tympanostomy tube placement drains the effusion and improves middle ear ventilation. This leads to resolution of mucosal edema and restoration of the patency of eustachian tube. Tympanostomy tubes get extruded spontaneously and the myringotomy closes soon after.

The mean time for spontaneous extrusion of short-term tympanostomy tubes (e.g. Goode, Shepard) is 6–9 months. Tubes designed for long-term retention (e.g. T-tube, Armstrong tube) last 12–18 months. Children with tympanostomy tubes should wear earplugs while swimming to avoid entry of water into the middle ear space. Complications after tympanostomy tube insertion, noted in 5–10% cases, include recurrent otorrhea, early extrusion, tube blockage and persistent perforation. Long-term tubes are associated with higher rates of complication.

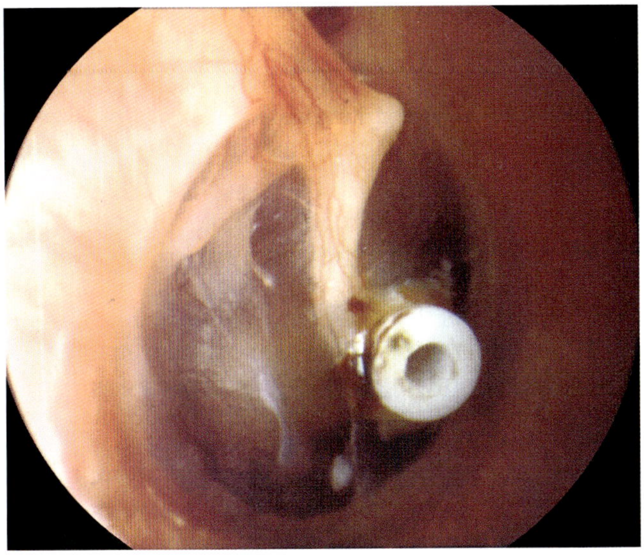

Fig. 14.3: Tympanostomy tube *in situ* in the anteroinferior quadrant of the tympanic membrane (*Courtesy:* Textbook of ENT, Hazarika)

Patients with adenoid hypertrophy should undergo adenoidectomy to avoid obstruction of the eustachian tube openings, particularly in cases with recurrence after tympanostomy tube extrusion. Isolated tonsillectomy or myringotomy should not be performed to treat otitis media with effusion. Patients with persistent otitis media with effusion and hearing loss should be offered hearing amplification with hearing aid, if surgery cannot be performed.

*Prevention:* The incidence of acute otitis media and otitis media with effusion is reduced with exclusive breast-feeding for the first 6 months of life, avoiding bottle feeding in supine position and use of pacifiers, eliminating passive smoking, and vaccination against pneumococci and *Hemophilus* spp.

### Chronic Otitis Media

Chronic otitis media is defined as chronic inflammation of the middle ear space and mastoid air cells. It may result in perforation of the tympanic membrane, tympanosclerosis, retraction pocket in the tympanic membrane, ossicular damage or cholesteatoma leading to ear discharge and/or hearing loss. Chronic suppurative otitis media (CSOM) is diagnosed in the presence of an ear discharge persisting for longer than 6 weeks.

*Risk factors:* Perforations in the tympanic membrane following otitis media or tympanostomy tube placement may not heal due to persistent infection, leading to chronic otitis media. Factors preventing resolution of otitis media include recurrent infections through a perforated tympanic membrane, ascending infection from nasopharynx through the eustachian tube and colonization of middle ear by bacteria. Commonly isolated organisms include *P. aeruginosa*, *S. aureus*, *Proteus*, *E. coli* and anerobes.

*Presentation and classification:* Patients usually present with mucoid or mucopurulent ear discharge and/or hearing loss that is chiefly mild to moderate and of conductive type. Chronic otitis is broadly categorized into two types. Simple central perforations of the pars tensa are classified as *tubotympanic*. Disease affecting the attic and posterosuperior region, especially if associated with cholesteatoma, retraction pockets or persistent granulation, is classified as *atticoantral*. Atticoantral disease, associated with high risk of intracranial and intratemporal complications, is termed unsafe chronic otitis media and tubotympanic disease is considered *safe*. The incidence of complications very significantly lower with tubotympanic disease.

Perforations in the tympanic membrane are described based on their size and location. Those involving the pars tensa and not affecting the bony margin are central perforations (Fig. 14.4). Perforations affecting the posterosuperior tympanic membrane and marginal perforations (i.e. those reaching the margin of the membrane) are associated with retraction pockets and cholesteatoma formation.

*Management:* Medical therapy chiefly consists of topical antibiotics and aural toilet. Parents are instructed to avoid water ingress. Topical quinolones are effective and safe. Complicated infections and/or signs of systemic involvement merit the use of systemic antibiotics. Secondary fungal otitis externa may develop as a complication of topical antibiotic therapy. Otolaryngology referral is necessary to rule out cholesteatoma. Surgery is indicated in cases that do not respond to conservative treatment, and involves repair of the tympanic membrane perforation (tympanoplasty) with or without mastoidectomy.

### Cholesteatoma

This term refers to a sac of squamous epithelium extending from the tympanic membrane into the middle ear. It is usually acquired and related to eustachian tube dysfunction. Cholesteatoma may arises from extension of a tympanic membrane retraction pocket, or from aberrant inward migration of normal epithelium. Cholesteatoma

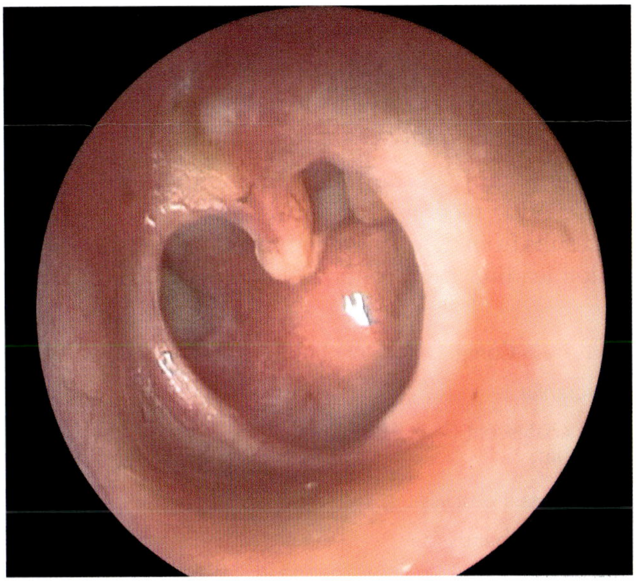

Fig. 14.4: Otoscopy in a child with chronic suppurative otitis media showing subtotal central perforation and purulence in the middle ear (*Courtesy:* Textbook of ENT, Hazarika)

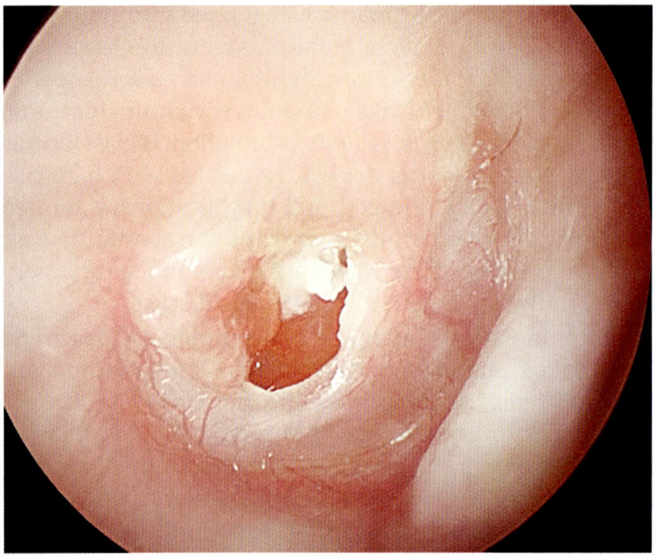

Fig. 14.5: Keratin debris and granulation seen arising from the posterosuperior margin of the perforation and extending into the middle ear suggestive of cholesteatoma

can cause serious complications by its slow expansion and destruction of surrounding bone.

*Diagnosis:* Patients with cholesteatoma present with a chronically draining ear and hearing loss. Diagnosis is made by visualization of keratin debris/flakes in the middle ear or pars flaccida (Fig. 14.5). Computed tomography (CT) of temporal bone outlines the extent of cholesteatoma in the middle ear, mastoid air cells and beyond, and thus helps in planning the management.

*Treatment:* Patients with otitis media and cholesteatoma require mastoidectomy and removal of the cholesteatoma. The goal of therapy is to create a safe ear by removing the cholesteatoma and to achieve dry ear. Hearing restoration is a secondary goal.

### Complications of Otitis Media

Untreated otitis media may cause serious complications that are classified as extracranial or intracranial (Table 14.2). Complications of acute otitis media usually occur in young children, while complications of chronic otitis with cholesteatoma are common in older children.

*Hearing loss:* It is the most common complication of chronic otitis media. Hearing loss is usually conductive and results from tympanic membrane perforation, ossicular erosion leading to discontinuity and discharge in middle ear. Sensorineural hearing loss may occur, either due to involvement of the labyrinth by infection or inflammation and cholesteatoma eroding the labyrinth. Bilateral hearing loss affects speech and language development in early childhood and academic performance in school going kids.

*Acute coalescent mastoiditis:* It results from spread of infection into the mastoid air cells and erosion of bony septations. It presents with post-auricular erythema, tenderness and edema, with the auricle displaced inferiorly and laterally. The entity should be differentiated radiologically from fluid effusion within mastoid air cells that is commonly associated with acute or chronic otitis media. Untreated coalescent mastoiditis may erode the mastoid cortex, leading to subperiosteal abscess in postauricular, temporal or zygomatic area (Fig. 14.6). The ruptured subperiosteal abscess may track along neck muscles leading to deep neck abscesses. Findings on CT include fluid in the mastoid air cells and loss of bony septa between these cells. Initial therapy should be with parenteral antibiotics covering against gram-negative and anerobic pathogens when mastoiditis is superimposed on a chronically draining ear. Surgery is indicated in patients with unsatisfactory response to parenteral antibiotics, subperiosteal or neck abscesses, intracranial complications and for mastoiditis with CSOM. Cortical mastoidectomy with/without tympanostomy tube insertion is adequate in the backdrop of acute otitis media, whereas canal wall down mastoidectomy, cholesteatoma removal and tympanoplasty is considered for CSOM.

*Labyrinthine fistula:* It may form due to inner ear erosion by cholesteatoma, and presents with vertigo and sensorineural hearing loss. Cholesteatoma-induced labyrinthine fistula and labyrinthitis (inflammation or infection of the inner ear) requires urgent surgical intervention in the form of mastoidectomy along with antibiotics.

*Facial nerve paralysis* secondary to otitis media is treated with antibiotics, but surgery is often indicated. During the early phase of acute otitis media, myringotomy to release pus from the middle ear may suffice, whereas cases

Table 14.2: Complications of otitis media

| *Extracranial* | *Intracranial* |
|---|---|
| Acute coalescent mastoiditis | Meningitis |
| Subperiosteal abscess | Epidural abscess |
| Facial nerve paralysis | Venous (sigmoid sinus) thrombosis |
| Labyrinthitis or labyrinthine fistula | Brain or subdural abscess |
| | Otitic hydrocephalus |

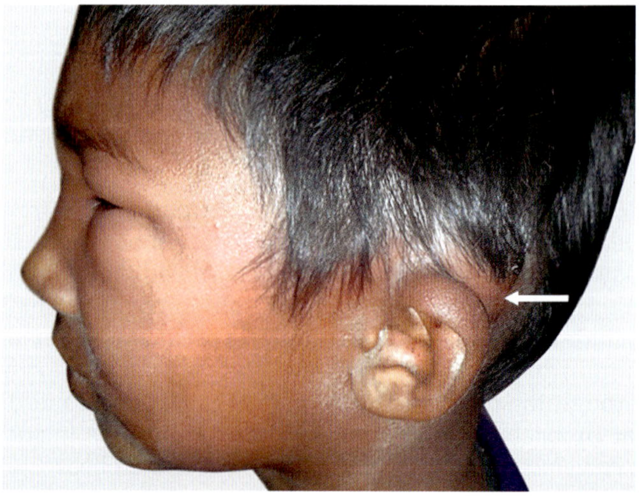

Fig. 14.6: An 8-year-old boy with left-sided chronic suppurative otitis media associated with post-auricular abscess (arrow). Note the swelling at the root of zygoma and periorbital puffiness

presenting later with accompanying mastoiditis require cortical mastoidectomy and facial nerve exploration. Facial nerve paralysis secondary to cholesteatoma requires modified radical mastoidectomy and facial nerve decompression.

*Meningitis:* It is the most common intracranial complication of both acute and chronic otitis media. Acute otitis media is also the chief cause of secondary meningitis and pneumococcal meningitis is the most common cause of acquired sensorineural hearing loss in children. The morbidity and mortality associated with meningitis has decreased significantly following use of appropriate antibiotics, and pneumococcal vaccines.

*Brain abscess:* It is a potentially lethal complication. Unlike meningitis, which is more commonly associated with acute otitis media, brain abscess is almost exclusively a complication of CSOM. Therapy with broad-spectrum parenteral antibiotics is begun immediately and surgical drainage is considered to relief compressive features.

*Thrombosis of the sigmoid or transverse sinus:* It is an important intracranial complication. Patients present with headache, malaise and high spiking fever. Treatment is with parenteral antibiotics and mastoidectomy surgery.

In the setting of otitis media, the warning signs of possible complications are mentioned in Table 14.3. When suspected the patient should be promptly referred to a specialist after initiation of medical treatment.

### Otitis Externa

*Acute otitis externa (swimmer's ear):* It presents with itching, pain and fullness of the ear, with or without otorrhea. Erythema and edema of the ear canal and tenderness on moving the pinnae or tragus are diagnostic. Risk factors include swimming, impacted cerumen, use of hearing aid, eczema and trauma to the ear canal. Chief pathogens include *P. aeruginosa*, *Staphylococcus*, *Proteus*, *E. coli* and *Aspergillus* or *Candida* sp. Management with aural toileting and topical antibiotic drops is associated with clinical cure rates of up to 80%. If edema is significant, a ribbon gauze or wick may be placed in the external auditory canal to keep it patent and allow delivery of topical ear

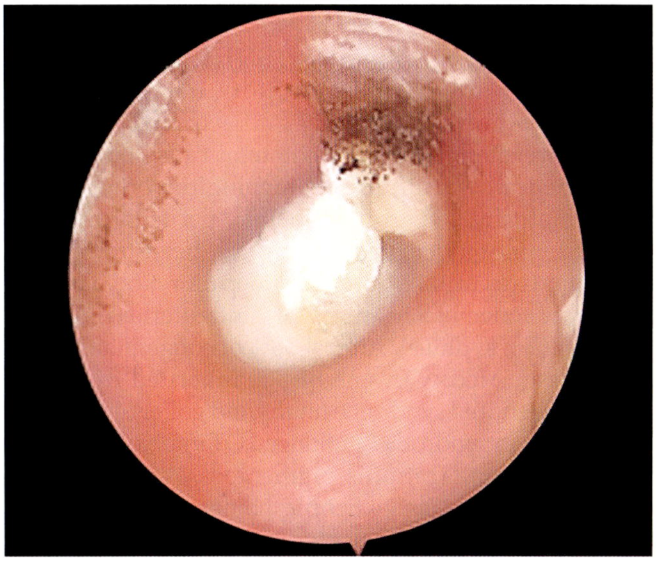

**Fig. 14.7:** Cream-colored discharge (*Candida* infection) and black spores (*Aspergillus niger*) seen in otomycosis

drops. Oral antibiotics are reserved for cases who fail to improve or are complicated.

*Otomycosis or fungal otitis externa:* It is common in humid weather or following treatment of a bacterial infection. Patients present with ear pain and pruritus; *Aspergillus* and *Candida* spp. are common pathogens. Otoscopy reveals thick cream-colored discharge associated with fungal spores and filaments (Fig. 14.7). The condition is managed with aural toilet and topical antifungal (e.g. clotrimazole) drops.

*Otic furunculosis:* It is a very painful, superficial abscess in the outer portion of the ear canal, typically due to *S. aureus*. Oral antibiotics and analgesics ensure relief; incision and drainage is rarely required.

*Eczematous or psoriatic otitis* externa refers to inflammatory conditions characterized by ear discharge, pruritus and/or scaling of skin of the ear canal. Contact, atopic or seborrheic dermatitis is usually present.

### Hearing Loss

Hearing loss in children may be congenital or acquired. Based on the pathology, it is categorized as conductive, sensorineural or mixed. Early detection of hearing loss in children is important as untreated hearing loss interferes with development of speech, language and cognitive skills.

#### Conductive Hearing Loss

Any pathology that interferes with the conduction of sound through the ear canal, tympanic membrane or middle ear ossicles may cause conductive hearing loss (CHL). CHL is usually acquired and mild to moderate in severity. Common causes include impacted cerumen, otitis media with effusion, tympanic membrane perforation, tympanosclerosis and cholesteatoma. Less commonly, CHL is congenital, associated with congenital ossicular fixation or discontinuity and atresia of the ear canal. CHL with middle ear abnormalities may be seen in syndromic conditions, e.g. Apert, Crouzon and Treacher Collins syndromes.

| **Table 14.3:** Red flag signs of complicated otitis media |
|---|
| Fever, otalgia, thick purulent and malodorous discharge with: |
| • Fever |
| • Painful swelling behind the ear |
| • Facial weakness |
| • Sudden hearing loss |
| • Dizziness |
| • Headache with/without vomiting |
| • Stiffness of neck |
| • Seizures |
| • Ataxia |
| • Disorientation or loss of consciousness |

### Sensorineural Hearing Loss

Sensorineural hearing loss (SNHL) is caused by pathology in the cochlea, auditory nerve or central auditory pathway. Congenital and acquired SNHL are equally prevalent. The most common cause of acquired sensorineural hearing loss is meningitis; other causes are prematurity, hyperbilirubinemia, perinatal hypoxia, acquired immunodeficiency syndrome, head trauma and medications (e.g. aminoglycosides, loop diuretics). The chief etiology of congenital hearing loss is intrauterine infections (e.g. TORCH, syphilis). Almost 30% of congenital hearing loss is associated with one of 300 inherited disorders, including Pendred syndrome (euthyroid goiter), Jervell and Lange-Nielsen syndrome (prolonged QT interval, syncope), Usher syndrome (retinitis pigmentosa and blindness), Alport syndrome (microscopic hematuria and kidney failure), branchio-otorenal syndrome, neurofibromatosis and Waardenburg syndrome.

Over 65 genes are associated with inherited hearing loss. Mutations in *GJB2*, encoding for connexin 26 (expressed in the inner ear and involved in cochlear homeostasis) account for one-half of patients with autosomal recessive non-syndromic hearing loss.

### Screening for Hearing Loss

Significant hearing loss is present in 1–3 per 1000 newborns, particularly in babies requiring neonatal intensive care. Hearing loss has significant impact on development of speech, language and cognitive skills. Effective rehabilitation with hearing aids and cochlear implants is now routinely anticipated, and its immense success has resulted in financial support for cochlear implants from government agencies and schemes. When applied early in life and supplemented with auditory training, such rehabilitation can lead to near-normal hearing, good acquisition of speech and language, and integration into normal schooling. Hence, most developed countries have adopted programs for universal neonatal hearing screening for all newborns. The Indian Academy of Pediatrics and the Indian Academy of Otolaryngologists & Head-Neck Surgery recommend universal screening for hearing loss in newborn period, but this is not yet uniformly adopted across India and most developing countries.

An important guideline in infant hearing screening and intervention program is the '1-3-6' rule. This recommends screening all newborns for hearing loss by 1 month of age, completing secondary diagnostic testing for infants who fail the first screening by 3 months, and ensuring early intervention for diagnosed hearing loss by 6 months, thus enabling language and social development in line with physical development.

Strategies for neonatal hearing screening may be based on subjective response to spoken loud sounds, rattles, and spoken speech, but this is significantly inferior to objective testing by instrumentation. Screening by instrumentation may be undertaken by otoacoustic emissions (OAE) or by automated auditory brainstem responses (AABR). Children failing the hearing screen need further confirmation by definitive tests. Table 14.4 lists the screening tests and further confirmatory tests used to assess hearing sensitivity as the child progresses in age and ability to cooperate with testing.

In countries where neonatal hearing screening is not routine, hearing loss is usually detected by 18–36 months when testing is undertaken for parental concern for hearing or speech, poor language development or decline in language skills, ear infections, difficulty in understanding conversation or inappropriate response to commands. Some forms of early-onset hearing loss may also not manifest at birth, but at a later age.

### Management of Hearing Loss

Management of hearing loss is based on the extent of deficit and the underlying pathology. For mild to moderate conductive hearing loss, options include tympanostomy tube for otitis media with effusion, tympanoplasty for tympanic membrane perforation, mastoidectomy and tympanoplasty for cholesteatoma and canaloplasty for canal atresia. Conventional hearing aid, bone conduction hearing aid or middle ear implants are considered in patients with conductive hearing loss when the pathology cannot be surgically corrected.

Treatment of mild sensorineural hearing loss may consist simply of preferential seating in school. Bilateral or occasionally unilateral hearing aid usage is advised for mild to moderate sensorineural hearing loss, while children with severe to profound loss who do not benefit significantly from hearing aid are considered for cochlear implantation. Bilateral rehabilitation by hearing aids is routine and bilateral use provides improved sound localization and

**Table 14.4:** Tools for screening of hearing

| *Test* | *Principle* | *Age of child* |
|---|---|---|
| Automated otoacoustic emissions | Evaluates cochlear function; also affected by ear canal obstruction or middle ear effusion | Any age; neonatal screening |
| Automated auditory brainstem response | Measures integrity of cochlea, auditory nerve and brainstem | Any age; neonatal screening |
| Auditory brainstem response—full test battery | Measures integrity of cochlea, auditory nerve and brainstem | Any age; confirmatory test for screening failed infants |
| Free field audiometry | Sound booth based conditioned hearing | 6 months to 2.5 years |
| Play audiometry | Play/game reinforced hearing evaluation | >2.5 years |
| Audiometry | Ear and frequency specific hearing assessment | >4 years |

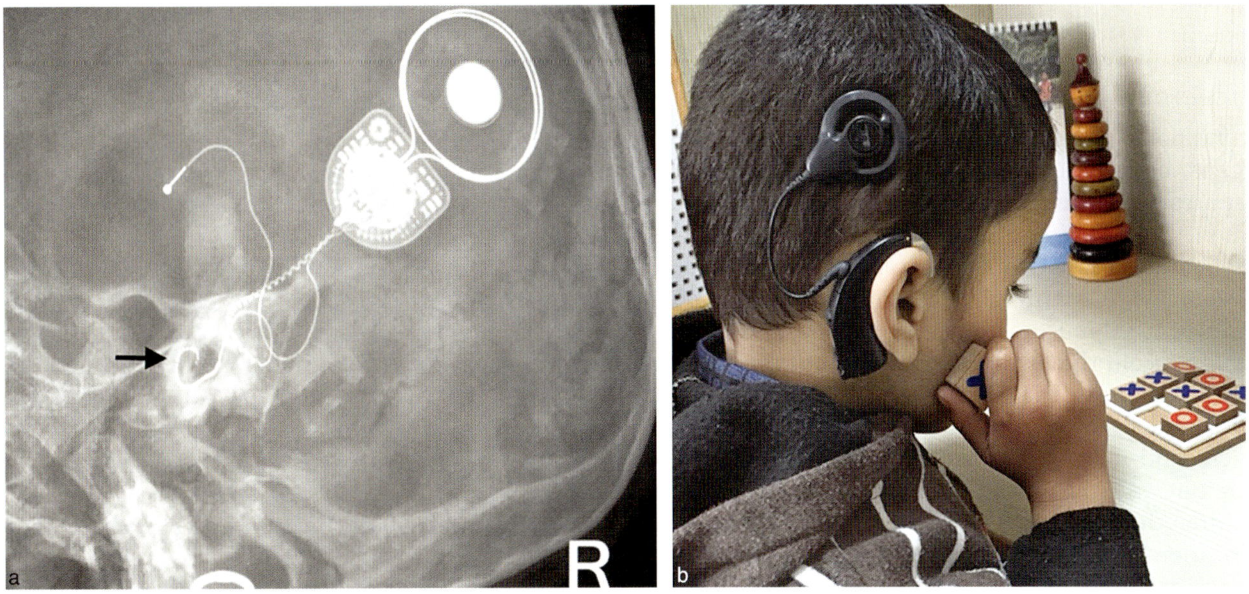

Fig. 14.8: (a) X-ray (modified Stenvers view) of the mastoid showing cochlear implant with multichannel stimulating electrodes along the cochlear turn (arrow). Note the other internal components of cochlear implant (receiver stimulator component placed posterosuperiorly and the ball/ground electrode located superiorly; (b) Cochlear implantee in a rehabilitation session. Note the external component, including a microphone and sound processor behind the pinna and a transmitter superiorly over the mastoid that transmits amplified sound to the internal receiver stimulator complex transcutaneously

speech understanding in noise. Cochlear implantation is usually undertaken as a unilateral procedure, but bilateral implantation is preferred for the same advantages.

If cochlear implantation is not feasible [late age of presentation (>5 years); financial constraints], communication necessarily has to then be by sign language and enrolment in deaf education programs. This should, however, be rare with current advances and access to medical care.

*Pediatric Cochlear Implantation*

Cochlear implant directly stimulates the residual cochlear nerve cells in the spiral ganglion (cochlea). The US FDA approved pediatric cochlear implantation for children with bilateral severe to profound sensorineural hearing loss (≥70 dB hearing loss) with unsatisfactory benefit from hearing aid use for at least 3–6 months. As early introduction of sound is crucial to develop processes for sound awareness and speech development in the auditory cortex, and hence hearing should be aided as early as possible. The minimum age for cochlear implant has been reduced to 9 months by US FDA. Evaluation before surgery includes computed tomography and magnetic resonance imaging to assess anatomy of the inner ear and to confirm the presence of cochlear nerve. Multielectrode implants that provide information across various frequencies are positioned sequentially along the cochlea to allow sound to be coded and transmitted for the entire sound spectrum (Fig. 14.8). The implant risks damage with strong magnetic fields and caution is advised with MR scanning. Most current implants are safe for MR scanners up to 3.0 Tesla.

### Suggested Reading


1. Liming BJ, Carter J, Cheng A, et al. International Pediatric Otolaryngology Group consensus recommendations: Hearing loss in the pediatric patient. Int J Pediatr Otorhinolaryngol 2016; 90: 251–58.
2. Siddiq S, Grainger J. The diagnosis and management of acute otitis media: American Academy of Pediatrics Guidelines 2013. Arch Dis Child Educ Pract Ed 2015; 100:193–97.
3. Standard treatment workflow for the management of otorrhoea, ICD-10-H92.10 and hearing impairment in pediatric age group (0-12 years), ICD 10 H90.5 in Standard Treatment Workflows of India. Ministry of Health and Family Welfare, Govt of India; 2019.
4. Paul A, Prasad C, Kamath SS, et al. On behalf of the IAP Newborn hearing screening. Indian Pediatr 2017; 54:647–51.
5. Rosenfeld RM, Shin JJ, Schwartz SR, et al. Clinical practice guideline: Otitis media with effusion (update). Otolaryngol Head Neck Surg 2016; 154:S1–S41.


*Competencies:* **PE28.13; PE28.14; PE28.17**

## DISEASES OF NOSE AND SINUSES

### Rhinitis

Inflammation of the mucosa lining the nose may occur alone (rhinitis) or with paranasal sinuses (rhinosinusitis).

*Viral Rhinitis*

Viral rhinitis (common cold) is the most frequent cause of nasal obstruction and rhinorrhea in children, occurring up to 6–8 times a year, usually due to infection with rhinovirus, influenza or adenovirus. Symptoms include malaise, low to moderate grade fever, nasal congestion and rhinorrhea, with or without sore throat. Antipyretics, saline nasal drops, oral decongestants and antihistamines provide symptomatic relief. Annual influenza vaccination reduces the incidence of severe cases. Less than 5% affected children develop superimposed bacterial rhinosinusitis and suppurative otitis media.

Competencies: **PE31.1; PE31.2**

### Allergic Rhinitis

The condition is due to an IgE-mediated reaction to specific allergens, commonly inhaled house dust mite, pollen and spores. Coexisting atopic dermatitis and asthma are common. Presentation is with sneezing, itching, nasal obstruction and clear rhinorrhea that are seasonal (hay fever) or perennial with intermittent exacerbations. Examination shows pale nasal mucosa, hypertrophied nasal turbinates and thin mucoid rhinorrhea with or without conjunctival itching and redness. Diagnosis is clinical. Supportive tests such as eosinophilia on nasal smear, skin tests for common allergens and increased serum total or allergen specific IgE are not essential. Further, skin tests may be negative in children during the first 1–2 years of illness while the sensitization is confined to nose and sinuses. Differential diagnosis includes food allergy (egg protein, cow milk, sea food). Management comprises of allergen avoidance. Topical corticosteroid sprays provide symptomatic relief. Long-term topical decongestants are discouraged due to the risk of rebound congestion and rhinitis medicamentosa.

### Bacterial Rhinosinusitis

Four pairs of paranasal sinuses surround the nose and help humidify the inspired air. The maxillary and ethmoid sinuses are present at birth and get easily infected in childhood. Sphenoid and frontal sinuses develop at approximately 9–10 months and 7–8 years of age, respectively, and rarely get infected alone.

***Acute bacterial rhinosinusitis:*** Rhinosinusitis is termed acute, if symptoms are for less than 12 weeks. It usually follows viral rhinitis but may develop *de novo* and recurrently in the presence of predisposing factors such as allergic rhinitis, adenoid inflammation and hypertrophy, cystic fibrosis, immunodeficiency, ciliary dyskinesia, daycare attendance, exposure to tobacco smoke and gastroesophageal reflux. Viral infections cause mucosal edema and ciliary hypoactivity causing obstruction of sinus ostia (openings of sinuses into the nasal cavity) and stasis of secretions. Obstructed sinuses are likely to get infected by bacteria from the nasopharynx, usually *S. pneumoniae*, *H. influenzae* and *M. catarrhalis*.

Persistent fever, facial pain or heaviness, nasal obstruction or purulent discharge, cough, dental pain and earache or fullness beyond 7–10 days of upper respiratory tract infection suggest the diagnosis of infective rhinosinusitis.

Periorbital edema, proptosis, diplopia, severe headache, vomiting, seizures or focal neurological deficits suggest ocular or central neurological system involvement, requiring computed tomography for confirmation. Orbital extension, contributing to 90% of complications, follows direct extension of infection from the ethmoid sinuses, and is graded as inflammatory edema, orbital or preseptal cellulitis, subperiosteal abscess, orbital abscess and cavernous sinus thrombosis **(Fig. 14.9)**. Ophthalmoplegia, vision loss and toxemia indicate infection of cavernous sinuses. Intracranial complications, including meningitis and brain abscesses, are common with frontal and sphenoid sinusitis.

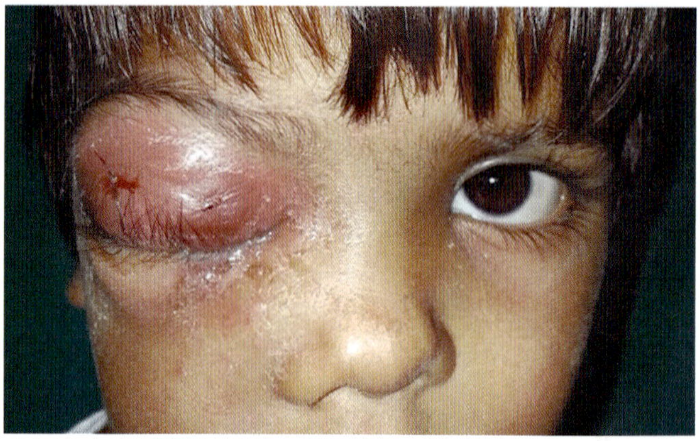

**Fig. 14.9:** Acute bacterial rhinosinusitis with orbital cellulitis. Note the marked lid edema, congestion and proptosis

Therapy with oral antibiotics (amoxicillin, coamoxiclav for 10–14 days) is preferred. Longer courses and/or second-line antibiotics may be indicated based on organism sensitivity and nature of illness. Measures, such as oral or topical decongestants, mucolytics and nasal saline drops/sprays/irrigation provide early symptomatic relief. Patients with complications require parenteral antibiotics with or without endoscopic sinus surgery and abscess drainage.

***Chronic bacterial rhinosinusitis:*** When symptoms of rhinosinusitis persist for >12 weeks, infection with *S. aureus*, anerobes and even fungi should be considered apart from usual bacterial pathogens. Nasal obstruction, purulent discharge, chronic cough, facial heaviness, dental pain, malaise and headache are common features. Young children may be just irritable. Prolonged inflammation causes formation of polypi in paranasal sinuses, ethmoid sinuses being most commonly affected.

Chronic bacterial rhinosinusitis is treated with a broad-spectrum antibiotic (co-amoxiclav, broad-spectrum cephalosporin or fluoroquinolone) for 3–6 weeks. Oral decongestants and topical corticosteroid sprays (e.g. mometasone or fluticasone) lead to faster symptomatic relief by reducing mucosal edema, improving patency of sinus ostia. Nasal steroid sprays are safe and do not impact facial or body growth. Saline irrigation decreases mucosal edema and improves mucociliary clearance of the nose and paranasal sinuses. Managing underlying gastroesophageal reflux with proton pump inhibitors may defer the need for surgery. Computed tomography and referral to a specialist is recommended in patients refractory to 3–6 weeks of medical management and those with complications.

### Allergic Fungal Rhinosinusitis

Allergic fungal rhinosinusitis is increasingly recognized in atopic immunocompetent children, chiefly adolescents, but is less common than in adults. It is caused by hypersensitivity to fungal antigens. Patients present with nasal obstruction, discharge and headache. Evaluation shows unilateral or bilateral nasal polypi. Proptosis and telecanthus suggest extensive disease with expansion of the ethmoid (lateral displacement of orbit) **(Fig. 14.10a)**

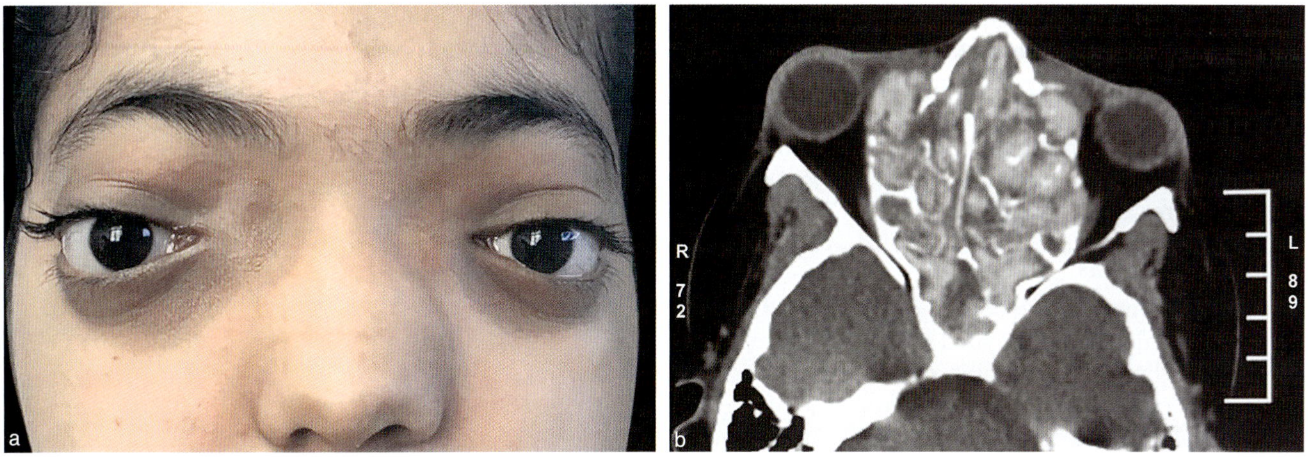


Fig. 14.10: (a) 13-yr-old girl with bilateral proptosis and telecanthus as a result of allergic fungal sinusitis; (b) CT of nose and paranasal sinuses showing soft tissue density with intermittent areas of hyperdensities (due to heavy metal content of the allergic mucin) seen in the expanded nasal cavity and sinuses with resultant bulging and lateral displacement of the eyeballs



or frontal sinuses (inferolateral displacement of orbit). CT imaging shows characteristic non-erosive expansion of sinuses with opacification and intermittent hyperdensities (Fig. 14.10b). Management consists of endoscopic removal of polypi and widening of sinus ostia. Topical steroid sprays reduce mucosal edema and prevent as well as delay recurrence.

## Nasal Obstruction

Apart from chronic rhinosinusitis, common and important causes of chronic nasal obstruction are adenoid hypertrophy and deviated nasal septum.

### *Adenoid Hypertrophy*

Adenoids are the lymphoid tissue located in the roof and posterior wall of nasopharynx that protects the upper aerodigestive tract against inhaled antigens. Adenoids usually grow until the age of 5 years due to heightened immunologic activity, often causing some airway obstruction following which it gradually shrinks. Chronic bacterial infection, gastroesophageal reflux and passive smoking may cause persistent adenoidal hypertrophy, leading to nasopharyngeal obstruction. An obstructed nasopharyngeal airway leads to chronic mouth breathing and dental malocclusion, while dysfunction of eustachian tube causes otitis media with effusion and conductive hearing loss. When associated with tonsillar hypertrophy, patients may show features of obstructive sleep apnea. Diagnosis is based on examination and endoscopic evaluation. Lateral radiograph of the neck reveals enlarged soft tissue in nasopharynx, occluding the airway (Fig. 14.11).

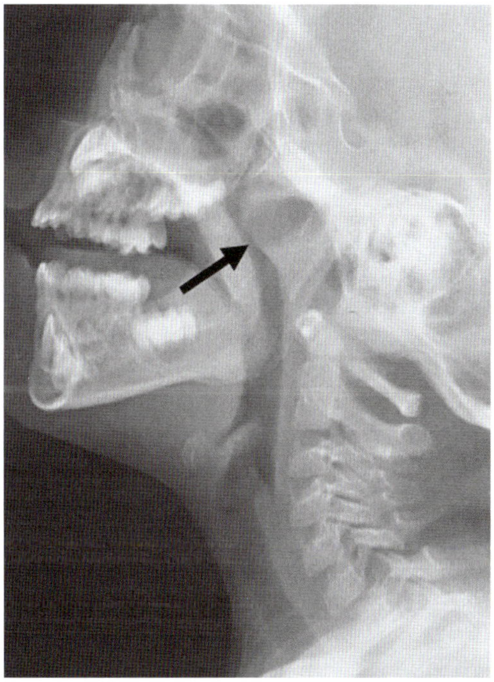

Fig. 14.11: Lateral radiograph of the neck showing adenoid hypertrophy occluding the nasopharyngeal airway in a 7-year-old girl with complaint of mouth breathing

Pubertal growth of the midface and regression of adenoids provide symptomatic relief of adenoid-related nasal obstruction beyond the age of 9-year. Medical management of symptomatic adenoid hypertrophy includes courses of antibiotics, prolonged use of aqueous nasal steroid spray and treatment of gastroesophageal reflux with proton pump inhibitors. Adenoidectomy is recommended in the presence of adenoid hypertrophy that is associated with persistent or recurrent otitis media with effusion, failure of medical management for obstructive sleep apnea, chronic adenoiditis, craniofacial growth abnormalities due to prolonged airway obstruction and chronic rhinosinusitis. When indicated, limited adenoidectomy is done for patients with concomitant cleft palate or submucous cleft palate so as to avoid uncovering symptoms of velopharyngeal insufficiency, such as nasal regurgitation of fluids and hypernasal speech that are masked due to compensation by hypertrophied adenoids.

### *Deviated Nasal Septum*

Deviation of septum (bony, cartilaginous or both) may be developmental or following trauma at birth or in later life. The space in nasal cavity is reduced on the convex side. Patients may experience bilateral nasal obstruction due to compensatory inferior turbinate hypertrophy on the concave side and/or rhinitis. To avoid injury to the growth centers, surgical correction of the deviated septum is planned after the age of completion of facial growth and development (approximately 14–16 years). Septoplasty may be considered in pediatric age only in cases of bothersome symptoms not relieved by medical management or septal spur causing recurrent epistaxis.

### Congenital Disorders

Developmental nasal anomalies include nasal dermoid, glioma, encephalocele and choanal atresia. While dermoids present as midline pit or swelling (with protruding hair strands in majority of them) anywhere from root of the nose to nasal tip, glioma and encephaloceles present as intranasal or extranasal mass. Following radiological evaluation, surgical excision is planned.

#### *Choanal Atresia*

This term refers to congenital failure of the nasal cavities to open into the nasopharynx. Unilateral or bilateral choanal atresia or stenosis is hypothesized to be caused by complete or partial persistence of buccopharyngeal membrane (separating oral cavity from pharynx) or nasobuccal membrane (separating nose from oral cavity) or due to abnormal neural crest cell migration. As infants are obligate nasal breathers, bilateral choanal atresia manifests immediately after birth with respiratory distress and intermittent cyanosis, precipitated by suckling that improves when the child cries. Bilateral atresia can be associated with CHARGE syndrome (coloboma, heart abnormalities, choanal atresia, retardation of growth and development, genitourinary defects and ear anomalies). The presentation of unilateral atresia is less dramatic and usually delayed. Patients present with persistent unilateral nasal discharge or blockage, typically when the opposite nasal passage is blocked due to rhinitis or adenoid hypertrophy.

The diagnosis of choanal atresia is considered when a 6F feeding catheter cannot be passed through the nose into the nasopharynx at birth. Flexible nasal endoscopy and CT confirm the diagnosis (Fig. 14.12). Patients with bilateral atresia require facilitation of oral breathing by keeping the mouth open and pulling the tongue forward manually by oral digital manipulation, followed by placement of plastic oropharyngeal airway or McGovern open-tip nipple. Surgical creation of posterior choanal patency is often followed by temporary stent placement to avoid restenosis.

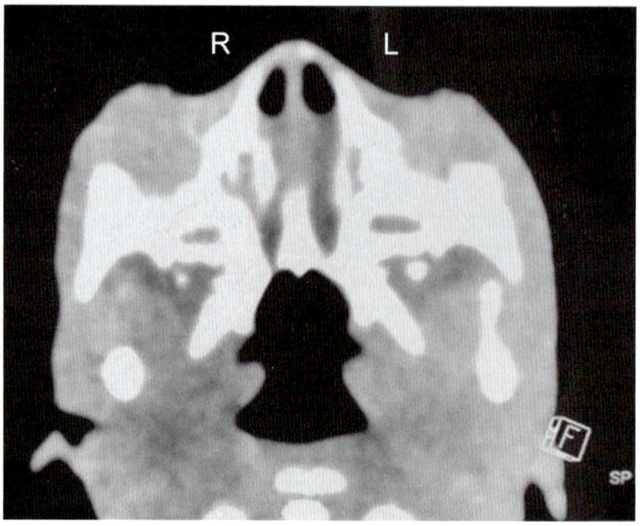

**Fig. 14.12:** Axial computed tomography of paranasal sinuses showing right (R)-sided bony and membranous choanal atresia and left (L)-sided complete bony atresia

### Epistaxis

Bleeding from the nose is frequent in children and usually follows injury to the anterior portion of the nasal septum in Little's area, the location of Kiesselbach arterial plexus. Bleeding follows local trauma, especially by nose picking during hot summer days, when reduced ambient humidity causes crusting in the anterior nasal cavity. Examination reveals prominent vessels that bleed promptly when touched with a cotton-tipped probe or a dried clot over Little's area. Avoidance of nose picking, use of lubricating ointment and pinching the nose to stop the bleeding in a head down position are taught to the child and parents. Refractory cases require chemical (topical silver nitrate) or electrocautery.

**Table 14.5:** Warning signs in patients with epistaxis that warrant referral to specialist

| |
|---|
| Features suggestive of neoplasia:<br>• Unilateral recurrent epistaxis<br>• Nasal blockage<br>• Visual/orbital symptoms (reduced vision, visual blurring, diplopia, proptosis)<br>• Obvious mass/growth visualized in the nasal cavity |
| Persistent bleeding despite nasal packing |
| Abnormal coagulation profile, blood counts |
| Recurrent epistaxis following trauma to head and neck |

Coagulopathy should be ruled out in children with similar family history, bleeding from other sites and refractory or severe epistaxis. Uncommon causes of recurrent epistaxis include juvenile nasopharyngeal angiofibroma (JNA) and hereditary hemorrhagic telangiectasia (Osler-Weber-Rendu syndrome). While JNA presents as unilateral nasal obstruction, recurrent epistaxis in prepubertal boys, the latter is associated with severe recurrent epistaxis, gastrointestinal bleeding and pulmonary hemorrhage. In the presence of red flag signs (Table 14.5), patients should be referred to specialist for further evaluation.

### Suggested Reading

1. Sagar P, Singh S. Pediatric sinonasal disorders: Surgical perspective. In: Bhalla AS, Jana M (Eds). Clinico-Radiological Series: Sinonasal Imaging. New Delhi: Jaypee; 2018.
2. Siddiqui Z, Tahiri M, Gupta A, et al. The management of pediatric rhinosinusitis. Int J Pediatr Otorhinolaryngol 2021 Aug;147:110786.
3. Standard Treatment Workflow for the management of Epistaxis, ICD-10-R04.0 in Standard Treatment Workflows of India by Ministry of Health and Family Welfare, Govt of India, 2019.

## DISEASES OF ORAL CAVITY AND PHARYNX

### Inflammatory Disorders

***Recurrent aphthous stomatitis*** presents as variable-sized painful white ulcers with surrounding erythema, located on the oral mucosa and/or tongue. The precise etiology is unknown. Minor (<1 cm) ulcers resolve spontaneously over several days. Major ulcers (>1 cm) are less common, may affect the soft palate or tonsils, and heal slowly (4–6 weeks) sometimes with scarring. Though most cases are idiopathic, recurrent ulcers are seen in Behcet disease and cyclic neutropenia. Symptomatic management includes local application of protective and analgesic pastes or anesthetic gels, failing which topical or, rarely, systemic steroids may be tried.

***Herpetic stomatitis,*** caused by herpes simplex virus type 1, is highly contagious. Erythematous gingiva and mucosal hemorrhage are associated with clusters of painful vesicles, evolving to gray pseudomembranous mucosal ulcers. Symptomatic treatment includes analgesics and oral or intravenous hydration. While oral acyclovir hastens recovery, lesions usually heal spontaneously in 10–14 days.

***Oral candidiasis (thrush),*** caused by *Candida*, appears as small white curd-like lesions on tongue and oral mucosa. While common in infants <6 months of age, the condition is often seen in patients receiving prolonged antibiotics or corticosteroids. Other risk factors include poor oral hygiene, xerostomia, diabetes, leukemia or immunodeficiency. Topical nystatin solution application multiple times a day or oral fluconazole are effective.

### Congenital Disorders

#### *Ankyloglossia (tongue tie)*

It refers to limitation of anterior tongue mobility due to congenitally short lingual frenulum. Mild forms are common, do not affect speech and improve as the patients grow. A very short and tight frenulum might restrict tongue protrusion beyond the lips, and may be associated with clefting of the tongue tip. Interference with feeding and speech may necessitate surgical correction of the tongue tie.

#### *Cleft Lip and Cleft Palate*

Cleft lip and cleft palate occur due to incomplete fusion of the developing maxillary and nasal processes. The cleft may be unilateral or bilateral, and incomplete. 40% cases of cleft lip or palate are associated with other congenital anomalies; syndromic associations include Goldenhar and Treacher Collins syndrome. Cleft palate leads to feeding difficulty, abnormal nasal breathing, abnormal speech, hearing impairment and impaired dentofacial growth. Staged surgical reconstruction of the lip and palatal defects is performed.

#### *Micrognathia*

Micrognathia refers to a disproportionately small mandible. Congenital micrognathia may be isolated or associated with Pierre Robin sequence (with cleft palate and glossoptosis). Unilateral mandibular hypoplasia may present with other features of hemifacial macrosomia. Micrognathia may cause difficulty in feeding, dental overcrowding and in severe cases where the tongue is displaced posteriorly, breathing difficulty. Milder cases resolve spontaneously. Neonates with breathing difficulty require prone nursing and/or oropharyngeal airway.

#### *Macroglossia*

Macroglossia refers to disproportionately large tongue compared to other structures of the oral cavity. Cases may be idiopathic or syndromic, associated with Down or Beckwith-Wiedemann syndromes, neurofibromatosis or congenital hypothyroidism. Macroglossia may be acquired, due to infections, trauma, tumor or vascular malformation. The condition may lead to drooling, speech impairment, feeding difficulty, abnormal growth of alveolus and dentition, or airway obstruction. Speech rehabilitation and/or surgical reduction may be needed.

### Stuttering or Stammering

Stuttering or stammering is dysfluency of speech characterized by abnormal repetition of syllables and prolonged interruptions. The most common pattern is developmental stuttering, appearing usually at 3–4 years, when there is inappropriate stuttering for the level of language development. Acquired stuttering is uncommon and may follow emotional trauma or neurological illness. Stuttering is usually not associated with structural orofacial anomalies like tongue tie or adenotonsillar hypertrophy. Mild forms of dysfluency improve spontaneously; persistent stammering requires speech and language therapy starting in preschool years. Delayed intervention is associated with persistent stammering into adulthood and psychosocial morbidity.

*Competencies:* **PE28.1; PE28.2; PE28.3**

### Sore Throat

***Viral pharyngitis:*** It is common and caused by rhinovirus, influenza or parainfluenza virus, adenovirus or coxsackie virus. Patients present with fever, sore throat, dysphagia, rhinorrhea, nasal obstruction, cough and malaise. Examination shows non-exudative erythema of pharynx and tonsils and tender cervical lymphadenopathy. Supportive treatment with analgesics, saline gargles and saline nasal drops is sufficient. Antibiotics are required in cases of secondary bacterial infection.

***COVID 19 illness:*** SARS CoV 2 infection in children, though assumed to be less frequent than adults, should be considered during the ongoing pandemic, especially with history of exposure. Almost one-half of the children may be asymptomatic. Fever with cough is the most common presentation of COVID-19 infection. The presentation is very similar to influenza (runny nose, fever), streptococcal pharyngitis (fever, sore throat) and allergic rhinitis (sneezing, runny nose and nasal obstruction). Smell and taste disturbances can also be reported by older children, similar to adults. Most children experience mild form of illness and are to be managed symptomatically. Vaccination against COVID-19 is reported to reduce the incidence of severe disease in adults.

***Infectious mononucleosis***, caused by Epstein-Barr virus, affects teenagers and is transmitted via body fluids, commonly saliva. Patients present with fatigue, high fever, malaise, sore throat, dysphagia and odynophagia.

Examination shows enlarged tonsils, edema of soft palate, palatal petechiae, significant cervical lymphadenopathy, hepatosplenomegaly, and a fine rash over arms or trunk. Differential leukocyte count indicates lymphocytosis and more than 10% lymphocytes have an atypical appearance. The presence of anti-VCA IgM antibody confirms the diagnosis. Management is supportive, comprising of hydration, bed rest, analgesics and antipyretics. Patients with respiratory difficulty or extreme dysphagia due to enlarged tonsils may require corticosteroids. Ampicillin may cause generalized itchy maculopapular rash and should be avoided. In rare scenario, severe airway obstruction may necessitate tonsillectomy or tracheotomy.

***Diphtheria:*** Though its incidence has declined significantly following immunization, early diagnosis of this potentially lethal condition is critical. The patient appears ill and toxic. Examination shows exudative tonsillopharyngitis with a thick gray membrane over the tonsils which may extend to palate, pharynx and occasionally larynx. Attempt to remove the membrane leads to bleeding. Cervical lymphadenopathy is common. Albert staining and culture of throat swab confirms infection with the causative gram-positive bacillus *Corynebacterium diphtheriae*. Clinical suspicion is enough to warrant immediate treatment with diphtheria antitoxin without awaiting microbiological confirmation. Therapy is with high dose penicillin or erythromycin. Airway obstruction is managed with tracheotomy.

***Acute bacterial pharyngotonsillitis:*** It is usually caused by group A β-hemolytic streptococci (GABHS). Less common pathogens include non-group A streptococci, *S. aureus*, *H. influenzae*, *M. catarrhalis*, diphtheria, gonococci, *Chlamydia* and *Mycoplasma* spp. Pharyngitis presents with fever, throat pain, odynophagia and occasionally, headache, abdominal pain, nausea and vomiting. Enlarged erythematous bilateral tonsils with yellow follicles are typical (Fig. 14.13). Severe cases show purulent exudation with or without membrane formation on tonsils, and cervical lymphadenopathy. A rapid strep test helps distinguish viral from streptococcal pharyngotonsillitis; negative results should be confirmed by throat culture. If strongly suspected, therapy against *Streptococcus* should begin without awaiting microbiological confirmation. Initial therapy is with amoxicillin for 10 days. Coamoxiclav, third generation cephalosporin (cefdinir, cefpodoxime), clindamycin or azithromycin are considered in refractory cases. Complications include bacteremia, peritonsillar, parapharyngeal or retropharyngeal abscesses; non-suppurative complications are scarlet fever, acute rheumatic fever and poststreptococcal glomerulonephritis.

For the clinical differentiation of viral pharyngitis from GABHS pharyngitis, the modified Centor scoring (Table 14.6) may be helpful. Timely initiation of antibiotics may avoid the above-mentioned complications.

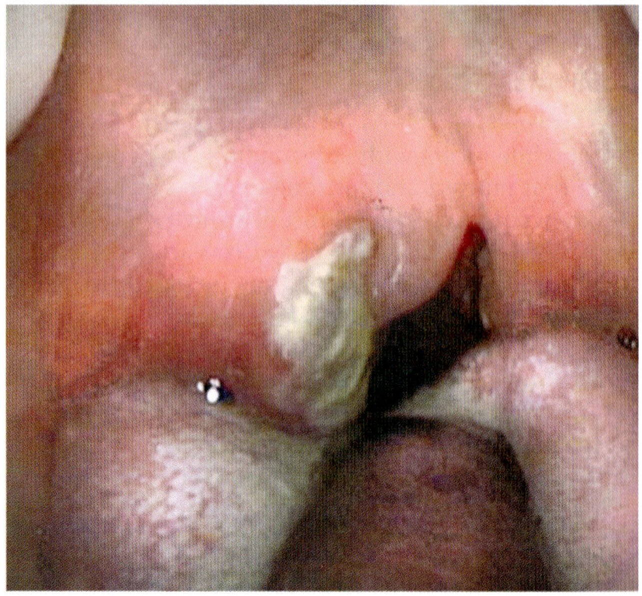

**Fig. 14.13:** Acute staphylococcal pseudomembranous tonsillitis with unilateral hypertrophy of the right tonsil. This condition has to be differentiated from other causes of white patch on the tonsil (*Courtesy:* Textbook of ENT, Hazarika)

**Table 14.6:** Centor criteria to identify patients with streptococcal pharygitis (GABHS)

**Patient with sore throat**

↓

**Apply Centor Score**

| Criteria | | Points |
|---|---|---|
| Absence of cough | | 1 |
| Swollen, tender anterior cervical nodes | | 1 |
| Temperature >100.4°F (38°C) | | 1 |
| Tonsillar exudates/swelling | | 1 |
| Age | 3–14 years | 1 |
| | 15–44 years | 0 |
| | 45 years or older | –1 |

| Score 0–1 | Score 2–3 | Score ≥4 |
|---|---|---|
| Risk of GABHS pharyngitis low | Risk of GABHS pharyngitis moderate | Risk of GABHS pharyngitis high |
| No further testing or antibiotics indicated | Throat culture or rapid antigen test | **Empiric treatment with antibiotics** |

Throat culture or rapid antigen test → **Negative** – **No antibiotics required**; **Positive** – **Treat with antibiotics**

## Tonsillectomy

Indications for tonsilloadenoid resection include adenotonsillar hypertrophy causing obstructive sleep apnea, speech defects, craniofacial growth abnormality, dysphagia, failure to thrive or cor pulmonale. Other indications for tonsillectomy are recurrent acute tonsillitis, recurrent tonsillitis associated with valvular heart disease or recurrent febrile seizures, recurrent peritonsillar abscess, infectious mononucleosis with severely obstructing tonsils refractory to medical management, and suspected tonsillar neoplasia.

### Obstructive Sleep Apnea

Obstructive sleep apnea is characterized by partial or complete upper airway obstruction during sleep. The chief etiology is adenotonsillar hypertrophy. Disease associations include obesity, allergic rhinitis, laryngomalacia, mucopolysaccharidoses, Down syndrome, craniofacial syndromes, cerebral palsy, hypothyroidism and nasal masses. Sequelae of obstructive sleep apnea are hypoxemia, hypercapnia and acidosis that contribute to behavioral and neurocognitive impairment with poor learning, attention deficit and hyperactivity, cardiovascular sequelae (systemic and pulmonary hypertension and cor pulmonale), and metabolic complications such as reduced insulin sensitivity, failure to thrive and dyslipidemia.

Parents complain of snoring, choking, breath holding, frequent arousal episodes during sleep, excessive daytime sleepiness, morning headaches and/or enuresis. Other daytime symptoms include hyperactivity and inattention, moodiness and poor scholastic performance. Examination reveals obesity, sleepiness, adenotonsillar hypertrophy, high arch palate, large tongue, long face and/or retrognathia. The diagnosis is ascertained by polysomnography (sleep study) and continuous video monitoring in the sleep laboratory. The apnea-hypopnea index, that estimates the number of apnea and hypopnea events per hour of sleep, indicates the severity of sleep apnea; value >10 suggests severe obstructive apnea. Sleep study also helps differentiate between this condition and central apnea, periodic breathing and central hypoventilation syndromes.

Adenotonsillectomy is the treatment of choice for severe obstructive sleep apnea. Tracheotomy may be considered in the most severe cases. Children younger than 3 years and those with severe apnea, obesity, cardiac complications or neuromuscular disorders require careful monitoring.

*Competencies:* **PE28.5; PE28.6; PE28.7; PE28.8; PE28.9; PE28.17**

## DISEASES OF THE LARYNX AND TRACHEA

### Stridor

The term stridor refers to audible respiratory noise produced by turbulent airflow through an obstructed upper airway. It should be differentiated from stertor that refers to snoring-like noise produced from obstructed nasopharynx or oropharynx.

X-ray of chest or lateral neck may suggest retropharyngeal abscess, epiglottitis, croup or tracheal stenosis. Computed tomography may be required to rule out extrinsic vascular compression, but is rarely required in an acute scenario. Flexible endoscopy helps assess nasal cavity, nasopharynx, oropharynx, supraglottis and glottis during dynamic respiration without need for general anesthesia, but is avoided, *if acute epiglottitis is suspected.* Rigid laryngotracheobronchoscopy, performed under general anesthesia, is the gold standard when evaluating a child with stridor. Apart from enabling diagnosis, it may be therapeutic, allowing removal of foreign body, release of a web or excision of papilloma. Common etiologies of airway obstruction and stridor are discussed below.

*Acute laryngotracheobronchitis (croup)* is a viral upper respiratory tract infection that affects children, 6 months to 3 years of age. Patients present with biphasic stridor, barking cough and low-grade fever after an episode of common cold. Symptoms may evolve over several days. Chest X-ray reveals characteristic narrowing of the subglottic region, known as the 'steeple' sign **(Fig. 14.14)**. Most cases of croup are mild and resolve in 1–2 days with conservative management, including reassurance, cool mist and oral hydration. Nebulized epinephrine (1:1000, at doses of 0.1–0.5 mL/kg, to a maximum of 5 mL) provides symptomatic relief. A single dose of dexamethasone (0.3–0.6 mg/kg, intramuscular) reduces severity, if given within the first 24 hours. Inhaled budesonide (1 mg twice a day for two days) also shows satisfactory results. Antibiotics against *Staphylococcus* and *H. influenzae* are indicated, if the child fails to improve and/or purulent secretions are present.

*Acute epiglottitis (supraglottitis)*, due to infection with *H. influenzae* type B, is less common but a more severe illness than croup. The incidence has declined following improving immunization against *Hemophilus*. Patients, usually 3–6 years of age, present with acute sore throat, high fever, muffled voice, inspiratory stridor, marked dysphagia and drooling. Unlike croup, cough is usually absent. The patient looks toxic and prefers to sit in a leaning forward, 'tripod' position that helps them breathe better. Lateral neck X-ray reveals a characteristic thickening of the epiglottis ('thumbprint' sign). Maneuvering of the oropharynx or larynx is not advised as it might precipitate fatal laryngospasm. Rapid airway management is crucial and includes intubation by skilled personnel or rigid bronchoscopy followed by tracheotomy. In atypical presentations, a skilled physician might try flexible endoscopy, which shows significant edema and erythema of the supraglottic structures compromising the airway. IV cefotaxime or ceftriaxone are administered for 7 days.

*Bacterial tracheitis* typically caused by *S. aureus*, affects younger children and follows a viral upper respiratory tract infection. The child appears toxic and has brassy cough with biphasic or expiratory stridor. X-ray neck shows an

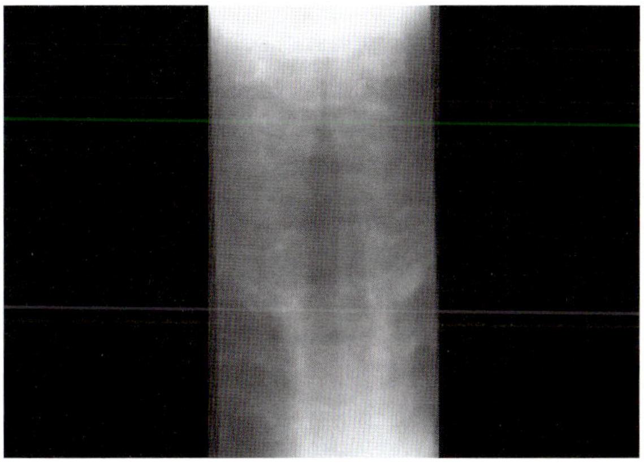

**Fig. 14.14:** Laryngotracheobronchitis (croup). 'Steeple' sign

irregular tracheal wall. Bronchoscopy is diagnostic and allows culture and removal of purulent tracheal secretions.

*Retropharyngeal abscess* is a suppurative complication of bacterial pharyngitis or dental infection, with abscess formation in lymph nodes between the pharynx and prevertebral fascia. Patients appear toxic with high fever, stridor, drooling and reduced neck mobility. Spread of infection into the mediastinum can be fatal. The diagnosis is confirmed by lateral neck radiograph and contrast CT. Management comprises parenteral antibiotics and surgical drainage of abscess by transoral or transcervical approach. Tracheotomy may be necessary to secure the airway.

*Laryngomalacia* is the most frequent congenital laryngeal anomaly and the chief cause of chronic stridor in infancy. The condition is characterized by inspiratory stridor that increases when the child is supine or crying, and decreases in a prone position. Flexible endoscopy reveals omega-shaped epiglottis, short aryepiglottic folds and partial collapse of a flaccid supraglottic airway with inspiration (Fig. 14.15). Laryngomalacia is generally benign and self-limited, with most cases resolving by 18 months of age. Concomitant gastroesophageal reflux should be managed medically. Surgical intervention, in form of supraglottoplasty and less commonly temporary tracheotomy is considered in less than 10% of cases due to significant respiratory distress, apneic spells, failure to thrive and feeding difficulties.

*Vocal cord paralysis* is the second most common congenital laryngeal anomaly. Bilateral vocal cord paralysis presents with high-pitched inspiratory stridor and cyanosis. It is usually caused by palsy of the recurrent laryngeal nerve due to excessive stretching of the neck during vaginal delivery. The condition may be idiopathic or associated with Arnold-Chiari malformation, hydrocephalus or hypoxia. Aspiration may occur, if cord immobility is due to vagus nerve paralysis at the skull base, as then the superior laryngeal nerve (that carries laryngeal mucosal sensation) is also affected. Diagnosis is made on fiberoptic laryngoscopy, which reveals bilateral vocal cord immobility. Plain radiograph of neck may reveal a dilated ventricular space between the true and false vocal cords without any other airway abnormalities (Fig. 14.16). Laser-assisted cordotomy and cordectomy and posterior cricoid expansion by a costal cartilage graft lead to widening of the glottis and airway restoration.

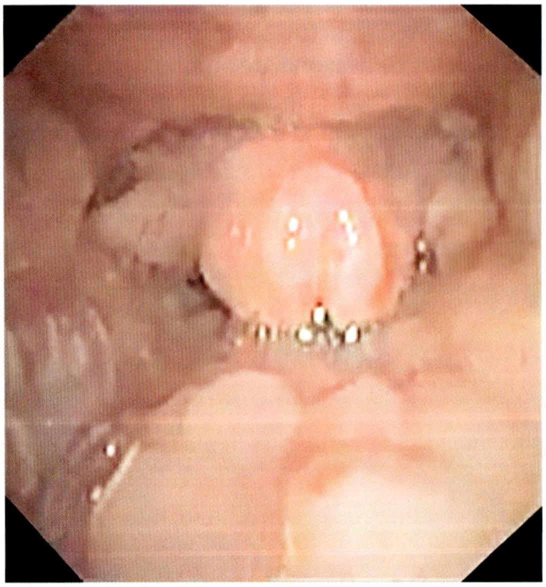

Fig. 14.15: Fiberoptic laryngoscopic view showing omega-shaped epiglottis obstructing the laryngeal inlet during inspiration suggestive of laryngomalacia in a 7-month-old child

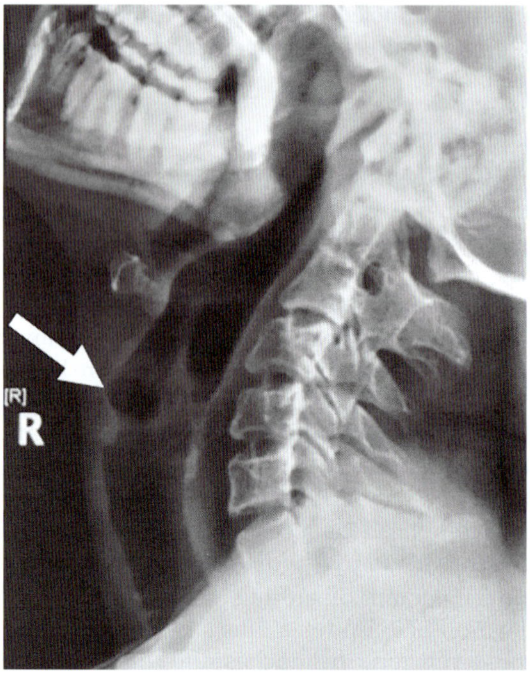


Fig. 14.16: Dilated ventricular sign (white arrow) seen in bilateral abductor cord palsy

*Acquired subglottic stenosis* is the most common cause of acquired stridor, and usually follows long-term endotracheal intubation. A snugly fitting endotracheal tube may cause mucosal trauma and inflammation in the subglottis, the narrowest part of the larynx leading to scarring. Patients present with progressive biphasic stridor a few days after extubation and are diagnosed by radiology along with endoscopic evaluation of the laryngotracheal airway (Fig. 14.17). Minor stenosis requires careful observation; severe stenosis requires release of stenosis with $CO_2$ laser and dilatation, widening with cartilage grafts or excision of stenotic segment, with tracheotomy. Special T-shaped silicone tracheostomy tubes are used for temporary stenting until complete healing. If prolonged intubation is expected, early tracheotomy prevents the complication of post-intubation subglottic stenosis. Cuffed tracheostomy tubes should be avoided in children; if a cuffed tube is essential, intermittent deflation is advised.

Another complication of prolonged intubation is laryngeal granuloma, typically located in the posterior part of the vocal cord. Small granulomas cause hoarseness while large lesions present with breathing difficulty. They are diagnosed by endoscopy, followed by endoscopic removal.

### Foreign Body Aspiration

Foreign body aspiration should always be considered in children presenting with acute onset stridor and airway

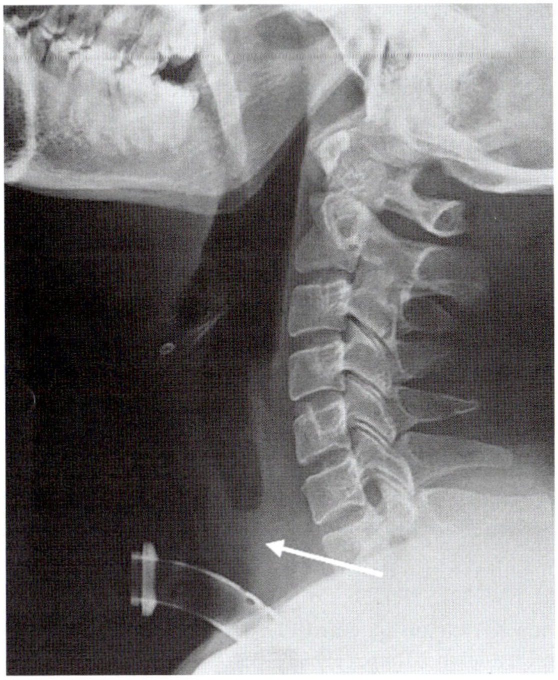

Fig. 14.17: Subglottic stenosis (white arrow) and tracheostomy tube *in situ*

obstruction (Fig. 14.18). If a foreign body is not expelled by coughing, it migrates into the lower airway lodging most commonly in the subglottis, the narrowest lumen in the airway leading to breathing difficulty. Objects such as balloons pose the greatest risk of choking to death, followed by round objects such as balls or marbles. Rigid bronchoscopy and removal of foreign body by an experienced surgeon is urgently required. Small foreign bodies may lodge in secondary bronchioles and present later with pneumonia. Management comprises bronchoscopy for foreign body removal, lavage and physiotherapy to clear up secretions and antibiotics. Occasionally, thoracotomy may be required for foreign bodies that cannot be retrieved endoscopically.

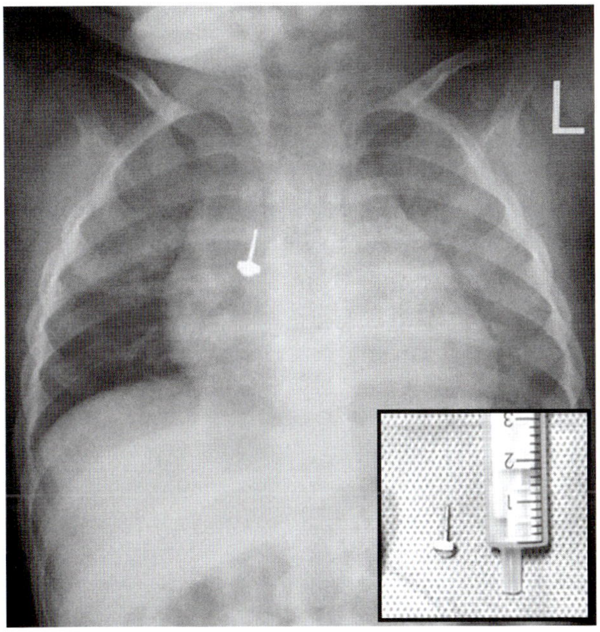


Fig. 14:18 Foreign body lodged in right main bronchus

## Tracheostomy

The requirement of prolonged ventilatory support, neurologic dysfunction causing aspiration, and need for pulmonary toileting are indications for tracheostomy. Carers should be explained about the implications of tracheostomy, including the inability of patients to vocalize and the care required. Tracheostomy is performed under general anesthesia with mechanical ventilation provided through an endotracheal tube or laryngeal mask. The trachea is opened at the level of the third or fourth ring by a vertical incision that is kept patent using two non-absorbable sutures placed on either side of the incision. Usually, an uncuffed tracheostomy tube is placed in children unless there is concern of aspiration, in which case a cuffed tube may be used. Care after tracheostomy includes repeated suctioning to maintain patency, change of tube every 5–7 days, chest physiotherapy and peristomal skin care. When tracheostomy is performed in infancy and kept for long, speech and language development may be delayed or impaired.

## Hoarseness

***Vocal nodules*** are the chief cause of hoarseness in children. Caused by vocal abuse, these are seen most often in children who scream habitually. The severity of hoarseness fluctuates, worsening with vocal abuse and improving with rest. Endoscopy reveals small, bilateral, opposing nodules at the junction of anterior and middle-thirds of the vocal cord. Speech therapy is advised; surgery is rarely indicated.

***Unilateral vocal cord palsy*** following an episode of upper respiratory viral infection or surgical ligation of patent ductus arteriosus is not uncommon. The resultant hoarseness usually improves over time and with speech therapy. Surgery is rarely indicated.

***Reflux*** is implicated in occurrence of laryngitis, subglottic stenosis, chronic sinusitis and otitis media with effusion. Diagnosis is established with 24-hour pH monitoring. Patients respond to lifestyle changes and use of proton pump inhibitors; fundoplication is required in severe cases.

***Hypothyroid myxedema*** may occasionally cause vocal fold edema, presenting as hoarseness or stridor.

***Laryngotracheal cleft*** is a rare congenital defect in the posterior part of cricoid cartilage of the larynx. The condition may be associated with Opitz-Frias or Pallister-Hall syndrome. Symptomatic clefts require multilayer repair, either by endoscopy or using transcervical approach.

## Suggested Reading


1. Bagwell T, Hollingsworth A, Thompson T, et al. Management of croup in the emergency department: The role of multidose nebulized epinephrine. Pediatr Emerg Care 2017; doi: 10.1097/PEC.0000000000001276.
2. Marchese A, Langhan ML. Management of airway obstruction and stridor in pediatric patients. Pediatr Emerg Med Pract 2017; 14:1–24.
3. McCaffer C, Blackmore K, Flood LM. Laryngomalacia: Is there an evidence base for management? J Laryngol Otol 2017; 131:946–54.

## DISEASES OF THE SALIVARY GLANDS

### Infections

*Bacterial parotid sialoadenitis* is frequent in young children and presents with painful unilateral parotid swelling. Purulent material can be expressed intraorally from the parotid duct upon parotid massage. Management involves oral antibiotics, hydration, sialogogues, parotid gland massage and warm compresses.

*Mumps:* Patients usually present with bilateral painful parotid enlargement and mild fever, and rarely, with acute unilateral hearing loss or vestibular weakness. Therapy comprises adequate hydration and analgesics.

*Tuberculosis* may affect the parotid or other salivary glands with or without lung involvement. Sarcoidosis may present with unilateral or bilateral parotid swelling, systemic symptoms and peripheral lymphadenopathy. HIV infection commonly involves the parotid glands, presenting as bilateral intraglandular cysts that recur after needle aspiration.

### Drooling

Drooling (sialorrhea) is common in infancy but persists beyond 2–3 years in children with neuromuscular disorders and in mouth breathers. Common causes of drooling are dental malocclusion, adenoid hypertrophy, cerebral palsy and lip incompetency. Chronic drooling may lead to skin excoriation, dyselectrolytemia, social isolation, learning difficulties and, in severe cases, aspiration pneumonia. Initial treatment is conservative and includes correcting the posture, orodental rehabilitation, oromotor training and anticholinergic agents like glycopyrrolate. Injection of botulinum toxin (Botox) into the salivary glands provides relief for 3–6 months. Refractory patients, >5 years old, are considered for surgery; bilateral submandibular duct rerouting is a simple and effective surgical procedure.

### Suggested Reading

1. Dritsoula AK, Greenstreet D, Thevasagayan MS. The drooling child. BMJ 2015;350:h38.
2. Wilson KF, Meier JD, Ward PD. Salivary gland disorders. Am Fam Physician 2014;89(11):882–88.

Chapter 15

# Disorders of Respiratory System

Sushil K Kabra

## DEVELOPMENTAL PHYSIOLOGY

Newborn has to contend with sudden transition from fetal life to extrauterine existence at the time of birth. In childhood, the lungs have to keep pace with the ordered growth of the body. During fetal life, the placenta helps in the gas exchanges. Therefore, the fetal oxygen tension remains constant, independent of the maternal levels of oxygen. As the lungs are fluid filled, there is no air fluid interface.

By the 24th week of gestation, the surfactant precursors appear as inclusion bodies in the alveolar lining cells. Prior to 28–32 weeks of gestation, the lungs have an inherent tendency to collapse. They are unable to retain any air. The surfactant, a protein in the alveolar lining layer decreases the alveolar surface tension and imparts finite elasticity to the interface. As a result, less pressure is needed to distend the lungs. When the lung is inflated from a small or negligible volume such as in atelectasis or from a situation when the alveoli are filled with liquid as happens during the first breath at birth, lesser force is required to open up the alveoli, if there is low surface tension at the air–liquid interface and if the radius of the terminal units of the lung is adequate.

Although surfactant can be detected in the lung exudate from the human fetuses as early as 24 weeks, the quantity increases greatly towards the end of the term gestation. Deficiency of surfactant leads to respiratory distress syndrome.

### Gas Transport from Fetal Life to Postnatal Period

Carbon dioxide tension falls from 35.5 mm Hg at 10 weeks of gestation to 28 mm Hg at the full term. The difference in the oxygen dissociation curves and increase in the hemoglobin concentration enable the fetus to carry out effective oxygenation of the tissues. It has been found that 2,3-diphosphoglycerate (2,3-DPG) in the surrounding medium seems to increase its affinity for oxygen. Fetal hemoglobin appears to be insensitive to this 2,3-DPG, hence its affinity for oxygen is not affected by the presence of 2,3-DPG. The uptake of $CO_2$ also shifts the oxygen dissociation curve to the right and, therefore, adequate $O_2$ delivery is ensured by the high tissue levels of $CO_2$. Relative hypoxia in a newborn is corrected in 5 minutes, hypercapnia by 20 minutes and acidosis in 24 hours after birth. The initial acidosis is partly metabolic in origin, due to the elevated blood lactate levels. The higher hemoglobin concentration in the newborn, and the shift to the left of the $O_2$ dissociation curve allow the newborn baby to carry higher concentration of oxygen than in the adult.

### Onset of Respiration

The mechanisms of the onset of respiration at birth are multifactorial. Hypoxia, hypercapnia (more $CO_2$ in blood) and sudden increase in the sensitivity of chemoreceptor due to increased sympathetic activity after the cord is clamped, appear to be the main factors responsible for initiation of respiration at birth.

### Respiratory Function in the Newborn

Before birth, the lungs are filled with fluid. This has to be replaced by air. Some of the fluid is extruded from the mouth and some is absorbed by the lymphatics. Intrapleural negative pressure required for the first breath is 40 to 100 cm $H_2O$. This pressure is higher initially, because of the low compliance of the newborn lung (1.5 mL/cm $H_2O$ at birth). The compliance of the lungs increases in the first few hours to 6 mL/cm $H_2O$ and resistance to the air flow decreases. The tidal volume of a 3 kg infant is approximately 16 mL at about 28 breaths per minute. Resting lung volume also gradually increases in the first few hours and reaches a maximum of 80 mL within 24 hours.

### Gas Exchange in Newborn

The normal newborn requires about 7 mL of oxygen/minute/kg. This is almost double the $O_2$ requirements of an adult on a relative weight basis.

The uptake of oxygen is a complex process involving transport across the alveolar capillary membrane. This process known as diffusion is virtually the same as in the adult in relation to the surface area. The dead space of the newborn in about 2 mL/kg with the resting tidal volume being 20 mL; 35% of the breath is wasted as compared to 30% in the adults. Persisting fetal channels and the ventilation perfusion problems in a newborn lead to increase in the right-to-left shunt.

### Mechanical Function throughout Childhood

The total lung capacity in a newborn is 150 mL as compared to that in an adult which is around 5000 mL. With the growth of the lungs, there is multiplication of the alveoli and increase in the size of alveoli and airways. Pores of Cohn or interalveolar communications also develop, with increasing age. There is a large increase in compliance and a fall in resistance. The reciprocal of resistance, i.e., conductance rises in proportion to the increase in the lung volumes. Increase in minute ventilation reflects the increase in the metabolic rate. The dead space, the tidal volume and the frequency changes reflect changes in the mechanics of the lungs.

### Gas Transport in Childhood

The rise of pH and $PCO_2$ together means that the buffer base of the blood also increases. Bicarbonate rises from 19 mEq/L at the age of 2 years to 24 mEq/L at 16 years of age. Arterial $PaO_2$ is about 75 mm Hg in the newborn period and around the age of 5 years, it reaches the adult level of 95 mm Hg.

### Suggested Reading


1. Warburton D. Conserved mechanisms in the formation of the airways and alveoli of the lung. Front Cell Dev Biol 2021;9:662059.


*Competencies:* **PE28.9; PE28.13**

## COMMON RESPIRATORY SYMPTOMS

### Cough

Cough is an important defense mechanism of the respiratory system and helps to bring out the infected secretions from the trachea and bronchi. Cough should not be suppressed in younger children as retention of secretions in their lungs may result in atelectasis and pulmonary complications.

A bout of cough is produced by maximal inspiration, the air is suddenly released through the partially closed glottis, because of forceful contraction of the expiratory muscles. Irritation of the pharynx, larynx, trachea, bronchi and pleura transmit the afferent impulses through the vagus or glossopharyngeal nerves to the center in medulla. Efferent pathways are in the nerve supply to the larynx and respiratory muscles.

On the other hand, persistent cough interferes with the sleep and feeding. A balanced approach is necessary in the management of cough. Information in relation to cough that may help in finding underlying illness include: Duration, nature (spasmodic/non-spasmodic), wet/dry, postural relation, diurnal variation, associated expectoration, relieving and aggravating factors and associated fever, respiratory difficulty, and wheeze.

#### Causes of Acute Cough

- Upper respiratory tract infection. Common cold, postnasal discharge due to sinusitis (in older children), rhinitis, hypertrophied tonsils and adenoids, pharyngitis, laryngitis, and tracheobronchitis
- Nasobronchial allergy and asthma
- Bronchiolitis, pneumonia and pulmonary suppuration
- Measles
- Whooping cough
- Foreign body in the air passages
- Empyema

#### Causes of Chronic and Recurrent Cough

- Inflammatory disorders of airway
  - Asthma and Loeffler syndrome
  - Infection—viral, bacterial, chlamydia, mycoplasma, tuberculosis, parasitic
  - Inhalation of environmental irritants, e.g. tobacco smoke, dust, etc.
- Suppurative lung disease
  - Bronchiectasis, cystic fibrosis
  - Foreign body retained in bronchi
  - Congenital malformations, sequestrated lobe, bronchomalacia
  - Immune deficiency, primary ciliary dyskinesia (PCD)
- Anatomic lesions—tumors, tracheal stenosis, H-type tracheoesophageal fistula
- Psychogenic, habit cough
- Post-nasal discharge, sinusitis
- Gastroesophageal reflex disease (GERD)
- Interstitial lung disease

### Expectoration

Children as such are not able to expectorate. They swallow the respiratory secretions. Older children with chronic respiratory problems may be able to bring out expectoration. Common causes of significant expectoration include bronchiectasis due to various causes, lung abscess, bronchitis, asthma, and tuberculosis. The amount and nature of expectoration may give clue about the cause of respiratory disease. Further investigation such as cell count, Gram stain and culture or stain for AFB and culture may help in diagnosis and guide for treatment.

### Hemoptysis

Hemoptysis is defined as blood-stained expectoration. Children are not able to bring out expectoration, therefore, hemoptysis as a clinical symptom in children is less common. Causes of hemoptysis may be necrotizing pneumonia, foreign body aspiration, bleeding diathesis, cavitatory tuberculosis, idiopathic pulmonary hemosiderosis, mitral stenosis, dilated cardiac myopathy, Goodpasture syndrome, and vasculitis syndromes.

### Respiratory Noises

Various types of sounds originating from respiratory system may be heard with or without the help of stethoscope. The intensity and pitch of these sounds alter depending on their site of origin within the respiratory tract. The pitch of the sound keeps on increasing and the intensity keeps on decreasing as one goes down lower into the respiratory tract. For example, snoring is a highly intensive but low-pitched sound because it results from the region of oropharynx. On the other hand, wheeze is a high-pitched, less intense sound originating from lower airway obstruction. Various sounds as given below are recognized (Table 15.1). As a rule, extrathoracic airway obstruction produces inspiratory sounds; intrathoracic major airway produces inspiratory as well as expiratory sounds; while distal airway obstruction predominantly produces expiratory sounds.

### Rattling

Rattling is due to excessive secretions in the pharynx or tracheobronchial tree during breathing. It is present in asthma, bronchitis and tracheobronchial stenosis. Aspiration of gastrointestinal content into the tracheobronchial tree can also result in rattling. Some normal infants may have transient rattling but prolonged rattling is always pathological.

### Wheezing

Wheezing refers to high-pitched whistling sounds audible without auscultation by the stethoscope. Wheezing causes considerable anxiety to the parents. Sufficient air must flow through the narrowed airway to produce the wheezing sound. This may be due to causes within the lumen or in the walls of the bronchi. Pressure from outside the bronchi may also be responsible for localized wheezing. Common causes of wheezing include:

- *Wheeze-associated lower respiratory tract infection (WLRI) or viral infection-associated wheeze:* All that wheezes are not asthma. Wheezing is most often due to heightened sensitivity of the respiratory tract. Infections of the lower respiratory passages may cause bronchospasm in these patients. Attacks of wheezing are always preceded by a cold or acute respiratory disease. These are most frequent below 5 years of age and become less frequent thereafter. These attacks are relieved by simple antispasmodic drugs.
- *Bronchiolitis*
- *Bronchial asthma*
- *Tropical eosinophilia:* It is an unusual form of infection with filariasis, e.g. *Dirofilaria imitis*, *W. bancrofti*, *B. malayi*. Clinical features simulate chronic recurrent asthma. X-ray films of the lungs show fine infiltration with snowflake-like appearance. This should be distinguished from miliary tuberculosis. The leukocyte count shows eosinophilia. Patients are treated with diethylcarbamazine (10 mg/kg) in three divided doses orally for 3 weeks. Some patients may require 2–3 spaced courses.
- *Loeffler syndrome:* The pulmonary phase of migration of ascaris larvae may cause transient wheezing, pulmonary problems and eosinophilia.
- *Hypersensitivity pneumonitis*

*Rare causes*

- Inhaled foreign bodies cause unilateral localized wheeze which begins suddenly. Wheezing is continuous, and worsens with crying, during excitement and with cold.
- Pressure from enlarged mediastinal nodes due to tuberculosis or neoplasm.
- Pressure from anomalous pulmonary artery compressing the right main bronchus.
- Cystic fibrosis: Recurrent wheezing, productive cough and malabsorption are the usual features. Some patients have history of meconium ileus in the neonatal period.
- Pulmonary hemosiderosis.

*Competency:* **PE28.7**

### Stridor

Stridor indicates upper respiratory obstruction and is usually accompanied by hoarseness, brassy cough, dyspnea, retraction of the chest during inspiration and restlessness. Accessory muscles of respiration are usually working.

Stridor is frequently seen in infants and is attributed to: (i) small size of the larynx, (ii) loose submucous connective tissue around the glottic region, and (iii) rigid cricoid cartilage encircling the subglottic zone.

#### *Acute Stridor*

Acute upper airway obstruction occurring in the region of glottis, which is produced by inflammation and edema may be life-threatening. The obstruction may either be supraglottic (e.g. epiglottitis) or may be subglottic (e.g. infectious croup) (Table 15.2).

#### *Chronic Stridor*

***Congenital laryngeal stridor:*** This is caused by flaccidity (laryngomalacia) or easy collapsibility of the aryepiglottic folds or epiglottis. This condition usually manifests by

**Table 15.1:** Respiratory sounds

| Sound | Causes | Character |
|---|---|---|
| Snoring | Oropharyngeal obstruction | Inspiratory, low pitched irregular |
| Grunting | Partial closure of glottis | Expiratory, occurs in young infants |
| Rattling | Secretions in trachea/bronchi | Inspiratory, coarse. This sound can also be felt by placing hands over the chest |
| Stridor | Obstruction larynx/trachea | Inspiratory sound, may be associated with an expiratory component |
| Wheeze | Lower airway obstruction | Continuous musical sound predominantly expiratory |

**Table 15.2:** Distinguishing stridor due to supraglottic and tracheal obstruction

| *Clinical features* | *Supraglottic obstruction* | *Tracheal obstruction* |
|---|---|---|
| Stridor | Inspiratory and often less serious | Usually expiratory or biphasic and more serious |
| Cry | Muffled | Normal |
| Dyspnea | Less severe | More marked |
| Cough | Less marked | Deep barking or brassy |

the end of the first week or during the second week after birth. The stridor is characteristically intermittent, and is aggravated by crying or feeding. It is modified in sleep or by the change of posture. The loud inspiratory sound frightens the parents but the infant is relatively less symptomatic. Respiratory distress and chest retraction are absent or minimal. Feeding behavior and activity of the infant are generally normal. Breathing difficulty may be significant, if micrognathia and cleft palate are also associated. Congenital laryngeal stridor disappears spontaneously by the age of six months to one year. These infants are more prone to develop aspiration of feeds and frequent lung infection.

***Congenital laryngeal tracheal stenosis or web:*** Cry of the infant is weak and hoarse, breathing is labored and the air entry in the lungs is reduced. In subglottic tracheal stenosis, the cry is unaffected and the stridor is both inspiratory and expiratory.

***Laryngeal cysts or neoplasm:*** Angioma, papilloma, lymphangioma and retention cysts may be responsible for the stridor.

### Neurogenic Stridor

***Bilateral vocal cord paralysis:*** This results from brainstem injury. Unilateral paralysis is due to the involvement of the recurrent laryngeal nerve. The latter is more common on the left side, because the left recurrent laryngeal nerve has a longer course and hooks around the aorta from the front to back. Stridor is common in hydrocephalic infants and those with Down syndrome.

### Extrinsic Obstruction

***Vascular rings:*** Stridor is intermittent and becomes worse when the neck is flexed. The infant prefers to keep the head in the position of hyperextension.

***Tumors of neck*** such as mediastinal goiter, lymphangioma and thyroglossal duct cyst. Congenital goiters, which cause respiratory obstruction and stridor are due to maternal intake of antithyroid drugs and iodides during pregnancy. Goiter of neonatal hypothyroidism and due to defect in synthesis of thyroid hormones usually do not cause stridor.

### Treatment of Stridor

The diagnosis of congenital laryngeal stridor is made on direct laryngoscopy. Barium swallow should be done to rule out the extrinsic causes of obstruction, if there is feeding problem. Tumors and cysts require surgical excision. Corticosteroids hasten the recovery in laryngeal edema. Congenital laryngeal stridor does not require treatment in majority. Gavage feeding is done, if the respiratory distress is marked. Congenital goiter caused by intake of antithyroid drugs or iodides by the mother during pregnancy is treated with tri-iodothyronine and Lugol iodine.

## Dyspnea

Tachypnea means abnormally rapid respiration. Dyspnea means labored or difficult breathing, usually accompanied by pain and air hunger.

### Causes of Dyspnea

#### *Respiratory system*

***Newborn:*** Respiratory distress syndrome; hypoplastic lung; diaphragmatic hernia and eventration; meconium aspiration; pulmonary edema; congenital heart disease, pneumonia; central nervous system depression.

***Infants and childhood:*** Pneumonia, bronchiolitis; bronchial asthma; aspiration; pneumothorax; pleural effusion; obstructive emphysema; pulmonary edema.

#### *Cardiovascular system*

Myocarditis; pulmonary edema; pericarditis; cardiac failure.

#### *Miscellaneous*

Anemia; pickwickian syndrome; chest deformities; fractured ribs or pleuritis; acidosis, diabetes and uremia; drugs (salicylate); smoke inhalation; and myasthenia gravis.

## Epistaxis

Epistaxis or bleeding from the nose is rare in children below the age of 3 years. It may occur due to local or systemic causes. Local causes include: (i) Trauma to nose caused by nose picking, (ii) capillary malformations in the Little's area, (iii) foreign body, (iv) bleeding polyps of the septum (v) allergic rhinitis and nasal diphtheria.

Systemic causes are: (i) Hypertension, (ii) blood dyscrasia, and (iii) pertussis (whooping cough).

***Treatment:*** Pressure on alae nasi for 10 minutes controls bleeding in most cases. In resistant cases, the nasal mucosa is plugged with gauze piece soaked in 1:10,000 solution of adrenaline hydrochloride as a temporary measure. Plugging of the nose for a prolonged period (>48 hours) is best avoided. The bleeding points should be identified and cauterized with silver nitrate solution. Cases due to systemic causes should be evaluated and treated appropriately. The child might need iron supplements to treat anemia. Profuse bleeding is more likely to be from the posterior aspect from sphenopalatine vessels. Cauterization is ineffective in these vessels. Firm anterior and posterior packing is done. Blood dyscrasia, if present, should be appropriately treated.

## Suggested Reading


1. Kendigelen P. The anesthetic consideration of tracheobronchial foreign body aspiration in children. J Thorac Dis 2016;8:3803–07.
2. Lands LC. Dyspnea in children: What is driving it and how to approach it. Pediatr Respir Rev 2017;24:29–31.
3. Michaudet C, Malaty J. Chronic cough: Evaluation and management. Am Fam Physician 2017;96:575–80.

## DIAGNOSIS OF RESPIRATORY ILLNESSES

### Imaging

X-ray film and newer imaging like computerized tomography are non-invasive diagnostic methods. X-ray films help in diagnosis of soft tissue and bony abnormalities. This is the most commonly used modality for making a diagnosis of pulmonary infection. A particular pattern of pneumonia may suggest the etiological agent. Lobar consolidation suggests infection due to *Streptococcus pneumoniae* (Fig. 15.1), while evidence of hilar or mediastinal adenopathy suggests the possibility of tubercular infection. Pneumatoceles may be seen in pneumonia due to *Staphylococcus* (Fig. 15.2). Generalized hyperinflation with minimal parenchymal lesions suggests acute bronchiolitis (Fig. 15.3). Computerized tomographic scans are used for visualization of lymph nodes, tumors, bronchiectasis and pleural pathologies.

### Bronchoscopy

Bronchoscopy can be of two types—flexible fiberoptic and rigid. Fiberoptic bronchoscopy is done under local anesthesia and sedation. This is used for diagnosis of structural abnormality of airways, diagnosis of foreign body in respiratory tract and for obtaining bronchoalveolar lavage samples to identify cell type, infective etiology from lower respiratory tract, and biopsies. Rigid bronchoscopy can be used in place of fiberoptic bronchoscopy especially when used for removal of foreign bodies from airways or obtaining biopsy from airway tumors.

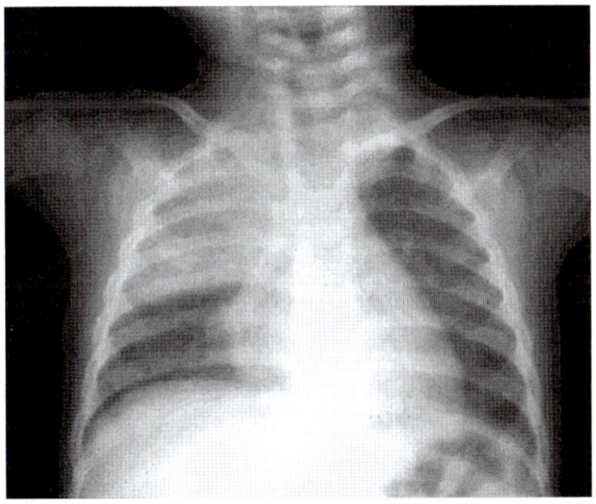


**Fig. 15.1:** Consolidation of right upper lobe due to infection with *Strepococcus pneumoniae*

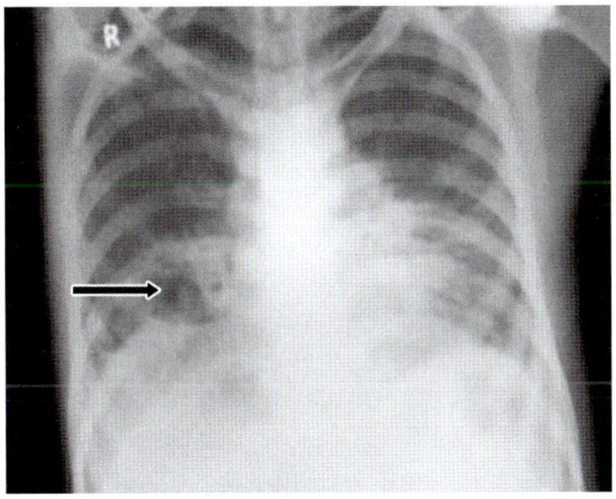

**Fig. 15.2:** Multiple pneumatoceles (black arrow) due to staphylococcal pneumonia

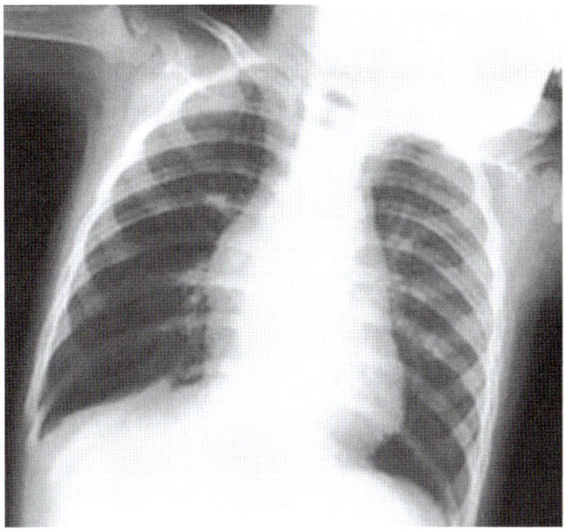

**Fig. 15.3:** X-ray chest in a 1-yr-old with acute bronchiolitis. Note hyperinflation on both sides, and few infiltrates

### Pulmonary Function Test

Pulmonary function tests are important tools for monitoring of a patient with chronic respiratory illness. Flow rates and lung volumes are measured. These tests may be performed in children above the age of 5–7 years. Commonly a flow volume loop is generated by asking the child to take tidal breathing followed by exhalation fast and complete. Configuration of the curve generated give an idea about type of illness (obstructive or restrictive) (Fig. 15.4). Precise assessment can be carried out by using data generated by spirometer. Commonly used parameters include: Forced expiratory volume in first second (FEV1), forced vital capacity (FVC), mid-expiratory flow rate (FEF25-75) and ratio of FEV1/FVC. Normal FEV1/FVC ratio is between 0.8 and 1.0. In obstructive diseases (asthma), the ratio is reduced. In restrictive lung diseases (interstitial lung disease), the ratio of FEV1/FVC is normal but FVC is reduced below 80% of predicted.

### Blood Gas Analysis

Estimation of pH and partial pressures of oxygen and carbon dioxide in blood gives a fair idea about pulmonary functions. Arterial blood gas analysis is used for making a diagnosis of respiratory failure, and subsequent monitoring. Partial pressures of oxygen less than 60 mm Hg and of carbon dioxide more than 50 mm Hg suggest respiratory failure.

### Sweat Chloride Test

Sweat chloride is estimated by quantitative pilocarpine iontophoresis. Chloride in sweat is increased in children suffering from cystic fibrosis. In normal children, sweat chloride values are less than 40 mEq/L. In children with cystic fibrosis, it is more than 60 mEq/L. A value of 40–60 mEq/L is borderline and should be repeated.

## Suggested Reading

1. Elenius V, Chawes B, Malmberg PL, et al; EAACI Preschool Wheeze Task Force. Lung function testing and inflammation markers for wheezing preschool children. Pediatr Allergy Immunol 2021;32:501–13.
2. Jana M, Bhalla AS, Gupta AK. Approach to pediatric chest radiograph. Indian J Pediatr 2016;83:533–42.
3. Piccione J, Hysinger EB, Vicencio AG. Pediatric advanced diagnostic and interventional bronchoscopy. Semin Pediatr Surg 2021;30:151065.


*Competencies:* **PE28.1; PE28.14**

## RESPIRATORY TRACT INFECTIONS

### Common Cold or Nasopharyngitis

Common cold is the most frequent medical problem in childhood and is usually due to infection of the upper respiratory tract with adenoviruses, influenza, rhinovirus, parainfluenza or respiratory syncytial viruses. These are spread by droplet infection. Rhinitis could also be due to allergy.

#### Clinical Features

These include fever, thin nasal discharge and irritability. Cervical lymph nodes may enlarge. Nasopharyngeal congestion causes nasal obstruction and respiratory distress. The later is more pronounced in young infants. Eustachian tube opening may be blocked leading to serous otitis media and congestion of tympanic membrane. In allergic rhinitis, there is a clear mucoid discharge with sneezing. There is no contact with an infected patient and history of allergy is usually present. Wheezing may occur in a significant proportion of cases with upper respiratory tract disease.

Narrowing of the airway and pharyngeal irritation causes dry hacking cough. Excessive lacrimation due to the blocked lacrimal ducts in the nose. Purulent discharge does not necessarily mean secondary infection as it can result from shedding of epithelial and inflammatory cells resulting from viral infection itself. The illness usually lasts for three days but cold may persist up to 2 weeks. Rhinitis and stuffy nose could become chronic and last for several weeks.

*Complications:* Otitis media, laryngitis, sinusitis, bronchiolitis, exacerbation of asthma and bronchopneumonia.

#### Differential Diagnosis

*Foreign body:* Unilateral serosanguineous or purulent discharge from the nose indicates presence of foreign body.

*Drugs:* Intermittent use of rifampicin may cause flu-like syndrome in some children. Drugs like reserpine and prochlorperazine cause nasal stuffiness.

*Snuffles:* Clear mucoid discharge from the nose in the first few weeks of life is called snuffles. The cause is unknown. There is no evidence for allergy or infections. "Snuffles" of congenital syphilis is severe rhinitis with bilateral serosanguineous discharge commonly excoriating the upper lip and leaving fine scars. Nasal strictures may ulcerate leaving a flat nasal bridge.

#### Treatment

*To relieve nasal congestion:* Nose drops of saline may give symptomatic relief. Nasal decongestants (ephedrine, xylometazoline) may cause rebound congestion. These should not be used routinely, and advised only in refractory cases for limited duration. Antihistaminics are increasingly being used for allergic colds. These are best avoided in the first six months of life. Antihistaminics dry up the thin secretions and relieve sneezing. Newer non-sedating antiallergic drugs include loratidine and cetirizine may be useful in allergic rhinitis. Terfenadine should not be prescribed to children because of potential cardiotoxicity.

*Fever* is controlled by antipyretics such as paracetamol (acetaminophen).

*Do not give cough syrups:* If the cough is suppressed in infants and young children, mucoid secretions may be retained in the bronchi, and may predispose to spasmodic cough wheezing, atelectasis and infection.

*Antibiotics* are of little value in viral infections. These are used with purulent secretions, persistent or recurrence of fever or if complicated by bronchopneumonia. There is no conclusive evidence that large doses of vitamin C or other micronutrients including zinc are helpful.

*Nursing:* The children should be protected from sudden exposure to chills and kept warm during the winter months. Feeding should be continued to maintain their hydration.

*Competencies:* **PE28.2; PE28.3**

### Acute Tonsillopharyngitis (Sore Throat)

Sore throat is due to acute inflammation of the pharynx and tonsils. Most often, it is associated with the viral infections of the upper respiratory tract such as adenovirus, influenza, parainfluenza virus, enterovirus and Epstein-Barr virus. It may, however, be a prodrome of measles and rubella or caused by *Streptococcus pyogenes* especially group A beta-hemolytic streptococci. *Mycoplasma pneumoniae* and *Candida albicans* have also been incriminated. Irritant fumes and smoke also cause irritation of the throat.

#### Clinical Features

Clinical features include fever, malaise headache, nausea, and sore throat. It is difficult to distinguish the clinical syndromes due to viral or streptococcal infections. Hoarseness, cough and rhinitis are more common in viral infection. In these, the onset is gradual and there is less toxemia. In streptococcal infections, cervical lymph nodes are enlarged and illness is more acute with high fever, exudates may be seen over tonsillar surface and there may be absence of nasal discharge or conjunctivitis.

Tonsils become swollen and covered with exudates in both types of infections. Younger children may not complain of sore throat but often refuse to feed normally.

#### Complications

Acute glomerulonephritis, rheumatic fever, otitis media, sinusitis, peritonsillar and retropharyngeal abscesses. The infection may spread down the tracheobronchial tree and cause tracheobronchitis and pneumonia.

### Diagnosis

The possibility of acute pharyngitis due to group A beta hemolytic streptococci is considered in patients with exudates in the throat, tender enlarged cervical nodes and absence of nasal or conjunctival congestion. Throat swab culture helps in the definitive diagnosis. Neutrophil count in the peripheral blood is elevated. Rapid diagnostic test for identification of group A beta hemolytic streptococci may give the result within 10 minutes.

### Differential Diagnosis

*Herpangina:* Herpangina is an acute febrile illness due to the group A Coxackie virus. Patients have dysphagia, sore throat and papulovesicular lesions surrounded by erythema over the tongue, pharynx, anterior tonsillar pillars and soft palate. Pharynx appears congested.

*Diphtheria:* There is mild to moderate fever, severe toxemia, sore throat and membrane formation over the fauces or palate. The diagnosis should be confirmed by a smear examination from the throat swab.

*Pharyngoconjunctival fever:* Patients have fever, conjunctivitis, pharyngitis and cervical lymphadenitis due to infection with adenovirus type III.

*Infectious mononucleosis:* The illness is characterized by lymphadenopathy, morbilliform rash, hepatosplenomegaly and sometimes aseptic meningitis.

### Treatment

*Symptomatic:* Warm saline gargles are prescribed for older children. Younger children are encouraged to sip warm tea or other home made drinks. Paracetamol is administered for fever. Soft food such as custard or rice and lentil gruel is given because swallowing is painful. Rest in bed accelerates recovery.

*Specific:* Antibiotics are not used for viral infections. Infections with beta hemolytic streptococci are treated with penicillin V orally, injections of procaine penicillin or oral amoxicillin or macrolides in adequate doses for at least 10 days. Parents are likely to stop medication after 2 to 3 days as the child begins to improve clinically. If compliance is a problem, a single dose of benzathine penicillin given IM is preferred. Cotrimoxazole, which is commonly used for sinusitis and otitis media, should *not* be used for sore throat.

### Recurrent Attacks of Sore Throat

Parents often seek advice for treatment of recurrent sore throat in their children. A detailed history is obtained and physical examination conducted. Paranasal sinuses and ears should be examined for the foci of infection, and adequately treated. Smoky and dusty atmosphere should be avoided. Dampness in the environment and overcrowding predispose children to recurrent upper respiratory tract infections. The general health should be improved by good nutritious diet.

Every episode of bacterial pharyngitis should be treated with adequate doses of antibiotics for at least 10 days, so that no residua of infection are left. A single dose of benzathine penicillin by IM route or penicillin V orally are the drugs of choice. Presence of beta lactamase producing bacteria in the pharynx may inactivate penicillin and lead to recurrent sore throat. This should be treated with amoxycillin plus clavulanic acid. Clindamycin is an effective agent to eradicate the carrier state. In resistant cases, long-term penicillin prophylaxis should be carried out, especially if group A beta hemolytic streptococcal infection is present.

Tonsillectomy is often recommended for recurrent attacks of sore throat. It does not prevent recurrence of pharyngeal infections. Tonsillectomy should be advised, only if there are more than seven documented attacks of tonsillitis in a year, or more than 5 episodes in two consecutive years or for tonsillar or peritonsillar abscess. It may reduce the incidence of group A beta hemolytic streptococcal infection. Tonsillectomy is also recommended in diphtheria carriers, and retention cysts in tonsils and tonsilloliths. Tonsils may be removed, only if these are acting as foci of infection for suppurative otitis media. Tonsillectomy should not be done during epidemics of poliomyelitis. There is no indication for tonsillectomy after rheumatic fever or glomerulonephritis.

### Suggested Reading

1. Kumar P, Medigeshi GR, Mishra VS, et al. Etiology of acute respiratory infections in infants: A prospective birth cohort study. Pediatr Infect Dis J 2017;36:25–30.
2. Tenenbaum T. Respiratory tract infections in children. Pathogens 2021;10:1596.

## ACUTE LOWER RESPIRATORY TRACT INFECTIONS

Acute lower respiratory tract infections are the leading cause of death in children below 5 years of age. The diseases included under this heading include: Croup syndromes, bronchitis, bronchiolitis and pneumonia.

*Competency:* **PE28.6**

### Croup

The term croup is used for a variety of conditions in which a peculiar brassy cough is the main presenting feature. Inspiratory stridor, hoarseness or respiratory distress may not always be associated with croup. The diseases include acute epiglottitis, laryngitis, laryngotracheobronchitis and spasmodic laryngitis.

#### Epiglottitis

Supraglottitis includes both epiglottitis and inflammatory edema of the hypopharynx. *Hemophilus influenzae* type B is the most frequent causative agent. This condition is discussed in Chapter 14.

#### Laryngitis and Laryngotracheobronchitis (Infectious Croup)

These conditions are nearly always caused by viral infections, usually parainfluenza type 1. Other viruses incriminated include respiratory syncytial and parainfluenza types

| Table 15.3: Assessment of severity of acute laryngotracheobronchitis | | | |
|---|---|---|---|
| | *Mild* | *Moderate* | *Severe* |
| General appearance | Happy, feeds well, interested in surroundings | Irritable but comforted by parents | Restless, agitated or altered sensorium |
| Stridor | Stridor on coughing, no stridor at rest | Stridor at rest; gets worse when agitated | Stridor at rest and worsens on agitation |
| Respiratory distress | No distress | Tachypnea and chest retractions | Marked tachypnea with chest retractions |
| Oxygen saturation | >92% in room air | >92% in room air | <92% in room air, may be cyanosed |

2 and 3, influenza virus, adenovirus and rhinovirus. Bacterial etiology or bacterial superinfection is unusual. In infectious croup, the onset of the illness is more gradual. Usually, there is a mild cold for a few days before the child develops a brassy cough and mild inspiratory stridor. As the obstruction increases, the stridor becomes more marked and the suprasternal and sternal recession with respiration become manifest. *See* Chapter 14; **Fig. 14.14**. Child with acute laryngotracheobronchitis should be assessed for severity of illness on basis of general appearance, stridor (audible with or without stethoscope), oxygen saturation and respiratory distress (Table 15.3).





### Spasmodic Croup

It occurs in children between the age of 1 and 3 years. There may not be preceding coryza. The child wakes up suddenly in the early hours of the morning with brassy cough and noisy breathing. The symptoms improve within a few hours. The illness may recur on subsequent days. The course is generally benign and patients recover completely. The cause is unknown. Humidification of the room in which the child is nursed is all that is necessary.

### Differential Diagnosis

The syndromes of croup should be distinguished from each other and also from the croup associated with diphtheria in which a membrane is seen on laryngoscopy or occasionally with measles. Rarely the croup may result from angioneurotic edema. A retropharyngeal abscess may cause respiratory obstruction. Aspiration of a foreign body is an important cause of obstruction. It may be rarely confused with wheezing in asthma.

### Suggested Reading

1. Petrocheilou A, Tanou K, Kalampouka E, et al. Viral croup: Diagnosis and a treatment algorithm. Pediatr Pulmonol 2014;49:421–29.

## Pneumonia

Pneumonia may be classified anatomically as lobar or lobular pneumonia, bronchopneumonia and interstitial pneumonia. Pathologically, there is a consolidation of alveoli or infiltration of the interstitial tissue with inflammatory cells or both.

### Etiology

***Viral:*** Viral pneumonia caused by RSV, influenza, parainfluenza, adenovirus, corona virus may be responsible for about 40% of the cases.

***Bacterial:*** In over 40–60% of the cases, common bacteria cause pneumonia. In first 2 months, the common agents include gram-negative bacteria such as *Klebsiella*, *E. coli* and gram-positive organisms like pneumococci and staphylococci. Between 3 months and 3 years, common bacteria include *S. pneumoniae*, *H. influenzae* and staphylococci. After 3 years of age, common bacterial pathogens include pneumococci and staphylococci. Gram-negative organisms cause pneumonia in early infancy, severe malnutrition and immunocompromised states.

***Atypical organisms:*** *Chlamydia* and *Mycoplasma* spp may cause community-acquired pneumonia in adults and children.

***Pneumocystis jirovecii:*** This organism causes pneumonia in immunocompromised children.

***Fungi:*** Histoplasmosis and coccidioidomycosis may cause pneumonia in immunocompromised children.

***Miscellaneous causes*** include ascariasis (Loeffler syndrome), aspiration of food, oily nose drugs, kerosene and hypersensitivity pneumonitis. The etiology remains unknown in one-third of the cases of pneumonia.

### Clinical Features

Risk factors for pneumonia include low birth weight, malnutrition, vitamin A deficiency, lack of breastfeeding, passive smoking, large family size, family history of bronchitis, advanced birth order, crowding, young age and air pollution. Onset of pneumonia may be insidious starting with upper respiratory tract infection or may be acute with high fever, dyspnea and grunting respiration. Respiratory rate is always increased.

Rarely, pneumonia may present with symptoms of acute abdominal emergency. This is attributed to referred pain from the pleura. Apical pneumonia may sometimes be associated with meningismus and convulsions. On examination, there is flaring of alae nasi, retraction of the lower chest and intercostal spaces. Signs of consolidation are observed in lobar pneumonia.

### Pneumococcal Pneumonia

Respiratory infections due to *Streptococcus pneumoniae* are transmitted by droplets and are more common in the winter months. Overcrowding and diminished host resistance predispose the children to infection with pneumococci.

***Pathology:*** Bacteria multiply in the alveoli and an inflammatory exudate is formed. Scattered areas of consolidation occur, which coalesce around the bronchi and later become lobular or lobar in distribution. Pathological process passes from the stage of congestion to red and gray hepatization before the final stage of resolution.

*Clinical features:* Incubation period is 1 to 3 days. The onset is abrupt with headache, chills, cough and high fever. Cough is initially dry but may be associated with thick rusty sputum. Child may develop chest pain, that may be referred to the shoulder or abdomen. Respiration is rapid. In severe cases, there may be grunting, chest indrawing, difficulty in feeding and cyanosis. Percussion note is impaired, air entry is diminished, crepitations and bronchial breathing may be heard over areas of consolidation. Meningismus may be present in apical pneumonia.

*Diagnosis:* The diagnosis is based on history, physical examination, X-ray findings of lobar consolidation **(Fig. 15.1)** and leukocytosis. Bacteriological confirmation is difficult, but sputum may be examined by Gram stain and culture. Blood culture may be positive in 5–10% of cases. Demonstration of polysaccharide antigen in urine and blood is an attractive investigation, but does not have sufficient specificity for confirming pneumococcal pneumonia as it may also be positive in children with colonization in throat.

*Treatment:* Penicillin G 50,000 units/kg/day is given intravenously or intramuscular in divided doses for 5–7 days. In patients allergic to penicillin, alternative agents are chloramphenicol or cephalosporins (ceftriaxone, cefotaxime). The latter should be given with caution as cross sensitivity to penicillin may occur. In communities with high prevalence of significant penicillin resistance, higher doses of penicillin or ampicillin may be required. Oxygen should be given, if cyanosis and respiratory distress are present.

### Staphylococcal Pneumonia

Staphylococcal pneumonia occurs in infancy and childhood. The pulmonary lesion may be primary infection of the parenchyma; or may be secondary to generalized staphylococcal septicemia. It may be a complication of measles, influenza and cystic fibrosis of the lungs or may follow minor staphylococcal pyoderma. Debilitating conditions including malnutrition, diabetes mellitus and macrophage dysfunction predispose to infection with staphylococci.

*Pathology:* In infants, the pneumonic process is diffuse initially, but soon the lesions suppurate, resulting in bronchoalveolar destruction. Multiple microabscesses are formed, which erode the bronchial wall and discharge their contents in the bronchi. During inspiration, the air enters the abscess cavity because the bronchi are dilated. The bronchioles collapse during expiration and, therefore, the air cannot easily move out. Thus the abscess is progressively inflated, resulting in pneumatoceles, which are pathognomonic of staphylococcal pneumonia. Several pneumatoceles may form and they may fluctuate in size over the time, ultimately resolving and disappearing within a period of few weeks to months. Staphylococcal abscesses in the lungs may erode into the pericardium causing purulent pericarditis. Empyema in a child below two years of age is nearly always staphylococcal in etiology.

*Clinical features:* The illness usually follows upper respiratory tract infection, pyoderma or other associated purulent disease. Besides the usual features of pneumonia, i.e. grunting respiration, the child has fever and anorexia, is listless and irritable. Cyanosis may be present. Progression of the symptoms and signs is rapid. Sometimes pulmonary infection may be complicated by disseminated disease, i.e. involvement of more than two anatomically different sites. This may manifest as metastatic abscesses in joints, bone, muscles, pericardium, liver, mastoid or brain.

*Diagnosis:* The diagnosis of staphylococcal pneumonia is suspected in a newborn or an infant with respiratory infection who has evidence of staphylococcal infection elsewhere in the body. The characteristic complications of pyopneumothorax and pericarditis are highly suggestive of the diagnosis. Pneumatoceles are present in X-ray films of the lung **(Fig. 15.2)**, characteristically in pneumonia due to staphylococci and *Klebsiella*. These pneumatoceles persist as thin-walled asymptomatic cysts for several weeks. Often staphylococci can be grown from the blood.

*Treatment:* The child should be immediately hospitalized and isolated to prevent the spread of resistant staphylococci to the other patients. Fever is controlled with antipyretics and hydration is maintained by intravenous fluid. Oxygen is administered to relieve the dyspnea and cyanosis.

Empyema is aspirated and the pus is sent for culture and sensitivity to antibiotics. Appropriate antibiotic therapy is carried out using coamoxiclav or ceftriaxone with cloxacillin. If the patient does not respond soon, vancomycin or teicoplanin may be added, in place of cloxacillin. Therapy should continue till all the evidence of the disease disappears both clinically and radiologically. Usually child improves in 7–10 days. However, oral antibiotics may be required up to 4–6 weeks. Prolonged therapy is desirable as the bacteria persist in the necrotic area.

*Complications:* Pneumatoceles do not require specific measures. Empyema and pyopneumothorax are treated by intercostal drainage under water seal or low pressure negative suction. Metastatic abscesses require surgical drainage. Significant pleural thickening that is preventing complete expansion of underlying lung may require decortication. It can be done by open thoracotomy or by video-assisted thoracoscopic surgery. Early thoracoscopic drainage of empyema may help in prevention of pleural thickening. Instillation of streptokinase or urokinase in pleural cavity with loculated pleural effusion may help in prevention of pleural thickening.

### Hemophilus Pneumonia

*Hemophilus influenzae* infections occur usually between the age of three months and three years. Infection with *H. influenzae* usually begins in the nasopharynx and spreads locally or through the bloodstream. Most nasopharyngeal infections are mild and confer immunity from subsequent serious illness after the early months of life.

*Clinical features:* The onset of the illness is gradual with nasopharyngeal infection. Certain viral infections probably act synergistically with *H. influenzae*.

The child has moderate fever, dyspnea, grunting respiration and retraction of the lower intercostal spaces. Complications of *H. influenzae* pneumonia include bacteremia, pericarditis, empyema, meningitis and polyarthritis.

***Treatment:*** *H. influenzae* pneumonia is best treated with cefotaxime (100 mg/kg/day) or ceftriaxone (50–75 mg/kg/day) intravenously for 7–10 days.

### Streptococcal Pneumonia

Streptococcal infection of the lungs by group A beta hemolytic streptococci is usually secondary to measles, chickenpox, influenza or whooping cough. Group B Streptococcus is an important cause of respiratory distress in newborns. Pathologically, it causes interstitial pneumonia, which may at times be hemorrhagic. Tracheobronchial mucosa may be ulcerated. Lymph nodes are enlarged. Serosanguineous or thinly purulent pleural effusion is frequently associated.

***Clinical features:*** The onset is abrupt with fever, chills, dyspnea, rapid respiration, blood streaked sputum, cough and extreme prostration. Signs of bronchopneumonia are less pronounced, as the pathology is usually interstitial.

***Complications:*** Thin serosanguineous or purulent empyema is a usual complication. Pulmonary suppuration is less frequent. When pneumatoceles are present, the condition mimics staphylococcal pneumonia.

***Diagnosis:*** X-ray film shows segmental involvement, diffuse peribronchial densities or an effusion.

***Treatment:*** Penicillin G (or ampicillin 100 mg/kg/day in 3-divided doses) should be given for 7–10 days. The response is gradual but recovery is generally complete. Empyema is treated by closed drainage with indwelling intercostal tube.

### Primary Atypical Pneumonia

The etiological agent is *Mycoplasma pneumoniae*; other pathogens include *Chlamydia* and *Legionella* spp. It occurs in epidemics chiefly in the winter months. Children living in overcrowded environments are more prone to develop pneumonia. The disease due to *Mycoplasma* is uncommon in below the age of four years, although subclinical and mild infections have been reported in infants. *Chlamydia* and *Legionella* pneumonia may occur in all age groups.

***Pathology:*** Primary atypical pneumonia involves the interstitial tissue of the lungs, in which round cell infiltration is seen. The alveolar septa become edematous. The mucosa of the bronchioles is inflamed, necrotic and may ulcerate. The obstruction of the terminal bronchioles causes emphysema and atelectasis. Pleura may show patchy fibrinous exudates.

***Clinical features:*** Incubation period is 12 to 14 days. Onset may be insidious or abrupt. Initial symptoms are malaise, headache, fever, sore throat, myalgia and cough. Cough is dry at the beginning, but later it is associated with mucoid expectoration that may be blood streaked. Dyspnea is unusual. There are very few physical signs, except mild pharyngeal congestion, cervical lymphadenopathy and a few crepitations. Extrapulmonary manifestations include hemolytic anemia.

X-ray findings are more extensive than suggested by the physical findings. Poorly defined hazy or fluffy exudates radiate from the hilar regions. Enlargement of the hilar lymph nodes and pleural effusion have been reported at times. Infiltrates involve one lobe, usually the lower.

***Diagnosis:*** It is difficult to distinguish *Mycoplasma* pneumonia from viral or rickettsial pneumonia. The leukocyte count is usually normal. Cold agglutinins are elevated in 1/3 to 3/4 of the patients. *Mycoplasma pneumoniae* may be recovered from the pharynx and sputum. The diagnosis is made rapidly by demonstration of IgM and IgG antibody by ELISA during the acute stage. More recently diagnosis is confirmed by polymerase chain reaction on throat swab samples.

***Treatment:*** Patients are treated with macrolide antibiotics (erythromycin, azithromycin or clarithromycin) or tetracycline for 7 to 10 days.

### Pneumonia due to Gram-Negative Organisms

The etiological agents are *E. coli*, *Klebsiella* and *Pseudomonas*. These organisms affect small children (<2 months of age) or children with malnutrition and poor immunity. *Pseudomonas* may colonize airways of patients with cystic fibrosis and cause recurrent pulmonary exacerbations.

***Clinical features:*** Onset is gradual and assumes life-threatening proportions during its course. Signs of consolidation are minimal, particularly in infants. Constitutional symptoms are more prominent than respiratory distress.

***Diagnosis:*** Radiological signs are extensive in a form of massive consolidation. *E. coli* or *Klebsiella pneumoniae* may have pneumatoceles.

***Treatment:*** Intravenous use of a third generation cephalosporin (cefotaxime or ceftriaxone, 75–100 mg/kg/day) with or without an aminoglycoside is recommended for 10 to 14 days. In case of suspected *Pseudomonas* infection, ceftazadime or a carbapenem may be the drug of choice.

### Viral Pneumonias

Respiratory syncytial virus is the most important cause in infants under 6 months of age. At other ages, influenza, parainfluenza, corona and adenoviruses are common. Either the bronchial tree or alveoli are involved resulting in extensive interstitial pneumonia. Clinical manifestations are variable. There is no evidence of consolidation clinically. Radiological signs consist of perihilar and peribronchial infiltrates. CT chest may show peripherally placed ground glass haziness.

### Pneumonia due to Inhalation of Aliphatic Hydrocarbons as Kerosene

Kerosene exerts its toxic effects on the lungs and the central nervous system. It is poorly absorbed from the gastrointestinal tract. Milk and alcohol promote its absorption. It has low viscosity and less surface tension and, therefore, diffuses quickly from the pharynx into the lungs. Clinical features of hydrocarbon pneumonia include cough, dyspnea, high fever, vomiting, drowsiness and coma. Physical signs in lungs are minimal. X-ray film of the chest shows ill-defined homogeneous or patchy opacities. Picture may resemble miliary mottling of the lungs.

*Treatment:* Vomiting is not induced. Gastric lavage is usually avoided to prevent inadvertent aspiration. The patient is kept on oxygen. Corticosteroids have little beneficial effect (*see* Chapter 28).

### Loeffler Syndrome

Larvae of many nematodes (intestinal parasites) during their life cycle enter the portal circulation, liver and then they pass through the hepatic vein and inferior vena cava into the heart and lungs. In the lungs, the larvae penetrate the capillaries, enter the alveoli, plug the bronchi with mucus and eosinophilic material due to allergic reaction. There are fleeting patchy pulmonary infiltrations. Some cases may be due to drug reaction to aspirin, penicillin, sulfonamide or imipramine.

*Clinical features:* These include cough, low fever, feeling of being unwell and scattered crepitations. There is eosinophilia in the blood and X-ray plate of the lungs shows pulmonary infiltrates of varying size that may superficially resemble miliary tuberculosis. Treatment is symptomatic.

### Suggested Reading


1. Ginsburg AS, Klugman KP. Antibiotics for pediatric community-acquired pneumonia in resource-constrained settings. Eur Respir J 2020;56:2002773.
2. Lodha R, Kabra SK, Pandey RM. Antibiotics for community-acquired pneumonia in children. Cochrane Database Syst Rev 2013; (6): CD004874.
3. Lodha R, Randev S, Kabra SK. Oral antibiotics for community acquired pneumonia with chest indrawing in children aged below five years: A systematic review. Indian Pediatr 2016; 53: 489–95.


## Acute Respiratory Tract Infection (ARI) Control Program

Acute lower respiratory tract infection (LRTI) is a leading cause of mortality in children below 5 years of age. It has been shown in various studies from developing countries that the etiological agent in LRTI is bacterial in 50–60% of children. Common bacteria causing LRTI in preschool children include *H. influenzae*, *S. pneumoniae* and staphylococci. All these are sensitive to antimicrobial agents, including cotrimoxazole and amoxicillin. Judicious use of cotrimoxazole in children suffering from LRTI may prevent death due to pneumonia. The WHO has recommended clinical criteria for diagnosis of pneumonia in children at primary health care level for reducing LRTI deaths in countries where the infant mortality is more than 40/1000 live births.

The clinical criteria for diagnosis of pneumonia include rapid respiration with or without difficulty in respiration. Rapid respiration is defined as respiratory rate of more than 60, 50 or 40/minute in children below 2 months of age, 2 months to 1 year, and 1 to 5 years of age, respectively.

Difficulty in respiration is defined as lower chest indrawing. The WHO recommends that in a primary health care setting if a child between 2 months and 5 years of age present with cough, he should be examined for rapid respiration and difficulty in breathing along with presence of cyanosis or difficulty in feeding (Table 15.4). If the respiration is normal, and there is no chest indrawing and he/she is feeding well, child is considered to have an upper respiratory tract infection and can be managed symptomatically at home. If the child has rapid respiration and chest indrawing but no evidence of hypoxia (oxygen saturation is normal), feeding well and does not have any danger signs, he/she may be treated on ambulatory basis with oral amoxicillin for 5 days.

If child has severe chest indrawing, has clinical evidence of hypoxia or danger signs like lethargy, cyanosis, poor feeding and convulsions, he/she is considered to have severe pneumonia. Such children are admitted in hospital and treated with IV penicillin or ampicillin with gentamicin along with supportive care.

In children below 2 months of age, presence of any of the following indicates severe disease: Fever (38°C or more), convulsions, abnormally sleepy or difficult to wake, stridor in calm child, wheezing, not feeding, tachypnea, chest indrawing, altered sensorium, central cyanosis, grunting, apneic spells or distended abdomen. Such children should

**Table 15.4:** Children aged 2 months to 5 years with cough or difficult breathing: Clinical classification to facilitate treatment decisions

| *Category* | *Essential features* | *Treatment category* |
|---|---|---|
| Cough, cold | No fast breathing, and no indicators of severe or very severe pneumonia | Home care: Remedy for cough, paracetamol for fever |
| Pneumonia with/without lower chest indrawing | Fast breathing:<br>• 2–12 months: ≥50<br>• 12 months–5 years: ≥40<br>Lower chest indrawing but normal oxygen saturation | Home care: Oral amoxicillin<br>40–50 mg/kg/day in 2–3 divded doses for 5 days |
| Severe pneumonia | • Lower chest indrawing<br>• Unable to drink or breastfeed, or convulsions, or lethargy, or unconsciousness, or severe respiratory distress<br>• Central cyanosis | Inpatient care<br>• IM, IV Benzyl penicillin 50000 U/kg every 6-hr or ampicillin 50 mg/kg every 6 hr and gentamicin 7.5 mg/kg once a day for 5 days<br>• Supportive care |

Ceftriaxone may be used as second-line agent for severe pneumonia

be referred to hospital for admission and they are treated with injection ampicillin and gentamicin along with supportive care.

### Suggested Reading

1. Revised WHO classification and treatment of childhood pneumonia at health facilities: evidence summaries. http://apps.who.int/iris/bitstream/10665/137319/1/9789241507813_eng.pdf

## ACUTE BRONCHIOLITIS

It is one of the common serious acute lower respiratory infections in infants. Affected infants are between the ages of 1 and 6 months, but the disease can affect children up to their second birthday. Disease usually occurs in winter and spring. Respiratory syncytial virus (RSV) is implicated in most cases. Other causative organisms include parainfluenza virus, adenovirus, influenza viruses and rarely *Mycoplasma pneumoniae*.

Protection against RSV is mediated by antibodies of IgG3 subclass. These antibodies have shorter half life and do not cross the placenta in substantial amount so as to offer protection to the infant. High quantities of secretory IgA antibodies to RSV are present in the colostrum, and breastfeeding reduces the likelihood of an infant being hospitalized with acute bronchiolitis. Inflammatory mediators such as leukotrienes also play a role in the disease.

### Pathogenesis

The inflammation of the bronchiolar mucosa leads to edema, thickening, formation of mucus plugs and cellular debris. Bronchiolar spasm occurs in some cases. The bronchial lumen, which is already narrow in the infants, is further reduced. As airway resistance is inversely related to the fourth power of the radius of the bronchiolar lumen, even slight narrowing causes marked increase in airway resistance and reduction of airflow, during inspiration and expiration. During expiration, the bronchioles are partially collapsed and egress of air from the lungs is reduced resulting in emphysematous changes. When obstruction becomes complete, the trapped air in the lungs may be absorbed causing atelectasis.

Due to diminished ventilation and diffusion, hypoxemia is produced in severe disease. In severely hypoxemic infants, retention of carbon dioxide leads to respiratory acidosis. In the milder cases, compensation occurs due to hyperventilation of the normal alveoli.

### Clinical Manifestations

The disease starts with an upper respiratory tract infection. After a few days, the breathing becomes fast and respiratory distress develops. Majority of infants show mild symptoms and recover in 3–7 days. Those with severe disease may develop retraction of lower intercostal spaces and suprasternal notch on 3–5 days.

In severe infection, the infant pants for breath and may appear cyanosed. The fever is moderately high. Accessory muscles of respiration are working. Expiration is prolonged, fine crepitations and rhonchi are auscultated. Breath sounds may be faint, or inaudible in severe cases. Respiratory distress is out of proportion to the extent of the physical signs in the lungs.

As the air is trapped in the lungs leading to emphysema, the liver and spleen are pushed down. When the chest becomes over inflated, the anteroposterior diameter of the chest is increased, and hyperresonance is noted on percussion.

### Investigations

X-ray chest shows hyperinflation and minimal infiltrates (Fig. 15.3). Diaphragm is pushed down. The lung fields appear abnormally translucent. The leukocyte count is normal or slightly elevated. A rapid test using monoclonal antibodies against respiratory syncytial virus on nasopharyngeal aspirate can rapidly identify RSV.

### Course and Prognosis

Bronchiolitis is generally a self-limiting illness. The symptoms subside in 3 to 7 days. Death may occur in one percent of the severely ill patients due to respiratory failure. The relationship of bronchiolitis to bronchial asthma in later life has been observed in about one-fourth of the cases. Bronchial asthma is more likely in children with personal or family history of an allergic illness.

### Differential Diagnosis

#### *Bronchial Asthma*

Bronchiolitis is often confused with bronchial asthma. The latter is unusual below the age of one year. There is often a family history of asthma. Several attacks occur in the same patient. Bronchial asthma may occur without a preceding respiratory infection. Response to bronchodilators is more consistent in children with asthma as compared to children with bronchiolitis.

#### *Congestive Heart Failure*

Congestive heart failure is suggested, if there is cardiomegaly on X-ray film of chest, tachycardia, large tender liver, raised JVP, edema and rales in the bases of the lungs.

#### *Foreign Bodies in Trachea*

These are diagnosed by the history of aspiration of foreign body, localized wheeze, and signs of collapse or localized obstructive emphysema.

#### *Bacterial Pneumonia*

In bacterial pneumonia, the signs of obstruction are less pronounced, fever is high and adventitious sounds in the lungs are prominent.

### Treatment

Treatment of bronchiolitis is essentially symptomatic. The child should be nursed in a humid atmosphere preferably in sitting position at angle of 30° to 40° with head and neck elevated. Infants with mild disease can be cared for at home in a humidified atmosphere. If respiratory distress increases or feeding problems appear, the child should be hospitalized.

In hospital, moist oxygen inhalation remains the mainstay of treatment. It is administered continuously even in the absence of cyanosis. Fluids and electrolyte balance should be maintained. Very sick infants may need a concentration of 60% oxygen given through a hood. Pulse oximetry should be performed regularly to keep oxygen saturation of more than 92%.

Antibiotics have no role. Ribavirin, an antiviral agent has no role in the treatment of infants who were previously healthy. Ribavirin, however, shortens the course of illness in infants with underlying congenital heart disease, chronic lung disease and immunodeficiency. Ribavirin is delivered by a nebulizer 16 hours a day for 3–5 days in such cases.

Bronchodilators, inhaled or systemic steroids have not been found to be useful in infants with acute bronchiolitis. Similarly inhaled epinephrine has not been found to give consistent benefits. If a patient show improvement, after first dose of bronchodilators/epinephrine, therapy may continue every 4–6 hourly. Initial evidence support use of inhaled hypertonic saline in infants with acute bronchiolitis. Continuous positive airway pressure (CPAP) or assisted ventilation may be required to control respiratory failure in severe cases. Extracorporeal membrane oxygenation is effective, when respiratory failure is not controlled by mechanical ventilation.

### Suggested Reading


1. Caffrey Osvald E, Clarke JR. NICE clinical guideline: Bronchiolitis in children. Arch Dis Child Educ Pract Ed 2016; 101: 46–48.
2. Kirolos A, Manti S, Blacow R, et al. RESCEU investigations. A systematic review of clinical practice guidelines for the diagnosis and management of bronchiolitis. J Infect Dis 2020;222 (supp):S672–79.
3. O'Brien S, Borland ML, Cotterell E, et al. Australasian bronchiolitis guideline. J Paediatr Child Health 2019; 55: 42–53.


*Competencies:* **PE28.19; PE28.20; PE31.5; PE31.6; PE31.7; PE31.8; PE31.9**

## BRONCHIAL ASTHMA

### Definition

Bronchial asthma is a group of disorders characterized by an increased responsiveness of the airways to various stimuli. It manifests by widespread narrowing of the airways causing paroxysmal dyspnea, wheezing or cough. The obstruction to airflow is reversible in the majority of cases, either spontaneously or in response to treatment. Bronchial reactivity is a necessary component of asthma.

### Pathophysiology

Airway obstruction in asthma is caused by (i) edema and inflammation of mucous membrane lining the airways, (ii) excessive secretion of mucus, inflammatory cells and cellular debris, and (iii) spasm of the smooth muscle of bronchi. Obstruction is diffuse but not uniform.

Asthma has been classified as atopic (extrinsic; IgE mediated, triggered by allergens), non-atopic (intrinsic; non-IgE mediated, triggered by infection), mixed, exercise induced, or aspirin induced. Inhalation of an allergen leads to a biphasic response with early and late reactions ultimately causing bronchoconstriction.

The **early reaction** starts within 10 minutes of the exposure to allergen. It is characterized by release of histamine, leukotrienes C, D, E, prostaglandins, platelet activating factor and bradykinin from the mast cells following the interaction of allergen with specific mast cell bound IgE. All these substances cause bronchoconstriction, mucosal edema and mucus secretion which manifests as airway obstruction. This phase is inhibited by $\beta_2$ agonist drugs.

The **late phase** occurs in about two-thirds of patients. It develops 3–4 hours later with peak at 8–12 hours. Again there is a release of mast cell mediators. This phase is not prevented by premedication with $\beta_2$ agonist drugs. However, it is inhibited by premedication with steroids suggesting that airway narrowing is mainly due to an inflammatory reaction and mucosal edema. This phase presents as clinical asthma.

Airway resistance is increased more so during exhalation because airways close prematurely during expiration. As a result, lungs are hyperinflated; elasticity and frequency-dependent compliance of the lungs are reduced. Breathing involves more work resulting in dyspnea. Perfusion of inadequately ventilated lungs causes low $PaO_2$. In early stages of illness, $PaCO_2$ also falls because of hyperventilation caused by dyspnea. When obstruction becomes more severe, alveolar hypoventilation supervenes. This leads to retention of $CO_2$ with a rise of $PaCO_2$. With the exhaustion of buffer mechanisms, pH of blood falls (respiratory acidemia).

### Pathology

Airway inflammation is now considered to be the basic pathology in asthma. This is initiated by degranulation of mast cells. Degranulated mast cells release various mediators of inflammation as discussed earlier. These mediators damage the wall of the airways leading to epithelial shedding and mucus secretion. Inflammatory mediators also influence reactivity via neural mechanisms.

### Triggers of an Attack of Asthma

#### *Viral Infections*

Viral infections in the young children and exercise in older child or adult appear to be frequent triggers of airway narrowing. Exact mechanism by which viral infections (mainly rhinovirus, RSV) induce temporary bronchoconstriction is not clear. Viral infections may interfere with the integrity of mucosal surface by opening up the tight intraepithelial cell junctions, inducing the shedding of epithelium. It results in mucosal edema and mucus secretion.

#### *Exercise*

Exercise-induced asthma occurs in genetically susceptible individuals with hyper-reactive airways because of the loss of water and heat from the respiratory tract following exercise. Water loss induces mucosal hyperosmolarity, which stimulates mediator release from mast cells.

#### Weather Change

Sudden weather change may result in (i) loss of heat and water from lower airways, and (ii) sudden release of airborne allergens in atmosphere, resulting in exacerbation of asthma.

#### Emotional Factors

Emotional stress operated through the vagus nerve might initiate contraction of bronchial smooth muscles.

#### Food

Allergy to food proteins or food additives plays an insignificant role in the pathogenesis of asthma. These should be incriminated only on a very strong association with the illness.

#### Endocrine Factors

Children may show increase in symptoms during puberty.

### Clinical Features

The clinical features of asthma are variable. Symptoms vary from simple recurrent cough to severe wheezing. Children may present with recurrent cough with or without wheezing. The symptoms occur with change in season, aggravated by exercise and more in nights. Acute asthma may usually begin with a cold, or bouts of spasmodic coughing more so at night. In early phase of the attack, cough is non-productive. The patient becomes dyspneic, with prolonged expiration and wheezing. Accessory muscles of respiration are excessively used. The child sweats profusely, may develop cyanosis and becomes apprehensive and restless, and appears fatigued.

In severe episodes, the child may show air hunger. The chest is hyperresonant because of air trapping. As the obstruction becomes severe, the airflow decreases markedly. As a result, the breath sounds become feeble. Wheezing which was earlier audible may disappear. Absence of wheezing in the presence of cyanosis and respiratory distress should not be considered as an evidence of clinical improvement. As the child starts improving clinically, the airflow increases, and wheezing may reappear.

Severe hypoxemia in asthma results in cyanosis and cardiac arrhythmias. Pulsus paradoxus indicates severe illness. Mucus plugs occluding the bronchi may cause collapse of small segments of the lung. Persistence of hyperinflation of the chest even after subsidence of asthmatic attack signifies that the apparent relief from bronchospasm will be short lived. In chronic intermittent cases, the chest becomes barrel shaped. Clubbing of fingers, however, is unusual in uncomplicated bronchial asthma.

### Diagnosis

Recurrent attacks of wheezing indicate bronchial asthma. Although intermittent attacks of coughing may be due to recurrent viral infections, diagnosis of bronchial asthma must be considered. Cough, which is associated with asthma generally, worsens after exercise. Sputum is generally clear and mucoid but expectoration of yellowish sputum does not exclude the diagnosis of asthma. This may be attributed to large number of eosinophils in the sputum. Chronic spasmodic cough may suggest occult asthma.

### Investigations

#### Pulmonary Function Test (PFT)

The diagnosis of asthma is clinical in most cases, however, it is desirable to document variable/reversible airflow obstruction. PFT plays an important role in diagnosis of doubtful cases and in monitoring of response to treatment. The important parameters in spirometry include PEFR, FEV1, FVC and FEV25-75. All parameters are decreased in asthma. FEV1 is commonly used parameter for documentation of severity of asthma. FEV25-75 is effort independent and is probably more sensitive indicator of airway obstruction. PEFR can be measured easily with peak expiratory flow meter; for other parameters, spirometry is required. Abnormalities in PEFR suggestive of asthma include: A diurnal variation of more than 20%, $\leq$80% of predicted and improvement of $\geq$20% after bronchodilator therapy.

#### Absolute Eosinophil Counts

Significance of eosinophilia for distinguishing between allergic, vasomotor or infectious nature of the chronic respiratory obstructive disease is limited. When eosinophilia is present, bronchial obstruction generally responds well to antispasmodic and anti-inflammatory therapy and the condition is often reversible. The eosinophil count may be low in cases associated with infection.

#### Chest X-Ray

The X-ray may be normal or show bilateral and symmetric air trapping. Patches of atelectasis of varying sizes due to mucus plugs are not unusual. Bronchial cuffing may occur due to the presence of edema fluid in perivascular and peribronchial interstitial space. Extensive areas of collapse or consolidation should suggest an alternative diagnosis.

#### Allergy Test

Skin test and RAST (radioallergosorbent allergen specific IgE) have limited usefulness. Blood IgE may be raised in children with atopic asthma and will be normal in non-atopic asthma. Unlike adults, all children may not have atopic asthma, therefore, it cannot be used as diagnostic test. A few children need skin tests to identify sensitivity to different antigens, since the role of desensitization in therapy is not fully established.

### Differential Diagnosis

#### Bronchiolitis

Bronchiolitis always occurs within the first 2 years, usually within the first 6 months of life. It is commoner in winter or spring months. Generally, there is a single attack. Repeated attacks indicate viral infection associated wheeze or asthma. Hyperinflation of chest with scattered areas of infiltration may be seen in chest X-ray. On the other hand, asthma may start at any age; more than 3 episodes are usual and wheezing is prominent. Infants diagnosed as bronchiolitis who present with family history of allergy have eczema or whose IgE levels are elevated, are most likely candidates for developing asthma.

### Congenital Malformation

Congenital malformation causing obstruction, viz. vascular rings such as aberrant right subclavian artery or double aortic arch, bronchogenic cysts and tracheomalacia should be excluded in differential diagnosis.

### Aspiration of Foreign Body

Wheeze, if present, is generally localized. The history of foreign body aspiration may be forgotten. An area with diminished air entry, with or without hyperresonance, may be due to obstructive emphysema. Most children develop frequent infections in the lung around the foreign body.

### Hypersensitivity Pneumonitis

An acute or chronic lung disease may develop following inhalation of organic dust such as molds, wood or cotton dust, bird droppings, fur dust, grain, or exposure to chemicals or drugs such as epoxy resins, PAS and sulfonamide. In the acute form, these children show fever, chills, dyspnea, malaise, aches and pain and inspiratory rales at bases of lung, and weight loss. X-ray of the chest shows interstitial pneumonia. Bronchial markings are prominent. The levels of IgE antibodies to the specific antigen are increased. The skin test shows Arthus phenomenon with local hemorrhage, edema and local pain within 8 hours. Diagnosis is established by lung biopsy.

### Cystic Fibrosis

Children with cystic fibrosis may present with recurrent wheezing but over a period of time they develop clubbing, and features of malabsorption. X-ray film may show hyperinflation, peribronchial cuffing and pneumonia. Diagnosis is established by sweat testing.

Competency: **PE31.10**

## Management of Bronchial Asthma

The goals of therapy are: (i) Maintenance of near normal pulmonary function, (ii) maintenance of near normal physical activity, (iii) prevention of night-time cough or wheezing with minimal chronic symptoms, (iv) prevention of exacerbations and (v) avoiding adverse effects of medications.

Effective long-term management of asthma involves three major areas:

i. Identification and elimination of exacerbating factors
ii. Pharmacological therapy
iii. Education of patient and parents about the disease, and steps to avoid exacerbations.

### Identification and Elimination of Exacerbating Factors

Common factors associated with development and precipitation of asthma include passive smoking, allergic disorders, inadequate ventilation at home leading to dampness, cold air, cold food, smoke, dust, and pets in the family. Acute respiratory infection due to viruses is the commonest cause of exacerbation of asthma.

*Following measures may help in decreasing the triggers:*

1. The bedroom of the child should be kept clean and as free from dust as possible. Wet mopping of the floor should be done because dry dusting increases exposure of the child to house dust.
2. Heavy tapestry attracts dust and, therefore, light plain cloth sheets should be used as curtains in the child's room.
3. Carpets, stuffed furniture, loose clothing, wall hangings, calendars and books attract lot of dust and should be regularly cleaned at periodic intervals.
4. The bed of the child should be made of light material and should be aired regularly.
5. Caressing of animal pets should be discouraged, as the child may be sensitive to their fur.
6. It is not necessary to restrict the diet, because bronchial asthma due to food allergy is unusual.
7. Adolescent patients should be advised to refrain from smoking.
8. Exposure to strong or pungent odors such as wet paint, disinfectants and smoke should be minimized.
9. The child with asthma should avoid attics or basements, especially if these were unoccupied and kept closed for some days.

### Pharmacotherapy

The pharmacological therapy of bronchial asthma involves use of drugs that relax smooth muscle and dilate the airways and drugs that decrease inflammation and thereby prevent exacerbations. The medications used for long-term treatment of asthma include bronchodilators, steroids, mast cell stabilizers, leukotriene modifiers and theophylline (Table 15.5).

***Bronchodilators:*** This group of drugs provides immediate symptomatic relief. They may be short acting and long acting. The commonly used short-acting bronchodilators are adrenaline, terbutaline and salbutamol. All of these have quick onset of action. Adrenaline stimulates $\alpha$ and both $\beta$ receptors; thus causes cardiac side effects. Terbutaline and salbutamol are specific $\beta_2$ agonists and hence, have minimum cardiac side effects. Adrenaline is given subcutaneously. The other two agents can be administered by oral/inhalation or parenteral route. Inhalation route is preferred because of quick onset of action and fewer side effects.

Long-acting beta agonists include salmeterol and formoterol. Both these drugs are specific $\beta_2$ agonist and have a longer duration of action of 12–24 hours. The onset of action is delayed by ½–1 hour. Their safety and efficacy have been demonstrated in children above four years of age. A recent guideline suggests the use of single maintenance and reliever therapy (SMART) with combination of formoterol and budesonide. Patient may take this inhaler as reliever also (up to 12 puffs a day).

***Corticosteroids:*** Asthma is a chronic inflammatory disease of airways. Corticosteroids being potent anti-inflammatory agent, are the cornerstone of long-term treatment of asthma.

Table 15.5: Medications for long-term treatment of asthma

| *Medication, route of administration* | *Side effects* | *Dose* | *Comments* |
|---|---|---|---|
| **Bronchodilators**<br>***Salbutamol*** 100 µg/puff MDI<br><br>Respirator solution 5 mg/mL<br>Respules 2.5 mg/3 mL<br>Dry powder capsules 200 µg/cap (Rotacap)<br>***Terbutaline*** 250 µg/puff MDI | Tachycardia, tremors, headache, hypokalemia hyperglycemia | 1–2 puff 4–6 hourly<br><br>0.15–0.2 mg/kg/dose nebulization<br>1 dry powder cap 4–6 hourly<br>1–2 puff 4–6 hourly | • Drug of choice for acute attack<br>• Prior to exercise to prevent exercise induced bronchospasm |
| ***Salmeterol*** 25 µg/puff MDI<br>Dry powder capsules 50 µg/cap (Rotacap) | Tachycardia, tremors, headache, hypokalemia, hyperglycemia | 1–2 puffs 12–24 hourly<br>1 dry powder cap inhalation 12–24 hourly | • Long-term prevention of symptoms<br>• Useful for nocturnal symptoms and exercise-induced bronchospasm |
| ***Formoterol*** 6, 12 µg/puff MDI<br>Dry powder capsules 12 µg/cap (Rotacap) | | 1–2 puffs 12–24 hourly<br>1–2 dry powder cap inhalation 12–24 hourly | • Not for treatment of acute symptoms<br>• Use with anti-inflammatory therapy; not as substitute<br>• Single maintenance and reliever therapy (SMART) contains two medications: Budesonide and formoterol; patients may take this inhaler (up to 12 puffs a day) |
| ***Theophylline*** 100, 150, 200, 300 mg tablets | Toxicity at >20 µg/mL; nausea, headache, tachycardia, drowsiness, seizures | 5–15 mg/kg/day<br>2 divided doses | • Drug interaction (antitubercular, anti-convulsants, ciprofloxacin)<br>• May be used in step II when inhalation route is not possible |
| **Mast cell stabilizers**<br>***Sodium cromoglycate*** 5 mg/puff MDI<br><br>***Ketotifen*** Tab 1 mg and Syrup 1 mg/5 mL | Medicinal taste; reflex coughing<br>Bitter taste, cough<br>Sedation, weight gain | 1–2 puffs 3–4 times a day<br><br>1 mg twice a day | • Continuous prophylaxis for control of symptoms; may take 4–6 weeks for clinically evident effect<br>• Safe medication for oral use |
| **Inhaled corticosteroids**<br>***Beclomethasone*** 50, 100, 200, 250 µg/puff<br>***Budesonide*** 50, 100, 200 µg/puff MDI<br>Respules 0.5 and 1 mg /mL<br>Rotacaps 100, 200, 400 µg/cap<br>***Fluticasone*** 25, 50, 125 µg/puff MDI<br>Dry powder capsules: 50, 100, 250 µg/ cap<br>Respules 0.5 and 1 mg/mL<br>***Ciclesonide*** 80 and 160 µg/puff | Cough, dysphonia, oral thrush (gargling, spacer use minimizes effects)<br>Negligible side effects at dose of <400–800 µg/day | Low dose 100–200 µg/day in 2 divided doses<br>Medium dose 400 µg/day in 2 divided doses<br>High dose ≥800 µg/day in 2 divided doses | • Not recommended as relievers<br>• Budesonide, fluticasone are completely inactivated during first pass metabolism; thus have minimal systemic side effects<br>High dose for long duration may cause systemic side effects like growth suppression, adrenal suppression, skin thinning<br>Use minimum required dose preferably on alternate days<br><br>Not cleared for use in children below 12 years of age |
| **Montelukast** 4, 5, 10 mg tabs | Generally well tolerated<br>Churg-Strauss syndrome reported | 2–5 years: 4 mg/day<br>5–12 years: 5 mg/ day<br>>12 years: 10 mg/day | • Exercise-induced asthma<br>• Alternative to long acting β-agonist |

Systemic glucocorticoids used early in the treatment of acute exacerbation reduce the need for visits to emergency department and hospitalization. Inhaled corticosteroids allow application of these medication to the sites where it is specifically needed, reducing the risk for systemic adverse effects.

The commonly used inhaled steroids include beclomethasone, budesonide and fluticasone. The main concern with the use of inhalation steroids is the effect on growth. An approximately 20% reduction in the growth velocity during the first year of treatment with inhaled steroids is reported. Subsequently, the growth velocity recovers and children ultimately attain predicted adult height.

***Mast cell stabilizers:*** Medications include cromolyn sodium, nedocromil sodium and ketotifen. These drugs have limited use in current treatment algorithms.

*Leukotriene modifiers:* Leukotriene inhibitors are useful for the treatment of mild to moderate persistent asthma and exercise-induced asthma. Leukotriene inhibitors act either by decreasing the synthesis of leukotrienes (zileuton) or by antagonizing the receptors (montelukast and zafirlukast).

Montelukast and zafirlukast have received approval for use in pediatric asthma. The former can be used in children above one year of age, while the latter is recommended above 12 years of age.

*Theophylline:* Theophylline has concentration-dependent bronchodilator effects. In addition, theophylline has anti-inflammatory and immunomodulatory effects at therapeutic serum concentrations that are distinct from its bronchodilator properties. Most recent guidelines recommend theophylline as an alternative second-line therapy in combination with inhaled glucocorticoids in moderate persistent asthma in children older than 5 years, as second-line therapy for mild persistent asthma in older children and adults, and as adjunctive therapy (largely for control of nocturnal symptoms) in moderate or severe persistent asthma.

*Long-acting muscarinic antagonists (LAMA):* This group of drug is being used in children who do not respond to inhaled steroids with long-acting beta agonists. Tiotropium has been approved for use in children above 12 years of age.

*Biological agents:* In asthma, a complex interaction of various cytokines is involved that result in airway inflammation. Various monoclonal antibodies are used the pathways of inflammation. These include anti-IgE (omalizumab), and anti-IL5 (mepolizumab, reslizumab). Omalizumab is commonly used drug for difficult to treat asthma above 6-year-old. The other drugs are cleared for use in young adults.

#### *Immunotherapy*

This consists of giving gradually increasing quantities of an allergen extract to a clinically sensitive subject, so as to ameliorate the symptoms associated with subsequent exposure to causative allergen. This is considered only occasionally in highly selected children who are sensitive to a specific allergen such as grass pollen, mites, etc. It is done only under specialist supervision and usually given for 3 years.

### Pharmacological Management

For optimal use of pharmacological agents, one should go in a stepwise manner. That can be achieved by the following:

i. Assessment of symptom control
ii. Assessment of risk of exacerbation
iii. Selection of medications
iv. Selection of appropriate inhalation device
v. Monitoring

#### *Assessment of Symptom Control*

Successful management of asthma requires grading the control of disease according to the frequency and severity of symptoms and functional impairment. Based on the assessment, children can be classified as controlled, partially controlled and uncontrolled (Table 15.6).

#### *Assessment of Risk of Exacerbations*

Based on history, children with risk factors (modifiable or non-modifiable) can be assessed (Table 15.7). Appropriate treatment to children who are at risk of exacerbation may help in prevention of exacerbation.

#### *Selection of Medication*

After assessment of control of asthma and review of factors for exacerbation, appropriate anti-asthma medications are selected (Table 15.8).

Recent guidelines recommend use of inhaled steroids along with salbutamol even for as and when required (SOS).

**Table 15.6:** Assessment of symptom control of asthma

| *Characteristics* | *Controlled (all of the following)* | *Partially controlled (any measure present in any week)* | *Uncontrolled* |
|---|---|---|---|
| Daytime symptoms | None (twice a week or less) | More than twice per week | Three or more features of partly controlled asthma present in any week |
| Limitation of activity | None | Any | |
| Nocturnal symptoms, awakening | None | Any | |
| Need for reliever or rescue drugs | None (less than twice a week) | More than twice per week | |

**Table 15.7:** Assessment of risk of exacerbation

| | *Risk factors* |
|---|---|
| Modifiable | • Uncontrolled asthma symptoms<br>• One or more severe exacerbation in previous year<br>• Start of the child's usual 'flare-up' season<br>• Exposures: Tobacco smoke; indoor, outdoor air pollution; indoor allergens (house dust mite, cockroach, pets, mold)<br>• Major psychological or socioeconomic problems<br>• Poor adherence with controller medication; incorrect inhaler technique<br>• Co-morbidities: Obesity, rhinosinusitis, food allergy |
| Not modifiable | • Ever intubated; PICU admissions<br>• >1 severe exacerbation requiring hospitalization in last 12 months |

Table 15.8: Initial treatment of asthma

| *Symptom control* | *First choice* | *Other choice* |
|---|---|---|
| Infrequent symptoms (not uncontrolled or partly controlled and no risk factors) | No controller medications. As and when required short-acting beta agonists with inhaled steroids | — |
| Asthma (even if infrequent symptoms) with any risk factors for exacerbations<br>Asthma symptoms more than twice a month<br>Waking due to asthma more than once a month | Low dose inhaled steroids<br>As and when required short-acting beta agonists | Montelukast |
| Troublesome symptoms on most days<br>Waking once a week or more or medium dose inhaled steroids | Low dose inhaled steroids + long-acting beta agonists; or medium dose inhaled steroids | Low/medium dose inhaled steroids + LTRA or sustained release theophylline |
| Severely uncontrolled symptoms | Medium to high dose Inhaled steroids + long-acting beta agonists | Short course oral steroids and high dose inhaled steroids; or moderate dose inhaled steroids and long-acting beta agonists |

LTRA leukotriene receptor antagonists





### Selection of Appropriate Inhalation Device

Drugs used by the inhalation route are more effective, i.e. have a rapid onset of action, and have fewer side effects. Most important in the delivery of effective therapy to asthmatic children is the optimal use of appropriate inhalation devices, which include:

i. Metered dose inhaler (MDI)
ii. MDI with spacer
iii. MDI with spacer with face mask
iv. Dry powder inhaler
v. Nebulizer

*Metered dose inhaler* (Fig. 15.4): An MDI is a device, which delivers a fixed amount of medication in aerosol form each time it is activated. It can be used for exacerbation and maintenance therapy. They are effective but require considerable coordination, i.e. press-and-breath coordination. This may not be possible in young children. After actuation, the drug comes out at a pressure and a significant amount of the drug gets deposited in the oropharynx. To overcome this problem, MDI is combined with a spacer. MDIs continue to work past the labeled number of doses because of excess propellant. Therefore, a track of number of actuations should be kept to ensure that children receive adequate therapy when needed.

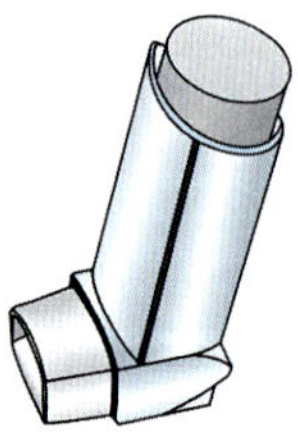

1. Remove cap and shake inhaler in vertical direction
2. Breathe out gently
3. Put mouthpiece in mouth and at start of inspiration that should be slow and deep, press canister down and continue to inhale deeply
4. Hold breath for 10 seconds or as long as possible then breathe out slowly
5. Wait for a few seconds before repeating steps 2–4

Fig. 15.4: Using a metered dose inhaler

*Metered dose inhaler with spacer* (Fig. 15.5): Use of spacer inhalation device with an MDI should be encouraged as it results in a larger proportion of the medication being deposited in the lung, with less impaction in the oropharynx. They also overcome the problems of poor technique and coordination of actuation and inspiration. Furthermore, use of spacer allows MDI to be used for the young patient. MDI used with spacer has been found to be comparable to nebulizer in delivering salbutamol in acute exacerbation of asthma in children. Spacers have the limitation of being bulky, relatively costly and cannot be used in young infants and toddlers.

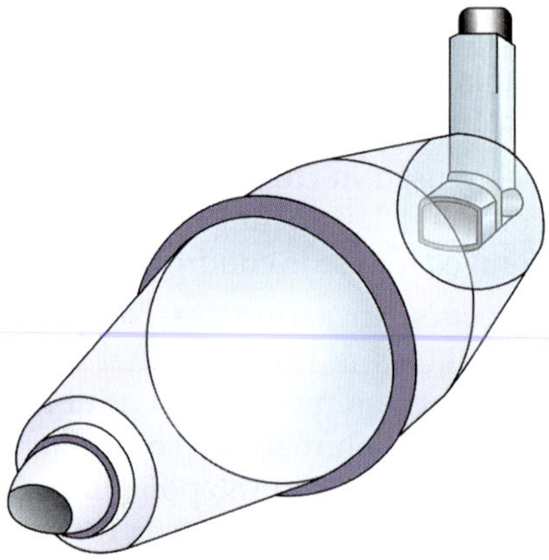

1. Remove cap, shake inhaler and insert into spacer device
2. Place mouthpiece of spacer in mouth
3. Start breathing in and out gently and observe movements of valve
4. Once breathing pattern is established press canister and continue to breath 5–10 times (tidal breathing)
5. Remove the device from mouth and wait for 30 seconds before repeating steps 2–4

Fig. 15.5: Using a metered dose inhaler with spacer

*Metered dose inhaler with spacer with facemask* (Fig. 15.6): Attaching a facemask to the spacer facilitates their use in children below 2–3 years of age.

*Dry powder inhaler (DPI)*: These are breath-activated devices like Rotahaler (Fig. 15.7), Diskhaler, Spinhaler, Turbohaler and Acuhaler. They can be used in children above 4–5 years of age. They have the advantage of being portable and eliminate the need to coordinate actuation with breathing. In addition, they are environmental friendly,

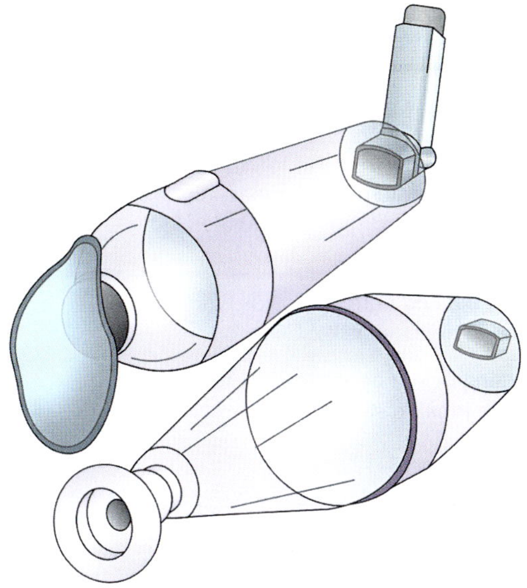

1. Attach baby mask to the mouth end of spacer
2. Shake MDI; insert it in the MDI end of spacer device
3. Cover baby's mouth and nose with baby mask
4. Press canister and encourage the child to take tidal breathing with mouth open (if possible) 5–10 times
5. Remove baby mask and wait for 30–60 seconds before repeating steps 2–4

**Fig. 15.6:** Using a metered dose inhaler with spacer and baby mask

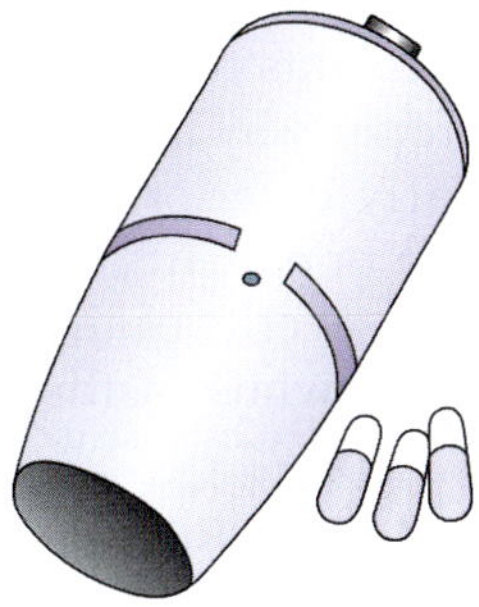

1. Hold Rotahaler vertically and insert capsule (clear end first) into square hole, make sure that top of the capsule is level with top of hole
2. Hold Rotahaler horizontally, twist barrel in clockwise and anti-clockwise direction, this will split the capsule into two
3. Breathe out gently; put mouth end of Rotahaler in mouth and take deep inspiration
4. Remove Rotahaler from mouth; hold breath for 10 seconds

**Fig. 15.7:** Using a rotahaler

as they do not contain CFC. However, the effect of DPI depends upon the inspiratory flow rate and there is reduced efficacy during episodes of acute wheezing or in children with low pulmonary function.

*Nebulizers* (Fig. 15.8): Nebulizers with air compressors are bulky and inefficient aerosol delivery systems. With the advent of efficient spacer systems, the need for nebulizers has diminished. There is a place for the use of nebulized β-agonist in acute severe asthma in young irritable and hypoxic children, who do not tolerate MDI with spacer and facemask, because this allows the delivery of a large dose.

The following measures can improve the amount of drug delivered to the airways: (i) the total fill volume should be about 3–5 mL; (ii) tapping the side of nebulizer chamber

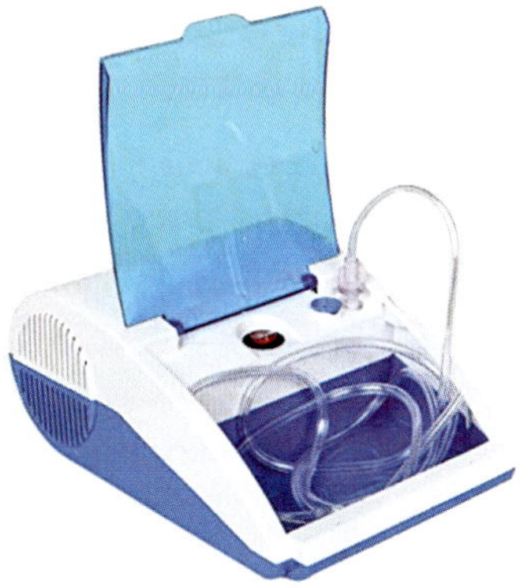

1. Connect nebulizer to mains
2. Connect output of compressor to nebulizer chamber by the tubings provided with nebulizer
3. Put measured amount of drug in the nebulizer chamber and add normal saline to make it 2.5–3 mL
4. Switch on the compressor and look for aerosol coming out from other end of nebulizer
5. Attach face mask to this end of nebulizer chamber and fit it to cover nose and mouth of the child
6. Encourage child for tidal breathing with open mouth

**Fig. 15.8:** Using a nebulizer

during operation induces the droplets on the sides to fall back into the reservoirs, minimizing the loss; (iii) the optimal flow rate is 6–12 L/min, since at this flow, 30–50% of aerosol is in the respirable range of 1–5 μm; (iv) slow, deep inhalations and breath holding can improve delivery.

It is very important to select an appropriate device by which the maintenance medication has to be administered. Inhalation method should be chosen on individual basis but a rough guideline is as follows.

- *Children below 4 years of age:* MDI with spacer with facemask can be used successfully.
- *For children above 4 years of age:* MDI with spacer is preferred.
- *For children above 12 years of age:* MDI may be used directly. However, use of spacer improves drug deposition in airways.

### Monitoring and Modification of Treatment (Step-up, Step-down)

After starting appropriate treatment, patients should be seen every 4–12 weeks. On each visit, a detailed history regarding frequency of symptoms, sleep disturbance, physical activity, school absenteeism, visit to a doctor, need for bronchodilators, and PEFR is recorded. The patient or parents should be encouraged to maintain a symptom diary. The patient is assessed as being controlled, partially controlled, or uncontrolled (Table 15.6).

If the disease is partially controlled or uncontrolled, the causes could be: Poor compliance, wrong technique of inhalation, continued use of empty canister, inappropriate doses, infection (otitis media, sinusitis, pneumonitis), continued exposure to allergens, or under assessment of illness. Many asthmatic children have allergic rhinitis and its treatment has a beneficial effect on asthma. Asthmatic children also have a higher incidence of sinusitis, which may trigger asthma. Bronchial hyperresponsiveness and symptoms improve following therapy for these upper respiratory diseases.

**Table 15.9:** Stepwise treatment of asthma

| | *Symptoms* | *Treatment* | |
|---|---|---|---|
| Step 4: Severe persistent | Continuous<br>Limited physical activity | High dose inhaled steroids + long-acting beta agonists | Refer to specialist for consideration of omalizumab and tiotropium |
| Step 3: Moderate persistent | Daily use $\beta_2$ agonist; daily episodes affect activity | Low dose inhaled steroids + long-acting beta agonists or medium dose inhaled steroids | |
| Step 2: Mild persistent | Low grade symptoms twice a month, or once night-time awakening per month | Low dose inhaled corticosteroids with short-acting beta agonists SOS | |
| Step 1: Intermittent | Infrequent<br>Asymptomatic and normal PEFR between attack | Short-acting beta-2 agonists (SABA) along with inhaled steroids SOS | |



If no cause is found, a step-up, i.e. increase in dose and frequency of medication, is required. Step-down, if control is sustained for 3–6 months and follow a gradual reduction in treatment (Table 15.9).

### Exercise-induced Bronchoconstriction

Some children in addition to varying severity of asthma may develop bronchoconstriction after exercise. To avoid unpleasant experience, they avoid participation in outdoor games. These children may be treated with appropriate stepwise management, may require additional medications like short- and long-acting beta agonists or leukotriene modifiers. Short-acting beta agonists should be taken before going for exercise, as their duration of action is short. Long-acting beta agonists can be taken in the morning and they continue to prevent exercise-induced bronchoconstriction throughout daytime, hence preferable in children who find it difficult to take short-acting beta agonists before exercise in school. Leukotriene modifiers are alternative to long-acting beta agonists.

### Seasonal Asthma

A small proportion of children get symptoms of asthma for a short period in a particular season. They remain asymptomatic for the rest of the year. These children can be started on maintenance treatment 2 weeks in advance. Medications are selected according to severity of asthma. These children should be examined again after discontinuing the medications after the season is over.

### Personalized Medicines

Asthma is group of disorders, a single treatment algorithm may not work for all. Children who do not respond to the above treatment, should be referred to specialist for feasibility of biological agents following appropriate investigations (eosinophils in blood and sputum, serum total IgE, exhaled NO). Children with high IgE may benefit with omalizumab. Children with peripheral blood or sputum eosinophilia may benefit with mepolizumab or reslizumab.

## Education of Parents

Education of parents is an important aspect of asthma treatment. A description of the pathogenesis of asthma in plain language should be explained.

Parents should be asked to maintain a record of daily symptoms such as cough, coryza, wheeze and breathlessness. A record of sleep disturbances, absence from school due to illness and medication required to keep the child symptom free is advised. These records help in stepping up or down the pharmacotherapy.

The parents should understand how various medications work, routes of administration including the use of spacer, and the potential harmful effects. Parents concerned about the use of steroids need to be reassured that in the conventional inhalation dosage, the risk of serious asthma outweights their side effects. Peak flow monitoring done properly by informed parents can help by: (i) Detecting early deterioration in lung function; (ii) managing asthma in patients who have difficulty in sensing the changes in severity of airway obstruction; and (iii) managing patients whose asthma severity changes very rapidly.

An important part of health education is instructing the parent/patient on how to recognize and manage acute exacerbation of asthma at home. A written action plan should be given to them.

## Home Treatment of Acute Exacerbation

Acute exacerbation can be identified by increase in cough, wheeze and breathlessness. PEFR, if measured, may be decreased by 20% from the baseline. For acute exacerbation parents should administer short acting $\beta_2$ agonists with inhaled steroids by MDI with or without spacer and facemask, one puff at a time, repeated every 30–60 seconds up to a maximum of 10 puffs with monitoring of symptoms. If symptoms are relieved and PEFR is increased at the end of inhalation, the child can be continued on salbutamol/terbutaline every 4–6 hours and a visit to treating physician is planned. If there is no improvement or partial improvement or there are symptoms of life-threatening attack at any time, the child should be immediately transferred to a hospital.

A single dose of prednisolone (1–2 mg/kg) may be administered before going to the hospital in a child with symptoms of life-threatening asthma, or who does not show satisfactory improvement after inhalation therapy at home.

## MANAGEMENT OF ACUTE EXACERBATION OF ASTHMA

Increase in the symptoms in form of cough, wheeze and/or breathlessness is termed as exacerbation of asthma. The severity of exacerbation is variable and can be classified as mild, moderate, severe or life-threatening on the basis of physical examination, measurement of PEFR/FEV1 and oxygen saturation (Table 15.10).

### Life-Threatening Asthma

Presence of any of the following indicates a life-threatening asthma: Cyanosis, silent chest, poor respiratory efforts, exhaustion/fatigue, altered sensorium, PEFR <30% of predicted and oxygen saturation of <90%.

Such patients should immediately receive oxygen inhalation; injection of terbutaline or adrenaline is given subcutaneously, and inhalation of salbutamol or terbutaline and ipratropium is started. An injection of hydrocortisone 5 mg/kg is given and an arrangement is made to transfer the patient to ICU preferably with an accompanying physician. In ICU, if patient shows improvement, the salbutamol/terbutaline inhalation is continued every 20– 30 minutes, hydrocortisone (2–3 mg/kg) is continued every 6–8 hourly till patient starts accepting orally. If the patient does not improve or deteriorates, a slow intravenous infusion of magnesium sulfate (50 mg/kg) may be given. Alternatively, a loading dose of theophylline is infused. If there is no improvement with this management, patient is prepared for mechanical ventilation. Patient is also screened for causes of poor response such as acidosis, pneumothorax, electrolyte imbalance and infection, and treated accordingly.

### Mild Acute Asthma

Patients with mild exacerbation have cough, rapid respiration and some wheezing but no chest indrawing and are able to speak and drink well. PEFR, if can be measured is >80% of predicted and oxygen saturation is more than 95% in room air.

Such patients should be given beta-2 agonists by nebulizer or MDI with a spacer and with or without face mask. If the latter is used, then one puff of medicine is repeated every minute up to 10 puffs. If case of significant improvement, the patient can be sent home on inhalation or oral beta agonists every 6–8 hours and called back after 1–2 weeks for reassessment and long-term treatment. In case of no response or poor response, the patient should be treated as moderate exacerbation.

### Acute Moderate and Severe Asthma

These patients have rapid respiration, chest indrawing, wheezing, pulsus paradoxus, difficulty in speech and feeding, PEFR and oxygen saturation is decreased. The sensorium is normal.

Such patients should be treated with inhaled beta-2 agonists as described in treatment of mild asthma. It is repeated every 20 minutes, oxygen inhalation is started and oral dose of prednisolone 1–2 mg/kg is given. At end of one hour, the patient is assessed for improvement. In case of improvement, the child is continued on inhalation of beta-2 agonists every 30 minutes and the interval is gradually increased to every 4–6 hourly. Oxygen inhalation is stopped, if able to maintain oxygen saturation of >95%. Prednisolone is continued once daily for 5–7 days and then stopped without tapering. The patient can be discharged from hospital when the need for bronchodilators is every 4–6 hourly, able to feed and speak well, maintains oxygen saturation of >95% in room air and the PEFR is >75% of predicted. These patients should be educated about the disease, need for regular follow-up and avoidance of triggers. They should be assessed for long-term treatment.

In case of no improvement at end of one hour, the inhalation of salbutamol is continued and ipratropium 250 µg is also added every 20 minutes. An injection of hydrocortisone 5 mg/kg is given and reassessed at end of two hours. If good response, the patient is treated like the early responders. If case of no response; injectable theophylline bolus followed by continuous infusion is started. Such patients may respond well to magnesium infusion at doses of 50 mg/kg dissolved in dextrose over 30 minutes. If there is no improvement, these patients should be prepared for possible mechanical ventilation.

#### *Monitoring the Treatment*

Monitoring of vital signs (heart rate, respiratory rate, chest indrawing, oxygen saturation, sensorium) is necessary.

**Table 15.10:** Grading of severity of acute asthma

| *Clinical parameter* | *Mild* | *Moderate* | *Severe* |
|---|---|---|---|
| Color | Normal | Normal | Pale |
| Sensorium | Normal | Anxious | Agitated |
| Respiratory rate | Increased | Increased | Increased |
| Dyspnea | Absent<br>Can speak sentences | Moderate<br>Can speak in phrases | Severe<br>Difficulty in speech |
| Accessory muscles | Nil or minimal | Chest indrawing | Chest indrawing, flaring of ala nasi |
| Pulsus paradoxus | <10 mm | 10–20 mm | >20 mm |
| Rhonchi | Expiratory | Expiratory, inspiratory | Expiratory or absent |
| PEFR | >80% | 60–80% | <60% |
| $SaO_2$ | >95% | 90–95% | <90% |

### When to Discharge from the Hospital

Patient should have been on discharge medication for 24 hours and had inhaler technique checked and recorded. Treatment should include steroids tablets and inhaled steroids in addition to the bronchodilator. The patient should given a self-management plan or instructions should be given to the parents.

## Recurrent Wheezing in Children below 5 Years of Age

There are multiple phenotypes of wheezing in young children and can be classified as follows.

1. Episodic wheezing due to repeated viral infections. The episodes decrease by age of 5 years with decline in incidence of viral infection in these patients.
2. Multitrigger wheezing: Children with this phenotype may get wheezing with viral infection as well as other triggers. Children may get some symptoms in between the viral infections. These children respond well to bronchodilators. Some of these patients may continue to get wheezing even after 5 years of age and are treated as asthma.

### Management

Each episode should be treated with inhaled salbutamol and in severe cases, a short course of systemic steroids may be given. Children getting frequent episodes of wheezing should be started on low dose inhaled corticosteroids for 8–12 weeks. If good response, inhaled steroids are stopped and child is followed for recurrence of symptoms. Initial response and recurrence of symptoms after stopping treatment, suggest the diagnosis of bronchial asthma.

### Suggested Reading


1. 2021 GINA Report, Global Strategy for Asthma Management and Prevention. https://ginasthma.org/gina-reports/
2. Fanta CH. Advances in evaluation and treatment of severe asthma. Med Clin N Am 2022;106(6):971–86.
3. Martin J, Townshend J, Brodie M. Diagnosis and management of asthma in children. BMJ Pediatrics Ogan 2022;6:e001277.


## FOREIGN BODY ASPIRATION

Young children between 1 and 4 years of age are especially prone to aspirate small objects in their air passages. Unless recognized and treated, these children have significant respiratory morbidity, such as recurrent wheezing, cough and pneumonia. Immediate response to foreign body aspiration is a choke, gag, cough or localized wheeze. After the initial episode, symptoms may improve for some time and the whole episode may be forgotten.

Subsequently, the course of illness depends on the nature of foreign body, its size, extent and the site of obstruction. Foreign bodies of organic or vegetable source swell up and cause more symptoms. A partial obstruction may cause ball valve type effect leading to localized hyperinflation. The overlying chest wall may show hyperresonance, diminished vocal resonance and poor air entry. In small children, it may be difficult to elicit hyperresonance. Thus a localized area of poor air entry in a child with chronic respiratory illness should arouse suspicion of a foreign body. Complete obstruction and surrounding inflammation cause distal atelectasis and suppuration of the surrounding parenchyma of the lungs result in bronchiectasis.

These children are treated by removal of foreign body through a rigid bronchoscope. Appropriate antibiotics are given for secondary infection. Bronchoscopy should be undertaken, if the clinical and radiological picture suggests the diagnosis even when the history of foreign body aspiration is not forthcoming.

### Suggested Reading


1. Foltran F, Ballali S, Passali FM, et al. Foreign bodies in the airways: a meta-analysis of published papers. Int J Pediatr Otorhinolaryngol 2012; 76 Suppl 1:S12–19.


## LUNG ABSCESS

Lung abscess in children is most frequently a complication of bacterial pneumonia especially those due to *Staphylococcus aureus*, and *Klebsiella pneumoniae*. It may also develop in sequestration of lung tissue or in association with foreign bodies, bronchial cysts or stenosis. Staphylococcal lung abscesses are often multiple, while those complicating aspiration are solitary. The abscess may rupture into the pleural space leading to pyopneumothorax. The main pathological changes are of necrosis and liquefaction with inflammation in the surrounding lung tissue.

### Clinical Features

The patient has fever, anorexia, lethargy, pallor, and cough with foul smelling expectoration. Physical signs may be minimal. Amphoric breath sounds, coarse crepitations and whispering pectoriloquy are characteristic but often not elicitable. The diagnosis is confirmed by plain X-ray film of the chest and ultrasound or CT scan of chest.

### Treatment

Appropriate antibiotics to which the organisms isolated from the sputum or bronchoscopic aspirate are sensitive, are administered for 4 to 6 weeks. Physiotherapy is carried out for effective drainage of the pus. Surgical resection of the involved area of lung is indicated, if medical therapy is not effective.

## BRONCHIECTASIS

Bronchiectasis is a chronic suppurative disease characterized by destruction of the bronchial and peribronchial tissues, dilatation of the bronchi and accumulation of infected material in the dependent bronchi.

Most cases follow recurrent episodes of respiratory infections such as bronchitis, bronchiolitis, post-measles or post-pertussis pulmonary infections, cystic fibrosis, and pneumonia in infancy and early childhood. Infections damage the bronchial wall and cause segmental areas of collapse, which exert a negative pressure on the damaged bronchi, causing them to dilate. The bronchial dilation is widespread and patchy. The bronchi may show cylindrical, fusiform or saccular dilatation.

*Congenital disorders* of bronchi such as bronchomalacia, communicating type of bronchial cyst or sequestrated lung may be the cause of bronchiectasis in some cases.

*Kartagener syndrome* is characterized by bronchiectasis, situs inversus and sinusitis, and is attributed to disorder to ciliary motility (primary ciliary dyskinesia).

*Cystic fibrosis* is characterized by recurrent lower respiratory infections associated with malabsorption. These patients may give history of meconeum ileus during neonatal period.

*Immunodeficiency syndromes* may be responsible for recurrent pulmonary infections and bronchiectasis. *Young syndrome* patients have sinusitis, bronchiectasis and azoospermia (detected later in life).

*Forgotten foreign bodies* may lead to recurrent infection resulting in localized bronchiectasis.

### Clinical Manifestations

Clinical features depend on extent, duration, and underlying illness. The respiratory infections tend to persist longer and recur frequently with waxing and waning. Often the illness can be traced back to an episode of measles or whooping cough. A history of inhalation of foreign body is usually not forthcoming as it is often forgotten. The most prominent symptom is morning cough with copious mucopurulent expectoration. In the course of illness, the sputum may become blood streaked or even frank hemoptysis may occur. In chronic cases, clubbing of fingers is seen. The general health is poor, with recurrent infections. The patient complains of loss of appetite, irritability and poor weight gain.

### Investigations

X-ray film of the chest shows honeycombing of the involved area indicating multiple small abscess cavities. High resolution computerized scan is the gold standard for making a diagnosis of bronchiectasis. Bronchoscopy is undertaken where there is a possibility of surgical intervention. Sputum should be sent for culture and sensitivity. Tuberculin reaction is done to exclude tuberculosis. Pilocarpine iontophoresis is done for estimating sweat chloride in cases with suspected cystic fibrosis.

### Management

During acute exacerbations, bacterial infections should be controlled and airway kept clear of secretions. This is facilitated by effective cough at regular intervals and chest physiotherapy. Assistance by a specially trained pulmonary physiotherapist may be useful. Surgical resection of the involved area is undertaken in children with marked symptoms and localized disease. Extrinsic compression of bronchi by mediastinal masses requires surgical intervention. If the child cannot cooperate in postural coughing, segmental or lobar collapse may occur in the postoperative period and new bronchiectatic lesions may appear. Children with generalized disease may improve clinically with medical treatment alone during adolescence.

### Suggested Reading


1. Chang AB, Grimwood K, Boyd J, et al. Management of children and adolescents with bronchiectasis: Summary of the ERS guidelines. Breathe (Sheff) 2021;17:210105.
2. Gupta AK, Lodha R, Kabra SK. Non cystic fibrosis bronchiectasis. Indian J Pediatr 2015; 82: 938–44.
3. Kaehne A, Milan SJ, Felex LM, et al. Head-to-head trials of antibiotics for bronchiectasis. Cochrane Database Syst Rev 2018;9:CD012590.


## EMPYEMA THORACIS

Empyema thoracis is defined as collection of pus in the pleural cavity. This is commonly caused as a complication of pneumonia or rupture of subdiaphragmatic or liver abscess in the pleura.

### Etiology

Commonly it is sequelae of staphylococcal pneumonia. It can occur secondary to pneumonia due to other organisms including *S. pneumoniae*, gram-negative bacilli and *Mycoplasma*. Tuberculous empyema is rare, compared with pleural effusions.

### Clinical Features

These include fever, breathing difficulty and toxic appearance of child. There is decreased movement of respiration with reduced air entry and vocal resonance. Occasionally, it may manifest as a pulsatile swelling over chest, called empyema necessitans.

### Diagnosis

X-ray film of chest shows shift of the mediastinum with obliteration of costophrenic angle and varying degree of opacification. A pleural tap shows purulent material full of leukocytes with high protein and low sugar. Gram stain and culture may show causative agent. Empyema should be differentiated from other causes of pleural effusion including tuberculous and neoplastic.

### Treatment

This includes administration of antibiotics that are effective against *Staphylococcus*. Empyema is managed by continuous intercostal drainage through underwater seal. If facilities exist, one time drainage of the fluid is done by thoracoscopy. After antibiotics and drainage, if lung is not expanding or there are loculations in the pleura, CT scan of chest is done for evidence of thickening of pleura or loculated empyema. Such patients may need decortication by thoracotomy, or thoracoscopy.

### Suggested Reading


1. Brims FJ, Lansley SM, Waterer GW, Lee YC. Empyema thoracis. Eur Respir Rev 2010; 19: 220– 28.


## CYSTIC FIBROSIS

Cystic fibrosis (CF) is the most common life-limiting recessive genetic disorder in Caucasians with an incidence of approximately 1 in 2500 children born in the United

Kingdom. It is less common in African Americans (1 in 15000) and in Asian Americans (1:31000). It also affects other ethnic groups such as black population with an incidence of 1 in 17,000 and the native American population with an approximate incidence of 1 in 80,000. The incidence in the migrant Indian population in the UK is between 1 in 10000 to 12000. The precise incidence of the condition in India is not known.

### Molecular Genetics

The basic defect in CF is a mutation in the gene for chloride conductance channel, i.e. cystic fibrosis transmembrane conductance regulator (*CFTR*). The failure of chloride conductance by epithelial cells leads to dehydration of secretions that are too viscid and difficult to clear. The defective gene is located on the long arm of chromosome 7. Till now more than 2000 mutations in the gene are recognized, the commonest being delta F508.

### Clinical Manifestations

The clinical features depend on age at diagnosis, supportive care received and treatment. Common clinical features include meconium ileus in neonatal period, recurrent bronchiolitis in infancy and early childhood, recurrent lower respiratory tract infections, chronic lung disease, bronchiectasis, steatorrhea and with increasing age pancreatitis, and azoospermia. Pancreatic insufficiency is present in >85% of patients (Table 15.11).

### Diagnosis

The diagnosis is suspected by presence of a typical phenotype or family history, and confirmed by the demonstration high sweat chloride (>60 mEq/L) on at least two occasions, and/or identifying mutations in both copies of *CFTR*. Nasal potential difference measurements can be used as an adjunct to sweat test, but are not widely available.

**Table 15.11:** Common clinical features of cystic fibrosis (%)

| | |
|---|---|
| **0–2 years** | |
| Meconium ileus | 10–15 |
| Obstructive jaundice | |
| Hypoproteinemia, anemia | |
| Bleeding diathesis | |
| Heat prostration, hyponatremia | |
| Undernutrition | |
| Steatorrhea | 85 |
| Rectal prolapse | 20 |
| Bronchitis, bronchiolitis | |
| Staphylococcal pneumonia | |
| **2–12 years** | |
| Malabsorption | 85 |
| Recurrent pneumonia | 60 |
| Nasal polyposis | 6–36 |
| Intussusception | 1–5 |
| **>13 years** | |
| Chronic pulmonary disease | 70 |
| Clubbing | |
| Abnormal glucose tolerance | 20–30 |
| Diabetes mellitus | 7 |
| Chronic intestinal obstruction | 10–20 |
| Focal biliary cirrhosis | |
| Portal hypertension | 25 |
| Gallstones | 4–14 |
| Azoospermia | 98 |

### Management

Therapy of CF includes respiratory management, nutritional care, anticipation and early diagnosis of liver disease, diabetes and other organ dysfunction.

#### *Respiratory Management*

The principal components of care include airway clearance techniques, antibiotics and anti-inflammatory agents. CFTR modulators help the function of the defective CFTR protein, their role in therapy of CF is being examined.

#### *Nutritional Management*

Nutritional management of CF includes:

i. Increasing caloric intake by encouraging parents to feed the child more frequently. If appetite is poor due to persistent infection, feeding may be given by nasogastric route or by gastrostomy.
ii. Supplement fat soluble vitamins: Pancreatic insufficiency results in deficiency of fat soluble vitamins. Vitamins A, D and E are supplemented at twice the recommended doses, given along with food and enzymes.
iii. Replace pancreatic enzymes: Enteric coated tablets or spherules of pancreatic enzymes are given with each feed. Enzymes are started at the doses of 1000–2000 IU of lipase/kg in divided doses, and increased based on improvement in weight gain, nature of stools and abdominal symptoms.

### Suggested Reading


1. da Silva Filho LVRF, Zampoli M, Cohen-Cymberknoh M, Kabra SK. Cystic fibrosis in low and middle-income countries (LMIC): A view from four different regions of the world. Pediatr Respir Rev 2021;38:37–44.
2. Kaur H, Pandey S, Jat KR, et al. Predictors of mortality in children with cystic fibrosis in India. Pediatr Pulmonol 2021. doi: 10.1002/ppul.25766.


## ACUTE RESPIRATORY DISTRESS SYNDROME (ARDS)

ARDS is defined as pulmonary edema not originating from the heart. The chief cause is severe pneumonia followed by sepsis. Predisposing factors include shock, tissue injury, aspiration, toxins, microthrombi, intravascular coagulation, uremia and increased intracranial pressure.

### Pathogenesis

There is increased permeability of alveolar capillary membrane leading to aggregation of leukocytes in pulmonary circulation. Mediators such as free oxygen radicals and platelet activating factors are released and injure vascular epithelium. In the acute stage, there is edema and hyaline membrane formation, followed by fibrosis. Microthrombi in vessels contributes to increased pulmonary vascular resistance and right-to-left shunting.

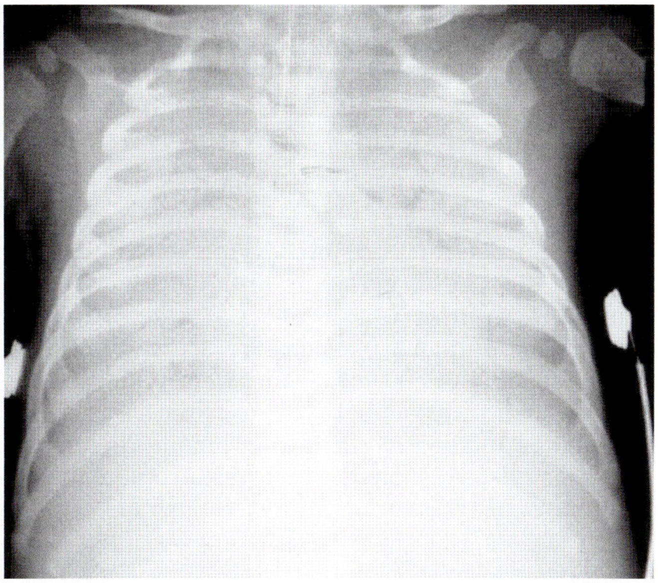

Fig. 15.9: X-ray film of chest showing diffuse opacities bilaterally, compatible with acute respiratory distress syndrome

### Clinical Features

ARDS can occur at any age. Initially symptoms are less and lungs are clear. Later on within 6–8 hours, patient becomes breathless. After 12 hours of insult, refractory hypoxia occurs followed by hypercapnia. Radiologically most lung fields are affected with reticular opacities (Fig. 15.9). Mortality is very high, approaching 50–60%.

### Treatment

Patient should be managed in an intensive care unit with cardiorespiratory monitoring and artificial ventilation. Ventilation is achieved by high PEEP or inverse ratio ventilation. The cause of ARDS should be treated simultaneously.

### Suggested Reading


1. Gupta S, Sankar J, Lodha R, Kabra SK. Comparison of prevalence and outcomes of pediatric acute respiratory distress syndrome using Pediatric Acute Lung Injury Consensus Conference Criteria and Berlin Definition. Front Pediatr 2018 Apr 9;6:93.


## CHRONIC COUGH

Chronic cough can be quite distressing. Parents are concerned and often seek consultation. The diagnosis is made by careful analysis of the following: Age of the child (Table 15.12); nature of cough and sputum; relationship to the time or posture; presence of wheezing or stridor; effect of season; response to previous therapy; state of nutrition; physical signs in the chest and presence or absence of clubbing of fingers.

### Type of Cough

Staccato paroxysms of cough suggest whooping cough or *Chlamydia* infection. Barking or brassy cough associated with changes in the voice indicate laryngotracheal disease. In case of post-nasal drip, cough appears to be like an attempt to clear the throat and is described as hawking. Cough of psychogenic nature has a honking character.

*Sputum:* Purulent sputum indicates the presence of suppurative lung disease. Although sputum is mucoid in cases of asthma, yellow sputum may indicated the presence of a large number of eosinophils. Hemoptysis suggests the possibility of bronchiectasis, tuberculosis, mitral stenosis, cystic fibrosis or foreign body.

*Seasonal cough:* Wheezing is indicative of asthma. Chronic cough, which is more common in certain seasons, should arouse the suspicion of asthma. Chronic cough occurring in winter months is indicative of viral etiology.

*Undernutrition:* Undernutrition in association with chronic cough is found in tuberculosis, bronchiectasis, pertussis, cystic fibrosis, severe chronic asthma or immune deficiency.

### Investigations

Investigations are required, if child is not growing well, has chronic wet cough or gets severe illness requiring admission. Chest X-ray film, examination of the sputum, blood counts and tuberculin test may be necessary. Bronchoscopy or CT scan of the chest is required in some cases.

### Management

Bronchial asthma should be excluded before evaluating for other causes of cough.

*Non-specific therapy:* Cough suppressants are preferably avoided in children. These are indicated only, if the cough is dry and exhausting, or if it disturbs sleep and prevents adequate nutrition, e.g. in whooping cough. Dextromethorphan is an effective cough suppressant and is non-habit forming.

*Bronchodilators* are useful in the treatment of children with cough due to occult asthma because of retained tracheobronchial secretions. Mucociliary transport of secretions is helped by the beta-adrenergic agonists and the

Table 15.12: Diagnosis of chronic cough in relation to age

| *Onset of cough* | *Causes* |
|---|---|
| Onset from birth | Laryngeal webs, vascular rings, H type tracheoesophageal fistula |
| First month | Congenital infections (rubella, CMV) leading to interstitial pneumonia; primary ciliary dyskinesia |
| Early infancy | Gastroesophageal reflux leading to vomiting and aspiration of milk, saliva, gastric contents |
| Late infancy | Bronchitis, asthma, cystic fibrosis, whooping cough |
| Preschool age | Recurrent bronchitis, allergic bronchitis, asthma, foreign body, chronic suppurative lung disease, pulmonary eosinophilia |
| All ages | Asthma, whooping cough, viral bronchitis, tuberculosis, foreign body aspiration |

xanthine group of drugs both in the asthmatic as well as in non-asthmatic children with chronic bronchitis.

*Physiotherapy*, e.g. chest clapping, vibrations and postural drainage are useful in facilitating removal of bronchial secretions.

### Suggested Reading


1. Cheng ZR, Chua YX, How CH, Tan YH. Approach to chronic cough in children. Singapore Med J. 2021; 62:513–19.


## PULMONARY MANIFESTATIONS OF HIV INFECTION

Pulmonary diseases are an important cause of morbidity and mortality in HIV-infected children. These illnesses include recurrent upper respiratory tract infections, serious bacterial infections, opportunistic infections and lymphoid interstitial pneumonitis. The use of highly active antiretroviral therapy has improved the quality of life and survival in HIV-infected children.





### Recurrent Bacterial Infections

Children living with HIV (CHLHIV) may get recurrent bacterial infections due to usual and unusual organisms. The common pathogens for community-acquired pneumonia in these children are *Streptococcus pneumoniae*, *Hemophilus influenzae*, and *Staphylococcus aureus*. However, in children with severe immunosuppression and in hospital-acquired infections, gram-negative organisms, e.g. *Pseudomonas aeruginosa* gain importance.

The clinical features of pneumonia in HIV-infected children are similar to those in uninfected children. However, in severely immunocompromised children, the signs may be subtle. Often, the response to therapy is slow and the relapse rates are high. Bacteremia may be more common, seen in up to 50%.

Sick children with pneumonia should be treated with parenteral antibiotics: The initial choice is a combination of third generation cephalosporin and an aminoglycoside. Children with non-severe pneumonia may be managed on outpatient basis using a second or a third generation cephalosporin or coamoxiclav. Very often, in sick children, possibility of *Pneumocystis jirovecii* pneumonia cannot be excluded; cotrimoxazole should be added in such cases.

### Tuberculosis

The overall relative risk of active tuberculosis in children infected with HIV is at least 5- to 10-fold higher than that in children not infected with HIV. In absence of significant immunosuppression, the clinical manifestations are not much different from that in otherwise healthy children. In patients with low CD4 counts, the pulmonary lesions are more extensive. Mediastinal adenopathy is also more frequently seen. Pleural effusions are uncommon.

The diagnosis of tuberculosis in infected children poses a challenge. Even with the use of a lower cut-off of 5 mm, the tuberculin test is often negative, particularly in children with severe immunosuppression. In extensive disease, the bacteriological confirmation rates are likely to be greater. All attempts should be made to isolate *Mycobacterium tuberculosis*.

All HIV-infected children with active tuberculosis should receive standard medications for 6 months followed by another 6 months of INH.

### Infection with *Mycobacterium avium-intracellulare* (MAI)

Pulmonary disease with MAI is uncommon in children with HIV infection. Common symptoms and signs include: Persistent fever, failure to thrive, night sweats, lymphadenopathy, organomegaly, and refractory anemia. The pulmonary lesions are usually limited to lymphadenopathy and localized parenchymal lesions. The diagnosis of disseminated disease primarily depends on isolation of the organism from blood. Therapy for disseminated MAI infection involves a combination of clarithromycin or azithromycin with ethambutol.

### *Pneumocystis jirovecii* Pneumonia (PCP)

PCP is the most common opportunistic infection in HIV-infected children. Children with PCP are sicker than the adults with this infection. The case fatality rates are also higher.

The onset may be acute in infants, but more indolent in older children. Clinical features include tachypnea, dyspnea and fever. Examination of the chest is unremarkable except for tachypnea and retractions. Asymmetric breath sounds, crepitations and rhonchi are uncommon. Hypoxemia is the hallmark of PCP.

Chest radiograph reveals diffuse interstitial lung disease without hilar adenopathy. Other patterns include localized infiltrates, hyperinflation, and non-cardiogenic pulmonary edema. The radiograph may be normal in less than 5% children. A markedly elevated (A-a)$DO_2$ and a high serum LDH level are often seen.

The diagnosis of PCP requires demonstration of cysts or organisms in lung secretions or tissue. Induced sputum, nasopharyngeal swab and BAL useful for detecting the organism.

The most effective therapy is contrimoxazole, at a trimethoprim dose of 20 mg/kg/day intravenously. In absence of the IV preparation, an oral preparation may be used. Other medications used include: Pentamidine, combination of primaquine and clindamycin, dapsone and trimethoprim, or atovaquone. Even with optimal therapy, response may be seen after 4–8 days. Therapy is given for 21 days, followed by secondary PCP–prophylaxis in all.

Therapy with corticosteroids is indicated, if the $PaO_2$ is less than 70 mm Hg or the alveolar-arterial oxygen gradient is more than 30 mm Hg. The doses used are 1–2 mg/kg/d of methylprednisolone or prednisone, for 10–20 days.

Even if a child develops PCP while on prophylaxis, therapy should be started with cotrimoxazole. This is because the prophylaxis may have failed because of poor compliance, or unusual pharmacokinetics.

### Viral Infections

In children with AIDS, disseminated CMV is a known opportunistic infection, but pneumonia is rare. Infections with influenza, herpes simplex and varicella viruses are uncommon.

### Fungal Infections

Pulmonary fungal infections usually present as a part of disseminated disease in immunocompromised children. Invasive disease usually presents as persistent pneumonia associated with nodules and cavitatory lesions. Diagnosis of invasive bronchopulmonary aspergillosis must be considered in a child with compatible clinicoradiologic picture and recovery of organism from BAL, and raised serum galactomannan. In children with advanced HIV infection, the disease runs an aggressive course.

Isolated pulmonary cryptococcosis, histoplasmosis and coccidioidomycosis are uncommonly seen.

### Lymphoid Interstitial Pneumonitis (LIP)

LIP is a distinctive marker for pediatric HIV infection and is included as a Class B condition in the revised CDC criteria for AIDS in children. LIP is usually diagnosed after infancy in children with perinatally acquired HIV infection. In contrast, PCP is diagnosed typically in the first year of the life. Most children with LIP are asymptomatic. Tachypnea, cough, wheezing and hypoxemia are usual signs; crepitations are uncommon. Clubbing is present in advanced disease.

The presence of a reticulonodular pattern, with or without hilar lymphadenopathy, that persists on chest radiograph for 2 months or greater and that is unresponsive to antimicrobial therapy is considered presumptive evidence of LIP. Care should be taken to exclude other etiologies. A definitive diagnosis of LIP is made on histopathology.

Early disease is managed conservatively. The effect of antiretrovirals on LIP is probably limited. Steroids are indicated, if children with LIP have symptoms and signs of chronic pulmonary disease, clubbing and/or hypoxemia. Treatment usually includes an initial 4–12 weeks course of prednisolone followed by long-term tapering, using oxygen saturation and clinical status as a guide to improvement.

### Suggested Reading


1. Benito N, Moreno A, Miro JM, Torves A. Pulmonary infections in HIV-infected patients. Eur Resp J 2012;39:730–45.
2. Nuttall JJC. Current antimicrobial management of community-acquired pneumonia in HIV-infected children. Expert Opin Pharmacother. 2019;20:595–608.
3. Theron S, Andronikou S, George R, et al. Non-infective pulmonary disease in HIV-positive children. Pediatr Radiol. 2009; 39: 555–64.

Chapter

16

# Disorders of the Cardiovascular System

R Krishna Kumar

Diseases of the cardiovascular system are an important cause of childhood morbidity and mortality. The majority of heart diseases presenting in early childhood are congenital, resulting from structural defects during development. Rheumatic heart disease continues to be prevalent in selected regions in India. Systemic hypertension is increasingly recognized in childhood and predisposes to cardiovascular morbidity in adulthood. A variety of other cardiovascular conditions may present in childhood. Infection or exposure to COVID-19 results in unique cardiovascular manifestations in children.

The management of children with cardiovascular diseases requires an integrated approach with inputs from various specialties. There have been substantial advances in the field of pediatric cardiology and pediatric cardiac surgery that have dramatically transformed the outlook of children with heart disease. This chapter seeks to provide contemporary basic information on diagnosis and management of cardiovascular disease in children.

## EPIDEMIOLOGY AND DISEASE BURDEN OF PEDIATRIC HEART DISEASE IN INDIA

Heart disease is a significant cause of death and disability in children. It is estimated that each year, 200–250,000 children in India are born with CHD, and of these nearly 100,000 are significant enough to need surgery or a catheter procedure early in life. The relative importance of CHD as a cause of infant deaths is increasing as infant mortality due to preventable condition declines. In states with low IMR, CHD is among the leading causes of deaths in infancy. While rheumatic fever (RF) and RHD has declined sharply with improvements in hygiene and access to health care, the disease persists among underprivileged and marginalized populations, particularly the rural poor. In these populations, children and adolescents with RHD may have significant valve damage and heart failure. The COVID-19 pandemic has had various cardiovascular manifestations that can be life-threatening.

Caring for the vast numbers of children with heart disease in India is challenging as the number of institutions with comprehensive pediatric heart programs are a few and largely limited to metropolitan cities. There are significant limitations in awareness on heart disease among care-givers, policymakers and general public. Figure 16.1 illustrates the challenges in care continuum for congenital heart disease that impact outcomes. The pediatrician has a very significant role in this care continuum by enabling timely detection, facilitating initial stabilization, ensuring timely referral including safe and expeditious transport when required and caring for the child after initial cardiac care.

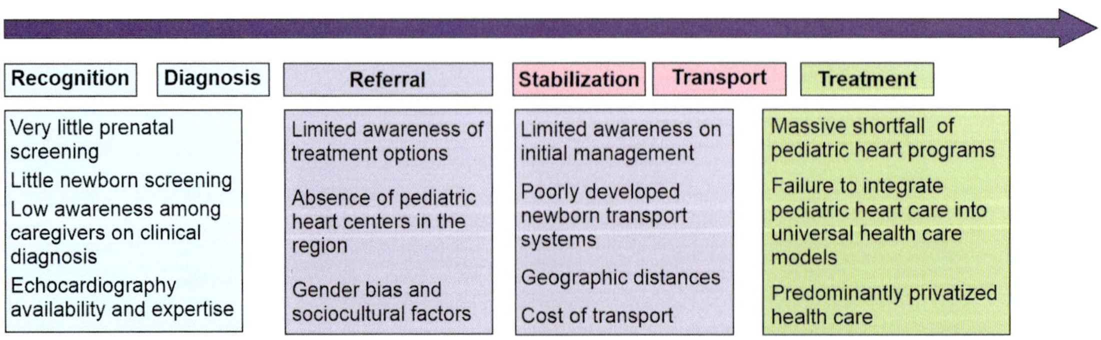


Fig. 16.1. Health system challenges that impact outcomes in congenital heart disease

In 2012, the Government of India started the Rashtriya Bal Swasthya Karyakram (RBSK), a national child health initiative for screening and treatment of childhood diseases and disabilities including CHD. This program, administered by the National Health Mission (within the Ministry of Health and Family Welfare), provides funding and technical assistance to individual states. As an example of achievements within the program, the Kerala government in its systematic plan named Hridyam, developed to address the state's burden of CHD under the RBSK scheme, brought about 40% reduction in deaths due to CHD as well as a 21% reduction in the overall IMR, which is now down to 7 per 1000 live births.

### Suggested Reading


1. Nair SM, Zheleva B, Dobrzycka A, Hesslein P, Sadanandan R, Kumar RK. A population health approach to address the burden of congenital heart disease in Kerala, India. Global Heart 2021;16:71.
2. National Health Mission, Ministry of Health and Family Welfare, Government of India. Rash triya Bal Swasthya Karyakram (RBSK).https://nhm.gov.in/index1.php?lang=1&level=4&sublinkid=11 90&lid=583.


*Competencies:* **PE23.3; PE23.7; PE23.8; PE23.9; 23;11**

## CONGESTIVE CARDIAC FAILURE

Congestive cardiac failure is the inability of the heart to maintain an output, at rest or during stress, necessary for the metabolic needs of the body (systolic failure) and inability to receive blood into the ventricular cavities at low pressure during diastole (diastolic failure). Thus, due to systolic failure it is unable to propel blood into the aorta and in diastolic failure, it receives inadequate amount of blood. Diastolic heart failure is recognized by clinical features of heart failure with evidence of increased filling pressures with preserved systolic function and in many instances, cardiac output. An increase in left-sided pressures results in dyspnea from pulmonary congestion. An increase in right-sided pressures results in hepatomegaly and edema. Besides hypertrophied ventricles, diastolic failure occurs in restrictive heart disease and constrictive pericarditis. While mitral and tricuspid valve stenoses result in elevated atrial pressure, they are not, in the strictest sense, diastolic heart failure.

### Etiopathogenesis

The common causes of diastolic failure are indicated in Table 16.1. The causes of congestive failure can be classified according to age (Table 16.2). Rheumatic fever and rheumatic heart disease is typically encountered beyond 5 yr age; its prevalence appears to be declining in many parts of the country.

Heart failure from congenital heart disease (CHD) typically happens within the first 1–2 yr of life. Patients with left-to-right shunts tend to develop CCF around 6 to 8 weeks of life. Unlike left-to-right shunts, congenital leakage of the mitral or the tricuspid valve can result in heart failure at an early age. Congenital tricuspid regurgitation (TR) manifests early because the elevated pulmonary artery pressures increase its severity. For the same reasons, TR may decline as pulmonary vascular resistance declines.

The age of occurrence of heart failure may point towards the underlying CHD (Table 16.3). Heart failure at an unexpectedly early age for a patient thought to have a simple shunt lesion should prompt the search for an associated condition such as coarctation.

Arrhythmias are an important cause of congestive cardiac failure in infancy. Heart rates above 180/min tend to precipitate heart failure. Any long-standing tachyarrhythmia can be associated with ventricular dysfunction that may mimic cardiomyopathy. Typical examples include ectopic atrial tachycardia and permanent junctional re-entrant tachycardia. Severe bradycardia, typically from complete heart block, can also result in heart failure.

With a normal heart, hemoglobin levels 5 g/dL can result in heart failure. In a heart compromised by disease,

**Table 16.1:** Heart failure due to diastolic dysfunction

| |
|---|
| Mitral or tricuspid valve stenosis* |
| Constrictive pericarditis |
| Restrictive cardiomyopathy |
| Acute ventricular volume overload (acute aortic or mitral valve regurgitation) |
| Myocardial ischemia# |
| Marked ventricular hypertrophy (hypertrophic cardiomyopathy, storage disorders, severe hypertension, severe aortic or pulmonary valve stenosis) |
| Dilated cardiomyopathy# |

*Elevated atrial pressures with normal ventricular diastolic pressures
#Often have combined systolic and diastolic dysfunction

**Table 16.2:** Causes of congestive cardiac failure

**Infants**

- Congenital heart disease
- Myocarditis and primary myocardial disease
- Tachyarrhythmias, bradyarrhythmias
- Kawasaki disease with coronary occlusion
- Pulmonary hypertension (persistent pulmonary hypertension of the newborn; primary pulmonary hypertension; hypoxia, e.g. upper airway obstruction)
- Miscellaneous causes
  - Anemia
  - Hypoglycemia
  - Infections
  - Hypocalcemia
  - Neonatal asphyxia (myocardial dysfunction, pulmonary hypertension)

**Children**

- Rheumatic fever, rheumatic heart disease
- Congenital heart disease complicated by anemia, infection or endocarditis
- Systemic hypertension
- Myocarditis, primary myocardial disease
- Pulmonary hypertension (primary, secondary)

**Table 16.3:** Time of onset of congestive failure

| *Age* | *Lesion* |
|---|---|
| Birth–1 week | Duct-dependent systemic circulation (hypoplastic left heart syndrome, critical aortic stenosis, severe coarctation, arch interruption); total anomalous pulmonary venous return (obstructed), congenital mitral and tricuspid valve regurgitation, neonatal Ebstein anomaly |
| 1–4 weeks | Patent ductus arteriosus (PDA) in preterms, ventricular septal defect (VSD) with coarctation, persistent truncus arteriosus, transposition with large VSD or PDA, severe coarctation, critical aortic stenosis, congenital mitral or tricuspid regurgitation, single ventricle physiology with unrestrictive pulmonary blood flow |
| 1–2 months | Transposition with VSD or PDA, endocardial cushion defects, VSD, PDA, severe coarctation; total anomalous pulmonary venous return, anomalous left coronary artery from pulmonary artery, single ventricle physiology with unrestrictive pulmonary flow |
| 2–6 months | VSD, PDA, endocardial cushion defect; anomalous left coronary artery from the pulmonary artery, coarctation, single ventricle physiology with unrestrictive pulmonary blood flow |



failure may be precipitated even with hemoglobin levels of 7–8 g/dL. Younger infants are more susceptible to develop failure with anemia.

## Clinical Features

***Symptoms:*** Slow weight gain results from inadequate feeds because of easy fatigability together with excessive loss of calories from increased work of breathing. Uncommonly, there may be an unusual short-term gain in weight due to collection of water, manifesting as facial puffiness or rarely as edema on the feet. The difficulty in feeding may manifest itself as 'poor feeder', a complaint that the baby does not take more than one to two ounces of milk at a time because of fatigue or shortness of breath. The baby then gets hungry within a few minutes after taking a small feed. The history is often of an irritable infant crying all the time. Often, a mother may state that the baby breathes too fast while feeding or that the baby is more comfortable and breathes better when held against the shoulder—which is the equivalent of orthopnea in older children. Not infrequently, the baby is brought with persistent hoarse crying, wheezing, and excessive perspiration and less commonly, because of facial puffiness (Table 16.4).

***Signs:*** Left-sided failure is indicated by tachypnea and tachycardia. Persistent cough, especially on lying down, hoarse cry and wheezing are other evidences of left-sided failure; basal rales in the chest are usually not audible. Right-sided failure is indicated by hepatomegaly and facial puffiness. Examination of the neck veins in small babies is not helpful. Firstly, it is difficult to evaluate the short neck with baby fat and secondly, hemodynamic studies show that right atrial mean pressures stays normal in many infants with congestive failure. Edema on the feet occurs late. Common to both left- and right-sided failures is the presence of cardiac enlargement, third sound gallop and poor peripheral pulses with or without cyanosis (Table 16.5).

**Table 16.4:** Symptoms of cardiac failure

| |
|---|
| Poor weight gain |
| Difficulty in feeding |
| Breathes too fast; breathes better when held against the shoulder |
| Persistent cough and wheezing |
| Irritability, excessive perspiration and restlessness |
| Pedal edema |

**Table 16.5:** Signs of congestive cardiac failure

| *Left-sided failure* | *Failure of either side* | *Right-sided failure* |
|---|---|---|
| Tachypnea | Cardiac enlargement | Hepatomegaly |
| Tachycardia | Gallop rhythm (S3) | Facial edema |
| Cough | Peripheral cyanosis | Jugular venous engorgement |
| Wheezing | Small volume pulse | |
| Rales in chest | Lack of weight gain | Pedal edema |

## Treatment

Management of heart failure is a four-pronged approach for correction of inadequate cardiac output. They include: (i) Reducing cardiac work, (ii) augmenting myocardial contractility, (iii) improving cardiac performance, (iv) correcting the underlying cause. *Identification of the cause is most important since it has direct bearing on survival. The focus of heart failure management has entirely shifted towards correcting the cause as early as possible.*

### *Reducing Cardiac Work*

The work of the heart is reduced by restricting patient activities, treatment of fever, anemia, obesity, and by vasodilators. Mechanical ventilation helps when heart failure is severe by eliminating the work of breathing.

Neonates with heart failure are nursed in an incubator. They are handled minimally. The baby is kept propped up at an incline of about 30°. The pooling of edema fluid in the dependent areas reduces the collection of fluid in lungs, thus reducing the work of breathing. At a temperature of 36–37°C, the overall circulatory and metabolic needs are minimal, thus reducing work of heart. Humidified oxygen to maintain a concentration of 40 to 50%, improves impaired oxygenation secondary to pulmonary congestion. Oxygen should not be used indiscriminately. There are situations with left-to-right shunts where oxygen can worsen heart failure by inappropriately increasing pulmonary blood flow at the cost of systemic perfusion.

If the infant or the child is restless or dyspneic, cautious sedation may be appropriate in very select circumstances.

Fever, anemia or infection also increase the work of the heart and must be treated.

*Anemia* imposes stress on the heart because of the decreased oxygen carrying capacity of blood. Anemia results in tachycardia and in a hyperkinetic circulatory state. Correction of anemia will result in decreased cardiac work. If transfusion is indicated, packed red cells can be administered. Typically packed cell volumes of 10–20 mL/kg are required to correct severe anemia; a single dose of furosemide IV is often given prior to the transfusion.

*Vasodilators* counteract the compensatory mechanisms in heart failure and improve cardiac output (Fig. 16.2). Arteriolar and venous vasoconstriction is mediated through catecholamines. Arteriolar constriction maintains blood pressure by increasing the systemic vascular resistance, which increases the work of heart (Fig. 16.3). Venoconstriction results in decreased venous capacitance and increased venous return, increasing the filling pressures of the ventricles to increase the cardiac output. Since compensatory mechanisms are inappropriately excessive, vasodilators, by reducing the arteriolar and venous vasoconstriction, reduce the work of heart. Nitrates are used as preferential venodilators.

ACE inhibitors (captopril, enalapril) are effective for treating heart failure in infants and children. These agents

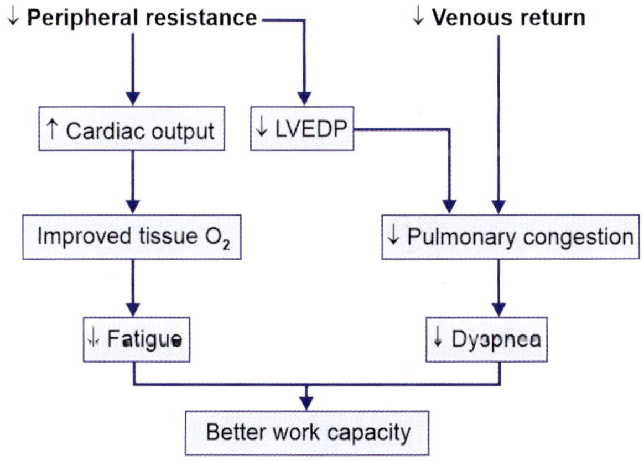


Fig. 16.2: By reducing the systemic vascular resistance and decreasing the venous tone, vasodilators provide better work capacity. LVEDP left ventricular end-diastolic pressure

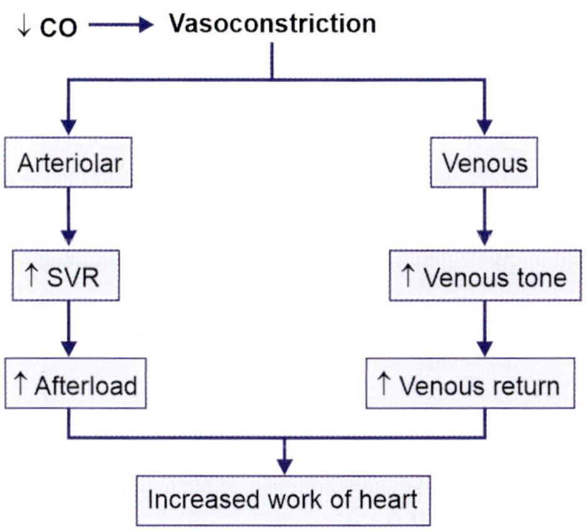


Fig. 16.3: Low cardiac output (CO) results in vasoconstriction, increasing systemic vascular resistance (SVR) and venous tone leading to increase in the work of heart

suppress renin–angiotensin–aldosterone system thereby reducing vasoconstriction and salt and water retention. They are clinically the most useful oral vasodilators. By suppressing catecholamines, they prevent arrhythmias and other adverse effects on the myocardium. The major side effect of ACE inhibitors is cough, which, if persistent, may necessitate the use of angiotensin receptor blockers, such as losartan. Initially, it is necessary to monitor the blood levels of creatinine and electrolytes every 1–2 weeks for 4–6 weeks. To avoid first-dose hypotension, the first dose should be one-quarter of the calculated dose. ACE inhibitors should be withheld in settings of dehydration and avoided in neonates because of the risk of acute kidney injury.

Although beta-blockers might precipitate CCF, they improve symptoms, especially in patients with dilated cardiomyopathy, who continue to have tachycardia. Useful agents include metoprolol and carvedilol. The latter is preferred since it has properties of beta-blockers with peripheral vasodilation; treatment is started at low dose and increased depending on tolerability (0.08 to 0.4 mg/kg/day, maximum 1.0 mg/kg/day). Calcium channel blockers have adverse effects in heart failure and should be avoided, unless indicated for systemic hypertension.

In the acute care setting, sodium nitroprusside is used as a vasodilator, since it acts on the venous and arterial systems. Phosphodiesterase inhibitors such as milrinone and calcium sensitizers (levosimendan) have become popular especially in postoperative period. These agents have powerful vasodilatory and inotropic effects. Specific indications for use of vasodilators include acute mitral or aortic regurgitation, ventricular dysfunction resulting from myocarditis, anomalous coronary artery from pulmonary artery and in the early postoperative setting.

### Augmenting Myocardial Contractility

Inotropic agents, like digoxin, improve cardiac output by augmenting myocardial contractility. It has a rapid onset of action and is eliminated quickly. It is available for oral and parenteral administration. Oral digoxin is available as 0.25 mg tablets and as digoxin elixir (1 mL = 0.05 mg) (Table 16.6). Parenteral digoxin (0.5 mg/2 mL) is available; its dose is 70% of the oral dose. Digoxin is beneficial for symptom relief and is advised in patients with mild, moderately severe or severe congestive failure, with or without sinus rhythm. Digoxin can be combined with

Table 16.6: Dosage of digoxin and diuretics

| | *Digitalizing dose, mg/kg* | *Maintenance dose mg/kg/day* |
|---|---|---|
| **Digoxin** | | |
| Premature, neonates | 0.04 | 0.01 |
| 1 month to one year | 0.08 | 0.02–0.025 |
| 1 to 3 years | 0.06 | 0.015–0.02 |
| Above 3 years | 0.04 | 0.017 |
| **Diuretics** | | |
| Furosemide | 1–3 mg/kg per day orally or 1 mg/kg per dose IV | |
| Spironolactone | 1 mg/kg orally every 12 hours | |

ACE inhibitors for synergistic effect. By increasing cardiac output, digoxin lowers systemic impedance indirectly, unloading the ventricles.

The use of digoxin for heart failure has declined considerably in the recent years.

***Intravenous inotropic agents:*** These agents belong to three groups: (i) Catecholamine inotropes, like dopamine, dobutamine and adrenaline; (ii) phosphodiesterase inhibitors like amrinone and milrinone, which combine inotropic effects with peripheral vasodilation (inodilators); and (iii) levosimendan, a calcium sensitizer that has become popular in acute care settings as a potent inodilator with systemic and coronary vasodilatation. Unlike milrinone, it does not increase risk of rhythm disturbances.

If blood pressure is low, dopamine can be used, as an intravenous infusion. At a dose of less than 5 μg/kg/min, dopamine causes peripheral vasodilation and increases myocardial contractility. Renal blood flow improves, resulting in natriuresis; higher doses result in peripheral vasoconstriction. The dose of dobutamine is 2.5–15 μg/kg/min; the dose should be increased gradually until the desired response is achieved. In patients with dilated cardiomyopathy, dobutamine can be used as 24 hr infusion once or twice a week and retains its effectiveness for varying lengths of time. Milrinone is given in infusion 0.3–0.7 μg/kg/min following a loading dose of 50 μg/kg. The loading dose is often not given, if there are concerns of hypotension. The usual dose of levosimendan is 6 to 12 μg/kg loading dose over 10 minutes followed by 0.05–0.2 μg/kg/min as a continuous infusion.

### *Improving Cardiac Performance by Reducing Venous Return (Preload)*

Diuretics reduce the blood volume, decrease venous return and ventricular filling. Diuretics reduce the total body sodium thereby, reducing blood pressure and peripheral vascular resistance. This helps in increasing the cardiac output and reducing the work of the heart. Diuretics are the first line of management in congestive failure. The action of oral furosemide starts within 20 min. Furosemide should be used in combination with a potassium sparing diuretic (triamterene, spironolactone, amiloride) instead of using potassium supplements. The combination prevents potassium and magnesium loss and reduces the risk of arrhythmias. Furosemide activates the renin–angiotensin–aldosterone axis, which is responsible for vasoconstriction and sodium and water retention. When furosemide is combined with ACE inhibitors, the combination suppresses the axis and is, therefore, synergistic.

Sodium restriction is recommended but difficult to implement in infants and young children. Low sodium diets should be used only if the heart failure cannot be controlled with digitalis, diuretics and ACE inhibitors. However, it is prudent to advise such patients to avoid salt-rich foods such as chips and pickles. Since heart failure increases calorie requirements, adequate intake is advised.

### *Correcting the Underlying Cause*

The focus of management of CHF has shifted entirely towards identifying and correcting the underlying cause. It is now possible to rapidly identify the cause of CHF in most children with suspected heart disease. Many of these are managed by curative or palliative operations. A diagnosis of idiopathic dilated cardiomyopathy requires exclusion of conditions that are known to cause ventricular dysfunction. The conditions that might be missed are sustained tachyarrhythmias, coarctation of aorta and obstructive aortitis, anomalous origin of the left coronary artery from pulmonary artery and hypocalcemia. It is important to look for subtle evidence of sustained tachyarrhythmias. Anomalous origin of the left coronary artery is treated surgically.

The presence of CCF in a child with rheumatic heart disease does not necessarily mean presence of active carditis. In any patient of rheumatic heart disease, if active carditis has been excluded and an adequate trial has been given to medical management, operative treatment should be considered. Uncommon causes of CCF in infants and children include upper respiratory obstruction, hypoglycemia, neonatal asphyxia and hypocalcemia.

A practical management plan based on clinical risk status is presented in **Fig. 16.4**. This generally works in most clinical circumstances.

## Suggested Reading


1. Shaddy RE, George AT, Jaecklin T, et al. Systematic literature review on the incidence and prevalence of heart failure in children and adolescents. Pediatr Cardiol 2018;39:415–36.


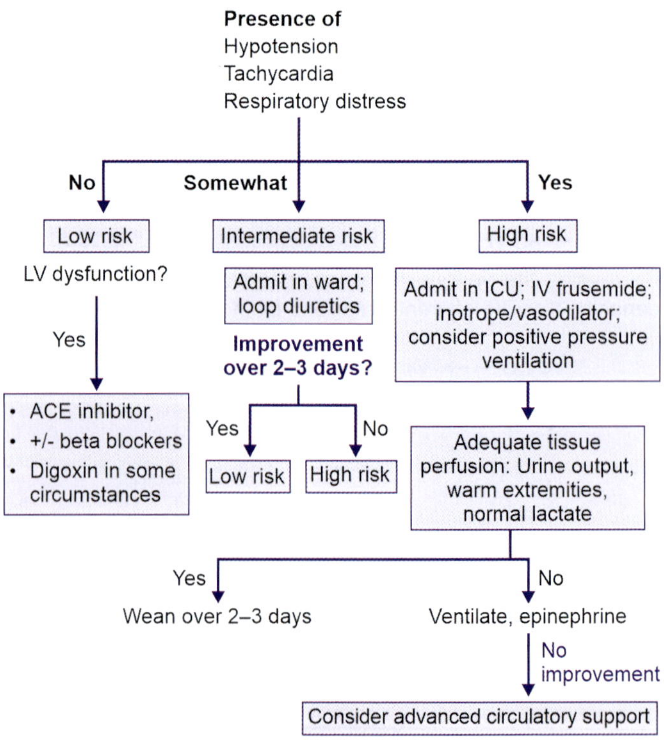


**Fig. 16.4:** Management algorithm for heart failure

Competencies: **PE23.1; PE23.7; PE23.8; PE23.9; PE23.16; PE23.17**

## CONGENITAL HEART DISEASE

Congenital heart disease (CHD) encompasses a broad and diverse range of conditions that manifest from prenatal period to late adulthood. In common terms, CHD refers to structural heart defects that are present at birth. Diagnosis requires a systematic approach starting from history, physical examination, chest X-ray, ECG and echocardiography.

A substantial proportion of patients with CHD have significant problems involving other organ systems, or specific chromosomal and single gene disorders. Pediatricians need to identify associated conditions, since they might have significant bearing on outcomes. It is important to recognize that, in spite of significant recent advances that have substantially improved overall the outlook of children with CHD, long-term concerns after palliation and corrective surgery are significant and many children need lifelong follow-up.

### Epidemiology and Etiology

CHD accounts for nearly one-third of all major congenital anomalies. The prevalence of CHD in infancy is estimated at 6–8 per 1000 live births; 25% are life-threatening and require early intervention. A proportion of patients with CHD have an identifiable genetic basis (Table 16.7). Table 16.8 shows the association of CHD with acquired disorders and teratogens. Over the past 2–3 decades, the rank order of CHD as a cause of infant mortality has increased steadily and it is among the top 5 causes of deaths in infants between 30 days and 1 year in most parts of the world including many parts of India.

### Pathophysiology

#### *Pressure, Flow and Resistances*

The pressures and resistances in the pulmonary and systemic circulations are indicated in Table 16.9. The pulmonary and systemic flows are equal, if there are no abnormal communications between the two sides.

According to Poiseuille's equation, modified for application to blood flow through vessels.

$$\text{Pressure} = \text{Flow} \times \text{Resistance}$$

The pressure is measured in mm Hg, flow in liters/min and resistance in dynes/sec/$cm^5$ or units (80 dynes/sec/$cm^5$ = 1 unit).

Although this equation is not strictly accurate when applied to flow of blood in pulmonary and systemic circuits, it does serve a useful purpose in understanding the hemodynamics. Thus,

$$\text{Systemic pressure} = \text{Systemic flow} \times \text{Peripheral vascular resistance}$$

$$\text{Pulmonary arterial pressure} = \text{Pulmonary flow} \times \text{Pulmonary vascular resistance}$$

It is thus obvious that the pressure in a vessel is dependent on the *flow* through the vessel and the resistance, offered by the vessel to the flow of blood. It is possible to increase the pressure in a vessel either by increasing the flow or by increasing the resistance. Increase in flow through the pulmonary artery means a left-to-right shunt, as occurs in atrial or ventricular septal defect or patent ductus arteriosus. Generally, this increase in flow is not associated with a proportionate increase in pressure as the *resistance falls* or *remains the same*. The distensibility characteristics of the pulmonary artery are such that it can accommodate almost three times the normal flow without a significant increase in pressure. Hence, *large left-to-right shunts can*

**Table 16.7:** Inherited syndromes associated with congenital heart disease

| *Syndrome* | *Genetic mutation; inheritance* | *Cardiac lesions* | *Other features* |
|---|---|---|---|
| CATCH 22 | Microdeletion in 22q; autosomal dominant | Interrupted aortic arch, TOF, VSD, persistent truncus arteriosus, double outlet right ventricle | Cleft palate, hypocalcemia, thymic hypoplasia, nasal regurgitation, gastroesophageal reflux, learning disability |
| Williams-Beuren | Microdeletion in *elastin* (7q11.23); AD | Supravalvar aortic stenosis, pulmonary stenosis, hypertension | Elfin facies, mental retardation, hypersocial personality, short stature, hypercalcemia |
| Down | Trisomy 21; Robertsonian translocation or mosaicism | AV canal defect, perimembranous VSD, TOF | Characteristic facies, clinodactyly, mental retardation; hypotonia |
| Turner | 45XO or 46/45XO mosaic | Bicuspid aortic valve, coarctation | Short stature, gonadal dysgenesis lymphedema |
| Noonan | *PTPN11*; AD | Pulmonic stenosis, hypertrophic cardiomyopathy, ASD | Short stature, dysmorphic facies, webbed neck, developmental delay, cryptorchidism |
| VATER association | Sporadic | VSD, TOF | Vertebral, renal and limb defects, anal atresia, tracheoesophageal fistula |
| Holt-Oram | *TBX5*; AD | Ostium secundum ASD; VSD | Radial ray anomalies |
| CHARGE association | *CHD7*; often de novo | Branch pulmonary artery stenosis, TOF, VSD | Coloboma, growth failure, choanal atresia, genital hypoplasia, ear anomalies |
| Alagille | *JAG1*; most cases are *de novo* | Pulmonary stenosis, TOF | Dysmorphic facies, cholestatic jaundice, butterfly vertebrae, renal anomalies |

AD autosomal dominant; AV atrioventricular; ASD atrial septal defect; TOF tetralogy of Fallot; VSD ventricular septal defect

| Table 16.8: Prenatal exposures that increase risk of congenital heart disease |
|---|
| Gestational diabetes (transposition, atrioventricular septal defects, hypoplastic left heart, cardiomyopathy, PDA) |
| Febrile illness in first trimester (increased risk) |
| Rubella (PDA, peripheral pulmonary stenosis, VSD) |
| Lupus (complete heart block) |
| Phenylketonuria (VSD, TOF, PDA, single ventricle) |
| Vitamin deficiency (increased risk of heart disease) |
| Teratogens (first trimester), e.g. anticonvulsants, NSAIDs, cotrimoxazole, thalidomide, retinoic acid |
| Exposure to organic solvents, herbicides, pesticides, ionizing radiation |

NSAIDs nonsteroidal anti-inflammatory drugs; PDA patent ductus arteriosus; TOF tetralogy of Fallot; VSD ventricular septal defect

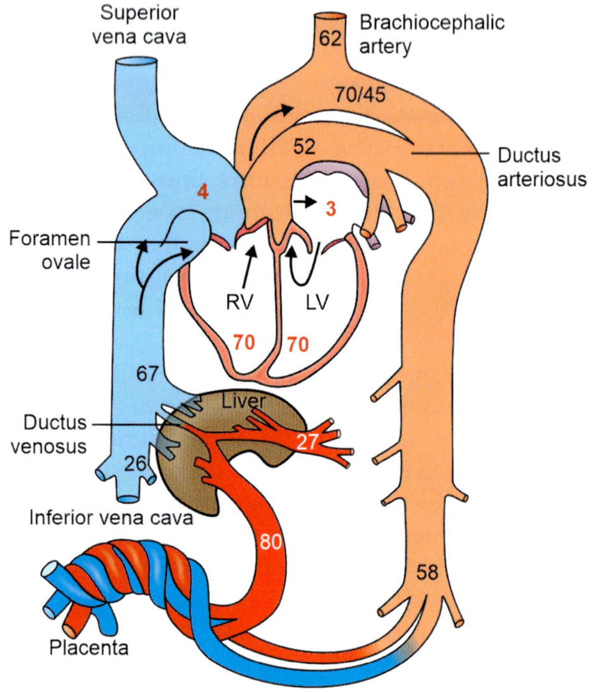


**Fig. 16.5:** Fetal circulation: Details of the circulation are provided in the text. Saturations of blood (%) in various chambers and vessels are indicated in black font and pressures (mm Hg) are indicated in red font

*take place without an substantial increase in pressure*. This particularly applies to pre-tricuspid shunts such as ASD.

*Increase in pulmonary vascular resistance means obstructive disease* in the pulmonary circuit. The total cross-sectional area of pulmonary vessels is reduced and individual arterioles develop medial hypertrophy and later intimal changes are added, to further obstruct the flow of blood through the pulmonary circulation. After a certain stage, it is an irreversible process. The increase in resistance in the pulmonary circuit is associated with reduction in flow. The increase in pressure in the pulmonary artery associated with normal resistance is called *hyperkinetic pulmonary arterial hypertension*. If the pressure is increased due to increase in pulmonary vascular resistance, it is called *obstructive pulmonary arterial hypertension*. Clinically both situations are seen and can be separated from each other at the bedside.

### *Fetal Circulation* (Fig. 16.5)

The heart assumes its normal four-chambered shape by the end of 6 weeks of intrauterine life. Thereafter, only minor changes occur and consist mainly in the growth of the heart as a whole with increasing age of the fetus. For the exchange of gases, the fetus is dependent on placental circulation, whereas the neonate is dependent on the lungs. Immediately following birth, with the first inspiration, the lungs expand with air and the gas exchange function is transferred from the placenta to the lungs. This necessitates circulatory adjustments following birth to transform the fetal circulation to the postnatal circulation.

Blood oxygenated in the placenta is returned by way of umbilical veins, which enter the fetus at the umbilicus and join the portal vein (Fig. 16.5). The ductus venosus provides a low resistance bypass between the portal vein and the inferior vena cava. Most of the umbilical venous blood shunts through the ductus venosus to the inferior vena cava. Only a small proportion mixes with the portal venous blood and passes through the liver. Blood from inferior vena cava comprising that from hepatic veins, umbilical veins and that from lower extremities and kidneys enters the right atrium. On reaching the right atrium, the bloodstream is divided into two by the inferior margin of septum secundum—the crista dividens. About one-third of the inferior vena cava blood enters the left atrium, through the foramen ovale, the rest two-thirds mixes with the venous return from the superior vena cava to enter the right ventricle.

The blood reaching the left atrium from the right atrium mixes with small amount of blood reaching the left atrium through the pulmonary veins and passes to the left ventricle. The left ventricle pumps out the blood into the ascending aorta for distribution to the coronaries, head and upper extremities. The superior vena cava stream, comprising blood returning from the head and arms, passes almost directly to the right ventricle. The right ventricle pumps

**Table 16.9:** Systolic and diastolic pressures and resistance in the pulmonary and systemic circuits

| *Chamber/vessel* | *Pressure (mm Hg)* | *Chamber/vessel* | *Pressure (mm Hg)* |
|---|---|---|---|
| Superior vena cava | 0–6 | Pulmonary vein | 6–10 |
| Right atrium | 0–6 | Left atrium | 6–10 |
| Right ventricle | 25/0–6 | Left ventricle | 80–120/5–10 |
| Pulmonary artery | 25/10 | Aorta | 80–120/60–85 |
| Resistance, dynes/sec/$cm^5$<br>Pulmonary vascular | 80–240 | Systemic vascular | 800–1600 |

out blood into the pulmonary trunk. A small amount of this blood enters the pulmonary circulation, the rest passes through the ductus arteriosus into the descending aorta to mix with the small amount of blood reaching the descending aorta from the aortic arch (derived from the left ventricle).

The main differences between the fetal and postnatal circulation are: (i) Presence of placental circulation, which provides gas exchange for the fetus; (ii) absence of gas exchange in the collapsed lungs—this results in very little flow of blood to the lungs and thus little pulmonary venous return to left atrium; (iii) presence of ductus venosus, joining the portal vein with the inferior vena cava, providing a low resistance bypass for umbilical venous blood to reach the inferior vena cava; (iv) widely open foramen ovale to enable oxygenated blood (through umbilical veins) to reach the left atrium and ventricle for distribution to the coronaries and the brain; and lastly (v) wide open ductus arteriosus to allow right ventricular blood to reach the descending aorta, since lungs are non-functioning.

### *Circulatory Adjustments at Birth—Transitional Circulation*

Circulatory adjustments continue to occur for a variable period following birth. This change is brought about because of a shift from placental dependence for gas exchange in the fetus to pulmonary gas exchange in the neonate. Loss of placental circulation and clamping of the umbilical cord, after birth, results in a sudden increase in systemic vascular resistance with the exclusion of the low resistance placental circulation. This tends to increase the aortic blood pressure and the left ventricular systolic pressure. The left ventricular diastolic pressure also tends to rise and increases the left atrial pressure. The loss of placental circulation results in a sudden reduction of flow through the ductus venosus that closes off. Flow through the ductus venosus disappears by the 7th day of postnatal life. The loss of placental flow results in a decrease in the volume of blood returning to the right atrium. The right atrial pressure decreases. The left atrial pressure becomes higher than the right atrial pressure and the septum primum, which acts as a valve of the fossa ovalis, approximates with the septum secundum to close off the foramen ovale. Functional closure of the foramen ovale occurs relatively quickly. Over a period of months to years, the septum primum and septum secundum become firmly adherent resulting in anatomical closure of the foramen ovale.

Sudden expansion of lungs with the first few breaths causes a fall in pulmonary vascular resistance and an increased flow into the pulmonary trunk and arteries. The pulmonary artery pressure falls due to lowering of pulmonary vascular resistance. The pressure relations between the aorta and pulmonary trunk are reversed so that the flow through the ductus is reversed. Instead of blood flowing from the pulmonary artery to aorta, the direction of flow through the ductus, is from the aorta to pulmonary trunk. The increased oxygen saturation following birth causes the ductus arteriosus to constrict and close. Some functional patency and flow can be demonstrated through the ductus arteriosus for a few days after birth. The ductus arteriosus closes anatomically within 10 to 21 days.

This results in the establishment of the postnatal circulation. Over the next several weeks, the pulmonary vascular resistance continues to decline with a decline in the pulmonary artery and right ventricular pressures. The adult relationship of pressures and resistances in the pulmonary and systemic circulations is established by the end of approximately 2 to 3 weeks (Fig. 16.6).

## Hemodynamic Classification of Congenital Heart Disease

CHD has been broadly classified as cyanotic and acyanotic heart disease (Table 16.10). While broad classifications work for most situations, there are patients who cannot be classified into common physiologic categories. Additionally,

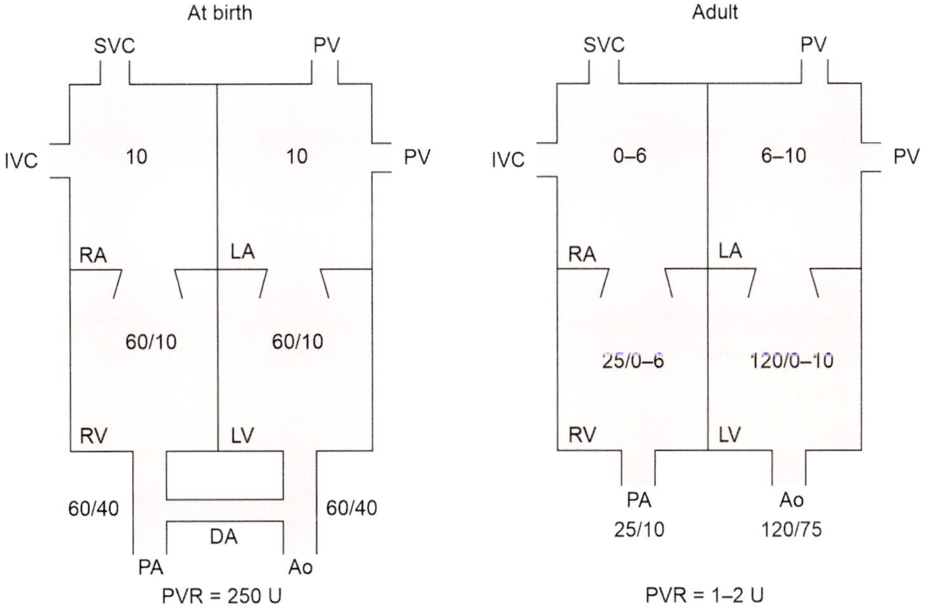


**Fig. 16.6:** Pressure and resistance in the right- and left-sided chambers and vessels at birth compared to adults. Ao aorta; DA ductus arteriosus; IVC inferior vena cava; LA left atrium; LV left ventricle; PA pulmonary artery; PV pulmonary vein; PVR peripheral vascular resistance; RA right atrium; RV right ventricle; SVC superior vena cava

**Table 16.10:** Broad physiologic categories of congenital heart disease

| **Acyanotic heart disease: Left-to-right shunts** |
|---|
| • Pretricuspid: Partial anomalous pulmonary venous drainage, atrial septal defect<br>• Ventricular: Ventricular septal defect (VSD)<br>• Great artery: Aortopulmonary window, patent ductus; ruptured sinus of Valsalva<br>• Both pre- and post-tricuspid: Atrioventricular septal defect, left ventricle to right atrial communications |
| **Acyanotic heart disease: Obstructive lesions** |
| • *Inflow:* Cor-triatriatum, obstructive lesions of the mitral valve<br>• *Right ventricle:* Infundibular stenosis, pulmonary valve stenosis, branch pulmonary artery stenosis<br>• *Left ventricle:* Subaortic membrane, valvar aortic stenosis, supravalvar aortic stenosis, coarctation of aorta |
| **Acyanotic heart disease: Miscellaneous lesions** |
| Coronary artery abnormalities, congenital mitral and tricuspid valve regurgitation |
| **Cyanotic heart disease** |
| *Reduced pulmonary blood flow*<br>• *Intact interventricular septum:* Pulmonary atresia with intact ventricular septum, critical pulmonic stenosis with right-to-left shunt at atrial level, Ebstein anomaly; isolated right ventricular hypoplasia<br>• *Unrestrictive ventricular communication:* All conditions listed under VSD with pulmonic stenosis<br>*Increased pulmonary blood flow*<br>• *Pre-tricuspid:* Total anomalous pulmonary venous communication, common atrium<br>• *Post-tricuspid:* All single ventricle physiology lesions without pulmonic stenosis, persistent truncus arteriosus, transposition of great vessels<br>*Pulmonary hypertension*<br>Pulmonary vascular obstructive disease (Eisenmenger physiology)<br>*Miscellaneous*<br>Pulmonary arteriovenous malformation, anomalous drainage of systemic veins to LA |

This classification is useful but there is overlap between cyanotic and acyanotic conditions

there are often specific issues, such as valve regurgitation, that determine the clinical manifestations. The following physiological concepts are important to understand common congenital malformations:

i. Pre-tricuspid versus post-tricuspid shunts
ii. The VSD-PS physiology
iii. Single ventricle physiology
iv. Duct dependent lesions
vi. Unfavorable streaming and parallel circulation

### *Pre-Tricuspid versus Post-Tricuspid Shunts*

Acyanotic heart disease with left-to-right shunts is traditionally classified as pre-tricuspid and post-tricuspid shunts. There are important differences in physiology that impact clinical manifestations and natural history. Left-to-right shunts at or proximal to the level of the atria are known as pre-tricuspid shunts. They include atrial septal defects (ASD) and partial anomalous pulmonary venous connection. The left-to-right shunt and the consequent excessive pulmonary blood flow is dictated by relative stiffness of the two ventricles. Since the right ventricle is relatively stiff (non-compliant) at birth and during early infancy, the shunt is small. Over the years, the pulmonary vasculature becomes capacious and right ventricle progressively enlarges to accommodate the excessive pulmonary blood flow. This explains why ASD seldom manifest with symptoms of pulmonary over-circulation during infancy and childhood. The clinical signs are also easily explained by the physiology of pre-tricuspid shunts. The diastolic flow murmur of ASD is across the much larger tricuspid valve and is, therefore, relatively subtle or even inaudible. The excessive blood in the right ventricle is ejected into the pulmonary artery resulting in an ejection systolic murmur. The second heart sound splits widely and is fixed because of the prolonged right ventricular ejection time and prolonged "hang-out" interval resulting from increased capacitance of the pulmonary circulation. Pulmonary arterial hypertension (PAH) is typically absent or, at most, mild. The presence of moderate or severe PAH in ASD is uncommon but worrisome and may suggest the onset of irreversible changes in the pulmonary vasculature.

Post-tricuspid shunts are different in that there is direct transmission of pressure from the systemic to the pulmonary circuit at the ventricular level (VSD) or great arteries (PDA and aortopulmonary window). The shunted blood passes through the lungs and finally leads to a diastolic volume overload of the left ventricle. The hemodynamic consequences are dictated by the size of the defect. For patients with large post-tricuspid shunts, symptoms begin in early infancy, typically after some regression of elevated pulmonary vascular resistance in the newborn period together with progressive development of the pulmonary vascular tree.

The excessive pulmonary blood flow returns to left atrium and flows through the mitral valve resulting in apical diastolic flow murmur that is a consistent marker of large post-tricuspid shunts. The left atrium and ventricle are dilated as a result of this extra volume. Elevated pulmonary artery pressure is an inevitable consequence of large post-tricuspid shunts, and is labeled hyperkinetic PAH. This needs to be distinguished from elevated pulmonary vascular resistance that results from long-standing exposure to increased pulmonary blood flow. Correction of large post-tricuspid shunts result in rapid and dramatic reduction in elevated pulmonary artery pressures because of cessation of increased pulmonary blood flow.

### *VSD-PS Physiology (Fallot Physiology)*

This situation is characterized by a large communication at the ventricular level together with varying degrees of obstruction to pulmonary blood flow. Typically, this is in the form of subvalvar (infundibular), valvar, annular (small annulus) and occasionally supravalvar stenosis. The free communication between the two ventricles results in equalization of pressures. Severity of PS dictates the volume of blood flowing through pulmonary arteries and, therefore, amount of oxygenated blood returning via pulmonary veins. Severe PS results in right-to-left shunt across the VSD with varying degrees of hypoxia and, consequently, cyanosis. Cyanosis is directly proportionate to the severity of PS. Because the right ventricle is readily decompressed by the large VSD, heart failure is unusual. The best example of VSD-PS physiology is tetralogy of Fallot (TOF). In its least severe form, TOF is often not associated with cyanosis (pink TOF). Here PS is significant enough to result in a large pressure gradient across the right ventricular outflow tract (RVOT), but not severe enough to result in a reduction in pulmonary blood flow. Pink TOF is typically associated with a loud ejection systolic murmur because of a reasonable volume of blood flowing across the RVOT. As the severity of PS increases, pulmonary blood flow declines and the intensity and the duration of systolic murmur declines progressively. Identical symptoms and physical findings are present in: (i) Complete transposition of great arteries with VSD and pulmonic stenosis, (ii) double outlet right ventricle with pulmonic stenosis and a large subaortic VSD, (iii) tricuspid atresia with diminished pulmonary blood flow, (iv) single ventricle with pulmonic stenosis, and (v) corrected transposition of great arteries with VSD and pulmonic stenosis.

#### *Single Ventricle Physiology*

This refers to a group of conditions where there is complete mixing of pulmonary and systemic venous returns. In addition to single ventricle (double inlet ventricle), a variety of conditions come under the category of single ventricular physiology. Atresia of one of the AV valves, severe hypoplasia of one of the ventricles, severe straddling of one of the AV valves over a large VSD are all examples of situations where there is mixing of pulmonary and systemic venous returns. The clinical manifestations are dictated by the whether or not there is PS. In absence of PS, there is excessive pulmonary flow especially in infants because of the relatively lower pulmonary vascular resistance. The proportion of oxygenated blood from pulmonary veins that mixes with the systemic venous return is high. Cyanosis is minimal and measured oxygen saturation may be in the 90s. However, the price for preserved oxygenation is heart failure initially and, eventually, permanent elevation of pulmonary vascular resistance (pulmonary vascular obstructive disease or PVOD). If the child survives infancy, pulmonary vascular resistance progressively increases with increasing cyanosis.

Single ventricle and its physiologic variants can be associated with varying degrees of PS. The features are similar to VSD-PS physiology except for relatively severe hypoxia because of free mixing of systemic and pulmonary venous return.

Palliative operations are the only option for the large number of conditions that come under the category of single ventricle physiology. Single ventricle palliation is done in stages. The final procedure is the Fontan operation that allows separation of systemic venous return from pulmonary venous return thereby, eliminating cyanosis.

#### *Duct-Dependent Lesions*

An infant or a newborn with CHD that is dependent on the patency of the ductus arteriosus for survival can be termed as having a duct-dependent lesion. These are newborns where the systemic blood supply is critically dependent on an open PDA (duct-dependent systemic circulation, DDSC) or pulmonary blood flow is duct dependent (duct-dependent pulmonary circulation, DDPC). Closure of the PDA in DDSC results in systemic hypoperfusion (often mistaken as neonatal sepsis), as in hypoplastic left heart syndrome where the entire systemic circulation is supported by the right ventricle through the PDA and interrupted aortic arch where the descending aortic flow is entirely through the PDA. Severe coarctation and critical aortic stenosis are also examples of DDSC. Closure of PDA in DDPC results in severe hypoxia and cyanosis in neonates; examples include all forms of pulmonary atresia (irrespective of underlying heart defect) where the PDA is the predominant source of pulmonary blood flow. Patients with pulmonary atresia, where pulmonary blood supply is from major aortopulmonary collaterals, may survive even after the PDA closes. Critical PS can present as duct dependent pulmonary blood flow. Newborns with severe Ebstein anomaly can also present as DDPC (physiologic pulmonary atresia) even though the pulmonary valve is anatomically normal because of inability of the right ventricle to function effectively.

Neonates with duct dependent physiology require prostaglandin $E_1$ ($PGE_1$) for survival. Early recognition of a duct-dependent situation allows early initiation of $PGE_1$ and stabilization until definitive procedure is accomplished.

#### *Unfavorable Streaming and Parallel Circulation*

Unfavorable streaming refers to a situation where oxygen-rich pulmonary blood flow is directed towards the pulmonary valve and poorly oxygenated blood towards the aortic valve. The best example of unfavorable streaming is the parallel circulation in transposition of great arteries (TGA) with intact ventricular septum. Here survival is dependent of the presence of a communication (ideally at atrial level) that allows mixing of pulmonary and systemic venous return. The presence of a VSD may improve the situation in TGA but significant cyanosis is usually present unless the pulmonary blood flow is torrential.

### Recognition and Diagnostic Approach

While it is often easy to recognize the presence of CHD in older children, manifestations of heart disease can often be subtle in newborns and young infants. Conditions that do not primarily involve the cardiovascular system can result in clinical manifestations that overlap with those resulting from CHD in the newborn. Nonetheless, careful clinical evaluation is often rewarding and allows identification of CHD in most infants and many newborns. The following clinical features should alert the pediatrician regarding the presence of CHD.

***Cyanosis:*** Parents seldom report cyanosis unless it is relatively severe (saturation <80%). It is often easier for them to notice episodic cyanosis (when the child cries or exerts).

*Difficult feeding and poor growth:* The parent of an infant with CHD may complain that the child has difficulty with feeds. This is usually a feature of an infant with congestive heart failure resulting from CHD. The history may be of slow feeding, small volumes consumed during each feed, tiring easily following feeds and requirement of periods of rest during feeds. Excessive sweating involving forehead or occiput is a common accompaniment. Not infrequently, no history of feeding difficulty may be obtained, but the child's growth rate is not appropriate for age. A recent decline in growth rate (falling off the growth curve) or weight that is inappropriate for age (<5th centile) may result from a large left-to-right shunt. Characteristically, growth retardation affects weight more than height.

*Difficult breathing:* Tachypnea (respiratory rates more than 60/min in infants <2 months; >50/min in older infants; >40/min after 1 yr) is a characteristic manifestation of heart failure in newborns. For infants, subcostal or intercostal retractions together with flaring of nostrils are frequently associated with tachypnea.

*Frequent respiratory infections:* The association of respiratory infections that are frequent, severe and difficult to treat with large left-to-right shunts is frequent but not a specific feature.

*Specific syndromes:* The presence of chromosomal anomalies or other syndromes that are associated with CHD should alert the clinician to the presence of specific cardiac defects. Trisomy 21 is the commonest anomaly associated with heart disease; others include trisomy 13 and 18, Turner and Noonan syndromes, and velocardiofacial and DiGeorge syndromes (Table 16.7).

### Nadas' Criteria

The assessment for presence of heart disease can be done using the Nadas' criteria. Presence of one major or two minor criteria is essential for indicating the presence of heart disease (Table 16.11). It is important to recognize that these criteria are of limited use in newborns, where clinical signs are subtle.

#### *Major Criteria*

*i. Systolic murmur grade III or more in intensity:* A pansystolic murmur is always abnormal no matter what is its intensity. There are only three lesions that produce a pansystolic murmur, and these are (i) VSD, (ii) mitral regurgitation and (iii) tricuspid regurgitation. An ejection systolic murmur may be due to an organic cause or it may be functional. An ejection systolic murmur associated with a thrill is an organic murmur. Grade III ejection systolic murmur of a functional type may be heard in anemia or high fever especially in small children.

A number of children around the age of 5 yr may have a soft, short ejection systolic murmur. If it is accompanied with a normal second sound then it is unlikely to be significant. Before labeling a murmur as innocent, it may be necessary to reassess after an interval. Typically, innocent murmurs are often detected during a febrile illness and often disappear with the fever. It may be necessary to obtain an ECG and an echocardiogram to rule out heart disease and allay parental anxiety.

*ii. Diastolic murmur:* The presence of a diastolic murmur almost always indicates the presence of organic heart disease.

*iii. Central cyanosis:* Central cyanosis suggests that either unoxygenated blood is entering the systemic circulation through a *right-to-left shunt* or the *blood passing through the lungs is not getting fully oxygenated*. While normally, saturations are > 98% in infants, the threshold for classifying desaturation is <95%. If the blood is not getting fully oxygenated in the lungs, it is called *pulmonary venous desaturation* and indicates severe lung disease. Cyanosis due to a right to left cardiac shunt indicates presence of heart disease. Central cyanosis is present in fingers and toes as well as in the mucous membranes of mouth and tongue. It results in *polycythemia and clubbing*.

Peripheral cyanosis does not imply the presence of heart disease. *Peripheral cyanosis is the result of increased oxygen extraction from the blood by the tissues*. It is seen in fingers and toes but not in mucous membrane of mouth and tongue. The arterial oxygen saturation is normal. Presence of central cyanosis always indicates presence of CHD, if lung disease has been excluded. However, cyanosis that is obvious clinically usually results from significant desaturation (typically <85%). Poor lighting, anemia, dark skin complexion may further mask hypoxia. Routine use of the pulse oximeter allows detection of milder forms of hypoxia. Saturations of 95% or lower while breathing room air are abnormal.

*iv. Congestive cardiac failure:* Presence of congestive cardiac failure indicates heart disease except in neonates and infants, who might show cardiac failure due to extracardiac causes, including anemia and hypoglycemia.

#### *Minor Criteria*

*i. Systolic murmur less than grade III:* It is emphasized that soft, less than grade III murmurs by themselves do not exclude heart disease.

*ii. Abnormal second sound:* Abnormalities of the second sound always indicate presence of heart disease. It has been included as a minor criterion only because auscultation is an individual and subjective finding. However, with practice, the second heart sound can become an extremely useful bedside tool to identify and classify heart disease.

*iii. Abnormal electrocardiogram:* Electrocardiogram is used to determine the mean QRS axis, right or left atrial

**Table 16.11:** Nadas' criteria for clinical diagnosis of congenital heart disease

| *Major* | *Minor* |
|---|---|
| Systolic murmur grade III or more | Systolic murmur grade I or II<br>Abnormal second sound |
| Diastolic murmur | Abnormal electrocardiogram |
| Cyanosis | Abnormal X-ray |
| Congestive cardiac failure | Abnormal blood pressure |

hypertrophy and right or left ventricular hypertrophy. Criteria for ventricular hypertrophy, based only on voltage criteria are not diagnostic of heart disease. The voltage of the QRS complexes can be affected by changes in blood viscosity, electrolyte imbalance, position of the electrode on the chest wall and thickness of the chest wall.

*iv. Abnormal X-ray:* The reason for considering abnormal X-ray as a minor criterion is twofold. In infants and smaller children, the heart size varies considerably in expiration and inspiration. If there is cardiomegaly on a good inspiratory film, it suggests presence of heart disease. The second reason is the presence of thymus in children up to the age of two years, which might mimic cardiomegaly.

*v. Abnormal blood pressure:* It is difficult to obtain accurate blood pressure in smaller children. It is important to use appropriate sized cuffs while measuring blood pressure.

### Diagnostic Implications of the Second Heart Sound

Auscultation of the heart provides important diagnostic information. Of the various heart sounds and murmurs, the most important is the assessment of the second heart sound (Fig. 16.7). The normal second heart sound can be described in three parts:

i. It has two components: Aortic closure sound (A2) and pulmonary closure sound (P2).
ii. During quiet breathing, both the components are superimposed on each other during expiration, thus only a single second sound is heard. During inspiration, the aortic component comes early whereas the pulmonary component is delayed, resulting in a split in which the A2 precedes the P2.
iii. The aortic component is louder than the pulmonary component, except in young infants.

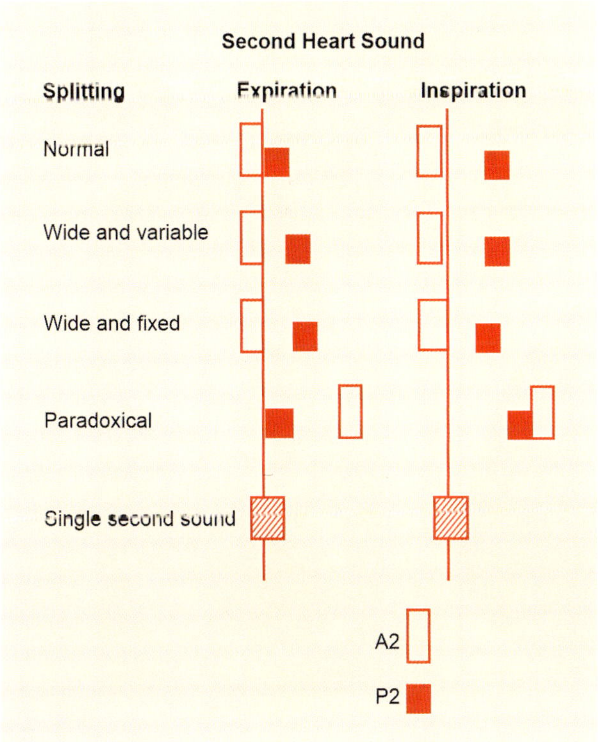


**Fig. 16.7:** Second sound (S2): The relationship of aortic (A2) and pulmonic component (P2) in inspiration and expiration. Single S2 means that it may be either A2 or P2 or a combination of both

When we say that the second sound is normal, it is in context of the above three aspects. Abnormalities of the second sound might occur in each of these aspects.

### Abnormalities of Aortic Component of the Second Sound

The A2 may be accentuated or diminished in intensity. It can also occur early or late in timing. The A2 is accentuated in systemic hypertension from any cause and in AR, and diminished or may be absent when the aortic valve is immobile because of fibrosis or calcification or if absent, as in aortic valve atresia.

The A2 is delayed when the left ventricular ejection is prolonged as in aortic valvar or subvalvar stenosis, patent ductus arteriosus with a large left-to-right shunt, AR, left bundle branch block and left ventricular failure. The A2 occurs early in VSD, mitral regurgitation and constrictive pericarditis.

### Abnormalities of Pulmonic Component of the Second Sound

The P2 may be accentuated or diminished in intensity or delayed in timing. Although it may be occurring early in tricuspid regurgitation, it is not recognized as such on the bedside since tricuspid regurgitation as an isolated lesion (without pulmonary arterial hypertension) is rare. Accentuated P2 is present in pulmonary arterial hypertension from any cause. The P2 is diminished in intensity in pulmonic stenosis. It is absent when the pulmonary valve is absent as in pulmonary valvar atresia. The P2 is delayed in pulmonic stenosis, atrial septal defect, right bundle branch block, total anomalous pulmonary venous connection and WPW syndrome with a left-sided accessory pathway.

### Abnormalities in Splitting of the Second Sound (S2)

As indicated above, the normal S2 is single (or closely split, <0.03 sec) in expiration and split in inspiration with the louder A2 preceding P2. Wide splitting of the second sound is defined as splitting during expiration due to an early A2 or late P2 or the A2–P2 interval of 0.03 sec or more during expiration. If the interval increases during inspiration, it is called wide variable splitting, but if it is the same in expiration and inspiration, it is defined as widely split and fixed second sound. Wide and variable splitting of S2 is seen in pulmonic stenosis, mitral regurgitation and VSD. In pulmonic stenosis, it is due to a delay in P2 whereas in mitral regurgitation and VSD, it is due to an early A2. Wide and fixed splitting of the S2 occurs in atrial septal defect, right bundle branch block and total anomalous pulmonary venous connection and is due to a delay in P2.

The delay in A2 results in closely split, single or paradoxically split S2. In paradoxically split S2, the split is wide in expiration but narrows during inspiration (Fig. 16.7). A single second sound means that it is either A2 or P2 or a combination. The decision, whether it is aortic or pulmonic or a combination, depends not on the location or intensity of the single second sound, but on the clinical profile. In tetralogy of Fallot, only a single S2 is heard and it is the A2 since the pulmonic component is delayed and so soft that it is inaudible. In VSD with pulmonary arterial hypertension and right-to-left shunt (Eisenmenger complex), again a single S2 is heard and represents a combination of A2 and P2. While based on auscultation alone, it may sometimes be difficult to differentiate between tetralogy of Fallot and Eisenmenger complex, the history and thoracic roentgenogram can easily distinguish between these conditions. Thus, the interpretation of single second sound is not dependent on auscultation alone.

### Imaging Studies

***Echocardiography* (Fig. 16.8):** Echocardiography has revolutionized the diagnosis of CHD and its high diagnostic yield makes this investigation cost-effective. This is particularly true for infants and newborns in whom excellent images are readily obtained. Transesophageal echocardiography can supplement transthoracic studies in selected older children.

***Cardiac magnetic resonance imaging:*** Cardiac magnetic resonance imaging is an important modality for evaluation of CHD, especially in older patients and for postoperative evaluation. Magnetic resonance imaging can also clearly define extracardiac structures such as branch pulmonary arteries, pulmonary veins and aortopulmonary collaterals. Very useful physiologic data (especially blood flow calculations at a number of locations; accurate estimates of ventricular function) is also obtained. Limitations include lack of expertise for interpretation and requirement of general anesthesia to enable breath-holding.

***Computed tomography (CT):*** CT overcomes some of the limitations of magnetic resonance imaging because it has a much lower image acquisition time. However, exposure to ionizing radiation is a major concern.

***Diagnostic cardiac catheterization:*** The role of diagnostic cardiac catheterization for patients with CHD has declined with the availability of high quality echocardiography, MRI and CT. Since cardiac catheterization is an invasive

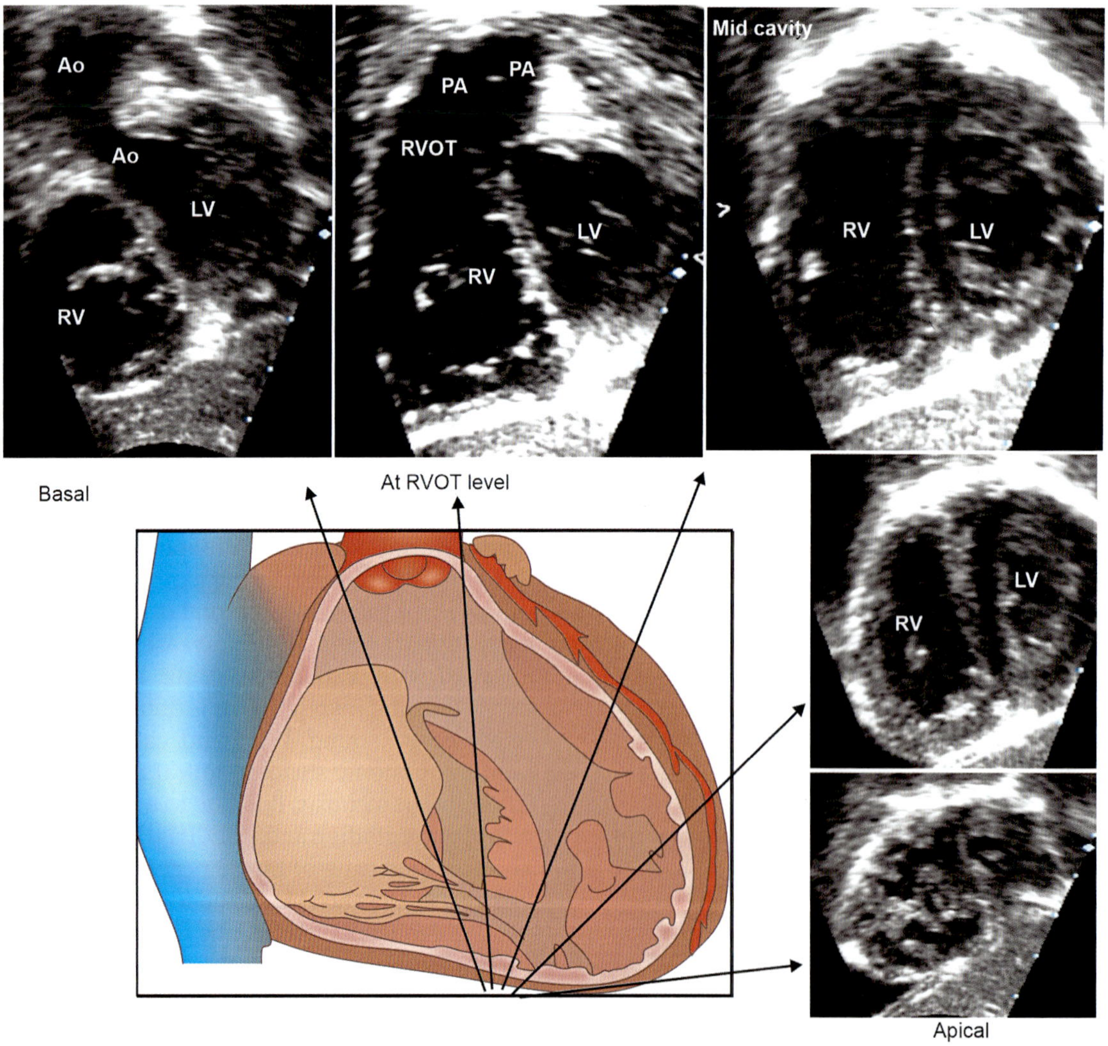


Fig. 16.8: Two-dimensional echocardiography. An illustrative example of how the ventricular septum can be sectioned at different levels to screen for ventricular septal defects. The lines with arrows represent levels at which cross-sectional images are obtained. The still frames of the respective echocardiograms are shown in relation to each of the level at which a section is obtained. Ao aorta; LV left ventricle; PA pulmonary artery; RV right ventricle; RVOT right ventricular outflow tract

procedure, its performance requires careful planning so that the information desired may be obtained with minimum risk to the patient. Diagnostic cardiac catheterization should be advised, if non-invasive investigations do not provide information that is required for surgery. Accurate estimation of filling pressures and pulmonary artery pressures, determination of blood flow and vascular resistance and definition of coronary arteries are best done through cardiac catheterization.

### Definitive and Palliative Treatment

To ensure the best possible results of management of CHD, it is necessary to assemble a team of qualified individuals who are a part of a comprehensive pediatric heart program. Definitive treatment for CHD requires the collaborative use of surgery and catheter-based interventions.

#### Surgery

Surgery is still the best option for definitive treatment or palliation of most CHD. Surgeries for CHD are broadly classified as open heart (requiring use of cardiopulmonary bypass—CPB) and closed heart (not requiring CPB). Most corrective operations and many palliative operations fall under the former category. These procedures are generally a more significant and expensive undertaking because of the use of the CPB circuit and a substantially larger number of disposable items. The morbidity of open heart operations is proportionate to the duration of exposure to CPB and the cross-clamp time (the period of time when heart beating is deliberately brought to a standstill through the use of cardioplegia).

*Corrective operations:* Corrective surgery is possible for atrial and ventricular septal defects, with no significant long-term concerns. If the repair of TOF does not result in pulmonary valve incompetence, long-term concerns are minimal. Certain operations require careful long-term follow-up because long-term concerns are substantial, especially after 10–20 years follow-up. These include the Senning operations (atrial switch) for transposition where the right ventricle continues to support the systemic circulation, TOF repair where the pulmonary valve is rendered incompetent through a transannular patch and operations that require the placement of a right ventricle to pulmonary artery conduit. Corrective surgeries associated with excellent long-term survival include the arterial switch operations, repair of total anomalous pulmonary venous connection and coarctation.

*Surgery for single ventricle physiology:* This category includes all anatomic examples of single ventricle. In addition, this includes situations when one atrioventricular valve is atretic or one of the ventricles is hypoplastic. The surgical management of single ventricle physiology is performed in stages. The first stage involves early pulmonary arterial band (usually under the age of 3 months) for patients who have increased pulmonary blood flow and the modified Blalock-Taussig shunt or stenting of the PDA for those who have reduced pulmonary blood flow with cyanosis. The second operation is the bidirectional Glen shunt. The superior vena cava is anastomosed to the right pulmonary artery. This operation allows effective palliation until the age of 4–6 years, sometimes longer. The Fontan operation is finally required for elimination of cyanosis. All the systemic venous return is routed to the pulmonary artery. Several requirements should be fulfilled before this operation can be successfully undertaken. This is a palliative procedure and there are a wide range of important long-term issues in a substantial proportion of the survivors.

#### Catheter Interventions

Catheter interventions are possible in many patients with CHD. Many simple defects such as selected secundum ASD, PDA and selected muscular and membranous VSD can now be closed in the catheterization laboratory. Additionally, balloon valvotomy is now the first line of treatment for congenital stenosis of the pulmonary and aortic valves. Additional details of catheter intervention procedures are shown in Table 16.12. Catheter-based interventions have a limited scope but are far less traumatic than surgery, accomplished with ease and allow rapid recovery.

### Complications of Congenital Heart Disease

A number of complications occur in patients with CHD.

*Pulmonary arterial hypertension (PAH):* Lesions that have the greatest likelihood of developing PAH include cyanotic heart disease with increased pulmonary blood flow. Here irreversible changes in pulmonary vasculature develops rapidly often during infancy. It is particularly important to correct or appropriately palliate these lesions early (ideally within the first few months of life). Large acyanotic post-tricuspid shunts are also prone to early development of PAH and should be ideally corrected early, preferably within the first year. In pre-tricuspid shunts, PAH develops slowly and unpredictably. While most patients with ASD will have mild or no PAH throughout their lives, a small proportion develop accelerated changes in the pulmonary vasculature. Some of the key features associated with the development of PAH include: Large size of the defect; presence of pulmonary venous hypertension; airway obstruction or syndrome association, (e.g. trisomy 21); prolonged duration of exposure to increased pulmonary blood flow; and residence at high altitude.

*Infective endocarditis or endarteritis (IE):* Endocarditis can complicate CHD, especially in patients with significant turbulence created by high-pressure gradients, e.g. restrictive VSD and PDA, tetralogy of Fallot, and left ventricular outflow tract obstruction. Some surgical operations (such as the Blalock-Taussig shunt) are also associated with increased risk of IE or endarteritis. Lesions with little or no turbulent flows, such as ASD are not associated with increased risk. The risk of endocarditis increases after dentition, hence the importance of good dental hygiene in patients with CHD cannot be overemphasized.

*Growth and nutrition:* This is affected in all forms of CHD and is particularly striking in large left-to-right shunts. Children with CHD show high prevalence of malnutrition,

**Table 16.12:** Congenital heart defects amenable to catheter-based interventions

| *Lesion* | *Procedure* | *Comments* |
|---|---|---|
| Atrial septal defect | Device closure | Amenable to device closure, if the defect is in the fossa ovalis and has sufficient margins |
| Patent ductus arteriosus (PDA) | Coil or device closure | Majority can be closed by catheter interventions, except large PDA in infants |
| Muscular ventricular septal defect (VSD) | Device closure | Device closure is an option for older infants (>8 kg) |
| Membranous VSD | Device closure | Controversial; carries a small risk of heart block |
| Pulmonary valve stenosis | Balloon pulmonary valvotomy | Treatment of choice for most forms except dysplastic valves in Noonan syndrome |
| Aortic valve stenosis | Balloon aortic valvotomy | Initial treatment of choice at all ages; however, dilated aortic valves eventually need surgery |
| Branch pulmonary artery stenosis | Balloon dilation with stenting | Stenting preferred to surgery |
| Coarctation of aorta | Balloon dilation with or without stenting | Neonates: Surgery preferred due to high risk of recurrence<br>Older infants: Balloon dilatation satisfactory<br>Children >10 years: Dilatation with stenting is curative |
| Coronary artery fistula | Coil or device closure | Treatment of choice |
| Pulmonary arteriovenous malformations | Coil or device closure | Treatment of choice when discrete; surgery preferred for diffuse malformations |
| Duct-dependent pulmonary circulation | Stenting of the PDA | Offered, in selected cases, as an alternative to Blalock-Taussig shunt |
| Pulmonary atresia with intact ventricular septum | Valve perforation followed by balloon dilation | Preferred procedure in some centers |
| Ruptured sinus of Valsalva aneurysm | Device closure | Preferred option in selected cases |
| Transposition of great arteries | Balloon atrial septostomy | For palliation before definitive surgery |

which improves after correction of the underlying condition. Catch up growth is slow, if CHD is corrected late.

*Myocardial dysfunction:* Chronic volume overload results in ventricular enlargement and ventricular dysfunction that is typically reversed after correction. A small proportion of patients with severe hypoxia also develop severe dysfunction involving both ventricles. Heart failure is mostly the result of hemodynamic consequences of increased pulmonary blood flow, mitral or tricuspid valve regurgitation and severe myocardial hypertrophy. Systolic dysfunction is a relatively less common cause.

*Neurologic and neurodevelopmental consequences:* Chronic hypoxia, *in utero* hypoxia and hypoperfusion and open-heart surgery contribute substantially to morbidity. Brain abscess is uniquely associated with cyanotic heart disease (typically beyond the age of 2 years) where the right-to-left shunt bypasses the pulmonary filter.

*Erythrocytosis:* Older children with cyanotic CHD are prone to complications from a chronically elevated red cell turnover. These include symptoms of hyperviscosity, gout, renal failure and gallstones.

*Rhythm disorders and sudden death:* Chronic enlargement of heart chambers predisposes to tachyarrhythmia. Chronic right atrial enlargement (such as atrial septal defect, Ebstein syndrome, severe tricuspid regurgitation) predisposes to atrial flutter, which might be persistent and refractory. Chronic right ventricular enlargement predisposes to ventricular tachycardia and may precipitate sudden cardiac arrest. This is a significant long-term concern after TOF repair where the pulmonary valve is rendered incompetent. Similarly left ventricular hypertrophy and dysfunction are associated with higher risk of ventricular tachycardia.

*Cyanotic spells:* Patients with the VSD-PS physiology are prone to cyanotic spells. Cyanotic spells are due to an acute decrease in pulmonary blood flow, increased right-to-left shunt and systemic desaturation due to: (i) Infundibular spasm due to increase in circulating catecholamines, during feeding or crying; (ii) activation of mechanoreceptors in right ventricle (due to decrease in systemic venous return) or in left ventricle (due to decrease in pulmonary blood flow), leads to peripheral vasodilatation and fall in systemic vascular resistance producing increased right-to-left shunt and systemic desaturation.

A cyanotic spell is an emergency, which requires prompt recognition and intervention to prevent disabling cerebrovascular insults or death. The spell needs to be taken seriously not just because of the immediate threat but also because it indicates the need for early operation. It is commonly seen below 2 years (peaks between 2 and 6 months). The onset is spontaneous and unpredictable and occurs more often in early morning, although it can occur at anytime in the day. The infant cries incessantly, is irritable and inconsolable. Tachypnea is prominent feature; there is deep and rapid breathing without significant subcostal recession. Cyanosis deepens as the spell progresses. Later

Table 16.13: Spontaneous closure of heart defects

| Variable | Likelihood of spontaneous closure |
|---|---|
| Age at evaluation | More likely in younger patients; most ASD and VSD that finally close or become very small do so by the age of 3 years; PDA either close in the first 2–4 weeks or not at all, particularly in preterm infants |
| Size of the defect | Larger defects are unlikely to close spontaneously, such as ASD >8 mm and large unrestrictive VSD |
| Location of the defect | Fossa ovalis ASD tend to close spontaneously; ostium primum and sinus venosus defects do not close; muscular VSD have high likelihood of spontaneous closure; perimembranous VSD can also close spontaneously; outlet (subpulmonic) VSD may close by prolapse of the aortic valve, resulting in aortic regurgitation; inlet VSD and malaligned VSD (as in tetralogy of Fallot) do not close spontaneously |

ASD atrial septal defect; PDA patent ductus arteriosus; VSD ventricular septal defect

gasping respiration and apnea ensues, which leads to limpness and ultimately anoxic seizures. Spells can last from minutes to hours. Auscultation reveals softening or disappearance of pulmonary ejection murmur. The management is summarized in Table 16.15.

### Natural History

Some defects have a tendency towards spontaneous closure and this can influence the timing of intervention. The defects known to close spontaneously are atrial and ventricular septal defects, and patent ductus arteriosus. The variables influencing the likelihood of spontaneous closure include: Age at evaluation (lower likelihood of closure with increasing age), size of the defect (smaller defects more likely to close) and location of the defects (fossa ovalis ASD and perimembranous and muscular VSDs can close on their own) (Table 16.13).

A review of natural history of common forms of CHD shows that without correction, many children with CHD (especially those with cyanotic CHD) will not survive beyond early childhood. The outcomes are improved by correction through surgery and, in some situations, through catheter interventions. Despite curative surgery, some patients have important long-term sequelae. For example, patients with tetralogy of Fallot who have undergone "corrective" repair might show progressive right ventricular dilation with increased risk of late heart failure and sudden cardiac death. There are long-term concerns after the arterial switch operation (aortic root dilation, silent coronary occlusion), AV canal repair (AV valve regurgitation) and coarctation (residual hypertension, aortic aneurysm). Operations that involve placement of conduits (pulmonary atresia, Rastelli operations) require replacement upon growth of the child. Conditions associated with near normal long-term survival include small left-to-right shunts and bicuspid aortic valves. Survival is also satisfactory for many patients with atrial septal defect, coarctation of aorta, pink TOF, mild Ebstein anomaly and some forms of corrected transposition of great arteries.

### Prevention of CHD

Education of lay public on the risks associated with consanguinity, drugs and teratogens in the first trimester of pregnancy and widespread immunization against rubella has limited role in preventing CHD. Folate supplementation during periconceptional period can also reduce CHD risk to a small extent. However, most CHD do not have an identifiable etiology and there is no effective strategy for their prevention in the periconceptional period.

Fetal echocardiography is emerging as a modality for early diagnosis of CHD. Conditions that involve major chamber discrepancy (such as hypoplastic left heart syndrome), single ventricles and common AV canal can be identified by routine four-chamber view screening as early as 14–16 weeks gestation. With some refinement, additional conditions such as tetralogy of Fallot, large VSD, transposition of great vessels and persistent truncus arteriosus can be detected. Once a serious CHD is identified, it is vital to counsel the families about postnatal manifestations, natural history, surgical options and their long-term outlook. Before 20 weeks of gestation, medical termination of pregnancy is an option. Detection of serious defects through fetal echocardiography enables delivery at a center with comprehensive pediatric heart program. While echocardiography is recommended for future pregnancies after diagnosis of serious CHD in a child, this practice has low yield because only 2–8% CHD recur. The highest chance of recurrence is with obstructive lesions of the left heart.

*Competencies:* **PE23.1; PE23.14; PE23.15**

## ACYANOTIC CONGENITAL HEART DEFECTS

### Atrial Septal Defect

Atrial septal defect (ASD) accounts for as an isolated anomaly 5–10% of all CHD. Based on anatomy, ASD is classified as follows (Fig. 16.9).

*Fossa ovalis ASD:* They are located in the central portion of atrial septum, in the position of foramen ovale. Some of these defects are amenable to closure in the catheterization laboratory.

*Sinus venosus ASD:* These are located at junction of superior vena cava and right atrium. These defects do not have a superior margin because the superior vena cava straddles the defect. These defects are associated with anomalous drainage of one or more right pulmonary veins.

*Ostium primum ASD:* These defects are created by failure of septum primum, and are in lower part of the atrial septum; inferior margin of ASD is formed by the atrioventricular valve.

*Coronary sinus ASD:* An unroofed coronary sinus is a rare communication between the coronary sinus and the left atrium, which produces features similar to other types of ASD.

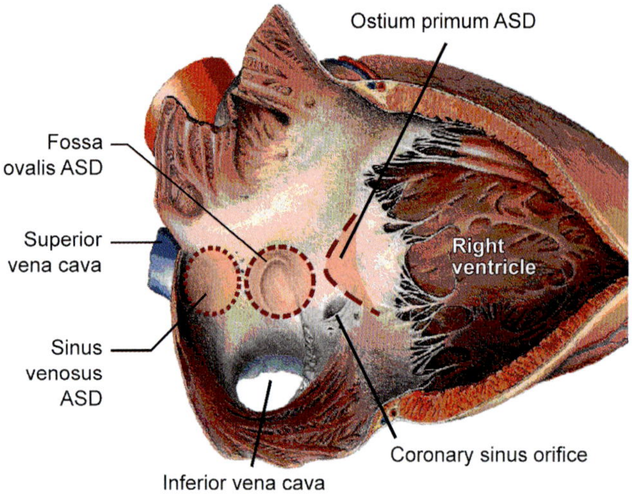


**Fig. 16.9:** Right-sided cardiac chambers showing the three commonest types of atrial septal defects (ASD)

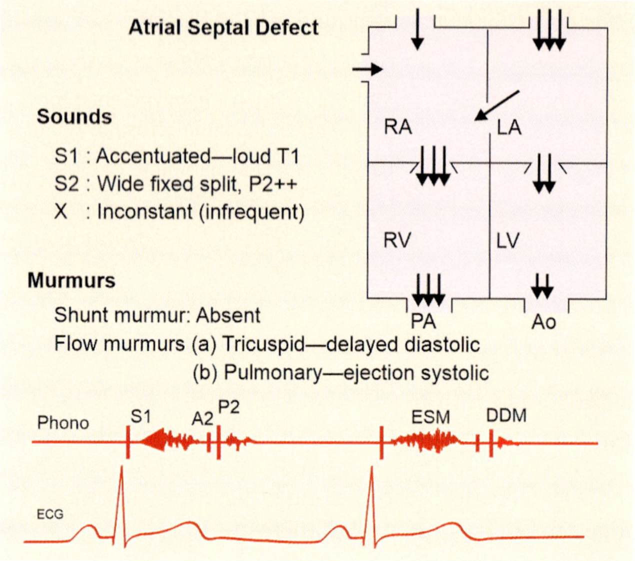


**Fig. 16.10:** Summary of auscultatory findings in the atrial septal defect. Ao aorta; A2 aortic component of the second sound; ESM ejection systolic murmur; LA left atrium; LV left ventricle; PA pulmonary artery; P2 pulmonic component of the second sound; RA right atrium; RV right ventricle; S1 first sound; S2 second sound; X click

### *Physiology and Findings*

The physiology of ASD is that of a pre-tricuspid shunt. The enlarged right ventricle results in a parasternal impulse. The ejection systolic murmur originates from the pulmonary valve because of the increased blood flow. An increased flow through the tricuspid valve may result in a soft delayed diastolic rumble at the lower left sternal border. The overload of the right ventricle due to an increase in venous return prolongs the time required for its emptying resulting in delayed P2. This delay also results from the prolonged 'hang-out' interval because of very low resistance in the pulmonary circulation. Additionally, since the two atria being linked via the large ASD, inspiration does not produce any net pressure change between them and respiration related fluctuations in systemic venous return to the right side of the heart are abolished; thereby the fixed S2 (Fig. 16.10).

The *electrocardiogram* of ostium secundum ASD is characterized by right axis deviation and right ventricular hypertrophy. The characteristic configuration of the lead V1 is rSR' seen in almost 90% patients (Fig. 16.11). Presence of left axis deviation beyond –30° suggests ostium primum ASD (Fig. 16.12). The chest X-ray (Fig. 16.13) shows mild to moderate cardiomegaly, right atrial and right ventricular enlargement, prominent main pulmonary artery segment, a relatively small aortic shadow and plethoric lung fields. The left atrium does not enlarge in size in atrial septal defect, unless associated with other anomalies like mitral regurgitation. Echocardiogram shows increased size of the right ventricle with paradoxical ventricular septal motion. 2D echo in subcostal view often best identifies the defect. The echocardiogram allows decision regarding suitability of catheter closure, based on measurements of the defect and the adequacy of margins (Fig. 16.14).

### *Assessment of the Severity*

The size of the left-to-right shunt is directly proportional to the intensity of the murmurs and heart size. The larger the shunt, the more the cardiomegaly and the louder the pulmonary and tricuspid murmurs.

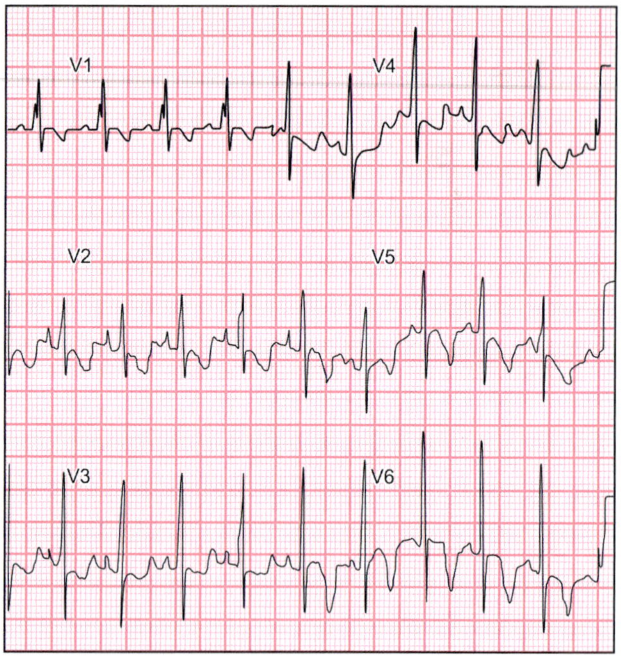


**Fig. 16.11:** Electrocardiogram of atrial septal defect of the secundum type showing rSR' pattern in lead V1

### *Natural History and Complications*

Heart failure is exceptional in infancy. A small proportion of patients might develop pulmonary hypertension, by the second or third decade. Closure of ASD is recommended during childhood (ideally between 3 and 5 years) to prevent complications of atrial arrhythmias and heart failure in late adulthood.

### *Treatment*

Most fossa ovalis defects with good margins can be closed percutaneously in the catheterization laboratory

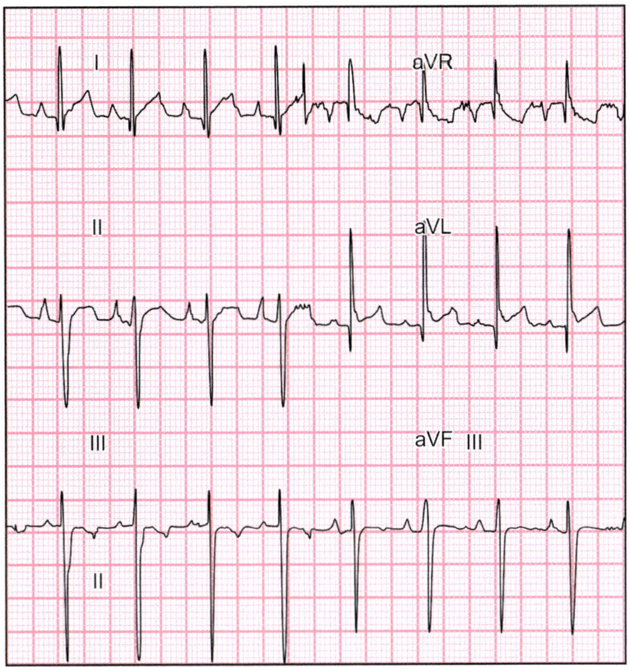


**Fig. 16.12:** Electrocardiogram of atrial septal defect of the primum type associated with endocardial cushion defect. The mean QRS axis is–60°

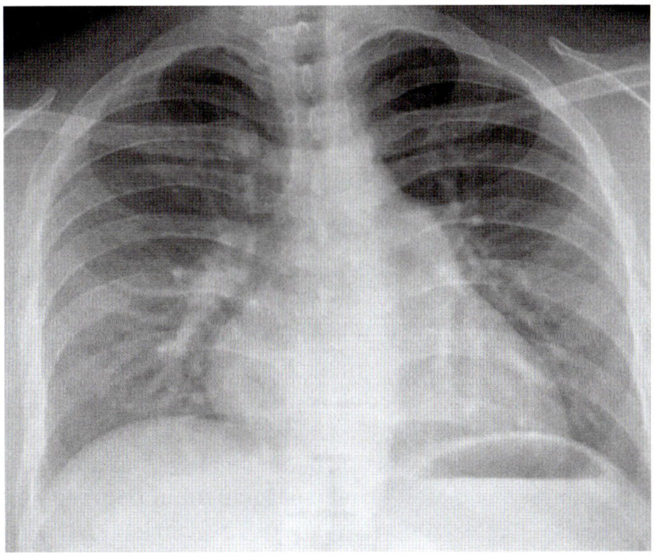

**Fig. 16.13:** This is a chest X-ray of an 18-year-old with a large atrial septal defect. Note the dilated right atrium, prominent main pulmonary artery and increased pulmonary blood flow

with occlusive devices. Others require surgical closure. Closure is recommended before school entry to prevent late complications. Small defects (<8 mm) can be observed. Spontaneous closure is well recognized in small defects that are diagnosed in infancy or early childhood.

### Ventricular Septal Defect (VSD)

This is the most common congenital cardiac lesion identified at birth accounting for one-quarter of all CHD. VSD is a communication between the two ventricles; 90% are located in the membranous part of the ventricular septum with variable extension into the adjacent muscular septum.

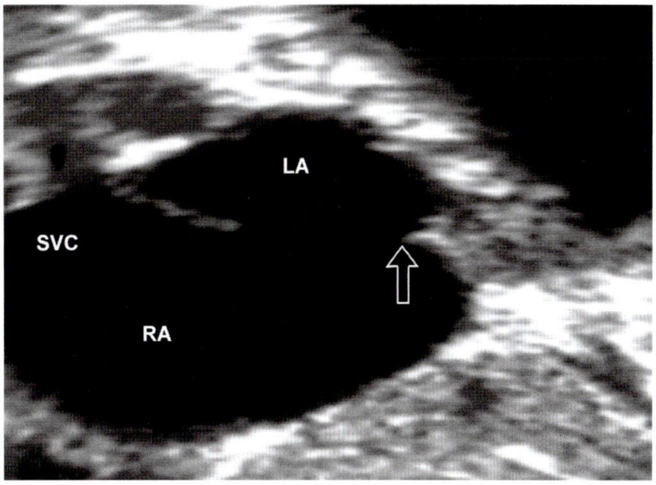


**Fig. 16.14:** Echocardiogram of atrial septal defect. Subxiphoid short axis view of the atrial septum shows deficient posterior inferior rim (arrow). LA left atrium; RA right atrium; SVC superior vena cava

Others are located in the muscular, inlet or outlet septum and can be multiple (Fig. 16.15).

#### *Hemodynamics*

VSD results in shunting of oxygenated blood from the left to the right ventricle. The left ventricle starts contracting before the right ventricle. The flow of blood from the left ventricle to the right ventricle starts early in systole. When the defect is restrictive, a high pressure gradient is maintained between the two ventricles throughout the systole. The murmur, starts early, masking the first sound and continues throughout the systole with almost the same intensity appearing as a pansystolic murmur on auscultation and palpable as a thrill. Toward the end of systole, the declining left ventricular pressure becomes lower than the aortic pressure. This results in closure of the aortic valve and occurrence of A2. At this time, however, the left ventricular pressure is still higher than the right

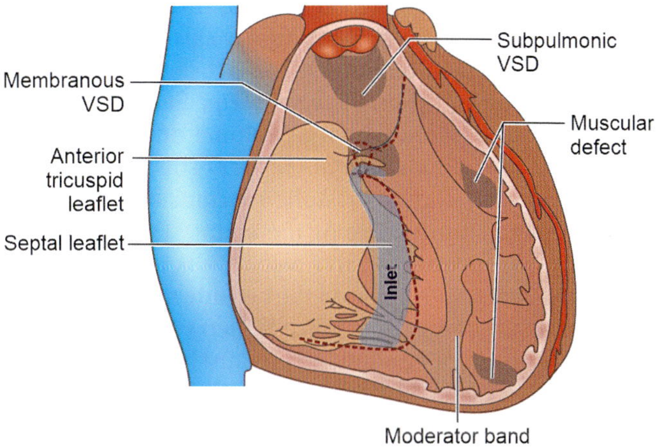


**Fig. 16.15:** Common locations of ventricular septal defects (VSD). Membranous septum is the commonest location. Subpulmonic VSD, located in the outlet septum, have a high risk of aortic valve prolapse. Muscular VSD can occur anywhere in the muscular part of septum (diagrammatic)

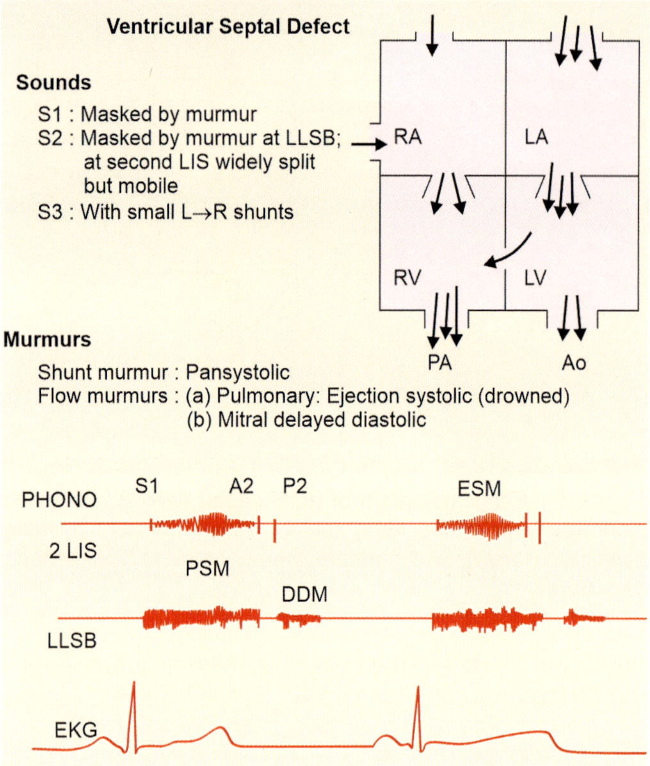


**Fig. 16.16:** Summary of auscultatory findings in ventricular septal defect. 2 LIS second left interspace; LLSB lower left sternal border; PSM pansystolic murmur; DDM delayed diastolic murmur; ESM ejection systolic murmur

ventricular pressure and the left-to-right shunt continues. The pansystolic murmur, therefore, ends beyond A2 completely masking it (Fig. 16.16).

The left-to-right ventricular shunt occurs during systole at a time when the right ventricle is also contracting and its volume is decreasing. The left-to-right shunt, therefore, streams to the pulmonary artery more or less directly. This flow of blood across the normal pulmonary valve results in an ejection systolic murmur at the pulmonary valve. On the bedside, however, the ejection systolic murmur cannot be separated from the pansystolic murmur.

The large volume of blood passing through the lungs is recognized in the chest X-ray as *pulmonary plethora*. The increased volume of blood finally reaches the left atrium and may result in *left atrial enlargement*. Passing through a normal mitral valve the large volume of blood results in a *delayed diastolic murmur at the apex*. The intensity and duration of the delayed diastolic murmur at the apex is directly related to the size of the shunt. The large flow across the normal mitral valve also results in accentuated first sound, not appreciable on the bedside as it is drowned by the pansystolic murmur. Since the left ventricle has two outlets, the aortic valve allowing forward flow and the VSD resulting in a backward leak, it empties relatively early. This results in an early A2. Since the ejection into the right ventricle and pulmonary artery is increased because of the left-to-right shunt, the P2 is delayed. Therefore, the second sound is widely split but varies with respiration in patients with VSD and a large left-to-right shunt. There is also an increase in the intensity of the P2.

### *Clinical Features*

Patients with VSD can become symptomatic around 6 to 10 weeks of age with congestive cardiac failure. Premature babies with a VSD can become symptomatic even earlier. Palpitation, dyspnea on exertion and frequent chest infection are the main symptoms in older children. The precordium is hyperkinetic with a systolic thrill at the left sternal border. The heart size is moderately enlarged with a left ventricular type of apex. The first and the second sounds are masked by a pansystolic murmur at the left sternal border. The second sound can, however, be made out at the second left interspace or higher. It is widely split and variable with accentuated P2. A third sound may be audible at the apex. A loud pansystolic murmur is present at the left sternal border. The maximum intensity of the murmur may be in the third, fourth or the fifth left interspace. It is well heard at the second left interspace but not conducted beyond the apex. A delayed diastolic murmur, starting with the third sound, is audible at the apex (Fig. 16.18).

The electrocardiogram in VSD is variable. Initially all patients with VSD have right ventricular hypertrophy. Because of the delay in the fall of pulmonary vascular resistance due to the presence of VSD, the regression of pulmonary arterial hypertension is delayed and right ventricular hypertrophy regresses more slowly. In small- or medium-sized VSD, the electrocardiogram becomes normal. In patients with VSD and a large left-to-right shunt, without pulmonary arterial hypertension, the electrocardiogram shows left ventricular hypertrophy by the time they are six months to a year old. There are, however, no ST and T changes suggestive of left ventricular strain pattern. Patients of VSD who have either pulmonic stenosis or pulmonary arterial hypertension may show right as well as left ventricular hypertrophy or pure right ventricular hypertrophy. The mean QRS axis in the frontal plane generally lies between +30° and +90°.

The cardiac silhouette on chest X-ray is left ventricular type with the heart size determined by the size of the left-to-right shunt (Fig. 16.17). The pulmonary vasculature is increased; aorta appears normal or smaller than normal in size. There may be left atrial enlargement in patients with large left-to-right shunts. Patients of VSD can have a normal sized heart because the ventricular defect is small or because of the associated pulmonic stenosis or pulmonary arterial hypertension. Echocardiogram shows increased left atrial and ventricular size. Echocardiography can identify the number, site and size of defect almost all cases (Fig. 16.18), presence or absence of pulmonic stenosis or pulmonary hypertension and associated defects.

### *Assessment of Severity*

If the VSD is small, the left-to-right shunt murmur continues to be pansystolic but since the shunt is small, the second sound is normally split and the intensity of P2 is normal. There is also absence of the delayed diastolic mitral murmur. If the VSD is very small, it acts as a stenotic area resulting in an ejection systolic murmur. This is a relatively common cause of systolic murmurs in young infants that disappear because of the spontaneous closure.

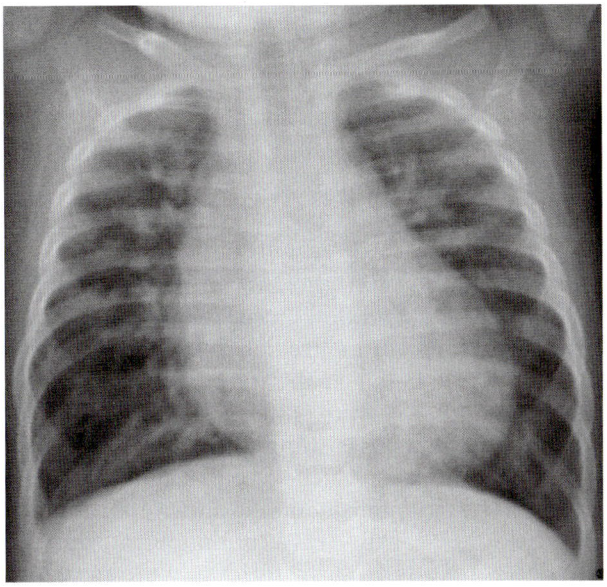

Fig. 16.17: Chest X-ray in ventricular septal defect. Note the cardiac enlargement mainly involving the left ventricle together with increased lung vasculature as suggested by the size and increased number of end-on vessels in the lung fields

If the VSD is large, it results in transmission of left ventricular systolic pressure to the right ventricle. The right ventricular pressure increases and the difference in the systolic pressure between the two ventricles decreases. The systolic left-to-right shunt murmur becomes shorter and softer and on the bedside appears as an ejection systolic murmur.

Patients of VSD may have either hyperkinetic or obstructive pulmonary arterial hypertension. The P2 is accentuated in both. In the former, there is large left-to-right shunt whereas the latter is associated with a small left-to-right shunt. In hyperkinetic pulmonary arterial hypertension, the cardiac impulse is hyperkinetic with a pansystolic murmur and thrill, widely split and variable S2 with accentuated P2 and a mitral delayed diastolic murmur. Obstructive pulmonary arterial hypertension is associated with a forcible parasternal impulse, the thrill is absent or faint, the systolic murmur is ejection type, the S2 is spilt in inspiration (closely split) with accentuated P2 and there is no mitral murmur.

Thus, on the basis of the assessment of physical findings, it is possible to separate very small, small, medium sized and large VSD. It is also possible to decide whether there is associated pulmonic stenosis or pulmonary arterial hypertension of the hyperkinetic or obstructive variety.

Echocardiography allows further refinement of clinical evaluation. Left atrial and left ventricular enlargement is consistent with a large shunt. The size of the defect can be measured; Doppler echo estimates the gradient between the left and right ventricles, thus helping in the assessment of right ventricular and pulmonary artery pressure. Flow direction across the defect is indicative of the pulmonary vascular resistance. A predominantly left to right flow is often indicative of operable status.

### *Course and Complications*

Patients with VSD have a very variable course. They may develop congestive cardiac failure in infancy which is potentially life-threatening. It has been estimated that almost 70% of all ventricular defects become smaller in size. A smaller proportion will disappear entirely. In almost 90% of patients who have spontaneous closure of the defect, it occurs by the age of three years, though it may occur as late as 25 years or more. Muscular VSD have the highest likelihood of spontaneous closure. Perimembranous VSD close with the help of the septal leaflet of the tricuspid valve and subpulmonic VSDs often become smaller as the aortic valve prolapses through it. However, this is not a desirable consequence and is often an indication for surgical closure.

Patients born with an uncomplicated VSD may develop *pulmonic stenosis* due to hypertrophy of the right ventricular infundibulum, develop *pulmonary arterial hypertension* or rarely develop aortic regurgitation due to prolapse of the

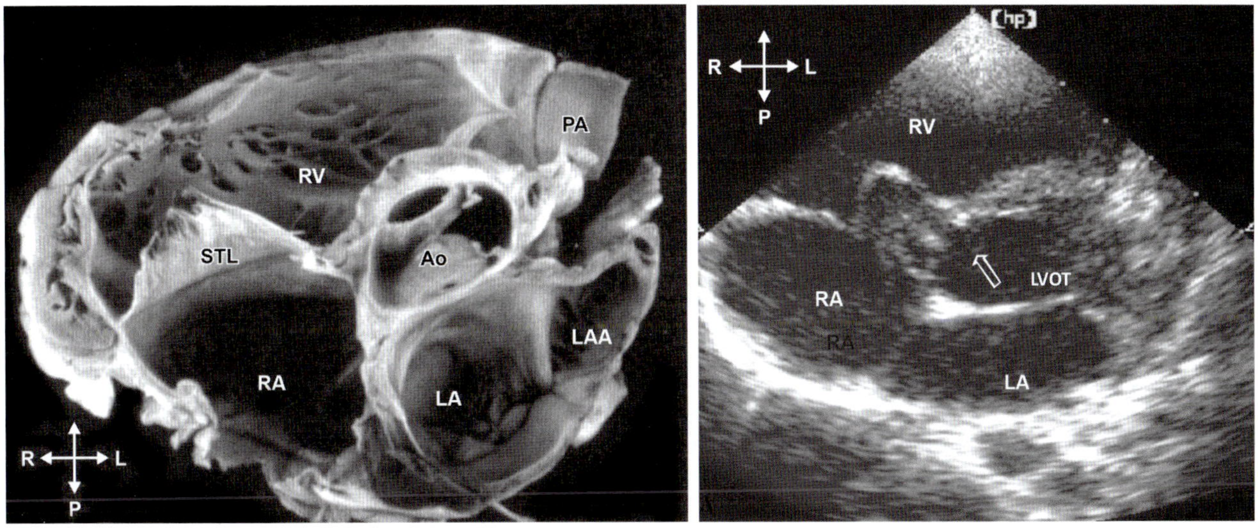


Fig. 16.18: Echocardiogram (right frame) with anatomic correlates (left) in membranous ventricular septal defects. This view is a parasternal short axis view. Arrow points to the VSD that is partly closed by aneurysm of septal leaflet of the tricuspid valve. Ao aortic root; LA left atrium; LVOT left ventricular outflow tract; RA right atrium, RV right ventricle; LAA left atrial appendage; STL septal tricuspid leaflet; PA pulmonary artery

right coronary or the non-coronary cusp of the aortic valve. Development of pulmonary arterial hypertension as a result of elevated pulmonary vascular resistance is a dreaded complication as the patient may then become inoperable.

A patient with a relatively small VSD often lives a life time without any symptoms or difficulty. Lastly, the VSD is the *commonest congenital lesion complicated by infective endocarditis*. The incidence of infective endocarditis has been estimated as 2/100–200 patients in a follow-up of 10 years, that is 1/500–1000 patient years. The incidence of infective endocarditis is small enough that it is not an indication for operation in small defects. However, it is important to emphasize good oral-dental hygiene in all patients with VSD.

#### Treatment

*Medical management* consists in control of congestive cardiac failure, treatment of repeated chest infections and prevention and treatment of anemia and infective endocarditis. The patients should be followed carefully to assess the development of pulmonic stenosis, pulmonary arterial hypertension or aortic regurgitation.

*Surgical treatment* is indicated if: (i) Congestive cardiac failure occurs in infancy; (ii) the left-to-right shunt is large (pulmonary flow more than twice the systemic flow); and (iii) if there is associated pulmonic stenosis, pulmonary arterial hypertension or aortic regurgitation. Surgical treatment is not indicated in patients with a small VSD (with the exception of subpulmonic defects with aortic valve prolapse) and in those patients who have developed severe pulmonary arterial hypertension and significant right-to-left shunt.

*Operative treatment* consists of closure of VSD with the use of a patch. The operation is performed through the right atrium. The operation can be done as early as a few months after birth, if congestive failure cannot be controlled with medical management. With evidence of pulmonary hypertension, the operation should be performed as early as possible. Modern centers prefer to close VSD surgically in young infants. It is unwise to make the sick infants to wait for a certain weight threshold because most infants with large VSD do not gain weight satisfactorily. Episodes of respiratory infections require hospitalization and are particularly difficult to manage. For sick infants with pneumonia who require mechanical ventilation, surgery is considered after initial control of the infection. Major complications of surgery are: (i) Complete heart block, (ii) tricuspid regurgitation, and (iii) residual VSD. These complications are rare and risk of surgery in uncomplicated defects is less than 1% in most centers.

Catheter closure of VSD is best suited for muscular defects in relatively older children (>8–10 kg). Perimembranous defects can also be closed in the catheterization laboratory. However, the risk of complete heart block as well as injury to the adjacent aortic valve with the membranous VSD closure is real and can occur late after implantation. Catheter closure of membranous VSD should be reserved for carefully selected older patients (>8 kg) with moderate shunts.

### Patent Ductus Arteriosus

Patent ductus arteriosus (PDA) is a communication between the pulmonary artery and the aorta. The aortic attachment of the ductus arteriosus is just distal to the left subclavian artery. The ductus arteriosus closes functionally and anatomically soon after birth; its persistence is called PDA.

#### Hemodynamics and Clinical Features

PDA results in a left-to-right shunt from the aorta to the pulmonary artery. The flow occurs both during systole and diastole as a pressure gradient is present throughout the cardiac cycle between the two great arteries, if the pulmonary artery pressure is normal. The flow of blood results in a murmur that starts in systole, after the first sound, and reaches a peak at the second sound. The murmur then diminishes in intensity and is audible during only a part of the diastole. Thus, it is a continuous murmur.

The PDA results in a systolic as well as diastolic overloading of the pulmonary artery. The increased flow after passing through the lungs reaches the left atrium. To accommodate the flow, the left atrium enlarges in size. The increased volume of blood reaching the left atrium enters the left ventricle in diastole, across a normal mitral valve. The passage of this increased flow across the mitral valve results in an accentuated first sound as well as mid-diastolic murmur from flow across the mitral valve. The large volume of blood in the left ventricle causes a prolongation of the left ventricular systole and an increase in the size of the left ventricle to accommodate the extra volume. The prolonged left ventricular systole results in delayed closure of the aortic valve and a late A2. With large left-to-right shunts, the S2 may be paradoxically split.

The large left ventricular volume ejected into the aorta results in dilatation of the ascending aorta. A dilated ascending aorta results in an aortic ejection click, and precedes the start of the continuous murmur. The large volume of blood from the left ventricle passing through a normal aortic valve results in an aortic ejection systolic murmur, however, it is drowned by the loud continuous murmur and is usually not made out as a separate murmur.

Patients with PDA may become symptomatic in early life and develop congestive cardiac failure around 6–10 weeks of age. Older children give history of effort intolerance, palpitation and frequent chest infections. The flow from the aorta to the pulmonary artery is a leak from the systemic flow. This results in a wide pulse pressure and many of the signs of wide pulse pressure are present in patients who have a PDA. On the bedside, presence of prominent carotid pulsations in a patient with features of a left-to-right shunt suggests the presence of PDA. The cardiac impulse is hyperkinetic with a left ventricular type of apex. A systolic or a continuous thrill may be palpable at the second left interspace. The first sound is accentuated and the second narrowly or paradoxically split with large left-to-right shunts. With small shunts, the second sound is normally split. The P2 is louder than normal. It is difficult to evaluate the S2 in patients with PDA, since the maximum intensity of the continuous murmur occurs at S2. The continuous murmur indicates presence of both a systolic as well as a diastolic difference in pressure between the aorta and pulmonary artery, thus excluding significant pulmonary arterial hypertension. The murmur starts after the first sound and reaches the peak at the second sound. The murmur then diminishes in intensity and is audible only during a part of the diastole. The peak at the second sound differentiates the PDA murmur from other causes of a continuous murmur. Additionally, the systolic portion of the murmur is very grating and rough. It appears to be broken into multiple systolic sounds—the multiple clicks. The murmur is best heard at the second left interspace and is also well heard below the left clavicle where it maintains its continuous character. There is a third sound at the apex, followed by a delayed diastolic murmur in large shunts (Fig. 16.19).

The electrocardiogram shows normal axis with left ventricular dominance or hypertrophy. Deep Q waves in left chest leads with tall T waves are characteristic of volume overloading of left ventricle. The roentgenogram (Fig. 16.20) exhibits cardiac enlargement with a left ventricular silhouette; cardiac size depends on the size of the left-to-right shunt. There may be left atrial enlargement. The ascending aorta and the aortic knuckle are prominent; pulmonary vasculature is plethoric. 2D echocardiogram confirms the diagnosis and measures size of PDA and identify its hemodynamic consequences. It is possible to obtain a semiquantitative assessment of shunt size and assess pulmonary artery pressure (Fig. 16.21).

### *Assessment of Severity*

The evaluation of the size of the left-to-right shunt depends on a number of features: (i) The larger the heart size the larger the left-to-right shunt; (ii) absence of the third sound

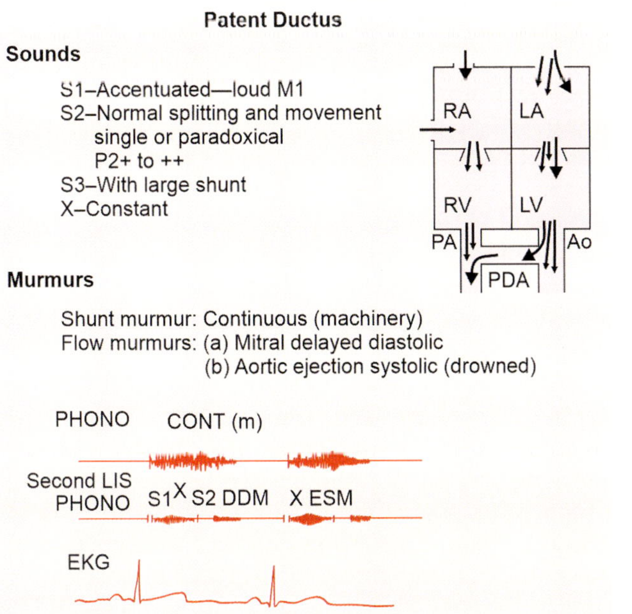


**Fig. 16.19:** Summary of auscultatory findings in patent ductus arteriosus (PDA). CONT continuous; DDM delayed diastolic murmur; ESM ejection systolic murmur; M1 mitral component of first sound

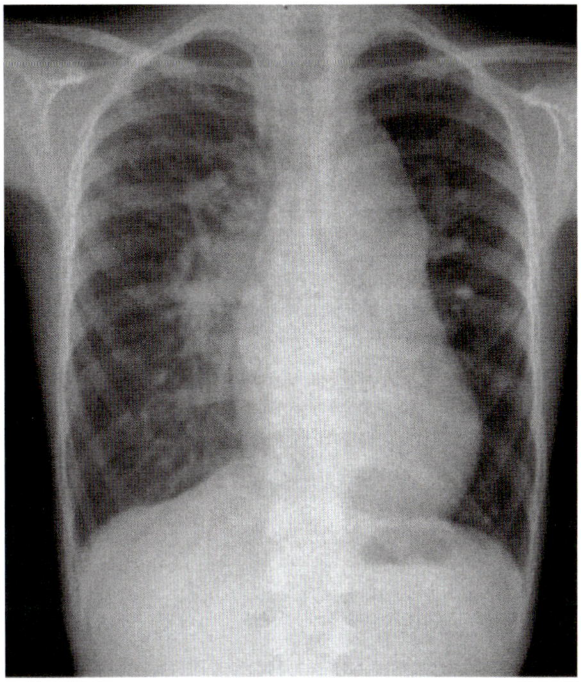

**Fig. 16.20:** Chest X-ray in an adolescent with a large patent ductus arteriosus. Note the enlargement of the aorta with a prominent aortic knuckle, large main pulmonary artery-left pulmonary artery and increased vasculature. There is no X-ray evidence of cardiac enlargement

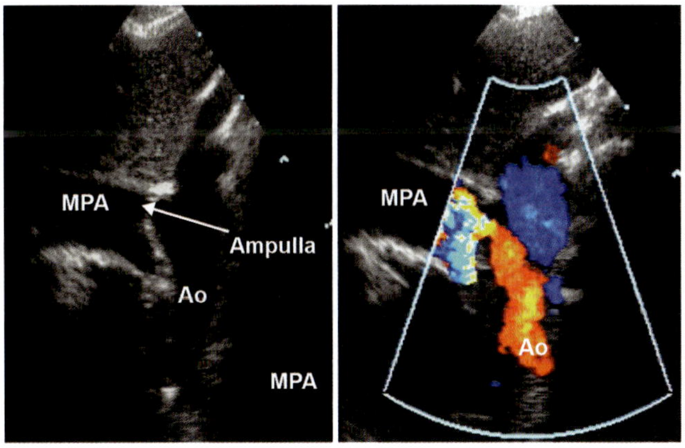


**Fig. 16.21:** Echocardiography in patent ductus arteriosus (PDA). The frame on the left is a cross-sectional two-dimensional view of the PDA and the frame on the right is a color flow image. The red flow represents flow reversal in the descending thoracic aorta as a result of a left-to-right shunt across the PDA. Ao aorta; MPA main pulmonary artery

and delayed apical diastolic murmur indicates a small left-to-right shunt. Presence of the third sound indicates a moderate left-to-right shunt whereas an audible delayed diastolic murmur suggests a large left-to-right shunt; (iii) the wider the pulse pressure the larger the shunt.

### *Course and Complications*

Neonates and infants have pulmonary hypertension at birth. The regression of pulmonary hypertension occurs slowly in the presence of PDA. The PDA murmur, therefore, is an ejection systolic murmur to start with (like in VSD) and assumes the continuous character only some weeks or months later. Congestive cardiac failure may occur within the first 6 weeks of life; cardiac failure can be controlled medically in uncomplicated patients. Patients with PDA develop pulmonary arterial hypertension earlier than VSD.

PDA may be associated with hyperkinetic or obstructive pulmonary arterial hypertension as in VSD. In both situations, the murmur tends to lose the diastolic component and the P2 is accentuated. The hyperkinetic pulmonary hypertension is associated with a large heart and mitral delayed diastolic murmur whereas the obstructive variety is accompanied with a normal heart size and absence of the mitral diastolic murmur. With severe pulmonary arterial hypertension and a right-to-left shunt through a PDA, the normal splitting of S2 is maintained but the murmur disappears and the patients develop differential cyanosis.

### Differential Diagnosis

The differential diagnosis of PDA includes conditions capable of giving a continuous murmur over the precordium. In addition, combination of a pansystolic murmur of a VSD with an early diastolic murmur of AR, which are partly superimposed on each other, may simulate a continuous murmur over the precordium. Differential diagnosis of a continuous murmur includes: (i) Coronary arteriovenous fistula; (ii) ruptured sinus of Valsalva fistulae into the right side, (iii) aortopulmonary window; (iv) systemic arteriovenous fistula over the chest; (v) aortopulmonary collateral murmurs; (vi) pulmonary arteriovenous fistula; (vii) peripheral pulmonic stenosis; (viii) venous hum including that associated with total anomalous pulmonary venous connection; and (ix) small atrial septal defect associated with mitral stenosis (Lutembacher syndrome).

### Treatment

A large PDA is better tolerated by term newborns when compared to premature newborns. Premature newborns with hemodynamically significant PDA that results in heart failure, respiratory distress or necrotizing enterocolitis require prompt management. Indomethacin, ibuprofen or paracetamol are likely to be effective before the age of 2 weeks in preterm newborns and is unlikely to be useful in term babies. Hepatic or renal insufficiency and bleeding tendency merit caution with indomethacin or ibuprofen. Newborns not responding to these agents require surgical ligation or in very selected instances, catheter closure. The PDA in term infants may close spontaneously as late as one month after birth and it is worth waiting, if the duct is large unless the heart failure is refractory.

Large PDA may result in congestive cardiac failure in infancy. Echocardiography allows ready confirmation of the diagnosis and estimation of hemodynamic severity of the PDA. Catheter-based treatment (occlusive devices or coils) is now realistic in most patients with PDA (Fig. 16.22). They are technically challenging in small infants especially those <5 kg and should be performed in centers with experience. Indications for surgery for PDA include small infants with large ducts, and ducts that are larger than the size of available devices.

Patients who have a PDA with pulmonary arterial hypertension are considered inoperable, if a right-to-left shunt has appeared because of pulmonary arterial hypertension. Since the right-to-left shunt through the PDA flows down the descending aorta, cyanosis is present in toes but not in fingers. This is called differential cyanosis and is characteristic of PDA with pulmonary arterial hypertension and right-to-left shunt.

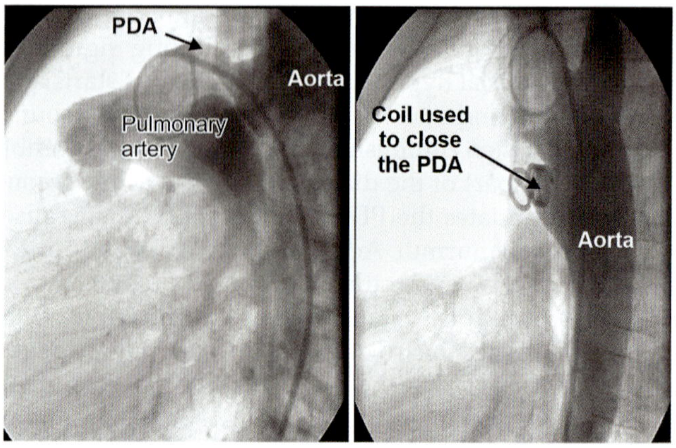


Fig. 16.22: Angiograms (aortogram) obtained before and after coil occlusion of a moderately large patent ductus arteriosus (PDA) showing complete occlusion

*Competencies:* **PE23.2; PE23.14; PE23.15**

## CYANOTIC HEART DISEASE

### Tetralogy of Fallot

Among cyanotic CHD, tetralogy of Fallot (TOF) has a relatively favorable natural history that allows survival beyond infancy in about 75% of cases. As a result, it is the most common cyanotic CHD encountered beyond the age of 1-yr constituting almost 75% of all blue patients. The physiology is that of VSD with pulmonic stenosis, as described above. Anatomically, it is characterized by the classic tetrad: Severe right ventricle outflow obstruction, large VSD, aorta that overrides the VSD and right ventricular hypertrophy. Multiple anatomical variations of TOF exist, which have a bearing on treatment (Table 16.14).

#### Hemodynamics

Physiologically, the pulmonic stenosis causes concentric right ventricular hypertrophy without cardiac enlargement and an increase in right ventricular pressure (Fig. 16.23). When the right ventricular pressure is as high as the left ventricular or the aortic pressure, a right-to-left shunt appears to decompress the right ventricle. Once the right and left ventricular pressures have become identical, increasing severity of pulmonic stenosis reduces the flow of blood into the pulmonary artery and increases the right-to-left shunt. As the systolic pressures between the two ventricles are identical, there is little or no left-to-right shunt and the VSD is silent. The right-to-left shunt is also silent since it occurs at insignificant difference in pressure between the right ventricle and the aorta. The flow from the right ventricle into the pulmonary artery occurs across the pulmonic stenosis producing an ejection systolic murmur. The more severe the pulmonic stenosis, the less the flow

**Table 16.14:** Anatomic variations in tetralogy of Fallot

| *Structure* | *Common variation* | *Implications* |
|---|---|---|
| Right ventricular outflow tract | Degree of stenosis at various levels: infundibulum, valve, pulmonary annulus, main pulmonary artery stenosis | Severe stenosis manifests early; annular narrowing requires correction with transannular patch with significant late sequelae; predominant valvar stenosis may allow palliation with balloon valvotomy in selected cases |
| Branch pulmonary arteries (PA) | Stenosis of left pulmonary artery (LPA), absence of either branch PA, hypoplastic | Small branch PA may not allow surgical correction at early age; absent branch PA require placement of PA conduit |
| Pulmonary valve | Absent pulmonary valve with aneurysmal branch PA | Severe airway compression; manifestations chiefly respiratory |
| Ventricular septal defect (VSD) | VSD extended to inlet or outlet septum; restrictive VSD with severe right ventricular hypertrophy; additional muscular VSD | Surgical approach needs to be tailored |
| Coronary arteries | Origin of left anterior descending artery | Abnormal vessel comes in way of corrective surgery |
| Atrial communication | Atrial septal defects, patent foramen ovale | Patent foramen ovale often helpful in early post-operative period; enables recovery |
| Aortopulmonary collaterals | Large major aortopulmonary collaterals | Collaterals need to be defined and closed, if their supply overlaps with the native pulmonary artery supply |

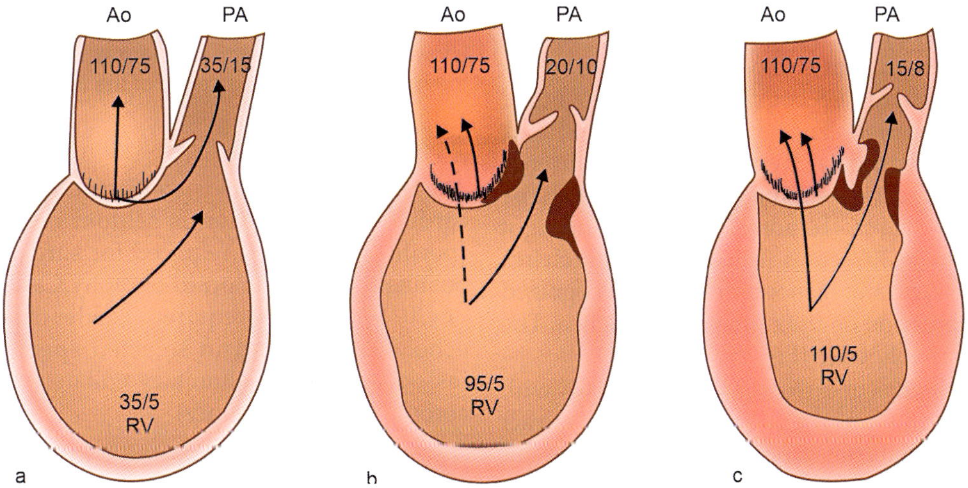


**Fig. 16.23:** Diagrammatic portrayal: (a) Ventricular septal defect; (b) Ventricular septal defect with moderate pulmonic stenosis; and (c) Fallot's tetralogy. (a) In the absence of pulmonic stenosis, the right ventricular (RV) and the pulmonary artery (PA) pressures are normal or slightly elevated. Since the left ventricular (LV) pressure is higher, there is a systolic flow of blood from the LV into the PA through the RV. (b) If a VSD is associated with moderate pulmonic stenosis, the RV systolic pressure increases and there is RV hypertrophy. The left-to-right shunt decreases and the VSD murmur becomes softer. The pulmonic stenosis murmur, however, is loud. (c). In Fallot's tetralogy, the RV and LV pressures are identical. There is no left-to-right shunt and as such the VSD is silent. The flow from RV to PA decreases, decreasing the intensity of pulmonic stenosis murmur. A right-to-left shunt occurs from RV to aorta (Ao) at identical pressures. As such the right-to-left shunt is silent

into the pulmonary artery and the bigger the right-to-left shunt. Thus the severity of cyanosis is directly proportional to the severity of pulmonic stenosis, but the intensity of the systolic murmur is inversely related to the severity of pulmonic stenosis. The VSD of TOF is always large enough to allow free exit to the right-to-left shunt. Since the right ventricle is effectively decompressed by the VSD, congestive failure seldom occurs in TOF. The exceptions to this rule are: (i) Anemia; (ii) infective endocarditis; (iii) systemic hypertension; (iv) right ventricular dysfunction from long-standing severe hypoxia; and (v) aortic or tricuspid valve regurgitation.

The right ventricular outflow obstruction results in a delay in the P2 (Fig. 16.24). Since the pulmonary artery pressure is reduced, the P2 is also reduced in intensity. The late and soft P2 is generally inaudible in TOF. The S2 is, therefore, single and the audible sound is A2. Since the aorta is somewhat anteriorly displaced, the audible single A2 is quite loud. The ascending aorta in TOF is large and may result in an aortic ejection click. On auscultation, the diastolic interval is completely clear in TOF as there is no third or fourth sound or a diastolic murmur.

Concentric right ventricular hypertrophy reduces the distensibility of the right ventricle during diastole. The right atrial contraction at the end of diastole causes a relatively large 'a' waves. Although the 'a' waves are prominent in the jugular venous pulse, they are not too tall unless right ventricular dysfunction is present.

### Clinical Features

Patients with TOF may become symptomatic any time after birth. Neonates as well as infants may develop anoxic spells (paroxysmal attacks of dyspnea). Cyanosis may be present from birth or make its appearance some years after birth. The commonest symptoms are dyspnea on exertion and exercise intolerance. The patients assume a sitting posture—squatting—as soon as they get dyspneic. Although squatting is not specific for TOF, it is the commonest congenital lesion in which squatting is noted. Anoxic spells occur predominantly after waking up or following exertion. The child starts crying, becomes dyspneic, bluer than before and may lose consciousness. Convulsions may occur. The frequency varies from once in a few days to numerous attacks everyday.

Physical examination discloses cyanosis, clubbing, slightly prominent 'a' waves in the jugular venous pulse, normal sized heart with a mild parasternal impulse, normal first sound, single second sound and an ejection systolic murmur which ends before the audible single second sound **(Fig. 16.24)**. The electrocardiogram in TOF shows right axis deviation with right ventricular hypertrophy. The 'T' waves are usually inverted in right precordial leads; *P pulmonale* may be present, but is uncommon. V1 may show pure 'R' but transition to R/S complex occurs at V2. The chest X-ray shows a normal sized heart with upturned apex suggestive of right ventricular hypertrophy. The absence of main pulmonary artery segment gives it the shape described as *Coeur en Sabot*. The aorta is enlarged and right aortic arch is present in 30% cases. The right aortic arch in a posteroanterior thoracic roentgenogram is easily recognized by its concave impression on the right side of trachea. The pulmonary fields are oligemic **(Fig. 16.25)**.

The murmur shortens and the cyanosis increases with increasing severity of the right ventricular outflow tract obstruction. Paroxysmal attacks of dyspnea can be present with mild as well as severe TOF. However, effort intolerance is directly related to the severity.

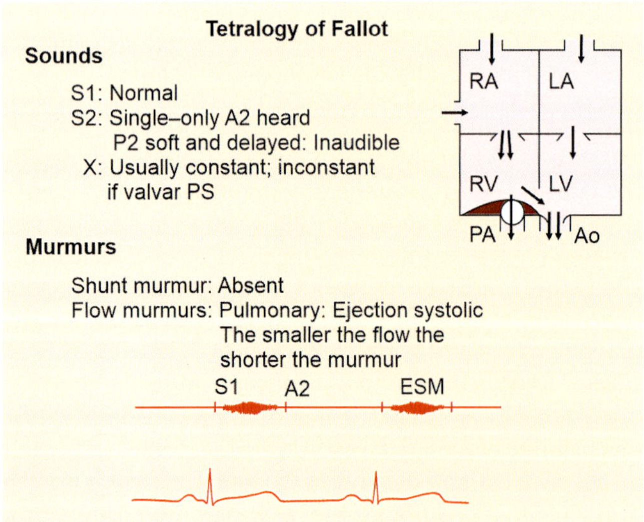


**Fig. 16.24:** Summary of auscultatory findings in tetralogy of Fallot. X systolic click; PS pulmonic stenosis

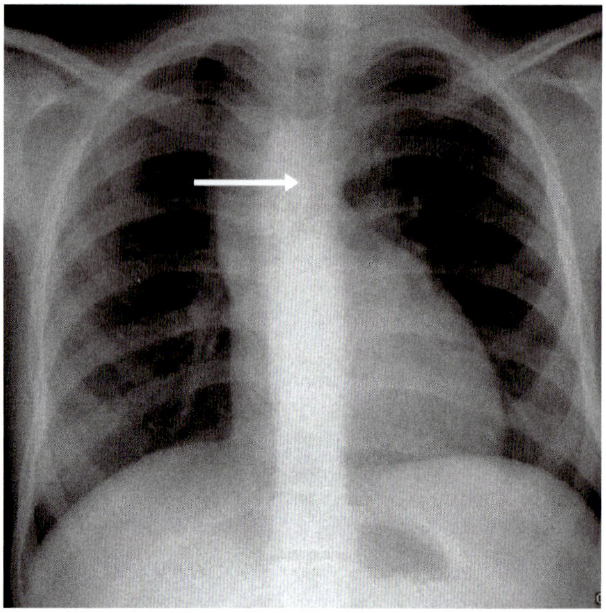

**Fig. 16.25:** Chest X-ray in tetralogy of Fallot with right aortic arch. The key findings are reduced lung vasculature as suggested by the dark lung fields, normal heart size, concavity in the region of the main pulmonary artery (pulmonary bay). This X-ray also shows a right aortic arch. The arrow indicates the indentation of the right arch on the right side of the trachea

### Diagnosis

The diagnosis of TOF is confirmed by echocardiography; cardiac catheterization is seldom necessary. Additional specific information required for surgical decision is also obtained through echocardiography. Cardiac catheterization or CT/MRI may be required in older children with limited echo windows and in selected specific circumstances (associated aortopulmonary collaterals, uncertainties in coronary artery anatomy)

### Course and Complications

Patients with TOF are subject to many difficulties. The pulmonic stenosis becomes progressively severe with age. The dyspnea and increasing exercise intolerance limit patient activities. Each attack of anoxic spell is potentially fatal. Anemia, by decreasing the oxygen carrying capacity of blood, reduces the exercise tolerance still further. Patients are prone to infective endocarditis.

***Neurological complications occur frequently:*** Anoxic infarction in the central nervous system may occur during an anoxic spell and result in hemiplegia. Anemia increases the propensity towards strokes by reducing red blood cell deformability. *Paradoxical embolism* to central nervous system and venous thrombosis due to sluggish circulation from polycythemia can also result in *hemiplegia*. *Brain abscess* is not an infrequent complication. It should be suspected in any cyanotic patient presenting with irritability, headache, convulsions, vomiting with or without fever and neurological deficit.

### Treatment

The medical management of TOF is limited to prevention and management of complications and correction of anemia.

Oral beta-blockers help prevent cyanotic spells. Maximally tolerated doses of propranolol ranging from 0.5–1.5 mg/kg/dose should be administered. Iron supplementation is recommended for all infants and young children with TOF. The management of anoxic spells is indicated in Table 16.15.

Definitive surgery for TOF involves closure of the VSD and relief of the RVOT obstruction. Most surgeons today seek to avoid the transannular patch. This "valve sparing" correction of TOF is often easier in infants. If the pulmonary valve annulus is very small, placement of a transannular patch across the pulmonary valve and the resultant severe pulmonary regurgitation is unavoidable.

Although definitive operation is feasible in young infants, some centers opt for palliative options initially. This is typically done through the Blalock-Taussig shunt, which consists of subclavian artery-pulmonary artery anastomosis using a Goretex graft. Alternatives include balloon dilation of the pulmonary valve or stenting of the patent arterial duct (if present). In a few selected instances, it may be possible to stent the RVOT as an initial palliation. A number of long-term concerns have emerged in survivors of TOF repair 2–3 decades after the operation. These include heart failure and risk of ventricular tachyarrhythmias as a result of right ventricular dilation that results from chronic pulmonary regurgitation, as well as the scar on the right ventricle, if ventriculotomy has been done during operation.

**Table 16.15:** Management of hypercyanotic spells

**Immediate steps**
- Check airway; deliver oxygen by face mask or nasal cannula
- Knee chest position
- Sedate with morphine (0.2 mg/kg SC or ketamine 3–5 mg/kg/dose IM)
- Sodium bicarbonate at 1–2 mL/kg (diluted 1:1 or in 10 mL/kg N/5 in 5% dextrose)
- Correct hypovolemia (10 mL/kg of dextrose normal saline)
- Transfuse packed red cell, if anemic (hemoglobin <12 g/dL)
- Metoprolol at 0.1 mg/kg IV slowly over 5 min; repeat every 5 min; for maximum 3 doses; may be followed by infusion at 1–2 μg/kg/min
- Monitor saturation, heart rates and blood pressure; keep heart rate below 100/minute

**Persistent desaturation and no significant improvement**
- Consider vasopressor infusion: Methoxamine 0.1–0.2 mg/kg/dose IV or 0.1–0.4 mg/kg/dose IM, or phenylephrine 5 μg/kg as IV bolus and 1–4 μg/kg/min as infusion
- If spells persist: Paralyze the patient, electively intubate and ventilate; plan for palliative or corrective surgery
- Seizures are managed with diazepam at 0.2 mg/kg IV or midazolam at 0.1–0.2 mg/kg/dose IV

**Following a spell**
- Conduct a careful neurological examination; CNS imaging, if focal deficits are present
- Initiate therapy with beta-blocker at the maximally tolerated dose (propranolol 0.5–1.5 mg/kg q 6–8 hr); helps improve resting saturation and decreases frequency of spells
- Ensure detailed echocardiography for disease morphology
- Plan early corrective or palliative surgery
- Administer iron in therapeutic (if anemic) or prophylactic dose

**Prevention**
- Counsel parents regarding the possibility of recurrence of spells and precipitating factors (dehydration, fever, pain)
- Encourage early surgical repair

### Tricuspid Atresia

Congenital absence of the tricuspid valve is called tricuspid atresia (Fig. 16.26). The right ventricle is hypoplastic. The inflow portion is absent. The hemodynamics is described above; *see* Single Ventricle Physiology.

#### *Clinical Features*

Clinical presentation depends on the state of pulmonary flow that may be diminished or increased. Clinically, patients who have diminished pulmonary blood flow constitute 90% and symptoms and physical signs are more or less identical to TOF. Features suggesting tricuspid atresia are: (i) Left ventricular type of apical impulse; (ii) prominent large 'a' waves in jugular venous pulse; (iii) enlarged liver with presystolic pulsations (a waves); and (iv) the electrocardiogram which is characterized by left axis deviation and left ventricular hypertrophy. The mean QRS axis is around –45°. Patients with tricuspid atresia and increased pulmonary blood flow cannot be diagnosed accurately clinically.

#### *Course*

Patients with tricuspid atresia follow a course similar to TOF. They are cyanosed at birth. Anoxic spells and squatting may be present; patients are relatively sicker than TOF.

#### *Treatment*

Tricuspid atresia is categorized as 'single ventricle physiology' and management is on similar lines.

### Ebstein Anomaly

An unusual and rare cyanotic congenital heart disease with diminished pulmonary blood flow results from an abnormality of the tricuspid valve. The posterior as well as the septal leaflet of the tricuspid valve is displaced downwards to a variable extent. The result is an attachment to the posterior wall of the right ventricle. In addition, the leaflets are malformed and fused resulting in obstruction to flow of blood into the right ventricle. The portion of the right ventricle above the leaflet attachment thins out and is called atrialized right ventricle. There is a particularly high prevalence of accessory pathways on the right side that result in a high likelihood of re-entrant supraventricular tachycardia.

#### *Hemodynamics*

The tricuspid valve anomaly results in obstruction to forward flow of blood as well as regurgitation of blood from the right ventricle into the right atrium. In addition, there is a large part of the right ventricle that is atrialized as a result of downward displacement of the tricuspid valve attachment. This atrialized right ventricle contracts with the rest of the ventricle and does not allow effective forward flow into the pulmonary circulation. The right atrium

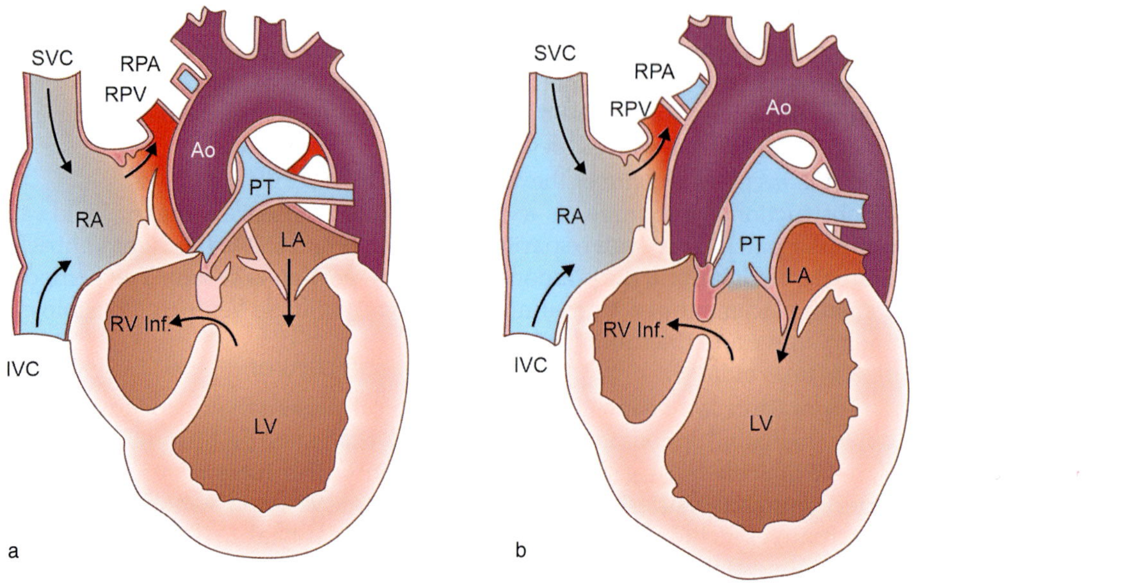


**Fig. 16.26:** Tricuspid atresia: (a) Normally related great arteries. Systemic venous blood reaching the RA through the superior (SVC) and inferior vena cava (IVC) reaches the LA through an atrial defect (or patent foramen ovale). There is complete mixing of the systemic and pulmonary venous blood in the LA. The LV is large. Aorta (Ao) arises from the LV. A muscular ventricular septal defect is the only route through which blood can reach the hypoplastic right ventricle (RV Inf.). The pulmonary trunk (PT) arises from the right ventricle. RPV and LPV right and left pulmonary veins; (b) Transposed great arteries with tricuspid atresia. The PT is arising from the LV whereas the Ao is arising from RV. LA left atrium; RA right atrium; RPA and LPA right and left pulmonary artery; RV Inf right ventricular infundibulum; RV and LV right and left ventricle; SVC and IVC superior and inferior vena cava

progressively dilates, to accommodate the extra volume. The foramen ovale may be patent or there is an atrial septal defect allowing a right-to-left shunt to occur. This results in cyanosis. The greater the tricuspid valve displacement, the more the cyanosis.

### *Clinical Features and Diagnosis*

Patients present with history of cyanosis, effort intolerance and fatigue. They may also give history suggestive of paroxysmal attacks of tachycardia. Cyanosis varies from slight to severe; clubbing is often present. The jugular venous pulse may show a dominant 'V' wave but there is usually no venous engorgement because of a capacious right atrium. The precordium is quiet. The first sound is split, however, the tricuspid component often cannot be made out, resulting in a single, normally audible first sound. The abnormal tricuspid valve may produce a midsystolic click. The second sound is widely split, but variable with a soft pulmonic component. A right ventricular third sound and/or a right atrial fourth sound may be audible. Thus, triple or quadruple sounds are usually heard. The systolic murmur may be a mid-systolic ejection murmur or a loud pansystolic murmur. There is also a short tricuspid delayed diastolic murmur. The combination of sounds clicks and murmurs result in a characteristic auscultatory cadence.

The electrocardiogram is characteristic in that it shows prominent 'P' waves and right bundle branch block. Characteristically the 'R' wave in V1 does not exceed 7 mm. Wolff-Parkinson-White type of conduction abnormality may be seen in the electrocardiogram (Fig. 16.27). The X-ray shows cardiac enlargement due to right atrial and right ventricular enlargement. The main pulmonary artery segment may be prominent and the aortic knuckle small (Fig. 16.28). The pulmonary vasculature is diminished. The echocardiogram is diagnostic as it outlines the displaced tricuspid valve and its physiological consequences (Fig. 16.29).

### *Treatment*

Surgical treatment consists of obliterating the atrialized portion of the right ventricle and repairing the tricuspid valve. The "cone repair" of tricuspid valve is increasingly popular for Ebstein anomaly. It involves extensive mobilization of the displaced tricuspid annulus and repositioning the valve at the level of the normal annulus. The age for surgical correction is unclear but there is an increasing emphasis on early repair even in the absence of symptoms to enable RV remodeling after surgery.

Tachyarrhythmias are common and require anti-arrhythmic medication followed by radiofrequency ablation.

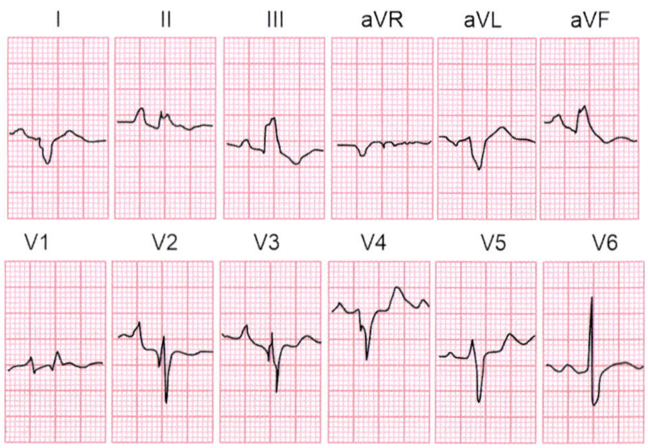


**Fig. 16.27:** Electrocardiogram typical of Ebstein anomaly. Right bundle branch block with 'R' of less than 7 mm is present

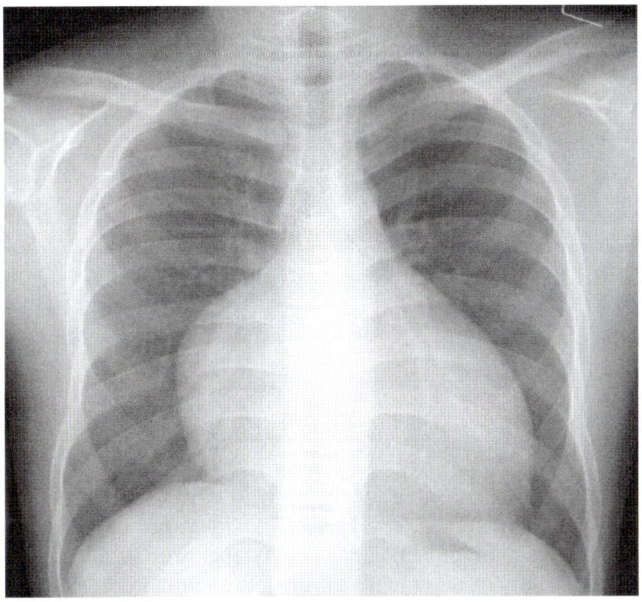

Fig. 16.28: Chest X-ray in Ebstein anomaly. There is considerable enlargement of the right atrium. The lung vascularity is reduced

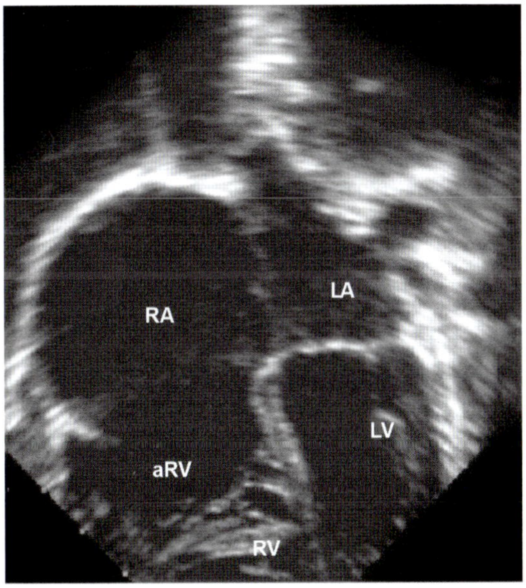


Fig. 16.29: Apical four-chamber view from a patient with Ebstein anomaly. Note the downward displacement of the septal leaflet of the tricuspid valve (arrow). aRV atrialized right ventricle; LA left atrium; LV left ventricle; RA right atrium; RV right ventricle

## Transposition of Great Vessels

In transposition of great vessels (TGA), the aorta arises from the right ventricle and pulmonary artery from the left ventricle. The aorta generally lies anterior and to the right of the pulmonary artery. For this reason, this is also referred to as D-TGA. Since the systemic and pulmonary circulations are separate, survival depends on the presence of atrial, ventricular or aortopulmonary communications.

TGA is classified into: (a) With intact ventricular septum, and (b) with VSD. The latter group is further subdivided into cases with and without pulmonic stenosis. Patients with TGA, VSD and pulmonic stenosis in some ways present like tetralogy physiology except that they have more intense cyanosis.

In patients with TGA, oxygenated pulmonary venous blood recirculates in the lungs whereas systemic venous blood recirculates in the systemic circulation. The pulmonary artery saturation is thus always higher than the aortic saturation. Survival depends on the mixing between the two circulations. In patients with intact ventricular septum, the best mixing site is the atrial communication. Generally, the atrial communication is the patent foramen ovale and this being small, the mixing is very poor (Fig. 16.30). Neonates become symptomatic due to severe hypoxemia soon after birth.

Presence of a VSD of adequate size improves mixing. As the fetal pulmonary vasculature regresses, the pulmonary blood flow increases and results in congestive failure around 4–10 weeks of age. The failing left ventricle as well as the markedly increased pulmonary blood flow increases the left atrial pressure with resultant pulmonary venous hypertension. Those who survive the heart failure often develop pulmonary vascular obstructive disease (Eisenmenger physiology) relatively early in life.

### Clinical Features

Patients of complete TGA with intact ventricular septum are cyanotic at birth. Since the interatrial communication results in poor mixing, the neonates present with rapid breathing and congestive failure secondary to hypoxemia within the first few days of life. Physical examination shows severe cyanosis, congestive failure, normal first sound, single second sound and an insignificant grade one to two ejection systolic murmur. The electrocardiogram shows right axis deviation and right ventricular hypertrophy. The thoracic roentgenogram shows cardiomegaly with a narrow base and plethoric lung fields. The cardiac silhouette can have an "egg on side" appearance: The thymic shadow is often absent (Fig. 16.31).

Patients of TGA with VSD have increased pulmonary blood flow; mixing at the ventricular level determines the severity of cyanosis. They develop congestive failure around 4–10 weeks of age. Physical findings consist of

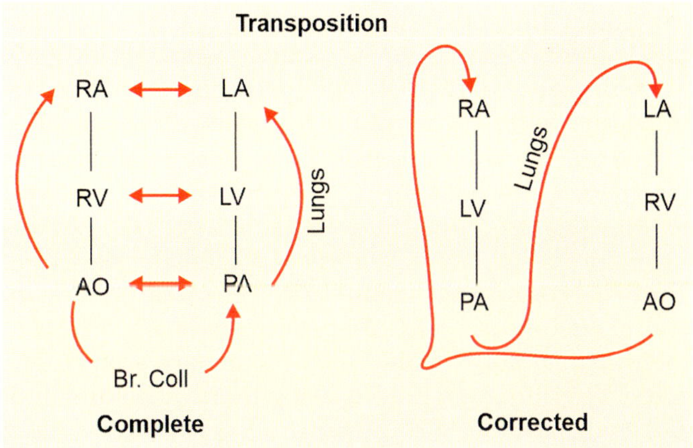


Fig. 16.30: The route of blood flow in complete TGA results in two separate circulations and survival depends on mixing. The mixing can occur at the atrial, ventricular or great vessel level. Bronchial collaterals (Br. Coll.) also increase pulmonary blood flow: In corrected TGA, the route of blood flow is normal. Hemodynamics depend on associated anomalies

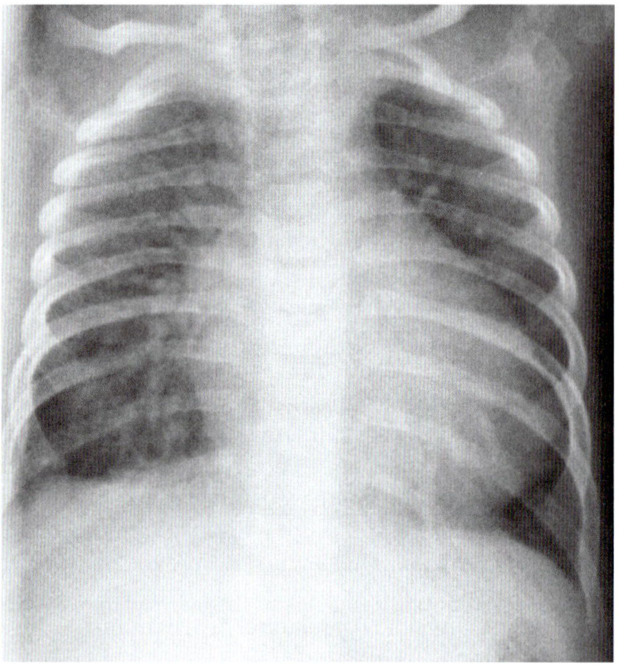

Fig. 16.31: Egg on side appearance in transposition. This characteristic appearance is seen only in about one-third cases and results from a narrow pedicle of the heart because of malposition of great vessels

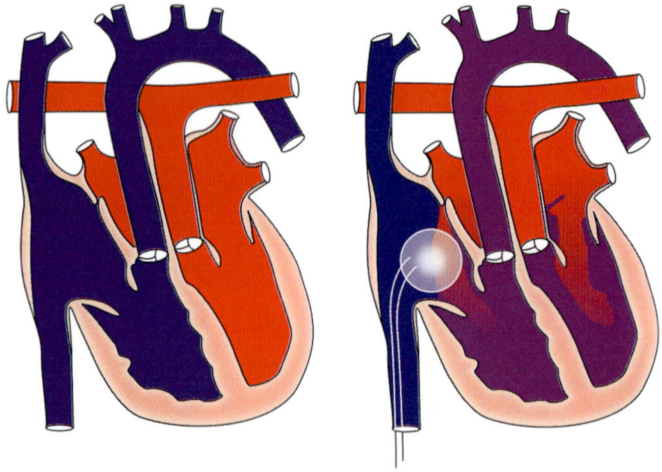

Fig. 16.32: Balloon atrial septostomy; this cartoon shows how a balloon atrial septostomy works. The figure on the left shows the physiology of transposition. The parallel circulation with poor intercirculatory mixing results in very low saturations in the aorta. Balloon atrial septostomy (right) creates an opening in the atrial septum and allows better intercirculatory mixing with improved saturation that is often life saving

cyanosis, cardiomegaly, congestive failure, normal first sound, single or normally split second sound and grade II–IV ejection systolic murmur. Apical third sound gallop or a mid-diastolic rumble may be present. Electrocardiogram shows right axis deviation with biventricular, right ventricular or left ventricular hypertrophy. Chest X-ray shows cardiomegaly, plethoric lung fields and features of pulmonary venous hypertension.

#### Treatment

Prostaglandin $E_1$ can help reduce cyanosis in selected cases by keeping the PDA open. Interim palliation can be accomplished through a balloon atrial septostomy **(Fig. 16.32)**. This procedure can be accomplished in catheterization laboratory or in the ICU under echocardiographic guidance. Septostomy is successful only up to the age of 6–12 weeks and gives temporary relief by providing better mixing and reducing left atrial pressure.

The *arterial switch operation* is now well established as the treatment of choice for TGA and most centers endeavor to offer this procedure for all infants with TGA. In this operation, the pulmonary artery and aorta are transected. The distal aorta is anastomosed to the proximal pulmonary stump (neo-aortic root) and the pulmonary artery to the proximal aortic stump (neo-pulmonary artery). The coronary arteries are moved along to the neo-aortic root along with a cuff of aortic tissue to allow suturing without compromise of coronary blood flow. Most modern pediatric cardiac centers strive to achieve excellence with the neonatal arterial switch operation because the long-term results are very satisfying. There is a limited window of time for performing the arterial switch for TGA. Infants with TGA and intact septum should ideally undergo this procedure within the first 4 weeks of life. As pulmonary vascular resistance falls after birth, the left ventricle regresses rapidly. In the first 1–2 months, the left ventricle has the ability to adjust to the elevated systemic vascular resistance after the arterial switch through hyperplasia of the available muscle. After this, it is difficult for the left ventricle to adapt to an arterial switch. Later in infancy, the *atrial switch operation* (Senning operation) may be considered for TGA with intact ventricular septum. This is not an ideal long-term option because the right ventricle remains as the systemic ventricle for life. Over time, right ventricle dysfunction and severe tricuspid regurgitation sets in. Additionally, extensive restructuring of atria predisposes to atrial rhythm disturbances. Alternatively, the left ventricle may be trained over 1–2 weeks through a ductal stenting or pulmonary artery band with a BT shunt and an arterial switch may then be performed.

In the presence of a sizable PDA or VSD, there is no fear of early regression of LV because the PA pressures are elevated. Nevertheless, the window of time for operation of TGA-VSD and TGA-PDA is still limited. This is because there is accelerated development of pulmonary vascular obstructive disease in these patients. Surgical correction involves the arterial switch operation with closure of the VSD or PDA. This should ideally be accomplished within 2–3 months of age. Beyond this age, an increasing proportion of infants show irreversible changes in the pulmonary vasculature. Consequently, postoperative recovery may be complicated by pulmonary hypertensive crisis and long-term results are unsatisfactory. Most centers seek to operate these infants in the first month itself.

Many centers are able to perform arterial switch operations with operative mortality of <3%. Twenty-year survival is >90%. Long-term concerns after surgery include development of aortic root dilation and aortic regurgitation, right ventricular outflow tract obstruction and coronary artery occlusion.

### Corrected TGA

In corrected TGA, the right atrium is connected to the left ventricle and vice-versa. The left ventricle gives rise to the pulmonary artery and right ventricle to the aorta. The aorta lies anterior and to the left of the pulmonary artery (hence the term L-TGA). The ascending aorta forms the left upper border of the cardiac silhouette. Since the route of blood flow is normal, it is the associated anomalies that determine the clinical features. The commonest anomalies include: (i) A VSD with or without pulmonic stenosis; (ii) left-sided Ebstein anomaly of the tricuspid valve (clinically simulates mitral regurgitation); and (iii) atrioventricular conduction abnormalities including complete atrioventricular block, each in approximately 65% cases. The precordial leads V4R, V1, and V2 may show a 'Q' wave that is absent in the left precordial leads. Chest X-ray shows a smooth left upper border corresponding to the ascending aorta. The diagnosis depends on echocardiographic identification of ventricular inversion as well as the additional anomalies. Management depends on the type of associated anomalies. The need to retain the morphologic left ventricle as the systemic ventricle makes the surgical management of corrected transposition rather complex.

### Total Anomalous Pulmonary Venous Connection (TAPVC)

Here, all the pulmonary veins instead of joining the left atrium are connected anomalously to result in the total pulmonary venous blood reaching the right atrium. The anatomical classification of TAPVC is into supracardiac, cardiac, infracardiac and mixed varieties. In the supracardiac TAPVC, the pulmonary veins join together to form a common pulmonary vein that may drain into the left innominate vein or the right superior vena cava. In the cardiac TAPVC, the veins join the coronary sinus or enter the right atrium directly. In the infracardiac variety, the common pulmonary vein drains into the portal vein. The key determinant of age at presentation is whether or not the pulmonary venous drainage via the common pulmonary vein is obstructed.

#### *Hemodynamics*

TAPVC results in the pulmonary venous blood reaching the right atrium, which also receives the systemic venous blood. This results in almost complete mixing of the two venous returns. The blood flow to the left atrium is the right-to-left shunt through a patent foramen ovale or atrial septal defect. The oxygen saturation of the blood in the pulmonary artery is often identical to that in the aorta because of mixing of the blood in the right atrium. Physiologically, TAPVC can be divided into: (a) Patients with pulmonary venous obstruction, and (b) patients without pulmonary venous obstruction. Pulmonary venous obstruction invariably results in pulmonary arterial hypertension as well as restriction to pulmonary blood flow and often presents in the first few weeks after birth. In the absence of pulmonary venous obstruction, pulmonary blood flow is large and results in cardiac failure between 4 and 10 weeks of age. TAPVC of the infracardiac type is always obstructive whereas cardiac and supracardiac types may or may not have pulmonary venous obstruction.

#### *Clinical Picture*

TAPVC of the non-obstructive type present with cyanosis and congestive failure as the fetal pulmonary vasculature regresses. The onset of congestive failure is around 4 to 10 weeks of age. Occasionally, with large pulmonary blood flow, the cyanosis may be minimal or clinically not recognizable. The patients are irritable and have failure to thrive. Besides features of congestive failure, the patients have cardiomegaly, hyperkinetic precordium normal or accentuated first sound, widely split and fixed second sound with accentuated pulmonic component, a grade two to four pulmonary ejection systolic murmur and a tricuspid flow murmur. The physical findings are identical to that of an atrial septal defect. Presence of systemic desaturation and congestive failure at this age suggests TAPVC. A continuous venous hum may rarely be audible at the upper left or right sternal border or in the suprasternal notch.

Patients with *obstructive* TAPVC present with marked cyanosis and congestive failure typically within the first one to two weeks of life. The condition is often fatal without specific treatment. The physical findings consist of parasternal heave, normal first sound, accentuated pulmonic component of S2 and insignificant murmurs. Tricuspid regurgitation can occur and results in cardiomegaly. These infants are severely compromised and need admission in an intensive care unit and emergency corrective surgery.

The electrocardiogram in TAPVC with or without pulmonary venous obstruction shows right axis deviation and right ventricular hypertrophy. Chest roentgenogram shows cardiomegaly with plethoric lung fields in non-obstructive TAPVC. The characteristic pattern of the "snowman" or figure of '8' configuration in the supracardiac TAPVC draining to left innominate vein is seen only after the age of 2 years (Fig. 16.33). The characteristic X-ray of the obstructive TAPVC consists of a normal sized heart with severe pulmonary venous hypertension resulting in

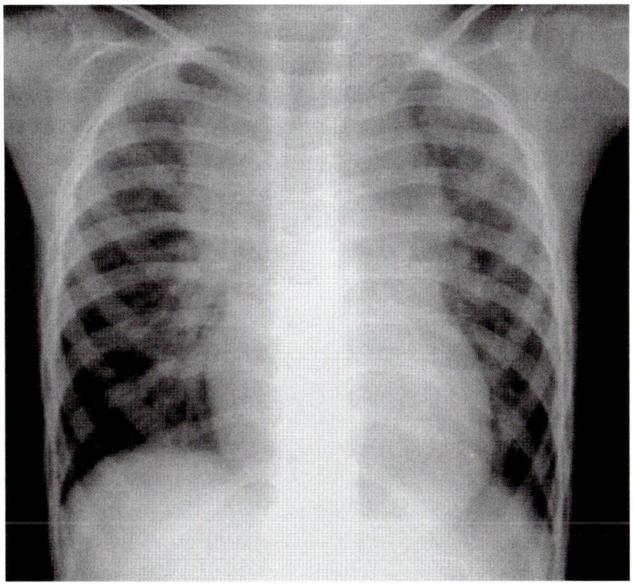

**Fig. 16.33:** Chest X-ray in unobstructed supracardiac total anomalous pulmonary venous connection to the innominate vein via the left vertical vein in an 8-year-old child. This is the characteristic figure of '8' sign or the snowman's sign

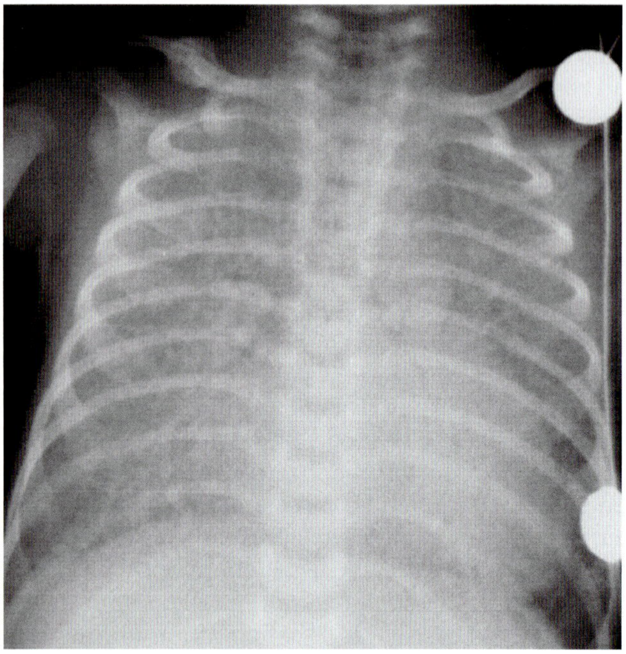

Fig. 16.34: Chest X-ray from a newborn with obstructed infracardiac total anomalous pulmonary venous connection. Note the characteristic ground glass appearance

"ground glass" appearance of the lungs very much like that of hyaline membrane disease (Fig. 16.34). Echocardiogram allows confirmation of the diagnosis, definition of the individual pulmonary veins and assessment of the site of obstruction. In addition, the pulmonary artery pressure can be quantified. In most situations, echo alone is adequate for surgical planning.

The diagnosis of the obstructive TAPVC is made in a neonate with cyanosis and normal sized heart with "ground glass" lung fields. The diagnosis of non-obstructive TAPVC should be suspected, if the auscultatory features of atrial septal defect are associated with cyanosis with or without congestive failure in the first 2 to 3 months of life.

#### *Management*

Operation is indicated as early as possible since 80% of infants die within the first 3 months of life without surgical help. Obstructed TAPVC needs surgery at short notice. The results of surgery for both forms of TAPVC are good in most modern centers but newborns and infants with obstructed TAPVC sometimes need a long time to recover after surgery. A small proportion of infants develop progressive pulmonary venous obstruction after repair of TAPVC that is often not easy to correct.

### Additional Conditions with Cyanosis and High Pulmonary Flow

Apart from transposition of great vessels and total anomalous pulmonary venous connection, single ventricle without obstruction to pulmonary blood flow, persistent truncus arteriosus, tricuspid atresia with absence of obstruction to pulmonary blood flow and double outlet right ventricle without pulmonic stenosis present with cyanosis and increased pulmonary blood flow. Clinically patients present with congestive failure in the neonatal period and are characterized by cyanosis, cardiomegaly and failure to thrive. Almost 80% die within 3 months of life due to congestive cardiac failure or pulmonary infection. Those who survive develop pulmonary arterial hypertension due to pulmonary vascular obstructive disease. Echocardiography is necessary to arrive at the specific diagnosis. Since the mortality of unoperated patients is high and patients develop Eisenmenger syndrome early in life, it is necessary that patients presenting with cyanosis and increased pulmonary blood flow be referred to specialized centers as early as possible. Surgical treatment is dictated by the specific anatomy.

### Cyanotic Heart Disease with Pulmonary Arterial Hypertension

Patients with Eisenmenger syndrome have severe pulmonary arterial hypertension resulting in a right-to-left shunt at the atrial, ventricular or pulmonary arterial level. Eisenmenger complex consists of pulmonary arterial hypertension with a VSD providing the right-to-left shunt.

#### *Hemodynamics*

The pulmonary arterial hypertension is due to pulmonary vascular obstructive disease. If a communication is present at the pulmonary arterial level or the ventricular level, the right ventricular pressure cannot go beyond the systemic pressure. The right-to-left shunt decompresses the right ventricle. The right ventricle has only concentric hypertrophy without significant increase in the size. In patients who have a PDA or VSD, there is only a mild parasternal impulse without significant heave. In patients who do not have a VSD or PDA, the right ventricle also dilates. The right-to-left shunt at the atrial level is an indication of right ventricular failure to accommodate this volume and push into the pulmonary artery. Patients of Eisenmenger syndrome with communication at the atrial level only, exhibit a parasternal heave and cardiac enlargement. The right ventricular pressure may even be higher than the systemic pressure.

A right-to-left shunt at the atrial level or the ventricular level reaches the ascending aorta and is thus distributed to the whole systemic circulation. This results in equal cyanosis of fingers and toes. A right-to-left shunt through a PDA is directed downwards into the descending aorta, which results in differential cyanosis affecting lower limbs, with pink upper limbs.

#### *Clinical Features*

Patients present with history of cyanosis, fatigue, effort intolerance and dyspnea. There may also be history of repeated chest infections in childhood. On physical examination, they have cyanosis and clubbing. Differential cyanosis separates patients who have a PDA from those who have a VSD or atrial septal defect. The features indicative of pulmonary arterial hypertension consist of parasternal impulse and palpable second sound. The pulmonary component of the second sound is accentuated and louder than the aortic component. The splitting of the second sound remains wide and fixed in atrial septal defect. Due to superimposition of A2 and P2, the second sound is single in patients who have a VSD. Patients who have a PDA continue to have a normally split second sound. A constant pulmonary ejection click, unlike in patients of valvar pulmonic stenosis, is well heard both during inspiration and expiration at the second left interspace. A harsh, high-pitched, early diastolic pulmonary regurgitation murmur can be present along the left sternal border. Patients with atrial septal defect, in whom Eisenmenger physiology is uncommon, can develop tricuspid regurgitation (Fig. 16.35).

The electrocardiogram reveals right axis deviation and right ventricular hypertrophy, *P pulmonale* may be present. The chest radiograph is characteristic, showing prominence of the pulmonary arterial segment and large right and left main pulmonary arteries and their branches. The peripheral lung fields are oligemic. Thus the hilar area suggests pulmonary artery enlargement whereas the peripheral lung fields suggest pulmonary oligemia (Fig. 16.36).

#### Treatment

Ideally pulmonary vascular obstructive disease should be prevented. This means early diagnosis and correction of all CHD associated with increased pulmonary blood flow. Patients with cyanosis and increased pulmonary blood flow develop Eisenmenger physiology very early and often need to be operated by 2–3 months of age. Medications are available for the management of pulmonary hypertension (see later section on pulmonary hypertension) and they may help reduce symptoms as well as improve survival in patients with Eisenmenger syndrome.

*Competencies:* **PE23.14; PE23.15**

## OBSTRUCTIVE LESIONS

### Aortic Stenosis

Pathologically, the site of obstruction may be at valve level, above the valve (supravalvar) or below the valve (subvalvar). At the valve level, the aortic stenosis results

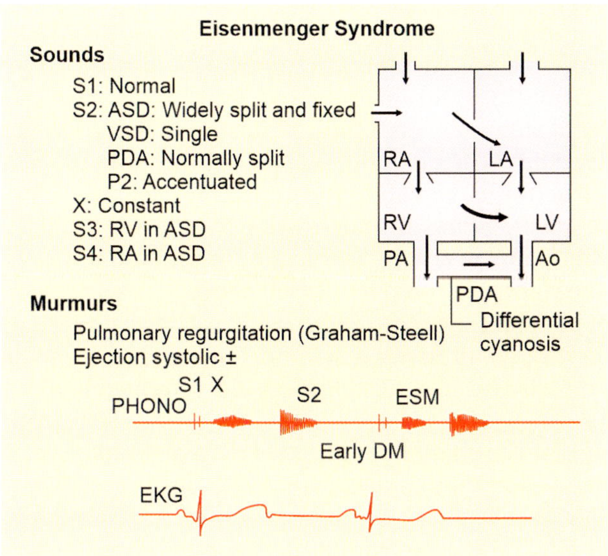


Fig. 16.35: Summary of auscultatory findings in Eisenmenger syndrome

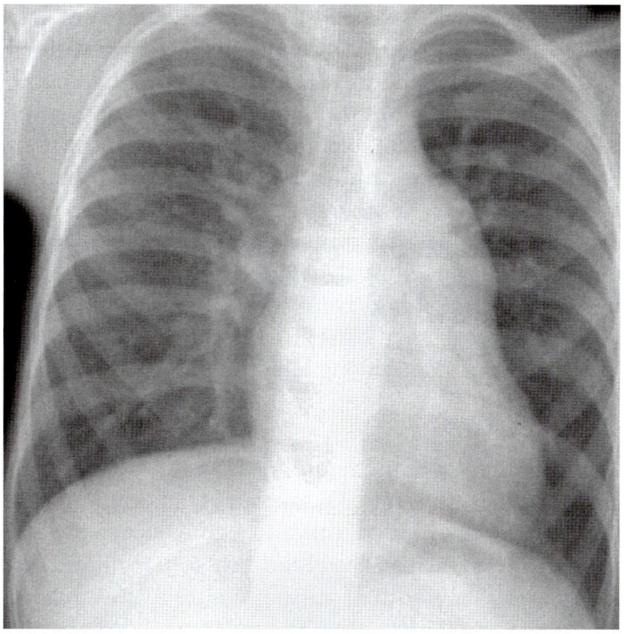

Fig. 16.36: Chest X-ray in Eisenmenger syndrome following ventricular septal defect. The proximal right pulmonary artery is enlarged. There is a relative paucity of vasculature in the periphery with a sudden tapering of caliber of the right pulmonary artery (pruning)

from either a unicuspid or a bicuspid aortic valve. Rarely the aortic valve annulus may itself be small. *Supravalvar aortic stenosis* results from obstruction in root of aorta, above the aortic valve, as in Williams syndrome. *Subvalvar aortic stenosis* may be discrete (membranous), fibromuscular or muscular (hypertrophic obstructive cardiomyopathy).

#### Hemodynamics

Valvar obstruction is overcome by raising the systolic pressure of the left ventricle. This is brought about by concentric hypertrophy of the left ventricle. Because of a powerful, muscular left ventricle, the emptying of the left ventricle is complete but the duration of the systole is prolonged. The prolongation of left ventricular ejection time causes delayed closure of the aortic valve resulting in delayed A2. The flow across the obstruction results in the aortic ejection systolic murmur that is typically diamond-shaped, starting after the first sound and ending before the aortic component of the second sound with a mid-systolic peak. The systolic murmur is always palpable as a thrill at the second right interspace, suprasternal notch and the carotid vessels. The powerful left ventricle can maintain a normal forward cardiac output. The prolonged ejection results in the characteristic pulse that can be best described as slowly rising to a peak that is sustained and then has a slowdown-slope. The peak is low so that the pulse is of low amplitude and prolonged duration.

Concentric hypertrophy of the left ventricle results in decreased distensibility of the left ventricle in diastole-reduced compliance. In severe aortic stenosis (AS), with marked left ventricular hypertrophy, the left ventricular diastolic pressure also rises. With increase in left ventricular diastolic pressure, the left atrial pressure must increase to be able to fill the left ventricle during diastole. Hence, with severe AS accompanied with marked left ventricular hypertrophy, a forceful left atrial contraction results in a palpable as well as audible fourth sound (S4). When the left ventricle starts failing in AS, besides hypertrophy, dilatation also appears and causes increase in heart size. With left ventricular failure, a third sound (S3) becomes audible. In valvar AS, there is post stenotic dilatation of ascending aorta, seen on posteroanterior chest radiograph. In supravalvar and subvalvar AS, this is absent. In valvar stenosis, the first sound is followed by an aortic ejection click that precedes the starts of the murmur; the click is heard at the apex, and along left sternal border.

### Clinical Features

Patients with mild to moderate AS are asymptomatic. With severe stenosis, the initial symptom is generally dyspnea on exertion. These patients may also give history of angina on effort and syncope. The blood pressure is normal with mild disease; the width of pulse pressure relates inversely with severity of AS resulting in low amplitude prolonged duration pulse. The cardiac size remains normal unless left ventricular failure is present. The apical impulse is forcible or heaving. In severe AS, the fourth sound may be palpable. If left ventricular failure is present, the third sound may be palpable. A systolic thrill is palpable at the second right interspace, suprasternal notch and the carotid arteries. The first sound is normal and followed by an ejection click in valvar aortic stenosis. The aortic component of the second sound (A2) is delayed but not diminished in intensity in AS. The delay results in closely split, single or paradoxically split second sound according to the severity of obstruction. With severe AS, S4 is audible, while in patients with left ventricular failure, S3 is palpable and audible. The ejection systolic murmur starting after the ejection click reaches a peak in mid-systole (Fig. 16.37). With increasing severity, the peak gets delayed so that the maximum intensity of the murmur is closer to the end rather than being mid-systolic. With immobile valves, either due to severe fibrosis or calcification, the systolic click as well as the A2 diminish in intensity and may become inaudible (Fig. 16.38).

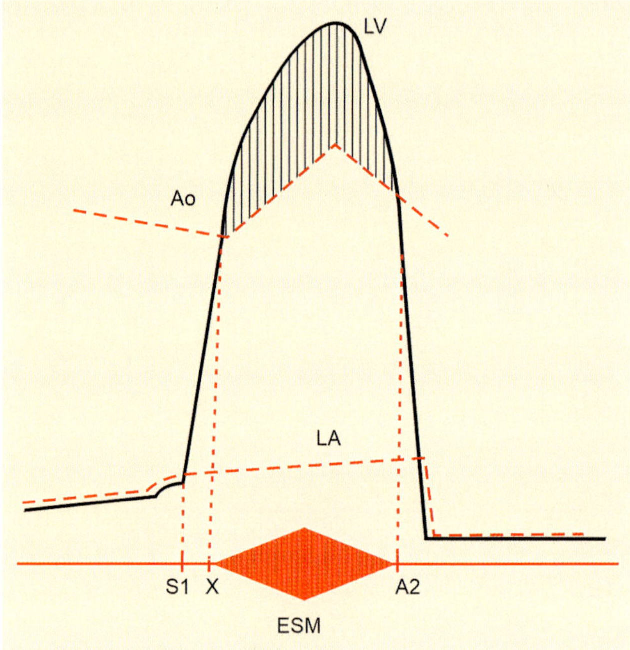


Fig. 16.38: Aortic stenosis: Diagrammatic portrayal of the hemodynamic basis for aortic stenosis murmur. The first sound (S1) occurs as the left ventricular (LV) pressure increases above left atrial (LA) pressure. This is followed by the ejection click (X) occurring after the aortic valve opens. The shape of the gradient between LV and aorta (Ao) corresponds to the shape of the aortic ejection systolic murmur (ESM). The murmur ends before the aortic components of the second sound (A2)

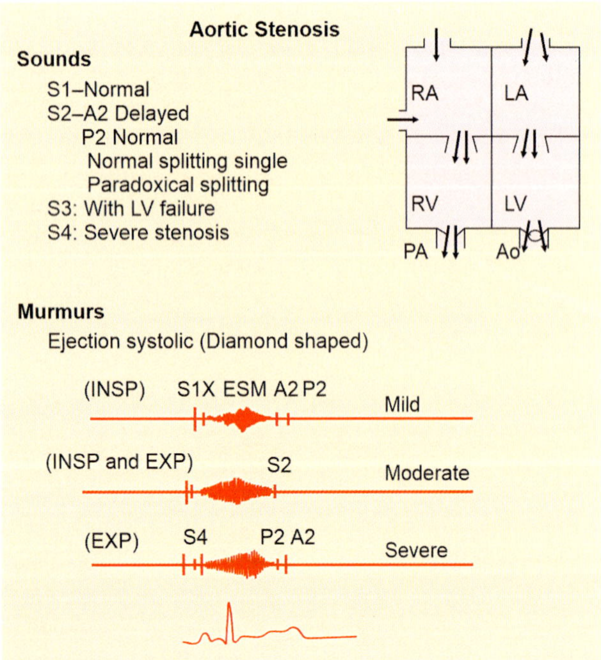


Fig. 16.37: Summary of auscultatory findings in aortic stenosis. S4 fourth sound; X aortic click

Subvalvar AS is differentiated from valvar lesions by absence of ejection click and the post stenotic dilatation of the ascending aorta in the thoracic roentgenogram. An aortic regurgitation murmur may be audible. The maximum intensity of the systolic murmur and thrill may be in the third or fourth left interspace.

Supravalvar AS may be associated with Williams syndrome (elfin facies, mental retardation, dental abnormalities, strabismus and peripheral pulmonary arterial stenosis). Since the obstruction is above the aortic valve, the pressure in the segment of the aorta before the obstruction is elevated and results in loud A2. The jet through the supravalvar narrowing may be directed toward the innominate artery resulting in higher systolic pressure in the right arm compared to left arm.

The electrocardiogram reveals left ventricular hypertrophy. Presence of ST and T wave changes suggest severe disease (Fig. 16.39). It should be remembered that a normal electrocardiogram does not exclude severe aortic stenosis. The chest X-ray shows a normal sized heart with dilated ascending aorta in valvar AS. In supravalvar and subvalvar stenosis, the thoracic roentgenogram may be normal. Presence of cardiac enlargement indicates severe AS. Echocardiogram can identify the site of stenosis, and assess the gradient across the obstruction fairly accurately.

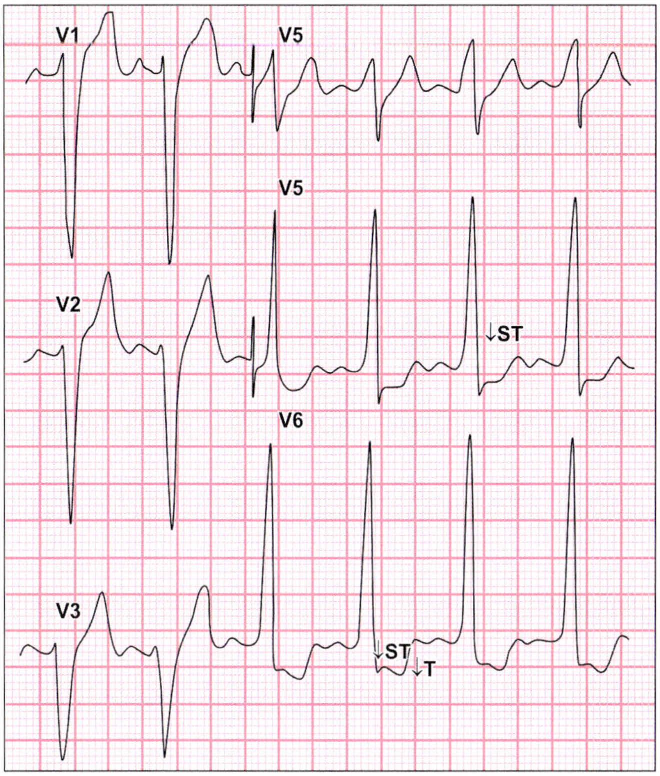


**Fig. 16.39:** Electrocardiogram from a patient with severe aortic stenosis showing prominent left ventricular voltages together with ST segment depression and T wave inversion in lateral leads (strain pattern)

### Assessment of Severity

The severity of AS should be determined, based on the following:

i. Symptomatic patients have severe AS; lack of symptoms does not exclude severe disease.
ii. Narrower the pulse pressure, the more severe the AS.
iii. Systolic thrill at second right interspace suggests at least moderately severe AS.
iv. The later the peak of the ejection systolic murmur, the more severe the narrowing.
v. The delay in A2 correlates well with severity. With mild AS, the S2 is normally split; with moderate AS, it is closely split; with severe or critical AS, it is single or paradoxically split.
vi. Presence of S4 is indirect evidence for severe AS.
vii. Presence of S3 indicates severe AS and systolic ventricular dysfunction often with heart failure.
viii. ST and T changes in the lateral leads of electrocardiogram suggest severe stenosis.
ix. Cardiac enlargement on chest radiograph indicates severe AS with left ventricular failure.
x. Doppler can quantitate the gradient across the aortic valve accurately. Two-dimensional echo reveals concentric left ventricular hypertrophy; ventricular dysfunction is associated with heart failure.

### Treatment

Patients with AS should be followed closely, with 6–12 monthly electrocardiogram. Symptoms should be carefully evaluated. Doppler echo can be used to quantitate the gradient at each visit and ventricular function should be monitored. Severe AS is risk for *sudden death*. Patients should be discouraged from outdoor games, athletics, competitive sports and strenuous exercises, if AS is significant (gradient of 50 mm Hg or more).

Balloon aortic valvuloplasty is the procedure of choice for valvar AS. A balloon introduced through the femoral artery can be placed at the aortic valve and inflated to tear the valve along the commissure. It is indicated, if the peak gradient is above 75 mm Hg. Supravalvar and subvalvar AS do not respond to balloon dilation; the procedure should also be avoided in patients with significant aortic regurgitation. Surgical options include aortic valve repair and replacement with a prosthetic valve. Patients need to be administered anticoagulants, if they have a prosthetic valve replacement and careful follow-up to prevent/detect complications, such as restenosis, thrombus or pannus formation and infective endocarditis.

## Coarctation of the Aorta

Coarctation of the aorta is located at the junction of the arch with the descending aorta. It is a sharp indentation involving the anterior, lateral and posterior wall of the aorta; the medial wall is spared. It may be distal or proximal to the ductus or ligamentum arteriosus and also the left subclavian artery. A bicuspid aortic valve is a common association.

### Hemodynamics

In fetal life, the right ventricular output passes down the descending aorta through a wide ductus arteriosus. The left ventricular output empties into the innominate, left carotid and left subclavian arteries and little output reaches the descending aorta. The portion of the aorta distal to the left subclavian and before the portion where the ductus arteriosus joins is called the isthmus. At birth, the isthmus is the narrowest part of the aorta. Following closure of the ductus arteriosus, the descending aorta must receive its total supply from the left ventricle via the ascending aorta. Neonates with severe coarctation, therefore, become symptomatic immediately as the duct starts to close. However, a significant proportion present late.

The exact mechanism for the production of systemic hypertension in coarctation is not known. The aortic obstruction is certainly partly responsible for it. The narrow pulse pressure in the descending aorta distal to the coarctation has been implicated in the renal mechanism for the causation of hypertension in coarctation. The obstruction stimulates growth of collateral vessels between the proximal and distal segments. The intercostal vessels also participate in decompressing the hypertensive upper segment. They enlarge and become palpable at the lower borders of the ribs often later in childhood or adolescence. Palpable collaterals are also felt at the medial and inferior angle of scapula. Because of the decompression of the upper segment by the collaterals, the resting blood pressure in upper extremities may even be normal, but rises on exercise.

### Clinical Features

Coarctation has a continuum of severity and the age at presentation is linked to severity. Newborns with severe coarctation presents as soon as the duct start to close (see duct dependent circulation). Infants with coarctation occasionally present with left ventricular dysfunction and heart failure. It is important to examine femoral pulses in newborns and infants with heart failure. Later in life, coarctation is often not associated with symptoms.

The only symptoms in uncomplicated coarctation may be intermittent claudication, pain and weakness of legs and dyspnea on running. Examination shows delayed and weak femorals compared to strong brachial arteries. The heart size remains normal with a forcible or heaving left ventricular apex. A systolic thrill may be palpable in the suprasternal notch. There are prominent arterial pulsations in the suprasternal notch and the carotid vessels. The first sound is accentuated and sometimes followed by a constant ejection click. The second sound is normally split with a loud aortic component. A variable intensity ejection systolic murmur is heard with the point of maximum intensity over the back in the interscapular area. The murmur starts late in systole after a considerable gap from the first sound and click. It may appear to go through the second sound suggesting a continuous murmur. This is because of delay in the transmission of pulse from the heart to the site of coarctation. Continuous murmurs may be audible over collaterals in the chest wall but are uncommon. An aortic ejection systolic murmur and/or an aortic regurgitation murmur may also be present because of the commonly associated bicuspid aortic valve (Fig. 16.40).

The electrocardiogram shows left ventricular hypertrophy; ST and T wave changes below the age of 15 yr suggests additional aortic stenosis or endocardial fibroelastosis. Chest X-ray shows a normal sized heart with prominent ascending aorta and the aortic knuckle. In an overpenetrated film, the site of coarctation can be localized as the proximal segment is dilated and there is post stenotic dilatation of the distal segment. The characteristic notching of the lower borders of ribs tends to appear beyond the age of 10 yr. Using suprasternal approach, coarctation can be seen on echocardiogram and the gradient estimated. Additionally, the descending aortic flow pattern is altered from phasic systolic flow to continuous low amplitude, systolic-diastolic flows. The echocardiogram also enables measurement of the transverse arch and isthmic diameters. Older children and young adults sometimes require a CT scan to evaluate anatomic details.

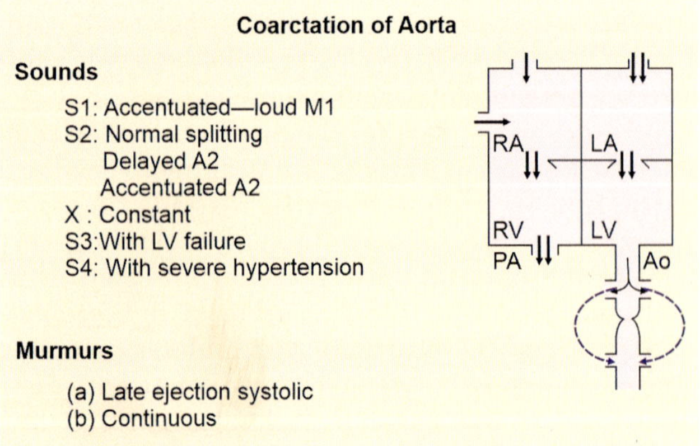


**Fig. 16.40:** Summary of auscultatory findings in coarctation of the aorta. S3 third heart sound, S4 fourth heart sound

### Course and Complications

Coarctation may result in congestive failure in infancy. If congestive failure does not occur in infancy, it is unlikely to occur throughout the pediatric age group. The complications of coarctation include rupture of berry intracranial aneurysm and dissection of aorta. These complications are rare in children. Infective endarteritis may occur in the wall of aorta distal to coarctation or there could be endocarditis involving the bicuspid aortic valve.

### Treatment

Relief of coarctation is recommended as soon as diagnosis is made when coarctation is severe. In newborns and infants, surgery is preferred. In older children, adolescents and adults, balloon dilation with or without stenting is often undertaken. The recurrence rate of balloon dilation in newborns is over 90% and this procedure should only be done as interim palliation in the face of heart failure and severe ventricular dysfunction. Prostaglandin $E_1$ is used to maintain ductal patency prior to surgery in the first few weeks of life.

It is likely that coarctation is not a localized disease at the junction of arch and descending aorta and there is perhaps generalized weakness of the arterial media. Resection of coarctation does not guarantee freedom from complications like dissection of aorta. Systemic hypertension can persist following operation and re-coarctation of aorta can also occur, requiring repeat balloon angioplasty.

## Pulmonic Stenosis (Pure Pulmonic Stenosis or Pulmonic Stenosis with Intact Ventricular Septum)

Pulmonic stenosis (PS) is usually valvar or subvalvar (infundibular PS). Uncommonly pulmonic stenosis may be in the pulmonary artery above the valve or in the main right or left branches or the peripheral branches.

### Hemodynamics and Clinical Features

Flow across the narrow pulmonary valve results in a pulmonary ejection systolic murmur and a thrill in the left second interspace. To keep the flow normal, the right ventricle increases its systolic pressure and develops concentric right ventricular hypertrophy. The pulmonary artery beyond the obstruction shows post-stenotic dilatation visible on the thoracic roentgenogram as a dilated pulmonary arterial segment. Because of the obstruction, the right ventricular systole is prolonged resulting in delayed closure of the pulmonic component (P2) of second sound. The delay in P2 results in a wide and variably split second sound. In valvar PS, a pulmonary ejection click is audible, soon after S1 and just before the onset of murmur, during expiration but disappears or becomes softer during inspiration. With increasing severity of stenosis, the duration and intensity of the murmur increase and the peak gets delayed; the click disappears and P2 becomes softer. With moderate PS, the murmur ends just short of the aortic component of the second sound. The concentric right ventricular hypertrophy results in maintaining a normal heart size, but reduces its distensibility. In severe PS with marked right ventricular hypertrophy, the ventricular diastolic pressure also increases. The right atrial pressure increases to be able to fill the right ventricle and results in a fourth heart sound (S4) as well as prominent 'a' waves in the JVP (**Fig. 16.41**).

Patients with mild to moderate PS are asymptomatic; with severe stenosis, dyspnea on effort appears. If foramen ovale is patent, a right-to-left shunt at the atrial level may occur in severe PS and result in cyanosis. Palpitation, easy fatigability and rarely chest pain may occur. Features of Noonan syndrome should be looked for. The cardiac size is normal and the hypertrophied right ventricle results in left parasternal heave. If the right ventricle fails, a right ventricular third sound may be audible. Rarely with right ventricular failure, tricuspid regurgitation may appear. Since the right atrium offers less resistance to flow of blood than obstruction at the pulmonary valve, the flow through the pulmonary valve diminishes reducing the intensity as well as the duration of ejection systolic murmur.

Infundibular stenosis is distinguished from valvar PS by: (i) Absence of click; (ii) absence of post stenotic dilatation; and (iii) a relatively lower point of maximum intensity of systolic murmur in 3–4th left interspace. Isolated pure infundibular PS is relatively rare.

The electrocardiogram shows right axis deviation and right ventricular hypertrophy. PS results in systolic overload for the right ventricle, suggested by pure 'R' or

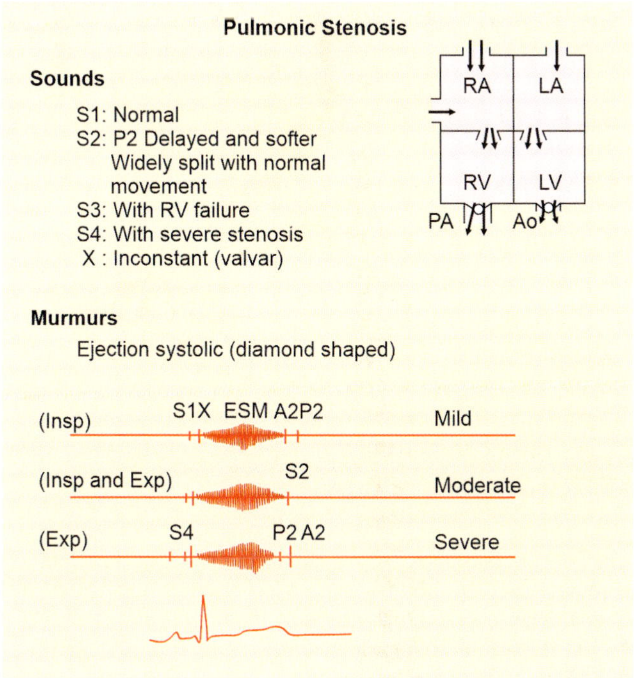


**Fig. 16.41:** Summary of auscultatory findings in pulmonic stenosis

'qR' complex in V4R and V1 leads. P pulmonale suggests severe PS. Chest X-ray shows a normal sized heart with normal pulmonary vasculature in mild, moderate as well as severe PS. Pulmonary oligemia occurs, if the patients develop a right-to-left shunt at the atrial level in severe or critical PS. The main pulmonary artery exhibits post-stenotic dilatation. Echocardiography can identify the site and severity of obstruction and helps in planning catheter intervention.

### *Treatment*

Valvar PS generally does not increase in severity with time unless it is severe or diagnosed in the newborn period. Patients with mild PS (gradients of 50 mm Hg or less) need annual review. Balloon pulmonary valvuloplasty is the treatment of choice for isolated valvar PS. The procedure is sometimes technically challenging in newborn with critical PS. Surgical treatment is indicated only if balloon valvotomy is unsuccessful, as in patients with dysplastic valves or small pulmonary valve annulus. Infundibular PS requires surgical resection.

### Suggested Reading

1. Kumar RK, Prabhu SS, Jain S, et al. IAP Specialty Textbook of Pediatric Cardiology. Jaypee Brothers, New Delhi, 3rd edition, 2021, ISBN 81-8448-273-6.
2. Wernovsky G, Anderson RH, Kumar K, et al. Anderson's Pediatric Cardiology. Elsevier, 4th edn 2019, ISBN 978-0-7020-7608-4.

*Competencies:* **PE23.4; PE23.5; PE23.13; PE23.14; PE23.15**

## RHEUMATIC FEVER AND RHEUMATIC HEART DISEASE

### Rheumatic Fever

Rheumatic fever is an immunological disorder initiated by group A beta hemolytic streptococci. Cell mediated and humoral immunity directed against selected streptococcal cell wall proteins and sugars react with the connective tissues of the body as well as the heart and result in rheumatic fever. There is no single test for the confirmation of diagnosis. There is a strong relationship with streptococcal infection and it is possible to prevent rheumatic fever by prompt treatment of streptococcal infections with penicillin.

#### *Epidemiology*

Rheumatic heart disease (RHD) constitutes a variable proportion of cardiac patients in Indian hospitals. Selected parts of India that have experienced improved human development are now reporting a significant decline in incidence of rheumatic fever. Surveys conducted at Chandigarh, Indore, Cochin and Vellore involving more than 100,000 children (2004 to 2007) indicate that the prevalence has dropped to between 0.5 and 1/1000. Surveys using echocardiography alone have suggested a higher prevalence of RHD in selected regions (as high as 20/1000).

*Age and sex:* The incidence of rheumatic fever following streptococcal throat infection is 0.3% in the general population and 1 to 3% in presence of epidemics of streptococcal sore throat. The commonest age group involved is 5–15 years, and first episodes of RF are rare before 3 years or after 30 years age. Although the sexes are nearly equally affected, mitral valve disease and chorea is more common in girls whereas aortic valve involvement is more often seen in boys.

***Predisposing factors:*** Poor socioeconomic conditions, unhygienic living conditions and overcrowded house holds predispose to streptococcal infections. However, an epidemic in United States occurred in upper middle class families in the absence of overcrowding and with good medical facilities in the mid-1980s.

### Etiopathogenesis

A strong association with beta hemolytic streptococci of group A is indicated by a number of observations:

i. History of preceding sore throat is often encountered.
ii. Epidemics of streptococcal infection are followed by higher incidence of rheumatic fever.
iv. In patients with established RHD, streptococcal infection is followed by recurrence of acute rheumatic fever.
v. Penicillin prophylaxis for streptococcal infection prevents recurrences of rheumatic fever in those patients who have had it earlier.
vi. More than 85% of the patients with acute rheumatic fever show elevated levels of anti-streptococcal antibody titer.

Streptococci have never been isolated from rheumatic lesions in joints, heart or the bloodstream. Considerable evidence suggests that rheumatic fever is an immune-mediated reaction. Following streptococcal sore throat, there is a latent period of 10 days to several weeks before the onset of rheumatic fever. This latent period is similar to other antigen-antibody diseases like serum sickness. Streptococcal cell wall proteins as well as carbohydrates have the capacity to produce antibodies capable of reacting with human connective tissue, resulting in rheumatic fever. Rheumatic fever appears to be the result of the host's unusual response at both the cellular and humoral levels to *Streptococcus*. There is no marker that consistently identifies genetic susceptibility to rheumatic fever.

Only heart valves are permanently damaged during an episode of rheumatic fever. All other affected tissues typically heal without residua: Pericarditis, chorea and arthritis resolve completely without constriction, long-term neurologic consequences or joint disability, respectively. Concepts about the pathogenesis of rheumatic fever and RHD are summarized in Fig. 16.42.

### Clinical Features

The clinical features of rheumatic fever consist of streptococcal sore throat with fever followed 10 days to a few weeks later by recurrence of fever and the various manifestations of acute rheumatic fever. The history of sore throat is available in less than 50% of the patients.

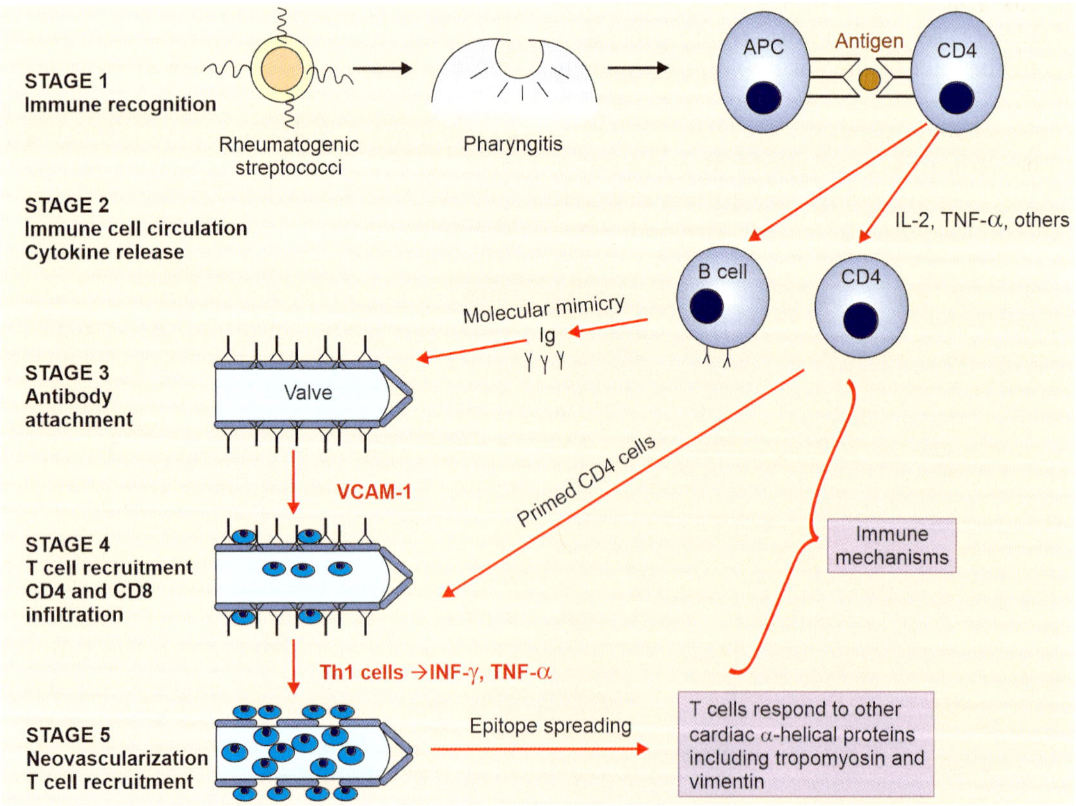


**Fig. 16.42:** Presumed pathogenesis of rheumatic fever; It is likely that the endothelium suffers initial damage due to a humoral immune response, the damage resulting in vascular cell adhesion molecule 1 (VCAM-1) being expressed on the endothelium. This is followed by activation of cellular immune response. As a result CD4+, CD8+, T lymphocytes and macrophages get attached to the valvar endothelium and migrate to the connective tissue core. This sets up an inflammatory response. The inflammation is accompanied by neovascularization of the valve substance

GAS group A streptococcus; INF-γ gamma interferon; TNF-α tumor necrosis factor alpha; Th1 T helper cells 1

**Table 16.16:** Revised Jones criteria for acute rheumatic fever (2015)

| American Heart Association and World Heart Federation | |
|---|---|
| **For all populations**<br>• Initial episode of acute rheumatic fever: Two major or one major + two minor criteria<br>• Recurrent episodes of acute rheumatic fever: Two major, one major + two minor, or three minor<br>• Essential criteria: Previous evidence of group A beta hemolytic streptococcal infection | |
| **Low-risk populations**<br>Incidence <2/100,000 in school-going children; rheumatic heart disease prevalence <1/1000 | **Moderate, high-risk populations** |
| ***Major criteria***<br>Carditis: Clinical or subclinical<br>Arthritis: Polyarthritis only<br>Chorea<br>Erythema marginatum<br>Subcutaneous nodules | ***Major criteria***<br>Carditis: Clinical or subclinical<br>Arthritis: Polyarthritis, monoarthritis<br>Polyarthralgia<br>Chorea<br>Erythema marginatum<br>Subcutaneous nodules |
| ***Minor criteria***<br>Polyarthralgia<br>Fever (>38.5°C)<br>ESR ≥60 mm in the first hour; CRP ≥3.0 mg/dL<br>Prolonged PR interval, after accounting for age variability (unless carditis is a major criterion) | ***Minor criteria***<br>Monoarthralgia<br>Fever (>38.0°C)<br>ESR ≥30 mm in the first hour; CRP ≥3.0 mg/dL<br>Prolonged PR interval, after accounting for age variability (unless carditis is a major criterion) |

Gewitz MH, et al. Revision of the Jones criteria for the diagnosis of acute rheumatic fever in the era of Doppler echocardiography. Circulation 2015;131: 1806–18.

Guidelines for the clinical diagnosis of acute rheumatic fever, originally suggested by T. Duckett Jones have been revised by the American Heart Association and WHO. The most recent guidelines have been endorsed by the World Heart Federation. These guidelines are different for low-risk population (RHD prevalence of <1/1000) versus moderate or high-risk population. The guidelines consist of major, minor and essential criteria (Table 16.16). Two major or one major and two minor criteria are required in the presence of essential criteria to diagnose the first episode of acute rheumatic fever. Additionally, for RF recurrences, three minor criteria are sufficient. It is important to emphasize that these guidelines are meant to help a physician in making a firm diagnosis of rheumatic fever and do not mean that a physician should not use his or her clinical judgment in making a diagnosis in the absence of these criteria.

### Major Criteria

These include:

***i. Carditis:*** It is an *early* manifestation of rheumatic fever. Studies utilizing echocardiography indicate that carditis occurs in almost 90% patients. In 60–70%, it is clinically obvious whereas in the remaining, the diagnosis is based on echocardiographic findings labeled as subclinical carditis. Rheumatic carditis is designated as a pancarditis involving the pericardium, myocardium and endocardium, although studies indicate limited myocardial component. Almost 80% of those patients who develop carditis do so within the first two weeks of onset of rheumatic fever.

Pericarditis results in precordial pain that may be quite severe. On auscultation, a friction rub is present. Clinical pericarditis is seen in approximately 15% of those who have carditis. The electrocardiogram may show ST and T changes consistent with pericarditis. As a rule, the rheumatic pericarditis is associated with only small effusions and does not result either in tamponade or constrictive pericarditis. A patient of rheumatic pericarditis always has additional mitral or mitral and aortic regurgitation murmurs.

Other features of carditis are (i) cardiac enlargement, (ii) soft first sound, (iii) protodiastolic (S3) gallop, (iv) congestive cardiac failure and (v) Carey Coombs' murmur. This is a soft delayed diastolic mitral murmur heard transiently during the course of acute rheumatic fever possibly as a result of flow across the inflamed and thickened mitral valve.

Endocarditis is represented by a pansystolic murmur of mitral regurgitation with or without an associated aortic regurgitation murmur. Pathologically, mitral valve is involved in all cases of rheumatic fever with carditis. Clinically, however, 5–8% patients may present as pure aortic regurgitation. Thus almost 95% patients will have mitral regurgitation murmur, a quarter of them also have an aortic regurgitation murmur and only 5% present as pure aortic regurgitation. Tricuspid valvulitis resulting in tricuspid regurgitation occurs in 10–30% of cases; always in association with other valves. The acute hemodynamic overload resulting from acute mitral regurgitation and/or aortic regurgitation leads to left ventricular failure and is the main reason for the morbidity and mortality of rheumatic fever and RHD.

***Subclinical carditis:*** It is now well accepted that carditis may be clinically silent and only identifiable through echocardiography. The most common echocardiographic manifestation of rheumatic carditis is mitral regurgitation. This may be accompanied by morphological changes in the valve (see below).

*ii. Arthritis:* Rheumatic arthritis is a polyarthritis involving large joints that include knees, ankles and elbows. Uncommonly smaller joints may also be involved. It is a migratory polyarthritis with the affected joints showing redness, warmth, swelling, pain and limitation of movement. It is an *early* manifestation and occurs in 70–75% of cases according to western literature. However, the figures from India indicate that arthritis is seen in 30 to 50% of patients. The pain and swelling appear rather quickly, last 3 to 7 days and subside spontaneously to appear in some other joint. There is no residual damage to the joint. Arthritis tends to be commoner in older patients.

*iii. Subcutaneous nodules:* Subcutaneous nodules appear on bony prominences like elbows, shins, occiput and spine. They vary in size from pinhead to an almond. They are non-tender. Subcutaneous nodules are a *late* manifestation and appear around 6 weeks after the onset of rheumatic fever though they have been described as early as 3 weeks from the onset. They occur in about 3 to 20% cases of rheumatic fever in India. Patients who have subcutaneous nodules almost always have carditis. They last from a few days to weeks but have been known to last for almost a year.

*iv. Chorea:* Sydenham's chorea is also a *late* manifestation occurring about 3 months after the onset of acute rheumatic fever. Generally, by the time a patient manifests chorea, the signs of inflammation usually subside. Chorea consists of semi-purposeful, jerky movements resulting in deranged speech, muscular incoordination, awkward gait and weakness. The affected child is emotionally disturbed and drops things she or he is carrying. It is three to four times more common in females as compared to males. Untreated, it has a self-limiting course of 2 to 6 weeks.

*v. Erythema marginatum:* It is an early manifestation, predominantly seen over the trunk. The rash is faintly reddish, not raised above the skin and non-itching. It starts as a red spot with a pale center, increasing in size to coalesce with adjacent spots to form a serpiginous outline. We believe that the inability to recognize erythema marginatum is not because it does not occur but because of the dark complexion of the skin.

### Minor Criteria

These include:

*Clinical criteria*

a. *Fever:* Rheumatic fever is almost always associated with fever. The temperature rarely goes above 39.5°C.
b. *Arthralgia:* Arthralgia is defined as subjective pain whereas arthritis means subjective symptoms as well as objective signs of joint inflammation. Whereas arthritis is a major manifestation, arthralgia is a minor manifestation. Figures from India indicate that arthritis and arthralgia together occur in about 90% of the patients
c. *Previous rheumatic fever or rheumatic heart disease:* This minor criterion is applicable only for a second attack of rheumatic fever.

### Laboratory Manifestations

*Acute phase reactants* consist of increased sedimentation rate and C-reactive protein. The leukocyte count usually lies between 10,000 and 15,000/cu mm. The sedimentation rate is elevated during acute rheumatic fever and remains so for 4 to 10 weeks in almost 80% of patients. In a small proportion of patients, it may remain elevated even beyond 12 weeks. Although congestive cardiac failure tends to bring the sedimentation rate down toward normal, it is unlikely that a patient of acute rheumatic fever in congestive cardiac failure will have a normal sedimentation rate. C-reactive protein is increased in all patients of acute rheumatic fever. It subsides rapidly, if the patient is on steroids. While absence of C-reactive protein is strongly against the diagnosis of acute rheumatic fever, its presence is non-specific.

*Prolonged PR interval in the electrocardiogram:* Prolonged PR interval is a not diagnostic criterion since it can get prolonged in many infections. It is also not diagnostic of carditis. Higher grades of block like second degree atrioventricular block especially of the Wenckebach type may also be seen. Complete atrioventricular block is extremely rare.

### Essential Criteria

These include evidences of recent streptococcal infection. The commonest in use is the antistreptolysin'O' titer (ASO). Elevated levels of ASO only indicate previous streptococcal infection and not rheumatic fever. Although generally the higher the level the more likely one can conclude a recent streptococcal infection, lower levels considered "normal" do not necessarily exclude a recent streptococcal infection. If the basal ASO titer of an individual is 50 units and it goes up to 250 units, it is indicative of recent streptococcal infection. Rising titer of ASO is a strong evidence for a recent streptococcal infection.

Positive throat culture for streptococci is relatively uncommon, when a patient presents with acute rheumatic fever. Positive throat culture can also not be equated with the diagnosis of rheumatic fever. Positive throat culture means that streptococci are present in the throat. The patient may or may not have rheumatic fever.

The third feature suggestive for the diagnosis of recent streptococcal infection is the presence of residua of scarlet fever. The desquamation of skin of palms and soles indicates that the patient has had scarlet fever within the previous 2 weeks. Scarlet fever is rare in India.

*Echocardiography:* The most recent revision of Jones criteria now includes echocardiographic findings for the diagnosis of carditis. This is a sensitive investigation for diagnosis of rheumatic carditis. The features indicative of rheumatic carditis consist of annular dilatation, elongation of the chordae to the anterior leaflet of the mitral valve causing a prolapse and lack of coaptation of the two leaflets resulting in mitral regurgitation. There is focal nodular thickening of the tips of the mitral leaflets, which do not have an independent chaotic movement seen with infective endocarditis. In addition, there is variable degree of increase in the left atrial and ventricular size. Involvement of the aortic valve is recognized as aortic regurgitation. Occasionally, the leaflet tip of the mitral valve becomes flail during an episode of rheumatic fever because of chordal rupture resulting in severe mitral regurgitation.

Echocardiography has improved recognition of the presence of carditis, which at times is not possible clinically by auscultation. This has lead to the recognition of the entity of subclinical carditis in which although there are no clinical findings to suggest mitral regurgitation, the echocardiographic findings indicate mitral regurgitation. While the course of patients with subclinical carditis is not clear, long-term penicillin prophylaxis is recommended. Recently, it has been demonstrated that prophylactic long-acting penicillin prevents the progression of subclinical RHD.

### Treatment

Management is symptomatic combined with suppressive therapy.

*Bed rest:* Bed rest is generally recommended for acute rheumatic fever. Prolonged bed rest (>2–3 weeks) is seldom necessary unless there is clinically apparent carditis with heart failure.

*Penicillin:* After obtaining throat cultures, the patient should receive penicillin. A single injection of benzathine penicillin can be administered when the diagnosis of rheumatic fever is made. Penicillin V (250 mg four times a day for 10 days) is another alternative; Azythromycin can be administered for those with penicillin allergy.

*Suppressive therapy:* Aspirin or steroids are given as suppressive therapy. Since untreated rheumatic fever subsides in 12 weeks in 80% of the patients, either of the two suppressive agents is given for 12 weeks. Steroids are a more potent suppressive agent as compared to aspirin. However, there is no proof that the use of steroids results in less cardiac damage as compared to aspirin. A number of observations indicate that steroids act faster and are superior at least in the initial phases. Pericardial friction rub tends to disappear within 3 to 5 days after starting the steroids and a new friction rub does not appear. Subcutaneous nodules tend to disappear faster with the use of steroids as compared to aspirin. Patients who have carditis with congestive cardiac failure have a higher mortality, if aspirin is used compared to steroids. In selecting the medication, the following guidelines are followed:

- Carditis with congestive cardiac failure: Use steroids
- Carditis without congestive cardiac failure: One may use either steroids or aspirin, however, steroids are often preferred.
- If the patient does not have carditis, it is preferable to use aspirin.

The total duration of course for the suppressive agent, aspirin or steroids, is 12 weeks. Aspirin is given at a dose of 90–120 mg/kg/day (in 4 divided doses) for 10 weeks, and then tapered in the next two weeks. Alternatively, prednisolone (2 mg/kg daily; maximum dose 60 mg) is given for three weeks and then tapered gradually in next 9 weeks. The management of congestive cardiac failure is based on principles discussed above.

Surgical replacement of the mitral and/or aortic valve is sometimes indicated, if the patient is deteriorating despite aggressive decongestive measures. Acute hemodynamic overload due to mitral or aortic regurgitation is the main cause of mortality due to rheumatic fever.

*Management of chorea:* The patient as well as the parents should be reassured and told about the self-limiting course of the disease. The signs and symptoms of chorea do not respond well to anti-inflammatory agents or steroids. Supportive measures such as rest in a quiet room and medications such as pimozide, haloperidol, diazepam and carbamazepine are effective.

### Prevention of Rheumatic Fever

*Primary prevention* requires identification of streptococcal sore throat and its treatment with penicillin. For primary prevention, it is necessary to educate the community regarding the consequences of streptococcal sore throat. Logistically, it is difficult since it requires: (i) Identification of sore throat that is dependent on education of parents, (ii) rapidly confirming that sore throat is streptococcal: requires availability of microbiological facilities; and (iii) medical help and availability of penicillin. Data from recent epidemics of rheumatic fever indicates that anywhere from 30 to 80% of sore throats resulting in rheumatic fever can be asymptomatic. Because asymptomatic streptococcal pharyngitis can result in rheumatic fever, primary prevention can only be possible by using an anti-streptococcal vaccine, which is not available.

*Secondary prevention* consists of giving long-acting benzathine penicillin. The dose is 1.2 million units once every 3 weeks or 0.6 million units every alternate week. The injection is painful and since some patients get fever for 24 to 36 hr following the injection, it is preferable to give the injection on a weekend to avoid school absence. While the responsibility of continuing penicillin prophylaxis is on parents, the physician should explain the seriousness of the problem and the need for prolonged treatment (Table 16.17).

*Duration of secondary prophylaxis:* Recommendations of the WHO are widely accepted. Patient without proven carditis should receive prophylaxis for 5 years after the last episode, or until they are 18-year-old (whichever is longer). Patient with carditis (mild mitral regurgitation or healed carditis) should receive prophylaxis for 10 years after the last episode, or at least until they are 25-year-old (whichever is longer). Patients with established RHD disease or following valve surgery or balloon mitral valvotomy should receive lifelong prophylaxis or at least until the age of 40 after which recurrence of RF is rare.

**Table 16.17:** Secondary prophylaxis following an episode of rheumatic fever

| *Antibiotic* | *Mode of administration, dose* |
|---|---|
| Benzathine penicillin | Single intramuscular injection every 3 to 4 weeks*, 1200 000 units for patients >30 kg; and 600 000 units for <30 kg |
| Penicillin V | 250 mg orally twice daily |

*In high prevalence regions, 3 wk injections are recommended for prophylaxis, in patients >30 kg and often every 2 weeks in patients <30 kg

## Rheumatic Heart Disease

The sequelae of rheumatic fever consist of mitral, aortic and tricuspid valve disease. Mitral valve involvement manifests predominantly as mitral regurgitation (MR) and less commonly as mitral stenosis (MS). Aortic valve and tricuspid valve involvement presents as aortic (AR) and tricuspid regurgitation (TR), respectively. Rheumatic aortic stenosis (AS) is very rare in childhood or adolescence.

## Mitral Regurgitation

Mitral regurgitation (MR) is the commonest manifestation of acute as well as previous rheumatic carditis. In our study of 850 patients of RHD below the age of 12 years, 750 had pure or dominant MR.

### *Hemodynamics*

Mitral regurgitation results in a systolic leak of blood to the left atrium. The regurgitant volume of blood reaches the left atrium during ventricular systole at almost systolic pressure. However, during diastole, it can pass freely across the mitral valve. Thus, although the left atrial pressure increases during systole, it drops during diastole. The mean left atrial pressure, therefore, stays normal or is only slightly increased. There is thus only a minimal increase in pulmonary venous pressure and no pulmonary congestion unless MR happens acutely over a short period. The increased volume of blood handled by the left atrium and left ventricle results in an increase in the size of both these chambers. Mitral regurgitation provides two exits for the left ventricular blood—the forward flow through the aortic valve into the systemic circulation and the backward leak into the left atrium. The forward output becomes insufficient during exertion. This decrease in the systemic output results in fatigue, the commonest symptom of significant MR. Absence of pulmonary congestion prevents occurrence of dyspnea unless the MR is severe or the left ventricular myocardium is failing. With failing left ventricle, the left ventricular diastolic pressure increases, the left atrial and pulmonary venous pressures increase and pulmonary congestion appears. There is an increase in pulmonary arterial pressure and features of pulmonary arterial hypertension appear. Thus presence of features of pulmonary arterial hypertension in a patient having pure MR suggests (i) severe MR or (ii) failing left ventricular myocardium.

MR developing during acute rheumatic fever is of sudden onset. It results in an acute hemodynamic overload over the left ventricle. The features of left ventricular failure can occur even with relatively moderate leaks during the acute illness. The size of the left atrium also plays a significant role in MR. With acute MR, the left atrial size is normal and the increased volume reaching the left atrium increases the left atrial and the pulmonary venous pressure, resulting in pulmonary congestion and features of left ventricular failure. With long-standing MR the left atrium increases in size to accommodate the regurgitant volume without increasing the left atrial pressure and features of left ventricular failure are absent. Another important adjustment consists of decrease in the systemic vascular resistance to help increase the forward flow. The maximum ejection of blood into the aorta takes place during early systole. The combination of these two factors results in an increased systolic and decreased diastolic pressure in the systemic circuit. The pulse pressure is, therefore, mildly increased in MR.

### *Clinical Features*

The resting pulse rate is increased to maintain an adequate cardiac output. In absence of pulmonary congestion the respiratory rate is normal. Features of left ventricular failure are often absent and appear late unless the MR is acute, severe or left ventricular myocardium is failing. The heart size is dependent on the severity of MR as well as the status of the left ventricular myocardium. The cardiac apex is displaced downward and outward with forcible apex and hyperkinetic precordium. Less than 10% of patients have a systolic thrill because of posterior direction of the regurgitant stream. The first sound may be soft as it is masked by the systolic murmur. The second sound is normally split with mild MR. With moderate or severe MR, the second sound is widely and variably split. The wide split is due to an early aortic component of the second sound. With failing left ventricle, the wide splitting disappears. Except with very mild MR, a third sound is audible at the apex and indicates increased early rapid filling of the left ventricle. With severe MR, a delayed diastolic mitral murmur starting with the third sound is audible. The delayed diastolic murmur is secondary to a large flow across the mitral valve during diastole. In pure MR, the delayed diastolic murmur always ends somewhere in mid-diastole and there is no late diastolic (presystolic) accentuation. The classical diagnostic sign is the pansystolic murmur, best heard at the apex and widely radiating to the axilla and back as well as to the left sternal border **(Fig. 16.43)**.

The electrocardiogram shows sinus tachycardia and a normal axis. Signs of left ventricular hypertrophy may be present with long-standing and severe MR. The thoracic roentgenogram shows cardiac enlargement secondary to left ventricular enlargement, the size depending on the severity of MR. Left atrial enlargement may be inferred from the elevation of left bronchus. In the absence of left ventricular failure, there is absence of prominence of pulmonary veins as well as features of pulmonary congestion. Echocardiogram shows enlarged left atrium and ventricle. The specific findings of pathology of mitral valve affliction can be demonstrated vividly by two-dimensional and three-dimensional echocardiography, and this is essential to plan treatment. Color Doppler can quantify MR non-invasively **(Fig. 16.44)**.

### *Differential Diagnosis*

Other causes of MR in childhood include: (i) Atrial septal defect of the primum variety; (ii) coarctation of the aorta with MR (congenital); (iii) left ventricular fibroelastosis; (iv) congenital corrected transposition of great arteries; (v) papillary muscle dysfunction in dilatation of left ventricle from any cause including myocarditis; (vi) atrial septal defect of the secundum type with floppy mitral valve; (vii) Marfan and Hurler syndrome,

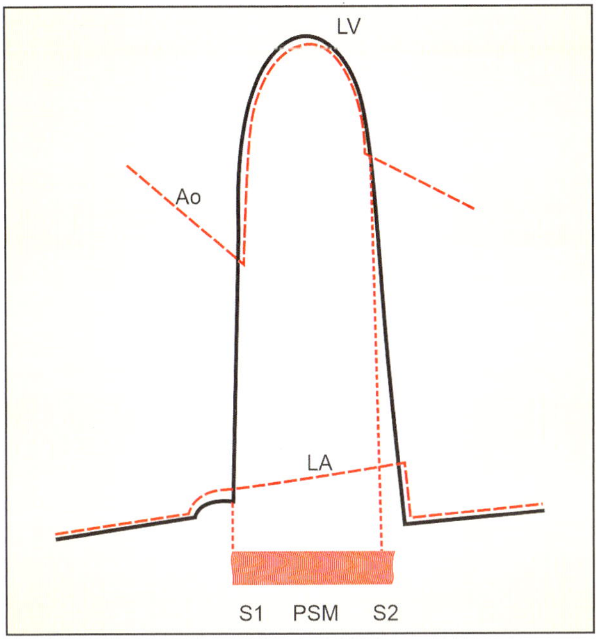


**Fig. 16.43:** The characteristic pansystolic murmur. As the left ventricular (LV) pressure exceeds the left atrial pressure (LA), the first sound (S1) occurs. However, the murmur of mitral regurgitation will also start at the same time masking the S1. Since the maximum difference in the LV and LA pressure is quickly reached and maintained throughout systole, the murmur maintains the same intensity throughout systole appearing pansystolic. Finally as the LV pressure drops below the aortic (Ao) pressure, A2 occurs. The LV pressure is higher than LA pressure at this time and the murmur goes beyond, A2 thus masking both the S1 and A2. PSM pansystolic murmur

and (viii) anomalous origin of left coronary artery from pulmonary artery.

### *Treatment*

Mild to moderate MR is well tolerated for long periods. However, its severity increases with time. Medical management consists of the use of digitalis and diuretics besides penicillin prophylaxis for prevention of recurrences. The role of systemic vasodilators, most commonly ACE inhibitors and calcium channel blockers, to reduce afterload in isolated MR and aortic regurgitation is controversial. An important additional consideration in RHD is the presence of varying degrees of mitral stenosis that accompanies MR.

There are no clear guidelines for the timing of mitral valve surgery (particularly replacement) in children. The natural history of MR is quite different in children and standard guidelines for mitral valve surgery in adults might not apply to children. Persistent symptoms, in spite of maximally tolerated medications, warrant consideration of surgery especially in the presence of pulmonary artery hypertension. For an asymptomatic child, evidence of even the slightest ventricular dysfunction merits consideration for surgery. The treatment of choice is mitral valve repair. Prosthetic valve replacement is reserved for those situations where the valve is deemed unsuitable for repair. It is necessary to emphasize that valve replacement is not a cure and patients need to receive anticoagulants on the long-term, which is a significant challenge in young children.

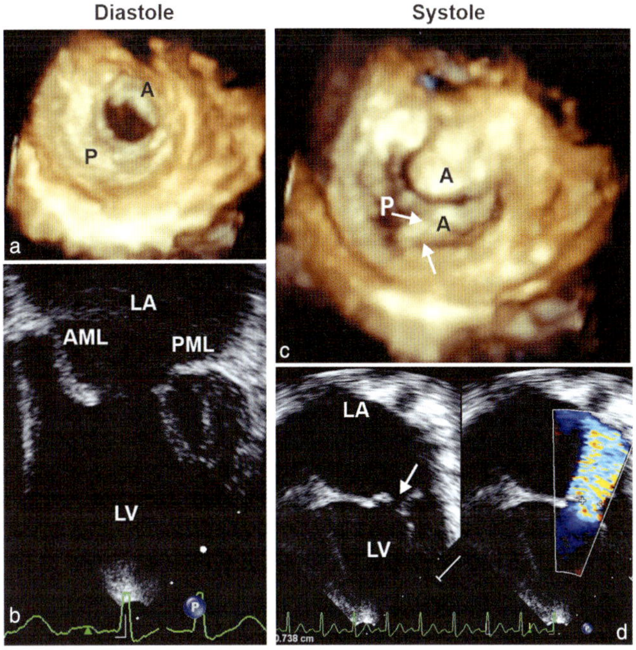


**Fig. 16.44:** Rheumatic mitral valve disease with mitral stenosis and regurgitation. These frames are from a 10-yr-old child with rheumatic heart disease with severe affliction of the mitral valve. Although the predominant lesion is mitral regurgitation, there is also some mitral stenosis. Three-dimensional (3D) echocardiograms are shown in the upper panel and equivalent two-dimensional frames obtained from apical four-chamber views are in the lower panel; (a) The diastolic frame in the 3D image shows the mitral valve from its left atrial aspect. Note that the leaflet substance is seen in diastole; (b) Equivalent diastolic frame on 2D shows several features rheumatic affliction. The anterior mitral leaflet (AML) is thickened. The tip of the AML is oriented horizontally and does not point downwards suggesting restriction of mobility of diastolic motion. The posterior mitral leaflet (PML) is also thickened and mobility is restricted to a greater degree. The chordae tendinae beneath the PML are visibly thickened; (c) During systole, the PML stays in a relatively fixed position. The free edge of the AML moves to a position above the optimal zone of coaptation between the two leaflets. The resultant regurgitation orifice is shown by white arrows in both the 3D and 2D frames. This orifice is typically crescentic and extends along the length of the AML; (d) The resultant color Doppler jet of mitral regurgitation is directed posteriorly and laterally

## Rheumatic Mitral Stenosis (MS)

Rheumatic MS is less common than MR in children. Juvenile MS (<18 yr) is typically seen in regions with high prevalence of RHD.

### *Hemodynamics* (Fig. 16.45)

MS results in obstruction to flow of blood across the mitral valve during left ventricular diastole. The left atrium compensates for this obstruction by increasing its pressure. This increase in pressure results in hypertrophy of the left atrial wall. Unfortunately, the left atrium is a thin-walled chamber and the capacity for hypertrophy of the left atrial wall is limited. The increase in left atrial pressure maintains blood flow across the mitral valve. The increased left atrial pressure is transmitted to pulmonary veins and results in pulmonary capillary engorgement and pulmonary

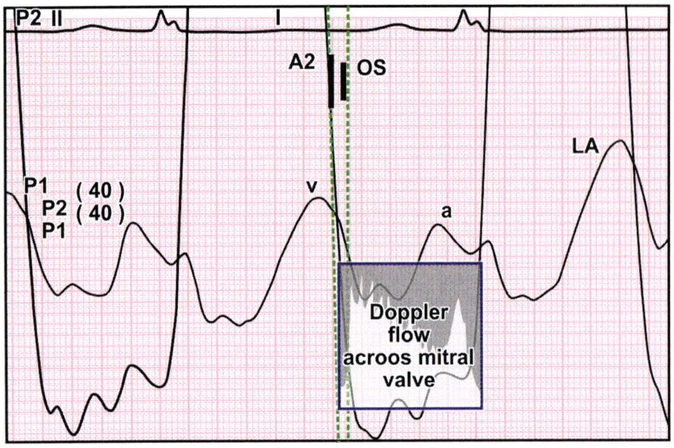


Fig. 16.45: Hemodynamics of mitral valve stenosis: A cardiac catheterization tracing with simultaneous recording of left atrial (LA) with 'a' and 'v' waves and left ventricular (LV) waveforms is shown. A continuous wave Doppler record is superimposed during diastole; note the two peaks in flow acceleration-the second peak coincides with pre-systolic accentuation. The flow patterns reflect the pressure gradients across the mitral valve in diastole. A2 aortic component of second heart sound; OS opening snap

congestion, which produces dyspnea, the commonest symptom of MS. The pulmonary arterial pressure increases to maintain forward flow from the pulmonary artery to the left side of the heart. In the absence of tricuspid regurgitation, the right ventricular hypertrophy is concentric without an increase in the size of right ventricular chamber. The heart size usually stays normal.

With mild or moderate MS, the forward flow through the mitral valve remains normal. With severe obstruction, the forward flow is diminished with reduced cardiac output resulting in a small volume pulse and cold extremities.

### Clinical Features

Boys are twice as commonly affected as girls in the age group up to 12 yr. Juvenile rheumatic MS has been described in children as young as 5 years and is now largely limited to high RHD prevalence regions. Patients with MS give history of shortness of breath on exertion or even at rest depending on the severity. Other important symptoms consist of cough, hemoptysis, paroxysmal nocturnal dyspnea, attacks of acute pulmonary edema and atypical angina. On examination, the pulse volume is small. Depending on the severity, there may or may not be signs of right-sided congestion, in the form of engorged neck veins and enlarged tender liver. The liver may have systolic pulsations, if there is associated tricuspid regurgitation; the jugular venous pulse shows prominent 'a' waves. If tricuspid regurgitation is present, the jugular veins show dominant 'V waves. With moderate or severe MS, signs of pulmonary congestion in the form of rales are present.

Examination of the precordium reveals a normal sized heart with a palpable first heart sound, parasternal impulse and an apical diastolic thrill. The second sound may be palpable at the second left interspace. On auscultation, the first sound is accentuated, the second sound normally split with a loud pulmonary component. An opening snap of the mitral valve is best audible just medial to the apex. The delayed diastolic mitral murmur starts immediately following the opening snap, diminishes somewhat in intensity during mid-diastole and accentuates again at the end of diastole. The late diastolic accentuation is always present in the presence of MS. Absence of late diastolic accentuation of murmur is against the diagnosis of dominant MS.

The electrocardiogram shows right axis deviation with right ventricular hypertrophy. In addition, there is evidence for P mitrale. Thoracic roentgenogram shows a normal sized heart with features of pulmonary venous and arterial hypertension, as well as left atrial enlargement. Echocardiogram shows decreased movement of the anterior leaflet, paradoxical posterior leaflet motion, left atrial enlargement and pulmonary arterial hypertension. 2D echo can identify the narrowed mitral opening and accurately quantify the mitral valve area. Doppler echo provides accurate information on transmitral gradient.

*Assessment of severity:* The minimum criteria for the clinical diagnosis of MS are accentuated first sound, the mitral opening snap and delayed diastolic murmur with late diastolic accentuation. The closer the openings snap to the second sound, the more severe the mitral obstruction. The intensity or the duration of the diastolic murmur does not correlate with the severity since mild as well as severe MS may result in very soft murmurs. The duration of the murmur depends on the heart rate. Severe pulmonary arterial hypertension can occur only with severe mitral obstruction. Echocardiogram (determination of cross-sectional area) combined with Doppler gradient gives more precise assessment of severity. Atrial fibrillation is rare in the pediatric age group.

### Differential Diagnosis

Very few conditions can be considered in the differential diagnosis in children. Isolated congenital MS is uncommon. The opening snap is unusual in congenital MS. Cor triatriatum, obstruction of individual pulmonary veins and left atrial myxoma should be considered in the differential diagnosis.

### Treatment

The management of MS is essentially catheter based or surgical. Beta blockers or digoxin work equally well by reducing resting and exercise heart rates thereby improving diastolic filling. Diuretics help by reducing pulmonary venous congestion. Balloon mitral valvotomy (BMV), also known as percutaneous trans-septal mitral commissurotomy (PTMC) has largely replaced closed or open mitral commissurotomy for MS in children. Improvement in mitral valve area following these procedures largely results from splitting of the fused commissures. The subvalvar pathologic abnormalities of MS remain after valvotomy, so the mitral valve area does not normalize. The balloon, introduced through the femoral vein is passed through the atrial septum, positioned in the mitral valve and inflated to open the stenotic valve.

Long-term follow-up after valvotomy is mandatory because of significant risk of restenosis with time. Restenosis is typically associated with significant residual MS following balloon mitral valvotomy. A repeat procedure is an option for restenosis and helps postpone mitral valve surgery. Closed mitral valvotomy (CMV) is an inexpensive and equally effective surgical alternative to BMV but is seldom performed today.

### Aortic Regurgitation (AR)

Aortic valve involvement in RHD results in AR. Clinically pure AR, without associated mitral valve disease, is rare and occurs in 5 to 8% patients. Pathologically, pure rheumatic aortic valve disease is almost unknown.

#### *Hemodynamics*

AR is a backward leak from the aorta into the left ventricle during diastole. This increases the volume of blood reaching the left ventricle. The left ventricle increases in size to accommodate the extra volume. The size of the left ventricle is thus directly related to the degree of aortic leak, unless there is myocardial disease. Because of the backward flow of blood, the forward flow is impaired. This is compensated by peripheral vasodilatation as well as increased ejection from the left ventricle during early part of the systole. However, significant AR results in low forward output. Signs of wide pulse pressure in the form of exaggerated arterial and arteriolar pulsations are present unless the AR is mild. Slowing of heart rate increases the diastolic period and increases the regurgitant volume of blood in AR. With good left ventricular myocardial function, even moderate AR is tolerated well for long periods. If the left ventricular myocardium is failing, the left ventricular diastolic pressure goes up and results in an increase in left atrial pressure and pulmonary congestion.

#### *Clinical Features*

Aortic valve disease is more common in boys compared to girls. The main symptom is palpitation, related to the large stroke volume. With mild to moderate AR, the forward flow can be raised effectively on exercise. Thus fatigue is not an early symptom.

The pulse pressure is wide. The wider the pulse pressure, the more severe the aortic leak. The diastolic blood pressure may be recorded as zero with severe AR. Prominent carotid pulsations (*Corrigan sign*), visible arterial pulsations over extremity vessels (*dancing peripheral arteries*) and visible pulsations of the abdominal aorta are evidences of wide pulse pressure from any cause. Holding the middle of the forearm or leg and elevating it, discloses a sharply rising and abruptly falling pulse (*Corrigan pulse* or *water hammer pulse*). Nodding of head may be present with each systole (*de Musset sign*) due to sudden filling of carotid vessels in severe AR. Arteriolar pulsations may be seen over the nail bed, uvula, lips, ear lobes and in the eye grounds. There is also exaggeration of the systolic pressure difference between the brachial and femoral arteries (*Hill sign*). Normally, the difference between the pressures in brachial artery and femoral artery is less than 20 mm Hg, the femoral systolic pressure being higher. Systolic pressure difference between 20 to 40 mm Hg suggests mild AR, 40 to 60 mm Hg moderate AR, and more than 60 mm Hg severe AR. If a stethoscope is put over the brachial or the femoral artery without applying pressure, *pistol shot sounds* may be heard in severe AR. A systolic murmur may be heard, if pressure is applied to partially occlude the artery proximal to the chest piece, and diastolic murmur if pressure is applied distally; the combination of systolic and diastolic murmurs is the *Duroziez sign*.

The apex is displaced downward and outward and is forcible or heaving. A diastolic thrill is unusual. The first sound is soft and the aortic component of the second sound may be audible or may be masked by the regurgitant diastolic murmur. The murmur of AR is a high-pitched, decrescendo diastolic murmur starting with the aortic component of the second sound. The intensity and the length of the murmur do not correlate with the severity of AR. The murmur is heard along the left sternal border and may radiate to the apex. With large aortic leaks, there is also an ejection systolic murmur at the second right interspace, conducted to the neck and not infrequently associated with a systolic thrill. The systolic murmur is the result of a large stroke volume, passing across rough valves. It does not indicate aortic stenosis, if the pulse pressure is wide and the carotid upstroke is brisk.

The electrocardiogram shows increase in left ventricular voltages with deep S waves in V1 and tall R waves in V6. There are also deep Q waves in left chest leads accompanied with tall T waves; this is called diastolic overload pattern of the left ventricle. The thoracic roentgenogram shows cardiac enlargement of the left ventricular type and dilated ascending aorta. Echocardiogram identifies enlarged left ventricle, dilated aorta and flutter of anterior mitral leaflet. Doppler echo can quantitate the severity of AR.

#### *Differential Diagnosis*

The differential diagnosis of rheumatic AR includes two sets of conditions: (i) *Conditions associated with a wide pulse pressure* like patent ductus arteriosus, arteriovenous fistulae, ventricular septal defect with AR, ruptured sinus of Valsalva, anemia and thyrotoxicosis, and (ii) *conditions associated with a non-rheumatic regurgitant diastolic murmur* like pulmonary regurgitation, AR with ventricular septal defect, ruptured sinus of Valsalva and congenital aortic valve disease. As a rule, congenital aortic valve disease is either a leaking bicuspid aortic valve or aortic stenosis. Pure congenital AR is extremely rare. Other conditions that may result in AR include Marfan syndrome, Hurler syndrome and Takayasu aortoarteritis.

#### *Management*

Mild to moderate AR is well tolerated for years. Significant AR, if associated with either chest pain or left ventricular failure, should be treated surgically. Surgical treatment consists of aortic valve replacement either by homograft or prosthetic valve; valve repair is not feasible for rheumatic AR. Better surgical results are obtained before onset of significant ventricular dysfunction.

Patients planned for valve replacement should be screened for: (i) Rheumatic activity; (ii) ability of the patient and the family to monitor lifelong anticoagulation. Aortic valve replacement has fewer long-term complications when compared to mitral valve replacement.

### Tricuspid Regurgitation (TR)

Features indicative of TR are seen in 20 to 50% patients of RHD in children in our country. It is often difficult to determine whether TR is organic (due to involvement of the tricuspid valve by the rheumatic process) or functional (due to pulmonary hypertension).

#### *Hemodynamics and Clinical Features*



TR results in a systolic backflow of blood from the right ventricle to the right atrium. The systolic leak thus results in a systolic murmur and a volume load of the right atrium as well as the right ventricle. Most patients who have TR also have features of pulmonary arterial hypertension. The systolic backflow under pressure results in a prominent systolic wave, the V wave, in the jugular venous pulse as well as the liver. Both the systolic as well as the diastolic murmurs at the tricuspid valve become louder during inspiration. In patients of rheumatic heart disease, the TR may be associated either with MS or with MR.



There are no specific symptoms of TR. It is possible that with onset of TR the dyspnea may be relieved to some extent in patients of MS. The patients may give history of pain in right hypochondrium due to a congested liver and of fatigue due to a decrease in systemic output. In addition to features of TR, there are signs of pulmonary arterial hypertension and those of mitral valve disease. In association with MS, severe TR may result in marked dilatation of the right ventricle and the whole of the anterior surface, including the apex may be formed by the right ventricle. Patients of TR of this severity almost always show severe right ventricular hypertrophy in the electrocardiogram. Echocardiography and color Doppler can document and identify the nature (organic vs. functional) and quantitate severity of TR.

#### *Management*

Decongestive measures will help in reducing the severity of TR. Further management depends on the associated mitral valve lesion. TR may resolve following mitral valvotomy. In those patients undergoing surgery for the MR, the tricuspid valve can be inspected and tricuspid annuloplasty or repair performed, if needed.

### Clinical Problems in Patients with Rheumatic Heart Disease

Two major problems that clinicians face in patients of RHD are discussed below.

#### *Active or Inactive Rheumatic Fever?*

A lot of 'judgment' or personal bias is generally involved in this decision. For the diagnosis of activity, one has to fall back on the Jones criteria. Presence of cardiac involvement cannot be used as a major criterion since the carditis may be the result of a previous attack of rheumatic fever. However, presence of a pericardial friction rub is evidence of active carditis. If the patient has well documented cardiac findings, then the appearance of a new murmur or a significant increase in a pre-existing murmur is very suggestive for active rheumatic fever. History of arthralgia or arthritis within a period of less than 12 weeks is suggestive of active rheumatic fever, specially if associated with elevated sedimentation rate and ASO titer. Despite congestive cardiac failure, it is unusual for the sedimentation rate to be normal in a patient of active rheumatic fever. All patients of RHD should show elevated ASO titer before they can be labeled as active rheumatic fever. The difficulty arises in those patients who have relatively low levels of the ASO titer. In such cases, unless serial serum samples are available, it is difficult to decide whether there is rise in level of ASO titer.

#### *In a Febrile Patient, Is it Active Rheumatic Fever or Infective Endocarditis?*

At times separation of rheumatic activity from infective endocarditis can be very difficult. The arguments used above for separating active from inactive rheumatic fever can be used for diagnosis of active rheumatic fever. A detailed description of endocarditis follows.

### Suggested Reading


1. Bland EF, Jones TD. Rheumatic fever and rheumatic heart disease. A twenty year report on 1000 patients followed since childhood. Circulation 1951; 42:836.
2. Dougherty S, Mayosi B, Carapetis J, Wilson N. Acute rheumatic fever and rheumatic heart disease. Elsevier, 2020.
3. Gewitz MH, Baltimore RS, Tani LY, et al; on behalf of the American Heart Association Committee on Rheumatic Fever, Endocarditis, and Kawasaki Disease. Revision of the Jones criteria for the diagnosis of acute rheumatic fever in the era of Doppler echocardiography: A scientific statement from the American Heart Association. Circulation 2015;131:1806–18.
4. Kumar RK, Antunes MJ, Beaton A, et al; American Heart Association Council on Lifelong Congenital Heart Disease and Heart Health in the Young. Contemporary diagnosis and management of rheumatic heart disease. A scientific statement from the American Heart Association. Circulation 2020;142: e337–57.


*Competencies:* **PE23.6; PE23.13; PE23.15**

## INFECTIVE ENDOCARDITIS

Infection of the endocardial lining of the heart is called infective endocarditis, and may involve the endocardium of the valves, the mural endocardium or the endothelium of blood vessels (infective endarteritis). The commonest site of infection is a diseased valve from where the infection can spread along the endothelium.

### Etiopathogenesis

Infective endocarditis (IE) predominantly occurs in a diseased heart. The commonest substrate is a damaged endothelium or endocardium resulting from contact with a high velocity jet together with the presence of a significant bacteremia. Endocarditis can occur following a surgical shunt as in Blalock-Taussig shunt. Other congenital lesions, associated with endocarditis are VSD, PDA, tetralogy of Fallot, aortic stenosis and mitral regurgitation. Examples of conditions seldom associated with IE include atrial septal defect and isolated pulmonary valve stenosis.

Infective endocarditis occurs over the mitral valve or the aortic valve in patients with rheumatic heart disease. Patients with prosthetic valves or those who have had a recent cardiac operation are also especially prone to endocarditis. Infections anywhere in body like boils or furuncles, tooth abscess, ear infection, urinary tract infection or osteomyelitis may result in endocarditis. Although interventions like dental procedures, genitourinary procedures or bronchoscopy can be followed by IE, it is uncommon to be able to identify the predisposing event. Perhaps the most important preventable cause of endocarditis is poor dental hygiene. Parenteral drug abuse is a frequent cause of right-sided endocarditis involving the normal tricuspid or the pulmonary valve. Occasionally, it can result in mitral and/or aortic valve disease as well.

## Pathogenesis

The pathogenesis of endocarditis depends on the invasiveness and virulence of the infective organisms. The infection generally starts at a jet lesion, where the high-pressure jet strikes the endocardium or the endothelium. The tricuspid valve in membranous VSD, aortic endothelium, coarctation of the aorta, ventricular surface of the aortic valve in AR and subaortic obstruction are the usual sites. Endocarditis results in immune-mediated vasculitis and thrombocytopenia.

Bacteremia resulting from an infection such as a boil, furuncle, otitis media or initiated by an intervention such as cardiac or urinary catheterization or dental extraction is necessary for initiation of endocarditis. Bacteremia may also result from simple events such as brushing teeth. Bacteria that are deposited on the endocardium are covered by fibrin and platelets forming vegetations. Almost any species of bacteria and some species of fungi can cause endocarditis. *Streptococcus viridans*, *S. aureus*, enterococci, *P. aeruginosa* and some gram negative bacilli are responsible for most episodes. Fungal endocarditis typically results in the setting of chronic hospitalization with indwelling central venous catheters.

## Diagnosis

Any fever in a patient with known heart disease raises the question of endocarditis. The minimum criteria for the diagnosis of endocarditis consist of unexplained fever of 7 to 10 days duration in a patient with known heart disease. If this is associated with other clinical manifestations of endocarditis, the diagnosis becomes more likely.

Endocarditis has been subdivided into acute and sub-acute types, depending on whether the patient presented with a chronic illness or as septicemia. Endocarditis is also identified by the infective organism, for example viridans endocarditis, staphylococcal endocarditis and enterococcal endocarditis. *S. viridans* results in the subacute form of illness while *S. aureus* and other pyogenic organisms cause a fulminant (acute) and rapidly progressive illness. It is possible, for an organism like *Staphylococcus* to cause a subacute or acute type of illness. Identification of the organism is necessary, as it helps determine the choice of antibiotics.

### Clinical Features

Infective endocarditis is uncommon below the age of two years. The clinical features of endocarditis may be grouped into those: (i) Indicating the presence of an infection; (ii) indicating involvement of the cardiovascular system; and (iii) indicating the presence of an immunological reaction to infection. The features indicating the presence of infection consist of fever, chills, rigors, night sweats, general malaise, and weakness, loss of appetite, weight loss and amenorrhea in females. Loss of appetite is a very persistent and important symptom. Arthralgia and diffuse myalgia can occur, however, arthritis does not occur except in acute endocarditis as part of septicemia when it is likely to be monoarticular.

Features indicative of the involvement of the cardiovascular system may be absent in the initial stages. Appearances of left or right heart failure, development of a new murmur or change in a pre-existing murmur, presence of embolic episodes to various parts of the body (like stroke from central nervous system embolism, hematuria from renal infarct, left flank pain from splenic infarct, gastrointestinal hemorrhage from mesenteric embolism, etc.) indicate involvement of the cardiovascular system. As damage to the valve tissue occurs, regurgitant lesions appear. These regurgitant lesions, aortic, mitral or tricuspid, progress rapidly causing hemodynamic changes that result in congestive failure.

Features of immunological response presenting as vasculitis consist of arthralgia, myalgia, clubbing, splenomegaly and microscopic hematuria. Splinter hemorrhages are hemorrhagic spots under the nails, though suggestive, are not specific for endocarditis as they can result from minor injuries. Petechiae over the skin or mucous membranes and conjunctiva are seen in about 50% patients. Petechiae in the retina are called Roth spots. Osler nodes are tender erythematous nodules over the pulp of fingertips, but are relatively rare. Janeway lesions are non-tender erythematous patches on the palms and soles. Clubbing and splenomegaly tend to appear 3 weeks after the onset of endocarditis.

In the acute form, the symptoms appear early and progress rapidly with hectic fever, chills and rigors. Perforation of valve cusps may result in appearance of acute regurgitant lesions like acute tricuspid, aortic or mitral regurgitation. With inadequate treatment, the course is downhill and death within 6 weeks from the onset. Metastatic lesions causing abscesses in the central nervous system, spleen, mesentery, bones and joints are common. Metastatic abscesses are rare in subacute endocarditis.

Patients with endocarditis of the right side, such as tricuspid or the pulmonary valve, throw emboli to the lungs. The embolic episodes to lungs may present as repeated episodes of pneumonitis or septic infarcts resulting in lung abscesses. It is more common in patients with indwelling central catheters, intravenous drug abuse and with VSD. Some of these patients remain afebrile for several days at a time and yet have large vegetations and elevated acute phase reactants.

***Postoperative endocarditis:*** Postoperative endocarditis is classified as early (<12 months) and late. Early endocarditis is usually due to pyogenic organisms such as *Staphylococcus*, *Pseudomonas* or gram-negative bacilli introduced at the time of operation. These patients have high fever with chills and rigors and features of septicemia. Late endocarditis is more like native valve endocarditis and the commonest organisms are *S. viridans* and gram-negative bacilli; these patients have a subacute course. Cardiac operations are an important predisposing factor for gram-negative endocarditis. Prosthetic valve endocarditis may also be early or late and behaves as above.

***Fungal endocarditis:*** With extensive use of broad-spectrum antibiotics, yeast and fungal infections occur more frequently than before specially following cardiac operations and in intensive care settings. *Candida* is by far the commonest fungus responsible; others include *Histoplasma*, *Blastomyces*, *Aspergillus*.

***Cryptococcus and Mucor:*** The organism is easily cultured from the peripheral blood. Predisposing factors for fungal endocarditis include intravenous drug abuse, indwelling catheters, intensive antibiotic therapy, prolonged steroid administration, radiation, immunosuppressive therapy and prosthetic valves. Incidence of embolism is higher since the fungal vegetations tend to be very large. Despite intensive therapy, mortality is high.

#### Laboratory Diagnosis

Blood culture is essential for diagnosis. A positive blood culture in a patient with underlying heart disease, suspected to have endocarditis is confirmatory. Three sets of cultures, each containing adequate volumes of blood, taken every half-hour are appropriate and detect 95% cases. The commonest cause for negative cultures is prior antibiotic therapy or unsatisfactory culture technique. Infection with unusual organisms, anerobic organisms and fungi require special media and incubation for 2–3 weeks before declaring that the culture is negative. Arterial sampling does not offer any advantage over venous samples. Other investigations, which provide supportive evidence for the diagnosis, include:

i. Normocytic normochromic anemia
ii. Moderately elevated total leukocyte count
iii. Reduced platelet count
iv. Elevated sedimentation rate and C-reactive protein
v. Microscopic hematuria and albuminuria in more than 95%.

#### Echocardiography

Echocardiography is a valuable diagnostic tool, especially in patients with culture negative endocarditis. The investigation identifies complications like ruptured chordae, perforated cusps and flail cusps resulting from endocarditis. Vegetations more than 2 mm can be identified on echocardiography, but its sensitivity is dependent on the site of involvement. For aortic and mitral valves, the sensitivity is more than 90%, while for tricuspid and pulmonary valves, it is 70%. The presence of vegetations has high negative as well as positive predictive value for confirming the diagnosis of infective endocarditis. However, the procedure is highly operator dependent. Limitations of echocardiography can be overcome by transesophageal echocardiography, especially in patients with prosthetic valve endocarditis and if valve ring abscess is suspected.

### Complications

Damage to valve cusps or perforation, and rupture of chordae tendinae result in acute regurgitant lesions causing hemodynamic deterioration. Migration of vegetations may result in embolic neurological deficit, renal infarcts with hematuria, mesenteric infarct and melena, loss of fingers or toes due to obstruction of blood supply. Damage to the vasa vasorum of blood vessels due to vasculitis may result in the formation of mycotic aneurysms that can rupture and result in massive bleeding. The kidneys suffer from embolic infarct with hematuria and focal or diffuse membranoproliferative glomerulonephritis resulting in albuminuria and microscopic hematuria. The finding of IgG, IgM and complement deposits on the glomerular basement membrane indicate that it is an immune complex nephritis. Renal insufficiency tends to appear beyond three weeks of the onset of endocarditis and is progressive until the endocarditis is cured; hematuria can persist for 3 to 6 months. Even advanced renal insufficiency tends to regress and renal function returns to normal after the endocarditis has been cured.

### Treatment

The main principles in management consist of: (i) Identification of organism and its antibiotic sensitivity; and (ii) prompt, appropriate and prolonged antimicrobial treatment to cure and prevent relapse. If the blood culture is positive, the choice of antibiotics is dictated by the antibiotic sensitivity. If the culture is negative, empirical therapy covering a wide range of organisms is necessary. If the culture is positive, the culture plate should not perhaps be discarded. After starting the antibiotic treatment, patient's serum diluted to 1:8 parts or more should be used to determine if it inhibits the growth of the organism in subculture, to indicate the efficacy of treatment. Common organisms causing endocarditis, antibiotic of choice and duration of treatment is shown in Table 16.18. Over the last 2–3 decades, the threshold for surgery for treatment of endocarditis has been lowered considerably. Surgery is indicated, if response to antibiotics is suboptimal, in presence of large vegetation, damage to valve apparatus with severe or refractory heart failure and for fungal endocarditis.

***Fungal endocarditis:*** Fungal endocarditis is very resistant to treatment. After two to three weeks of appropriate antifungal treatment (amphotericin B), the patient should be operated to remove the fungal mass. Without surgery, fungal endocarditis is almost universally resistant to treatment. The antifungal agents should be continued

**Table 16.18:** Choice of antibiotics and duration of treatment for infective endocarditis

| Organism | Option I | Option II | Duration, weeks |
|---|---|---|---|
| *Streptococcus viridans* | Penicillin, aminoglycoside | Ceftriaxone, aminoglycoside | 4 |
| *Group A streptococci* | Penicillin, aminoglycoside | Ceftriaxone, aminoglycoside | 4 |
| *Streptococcus fecalis* | Ampicillin, aminoglycoside | Vancomycin, aminoglycoside | 4–6 |
| *Staphylococcus aureus* | Cloxacillin/cefazolin, aminoglycoside | Vancomycin, aminoglycoside | 6 |
| *Escherichia coli* | Ceftriaxone, aminoglycoside | Ampicillin, aminoglycoside | 6 |
| *Pseudomonas* spp. | Ticarcillin, aminoglycoside | Meropenem, aminoglycoside | 6 |
| Culture negative | Ampicillin, aminoglycoside | Ampicillin, aminoglycoside | 6 |

The choice of antibiotics should ideally be guided by culture results and organism sensitivity

postoperatively for a minimum period of 6 weeks. Relapse following apparently successful treatment can occur even up to 2 years.

*Culture negative endocarditis:* Patients with culture negative endocarditis need to be treated empirically. The choice of treatment is dictated by circumstances anticipating the most likely organism. If the patient seeks help late and has significant renal insufficiency, the treatment has to be modified.

### Prophylaxis

There have been major changes in the recommendations for prevention of endocarditis patients with congenital heart defects such as ventricular septal defect, bicommissural aortic valve and valvar pulmonary stenosis, do not routinely require prophylaxis. According to the new guidelines of the American Heart Association, since the absolute lifetime risk of endocarditis is small, prophylaxis is only recommended for patients with conditions associated with increased risk of adverse outcome from endocarditis (Table 16.19).

The focus of prophylaxis has shifted from prophylactic antibiotics for a dental procedure to the prevention of dental caries, which reduces the incidence of bacteremia from daily activities and is, therefore, more important. These guidelines need validation in low resource settings where oral hygiene is unsatisfactory and regular dental health screening is not instituted in the majority.

The antibiotic recommendations for those who need prophylaxis are as follows:

*Dental procedures:* Antibiotic prophylaxis is only indicated if the procedure involves breach of the oral mucosa such as tooth extraction, procedures involving manipulation of gingival tissue or the periapical region of teeth. Single dose of amoxicillin is given 50 mg/kg orally 30–60 minutes before the procedure.

**Table 16.19:** Conditions where antibiotic prophylaxis is definitely recommended

| |
|---|
| Prosthetic cardiac valve; prosthetic material used for valve repair |
| Past history of infective endocarditis |
| Uncorrected cyanotic heart disease, palliative shunts and conduits |
| During first 6 months following complete surgical repair of congenital heart disease |
| Repaired congenital heart disease with residual defects at or adjacent to the site of repair |
| Cardiac transplantation recipients with cardiac valvulopathy |

*Respiratory tract:* Antibiotic prophylaxis against *Streptococcus viridans* is recommended for invasive respiratory tract procedures such as incision on the respiratory mucosa (e.g. tonsillectomy, adenoidectomy). A single dose of amoxycillin is adequate here.

*Infected skin or musculoskeletal tissue procedures:* High-risk cardiac patients undergoing surgical procedure that involves infected skin, or musculoskeletal tissue should receive cover for staphylococci and beta-hemolytic streptococci. Vancomycin is recommended for known or suspected methicillin-resistant strains of *S. aureus*.

*Genitourinary and gastrointestinal tract procedures:* Endocarditis prophylaxis is no longer recommended for patients undergoing genitourinary or gastrointestinal tract procedures.

Infective endocarditis is a life-threatening disease with significant mortality and morbidity. The treating physician should advise patients and parents regarding prevention of endocarditis. The maintenance of good oral hygiene is encouraged. Careful attention to prophylaxis on the long-term is useful in preventing relapses.

### Suggested Reading


1. Wilson W, Taubert KA, Gewitz M, et al. Prevention of infective endocarditis. Guidelines from American Heart Association: A guideline from the American Heart Association Rheumatic Fever, Endocarditis, and Kawasaki Disease Committee, Council on Cardiovascular Disease in the Young, and the Council on Clinical Cardiology, Council on Cardiovascular Surgery and Anesthesia. Circulation 2007;116:1736–54.


*Competencies:* **PE23.14; PE23.15**

## MYOCARDIAL DISEASES

### Myocarditis

Myocarditis is usually caused by viral infections. The list of viruses include, echovirus, Coxsackie B, rubella, herpes and influenza viruses. Diphtheritic myocarditis is occasionally noted in South Asia. The presentation may be abrupt, with cardiovascular collapse, or insidious development of heart failure. Arrhythmias and conduction disturbances may be present. Examination shows cardiac enlargement, tachycardia, muffled heart sounds and features of congestive cardiac failure. The electrocardiogram shows low voltages, and nonspecific ST-T changes. Chest X-ray reveals cardiac enlargement with pulmonary venous congestion.

Treatment includes management of congestive failure. Digoxin should be used cautiously, preferably in half to three quarters of the standard dose. Steroids are of uncertain value and perhaps should be avoided in the acute phase of viremia. ACE inhibitors are a useful adjunct to therapy. The utility of IV immunoglobulin infusion is not proven. Advanced heart failure may require admission in an intensive care unit and mechanical ventilation. A variable proportion of children with myocarditis may recover completely, especially if the heart failure is acute and severe.

## Cardiomyopathies

The term cardiomyopathy is an intrinsic disease of the myocardium which is not associated with a structural deformity of the heart. It is considered primary cardiomyopathy when the etiology is unknown, and secondary, if the myocardial disease is attributed to a systemic disease. Myocardial diseases are classified clinically as: (i) dilated, (ii) restrictive, and (iii) hypertrophic type of cardiomyopathy.

A significant proportion of patients have correctable causes of left ventricular dysfunction that mimics dilated cardiomyopathy (Table 16.20). A diagnosis of idiopathic dilated cardiomyopathy can only be made after these causes are excluded.

### *Dilated Cardiomyopathy (DCM)*

Dilated cardiomyopathy is the commonest form of myocardial disease. The onset of cardiac failure may be acute or insidious. Cardiomegaly and S3 gallop are present. Murmur of MR may be present. The patients are prone to embolic phenomena. The electrocardiogram may show nonspecific ST and T changes with or without left ventricular hypertrophy, conduction disturbances, arrhythmias or pseudo-infarction pattern. Chest X-ray shows cardiomegaly with pulmonary venous hypertension. Echocardiogram confirms dilated ventricular cavity without hypertrophy of the free wall of the left ventricle or the septum. The left ventricular contractility is reduced.

Treatment consists of decongestive therapy with vasodilators, especially ACE inhibitors. Beta-blockers control the heart rate, reduce vasoconstriction caused by catecholamines and upgrade beta-receptors. These agents are expected to prevent or retard myocardial damage related to high catecholamine levels. Carvedilol, a beta-blocker with peripheral vasodilator effect, has shown utility in the management of CCF. Though evidence of benefit in children is limited, it should be considered in presence of disproportionate tachycardia. The starting dose is 0.1 mg/kg/day once daily, which is gradually increased up to 0.5 mg/kg/day.

Gradual improvement occurs in a significant proportion of patients. The prognosis for individual patients cannot be predicted and treatment should continue for prolonged periods.

Despite aggressive therapy, about one-third of children with cardiomyopathy continue to deteriorate with time

**Table 16.20:** Correctable causes of left ventricular dysfunction in children

| *Condition* | *Clues to diagnosis* |
|---|---|
| **Congenital cardiovascular diseases** | |
| Anomalous left coronary artery from pulmonary artery | ECG changes of myocardial infarction in I, aVL, V4-6; 2D, Doppler echocardiography |
| Severe coarctation of aorta | Weak femoral pulses; echocardiography |
| Critical aortic stenosis | Auscultation; echocardiography |
| **Acquired cardiovascular diseases** | |
| Takayasu arteritis | Asymmetric pulses, bruit, Doppler, scintigraphy, angiography |
| Tachyarrhythmia | Disproportionate tachycardia |
| Ectopic atrial tachycardia | ECG |
| Permanent junctional re-entrant tachycardia | Esophageal electrophysiology |
| Chronic atrial flutter | |
| Severe hypertension | Blood pressure; fundus examination |
| **Metabolic and nutritional causes** | |
| Hypocalcemia | Setting (newborns; severe hypoparathyroidism); Chvostek, Trousseau signs; prolonged QTc on ECG |
| Infantile beri-beri | Prominent edema, diarrhea and vomiting; documented thiamine deficiency in mother (if breastfed) |
| Carnitine deficiency | Hypoglycemia, congestive heart failure; coma; ventricular hypertrophy; high ammonia, low carnitine |
| Hypophosphatemia | Poorly controlled diabetes; following hyperalimentation, nutritional recovery syndrome; recovery from severe burns; hyperparathyroidism; vitamin D deficiency; hypomagnesemia, Fanconi syndrome; malabsorption |
| Selenium deficiency | Keshan disease (endemic in parts of China); chronic parenteral nutrition, AIDS |

and eventually become refractory. Intermittent (weekly or bi-weekly) dobutamine or levosimendan infusions may be used effectively in some patients. It is important to consider a number of correctable conditions that can masquerade as cardiomyopathy **(Table 16.23)** and correct them.

Clues to presence of these conditions may be obtained from clinical examination, laboratory profile or ECG **(Fig. 16.46)**.

### *Anomalous Left Coronary Artery from Pulmonary Artery (ALCAPA)*

ALCAPA needs specific mention in the context of suspected cardiomyopathy. The diagnosis is likely in a patient with heart failure with or without a murmur suggesting MR and a pattern on electrocardiogram that suggests anterolateral myocardial infarction **(Fig. 16.47)**. Echocardiography shows a large right coronary artery and absence of the origin of left coronary artery from the aorta. The left coronary artery is seen to arise from the pulmonary artery and shows flow in the reverse direction in the left anterior descending artery and the left circumflex artery. This flow reversal results from collateral flow into the left coronary system from the right coronary artery. Angiography is rarely necessary for the diagnosis. The treatment is surgical and requires mobilization and translocating the origin from pulmonary artery to aorta.

### *Restrictive Cardiomyopathy (RCM)*

It is relatively uncommon in children. Restriction to ventricular filling is usually associated with either endomyocardial fibrosis or endocardial fibroelastosis with a normal or smaller than normal left ventricle. Endomyocardial fibrosis was previously endemic in the state of Kerala and is now quite rare anywhere in the country. Pathologically, there is dense fibrosis in the apical and inflow regions of the left and right ventricles. Fibrosis restricts the ventricular filling in diastole. Papillary muscles and chordae may be tethered by the connective tissue, resulting in severe mitral or tricuspid regurgitation.

Patients with predominant left-sided involvement have symptoms of dyspnea, orthopnea, and embolic phenomena. On examination, there is cardiomegaly with or without findings of MR. Cardiac output is low and there are features of pulmonary venous and arterial hypertension. With predominant right-sided involvement, patients present with fatigue, pedal edema and ascites. There is cardiomegaly with prominent cardiac pulsations in the second, third and fourth left interspace from a dilated right ventricular outflow. S3 gallop and tricuspid regurgitation murmur may be present. The electrocardiogram and chest X-ray do not show specific changes. Treatment consists of decongestive therapy. Decortication or stripping of the endocardium with mitral valve replacement has been tried with very limited success.

Restrictive cardiomyopathy of other uncommon varieties is characterized by a combination of features of left and right-sided failure with a normal sized heart. Clinically, or even following cardiac catheterization, it may be difficult to distinguish it from constrictive pericarditis. However, children with restrictive cardiomyopathy tend to have dominant left-sided involvement and disproportionate pulmonary hypertension. Echocardiogram can be useful in excluding constrictive pericarditis. Treatment is often supportive with diuretics and prognosis is poor without transplantation.

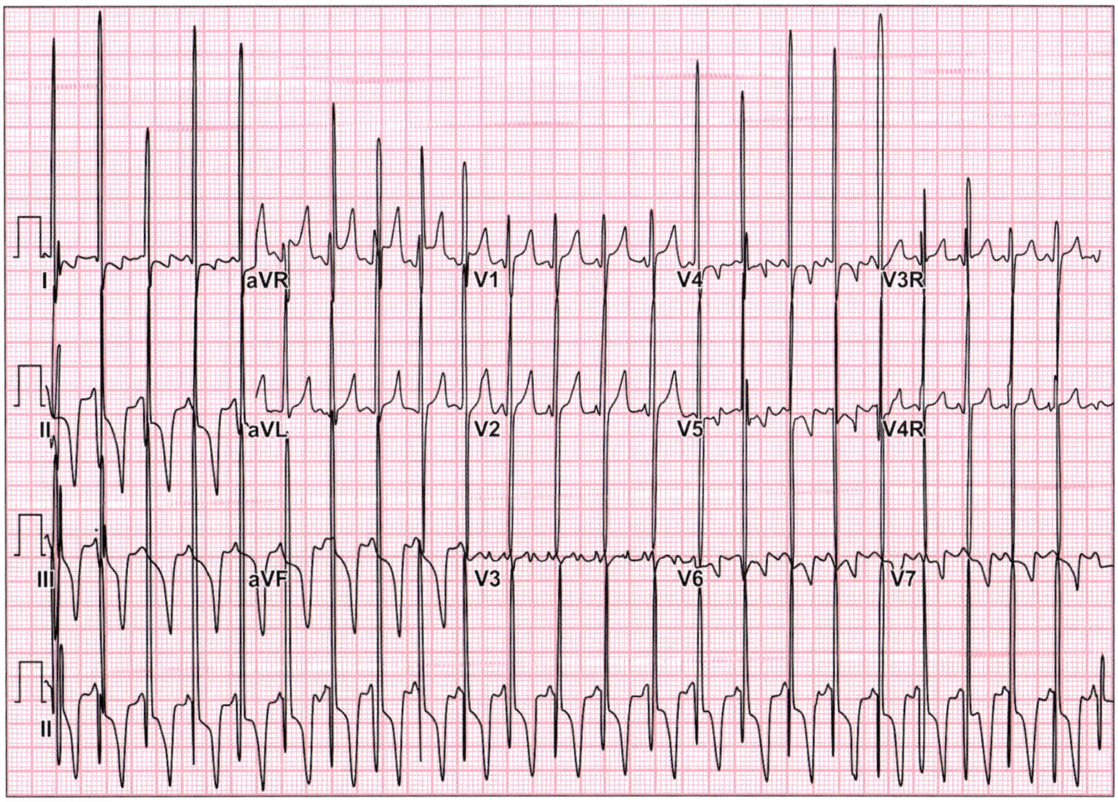


**Fig. 16.46:** Pompe disease; Note the characteristically tall QRS voltages and very short PR interval

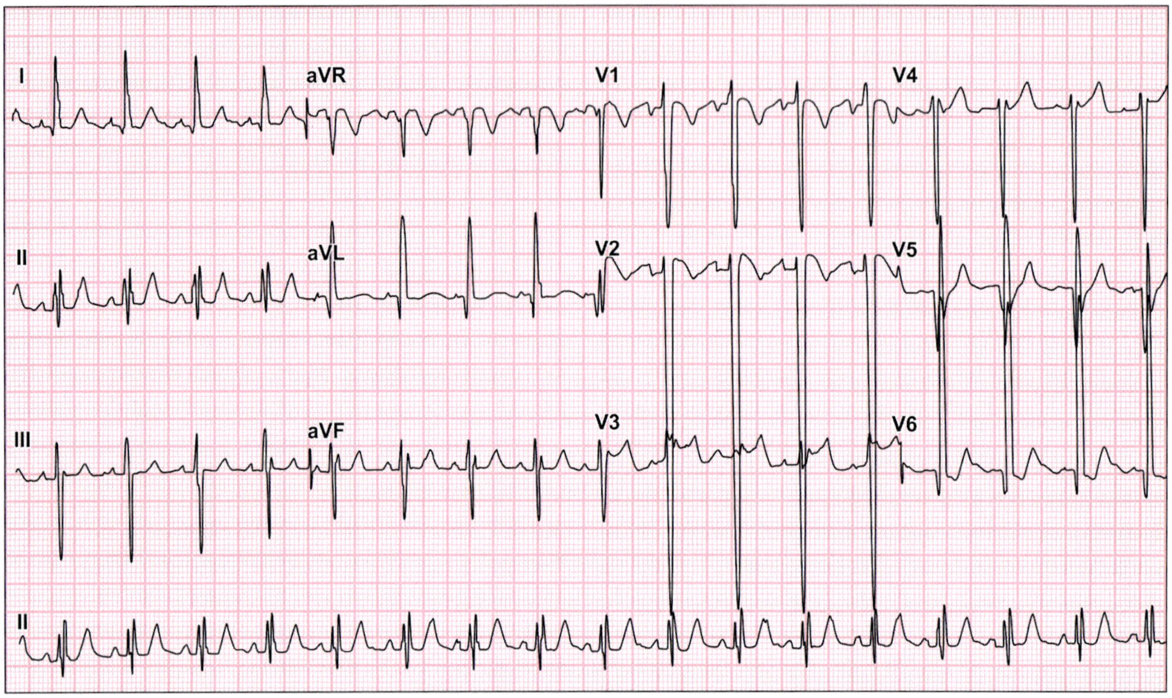


**Fig. 16.47:** ECG obtained from an infant with heart failure and ventricular dysfunction. He was labeled as having dilated cardiomyopathy. The leads I, aVL and V6 show 'q' waves suggesting of myocardial infarction. There is subtle ST segment elevation in lead aVL. The echocardiographic diagnosis of anomalous left coronary artery from pulmonary artery was confirmed at surgery. The ventricular function recovered over the next 3 months

### *Hypertrophic Cardiomyopathy*

Hypertrophic cardiomyopathy (HCM) may occur (a) without outflow obstruction, or (b) with outflow obstruction. In the obstructive variety, the ventricular septum bulges into the left ventricle, and the anterior mitral valve leaflet causes obstruction in the left ventricular outflow during systole. Uncommonly, there is right ventricular outflow obstruction as well.

Hypertrophic cardiomyopathy in adults occurs almost exclusively due to pathogenic variants in the sarcomeric proteins. In contrast, the genetic profile of children with HCM is more heterogenous with metabolic disorders and malformation syndromes including rasopathies reported more frequently.

Patients with obstructive HCM usually present with exertional dyspnea, anginal chest pain, palpitation and syncope; sudden death can occur. The pulse has a sharp upstroke with a bisferiens character. The apex beat is forcible or heaving. The fourth sound may be palpable at the apex. Double or triple apical impulse may be present. The second sound may be normally split, single or paradoxically split, depending on the severity of the left ventricular outflow obstruction. An ejection systolic murmur of varying intensity is heard at left sternal edge. A pansystolic murmur or MR and a fourth sound may be heard at the apex.

The ejection systolic murmur increases in intensity with maneuvers which increase the myocardial contractility or decrease the volume of the left ventricle. The murmur decreases in intensity with procedures that increase left ventricular volume or decrease the myocardial contractility. Thus, sudden squatting tends to decrease the intensity of the murmur whereas standing upright from sitting position by decreasing the venous return tends to decrease the left ventricular size and increases the intensity of the ejection systolic murmur. The electrocardiogram shows left ventricular hypertrophy, with or without ischemic changes. Prominent initial R in right precordial leads and deep Q waves in the left chest leads may be present with or without a WPW pattern. Echocardiogram shows disproportionate hypertrophy of the ventricular septum, systolic anterior motion (SAM) of the anterior leaflet of the mitral valve and mid-systolic closure of the aortic valve.

There is morphological, functional and genetic heterogeneity of pediatric HCM and this clearly argues for the consideration of pediatric HCM as a distinct subset as compared to adult onset HCM with its unique clinical features and prognosis. A number of distinct genetic conditions manifest with an HCM-like picture in children. They include, Noonan's syndrome, Fabry's disease, storage disorders and, Fredreich's ataxia. Additionally, there are a wide variety of mutations that are associated with adult onset HCM that can also manifest in childhood.

The prognosis is variable; young age of onset predicts poor prognosis. The disease may be progressive and sudden death may occur in spite of medical and/or surgical treatment. Risk stratification for sudden cardiac death includes, careful documentation of family history, 24 hour Holter, echocardiography and genetic testing. Magnetic resonance imaging may help identify myocardial fibrosis and indirectly help in identifying patients at risk of sudden cardiac death.

Management includes the use of beta-blockers to decrease the myocardial contractility and thus decrease the obstruction. Additionally, selected patients at high risk of sudden cardiac death will need implantable cardioverter defibrillator. Surgery is indicated for patients with symptomatic severe outflow obstruction that is refractory to medical therapy.

### Suggested Reading


1. Krishna MR, Cardiomyopathy. In: IAP Specialty Textbook of Pediatric Cardiology. Eds. Kumar RK, Prabhu SS, Jain S, Venkatesh S, Ahamed Z.Jaypee brothers, New Delhi, India, 3rd edition, 2021, ISBN 81-8448-273-6;pp 801–21.


## CARDIOVASCULAR MANIFESTATIONS OF SARS-CoV-2 INFECTION

In the recent COVID pandemic, several children have been affected across the world with severe systemic hyperinflammation and shock where in there is evidence of exposure to COVID-19. This is now well characterized as multisystem inflammatory syndrome in children (MISC). The cardiovascular involvement in MISC is in the form of ventricular dysfunction, coronary artery dilation, rhythm disorders and thrombotic complications. Some degree of myocardial dysfunction with reduced ejection fraction is common. There is considerable overlap with Kawasaki disease. Rhythm disorders include complete heart block and sinus node dysfunction.

A small proportion of patients present with severe dysfunction that results in a clinical picture of cardiogenic shock. Investigations show evidence of hyperinflammation with elevated C-reactive protein, (CRP), procalcitonin (PCT), and erythrocyte sedimentationrate (ESR), ferritin and IL-6. Altered coagulation profile with a significant increase in D-dimer and fibrinogen are also invariably seen. Elevated brain natriuretic peptide (BNP), CK-MB and toponin are all markers of cardiac involvement.

The simultaneous presence of vasoplegia results in profound hypotension with multiorgan dysfunction warranting aggressive management. Intensive care, mechanical ventilation and inotropes need to be instituted quickly. Circulatory support in the form of extracorporeal membranous oxygenator (ECMO) may be needed when above measures fail to restore adequate perfusion. Timely institution of aggressive supportive therapy together with immunomodulation in the form of intravenous, immunoglobulin with or without steroids (high dose methyl-prednisolone) is often life-saving and most patients can be salvaged. The use of biologic drugs (tocilizumab, anakinra, infliximab) could be considered in severely ill children who do not respond to first line management. Anticoagulation and antiplatelet therapy need to be considered especially in severe cases. Children with abnormal coagulation profile (i.e. D-dimer ≥3 mg/mL), documented thrombosis, severe ventricular dysfunction and giant coronary artery aneurysm require to be on anticoagulation in the form of unfractionated or low molecular weight heparin followed by oral anticoagulants in selected cases.

Progress should be monitored through serial echo-cardiography and ECGs as delayed and incomplete recovery is described both with ventricular function and coronary artery dilation. Persistent coronary artery dilation merits long-term antiplatelet therapy.

### Suggested Reading


1. Sperotto F, Friedman KG, Son MBF, VanderPluym CJ, Newburger JW, Dionne A. Cardiac manifestations in SARS-CoV-2-associated multisystem inflammatory syndrome in children: A comprehensive review and proposed clinical approach. Eur J Pediatr 2021;180:307–22.


*Competency:* **PE23.15**

## PERICARDIAL DISEASE

Inflammatory diseases of the pericardium may present as acute pericarditis, pericarditis with effusion or chronic constrictive pericarditis (Table 16.21).

### Acute Pericarditis

Acute pericardial inflammation causes precordial pain, which may be dull, sharp or stabbing in character. Occasionally, the pain may be felt over the neck and shoulder and may worsen on lying down. The child becomes dyspneic and has cough. The pattern of fever and toxemia depends on the etiology. The bedside diagnostic physical sign is the presence of pericardial friction rub, which is a rough scratchy sound, with three components—a systolic, diastolic and a presystolic scratch. It can be heard anywhere over the precordium, is unrelated to the respiratory cycle and increases on pressing the chestpiece of stethoscope over the precordium. The electrocardiogram shows generalized ST elevation in the initial stages. Later the ST segment becomes isoelectric and T waves become inverted. Still later, the ST segment may be depressed. The thoracic roentgenogram is unremarkable at this stage.

If effusion develops, the cardiac silhouette increases in size. The heart sounds become muffled and evidence of peripheral congestion in the form of raised jugular venous pressure, hepatomegaly and edema may develop. The pericardial friction rub may persist or disappear. If the fluid accumulates rapidly, there is marked interference with cardiac filling resulting in features of cardiac tamponade such as: (i) Rising jugular venous pressure; (ii) paradoxical inspiratory filling of the neck veins; (iii) increasing heart rate; (iv) falling pulse pressure; and (v) appearance of pulsus paradoxus. The electrocardiogram shows non-specific generalized ST and T changes with low voltage tracings.

**Table 16.21:** Etiology of pericardial diseases

| *Acute* | *Chronic* |
|---|---|
| Bacterial | Constrictive pericarditis |
| Viral | Tuberculous |
| Tuberculous | Idiopathic |
| Rheumatic fever | Post-pyogenic |
| Collagen disorders | Post-traumatic |
| Uremic | |
| Postoperative | |
| Idiopathic | |

The chest X-ray shows cardiomegaly with smooth outline and blunting of the cardiophrenic angle. The lung fields are clear. Echocardiogram shows an echo-free space behind the posterior left ventricular wall.

Evidence of right atrial or right ventricular diastolic collapse indicates a hemodynamically significant effusion. Pericardiocentesis should be done to determine the etiology as well as to relieve cardiac tamponade, if present. Treatment is dictated by the etiology. Surgical drainage is indicated when pyopericardium is suspected.

### Chronic Constrictive Pericarditis

Constrictive pericarditis most commonly results as a consequence of tuberculous infection and less commonly from pyogenic bacterial infection. Fibrous thickening of both layers of the pericardium encases the heart and restricts filling of both the ventricles equally; calcification is rare in childhood. The myocardium is not involved initially, but the fibrous process later infiltrates the myocardium, making surgical correction difficult. Dyspnea, fatigue and progressive enlargement of the abdomen are common.

Jugular venous pressure is always elevated with equally prominent 'a' and 'v' waves and a prominent 'y' descent. Inspiratory filling of neck veins (Kussmaul sign) is seen frequently. Liver is enlarged and pulsatile; ascites with unilateral or bilateral pleural effusion is common. Splenomegaly may also be present. Pulse is fast and of low volume and pulsus paradoxus may be present. The precordium is quiet with a normal sized heart. First and second sounds are normal. An early third heart sound (pericardial knock) is commonly heard. The EKG often shows low voltage and non-specific ST-T changes in all cases. Normal electrocardiogram is against the diagnosis of constrictive pericarditis. Occasionally, there is right axis deviation or right ventricular hypertrophy pattern.

The chest X-ray shows normal sized heart, occasionally with ragged or shaggy borders and prominent superior vena cava shadow merging with the right atrial margin. The lungs may show pleural effusion and plate atelectasis. Fluoroscopy shows reduced cardiac pulsations and may help reveal pericardial calcification. Hemodynamic studies reveal elevation of right atrial mean pressure, right ventricular end-diastolic pressure, pulmonary artery diastolic pressure and the pulmonary artery wedge pressures, which are identical. The right ventricular end-diastolic pressure is more than one-third of the systolic pressure. The cardiac index may be normal or reduced, but the stroke volume is low.

Surgical decortication of the pericardium results in normalization of the hemodynamic abnormalities in most cases. Some cases of long-standing constrictive pericarditis with myocardial dysfunction may improve slowly or have residual myocardial dysfunction. A full course of antitubercular treatment often follows pericardiectomy, if the cause is not clear because of overall prevalence of tuberculosis.

Competency: **PE23.17**

## SYSTEMIC HYPERTENSION

Hypertension is a leading cause of adult morbidity and mortality. In recent decades, the prevalence of hypertension in children has increased, contributed chiefly by rising obesity. Approximately 3–4% of children and adolescents have hypertension and 10% have elevated blood pressure. While essential hypertension is more common in adolescents, severe hypertension in young children and adolescents is often secondary to an underlying disease. Pediatric hypertension tracks into adulthood and increases the risk of premature cardiovascular and kidney disease. Hence, early recognition and adequate management of hypertension in children are crucial.

### Etiology

The etiology of essential hypertension is multifactorial. Obesity, insulin resistance, activation of sympathetic nervous system, disorders in sodium homeostasis and renin–angiotensin system, vascular smooth muscle structure and reactivity, uric acid levels, genetic factors and fetal programming are implicated. There is often a history of hypertension in the parents.

Approximately 90% of secondary hypertension in children are due to kidney disorders or renovascular abnormalities. The major renal causes are chronic glomerulonephritis, reflux or obstructive nephropathy, polycystic or dysplastic kidney diseases, and renovascular hypertension. Coarctation of the aorta and Takayasu arteritis are leading vascular causes. Endocrine disorders such as hyperthyroidism, hypothyroidism, hyperparathyroidism, congenital adrenal hyperplasia, Cushing syndrome, primary aldosteronism, pheochromocytoma, and neuroblastoma are uncommon.

Transient or intermittent hypertension may be caused by postinfectious glomerulonephritis, rapidly progressive (crescentic) glomerulonephritis, IgA vasculitis, hemolytic uremic syndrome, acute tubular necrosis, and renal trauma. Raised intracranial pressure, Guillain-Barré syndrome, burns, Stevens-Johnson syndrome, porphyria, poliomyelitis, encephalitis, drugs (e.g. sympathomimetic agents, steroids, cyclosporine), heavy metal poisoning (e.g. lead, mercury) and vitamin D intoxication may result in acute elevation of blood pressure.

### Definition and Staging

The American Academy of Pediatrics (AAP) clinical practice guidelines for screening and management of high blood pressure in children and adolescents (2017) provide revised normative data on distribution of blood pressure in normal weight children. Hypertension is defined as average systolic blood pressure (SBP) and/or diastolic blood pressure (DBP) that is >95th percentile for age, sex and height on three different occasions. Elevated blood pressure is defined as SBP or DBP that is 90th percentile but <95th percentile. Various definitions and staging of clinical and ambulatory blood pressure are described in Table 16.22.

**Table 16.22:** Definition and staging of hypertension in children

| *Category* | *Children aged 1 to 13 years* | | *Children aged ≥13 years* | |
|---|---|---|---|---|
| **Clinic blood pressure**[#] | | | | |
| Normal blood pressure | <90th percentile | | <120/<80 mm Hg | |
| Elevated BP | >90th percentile to <95th percentile | | 120/<80 to <129/<80 mm Hg | |
| Stage I hypertension | >95th percentile to <95th percentile +12 mm Hg | | 130/80 to 139/89 mm Hg | |
| Stage II hypertension | >95th percentile +12 mm Hg | | ≥140/90 mm Hg | |
| **Ambulatory blood pressure** | | | | |
| | *Clinic SBP or DBP* | *Mean ambulatory SBP or DBP* | *Clinic SBP or DBP* | *Mean ambulatory SBP or DBP* |
| Normal | <95th percentile | <95th percentile, or adolescent cut points* | <130/80 mm Hg | <125/75 mm Hg 24-h, and <130/80 mm Hg wake, and <110/65 mm Hg sleep |
| White coat hypertension | ≥95th percentile | | ≥130/80 mm Hg | |
| Masked hypertension | <95th percentile | ≥95th percentile, or adolescent cut points* | <130/80 mm Hg | ≥125/75 mm Hg 24-h, or ≥130/80 mm Hg wake, or ≥110/65 mm Hg sleep |
| Ambulatory hypertension | ≥95th percentile | ≥95th percentile, or adolescent cut points* | ≥130/80 mm Hg | |

BP–blood pressure

[#]On the basis of age, sex, and height percentiles for systolic (SBP) and diastolic blood pressure (DBP)

*Including 24-hour, wake and sleep blood pressure

Ambulatory blood pressure monitoring (ABPM) is method in which multiple BP readings are obtained at regular intervals, over entire 24-hour while the child performs normal activities, including sleep. Compared to clinic monitoring, ABPM is a better predictor of target organ damage. In addition, ABPM is also valuable in diagnosing white coat and masked hypertension. White coat hypertension is diagnosed when clinic BP is in hypertensive range, but ambulatory pressure is normal; the reverse is the situation in masked hypertension (Table 16.22).

Figures 16.48 and 16.49 indicate blood pressure cut off for stage I and stage II hypertension in girls and boys with stature at median for age. Blood pressure cut-offs for identifying children in the outpatient who need further evaluation are provided in Table 16.23.

### Measurement of Blood Pressure

Blood pressure in children can be measured by auscultation, palpation, oscillometry and Doppler ultrasound. Auscultation or oscillometric determination is preferred. Children and adolescents should undergo blood pressure measurement only after a period of adequate rest (5 to 10 minutes). Blood pressure should be measured at least twice on each occasion in a child's right arm in the seated position. The stethoscope is placed over the brachial artery pulse, proximal and medial to the cubital fossa and below the bottom edge of the cuff. An appropriate selection of cuffs is necessary (Table 16.24). Cuffs should have a bladder width of approximately 40% of the arm circumference midway between the olecranon and the acromion. The inflatable bladder should cover at least two-thirds of the upper arm length and 80–100% of its circumference.

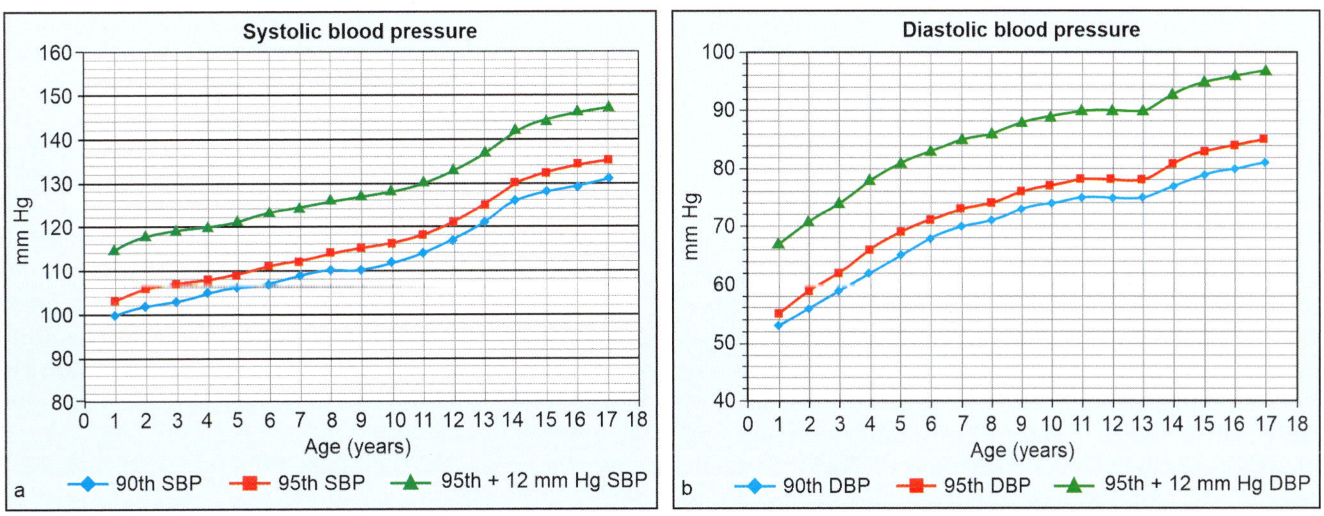


**Fig. 16.48:** Blood pressure levels for boys at 50th percentile for height. Chart depicting 90th (diamonds), 95th (squares) and 95th + 12 mm Hg (triangles) percentile values for (a) systolic and (b) diastolic blood pressures, representing cut off values for the diagnosis of elevated blood pressure, stage I and stage II hypertension, respectively. (Based on American Academy of Pediatrics Clinical Practice Guidelines for Screening and Management of High Blood Pressure in Children and Adolescents, 2017)

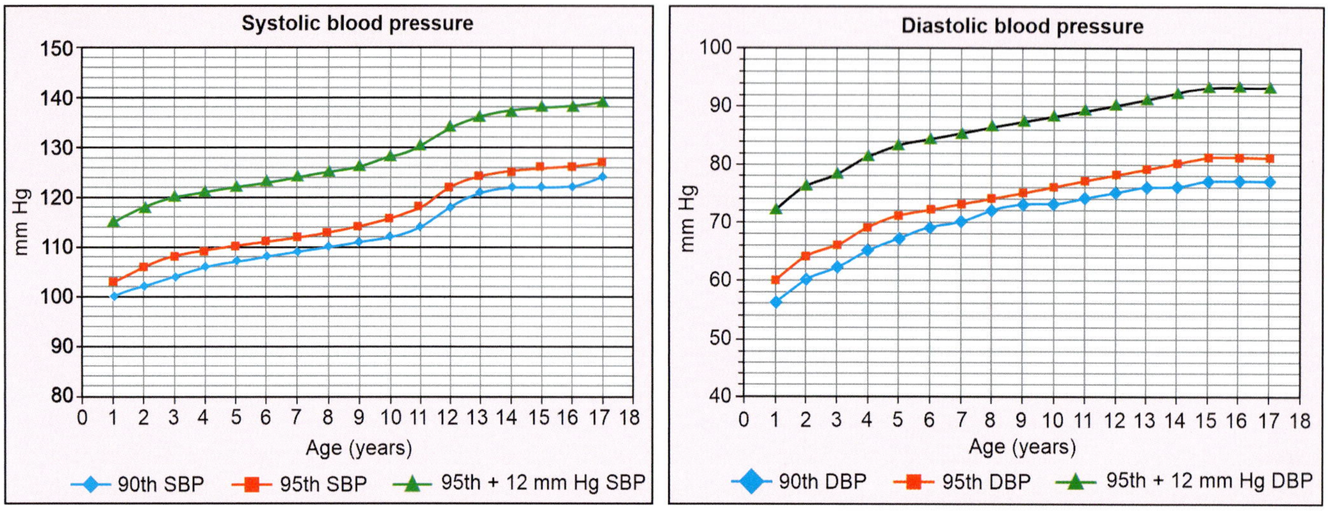


**Fig. 16.49:** Blood pressure levels for girls at 50th percentile for height. Chart depicting 90th (diamonds), 95th (squares) and 95th + 12 mm Hg (triangles) percentile values for (a) systolic and (b) diastolic blood pressures, representing cut off values for the diagnosis of elevated blood pressure and stage I and stage II hypertension, respectively. (Based on American Academy of Pediatrics Clinical Practice Guidelines for Screening and Management of High Blood Pressure in Children and Adolescents, 2017)

**Table 16.23:** Screening blood pressure cut-offs useful for screening for systolic (SBP) or diastolic (DBP), mm Hg hypertension

| *Age, yr* | | *1* | *2* | *3* | *4* | *5* | *6* | *7* | *8* | *9* | *10* | *11* | *12* | *>13* |
|---|---|---|---|---|---|---|---|---|---|---|---|---|---|---|
| *Girls* | SBP | 98 | 101 | 102 | 103 | 104 | 105 | 106 | 107 | 108 | 109 | 111 | 114 | 120 |
| | DBP | 54 | 58 | 60 | 62 | 64 | 67 | 68 | 69 | 71 | 72 | 74 | 75 | 80 |
| *Boys* | SBP | 98 | 100 | 101 | 102 | 103 | 105 | 106 | 107 | 107 | 108 | 110 | 113 | 120 |
| | DBP | 52 | 55 | 58 | 60 | 63 | 66 | 68 | 69 | 70 | 72 | 74 | 75 | 80 |

The cuff is inflated rapidly to occlude the brachial artery in the cubital fossa (at least 20–30 mm Hg above expected SBP). The cuff is deflated slowly at the rate of 2–3 mm Hg per second while auscultating at the cubital fossa. Systolic blood pressure is indicated by the appearance of Korotkoff sounds (phase I) and diastolic blood pressure by its complete disappearance (phase V). Environmental concern with regard to mercury has resulted in replacement of mercury with aneroid sphygmomanometers and oscillometric devices. Oscillometric techniques are easy to use but are susceptible to artifacts and require calibration. Improvement in technology has resulted in widespread use of oscillometric devices for measurement of blood pressure in infants and children.

**Table 16.24:** Recommended dimensions for blood pressure cuff bladders

| *Age group* | *Width (cm)* | *Length (cm)* | *Maximum arm circumference (cm)* |
|---|---|---|---|
| Newborn | 4 | 8 | 10 |
| Infant | 6 | 12 | 15 |
| Child | 9 | 18 | 22 |
| Small adult | 10 | 24 | 26 |
| Adult | 13 | 30 | 34 |
| Large adult | 16 | 38 | 44 |
| Thigh | 20 | 42 | 52 |

Maximum arm circumference is calculated such that the largest arm would still allow bladder to encircle arm by at least 80% (Adapted from Fourth Task Force report)

## Clinical Features

Hypertension in children is usually asymptomatic unless blood pressures are high or sustained. Symptoms are common with secondary hypertension. Headache, dizziness, irritability, epistaxis, anorexia, visual changes and seizures may occur with significant elevations of blood pressure. Marked increase in blood pressure may also result in cardiac failure, pulmonary edema and kidney dysfunction. Hypertensive encephalopathy usually presents with vomiting, high temperature, ataxia, stupor and seizures. Hypertensive emergency may present with decreased vision, symptoms of encephalopathy, cranial nerve palsies, cardiac failure and rapid worsening of kidney function. Eye examination may reveal papilledema or retinal hemorrhages. Subclinical target organ injury may occur in asymptomatic children and include left ventricular hypertrophy, increased carotid intima media thickness, retinopathy and microalbuminuria. Children with secondary hypertension due to chronic kidney disease may present with polyuria, polydipsia, pallor, weight loss and growth retardation.

## Evaluation

Children and adolescents with confirmed hypertension need evaluation to identify potential causes, co-morbidities and extent of target organ damage. The history should include sleep history, physical activity, treatment history, smoking and alcohol intake, drug abuse and family history. The examination should focus on identification of pallor, edema, syndromic facies, ambiguous or virilized genitalia, rickets, goiter, and skin changes (café au lait spots, neurofibromas, rash, striae). Examination of eyes is done for proptosis, extraocular muscle palsies and fundal changes. Cardiovascular examination is done for asymmetry of peripheral pulses, upper and lower limb blood pressures, cardiomegaly, heart rate, cardiac rhythm abnormalities, murmurs and pulmonary edema. Abdominal examination may reveal hepatomegaly, abdominal mass, or epigastric or renal bruit.

Laboratory evaluation includes estimation of blood levels of creatinine, pH and, electrolytes, and urinalysis. Kidney ultrasound may identify a mass, parenchymal scarring, congenital anomalies or disparate kidney size. Evaluation should include fasting lipid profile, HbA1c and glucose levels, especially in older children and adolescents. Children with history of sleep-disordered breathing may benefit from polysomnography. An echocardiogram is used to identify left ventricular hypertrophy and screen for coarctation of aorta. Investigations like plasma renin and aldosterone, plasma/urine steroid levels and plasma/urine catecholamines may be required in some instances. Children with suspected renal or renovascular hypertension are investigated by Doppler imaging and angiography.

### Treatment

The treatment of hypertension in children and adolescents has two components, i.e. therapeutic lifestyle interventions and pharmacotherapy. Weight reduction, increased physical activity and dietary modifications are the major lifestyle interventions. Weight reduction in overweight children results in significant reductions of blood pressure. Weight reduction also decreases other cardiovascular risk factors like dyslipidemia and insulin resistance. Physical activity recommendations for children include 30 to 60 minutes per day or more of moderate intensity aerobic exercise plus limitation of sedentary activity to less than two hours per day. Children with hypertension may benefit from a dietary increase in fresh fruits and vegetables, fiber, non-fat dairy, as well as a reduction in salt consumption. The recommendation for adequate sodium intake is 1.2 g per day for children 4 to 8-yr-old, and 1.5 g per day for older children.

Children with symptomatic essential hypertension, secondary hypertension, diabetes associated hypertension, evidence of target-organ damage (left ventricular hypertrophy), or failed non-pharmacologic interventions require pharmacologic therapy. Agents approved for management of hypertension include ACE inhibitors, angiotensin receptor blockers (ARB), beta blockers, calcium channel blockers and diuretics (Table 16.25). ACE inhibitors and calcium-channel blockers are commonly used in children. ACE inhibitors or ARB are preferred in patients with diabetes or proteinuria or chronic kidney disease.

The goal of therapy for pediatric hypertension should be to reduce blood pressure below 95th percentile, except in the presence of chronic kidney disease, diabetes or target organ damage, when the goal is to reduce blood pressure to less than 90th percentile. Pharmacotherapy is done in a stepped-care approach and usually starts with a low dose of a single agent (step 1). If blood pressure control is not achieved, the dose is titrated every 2-week until blood pressure goals are achieved or the maximum dosage for the drug is reached (step 2). If adequate blood pressure control is not achieved with a single agent, a second agent with a complementary mechanism of action should be added, and dose titrated until adequate control or dosage limit is reached (step 3). If adequate blood pressure control is not achieved with a two-drug regime, a third agent from a different drug class should be added (step 4).

In the case of hypertensive emergencies, the safest way is to lower blood pressure using an antihypertensive medication that is administered by continuous IV infusion in an intensive care unit, where the patient can be monitored appropriately. In general, the pressure should be reduced by up to 25% over the first 8 hr (~10% in the first hour), followed by a further gradual reduction in blood pressure over the next 24–36 hr. Too rapid a reduction in blood pressure may lead to cerebral ischemia. Drug choices include labetalol, nicardipine and sodium nitroprusside of which nicardipine is the preferred drug in children due to its efficacy and safety (Table 16.26). Many patients in hypertensive crisis are volume depleted because of a combination of decreased oral intake and pressure natriuresis. Volume repletion in such conditions will help restore tissue perfusion and prevent a precipitous fall in blood pressure.

### Prevention

Tracking of hypertension into adulthood is well accepted. Hence, prevention and control of hypertension in children is considered to reduce cardiovascular morbidity in adults. This may be achieved by preventing childhood obesity, regular physical activity, consumption of fruits and vegetables, moderation of salt intake, low consumption of processed food items and animal fats, and reducing sedentary activities.

### Suggested Reading

1. Flynn JT, Kaelber DC, Baker-Smith CM, et al; Subcommittee on Screening and Management of High Blood Pressure in Children. Clinical practice guideline for screening and management of high blood pressure in children and adolescents. Pediatrics. 2017;140:e20171904.
2. Flynn JT, Urbina EM, Brady TM. Ambulatory blood pressure monitoring in children and adolescents: 2022 Update: A Scientific Statement from the American Heart Association. Hypertension. 2022; 79:e114–e124.

*Competency:* **PE23.15**

## PULMONARY ARTERIAL HYPERTENSION

Pulmonary arterial hypertension (PAH) is defined as resting mean pulmonary arterial pressure greater than 25 mm Hg, or mean pulmonary artery pressure following exercise that exceeds 30 mm Hg. PAH occurs in an idiopathic form or in association with other etiologies. The condition is a critical

**Table 16.25:** Common antihypertensive medications for outpatient management

| *Agents* | *Dose; frequency* | *Comments* |
|---|---|---|
| **ACE inhibitors, angiotensin receptor blockers** | | |
| Captopril<br>Enalapril<br>Lisinopril<br>Ramipril<br>Irbesartan<br>Losartan | 0.3–6 mg/kg/day; tid<br>0.1–0.6 mg/kg/day; qd or bid<br>0.06–0.6 mg/kg/day; qd<br>6 mg/m$^2$; qd<br>4–5 mg/kg/day<br>0.7–1.4 mg/kg/day; qd | • Use cautiously if GFR <30 mL/min/1.73 m$^2$; avoid in renal artery stenosis<br>• Use smaller doses in neonates<br>• Monitor serum potassium, creatinine regularly<br>• Hyperkalemia, impaired renal functions; anemia, neutropenia, dry cough infrequent |
| **Calcium channel blockers** | | |
| Amlodepine<br>Nifedipine (extended release)<br>Isradipine | 0.05–0.5 mg/kg/day; qd-bid<br>0.25–3 mg/kg/day; qd-bid<br>0.15–0.8 mg/kg/day; tid | • Extended release nifedepine must be swallowed whole<br>• Side effects: Headache, flushing, dizziness, tachycardia; lower extremity edema, erythema |
| **Beta-blockers** | | |
| Atenolol<br>Metoprolol<br>Labetalol | 0.5–2 mg/kg/day; qd or bid<br>1–6 mg/kg/day; bid<br>10–40 mg/kg/day; bid or tid | • Decrease dose by 50% at GFR <50 mL/min/1.73 m$^2$; give on alternate days at GFR <10 mL/min/1.73 m$^2$; sleep disturbances with propranolol, metoprolol; hyperlipidemia; avoid in asthma, heart failure; blunt symptoms of hypoglycemia |
| **Alpha agonists** | | |
| Clonidine<br>Prazosin | 5–25 μg/kg/day; tid or qid<br>0.05–0.5 mg/kg/day; bid or tid | • Abrupt cessation may cause rebound hypertension; sedation<br>• May cause 'first dose' hypotension, syncope |
| **Vasodilators** | | |
| Hydralazine<br>Minoxidil | 1–8 mg/kg/day; qid<br>0.1–1 mg/kg/day; qd or bid | • Useful in hypertension refractory to other drugs<br>• Side effects: Headache, palpitation, fluid retention, congestive heart failure; pericardial effusions and hypertrichosis with minoxidil |
| **Diuretics** | | |
| Furosemide<br>Metolazone<br>Hydrochlorothiazide<br>Amiloride | 0.5–6 mg/kg/day; qd or bid<br>0.2–0.4 mg/kg/day; qd<br>1–3 mg/kg/day; qd<br>0.4–0.6 mg/kg/day; qd | • Monitor electrolytes, fluid status periodically<br>• Thiazides: Dyslipidemia, hyperglycemia, hyperuricemia, hypokalemia, hypomagnesemia<br>• Loop diuretics: Metabolic alkalosis<br>• Use cautiously with ACEI, angiotensin receptor blockers |

qd once daily; bid twice daily; tid thrice daily; qid four times qd

**Table 16.26:** Antihypertensive agents for management of severe hypertension

| *Medication* | *Onset* | *Duration of effect* | *Route* | *Dose* | *Side effects* |
|---|---|---|---|---|---|
| Sodium nitroprusside | 30 sec | <10 min | IV infusion | 0.5–8 μg/kg/min (made in 5% dextrose) | Nausea, vomiting, headache, tachycardia, cyanide toxicity (dizziness, confusion, seizures, jaw stiffness and lactic acidosis) |
| Labetalol | 5–10 min | 3–6 hr | IV infusion<br>IV bolus | 0.25–3 mg/kg/hr<br>0.2–1 mg/kg/dose q 5–10 min (max 40 mg) | Orthostatic hypotension, bradycardia, pallor, abdominal pain, diarrhea |
| Nicardipine | 1–10 min | 3 hr | IV infusion | 0.5–4 μg/kg/min (max 5 mg/hr) | Flushing, reflex tachycardia, phlebitis, nausea, increased intracranial pressure, headache |
| | | | IV bolus | 30 μg/kg (max 2 mg/dose) q 15 min | |
| Nitroglycerine | 2–5 min | 5–10 min | IV infusion | 1–3 μg/kg/min | Methemoglobinemia, headache, tachycardia |
| Phentolamine | 10 min | 30–60 min | IV bolus | 0.1–0.2 mg/kg (max 5 mg) q 2–4 hr if required | Reflex tachycardia, abdominal pain |
| Nifedipine | 10–30 min | 1–4 hr | Oral | 0.2–0.5 mg/kg (max 10 mg) q 4–6 hr | Excessive hypotension, peripheral edema |
| Clonidine | 15–30 min | 2–4 hr | Oral | 0.05–0.1 mg/dose, may repeat q hr; max 0.8 mg total dose | Somnolence, dry mouth |

determinant of morbidity and mortality in diverse pediatric cardiac, lung, hematologic, and other diseases.

### Etiology

PAH may be associated with a number of congenital heart diseases. Idiopathic PAH is rare in children. In a small proportion, mutations in the bone morphogenetic protein receptor type 2 (*BMPR2*) gene, the activin receptor-like kinase type 1 (*ACVRL1*), or endoglin are identified. Other causes of pulmonary hypertension in children include respiratory disease, upper airway obstruction, connective tissue disease and, advanced liver disease (hepatopulmonary syndrome). For an updated clinical classification, please see the references listed at the bottom of this section.

#### Persistent Pulmonary Hypertension of the Newborn (PPHN)

At birth, pulmonary vascular resistance is high, it normally falls rapidly throughout the first week of life. By 6 to 8 weeks, pulmonary vascular resistance usually has reached a normal adult level of 1 to 3 Wood units. These changes are accompanied by a gradual dilation of the smaller and then the larger muscular pulmonary arteries and development of new arteries and arterioles. PPHN develops when pulmonary vascular resistance remains elevated after birth, resulting in right-to-left shunting of blood through fetal circulatory pathways. The common associations include congenital diaphragmatic hernia, meconium aspiration syndrome and perinatal asphyxia. These newborn patients typically require mechanical ventilatory support and those with underlying lung disease may benefit from high-frequency oscillatory ventilation or extracorporeal membrane oxygenation (ECMO). Pulmonary vasodilators, such as inhaled nitric oxide, improve the outcome and reduce the need for ECMO. Sildenafil is increasingly used for PPHN as an alternative to inhaled nitric oxide.

### Clinical Manifestations

The clinical features of PAH are related to the degree of pulmonary hypertension and right ventricular function and status of the right ventricle. Most common symptom is exertional breathlessness due to the inability of the right ventricle to raise cardiac output with exercise. Other symptoms are hemoptysis, atypical chest pain, congestive heart failure, dizziness or syncope and arrhythmias. Cyanosis and its complications are seen in Eisenmenger patients but not otherwise unless there is a patent foramen ovale. A comprehensive evaluation is advised before a diagnosis of idiopathic PAH is made. It is essential to rule out cardiac (congenital heart disease), respiratory, upper airway obstruction (Down syndrome, adenoids), neurogenic causes (sleep apnea) and liver disease (portopulmonary hypertension).

### Management

Supplemental low-flow oxygen alleviates arterial hypoxemia in patients with pulmonary parenchymal disease. Patients with Eisenmenger syndrome or idiopathic PAH do not exhibit resting alveolar hypoxia and do not require oxygen unless significantly hypoxic. Children with severe right ventricular failure and resting hypoxemia may require continuous oxygen therapy.

*Diuretics* are useful in patients with symptomatic right heart failure. The right ventricle is highly preload dependent, and care should be taken to avoid excessive diuresis since this can lead to a fall in cardiac output and compromise other pharmacologic measures, such as vasodilators. Patients are at higher risk of thromboembolic events due to sluggish pulmonary circulation and dilated right-sided cardiac chambers. Anticoagulants may have a role in select cases when the risk for thromboembolism outweighs the likelihood of hemoptysis.

*The goal of vasodilator therapy* for PAH is to reduce pulmonary artery pressure and increase cardiac output without causing systemic arterial hypotension. Sildenafil and tadalafil are oral phosphodiesterase type 5 inhibitors that prevent the breakdown of cGMP and potentiate pulmonary vasodilation with endogenous nitric oxide synthesized by the vascular endothelium. Symptomatic patients with PAH, PPHN and postoperative PAH benefit with sildenafil. Oral endothelin-receptor antagonists (ERA) such as bosentan, ambrisentan and macetentan are now available in India. These new selective pulmonary vasodilators have improved the outlook of many forms of pulmonary hypertension in terms of symptoms and survival. Prostacyclin analogs have been administered intravenously or subcutaneously as a continuous infusion or through frequent inhalations and are not available in India. Recently, oral prostacycline analogs, such as selexipag, have become available in India.

*Surgery* combined heart lung transplantation, or lung transplantation alone has been performed successfully in patients with PAH. The major limitations to its widespread use include the limited number of centers with the expertise to perform the procedure and care for patients and the limited availability of suitable donors and significant cost.

### Prognosis

Prognosis is dictated by the underlying etiology and the right ventricular function. An overall 80% 5-yr survival has been reported in patients with Eisenmenger syndrome compared with a much lower mean survival after the diagnosis of idiopathic PAH.

### Suggested Reading


1. Abman SH, Ivy DD. Recent progress in understanding pediatric pulmonary hypertension. Curr Opin Pediatr 2011; 23:298–304.
2. Hansmann G, Koestenberger M, Alastalo TP, et al. 2019 Updated consensus statement on the diagnosis and treatment of pediatric pulmonary hypertension: The European Pediatric Pulmonary Vascular Disease Network (EPPVDN), endorsed by AEPC, ESPR and ISHLT. J Heart Lung Transplant 2019;38:879–901.
3. Simonneau G, Gatzoulis M, Adatia A, et al. Updated clinical classification of pulmonary hypertension. J Am Coll Cardiol 2013;62(25 Suppl):D34–41.

Competency: **PE23.14**

## RHYTHM DISORDERS

The recognition of cardiac arrhythmias in children is challenging and requires a high index of suspicion. It is important to arrive at a precise diagnosis since the treatment is dictated by the specific arrhythmia. In some situations, it may be possible to affect a complete cure.

### Clinical Features

These are listed in Table 16.27.

*Irregular heart rate:* The commonest cause of an irregular heart rate is physiological sinus arrhythmia. This can be recognized by an increase in heart rate with inspiration and decrease with expiration. Sinus arrhythmia is usual following a febrile illness and by drugs that increase vagal tone (such as digoxin). It is readily abolished by exercise. Irregularities of rhythm are commonly seen in premature infants especially bradycardia associated with periodic apnea. Common causes of heart rate irregularity in children include atrial and ventricular premature beats and conduction disturbances (Table 16.28).

*Inappropriate heart rate:* A heart rate that is inappropriately fast or slow for the clinical condition or physiological state should arouse the suspicion of an underlying arrhythmia. Inappropriately slow heart rate in a child with fatigue, giddiness or syncope should arouse the suspicion of complete heart block. Inappropriately fast rates suggest tachyarrhythmias such as SVT.

*Unexplained heart failure:* Incessant arrhythmias such as ectopic atrial tachycardia (EAT), permanent junctional re-entrant tachycardia (PJRT) and some forms of ventricular tachycardia can present as heart failure. At the time of initial evaluation, the heart rates may not be inappropriate for the degree of heart failure. Diagnosis may be missed and requires a high index of suspicion. These conditions should be considered in the differential diagnosis of childhood dilated cardiomyopathy, especially if the heart rate is relatively fixed.

*Underlying conditions:* A number of congenital and acquired heart diseases and certain systemic conditions are known to be associated with cardiac arrhythmias (Table 16.29). Ventricular and supraventricular arrythmias can follow cardiac surgery for correction of CHD. Operations resulting in scar formation in the right ventricle such as repair of tetralogy of Fallot are known to be associated with ventricular tachycardia. The Fontan operation for single ventricle physiology or the Senning or Mustard procedure for transposition is known to result in a particularly high incidence of re-entrant atrial arrhythmias. Organophosphate exposure, tricyclic antidepressant overdose, digoxin toxicity, antiarrhythmic drug treatment and substance abuse can be associated with a variety of arrhythmias.

*Syncope:* The commonest cause of syncope in children is mediated via the autonomic nervous system, known as the neurocardiogenic syncope or vasovagal syncope. A small fraction of syncopal episodes result from cardiac arrhythmias. Life- threatening ventricular tachycardia (VT), as associated with long QT syndrome characteristically results in syncope. It is important to differentiate them from vasovagal episodes. Vasovagal syncope occurs in specific situations like prolonged standing in a hot environment, sight of blood, painful stimulus, emotional stress or following a recent illness. Syncope secondary to arrhythmia are sudden, unpredictable, paroxysmal and usually have

| Table 16.27: Clinical features in arrhythmias |
|---|
| Irregular heart beat |
| Heart rate that is inappropriate for the clinical condition |
| Unexplained heart failure |
| Syncope, palpitations, chest discomfort |
| Underlying cardiac anomaly known to be associated with rhythm disorders |
| Family history of sudden cardiac events |

| Table 16.28: Causes of irregular heart beat |
|---|
| *Sinus arrhythmia* |
| **Other common and usually benign causes**<br>• Supraventricular (atrial and junctional) premature beats<br>• Ventricular premature beats<br>• Transient conduction disturbances (Wenckebach type), atrioventricular and sinoatrial blocks<br>• Transient bradycardia in a premature infant |
| **Uncommon but potentially serious causes**<br>• Mobitz type II heart block<br>• Ectopic atrial tachycardia; multifocal atrial tachycardia<br>• Polymorphic ventricular tachycardia and Torsades<br>• Atrial fibrillation, with or without WPW syndrome<br>• Atrial flutter with variable conduction |

| Table 16.29: Arrhythmias suggestive of specific congenital heart disease |
|---|
| **Sick sinus syndrome**<br>Sinus venosus, atrioventricular canal defect, Holt-Oram syndrome with atrial septal defect (ASD) and left isomerism |
| **Narrow QRS tachycardias**<br>• Ebstein anomaly; corrected transposition with Ebstein anomaly<br>• Atrioventricular canal defect, ASD, pulmonic stenosis, total anomalous pulmonary venous connection, tricuspid atresia |
| **Atrial fibrillation and flutter**<br>Congenital mitral stenosis, total anomalous pulmonary venous connection, coronary AV fistula |
| **WPW and pre-excitation syndromes**<br>Ebstein anomaly; corrected transposition |
| **Wide QRS tachycardias**<br>Anomalous left coronary artery from pulmonary artery, coronary AV fistula, arrhythmogenic right ventricle, atrioventricular conduction defects, corrected transposition of great arteries; Ebstein anomaly |
| **Postoperative patients**<br>Supraventricular, ventricular arrhythmias |

no predisposing cause or premonition. Duration of syncope depends upon the duration of arrhythmia. Some forms of long QT syndromes and catecholaminergic tachycardia are precipitated by exercise. Ventricular tachycardia secondary to Brugada syndrome may be precipitated during febrile illness. Syncope during exertion is potentially serious and may suggest specific arrhythmic substrates such as catecholaminergic ventricular tachycardia and long QT syndrome.

*Palpitations and chest discomfort:* Older children may complain of episodic palpitations. Not infrequently, they have a sensation of chest discomfort or pain during tachyarrhythmia.

### Basic Electrophysiology Concepts

Arrhythmia that originates at or above the bundle of His has narrow QRS morphology; that below this level (Purkinje fibers, ventricular muscles) have wide QRS morphology. Majority of tachycardia in children are regular. Common irregular tachycardias are ectopic atrial tachycardia, multifocal atrial tachycardia, atrial flutter with varying conduction, atrial fibrillation (rare in children) and ventricular fibrillation. During a regular narrow QRS tachycardia, if a P wave is identified and has normal morphology, axis and 1:1 P and QRS relation, it suggests sinus tachycardia. Absence of any of the three suggests supraventricular tachyarrhythmia.

*Re-entrant vs automatic tachyarrhythmias:* Tachyarrhythmia is generally considered to result from one of the three mechanisms—re-entry, increased automaticity and triggered activity. In children, the first two mechanisms account for most important arrhythmias. Clinical and EKG features together with response to certain medications and maneuvers help distinguish re-entrant tachyarrhythmias from those due to increased automaticity. Re-entrant arrhythmias characteristically have a relatively sudden onset and termination. Successful termination with DC cardioversion or overdrive pacing (pacing at rates faster than the arrhythmia rate) strongly suggests a re-entrant mechanism. Automatic arrhythmias characteristically have a relatively slow onset. Gradual acceleration (warm-up) to the peak rates may be demonstrable at onset and gradual deceleration (cool down) at termination is seen.

### Diagnostic Workup of Suspected Arrhythmia

Attempts should be made to answer all the questions listed in Table 16.30. This will allow the specific treatment strategy to be initiated. A 12-lead EKG should be obtained and cardiac rhythm monitoring should be initiated as quickly as possible.

**Table 16.30:** Initial assessment of arrhythmia

| |
|---|
| Can the clinical condition result from a cardiac arrhythmia? |
| Is there hemodynamic instability? |
| Is the arrhythmia incessant or episodic? |
| Is this a re-entrant arrhythmia or does it involve an automatic focus? |
| Where is the arrhythmic focus or circuit located? |
| Is there an underlying structural heart disease? |

### Management of Hemodynamic Instability

Extreme hemodynamic instability is relatively rare in childhood arrhythmias, particularly in absence of structural heart disease. Hemodynamic instability necessitates emergency treatment. Most unstable tachyarrhythmias are broad QRS. Unstable narrow QRS tachycardia are quite uncommon, especially in the absence of structural heart disease. Low energy (0.5–2 J/kg) synchronized DC cardioversion should be performed. If and when possible, cardioversion should always be preceded by administration of a short-acting benzodiazepine such as midazolam (0.1–0.2 mg/kg/dose). Emergency treatment options for bradyarrhythmias are shown in Table 16.31.

### Diagnosis and Management of Tachyarrhythmia

A combined strategy that simultaneously addresses both diagnosis and treatment is appropriate. This is determined by the QRS duration on the initial EKG and presence or absence of hemodynamic instability. Based on the QRS duration, arrhythmias can be classified as narrow and wide. This is a useful practical classification and serves as an excellent guide to initial treatment. Age specific normal values for QRS duration are given in Table 16.32. As a preliminary step, sinus tachycardia should be excluded. Rates as high as 240/min can occasionally be recorded during sinus tachycardia. There is always an underlying cause for sinus tachycardia and this is usually apparent during the initial evaluation. Fever, circulatory failure, extreme dehydration, accidental ingestion of drugs and toxic substances are common examples. Figure 16.50 depicts a useful treatment algorithm.

*Narrow QRS tachycardia:* Most narrow QRS tachycardias (Table 16.33) are reasonably well tolerated and allow a preliminary diagnostic workup (Table 16.34). If a patient is seen during an episode of tachyarrhythmia, all attempts should be made to obtain quality data before terminating the arrhythmia. Information that should be specifically sought include the P wave morphology and P-QRS relation ship. P waves that appear normal during the tachyarrhythmia

**Table 16.31:** Emergency treatment for bradyarrhythmias

| *Modality* | *Indication* | *Dose* |
|---|---|---|
| Atropine | Severe sinus bradycardia, AV block with narrow QRS (supraventricular) escape | 0.02 mg/kg IV bolus |
| Isoproterenol | Lack of response to atropine, AV block with wide QRS (ventricular) escape | 0.1–2 µg/kg/min IV infusion |
| Transcutaneous pacing | Severe symptomatic bradycardia, asystole (not suitable for infants, young children) | Twice the capture threshold |
| Transvenous pacing | Alternative to transcutaneous pacing for infants and young children | Twice the capture threshold |

**Table 16.32:** Normal QRS duration at various age groups

| *Age group* | *QRS duration in seconds* |
|---|---|
| 0–6 months | 0.03–0.07 (0.05) |
| 1–5 years | 0.04–0.08 (0.06) |
| 10–15 years | 0.04–0.09 (0.07) |
| >15 years | 0.06–0.09 (0.08) |

Values represent range (mean)

suggest sinus tachycardia. Ectopic atrial tachycardia is suggested by abnormal P wave morphology. Inverted P waves may be seen when atria are activated in a retrograde fashion as in the case of re-entrant tachyarrhythmias involving accessory pathways (AV re-entrant tachycardia) (Fig. 16.51). Often P waves are not clearly seen on baseline EKG but are unmasked by adenosine. Evidence of 2:1 AV conduction as suggested by a 2:1 P-QRS ratio during a narrow QRS tachycardia indicates atrial flutter (Fig. 16.52). Evidence of complete AV dissociation (no consistent P-QRS relationship) indicates junctional ectopic tachycardia.

***Adenosine*** administration acts by producing a marked slowing of AV node conduction (Table 16.32). The effect of adenosine lasts for a few seconds. Side effects are short-lived

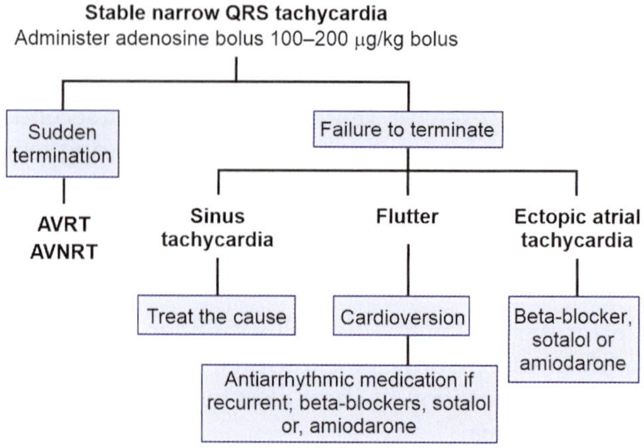


**Fig. 16.50:** Management algorithm for stable narrow QRS tachycardia. AVNRT atrioventricular nodal re-entrant tachycardia; AVRT atrioventricular re-entrant tachycardia

and include flushing, chest pain and dyspnea. Adenosine needs to be administered rapidly followed by rapid push of normal saline as a bolus. The recommended dose is 50–300 μg/kg. Most re-entrant tachycardias, where AV node is a part of the circuit (AV node re-entrant tachycardia, AV re-entrant tachycardia) will be terminated by adenosine.

**Table 16.33:** Causes of narrow QRS tachycardia

| *Site* | *Re-entrant arrhythmias* | *Automatic arrhythmias* |
|---|---|---|
| Sinus node | Sinus node re-entry | Sinus tachycardia |
| Atrium | Intra-atrial re-entrant arrhythmias following cardiac surgery (Fontan, Senning operations)<br>Atrial flutter<br>Atrial fibrillation | Ectopic atrial tachycardia<br>Multifocal atrial tachycardia |
| AV node | AV node re-entry | Junctional ectopic tachycardia |
| Accessory pathway | Atrioventricular re-entry involving concealed or manifest (WPW) pathway<br>Permanent junctional re-entrant tachycardia | |

**Table 16.34:** Differential diagnosis of narrow QRS tachycardia

| *Arrhythmia* | *P waves* | *P-QRS relationship* | *Response to adenosine* |
|---|---|---|---|
| Sinus tachycardia | Normal | 1:1 | Transient slowing; AV block |
| Sinus node-entry | Normal | Usually 1:1 | No effect or transient AV block |
| Ectopic atrial tachycardia | Abnormal and different from baseline | Usually 1:1 | No effect or transient AV block |
| Atrial flutter | Saw tooth appearance rates exceed 240/min | 2:1 or 1:1 | Transient AV block may unmask flutter waves; rarely arrhythmia terminates |
| Postoperative intra-atrial re-entry* | Slow atrial flutter, P waves different from baseline | Variable, often 1:1 | Transient AV block may unmask flutter waves; rarely arrhythmia terminates |
| Multifocal atrial tachycardia | Multiform | Usually 1:1 | No effect or transient AV block |
| Junctional ectopic tachycardia | Normal (AV dissociation) or inverted (1:1 retrograde conduction) | Complete AV dissociation is diagnostic | No effect on rate; transient retrograde VA conduction block unmasks AV dissociation |
| AV nodal tachycardia | Usually not visible (masked by RS complexes) | 1:1 | Sudden termination is characteristic |
| AV re-entrant tachycardia | Inverted (retrograde VA conduction) | 1:1 | Sudden termination |
| Junctional re-entrant tachycardia | Inverted (long VA conduction time) | 1:1 | No effect or transient termination |

*Postoperative intra-atrial re-entry may follow surgery that results in atrial scarring, e.g. Fontan operation, Senning operation

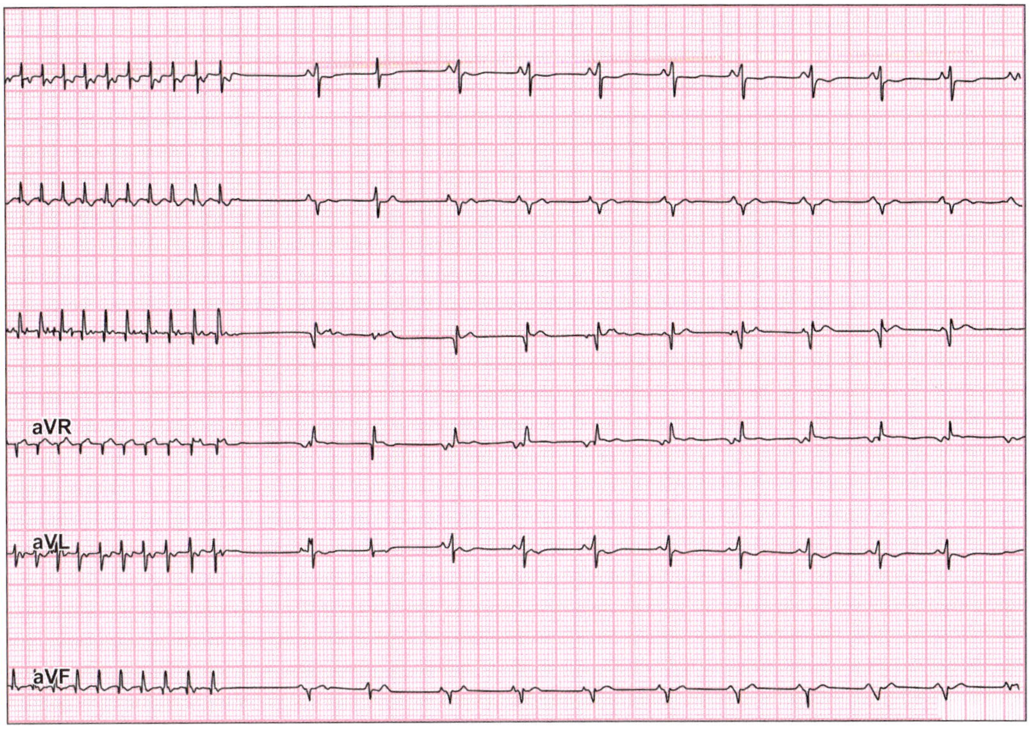


Fig. 16.51: Six-lead ECG. Adenosine was administered to a child with regular narrow QRS supraventricular tachycardia. Note the tachycardia terminates with a P wave. Note delta waves with short PR interval that is prominently seen in lead I. Adenosine administration was therapeutic in this case

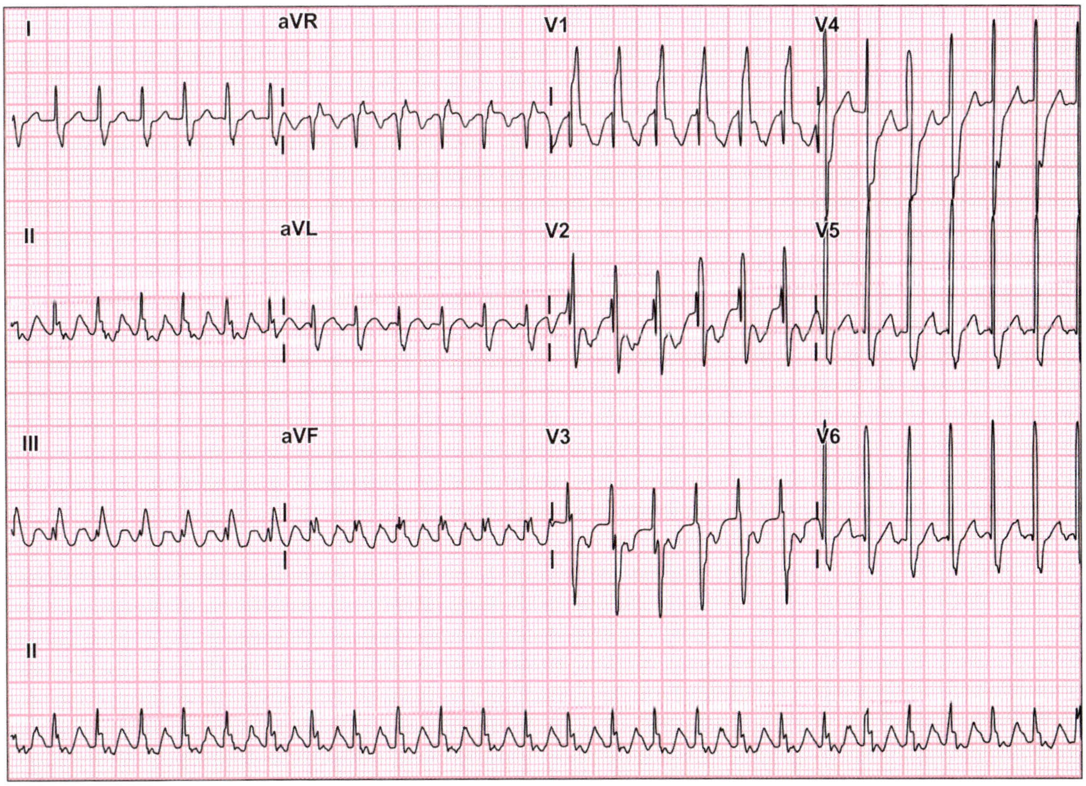


Fig. 16.52: Regular narrow QRS tachycardia at a heart rate of 150/min. Heart rate was fixed at 150/min for several hours that was suggestive of underlying arrhythmia. P waves were abnormally tall with a suggestion of a 'saw-tooth pattern' that points towards the possibility of underlying atrial flutter

*Atrial flutter is seldom terminated by adenosine:* The transient AV block that results from adenosine administration can unmask flutter waves on the EKG thereby confirming the diagnosis (Fig. 16.53). Similarly transient slowing of AV conduction can unmask ectopic atrial tachycardia. If adenosine is not available, vagal maneuvres can be attempted. For infants and young children, an ice-filled plastic bag placed on the face is the most effective vagal

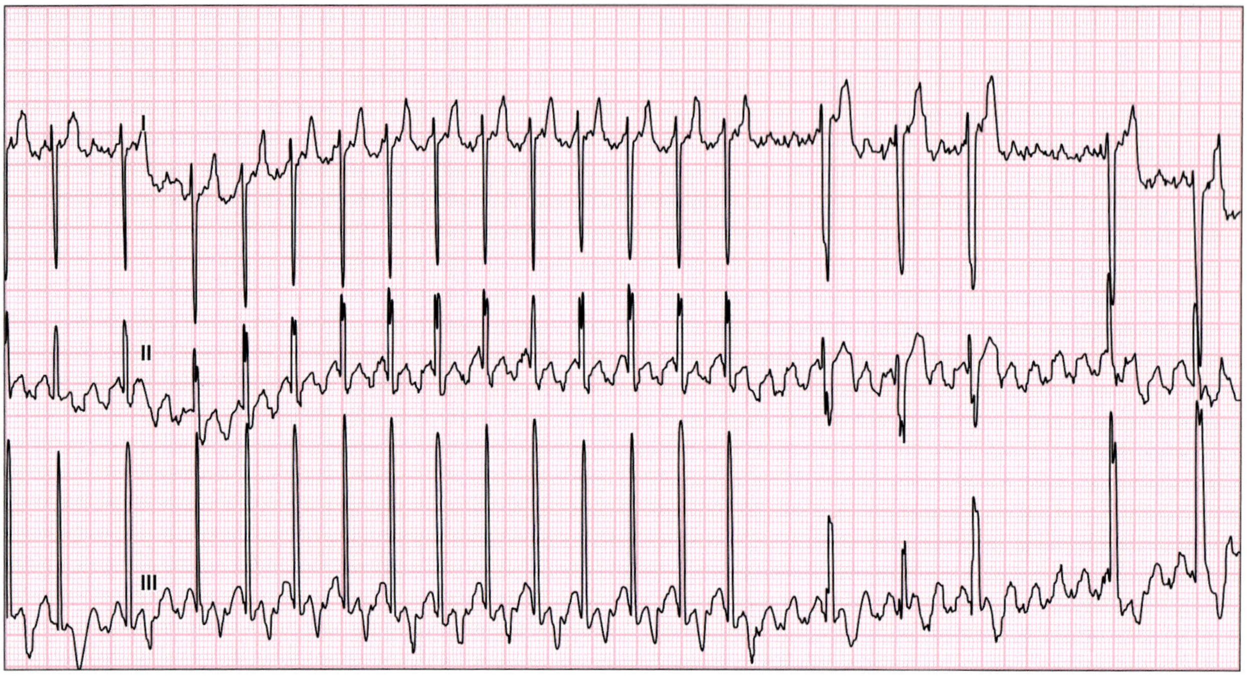


**Fig. 16.53:** Response to adenosine administration to a child with atrial flutter. Note the unmasking of flutter waves that are prominently seen in lead II and III. P rate was 300/min. Before administration of adenosine, there was 2:1 AV conduction. The blocked P waves were hidden within the QRS complexes. After administration of adenosine, AV block increased and AV conduction block increased to 4:1 unmasking the flutter waves

maneuver. Older children can be encouraged to perform the Valsalva maneuver or carotid sinus massage can be attempted. Eyeball pressure is contraindicated in infants.

### *Wide QRS Tachycardia*

Wide QRS complex tachycardias usually result from foci or circuits in the ventricles. Some supraventricular tachycardias can also result in a wide QRS configuration. The overall approach is quite similar to narrow QRS tachycardias, with identification of P waves, defining P-QRS relationship and determining the QRS axis configuration **(Fig. 16.54)**.

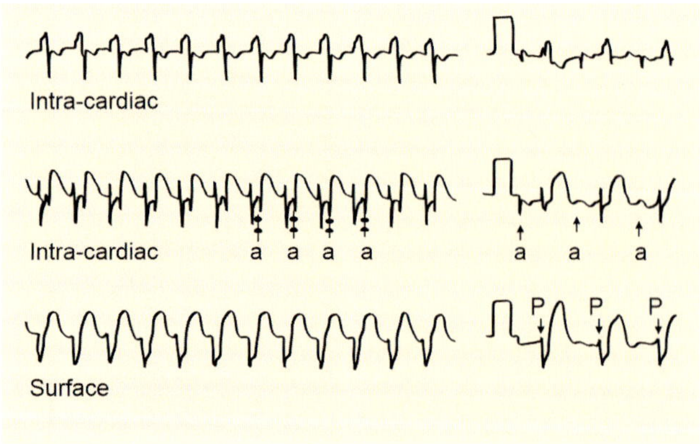


**Fig. 16.54:** Wide QRS tachycardia resulting from a re-entrant circuit involving an accessory pathway in a patient with right bundle branch block. Surface ECG, can be mistaken for ventricular tachycardia. ECG of the top two rows has been obtained directly from the atrium using postoperative atrial wires as electrodes. The bottom strip is the surface ECG from a monitoring lead. Conversion to sinus rhythm after adenosine is seen in the last four complexes on the right. a artial contraction, P p wave

Demonstrable AV dissociation (inconsistent P-QRS relation) suggests ventricular tachycardia (VT). In most situations, however, it is not easy to distinguish VT from SVT. If the patient is stable, administration of adenosine will terminate or unmask SVT. If there is no response, treatment for VT should be initiated. In stable patients, it is better to initiate pharmacologic treatment of VT before considering cardioversion since the response to initial treatment can help decide long-term therapy. Lignocaine is the initial choice, while procainamide is an effective alternative; others include amiodarone, sotalol, mexeletine and flecanide.

***Unstable wide QRS tachycardia:*** Wide QRS tachycardia with hemodynamic instability is a medical emergency. Synchronised cardioversion (0.5–2 J/kg) should be performed immediately. For pulseless patients, CPR should be initiated. Subsequent treatment should follow standard guidelines recommended for pulseless patients with VT **(Fig. 16.55)**.

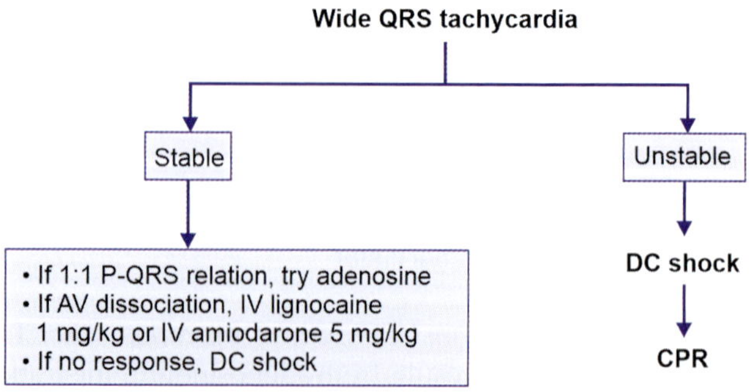


*CPR Cardiopulmonary resuscitation*

**Fig. 16.55:** Management of wide QRS tachycardia

*Irregular wide QRS tachycardia:* Sustained and irregular wide QRS tachycardia is uncommon and usually suggests a diagnosis of Wolf-Parkinson-White (WPW) syndrome with atrial fibrillation. In presence of hemodynamic instability, synchronized cardioversion (1–2 J/kg) is indicated.

Once the arrhythmia has been managed, recurrences need to be prevented. Most childhood arrhythmias warrant evaluation by a pediatric cardiologist for follow-up care and to plan definitive treatment. An echocardiogram and Holter test (24 hr ambulatory EKG recording) is often required. Invasive intracardiac electrophysiologic study is combined with radiofrequency (RF) ablation. Most accessory pathways are now treated by radiofrequency ablation, especially in older children (>4-yr-old). For younger children, RF ablation is reserved for refractory situations.

## PREVENTING ADULT CARDIOVASCULAR DISEASE

Major risk factors for cardiovascular disease in adulthood include cigarette smoking, hypertension, dyslipidemia, diabetes mellitus, obesity and physical inactivity. Some of these risk factors have genesis in childhood and are amenable to modification, contributing to primary prevention of cardiovascular disease.

### Childhood Obesity

Obesity influences major cardiovascular risk factors such as dyslipidemia, hypertension, glucose intolerance and inflammation. Emerging cardiovascular risk factors like carotid intima media thickness as well as carotid elasticity has also shown strong association with childhood obesity. Childhood obesity is managed by a combination of increased physical activity and dietary interventions.

#### *Hypertension*

Primary or essential hypertension is the most common form of hypertension in older children and adolescents. Childhood obesity is associated with hypertension in children, which often tracks into adulthood.

#### *Dyslipidemia*

Screening for dyslipidemia is recommended for children whose parents and/or grandparents required coronary artery bypass-surgery or balloon angioplasty before age 55, those with a family history of myocardial infarction, angina pectoris, peripheral or cerebral vascular disease, or sudden death before age 55 and those whose parents have dyslipidemia. Youth with dyslipidemia are treated with a diet low in total and saturated fats and cholesterol. The intake of complex carbohydrates is increased, whereas that of simple sugars is decreased. Drug therapy is used in patients with significantly elevated LDL-cholesterol.

#### *Diabetes Mellitus*

Diabetes mellitus is associated with cardiovascular complications, which develop early in childhood and adolescence. Endothelial dysfunction seen in both types of diabetes is recognized to aggravate cardiovascular risk in later life. Optimal daily and long-term glycemic control, maintenance of blood pressure and lipid levels in the normal values for age, regular exercise, healthy diet and avoidance of smoking are necessary.

#### *Tobacco Consumption*

Mechanisms by which smoking exerts its detrimental effects on cardiovascular system include endothelial dysfunction, increased oxidative stress, increased arterial stiffness, alterations in lipoprotein metabolism and induction of prothrombotic state. School based campaigns to prevent smoking and chewing tobacco are appropriate tools to contain this public health concern. Parents should be role models to children by avoiding or quitting smoking and chewing tobacco. Early atherosclerotic disease has been documented in certain conditions in children.

### Suggested Reading


1. Raj M. Obesity and cardiovascular risk in children and adolescents. Indian J Endocrinol Metab 2012;16:13–19.
2. Raj M, Sundaram KR, Paul M, et al. Obesity in children: Time trends and relationship with hypertension. Natl Med J India 2007; 20:288–93.

Chapter

17

# Disorders of Kidney and Urinary Tract

❍ Arvind Bagga ❍ Aditi Sinha ❍ RN Srivastava

## RENAL ANATOMY AND PHYSIOLOGY

Each kidney is composed of approximately a million nephrons, each consisting of a glomerulus and renal tubule. The glomerulus is made of a tuft of capillaries and a central region of mesangium. The capillaries arise from the afferent arteriole and join to form the efferent arteriole. The capillary wall consists of fenestrated endothelium, glomerular basement membrane and foot processes (podocytes) of visceral epithelial cells. The basement membrane is made of type IV collagen, laminin and heparan sulfate proteoglycan. The Bowman space leads into the proximal tubule that has an initial convoluted portion, then the straight segment, descending and ascending limbs of the loop of Henle and the distal tubule (Fig. 17.1). Six to eight distal tubules join to form the collecting ducts that finally enter the renal pelvis.

The early part of the distal tubule on its ascent from the medulla to the cortex lies near the glomerulus of the same nephron. The cells of the tubule in contact with the afferent arteriole are denser than the rest and called macula densa. The smooth muscle cells of the afferent arteriole, in this region, contain prominent cytoplasmic granules that are the site of renin activity. The juxtaglomerular apparatus (JGA) is composed of afferent and efferent arterioles, the macula densa and lacis cells located between these structures. The JGA is involved in systemic blood pressure regulation, electrolyte homeostasis and tubuloglomerular feedback.

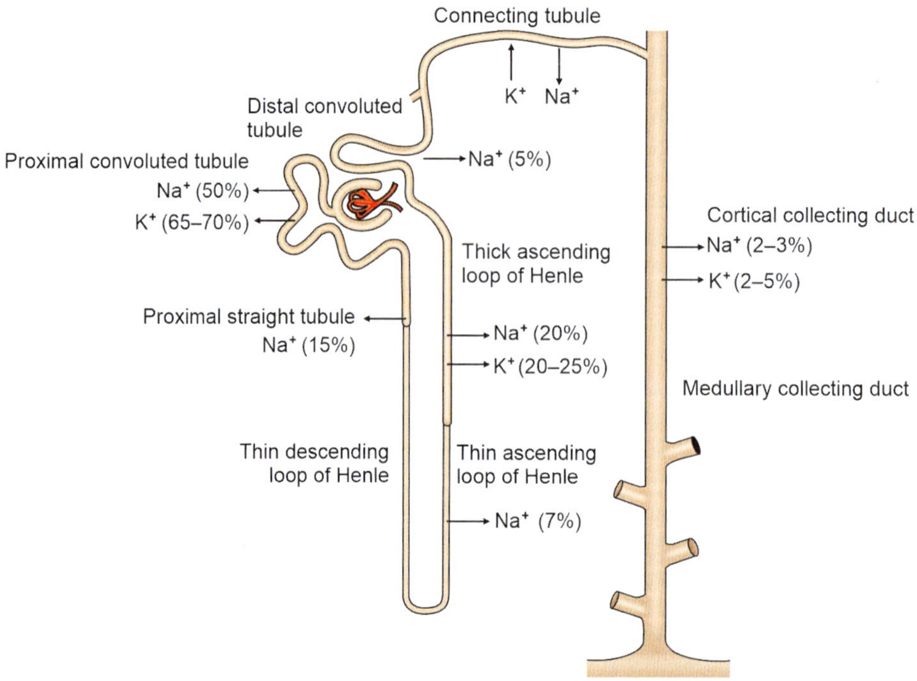


Fig. 17.1: Parts of the nephron, indicating renal tubular handling of sodium and potassium. The major sites of reabsorption are shown, with percentage of filtered cation in parenthesis

## Renal Physiology

Glomerular filtration depends upon the higher pressure in afferent arterioles. The filtration barrier is constituted by the endothelium with slit pores, basement membrane and podocytes of visceral epithelial cells. Filtration of solutes depends upon their molecular size, shape and electrical charge. The filtrate from the glomerular capillaries passes from the Bowman capsule into the renal tubule and collecting ducts. The filtrate contains all the substances that are diffused and ultrafiltered across the filtration barrier from the plasma. Small quantities of protein are present, but are reabsorbed in the proximal tubule. Bulk of the glomerular filtrate is reabsorbed into the peritubular capillaries and only 0.5% is excreted as urine.

### *Tubular Reabsorption*

The proximal tubules reabsorb ~80% of the glomerular filtrate. Approximately 65% of sodium is reabsorbed in the proximal tubule, through several active transport systems. Sodium transport is dependent on the parallel transport of bicarbonate, chloride, amino acids and glucose. Tubular reabsorption of sodium and other permeable solutes is also promoted by the phenomenon of solvent drag during transport of water across the tubular epithelium **(Fig. 17.1)**. The glomerular filtration rate is regulated by tubuloglomerular feedback, which depends upon the functional integrity of the JGA. Increased delivery of chloride to the macula densa results in activation of the renin–angiotensin–aldosterone pathway, which along with the prostaglandins and natriuretic peptides are involved in sodium handling. Potassium is completely reabsorbed in the proximal tubule; the amount in urine depends upon its secretion in the distal tubule.

Distal tubules and collecting ducts are responsible for urinary acidification, concentration and regulation of sodium balance. Exchange of potassium or hydrogen ions for sodium takes place in the distal tubules under the regulation of aldosterone. Antidiuretic hormone mediates absorption of water through insertion of 'water channels' (aquaporins) on the luminal surface of cells in the collecting tubules.

### *Renal Acidification*

The kidney helps in regulation of acid–base balance by maintaining plasma bicarbonate level at 22–26 mEq/L. Depending on dietary protein intake, children produce about 1–3 mEq/kg/day of nonvolatile acids. Filtered bicarbonate is almost completely reabsorbed, chiefly in the proximal tubules and partly in distal tubules and collecting ducts. Bicarbonate, consumed in the buffering of nonvolatile acids, is regenerated by the renal excretion of titrable acid and ammonia. Chronic acidosis augments the production of ammonia and thus elimination of acid. **Figures 17.2 and 17.3** demonstrate the mechanisms of reabsorption of bicarbonate and excretion of protons in the proximal and distal tubules, respectively, which is chiefly mediated by tubular secretion of hydrogen ions ($H^+$).

In the proximal tubule, filtered $HCO_3^-$ combines with $H^+$ to form $H_2CO_3$ that rapidly dissociates to $H_2O$ and $CO_2$ (catalyzed by brush border carbonic anhydrase) **(Fig. 17.2)**. $CO_2$ diffuses along its concentration gradient into the tubular cell, combining with $H_2O_3$ to generate $HCO_3^-$ that is absorbed by the capillaries. The proximal tubule thus reabsorbs 85–90% of the filtered $HCO_3^-$; the remainder is reabsorbed distally. In the distal tubule, the secreted

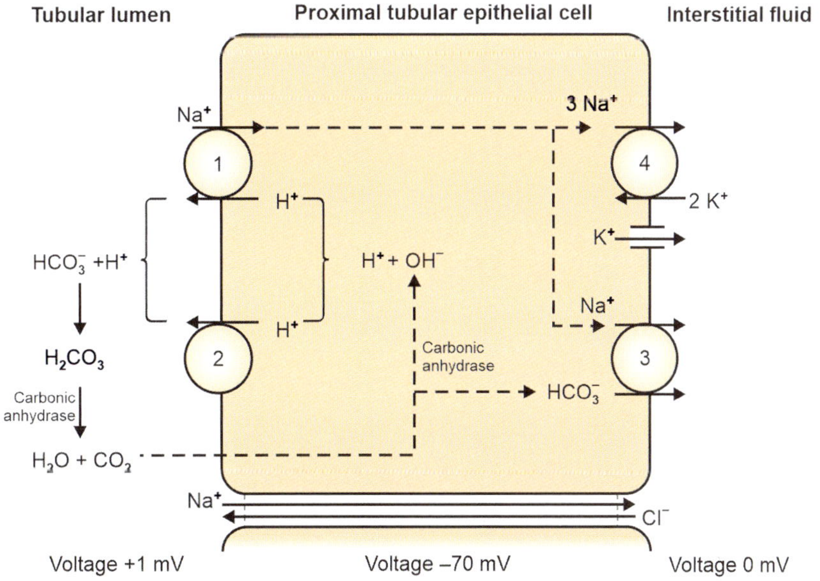


**Fig. 17.2:** Reabsorption of bicarbonate ($HCO_3^-$) in the proximal tubule. Protons ($H^+$) are secreted into the lumen chiefly through the actions of the sodium ($Na^+$) $H^+$ exchanger, NHE-3 (1) and less so, by the $H^+$ ATPase (2). Secreted $H^+$ combines with filtered luminal $HCO_3^-$ to form $H_2CO_3$, which, under the action of luminal membrane carbonic anhydrase, dissociates to form $H_2O$ and $CO_2$. The $CO_2$ travels across the membrane into the cell where it combines with $OH^-$ to generate $HCO_3^-$. The $HCO_3^-$ and $Na^+$ cross the basolateral membrane using the $Na^+/HCO_3^-$ symporter/exchanger, NBCe1 (3). $Na^+$ exits the cell via active transport by $Na^+/K^+$ ATPase (4). Electrogenic $H^+$ secretion generates a small lumen-positive voltage that promotes paracellular flow of cations. Proximal tubular cells are also the site of $Na^+$ coupled reabsorption of glucose, amino acids and $PO_4^{3-}$, the mitochondrial synthesis of $NH_4^+$, and its exit into the lumen, using NHE-3 (not shown)

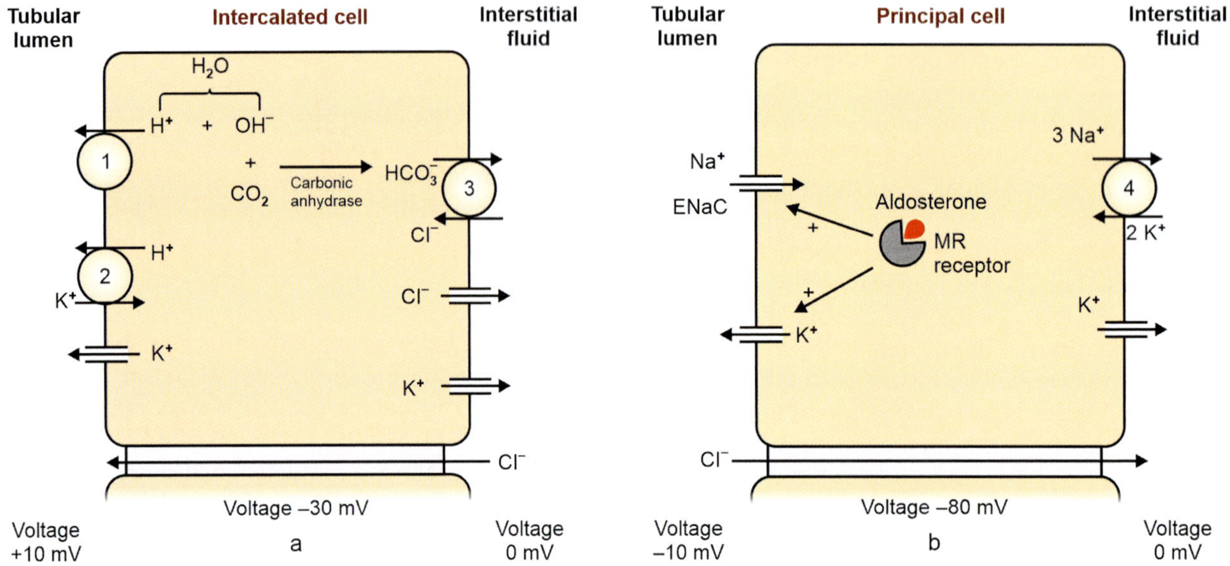


Fig. 17.3: Mechanism of acidification and potassium excretion in the distal renal tubules. (a) The α-intercalated cells of the cortical collecting ducts secrete $H^+$ through the $H^+$ ATPase (1) and $H^+/K^+$ ATPase (2), independent of $Na^+$ transport. The hydroxyl ($OH^-$) ion generated in the cell through dissociation of $H_2O$ combines with $CO_2$ to form $HCO_3^-$, which exits the cell by the $HCO_3^-/Cl^-$ exchanger (anion exchanger 1, AE1) (3). The secreted $H^+$ is buffered by luminal ammonia (to form $NH_4^+$) and phosphate ($HPO_4^{2-}$ to $H_2PO_4^-$; termed titratable acids), to prevent a drop in luminal pH that would prevent further $H^+$ secretion. (b) Principal cells mediate sodium ($Na^+$) absorption and potassium ($K^+$) secretion. Sodium is absorbed through the apical membrane by an amiloride-sensitive $Na^+$ channel (epithelial sodium channel, ENaC), and exits basolaterally via the $Na^+/K^+$ ATPase (4). Sodium transport creates a lumen negative transepithelial potential that increases the rate of $H^+$ secretion by intercalated cells. Aldosterone binds to the mineralocorticoid (MR) receptor and enhances $Na^+$ absorption through ENaC, and $H^+$ and $K^+$ secretion by the $H^+$ ATPase and renal outer medullary potassium (ROMK) channels, respectively. Proteins called WNK-kinases also influence sodium and potassium transport in these cells

$H^+$ ions combine with the major urinary buffers, sodium hydrogen phosphate ($Na_2HPO_4$) and ammonia ($NH_3$) to form $NaH_2PO_4$ and $NH_4^+$, respectively (Fig. 17.3). The distal nephron generates and maintains a steep pH gradient between the blood and urine, but its capacity to secrete $H^+$ ions is small. Thus, even a slight increase in distal $HCO_3^-$ delivery results in increase in urine pH. Extracellular fluid volume and potassium balance also regulate $H^+$ secretion and $HCO_3^-$ reabsorption.

## Suggested Reading

1. Alexander RT, Bitzan M. Renal tubular acidosis. Pediatr Clin North Am 2019; 66:135–57.
2. Bagga A, Sinha A. Renal tubular acidosis. Indian J Pediatr 2020; 87:733–44.
3. Cheng HM, Jusof F. Tubular function. In: Defining physiology: Principles, themes, concepts; 2018. Springer, Singapore. doi.org/10.1007/978-981-13-0499-6–12.
4. Wagner CA, Imenez Silva PH, Bourgeois S. Molecular pathophysiology of acid-base disorders. Semin Nephrol 2019; 39: 340–52.

## Development of Structure and Function

The fetal kidneys are lobulated structures that ascend from size between 12 and 40 weeks, with the renal length increasing from about 1.0 to 4.0 cm. The fetal bladder is visualized by 10–14 weeks, and its capacity increases steadily to about 50 mL at term. Beyond 16 weeks, the amniotic volume is principally dependent on urine production of gestation. These kidneys can be visualized on antenatal ultrasound by 12–13 weeks. The kidneys grow steadily in the pelvis to their normal position between 6 and 9 weeks.

### *Glomerular Filtration*

Glomerular filtration begins at 5–9 weeks' gestation, initiating urine formation. The fetal kidney receives about 2–4% of cardiac output, which increases in neonates to 15–18%. Serum creatinine level is high at birth, reflecting maternal values, but falls rapidly to 0.3–0.5 mg/dL by the end of first week. Most (92%) neonates pass urine within the first 48 hours. The GFR is low at birth (15–20 mL/min/1.73 m² in the first 3 days in term, 10–15 mL/min/1.73 m² in preterm infants) but increases to 35–45 mL/min/1.73 m² at 2 weeks and 75–80 mL/min/1.73 m² by 2 months.

### *Tubular Function*

Tubular function contributes to urine formation around 14 weeks' gestation. Postnatal tubular maturation follows a pattern similar to GFR, but the maturation is relatively delayed. Infants have reduced sodium and bicarbonate reabsorption, and limited ability for hydrogen ion excretion. The pH of urine in newborns is high for the degree of acidemia.

### *Urine Osmolality*

The capacity of the kidneys to concentrate or dilute urine is limited in neonates. An infant can concentrate his urine to a maximum of 700–800 mOsm/kg whereas the older child can achieve 1200–1400 mOsm/kg. Growing babies utilize most of the protein available for growth rather than catabolize to urea. Decreased production and excretion of urea result in a relatively hyposmolar interstitium and reduced urinary concentration. The newborn can dilute urine to a minimum of 50 mOsm/kg, like an older child. However, the time taken to excrete a water load is longer. Thus, delayed feeding and overdiluted or concentrated feeds are potentially harmful.

#### *Maturation of Renal Function*

Renal function continues to improve during the first two years of life, at the end of which, various parameters of renal function approach adult values, if corrected to standard surface area. Structural growth parallels the functional maturation.

### Suggested Reading


1. den Bakker E, Gemke RJBJ, Bökenkamp A. Endogenous markers for kidney function in children: A review. Crit Rev Clin Lab Sci 2018;55:163–83.
2. Iacobelli S, Guignard JP. Maturation of glomerular filtration rate in neonates and infants: An overview. Pediatr Nephrol 2021; 36: 1439–46.
3. van den Anker J, Allegaert K. Considerations for drug dosing in premature infants. J Clin Pharmacol 2021; 61:S141–S151.
4. Zimmerman KO, Benjamin DK, Becker ML. Neonatal therapeutics: Considerations for dosing. Am J Perinatol 2019; 36:S18–S21.


*Competencies:* **PE21.8; PE21.9; PE21.10; PE21.11; PE21.13**

## DIAGNOSTIC EVALUATION

### Clinical Features of Renal Disease

#### *Hematuria*

Gross hematuria in acute glomerulonephritis (GN) is typically smoky brown or cola colored. Bright red blood suggests a nonglomerular cause, as in kidney or vesical stones. Gross hematuria is rare in urinary tract infections (UTI). Other conditions, which might impart a red color to urine, include hemoglobinuria, myoglobinuria, porphyria and ingestion of beetroot.

#### *Edema*

Acute GN presents with facial puffiness and gross hematuria; the edema does not pit readily on pressure. If fluid intake is not restricted, the edema may increase and involve hands, feet and legs. In nephrotic syndrome, edema develops insidiously, starting with eyelid puffiness most noticeable in the morning. Over a period of several days, there is pitting edema over the feet and legs. Facial swelling is often mistaken for allergy or insect bite.

#### *Oliguria*

Oliguria, defined as urine volume less than 0.5 mL/kg/hr for more than 6-hr, commonly results from gastroenteritis and hypovolemia. Oliguria is an important feature of moderate or severe acute GN, acute tubular necrosis and conditions causing severe glomerular injury (hemolytic uremic syndrome—HUS, vasculitis).

#### *Abnormalities of Micturition*

A poor urinary stream in boys, especially in presence of a full bladder, suggests obstruction, most commonly due to posterior urethral valves. Persistent dribbling indicates abnormal ureteric insertion distal to bladder neck, or neurogenic bladder. Infants with meningomyelocele are evaluated for bladder dysfunction. Dysuria, flank pain and ureteric colic suggest UTI or urinary tract calculi.

#### *Polyuria, Polydipsia*

Impaired urinary concentration is a feature of obstructive uropathy and primary or secondary tubulointerstitial disorders. Polyuria is also present in conditions associated with deficiency or resistance to antidiuretic hormone, diabetes mellitus, hypokalemia (e.g. distal renal tubular acidosis) and hypercalcemia.

#### *Enuresis*

Primary monosymptomatic enuresis needs to be distinguished from patients with dysfunctional voiding. Most children with the former have no evidence of renal disease. Urine culture and detailed investigations are not necessary in these cases.

#### *Hypertension*

Assessment of blood pressure is necessary in all children, and especially those with disorders of the kidneys or urinary tract. Symptomatic hypertension is chiefly due to a renal parenchymal or renovascular cause. Screening of healthy asymptomatic children may detect primary hypertension.

#### *Growth Retardation, Anemia*

Growth retardation is a feature of advanced chronic kidney disease (CKD, stages 3–5) and tubular disorders. Normocytic normochromic anemia is striking in patients with advanced CKD. Patients with unexplained anemia should be evaluated for a renal disease.

#### *Abdominal Mass*

Multicystic dysplastic kidney, polycystic kidneys, renal vein thrombosis, hydronephrosis (due to pelviureteric or lower urinary tract obstruction) and Wilms' tumor may result in palpable masses.

### Examination of Urine

Urinalysis is an important step for diagnosis of kidney disease. Evaluation includes microscopic examination of the uncentrifuged as well as centrifuged specimen and semiquantitative or quantitative detection of different substances. While automated analysers using flow cytometry or image-based have replaced manual microscopy in many centers, these instruments have variable diagnostic accuracy. Most instruments have high specificity, detect red and white cells accurately, but may be inferior in discriminating crystals, casts and yeast. Hence, automated analysers are useful in ruling out abnormalities, but manual microscopy is essential in samples with specific abnormalities.

### Collection of Specimen

The first morning specimen is preferred since it is relatively concentrated. While a clean container is sufficient, specimens for culture should be collected in a sterile container. A clean-catch sample is preferred in older children. If facilities for immediate processing are not available, the specimen may be stored at 4°C for 12–18 hours.

It is difficult to obtain satisfactory specimens in children below 2 years old. Urine may be collected using a sterile bag that is applied after local cleaning and removed soon after the void. These specimens should not be used for culture. Other reliable ways for obtaining urine specimens in infants include percutaneous suprapubic aspiration or transurethral catheterization.

### Specific Gravity

Specific gravity is measured using either refractometer or hydrometer; the former is convenient, requires less volume of urine and gives accurate values. The early morning urine specific gravity should exceed 1.015.

### pH

Urine is collected in a closed container; pH is measured promptly. Urine pH is lowest (~5.3–5.5) in the fasting, early morning specimen and increases following meals.

### Protein

Proteinuria is an important marker of renal injury. Detection of 3–4+ albuminuria suggests glomerular disease. Low molecular weight proteinuria, including lysozyme, β2 microglobulin, neutrophil gelatinase associated lipocalin and retinol-binding protein, suggest tubular injury. Dipstick methods (Uristix) for proteinuria are convenient and reliable. Composite strips for pH, glucose, hematuria, leukocyte esterase and nitrite are also available. Proteinuria can also be semiquantitatively tested using the boiling and sulfosalicylic acid tests. Proteinuria is quantitated on early morning spot-, or timed urinary collection. Nephrotic syndrome is characterized by excretion of large amounts of albumin, associated with hypoalbuminemia and edema.

### Reducing Substances

Reducing substances are estimated by Benedict test, or dipsticks, the latter based on the glucose oxidase method. Both tests produce a graded color change, allowing semiquantitative assessment.

### Microscopic Examination

A fresh, well-mixed specimen is examined for cellular elements, crystals and casts. Alternatively, urine is centrifuged at 1500 rpm for 10 minutes; urine is decanted and the cell pellet resuspended in 0.3–0.5 mL urine. Evaluation for hematuria, defined as more than 5 red cells/hpf in a centrifuged specimen is abnormal. Red cell casts indicate glomerular inflammation (Fig. 17.4). Leukocytes may occasionally be absent despite significant bacteriuria. On the other hand, isolated presence of leukocytes is not specific for UTI, and may be noted in interstitial nephritis, GN, stones and high fever. Microscopic detection of bacteriuria in fresh, uncentrifuged urine is significant.

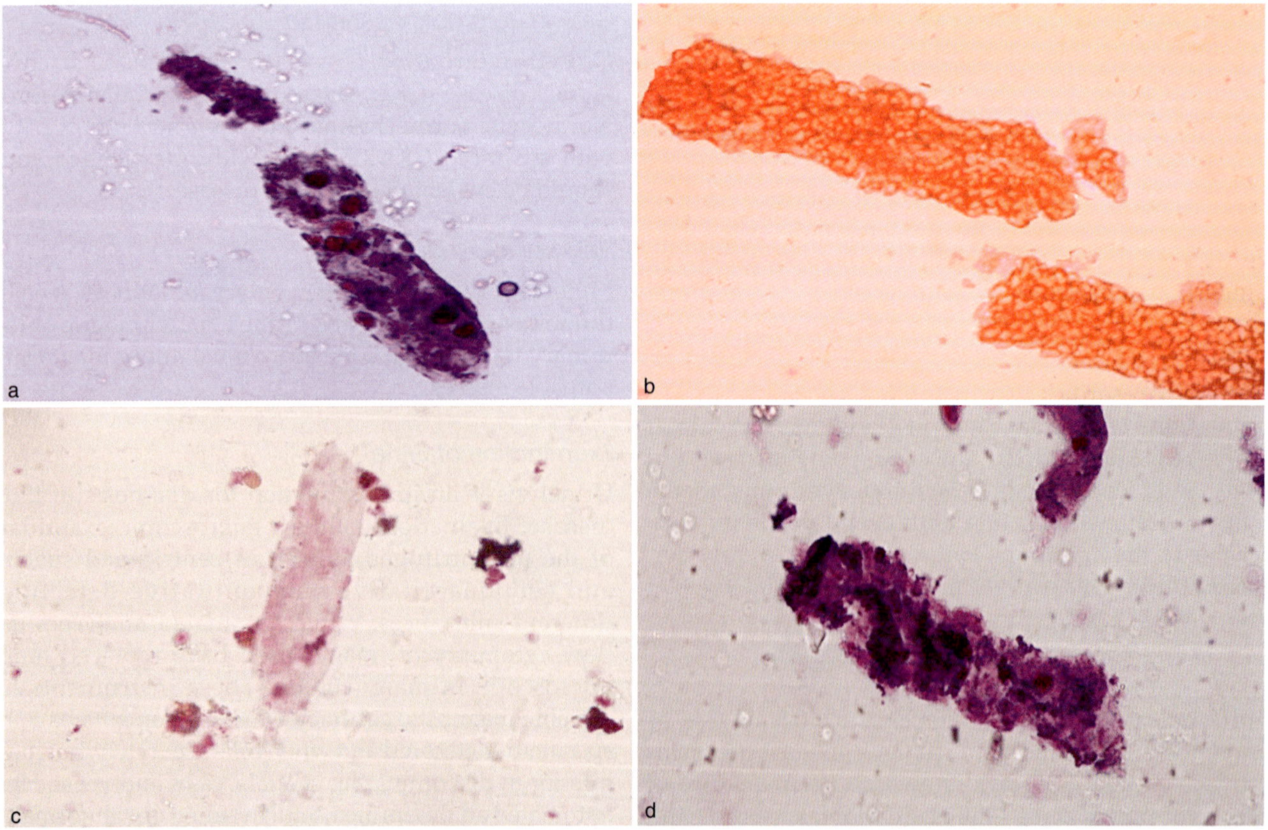


**Fig. 17.4:** Casts on urine microscopic examination: (a) White blood cell casts; (b) Red blood cells casts; (c) Hyaline cast with no cellular elements; (d) Granular cast with degenerated epithelial cells

## Blood Tests

Blood levels of creatinine and urea are used to assess renal function. The normal levels of serum creatinine are 0.2–0.5 mg/dL in children below 6 yr and 0.4–0.7 mg/dL in older children. Blood urea ranges between 20 and 30 mg/dL during childhood. However, it is important to realize the limitations of these investigations. Values of blood urea or creatinine do not increase even when glomerular filtration rate is reduced by 50%. The level of serum creatinine is dependent on muscle mass and is, therefore, low in malnutrition. Bilirubin may interfere with creatinine measurements. Blood urea levels are low on a protein deficient diet and high with tissue breakdown, trauma, hypovolemia, gastrointestinal bleeding and use of corticosteroids. Estimation of blood levels of cystatin C, which does not depend on the nutritional status, is considered a sensitive indicator of glomerular function.

Other specific investigations include albumin, cholesterol, antistreptococcal antibody titers, complement, immunoglobulins and autoantibodies. Estimation of blood pH, bicarbonate, electrolytes and osmolality is important in patients with tubular disorders and/or renal failure.

## Glomerular Filtration Rate (GFR)

While clearance of inulin is regarded as the reference for estimating GFR, the test is cumbersome. Measurement of the creatinine clearance is adequate for assessing GFR in most cases.

### Creatinine and Plasma Iohexol Clearance

Creatinine clearance depends on the body size; the values are normalized to surface area. The normal creatinine clearance is 80–120 mL/min/1.73 $m^2$. GFR can be estimated from serum creatinine (mg/dL) and patient height (cm), using the modified Schwartz formula. The value of *k* ranges between 0.41 and 0.43.

$$\text{GFR (mL/min/1.73 m}^2) = \frac{k \times \text{height (cm)}}{\text{Serum creatinine (mg / dL)}}$$

Plasma clearance of iohexol is used for reliable and accurate estimation of GFR.

### Radionuclide Clearance

Clearance curves of the radionuclides: $^{125}$I-iothalamate, $^{99m}$Tc-diethylenetriaminepentaacetic acid (DTPA) or $^{51}$Cr-ethylenediaminetetraacetic acid (EDTA), following IV injection, can be used to compute GFR.

## Tests of Tubular Function

Table 17.1 lists important evaluations useful in diagnosing disorders of tubular function.

### Water Deprivation Test

Following few hours of fluid deprivation, desamino-8-D-arginine vasopressin (DDAVP) is administered nasally (5–10 µg in neonates and infants, 20 µg in children) or by IM injection (0.4–1.0 µg in infants and young children, 2 µg in older children). Urine is collected every hr for the next 2–3 hr. Following administration of DDAVP, patients with nephrogenic diabetes insipidus fail to show a rise of urine osmolality that remains below 300 mOsm/kg (normal >800 mOsm/kg). Those with deficiency of the antidiuretic hormone concentrate urine appropriately following DDAVP administration.

**Table 17.1:** Investigations for evaluation of tubular diseases

| *Substrate* | *Test* |
|---|---|
| Phosphate | Tubular reabsorption of phosphate<br>Tubular maximum for reabsorption/GFR<br>Plasma parathyroid hormone |
| Glucose | Renal threshold and tubular maximum for glucose reabsorption |
| Amino acids | Clearance of amino acids |
| $\beta_2$ microglobulin | 24-hr urine $\beta_2$ microglobulin excretion |
| Bicarbonate | Plasma anion gap<br>Fractional excretion of bicarbonate |
| Hydrogen ions | Minimum urine pH<br>Urine anion gap; osmolal gap<br>Urine to blood (U–B) $CO_2$ gradient<br>Fludrocortisone furosemide test |
| Water | Maximum urine osmolality<br>Water deprivation test ± vasopressin challenge<br>Plasma antidiuretic hormone, copeptin |
| Sodium | Urinary sodium excretion<br>Fractional excretion of sodium<br>Plasma renin, aldosterone |
| Potassium | Spot urine potassium<br>Urine potassium to creatinine ratio (mEq/g)<br>Transtubular potassium gradient (TTKG) |
| Calcium | Spot urine calcium creatinine ratio (mg/mg)<br>24-hr urine calcium excretion |
| Magnesium | Fractional excretion of magnesium |
| Chloride | 24-hr or spot urine chloride<br>Thiazide test |
| Uric acid | 24-hr uric acid excretion |
| Oxalate | 24-hr oxalate excretion, plasma oxalate |

GFR glomerular filtration rate

*Competency:* **PE21.12**

## Imaging of the Urinary Tract

### Radiology

Ultrasonography is usually the first radiological investigation in patients with suspected kidney disease, and helps suggest or confirm various inherited or acquired conditions, including hydro(uretero)nephrosis, ectopic kidney, hypo- or dysplasia, nephrocalcinosis, nephrolithiasis, cystic kidney disease, tumor and abscesses. Antenatal ultrasonography is useful in detecting a variety of congenital anomalies of kidney and urinary tract that might be asymptomatic postnatally but require evaluation. Doppler evaluation detects renal vein thrombosis, renovascular stenosis, and nutcracker phenomenon. Plain radiograph of the abdomen might confirm constipation

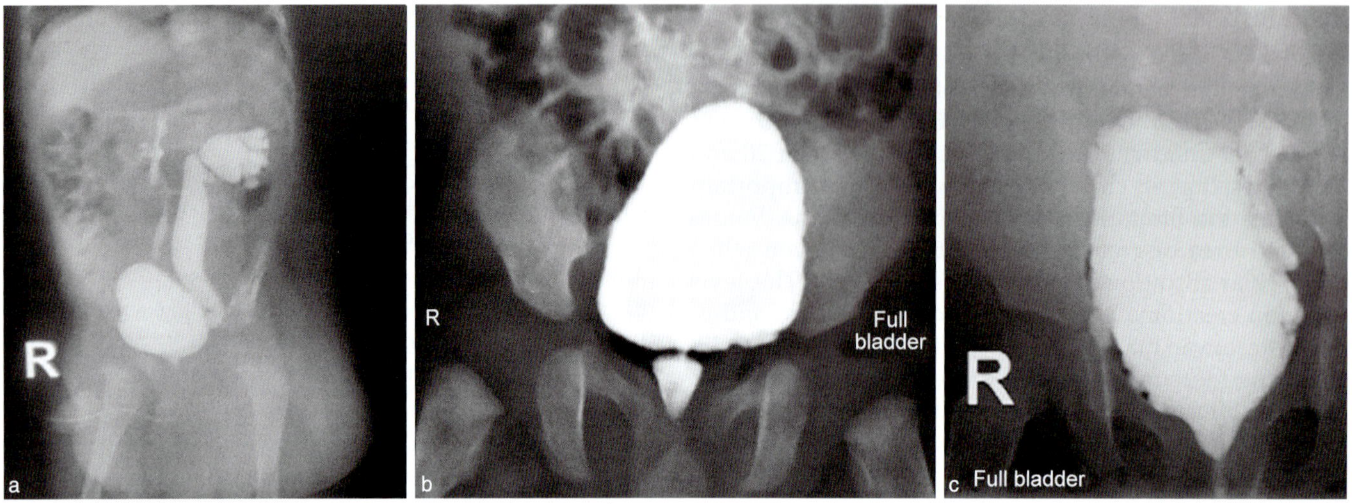


Fig. 17.5: Micturating cystourethrography (MCU) in diagnosis of congenital anomalies of the kidneys and urinary tract and neurogenic bladder: (a) Bilateral vesicoureteric reflux (VUR) of grade 3 on the right side and grade 5 on the left side. Note the dilatation and tortuosity of the left ureter with blunting of the calyces; (b) Dilated posterior urethra with trabeculated urinary bladder and an abrupt transition into a normal caliber urethra, indicating posterior urethral valve(s); (c) Elongated 'pine cone' appearance of the urinary bladder with trabeculations and diverticulae and spinning top urethra, indicating neurogenic bladder

(in suspected bladder bowel dysfunction), and detect spinal dysraphism and occasionally, nephrolithiasis or calcinosis. Micturating cystourethrography (MCU) is essential to diagnose vesicoureteric reflux (VUR) (Fig. 17.5a), posterior urinary valves (Fig. 17.5b), and neurogenic bladder (Fig. 17.5c). The use of high resolution ultrasonography obviates the need for computed tomography in most settings where it was conventionally indicated, including evaluation for nephrocalcinosis and cystic kidney disease. Magnetic resonance imaging and urography are reserved for selected cases, e.g. accurate calculation of total kidney volume in autosomal dominant polycystic kidney disease (ADPKD) and precise delineation of urinary tract anatomy prior to urological surgery, respectively.

### Radionuclide Imaging

Imaging of the kidney and urinary tract has been simplified by radionuclide methods. Radionuclide procedures are noninvasive, highly sensitive and expose patients to less radiation compared to radiocontrast studies. The compounds, labeled with radioactive $^{99m}$technetium, commonly used include dimercaptosuccinic acid (DMSA), DTPA and mercaptotriacylglycine (MAG-3).

DTPA is freely filtered by the glomeruli with no tubular reabsorption or excretion. A DTPA renogram is useful for evaluating perfusion and function of each kidney. Obstruction to the urine flow is diagnosed by studying the effect of IV frusemide. Normally, there is prompt washout of the radionuclide, but this clearing may not occur in subjects with upper urinary tract obstruction (Fig. 17.6a). Renal arterial narrowing results in reduced renal blood flow and an abnormal pattern on DTPA renogram. This effect is accentuated by administration of angiotensin-converting enzyme inhibitors, increasing its sensitivity in diagnosis of renal artery stenosis. MAG-3 is a versatile radionuclide since it provides satisfactory information on renal structure and function.

Following IV injection, DMSA attains high concentration in the cortex and provides high quality images of kidney morphology. This is useful in detection and follow-up of renal parenchymal defects associated with urinary tract infections (Fig. 17.6b).

$^{99m}$Tc-labeled radionuclide scan can be used instead of the radiocontrast MCU. The procedure is sensitive in detecting VUR with minimal radiation exposure (Fig. 17.6c). However, this procedure neither provides precise anatomic details of bladder and urethra to be used in evaluating patients with suspected urinary tract obstruction, nor does it allow grading of VUR.

### Genetic Testing

Inherited disorders contribute to almost 30% of chronic kidney diseases in children, including nephrotic syndrome, atypical hemolytic uremic syndrome, cystic kidney disease, tubulopathies, hematuric nephropathies, and congenital anomalies of the kidneys and urinary tract. Novel techniques of testing, including next-generation sequencing and multiplex ligation-dependent probe amplification are finding applications in genetic testing, in various kidney disorder, and help disease identification and classification, inform physicians and families regarding the disease prognosis and specific treatment if available, and facilitate prenatal genetic counseling and testing.

### Suggested Reading


1. Arora V, Anand K, Verma C. Genetic testing in pediatric kidney disease. Indian J Pediatr 2020; 87: 706–15.
2. Cavanaugh C, Perazella MA. Urine sediment examination in the diagnosis and management of kidney disease: Core curriculum 2019. Am J Kid Dis 2109; 73: 258–72.
3. Dhull RS, Joshi A, Saha A. Nuclear imaging in pediatric kidney diseases. Indian Pediatr 2018;55:591–97.
4. Pottel H, Schaeffner E, Ebert N, et al. Iohexol plasma clearance for measuring glomerular filtration rate. BMC Nephrol 2021; 22:166.

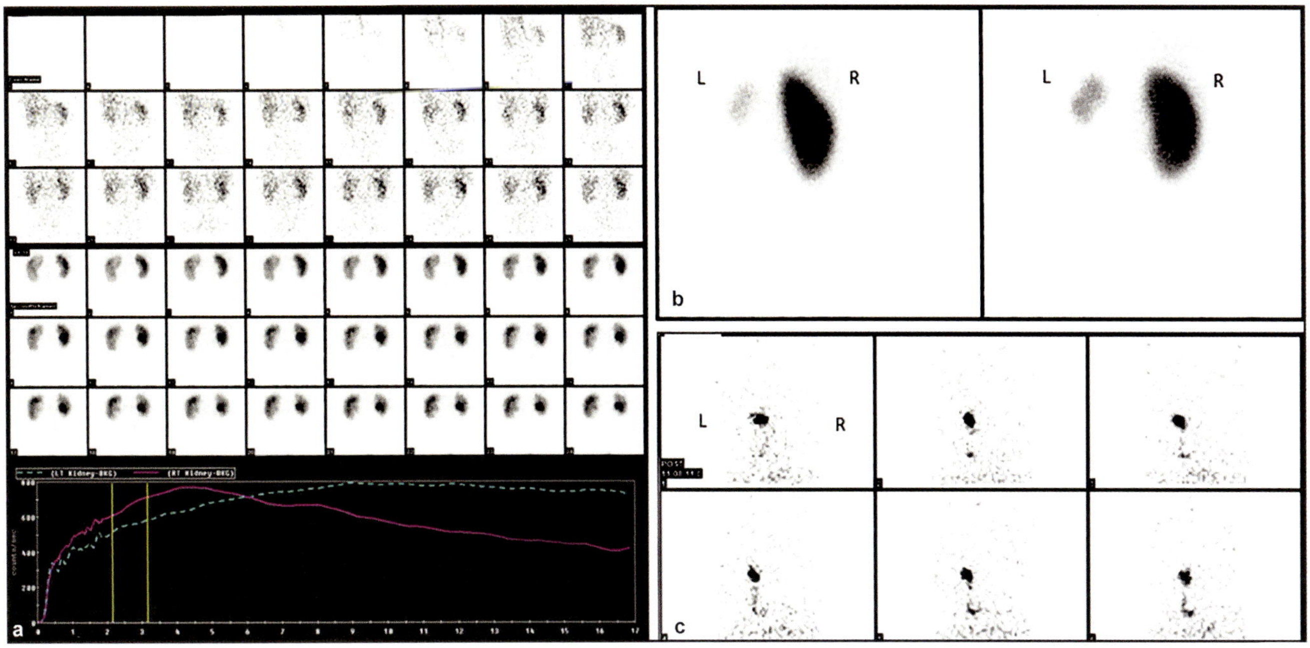


**Fig. 17.6:** Nuclear imaging in diagnosis of congenital anomalies of the kidneys and urinary tract: (a) $^{99m}$DTPA dynamic scan with diuretic was performed in a 6-week-old boy with isolated left hydronephrosis. The excretion of the tracer on the left kidney (LK) is delayed and unchanged with administration of diuretic, suggesting an obstructive pattern of excretion, as seen with pelviureteric junction obstruction; (b) $^{99m}$Tc-DMSA scintigraphy showing scarred left kidney with loss of volume, while the right kidney is normal; (c) Direct radionuclide cystography indicating vesicoureteric reflux into left ureter and kidney. Note: All images are taken from the back, hence the right side of images indicates the left kidney

5. Murray SL, Fennelly NK, Doyle B, Lynch SA, Conlon PJ. Integration of genetic and histopathology data in interpretation of kidney disease. Nephrol Dial Transplant 2020; 35: 1113–32.
6. Niyyar VD, O'Neill WC. Point-of-care ultrasound in the practice of nephrology. Kidney Int 2018;93:1052–59.

*Competencies:* **PE21.4; PE21.15; PE21.16**

## HEMATURIA

The presence of blood in urine imparts it a color, which includes various shades of deep red, smoky brown, cola-color and faint pink. Parents may mistake concentrated urine for that containing blood. Microscopic examination of urine will show red blood cells. Reagent-coated dipsticks detect free hemoglobin and myoglobin. Red urine may be present in porphyria and following beetroot ingestion. Urine appears orange-colored after administration of rifampicin or pyridium. Uric acid and xanthine crystals may also impart a pink tinge to the nappy. In children, the commonest cause of gross hematuria is postinfectious GN (Table 17.2). Urinary tract stones are not infrequent. Gross hematuria is rare in acute pyelonephritis, but may occur with viral cystitis.

Conditions that cause persistent microscopic hematuria include idiopathic hypercalciuria, infection related GN, IgA

**Table 17.2:** Causes of hematuria

| *Glomerular* | *Non-glomerular* |
|---|---|
| Infection related glomerulonephritis (GN) | Hypercalciuria |
| IgA nephropathy | Kidney stones |
| IgA vasculitis (Henoch-Schönlein purpura) | Urinary tract infection |
| C3 glomerulopathy | Hemorrhagic cystitis*[1] |
| Rapidly progressive GN | Trauma, exercise |
| | Nutcracker syndrome |
| | Cystic kidney disease |
| | Interstitial nephritis |
| *Uncommon* | *Uncommon* |
| Lupus nephritis | Vascular malformations |
| Other vasculitides, e.g. microscopic polyangiitis | Coagulation disorders |
| Membranous nephropathy | Thrombocytopenia |
| Alport syndrome | Renal or bladder malignancy |
| *MYH9* related disorders; rare familial nephropathies | Drug-induced crystalluria*[2] |

*MYH9* myosin heavy chain 9
*Common causes are: [1]adenovirus infection and IV cyclophosphamide; [2]amoxycillin, acyclovir and foscarnet

nephropathy, C3 glomerulopathy, Alport syndrome, and uncommon rare inherited nephropathies.

### Diagnostic Evaluation

A history of pain in the flank or suprapubic region, dysuria and edema should be obtained. Physical examination includes assessment of growth and features of acute or chronic kidney disease such as edema, hypertension, unexplained pallor, bony abnormalities and abdominal mass. An audiogram and a detailed eye examination may be needed. Figure 17.7 shows an algorithm for evaluation of patients with hematuria.

A fresh specimen is examined for red cells, red cell casts and protein. Absence of large number of red cells

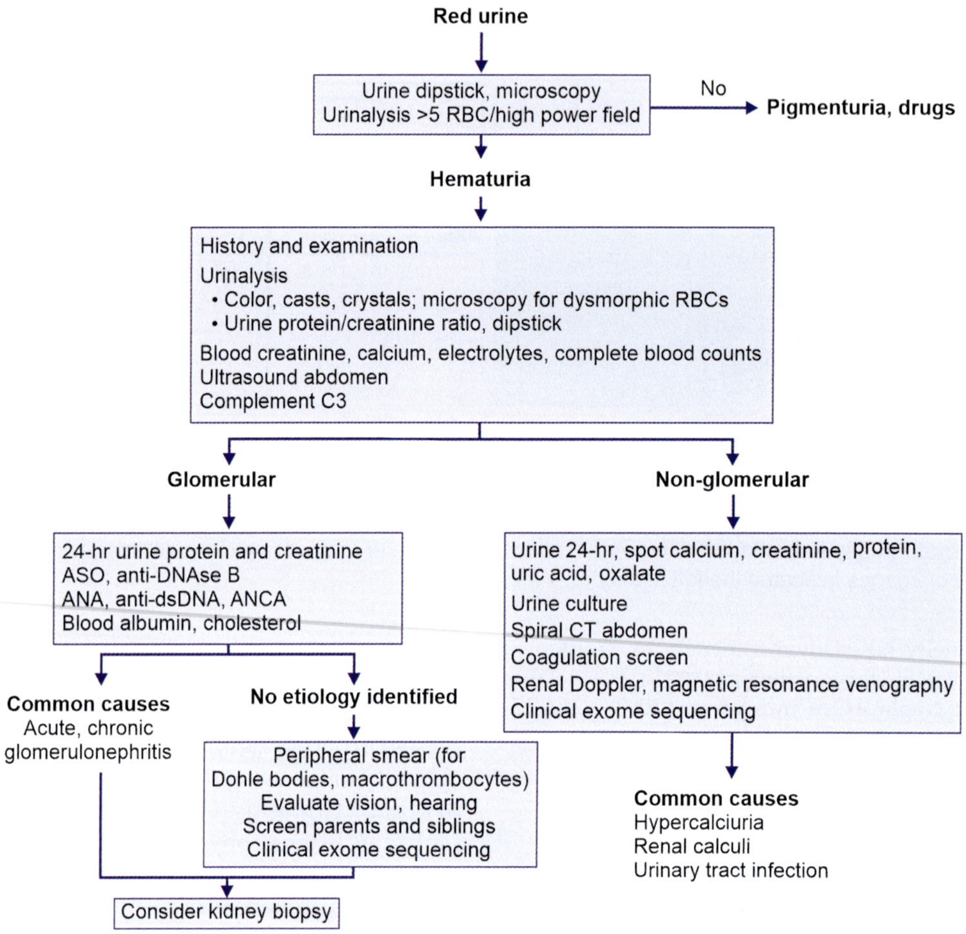


**Fig. 17.7:** Approach to evaluation of a patient with hematuria. The initial step in evaluation attempts to distinguish glomerular from non-glomerular causes of hematuria (*see* Table 17.3). Estimation of complement C3 is an important screening test for postinfectious glomerulonephritis. Patients with persistent glomerular hematuria require kidney biopsy and/or screening for familial causes. ANA antinuclear antibody; anti-dsDNA anti-double-stranded DNA antibody; ANCA antineutrophil cytoplasmic antibody; ASO antistreptolysin O

**Table 17.3:** Features that distinguish glomerular from non-glomerular hematuria

| *Features* | *Glomerular causes* | *Non-glomerular causes* |
|---|---|---|
| Dysuria | No | Suggests urethritis or cystitis |
| Systemic complaints | Edema, pharyngitis, rash, arthralgia | Fever (UTI), loin pain (calculi) |
| Family history | Deafness, kidney failure (Alport syndrome) | Calculi (hypercalciuria, uricosuria) |
| Hypertension, edema | Common | Rare |
| Association with exercise | Absent | Nutcracker syndrome |
| Abdominal mass | Absent | Wilms tumor, obstructive uropathy, polycystic kidney disease |
| Urine color | Brown, tea, or cola | Bright red, clots |
| Proteinuria | 2+ or more | Trace, 1+ |
| Dysmorphic red cells | >20% | <15% |
| Red cell casts | Common | Absent |
| Crystals | Absent | May suggest calculi |
| Hypercalciuria or hyperuricosuria | Absent | May suggest calculi |

UTI urinary tract infection

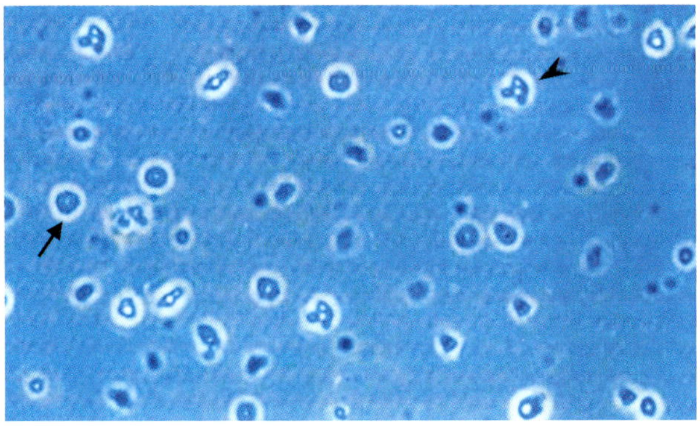

Fig. 17.8: Phase contrast microscopy showing dysmorphic red cells (arrowhead). Normal red cells are also seen (arrow)

in bloody urine suggests hemoglobinuria (intravascular hemolysis) or myoglobinuria. In glomerular disease, urine shows dysmorphic red cells, of different shapes, whereas in bleeding from renal pelvis or the lower urinary tract, the red cells maintain normal morphology (Fig. 17.8 and Table 17.3). Presence of significant proteinuria (2+ or more) and/or red cell casts suggests glomerular disease. Hypercalciuria is screened for determination of urinary calcium to creatinine ratio on one or more random samples.

A plain X-ray film of the abdomen and abdominal ultrasound is done to exclude major renal and urinary tract anomalies and calculi. Blood levels of creatinine are measured; specialized blood tests depend on the likely clinical etiology. Surgical conditions that cause hematuria can be diagnosed by appropriate imaging. Invasive procedures such as cystoscopy are rarely indicated. In a significant proportion, isolated microscopic hematuria spontaneously disappears over a period of several years. Other family members may have similar urinary abnormalities. If there is no family history, a renal biopsy is not urgently indicated and the patient kept under observation.

### Kidney Biopsy

Biopsy is advised, if hematuria is associated with persistent or heavy (≥3+) proteinuria, history of kidney disease in the family, or if features of CKD, renal impairment or hypertension are seen on follow up. A biopsy is also considered in children, if microscopic hematuria persists for 2 or more years, even in the absence of above features. This procedure is necessary to diagnose IgA nephropathy, and various primary and secondary GN.

The biopsy specimen should be evaluated by light, immunofluorescence and electron microscopy.

### Alport Syndrome

This condition is inherited in an X-linked manner, although autosomal transmission is known. Mutations in the gene encoding alpha subunit of collagen IV (*COL4A*) result in persistent microscopic hematuria, moderate proteinuria and progressive kidney failure. A significant proportion show high frequency sensorineural deafness; ocular defects (lenticonus, cataract, macular flecks) are often associated. Ultrastructural examination of renal biopsy shows variable thickness of glomerular basement membrane with lengths of marked attenuation to areas of lamination. Therapy is supportive, including the use of angiotensin-converting enzyme inhibitors. The majority of male patients (X-linked illness; hemizygous mutations in *COL4A5*) show progression to kidney failure. Progression of illness in patients with autosomal recessive illness (mutation in *COL4A3* or *COL4A4*) is also rapid. Patients with thin GBM disease are considered a spectrum of Alport syndrome, and should be appropriately counseled. Diagnosis has conventionally relied on demonstration of typical changes on electron microscopy (Fig. 17.9); non-invasive diagnosis is increasingly performed using clinical exome sequencing.

### Suggested Reading


1. Bignall ONR 2nd, Dixon BP. Management of hematuria in children. Curr Treat Options Pediatr 2018;4:333–49.
2. Kailash M, Rheault MN. Approach to persistent microscopic hematuria in children. Kidney 360 2020;1:1014–20
3. Luciano RL, Moeckel GW. Update on the native kidney biopsy: Core curriculum 2019. Am J Kidney Dis 2019;73:404–15.


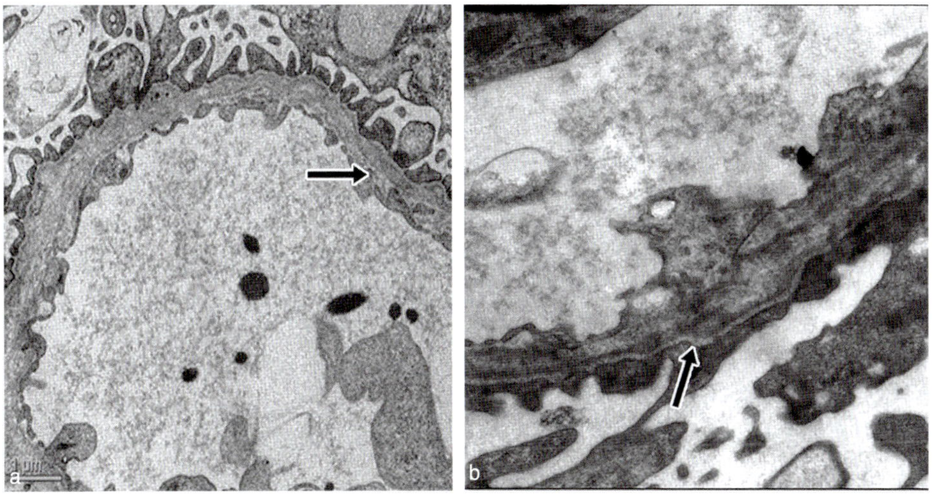

Fig. 17.9: Electron microscopy images: (a) A 12-yr-old boy with nephrotic syndrome and persistent microscopic hematuria showing 'basket weave' appearance (arrow) of glomerular basement membrane (GBM) with focal foot process effacement [uranyl acetate 2050x]; (b) A 10-yr-old boy with hematuria and proteinuria showing lamellation and rarefaction of GBM with tenting (arrow), reduced GBM thickness (100–180 nm) for age and focal foot process effacement [uranyl acetate 3000×]

4. Mantan M, Batra V. Renal biopsy in children. Indian Pediatr 2020;57:452–58.
5. Warady BA, Agarwal A, Bangalore S, et al. Alport syndrome: classification and management. Kidney Med 2020;2:639–49.

## PROTEINURIA

The glomerular capillaries provide an effective barrier to filtration of proteins. Small amounts of protein are filtered but almost completely reabsorbed by the proximal tubule. Detection of more than trace amounts of protein in the urine is abnormal. Massive proteinuria occurs in minimal change disease, in which glomeruli are normal or show mild changes. Persistent and heavy proteinuria, especially if associated with hematuria, should be promptly evaluated.

### Quantitation of Proteinuria

Protein excretion at 100–1000 mg/$m^2$/day indicates mild to moderate proteinuria; more than that is heavy (nephrotic range) proteinuria. Accurate quantitative measurement of 24-hour urinary protein is not needed, if semiquantitative tests are done on a concentrated specimen. Normally, the protein to creatinine ratio, in the first or second morning urine specimen, is below 0.2 mg/mg; a ratio of 0.2–2 mg/mg indicates mild to moderate and >2 mg/mg heavy proteinuria. The latter usually corresponds to 3+ or 4+ reaction on boiling or dipstick.

Important causes of asymptomatic proteinuria include orthostatic proteinuria, chronic glomerular diseases, reflux nephropathy, renal hypoplasia and renal tubular disorders (Table 17.4). In orthostatic (postural) proteinuria, protein is absent in urine specimen collected after overnight recumbence, but increases by the afternoon following upright posture.

Kidney biopsy is indicated in presence of persistent or heavy proteinuria. Long-term observation is necessary to monitor clinical course and renal function. The underlying cause is treated, where possible. Low salt diet and prolonged treatment with angiotensin-converting enzyme inhibitors or angiotensin receptor blockers are effective in reducing glomerular proteinuria.

**Table 17.4:** Conditions presenting with proteinuria

**Glomerular proteinuria**
- Nephrotic syndrome (minimal change disease, focal segmental glomerulosclerosis, congenital nephrotic syndrome)
- Membranous nephropathy
- Hepatitis B, C; HIV associated nephropathy
- Reflux nephropathy
- Amyloidosis, Fabry disease
- Associated with hematuria: Infection related GN, IgA nephropathy, IgA vasculitis, lupus nephritis, C3 glomerulopathy, hemolytic uremic syndrome, Alport syndrome, other familial hematuric nephropathies, malignant hypertension

**Nonglomerular proteinuria**
- Medication induced nephropathy (analgesics)
- Heavy metal nephropathy (e.g. gold, lead, cadmium)
- Dent disease, cystinosis, other causes of renal tubular acidosis
- Interstitial nephritis, pyelonephritis
- Intermittent or transient proteinuria
- Postural (orthostatic)
- Fever
- Exercise

### Suggested Reading

1. Larkins NG, Teixeira-Pinto A, Craig JC. A narrative review of proteinuria and albuminuria as clinical biomarkers in children. J Paediatr Child Health 2019;55:136–42.
2. Leung AKC, Wong AHC, Barg SSN. Proteinuria in children. Am Fam Physician 2017;95:248–54.
3. Viteri B, Reid-Adam J. Hematuria and proteinuria in children. Pediatr Rev 2018;39:573–587.

*Competencies:* **PE21.2; PE21.15; PE21.16**

## ACUTE GLOMERULONEPHRITIS

Acute glomerulonephritis (GN) is characterized by abrupt onset of hematuria, oliguria, edema and hypertension. The clinical severity varies: mild disease may go undetected; severe cases have anuria, hypertensive encephalopathy and heart failure. Poststreptococcal GN is the most common cause of acute GN in India (Table 17.5). Key investigations include blood urea and creatinine, urinalysis, serum complement C3 and titers of antistreptolysin. Therapy of skin and throat infections has resulted in decline of poststreptococcal GN, and increasing recognition of other infectious causes. Renal biopsy is required, if the presentation or course suggests a diagnosis other than poststreptococcal GN (Table 17.6).

### Poststreptococcal Glomerulonephritis

Acute GN following infection by group A beta-hemolytic streptococci is a common disorder. Streptococcal infection of the throat or skin precedes the onset of nephritis by 1 to 4 weeks. Only a few strains of streptococci are nephritogenic, e.g. types 4 and 12 causing pharyngitis and type 49 causing pyoderma.

**Table 17.5:** Etiology of the acute nephritic syndrome

**Infection related glomerulonephritis (IRGN)**
- *Postinfectious:* Streptococci, staphylococci, pneumococci, meningococci
- *Treponema pallidum*, *Salmonella*, *Leptospira*
- *Plasmodium malariae*, *P. falciparum*, toxoplasma, filariasis
- Hepatitis B & C, cytomegalovirus, parvovirus B19, Epstein-Barr virus, coxsackievirus, echovirus, varicella
- Severe infections: Infection of shunts, prostheses, bacterial endocarditis

**Systemic vasculitis**
- IgA vasculitis (Henoch-Schönlein purpura)
- Microscopic polyarteritis, polyangiitis with granulomatosis

**Others**
- C3 glomerulopathy
- IgA nephropathy
- Systemic lupus erythematosus
- Alport syndrome; *MYH9* related kidney disease

**Table 17.6:** Indications for kidney biopsy in acute glomerulonephritis (GN)

**Systemic features**
- Fever, rash, joint pain, pulmonary symptoms, heart disease; history of recurrences
- Absence of serologic evidence of streptococcal infection; normal C3 in acute stage of illness
- Features of both GN and nephrotic syndrome
- High blood urea and creatinine, or anuria requiring dialysis

**Delayed resolution**
- Oliguria, hypertension, azotemia beyond 7–10 days
- Gross hematuria persisting beyond 3–4 weeks
- Nephrotic range proteinuria beyond 2 weeks
- Low C3 levels beyond 12 weeks

### Pathology

On light microscopy, glomeruli are enlarged and ischemic and capillary loops narrowed, making glomeruli appear bloodless **(Fig. 17.10a)**; there is proliferation of mesangial cells and neutrophil infiltration. Immunofluorescence shows granular deposits of IgG and complement (C3) along capillary walls **(Fig. 17.10b)**. Electron microscopy shows deposits (humps) on the subepithelial side of the glomerular basement membrane.

### Clinical Features

Poststreptococcal GN affects school-age children, more commonly boys and is uncommon below 3-yr. Subclinical episodes are more common than overt disease, especially during epidemics. The onset is rapid, with puffiness around the eyes and pedal edema. Urine is cola-colored; hematuria is brief, often lasting only a few hours and does not persist beyond 1–2 weeks. While the degree of oliguria correlates with disease severity, anuria is uncommon. Hypertension, present in over half the patients, resolves with loss of edema. Atypical presentations include: (i) Convulsions due to hypertensive encephalopathy; (ii) left ventricular failure and pulmonary edema, due to malignant hypertension and hypervolemia; (iii) acute kidney injury; and (iv) nephrotic syndrome.

### Laboratory Findings

Urine shows 1–2+ protein with red cells, and red cell and granular casts. White cells may indicate inflammation within the glomeruli. Hemodilution may result in normocytic anemia; ESR is raised. Blood levels of urea and creatinine are elevated reflecting renal impairment; hyponatremia and hyperkalemia occur with continuing oliguria. Chest X-ray may show prominent vascular markings, suggesting hypervolemia.

Serologic evidence for streptococcal infection is present in most patients with pharyngitis, though antibiotic therapy may blunt this response. ASO titer is increased in more than 80% patients; anti-DNase B is elevated in cases of streptococcal skin infection. The titers decrease within 4–6 weeks. The level of serum C3 is low in 90% patients but normalizes by 8–12 weeks. Persistent low C3 levels indicate other forms of GN.

### Management

Patients with mild oliguria and normal blood pressure can be managed at home. Close attention to blood pressure and dietary intake is essential. Therapy with antibiotics has no effect on the course of the disease, but may be given, if active pharyngitis or pyoderma is present. The principles of management of patients with severe oliguria and acute kidney injury are discussed later.

***Diet:*** The intake of sodium, potassium and fluids is restricted until blood levels of creatinine reduce and urine output increases. Overhydration may increase the risk of hypertension and precipitate left ventricular failure. Patients with azotemia require accurate measurement of urine output and daily weight, and restriction of fluid

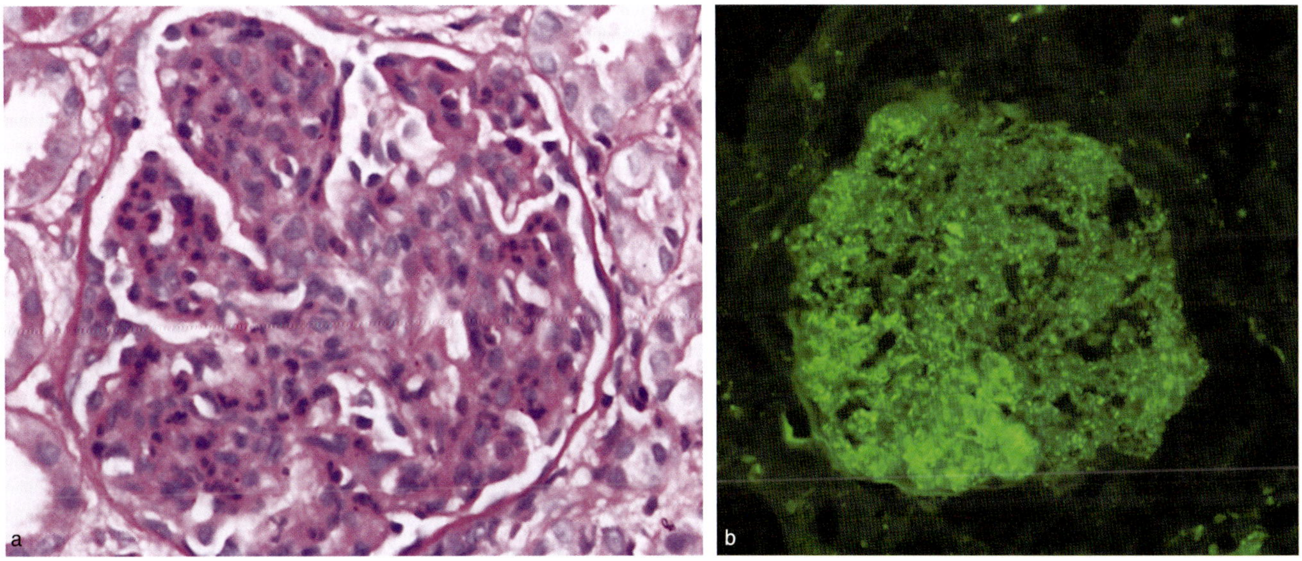


**Fig. 17.10:** Post-streptococcal GN: (a) Moderately severe proliferation and exudative changes with infiltration of neutrophils. A few open capillary lumina are seen; (b) Immunofluorescence stain shows extensive granular deposits of IgG along the capillary wall and mesangium, resulting in starry sky appearance

intake to an amount equal to insensible losses and 24 hr urine output.

***Diuretics:*** Patients showing modest edema are treated with oral frusemide at a dose of 1–3 mg/kg; the edema disappears with the return of renal function. Therapy with IV frusemide (2–4 mg/kg) is necessary in patients with pulmonary edema.

***Hypertension:*** Mild hypertension may be controlled by restricting salt and water intake. Effective antihypertensive agents include amlodipine, nifedipine or diuretics. Beta blockers and angiotensin-converting enzyme inhibitors carry risk of hyperkalemia. Patients with hypertensive emergencies need prompt treatment with IV nitroprusside or labetalol.

***Left ventricular failure:*** Hypertension should be controlled and IV frusemide given to induce diuresis, leading to improvement in heart failure. If diuresis is not noted, dialysis is initiated. Respiratory support with positive end-expiratory pressure may be needed.

***Prolonged oliguria:*** Treatment, as outlined above, should be continued and levels of blood urea, creatinine and electrolytes monitored. Dialysis is required in children with severe renal failure and prolonged oligoanuria, fluid overload and life-threatening electrolyte disturbances. Occurrence of secondary infections should be avoided.

### *Outcome and Prognosis*

Acute poststreptococcal GN has an excellent prognosis in childhood. The symptoms begin to resolve in the first week with loss of edema and fall in blood pressure. Gross hematuria and significant proteinuria disappear within 2 weeks, although microscopic hematuria and slight proteinuria may persist for several months. Hypertension subsides within 2–3 weeks, but rarely may persist for several weeks. Patients with acute GN of nonstreptococcal etiology have variable and unpredictable outcome. These cases need close follow-up over several years with periodic urinalyses and measurements of blood pressure.

***Kidney biopsy:*** A biopsy is rarely indicated in suspected poststreptococcal GN, except if there is rapidly deteriorating kidney function, nephrotic range proteinuria, features of a systemic illness (e.g. systemic lupus), or serum C3 remains depressed beyond 12 weeks (Table 17.6).

## Crescentic Glomerulonephritis

Rapidly progressive GN (RPGN) is defined as an acute nephritic illness accompanied by rapid loss of kidney function over days to weeks. The histopathological correlate is the presence of crescents involving 50% or more glomeruli (Fig. 17.11), indicating severe glomerular injury. The chief forms of the illness are: Immune complex crescentic GN (immunofluorescence showing IgG and C3 deposits; normal or low C3); pauci-immune crescentic GN (small vessel vasculitis; scant immune deposits; positive ANCA); and anti-glomerular basement membrane GN (with anti-GBM antibodies; linear IgG deposits).

There is satisfactory clinicopathologic correlation, and patients with extensive histological changes have poor outcomes. Renal biopsy should be performed in all patients with severe nephritic features, which do not resolve within 1–2 weeks.

The outcome is related to histological severity and prompt institution of therapy. Satisfactory results have been obtained with initial administration of IV and oral corticosteroids and IV cyclophosphamide, followed by maintenance immunosuppression for 2–3 years. Prompt institution of plasma exchanges is recommended for patients with anti-GBM antibodies, and dialysis dependent patients with pauci-immune crescentic GN. Patients with ANCA-associated small vessel vasculitis require the above therapy, along with additional use of other immunosuppressive agents, including rituximab.

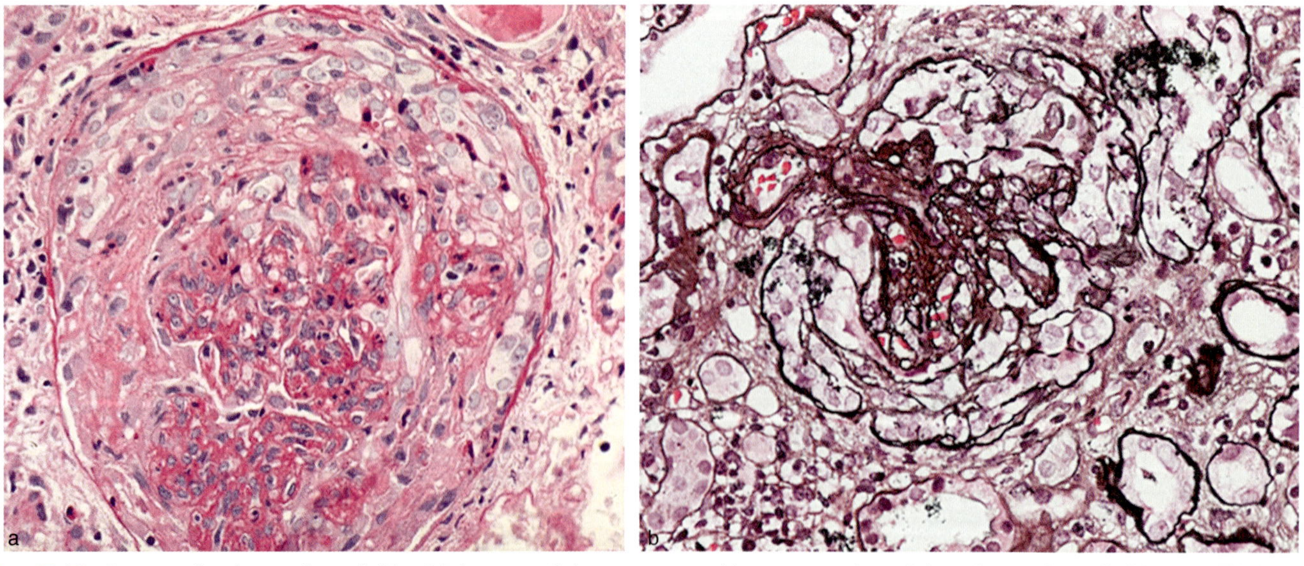


Fig. 17.11: Crescentic glomerulonephritis: (a) Large cellular crescent with compression of the glomerular tuft (Masson Trichome, 200×); (b) A cellular crescent with early fibrous stranding, without significant proliferation, and partial sclerosis of the underlying tuft (Jones silver methenamine 200×). (*Images courtesy:* Dr Geetika Singh, Department of Pathology, All India Institute of Medical Sciences, New Delhi, India)

#### Nephritis in IgA Vasculitis (Henoch-Schönlein Purpura)

IgA vasculitis is the most common vasculitis in children (Fig. 17.12), characterized by the triad of palpable purpura, abdominal pain and arthralgia involving large joints. One-third patients show mild kidney involvement, with microscopic hematuria and mild proteinuria, usually within 6–12 months of disease onset. Serum IgA levels may be elevated. Kidney biopsy shows variable mesangial proliferation with mesangial deposits of IgA. Most patients recover without any specific treatment. Long-term observation is necessary to detect insidious renal damage, especially in older children and adults.

Rarely a patient may present with nephritic or nephrotic syndrome, hypertension, azotemia or as rapidly progressive GN. Therapy with a combination of oral/IV corticosteroids and cyclophosphamide initially, followed by maintenance steroids and azathioprine is recommended. Long-term outcome depends on the severity of kidney manifestations; ~1% patients may show progressive loss of kidney function.

#### Immunoglobulin A Nephropathy

Predominant deposition of IgA in the glomeruli, chiefly in the mesangium and occasionally in capillary walls is characteristic. The usual clinical manifestation is recurrent episodes of gross hematuria following upper respiratory infections; each episode lasts for 3–7 days. An acute nephritic or nephrotic syndrome is rarely the initial manifestation. Kidney histology shows mesangial proliferation of varying severity. Patients with hematuria and non-nephrotic proteinuria are treated with angiotensin-converting enzyme inhibitors. Therapy with corticosteroids and alkylating agents is indicated for patients with nephrotic range proteinuria, deranged kidney function or those showing severe histological changes, including severe endocapillary proliferation or crescents.

#### Lupus Nephritis

Pediatric patients with systemic lupus erythematosus often present with asymptomatic proteinuria and/or hematuria, acute nephritic syndrome and nephrotic syndrome. Renal biopsy may show almost normal glomeruli, focal or diffuse proliferative GN or membranous nephropathy. Immunofluorescence studies show mesangial and capillary wall deposits of all immune reactants (full-house deposition). Antinuclear and double-stranded DNA antibodies are present in most cases with lupus nephritis; C3 and C4 levels are reduced.

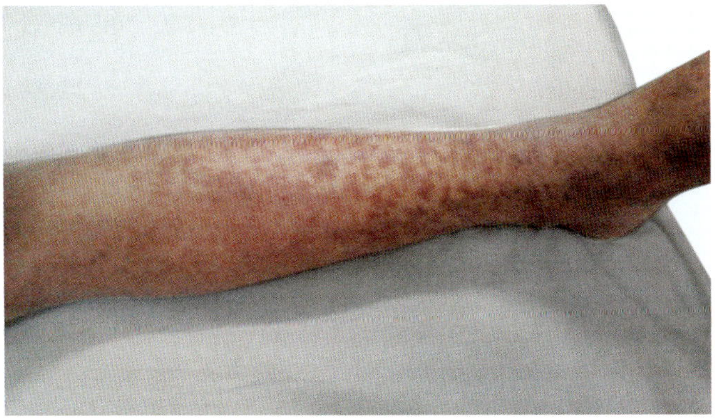

Fig. 17.12: IgA vasculitis in a 6-year-old girl with severe abdominal pain. Note the purpuric rash over the lower limbs

Therapy for lupus nephritis is based on the severity of the kidney disease, and is targeted at complete response (proteinuria <0.5–0.7 g/24 hours with normal glomerular filtration rate by 12 months). Hydroxychloroquine is recommended in all patients with regular ophthalmological monitoring. Patients with active proliferative nephritis should receive initial (induction) treatment with either intravenous cyclophosphamide (6 doses every 2–4 weeks) or high dose mycophenolate mofetil, combined with corticosteroids, initially as pulses of intravenous methylprednisolone, followed by oral prednisone (at 0.3–1 mg/kg/day). Maintenance treatment with MMF or azathioprine should continue along with low-dose prednisolone. Refractory cases may benefit from switch of induction regimens, IV rituximab or combination of MMF and tacrolimus. Patients with pure membranous lupus nephrotis (class V) with nephrotic-range proteinuria are treated with MMF and oral prednisolone; IV cyclophosphamide and tacrolimus are alternatives.

Patients require prolonged monitoring for kidney and extrarenal disease activity, and management of comorbidities. Repeat kidney biopsy is needed in cases with incomplete response or nephritic flares. Remissions and relapses, and progressive kidney damage can occur. Systemic infections and kidney failure are the chief cause of mortality.

#### C3 Glomerulopathy

C3 glomerulopathy (C3G) comprises glomerulonephritis secondary to uncontrolled activation of the alternate complement pathway, characterized histologically by predominant deposits of C3. In most cases, complement dysregulation is caused by the C3 nephritic factor, an autoantibody that binds to C3 convertase, stabilizing it against inactivation by factor H (FH). This results in uncontrolled activation of C3. Patients usually show a membranoproliferative pattern of injury, with lobulation and mesangial interposition with thickening of capillary walls, which appear split on silver methenamine staining. Immunofluorescence shows isolated or predominant C3 deposits in basement membrane, mesangium and/or capillaries. Based on electron microscopy, C3G is classified as dense deposit disease (ribbon-like electron dense material in the glomerular basement membrane) and C3 glomerulonephritis (C3GN; deposits in mesangium, subepithelial and/or subendothelial location).

Most patients present with proteinuria, gross or persistent microscopic hematuria, hypertension and/or renal failure. Diagnosis is suggested by renal histology and persistently low serum C3. Management comprises reduction of proteinuria and control of hypertension using ACE inhibitors. Immunosuppression with prednisolone and mycophenolate mofetil is proposed, but most patients show progressive renal disease. Therapy with complement inhibitors is being examined. There is a high risk of recurrence of C3G in the allografts.

### Suggested Reading


1. Coppo R. Treatment of IgA nephropathy in children: A land without KDIGO guidance. Pediatr Nephrol 2021;36:491–96.
2. Hunt EAK, Somers MJG. Infection-related glomerulonephritis. Pediatr Clin North Am 2019;66:59–72.
3. Khandelwal P, Govindarajan S, Bagga A. Management and outcomes of lupus nephritis in developing countries. Pediatr Nephrol 2022; doi: 10.1007/s00467-02205769-x.
4. Leung AKC, Barankin B, Leong KF. Henoch-Schönlein purpura in children: An updated review. Curr Pediatr Rev 2020; 16:265–276.
5. Parikh SV, Almaani S, Brodsky S, Rovin BH. Update on lupus nephritis: Core curriculum 2020. Am J Kidney Dis 2020;76: 265–81.
6. Plumb LA, Oni L, Marks SD, Tullus K. Pediatric ANCA-associated vasculitis: an update on renal management. Pediatr Nephrol 2018; 33:25–39.
7. Smith RJH, Appel GB, Blom AM, et al. C3 glomerulopathy: Understanding a rare complement-driven renal disease. Nat Rev Nephrol 2019;15:129–43.


*Competencies:* **PE21.15; PE21.16**

## NEPHROTIC SYNDROME

Nephrotic syndrome is defined by the presence of heavy proteinuria (>1 g/m²/day) and hypoalbuminemia (below 3 g/dL). Edema results due to fall in plasma oncotic pressure and hypovolemia, and stimulation of the renin–angiotensin–aldosterone axis with salt and water retention. The pathogenesis of edema may be different in other patients, who show primary sodium retention and an expanded intravascular volume. Hypoalbuminemia also induces hepatic synthesis of lipoproteins resulting in hypercholesterolemia. Some patients may show microscopic hematuria and hypertension.

More than 90% of childhood nephrotic syndrome is primary (or idiopathic). Other causes such as amyloidosis, vasculitis, systemic lupus erythematosus, and hepatitis B nephropathy are infrequent.

Nephrotic syndrome in children is broadly divided into two groups based on response to corticosteroids, steroid-sensitive nephrotic syndrome (80–85% cases) and steroid-resistant nephrotic syndrome (10–15%) cases. Based on histology, two categories are recognised: (i) A nonproliferative glomerulopathy popularly termed as minimal change disease or nephrotic syndrome (MCD or MCNS); and (ii) nephrotic syndrome with significant glomerular lesions (Table 17.7). The latter include focal segmental glomerulosclerosis (FSGS), mesangial proliferative GN, and C3 glomerulopathy; membranous nephropathy is uncommon.

Steroid-sensitive disease (usually MCNS) has satisfactory long-term outcome. In contrast, the steroid-resistant form (usually associated with significant glomerular lesions) has less satisfactory course and a proportion of patients show progressive kidney failure.

*Competencies:* **PE21.15; PE21.16**

## STEROID-SENSITIVE NEPHROTIC SYNDROME

MCNS accounts for 80% cases of nephrotic syndrome in children. Renal biopsy does not show significant abnormalities on light microscopy (Fig. 17.13a). Electron microscopy shows nonspecific effacement of epithelial foot processes (Fig. 17.13b). Immunofluorescence studies do not demonstrate deposition of immune reactants, except occasional mesangial IgM. Patients with FSGS, seen in less than 10–15% cases of steroid-sensitive disease, show evidence of sclerosis involving a segment of the glomerular tuft (Fig. 17.13c).

The pathogenesis of MCNS is obscure. There is evidence of perturbed cell-mediated immunity, which through undefined mechanisms alters the permselectivity of the glomerular filter, resulting in proteinuria. A significant proportion of patients, during relapses, show evidence of Th2 polarization, and some show disturbed T-regulatory/Th17 axis.

### Clinical Features

The onset is insidious with edema first noticed around the eyes and subsequently on legs. It is soft and pits easily on pressure. Gradually, edema becomes generalized with ascites, hydrothorax and hydrocele (Fig. 17.14). With increasing edema, urine output may fall. The blood pressure is normal; sustained elevation suggests the possibility of

**Table 17.7:** Features of idiopathic nephrotic syndrome

| *Features* | *Minimal lesion* | *Significant lesions* |
|---|---|---|
| Age at onset | 2–6 years | Older children |
| Sex | Higher in boys | Equal |
| Microscopic hematuria | Infrequent | Usual |
| Blood pressure | Normal | Normal or increased |
| GFR | Normal, high | Normal, reduced |
| Renal biopsy | Normal glomeruli; occasional IgM deposits | Varying changes; C3 and/or immunoglobulin deposits |
| Serum C3 | Normal | Low in C3 glomerulopathy |
| Selectivity of proteinuria | High | Low |
| Response to steroids | Remission in ~90% | Unsatisfactory; variable |
| Prognosis | Good; sustained remission by second decade in most | Variable risk of progressive kidney disease |

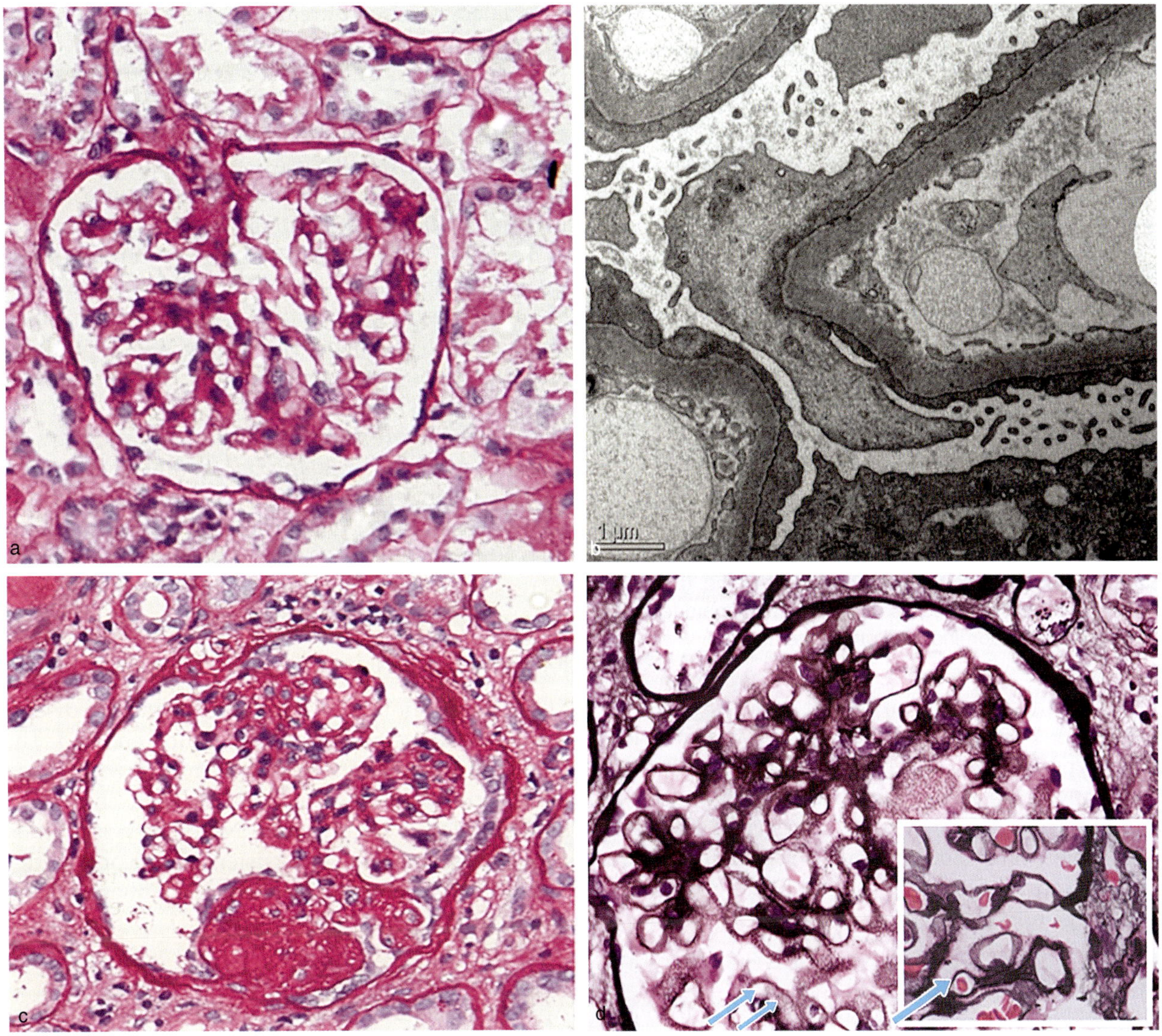


**Fig. 17.13:** Histology in childhood nephrotic syndrome: (a) Minimal change: Morphological unremarkable glomerulus (periodic acid-Schiff; 20×); (b) Transmission electron microscopy, in minimal change disease as well as other primary podocytopathies, is characterized by diffuse foot process effacement, actin condensation and microvillus transformation, the ultrastructural hallmarks of podocyte injury (uranyl acetate-lead citrate; 2550×); (c) Focal segmental glomerulosclerosis not otherwise specified (FSGS-NOS): The sclerotic segment at 6 o'clock is 'crowned' by epithelial cells. Note the irregularly thickened Bowman capsule (periodic acid-Schiff; 20×); (d) Membranous nephropathy: Note the prominent glomerular basement membrane with stiff capillary walls, a "spike" appearance (arrows) and numerous pinpoint "holes" (arrow in the inset) in tangential section, caused by the projections of basement membrane matrix towards the urinary space (silver methenamine; 40×). (*Images courtesy:* Dr Geetika Singh, Department of Pathology, All India Institute of Medical Sciences, New Delhi, India)

significant glomerular lesions. The bloated appearance and relative well-being of the child is misleading and after the loss of edema, severe muscle wasting is revealed. Infections may be present at the onset and during relapses.

### Laboratory Findings

Urinalysis shows heavy (3+ to 4+) proteinuria. Gross hematuria or persistent microscopic hematuria suggests the likelihood of significant glomerular lesions; hyaline and granular casts are present. Serum albumin is low, and values <1 g/dL are not uncommon. Blood urea and creatinine levels are within the normal range except if there is hypovolemia or AKI. Hypercholesterolemia may impart a milky appearance to the plasma. Blood levels of IgG are low; C3 level is normal.

Evaluation at onset of nephrotic syndrome includes: (i) Urinalysis for proteinuria, red cells, casts; (ii) spot protein to creatinine ratio; (iii) blood levels of urea, creatinine, albumin, cholesterol; (iv) complete blood counts; and (v) tuberculin test. Depending on clinical and laboratory findings, the following additional tests may be required: (i) C3 and antistreptolysin O (if gross or persistent microscopic hematuria); (ii) chest X-ray (positive tuberculin test or history of contact with tuberculosis); (iii) hepatitis B surface antigen (recent jaundice, raised levels of transaminases); (iv) antinuclear antibodies (suspected systemic lupus erythematosus); and (v) urine culture (suspected urinary tract infection).

A kidney biopsy is not required to confirm the diagnosis of MCNS prior to starting treatment. A biopsy is advised

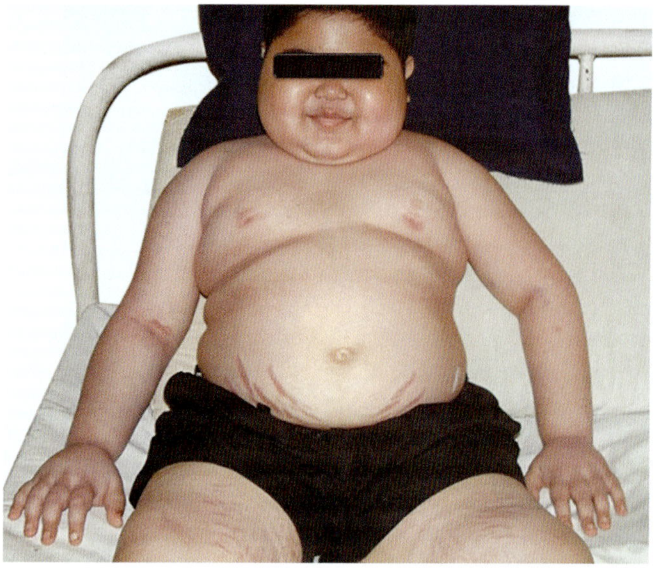

Fig. 17.14: An 8-year-old boy with steroid-dependent nephrotic syndrome. Anasarca is seen affecting upper limbs (including dorsa of hands), trunk and ascites. Note the cushingoid features and striae on lower abdominal wall and upper legs

in children with atypical features at onset (age below 12-month, gross or persistent microscopic hematuria, low blood C3, hypertension or impaired kidney function), or features of underlying systemic disease (IgA vasculitis, systemic lupus) (Fig. 17.15). Patients with steroid resistance (lack of complete remission despite 6 weeks daily therapy with prednisolone) require a biopsy to determine the underlying disorder (Fig. 17.15).

### Management of Initial Episode

The child should receive a high protein diet. Salt is restricted to the amount in usual cooking with no extra salt. Any associated infection is treated. Patients should be screened for tuberculosis. Diuretics are administered cautiously, only if edema is significant; overzealous fluid loss avoided. Frusemide (1–4 mg/kg/day in 2 divided doses) alone or with an aldosterone antagonist, spironolactone (2–3 mg/kg/day in 2 divided doses) is adequate. Corticosteroid therapy results in abolition of proteinuria (remission) usually by 10–14 days, diuresis and loss of edema.

The first episode of nephrotic syndrome should be treated adequately, both in terms of dose and duration of corticosteroids, since this is considered an important determinant of long-term course. Only prednisolone and prednisone are of proven benefit for the treatment of proteinuria. Either of these agents is given at a dose of 60 mg/m$^2$/day (or 2 mg/kg/day, maximum 60 mg) for 6 weeks, followed by 40 mg/m$^2$ (or 1.5 mg/kg, maximum 40 mg) as single morning dose on alternate days for the next 6 weeks (Fig. 17.15). Therapy with corticosteroids is then stopped. Extending initial therapy beyond 12 weeks increases the risk of steroid side effects without significant benefits, and is not recommended.

### Parent Education

The parents should be explained about the disease and the usual course and their cooperation ensured. They are taught how to examine urine for protein, which should be done periodically to detect a relapse. The child is advised a balanced and healthy diet. No dietary restrictions are necessary unless there is persistent edema or hypertension. The child is encouraged to participate in age-appropriate sports and physical activity.

### Subsequent Course

Approximately 20–25% patients have only a single episode of the illness, while the majority shows relapses. Some patients

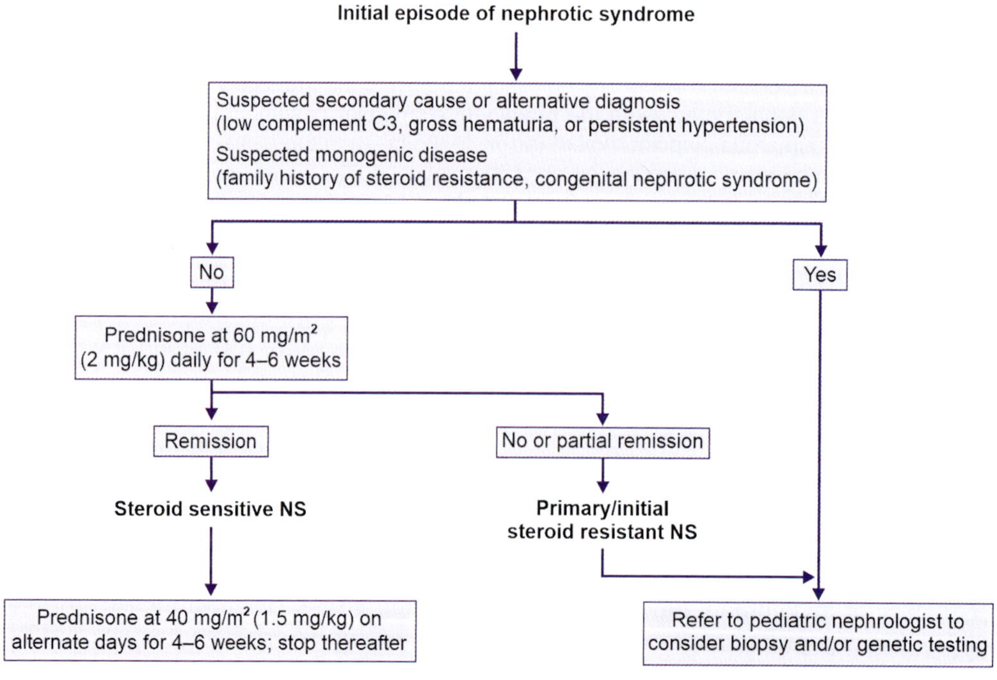


Fig. 17.15: Approach to management of the first episode of nephrotic syndrome. It is important to recognize atypical features and lack of complete remission to therapy, both of which merit referral to specialists

**Table 17.8:** Definitions for course of nephrotic syndrome (NS)

| Definition |
|---|
| *Remission:* Urine albumin nil or trace by dipstick for 3 consecutive days; urine protein <4 mg/m$^2$/hr; spot protein to creatinine ratio <0.2 mg/mg |
| *Relapse:* Urine albumin 3+ to 4+ for 3 consecutive days, or proteinuria >40 mg/m$^2$/hr or spot protein to creatinine ratio >0.2 mg/mg, having been in remission previously |
| *Frequent relapses:* Two or more relapses in first 6 months, or three or more relapses in any 12 months |
| *Steroid dependence:* Two consecutive relapses when on alternate day steroids or within 14 days of its discontinuation |
| *Steroid resistance:* Absence of remission despite therapy with prednisolone at a dose of 2 mg/kg (60 mg/m$^2$) per day for 6 weeks |
| *Congenital NS:* Nephrotic syndrome with onset within 3 months of birth |
| *Complicated relapse:* A relapse requiring hospitalization due to one or more of the following: Severe edema, symptomatic hypovolemia or AKI requiring IV albumin infusions, thrombosis, or severe infections (e.g. sepsis, peritonitis, pneumonia, cellulitis) |
| *Significant steroid toxicity:* New or worsening obesity (BMI >27 mg/m$^2$ equivalent of adult BMI); hyperglycemia; behavioral/ psychiatric disorders, slow growth (height velocity <25th percentile and/or height <3rd percentile); glaucoma, cataract; avascular necrosis |
| *Complete remission:* Negative or trace dipstick on three or more consecutive days, UPCR (based on first morning void or 24-hr urine sample) ≤0.2 mg/mg or <4 mg/m$^2$/hr |

have two or less relapses in a year (infrequent relapsers), while others have three or more (frequent relapsers) (Table 17.8). About 15–20% remain in remission while on prednisolone therapy, but relapse when the medication is reduced or within 2 weeks of its discontinuation (steroid dependent). About 10% patients either do not achieve remission despite adequate treatment with prednisolone, either at the onset (initial steroid resistance) or later in the disease course (late steroid resistance).

## Management of Relapse

Relapses are often triggered by minor infections. Symptomatic therapy of infectious illness might result in remission of low grade (1–2+) proteinuria. Persistence of 3–4+ proteinuria requires treatment for relapse. Prednisolone is given at a dose of 60 mg/m$^2$/day until protein is negative/trace for three consecutive days, and then on alternate days at a dose of 40 mg/m$^2$ for 4 weeks. Thus, treatment for a relapse usually lasts for 5–6 weeks (Fig. 17.16). The first 2–3 relapses are treated in the manner described above. Once the pattern of relapses is known, therapy is individualized. Patients with infrequent relapses continue to receive treatment for individual relapses as outlined above.

## Frequent Relapses and Steroid Dependence

Patients with frequent relapses or steroid dependence require prolonged treatment in order to maintain disease remission, without the risks of steroid side effects.

### *Long-term Alternate Day Prednisolone*

Following treatment of a relapse, the dose of prednisolone is tapered to maintain the patient in remission; usually a small dose is given on alternate days for 9–18 months (Table 17.9). This strategy is effective in maintaining remission in many patients with frequent relapses. Since infections precipitate relapses, administering the same small dose daily for 5–7

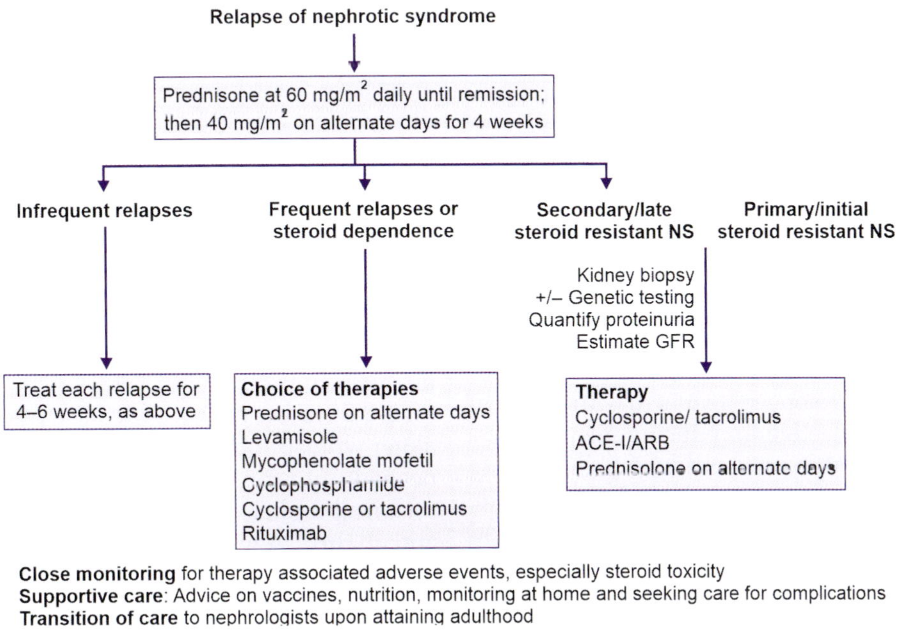


**Fig. 17.16:** Approach to the management of disease relapses in steroid-sensitive nephrotic syndrome and steroid-resistance. Patients with frequent relapses or steroid dependence require prolonged therapy with prednisolone on alternate days or steroid-sparing agents to prevent relapses and steroid toxicity. These patients and those with primary or late steroid resistance require specialist care in view of difficult disease course. Principles of management are similar for patients with initial and late steroid resistance, except that testing for monogenic etiology is considered only in the former. ACE-I angiotensin converting enzyme inhibitors; ARB angiotensin receptor blocker

**Table 17.9:** Therapy for frequent relapses or steroid dependent nephrotic syndrome

| *Agent* | *Dose* | *Duration* | *Adverse effects* |
|---|---|---|---|
| Prednisolone | 0.5–0.7 mg/kg on alternate days | 9–18 months | Cushingoid habitus, hypertension, short stature, cataract, hirsutism, osteoporosis |
| Levamisole | 2–2.5 mg/kg on alternate days | 1–2 years | Leukopenia, flu-like symptoms, ANCA positive vasculitis, raised transaminases |
| Cyclophosphamide | 2–2.5 mg/kg/day | 12 weeks | Leukopenia; alopecia; gonadal toxicity; nail discoloration; hemorrhagic cystitis; nausea and vomiting |
| Mycophenolate mofetil | 800–1000 mg/m²/day; 20–30 mg/kg/day | 1–3 years | Gastrointestinal discomfort, diarrhea; raised transaminases; leukopenia; weight loss; viral warts |
| Cyclosporine (CyA) | 4–5 mg/kg/day | 1–3 years | Acute and chronic nephrotoxicity, high transaminases (both agents)<br>Hirsutism, gum hyperplasia, hypertension, hyperlipidemia (CsA> Tac)<br>Hyperglycemia, neurotoxicity with headache and seizures (Tac>CsA) |
| Tacrolimus (Tac) | 0.1–0.2 mg/kg/day | | |
| Rituximab | 375 mg/m² body surface area IV once a week | 2 doses | Infusion reactions; serum sickness; neutropenia; poor response to vaccines; hypogammaglobulinemia; reactivation of hepatitis B |

days starting at onset of infections may prevent relapses. Patients with repeated relapses, while on long-term therapy, should be considered for treatment with a steroid-sparing agent **(Fig. 17.16)**.

### *Steroid-Sparing Agents*

The additional use of a medication **(Table 17.9)** should be considered in patients with: (i) Prednisolone threshold (for maintaining remission) higher than 0.5–0.7 mg/kg on alternate days, or (ii) features of corticosteroid toxicity (growth failure, hypertension, cataract).

***Levamisole:*** This medication is effective in reducing relapses in patients with frequent relapsing or steroid-dependent nephrotic syndrome. After inducing remission, levamisole is administered at a dose of 2–2.5 mg/kg on alternate days. Alternate day prednisolone is given in tapering doses and discontinued over 3–4 months. Treatment with levamisole is given for 1–2 years or longer. The chief side effect is leukopenia, which should be monitored for every 2 months.

***Cyclophosphamide:*** Treatment with cyclophosphamide and alternate day prednisolone is effective in patients with frequent relapsing or steroid-dependent nephrotic syndrome. A 12-week course of treatment may induce long-lasting remission in 30–40% cases. There is risk of gonadal toxicity and malignancies, although at the doses and duration used, these risks are minimal. However, a second course of treatment with the medication is not advised.

***Mycophenolate mofetil:*** Prolonged treatment with the agent is steroid sparing and effective in reducing relapse rates. The lack of renal, hemodynamic and metabolic toxicity makes it an alternative to calcineurin inhibitors. Chief side effects include gastrointestinal discomfort, diarrhea and leukopenia. Dose of the medication is 800–1000 mg/m²/day in two divided doses for 12–36 months. Monitoring of mycophenolic acid AUC is recommended to guide therapy, but not easily available. Tapering doses of prednisolone are given for 3–6 months.

***Cyclosporine and tacrolimus:*** Therapy with either of these agents is indicated in patients that fail to benefit with other steroid-sparing agents or show high steroid threshold with steroid toxicity. Cyclosporine A or tacrolimus is given, in two divided doses, for 12–24 months aiming for respective trough levels of 80–120 ng/mL and 3–7 ng/mL. Both have a strong steroid-sparing potential.

Adverse effects include acute and chronic nephrotoxicity. A renal biopsy is done after 2–3 years of therapy. Patients receiving cyclosporine have cosmetic side effects (hirsutism, gum hyperplasia), hypertension and hypercholesterolemia. Treatment with tacrolimus is associated with risk of hyperglycemia, elevated transaminases, diarrhea, tremors, headache and seizures.

***Rituximab:*** This monoclonal anti-CD20 antibody has been used successfully in patients with steroid dependent nephrotic syndrome, with remission lasting 6–18 months. Repeat courses of treatment may, therefore, be necessary. Treatment with rituximab should be limited to those who fail to respond to therapy with other steroid sparing agents. Patients should be screened for infection with hepatitis B/C and HIV prior to infusion. Monitoring for side effects, some of which may be serious, is required.

## Complications in Nephrotic Syndrome

The patient should be maintained in remission, as far as possible. Relapses should be promptly treated so that the child does not develop more than minimal edema.

### *Edema*

Edema is controlled with salt restriction and oral frusemide for 2–3 days. For massive edema, higher doses of frusemide along with spironolactone, and occasionally thiazides are needed. Infusion of albumin is necessary in cases where serum albumin levels are low causing poor renal perfusion and oliguria. Aggressive use of diuretics should, however, be avoided.

### *Infections*

Nephrotic syndrome and steroid therapy render children susceptible to infections. Infections with *S. pneumoniae*, gram-negative organisms and varicella are common. Children present with serious infections, e.g. peritonitis, cellulitis, pneumonia and meningitis. Peritonitis may manifest with low grade fever, diarrhea and abdominal discomfort. These patients require prompt diagnosis and therapy. Patients with varicella should receive oral acyclovir for 7 days; severe illness requires administration of IV acyclovir. Immunization with pneumococcal and varicella vaccines is advised once the patient is off steroids for 4 weeks.

#### Thrombotic Complications

Patients with nephrotic syndrome are at risk for thrombosis involving renal, pulmonary and cerebral veins. Aggressive use of diuretics, venepuncture of deep veins and hypovolemia increase the risk of this complication. Treatment with low molecular weight heparin followed by oral anticoagulants is recommended.

#### Hypovolemia and Acute Renal Failure

Hypovolemia may occur during a severe disease relapse or following administration of diuretics, particularly in children with poor oral intake, diarrhea and vomiting. Features include abdominal pain, lethargy, dizziness and leg cramps, tachycardia, hypotension, delayed capillary refill, low volume pulses and clammy distal extremities. Elevated ratio of blood urea to creatinine, high hematocrit, urine sodium <20 mEq/L, low fractional excretion of sodium (0.2–0.3%), and high urinary potassium index [urine $K^+$/ urine $K^+ + Na^+$] >0.6 suggest the presence of hypovolemia. Therapy with diuretics should be discontinued. Patients require infusion of normal saline (10–20 mL/kg) over 20–30 minutes. Those who do not respond to two boluses of saline should receive infusion of 5% albumin (10–15 mL/kg) or 20% albumin (0.5–1 g/kg).

#### Steroid Toxicity

Repeated and prolonged courses of steroids often result in significant toxicity, characterized by cushingoid features, short stature, hypertension, osteoporosis, raised intraocular pressure and cataract. Timely use of steroid-sparing agents (levamisole, alkylating agents, calcineurin inhibitors, mycophenolate) is recommended.

### Long-term Outcome

Children with MCNS usually have an excellent prognosis. The frequency of relapses decreases with time and ~85% patients achieve sustained remission by late adolescence. The illness persists longer in those with early onset of disease and frequent relapsing course.

*Competencies:* **PE21.15; PE21.16**

## STEROID-RESISTANT NEPHROTIC SYNDROME

Steroid resistance is diagnosed, if there is lack of remission despite treatment with prednisolone, at a dose of 2 mg/ kg/day (60 mg/m$^2$/d) for 6 weeks **(Figs 17.15 and 17.16)**. Nephrotic syndrome that does not respond to corticosteroids from the outset is termed initial (primary) steroid resistance, while that which becomes steroid resistant during therapy of a relapse is termed late (secondary) steroid resistance. All patients with steroid-resistance should undergo kidney biopsy. Histology is usually suggestive of FSGS or MCD. Rarely, particularly in older children, significant lesions such as membranous nephropathy may be found **(Fig. 17.13d)**.

Nephrotic syndrome with onset at a very early age (<3 months, termed congenital NS) is usually due to inherited defects of the podocyte, and should not be treated with steroids or other immunosuppressive drugs. About 20–30% children with sporadic initial steroid resistance, particularly those with onset in infancy, similar history in family members, or syndromic features, have homozygous, compound heterozygous or hemizygous variations in *NPHS*2 (podocin), *NPHS*1 (nephrin), *PLCE*1, *WT*1 and *COL4A*5. Rarely dominant mutations involving *CD2AP*, *TRCP*6, *ACTN*4 and *INF*2 may present with steroid resistance in childhood. Mutations in more than 80 genes are known to be associated with steroid resistance. Next-generation sequencing, using targeted gene or whole exome approach, is useful in screening. Patients with an underlying genetic cause are unresponsive to immunosuppressive medications, show progressive loss of kidney function, and unlike nongenetic FSGS (that recurs after transplantation), show low risk of recurrence.

Genetic studies should be done in patients with: (i) Congenital nephrotic syndrome (onset below 3 months of age), (ii) initial steroid resistance with onset in infancy; (iii) familial steroid resistance; (iv) syndromic forms of steroid resistance; and (v) initial steroid resistance that does not respond to therapy with calcineurin inhibitors.

Blood levels of creatinine, electrolytes, albumin and cholesterol are measured; estimation of proteinuria (24 hours quantitation) is made **(Fig. 17.16)**. Patients should be screened for secondary causes, including serologies for hepatitis, and HIV. Children with steroid resistance should undergo kidney biopsy before instituting specific treatment. While patients with minimal change disease show satisfactory response to therapy, the presence of FSGS with chronic tubulointerstitial changes is associated with less satisfactory outcomes.

### Management

The management of these patients is difficult, with patients showing a variable response to immunosuppression, adverse effects of prolonged therapy and risk of progressive renal damage. Patients with steroid-resistance secondary to minimal change disease, FSGS or mesangioproliferative GN are treated similarly. *The chief factor predicting renal outcome is the response of proteinuria to therapy, rather than the renal histology*. Therapy aims to induce and maintain remission of proteinuria, while avoiding medication-related side effects. Most regimens use the combination of an immunosuppressive agent with prednisolone and an angiotensin-converting enzyme (ACE) inhibitor **(Table 17.10)**. Satisfactory results are obtained with regimens combining cyclosporine or tacrolimus, tapering doses of prednisolone, and enalapril/ramipril. While the aim of therapy is complete remission, even partial remission (1–2+ proteinuria; spot urine protein to creatinine 0.2–2 mg/ mg) is acceptable. Patients who respond to treatment do so within 3–6 months.

**Table 17.10:** Agents for management of steroid-resistant nephrotic syndrome

| *Agent** | *Dose* | *Duration* | *Efficacy* | *Adverse effects* |
|---|---|---|---|---|
| **Calcineurin inhibitors** | | | | |
| Cyclosporine | 4–5 mg/kg/day | 12–36 months | 50–70% | *see* Table 17.9 |
| Tacrolimus | 0.1–0.2 mg/kg/day | 12–36 months | 60–80% | |
| **Cyclophosphamide** | | | | |
| Intravenous | 500–750 mg/m$^2$ | q monthly for 6 pulses | 40–45% | Leukopenia; alopecia; nausea and vomiting; nail discoloration; gonadal toxicity; hemorrhagic cystitis |
| **Rituximab** | | | | |
| Intravenous | 375 mg/m$^2$ body surface area q weekly | 2–4 doses | 25–30% | *see* Table 17.9 |

*Prednisolone given concomitantly with all agents in tapering doses; e.g. 1.5 mg/kg on alternate days × 4 weeks; 1.25 mg/kg × 4 weeks; 1 mg/kg × 4 months; 0.5–0.75 mg/kg × 6 months



Therapy with 6-pulses of IV cyclophosphamide and alternate day prednisolone may be used in patients where therapy with calcineurin inhibitors is not possible. However, results with this therapy are less satisfactory.

Adjunctive therapy with angiotensin-converting enzyme (ACE) inhibitors (e.g. enalapril 0.3–0.6 mg/kg/day, ramipril 6 mg/m$^2$/day) is associated with decrease in proteinuria and control of hypertension. Adverse effects include dry cough, hyperkalemia and decline in renal function. Angiotensin receptor blockers (e.g. losartan, valsartan) may be used in case of persistent dry cough with ACE inhibitors; combination with ACE inhibitors is usually not advised in view of increased adverse effects. Therapy with HMG coenzyme-A reductase inhibitors may be used in patients with persistently elevated low density lipoproteins (LDL).

### Congenital Nephrotic Syndrome

Congenital nephrotic syndrome presents in the first 3 months of life with anasarca, hypoalbuminemia and oliguria. The etiology of congenital nephrotic syndrome is heterogeneous. The 'Finnish' form, inherited in an autosomal recessive manner with mutations in *NPHS1* (encoding nephrin), is the most frequent. The characteristic renal histology with microcystic dilation of proximal tubules is seen after a few months of life, although ultrastructural abnormalities of the glomerular basement membrane are present at birth. Elevated levels of alpha-fetoprotein (AFP) in maternal serum and amniotic fluid enable antenatal screening. The clinical course is complicated by failure to thrive, recurrent infections, hypothyroidism and progression to renal failure by 2–3 years.

Patients with Denys-Drash syndrome show mutations in *WT1*, congenital nephrotic syndrome, male pseudohermaphroditism and high risk of bilateral Wilms' tumor. Renal histology is characterized by diffuse mesangial sclerosis; patients show progressive loss of kidney function. Other causes include congenital infections (syphilis, cytomegalovirus disease, toxoplasmosis) and mutations in *PLCE1* or *NPHS2*; rarely renal histology may be normal (minimal change nephrotic syndrome) or show FSGS.

There is no specific treatment. Management includes ensuring appropriate nutrition and reduction of proteinuria using ACE inhibitors and/or indomethacin. Most patients show hypothyroidism, due to loss of thyroid binding globulin, and benefit from oral thyroxine. Regular use of IV albumin infusions (every 2–3 weeks) avoids marked hypoalbuminemia, reducing the need for hospitalization for managing anasarca.

### Suggested Reading


1. Boyer O, Schaefer F, Haffner D, et al. Management of congenital nephrotic syndrome: consensus recommendations of the ERKNet-ESPN Working Group. Nat Rev Nephrol 2021;17:277–89.
2. Kidney Disease: Improving Global Outcomes (KDIGO) Glomerular Diseases Work Group. KDIGO 2021 Clinical Practice Guideline for the Management of Glomerular Diseases. Kidney Int. 2021;100:S1–S276.
3. Meena J, Bagga A. Current perspectives in management of edema in nephrotic syndrome. Indian J Pediatr 2020;87:633–40.
4. Sinha A, Bagga A, Banerjee S, Mishra K, Mehta A, Agarwal I, Uthup S, Saha A, Mishra OP; For Indian Society of Pediatric Nephrology. Steroid sensitive nephrotic syndrome: Revised guidelines. Indian Pediatr. 2021;58:461–81.
5. Sinha A, Bagga A. Clinical practice guidelines for nephrotic syndrome: Consensus is emerging. Pediatr Nephrol 2022;37: 2975–84.
6. Trautmann A, Boyer O, Hodson E, Bagga A, et al. IPNA clinical practice recommendations for the diagnosis and management of children with steroid-sensitive nephrotic syndrome. Pediatr Nephrol 2022 Oct 21. doi: 10.1007/s00467-022-05739-3.
7. Trautmann A, Vivarelli M, Samuel S, et al. IPNA clinical practice recommendations for the diagnosis and management of children with steroid-resistant nephrotic syndrome. Pediatr Nephrol 2020;35:1529–61.
8. Tullus K, Webb H, Bagga A. Management of steroid-resistant nephrotic syndrome in children and adolescents. Lancet Child Adolesc Health 2018;2:880–90.
9. Vasudevan A, Thergaonkar R, Mantan M, Sharma J, Khandelwal P, Hari P, Sinha A, Bagga A; Expert Group of the Indian Society of Pediatric Nephrology. Consensus guidelines on management of steroid-resistant nephrotic syndrome. Indian Pediatr 2021; 58:650–66.


*Competencies:* **PE21.15; PE21.16**

## CHRONIC GLOMERULONEPHRITIS

Chronic GN is not a single disease entity, but comprises advanced stages of several forms of GN. In most cases, the glomerular disease is primary, and not part of a systemic disorder. Chronic GN may occur in systemic lupus, microscopic polyarteritis, C3 glomerulopathy, familial nephropathies and nephropathies due to drugs and toxins. Variable glomerular deposition of immunoglobulin, complement and fibrin is found on immunofluorescence studies. Renal biopsy in early stages shows several patterns; later the histology is nonspecific with sclerosis of glomeruli, and changes in tubulointerstitium and vessels.

### Clinical Features

The patient may be asymptomatic and the disease detected on routine urine examination. Others show failure to thrive, persistent anemia, moderate to severe hypertension, edema, nocturia, microscopic or gross hematuria, bone pains and deformities.

### Differential Diagnosis

It might be difficult to distinguish chronic from acute GN. The presence of anemia, growth retardation, hypertensive retinopathy, left ventricular hypertrophy and radiological skeletal changes indicate impaired renal function of long duration. Examination of the renal biopsy is valuable.

Urinalysis shows proteinuria, hematuria, white cells and casts. Urine specific gravity is fixed and low (around 1.010). Blood urea and creatinine levels are raised and eGFR is less than 30 mL/min/1.73 $m^2$. Ultrasonography shows small kidneys with regular outline.

### Management

There is no specific treatment for chronic GN. Treatment with immunosuppressive drugs does not offer any benefit. The blood pressure should be controlled and infections treated. If kidney function is reduced, treatment is that of advanced chronic kidney disease.

*Competencies:* **PE21.15; PE21.16**

## INTERSTITIAL NEPHRITIS

This is focal or diffuse inflammatory reaction of renal interstitium with secondary involvement of tubules and rarely, glomeruli. Acute interstitial nephritis is usually due to infections or drugs (e.g. ampicillin, cephalosporins). Common causes of chronic interstitial nephritis include urinary tract obstruction and VUR. Interstitial nephritis may be a feature of a systemic disorder (e.g. systemic lupus, vasculitis, associated with uveitis); autoantibodies to tubular basement membrane are found in some cases.

Tubulointerstitial nephritis with uveitis (TINU) is a rare autoimmune entity, often with persistent and severe symptoms, that may mimic sarcoidosis. Therapy with systemic steroids is usually associated with favorable outcomes. Clinical features of interstitial nephritis are nonspecific, and include abdominal pain, anorexia, pallor, headache and edema. Hypertension is absent. The presence of progressive renal insufficiency associated with satisfactory urine output, and minimal urinary abnormalities suggest the diagnosis. Leukocytes and eosinophils are seen on urinalysis.

Kidney biopsy establishes the diagnosis and helps assess severity. Drug-related interstitial nephritis is treated by stopping use of the implicated medication; therapy with corticosteroids is beneficial. The treatment of chronic interstitial nephritis is symptomatic.

### Suggested Reading

1. Clive DM, Vanguri VK. The syndrome of tubulointerstitial nephritis with uveitis (TINU). Am J Kidney Dis 2018;72:118–28.
2. Ruebner RL, Fadrowski JJ. Tubulointerstitial nephritis. Pediatr Clin North Am 2019;66:111–19.

*Competencies:* **PE21.1; PE21.15; PE21.16**

## URINARY TRACT INFECTIONS

Urinary tract infection (UTI) is a common medical problem in children, affecting 3–10% girls and 1–3% boys. They are an important cause of morbidity and might result in kidney scarring, often in association with VUR. During infancy, UTIs are equally common in boys and girls because the route of infection is often hematogenous and boys have a higher incidence of urinary tract anomalies. Beyond infancy, the incidence is higher in girls.

### Microbiology

*Escherichia coli* constitute the predominant periurethral flora as well the most common organism associated with UTI. Infection with other organisms, including *Klebsiella*, *Enterobacter*, *Staphylococcus saprophyticus*, *Proteus* and *Pseudomonas*, may occur following obstruction or instrumentation, and suggest presence of anatomic abnormalities. *Candida* infection occurs in immunocompromised children or after prolonged antimicrobial therapy.

### Predisposing Factors

Recurrent UTIs are observed in 30–50% children, usually within 3 months of the first episode. Predisposing factors for recurrent UTI are female sex, age below 6 months, bladder bowel dysfunction (BBD), VUR, obstructive uropathy, and repeated catheterization. Bladder-bowel dysfunction and constipation are approximately twice as common in children with, versus those without, UTI. Children with malnutrition and those on immunosuppressive therapy are also susceptible.

### Clinical Features

Neonates show features of sepsis with fever, vomiting, diarrhea, jaundice, poor weight gain and lethargy. Older infants have unexplained fever, frequent micturition and occasionally, seizures. Gross hematuria is uncommon. The presence of crying or straining during voiding, dribbling, weak or abnormal urine stream and palpable bladder suggest urinary obstruction.

It is difficult to distinguish between infection localized to the bladder (cystitis) and upper tracts (pyelonephritis). The distinction is not necessary, since most UTI in children below 5 years of age involve the upper tracts. Patients with high fever (>39°C), systemic toxicity, persistent vomiting, dehydration, renal angle tenderness or raised creatinine are considered as *complicated*. Patients with low grade fever, dysuria, frequency and urgency and absence of symptoms of complicated UTI are considered to have *simple UTI*. This distinction is important for purposes of therapy.

Features on evaluation include straining during micturition, incontinence or poor urinary stream, and surgery for meningomyelocele or anorectal malformation. In toilet-trained children, one must exclude bladder bowel dysfunction (BBD), defined as the combination of lower urinary tract dysfunction and constipation. BBD leads to incomplete bladder emptying and is an important risk factor for recurrent UTI in children. Parents may report history of incontinence, voiding postponement, frequency, urgency, postures of voiding postponement (Vincent curtsy, crossing one's legs, squatting with heel at the perineum), constipation (hard infrequent stools, pain with defecation) and/or encopresis.

The external genitalia are examined for anatomic abnormalities that predispose to UTI, such as tight phimosis, hypospadias, labial adhesions and cloacal malformations. The following findings point to an underlying cause: Palpable kidney (obstructive uropathy), costovertebral angle tenderness (pyelonephritis), palpable bladder or suprapubic tenderness (obstructive uropathy or neurogenic bladder), palpable fecolith (constipation), sacral dimple, tuft of hair or lipoma, or abnormal neurological evaluation of the lower limbs and/or abnormal perineal sensations (occult meningomyelocele).

## Diagnosis

The diagnosis of UTI is based on growth of significant number of organisms of a single species in the urine. Significant bacteriuria is a colony count of $>10^5$/mL of a single species in a clean catch sample. A lower threshold (e.g. $10^4$ colonies per mL) is applied in young infants with unexplained fever, particularly in presence of leukocyturia. Urine may be obtained by suprapubic bladder aspiration or urethral catheterization in children below 2 years. A colony count of $>10^3$/mL on suprapubic aspiration and $>10^4$/mL on urethral catheterization are considered significant. Bag or diaper specimens should not be used for culture. The occurrence of significant bacteriuria in absence of symptoms is termed *asymptomatic bacteriuria*.

The presence of >10 leukocytes per $mm^3$ in fresh uncentrifuged sample, or >5 leukocytes per high power field in centrifuged sample is useful for screening. However, sterile pyuria may occur in patients with partially treated UTI, appendicitis, tuberculosis, or fungal, viral, or parasitic infections. Dipstick examination, combining leukocyte esterase and nitrite, has good sensitivity and specificity for UTI, and can be used for making presumptive diagnosis. Blood tests, such as complete blood counts and serum biochemistry are not routinely needed and may be performed, if sepsis, AKI or CKD is suspected.

## Treatment

Once UTI is suspected, a urine specimen is sent for culture and treatment started. Therapy should be guided by the age of the child, severity of the illness, site of infection (upper versus lower UTI), presenting symptoms, presence of underlying urological abnormalities and local antimicrobial susceptibility pattern (Fig. 17.17). Infants below 3 months of age, and sick children, such as those with poor oral intake, features of septicemia, or renal angle tenderness, should initially receive parenteral antibiotics. The choice of antibiotics is empiric and is modified once the culture report is available. While a third-generation cephalosporin is preferred, oral therapy with amoxycillin-clavulanic acid or parenteral therapy with once daily dose of aminoglycoside is also safe and effective (Table 17.11). Once oral intake improves and symptoms abate, usually after 48 hours, therapy is switched to an oral agent. The duration of treatment for infants with complicated UTI is 10–14 days. Older infants and patients with simple UTI should receive treatment with an oral antibiotic for 7–10 days. Adolescents with cystitis may receive shorter duration of antibiotics, lasting 72 hours. *Patients with asymptomatic bacteriuria do not require treatment.*

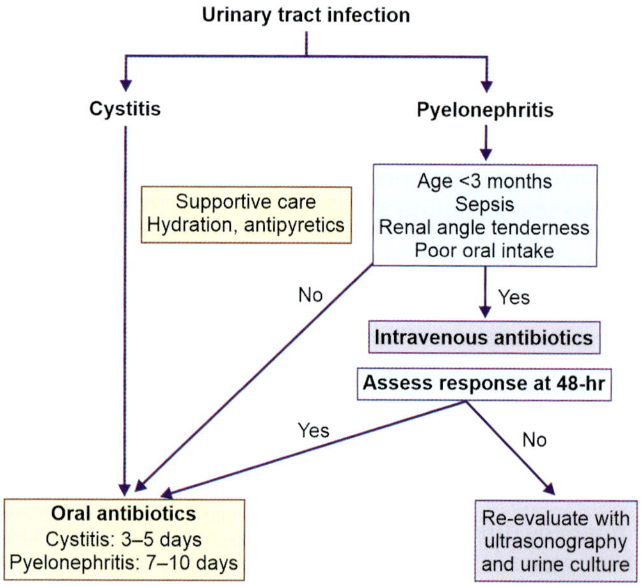


**Fig. 17.17:** Treatment of urinary tract infection. Infants below 3 months of age, and those with severe acute illness should initially receive parenteral antibiotics. Following initial IV antibiotic therapy, oral antibiotics usually suffice. In all other patients, oral therapy with cefixime or coamoxiclav is started empirically. Patients with cystitis can be managed with short course (3–5 days) of oral antibiotics; all others should receive therapy for 7–10 days

**Table 17.11:** Antimicrobials for treatment of UTI

| *Medication* | *Dose (mg/kg/day)* |
|---|---|
| **Parenteral** | |
| Ceftriaxone | 75–100, in 1–2 divided doses IV |
| Cefotaxime | 100–150, in 2 divided doses IV |
| Amikacin | 10–15, single dose IV or IM |
| Gentamicin | 5–6, single dose IV or IM |
| Coamoxiclav | 50–75 of amoxicillin, in 2 divided doses IV |
| **Oral** | |
| Cefixime | 8–10, in 2 divided doses |
| Coamoxiclav | 30–50 of amoxicillin, in 2 divided doses |
| Ciprofloxacin | 10–20, in 2 divided doses |
| Ofloxacin | 15–20, in 2 divided doses |
| Cephalexin | 75–100, in 3 divided doses |

All children with UTI are encouraged to take enough fluids and empty the bladder frequently. Routine alkalization of the urine is not necessary. With appropriate therapy, fever and systemic toxicity reduce and urine culture is sterile within 24–36 hours. Failure to obtain such results suggests either lack of bacterial sensitivity to the medication or presence of an underlying anomaly of the urinary tract. A repeat urine culture is not required during or following treatment, unless symptoms fail to resolve despite 72 hours of therapy, symptoms recur, or contamination of the initial culture is suspected.

### Imaging Studies

Following treatment of the first episode of UTI, the child should be evaluated for a cause for the infection. A detailed history should assess for presence of BBD. The aim of imaging studies has conventionally been to identify urologic anomalies that predispose to pyelonephritis, such as VUR or obstruction, and to detect evidence of renal scarring (Fig. 17.18). Renal ultrasonography is useful in detecting hydronephrosis or anomalies of the urinary bladder and must be performed in all children presenting with UTI. It may be performed during or following therapy for UTI.

MCU enables the diagnosis and grading of VUR (Fig. 17.19) and defines urethral and bladder anatomy. If indicated, this procedure is performed 2–4 weeks after treatment of the UTI. Renal cortical scintigraphy, using DMSA, detects cortical scars, which are regions of decreased uptake with loss of renal contours or presence of cortical thinning with decreased volume (Fig. 17.5a). In order to distinguish scars from reversible changes of pyelonephritis, this procedure should be done 4–6 months after therapy for UTI.

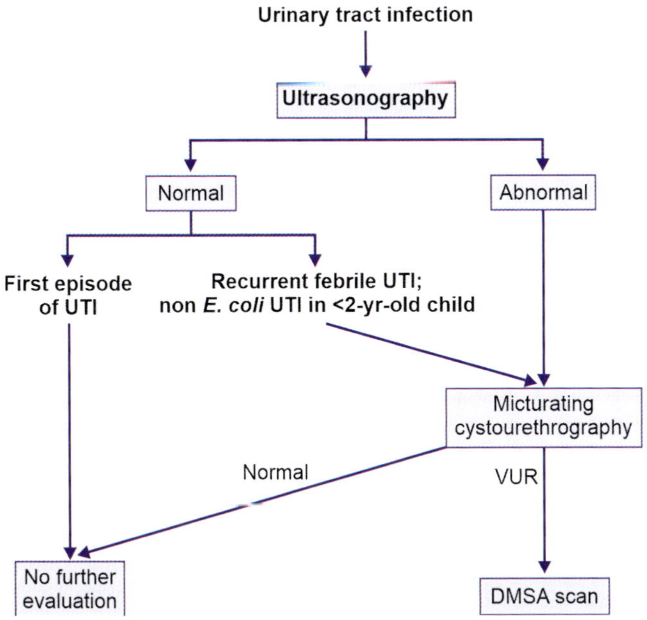


Fig. 17.18: Imaging evaluation following diagnosis of urinary tract infections. All patients should undergo ultrasonography following the first episode of UTI. A micturating cytourethrogram (MCU) is advised in patients with abnormal ultrasonogram, recurrent UTI, and/or infants with UTI due to an organism other than *E. coli*. Patients with VUR and/or recurrent UTI should undergo DMSA scintigraphy to screen for renal scarring

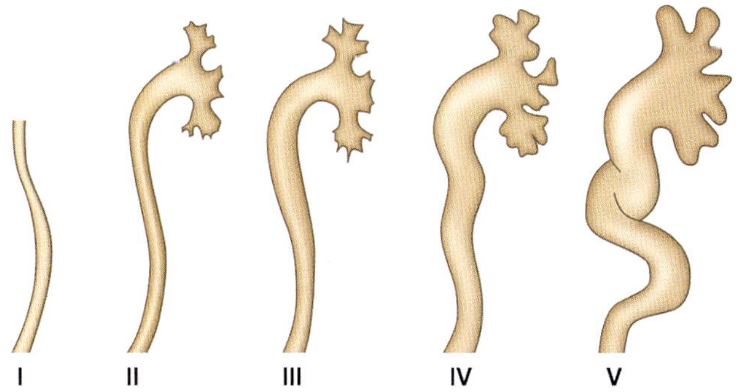


Fig. 17.19: Grading of vesicoureteric reflux (VUR) on micturating cystourethrogram. Grade I: VUR does not reach the renal pelvis; Grade II: VUR extending up to the renal pelvis without dilatation of pelvis or calyceal fornices; Grade III: VUR extending up to the kidney, with mild dilatation or tortuosity of the ureter and renal pelvis, and no or minor blunting of the calyceal fornices; Grade IV: Moderate dilatation or tortuosity of the ureter, renal pelvis and fornices, with complete obliteration of the sharp angles of the calyceal fornices, but normal appearance of the papillary impressions; Grade V: Gross dilatation and tortuosity of the ureter, renal pelvis and calyces, with loss of papillary impressions on calyces

Recommendations on UTI and VUR have been revised worldwide in keeping with the 'as low as reasonably achievable (ALARA)' principle of radioprotection. Apart from ultrasonography, the role of imaging in evaluating patients with UTI is less certain. Imaging is more aggressive in young infants with non-*E. coli* UTI, in whom high grade VUR and obstruction are more likely, and in patients with recurrent UTI, who require detailed evaluation for cause. The aggression in detecting VUR through the use of MCU has declined, since the procedure is invasive, carrying risks of discomfort, infection and radiation exposure, and the value of detecting VUR is increasingly uncertain.

VUR is common in young children, is usually low grade, abating spontaneously over time, and may not be associated with risk of cortical scarring; further, it is uncertain whether medical or surgical measures reduce the risk of scarring associated with VUR. Kidney scarring observed in association with VUR is chiefly congenital dysplasia rather than post-UTI scarring. Doing a DMSA scan during acute pyelonephritis (acute phase DMSA) does not increase the yield of MCU in detection of high-grade VUR, and is, therefore, not advised.

### Preventing Recurrent UTI

Medications used for prophylaxis should be narrow spectrum and effective against standard uropathogens, not alter the gut flora, have minimal adverse effects, and induce minimal bacterial resistance (Table 17.12). The medication is given as a single bedtime dose. Long-term prophylaxis is recommended in patients with high grade VUR, infants with low grade VUR, and in patients with recurrent febrile UTI, particularly in presence of BBD (Fig. 17.20). If initiated in infancy, prophylaxis is continued until two years of infancy and for at least one year beyond the last UTI. In older patients, prophylaxis may be continued until resolution of bladder bowel dysfunction.

Circumcision reduces the risk of recurrent UTI in infant boys, and might be beneficial in patients with high grade

**Table 17.12:** Antimicrobials for prophylaxis of urinary tract infections

| *Medication* | *Dose (mg/kg/day)* | *Remarks* |
|---|---|---|
| Cotrimoxazole | 1–2 of trimethoprim | Avoid in infants <3-month-old, glucose-6-phosphate dehydrogenase (G6PD) deficiency |
| Nitrofurantoin | 1–2 | May cause vomiting and nausea; avoid in <3-month-old, G6PD deficiency, renal insufficiency |
| Cephalexin | 10–12.5 | Drug of choice in first 3–6 months of life |
| Cefadroxil | 5 | Alternative agent in early infancy |

Usually given as a single bedtime dose

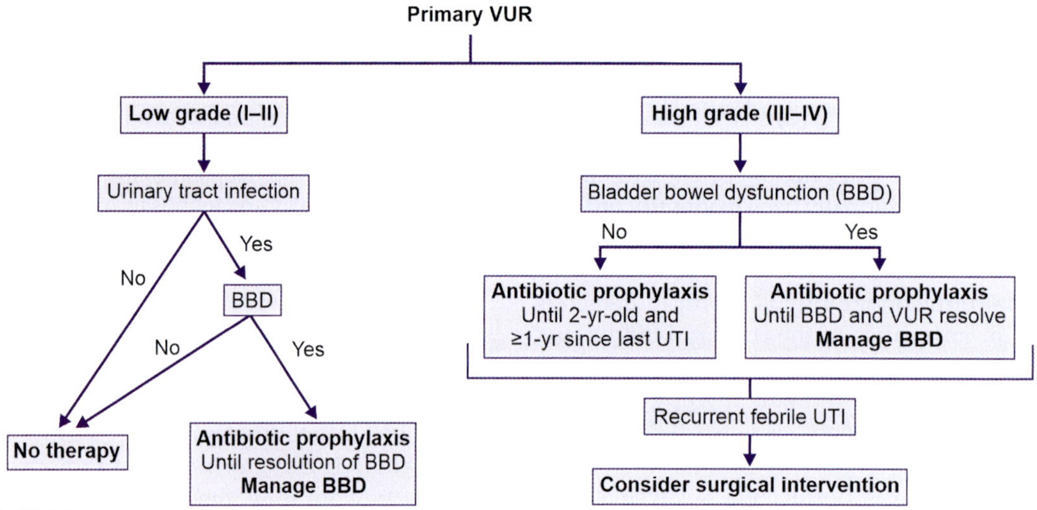


**Fig. 17.20:** Management of vesicoureteric reflux (VUR). Medical therapy is based on the principle that VUR resolves over time; prophylactic antibiotics maintain sterile urine and prevent UTI while awaiting spontaneous resolution. Reflux takes longer to resolve, in patients with bowel bladder dysfunction (BBD) or if high grade VUR is present; such patients require prolonged prophylaxis. Surgical correction of VUR is indicated, if breakthrough infections occur, since parenchymal injury may occur with pyelonephritis

VUR. Patients with recurrent UTI and/or VUR may have BBD and require appropriate advice. Constipation is managed with dietary modification and medications. Some patients require bladder retraining, anticholinergic medications, and/or clean intermittent catheterization.

## Suggested Reading


1. Diviney J, Jaswon MS. Urine collection methods and dipstick testing in non-toilet-trained children. Pediatr Nephrol 2021; 36:1697–1708.
2. Buettcher M, Trueck J, Niederer-Loher A, et al. Swiss consensus recommendations on urinary tract infections in children. Eur J Pediatr 2021;180:663–74.
3. Indian Society of Pediatric Nephrology. Revised statement on management of urinary tract infections. Indian Pediatr 2011; 48:709–17.
4. Mattoo TK, Shaikh N, Nelson CP. Contemporary management of urinary tract infection in children. Pediatrics 2021;147: e2020012138. doi: 10.1542/peds.2020-012138.
5. Okarska-Napierała M, Wasilewska A, Kuchar E. Urinary tract infection in children: Diagnosis, treatment, imaging - Comparison of current guidelines. J Pediatr Urol 2017;13: 567–73.
6. 't Hoen LA, Bogaert G, Radmayr C, et al. Update of the EAU/ESPU guidelines on urinary tract infections in children. J Pediatr Urol] 2021;17: 200–07.
7. Thergaonkar RW, Hari P. Current management of urinary tract infection and vesicoureteral reflux. Indian J Pediatr 2020;87: 625–32.


*Competencies:* **PE21.15; PE21.16**

## VESICOURETERIC REFLUX

VUR refers to the retrograde flow of urine from bladder to ureters and pelvis at rest or during micturition. Pathogenic organisms that might be present in the bladder can gain access to the renal parenchyma, initiate inflammation and renal scarring (*reflux nephropathy*). VUR may be an isolated anomaly (primary) or associated with other anomalies of the urinary tract (secondary).

VUR is present in 30–35% of children with febrile UTI and has conventionally been considered to be a major risk factor for acute pyelonephritis and reflux nephropathy. The latter may result in hypertension, renal insufficiency and cause morbidity during pregnancy.

Two techniques are commonly used to detect VUR. The radiocontrast MCU is commonly used since in addition to showing VUR it provides excellent anatomical details **(Fig. 17.5a)**. The severity of VUR is graded from I to V **(Fig. 17.19)**. Direct or indirect radionuclide cystography (DRCG, IRCG) is more sensitive for detecting VUR and causes less radiation exposure but provides fewer anatomical details **(Fig. 17.6c)**. Other techniques that are used to diagnose VUR, including contrast enhanced ultrasonography and magnetic resonance urography, require expertise and are not readily accessible.

### Management

The proposed guidelines for management of VUR are outlined in Fig. 17.20. Randomized trials suggest that antibiotic prophylaxis has a modest benefit in reducing the risk of recurrent UTI. Cotrimoxazole or nitrofurantoin is given as a bedtime dose. Since the risk of recurrent UTI and renal scarring is low after 4–5 years of age, prophylaxis may be discontinued in children older than 5 years with normal bowel and voiding habits, even if mild to moderate reflux persists. Other measures to be instituted include a liberal fluid intake, regular and complete bladder emptying and local toilet. Constipation should be avoided. A close follow-up is required for occurrence of breakthrough UTI.

The indications for surgical correction of primary VUR are limited and include poor compliance or intolerance to medical treatment. Patients with high grade (grades IV–V) VUR may be offered surgical repair, if they have breakthrough febrile UTI, or if parents prefer surgical intervention to prophylaxis, or in patients who show deterioration of renal function. Ureteric reimplantation has cure rates of 95–97%. The precise indication for endoscopic submucosal injection of dextranomer/hyaluronic acid copolymer (Deflux) at ureteric orifices is not defined. While results are satisfactory in centers with expertise, a significant proportion of patients, particularly those with BBD, may show persistence and/or recurrence of reflux.

#### *Follow-up*

Repeat imaging is required after 24–36 months in patients with grades III–V VUR. Radionuclide cystogram, with lower radiation exposure and higher sensitivity, is preferred for follow-up evaluation. Urinalysis and measurement of height, weight and blood pressure are done annually. Urine cultures are obtained, if the patient has symptoms of UTI.

#### *Screening of Siblings and Offspring*

VUR is inherited in an autosomal dominant manner with incomplete penetrance; almost one-third siblings and offspring of patients show VUR. Ultrasonography is recommended to screen for presence of reflux.

#### *Outcome*

Primary VUR tends to resolve by 6–10 years of age. Factors favoring resolution are younger age, lower grades, and unilateral VUR. The rate of resolution is 70–90% for grades I–III and 10–35% for higher grades of reflux.

### Reflux Nephropathy

This is characterized by renal cortical scarring, predominantly at the poles. The underlying calyces lose their normal concave shape and show clubbing. Such scarring occurs early in life when the kidneys are still growing. Reflux nephropathy is an important cause of hypertension and kidney failure in children.

### Suggested Reading

1. Austin PF, Bauer SB, Bower W, et al. The standardization of terminology of lower urinary tract function in children and adolescents: Update report from the standardization committee of the International Children's Continence Society. Neurourol Urodyn. 2016; 35: 471–81.
2. Edwards A, Peters CA. Managing vesicoureteral reflux in children: Making sense of all the data. F1000Res 2019; 8: F1000 Faculty Rev-29.
3. Meena J, Hari P. Vesicoureteral reflux and recurrent urinary tract infections. Asian J Pediatr Nephrol 2019;2:61–70.
4. Yang S, Chua ME, Bauer S, et al. Diagnosis and management of bladder bowel dysfunction in children with urinary tract infections: a position statement from the International Childern's Continence Society. Pediatr Nephrol. 2018;33:2207–19.

*Competencies:* **PE21.5; PE21.15; PE21.16**

## ACUTE KIDNEY INJURY

Acute kidney injury (AKI) denotes an acute impairment of kidney function resulting in retention of nitrogenous wastes and other metabolic derangements. Oliguria or anuria is a prominent feature, though rarely urine output may be normal. Incident AKI may be seen in 5–8% hospitalized children, and ~25–30% of those admitted to intensive care units. AKI is an independent risk factor for mortality. Given that this mortality could be reduced with time saving kidney replacement therapy (KRT), the International Society of Nephrology has resolved that there should be no preventable deaths due to AKI by 2025 (0 by 25 initiative).

### Definition and Classification

The term acute kidney injury (AKI) reflects the entire spectrum of the disorder. Patients are diagnosed to have AKI, if there is abrupt reduction in kidney function, defined as either: (i) Absolute increase in serum creatinine of more than or equal to 0.3 mg/dL over 48 hours, or a percentage increase of more than or equal to 50% from baseline in last 7 days, or (ii) reduction in urine output (less than 0.5 mL/kg/hr for >6 hours). The inclusion of both an absolute and a percentage change in creatinine allows for variations related to age, gender and body mass index. Table 17.13 shows the classification of AKI. Cohort studies show that patients with increasing stage of AKI show progressively rising mortality, compared to children with no AKI.

### Incidence and Etiology

The etiology of AKI is classified as prerenal, intrinsic renal or postrenal (Table 17.14). The chief causes of AKI include acute tubular necrosis (ATN) secondary to hypovolemia, sepsis and nephrotoxic agents, acute glomerulonephritis and hemolytic uremic syndrome (HUS). Postrenal failure is consequent to mechanical obstruction in the collecting system.

### Pathophysiology

Prerenal failure is secondary to systemic hypovolemia or renal hypoperfusion, where renal tubular injury leads to marked decline in glomerular filtration and renal blood flow, often by 50 to 75%. Leakage of glomerular filtrate back into the circulation across the damaged tubular epithelium and tubular obstruction from impaction of casts and cellular debris results in oliguria. While early stages are rapidly

Table 17.13: Staging of acute kidney injury (AKI), based on KDIGO criteria*

| Stage | Serum creatinine | Urine output |
|---|---|---|
| 1 | Increase in serum creatinine of ≥0.3 mg/dL over 48 hours, or ≥150 to 200% (1.5- to 2-fold) from baseline in last 7 days | Less than 0. 5 mL/kg per hour for >6 hr |
| 2 | Increase in serum creatinine to more than 200 to 300% (>2- to 3-fold) from baseline | Less than 0.5 mL/kg per hour for >12 hr |
| 3** | Increase in serum creatinine to more than 300% (>3-fold) from baseline (or serum creatinine ≥4.0 mg/dL with acute increase of ≥0.5 mg/dL) | Less than 0.3 mL/kg per hour for 24 hr, or anuria for >12 hr |

*Only one criterion (creatinine or urine output) should be fulfilled to qualify for a stage

**Patients receiving kidney replacement therapy, or children with eGFR <35 mL/min/1.73 $m^2$ are also considered in stage 3

KDIGO Kidney Disease Improving Global Outcomes

Table 17.14: Important causes of acute kidney injury (AKI)

**Prerenal AKI**

- Hypovolemia (dehydration, blood loss, diabetic ketoacidosis)
- Third space losses (septicemia, nephrotic syndrome)
- Congestive heart failure
- Perinatal asphyxia
- Medications (ACE inhibitors, diuretics)

**Intrinsic renal AKI**

- Acute tubular necrosis
- Prolonged prerenal insult (see above)
- Medications: Aminoglycosides, radiocontrast, NSAID
- Exogenous toxins: Diethylene glycol, envenomations
- Malaria, leptospirosis, typhus, dengue, hemorrhagic fevers, mucormycosis
- Intravascular hemolysis, hemoglobinuria
- Tumor lysis syndrome
- Hemolytic uremic syndrome: Shiga toxin associated; atypical
- Glomerulonephritis (GN)
  - Postinfectious GN
  - *Systemic disorders:* SLE, IgA vasculitis, microscopic polyangiitis
  - C3 glomerulopathy
- Interstitial nephritis (drug-induced, infections)
- Bilateral renal vessel occlusion (arterial, venous)

**Post-renal AKI**

- Posterior urethral valves, urethral stricture
- Urolithiasis
- Bilateral pelviureteric junction obstruction
- Ureteral obstruction (stenosis, stone, ureterocele)

NSAID nonsteroidal anti-inflammatory drug; SLE systemic lupus erythematosus

reversible by infusion of fluids, prolonged or severe ischemia may lead to acute tubular necrosis. Nephrotoxic agents cause uniform epithelial damage, especially in the proximal tubules, without disruption of tubular basement membrane.

In acute tubular necrosis, examination may be normal except for dehydration. The oliguric phase lasts about 3–10 days, during which period the biochemical and clinical abnormalities gradually worsen, more rapidly, if infection, trauma and bleeding are associated. Subsequently, urine output increases steadily. A diuretic phase may be observed, usually lasting for a week, during which large amounts of water and electrolytes may be lost.

## Approach to Evaluation

History provides clues to the underlying cause of AKI. It is important to examine for prerenal factors that lead to renal hypoperfusion. A history of diarrhea, vomiting, fluid or blood loss is taken and assessment of fluid intake in the previous 24 hours made. AKI may follow systemic infections, including malaria, dengue, leptospirosis and scrub typhus. In patients with exposure to nephrotoxic agents or intravascular hemolysis, urine output is often not diminished (non-oliguric renal failure).

Laboratory evaluation (Table 17.15) includes blood counts and levels of urea, creatinine, electrolytes, pH and bicarbonate, and urinalysis. In prerenal azotemia, the tubular function is intact and reabsorption of water and sodium is increased. The urine is concentrated with low sodium content. Impaired tubular function in acute tubular necrosis results in increased sodium excretion and failure to concentrate urine. Ultrasonography is a useful imaging tool in AKI since it allows visualization of the pelvicalyceal system and assessment of the renal size, structural anomalies and calculi.

The role of novel biomarkers (NGAL, KIM-18, IL-10, cystatin and others) for early diagnosis and aiding management of AKI is under investigation.

Most patients with AKI do not require a kidney biopsy. Indications for biopsy are: (i) Rapidly progressive or non-resolving GN; (ii) underlying systemic disorders, e.g. systemic lupus, IgA vasculitis; (iii) suspected interstitial nephritis; (iv) clinical diagnosis of acute tubular necrosis or HUS, if significant dysfunction persists beyond 2–3 weeks; (v) cause of AKI not apparent on clinical features and investigations. Patients with severe azotemia might require dialysis prior to biopsy to reduce the risk of bleeding.

Table 17.15: Investigations in patients with acute kidney injury

- Complete blood counts
- *Blood:* Urea, creatinine, sodium, potassium, calcium, phosphate, pH, bicarbonate
- Urinalysis; culture
- *Urine:* Sodium, osmolality, fractional excretion of sodium
- Chest X-ray (fluid overload, cardiomegaly)
- Abdominal ultrasonography

**Investigations to determine cause**

- Peripheral smear, platelet and reticulocyte count, complement C3, LDH levels; stool Shiga toxin (suspected HUS)
- Serology for malaria, dengue, leptospirosis
- Blood ASO, C3, antinuclear antibody, antineutrophil cytoplasmic antibody (suspected rapidly progressive GN)
- Doppler ultrasound (suspected arterial or venous thrombosis)
- Kidney biopsy (specific diagnosis feasible)

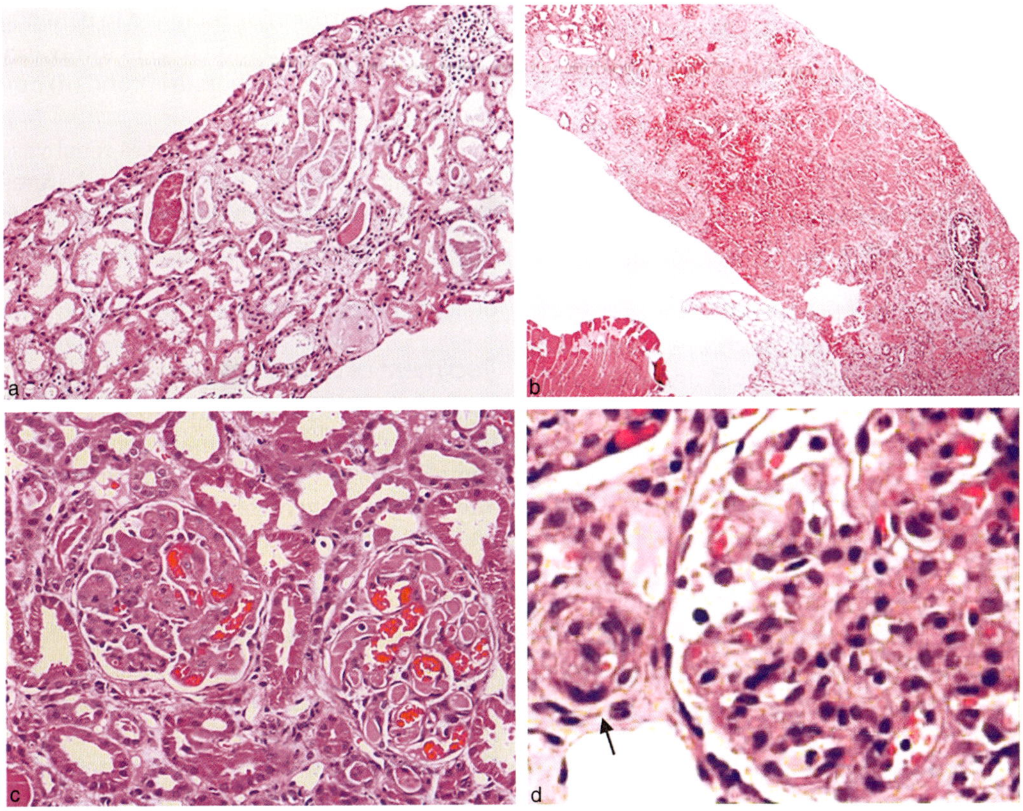

Fig. 17.21: Photograph of kidney biopsy showing: (a) Acute tubular necrosis/injury in form of simplification of proximal tubular epithelium along with fine granular casts in some tubular lumina (H & E, 200×); (b) Patch of acute cortical necrosis involving glomeruli, tubules and interstitium with adjacent relatively preserved cortical parenchyma (H & E, 40×); (c) Thrombotic microangiopathy, suggested by glomeruli with marked endothelial swelling, capillary lumina occluded by fibrin thrombi and mesangiolysis; (d) Thrombotic microangiopathy, suggested by glomeruli showing endothelial swelling and detachment, widened subendothelial spaces, and arterioles showing intimal hyperplasia, endothelial swelling and lumen occluded by platelet thrombi (arrow)

Figures 17.10, 17.11 and 17.21a–d show various diagnoses on histology.

Occasionally, a patient with undetected chronic kidney disease may present for the first time with acute onset of oliguria. History of previous renal disease may be present. The presence of the following suggests the possibility of chronic kidney disease: (i) Retarded physical growth, (ii) severe anemia, (iii) hypertensive retinopathy, (iv) hypocalcemia, hyperphosphatemia and high PTH, (v) radiologic features of mineral bone disease, and (vi) small kidneys on imaging.

## Management

Prompt clinical and laboratory evaluation is necessary. Management includes treatment of life-threatening complications, maintenance of fluid and electrolyte balance and nutritional support. Evaluation for complications includes measurement of blood pressure, search for signs of congestive heart failure, fluid overload, acidosis and anemia. Complications such as dehydration or fluid overload, hypertension, heart failure, severe anemia, hyperkalemia and acidosis require urgent treatment.

### *Fluid Repletion*

Prerenal AKI responds to fluid replacement with improved renal perfusion and increased urine output. Dehydration is corrected by infusion of 20–30 mL/kg of normal saline or Ringer's lactate over 45–60 min. If hemorrhage accounts for vascular collapse, blood transfusion should be given. Potassium should not be administered until urine flow is established, and care is taken to avoid overhydration. Patients with renal hypoperfusion, in whom the only reason for oliguria is intravascular volume depletion, respond to fluids with increase in urine output (~2 mL/kg over 2–3 hours). If oliguria persists despite correction of dehydration, frusemide (1–1.5 mg/kg IV) may be given. Patients who do not show urine output ~3 mL/kg over the next 4 hr, are predicted to have stage II–III AKI.

### *Fluid Restriction*

In patients with AKI, fluid retention may result from excessive oral or parenteral fluids, and leads to edema, hypertension and heart failure. Daily fluid requirement is restricted to insensible water losses (300–400 mL/m$^2$), urine output and extrarenal fluid losses. The amount is given orally; intravenous fluids are not required.

Intake–output monitoring, daily weight, physical examination and serum sodium guide fluid management. If fluid in an appropriate volume and composition is given, the patient should lose 0.5–1% of weight everyday and serum sodium should stay within normal range. A rapid weight loss and rising sodium suggest inadequate fluid replacement, while absence of weight loss and low serum sodium indicate fluid excess.

*Diet*

Patients with AKI have increased metabolic needs and are usually catabolic. Adequate nutritional support with maximization of caloric intake should be achieved as early as possible. A diet containing 1.0–1.2 g/kg of protein in infants and 0.8–1.2 g/kg in older children and a minimum of 60–80 Cal/kg is recommended. Energy requirements are met by addition of carbohydrates and fat in the diet. Vitamin and micronutrient supplements are provided. In patients with oligoanuria and fluid overload, daily caloric requirement cannot be met due to fluid restriction. Once dialysis is initiated, dietary protein, fluid and electrolyte intake should be increased.

*General Measures*

Patients with AKI are managed under intensive care conditions. Accurate records of intake and output, and daily weight should be maintained. Urine should be collected by condom drainage; bladder should preferably not be catheterized. The risk of infection is high and appropriate preventive measures are necessary. Prophylactic antibiotics are not recommended, but infections should be promptly managed.

Drugs that increase kidney damage, delay recovery of function or reduce perfusion, e.g. aminoglycosides, colistin, radiocontrast media, NSAID, amphotericin B, calcineurin inhibitors, ACE inhibitors and indomethacin should be avoided. Standard charts are used for modifying the dose and dosing interval of antibiotics, depending on the severity of kidney injury.

While diuretics may transiently improve urine output, they do not affect renal function or improve acute outcomes. The use of IV frusemide is limited to patients with: (i) Risk of intratubular precipitation (e.g. in intravascular hemolysis, hyperuricemia, myoglobinuria), and (ii) pulmonary edema awaiting dialysis.

Dopamine at low doses causes renal vasodilatation and may induce a modest natriuresis and diuresis. However, it has no beneficial effect on prevention or outcome of AKI, and may be associated with transient tachyarrhythmia or tissue ischemia. Hence, its use for prevention or treatment of acute tubular necrosis is not recommended.

*Treatment of Complications*

In a child with AKI, immediate attention is directed towards detection and management of life-threatening complications. Table 17.16 lists important complications and their management. Children with pulmonary edema and congestive cardiac failure may require endotracheal intubation and assisted ventilation. Severe acidosis is treated by administration of sodium bicarbonate, and, if persistent, dialysis.

Infections, including respiratory and urinary tract, peritonitis and septicemia, are important causes of death. Procedures should be performed with aseptic techniques, IV lines carefully watched, skin puncture sites cleaned, and long-term catheterization of the bladder avoided.

*Specific Therapy*

Immunosuppressive medications and plasma exchange are useful in dialysis-dependent patients with vasculitis, crescentic GN or systemic lupus erythematosus. Most patients with atypical HUS benefit from terminal complement blockade; these agents are not available in

**Table 17.16:** Management of complications

| *Complication* | *Treatment* | *Remarks* |
|---|---|---|
| Fluid overload | *Fluid restriction:* Replace insensible losses (400 mL/m²/day) as 5% dextrose, and urine output and other losses as N/5 saline | Monitor daily weight; plasma electrolytes<br>Prefer oral to parenteral fluids; consider dialysis |
| Pulmonary edema | Oxygen; frusemide 2–4 mg/kg IV | Monitor central venous pressure; consider dialysis |
| Hypertension | *Symptomatic:* Sodium nitroprusside 0.5–8 μg/kg/min infusion; frusemide 2–4 mg/kg IV; nifedipine 0.3–0.5 mg/kg oral/sublingual<br>*Asymptomatic:* Nifedipine, amlodepine, prazosin, labetalol, clonidine | In emergency, reduce blood pressure by one-third of the desired reduction during first 6–8 hours, one-third over next 12–24 hours and the final one-third slowly over 2–3 days |
| Metabolic acidosis | Sodium bicarbonate, if bicarbonate <18 mEq/L | Watch for fluid overload, hypernatremia, hypocalcemia; consider dialysis |
| Hyperkalemia | Calcium gluconate (10%) 0.5–1 mL/kg over 5–10 minutes IV<br>Salbutamol 5–10 mg nebulized<br>Dextrose (10%) 0.5–1 g/kg and insulin 0.1–0.2 U/kg IV<br>Sodium bicarbonate (7.5%) 1–2 mL/kg over 15 min<br>Calcium or sodium resonium (Kayexalate) 1 g/kg | Stabilizes cell membranes; prevents arrhythmias<br>Shifts potassium into cells<br>Requires monitoring of blood glucose<br>Shifts potassium into cells; less efficient<br>Given orally or rectally, can be repeated 4–8 hours |
| Hyponatremia | Fluid restriction; if sensorial alteration or seizures 3% saline 6–12 mL/kg over 30–90 min | Hyponatremia is usually dilutional; 12 mL/kg of 3% saline raises sodium by 10 mEq/L |
| Severe anemia | Packed red cells 3–5 mL/kg; exchange transfusion | Monitor blood pressure; fluid overload |
| Hyperphosphatemia | Phosphate binders (calcium carbonate or acetate; sevelamer carbonate) | Avoid high phosphate products: Milk products, high protein diets, sodas |

the country and most patients receive multiple plasma exchanges. If interstitial nephritis is suspected, the offending agent should be withdrawn and oral corticosteroids given.

### Dialysis

AKI requiring KRT can be managed with multiple modalities, including peritoneal dialysis, intermittent hemodialysis and continuous hemofiltration or hemodiafiltration. The purpose of dialysis is to remove endogenous and exogenous toxins and maintain fluid, electrolyte and acid–base balance until kidney function recovers.

Indications for dialysis include persistent hyperkalemia (>6.5 mEq/L), cumulative fluid overload exceeding 10% of body weight, uremic encephalopathy, severe metabolic acidosis (bicarbonate <10–12 mEq/L) and hyponatremia (<120 mEq/L) or hypernatremia. The decision to institute dialysis should be based on assessment of the patient, keeping in view the likely course of AKI. Dialysis should begin early to prevent life-threatening complications.

The choice of modality for KRT is influenced by several factors, including goals of dialysis, the advantages and disadvantages of each modality and institutional resources (Table 17.17).

#### *Peritoneal Dialysis*

Peritoneal dialysis does not require vascular access and sophisticated equipment and is easy to perform even in neonates. It is often the initial renal replacement therapy of choice in sick and unstable infants. Peritoneal access may be rapidly initiated using a stiff catheter and trocar; use of a soft silastic catheter is, however, preferred. Stiff polyurethane catheters need to removed after 48–72 hr, compared to the soft catheters that can stay for a longer duration. The use of automated cyclers has significantly reduced frequent manipulation and opening of the dialysis circuits, and changing dialysate bags after few cycles. The dialysate fluid is prewarmed to body temperature; accurate data on net dialysate balance is also maintained.

The abdominal skin is prepared as for a surgical procedure. Dialysis fluid is infused 30–50 mL/kg, left in the peritoneal cavity for 30–60 minutes and then drained using siphon effect (Fig. 17.22a). Initially, 30–40 cycles are carried out. Commercially available dialysates are lactate based and with a dextrose concentration of 1.7%. In patients with fluid overload, the concentration of dextrose is increased to 2.5–3% to facilitate faster ultrafiltration. Potassium is not added in the first 5–10 cycles, to enable correction of hyperkalemia. Later, 3 mEq/L potassium chloride is added to the dialysate. The results of peritoneal dialysis are gratifying. In acute tubular necrosis, often a single dialysis is adequate. The procedure can be repeated, if necessary.

The most important complication is bacterial peritonitis. Meticulous aseptic precautions and use of an automated cycler will minimize its incidence. Stiff catheters should be removed after 48–72 hours, beyond which the risk of infection is very high. The risk of injury to viscera and of infections is less with the soft silastic (Tenckhoff or Cook) catheters, which, therefore, may be used for longer periods. While the standard (double cuff) Tenckhoff catheter needs to be placed surgically, a temporary (peel away) catheter is inserted bedside.

#### *Hemodialysis*

Hemodialysis is highly efficient for correction of fluid and electrolyte abnormalities. However, it is expensive to institute, and requires expertise and skilled nursing. The procedure might not be suited for patients with hemodynamic instability, bleeding tendency and in young children with difficult vascular access.

Equipment required for hemodialysis includes the machine, pediatric dialyzer with tubings, and dialysate fluid (Fig. 17.22b). These dialyzers are available in different sizes (0.5–1.7 $m^2$) and selection depends upon patient size and ultrafiltrate properties. Vascular access is usually achieved using a double lumen catheter inserted into the internal jugular, femoral or subclavian veins. Most children are maintained on a hemodialysis regimen of 3–4 hours, three times a week. Sick patients with fluid overload might require daily dialysis initially. The chief complications include hemodynamic and autonomic instability, dialyzer reactions, and dialysis disequilibrium syndrome.

#### *Continuous Kidney Replacement Therapies (CKRT)*

CKRT is any extracorporeal blood purification therapy intended to substitute for impaired kidney function over an extended period of time and applied for 24 hours/day.

**Table 17.17:** Comparison of modalities of dialysis for kidney injury

| *Features* | *Peritoneal dialysis* | *Hemodialysis* | *Sustained low efficiency dialysis* | *Continuous kidney replacement therapy* |
|---|---|---|---|---|
| Availability; ease of performance | ++ | + | + | – |
| Technical expertise required | – | ++ | ++ | ++ |
| Vascular access required | – | + | + | + |
| Anticoagulation required | – | + | + | ++ |
| Slow and continuous removal of fluid and toxins without disequilibrium | + | – | + | ++ |
| Rapid clearance of toxins, fluid | – | ++ | - | + |
| Achieve desired fluid removal | +/– | + | + | ++ |
| Feasible in hemodynamically unstable patients | + | – | + | + |
| Cost | – | + | + | ++ |

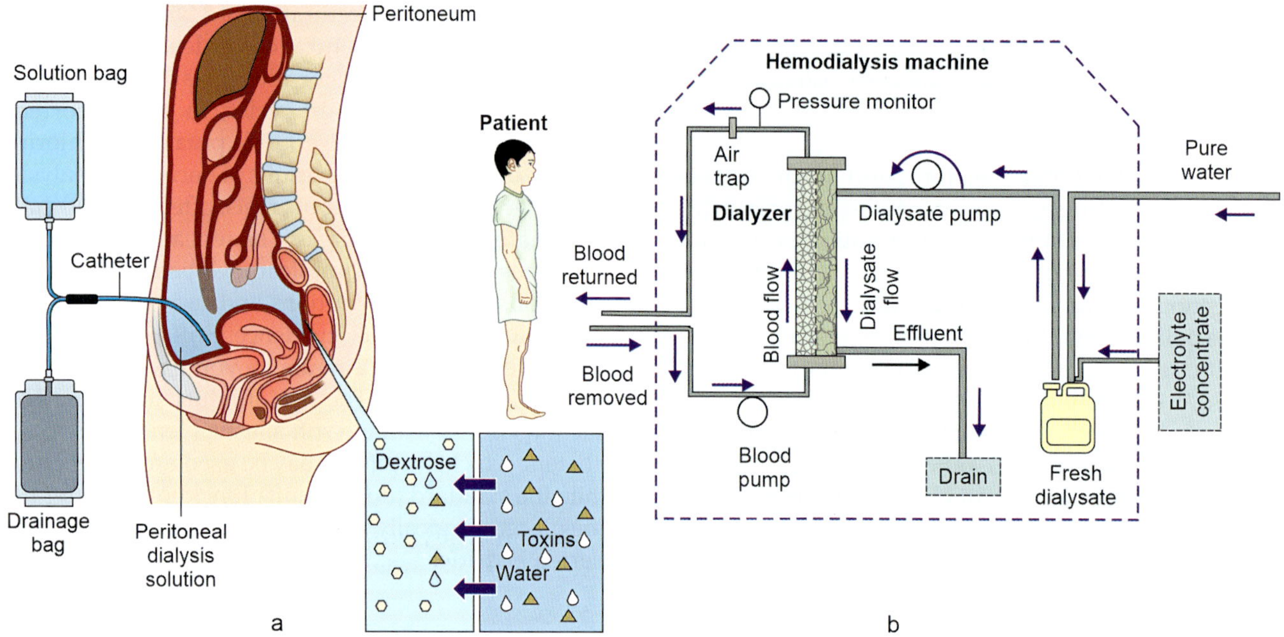


**Fig. 17.22:** Modalities of dialysis for acute kidney injury: (a) Peritoneal dialysis is based on solute exchange and water transfer across the peritoneal membrane, driven by the concentration gradient and high dextrose content of the dialysate; (b) Hemodialysis requires blood to be pumped outside the body through a large bore double lumen catheter, followed by the exchange of solutes and ultrafiltration of water across a synthetic hemodialyser membrane; the purified blood is then returned into the bloodstream through the same catheter. Two other extracorporeal modalities, namely sustained low-efficiency dialysis and continuous kidney replacement therapy, are preferred in hemodynamically unstable critically ill patients (not shown in this image)

Modalities include continuous venovenous hemofiltration (CVVH), continuous venovenous hemodialysis (CVVHD), continuous venovenous hemodiafiltration (CVVHDF), and slow continuous ultrafiltration (SCUF). These therapies are useful when ultrafiltration of solute clearance is required in sick and unstable patients. CKRT enables precise ultrafiltration and slow and continuous solute clearance. CVVH is preferred modality in AKI secondary to major surgical procedures, burns, heart failure and septic shock, especially when conventional hemodialysis or intermittent peritoneal dialysis is not possible. CKRT can be satisfactorily conducted in an intensive care unit; filters and tubing appropriate for young infants are available. The main disadvantages involve high expense and need for trained personnel, and the risks of bleeding.

#### *Slow Low Efficiency Dialysis (SLED)*

Sick patients often benefit from hybrid treatments that combine the advantages of CRRT and feasibility of hemodialysis. SLED is usually done daily for an extended but limited period (6–12 hours) using low blood and dialysate flow rates. With a slow ultrafiltration rate, SLED is able to achieve the volume target, at the same time minimizing the cost and technical complexities of CRRT. It can also be combined with hemofiltration to improve connective clearance.

### Outcome

AKI carries a mortality of 20–40%, chiefly related to the underlying etiology and duration of renal failure. Patients with septicemia and HUS with prolonged anuria are associated with poor prognosis. The outcome in crescentic GN and vasculitis depends on the severity of the renal injury and promptness in initiation of specific therapy. The outlook is satisfactory in acute tubular necrosis without complicating factors. Other factors associated with poor outcome include delayed referral, presence of complicating infections and cardiac, hepatic or respiratory failure. Maintenance of nutrition and prevention of infections is crucial in improving outcome.

### Acute Kidney Injury in Newborn

Newborns are at high risk of AKI. Chief causes include: (i) Perinatal hypoxemia, associated with birth asphyxia or respiratory distress syndrome; (ii) hypovolemia secondary to dehydration, intraventricular hemorrhage, heart disease and postoperatively, (iii) sepsis with hypoperfusion; (iv) delayed initiation and inadequacy of feeding in early neonatal period; (v) increased insensible losses (phototherapy, radiant warmers, summer heat), twin-to-twin transfusions and placental hemorrhage; (vi) nephrotoxic medications; maternal intake of ACE inhibitors; and (vii) renal vein thrombosis. AKI may be the first manifestation of an anomaly of the urinary tract.

Serum creatinine levels are high at birth (reflecting maternal levels) and decrease to below 0.5 mg/dL by 5–7 days of age. Failure of reduction or rise of serum creatinine indicates impaired renal function. AKI is present in presence of oliguria (urine output <1 mL/kg/hr for 6–12 hr), or serum creatinine increase of 0.3 mg/dL within 48-hr, or increase of 50% or higher from baseline within 7 days. Serum creatinine level >2.5 mg/dL represents stage 3 AKI.

The principles of management are similar to that for older children. Fluid should be limited to insensible (30 mL/kg/day for full-term, 50–100 mL/kg/day for preterm neonates), gastrointestinal and renal losses. Extremely premature neonates nursed in radiant warmers require extra fluids. Systolic blood pressure more than 95–100 mm Hg may need treatment.

Extra care should be taken while dialyzing neonates; peritoneal dialysis is technically easier and preferred. However, sudden distention of peritoneal cavity may cause respiratory embarrassment or apnea. Hypothermia should be avoided by carefully warming the dialysis fluid. A number of drugs are dialyzable and appropriate amounts should be added to supplement for their losses.

### Suggested Reading


1. Ciccia E, Devarajan P. Pediatric acute kidney injury: Prevalence, and management. Int J Nephrol Renovasc Dis 2017;10:77–78.
2. Che R, Quadri MM, Zhang A. Epidemiology and management of pediatric AKI in Asia. Semin Nephrol 2020;40:516–32.
3. de Galasso L, Picca S, Guzzo I. Dialysis modalities for the management of pediatric acute kidney injury. Pediatr Nephrol 2020;35:753–65.
4. Moore PK, Hsu RK, Liu KD. Management of acute kidney injury: Core curriculum 2018. Am J Kidney Dis 2018;72:1–13.
5. Ricci Z, Goldstein SL. Pediatric continuous renal replacement therapy. Contrib Nephrol 2016;187:121–30.
6. Sanderson KR, Harshman LA. Renal replacement therapies in the ICU. Curr Opin Pediatr 2020;32: 360–66.
7. Selewski DT, Goldstein SL. Role of fluid overload in prediction of outcome in acute kidney injury. Pediatr Nephrol 2018; 33:13–24.


*Competencies:* **PE21.15; PE21.16**

## HEMOLYTIC UREMIC SYNDROME

Hemolytic uremic syndrome (HUS) is a heterogeneous group of disorders that are a common cause of AKI in children. They are characterized by microangiopathic hemolytic anemia, thrombocytopenia and AKI. Two broad groups are recognized; the first is more common, occurs in young children and is associated with Shiga toxin producing enteropathogens, while the second is uncommon, affects children of all ages and is associated with abnormalities of the alternate complement pathway (atypical HUS). Similar features may be seen with systemic disorders (lupus, certain cancers), pregnancy, and following marrow transplant (secondary HUS).

### Shiga Toxin-Associated HUS

Verotoxin-producing *E. coli* (North America and Europe; commonly O157:H7; O104:H4) and *Shigella dysenteriae* 1 (south Asia) cause the diarrheal prodrome preceding HUS. Cytotoxin-mediated injury to endothelium in the renal microvasculature leads to localized coagulation and fibrin deposition. As red cells and platelets traverse, these damaged vessels, they are injured and sequestered. Though the brunt of the microvascular injury is on the kidney, other organs especially the brain may be affected. Since chiefly Shiga toxins 1 and 2 are implicated, the illness is also called Shiga toxin-associated HUS (STEC-HUS).

### Atypical HUS

This condition often lacks the prodromal history of diarrhea or dysentery, but may be triggered by minor respiratory infections. The onset may be insidious or as a rapidly progressive illness. Microangiopathic lesions chiefly affect interlobular arteries and result in severe hypertension and AKI. Causes include pathogenic variations in genes encoding proteins of the alternate complement or thrombotic pathway (*CFH, CFI, CFB, C3, MCP, MMAHC, THBD, PLG, DGKE*) and antibodies against factor H (anti-FH).

### Clinical Features

Children of all ages may be affected. Following a prodrome of acute diarrhea, dysentery or a febrile illness, patients show sudden onset of pallor and oliguria. Blood pressure is usually elevated. Focal or generalized seizures and alteration of consciousness, and mild jaundice may occur.

The blood film shows broken red cells (schistocytes), increased reticulocyte count, high blood LDH and reduced haptoglobin. Coombs' test is negative, except in *S. pneumoniae* or lupus-associated HUS. Thrombocytopenia is present, but rarely <30000/cu mm; neutrophil leukocytosis is seen in patients with shigellosis. Urine shows microscopic hematuria and variable proteinuria. The diagnosis of STEC-HUS requires growth of VTEC or *Shigella* spp on stool culture, and detection of Shiga toxin by PCR or ELISA. Serum complement C3 levels are low in some patients with atypical HUS. ELISA for anti-FH antibodies, flow cytometry for CD46, exome sequencing for variations in commonly associated genes, and MLPA for copy number variations in *CFHR1-5* is advised. HUS is diagnosed on clinical and laboratory features, and a kidney biopsy is rarely required (Fig. 17.21c, d).

### Treatment

Treatment includes management of complications of AKI, treatment of hypertension and correction of anemia. Proper nutrition must be ensured. Peritoneal or hemodialysis may be necessary for AKI. Shigellosis should be treated with appropriate antibiotics.

Therapy with complement inhibitor, eculizumab or ravulizumab, is the standard of care for patients with atypical HUS. While effective in ensuring hematological and renal remission, these medications are yet not available in the country. In absence of the above medications, plasma exchanges with infusion of fresh frozen plasma is recommended for patients with atypical HUS. The exchanges are initiated as early as possible, performed daily until hematological remission, and then less frequently for 3–4 weeks. Patients with anti-FH antibodies benefit from concomitant immunosuppression for 12–24 months. Long-term follow-up is recommended.

### Outcome

Mortality during the acute episode of STEC-HUS is low. However, on follow-up, 20–30% patients show varying degree of residual kidney damage. Factors suggestive of poor outcome include oligoanuria for >2 weeks, severe neurological involvement and presence of cortical necrosis.

The acute and long-term outcome in patients with atypical HUS is not satisfactory, especially since there is limited access to complement inhibitors. Almost 30–50% patients may show progressive kidney failure. Patients with atypical HUS may have relapses, including in the renal allograft.

### Suggested Reading


1. Bagga A, Khandelwal P, Mishra K, et al. Hemolytic uremic syndrome in a developing country: Consensus guidelines. Pediatr Nephrol 2019;34:1465–82.
2. Michael M, Bagga A, Sartain SE, Smith RJH. Hemolytic uremic syndrome. Lancet 2022; 400 (10364): 1722–40.
3. Puraswani M, Khandelwal P, Saini H, et al. Clinical and immunological profile of anti-factor H antibody associated atypical HUS. Frontiers Immunol 2019;10:1282.




*Competencies:* **PE21.6; PE21.15; PE21.16**

## CHRONIC KIDNEY DISEASE



Chronic kidney disease (CKD) is defined as kidney damage lasting for at least 3 months, characterized by structural or functional abnormalities of the kidney with or without decreased glomerular filtration rate (GFR). Abnormalities include structural malformations (e.g. hydronephrosis, single kidney), pathological conditions (e.g. focal segmental glomerulosclerosis) and markers of kidney damage such as abnormal urinalysis (hematuria, proteinuria) or biochemistry (persistently increased serum creatinine). CKD is divided into 5 stages, based on estimated GFR (Table 17.18). Since renal maturation increases from infancy to reach adult values at the age of 2 years, CKD stages apply to children beyond >2-yr-old. Important conditions resulting in CKD are listed in Table 17.19. Congenital abnormalities of the kidney and urinary tract (CAKUT) follwoed by glomerular diseases are the leading causes of childhood CKD.

### Pathophysiology and Clinical Features

The term CKD implies permanent decrease in renal function. Most children with CKD stage 1–3 (GFR more than 30 mL/min/1.73 m$^2$) are asymptomatic; reduction of GFR below this level is associated with symptoms. Regardless of the etiology, once there is a critical loss of nephron mass, the renal failure is progressive and manifests with similar symptoms. Loss of urinary concentrating ability results in frequency, nocturia and increased thirst. Anemia, that is normocytic and normochromic, is chiefly due to reduced erythropoietin production. Mild hemolysis and blood loss from gastrointestinal tract also contributes.

Resistance to the action of growth hormone, the levels of which are increased, is considered to be responsible for growth failure. Anorexia, malnutrition and skeletal deformities contribute to growth retardation. Abnormalities in metabolism of calcium and phosphate, lack of renal formation of 1,25-dihydroxyvitamin D, chronic acidosis and secondary hyperparathyroidism result in bone disease, classified as CKD-mineral bone disease.

The blood pressure may be increased and optic fundi show hypertensive retinopathy. Severe proximal muscle weakness, peripheral neuropathy, itching, purpura and pericarditis are late features. Infections are common and may acutely worsen renal function.

### Investigations

The patient should be investigated to find the cause of renal failure and detect reversible factors (e.g. urinary tract obstruction, UTI, severe hypertension, drug toxicity and dehydration). Appropriate imaging studies are done. Blood counts and levels of urea, creatinine, electrolytes, protein, albumin, pH, bicarbonate, calcium, phosphate, alkaline phosphatase and parathyroid hormone (PTH) are obtained. Levels of ferritin and transferrin saturation are obtained in patients with anemia. GFR is estimated based on serum creatinine and height.

### Management

Optimal management of CKD involves a team approach involving pediatric nephrologist and urologist, specialist nurse, dietitian, and social worker. The management of CKD focuses on the following: (i) Treating reversible conditions; (ii) retarding progression of kidney disease, with attention to hypertension and proteinuria; (iii) anticipating, preventing and managing complications, i.e. malnutrition, anemia, growth failure, mineral bone disease, metabolic acidosis; (iv) identifying children who require

**Table 17.18:** Stages of chronic kidney disease (CKD)

| *GFR, ml/ min/1.73 m$^2$* | *NKF-KDOQI stage* | *Description* | *KDIGO stage* | *Description* |
|---|---|---|---|---|
| >90 | 1 | Kidney damage with normal or increased GFR | G1 | Normal or high |
| 60–89 | 2 | Kidney damage with mild reduction of GFR | G2 | Mildly decreased |
| 45–59 | 3 | Moderate reduction of GFR | G3a | Mildly to moderately decreased |
| 30–44 | | | G3b | Moderately to severely decreased |
| 15–29 | 4 | Severe reduction of GFR | G4 | Severely decreased |
| <15 | 5 | Kidney failure | G5 | Kidney failure |
| <15, on dialysis | 5D | Kidney failure, dialysis dependence | | |

KDIGO kidney Diseases Improving Global Outcomes; NKF-KDOQI National Kidney Foundation and Kidney Disease and Outcome Quality Initiative

In the absence of evidence of kidney damage, GFR category G1 or G2 do not fulfil the criteria for CKD

Severity of disease is additionally expressed by etiology and albuminuria, categorized as follows: (i) A1: Normal to mildly increased (urine protein to creatinine ratio, Up/Uc <150 mg/g); (ii) A2: Moderately increased (Up/Uc 150–500 mg/g); (iii) A3: Severely increased (Up/Uc >500 mg/g)

**Table 17.19:** Common causes of chronic kidney disease

| |
|---|
| *Obstructive uropathy:* Posterior urethral valves, pelviureteric junction obstruction, renal stones |
| *Reflux nephropathy:* Primary, secondary |
| *Glomerulonephritis:* Focal segmental glomerulosclerosis; systemic lupus erythematosus, IgA nephropathy, microscopic polyarteritis, IgA vasculitis |
| *Developmental anomalies:* Bilateral renal hypoplasia, dysplasia |
| *Familial nephropathy:* Nephronophthisis, Alport syndrome, polycystic kidneys |
| *Others:* Hemolytic uremic syndrome, amyloidosis, renal vein thrombosis, cortical necrosis |

kidney replacement therapy (KRT); and (v) counseling and preparing the family.

Initially, management aims at maintaining nutrition and retarding progression of kidney failure. Later, treatment of complications and KRT in form of dialysis or transplantation is required.

### Treatment of Reversible Renal Dysfunction

Conditions with potentially recoverable kidney function include obstruction to the drainage, recurrent urinary tract infections with vesicoureteric reflux, and decreased renal perfusion due to renal arterial stenosis. Care is taken to avoid AKI that may follow therapy with nephrotoxic drugs, herbal medications and radiocontrast agents, dehydration, and following surgery.

### Retarding Progression of Renal Failure

Hypertension and proteinuria increase intraglomerular perfusion, adaptive hyperfiltration and progressive kidney injury. Hypertension should be controlled, aiming for systolic and diastolic pressures between 50th to 75th percentiles for age and sex. Therapy with angiotensin-converting enzyme inhibitors or angiotensin receptor blockers results in reduced proteinuria, retarding progression of kidney failure. Therapy with lipid lowering agents and correction of anemia is also beneficial.

### Diet

Careful attention to diet is essential. Recommended daily amounts of calories should be ensured. A diet high in polyunsaturated fats, such as corn oil and medium chain triglycerides and complex carbohydrates is preferred. Water restriction is usually not necessary, except in kidney failure or in presence of fluid overload. Excessive use of diuretics, overzealous salt restriction and gastroenteritis may lead to dehydration that requires correction.

***Proteins:*** Protein intake should be 1–2 g/kg/day; proteins consumed should be of high biologic value. Restriction of protein intake is not required as it is not shown to retard disease progression in childhood CKD and may be associated with growth faltering.

***Potassium:*** Renal regulation of potassium balance is maintained until very late, but the capacity to rapidly excrete a potassium load is reduced. Dietary items with large potassium content should be avoided.

***Calcium and phosphorus:*** Calcium supplements are given as calcium carbonate or acetate. Excessive consumption of dairy products is avoided to restrict phosphate intake.

***Sodium:*** Since renal regulation of sodium reabsorption is impaired, its dietary intake needs to be individualized. Some infants are polyuric and lose large amounts of salt and water, that must be supplemented. Salt and water restriction is advised in children with chronic glomerulonephritis.

***Vitamins:*** Thiamine, riboflavin, folic acid, pyridoxine and $B_{12}$ are supplemented.

### Hypertension

Hypertension in patients with proteinuria and glomerular filtration rate >30 mL/min/1.73 m$^2$ is preferably treated with angiotensin-converting enzyme inhibitors (e.g. enalapril). Thiazides, beta-adrenergic blockers, and calcium channel antagonists are also effective; the latter are the preferred initial choice in CKD stage 4–5 (GFR <30 mL/min/1.73 m$^2$). Treatment with loop diuretics is beneficial in those with fluid overload. Patients with severe hypertension, uncontrolled with the above medications, require additional therapy with clonidine and prazosin.

### Anemia

Anemia develops when GFR is <30 mL/min/1.73 m$^2$. Iron deficiency, indicated by low levels of transferrin saturation (<20%) and ferritin (<100 ng/dL), is often present. Therapy with iron (elemental iron 4–6 mg/kg per day) should be initiated. Iron replete patients should receive therapy with recombinant human erythropoietin 50–150 U/kg/dose given SC or IV, 2–3 times a week. Darbepoetin has a longer half-life and is given once in 1–2 weeks. The dose of erythropoietin should be adjusted to achieve target hemoglobin of 11–12 g/dL. Inadequate response to erythropoietin may occur due to iron, folate or vitamin $B_{12}$ deficiency, chronic infection, aluminum toxicity and severe hyperparathyroidism. Patients with hemoglobin <6 g/dL should receive leukocyte poor, packed red cell transfusions.

### Growth

Optimization of energy and protein intake and treatment of mineral bone disease is important. Recombinant human growth hormone, given at a dose of 0.024–0.070 mg/kg SC once a day, 6–7 times a week (max 0.35 mg/kg/week) improves growth velocity in children with CKD. Early recognition and management of malnutrition, mineral bone disease, metabolic acidosis and electrolyte disturbances take precedence over therapy with growth hormone.

### Mineral Bone Disease

Mineral bone disease (MBD) is a serious problem in children as it occurs during the period of active growth (Fig. 17.23). Reduced renal synthesis of 1,25-dihydroxyvitamin $D_3$ (calcitriol), the most potent metabolite of vitamin D, is important in the pathogenesis of secondary hyperparathyroidism. Studies show a high incidence of vitamin D deficiency among children with CKD. With reduction of renal function, phosphate balance is initially

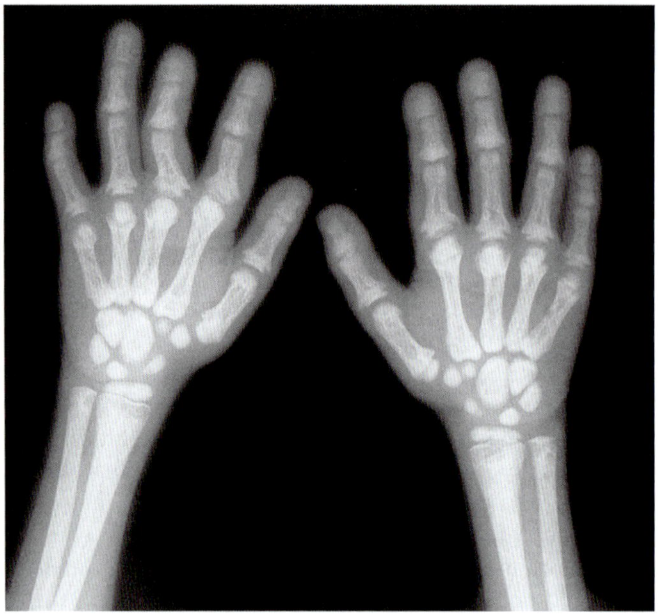

Fig. 17.23: Mineral bone disease with hyperphosphatemia and secondary hyperparathyroidism in a 12-year-old girl on chronic hemodialysis. Note the osteopenia and bone resorption in terminal phalanges

maintained by its increased excretion from the normal nephrons. However, when the GFR falls below 25%, blood phosphate levels rise.

The symptoms are vague and nonspecific. Bone pain, muscle weakness, growth retardation and skeletal deformities are prominent. Blood examination shows hypocalcemia, hyperphosphatemia and raised levels of alkaline phosphatase and PTH. X-rays reveal changes suggestive of rickets, and/or secondary hyperparathyroidism.

The goals of intervention are to maintain normal bone mineralization and growth, avoid hyperphosphatemia and hypocalcemia, and prevent or reverse increased PTH secretion. Treatment is based on dietary restriction of phosphate, and administration of phosphate binders and vitamin D. When serum phosphate exceeds the target range, phosphate containing foods (e.g. dairy products) are restricted. Oral phosphate binders, calcium carbonate or acetate (0.5–1 g/day with meals) reduce intestinal absorption of phosphate. Since aluminum accumulation may increase the risk of bone disease and encephalopathy, prolonged administration of aluminum hydroxide is avoided. Sevelamer carbonate, a calcium and aluminum free ion-exchange resin that binds phosphorus within the intestinal lumen, is a safe and effective phosphate binder.

The first steps in managing elevated levels of PTH in children with CKD are correction of underlying nutritional vitamin D deficiency and management of hyperphosphatemia. If the PTH is still elevated, therapy with activated vitamin D should be started. Vitamin D analogs with short half-life (calcitriol, 20–50 ng/kg/day or 1α-hydroxyvitamin $D_3$, 25–50 ng/kg/day) are preferred. Excessive vitamin D intake may cause hypercalcemia, hypercalciuria and high calcium phosphorus product.

Osteotomy may be required to correct bony deformities.

*Immunization*

Patients with CKD should receive all routine vaccines. Apart from regular immunization, children with CKD should also receive vaccines against pneumococcal, chickenpox and hepatitis A and B infections, especially if prepared for transplantation. Immunization with live vaccines should be completed prior to transplantation. Primary as well as booster doses of inactivated vaccines can be given 6 months after transplant.

### Long-Term Care

The rate of progression of CKD is variable. Some disorders (e.g. hemolytic uremic syndrome, crescentic GN) progress rapidly to stage V CKD while others (e.g. reflux nephropathy and some forms of chronic GN) show slow decline in renal function. Patients with a rapid deterioration of renal function are evaluated for reversible complications (infection, urinary outflow obstruction, fluid loss, hypertension and use of nephrotoxic drugs).

Urinary tract and other infections should be promptly treated with effective and least toxic drugs. The dosage of most drugs requires modification (reduction of dosage and/or increase in dosing interval), depending on the severity of kidney failure.

### Suggested Reading


1. Atkinson MA, Warady BA. Anemia in chronic kidney disease. Pediatr Nephrol 2018;33:227–38.
2. Drube J, Wan M, Bonthuis M, et al; European Society for Pediatric Nephrology Chronic Kidney Disease Mineral and Bone Disorders, Dialysis, and Transplantation Working Groups. Clinical practice recommendations for growth hormone treatment in children with chronic kidney disease. Nat Rev Nephrol 2019;15:577–89.
3. Harada R, Hamasaki Y, Okuda Y, et al. Epidemiology of pediatric chronic kidney disease/kidney failure: Learning from registries and cohort studies. Pediatr Nephrol 2022;37:1215–29.
4. McAlister L, Pugh P, Greenbaum L, et al. The dietary management of calcium and phosphate in children with CKD stages 2-5 and on dialysis-clinical practice recommendation from the Pediatric Renal Nutrition Taskforce. Pediatr Nephrol 2020;35:501–18.
5. Rees L. Protein energy wasting; what is it and what can we do to prevent it? Pediatr Nephrol 2021;36:287–94.
6. Shaw V, Polderman N, Renken-Terhaerdt J, et al. Energy and protein requirements for children with CKD stages 2-5 and on dialysis-clinical practice recommendations from the Pediatric Renal Nutrition Taskforce. Pediatr Nephrol 2020;35:519–31.


## KIDNEY REPLACEMENT THERAPY

Preparation of a child for support during kidney failure should be discussed in advance with the family members. The issues of finances and available family support should be addressed. Initiation of dialysis is considered when the glomerular filtration rate (GFR) falls below 12 mL/min/1.73 $m^2$ body surface area and is strongly recommended when the GFR is <8 mL/min/1.73 $m^2$. However, the well-being of the patient is more important than the estimated GFR for deciding when dialysis should begin. The presence of fluid overload, hypertension, gastrointestinal symptoms, growth retardation and neurological consequences of uremia influence the decision to initiate RRT.

The different forms of kidney replacement therapy are chronic peritoneal dialysis, hemodialysis and kidney transplantation. In children with ESKD, transplantation is the desired form of therapy. While chronic dialysis is life sustaining, it is inferior to transplant in providing replacement of kidney function. Transplantation is associated with significant survival advantage, decreased risks of hospitalization and improved quality of life.

### Chronic Peritoneal Dialysis (PD)

Chronic PD, done through a Tenckhoff catheter tunneled through the abdominal wall into the peritoneum, can be done manually (ambulatory PD) or with an automatic cycler (cyclic PD). The duration of dialysis is ~10–12 hr/day during which 4–6 cycles are performed. Chronic PD is preferred to chronic hemodialysis since it is done at home, without the need for hospital visits. Patients on chronic PD have less restriction of fluid and caloric intake; control of hypertension is better and hematocrit is maintained. The success of chronic PD relies upon the motivation of families to carry out the procedure.

### Chronic Hemodialysis (HD)

HD is mostly carried out in the hospital setting. These children require vascular access either as an arteriovenous fistula (preferred) or graft, or a double lumen indwelling catheter in a central vein (internal jugular vein preferred). Dialysis is done for 3–4 hr per session, with a frequency of 3 sessions/week. During a hemodialysis session, blood is circulated through an extracorporeal circuit that includes a hollow fiber dialyzer (artificial kidney) (Figs 17.22b and 17.24). Anticoagulation of the circuit is achieved by systemic heparinization. The procedure requires technical expertise and need for continuous monitoring.

### Kidney Transplantation

The feasibility and efficacy of kidney transplantation in children is well established. Advances in surgical skills, availability of immunosuppressive medications and ability to prevent and treat infections have improved the short- and long-term outcome. Immunosuppressive therapy is a combination of a calcineurin inhibitor (cyclosporin, tacrolimus), purine synthesis inhibitor (azathioprine, mycophenolate mofetil) and prednisone. Long-term allograft survival is better with live compared to deceased donors. Following successful kidney transplantation, the child can lead a normal life and resume physical activity and schooling. The allograft survival varies between 10 and 20 years.

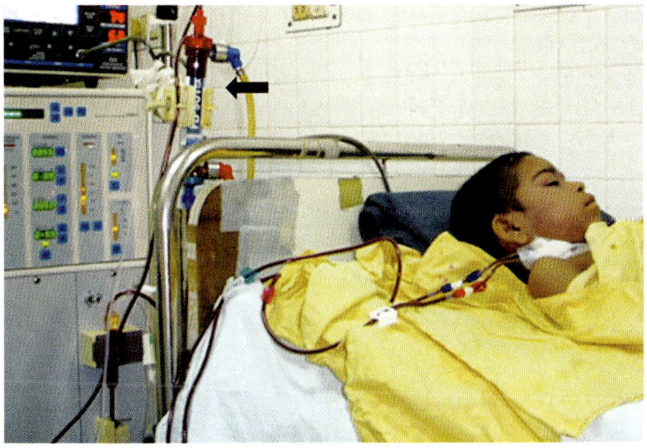

**Fig. 17.24:** Hemodialysis in a patient with end-stage kidney disease. Note the vascular access through a double-lumen catheter in the internal jugular vein, the hemodialysis machine and the dialyzer (solid arrow)

### Suggested Reading


1. Hataya H. Current state of peritoneal dialysis in children. Contrib Nephrol 2018;196:129–34.
2. Jacob H, Marlais M. Safeguarding children and young people requiring kidney replacement therapy: challenges and potential opportunities. Pediatr Nephrol. 2022;37:1007–15.
3. Lalji R, Francis A, Johnson DW, McCulloch M. Health disparities in access to kidney replacement therapy amongst children and adolescents with end-stage kidney disease in low- and lower-middle-income countries. Kidney Int 2020;97:463–65.
4. Leumann E. Renal replacement therapy in children and adolescents. Swiss Med Wkly. 2020; 150: w20371. doi: 10.4414/smw.2020.20371.


*Competencies:* **PE21.15; PE21.16**

## DISORDERS OF TUBULAR TRANSPORT

In comparison to glomerular diseases, tubular disorders are less common. Early and correct diagnosis is essential since specific management is possible in many cases. The diagnosis of a primary tubular disorder implies that there is no significant impairment of glomerular function or tubulointerstitial inflammation. A tubular disorder may be congenital or acquired and involve a single function of a tubule (renal glucosuria, nephrogenic diabetes insipidus) or multiple functions (Fanconi syndrome).

### Initial Evaluation

Children with primary defects in tubular function usually present during infancy (Table 17.20). Most tubular disorders can be diagnosed following careful interpretation of urine and plasma biochemistry. Key investigations are listed in Table 17.1.

### Renal Tubular Acidosis (RTA)

RTA includes conditions characterized by defective renal acidification, resulting in hyperchloremic metabolic acidosis and inappropriately high urine pH. Defects in tubular

| Table 17.20: Presenting features in tubular disorders |
|---|
| Stunting, undernutrition |
| Delayed gross motor milestones |
| Polyuria, excessive thirst |
| Recurrent episodes of dehydration, vomiting, fever |
| Refractory rickets, bone pains |
| Episodic muscle weakness |
| Constipation |
| Craving for salt and savory foods |

transport result in reduced proximal tubular reabsorption of bicarbonate ($HCO_3^-$), distal secretion of protons (hydrogen ion, $H^+$) or both, leading to impaired capacity for net acid excretion and metabolic acidosis. Plasma anion gap [$Na^+$–($Cl^-$ + $HCO_3^-$)] is in the normal range (8–12 mEq/L). The renal function is normal or only mildly impaired.

Two main forms are recognized: Distal RTA (type 1) and proximal RTA (type 2). Another variety (type 4), distinguished by the presence of hypoaldosteronism and hyperkalemia, is less common in children.

### *Distal RTA*

Distal (type 1) RTA is due to defective secretion of $H^+$ in the distal tubule, in the absence of significant decrease in glomerular filtration rate. Patients with distal RTA are unable to excrete ammonium ($NH_4^+$) ions adequately, and the urine pH cannot reach maximal acidity (i.e. remains >5.3) despite acidemia, indicating low $H^+$ concentration in the collecting duct. Hypokalemia is caused by increased urinary losses of potassium and aldosterone stimulation by urinary $Na^+$ loss and volume contraction, leading to further increase in tubular $K^+$ secretion.

The condition is sporadic, but may be inherited (dominant, recessive or X-linked). Important forms are listed in Table 17.21. The disease may be associated with systemic diseases (systemic lupus, Wilson disease) or secondary to renal disease (obstructive uropathy, reflux nephropathy) or drug toxicity (lithium, analgesics, amphotericin B).

**Table 17.21:** Inherited forms of renal tubular acidosis (RTA)

| *Type of RTA* | *Associated disorders (gene affected)* |
|---|---|
| Type 1 (distal) | • Hemolytic anemia (*SCL4A1*)<br>• Hearing loss (*ATP6V1B1, ATP6V0A4, FOXI1*)<br>• Normal hearing (*ATP6V1C2*)<br>• Dental enamel defects (*WDR72*) |
| Type 2 (proximal), isolated | Ocular abnormalities (band keratopathy, cataracts, glaucoma); intellectual impairment; basal ganglia calcification (*SCL4A4*) |
| Type 2, Fanconi syndrome | • Dent disease (*CLCN5*)<br>• Cystinosis (*CTNS*)<br>• Tyrosinemia type 1 (*FAH*)<br>• Fanconi-Bickel syndrome (*SLC2A2*)<br>• Fanconi renotubular syndrome type 1–5 (multiple genes)<br>• Glycogen storage disease type I (*G6PC, SLC37A4*)<br>• Wilson disease (*ATP7B*)<br>• Galactosemia (*GALT*)<br>• Hereditary fructose intolerance (*ALDOB*)<br>• Lowe syndrome (*OCRL1*)<br>• Arthrogryposis renal dysfunction cholestasis (ARC) syndrome (*VPS33B, VIPAS39*)<br>• Mitochondrial disorders (multiple genes) |
| Type 3 (combined) | Osteopetrosis (*CLCN7; TCIRG1*) |
| Type 4 (hyperkalemic) | • Congenital adrenal hyperplasia (*CYP21, CYP11B2*)<br>• Pseudohypoaldosteronism type 1 (*MR* or *NR3C2; SCNN1B*)<br>• Pseudohypoaldosteronism type 2 (*WNK4, WNK1, KLHL3, CUL3*) |

***Presenting features:*** Children show failure to thrive, polyuria, polydipsia, hypokalemic muscle weakness and rickets. Ultrasonography may show nephrocalcinosis (Fig. 17.25). Patients with incomplete distal RTA present with nephrolithiasis or incidentally detected nephrocalcinosis. Coexisting extrarenal findings may provide clues to diagnosis (Fig. 17.26a, b).

***Diagnosis:*** Biochemical abnormalities include hyperchloremic metabolic acidosis, hypokalemia, increased urinary excretion of calcium and decreased urinary citrate. Urinary net acid excretion (titratable acid and ammonium) is markedly reduced. Despite moderate to severe acidosis, patients cannot lower urine pH below 5.3. Measurement of the difference between urinary and blood $CO_2$, during the passage of alkaline urine, is a reliable indicator of distal tubular acidification. Normally, the difference is more than 20 mm Hg, provided the urine pH is >7.5. In children with distal RTA, the urine to blood $CO_2$ gradient is reduced below 10 mm Hg. Table 17.22 shows useful tests for the evaluation of patients with RTA. Hearing evaluation should be performed in all patients with idiopathic distal RTA.

Patients with incomplete forms of distal RTA show normal levels of serum pH and bicarbonate. The defect in distal acidification can be demonstrated by the fludrocortisone frusemide test that fails to show reduction in urine pH <5.3. Hypercalciuria and hypocitraturia are associated.

***Treatment:*** Hypokalemia should be treated before correction of acidosis. Acidosis is treated by administration of sodium bicarbonate (initially 2–3 mEq/kg in divided doses), its dose titrated to blood levels of bicarbonate. Alkali requirements decrease beyond 5 years of age. Treatment of acidosis reduces potassium losses and promotes growth and healing of rickets. Some patients require prolonged potassium replacement. Vitamin D supplements are not required.

### *Proximal (Type 2) RTA and Fanconi Syndrome*

Proximal RTA is due to reduced proximal tubular reabsorption of bicarbonate with marked bicarbonaturia.

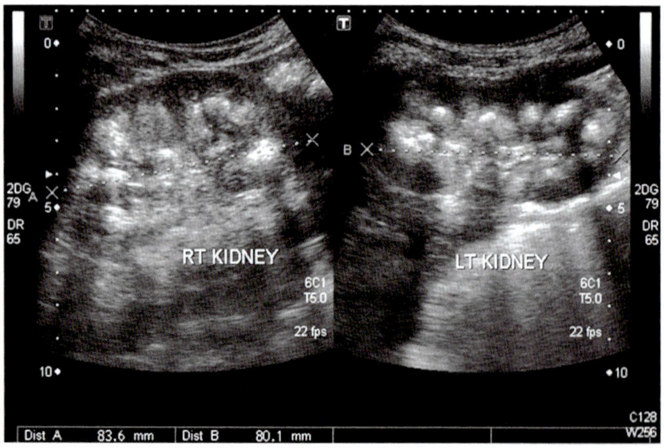


**Fig. 17.25:** Medullary nephrocalcinosis. Ultrasonography in a 3-year-old boy with distal renal tubular acidosis shows hyperechoic medulla in both kidneys

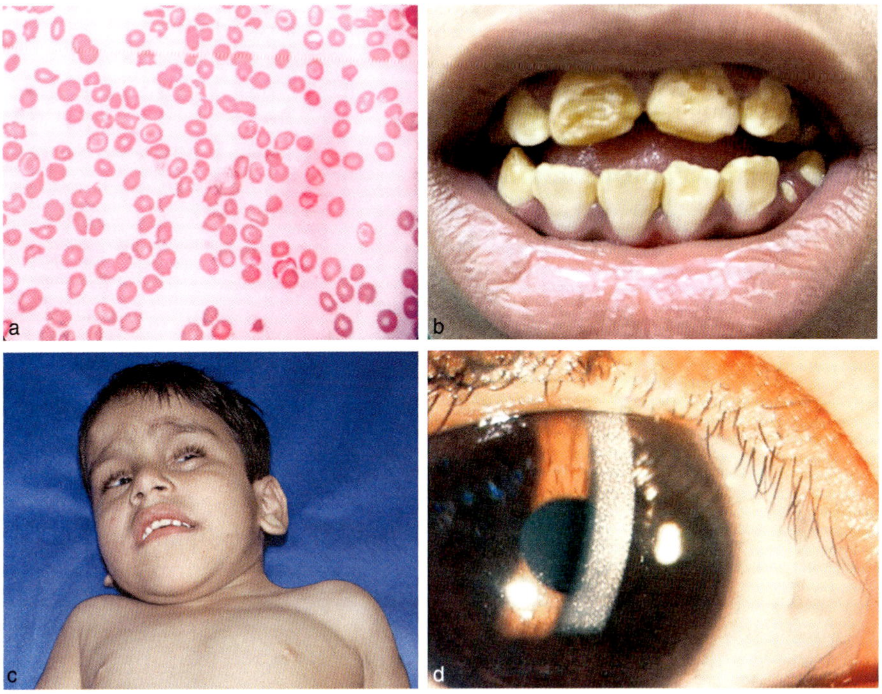


**Fig. 17.26:** Extrarenal findings in patients with renal tubular acidosis RTA: (a) Peripheral blood smear in a 4-yr-old boy with familial distal RTA showing schistocytes, acanthocytes, and spherocytes: The diagnosis of South Asian ovalocytosis was confirmed on next-generation sequencing to be secondary to a defect in anion exchanger 1 (*SLC4A1*); (b) Hypoplastic enamel with patchy enamel loss in a 10-yr-old boy with amelogenesis imperfecta associated with *WDR72* variation in distal RTA; (c) Facial dysmorphism with bilateral congenital glaucoma and cataract and intellectual disability is Lowe syndrome; (d) Slit-lamp examination of the cornea in a 4-year-old girl with cystinosis associated proximal RTA; diffuse crystal deposition is noted

**Table 17.22:** Investigations to differentiate types of renal tubular acidosis (RTA)

| | *Proximal RTA* | *Classic distal RTA* | *Type 4 RTA* |
|---|---|---|---|
| Plasma potassium | Normal or low | Normal or low | High |
| Urine pH (during acidosis) | <5.3 | >5.3 | <5.3 |
| Urine anion gap | Positive | Positive | Positive |
| Urine ammonium | Low | Low | Low |
| Fractional bicarbonate excretion | >10–15% | <5% | >5–10% |
| U-B $PCO_2$ mm Hg | >20 | <10 | >20 |
| Urine calcium | Normal | High | Normal or low |
| Other tubular defects | Often present | Absent | Absent |
| Nephrocalcinosis | Absent | Present | Absent |
| Bone disease | Common | Often present | Absent |

U-B $PCO_2$ urine to blood $PCO_2$ gradient

Once the plasma bicarbonate falls below 16 mEq/L, it is mostly reabsorbed. At steady state, daily acid loads are excreted successfully and the distal acidification mechanism is intact. Thus, children with proximal RTA have less severe acidosis than distal RTA.

***Pathophysiology:*** The primary defect in proximal RTA is reduced renal threshold for bicarbonate, resulting in bicarbonaturia. Proximal RTA may represent isolated or generalized proximal tubular dysfunction (Table 17.21). The latter, termed Fanconi syndrome, is characterized by tubular proteinuria and aminoaciduria and variable degrees of bicarbonaturia, phosphaturia, electrolyte wasting and glucosuria. Fanconi syndrome may be (i) idiopathic, or secondary to (ii) metabolic disorders (Table 17.21), (iii) drugs (ifosfamide, aminoglycosides, cisplatin), (iv) toxins (cadmium, lead, mercury) and (v) tubulointerstitial nephritis.

***Clinical features:*** Growth retardation is the chief clinical feature. Irritability, anorexia and listlessness may be present. Rickets is rare in isolated proximal RTA but common in Fanconi syndrome. Those with secondary Fanconi syndrome may have features of the underlying disorder. Nephrocalcinosis and urolithiasis are usually not seen. Symptoms of hypokalemia are less common.

***Diagnosis:*** Table 17.22 shows the features that allow proximal RTA to be distinguished from other forms of RTA. The blood pH and $HCO_3^-$ levels are low and urine pH is relatively alkaline. However, if blood $HCO_3^-$ is <14–16 mEq/L, urine pH falls <5.5. Urinary calcium and citrate excretion is normal. Demonstration of high fractional excretion of bicarbonate (>15%), at plasma bicarbonate level 20–22 mEq/L is confirmatory.

Evaluation of other proximal tubular functions includes assessment of phosphate excretion, and for aminoaciduria, glucosuria and low molecular weight proteinuria. Estimation of calcium excretion and examination for rickets are important. Disorders that are associated with Fanconi syndrome should be screened for, including cystinosis, Lowe syndrome, galactosemia and Wilson disease.

*Treatment:* Correction of acidosis requires 5–20 mEq/kg of alkali supplements daily. Part of the alkali is replaced as potassium citrate. Since administration of large amounts of alkali results in bicarbonate wasting, it is prudent to give a modest amount of sodium bicarbonate (5–8 mEq/kg/day in divided doses) along with restriction of dietary sodium. The latter causes contraction of extracellular fluid volume and increased proximal bicarbonate reabsorption. Children with Fanconi syndrome also need supplements of phosphate (neutral phosphate, Joulie solution). Treatment with vitamin D is necessary in children with rickets.

*Lowe syndrome:* This X-linked condition presents in the first few months of life with Fanconi syndrome, severe rickets, ocular defects (congenital cataract, buphthalmos, corneal degeneration, strabismus), neonatal or infantile hypotonia, rickets, seizures, developmental delay and mental impairment. Hypercalciuria may be prominent. Diagnosis is confirmed by genetic analysis for *OCRL* or measurement of the activity of the enzyme phosphatidylinositol bisphosphate 5-phosphatase in cultured fibroblasts. Chronic tubular injury leads to glomerulosclerosis and progressive renal insufficiency. Most children die in early childhood (Fig. 17.26c).

*Cystinosis:* This autosomal recessive disorder presents in infancy with features of severe Fanconi syndrome. The underlying defect is in the lysosomal membrane protein (cystinosin) that transports cystine from lysosomes into the cytosol. This leads to very high levels of free lysosomal cystine, which is deposited as crystals in the cornea, conjunctiva, bone marrow, leukocytes and lymph nodes. Tubular handling of cystine is normal. The most common form of cystinosis is the infantile nephropathic form in which patients present in early infancy. Later, patients show photophobia and enlarged liver and spleen; some have blond hair.

Diagnosis is indicated by the presence of cystine crystals in cornea on slit-lamp microscopy (Fig. 17.26d). Elevated levels of cystine in polymorphonuclear leukocytes or cultured fibroblasts and genetic testing to reveal significant homozygous or compound heterozygous variants in *CTNS* are confirmatory. Prenatal diagnosis requires measurement of cystine level in chorionic villi or cultured amniotic fluid cells. Correction of metabolic acidosis and replacement of electrolytes is essential. Early therapy with oral cysteamine may retard progression of systemic disease. Topical therapy is essential to prevent corneal deposits. Long-term complications include hypothyroidism and diabetes mellitus. If untreated, most patients show progression to kidney failure by late childhood.

### *Hyperkalemic (Type 4) RTA*

Hyperkalemia with distal RTA due to aldosterone resistance or deficiency is termed type 4 RTA. Aldosterone directly stimulates the proton pump, increases $Na^+$ absorption resulting in negative intratubular potential and increases urinary $K^+$ losses; and stimulates basolateral $Na^+/K^+$ ATPase. Aldosterone deficiency or resistance leads to hyperkalemia and acidosis. Maximally acidic urine (pH <5.5) can be formed, indicating the ability to establish a maximal $H^+$ gradient. However, the rate of ammonium excretion is low. Aldosterone deficiency without renal disease may occur with Addison disease, or following adrenal necrosis or tuberculosis. Aldosterone resistance may occur with chronic renal insufficiency such as obstructive uropathy or interstitial nephritis or with use of certain drugs (e.g. amiloride, spironolactone, ACE inhibitors, heparin, NSAIDs, calcineurin inhibitors).

The recessive form of pseudohypoaldosteronism (PHA type 1) should be considered in infants presenting with salt loss, hypotension, hyperkalemia and metabolic acidosis. Patients with PHA type 2 (Gordon syndrome) have hypertension, acidosis and hyperkalemia with hyporeninemic hypoaldosteronism.

## Nephrogenic Diabetes Insipidus

Congenital nephrogenic diabetes insipidus is an inherited disorder of water reabsorption, caused by resistance to the action of ADH on its receptor. Absorption of water in the distal tubules and collecting ducts is significantly impaired. The defect usually involves the arginine vasopressin receptor 2 (*AVPR2*) gene on X chromosome. Less commonly, the disease is inherited in an autosomal recessive manner due to mutations in the gene encoding aquaporin 2.

The usual history is of a boy who, within a few weeks of life, has excessive thirst, recurrent episodes of dehydration and unexplained fever. The infant has increased or normal urine output even when dehydrated. Constipation and growth retardation is common. Polyuria, polydipsia and enuresis are striking. Recurrent episodes of dehydration and rehydration might lead to neurological injury with intracranial calcification, seizures and psychomotor retardation.

Hypernatremia (sodium >170 mEq/L) with low urine sodium is characteristic. Correspondingly, serum chloride and osmolality are high. The urine osmolality is inappropriately low (usually below 150–200 mOsm/kg) for the elevated plasma osmolality. Furthermore, the urine osmolality does not increase despite administration of DDAVP. This allows nephrogenic diabetes insipidus to be distinguished from central diabetes insipidus. The latter show normal response to DDAVP with increase in urine osmolality to >600–800 mOsm/kg. Tubular unresponsiveness to ADH may occur as part of chronic pyelonephritis, obstructive uropathy, sickle cell disease, lithium toxicity, hypercalcemia, hypokalemia and tubulointerstitial disease.

Treatment consists of increased fluid intake and sodium restriction to reduce the osmolar load. Administration of hydrochlorothiazide (2–3 mg/kg/day), alone or in combination with amiloride (0.4–0.625 mg/kg/dose once daily; maximum dose 20 mg/1.73 $m^2$/day), reduces polyuria and leads to clinical improvement. Indomethacin may also reduce urine volume, but its use is limited beyond infancy.

### Renal Glucosuria

Renal glucosuria is an autosomal recessively transmitted, isolated defect of tubular glucose transport. It is recognized by the presence of glucose in the urine, despite normal blood glucose levels. Glucose metabolism and other renal tubular transport mechanisms are normal. Several members of a family may be affected. The disorder is asymptomatic and does not require treatment.

### Bartter Syndrome

Bartter syndrome is an autosomal recessive disorder characterized by hypokalemia and metabolic alkalosis, resulting from excessive chloride, potassium and sodium wasting in the thick ascending limb of the loop of Henle. Features include failure to thrive, polyuria, polydipsia and recurrent episodes of dehydration. Vomiting, constipation, muscle weakness and cramps are other manifestations. Patients show marked hypokalemia with high urinary potassium and hypochloremic metabolic alkalosis. Volume contraction leads to increase in levels of plasma renin and aldosterone. Elevated urinary levels of chloride (>20–30 mEq/L) are characteristic.

Several subtypes of Bartter syndrome are recognized, differing in their molecular basis and clinical severity. They are caused by mutations in six genes involved in the reabsorption of sodium in the thick ascending limb of Henle and/or the distal convoluted tubule.

The condition may occasionally present in the neonatal period with history of maternal polyhydramnios and postnatal polyuria, dehydration and nephrocalcinosis; some have sensorineural deafness.

Bartter syndrome should be differentiated from other conditions with hypokalemic metabolic alkalosis (e.g. cystic fibrosis, recurrent vomiting, monogenic forms of hypertension, and Gitelman syndrome) by the presence of normal blood pressure, and high urinary chloride and calcium excretion.

Therapy comprises replacement of urinary losses of fluid, sodium, potassium and chloride. Most patients require supplements of potassium chloride (1–3 mEq/kg/day); serum potassium might often not return to normal range. Use of prostaglandin synthase inhibitors (indomethacin 2–3 mg/kg or ibuprofen 20–30 mg/kg) is beneficial. Potassium sparing diuretics and ACE inhibitors have been used with modest benefit in correcting hypokalemia.

### Gitelman Syndrome

Hypokalemia, hypomagnesemia and metabolic alkalosis may be caused by Gitelman syndrome, an autosomal recessive condition characterized by a defect in the apical thiazide sensitive sodium chloride cotransporter (NCCT) in the distal tubules. Clinical and laboratory features are milder than in Bartter syndrome; hypomagnesemia and lack of hypercalciuria are characteristic. Patients present in adolescence with episodes of muscle weakness, cramps, tetany, vomiting or fatigue. Polyuria and failure to thrive are less pronounced.

### Suggested Reading


1. Bagga A, Sinha A. Renal tubular acidosis. Indian J Pediatr 2020; 87: 733–44.
2. Besouw MTP, Kleta R, Bockenhauer D. Bartter and Gitelman syndromes: Questions of class. Pediatr Nephrol 2020;35:1815–24.
3. Downie ML, Lopez Garcia SC, Kleta R, Bockenhauer D. Inherited tubulopathies of the kidney: Insights from genetics. Clin J Am Soc Nephrol 2021;16:620–30.
4. Do C, Vasquez PC, Soleimani M. Metabolic alkalosis pathogenesis, diagnosis, and treatment: Core curriculum 2022. Am J Kidney Dis 2022;80:536–51.
5. Kavanagh C, Uy NS. Nephrogenic diabetes insipidus. Pediatr Clin North Am 2019;66:227–34.
6. Kamel KS, Halperin ML. Use of urine electrolytes and urine osmolality in the clinical diagnosis of fluid, electrolytes, and acid-base disorders. Kidney Int Rep 2021;6:1211–24.


*Competencies:* **PE21.15; PE21.16**

## NEPHROLITHIASIS AND NEPHROCALCINOSIS

Renal calculi are uncommon in children and occur usually in the setting of an underlying metabolic abnormality. Symptoms include dysuria, hypogastric pain, hematuria and occasionally urinary infections. Nephrocalcinosis refers to formation of crystalline deposits within the renal parenchyma, presenting as enhanced renal echogenicity, which may be cortical, medullary or diffuse. Table 17.23 lists common underlying metabolic causes. Urinary tract infection, particularly with urease producing organisms like *Proteus*, favors precipitation of magnesium ammonium phosphate and calcium phosphate (struvite stones).

**Table 17.23:** Underlying metabolic abnormalities in children with nephrolithiasis or nephrocalcinosis

**Hypercalciuria with hypercalcemia**
- Vitamin D overdose
- Primary hyperparathyroidism
- Production of PTH related peptide (malignancy, sarcoidosis)

**Hypercalciuria with normal serum calcium**
- Idiopathic hypercalciuria
- Familial hypophosphatemia with hypercalciuria
- Distal renal tubular acidosis
- Dent disease
- Bartter syndrome with/without sensorineural deafness
- Autosomal dominant hypocalcemia with hypercalciuria
- Familial hypomagnesemia, hypercalciuria, nephrocalcinosis
- Lowe syndrome
- Frusemide use

**Miscellaneous causes**
- Primary hyperoxaluria (type I, type II)
- Cystinuria
- Abnormal purine, pyrimidine metabolism: Lesch-Nyhan syndrome, glycogenosis type 1, xanthinuria
- Melamine toxicity

### Evaluation

Ultrasonography detects most radiopaque and radiolucent calculi and nephrocalcinosis. High resolution computerized tomography (CT) detects even minute calculi.

A metabolic cause is found in ~50% patients. Initial investigations include renal function tests, pH, bicarbonate, calcium, phosphorus and uric acid. Presence of specific crystals in the urine might suggest an etiology (Fig. 17.27). Urine pH >5.5 in the morning sample suggests defective tubular acidification. Estimation of protein, calcium, oxalate and uric acid in timed urine collections evaluates their excretion, compared to normal individuals. Alternatively, their excretion is expressed as a ratio to creatinine in spot samples. Patients with hypercalciuria require evaluation for hypercalcemia (intact PTH, 25-hydroxyvitamin D) and for association with distal RTA, hypomagnesemia, hypophosphatemic rickets and abnormalities of thyroid hormone. Stone analysis is performed using X-ray diffraction or infrared spectroscopy.



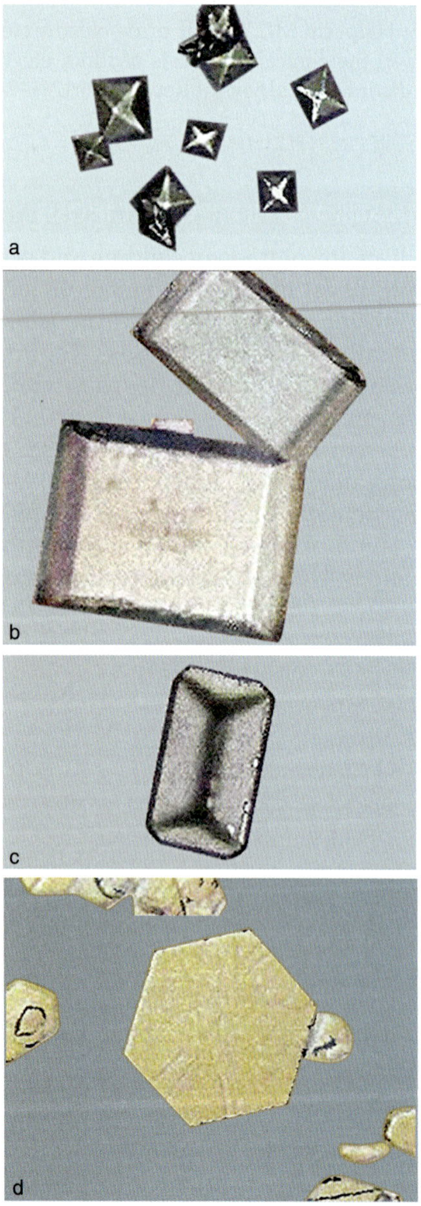


**Fig. 17.27:** Morphology of urine crystals may suggest etiology of renal stones: (a) Envelope-shaped oxalate dihydrate crystals (200×); (b) Rectangular uric acid crystal (400×); (c) Coffin lid-shaped triple phosphate (200×); (d) Hexagonal cystine crystals (200×)

### Idiopathic Hypercalciuria

This is the most common underlying cause in patients with nephrolithiasis, but may alternatively present with microscopic and gross hematuria. A family history of hematuria or nephrolithiasis is often present. Urinary calcium to creatinine ratio in the morning 'spot' urine serves as a screening test. The upper limit of normal in children over 2 years is 0.2 (mg/mg). The diagnosis is confirmed by measurement of 24-hour urinary calcium; values greater than 4 mg/kg/day are abnormal. Blood levels of calcium and magnesium are normal. A high fluid intake and diet low in animal protein and salt is advised. Therapy with thiazide diuretics, which reduces urinary calcium excretion, may be required.

### Endemic Vesical Calculi

Vesical calculi are usually single stones, detected in young boys (<5-year-old) in some regions of the country, e.g. Rajasthan, Andhra Pradesh and North-Eastern states, and in Pakistan and Afghanistan. These stones are composed of ammonium acid urate and calcium oxalate. Risk factors include consumption of a predominantly cereal (wheat or jowar) based diet, with low amount of calcium and phosphate and high oxalate. Recurrent diarrheal episodes contribute by causing dehydration and an acidic, concentrated urine. A high intake of dairy products and animal proteins has led to a decline in the prevalence of these stones. Treatment requires suprapubic cystolithotomy; these stones rarely recur.

### Primary Hyperoxaluria

Primary hyperoxaluria type 1 is an autosomal recessive disorder of glyoxylate metabolism with deficient activity of the liver-specific enzyme, alanine glyoxylate aminotransferase causing overproduction of endogenous oxalate that manifests as renal stones and/or nephrocalcinosis. Oxalosis also affects the eyes, heart, bones and bone marrow. The diagnosis is suggested by elevated oxalate in plasma and/or urine, and confirmed by deficient activity of the enzyme on liver biopsy and sequencing of *AGXT*. Treatment is supportive; some patients with partial deficiency benefit from pyridoxine supplementation.

Patients presenting in childhood progress to end-stage kidney disease by adolescence, and require combined liver kidney transplantation. Therapies that interfere with RNA synthesis appear promising. Lumasiran, which targets the hepatic enzymes glycolate oxidase, has been approved for the treatment of primary hyperoxaluria type 1 in USA and Europe. Nedosiran, which interferes with the RNA of lactate dehydrogenase A, is currently being examined in clinical trials.

### Cystinuria

This autosomal recessive disorder is characterized by impaired proximal tubular reabsorption of cystine and dibasic amino acids (ornithine, lysine and arginine). Supersaturation of urine with cystine crystals may lead to formation of recurrent radiopaque calculi. The diagnosis is suggested by presence of hexagonal urine crystals, excretion of specific amino acids (as above) and positive urine nitroprusside cyanide test. Confirmation requires quantification of cystine excretion (24-hr, spot sample), stone analysis or genetic testing. A high fluid intake and urinary alkalization help, since cystine is poorly soluble at normal pH but dissolves well at pH >8.0. Agents such as penicillamine and tiopronin prevent formation of calculi by cleaving disulfide bonds of cystine to form the more soluble homodimer, cysteine.

### Management of Renal Calculi

Stones less than 5–7 mm in size may pass spontaneously. Extracorporeal shock wave lithotripsy (ESWL) may suffice for small stones. Percutaneous nephrolithotomy is appropriate in patients with contraindication for ESWL or with stones that are too large for lithotripsy. Ureteroscopy is useful for distal and mid-ureteric calculi. Open surgery is necessary for stones >3 cm in size or those with pelviureteric junction obstruction.

UTI should be treated and an adequate fluid intake ensured. Patients with idiopathic hypercalciuria may benefit from a low salt intake; dietary calcium restriction is not necessary. Persistent hypercalciuria is treated with oral potassium citrate, an inhibitor of crystallization. Thiazide diuretics reduce urine calcium excretion; their long-term use, however, is restricted due to side effects. Prolonged alkali supplementation is necessary in patients with distal RTA.

### Suggested Reading

1. Desai M, Sun Y, Buchholz N, et al. Treatment selection for urolithiasis: percutaneous nephrolithomy, ureteroscopy, shock wave lithotripsy, and active monitoring. World J Urol 2017;35:1395–99.
2. Gupta A, Somers MJG, Baum MA. Treatment of primary hyperoxaluria type 1. Clin Kidney J 2022; 15 (Suppl 1): i9–i13.
3. Saadeh SA. Pediatric nephrolithiasis: Risk factors, evaluation, and prevention. Pediatr Ann 2020;49:e262–e267.
4. Singh P, Harris PC, Sas DJ, Lieske JC. The genetics of kidney stone disease and nephrocalcinosis. Nat Rev Nephrol 2022;18: 224–40.

*Competencies:* **PE5.8; PE21.15; PE21.16**

## ENURESIS

Enuresis is defined as normal, nearly complete evacuation of the bladder at a wrong place and time at least twice a month after 5 years of age. Enuresis should be differentiated from continuous or intermittent incontinence or dribbling. The bed is soaking wet in the former, compared to loss of urine without normal bladder emptying in the latter. Enuresis is usually functional while continuous or daytime incontinence is often organic.

More than 85% children attain complete diurnal and nocturnal control of the bladder by 5 years. The remaining 15% gain continence at approximately 15% per year, such that by adolescence only 0.5–1% children have enuresis. Up to 11 years, enuresis is twice as common in boys; thereafter, the incidence is similar or slightly higher in girls.

Enuresis is called primary when the child has never been dry and secondary when bed wetting starts after a minimum period of 6 months of dryness at night. It is termed monosymptomatic, if it is not accompanied by any lower urinary tract symptoms and nocturnal, if it occurs only during sleep. Children with *monosymptomatic nocturnal enuresis* require no further evaluation.

### Etiology

Maturational delay is the most likely cause of nocturnal enuresis, suggested by high spontaneous cure rates with increasing age. Other reasons include a lack of circadian rhythm of secretion of antidiuretic hormone (ADH), inadequate sleep arousal, urinary tract infections, bladder bowel dysfunction and stressful events.

### Evaluation

Less than 5% patients with nocturnal enuresis have an organic basis. History helps determine whether the enuresis is primary or secondary, and whether any daytime symptoms or voiding difficulty is present. In cases of secondary enuresis, history should be taken to rule out acute stressful conditions, polyuria and features of bladder irritability such as frequency and urgency. Physical examination should focus on spinal anomalies.

If the child has a normal urinary stream with no daytime symptoms suggestive of a voiding disorder and normal physical examination, the child does not require extensive evaluation. Clinical and neurological examination excludes an anatomical or neurological cause for incontinence.

A voiding diary with frequency and volume charting of urine output and fluid intake for at least 2 days, with a record of daytime accidents, bladder symptoms and bowel habits for at least 7 days is useful. It helps detect children with non-monosymptomatic enuresis or polydipsia, provides information on nocturnal polyuria (such children benefit from desmopressin) and helps monitor compliance to instructions and response to therapy. Urinalysis rules out infection, proteinuria and glucosuria. Additional diagnostic and invasive procedures, including ultrasonography and MCU, are limited to patients with suspected neurological or urological dysfunction.

### Treatment

The decision for treatment should be guided by the degree of concern and motivation on the part of the child rather than the parents. General advice should be given to all enuretic children, but active treatment need not begin before the age of 6 years. Caffeinated drinks like tea, coffee and sodas should be avoided in the evening. Adequate fluid intake, i.e. 40% in the morning, 40% in the afternoon and 20% in the evening, is recommended.

The first-line of therapy is non-pharmacological, comprising motivational therapy and use of alarm devices.

*Motivational therapy* alone is successful in 25% patients. The child is reassured and provided emotional support. The benign nature of the condition is explained to the child and parents, and the child is encouraged to assume active responsibility, including keeping a dry night diary, voiding before going to bed and changing wet clothes and bedding. Dry nights should be credited with praise and encouragement from the parents. Punishments and angry parental responses are avoided.

Behavioral modification is encouraged to achieve good bladder and bowel habits. The child is encouraged to void frequently enough to avoid urgency and daytime incontinence and to have a daily bowel movement. Bladder training exercises have not been shown to be useful in improving the functional bladder capacity.

*Alarm therapy* involves the use of a device to elicit a conditioned response of awakening to the sensation of a full bladder. The alarm device consists of a small sensor attached to the child's underwear, or a mat under the bed-sheet and an alarm attached to the child's collar or placed at the bedside. When the child starts wetting, the sensors are activated causing the alarm to ring. The child should awaken to the alarm, void in the toilet and reattach the alarm; a parent should ensure the child does not merely wake to switch off the alarm. The alarm is best used after 7 years of age and is successful in about two-thirds of children; one-third of children may relapse.

While alarm systems are available in India, the ordinary alarm clock may be used to wake the child to void in the toilet at a critical time when the bladder is full and the child is still dry. The combination of motivational and alarm therapy is successful in up to 60–70% of children.

*Pharmacotherapy* is considered, if enuresis persists despite institution of alarm, regular voiding habits, treatment of constipation and exclusion of postvoid residual urine or dysfunctional voiding. Cardiac arrhythmias are a rare but serious adverse event effect of tricyclic antidepressants, which are, therefore, not recommended. Anticholinergic drugs reduce uninhibited bladder contractions and are useful in children who have significant daytime urge incontinence besides nocturnal enuresis. The usual dose is 5 mg for oxybutynin or 2 mg for tolterodine at bedtime, given above 6 years of age. Desmopressin (DDAVP, 0.2–0.4 mg orally; oral melt 120–240 μg) works by reducing the volume of urine. Its rapid onset of action makes it a satisfactory choice for special occasions like staying out for the night. Relapse rates are high after stopping the medication.

### Suggested Reading


1. Nevéus T, Fonseca E, Franco I, et al. Management and treatment of nocturnal enuresis: An updated standardization document from the International Children's Continence Society. J Pediatr Urol 2020;16:10–19.
2. Rakowska-Silska M, Jobs K, Paturej A, Kalicki B. Voiding disorders in pediatrician's practice. Clin Med Insights Pediatr 2020; 14: 1179556520975035.
3. Van Herzeele C, Vande Walle J, Walle JV, Dhondt K. Recent advances in managing and understanding enuresis. F1000Res. 2017;6;1881.


*Competencies:* **PE21.15; PE21.16**

## CONGENITAL ABNORMALITIES OF KIDNEY AND URINARY TRACT

Congenital abnormalities of kidney and urinary tract (CAKUT) are common and account for about 25–30% of CKD.

### Single Kidney

In unilateral renal agenesis, one kidney fails to develop while the other is normal in size, position and function. Agenesis may occur due to primary failure of formation of the ureteric bud or its inability to engage with the renal mesenchyme. The condition may occur sporadically or as part of brachio-oto-renal, DiGeorge, Fanconi anemia, Fraser renal coloboma or Williams-Beuren syndromes. Various abnormalities of the female genital tract may be associated. Renal agenesis is asymptomatic, and usually detected incidentally on ultrasonography. Usually, there is compensatory hypertrophy of the normal kidney. A DMSA scan helps in ruling out scarring due to associated vesicoureteric reflux or an ectopic kidney. Children with single kidney should avoid contact sports that risk direct trauma to the kidneys. While patients do maintain glomerular function, they require annual monitoring for hypertension and proteinuria. Girls with single kidney should undergo pelvic ultrasonography, ideally after thelarche and before oneset of menarche, to rule out mesonephric anomalies leading to blind vagina or hemivagina and hemiuterus.

Fetuses with bilateral renal agenesis or hypoplasia rarely survive to term. Lack of fetal urine production leads to oligohydramnios and limb anomalies. Neonates show low set ears, flat nose, prominent epicanthic folds and small chin (Potter facies). Pulmonary hypoplasia is the usual cause of death.

### Renal Dysplasia

Renal dysplasia implies abnormal development of renal parenchyma. Primitive ducts surrounded by connective tissue, metaplastic cartilage, poorly differentiated glomeruli and dilated tubules are present. Bilateral total renal dysplasia is fatal in the neonatal period. The term cystic dysplasia denotes the presence of cyst(s) within an abnormal kidney (e.g. small kidney, loss of corticomedullary differentiation or increased parenchymal echogenicity).

*Multicystic dysplastic kidney:* A multicystic dysplastic kidney (MCDK) is an enlarged nonfunctioning kidney with cysts of varying sizes resulting from abnormal differentiation of the metanephros. Affecting 1 in 2400 to 4300 live births, it is the *most common* cystic renal malformation in children. Ultrasonography shows characteristic findings, including multiple thin-walled noncommunicating cysts of varying size, in an enlarged kidney without identifiable parenchyma or renal pelvis **(Fig. 17.28)**.

Most patients with MCDK have a normal contralateral kidney showing compensatory hypertrophy. However, 20–40% cases show abnormalities of the contralateral

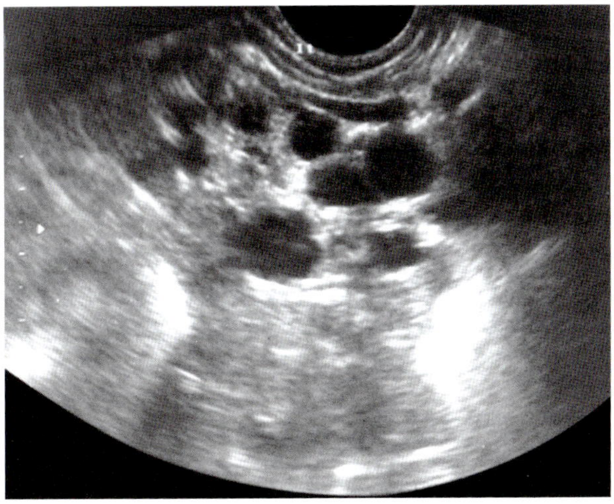

Fig. 17.28: Multicystic dysplastic kidney. Multiple, thin-walled and noncommunicating cysts involving the left kidney on postnatal ultrasound at one month age

genitourinary tract, such as vesicoureteric reflux or pelviureteric junction obstruction, and 15% have extrarenal anomalies. A DMSA scan confirms that the affected kidney is nonfunctional and rules out reflux-associated scarring of the contralateral kidney. However, given the high concordance between DMSA and ultrasonographic findings, nuclear scintigraphy is considered unnecessary, if ultrasound has been performed reliably.

Children with MCDK require 6-monthly monitoring by ultrasound that shows compensatory hypertrophy of the normal kidney and progressive involution of the MCDK by 5–7 years of age. Progressive renal impairment is seen only if other abnormalities are associated, compensatory hypertrophy is lacking, and in presence of proteinuria or hypertension. The risk of malignant transformation and of hypertension is negligible. Nephrectomy is usually not indicated.

### Obstructive Uropathy

Obstructive anomalies of the urinary tract are an important cause of irreversible renal damage in childhood. The common lesions include pelviureteric junction obstruction, vesicoureteric junction obstruction and posterior urethral valves. Diagnosis is suspected on antenatal ultrasonography or following presentations with dribbling of urine, poor urinary stream, fever and/or urinary tract infections. Chronic obstruction results in dysfunction of distal tubules with impaired urinary concentration and acidification, leading to polyuria, polydipsia, failure to thrive, refractory rickets and systemic acidosis.

*Pelviureteric junction (PUJ) obstruction:* Stenosis of the PUJ may be unilateral or, rarely, bilateral. Obstruction is more common in boys and in presence of ectopic, malrotated or horseshoe kidney. It may present as an asymptomatic flank mass, or with upper abdominal pain, UTI or hematuria. Ultrasonography shows a dilated renal pelvis without ureteric dilatation. Radionuclide (DTPA) renal scan shows impaired drainage of the affected kidney, which does not improve despite administration of frusemide. Where scintigraphy is not available, intravenous pyelography shows renal pelvis dilatation with an abrupt cut-off at the PUJ. Mild cases are followed up with ultrasound. Surgical treatment by pyeloplasty is indicated, if the relative function of the affected kidney is impaired. Nephrectomy may be required for a kidney with extremely poor function that does not improve despite temporary nephrostomy, severe hypertension or recurrent UTI.

*Posterior urethral valves:* These are an important cause of distal urinary tract obstruction in boys. The presenting features are dribbling, abnormal urinary stream, palpable bladder and recurrent UTI. The presence of severe obstruction *in utero* may lead to renal dysplasia, with mild to moderate renal dysfunction at birth. Antenatal ultrasound shows bilateral hydroureteronephrosis with or without a thick-walled bladder and oligohydramnios. The diagnosis is confirmed on MCU, which shows dilated posterior urethra and valves at its junction with the anterior urethra. The bladder is enlarged and may show diverticuli and trabeculations; secondary vesicoureteric reflux is common.

Endoscopic fulguration of the valves is performed as early as possible. Alternatively, temporary urinary diversion by vesicostomy or bilateral ureterostomies is necessary. Long-term follow-up is necessary since a significant proportion of patients show progressive kidney disease. Bladder dysfunction is common, with delayed continence or incontinence, poor bladder sensation and a poorly compliant low capacity bladder. If pharmacotherapy fails, patients may require clean intermittent catheterization and occasionally bladder augmentation.

*Phimosis:* Up to the age of 2 years, the prepuce cannot be fully retracted because of congenital adhesions with the glans. The diagnosis of phimosis should thus be made with caution in young children. Indications for therapy include recurrent balanoposthitis, forceful/difficult urination, paraphimosis or recurrent UTI.

*Ureterocele:* This is a congenital condition in which the terminal part of the ureter distends within the bladder to form a sac-like pouch. Symptoms include recurrent urinary infections, abdominal pain and urolithiasis. Ureteroceles are commonly associated with duplex systems, particularly in girls. Endoscopic deroofing is the treatment of choice.

### Miscellaneous

*Renal ectopia, renal fusion:* An ectopic kidney may lie in the pelvis or the iliac fossa. It may be structurally normal or hypoplastic. The patient may be asymptomatic, or have abdominal discomfort or dysuria. A horseshoe kidney results from fusion of identical poles of both kidneys. Patients with horseshoe kidney show VUR in 30% cases.

*Renal duplication:* A duplex (duplicated) system is a kidney with two pyelocalyceal systems. In patients with partial or incomplete duplication, either a single or bifid ureter is present; in those with complete duplication, two ureters from the affected side empty separately into the bladder. Evaluation consists of imaging of the upper tract (ultrasonography, DTPA renal scan, intravenous pyelography) to evaluate for obstruction and lower tract (MCU) for VUR.

Competencies: **PE21.15; PE21.16**

## ANTENATAL HYDRONEPHROSIS

Extensive use of antenatal ultrasonography has led to increasing detection of CAKUT. On antenatal ultrasound, hydronephrosis is identified in 4–5% pregnancies. The majority of cases of antenatal hydronephrosis resolve without sequelae, representing transient physiological obstruction or stasis. Patients require monitoring by ultrasound during the antenatal period for progressive worsening and association with oligohydramnios.

Patients with antenatally diagnosed hydronephrosis are advised postnatal ultrasound during the first week of life. Neonates with posterior urethral valves, solitary kidney or bilateral hydronephrosis and impaired renal function require prompt management. Neonates with significant unilateral or bilateral urinary tract dilatation and those with additional abnormalities should undergo an MCU at 4–6 weeks of life to detect VUR. If reflux is ruled out, a diuretic renal dynamic scan may be required to detect significant obstruction and evaluate differential kidney function.

Most cases with mild-to-moderate hydronephrosis require only ultrasound monitoring and show spontaneous resolution by 2–5 years of age. Surgery is indicated in presence of obstructive drainage pattern associated with low differential function, and/or recurrent UTI.

Parents of all infants with antenatal hydronephrosis should be counseled regarding the risk of urinary tract infections.

Figure 17.29 shows a proposed algorithm for postnatal evaluation and management of antenatally detected hydronephrosis.

### Suggested Reading


1. Nguyen HT, Phelps A, Coley B, et al. 2021 update on the urinary tract dilation (UTD) classification system: Clarifications, review of the literature, and practical suggestions. Pediatr Radiol 2022;52:740–51.
2. Sinha A, Bagga A, Krishna A, et al. Revised guidelines on the management of antenatally detected hydronephrosis. Indian Pediatr 2013;50:215–32.
3. Vincent K, Murphy HJ, Twombley KE. Urinary tract dilation in the fetus and neonate. Neoreviews 2022;23:e159–e174.


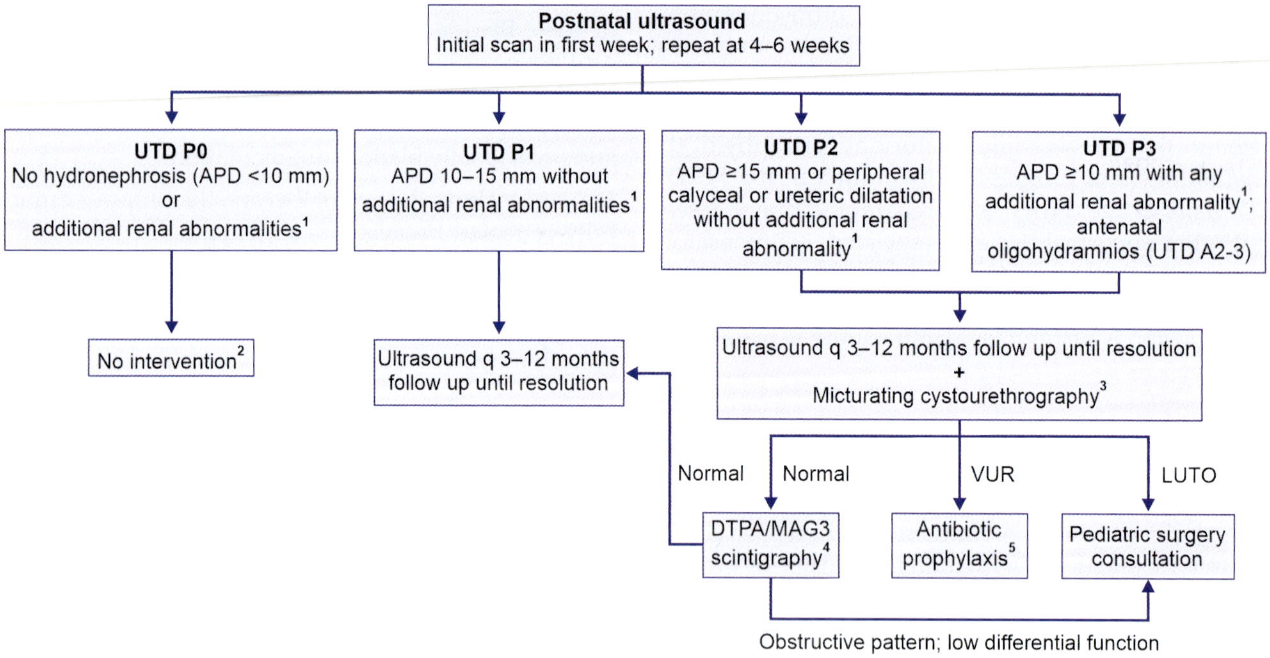


**Fig. 17.29:** Postnatal evaluation and management of antenatally detected hydronephrosis. Hydronephrosis is classified according to urinary tract dilatation (UTD) classification, antenatally (A0–3) and postnatally (P0–3). Postnatal management is based chiefly on findings on postnatal ultrasound. Infants with normal study should undergo a repeat study at 4–6 weeks. Patients with isolated mild hydronephrosis (unilateral or bilateral) should be followed with sequential ultrasounds, at 3–12 monthly intervals until resolution; those with worsening hydronephrosis require close evaluation. Patients with higher grades of hydronephrosis or additional abnormalities are screened for underlying obstruction or vesicoureteric reflux (VUR). Radionuclide renography is useful in detecting pelviureteric junction or vesicoureteric junction obstruction and determining the need for surgery.

[1]Includes abnormal parenchymal appearance (increased echogenicity; loss of corticomedullary differentiation) or thickness; peripheral calyceal dilatation; ureteric dilatation; or abnormal bladder.

[2]Infants with anteroposterior diameter (APD) of the renal pelvis between 7–10 mm require follow-up ultrasonography.

[3]Micturating cystourethrography (MCU) is performed early (<48-hr of life) if lower urinary tract obstruction (LUTO) is suspected, based on an abnormal bladder or antenatal oligohydramnios (UTD A3).

[4]Prefer DTPA/MAG-3 scintigraphy earlier than MCU if APD >20 mm, kidney is palpable or thin cortex without ureteric dilatation.

[5]Patients with low grade vesicoureteric reflux (VUR, grade 1–3) may be observed without prophylaxis

## CYSTIC KIDNEY DISEASES

Occasionally, one or both kidneys may show a few or multiple cysts. Unlike in adults, kidney cysts in children are usually part of an inherited disease. Most cases are ciliopathies, conditions caused by structural or functional alterations in the primary cilia that interfere with normal cellular signaling, and manifest as cysts along various parts of the nephron, interstitial fibrosis, and variety of extrarenal manifestations. Acquired causes include obstructive cystic dysplasia, dyselectrolytemia, and cysts acquired during renal replacement therapy. Polycystic kidney disease and nephronophthisis are relatively common conditions.

### Polycystic Kidneys

Autosomal dominant and autosomal recessive forms of polycystic kidneys have distinctive features.

*Autosomal recessive polycystic kidney disease (ARPKD),* caused by mutations in *PKHD1,* encoding fibrocystin or polyductin, is characterized by dilation of collecting tubules which are arranged radially from the cortex to medulla. Affected children often present in the neonatal period with oliguria, respiratory insufficiency and palpable kidneys. ARPKD is sometimes diagnosed in young children presenting with hypertension, renal insufficiency and enlarged kidneys, or with portal hypertension due to associated congenital hepatic fibrosis. Ultrasonography shows enlarged 'bright' kidneys, usually without visible cysts (Fig. 17.30a). High-resolution ultrasound reveals small elliptical cysts, oriented perpendicular to the cortex, located in the medulla alone or both medulla and cortex. Liver ultrasonography shows periportal echogenicity, intrahepatic bile duct dilatation, Caroli disease or cysts. Contrast-enhanced computerized tomography, if performed, reveals a characteristic striate pattern of contrast excretion on delayed films.

*Autosomal dominant polycystic kidney disease (ADPKD)* is caused by mutations in *ADPKD1* (chromosome 16) or *ADPKD2* (chromosome 4), encoding polycystins 1 and 2, respectively. These membrane proteins regulate tubular and vascular development in various tissues. The condition usually presents beyond the third decade of life with episodic hematuria, hypertension, palpable kidneys and gradual decline in renal function, but may be detected in childhood. Ultrasonography shows multiple cysts in each kidney (Fig. 17.30b). Associated findings include cysts in the liver, spleen and pancreas, mitral valve prolapse and fusiform berry aneurysms of the cerebral arteries. Ultrasonography often reveals cysts in the kidneys in one affected parent unless they are younger than 30 years, in which case grandparents my be screened; rare cases are due to *de novo* mutations. Therapy with angiotensin-converting enzyme inhibitors helps control hypertension and limits hyperfiltration and proteinuria. The role of inhibitors of the mTOR pathway (sirolimus and everolimus) and V2 receptor antagonists (tolvaptan) is being explored.

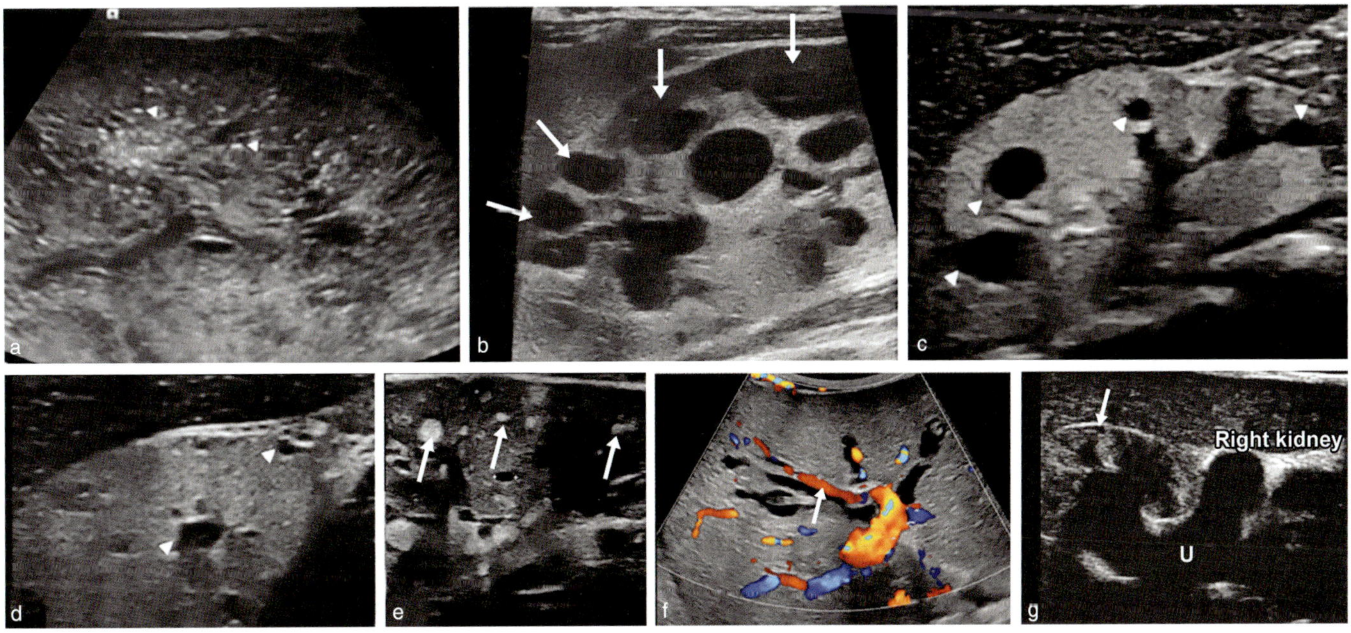


**Fig. 17.30:** Findings on high resolution ultrasonography in cystic kidney diseases: (a) Note bulky enlarged kidney with increased echogenicity, linear dilated collecting ducts in a radial distribution, and hyperechoic punctate foci (arrowheads) without posterior acoustic shadowing, in a child with autosomal recessive polycystic kidney disease; (b) Renal architecture is disorganized by multiple irregular rounded cysts (arrows) of varying size in autosomal dominant polycystic kidney disease; (c) Small kidney with increased cortical echogenicity, loss of corticomedullary differentiation, and cysts (arrowheads) chiefly in the cortex and corticomedullary junction, in a 1-yr-old girl with nephronophthisis; (d) Round cysts, located in the cortex and corticomedullary junction (arrowheads) in *HNF1*β-associated disease; (e) Multiple echogenic angiomyolipoms (arrows) and a tiny cyst (between cursors, below the central white arrow) in a 10-yr-old boy with tuberous sclerosis; (f) Hepatobiliary involvement in a 10-year-old child with ARPKD, seen as dilated intrahepatic biliary radicles and characteristic "central dot sign" (short arrow); (g) Dilated, tortuous right ureter (U), echogenic renal parenchyma, and small cysts (arrow) in a newborn with vesicoureteric reflux and cystic dysplasia

### Nephronophthisis

This group of recessively inherited cystic disorders constitutes the leading monogenic cause of kidney failure in the first three decades of life. Mutations in more than 50 genes are described, leading to alterations in cytosolic proteins, chiefly nephrocystins, that are localized to primary cilia. Conventionally, three clinical forms are recognized: Infantile, juvenile and adolescent onset, with a median age at kidney failure of 1, 12 and 15 years, respectively. Presentation is typically with polydipsia, polyuria or enuresis, growth retardation, acidosis and anemia. Extrarenal features may be present, including retinitis pigmentosa due to rod-cone dystrophy (Senor Loken, Bardet-Biedel and Joubert syndromes); ocular motor apraxia, hypotonia and cerebellar or midbrain abnormalities (Joubert syndrome); skeletal chondrodysplasia (Jeune asphyxiating thoracic dystrophy, Sensenbrenner syndrome); postaxial polydactyly (Bardet-Biedl and Meckel-Gruber syndromes), learning disabilities, obesity and hypogonadism or genital abnormalities (Bardet-Biedl syndrome); occipital meningoencephalocele (Meckel-Gruber syndrome); and phalangeal cone-shaped epiphyses. The diagnosis of nephronophthisis is supported by the ultrasound finding of small or normal-sized kidneys with cysts in corticomedullary junction or medulla, increased echogenicity, and loss of corticomedullary differentiation **(Fig. 17.30c)**. Renal histology shows cysts involving the collecting ducts lined by flattened or cuboidal epithelium, tubular dilatation with atrophy and interstitial fibrosis, and thickening of tubular basement membrane.

### Autosomal Dominant Tubulointerstitial Kidney Disease

ADTKD is an underrecognized entity, second only to ADPKD as a monogenic cause of CKD manifesting in adulthood. The diagnosis of ADTKD is suggested by ultrasound finding of normal to small-sized kidneys with multiple small cysts in the cortex, medulla or at the corticomedullary junction, associated with hyperuricemia and/or family history of hyperuricemia and cystic kidney disease with autosomal dominant inheritance. Genetic testing reveals pathogenic or likely pathogenic variations in *UMOD, MUC1, REN, HNF1β or SEC61A1*. Childhood onset ADPTKD is usually caused by mutations in *REN* or *HNF1B*.

***HNF1β-associated disease or HNF1β nephropathy:*** Mutations in the gene encoding hepatocyte nuclear factor β (*HNF1B*, also known as transcription factor 2) are associated with various kidney abnormalities, including uni- or bilateral cysts, hypo- or dysplasia and agenesis. *HNF1β* nephropathy is considered the single most common cause of hyperechogenic kidney(s) on antenatal ultrasonography and of kidney cysts in older children **(Fig. 17.30d)**. There may be coexisting genital malformations, e.g., vaginal and uterine anomalies, and/or atrophy and partial agenesis of pancreas. Mutations in *HNF1B* can occur in isolation or as part of 17q12 deletion syndrome. The diagnosis is suggested by family history of maturity-onset diabetes of the young (renal cysts and diabetes syndrome), gestational diabetes, hyperuricemia, or concurrent hypomagnesemia.

### Cysts in Systemic Disease

Kidney cysts may occur in various inherited diseases, including tuberous sclerosis **(Fig. 17.30e)**, von Hippel-Lindau disease, orofacial digital syndrome, and Beckwith-Wiedemann syndrome, and in certain metabolic diseases (bile acid synthesis defects, Zellweger syndrome, fatty acids oxidation disorders, multiple deficiency acyl-CoA dehydrogenase, carnitine palmitoyltransferase II deficiency). Cysts may be acquired during persistent hypokalemia, or with renal replacement therapy, vascular or lymphatic pathology or following infections.

### Glomerulocystic Kidney Disease

The predominant finding in glomerulocystic kidney disease (GCKD) is cysts involving glomeruli, diagnosed most definitely on renal biopsy. Ultrasonography shows small subcortical cysts with increased kidney echogenicity and loss of corticomedullary differentiation.

### Evaluation

The majority of kidney cysts in childhood are due to hereditary diseases rather than simple cysts or acquired cystic diseases, unlike in adults. The most common extrarenal finding is hepatic fibrosis, in presence of which the term hepatorenal fibrocystic kidney disease is used **(Fig. 17.30f)**. Acquired causes, including cystic dysplasia associated with VUR **(Fig. 17.30g)** or obstruction, dyselectrolytemia, and acquired cysts during KRT, can usually be ruled out based on history and ultrasonography.

The final diagnosis requires a multispecialty approach, including radiology, pathology, and genetics. High resolution ultrasonography is the modality of choice for diagnosis and follow-up of pediatric cystic kidney diseases, including for hepatobiliary tract abnormalities. An MRI may be occasionally indicated in patients with complex cysts, tuberous sclerosis or ADPKD.

### Suggested Reading

1. Gimpel C, Avni EF, Breysem L, et al. Imaging of kidney cysts and cystic kidney diseases in children: An international working group consensus statement. Radiology 2019;290:769–82.
2. Ma M. Cilia and polycystic kidney disease. Semin Cell Dev Biol 2021;110:139–48.
3. Raina R, Chakraborty R, Sethi SK, et al. Diagnosis and management of renal cystic disease of the newborn: Core curriculum 2021. Am J Kidney Dis 2021; 78:125–41.
4. Thomas CC, Jana M, Sinha A, et al. Ultrasound imaging of renal cysts in children. J Ultrasound Med 2021;40:621–35.

Chapter

18

# Endocrine and Metabolic Disorders

PSN Menon, Anurag Bajpai, Vandana Jain, Rajni Sharma

## GENERAL PRINCIPLES

Endocrine glands play a crucial role in the maintenance of body physiology and homeostasis. The hypothalamic–pituitary axis (HPA) regulates most endocrine organs, and growth, puberty, and mineral and water homeostasis.

### Structure and Mechanism of Action

Hormones are derived from amino acids (e.g. peptide hormones, glycoproteins, thyroxine and epinephrine) or cholesterol (e.g. steroid hormones, vitamin D, adrenal and gonadal steroids). The peptide hormones (e.g. parathyroid hormone, growth hormone and insulin) do not bind to circulating binding proteins resulting in their rapid elimination with a short half-life. The steroid hormones, on the other hand, bind to circulating proteins, and have a longer half-life.

The peptide hormones act via receptors on the cell membrane. Binding of hormone to its receptor results in the release of second messengers that induce structural changes in intracellular proteins, culminating in the hormone effect. Steroids and thyroxine act on intracellular receptors. The hormone–receptor complex binds to the hormone response elements in the target gene, resulting in regulation of transcription.

### Regulation and Metabolism

Hormone secretion is regulated by a feedback system that includes regulatory hormones, hormone levels, and their effects. The feedback operates at the level of the endocrine gland as well as the HPA. Plasma enzymes rapidly inactivate the peptide hormones, shortening their duration of action.

Activation of hormones (e.g. androgen to estrogen, testosterone to dihydrotestosterone and calcidiol to calcitriol) is vital for the action of some hormones. Inactivation of hormones at the site of their action prevents their excess effects (e.g. inactivation of cortisol by 11β-hydroxysteroid dehydrogenase prevents its action on mineralocorticoid receptor). Peripheral conversion also plays an important role in hormone function (e.g. conversion of thyroxine to triiodothyronine).

### Assessment of Hormone Action

Endocrine assessment relies on the estimation of basal hormone levels (e.g. for thyroid disorders), and in some cases on their metabolites (e.g. urinary metabolites in adrenal disorders), or their effects (e.g. insulin-like growth factor-1 (IGF-1) levels in growth hormone (GH) deficiency and urinary osmolality for diabetes insipidus). Stimulation tests are often needed in deficiency states (e.g. GH deficiency and adrenal insufficiency) and suppression tests in excess states (e.g. GH excess and Cushing syndrome).

The feedback mechanism also guides the assessment of endocrine disorders. For example, thyroid-stimulating hormone is elevated in primary hypothyroidism. Conversely, low or low-normal pituitary hormone levels with hormone deficiency suggest hypothalamic or pituitary dysfunction.

## DISORDERS OF THE PITUITARY GLAND

### Physiology

The principal hormones produced by the anterior pituitary are growth hormone (GH), thyroid-stimulating hormone (TSH), adrenocorticotropic hormone (ACTH), follicle-stimulating hormone (FSH), luteinizing hormone (LH) and prolactin (PRL). These hormones regulate the actions of their target organs. Their secretion in turn is regulated by hypothalamic peptides—growth hormone-releasing hormone (GHRH), growth hormone-inhibiting hormone (GHIH or somatostatin), dopamine, gonadotropin-releasing hormone (GnRH), corticotropin-releasing hormone (CRH) and thyrotropin-releasing hormone (TRH), and also by hormones produced by the target glands. Posterior pituitary hormones (arginine, vasopressin and oxytocin) are secreted by neurons in the hypothalamic nuclei.

## Growth Hormone Deficiency

Growth hormone deficiency (GHD) is caused by congenital malformations of central nervous system (CNS), genetic defects or acquired neurological insults (Table 18.1).

Children with congenital GHD usually have normal anthropometry at birth. Growth retardation becomes apparent by the age of one year. These children have an immature round facies with prominent forehead and midfacial hypoplasia (deep set eyes and depressed nasal bridge) (Fig. 18.1).

Micropenis and/or undescended testis and mild obesity are common clinical features. Body proportions are normal. The eruption of teeth is delayed. Bone age is delayed. Newborns and infants may occasionally present with hypoglycemic seizures due to severe GHD alone, and concomitant ACTH deficiency.

Resistance to GH action (GH insensitivity or Laron syndrome) presents with a similar phenotype with severe growth retardation and elevated baseline GH levels.

## Approach to Diagnosis of Short Stature and GHD

Growth failure may be a part of any long-standing systemic illness. Chronic systemic disorders and nutritional deficiencies have predominant effect on weight, and height is less affected initially, therefore, body mass index (BMI) is usually low. On the contrary, endocrine causes (GHD and hypothyroidism) mainly affect height with a relatively normal BMI (*see* Chapter 2).

### Evaluation

***History:*** Perinatal events, birth weight and length give clues about the etiology. Birth asphyxia, breech presentation, neonatal hypoglycemia, micropenis and prolonged jaundice suggest the possibility of GHD. Features of

**Table 18.1:** Etiology of growth hormone deficiency

| |
|---|
| **Congenital** |
| *Genetic defects* |
| Isolated GH deficiency |
| • Defect in *GH1* gene |
| – Type I: Autosomal recessive |
| – Type II: Autosomal dominant |
| – Type III: X-linked recessive |
| • Defect in *GHRHR* (GH-releasing hormone receptor) gene: Type IV |
| Multiple pituitary hormone deficiency |
| – Type I: Autosomal recessive |
| – Type II: X-linked recessive |
| *Developmental defects:* Pituitary aplasia or hypoplasia, holoprosencephaly, septo-optic dysplasia, anencephaly |
| **Acquired** |
| *Tumors:* Hypothalamic, pituitary or other intracranial tumors |
| *Irradiation* |
| *Infections:* Encephalitis, meningitis, tuberculosis, toxoplasmosis |
| *Infiltration:* Histiocytosis, hemochromatosis, sarcoidosis |
| *Injury:* Perinatal insult (breech), head injury, surgery |
| *Vascular:* Aneurysm, infarction |

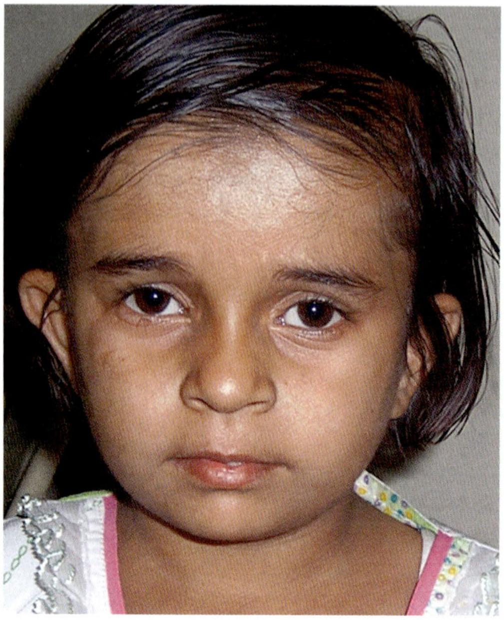

**Fig. 18.1:** A 6-year-old girl with short stature due to congenital growth hormone deficiency. Note the immature facies, midfacial hypoplasia and cherubic appearance

chronic infections, chronic systemic disorders especially cardiopulmonary disorders, malabsorption and raised intracranial tension should be looked for in all short children. Presence of polyuria and polydipsia suggests diabetes insipidus, diabetes mellitus and/or renal tubular acidosis. Constipation, delayed milestones, lethargy and cold intolerance indicate hypothyroidism. Family history of short stature and/or delayed puberty suggests the possibility of familial short stature (FSS) or constitutional delay of growth and puberty (CDGP).

***Examination:*** Anthropometry (weight, height, weight for height, BMI and head circumference) provides crucial inputs for the diagnosis. Body proportions help in identifying skeletal dysplasia—increased upper to lower segment (US:LS) ratio is observed in achondroplasia (Fig. 18.2) and rickets, while reduced US:LS ratio is seen in Morquio syndrome and spondyloepiphyseal dysplasia.

The clinician should also look for deformities and dysmorphism, and for specific phenotypes of an underlying etiology such as GHD, hypothyroidism (dull look, sallow complexion, dry skin, sparse hair, eyebrows and eyelashes, periorbital puffiness, and goiter in some cases), Turner syndrome (some girls may have webbed neck, cubitus valgus, low posterior hairline, etc.), and rickets. Pubertal staging (sexual maturity rating) is an essential part of evaluation.

***Investigations:*** Laboratory evaluation of short stature is guided by the history and examination, and best done by a stepwise application of diagnostic tests to determine the etiology (Fig. 18.3). Also *see* Chapter 2 (Table 2.10).

*Step 1:* Rule out common treatable causes such as malnutrition, chronic systemic illnesses and recurrent infections, and estimate the bone age of the child.

*Step 2:* Rule out hypothyroidism, celiac disease and Turner syndrome.

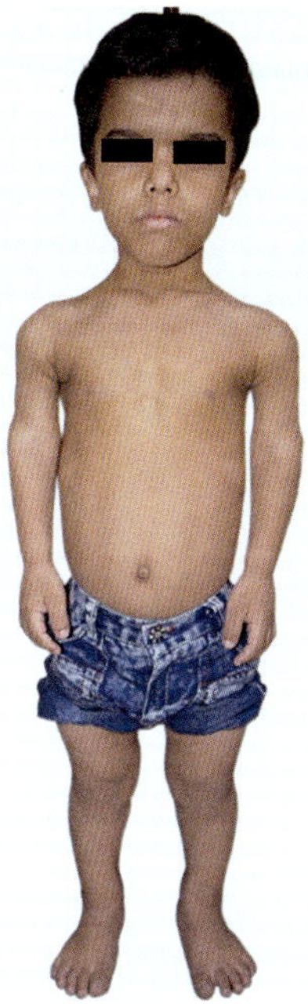

Fig. 18.2: Achondroplasia. Note the short stature with disproportionately short lower segment, short proximal limbs (rhizomelia) and characteristic facies (*Courtesy:* Dr. Neerja Gupta, AIIMS, Delhi)

*Step 3:* Evaluate for GH-IGF axis, after excluding common causes of short stature listed in steps 1 and 2. Measuring random or fasting blood GH level is not helpful as GH secretion is pulsatile. The diagnosis of GHD requires stimulation tests. GHD is suspected when the peak level of GH is less than 7 ng/mL following stimulation. The common provocative agents used are insulin, glucagon, clonidine or GHRH. IGF-1 and IGF binding protein-3 (IGFBP-3) are screening tests for the evaluation of GH-IGF axis, but are affected by malnutrition and systemic disorders. Low IGF-1 in the presence of high GH level suggests GH insensitivity (Laron syndrome).

GHD may be associated with other pituitary hormone deficiencies and investigations should be carried out to detect deficiency of these hormones, if GHD is present. Magnetic resonance imaging (MRI) of hypothalamic and pituitary region is essential to rule out developmental or acquired neurological lesions.

### Management

***General measures:*** Management of short stature involves correction of the underlying cause and provision of adequate nutrition. Nutritional deficiencies should be corrected, if present.

***Specific therapy:*** Specific treatment is effective in restoring growth in hypothyroidism (thyroxine), celiac disease (gluten-free diet) and renal tubular acidosis (bicarbonate supplements). A short course of testosterone helps boys with CDGP.

***Growth hormone:*** GH therapy results in increase in final height by 20–30 cm from pretreatment levels. The treatment is given as daily night-time injections (25–50 µg/kg/day) till epiphyses close. GH therapy is monitored by assessment of growth velocity and bone age. Lab parameters are not

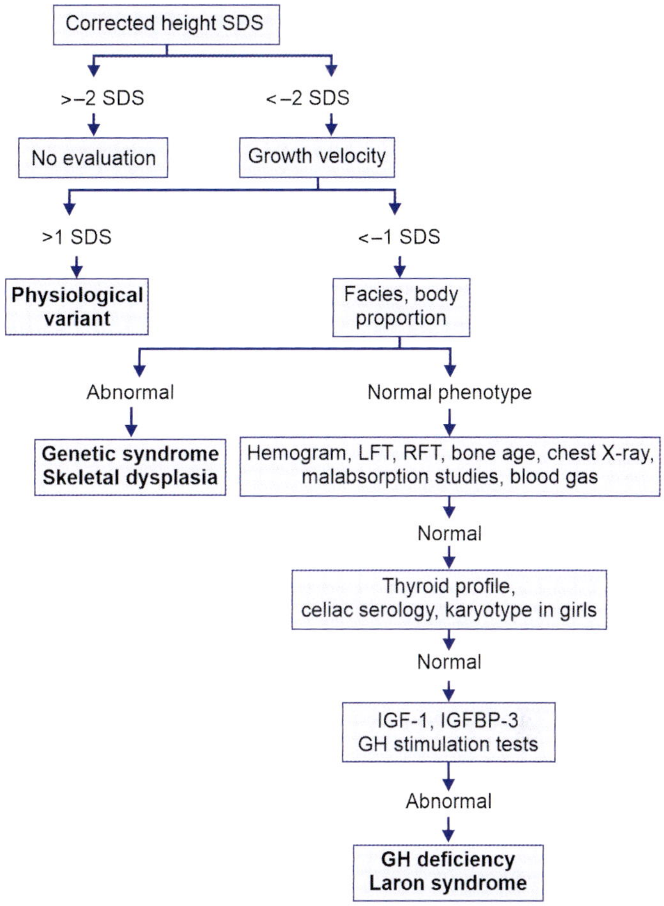


Fig. 18.3: Approach to a child with short stature. GH growth hormone; IGF-1 insulin-like growth factor-1; IGFBP-3 IGF binding protein-3; LFT liver function tests; RFT renal function tests; SDS standard deviation score

routinely used to monitor GH therapy. IGF-1 levels may be checked, if the response is suboptimal or the child is on a high dose. The treatment is expensive and all efforts should be made to ensure that treatment is given regularly. The role of GH is expanding with the increasing use in other disorders with short stature such as Turner syndrome, chronic renal failure, small for gestational age infants who fail to catch-up by 2 to 3 years of age, Russell-Silver syndrome, Prader-Willi syndrome and idiopathic short stature (Table 18.2).

## Growth Hormone Excess

Excess of GH during childhood may result in somatic overgrowth or gigantism. Increased GH secretion after

| Table 18.2: Indications for growth hormone therapy |
|---|
| Growth hormone deficiency in children and adults |
| Turner syndrome |
| Chronic renal insufficiency |
| Prader-Willi syndrome |
| Small for gestational age who fail to catch-up in growth by 2–3 years of age |
| *SHOX* gene mutations and Leri-Weill dyschondrosteosis |
| Noonan syndrome |
| Idiopathic short stature |

the fusion of skeletal epiphyses causes acromegaly (coarse features with prominent jaw, broad nose, large tongue, bushy eyebrows, thick skin and dorsal kyphosis). Headache and visual field defects (bitemporal hemianopia and enlargement of the blind spot) are common.

*Diagnosis:* IGF-1 is the best screening test for GH excess. Non-suppressible GH levels after a glucose challenge confirm the diagnosis. MRI of brain helps to confirm and determine the extent of the tumor.

*Management:* Resection of pituitary adenoma is the treatment of choice. Medical management involves the use of long-acting somatostatin analogs such as octreotide. The GH receptor antagonist, pegvisomant is also useful in treatment.





## Diabetes Insipidus

Polyuria (urine output above 5 mL/kg/hr or 2 L/m$^2$/day) may result from increased solute load or impaired renal concentrating capacity (Table 18.3). Diabetes insipidus (DI) is an important cause of polyuria. DI presents with low urine osmolality (<600 mOsm/kg) in association with high plasma osmolality (>300 mOsm/kg or serum sodium >146 mEq/L). DI may be due to decreased production of AVP (central DI) or its action (nephrogenic DI). Dehydration is unusual unless there is an abnormality of thirst mechanism. Infants are at a high risk of developing hypernatremic dehydration.

*Central DI:* This is commonly associated with an intracranial pathology (Table 18.3). Craniopharyngioma may present with DI, growth retardation and skull calcification. Germinoma located in the pituitary stalk may be missed on routine brain scans, and need repeat neuroimaging.

*Nephrogenic DI:* This results from inherited or acquired resistance to AVP. Congenital nephrogenic DI due to mutations in vasopressin receptor (V2) presents in infancy with failure to thrive, recurrent fever and dehydration. Hypokalemia and hypercalcemia are important causes of acquired nephrogenic DI.

**Table 18.3:** Causes of polyuria

**Increased fluid load**

Iatrogenic

Compulsive water drinking

**Increased solute load**

*Osmotic diuresis:* Diabetes mellitus, mannitol treatment

*Salt loss:* Adrenal insufficiency, diuretics, cerebral salt wasting, aldosterone resistance

**Impaired urinary concentration**

*Deficiency or inefficient action of AVP (diabetes insipidus, DI)*

- Central DI (neurogenic DI)
  - Genetic defects
  - Malformations: Septo-optic dysplasia, holoprosencephaly, anencephaly
  - CNS insults: Head trauma, neurosurgery, infection, brain death
  - Infiltrative disorders: Sarcoidosis, histiocytosis
  - Space occupying lesions: Craniopharyngioma, germinoma
- Nephrogenic DI
  - Genetic: X-linked (V2 receptor), AR and AD (aquaporin defect)
  - Acquired: Hypokalemia, hypercalcemia, obstructive uropathy, nephrocalcinosis

**Tubulopathy**

- Renal tubular acidosis
- Bartter syndrome
- Gitelman syndrome

AD autosomal dominant; AVP arginine vasopressin; AR autosomal recessive; CNS central nervous system; DI diabetes insipidus

### Evaluation

Urine output in excess of 2 L/m$^2$/day or 5 mL/kg/hr confirms polyuria (Fig. 18.4).

*Clinical:* Table 18.4 lists some pointers to the diagnosis of polyuria.

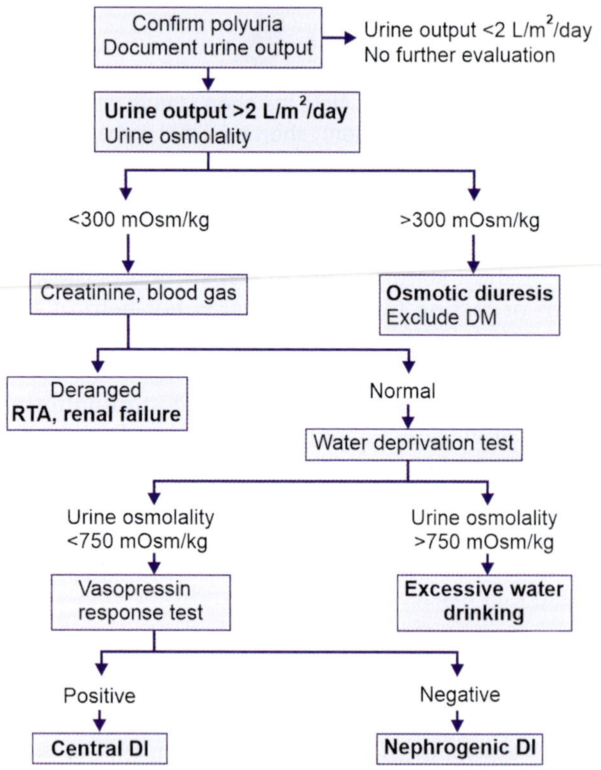


**Fig. 18.4:** Approach to a child with polyuria. DI diabetes insipidus; DM diabetes mellitus; RTA renal tubular acidosis

**Table 18.4:** Pointers to diagnosis of polyuria

| *Feature* | *Diagnosis* |
|---|---|
| Cleft lip, cleft palate | Hypopituitarism |
| Metabolic bone | Renal tubular acidosis (RTA), renal disease failure |
| Growth failure | Nephrogenic diabetes insipidus, RTA, congenital adrenal hyperplasia, Bartter syndrome |
| Rash, ear discharge | Histiocytosis |
| Pigmentation | Adrenal insufficiency |
| Genital ambiguity | Congenital adrenal hyperplasia |

***Investigations:*** Initial investigations include testing urine glucose and early morning urine specific gravity and osmolality. Blood gases, urea, electrolytes, glucose, calcium and creatinine should be estimated. High plasma osmolality (>300 mOsm/kg or sodium >146 mEq/L) with low urine osmolality (<300 mOsm/kg and urine specific gravity <1.005) suggest the diagnosis of DI, which needs further classification on the basis of response to AVP. Patients with normal plasma osmolality and low urine osmolality (<300 mOsm/kg) should undergo water deprivation test. Urinary osmolality >300 mOsm/kg (specific gravity >1.010) excludes the possibility of complete DI.

MRI of the hypothalamic–pituitary region and anterior pituitary hormone evaluation should be done in central DI. Evaluation of nephrogenic DI includes renal imaging and estimation of serum electrolytes.

***Water deprivation test:*** This test is indicated in children with polyuria with low urinary osmolality and normal plasma osmolality. The aim is to increase plasma osmolality above 300 mOsm/kg (or serum sodium above 146 mEq/L) to allow the opportunity for maximal renal concentration. Water deprivation test is not required in the presence of hypernatremia.

Water deprivation should be done on an inpatient basis as there is a risk for dehydration. It is started early in the morning. The child is weighed and target weight loss calculated (5% of total body weight). Body weight, urine output and urine and blood osmolality are monitored hourly. The test is stopped when urine osmolality increases above 750 mOsm/kg or specific gravity is more than 1.010, excluding DI. The test is also discontinued when serum sodium goes above 146 mEq/L (target achieved) or weight loss is more than 5% (risk of dehydration). Urine osmolality below 300 mOsm/kg in the presence of plasma osmolality above 300 mOsm/kg confirms DI and needs evaluation by a formal vasopressin test.

***Vasopressin response test:*** This test helps to differentiate central DI from nephrogenic DI. Urine osmolality is measured one hour after a vasopressin injection (0.1 unit/kg). An increase in urine osmolality by more than 50% of baseline level is diagnostic of central DI while a smaller increase suggests nephrogenic DI.

### Management

***Central DI:*** Central DI is managed with a vasopressin analog. Desmopressin (DDAVP), a vasopressin analog, has high potency and prolonged duration of action. It can be given by intranasal (2.5–10 μg 12 hourly), sublingual or oral (50–200 μg 12 hourly) route, to be titrated according to urine output. Patients with idiopathic DI should be monitored for an evolving brain tumor. Desmopressin is avoided in infants, as it may lead to hyponatremia.

***Nephrogenic DI:*** The combination of hydrochlorothiazide and amiloride reduces urine output by 40%. Addition of indomethacin to this regimen reduces urine output by 50–70%. This should be combined with salt restriction and reduction in solute load.

### Suggested Reading


1. Desai MP, Parikh R. Growth hormone deficiency and insensitivity. In: Desai MP, Menon PSN, Bhatia V, Seth A, (eds). Pediatric Endocrine Disorders, 4th edition. Hyderabad; Universities Press India Ltd. 2022; 94–109.
2. Godbole T, Menon PSN. Polyuria, diabetes insipidus and syndrome of inappropriate secretion of ADH. In: Gupta P, Menon PSN, Ramji S, Lodha R (eds). PG Textbook of Pediatrics, 3rd edn. New Delhi: Jaypee Brothers Medical Publishers (P) Ltd; 2021, pp 2678–82.
3. Grimberg A, DiVall SA, Polychronakos C, et al. Drug and Therapeutics Committee and Ethics Committee of the Pediatric Endocrine Society. Guidelines for growth hormone and insulin-like growth factor-I treatment in children and adolescents: growth hormone deficiency, idiopathic short stature, and primary insulin-like growth factor-I deficiency. Horm Res Paediatr 2016;86:361–97.
4. Patel R, Bajpai A. Evaluation of short stature in children and adolescents. Indian J Pediatr 2021;88(12):1196–1202.


## DISORDERS OF THE THYROID GLAND

### Physiology

Biosynthesis of thyroid hormones involves interactions of iodine, tyrosine, thyroglobulin and the enzyme, thyroid peroxidase. These processes are regulated by TSH, which is under the direct control of TRH and feedback control of thyroxine. Thyroid hormones bind to intracellular receptors and activate transcription factors. Most triiodothyronine ($T_3$) in the circulation is produced by peripheral conversion of thyroxine ($T_4$) by the enzyme monodeiodinase.

Thyroid hormones play an active role in the regulation of somatic and intellectual growth, intermediary metabolism and thermoregulation. There is a critical phase in the early neonatal period for the effect of thyroid hormone on intellectual development. This underscores the need for early diagnosis and management of congenital hypothyroidism. TSH levels increase immediately after birth, resulting in increase in $T_3$ and $T_4$ levels, and reach their peak by 24 hours. Their levels fall to normal in the next few weeks. TSH levels should thus be estimated after 48 hours of birth during neonatal screening for congenital hypothyroidism.

### Assessment of Thyroid Function

Thyroid function is assessed by serum TSH and $T_4$ and T3 levels. TSH is the most sensitive indicator of primary (thyroidal) hypothyroidism. Serum $T_4$ level is a better indicator of thyroid status than serum $T_3$ due to increased conversion of $T_4$ to $T_3$ during thyroid-depleted states. Considering the variability in the levels of circulating thyroxine-binding globulin (TBG), estimation of free thyroid hormones is superior to total hormone levels in the diagnosis of hypothyroidism. Low free $T_4$ ($FT_4$) and low or normal TSH suggest central hypothyroidism, while low $FT_4$ levels and high TSH indicate primary hypothyroidism. Persistent elevation of TSH in the presence of normal $FT_4$ suggests subclinical hypothyroidism. Elevated free $T_3$ ($FT_3$) and/or $FT_4$ and undetectable TSH levels imply a hyperthyroid state.

Competencies: **PE33.1; PE33.2; PE33.3**

## Hypothyroidism

Hypothyroidism results from defects in the hypothalamic–pituitary axis (central hypothyroidism), or thyroid gland (primary hypothyroidism) (Table 18.5). It may be congenital or acquired.

### *Congenital Hypothyroidism*

Congenital hypothyroidism (CH) is the most common preventable cause of intellectual disability, with an approximate prevalence of 1 in 2,000 newborns. The reported incidence in India is much higher.

*Etiology:* Thyroid dysgenesis is the most common cause of CH in India (75% of all cases) as well as most parts of the world. The disorder encompasses a spectrum ranging from agenesis to ectopic thyroid. Biosynthetic defects include disorders affecting iodine transport, peroxidation, thyroglobulin synthesis and deiodination. Pendred syndrome, a disorder of the pendrin gene, is associated with decreased intracellular transport of iodine and deafness. Nongoitrous CH is known to be associated with *TSHR*, *PAX8* and *TSHB* gene defects.

*Clinical features:* Features of CH are nonspecific and often difficult to identify in the neonatal period. They become prominent as the child grows older. Unfortunately, the window period for intervention would have elapsed in most children by that time. This underscores the need for universal neonatal screening for CH. Clinical manifestations in infancy include hoarse cry, facial puffiness, umbilical hernia, hypotonia, mottling of skin and lethargy (Fig. 18.5). Prolonged jaundice, constipation and unexplained hypothermia may also be present. Open posterior fontanel is an important indicator of CH (Table 18.6).

*Evaluation:* History of a maternal thyroid disease or ingestion of antithyroid medications to mother should be probed. Family history of hypothyroidism suggests dyshormonogenesis. Residence in iodine deficient area may suggest the diagnosis of iodine deficiency. Goiter is common in disorders of thyroid hormone biosynthesis. Hypoglycemia, micropenis and midline facial defects suggest a hypothalamic–pituitary etiology.

*Investigations:* Initial investigations in a neonate include serum TSH and $FT_4$ levels. Those with high TSH and low $FT_4$ levels need evaluation by radionuclide scan and ultrasound of thyroid to confirm agenesis, ectopia or dysgenesis of thyroid. Children with undetectable thyroid on radionuclear scan but normal thyroid on ultrasound may have defects in iodine transport, TSH receptor abnormalities or transplacental passage of TSH blocking antibody. Children with low TSH and $FT_4$ levels should be worked up for pituitary-hypothalamic defects.

**Table 18.5:** Etiology of hypothyroidism

| |
|---|
| **Primary** (thyroid, >95%)<br>*Autoimmune thyroiditis*<br>*Enzyme defects:* Trapping, organification, thyroglobulin synthesis, deiodination<br>*Iodine deficiency:* Endemic goiter<br>*Dysgenesis:* Aplasia, dysplasia, ectopia<br>*Thyroid injury:* Surgery, radiation, infection<br>*Goitrogens:* Thiocyanates, thionamides, lithium, amiodarone<br>*Transient causes:* Maternal TSH receptor blocking antibody, iodine excess, maternal antithyroid drug |
| **Secondary or tertiary** (hypothalamus or pituitary, <5%)<br>*Malformations:* Septo-optic dysplasia, holoprosencephaly<br>*Genetic defects*<br>*CNS insults:* Trauma, surgery, radiation, infection<br>*CNS tumors:* Craniopharyngioma, germinoma |
| **Peripheral** (extremely rare)<br>Resistance to thyroxine |

CNS central nervous system; TSH thyroid-stimulating hormone

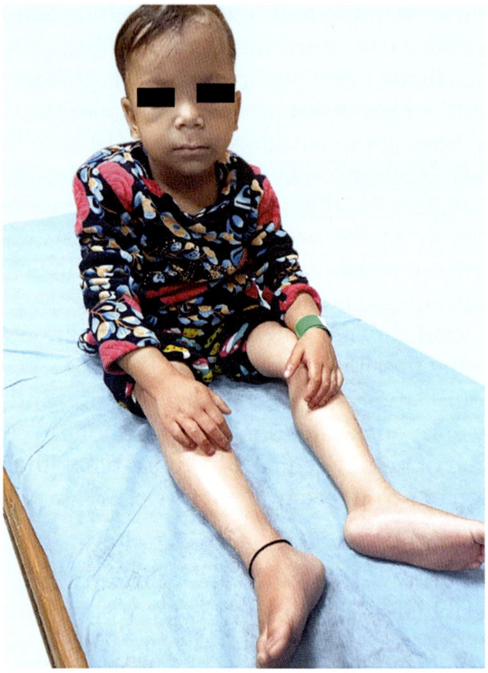

**Fig. 18.5:** A 7-year-old girl with untreated congenital hypothyroidism. Note the dull look, sallow complexion, puffiness around the eyes, sparse eyebrows, and 'edematous' lower limbs

**Table 18.6:** Clinical features of hypothyroidism

| *Congenital* | *Acquired* |
|---|---|
| Open posterior fontanel | Myopathy and pseudohypertrophy of limb muscles |
| Umbilical hernia | Enlarged sella |
| Delayed neurodevelopment | Pseudotumor cerebri |
| Large tongue | |
| **Common to both congenital and acquired forms** | |
| Growth retardation | |
| Sallow edematous facies | Pallor |
| Delayed skeletal maturation | Hypothermia |
| Delayed dental development | Rough dry skin |
| Delayed puberty | Hypotonia |
| Constipation | Protuberant abdomen |

18

Essential Pediatrics

*Management:* Thyroxine replacement is started immediately after diagnosis of CH. In central hypothyroidism, cortisol replacement should precede thyroid replacement as it may precipitate adrenal insufficiency. Thyroxine is initiated at a dose of 10–15 µg/kg/day. $FT_4$ and TSH levels are expected to normalize over one week and one month, respectively. $FT_4$ and TSH levels should be measured at each visit preferably every 2 months in the first year. Thyroxine dose should be adjusted to achieve $FT_4$ levels in the upper normal range for the age. Lifelong thyroxine replacement is required in most cases. In newborns with suspected transient CH, thyroxine replacement should be stopped for one month at the age of 3 years and retested. Treatment is not required, if follow-up thyroid functions are normal.

*Outcome:* Early diagnosis and treatment following neonatal screening has resulted in normal intellectual outcome. Outcome is, however, poor in children with CH who have been diagnosed beyond early infancy. Neurocognitive disability and short stature are common sequels.

*Screening:* Difficulty in early identification of CH and the disastrous consequences of delayed diagnosis have led to the practice of universal neonatal screening for CH. Screening programs use dried blood spot (DBS) sample collected at the postnatal age of 2 to 4 days. Cord blood is used, if postnatal DBS sample is not feasible. The most commonly used strategy screens first for TSH. TSH levels above 40 mU/L in the first week, 20 mU/L between 7 and 21 days and above 10 mU/L beyond 21 days suggest the need for treatment. Treatment should be started after sending a confirmatory venous sample for measurement of $FT_4$ and TSH. TSH-based screening has higher sensitivity compared to $T_4$-based approach. However, TSH-based approach may not identify central hypothyroidism. $T_4$-first approach can identify these children, but has the disadvantage of missing cases with compensated hypothyroidism

### Acquired Hypothyroidism

*Etiology:* Autoimmune thyroiditis (AIT), also called Hashimoto thyroiditis, is the most common cause of acquired hypothyroidism. Anti-thyroperoxidase (anti-TPO) antibodies are usually present. AIT may be associated with other autoimmune endocrinopathies (adrenal insufficiency, type 1 diabetes mellitus and hypoparathyroidism). Rarely, thyroid dysgenesis (ectopia) or an inborn error of thyroid hormone synthesis may become evident in older children and adolescents. Iodine deficiency and goitrogens are other causes of primary hypothyroidism in older children.

*Clinical features:* Features of acquired hypothyroidism are subtle compared to CH (Table 18.6). Often short stature may be the only manifestation. Cold intolerance, lethargy, constipation, delayed dentition and poor school performance may be present. Delayed puberty is common; uncontrolled long-standing hypothyroidism may present with peripheral sexual precocity due to functioning ovarian cysts in girls. Children with Down syndrome, Turner syndrome, celiac disease and type 1 diabetes should be periodically screened for hypothyroidism even in the absence of symptoms.

*Evaluation:* Severe short stature and intellectual disability suggest missed CH. A firm and non-nodular goiter implies iodine deficiency or a disorder of thyroid hormone synthesis; firm nodular goiter indicates AIT. Children with central hypothyroidism should be evaluated for other pituitary hormone deficiencies and MRI of the hypothalamic–pituitary region. Anti-TPO antibodies should be estimated in acquired primary hypothyroidism.

*Management:* Thyroxine in a dose of 100 µg/m²/day is recommended. In long-standing cases, treatment is started at 25–50% of the dose with a gradual build up every 3–4 weeks. Thyroxine is given on empty stomach in the morning, at least 30 minutes before breakfast, and at least 6 hours before iron or calcium supplements. Follow-up is done every 3 months during the first 2 years of therapy and six-monthly thereafter. The doses should be modified to maintain $FT_4$ and TSH levels in the normal range. Most children require lifelong therapy.

### Subclinical Hypothyroidism

Mild elevations of TSH (below 10 mU/L) with normal $FT_4$ levels are frequently observed in children especially with obesity. In most cases, these findings reverse over a period of 3 to 6 months. Treatment should be considered in children with thyromegaly, presence of anti-TPO antibodies, or family history of hypothyroidism.

## Goiter

Goiter refers to the enlargement of the thyroid gland.

*Etiology:* Goiter may be associated with diminished, normal or increased thyroid function. Thyroid enlargement may be diffuse or nodular, and may represent increase in size in response to compensatory TSH secretion (hypothyroidism), infiltration (AIT, neoplasms or hemochromatosis), or presence of TSH receptor stimulating antibodies (Graves disease) (Table 18.7). Important causes of congenital goiter include maternal antithyroid medications, dyshormonogenesis and iodine deficiency. AIT is the most common cause in older children, followed by iodine deficiency.

*Evaluation:* Goiter may be diffuse or nodular. Investigations should include thyroid function tests. Anti-TPO antibodies should be measured to identify AIT. Presence of anti-TPO antibodies indicate acquired hypothyroidism. Ultrasound and fine needle aspiration cytology may help in diagnosis.

*Management:* Treatment should be directed to the cause (antithyroid medications in Graves' disease; thyroxine in hypothyroidism). Suppressive thyroxine therapy for euthyroid goiter is of limited benefit and is best avoided. Surgery is indicated, only if goiter is large enough to cause respiratory embarrassment.

## Solitary Thyroid Nodule

Identification of solitary thyroid nodule in children should alert to the possibility of thyroid malignancy. A well-circumscribed, cystic nodule is usually benign. Pointers towards malignancy include a firm nodule with limited

**Table 18.7:** Causes of thyromegaly in children

**Diffuse**

- Thyroiditis
  - Autoimmune thyroiditis: Hashimoto thyroiditis, Graves disease
  - De Quervain's subacute thyroiditis, Reidel thyroiditis
- Environmental goitrogens: Iodine deficiency (endemic goiter), dietary goitrogens
- Dyshormonogenesis
  - Pendred syndrome
  - Mutations in genes encoding thyroid peroxidase, thyroglobulin
- Resistance to thyroid hormones
- Idiopathic

**Nodular**

- Multinodular goiter (due to long-standing simple goiter or autoimmune thyroiditis or dyshormonogenesis)
- Solitary nodule
  - Hyperfunctioning (toxic) nodule
  - Hypofunctioning (cold) nodule
    - ◊ Follicular adenoma
    - ◊ Cyst, abscess
    - ◊ Thyroid cancer



mobility and associated lymph node enlargement. Children with solitary thyroid nodule should undergo ultrasound-guided fine needle aspiration cytology to exclude an underlying malignancy.

*Competencies:* **PE13.8; PE13.9**

## Iodine Deficiency Disorders

The term 'iodine deficiency disorders (IDD)' refers to the wide-spectrum of effects of iodine deficiency on growth and development. These include endemic goiter, endemic cretinism and impaired mental function in children and adults with goiter and increased rates of stillbirths and perinatal and infant mortality. Correcting iodine deficiency can prevent these conditions. Endemic goiter is present when the prevalence of goiter in a defined population exceeds 5%. Endemic goiter is graded by the method suggested by World Health Organization (WHO) (Table 18.8). Screening of estimates of iodine intake are usually derived from 24-hour urinary iodine excretion values or urinary iodine concentration expressed in relation to creatinine concentration as given in Table 18.9.

**Table 18.8:** Estimation of thyroid size by palpation

| | |
|---|---|
| Stage 0 | No goiter |
| Stage 1A | Goiter detectable only by palpation and not visible even when the neck is fully extended |
| Stage 1B | Goiter palpable but visible only when the neck is fully extended (this stage also includes nodular glands, even if not goitrous) |
| Stage 2 | Goiter visible when the neck is in normal position; palpation not needed for diagnosis |
| Stage 3 | Very large goiter, which can be recognized at a considerable distance |

**Table 18.9:** Severity of iodine deficiency in a defined area

| *Iodine deficiency* | *None* | *Mild* | *Moderate* | *Severe* |
|---|---|---|---|---|
| Median urine iodine, μg/L | >100 | 50–99 | 20–49 | <20 |
| Goiter prevalence | <5% | 5–20% | 20–30% | >30% |
| Neonatal TSH, >5 mU/L whole blood | <3% | 3–20% | 20–40% | >40% |
| Cretinism | None | None | Present | Present |

WHO. Assessment of iodine deficiency disorders and monitoring their elimination: A guide for programme managers. 3rd edn. 2007.

*Endemic goiter:* This does not differ from nontoxic diffuse sporadic goiter and the diagnosis is established by epidemiologic criteria. Usually, TSH is elevated with low $T_4$ and $T_3$ levels.

*Endemic cretinism:* This is associated with endemic goiter and severe iodine deficiency. Two types of endemic cretinism are described. Neurological cretinism is characterized by deaf–mutism, squint, proximal spasticity and rigidity and severe intellectual disability. Myxedematous cretinism is characterized by less severe intellectual impairment, severe short stature, coarse facial features and myxedema. Iodine deficiency is also associated with poor school performance in children.

*Prevention and control:* Iodine deficiency disorders are best prevented as treatment is usually ineffective. Iodinated salt or iodized oil are highly efficacious in preventing iodine deficiency. Treatment of endemic cretinism may eliminate signs of hypothyroidism but neuromotor and intellectual deficiency are irreversible. Surgical removal of large goiters is indicated only to relieve airway obstruction or for cosmetic reasons.

The 'National Goiter Control Programme' of the Ministry of Health and Family Welfare in India began in 1962 with establishment of salt iodination plants. The program is directed towards control of iodine deficiency disorders and ensuring that only iodized salt is used in India. The recommended daily intake of iodine is 40–120 μg for children up to the age of 10 years, 150 μg for older children and adults and an additional 25 μg and 50 μg during pregnancy and lactation, respectively. Based on an assumption of a mean intake of salt of 5 g/day, the recommended level of iodination is one part of iodine in 25,000 to 50,000 parts of salt.

## Hyperthyroidism

Hyperthyroidism is relatively uncommon in children. It is most commonly seen in young girls, caused by Graves disease (Table 18.10).

*Clinical features:* Hyperthyroidism is suspected in children with weight loss with increased appetite, tremors, diarrhea, warm extremities, increased sweating and anxiety. Inability to concentrate, personality changes, mood instability and poor school performance are common. Examination reveals firm homogeneous goiter.

Eye signs are relatively uncommon compared to adults and are related to sympathetic overactivity (lid lag, ophthalmoplegia, absence of wrinkling) or autoimmune

**Table 18.10:** Etiology of hyperthyroidism

| |
|---|
| **Infancy** |
| • Transplacental passage of thyroid antibodies |
| • TSH receptor activating mutation |
| **After infancy** |
| • Graves disease (TSH receptor stimulating antibody) |
| • Toxic thyroid nodule, toxic multinodular goiter |
| • Pituitary resistance to T3 |
| *Transient:* |
| • Release of preformed thyroid hormone in viral or bacterial infections of the thyroid (acute or subacute thyroiditis) |
| • During early phase of Hashimoto thyroiditis (Hashitoxicosis) |
| • Iatrogenic |

infiltration (chemosis or proptosis). Tachycardia, cardiac arrhythmia and high output cardiac failure may occur.

*Diagnosis:* The diagnosis is confirmed by the demonstration of elevated serum $FT_4$ and $FT_3$ levels. The presence of goiter, infiltrative eye signs and hyperthyroidism are suggestive of Graves disease. Absence of goiter should raise the possibility of transient hyperthyroidism as part of AIT. Differentiating thyrotoxicosis from thyroiditis is important, as antithyroid drugs are not required in children with AIT who may progress to hypothyroidism. Diffusely increased radiotracer uptake is suggestive of Graves disease while reduced uptake is characteristic of AIT.

*Management:* Treatment should be started with methimazole (0.5–1.0 mg/kg/day) in 3–4 divided doses. Propylthiouracil is contraindicated in children due to hepatotoxicity. Beta-blockers (propranolol 2 mg/kg/day in 2–3 divided doses) are effective in ameliorating sympathetic symptoms. Prednisolone (1–2 mg/kg/day) inhibits peripheral conversion of $T_4$ to $T_3$ and is useful in treatment of hyperthyroid storm. Surgery and radioiodine ablation should be considered in patients with failure of medical management or relapse after stopping medication. Patients with large or toxic nodular goiter require partial or total thyroidectomy. Radioiodine ($^{131}I$) is now increasingly used in the management of childhood Graves disease.

### Neonatal Hyperthyroidism

One percent of babies born to mothers with Graves disease show fetal thyrotoxicosis and cardiac failure. This usually occurs within the first week of life but may be delayed, if mother is on antithyroid medications or has concomitant TSH receptor blocking antibody. Treatment should include antithyroid drugs, propranolol and corticosteroids.

## Suggested Reading


1. Desai MP, Sharma R, Riaz I, et al. Newborn screening guidelines for congenital hypothyroidism in India: Recommendations of the Indian Society for Pediatric and Adolescent Endocrinology (ISPAE)-Part 1: Screening and confirmation of diagnosis. Indian J Pediatr 2018;85:440–47.
2. Kahaly GJ, Bartalena L, Hegedüs L, et al. European Thyroid Association guideline for the management of Graves' hyperthyroidism. Eur Thyroid J 2018;7:167–86.
3. Sudhanshu S, Riaz I, Sharma R, et al. Newborn screening guidelines for congenital hypothyroidism in India: Recommendations of the Indian Society for Pediatric and Adolescent Endocrinology (ISPAE)-Part II: Imaging, treatment and follow-up. Indian J Pediatr 2018;85:448–53.


*Competency:* **PE13.12**

# DISORDERS OF BONE AND MINERAL METABOLISM

## Physiology

Serum calcium, especially free ionized calcium, plays an important role in cell membrane stability, myocardial function and neurotransmission. Calcium homeostasis involves interaction of gastrointestinal absorption, bone resorption and renal excretion. Parathyroid hormone (PTH), vitamin D and calcitonin are the key regulators of calcium metabolism (*see* Chapter 8; Fig. 8.3). These help to maintain serum total calcium in the range of 8–10 mg/dL and ionized calcium in 4.6–5.1 mg/dL.

The calcium-sensing receptors present in the parathyroid gland and kidney sense the extracellular calcium levels. Low serum calcium reduces the activity of these receptors leading to increased PTH secretion from the parathyroid glands and decreased calcium excretion from the kidneys. PTH increases serum calcium by three mechanisms:

1. Stimulates osteoclastic bone resorption and release of calcium from bone.
2. Stimulates the activity of renal 1α-hydroxylase enzyme with increased calcitriol production.
3. Inhibits renal calcium excretion from distal tubules.

At the same time, PTH increases phosphate excretion from the proximal renal tubules leading to low serum phosphate levels.

Calcitriol (1,25-dihydroxyvitamin D) is the active form of vitamin D (*see* Chapter 8: Vitamin D metabolism). It increases intestinal calcium and phosphate absorption. Vitamin D is activated first in the liver (25-hydroxylation) and then kidney (1α-hydroxylation) to produce calcitriol.

The diagnosis and management of calcium and magnesium disorders are also discussed in Chapter 6.

## Hypocalcemia

Hypocalcemia is defined as serum total calcium <8.5 mg/dL) and ionic calcium <4.4 mg/dL (<1.1 mmol/L).

### Clinical Features

In infancy, hypocalcemia is characterized by subtle clinical features like lethargy, jitteriness and poor feeding. Seizures are common and hypocalcemia is one of the most common biochemical abnormalities associated with neonatal seizures.

Beyond infancy, the commonest presentation is tetany. This is most commonly observed in hands (adduction of thumbs along with extension of interphalangeal joints) and feet (flexion and internal rotation of lower limbs) resulting in carpopedal spasm. Latent tetany is detected by tapping the facial nerve at the angle of jaw resulting in contraction of facial muscles (Chvostek sign). Inflating blood pressure cuff above the systolic blood pressure for more than 5 minutes triggers spasm of the hand muscles (Trousseau sign). Hypocalcemia should be considered in children with seizures, dilated cardiomyopathy and stridor (due to laryngospasm).

The diagnosis is supported by the demonstration of prolonged QT interval on ECG, as suggested by QTc more than 0.45 seconds, where $QT_c = Q_oT \div \sqrt{RR}$

($Q_oT$ = Interval from beginning of Q wave to beginning of T wave; RR = RR interval)

### Etiology

Hypocalcemia is most commonly caused by deficiency or inefficient action of PTH or vitamin D and occasionally by chelation of calcium (*see* Table 6.9).

***PTH related:*** Decreased production of PTH (hypoparathyroidism) and inefficient PTH action (pseudohypoparathyroidism) caused by receptor dysfunction are important causes of chronic hypocalcemia. These disorders are characterized by low serum calcium and high serum phosphate levels due to impaired phosphaturic action of PTH. Autoimmune hypoparathyroidism is the most common cause of acquired hypoparathyroidism in older children and is frequently associated with autoimmune polyendocrinopathy (APS type 1).

*DiGeorge syndrome* is an important cause of congenital hypoparathyroidism and is characterized by abnormal development of third and fourth pharyngeal pouches due to deletion of a part of chromosome 22q. Activating mutation of calcium-sensing receptor (CaSR) is associated with low PTH secretion, low serum calcium levels and paradoxically increased urinary calcium excretion (familial hypercalciuric hypocalcemia).

*Maternal hyperparathyroidism* may result in chronic fetal hypercalcemia, suppression of fetal parathyroid function and manifest as neonatal hypoparathyroidism after birth.

*Hypomagnesemia* should be excluded in children with refractory hypocalcemia.

***PTH resistance (pseudohypoparathyroidism, PHP):*** This is caused by an inactivating mutation in the gene encoding for stimulatory subunit of G protein (Gsα). This presents with clinical features of hypoparathyroidism but elevated PTH levels. PHP may be associated with the phenotype of Albright hereditary osteodystrophy (AHO) such as round facies, brachydactyly, short stature, obesity, short fourth and fifth metacarpals (brachymetacarpia), osteodystrophy and heterotopic ossification.

***Vitamin D related:*** Vitamin D deficiency (lack of sunlight, nutritional and malabsorption), increased inactivation of vitamin D (antiepileptic drugs), decreased 1α-hydroxylase action (renal failure and vitamin D-dependent rickets, VDDR type I), and calcitriol resistance (VDDR type II) are associated with hypocalcemia. In vitamin D related disorders, low serum calcium stimulates parathyroid glands to release PTH. Compensatory increase in PTH may raise the serum calcium levels to normal range when vitamin D deficiency is not severe. High PTH levels may also result in low serum phosphate levels due to increased renal phosphate excretion.

*Nutritional vitamin D deficiency* is the most common cause of hypocalcemia in children and is associated with clinical and biochemical findings of rickets (*see* Chapter 8). Maternal vitamin D deficiency results in reduced calcium and vitamin D stores in newborns at birth. As breastmilk is also low in vitamin D in mothers with vitamin D deficiency, it is recommended to supplement breastfed infants with vitamin D. Vitamin D-dependent rickets type I and II present with early onset severe hypocalcemia and rickets.

***Increased chelation:*** High serum phosphate levels due to renal failure or release of intracellular phosphate (due to hemolysis, tumor lysis or rhabdomyolysis) bind to serum calcium and result in extracellular deposition of calcium and low serum levels. Cow milk and certain commercial formulations have high phosphate loads that can chelate calcium and lead to hypocalcemia in the newborn period. Metabolic or respiratory alkalosis increases albumin binding of calcium resulting in low ionized calcium and features of hypocalcemia.

### Evaluation

***Clinical:*** Detailed history of the age of onset, presenting features, frequency of episodes of hypocalcemia and family history should be obtained. Neonates should be screened for prematurity, birth asphyxia, maternal hyperparathyroidism and initiation of top feeds. Congenital heart disease, towards recurrent infections and abnormal facies may point towards DiGeorge syndrome.

***Investigations:*** Initial evaluation should include serum phosphate levels, renal and liver function tests and serum alkaline phosphatase (Table 18.11). Phosphate regulation is dependent on PTH, and inefficient PTH action results in hyperphosphatemia. Hypocalcemia due to decreased vitamin D action is associated with secondary hyperparathyroidism and low phosphate levels. Thus hypocalcemia with hyperphosphatemia in the absence of phosphate load (exogenous or tissue lysis) and

**Table 18.11:** Laboratory features of common causes of hypocalcemia

| *Disorder* | *Phosphate* | *25-hydroxyvitamin D* | *Parathyroid hormone (PTH)* |
|---|---|---|---|
| Vitamin D deficiency | Low, normal | Low | High |
| Renal failure | High | Normal | High |
| Hypoparathyroidism | High | Normal | Low |
| Pseudohypoparathyroidism | High | Normal | High |
| Hypomagnesemia | Low, normal | Normal | Low |

normal renal function suggests parathyroid insufficiency. Hypomagnesemia should be considered in patients with refractory hypocalcemia and normal or low phosphate levels. 25-hydroxyvitamin D levels should be measured in children with rickets to identify vitamin D deficiency.

#### Management

In children with severe hypocalcemia, parenteral calcium should be administered (2 mL/kg of calcium gluconate, 9 mg calcium per mL) intravenously over 5–10 min after obtaining a blood sample for calcium. Care should be taken to administer the drug slowly under cardiac monitoring (to prevent cardiac arrhythmias) and avoid extravasation (to prevent skin necrosis).

Parenteral calcium should be started at a dose of 80 mg/kg/day and should be gradually tapered over 2 days. The management of nutritional and refractory rickets is given in Chapter 8.

### Hypercalcemia

Hypercalcemia (serum calcium >11 mg/dL) is rare in children. Its causes include increased bone resorption (hyperparathyroidism, malignancy and immobilization) or excessive vitamin D action (iatrogenic excess and increased 1α-hydroxylase activity).

*Etiology:* Hyperparathyroidism is the commonest cause of chronic hypercalcemia in children. Homozygous inactivating mutations of the calcium-sensing receptor present with severe neonatal hyperparathyroidism and hypocalciuria. Parathyroid adenoma is rare before the age of 10 years, but may be a feature of inherited endocrine disorders like multiple endocrine neoplasia type 1 (MEN type 1) especially with a positive family history. Rarely, hypercalcemia may be associated with other conditions, e.g. Williams syndrome (supravalvular aortic stenosis and abnormal facies) or hypophosphatasia (inactivating mutation of alkaline phosphatase). Vitamin D related hypercalcemia occurs in children receiving parental vitamin D or inadvertently high doses of oral vitamin D. Increased 1α-hydroxylase activity may occur in patients with granulomatous diseases (tuberculosis and sarcoidosis) or fat necrosis.

*Clinical features:* These are nonspecific, including muscular weakness, anorexia, nausea, vomiting, constipation, polydipsia and polyuria. Ectopic calcification in the kidney, basal ganglia and skin are common. Bony deformities and pathological fractures may be present. Infants present with failure to thrive, poor feeding, hypotonia and seizures.

*Diagnosis:* Serum total and ionized calcium levels are elevated with low levels of phosphate. Hyperparathyroidism is associated with elevated levels of PTH while the levels are low in vitamin D toxicity or malignancy.

*Management:* Treatment of acute hypercalcemia involves high fluid intake followed by diuresis (furosemide 1 mg/kg). Bisphosphonates are drugs which block osteoclastic bone resorption and decrease serum calcium. They are indicated, if there is no response to these measures. Hemodialysis may be required in refractory cases. Short course of glucocorticoids (prednisolone 2 mg/kg/day for 3 weeks) is indicated in children with iatrogenic vitamin D excess or increased 1α-hydroxylase action (fat necrosis or sarcoidosis).

#### Suggested Reading


1. Brandi ML, Bilezikian JP, Shoback D, et al. Management of hypoparathyroidism: Summary statement and guidelines. J Clin Endocrinol Metab. 2016;101:2273–83.
2. Chinoy A, Mughal Z, Padidela R. Hypocalcemia, hypercalcemia and disorders of the parathyroid glands. In: Desai MP, Menon PSN, Bhatia V, Seth A, eds. Pediatric Endocrine Disorders, 4th edn. Hyderabad: Universities Press (India) 2022;473–84.
3. Davies JH, Shaw NJ. Investigation and management of hypercalcemia in children. Arch Dis Child 2012;97:533–38.




## DISORDERS OF ADRENAL GLANDS

### Physiology

Adrenal cortex produces three important groups of hormones—glucocorticoids, mineralocorticoids and androgens. The process of steroidogenesis involves conversion of cholesterol to steroid hormones through a series of enzymatic processes (Fig. 18.6). Cholesterol is transferred into the mitochondria in a process mediated by the steroidogenic acute regulatory protein (StAR), an ACTH- dependent protein.

*Cortisol*, the major glucocorticoid hormone has an important role in intermediary metabolism causing increased blood glucose levels and enhanced catabolism of proteins and lipids.

*Aldosterone* acts on distal renal tubules and collecting ducts of kidneys to promote sodium and fluid reabsorption. Aldosterone deficiency causes urinary salt-wasting resulting in salt-wasting crisis (hyponatremia, hyperkalemia and metabolic acidosis).

*Adrenal androgens* are necessary for the development of pubic and axillary hair in girls.

*Regulation of adrenal cortical hormone synthesis:* ACTH is the major regulator of glucocorticoid and androgen synthesis. Aldosterone synthesis is regulated by intravascular volume, renin–angiotensin system and serum potassium levels. ACTH secretion is stimulated by hypothalamic CRH and suppressed by cortisol.

### Adrenocortical Hyperfunction—Cushing Syndrome

The most common disorder of adrenocortical hyperfunction is Cushing syndrome. The term Cushing disease refers to hypercortisolism caused by an ACTH-producing pituitary tumor. Classic features of Cushing syndrome such as central obesity, striae, moon facies and buffalo hump are less common in children (Fig. 18.7). Growth failure and obesity are more common; other features include hypertension, hirsutism, delayed puberty, behavioral problems, bone pain and muscle weakness.

*Etiology:* Cushing syndrome results from increased endogenous production or exogenous administration (Table 18.12). Prolonged steroid treatment is the commonest

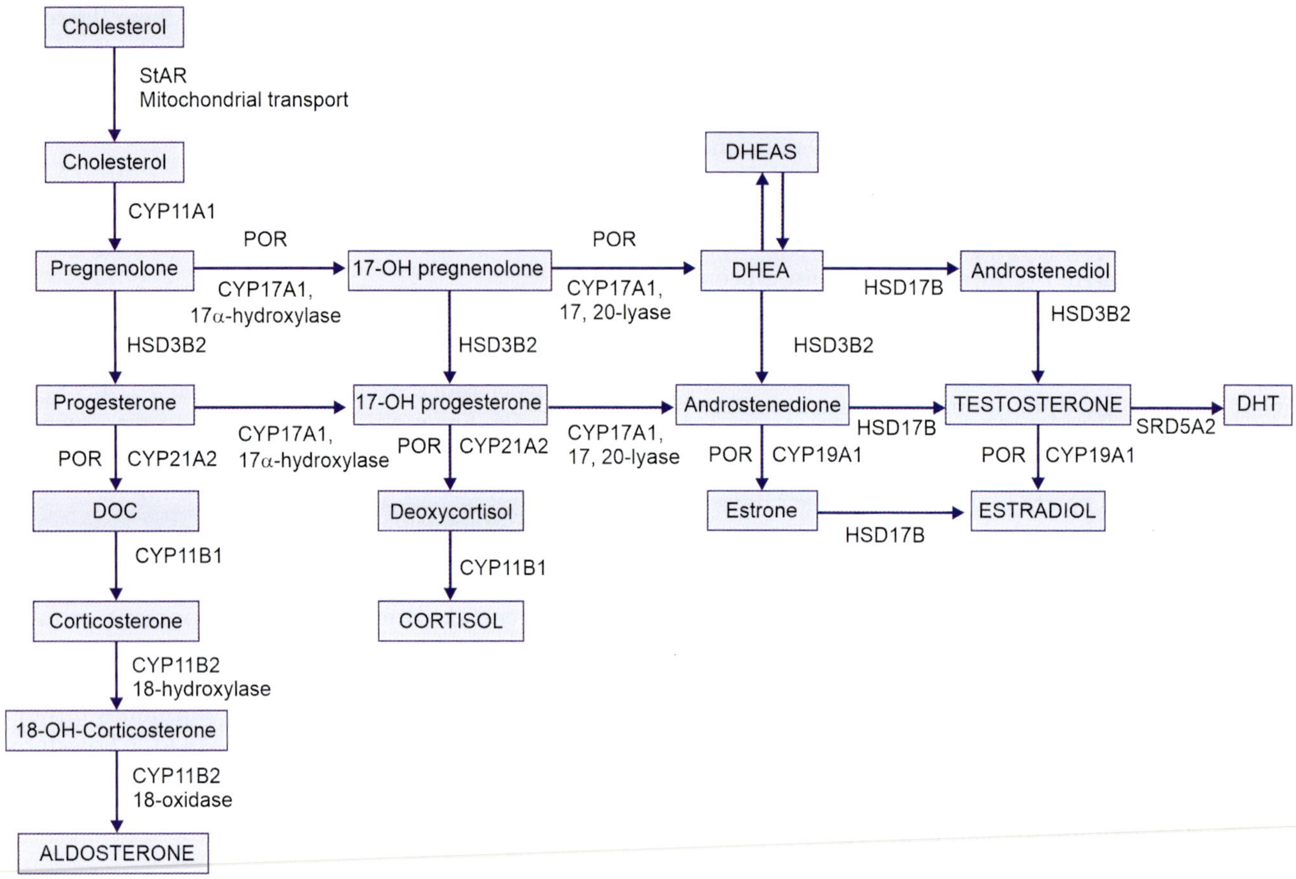


**Fig. 18.6:** Pathways of steroid biosynthesis. The key enzymes mediating synthesis of principal steroids are named according to their site of action and the nomenclature of cytochrome P450 enzymes. StAR steroidogenic acute regulatory protein; DOC deoxycorticosterone; DHEA dehydroepiandrosterone; DHEAS–DHEA sulfate; DHT dihydrotestosterone. The enzyme nomenclature: CYP11A1: P450 side chain cleavage enzyme, P450scc or 20,22-desmolase; HSD3B2: 3β-hydroxysteroid dehydrogenase type 2; CYP17A1: 17α-hydroxylase or17,20 lyase; CYP21A2: 21-hydroxylase; CYP11B1: 11β-hydroxylase; CYP11B2: This has 3 actions—11β-hydroxylase, 18-hydroxylase and 18-oxidase; POR: P450 oxidoreductase; CYP19A1: Aromatase; HSD17B: 17β-hydroxysteroid dehydrogenase; SRD5A2: 5α-reductase type 2

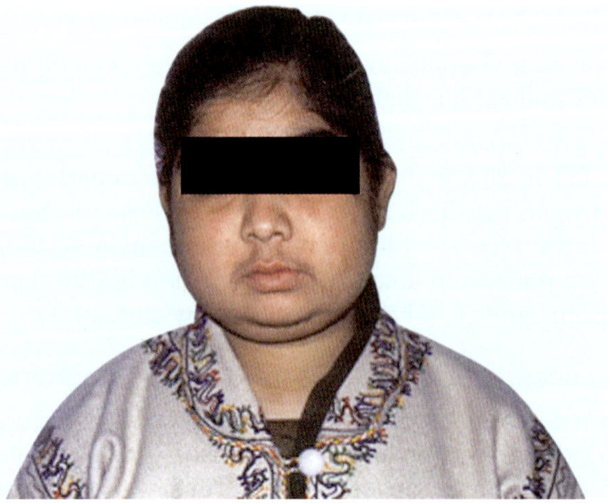

**Fig. 18.7:** Cushing disease secondary to pituitary adenoma. Note the moon face and hypertrichosis over forehead and upper lip

cause of childhood Cushing syndrome. Adrenal pathology is more likely in young children, while pituitary causes are more likely in older children and adolescents. Ectopic ACTH production is rare in children.

***Evaluation:*** Investigations are directed towards confirming the diagnosis of Cushing syndrome and finding the etiology.

**Table 18.12:** Etiology of Cushing syndrome

| |
|---|
| **ACTH-dependent causes** |
| • *Hypothalamic lesions:* Increased corticotropin production |
| • *Pituitary lesions:* Microadenoma, macroadenoma |
| • *Ectopic lesions:* Neuroblastoma, carcinoid tumor, Wilms tumor |
| **ACTH-independent causes** |
| • Adrenal carcinoma, adenoma |
| • Pigmented nodular hyperplasia |
| • McCune-Albright syndrome |
| **Exogenous administration** |
| • Glucocorticoids |
| • ACTH |

ACTH adrenocorticotropic hormone

Commonly used screening tests include assessment of diurnal cortisol rhythm, overnight single midnight dose of dexamethasone 0.03 mg/kg; maximum dose 1 mg) and 24-hour urine free cortisol (Table 18.13). The diagnosis is confirmed with low dose dexamethasone suppression test (serum cortisol after dexamethasone 5 μg/kg every 6 hours for two days).

The most important part of evaluation of a child with Cushing syndrome is to differentiate ACTH-dependent

**Table 18.13:** Screening tests for Cushing syndrome

| *Test* | *Sensitivity* | *Specificity* | *Cut-off level* | *Comments* |
|---|---|---|---|---|
| Morning cortisol | Low | Low | >10 μg/dL | Not recommended |
| Overnight dexamethasone suppression test | High | Low | >1.8 μg/dL | Screening test |
| Urine free cortisol | High | High | >75 μg/m²/day | Screening test* |
| Low dose dexamethasone suppression test | High | High | >1.8 μg/dL | Diagnostic test |

*Diagnostic of Cushing syndrome, if level is greater than 3 to 4 times the normal range

**Table 18.14:** Laboratory findings in common causes of Cushing syndrome

| *Disorder* | *Urinary free cortisol* | *High dose dexamethasone suppression test* | *Adrenocorticotropic hormone (ACTH)* |
|---|---|---|---|
| Adrenal lesion | High | Not suppressed | Low |
| Pituitary lesion | | | |
| Microadenoma | High | Suppressed | High |
| Macroadenoma | High | Not suppressed | High |
| Ectopic ACTH | High | Not suppressed | High |
| Exogenous | Low | Not suppressed | Low |

causes from autonomous adrenal steroid production (Table 18.14). ACTH levels differentiate ACTH-independent (ACTH levels <5 pg/mL) from ACTH-dependent conditions (ACTH levels >15 pg/mL). Ectopic ACTH production should be suspected in children with extremely high ACTH levels (>100 pg/mL). High dose dexamethasone suppression test is based on the principle that high doses of dexamethasone suppress ACTH production in individuals with pituitary lesions but not in those with ectopic ACTH production.

Adrenal tumors in children are usually large and identifiable on ultrasound. Magnetic resonance imaging of the hypothalamic–pituitary region should be performed in children with ACTH-dependent Cushing syndrome. Inferior petrosal sinus sampling can identify the source of ACTH production and should be performed in children with ACTH-dependent Cushing syndrome with normal neuroimaging.

*Management:* Resection of adrenal lesion is recommended for adrenal adenoma and carcinoma. Prolonged cortisol excess causes suppression of the normal contralateral adrenal gland. This mandates close monitoring for adrenal insufficiency in the perioperative period. Adrenal carcinoma is highly malignant and has a high rate of recurrence. Pigmented nodular hyperplasia should be treated with bilateral adrenalectomy. Trans-sphenoidal resection of pituitary adenoma is recommended for Cushing disease.

In refractory cases, medical management of Cushing syndrome with inhibitors of steroidogenesis (ketoconazole, aminoglutethimide, cyproheptadine, metyrapone and mitotane) has been tried with variable results.

## Aldosterone Excess

Hyperaldosteronism is associated with fluid and sodium retention along with increased urinary loss of potassium. The chief clinical features of primary hyperaldosteronism are hypertension and hypokalemic alkalosis. Primary hyperaldosteronism due to increased adrenal aldosterone production is extremely rare. Secondary hyperaldosteronism results from factors that activate the renin–angiotensin system (Table 18.15).

**Table 18.15:** Etiology of hyperaldosteronism

**Primary hyperaldosteronism**
- Adenoma, hyperplasia
- Glucocorticoid remediable hyperaldosteronism (chimeric fusion of promoter of CYP11B1 with coding region of CYP11B2, resulting in regulation of aldosterone synthesis by ACTH)

**Secondary hyperaldosteronism**
- Renal artery stenosis, renin-secreting tumor
- Cardiac failure, nephrotic syndrome, liver disease

**Other causes of excessive mineralocorticoid action**
- Apparent mineralocorticoid excess (deficiency of 11β-hydroxysteroid dehydrogenase type 2 in the kidneys)
- Liddle syndrome
- Congenital adrenal hyperplasia due to deficiency of 17α-hydroxylase or 11β-hydroxylase

*Evaluation:* Aldosterone excess should be suspected in a child with hypertension, hypokalemic alkalosis, and low plasma renin levels on investigations. High aldosterone level in this setting is suggestive of primary hyperaldosteronism or glucocorticoid remediable hyperaldosteronism (GRA). Decrease in aldosterone levels and resolution of clinical and laboratory features after dexamethasone suppression suggests GRA; no effect is seen in primary hyperaldosteronism. Diagnosis of primary hyperaldosteronism should be confirmed by adrenal imaging.

*Management:* Hyperaldosteronism should be managed with salt restriction and aldosterone antagonist (spironolactone or eplerenone). Physiological hydrocortisone replacement suppresses ACTH secretion in GRA. Surgery is the treatment of choice for adrenal adenoma.

## Pheochromocytoma

Pheochromocytoma is a catecholamine-secreting tumor, arising from chromaffin cells of adrenal medulla. It can also arise from the abdominal sympathetic chain, peri-adrenal area, or in the thoracic cavity. It is rare in children. Unlike adults, in children, pheochromocytoma is more likely to be bilateral, and associated with underlying genetic syndromes such as neurofibromatosis, von Hippel-Lindau disease and multiple endocrine neoplasia type 2 (MEN type 2).

*Clinical features:* Excessive secretion of catecholamines results in hypertension, which is usually sustained and occasionally paroxysmal. The clinical symptoms include headache, palpitation, pallor, sweating, nausea, vomiting, visual disturbances and occasionally convulsions.

*Evaluation:* It is important to rule out common causes of childhood hypertension such as renal parenchymal disorders, renal artery stenosis and coarctation of aorta. Diagnosis is established by demonstration of increased urinary excretion of catecholamines and their derivatives.

Ultrasound, CT scan, MRI scan and $^{123}$I metaiodobenzylguanidine (MIBG) scintigraphy are used for localization of the tumor. Occasionally, the tumors are multiple.

*Management:* Surgery is the treatment of choice. Transabdominal exploration of all the sites with removal of tumors is advocated. Preoperatively alpha-blockade is done using phenoxybenzamine and prazosin, followed by beta-blocking agents.

## Adrenal Insufficiency

Adrenal insufficiency may be related to adrenal defects (primary adrenal insufficiency; autoimmune destruction, infection, steroidogenic defects, hemorrhage), decreased ACTH production (secondary adrenal insufficiency) or ACTH resistance.

*Etiology:* Autoimmune adrenal dysfunction is the commonest cause of primary adrenal failure (Addison disease) beyond infancy. Autoimmune adrenal failure is often associated with autoimmune polyendocrinopathy (APS) types 1 and 2. Infections due to tuberculosis and human immunodeficiency virus (HIV) may result in primary adrenal failure. Adrenal hemorrhage in the setting of meningococcal and other bacterial infections (Waterhouse-Friderichsen syndrome) is an important cause of adrenal insufficiency. Tuberculosis is still an important cause of adrenal insufficiency (caseous necrosis of adrenals) in developing countries. Congenital adrenal hyperplasia (CAH) due to deficiency of 21-hydroxylase or 3β-hydroxysteroid dehydrogenase and deficient steroidogenesis due to defective steroidogenic acute regulatory protein (StAR; causing lipoid CAH) are the chief causes in the neonatal period. Adrenal hypoplasia congenita due to a defect in *DAX*1 gene causes early onset adrenal insufficiency with small adrenals. This is an X-linked condition, with affected infants often having unilateral or bilateral cryptorchidism presenting with hypogonadotropic hypogonadism later.

Secondary (central) adrenal insufficiency is caused by congenital malformations (holoprosencephaly and midline defects), genetic defects or acquired insults (neurosurgery, tumor or radiation). This is usually associated with other anterior pituitary hormone deficiencies as well. In secondary adrenal insufficiency, mineralocorticoid function is preserved, as ACTH does not regulate aldosterone secretion. Thus, salt-wasting is not observed. Prolonged steroid treatment is associated with suppression of the hypothalamic–pituitary axis resulting in adrenal insufficiency even after discontinuation of medications. Again, mineralocorticoid activity is preserved in these patients. ACTH resistance due to ACTH receptor defects (familial glucocorticoid deficiency) presents with isolated cortisol deficiency, pigmentation, and normal potassium levels.

*Clinical features:* Adrenal insufficiency presents with slowly progressive lethargy, vomiting, salt craving, fatigue, postural hypotension, hypoglycemia and episodes of shock during severe illness. The concomitant presence of shock, hyponatremia, hyperkalemia and hemoconcentration is characteristic of acute adrenal insufficiency and warrants immediate steroid replacement. Primary adrenal insufficiency is characterized by hyperpigmentation due to elevated levels of melanocyte-stimulating hormone (MSH). Hyperpigmentation is present in sun-exposed areas such as elbows and palmar creases and areas that are normally hyperpigmented such as areola and genitalia. Pigmentation is absent in children with secondary adrenal insufficiency.

*Evaluation:* All patients suspected to have adrenal insufficiency should undergo immediate testing for serum electrolytes and blood glucose. Basal levels of cortisol are low (<5 µg/dL), but these have low specificity, as they can be low even in healthy non-stressed individuals. The next step in evaluation of adrenal insufficiency is estimation of serum ACTH levels. In children presenting with salt-wasting and hyperpigmentation, presence of elevated plasma ACTH levels and low basal cortisol levels is sufficient to make the diagnosis of primary adrenal insufficiency. If plasma ACTH levels cannot be assessed due to nonavailability of the test, or are low, an ACTH stimulation test (cortisol estimation 60 minutes after 0.25 mg of intramuscular or intravenous ACTH injection) is the best test for adrenocortical reserve. Serum cortisol levels lower than 18 µg/dL are suggestive of adrenal insufficiency.

In children with low cortisol after ACTH stimulation test and low plasma ACTH levels, a pituitary defect is likely. Elevated plasma renin activity (PRA) indicates mineralocorticoid deficiency. Further evaluation of primary adrenal insufficiency includes abdominal CT scan and work-up for tuberculosis.

*Management:* The initial management of salt-wasting crisis includes correction of shock by fluid boluses. Hydrocortisone is given immediately in a dose of 50 mg/m$^2$, followed by 100 mg/m$^2$/day in four divided doses. Frequent monitoring of hemodynamic parameters, urine output and serum electrolytes are required. Once the child is hemodynamically stable, hydrocortisone is tapered to the physiological dose (10–12 mg/m$^2$/day given in three divided doses). Fludrocortisone acetate (0.1 mg/day once daily) is added when hydrocortisone dose is <50 mg/m$^2$/day.

Long-term management of adrenal insufficiency requires lifelong replacement of glucocorticoids and mineralocorticoids. Parents should be educated about the need for increasing the dose during periods of stress. The dose of glucocorticoid should be increased 2–3 times in conditions of minor stress (fever and mild infection) and 4–5 times in severe stress (severe infection or surgery). These doses should continue throughout the period of stress. Patients with secondary adrenal insufficiency require lower dose of glucocorticoids (6–10 mg/m²/day); mineralocorticoid replacement is not necessary.

### Congenital Adrenal Hyperplasia

Congenital adrenal hyperplasia (CAH), a group of autosomal recessive defects in steroid synthesis, is characterized by the deficiency of adrenocortical hormones on one hand and the excess of steroid precursors on the other (Fig. 18.6). CAH is the commonest adrenal disorder in childhood.

#### *21-hydroxylase Deficiency*

21-hydroxylase deficiency is the commonest form of CAH accounting for over 90% of all cases. This disorder is associated with diminished synthesis of the cortisol and aldosterone. Low cortisol levels stimulate ACTH synthesis. Elevated ACTH level causes accumulation of steroid precursors (e.g. dehydroepiandrosterone [DHEA], androstenedione and 17-hydroxyprogesterone [17-OHP]). Depending on the severity of enzyme deficiency, the disease forms a spectrum of presentations detailed below.

*Salt-wasting form:* These patients are the most severely affected due to almost absent enzyme activity and present in the neonatal period with salt-wasting and virilization. Abnormal genital appearance should prompt the diagnosis in girls. Diagnosis is often missed in boys as they lack specific clinical features and genital ambiguity. They present after second week of life with failure to thrive, polyuria, hyperpigmentation and shock. Early diagnosis is mandatory to prevent mortality. 21-hydroxylase deficiency should be suspected in neonates with ambiguous genitalia, polyuria, shock, recurrent vomiting and features of sepsis with negative septic screen. The diagnosis is confirmed by measurement of blood levels of 17-OHP.

*Simple virilizing form:* A subset of patients with 21-hydroxylase deficiency (25%) synthesizes enough aldosterone to prevent adrenal crisis. These patients have features of androgen excess in the form of virilization in girls and peripheral precocious puberty in boys (Fig. 18.8).

*Non-classic form:* This disorder is associated with partial 21-hydroxylase deficiency. Clinical manifestations are related to mild hyperandrogenism that presents with hirsutism, acne and menstrual irregularity in adolescents.

*Diagnosis:* Diagnosis of the salt-wasting form is established by demonstration of extreme elevations of 17-OHP levels (10000–20000 ng/dL, normal <200 ng/dL) in the presence of clinical and laboratory features of adrenal insufficiency. 17-OHP levels are elevated to a lesser extent in those with simple virilizing and non-classic forms. The best method of diagnosing these patients is the estimation of 17-OHP levels

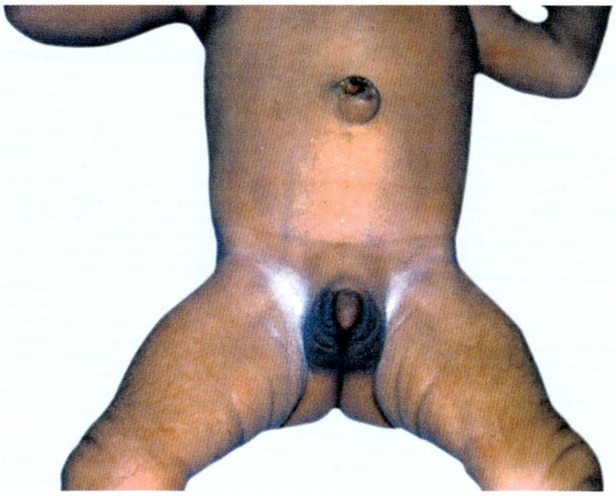

**Fig. 18.8:** Congenital adrenal hyperplasia secondary to 21-hydroxylase deficiency in a 46,XX newborn. Note the clitoral hypertrophy, hyperpigmentation and increased rugosity of the labial folds giving a male appearance to the female genitalia. Testes were absent.

before and 60 minutes after an intramuscular injection of ACTH (0.25 mg).

*Management:* These patients require lifelong steroid replacement therapy. Patients with salt-wasting and virilizing forms are treated with hydrocortisone (10–15 mg/m²/day) and fludrocortisone (0.1 mg/day). After completion of growth and pubertal development, long-acting glucocorticoid preparations (dexamethasone or prednisolone) can be used.

#### *Other Variants*

Enzyme deficiencies other than 21-hydroxylase deficiency account for less than 10% of cases of CAH (Table 18.16). Patients with 11-hydroxylase deficiency and 17- hydroxylase deficiency present with hypertension and are managed with hydrocortisone alone. Deficiencies of StAR and 3β-hydroxysteroid dehydrogenase manifest as salt-wasting crisis and require therapy with mineralocorticoid.

### Suggested Reading


1. Bajpai A, Menon PSN. Congenital adrenal hyperplasia. In: Gupta P, Menon PSN, Ramji S, Lodha R, Eds. PG Textbook of Pediatrics, 3rd edn. New Delhi; Jaypee Brothers, 2022; pp 2918–22.
2. Brandão Neto RA, de Carvalho JF. Diagnosis and classification of Addison disease. Autoimmune Rev 2014;13:408–11.
3. Greaves RF, Jevalikar G, Hewitt JK, Zacharin MR. A guide to understanding the steroid pathway: new insights and diagnostic implications. Clin Biochem 2014;47:5–15.
4. Speiser PW, Azziz R, Baskin LS, et al. Congenital adrenal hyperplasia due to steroid 21-hydroxylase deficiency: an Endocrine Society clinical practice guideline. J Clin Endocrinol Metab 2010;95:4133–60.


*Competencies:* **PE11.1; PE11.2; PE11.3; 11.4; PE11.5; PE11.6**

## OBESITY

The incidence of childhood obesity has increased rapidly in the last decade. The prevalence of overweight and/or obesity in urban Indian children is around 20% posing significant risk of lifestyle diseases in future.

**Table 18.16:** Comparison of common variants of congenital adrenal hyperplasia

| *Enzymes deficient* | *Androgen levels* | *Blood pressure* | *Clinical presentation* | | *Laboratory diagnosis* | *Treatment* |
|---|---|---|---|---|---|---|
| | | | *Boys* | *Girls* | | |
| **21-hydroxylase** | | | | | | |
| Salt-wasting | High | Low | Precocious puberty | Atypical genitalia | 17-OHP* | Hydrocortisone<br>Fludrocortisone |
| Simple virilizing | High | Normal | Precocious puberty | Atypical genitalia | 17-OHP* | Hydrocortisone<br>Fludrocortisone[@] |
| Non-classic | High | Normal | Normal | Hirsutism | 17-OHP* | Hydrocortisone |
| **11β-hydroxylase** | High | High/Normal[$] | Precocious puberty | Atypical genitalia | DOC | Hydrocortisone<br>Spironolactone |
| **3β-hydroxysteroid dehydrogenase** | Variable[#] | Low | Atypical genitalia | Atypical genitalia | ACTH stimulation test** | Hydrocortisone<br>Fludrocortisone |
| **17α-hydroxylase/ 17-lyase** | Low | High[$] | Atypical genitalia | Delayed puberty | DOC | Hydrocortisone[^] |
| **StAR** | Low | Low | Atypical genitalia | Delayed puberty | Low 17-OHP | Hydrocortisone<br>Fludrocortisone |

DOC deoxycorticosterone; StAR steroidogenic acute regulatory protein; 17-OHP 17-hydroxyprogesterone
*Basal and ACTH stimulated
[$]BP is high due to mineralocorticoid effect of DOC; however, BP may be normal
[#]Due to peripheral conversion of dehydroepiandrosterone (DHEA)
**Ratio of pregnenolone, progesterone, 17-hydroxypregnenolone to 17-OHP and DHEA to androstenedione following ACTH stimulation test
[@]Flurocortisone is useful in few patients with simple virilizing CAH, but not needed in most
[^]Few patients may need spironolactone

## Criteria for Diagnosis of Obesity

Obesity implies excessive fat and not merely excess weight. As methods of measuring body fat are cumbersome and expensive, several clinical and anthropometric parameters are used as markers of obesity.

*Body mass index:* Body mass index (BMI) is the most widely used parameter to define obesity. It takes into account weight as well as the height. It is calculated by the formula:

$$BMI = Weight\ (kg) \div Height\ (m^2)$$

BMI is a good indicator of body fat but is unreliable in short muscular individuals. As the aim of assessing BMI is to identify individuals at risk for metabolic complications, lower BMI cutoffs are recommended for Indian adults (23 kg/m$^2$ for overweight and 27 kg/m$^2$ for obesity). The IAP 2015 growth charts extrapolate 23rd and 27th adult equivalent centiles of BMI for diagnosis of overweight and obesity respectively, in children above 5 years of age. The 23rd adult equivalent centile corresponds to approximately 0.55 SDS (71st centile) for males and 0.67 SDS (75th centile) for females; while the 27th adult equivalent centile corresponds to 1.33 SDS (90th centile) and 1.63 SDS (95th centile), respectively, in males and females.

*Weight for height:* This compares the child's weight to the expected weight for his/her height and is useful in children below 5 years of age (*see* Chapter 2, Table 2.4).

In children below 5 years, the cutoffs, for overnutrition are based on WHO MGRS charts, are as follows:
***Overweight:*** Weight for length/height > +2 SDS
***Obesity:*** Weight for length/height > +3 SDS

*Skinfold thickness:* Skinfold thickness measured over the subscapular, triceps or biceps regions is an indicator of subcutaneous fat. Age-specific percentile cutoffs should be used.

*Waist circumference, waist–hip ratio and waist circumference to height ratio:* Waist circumference is a good indicator of abdominal adiposity. Waist circumference >75th centile for age or >80 cm in girls and >90 cm in boys is a good marker of risk for metabolic and cardiovascular effects of obesity. Waist circumference to height ratio of >0.5 is a better age-independent method to identify those at increased health risk.

## Etiology

In most children with obesity, lifestyle and hereditary factors play the major role (Table 18.17). A specific etiology is identified in a few cases (<5%).

*Constitutional or exogenous obesity:* Most children with obesity do not have an organic cause. Excessive weight gain is caused by an imbalance in energy intake and expenditure. They are tall for their age and with reference to their midparental height, a factor that differentiates them from pathological obesity.

*Endocrine causes:* Endocrine causes are rare (about 2–3%) in children referred for evaluation of overweight. An important clue to endocrine etiology is the deceleration or cessation of linear growth—height below the centile expected for the genetic potential. Cushing syndrome is characterized by central obesity, hypertension, and purple striae with delayed skeletal maturation. In GH deficiency and pseudohypoparathyroidism, growth retardation and

**Table 18.17:** Etiology of obesity

| |
|---|
| **Constitutional** |
| Environmental factors (95% cases) |
| **Pathological** |
| *Endocrine:* Cushing syndrome, growth hormone deficiency, hypothyroidism, pseudohypoparathyroidism |
| *Hypothalamic:* Head injury, infection, brain tumor, radiation, chemotherapy, following neurosurgery, ROHHAD(NET)* |
| *Drugs:* Antiepileptic drugs, steroids, antidepressants, estrogen |
| *Genetic syndromes:* Prader-Willi, Bardet-Biedl, Laurence-Moon, Beckwith-Wiedemann, Alström, Carpenter syndromes |
| *Monogenic disorders:* Leptin deficiency, or resistance (leptin receptor defect), abnormalities of melanocortin-4 receptor and proconvertase |
| *Psychological:* Personal or parental stress, binge eating |

*ROHHAD(NET) Rapid-onset obesity, hypothalamic dysfunction, hypoventilation, autonomic dysregulation, and neural crest tumors

hypocalcemia respectively are dominant clinical features and abdominal obesity is less prominent. Hypothyroidism is associated with mild weight gain, coarse skin and characteristic facies. However, mildly elevated TSH levels (up to 10 mU/L) seen in children with obesity, represent the effect and not the cause of obesity.

*Genetic syndromes:* Several genetic syndromes have obesity as their major clinical feature.

*Hypothalamic obesity:* CNS insults due to surgery, radiation, tumors and trauma result in rapid-onset obesity. Excessive appetite and features of CNS involvement and hypothalamic–pituitary defects are usually present. Rapid-onset obesity, hypothalamic dysfunction, hypoventilation, autonomic dysregulation (ROHHAD) is a rare disease that presents with rapid weight gain, most commonly between 2 and 4 years of age, with associated features, and neuroendocrine tumors in approximately 50% of affected children.

*Monogenic obesity:* Monogenic obesity is rare and more likely when the obesity is morbid, and has onset in infancy, with a strong family history of obesity. Leptin deficiency was the first monogenic cause of obesity identified. Inefficient leptin action (receptor deficiency or resistance) results in uncontrolled appetite and obesity. Melanocortin-4 receptor (*MC4-R*) defects are the commonest monogenic form of obesity and are associated with growth acceleration.

*Drugs:* Commonly used drugs associated with obesity include corticosteroids, antipsychotics (olanzapine and risperidone), antidepressants (paroxetine) and antiepileptics (valproic acid and lamotrigine).

### Evaluation

Initial evaluation is guided to differentiate exogenous (constitutional) from endogenous (pathological) obesity. Normal growth, generalized pattern of obesity and the lack of developmental delay or dysmorphism imply constitutional obesity.

*History:* Details of physical activity, dietary recall and sedentary habits help in diagnosis. Increased appetite in a child with recent-onset obesity may indicate the possibility of a hypothalamic lesion. Features of raised intracranial tension along with history of neurologic infection, head trauma or neurosurgery suggest an underlying neurologic cause for obesity. Intake of drugs linked with development of obesity should be probed.

*Examination:* Look for features of endocrinopathies, dysmorphic syndromes and complications such as hypertension and acanthosis nigricans (Fig. 18.9). Emphasis should be given to sexual maturity and ocular examination. Hypogonadism is an important feature of obese children with Laurence-Moon, Bardet-Biedl and Prader-Willi syndromes (Figs 18.10, 18.11 and Table 18.18). Parents of obese girls are often concerned about premature thelarche.

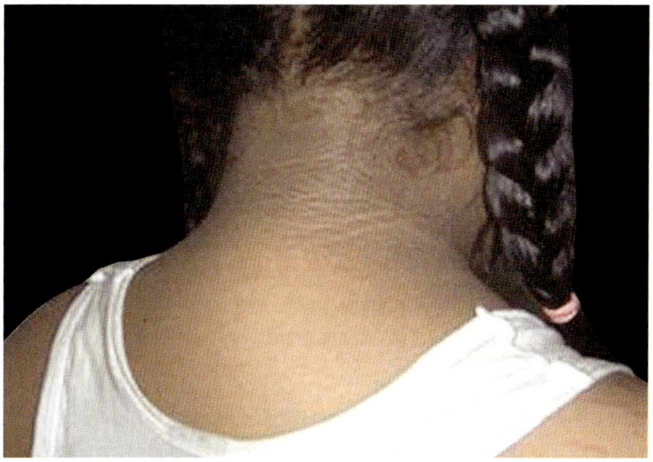

Fig. 18.9: Acanthosis nigricans on the back of neck in a girl with obesity

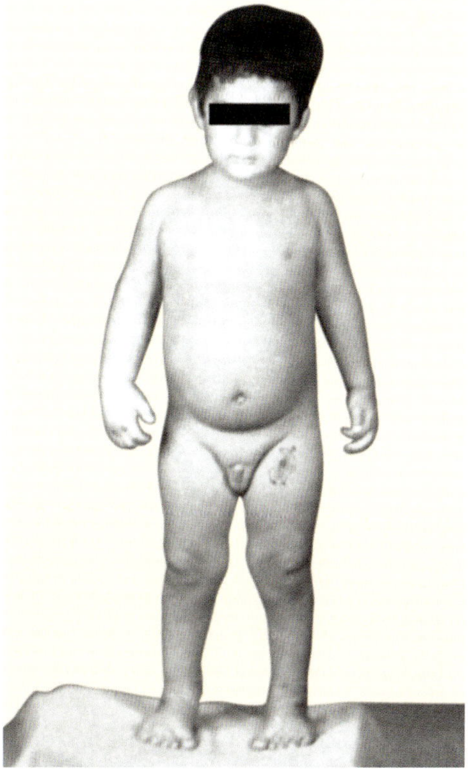

Fig. 18.10: Bardet-Biedl syndrome. Note the central obesity and hypoplastic genitalia

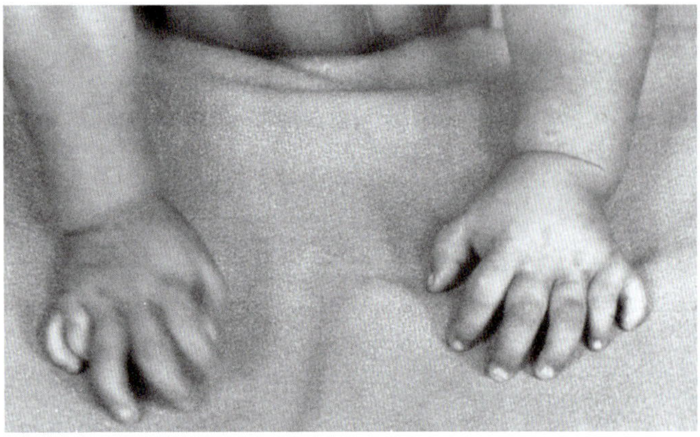

Fig. 18.11: Bardet-Biedl syndrome. Note the polydactyly

While this may reflect central isosexual precocious puberty caused by obesity, it is most likely due to increased fat. These conditions are distinguished by approximating the thumb and index finger around the nipple. Lack of resistance during this procedure indicates lipomastia while breast nodule can be felt as an area of resistance. Obese boys frequently present with concerns of small penile size. This is usually due to penis being buried in the suprapubic pad. Stretched penile length should be measured after pressing the suprapubic pad of fat to ascertain the actual size of penis.

*Investigations:* No workup for etiology is required in children with normal growth, facies and pubertal development. Thyroid profile and evaluation for Cushing syndrome should be done in the presence of growth failure and/or characteristic clinical features. Mildly elevated TSH levels with normal $FT_4$ are common in obese children. This is not the cause of obesity and should not be treated unless TSH is persistently elevated. Cortisol levels may be mildly elevated in obese children and should not be mistakenly diagnosed as Cushing syndrome. Genetic testing for Prader-Willi syndrome should be done in the presence of facial features, history of infantile hypotonia and growth failure. Monogenic causes of obesity should be considered only in the presence of clinical features or pointers to diagnosis.

### Complications

Childhood obesity is associated with significant complications. These are summarized in Table 18.19, and the more important ones are discussed below.

*Endocrine and metabolic:* Endocrine complications are the most important adverse effects of childhood obesity. Central to this is the development of insulin resistance caused by overspill of fat and its deposition in liver and skeletal muscle. Insulin resistance predisposes to development of type 2 diabetes, polycystic ovarian disease, metabolic syndrome and non-alcoholic fatty liver disease (NAFLD). Hyperandrogenism is a common feature in obese girls. Obesity has also been associated with accelerated growth, skeletal maturation and early puberty in girls.

*Cardiovascular system:* Children with obesity have a higher prevalence of dyslipidemia, hypertension and atherosclerosis. Childhood obesity is associated with increased risk of adult coronary disease.

*Non-alcoholic fatty liver disease (NAFLD):* It is present in up to 60% of children with obesity, and in a small proportion it can progress to steatohepatitis and fibrosis.

Table 18.18: Distinguishing features of endogenous causes of obesity

| *Disorder* | *Characteristic features* |
|---|---|
| Prader-Willi syndrome | Low birth weight, feeding difficulties, infantile hypotonia, hyperphagia starting around 1 year of age, almond-shaped eyes, short stature, acromicria (small hands and feet), hypogonadism, cognitive impairment and behavioral abnormalities |
| Bardet-Biedl (BB) and Laurence-Moon (LM) syndromes | Obesity by 1 year of age, visual impairment due to retinitis pigmentosa, polydactyly (BB), syndactyly (LM), notch between tragus and antitragus of ear (LM), spasticity (LM), hypogonadism, renal abnormalities and intellectual disability |
| Beckwith-Wiedemann syndrome | Macrosomia at birth, organomegaly, ear lobe creases, macroglossia, abdominal wall defects and hemihypertrophy |
| Alström syndrome | Obesity, short stature, retinal degeneration, sensorineural hearing loss, dilated cardiomyopathy, type 2 diabetes mellitus |
| Carpenter syndrome | Severe intellectual disability, syndactyly, brachydactyly, clinodactyly, lower limb deformities, undescended testes and cardiac defects |
| Cushing syndrome | Hirsutism, central obesity, growth retardation, striae, buffalo hump, hypertension and myopathy |
| Hypothyroidism | Growth retardation, coarse facies, dry skin and developmental delay |
| Pseudohypoparathyroidism with Albright hereditary osteodystrophy | Obesity, short stature, round face, short neck, short and wide long bones of hands, PTH resistance and hypocalcemic tetany |
| Leptin and leptin receptor deficiency | Infantile onset severe obesity, hyperphagia, hypogonadism, hypothalamic hypothyroidism and adult short stature |
| Mineralocortin-4 deficiency | Infantile onset severe obesity, hyperphagia, increased linear growth and bone mass and subclinical hypothyroidism |
| Hypothalamic obesity | History of brain tumor, radiation or chemotherapy, squint and pituitary hormone defects |

**Table 18.19:** Complications of obesity

| *Category* | *Complications* |
|---|---|
| Metabolic | Insulin resistance, type 2 diabetes, metabolic syndrome, hyperandrogenism |
| Cardiovascular | Hypertension, dyslipidemia, atherosclerosis |
| Gastrointestinal | Non-alcoholic fatty liver disease, gallstones, gastroesophageal reflux |
| Skeletal | Blount's disease, slipped capital femoral epiphysis, fractures |
| Respiratory | Obstructive sleep apnea, hypoventilation syndrome |
| Neurological | Benign intracranial hypertension |
| Psychological | Mood disorders, low self-esteem, risk of being bullied or teased, depression |

## Assessment of Complications

Table 18.20 summarizes the recommendations for screening for various complications of obesity in children.

## Prevention and Management of Overweight and Obesity

Prevention and management of obesity constitute a continuum of efforts aimed at reducing the imbalance between energy intake and output at one end to creating a negative energy balance at the other end. A stepwise approach is suggested, wherein the interventions are scaled up gradually, depending on the severity of obesity, presence of complications, and the response to interventions. The focus is on modifications in diet and lifestyle, but the intensity of the interventions (dietary and physical activity-related) increases at each successive level, with closer supervision, multi-disciplinary care with more frequent contacts with the healthcare team, and need for more committed involvement of the family (Table 18.21).

## Pharmacotherapy for Obesity

Orlistat is approved for use in children with obesity. The drug inhibits gastric lipase resulting in reduced absorption of fat. However, side effects like abdominal pain, bloating and steatorrhea lead to discontinuation of treatment by most patients. Glucagon-like peptide-1 (GLP1) analogs, e.g. liraglutide, have been recently approved for pediatric obesity and type 2 diabetes. Metformin should be used only in the presence of diabetes or polycystic ovarian disease. Overall, pharmacotherapy for obesity has limited utility.

## Specific Management

Specific treatment is initiated in children with hypothyroidism, GH deficiency and Cushing syndrome. Children with mildly elevated TSH level do not need treatment. Children with Prader-Willi syndrome and growth failure may benefit from GH therapy.

**Table 18.20:** Screening for complications of pediatric overweight and obesity

| *Complication* | *Age for screening* | *Tests and their interpretation* | | | |
|---|---|---|---|---|---|
| Prediabetes | Clinical screen at first visit, lab screen for >10 years | HbA1c 5.7 to <6.5%<br>Impaired fasting glucose: Fasting plasma glucose ≥100 but <126 mg/dL | | | |
| Diabetes | Older than 10 years | HbA1c ≥6.5%<br>Fasting plasma glucose ≥126 mg/dL<br>2 hr plasma glucose ≥200 mg/dL during an oral glucose tolerance test | | | |
| Dyslipidemia | First visit, then every 2 years | *Fasting lipids (mg/dL)* | *Normal* | *Borderline* | *Abnormal* |
| | | Triglycerides | | | |
| | | 0–9 years | <75 | 75–99 | ≥100 |
| | | 10–19 years | <90 | 90–129 | ≥130 |
| | | LDL-cholesterol | <110 | 110–129 | ≥130 |
| | | HDL-cholesterol | >45 | 40–45 | <40 |
| Hypertension | Children older than 3 years at every visit | BP is checked and compared against age, gender and height-based charts.<br>• Normal BP: <90th percentile for age and gender in 1–13-yr-old children, and <120/<80 mm Hg in adolescents ≥13 yr.<br>• Elevated BP: ≥90th to <95th percentile in 1–13-yr-old, and 120/<80 to 129/<80 mm Hg in adolescents ≥13 yr.<br>• Stage 1 hypertension: BP ≥95th to <95th percentile + 12 mm Hg in 1–13-yr-old children; and 130/80 to 139/89 mm Hg in ≥13 yr.<br>• Stage 2 hypertension: BP ≥95th percentile +12 mm Hg in 1–13-yr-old children, and ≥140/90 mm Hg in adolescents ≥13 yr. | | | |
| NAFLD | Older than 10 years | ALT >25 U/L (boys), >22 U/L (girls) are considered elevated.<br>Ultrasonography or fibroscan is used for screening for fatty liver. | | | |
| *Others* | *Testing to be done as per symptoms* | | | | |
| Sleep apnea | Polysomnography, if there is snoring, daytime somnolence, lethargy, difficulty in sleeping supine | | | | |
| Hyperandrogenism | Testosterone, LH, SHBG, if there is hirsutism, acne and menstrual irregularities in girls | | | | |
| Psychological | Psychological review, if features of depression, eating disorders, bullying, etc. | | | | |
| Musculoskeletal | Orthopedic review for bone pains, bowing, etc. | | | | |

ALT alanine transaminase; BP blood pressure; HDL high-density lipoprotein; LDL low-density lipoprotein; LH luteinizing hormone; SHBG sex hormone binding globulin; NAFLD non-alcoholic fatty liver disease

**Table 18.21:** Key interventions for prevention and management of obesity in children

| |
|---|
| **Dietary interventions** |
| • Exclusive breastfeeding for first 6 months<br>• Continued breastfeeding till 2 years<br>• Home-based complementary feeding starting at 6 months of life, with avoidance of sugar-sweetened beverages and packaged foods in the first 2 years<br>• Avoid force feeding, overfeeding, skipping of meals and frequent snacking<br>• Traffic light approach—green to be eaten often, yellow in moderation and red sparingly<br>– Green (low energy, high nutrient foods)—fruits and vegetables<br>– Yellow (moderate energy foods)—grains, pulses<br>– Red (high energy, low nutrient foods)—sweets, sweetened beverages, fried foods<br>• Structured and timely meals with appropriate portion size<br>• Increase water intake |
| **Physical activity** |
| • Reduction of sedentary habits<br>• At least 60 minutes/day of moderate to vigorous physical activity (sports, running, dancing, etc.) |
| **Behavioral interventions** |
| • Education to family about importance of healthy diet and activity<br>• Mindful eating, avoid distractions, and avoid grazing<br>• Sleep hygiene (adequate duration and without electronic devices)<br>• Role modeling of desirable behaviors by parents<br>• Positive reinforcements, praise and rewards<br>• Recognize and manage psychosocial co-morbidities (depression, anxiety, etc.)<br>• Limitation of non-academic screen time |





## Treatment of Complications

Complications should be treated early to avoid long-term adverse effects. Metformin is indicated in children with insulin resistance and type 2 diabetes, and polycystic ovarian disease. Statins are the drug of choice for children with persistent dyslipidemia. Children with symptomatic or stage 2 hypertension should receive antihypertensives (enalapril or amlodipine). Treatment of NAFLD includes the use of metformin, vitamin E and pioglitazone. Girls with polycystic ovarian syndrome may benefit from lifestyle modifications, metformin, oral contraceptives and antiandrogens. Medroxyprogesterone acetate is beneficial in children with obesity-hypoventilation syndrome while continuous positive airway pressure may be used in obstructive sleep apnea.

### *Surgical Management*

Bariatric surgery is considered in severe obesity when other measures fail. The intervention is preferred after achieving final height to avoid potential adverse growth effects. Laparoscopic adjustable banding is the recommended procedure in children.

## Suggested Reading

1. Mittal M, Jain V. Management of obesity and its complications in children and adolescents. Indian J Pediatr 2021;88:1222–34.
2. Ranjani H, Mehreen TS, Pradeepa R, et al. Epidemiology of childhood overweight & obesity in India: A systematic review. Indian J Med Res 2016;143:160–74.
3. Styne, Arslanian SA, Connor EL, et al. Pediatric obesity–Assessment, treatment and prevention: An Endocrine Society clinical practice guidelines. J Clin Endocrinol Metab 2017;102:709–57.

*Competencies:* **PE33.8; PE33.10**

# DISORDERS OF THE GONADS

## Puberty

Puberty is the phase of life when secondary sexual characteristics appear and mature, and the capability of reproduction is attained.

### *Physiology*

Puberty involves development of primary (testicular and penile growth in boys and ovarian and uterine growth in girls) and secondary sexual characteristics (pubic and axillary hair growth, change of voice in boys, acne and axillary odor). Sex hormones (estrogen in girls and testosterone in boys) play an important role in the development of primary sexual characteristics, while adrenal androgens are involved in the development of secondary sexual characteristics in girls.

Kisspeptin, a hypothalamic peptide, is the key regulator of puberty. Acting as the 'on-off switch' of puberty, kisspeptin initiates GnRH pulses. Initially, GnRH pulses occur only during nights followed by secretion during both day and night. This leads to increase in the levels of gonadotropins, and thereby, sex hormones. The hypothalamic– pituitary–gonadal axis is under feedback control. Thus secretion of LH is inhibited by testosterone produced by the Leydig cells in boys, and estrogen produced by the theca cells in girls. FSH is inhibited by inhibin produced by the Sertoli cells in boys, and granulosa cells in girls.

### Patterns of Pubertal Development

Puberty starts at around the age of 10 years in girls (range 8–12 years) and is completed over 3–5 years. Breast enlargement (thelarche) is the first event followed by the development of pubic hair (pubarche) and onset of menstrual cycles (menarche). Breast development may be asymmetrical in the initial phase. Menarche usually occurs 2 years after thelarche during stage III or IV. Average age at menarche in Indian girls is about 12 years.

Pubertal development is closely linked to the remaining growth potential of the child. Thus, a girl is expected to gain around 20 cm from breast stage II development and 6–10 cm after menarche. Discordant pubertal development (menarche within one year of thelarche) suggests a hyperestrogenic state with withdrawal bleeding.

In boys, puberty starts with testicular enlargement at 11.5 years (range 9 to 14 years). This is followed by penile enlargement and pubarche; spermarche occurs by 14 years. Peak growth velocity correlates to testicular volume of 10 mL.

### Assessment of Puberty

Pubertal development is assessed using Tanner staging system (*see* Chapter 5, Figs 5.1, 5.2). Breast development beyond Tanner II in girls and testicular volume equal or greater than 4 mL indicate the onset of puberty. Maximum growth spurt occurs during early puberty in girls (Tanner II–III) compared to boys where it occurs later (Tanner III–IV). Menstrual periods are irregular in the first few years before attainment of regular ovulatory cycles. It is important to differentiate adrenarche (pilosebaceous development related to increase in adrenal steroids causing pubarche and change in odor) from gonadarche (genital development related to increase in GnRH causing breast development) in girls.

## Precocious Puberty

Pubertal onset before the age of 8 years in girls and 9.5 years in boys is suggestive of precocious puberty. Precocious puberty may be due to stimulation of the hypothalamic– pituitary axis (gonadotropin-dependent or central precocious puberty) or autonomous sex hormone production (gonadotropin-independent or peripheral).

## Precocious Puberty in Girls

Precocious puberty is common in girls and may represent a normal variation in the age at onset of puberty. In most cases, puberty is slowly progressive with no long-term adverse effect. Endocrine workup should be restricted to girls with progressive forms of puberty.

***Gonadotropin-dependent precocious puberty (central precocious puberty, CPP)*** is much more common than gonadotropin-independent precocious puberty (Table 18.22). In more than 90% cases, no underlying cause is identified. It may be caused by a variety of pathologies of the central nervous system. Hypothalamic hamartoma, a neuronal migration defect, is the commonest cause of organic CPP. The disorder presents with early onset and rapid progression of puberty, seizures and uncontrolled laughter episodes (gelastic epilepsy).

**Table 18.22:** Etiology of precocious puberty in girls

| |
|---|
| **Gonadotropin-dependent or central precocious puberty** |
| *Idiopathic* (in more than 90%) |
| *Tumors:* Hypothalamic glioma |
| *Infections:* Neurotuberculosis, meningitis |
| *Injury:* Head trauma, neurosurgery, cranial irradiation |
| *Malformation:* Hypothalamic hamartoma, arachnoid cyst, hydrocephalus, septo-optic dysplasia |
| **Gonadotropin-independent or peripheral precocious puberty** |
| *Hypothyroidism* |
| *Ovarian estrogen:* McCune-Albright syndrome, cyst, tumor, aromatase excess |
| *Adrenal estrogen:* Estrogenic adrenal adenoma |
| *Exogenous estrogen exposure* |
| **Incomplete variants** |
| Isolated thelarche |
| Isolated pubarche (adrenarche) |
| Isolated menarche |

***Gonadotropin-independent precocious puberty (peripheral precocious puberty, PPP)*** is rare and usually caused by estrogenic ovarian cysts. Fluctuating pubertal development and early vaginal bleeding (due to hyperestrogenic state) is common. Recurrent ovarian cysts should raise the possibility of McCune-Albright syndrome, a somatic activating mutation of stimulatory G protein, which presents with a constellation of cutaneous (multiple café au lait spots), skeletal (multiple fibrous dysplasia) and endocrine abnormalities (hyperthyroidism, rickets and GH excess). Precocious puberty occurs at an early age and is rapidly progressive. Prolonged untreated primary hypothyroidism may induce early puberty due to action of TSH on FSH receptor. Delayed bone age and growth are characteristic features.

### Evaluation

***Clinical:*** History should include the onset, progression and extent of puberty. Exposure to steroids, estrogens and androgens should be enquired. Family history of precocious puberty and early menarche points towards idiopathic CPP. Features of hypothyroidism should be assessed. Advanced growth is characteristic of precocious puberty; growth retardation indicates hypothyroidism or concomitant GH deficiency (Fig. 18.12).

Abdominal examination for adrenal or ovarian mass should be done. Features of McCune-Albright syndrome include café au lait spots, polyostotic fibrous dysplasia, bony deformities and polyendocrinopathy.

***Investigations:*** Assessment of pubertal status is based on basal or stimulated gonadotropin levels. Pooled gonadotropin levels are preferred due to their pulsatile secretion. LH is a better indicator compared to FSH, since the former increases significantly during puberty. LH levels in the pubertal range (basal >0.3 mU/L or stimulated >6 mU/L with LH/FSH ratio >1) is suggestive of development of puberty.

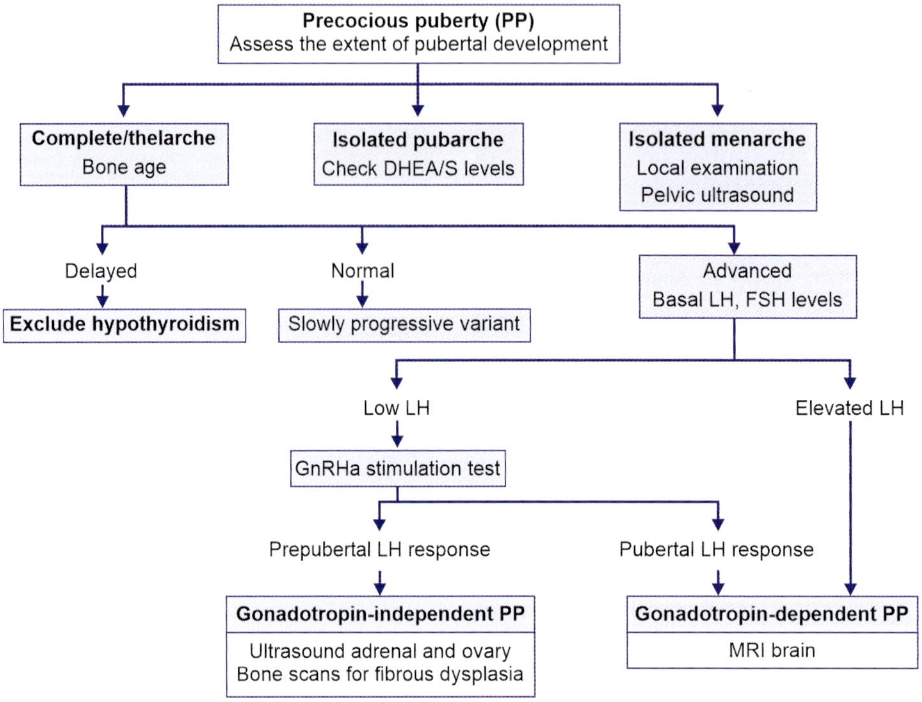


**Fig. 18.12:** Approach to precocious puberty in girls. DHEA/S dehydroepiandrosterone sulfate; FSH follicle-stimulating hormone; GnRHa gonadotropin-releasing hormone agonist; LH luteinizing hormone; MRI magnetic resonance imaging

Bone age is typically advanced, and helps in assessing the height compromise and in predicting final height. Short stature with delayed skeletal maturation suggests the possibility of hypothyroidism and associated GH deficiency. Thyroid function should be assessed to rule out hypothyroidism in these girls.

MRI of brain should be done in girls with onset of puberty before 6 years of age, rapid progression and associated neurological features. Ultrasound of abdomen and pelvis helps in diagnosing follicular cysts and ovarian and adrenal mass. Girls with prepubertal LH levels should undergo ultrasound of ovary and adrenals (for ovarian cyst and adrenal tumor) and skeletal survey (to assess for fibrous dysplasia).

### Management

Aims of management include treatment of underlying cause, management of associations, puberty suppression and achievement of target height potential. The significant long-term consequence of rapidly progressive precocious puberty is short stature. Growth is accelerated at presentation. This is associated with disproportionately advanced bone age resulting in premature epiphyseal fusion culminating in compromised final height.

*CPP:* Long-acting GnRH analogs are effective in improving height outcome in CPP. They cause sustained stimulation and desensitization of pituitary leading to reversal of pubertal changes. GnRH analogs should be considered in girls with early onset (before 6 years of age) rapidly progressive puberty and height compromise (predicted adult height below the target height range). The treatment is discontinued at the chronological age of 11 years and bone age of 12.5 years.

Other drugs used for pubertal suppression include depot medroxyprogesterone acetate (MPA), and cyproterone. MPA does not improve height outcome and may be considered in girls with intellectual disability as a temporary measure to stop or postpone menstruation.

*PPP:* Thyroxine replacement reverses the pubertal changes of hypothyroidism. Treatment for McCune-Albright syndrome is directed towards inhibiting estrogen production (aromatase inhibitors—anastrazole, letrozole) or estrogen action (estrogen receptor antagonist—tamoxifen, fulvestrant). Size and morphological features guide treatment of ovarian cysts.

### Incomplete Variants of Precocious Puberty

These disorders represent normal variants and do not require specific treatment. Their identification helps in restricting the extent of diagnostic workup and counseling.

*Isolated thelarche:* Isolated breast development may represent isolated thelarche or first manifestation of CPP. Bone age, gonadotropin levels and pelvic ultrasound help in differentiating the two conditions. Normal growth, prepubertal LH, age-appropriate bone age and small uterine size suggest isolated thelarche. These children usually present around the age of 1–2 years and show gradual regression of thelarche by 5 years of age.

*Isolated adrenarche:* Premature adrenarche refers to development of pubic hair and acne in the absence of breast development or menarche. Most cases are physiological variants. Rarely, androgen excess due to adrenal (21-hydroxylase deficiency, 11β-hydroxylase deficiency and adrenal tumor) or ovarian (tumor and polycystic ovarian disease) causes may be identified. DHEAS levels above 150 µg/dL suggest a pathological cause. Normal bone age and absence of virilization suggest premature adrenarche and no treatment is required.

*Isolated menarche:* Vaginal bleeding in the absence of thelarche is against the diagnosis of CPP. Vaginal bleeding occurs early in course of estrogen excess states like ovarian cysts, hypothyroidism and McCune-Albright syndrome. Vaginal bleeding without breast development requires evaluation of local causes (infection, foreign body, sexual abuse or tumors).

## Precocious Puberty in Boys

Precocious puberty is less common in boys, but when present is usually associated with a significant pathology. This mandates prompt evaluation and treatment of all boys with precocious puberty.

### Etiology

Gonadotropin-dependent and independent precocious puberty accounts for similar number of cases (Table 18.23).

*CPP:* The etiology is similar to girls, except that organic neurologic causes are common. Hypothalamic hamartoma, glioma, hydrocephalus and tubercular meningitis are important causes (Figs 18.13 and 18.14). These disorders are associated with an increase in testicular volume and elevated basal and GnRH-stimulated LH.

*PPP:* This results from increased androgen production by testes and adrenals, with prepubertal LH levels. Adrenal overproduction due to CAH due to 21-hydroxylase deficiency is a common cause of PPP in boys; adrenal tumors are rare. Human chorionic gonadotropin (hCG) secreting tumors of the liver, mediastinum or brain may present with precocious puberty. Testotoxicosis (familial male-limited precocious puberty), associated with constitutional activation of LH receptor, presents with early onset PPP. Androgen-secreting testicular tumors present with precocious puberty and unilateral testicular enlargement.

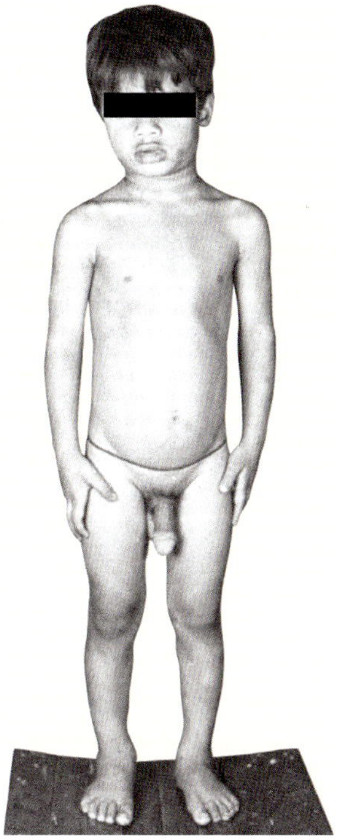

Fig. 18.13: Central precocious puberty secondary to hypothalamic hamartoma

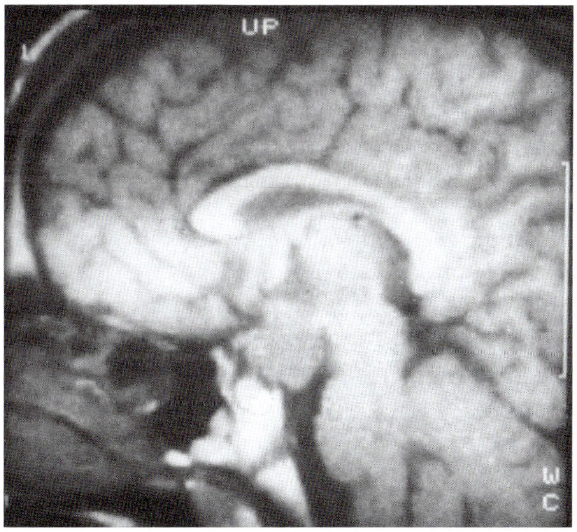


Fig. 18.14: MRI scan showing an isointense mass suggestive of hypothalamic hamartoma

### Evaluation

Evaluation is directed towards confirming the diagnosis and establishing the underlying cause.

*Clinical:* History should include the age at onset and progression of puberty, neurological features, family history of precocious puberty and androgen exposure. Detailed anthropometric and neurological examination is performed. Features of CAH (hyperpigmentation and hypertension) should be identified. Estimation of testicular volume is an integral part of assessment. Prepubertal testicular volume (<4 mL) is characteristic of PPP due to CAH and adrenal tumors; unilateral enlargement is seen in testicular tumors.

*Investigations:* Initial investigations include baseline LH, FSH and testosterone levels, stimulated LH (if required) and bone age. All patients with pubertal LH levels should undergo MRI of brain. In the presence of prepubertal LH levels, imaging for adrenals (preferably CT scan) and 17-OHP levels should be done. The levels of hCG should be estimated, if these investigations are noncontributory (Fig. 18.15).

Table 18.23: Etiology of precocious puberty in boys

| |
|---|
| **Gonadotropin-dependent or central precocious puberty** |
| Idiopathic |
| *Central nervous tumors:* Craniopharyngioma, glioma |
| *Infections:* Tubercular meningitis |
| *Injury:* Head trauma, surgery, radiation |
| *Malformation:* Hamartoma, arachnoid cyst, hydrocephalus |
| **Gonadotropin-independent or peripheral precocious puberty** |
| *Congenital adrenal hyperplasia:* 21-hydroxylase deficiency, 11β-hydroxylase deficiency |
| *Adrenal tumors:* Adenoma, carcinoma |
| *Testicular tumors:* Seminoma, germinoma |
| *Testotoxicosis:* Activation of LH receptor |
| *hCG secreting tumor:* Germinoma, hepatoblastoma |
| *Exogenous androgen exposure:* Testosterone cream |

hCG human chorionic gonadotropin, LH luteinizing hormone

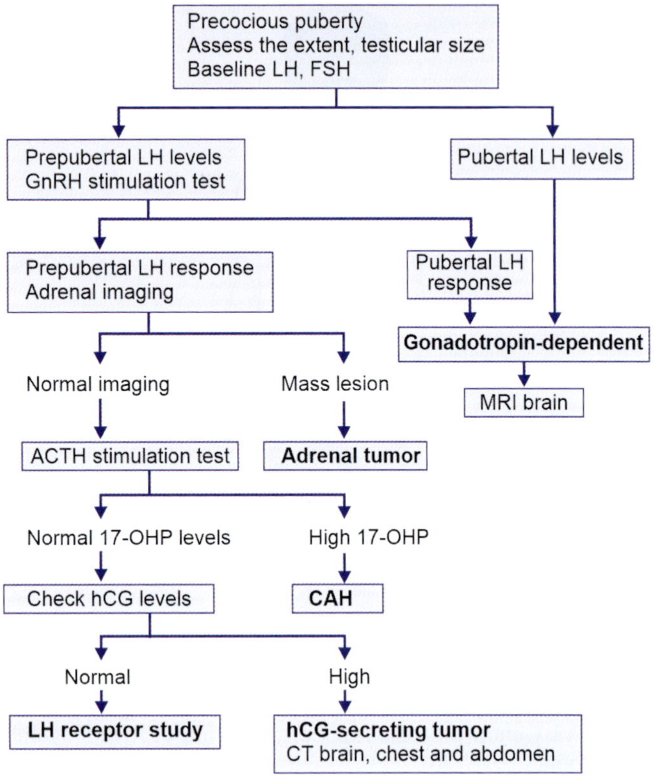


**Fig. 18.15:** Approach to precocious puberty in boys. ACTH adrenocorticotropic hormone; CAH congenital adrenal hyperplasia; CT computed tomography; FSH follicle-stimulating hormone; GnRH gonadotropin-releasing hormone; hCG human chorionic gonadotropin; LH luteinizing hormone; MRI magnetic resonance imaging; 17-OHP 17-hydroxyprogesterone

### *Management*

Management of CPP includes treatment of the underlying pathology and GnRH analog therapy. GnRH analog should be continued till the age of 12 years. CAH is managed with hydrocortisone and fludrocortisone. Surgery is the treatment of choice for adrenal and testicular tumors, while radiotherapy is effective in hCG-secreting tumors. Aromatase inhibitors and antiandrogens are indicated in testotoxicosis.

## Delayed Puberty

Delayed puberty is more common in boys than in girls. Most children with delayed puberty have constitutional delay emphasizing the need for watchful monitoring and a conservative approach.

## Delayed Puberty in Girls

Delayed puberty in girls is defined as lack of secondary sexual characteristics by the age of 13 years. Absence of menarche by the age of 16 years, or 5 years after onset of puberty indicates pubertal delay.

### *Etiology*

Delayed puberty may be caused by defects in the hypothalamic–pituitary axis, ovaries or genital tract (Table 18.24). Defects in the hypothalamic–pituitary axis are associated with low gonadotropin levels (hypogonadotropic hypogonadism). This may be related to reversible causes such as systemic diseases, malnutrition, eating disorders, hyperprolactinemia and hypothyroidism or a self-limited form that improves over time. Irreversible defects include destruction of the hypothalamic–pituitary axis by infection, surgery, radiation or tumor. Defective smell sensation, low GnRH levels and hypogonadotropic hypogonadism characterize Kallmann syndrome, a neuronal migration

**Table 18.24:** Etiology of delayed puberty

**Hypogonadotropic hypogonadism**

***Transient***

- *Self-limited delayed puberty (constitutional delay): Most common cause in boys, less frequent in girls*
- *Systemic disorders:* Renal failure, liver disease, celiac disease, renal tubular acidosis, cystic fibrosis
- *Nutritional disorders:* Malnutrition, anorexia nervosa
- *Endocrine disorders:* Hypothyroidism, hyperprolactinemia, type 1 diabetes

***Permanent***

- *Isolated hypogonadotropic hypogonadism*
  - *Genetic: KAL1, GnRH* receptor, *LH, FSH, CHD7, DAX1 gene mutations*
  - *Dysmorphic syndromes:* CHARGE, Prader-Willi, Laurence-Moon, Bardet-Biedl
- *Multiple pituitary hormone deficiencies*
  - *Malformations:* Holoprosencephaly, septo-optic dysplasia, midline defects
  - *Genetic disorders: PROP1, LH* gene deletions
  - *Brain tumors:* Craniopharyngioma, germinoma, glioma
  - *Brain injury:* Surgery, infection, radiation, trauma
  - *Infiltrative disorders:* Histiocytosis, autoimmune disorders

**Hypergonadotropic hypogonadism**

***In girls***

- *Gonadal dysgenesis:* Turner syndrome, 46,XY with *SRY* deletion, trisomy 18, 13, 21
- *Steroidogenic defects:* StAR, 17α-hydroxylase, 17β-hydroxysteroid dehydrogenase or aromatase deficiency
- *Ovarian insults:* Surgery, radiation, alkylating agents, infections
- *Autoimmune ovarian failure:* Autoimmune polyendocrinopathy
- *Gonadotropin resistance:* LH and FSH receptor mutations

***In boys***

- *Chromosomal abnormalities:* Klinefelter syndrome, gonadal dysgenesis
- *Steroidogenic defects:* StAR, 17α-hydroxylase, 17β-hydroxysteroid dehydrogenase deficiency, Smith-Lemli-Opitz syndrome
- *Testicular insults:* Radiotherapy, chemotherapy, trauma, torsion, infections
- *Malformations:* Vanishing testis syndrome, cryptorchidism
- *Inefficient testosterone action:* 5α-reductase deficiency
- *Resistance to testosterone action:* Androgen insensitivity syndrome

**Isolated amenorrhea in girls**

- *Structural malformations:* Müllerian agenesis, vaginal septum, imperforate hymen
- *Inefficient androgen action:* 46,XY with complete androgen insensitivity syndrome

*DAX1* dosage sensitive sex reversal; FSH follicle-stimulating hormone; GnRH gonadotropin-releasing hormone; LH luteinizing hormone; *KAL1* kallmann syndrome gene 1; StAR steroidogenic acute regulatory protein; *SRY* sex determining region on Y chromosome

defect due to mutation in one of the several genes associated with this syndrome. Hypergonadotropic hypogonadism is associated with defective estrogen production by ovaries and elevated gonadotropin levels. Causes include Turner syndrome, ovarian failure and enzymatic defects in estrogen synthesis.

### Evaluation

Goals of evaluation include identification of constitutional delay, organic etiology requiring neuroimaging and decision regarding treatment.

*Clinical:* Family history of delayed puberty provides a clue to constitutional delay in puberty. Patients are screened for chronic systemic or neurological diseases, Turner syndrome or hypothyroidism, and poor olfactory sensation. Amenorrhea with normal secondary sexual characteristics indicates anatomical defects.

*Investigations:* Workup is directed towards screening for systemic disorders (liver, renal or gastrointestinal disease), followed by estimation of FSH levels and karyotype. Steroidogenic defects are likely, if karyotype and pelvic ultrasound are normal. In patients with low/normal FSH levels, prolactin and thyroid profile is measured to exclude reversible causes. Neuroimaging and pituitary function tests should be done, if these levels are normal.

### Management

All patients with hypergonadotropic hypogonadism and irreversible hypogonadotropic hypogonadism need hormone replacement. Hormone replacement should be deferred till the bone age of 12 years to avoid deleterious effects on height. The goal of treatment is to initiate and maintain sexual characteristics and to prevent osteoporosis. Treatment should be started with low dose estrogens (2 µg ethinyl estradiol, 0.3 mg conjugated estrogen or 0.25 mg estradiol valerate everyday) and gradually increased every 3 months till adult doses (20 µg of ethinyl estradiol, 1.25 mg of conjugated estrogen or 2 mg estradiol valerate daily by 2 years) are reached. Medroxyprogesterone acetate (5–10 mg from day 11 to 21) should be added two years after initiation of treatment or when withdrawal bleeding occurs.

## Delayed Puberty in Boys

Delayed puberty is more common in boys than girls and is usually due to a constitutional delay. Lack of pubertal changes by the age of 14 years is suggestive of delayed puberty in boys.

### Etiology

*Constitutional delay in growth and puberty* is the commonest cause of delayed puberty in boys (Table 18.25). They have growth retardation and delayed bone age. Family history of delayed puberty is present. Gonadotropin levels are prepubertal similar to hypogonadotropic hypogonadism.

*Hypogonadotropic hypogonadism:* This may be reversible due to systemic illnesses or permanent due to neurological insult (e.g. infection, surgery, radiation or tumor). Kallmann syndrome is an important cause of isolated gonadotropin deficiency and presents with impaired smell sensation.

**Table 18.25:** Features suggestive of Turner syndrome

| *Age group* | *Features* |
|---|---|
| Intrauterine period | Increased neck translucency, cystic hygroma |
| Infancy | Cystic hygroma, lymphedema, coarctation of aorta, partial anomalous pulmonary venous return (PAPVR) |
| Childhood and adolescence | Growth failure, hearing defect, delayed puberty, skeletal abnormalities |
| Adulthood | Secondary amenorrhea, infertility |

*Hypergonadotropic hypogonadism* (testicular failure) may be due to chromosome abnormalities (e.g. Klinefelter syndrome), partial gonadal dysgenesis, steroidogenic defects and acquired testicular injury (infection, radiation, or chemotherapy) (Fig. 18.16).

### Evaluation

*Clinical:* Family history of delayed puberty suggests constitutional delay in puberty. History of delayed growth spurt with continued growth in adult years and late onset of shaving in father and brothers is common. Patients are examined for features of systemic disease(s); history of head injury, neurosurgery and intracranial space occupying lesions suggest a defect in the hypothalamic–pituitary axis.

*Investigations:* Initial step includes estimation of LH, FSH and testosterone levels. Elevated gonadotropin levels (hypergonadotropic hypogonadism) should be followed by karyotype (Klinefelter syndrome) and evaluation for biosynthetic defects. Boys with low LH and FSH levels may have constitutional delay in puberty

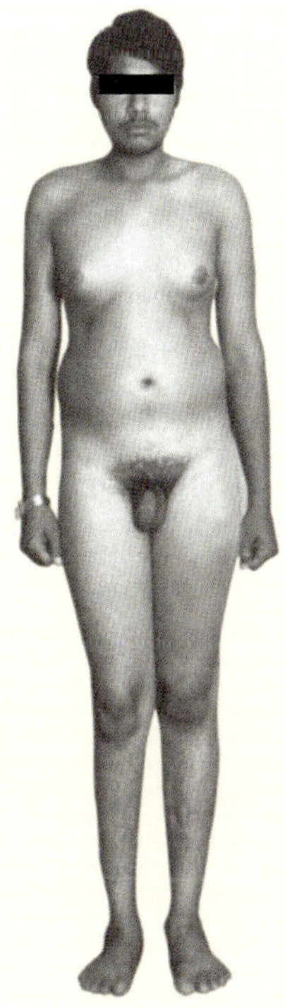

**Fig. 18.16:** Klinefelter syndrome. Note the tall stature and gynecomastia

or hypogonadotropic hypogonadism. Testicular volume below 1 mL points towards a permanent form of delayed puberty, while serum Inhibin B levels above 100 pg/mL are suggestive of constitutional delay. Adolescents with constitutional delay are likely to show a response on stimulation testing with hCG or GnRH. However, these tests are nondiscriminatory in most cases and follow-up after a course of testosterone is the best strategy. Patients with hypogonadotropic hypogonadism should undergo evaluation of hypothalamic–pituitary axis and neuroimaging.

#### *Management*

Testosterone treatment should be deferred till the age of 14 years and bone age of 13.5 years. Boys with suspected constitutional delay in puberty should receive three-monthly injections of testosterone enanthate (50 mg). This should be repeated, if adequate response is not achieved. Serum testosterone levels should be estimated three months after the last dose of the drug. Low testosterone levels indicate hypogonadotropic hypogonadism and the need for continued treatment. Gonadotropin treatment is effective in inducing fertility in hypogonadotropic hypogonadism.

### Turner Syndrome

Turner syndrome is the most important cause of hypergonadotropic hypogonadism in girls. The disorder affects 1 in 2500 newborn phenotypic females. Features in childhood include cubitus valgus (wide carrying angle), shield chest with widely spaced nipples, web neck and short fourth metacarpal (Table 18.25). Cardiac associations such as coarctation of aorta, mitral valve prolapse and aortic stenosis are common. Renal malformations such as horseshoe kidney, duplication of renal pelvis and agenesis may be present. Endocrine associations include hypothyroidism and diabetes mellitus (Table 18.26). The condition is discussed in detail in Chapter 23.

### Suggested Reading


1. Bangalore KK, Fuqua JS, Rogol AD, et al. Use of gonadotropin-releasing hormone analogs in children: Update by an international consortium. Horm Res Pediatr 2019;91:357–72.
2. Fuqua JS. Treatment and outcomes of precocious puberty: an update. J Clin Endocrinol Metab 2013;98:2198–207.
3. Menon PSN, Paulose A. Precocious puberty. In: Desai MP, Menon PSN, Bhatia V, Seth A (eds). Pediatric Endocrine Disorders, 4th edn. Hyderabad: Universities Press Pvt Ltd; 2022, pp 153–69.
4. Watson S, Fuqua JS, Lee PA. Treatment of hypogonadism in males. Pediatr Endocrinol Rev 2014;11(Suppl 2):230–39.


*Competencies:* **PE33.7; PE33.8**

## DIFFERENCES IN SEX DEVELOPMENT

Disorders or differences in sex development (DSD), previously termed as intersex disorders, are rare disorders of aberrant anatomical sexual differentiation.

### Physiology

*In utero*, normal sexual development proceeds in an orderly manner from genetic to gonadal to genital differentiation. Foremost, the sexual differentiation is determined by the karyotype of the fetus. The Y chromosome contains the SRY gene (sex-determining region of the Y chromosome), which encodes a transcription factor that is essential for the development of testes.

***Gonadal differentiation:*** Germ cells arise from the celomic epithelium of hindgut and migrate to the gonadal ridge at 4–6 weeks of gestation. These cells combine with somatic cells to give rise to the undifferentiated gonad that is bipotential and can develop into testes or ovary. Certain genes such as Wilms tumor gene 1 (*WT1*) and steroidogenic factor 1 (*SF1* or *NR5A1*) are needed for gonadal differentiation in both males and females. In the presence of Y chromosome and SRY, testes development ensues. Other genes act in conjunction with *SRY*, namely, *SOX9* (a transcription factor on X

**Table 18.26:** Associations of Turner syndrome and their evaluation

| *System* | *Association* | *Intervention* |
|---|---|---|
| Growth | Growth failure | GH, oxandrolone |
| Puberty | Delayed puberty, secondary amenorrhea, infertility | FSH estimation at 12 years, hormone replacement |
| Cardiovascular system | Coarctation of aorta, bicuspid aortic valve, partial anomalous pulmonary venous return (PAPVR), aortic dissection | Four limb blood pressure, ECG, ECHO at baseline, MRI at 18 years, imaging every 5 years |
| Ear | Otitis media, conductive and sensorineural hearing loss | Hearing assessment, otoscopic examination, hearing aid |
| Eye | Strabismus, ptosis, color blindness | Fundoscopy |
| Orthopedics | Scoliosis, lordosis, reduced cortical density, congenital dislocation of hip | Orthopedic review |
| Renal system | Collecting duct abnormality, horseshoe kidney, positional abnormality | Ultrasound kidney |
| Autoimmune disorders | Hypothyroidism, celiac disease | Thyroid function, tissue transglutaminase antibodies |
| Skin | Pigmented nevi | Monitoring for size |

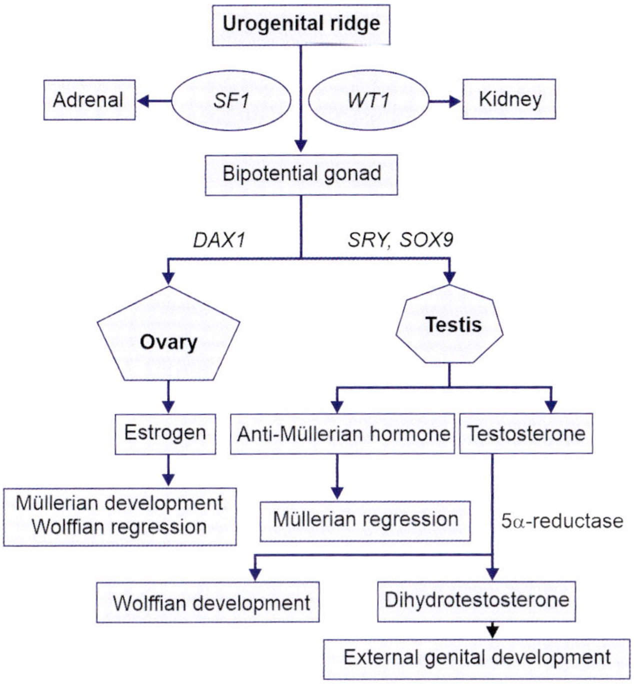


**Fig. 18.17:** The process of sex development (DSD) and its disorders. *DAX1* dosage sensitive sex reversal gene; *SF1* steroidogenic factor 1; *SOX9* transcription factor related to SRY; SRY sex-determining region on the Y chromosome; *WT1* Wilms tumor 1 gene

chromosome) and *DAX1* gene (dosage-sensitive sex reversal) to induce testes development (Fig. 18.17). In the absence of *SRY*, the bipotential gonad develops into ovary. Gonadal differentiation is complete by 7–8 weeks of gestation.

***Genital differentiation:*** The testes secrete anti-Müllerian hormone (AMH) and testosterone. AMH, produced by the Sertoli cells, leads to regression of Müllerian ducts. Testosterone produced by the Leydig cells is responsible for differentiation of Wolffian ducts into vas deferens and seminiferous tubules. Dihydrotestosterone (DHT), produced by the action of 5α-reductase on testosterone, is responsible for male external genital development (testicular descent, scrotal fusion and penile enlargement).

In the absence of testes and AMH production, Müllerian ducts differentiate into fallopian tubes, uterus and the upper two-thirds of the vagina. In the absence of testosterone, Wolffian ducts regress and external genitalia remain undifferentiated. Labioscrotal swellings and urethral folds do not fuse and give rise to labia majora and minora, respectively. The genital tubercle forms the clitoris while canalization of the vaginal plate creates the lower portion of the vagina. Prenatal exposure to androgens may lead to labioscrotal fusion, while exposure thereafter usually causes clitoromegaly alone and no labial fusion.

### Classification

DSD is defined as a discrepancy among the chromosomal, gonadal and genital sex. DSD is classified based on the karyotype as sex chromosomal DSD, 46,XY DSD and 46,XY DSD (Table 18.27).

**Table 18.27:** Karyotype based classification of differences in sex development (DSD)

**46,XX DSD**

- Androgen excess
  - Congenital adrenal hyperplasia
    - o 21-hydroxylase deficiency
    - o 11β-hydroxylase deficiency
    - o 3β-HSD deficiency
    - o POR deficiency
  - Placental aromatase deficiency
  - Maternal virilizing tumors
  - Maternal ingestion of androgenic drugs
- Abnormal gonadal developments
  - Ovotesticular DSDs
  - 46,XX testicular DSD (*SRY+*, *SOX9* duplication)

**46,XY DSD**

- Disorders of androgen synthesis or actions
  - *LHCGR* gene mutations
  - Congenital adrenal hyperplasia
    - o StAR deficiency
    - o 3β-HSD deficiency
    - o 17-hydroxylase/17,20-lyase deficiency
    - o POR deficiency
  - 17β-HSD deficiency
  - 5α-reductase deficiency: Types I and II
  - Androgen insensitivity syndrome: Complete or partial Smith-Lemli-Opitz syndrome
- Abnormal gonadal development
  - Gonadal dysgenesis: Complete or partial
  - Gonadal regression
- Other conditions
  - Persistent Müllerian duct syndrome

**Sex chromosomal DSD**

45,X (Turner syndrome and variants)
47,XXY (Klinefelter syndrome and variants)
45,X/46,XY (mixed gonadal dysgenesis)
46,XX/46,XY (chimeric, ovotesticular DSD)

HSD hydroxysteroid dehydrogenase; LHCGR luteinizing hormone/choriogonadotropin receptor; POR P450 oxidoreductase; StAR steroidogenic acute regulatory protein

#### *Sex Chromosomal DSD*

Sex chromosomal DSD includes patients with abnormal karyotype including mixed gonadal dysgenesis (mosaic karyotype 45,X/46,XY).

#### *XY DSD*

Among 46,XY individuals, defects in testicular differentiation (gonadal dysgenesis) androgen production or action may result in DSD.

***Disorders of gonadal differentiation:*** These disorders are associated with abnormal gonadal development. The gonad is usually a streak (no functional gonadal tissue, also called complete gonadal dysgenesis) or partially functional (partial gonadal dysgenesis). *SRY* gene deletion in a 46,XY male results in development of ovary and female phenotype. Causes of gonadal dysgenesis include mutations in genes involved in the testicular differentiation (*WT1*, *SF1*, *SOX9*, and *DAX1*). These disorders are associated with renal (*WT1* mutation), skeletal (*SOX9*) and adrenal abnormalities (*DAX1*). 46,XY gonadal dysgenesis is associated with the risk of development of gonadal malignancy (gonadoblastoma).

Vanishing testes syndrome consists of absent testes with normal or undervirilized external genitalia. The exact etiology of this condition is not known but postulated to be *in utero* ischemic insult to the testes.

*Inefficient androgen production:* Testosterone biosynthetic defects include deficiency of enzymes involved in steroid and androgen production like StAR, 3β-hydroxysteroid dehydrogenase, 17α-hydroxylase and 17β-hydroxysteroid dehydrogenase. These disorders may be associated with adrenal insufficiency depending on the enzyme that is deficient. Patients have low testosterone levels and testes fail to produce adequate testosterone after hCG injection.

*Inefficient androgen action:* These disorders result from decreased action of androgens. Androgen insensitivity syndrome (AIS) is an X-linked disorder that results from *AR* gene mutation and is characterized by absent or dysfunctional androgen receptor. AIS forms a clinical spectrum ranging from complete feminization to a boy with hypospadias, to a male with infertility. Children with complete AIS have feminized genitalia and may be diagnosed in childhood due to the presence of inguinal mass (palpable testes) or present at puberty with primary amenorrhea. These patients have normal thelarche (due to estrogen formed from high testosterone levels) but absent or sparse pubic and axillary hair.

Patients with 5α-reductase enzyme deficiency have normal testosterone but low levels of DHT leading to undermasculinization. The presentation ranges from female-looking genitalia to variable degrees of undermasculinization (micropenis, undescended testes, incomplete fusion of scrotum or hypospadias). Most children with 5α-reductase deficiency virilize during puberty due to increased testosterone levels. In classical cases, a 46,XY individual with 5α-reductase deficiency reared as a girl presents with spontaneous virilization and gender change at puberty.

#### 46,XX DSD

Increased androgen production during the critical period of fetal development can result in virilization of a 46,XX individual, the most common cause being CAH due to 21-hydroxylase deficiency. It is characterized by deficiency of glucocorticoids and mineralocorticoids with excess androgens levels. Delay in diagnosis may result in fatal salt-wasting crisis, underscoring the importance of early detection. 11β-hydroxylase deficiency, 3β-hydroxysteroid dehydrogenase deficiency and P450 oxidoreductase deficiency (POR) are the other forms of CAH that present with virilization of a 46,XX infant.

Rarely, transplacental transfer of androgens due to maternal medications or hyperandrogenism may lead to fetal virilization. These disorders are readily identifiable by history of virilization in mother. Placental aromatase enzyme converts fetal adrenal androgens to estrogen and deficiency of this enzyme may result in high levels of fetal androgens, virilization of mother during pregnancy and DSD in the newborn.

Other rare causes of 46,XX DSD include gonadal dysgenesis due to genes involved in gonadal development (*WT1* or *SF1*). These patients have normal female external genitalia but fail to undergo normal puberty due to lack of ovaries. Occasionally, an aberrant *SRY* gene translocation in a 46,XX individual can result in testicular development and typical male genitalia.

Ovotesticular DSD (previously called true hermaphroditism) is a condition in which both testes and ovary are present in the same individual. It results from mutations in certain genes involved in gonadal development. The most common karyotype is 46,XX and rarely 46,XY/46,XX or 46,XY/46,XXY chimerism. These patients have a variable presentation ranging from atypical genitalia to abnormal pubertal development.

### Evaluation

The main clinical presentation of DSD consists of atypical genitalia generally noticed at birth (Table 18.28). Sometimes, the genitalia may be normal-looking but the child may present at a later age with inguinal masses (probable AIS) or atypical pubertal development: Virilization in children raised as girls (possible 5α-reductase deficiency), delayed puberty (probable gonadal dysgenesis) or primary amenorrhea (probable complete AIS).

*Clinical:* Family history of genital ambiguity is suggestive of genetic disorders such as 21-hydroxylase deficiency, 5α-reductase deficiency or AIS. CAH is likely, if there is a history of fetal losses and sibling deaths and family history of consanguinity. On the other hand, history of similar disorder in healthy 'genetically male' relatives (brothers, maternal uncles and sons of maternal aunts) is suggestive of an X-linked disorder such as AIS.

Intake of progestational drugs during first trimester and features of virilization in mother should be searched. Failure to thrive, polyuria and lethargy indicate 21-hydroxylase deficiency (Table 18.29). Virilization during puberty is suggestive of 5α-reductase deficiency, while feminization (gynecomastia) indicates AIS.

General examination should include assessment for facial dysmorphism and hyperpigmentation. Maternal

| Table 18.28: Definition of atypical genitalia in a newborn |
|---|
| • Apparent female with clitoromegaly >1 cm |
| • Apparent female with inguinal masses |
| • Apparent male with bilateral cryptorchidism |
| • Apparent male with micropenis (stretched penile length <2.5 cm) |
| • Apparent male with isolated severe degree of hypospadias (penoscrotal or perineal) |
| • Any degree of hypospadias associated with micropenis or undescended testes |

**Table 18.29:** Clinical pointers to etiology of differences in sex development (DSD)

| *Pointer* | *Likely diagnosis* |
|---|---|
| Pigmentation | Congenial adrenal hyperplasia, *SF1* defect, StAR defect |
| Polydactyly | Smith-Lemli-Opitz syndrome |
| Skeletal dysplasia | *SOX9* defect |
| Genital asymmetry | Mixed gonadal dysgenesis, ovotesticular DSD |
| Hypertension | 11β- or 17α-hydroxylase defect |
| Hemihypertrophy | *WT1* mutation |
| Renal failure | Denys-Drash syndrome |

examination for features of hyperandrogenism such as hirsutism, acne and change in voice should be done.

*Genital examination:* The most important step is identification of gonads. Bilaterally rounded structures below the inguinal canal are most likely testis. If they are present, the position of the testes (inguinal or scrotal) should be noted. Unilateral gonads are suggestive of mixed gonadal dysgenesis. The labioscrotal region should be evaluated for the extent of fusion and the presence of separate urethral and vaginal openings. The length of phallus and the position of urethra should be recorded for the presence of hypospadias. In virilized females, the genitalia is staged according to the classification proposed by Prader from grades I to V, with grade I representing female with clitoromegaly and V male-looking genitalia with cryptorchidism. Müllerian structures may be confirmed by rectal examination.

*Investigations:* Initial investigations for a child with DSD presenting with atypical genitalia should include karyotyping, estimation of serum electrolytes and 17-OHP, and pelvic ultrasound. Fluorescent *in situ* hybridization (FISH) is used to confirm the presence of Y chromosome. Ultrasound of pelvis helps to identify intra-abdominal gonads and Müllerian structures.

In girls with common urogenital sinus, a genitogram is helpful to determine the level of fusion of the vagina with the common urogenital sinus, which is of surgical importance. Further investigations are guided by clinical and laboratory evaluation.

Presence of clitoromegaly and no palpable gonads in a child with 46,XX karyotype as well as Müllerian structures on ultrasound indicate an androgen excess state and the need for estimation of serum 17-OHP to rule out CAH. Similarly absence of Müllerian structures in a child with 46,XY karyotype is suggestive of inefficient testosterone production or action with normal sertoli cell function and should be evaluated with estimation of testosterone and DHT. The presence of both Müllerian structures and palpable gonads indicates gonadal dysgenesis or ovotesticular DSD. Absent gonads and Müllerian structures may be caused by vanishing testis syndrome or dysfunctional intra-abdominal testis. Estimation of levels of AMH and hCG stimulation test are helpful in differentiating these two conditions. Children with vanishing testis will have low levels of AMH and low testosterone response to hCG stimulation.

## Management

Management involves parental counseling, decision about sex of rearing, timing of surgical correction and gonadectomy.

*Parental counseling:* Birth of a child with DSD generates significant parental anxiety and stress. The most important aspect of counseling is reassurance of parents that the child is healthy and can be managed with appropriate surgical and/or medical treatment. Gender-specific connotation ('he or she', 'his or her', 'testis or ovary') should be avoided and neutral terms like 'child' or 'baby' and ' gonads' and 'phallus' be used during counseling.

*Decision about gender of rearing:* Gender assignment should depend on the potential for future sexual and reproductive function, anatomical status, feasibility of reconstructive surgery and social acceptance and norms. 46,XX girls with virilization disorders usually have potential for fertility and should be reared as females. Individuals with complete AIS should also be reared as females. Decision of gender of rearing is difficult in disorders of inefficient androgen production and action. This should depend on genital appearance, surgical feasibility and psychological evaluation.

*Surgery:* In virilized girls with CAH, most centers perform clitoroplasty at the age of 1 year with vaginoplasty later during puberty for girls with vaginal stenosis. Gonadectomy should be done in gonadal dysgenesis or ovotesticular DSD, if a Y cell line is present, as there is a risk of gonadal malignancy. In undervirilized males, hypospadias repair and chordee correction are generally done in early childhood.

## Cryptorchidism (Undescended Testes)

Cryptorchidism is present in about 3% of full-term infants and 20% of premature infants. In most of these cases, testes descend spontaneously by the age of one year with a decrease in the prevalence to 1%. Spontaneous testicular descent is unlikely after the age of one year and the prevalence in adult population is 0.8%.

### Etiology

Most children with undescended testis do not have an identifiable underlying cause. Endocrine causes account for only a small proportion. The possibility of salt-wasting 21-hydroxylase deficiency presenting with sex reversal should be considered in newborns with bilateral cryptorchidism. Undescended testis may be associated with hypopituitarism, dysmorphic syndromes and disorders of androgen production and action.

### Evaluation

It is important to differentiate true undescended testis from retractile or ectopic testis due to therapeutic and prognostic implications. Poorly developed scrotum and inability to bring down the testis to the scrotal sack suggests true undescended testis. Retractile testis is an otherwise fully descended testis that has an active cremasteric reflex, which retracts it into the groin.

Penoscrotal hypospadias and genital ambiguity are suggestive of disorders of androgen production or action. The hCG stimulation test and serum AMH levels should be done in boys with bilateral nonpalpable testis to differentiate abdominal testis from anorchia.

#### Management

Undescended testis is associated with significant complications like torsion, trauma, inguinal hernia, testicular dysfunction and development of malignancy. These children should be treated early because of the increased risk for malignancy and infertility in later life. Surgery is the only approved therapy for undescended testis due to potential adverse effects of hCG on germ cells. Surgery should be done within the first year of life.

18

Essential Pediatrics

### Micropenis

A penis whose length in stretched position is less than 2 SD below the mean for the age is termed micropenis. Most often it is the result of primary or secondary testicular failure.

#### Etiology

Micropenis results from decreased androgen action during fetal life. It may be due to hypogonadotropic hypogonadism as in Kallmann syndrome, Prader-Willi syndrome, septo-optic dysplasia, or Klinefelter syndrome. It may also be a manifestation of partial androgen insensitivity syndrome or testosterone biosynthetic defects.

#### Evaluation

Penile length should be measured in a fully stretched state by grasping the glans between thumb and forefinger. A firm ruler or caliper should be pressed against the pubic ramus to depress the suprapubic fat pad. The measurement should be made along the dorsum to the tip of the glans penis excluding the length of foreskin. Penile size is often underestimated in boys with obesity (due to the suprapubic fat) and hypospadias (due to chordae). Investigations should include estimation of gonadotropins and testosterone levels, if the child has been evaluated during mini-puberty of infancy (between 3 weeks to 8 months of age) or puberty. Otherwise, between the age of 1 to 10 years, these levels are physiologically low, and will require stimulation testing for further interpretation. Low gonadotropins and testosterone levels indicate hypogonadotropic hypogonadism.

#### Management

All boys with micropenis are treated with a course of low dose testosterone (25 mg testosterone enanthate or cypionate monthly for three doses). The aim of this short course of testosterone treatment is to increase penile length and not to induce puberty. Boys with micropenis should be reared as males as normal sexual function is usually attainable with early intervention.

### Suggested Reading


1. Ahmed SF, Achermann JC, Arlt W, et al. UK guidance on the initial evaluation of an infant or an adolescent with a suspected disorder of sex development. Clin Endocrinol. 2011;75:12–26.
2. Penson D, Krishnaswami S, Jules A, McPheeters ML. Effectiveness of hormonal and surgical therapies for cryptorchidism; a systematic review. Pediatrics 2013;131:e1897–1907.
3. Rey RA, Grinspon RP. Normal male sexual differentiation and etiology of disorders of sex development. Best Pract Res Clin Endocrinol Metab 2011;25:221–38.


*Competencies:* **PE33.4; PE33.5**

## DIABETES MELLITUS

Diabetes mellitus is a metabolic disorder characterized by hyperglycemia and glycosuria. The factors that contribute to hyperglycemia include decreased insulin secretion and its action as well as increased glucose production. Hyperglycemia resulting from diabetes mellitus causes damage to several organs and body systems, including the kidneys, eyes and cardiovascular system. While type 1 diabetes caused by insulin deficiency remains the predominant form in children, type 2 diabetes has emerged as an important entity in adolescents with obesity.

### Diagnostic Criteria

The definition of diabetes in children is similar to adults. Fasting blood glucose more than 126 mg/dL (7 mmol/L), postprandial blood glucose (two hours after an oral glucose load of 75 g) of more than 200 mg/dL (11.1 mmol/L) or random blood glucose greater than 200 mg/dL with classical symptoms is diagnostic of diabetes mellitus.

Glycated hemoglobin or hemoglobin A1c (HbA1c) is now accepted as a diagnostic criterion for diabetes in adults with levels greater than 6.5% indicating diabetes. The validity of HbA1c as the sole diagnostic criteria in children and adolescents is still disputed. Most children with type 1 diabetes have blood glucose level substantially higher than 200 mg/dL and do not need a glucose tolerance test (GTT). Tolerance testing is restricted to children with obesity and suspected type 2 diabetes. The test is performed after adequate carbohydrate intake for three days (150 $g/m^2$/day) and overnight fast. The child is given glucose (1.75 g/kg, maximum 75 g) as a chilled liquid with blood glucose measurements done at 0 and 120 minutes.

### Classification

Most children with diabetes have type 1 diabetes caused by damage to beta cells of pancreas (Table 18.30). Type 2 diabetes is an important cause in adolescents with obesity. Other forms of childhood diabetes include genetic forms of diabetes (monogenic diabetes of young, MODY) and neonatal diabetes.

In most situations, the type of diabetes is evident on clinical presentation and extensive diagnostic workup is not required. Investigations for classification of diabetes are reserved for children with onset after puberty (likely to be type 2 diabetes or MODY), no ketoacidosis at diagnosis (likely to be type 2 diabetes or MODY), those with obesity and acanthosis nigricans (likely to be type 2 diabetes) or in the presence of abdominal pain and steatorrhea (exocrine pancreatic disorder).

Investigations for classification for diabetes include ultrasound abdomen (for pancreatic calcification), levels

**Table 18.30:** Classification of diabetes mellitus (American Diabetes Association 2014)

| |
|---|
| **Type 1 diabetes mellitus**<br>Absolute insulin deficiency due to beta cell destruction: Up to 95% of all pediatric diabetes<br>1. IA (autoimmune)<br>2. IB (non-autoimmune) |
| **Type 2 diabetes mellitus**<br>Insulin resistance with relative insulin deficiency: 10–50% of diabetes in adolescents depending on ethnicity served |
| **Other specific types of diabetes mellitus**<br>• *Genetic defects of beta cell function:* Maturity onset diabetes of the young (MODY), neonatal diabetes, mitochondrial disorders, Wolfram syndrome<br>• *Genetic defects in insulin action:* Insulin receptor defects, lipodystrophy, type A insulin resistance, Rabson-Mendenhall syndrome<br>• *Diseases of exocrine pancreas:* Pancreatitis, trauma pancreatectomy, cystic fibrosis, fibrocalcific pancreatic disease, hemochromatosis<br>• *Endocrinopathies:* Growth hormone excess, Cushing syndrome, hyperthyroidism<br>• *Drug or chemical induced:* Steroids, L-asparaginase, cyclosporine, tacrolimus, interferon, pentamidine, thiazides, diazoxide, phenytoin<br>• *Infections:* Congenital rubella, cytomegalovirus<br>• *Uncommon forms:* Stiff-man syndrome, anti-insulin receptor antibodies |
| **Gestational diabetes**<br>Diabetes diagnosed in the second and third trimesters of pregnancy that is clearly not overt diabetes |

of C-peptide (a marker of beta cell function), glutamic acid decarboxylase (GAD) and insulin autoantibodies (indicators of autoimmune nature of type 1 diabetes) and genetic analysis for MODY (Table 18.31). The disease classification is often challenging as C-peptide levels may be low due to glucotoxicity in the initial stage of type 2 diabetes and autoantibodies are positive in only 60% of Indian children with type 1 diabetes.

## Type 1 Diabetes Mellitus

Type 1 diabetes is the commonest form of childhood diabetes characterized by insulin deficiency due to damage to beta cells of pancreas. The disorder requires lifelong insulin replacement.

### *Epidemiology*

There is a significant geographic variation in the incidence of type 1 diabetes. Scandinavia has the highest incidence, with Finland having the incidence of 35/100,000/year. Indian data suggest an incidence of 10.5/100,000/year. Type 1 diabetes can occur at any age but has two discernible age peaks of higher incidence. The first peak occurs around 5 to 7 years is related to exposure to viral infections, while the second peak around puberty is linked to increase in GH and sex steroids.

### *Pathogenesis*

Children born to parents with type 1 diabetes have a higher risk of developing the disease. The risk is higher, if the affected parent is father (7% compared to 4%, if mother is affected). If a sibling is affected, the risk is 6% when the onset is before 10 years of age and 3% thereafter. The role of heredity is less significant in type 1 diabetes compared to type 2. In studies on identical twins, concordance rates of only 30–40% have been reported for type 1 diabetes suggesting that factors other than heredity play an important role in the pathogenesis.

The most important genetic focus for type 1 diabetes lies on chromosome 6 and is linked with expression of HLA antigens. HLA-DR3 and DR4 are important determinants of developing type 1 diabetes. The genes implicated in pathogenesis include insulin gene and cytotoxic T lymphocyte antigen 4 (*CTLA4*). Together these genes can explain around 60% heritability of type 1 diabetes. Protection against the disease is provided by the HLA-DR2 haplotype.

Infections predisposing to type 1 diabetes include mumps, coxsackievirus, cytomegalovirus and rubella (congenital rubella syndrome). There is increasing evidence

**Table 18.31:** Differentiating features of common causes of diabetes in children

| *Feature* | *Type 1 diabetes mellitus* | *Type 2 diabetes mellitus* | *Maturity onset diabetes of the young (MODY)* |
|---|---|---|---|
| Age at onset | Any age; most common in children | Adults and adolescents | Adults and adolescents |
| Onset of disease | Acute | Insidious | Insidious |
| Diabetic ketoacidosis at onset | 30–60% | 5–25% | Less than 5% |
| Family history of diabetes | 5–10% | 75–90% | 100% |
| Obesity | Around 20% | More than 90% | Unusual |
| Acanthosis nigricans | Absent | Usually present | Absent |
| Insulin requirement | Universal | Variable | Variable |
| C-peptide levels | Low | High or normal | Low-normal |
| Insulin sensitivity | Normal | Low | Normal |
| Islet cell antibodies | 40–70% | Unusual | Negative |
| Management | Insulin | Diet, metformin | Diet, sulfonylurea |

that early introduction of cow milk protein may be an important factor in the subsequent development of diabetes in genetically susceptible infants.

There is substantial evidence for autoimmunity in type 1 diabetes. Lymphocytic infiltration around the beta cells is found on autopsy of individuals of type 1 diabetes who die due to incidental causes. At diagnosis, 70–80% of children with type 1 diabetes have antibodies against one or more of the several islet cell antigens (ICA). These antibodies usually predate the clinical presentation of insulin-dependent diabetes mellitus by a few months or years. This suggests that they play a major role during the initial pathogenesis of the disease.

### Clinical Features

Children and adolescents usually present with symptoms of diabetes that are ongoing for a month or two prior to seeking physician's contact, with an acute increase in symptoms over the previous week. Symptoms of type 1 diabetes include polyuria, nocturia, enuresis, polydipsia, recent weight loss, polyphagia and fatigue. Recent acute infection is often noted at presentation. Unfortunately, these symptoms are often ignored resulting in delayed diagnosis.

### Course of Illness

Insulin is the mainstay of therapy. Once insulin is initiated, blood glucose levels gradually decline. Often, after few weeks of insulin therapy, the need for exogenous insulin declines, due to a transient recovery of insulin secretion. This phase is called the "honeymoon phase of diabetes". Some children may be completely insulin-free during this time. This phase lasts from a few weeks to months, and rarely to one year, after which the need for insulin gradually increases.

### Ambulatory Care

Day-to-day management of type 1 diabetes involves management of glycemic control, and avoidance of acute complications and prevention of chronic complications on one hand and achieving social, scholastic and psychological goals of the child on the other. Comprehensive education and ongoing involvement with the family is mandatory. Teamwork approach with pediatrician/endocrinologists, diabetic nurse educator, social worker and nutritionist is essential.

### Insulin

Insulin is the cornerstone of type 1 diabetes management. The body secretes insulin at a basal rate with intermittent secretion with meals. The aim of management is to mimic this pattern as best as possible.

***Dose:*** Insulin dose is guided by pubertal status with lower dose for prepubertal children (0.6 unit/kg/day) compared to pubertal (1.0–1.2 unit/kg/day) and post-pubertal children (1.0 unit/kg/day). In the post-ketoacidosis phase, the dose may be as high as 2–2.5 unit/kg/day.

***Preparations:*** Chemical modifications of insulin alter their action profile providing flexibility in tailor made insulin regimen. Currently all available forms of insulin are derived by recombinant DNA technology (Table 18.32).

***Short-acting (regular) insulin:*** Regular insulin that is structurally the same as natural insulin, is the agent of choice for IV infusion while managing diabetic ketoacidosis (DKA). On subcutaneous administration, the medication forms hexamers in the skin, delaying onset of action by 30–60 minutes. Regular insulin should hence be given 30 minutes before a meal, which may be a problem in young children and toddlers with unpredictable eating patterns. The longer duration of action is helpful, if there is a substantial gap between meals especially in school-going children who have early breakfast and late lunch.

***Rapid-acting insulins (lispro, aspart, glulisine, and fast-acting aspart):*** These insulins do not form hexamers after injection and have immediate onset of action. They are ideal for toddlers with irregular eating patterns and can be given even after a meal. They provide better post-meal glycemic control compared to regular insulin and reduce the risk of hypoglycemia.

***Intermediate-acting insulin (NPH):*** NPH is a chemically modified insulin (protamine) with prolonged duration of action of 12–18 hours. It is traditionally used with short-acting insulin for split-mix regime, but has significant intra-individual variability in absorption resulting in fluctuating glycemic control.

***Long-acting insulin (glargine, detemir and degludec):*** These long-acting forms provide peakless cover for 18–36 hours. They are useful as basal insulin in basal-bolus regimen.

**Table 18.32:** Pharmacokinetic profile of insulin preparations

| *Preparation* | *Onset* | *Peak* | *Duration* | *Indications* |
|---|---|---|---|---|
| *Rapid-acting*<br>Lispro, Aspart, Glulisine | 5–10 min | 1–3 hr | 3–4 hr | For use with insulin pump, as the bolus insulin in multiple daily injections (MDI) regimes |
| *Short-acting*<br>Regular | 30–60 min | 2–4 hr | 5–8 hr | Diabetic ketoacidosis (DKA), mix-split regimen |
| *Intermediate-acting*<br>NPH | 1–2 hr | 2–8 hr | 16–24 hr | Mix-split regimen, basal bolus regimen |
| *Long-acting* | | | | |
| Glargine | 2–4 hr | Peakless | 20–24 hr | Basal insulin |
| Detemir | 1–2 hr | 6–12 hr | 20–24 hr | Basal insulin, mix-split regimen |
| Degludec | 0.5–1 hr | Peakless | >24 hr | Basal insulin |

### Insulin Regimen

The decision about the choice of insulin regimen is dependent on age, socioeconomic status and level of glucose control of a child. A physiological regimen with multiple daily injections is preferred in most children with the exception in a resource-poor setting where a conventional regimen is more practical.

***Basal-bolus regimen:*** Basal-bolus regimen tries to mimic physiological insulin secretion with the use of a long-acting basal insulin (detemir or glargine, 40–50% of total daily dose in older children, and 25–30% in children below 5–6 years of age) and mealtime rapid-acting analog (aspart, glulisine or lispro, remaining total daily dose, Fig. 18.18). The mealtime dose is distributed over 3–5 times a day depending on the diet pattern of the child. This regimen offers flexibility, as changes in mealtimes do not cause significant fluctuations in glycemic control. The risk of hypoglycemia is also lower compared to split-mix regimen.

***Mix-split regimen (two or three injections per day, Fig. 18.19):*** This involves the combination of short- and intermediate-acting insulins mixed at the time of injection. The injections are given 30 minutes before breakfast (two-thirds of daily dose) and 30 minutes before dinner (one-third of daily dose). The ratio of short- to intermediate-acting insulin is 1 to 2. This regimen has the advantage of less frequent injections and lower cost. The regimen requires rigid dietary control and strict lifestyle with regular mealtimes and snacks. In a variation of the regimen, another dose of regular injection is given before lunch. In yet another variation, the intermediate-acting insulin is shifted to bedtime to prevent nocturnal hypoglycemia and morning hyperglycemia (Fig. 18.20).

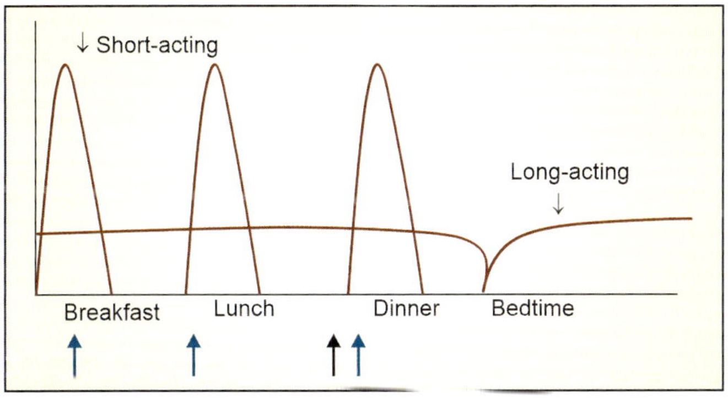


**Fig. 18.18:** Basal-bolus regimen. Intermediate- (NPH) or long-acting insulin (glargine or detemir) is given before dinner or at bedtime (40–50% of total daily dose; black arrow). Rapid- or short-acting insulin (aspart or lispro) is given before each meal (50–60% of total daily dose; blue arrows)

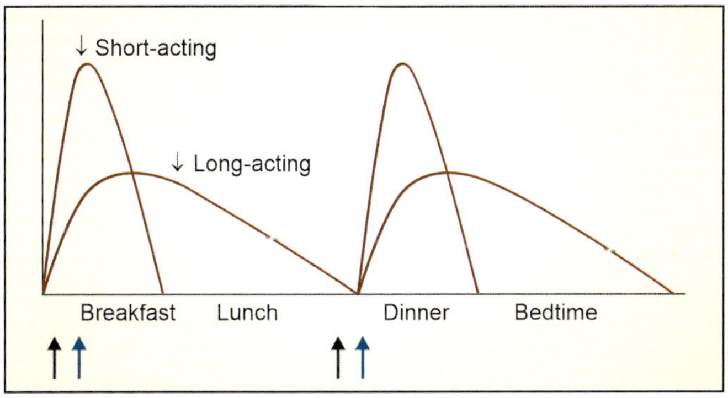


**Fig. 18.19:** Split-mix regimen. Insulin is given before breakfast (two-thirds of daily dose) and dinner (one-third of daily dose). Each injection is a combination of intermediate- or long-acting (NPH or detemir; two-thirds of the total dose; black arrows) and short- (regular) or rapid-acting insulin (lispro or aspart, one-third of the total dose; blue arrows). Regular meal pattern is required to prevent hypoglycemia

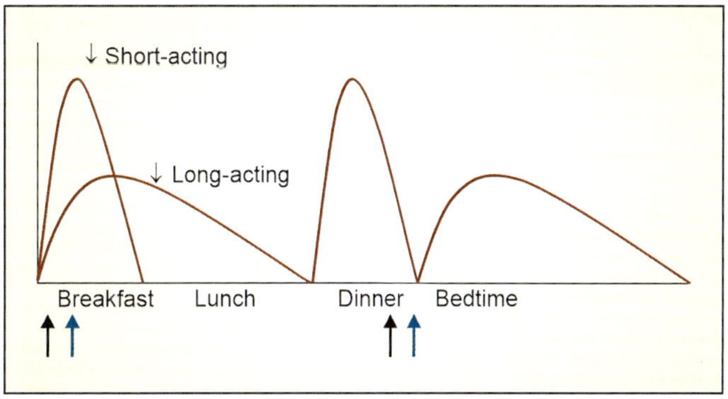


**Fig. 18.20:** Modified mix-split regimen. The night-time intermediate-acting insulin has been shifted from before dinner to bedtime. This is indicated in the presence of nocturnal hypoglycemia and high pre-breakfast blood glucose levels. Delayed administration and thereby peak of intermediate-acting insulin reduces the risk of nocturnal hypoglycemia on one hand while providing reasonable cover for morning hyperglycemia

***Continuous subcutaneous insulin infusion (CSSI) or insulin pump:*** Insulin pump is an external device that infuses insulin at a predetermined rate with additional boluses given at mealtime. The basal dose can be adjusted for different times of the day and boluses tailored to different amount and types of meals to provide good glycemic control with limited glycemic variability. Insulin pump is superior to basal-bolus regimen in terms of insulin requirement, glycemic variability and weight gain. Closed loop systems and insulin pumps with capability to detect blood glucose levels and infusing desired amount of insulin have also been introduced, and provide a more physiological glycemic control.

### Diabetes Education

Structured diabetes education is mandatory for the management of diabetes in children. Key areas to be covered in the program include pathophysiology of diabetes, insulin use, sick day management, hypoglycemia, nutrition, physical activity and social issues (Table 18.33).

### Nutritional Management

The key to successful nutritional management in type 1 diabetes is flexibility. Overzealous control is associated with rebellious behavior and dietary indiscretion. There is no 'diabetic diet' for children and they should be encouraged to have a normal healthy diet. Importance should be given to consistency of meal timings. Dietary exchanges and a 'nutritional pyramid approach' are useful in providing variety for children. Occasional treats during

**Table 18.33:** Diabetes education in children with type 1 disease

| *Category* | *Should know* | *May know* | *Optional* |
|---|---|---|---|
| Disease | Diabetes is a lifelong disease | Role of insulin as life-saving therapy | Glucose homeostasis |
| | Normal outcome is possible with appropriate therapy | Differences of type 1 vs. 2 diabetes | Disease classification |
| | | Pathophysiology of diabetes | Role of autoimmunity |
| | | Complications | Disease associations |
| Treatment | Insulin is the only mode of treatment | Insulin preparations | Insulin regimens |
| | Daily injections are a must | Time course of injections | Insulin pumps |
| | Physical activities | Injection devices | Newer insulins |
| | No alternative medicine | Exercise and sports | Competitive sports |
| Skills | Insulin storage | Glycemic targets | Ketone monitoring |
| | Drawing up and mixing of insulin | Insulin changes | Glucagon injection |
| | Insulin injection techniques | Ketone monitoring | |
| | Self-monitoring of blood glucose | | |
| | Diabetes diary and log | | |
| Nutrition | Healthy eating | RDA for age | Carbohydrate counting |
| | Avoid simple sugars | Food exchanges | Insulin to carb ratio |
| | Mid-meal snacks | High fiber intake | Glycemic index |
| Follow-up | Honeymoon phase | Role of HbA1c | CBGM |
| | Hypoglycemia | Complications; DKA prevention | Transplantation |
| | Sick day guidelines | Physical activity | Career counseling |

CBGM continuous blood glucose monitoring; DKA diabetic ketoacidosis; RDA recommended dietary allowances

**Table 18.34:** Nutritional guidelines for type 1 diabetes

| *Component* | *Recommendation* | *Implication* |
|---|---|---|
| Energy | 100% of RDA | No restriction |
| Carbohydrate | 50–55% of calories<br>Low GI carbohydrate | No restriction<br>Reduced sugar intake |
| Fat<br>• Saturated<br>• Polyunsaturated<br>• Monounsaturated<br>• Cholesterol | 25–40% of energy<br><10% of total energy<br><10% of total energy<br>>10% of total energy<br><300 mg/day | Less saturated fat<br>Less red meat, whole milk |
| Protein | 10–15% of calories | No restriction |
| Fiber | More than 10 g/day | More fruits, vegetables |

GI glycemic index; RDA recommended daily allowance

special occasions and eating out are allowed, if covered appropriately with insulin (Table 18.34).

### Monitoring

***Self-monitoring of blood glucose (SMBG):*** SMBG is critical for management of type 1 diabetes. It should ideally be done before each meal and at bedtime. Post-meal and midnight blood glucose levels are measured as required, adjusted according to the patient age (Table 18.35). In children with significant glycemic variability, continuous glucose monitoring system (CGMS) provides information about glycemic control every 5 minutes over a 72-hour period to help decide about insulin adjustment.

**Table 18.35:** Age-related glycemic targets for self-monitoring of blood glucose

| *Target* | *<6 years* | *6–12 years* | *>12 years* |
|---|---|---|---|
| Blood glucose | | | |
| Premeal | 100–180 mg/dL | 70–180 mg/dL | 70–130 mg/dL |
| Bedtime | 110–200 mg/dL | 100–180 mg/dL | 90–140 mg/dL |
| HbA1c | Less than 8% | Less than 7.5% | Less than 7% |

***Hemoglobin A1c:*** HbA1c is a marker of glycemic control over previous 3 months and is the best predictor of long-term complications. Target levels for HbA1c are less than 7% in children and adolescents. These levels may be falsely low in children with sickle cell disease and increased red cell turnover as in hemolytic anemia. Falsely elevated HbA1c levels are seen with uremia and high dose aspirin treatment.

#### Follow-Up

Children with diabetes should be followed every three months or more frequently as needed. Clinical assessment should include assessment of growth, puberty, blood glucose levels, and examination of injection sites and care of feet. Children with unexplained hypoglycemia should be evaluated for adrenal insufficiency, hypothyroidism and celiac disease. Puberty is associated with an increase in insulin requirement. The requirement further increases in adolescents with obesity.

#### Sick Day Care

Key aspects of sick day management include frequent self-monitoring of glucose, regular fluid intake and treatment of the intercurrent illnesses. Insulin requirement usually increases during a febrile illness but may decrease with vomiting and diarrhea. Basal insulin should never be omitted in sick children with type 1 diabetes. In children with blood glucose less than 80 mg/dL, rapid-acting insulin should be withheld and the dose of intermediate-acting insulin is reduced by 20–30%. No extra insulin is required in children with febrile illness and blood glucose between 80 and 270 mg/dL. Blood or urine ketones should be measured, if blood glucose is more than 270 mg/dL. Children with moderate ketosis (blood ketones between 1 and 1.5 mmol/L) should be given extra regular insulin (10% of total daily dose). Impending DKA (blood ketone >1.5 mmol/L) is managed with extra doses of regular insulin (15–20% of total daily) and hourly blood glucose monitoring (Fig. 18.21). The child should be hospitalized, if recurrent vomiting, poor oral intake and persistent hyper- or hypoglycemia are present.

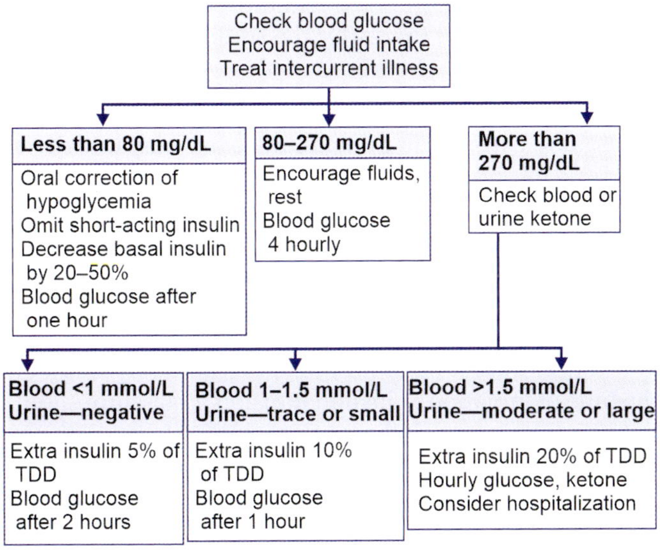


**Fig. 18.21:** Guidelines for sick day management in children with type 1 diabetes mellitus. TDD total daily dose

### Acute Complications of Type 1 Diabetes

#### Hypoglycemia

In patients with diabetes, hypoglycemia is defined as blood glucose <70 mg/dL. It is quite common in children and is an impediment to optimal glycemic control. It should be considered in the presence of autonomic (e.g. sweating, palpitations, tremor, and hunger) or neuroglycopenic symptoms (e.g. headache, confusion, drowsiness and seizures). Children with hypoglycemia should immediately receive 0.3 g/kg rapidly absorbed glucose (upto 15 g), followed by long-acting carbohydrate. Severe hypoglycemia is a medical emergency and should be treated with injectable glucagon (0.5 mg for weight <25 kg; 1 mg for weight >5 kg) or intravenous dextrose.

#### Diabetic Ketoacidosis (DKA)

DKA is the most severe acute complication of diabetes mellitus. Previously believed to be limited to subjects with type 1 diabetes, DKA is increasingly observed in type 2 diabetes and MODY. Early identification and management are essential to limit the extent of mortality and morbidity associated with DKA. Thirty to forty percent of newly diagnosed children with type 1 diabetes present with DKA. Although epidemiological data from India is lacking, the figure is higher than the developed countries.

***Pathophysiology:*** DKA is the end result of absolute or relative insulin deficiency combined with excess of counter-regulatory hormones such as glucagon, catecholamines, cortisol and GH. DKA is usually precipitated by infection, stress and trauma, and conditions associated with increased insulin requirement and higher level of counter-regulatory hormones. These hormonal alterations result in hyperglycemia and lipolysis resulting in increased free fatty acid production. Oxidation of fatty acids in liver generates β-hydroxybutyrate and acetoacetic acid (ketones). Accumulation of ketoacids produces acidosis resulting in Kussmaul breathing (acidosis), abdominal pain (acidosis) and fruity odor of breath (acetone). Hyperglycemia results in increased urinary water losses due to osmotic diuresis and dehydration. Acidosis causes shift of intracellular ions, most importantly potassium and phosphate, to the extracellular compartment. However, serum levels of potassium are variable, depending on the stage of DKA. Initially, serum potassium levels are high; as therapy with insulin is initiated, the patient becomes hypokalemic. Hyperglycemia also falsely lowers serum sodium resulting in pseudohyponatremia; each 100 mg/dL elevation in blood glucose lowers sodium by 1.6 mEq/dL.

***When to suspect:*** There is need for high index of suspicion for DKA and it should be considered in the differential diagnosis of the following:

- *Encephalopathy:* CNS infections, severe malaria, poisoning
- *Acute abdomen:* Pancreatitis, appendicitis
- *Dehydration:* Gastroenteritis
- *Tachypnea:* Bronchial asthma, pneumonia

- *Hyperglycemia with acidosis without ketosis:* Renal failure, septicemia
- *Ketoacidosis without hyperglycemia:* Starvation, salicylate poisoning, organic acidemia

***Criteria for diagnosis:*** DKA should be diagnosed in presence of all of the following:

i. Hyperglycemia (blood glucose >200 mg/dL);
ii. Metabolic acidosis (pH <7.3, bicarbonate <15 mEq/L); and
iii. Ketosis (blood ketone >1.5 mmol/L, or urine ketone >2+).

***Management:*** DKA is a life-threatening condition and should be managed in a hospital equipped with facilities for intravenous infusion and measurement of blood gas and electrolytes. Children younger than 2 years of age and those with severe DKA should be managed in an ICU.

*Evaluation*

***Clinical:*** Initial evaluation should be guided towards assessment of adequacy of airway, breathing and circulation. Level of dehydration is ascertained along with hemodynamic status. Careful neurological evaluation including assessment of level of consciousness, pupils (dilated fixed in presence of cerebral herniation), cranial nerves (sixth nerve palsy suggests cerebral edema) and deep tendon reflexes (brisk if raised intracranial tension) is mandatory.

*Investigations*

***Serum sodium:*** There is usually a significant sodium deficit (4–6 mEq/kg). The sodium levels are falsely reduced in hyperglycemia mandating the need to use corrected sodium. Rapid decline in serum sodium is a risk factor for cerebral edema.

***Serum potassium:*** There is substantial intracellular potassium deficit (3–6 mEq/kg). Serum levels are, however, normal or high due to extrusion of intracellular potassium due to acidosis and insulin deficiency. Treatment of DKA is associated with the risk of hypokalemia due to its intracellular shift following reversal of metabolic acidosis and correction of insulin deficiency.

***Serum phosphate:*** Usually there is significant phosphate deficit. Treatment is required, if phosphorus level is below 1 mg/dL.

***Infection screening:*** Transient leukocytosis is common; infection should be considered in the presence of persistent leukocytosis and fever.

***Renal function tests:*** High blood urea usually indicates severe DKA.

***Electrocardiography:*** This is often done to screen for hypo- or hyperkalemia.

*Management*

***Initial stabilization:*** The child should be assessed for adequacy of airway, breathing and circulation. Initial fluid bolus of 10 mL/kg normal saline over 1-hour should be given in children with dehydration. Oxygen and respiratory support should be provided, if required. The child should be kept nil by mouth with insertion of nasogastric tube and urinary catheter, if unconscious. Intubation should be deferred as it may worsen CNS acidosis.

***Fluid therapy:*** Fluid therapy is the mainstay of treatment for DKA. However, rapid and excessive fluid intake is a risk factor for developing cerebral edema. The aim is to provide maintenance requirement and deficit evenly over 48 hours (72 hours for children with high plasma osmolality). In most children, the fluid deficit is 5–10%. Fluid requirement is usually around 3–3.5 L/m$^2$/day. Care is taken to avoid fluid administration of more than 4 L/m$^2$/day due to risk of cerebral edema. The amount of fluids given at other centers prior to referral should also be considered while calculating fluid requirements.

***Insulin:*** Insulin should be administered after initial hydration as blood glucose levels fall rapidly even without insulin. Early insulin treatment is associated with drastic fall in plasma osmolality, hypokalemia and increased risk of cerebral edema.

***Continuous intravenous infusion*** is the preferred route. The intravenous tubing should be flushed with insulin as insulin binds to plastic tube. There is no role of initial insulin bolus. In infants and mild DKA, the insulin infusion rate should be kept at 0.05 unit/kg/hr. The dose should be increased, if the fall in glucose is less than 50 mg/dL/hr, or if the acidosis is not resolving satisfactorily. The dose is increased in quantum of 0.02 unit/kg/hr. The insulin infusion rate should be reduced only after resolution of acidosis.

If facility for intravenous insulin is not available, intramuscular regular insulin may be used. The first dose is 0.3 unit/kg followed by 0.1 unit/kg hourly. Recurrent intravenous boluses of insulin should be avoided due to the risk for cerebral edema. Subcutaneous insulin is not recommended due to decreased absorption in the setting of poor perfusion.

***Serum sodium:*** Most patients have significant sodium deficits (4–6 mEq/kg). Slow rise in sodium in patients with rapid fall in glucose is a risk factor for cerebral edema. Normal saline (154 mEq/L) should be used in the first 6 hours of therapy; thereafter the sodium content should be between 77 and 154 mEq/L.

***Serum potassium:*** Although there is deficit in total body potassium, extracellular potassium levels may initially be high due to acidosis and insulin deficiency. There is a risk of life-threatening hypokalemia following correction of insulin deficiency and resolution of metabolic acidosis. In patients with initial potassium levels less than 3.5 mEq/ L, potassium replacement should precede administration of insulin. In other situations, potassium replacement is begun, at a concentration of 40 mEq/L, after initial hydration at the time of initiation of insulin infusion. Potassium should not be administered, if the level is >6 mEq/L, the patient is anuric or ECG changes of hyperkalemia are present.

***Dextrose:*** Hyperglycemia resolves prior to correction of acidosis. Decreasing insulin infusion rate with lowering of blood glucose is not recommended since that would prolong the duration of acidosis. Dextrose (5%) is, therefore, added to intravenous fluids once blood glucose levels fall below <270 mg/dL.

*Acid–base management:* Alkali treatment should be avoided as it poses risks for cerebral edema, lactic acidosis and hypokalemia. It is considered only if pH is less than 6.9 with hemodynamic compromise or if there is severe hyperkalemia (serum potassium >6.5 mEq/L with ECG changes).

*Monitoring:* Careful clinical and laboratory monitoring is necessary. This should include hourly monitoring of neurological status, heart rate, blood pressure and fluid input/output. Laboratory monitoring includes hourly blood glucose and four-hourly blood ketone, pH, bicarbonate and electrolytes (Table 18.36).

*Discontinuation of acute treatment:* Subcutaneous insulin should be considered once the patient is conscious, ready to accept feeds orally and has resolution of acidosis. Regular or rapid-acting insulin (0.25 unit/kg) should be given 30 minutes before eating. Alternatively, the child may be started on a basal-bolus or mix-split regime. Insulin infusion should be stopped only 30 minutes after insulin to provide overlap, and avoid recurrence of hyperglycemia.

*Complications of DKA:* DKA is a life-threatening condition with potential for significant long-term morbidity. Timely identification and treatment of these complications are essential.

*Cerebral edema:* Cerebral edema is the most serious complication of DKA and the most common cause of death. Risk factors include age less than 5 years, severe acidosis, insulin bolus, excessive hydration, $CO_2$ levels less than 10 mmol/L, and alkali treatment. Cerebral edema usually presents at 4–12 hours following treatment, but may be present at diagnosis. The condition is suspected in the presence of persistent hemodynamic instability or worsening in clinical condition after initial improvement. Early pointers include headache, vomiting, drowsiness, irritability, and hypertension with bradycardia. Severe cerebral edema is indicated by unconsciousness, focal neurological deficits, papilledema and fixed dilated pupils. The diagnosis is clinical. Children with suspected cerebral edema should be immediately treated with intravenous mannitol (5 mL/kg) followed by fluid restriction and head end elevation.

*Infections:* Bacterial and fungal infections are common. Indicators include persistent fever, leukocytosis, black nasal discharge (rhinocerebral mucormycosis) and hemoptysis (pulmonary aspergillosis).

### Long-term Complications of Type 1 Diabetes

Regular screening for long-term complications is essential for their early identification, prevention and appropriate treatment (Table 18.37). Screening for complications should

**Table 18.36:** Laboratory parameters and response to treatment in DKA

| *Parameter* | *Expected* | *Concern* | *Action* |
|---|---|---|---|
| Blood glucose | Decrease by 50–100 mg/dL/hour | Decline >100 mg/dL/hour<br>Decline <50 mg/dL/hour | Add dextrose to IV hydration fluid<br>Prepare fresh infusion, flush tubing with insulin |
| Blood pH | Resolution by 12 hours | Persistent at 12 hours | Exclude infection, shock, lactic acidosis |
| Serum sodium | Increase | Increase <2 mmol/L/hour | Increase sodium concentration in IV fluid |
| Serum potassium | Gradual decrease | Hypokalemia | Increase potassium concentration in IV fluid |
| Anion gap | Resolution by 12 hours | Elevated at 12 hours | Exclude lactic acidosis, consider infection |
| Plasma osmolality | Stable | Decrease by >2 mOsm/kg/hour | Increase sodium concentration, decrease fluid rate |
| Blood urea | Decrease | Persistently elevated | Exclude renal failure |

**Table 18.37:** Screening for complications in children with type 1 diabetes mellitus

| *Complications* | *Indications* | *Procedures* | *Management* |
|---|---|---|---|
| *Retinopathy*<br><br>Prepubertal<br>Pubertal | First eye examination after 3 months of diagnosis; screening after 11 years<br>Duration of diabetes >5 years from onset<br>Duration of diabetes >2 years from diagnosis | Initial examination of dilated fundus | Improvement in diabetes control<br>Laser treatment for visual loss |
| *Nephropathy*<br>Prepubertal<br>Pubertal | Annual screening after 11 years<br>Duration of diabetes >5 years from onset<br>Duration of diabetes >2 years from diagnosis | Annual screening for microalbuminuria: Albumin excretion rate (AER) 20–200 μg/min or AER 30–300 mg/day | Improvement in diabetes control<br>Control of blood pressure<br>ACE inhibitors to reduce proteinuria |
| *Hypothyroidism* | At diagnosis; thereafter every 2 years | Serum TSH and $FT_4$ estimation<br>Thyroid autoantibodies | Thyroxine therapy |
| *Hyperlipidemia*<br>Prepubertal<br>Pubertal | Annual screening after 12 years<br>At diagnosis; thereafter every 5 years<br>At diagnosis; thereafter every 2 years | Serum lipid profile | Strict diet control<br>Statins |

be started after 5 years of diagnosis, if the onset of diabetes is before puberty, and 2 years, if diagnosed in puberty.

Lipodystrophy manifests as fat atrophy or hypertrophy at the injection sites. This can be prevented by rotation of injection sites. Limited joint mobility is due to flexion contractures of metacarpophalangeal and proximal interphalangeal joints, typically noted in the hands.

Growth failure occurs in children whose diabetes is not well controlled. Mauriac syndrome occurs with poor control of diabetes and is characterized by hepatomegaly, pale skin and extreme short stature. Delayed puberty is associated with inadequate control of diabetes and delayed bone age.

Hypoglycemic unawareness is caused by frequent hypoglycemia associated with tight metabolic control of diabetes. It is due to impaired counter-regulatory hormone response to hypoglycemia. Raising blood glucose targets and prevention of hypoglycemia usually causes reversal of hypoglycemic unawareness.

Retinopathy is characterized by microaneurysms and proliferative disease. Ophthalmologic examination should be conducted when the child is more than 10-year-old and has had diabetes for 3–5 years. Annual follow-up is suggested.

Peripheral neuropathy is unusual in children and adolescents. This results in decreased nerve conduction velocity and sensory changes. An abnormality in vibration perception may be the first clinical finding.

Nephropathy is defined by presence of albumin in the urine. Annual screening for microalbuminuria is initiated when the child is 10 years of age or has had diabetes for 5 years. Patients with significant microalbuminuria should receive ACE inhibitors to delay the progression of nephropathy.

***Dyslipidemia:*** Fasting lipid profile is performed on all children more than 2 years of age at the time of diagnosis (after glucose control is achieved), or if there is family history of high cholesterol (>240 mg/dL) and/or a cardiovascular event before the 55 years. If there are no concerns of hyperlipidemia in the family, screening is performed after onset of puberty (>12 years). For pubertal children (>12-year- old), a fasting lipid profile is performed at diagnosis after glucose control is achieved. If LDL is <100 mg/dL, lipid profile is repeated every 5 years. Intervention is needed, if fasting LDL >100 mg/dL, initially by dietary modification with decrease in saturated fat in diet. A pharmacologic agent is added for LDL >160 mg/ dL, and in patients at risk of cardiovascular disease and LDL values 130–159 mg/dL after initiation of dietary changes and lifestyle intervention. The goal of therapy is LDL level <100 mg/dL.

### Type 2 Diabetes Mellitus

Type 2 diabetes in children and adolescents is increasing rapidly with the advent of childhood obesity epidemic. The disorder presents with milder symptoms than type 1 diabetes though DKA can develop occasionally. Diagnosis is established based on the presence of obesity, acanthosis nigricans, elevated insulin levels, normal C-peptide, and lack of GAD antibodies. Lifestyle measures and metformin are the mainstay of treatment. Adolescent type 2 diabetes, however, has an aggressive course compared to adult type 2 diabetes, with faster loss of cell function. Children who present with ketosis are treated with insulin initially and transitioned to metformin when endogenous glucose secretion recovers. GLP1 receptor analog, liraglutide has recently been approved in adolescents with type 2 diabetes. These children and adolescents should be evaluated for hyperlipidemia, diabetic retinopathy and nephropathy at diagnosis. It is recommended that children at risk of type 2 diabetes be regularly screened for diabetes.

### Maturity Onset Diabetes of Young (MODY)

MODY represents a group of inherited conditions due to monogenic defects (single gene mutations) characterized by impaired glucose sensing (glucokinase, *GCK*) or insulin secreting capacity of beta cells (*HNF1A* and *HNF4A* and *HNF*1B). The disorder presents with relatively mild, non-ketotic diabetes in a lean individual with strong family history of diabetes affecting three generations. The condition responds to lifestyle measures and low doses of sulfonylurea.

### Neonatal Diabetes Mellitus

Onset of diabetes before 6 months of age suggests neonatal diabetes due to inherited monogenic causes. The disease represents transient cell dysfunction (transient neonatal diabetes), permanent insulin secretion defect (permanent neonatal diabetes) or congenital insulin resistance syndrome. The most common cause of permanent neonatal diabetes is activating mutation in *ABCC8* or *KCNJ11* genes, that encode for one of the two sub-units of KATP channel, the on-off button for insulin secretion. These disorders are amenable to treatment with sulfonylureas.

### Suggested Reading


1. American Diabetes Association. Children and Adolescents: Standards of Medical Care in Diabetes-2021. Diabetes Care 2021;44(Suppl 1): S180-S199.
2. DiMeglio LA, Acerini CL, Codner E, et al. ISPAD Clinical Practice Consensus Guidelines 2018: Glycemic control targets and glucose monitoring for children, adolescents, and young adults with diabetes. Pediatr Diabetes. 2018;19(Suppl 27):105–14.
3. Glaser N, Fritsch M, Priyambada L, et al. ISPAD clinical practice consensus guidelines 2022: Diabetic ketoacidosis and hyperglycemic hyperosmolar state. Pediatr Diabetes 2022;23:835–56.
4. Gregory JW, Cameron FJ, Joshi K, et al. ISPAD Clinical Practice Consensus Guidelines 2022: Diabetes in adolescence. Pediatr Diabetes 2022;23:857–71.
5. Mayer-Davis EJ, Kahkoska AR, Jefferies C, et al. ISPAD Clinical Practice Consensus Guidelines 2018: Definition, epidemiology, and classification of diabetes in children and adolescents. Pediatr Diabetes 2018;19(Suppl 27):7–19.
6. Shah AS, Zeitler PS, Wong J, et al. ISPAD Clinical Practice Consensus Guidelines 2022: Type 2 diabetes in children and adolescents. Pediatr Diabetes. 2022;23:872–902.

Chapter

19

# Diseases of Central Nervous System

Rashmi Kumar

*Competencies:* **PE30.17; PE30.18; PE30.19**

## NEUROLOGICAL DIAGNOSIS

### History

An accurate history gives insight into the disease process. Vascular events often have the most acute onset, symptoms being worst at the onset with improvement soon after. Acute inflammatory processes like infections and acute disseminated encephalomyelitis are not as sudden in onset as vascular events. Subacute onset is typical of infections like tuberculous meningitis, brain abscess and some brain tumors. A relapsing remitting course is seen in multiple sclerosis and metabolic diseases. A subacute or chronic progressive downhill course is seen in degenerative disorders and neoplasms. A history of consanguineous marriage or similar disorder in the family suggests a hereditary disorder.

### Development History

Neurological disorders are often associated with abnormal development. Age of onset of developmental deviation may pinpoint the onset of disease. Development may be abnormal in all or some domains or may regress after a period of normal development. Acute insults lead to sudden regression of development followed by improvement.

### Clinical Examination

Methods of examination are modified according to the age of the child, from adult scheme in older cooperative children, to play method in younger children, and to observation in young infants. Full examination cannot be done in unconscious or small children who are unable to cooperate. Tools required for examination are colored toys and cubes, bell, torch, reflex hammer, measuring tape, small objects for testing stereognosis, two-point discriminator, tuning forks (128 Hz and 256 Hz), development testing kit and ophthalmoscope.

It is important to observe posture, behavior, gait, activity and interest in surroundings, and examine for hyperkinesis, involuntary movements and dysmorphic features of the face, such as epicanthal folds, mongoloid or antimongoloid slant, high arched palate or malformed ears. Skin should be examined for neurocutaneous markers: Adenoma sebaceum and ash leaf macules of tuberous sclerosis, and café au lait spots of neurofibromatosis.

The Glasgow Coma or Alert-Verbal-Pain-Unresponsive (AVPU) scales may be applied for state of consciousness. The former is modified for children below 2 years of age. If conscious, higher functions can be examined in terms of orientation, memory, intellect, speech, hallucinations and delusions and affect. Skull is examined for size, shape, symmetry, sutures and fontanelles. The cranium can be oddly shaped in craniosynostosis because of premature fusion of sutures. McEwen's or cracked pot sign on percussion of the skull is abnormal, if present after closure of the fontanelles. Auscultation of the skull is useful when a cranial arteriovenous malformation is suspected. Spine should be inspected for any scoliosis, kyphosis or pilonidal sinus, tuft of hair or overlying lipoma. Palpation and percussion of the spine may be done to elicit tenderness. Meningeal signs should be looked for, especially beyond infancy. Gait and posture should be carefully observed.

Cranial nerve examination should be attempted but may have to be limited in younger children who cannot cooperate. The first cranial nerve (olfactory) is tested by closing the child's eyes and asking him to identify familiar odors like orange, rose water, and cardamom. Irritating substances should be avoided. The second or optic nerve is tested in terms of vision or visual acuity, field of vision, color vision and fundus examination. Visual acuity is 6/45 in a term newborn and reaches adult level of 6/6 by 6–7 years of age. Presence of vision can be tested in a young child after about 12 months of age by the visual menace reflex. Later, the infant's following of coloured objects or toys may indicate presence of vision. Field of vision can be tested by 'confrontation method' in an older cooperative child and informally in a young baby by moving toys into his field of vision. Colour vision is usually tested in children beyond 3 years of age.

The 3rd, 4th and 6th cranial nerves are tested together. Ptosis, squint and nystagmus are looked for, then eye movements are tested by moving objects through the field of vision of the child. In a comatose child, the doll's eye reflex can be used for testing the medial and lateral movements. Finally, direct and consensual pupillary reflexes are checked.

The 5th cranial nerve (trigeminal) has motor and sensory components. The motor component supplies the temporalis and masseter muscles which can be tested by feeling them on clenching the jaw. Medial and lateral pterygoids can be tested in an older child by sideways movements of the lower jaw with mouth open. All sensations of the face from the vertex to the chin are carried by the 5th nerve. The corneal reflex is also a test of the 5th nerve.

The 7th cranial (facial) nerve can be tested by looking closely for any asymmetry of the face and flattening of the nasolabial fold. In a conscious cooperative child, five manoeuvres, namely looking upward and observing for asymmetry in forehead creases, eyeballs rolling upwards on closing eyes tightly (Bell sign), blowing out cheeks, whistling, and showing teeth, are performed. In upper motor neuron lesions of the facial nerve, the forehead is spared because of bilateral innervation. In unilateral facial palsy, mouth is deviated to the opposite side. In a smaller or comatose child, asymmetry may be brought out by stimulating him to smile or cry.

The 8th or vestibulocochlear nerve can be tested in an older cooperative child by asking him to repeat some words whispered from behind him. A younger child may respond to sudden sounds by some change in stance or expression or may turn head to the sound.

Ninth, 10th and 11th cranial nerves are tested together. Paralysis may cause noisy stertorous breathing because of pooling of secretions in the pharynx. The gag reflex is checked by inserting a tongue depressor to touch the anterior tonsillar pillar, and observing the position of the uvula, for palatal movements, and for nasal twang. The older child may be asked to swallow some water, for evidence of nasal regurgitation. The spinal part of the 11th (accessory) nerve is tested by asking the child to shrug or turn his head against resistance. Weakness on one side may result in torticollis or drooping of one shoulder.

The 12th (hypoglossal) nerve is tested by asking the child to protrude the tongue. A paralysed nerve causes deviation toward the paralysed side. Atrophy or fasciculations are also looked for.

Motor examination comprises examination for muscle mass, muscle tone, muscle power, coordination and abnormal movements. If any unilateral or local decrease in muscle mass is suspected, the circumference of the limb in relation to fixed bony points should be measured.

Muscle tone should be evaluated by observing posture (frog leg posture with decreased tone, scissoring of lower limbs with increased tone), palpating the muscles, moving the limbs across joints to feel the resistance to motion, flappability and extensibility across joints. Tone is physiologically increased in the term newborn. Muscle power is graded according to the Medical Research Council grading (0 = no movement; 1 = flicker of movement; 2 = movement with gravity eliminated; 3 = movement against gravity; 4 = movement against mild resistance; 5 = full power). In young children, it may not be possible to test against resistance as this requires cooperation.

Early handedness in a child below 3 years of age may suggest weakness in the other arm. Again, in unconscious children, it may not be possible to formally test power but response to stimulation may be observed and difference on the two sides can be appreciated. Abnormal movements may be classifiable as chorea (sudden, jerky, nonrepetitive, quasipurposive), athetosis (slow, writhing, distal), myoclonus (sudden, shock like involving different muscle groups), hemiballismus (large amplitude, flinging of whole limb), tremors (small amplitude, distal, around an axis) and tics (repetitive movements on one part of the body, suppressible) or unclassifiable. Dystonia refers to involuntary, sustained muscle contraction leading to abnormal twisted postures. All types of extrapyramidal movements usually disappear during sleep. Coordination can only be tested when full power is present and cooperation can be obtained. Tests for coordination include finger nose test, dysdiadokokinesis, heel shin test, past pointing and ataxia.

Sensory examination includes testing for both spinal and cortical sensations. Spinal sensations are those of touch, pain, temperature, vibration and position sense. The former three are carried by the spinothalamic tracts while the latter two are posterior column sensations. Except for touch and pain, testing requires cooperation from the child. The child's eyes should be covered while testing, after explaining the procedure. Cortical sensations include tactile localization, two-point discrimination, stereognosis, and graphesthesia.

Superficial reflexes tested are the corneal reflex, abdominal reflexes, cremasteric (in boys) and plantar reflex. Plantar reflexes may normally be extensor till the child starts walking. Abdominal reflexes are tested by stroking the skin in the four quadrants of the abdomen towards the umbilicus. Cremasteric reflex is tested by stroking upward on the skin of the upper inner thigh. Abdominal and cremasteric reflexes are lost in both upper and lower motor neuron lesions but are later regained in upper motor neuron lesions. Deep reflexes may be normally brisk in school aged children. Ill sustained ankle clonus with 3-6 jerks may normally be elicited till about 2 months of age. To elicit deep reflexes, the muscle should be exposed so that contraction can be observed.

### Developmental Testing

The neurological examination in a child should always be considered in context of the developmental examination. A detailed history of developmental milestones should be asked for (Chapter 3).

Gross motor development is tested in infancy in supine posture, pull to sitting, prone, ventral suspension, sitting and standing positions. Developmental and postural reflexes are tested. These are primitive reflexes most of which disappear as the child develops. Vision and hearing are tested by visual and auditory tracking.

Muscle tone in newborn period and infancy are also tested by measuring adductor angle, popliteal angle and ankle dorsiflexion angle by a goniometer for passive tone, traction response and recoil for active tone, and joint mobility (Chapter 9). Passive tone increases in a cephalocaudal direction from 28 to 40 weeks gestational age so that a term newborn has maximum physiologic hypertonia. It then decreases in a caudocephalic direction in the first year.

## Localization of Neurological Lesion

Neurological lesions are broadly divided into upper and lower motor neuron lesions (Table 19.1). Any lesion at or below the anterior horn cell of the spinal cord is a lower motor neuron lesion. The distribution of weakness suggests the level of lesion. A spinal lesion results in paraplegia or quadriplegia below the level. Lesions in the brainstem usually cause crossed paralysis, i.e., ipsilateral cranial nerve palsy with contralateral limb weakness. Lesions in the internal capsule cause dense contralateral hemiplegia affecting the arm more than the leg along with contralateral upper motor neuron facial palsy. Lesions in the cortex often cause seizures and more localized weakness, such as monoplegia. Acute destructive upper motor neuron lesions, as occurs with stroke, may cause flaccidity.

In lesions of the spinal cord, reflexes are usually lost at the level of the lesion. Sudden acute transverse lesions of the cord may cause complete loss of all function below that level which may last for a few weeks (spinal shock). Chronic lesions of the anterior horn cells give rise to fasciculations. Peripheral neuropathy causes weakness with early and complete loss of reflexes. Neuromuscular junction disorders, like myasthenia, cause weakness of extraocular and pharyngeal muscles towards the later part of the day. Muscle weakness may cause depressed but elicitable reflexes and positive Gower sign, if proximal muscles are involved.

**Table 19.1:** Localization of neurological disorder

| | |
|---|---|
| *Upper motor neuron (UMN)* | |
| Cortex | Contralateral UMN hemiplegia or monoplegia with UMN facial palsy; with/without seizures; spasticity; brisk deep tendon reflexes |
| Internal capsule | Contralateral dense UMN hemiplegia with UMN facial palsy; spasticity; brisk reflexes |
| Brainstem | Contralateral UMN hemiplegia with ipsilateral LMN cranial nerve palsy; spasticity; brisk reflexes |
| Spinal cord | Quadriplegia or paraplegia |
| *Lower motor neuron (LMN)* | |
| Anterior horn cells | LMN type weakness in spinal segment; loss of reflexes; fasciculation |
| Neuropathy | LMN type weakness in nerve distribution; early and complete loss of reflexes |
| Neuromuscular junction | Weakness and fatigue of ocular and pharyngeal muscles |
| Muscle | Weakness, especially proximal; Gower sign; depressed deep tendon reflexes |

*Competencies:* **PE30.20; PE30.21; PE30.22**

## Investigations

### *Lumbar Puncture*

Examination of cerebrospinal fluid (CSF) is required for the diagnosis of CNS infections. The normal CSF is clear, colorless and sterile with less than 5 cells (lymphocytes)/mm$^3$, protein 20–40 mg/dL and sugar level approximately two-thirds of concomitant blood sugar. CSF may be examined for antibody levels, culture and sensitivity, microbial DNA/RNA by polymerase chain reaction (PCR), myelin basic protein (in demyelinating disorders), and specific metabolites like lactate (in neurometabolic disorders). Lumbar puncture should be deferred in presence of raised intracranial tension (risk of brain herniation), circulatory failure, overlying local infection or severe bleeding disorder.

### *Cranial Ultrasonography*

This bedside procedure is especially useful for newborn and infants with open fontanelle. The ventricles, periventricular tissues and parts of the cortex are well-visualized, whereas the peripheral cortex, subdural spaces and posterior fossa are poorly seen.

### *Computerized Tomography (CT)*

This is relatively quick and inexpensive compared to magnetic resonance imaging. Calcification and bleeding are well visualized. Posterior fossa and temporal lobes are not visualized well, nor are myelination, migration disorders and small cortical dysplasias.

### *Magnetic Resonance Imaging (MRI)*

This offers better anatomic detail than CT especially for myelination and migration disorders, and vascular and congenital abnormalities. Sagittal and coronal views provide important information on midline, posterior fossa and temporal lobe structures. There is no risk of exposing the brain to harmful ionizing radiations.

## Genetic Tests

Genomic imbalances or copy number variations are increasingly recognized as a cause of intellectual disability. Techniques used include fluorescent *in situ* hybridization, multiplex ligation dependent probe amplification (MLPA) and chromosomal microarray. While MLPA has a yield of 5–10%, microarray, which examines the whole genome, yields diagnosis in up to 20% patients with intellectual disability with or without dysmorphism. Next generation sequencing allows detection of single nucleotide changes through the whole genome/exome.

## Suggested Reading

1. Menkes JH, Moser FG. Neurologic examination of the child and infant. In: Child Neurology, 7th edn. Eds. Menkes JH, Sarnat

HB, Maria BL. Lippincott Williams Wilkins, Philadelphia; 2006, pp 1–29.
2. Swaiman Pediatric Neurology: Principles and Practice, 6th edn. Eds. Swaiman KF, Ashwal S, Ferriero DM, Schor NF. Elsevier, Philadelphia, 2012; pp 15–32.

## CONGENITAL MALFORMATIONS

### Normal Development of Nervous System

Very early in development, a thickening of the ectoderm overlying the notochord forms the neural plate. This invaginates to form the neural groove. Fusion of the two sides of the groove results in formation of the neural tube. The rostral end and caudal end of this tube then fuse. The rostral end develops three dilatations—the prosencephalon, mesencephalon and rhombencephalon. The cerebral cortex, basal ganglia, thalamus and hypothalamus develop from the prosencephalon. Mesencephalon is the later midbrain. Pons, cerebellum and medulla develop from the rhombencephalon. The neural tube within these structures later forms the lateral and 3rd ventricles, aqueduct and 4th ventricles. At about 6 weeks gestation, neurons at the subependymal germinal matrix migrate to their final site, along radial glial fibres. After migration of the first layer, layers 2–6 migrate in an 'inside out' manner.

*Competency:* **PE30.3**

### Congenital Hydrocephalus

Hydrocephalus or excessive accumulation of cerebrospinal fluid in the brain can be congenital or acquired. Congenital causes include X-linked aqueductal stenosis, Dandy-Walker cyst, Arnold-Chiari malformation (herniation of cerebellum and brainstem into cervical spinal canal), intrauterine infections (toxoplasmosis, rubella, cytomegalovirus), and arteriovenous malformations. Hydrocephalus may be detected *in utero* by ultrasound. As the sutures are open, head size enlarges to accommodate the excess fluid. A large head may cause difficulty in delivery, making Cesarian section necessary. A postnatal increase in head circumference by more than 1 cm every fortnight, separation of sutures by more than 0.5 cm after the first 2 weeks, large anterior fontanelle and persistent widening of the squamoparietal sutures should raise the suspicion of hydrocephalus. In advanced cases, eye pupils are turned downward (sunset sign) and scalp veins may be prominent. Diagnosis can be confirmed by imaging, including cranial ultrasound, CT scan or MRI of the brain. The latter also may give the precise cause and associated malformations. Treatment is generally by shunt surgery, which usually remains for life and requires revisions as the child grows older. Endoscopic third ventriculostomy procedure is another option. Prognosis is guarded.

*Competency:* **PE30.4**

### Microcephaly

This is defined as occipitofrontal circumference more than 2 standard deviations below the mean for age, gender and sex. Primary or genetic microcephaly may be inherited as autosomal dominant or recessive, or associated with Down, Edward, Cri-du-chat, Cornelia de Lange, Rubinstein Taybi or Smith-Lemli-Opitz syndromes. Secondary or nongenetic microcephaly follows insults such as congenital infections (rubella, cytomegalovirus, toxoplasmosis, and syphilis), fetal alcohol syndrome, radiation, fetal hydantoin syndrome, maternal diabetes, malnutrition and hypoxic ischemic encephalopathy. Postnatally, severe hypoglycemia, Rett syndrome and human immunodeficiency virus infection can result in microcephaly. A receding forehead, overriding cranial sutures and intellectual disability are usually present. There is no known treatment.

*Competency:* **PE30.5**

### Neural Tube Defects (NTDs)

These are disorders in the closure of the neural tube. They are one of the most common congenital anomalies with occurrence in 1.5/1000 live births. Risk in subsequent sibling is 3–4/1000. A wide spectrum from spina bifida occulta, meningocele, meningomyelocele and encephalocele may occur.

Spina bifida occulta refers to failure of bony fusion of the vertebral column. The defect is covered by skin. An overlying tuft of hair **(Fig. 19.1a)**, lipoma or sinus may be markers of underlying spina bifida. A sinus carries the risk of recurrent meningitis and should be excised. A meningocele means the bulging out of meninges through the bony defect, which may or may not be covered by skin. The infant is born with a soft mass in the lumbar or sacral region through which cerebrospinal fluid may exude. The open meninges may get infected. Early repair is essential. A meningomyelocele refers to herniation

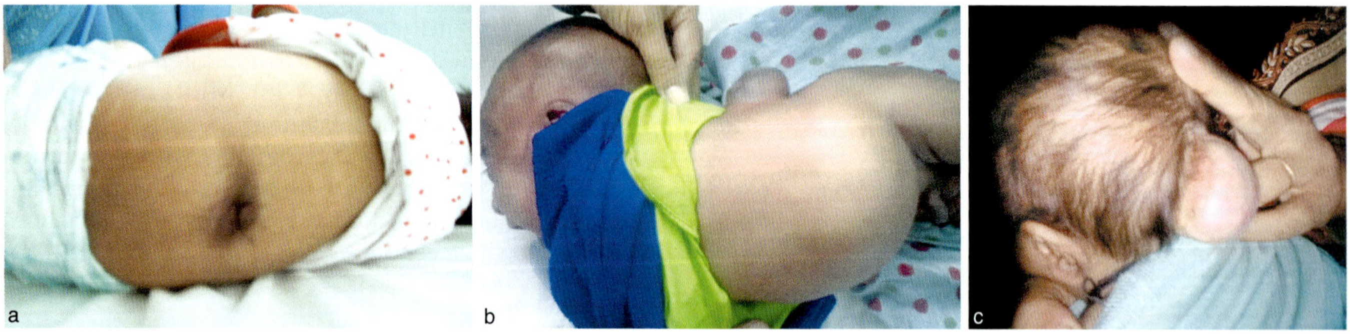


**Fig. 19.1:** Neural tube defects: (a) Tuft of hair overlying spina bifida occulta; (b) Dorsolumbar meningomyelocele; (c) Occipital encephalocele

of both meninges and neural tissue through the defect (Fig. 19.1b). There is associated neurological deficit, the extent of which depends on the level of the defect. Usually there is lower motor neuron type of paraplegia with bladder and bowel dysfunction and perineal anesthesia. Most cases have type II Arnold Chiari malformation, and half of the cases are associated with aqueductal stenosis, resulting in hydrocephalus. Club feet and dislocated hips may be present. An encephalocele is a midline bony defect in the calvaria with herniation of brain and meninges (Fig. 19.1c).

Management of severe defects is difficult and multidisciplinary. Many would develop hydronephrosis and renal failure due to neurogenic bladder. A series of surgical procedures may be required. Ambulatory potential depends on the level and degree of neurological deficit.

Antenatal diagnosis of neural tube defects can be made by ultrasound and raised α-fetoprotein and acetylcholinesterase levels in amniotic fluid and maternal serum. The risk of defects is reduced by about 72% by intake of 0.4 mg/day of folic acid periconceptionally.

### Neuronal Migration Defects

These occur when neurons fail to migrate to their intended destination.

*Heterotopia:* This is said to occur when gray matter lies within white matter. This can be periventricular or subcortical. Intractable seizures may occur.

*Lissencephaly:* This term means smooth brain. The cerebral convolutions are not formed. Patients present with developmental delay, microcephaly, eye abnormalities and intractable spasms. Pachygyria is a milder malformation in which areas of normal organization are seen.

*Schizencephaly:* This refers to clefts within the cerebral cortex which may extend from the ventricular wall to the cortical surface. The cleft is lined by heterotopic gray matter. Affected children may have seizures, hemiparesis, hypotonia or spasticity (Fig. 19.2a).

*Holoprosencephaly:* Here the two cerebral hemispheres appear fused because of failure of cleavage in the midsagittal plane. The most severe form is characterized by a single ventricle with absent falx (Fig. 19.2b). Causes include chromosomal defects and maternal diabetes. Midline facial defects like cyclopia (single midline eye), and cleft lip and palate, may occur. Hypothalamic and pituitary involvement may result in endocrine disturbances.

*Porencephaly:* This is cyst in the cerebral hemisphere which may communicate with the ventricle or extend upto the brain surface (Fig. 19.2c). It is usually the result of cystic degeneration of a perinatal infarct.

#### Agenesis of Corpus Callosum

This anomaly is seen in about 2% of the population. It may occur in isolation or associated with other brain malformations. It may be partial or complete. Secondary destruction of the corpus callosum can occur with hypoxic ischemic encephalopathy or infarcts. Patients may be asymptomatic or have epilepsy, cognitive defects or learning disabilities. Aicardi syndrome is an association of agenesis of corpus callosum, retinal colobomas, intellectual disability and infantile spasms in girls. Neuroimaging reveals parallel lateral ventricles with associated anomalies like interhemispheric cysts, intracranial lipomas, and disorders of neuronal migration, including neuronal heterotopias, lissencephaly, pachygyria, and schizencephaly.

### Arnold-Chiari Malformation

These are of two types. In Chiari I malformation, the cerebellar tonsils are displaced downward 3–5 mm through the foramen magnum into the upper cervical canal. Patients may be asymptomatic or present with headache, dizziness, vertigo, torticollis, downgaze nystagmus and drop attacks. In type II malformation, the pons, medulla, vermis and elongated 4th ventricle are displaced into the upper cervical canal. Neural tube defects occur in almost all cases. Cerebellar, brainstem and cortical abnormalities may be associated.

### Dandy-Walker Malformation

This is caused by failure of the foramen of Magendie to open resulting in ballooning of the posterior wall of the 4th ventricle to form a cyst in the posterior fossa. It is associated with other cerebellar and cerebral anomalies. Infants present with increase in head size with occipital prominence.

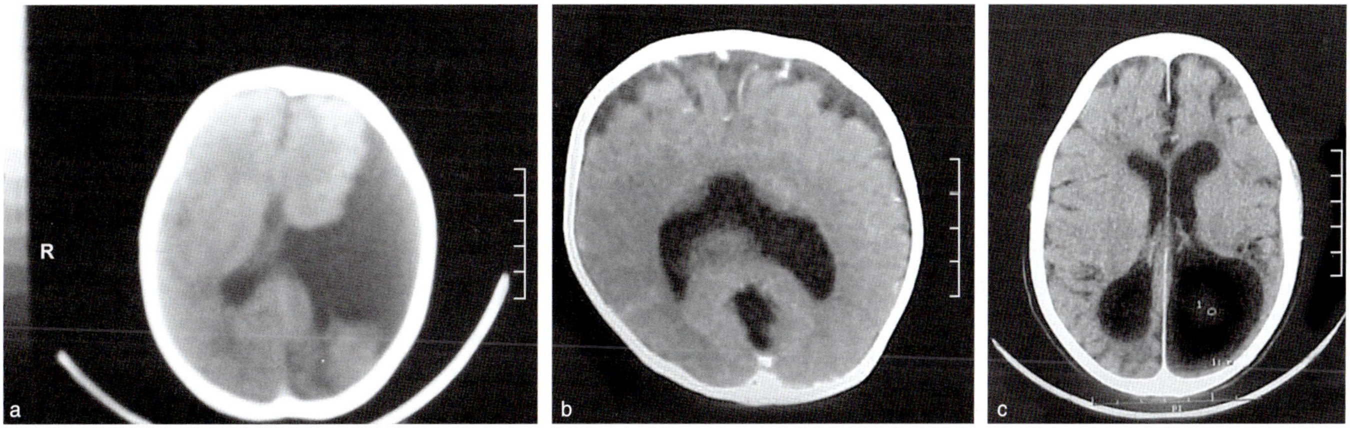


Fig. 19.2: Neuronal migration defects. Computed tomography of the brain with axial sequences showing: (a) Left hemispheric schizencephaly; (b) Anterior fusion of cerebrum and absent corpus callosum, suggesting holoprosencephaly; (c) Cystic structure in left parieto-occipital cortex, suggestive of left cerebral porencephalic cyst

Delayed development, cerebellar ataxia and spasticity are usually present. Treatment is that of hydrocephalus.

### Syringomyelia and Hydromyelia

These refer to a fluid-filled cavity or syrinx within the spinal cord. It may be an isolated developmental anomaly or associated with the Chiari malformation, tumor, infarction or trauma. Manifestations are dissociated sensory loss in 'cape-like'distribution, atrophy of hand muscles and spasticity in lower limbs. Treatment is decompression by laminectomy and syringotomy.

### Suggested Reading


1. Ravi KS, Divasha, Hassan SB, et al. Neural tube defects: Different types and brief review of neurulation process and its clinical implication. J Family Med Prim Care 2021;10:4383–90.
2. Roberts B. Neuronal migration disorders. Radiol Technol 2018; 89:279–95.
3. Saletti V, Farinotti M, Peretta P, et al. The management of Chiari malformation and syringomyelia in children. Neurol Sci 2021; 42:4965–95.
4. Vriend I, Oegema R. Genetic causes underlying grey matter heterotopia. Eur J Paediatr Neurol 2021;35:82–92.




## NEUROCUTANEOUS SYNDROMES

These are a group of disorders which affect both the nervous system and skin. One of the common manifestations is a tendency to form benign and sometimes malignant tumors in various parts of the body.

### Neurofibromatosis (NF)

This is the most common of the neurocutaneous syndromes. There are two types: NF1 or von Recklinghausen disease caused by deletion of NF on chromosome 17, and NF2 or central NF, with NF2 located on chromosome 22. Both are autosomal dominant with highly variable penetration. Diagnostic criteria for NF1 are given in Table 19.2. Nervous system abnormalities include optic glioma, intraspinal neurofibroma, aqueductal stenosis and dural ectasia. MRI brain may show areas of increased signal intensity in basal ganglia, cerebellum, brainstem and subcortical white matter. Treatment is supportive.

### Tuberous Sclerosis Complex (TSC)

This disorder is caused by variations in either *TSC1* (chromosome 9q34) or *TSC2* (chromosome 16 p13.3). Inheritance is autosomal dominant with complete penetrance but variable expression. Central nervous system manifestations are developmental delay, intellectual disability, seizures (often epileptic spasms), autism and attention deficit hyperactivity disorder. Subependymal nodules **(Fig. 19.3a)** and cortical tubers **(Fig. 19.3b)** are seen on neuroimaging. The former may undergo malignant transformation as glial tumours. Skin manifestations, which increase with age include ash leaf macules **(Fig. 19.3c)**, adenoma sebaceum **(Fig. 19.3d)**, café au lait spots and shagreen patches. TSC is a multisystem disease affecting kidneys (angiomyolipomas), lungs (lymphangiomyomatosis), heart (rhabdomyoma) and retina (hamartomas). Diagnostic criteria are listed in Table 19.3. Regular screening should be done for renal, lung, heart and retinal tumors. Treatment is supportive with anticonvulsants, and surgery for tumors. mTOR inhibitors, e.g., everolimus are shown to control growth of affected tissues and everolimus is approved by US FDA to treat brain and kidney tumors.

**Table 19.2:** Revised diagnostic criteria for neurofibromatosis type 1 (2021)

| |
|---|
| Six or more café-au-lait macules over 5 mm in greatest diameter in prepubertal individuals and over 15 mm in greatest diameter in postpubertal individuals[1] |
| Freckling in the axillary or inguinal region[1] |
| Two or more neurofibromas of any type or one plexiform neurofibroma |
| Optic pathway glioma |
| Two or more iris Lisch nodules identified by slit lamp examination or two or more choroidal abnormalities, defined as bright, patchy nodules imaged by optical coherence tomography or near-infrared reflectance imaging |
| A distinctive osseous lesion such as sphenoid dysplasia[2], anterolateral bowing of the tibia, or pseudarthrosis of a long bone |
| A heterozygous pathogenic NF1 variant with a variant allele fraction of 50% in apparently normal tissue such as white blood cells |

**Diagnosis**

- *If neither parent has been diagnosed with NF1:* Two or more criteria should be met
- *If either parent diagnosed with NF1 (meets two or more diagnostic criteria):* One or more of the criteria should be met

[1]At least one of the two pigmentary findings (café au lait macules or freckling) should be bilateral.

[2]Sphenoid wing dysplasia is not a separate criterion in case of an ipsilateral orbital plexiform neurofibroma.

**Table 19.3:** Clinical criteria for the diagnosis of tuberous sclerosis complex

| *Major criteria* | *Minor criteria* |
|---|---|
| Hypomelanotic macules (≥3, ≥5 mm in diameter) | "Confetti" skin lesions |
| Angiofibromas (≥3) or fibrous cephalic plaque | Dental enamel pits (>3) |
| Ungual fibromas (≥2) | Intraoral fibroma (≥2) |
| Shagreen patch | Retinal achromic patch |
| Multiple retinal hamartomas | Multiple renal cysts |
| Cortical dysplasia | Nonrenal hamartomas |
| Subependymal nodules | |
| Subependymal giant cell astrocytoma | |
| Cardiac rhabdomyoma | |
| Lymphangioleiomyomatosis | |
| Angiomyolipomas (≥2) | |

**Diagnosis**

*Definite:* Presence of two major features, or one major feature with ≥2 minor features

*Possible:* Either one major feature or ≥2 minor features

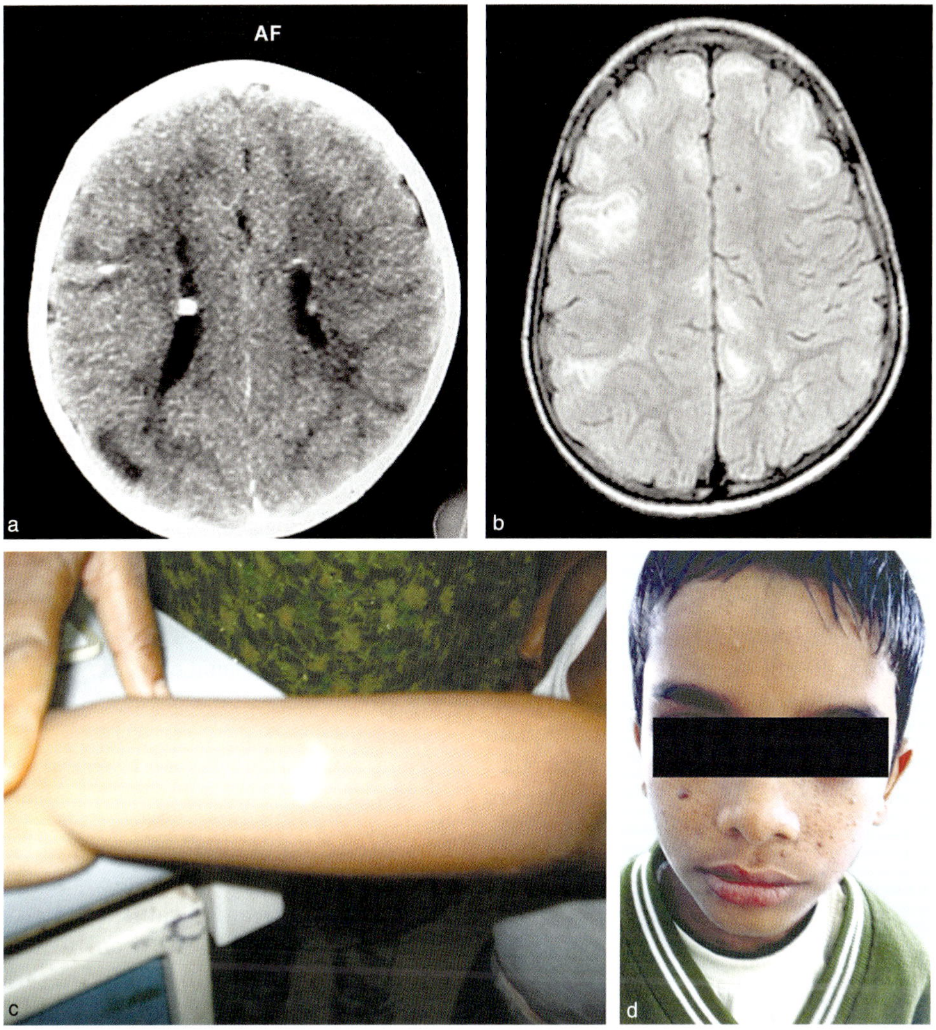


Fig. 19.3: Findings in tuberous sclerosis include: (a) Subependymal nodule on non-contrast CT of brain; (b) Cortical tubers on axial FLAIR magnetic resonance imaging; (c) Hypopigmented ash leaf macule; (d) Hyperpigmented maculopapular facial rash (adenoma sebaceum)

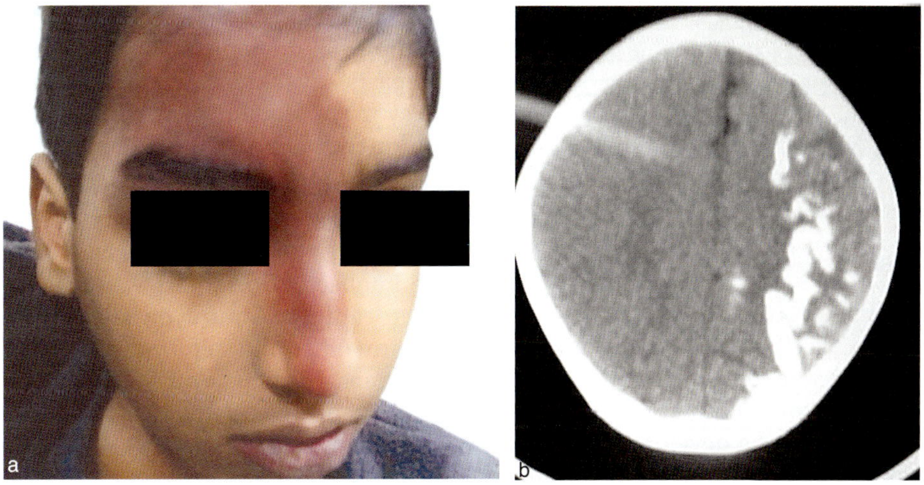

Fig. 19.4: Features of Sturge-Weber syndrome include: (a) Hemifacial angioma or port-wine stain; (b) Intracranial calcifications in left hemisphere on computed tomography

### Sturge-Weber Syndrome

This is a sporadic disorder characterized by a facial nevus or 'port wine stain' **(Fig. 19.4a)** in the distribution of the first branch of the trigeminal nerve along with an ipsilateral 'rail road pattern' of intracranial calcification **(Fig. 19.4b)** and glaucoma. The major manifestation is contralateral hemiplegia and intractable focal seizures which may lead to intellectual disability. Control of seizures may require surgery. Regular eye evaluation is necessary to monitor for glaucoma.

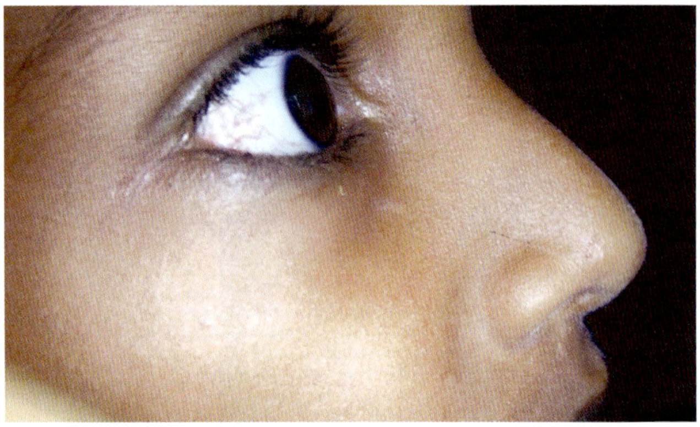

Fig. 19.5: Bulbar conjunctival telangiectasia in a child with ataxia telangiectasia

### Ataxia Telangiectasia

This is an autosomal recessive disorder due to mutations in *ATM* located on chromosome 11q. There is slowly progressive truncal ataxia starting in infancy. Choreoathetosis and oculomotor apraxia are usually present. Skin manifestations start after age 2–3 years with cutaneous (at flexures) and ocular (bulbar conjunctiva) telangiectasia (Fig 19.5). In addition, there is an immunodeficiency leading to frequent pulmonary and sinus infections and risk of lymphoreticular malignancies. Alpha-fetoprotein is raised in 90% and serum immunoglobulins (especially IgA and IgG2) are low in 80%.

### Von Hippel-Lindau Disease

This autosomal dominant disorder is characterized by cerebellar and retinal hemangioblastomas, spinal cord angiomas, and cystic tumors of the kidneys and pancreas. Cerebellar signs and raised intracranial tension are the usual manifestations.

### Suggested Reading


1. Little H, Kamat D, Sivaswamy L Common neurocutaneous syndromes. Pediatr Ann 2015;44:496–504.
2. Luo C, Ye WR, Shi W, et al. Perfect match: mTOR inhibitors and tuberous sclerosis complex. Orphanet J Rare Dis 2022;17(1):106.
3. Portocarrero LKL Tuberous sclerosis complex: review based on new diagnostic criteria. An Bras Dermatol 2018;93:323–31.
4. Sur mL, Armat I, Sur G, et al. Neurofibromatosis in children: Actually and perspectives. Children (Basel) 2022;9:40.


*Competencies:* **PE3.8; PE30.11**

## CEREBRAL PALSY

Cerebral palsy refers to permanent, nonprogressive and occasionally evolving disorders of tone, movement or posture, caused by an insult to the developing brain. It is the most common chronic motor disability in childhood, affecting 2–3 infants per 1000 live births. While perinatal asphyxia was considered the most common cause, it accounts for less than 10% of cases. Various causes are listed in Table 19.4.

Table 19.4: Causes of cerebral palsy

**Genetic or prenatal factors**
- Genetic disorders
- Inborn errors of metabolism
- Structural malformations of nervous system
- Congenital or intrauterine infections
- Teratogens
- Maternal or obstetric complications

**Perinatal causes**
- Birth asphyxia
- Prematurity
- Low birth weight
- Birth trauma
- Neonatal infection
- Neonatal seizures
- Neonatal hypoglycemia
- Intracranial hemorrhage
- Neonatal hyperbilirubinemia

**Postnatal causes**
- Infections of the central nervous system
- Hypoxia
- Trauma
- Drugs, toxins, and metabolic disorders

### Clinical Features

The most common presentation is with developmental delay. Physical findings are persistence of neonatal reflexes, increased tone, fisting with cortical thumb, scissoring of legs, toe-walking, abnormal posture and gait, abnormal movements and/or hyperreflexia. Common comorbidities include intellectual disability, microcephaly, seizures, behavioral problems, difficulty in speech, language, swallowing or feeding, blindness, deafness, squint, malnutrition, sleep disturbances and excessive drooling. Contractures may develop that are initially dynamic and later fixed.

### Classification

Cerebral palsy is classified topographically as quadriplegic, hemiplegic, monoplegic or diplegic, and physiologically as spastic, dyskinetic, ataxic or mixed (Table 19.5). Spastic palsy may be quadriplegic, diplegic or hemiplegic, while dyskinetic palsy may be choreoathetoid or dystonic.

***Spastic quadriplegia*** is the most common type of cerebral palsy in India. It is often caused by perinatal asphyxia or neonatal illness. Common comorbidities are intellectual disability, seizures, pseudobulbar palsy, microcephaly, squint or visual disturbances, speech abnormalities and deformities. Neuroimaging may show cystic encephalomalacia.

***Spastic diplegia*** is the second most common type, and is linked to prematurity. Intellect is often preserved. Neuroimaging shows periventricular leukomalacia.

***Spastic hemiplegic palsy*** usually results from a vascular insult or perinatal stroke. Early hand preference is a clue. Neuroimaging usually reveals focal changes or a porencephalic cyst. These children are usually mobile. They may have preserved or impaired intellect.

***Dyskinetic or extrapyramidal palsy*** may result from asphyxia or kernicterus. Rigidity, dystonia, dyskinesia

Table 19.5: Types of cerebral palsy and their characteristics

| *Type and distribution* | *Antecedent cause(s)* | *Clinical signs; comorbidity* | *Radiological findings* |
|---|---|---|---|
| Spastic quadriplegia | Perinatal asphyxia | Intellectual disability, seizures, microcephaly, pseudobulbar palsy, squint, visual disturbances, speech abnormalities | Cystic encephalomalacia |
| Spastic diplegia | Prematurity | Intellect often preserved; toe walking | Periventricular leukomalacia |
| Spastic hemiplegia | Vascular event | Preserved or impaired intellect; usually ambulatory | Porencephaly |
| Extrapyramidal | Asphyxia, kernicterus | Rigidity, dystonia, dyskinesia and drooling are prominent; intellect is usually preserved | Basal ganglia abnormalities |
| Ataxic | Cerebellar malformation | Cerebellar signs | Cerebellar malformation |
| Mixed | Asphyxia | Both spastic and dystonic features | |

and drooling are prominent while intellect is relatively preserved. Radiology may indicate abnormalities in basal ganglia or thalamus.

*Ataxic palsy* is caused by cerebellar malformations and is associated with other cerebellar signs.

*Mixed cerebral palsy* refers to a presentation including both spastic and extrapyramidal features.

### Evaluation

A detailed history is taken to detect various manifestations and antecedent events. Physical and neurologic examination should include assessment of development and evaluation for dysmorphism and neurocutaneous markers. Spasticity is classified using tools such as Gross Motor Function Classification System and Modified Ashworth Scale.

### Management

Management requires multidisciplinary inputs from the pediatrician, occupational therapist, physiotherapist, clinical psychologist, orthopedic surgeon, speech therapist, ophthalmologist, ENT specialist, social worker and special educator. Generalized spasticity is managed by physiotherapy and drugs such as diazepam, baclofen, tinazidine or dantrolene. Intrathecal baclofen therapy uses an implantable pump to deliver the muscle relaxant drug baclofen, into the cerebrospinal fluid. Dystonia is managed with trihexiphenidyl, levodopa or botulinum toxin injections. Localized spasticity can be effectively treated with injection of botulinum A toxin. Some patients may require tendon release or tendon lengthening. Orthotic devices such as braces, splints, wedges, and special chairs help to compensate for muscle imbalance and increase independent mobility.

### Suggested Reading


1. Gulati S, Sondhi V. Cerebral palsy: An overview. Indian J Pediatr 2018; 85: 1006–16.
2. Stavsky M, Mor O, Mastrolia SA, et al. Cerebral palsy: Trends in epidemiology and recent development in prenatal mechanisms of disease, treatment, and prevention. Frontiers Pediatr 2017;5:21 doi:10.3389/fped.2017.00021.
3. www.cdc.gov>cp>facts


*Competencies:* **PE30.8; PE30.9**

## SEIZURES AND EPILEPSY

A seizure is an abnormal paroxysmal electrical activity in the brain with motor, sensory, behavioral or autonomic manifestations. About 5% children experience a seizure in the first 5 years of life. A detailed account of the sequence of events should be taken. Table 19.6 lists the chief causes of seizures.

### Acute Symptomatic Seizures

A seizure occurring within a week of acute neurological injury, such as stroke, trauma, anoxia, active inflammation and infection, and within 24 hours of acute metabolic derangements, requires evaluation with serum electrolytes, lumbar puncture and neuroimaging, if indicated clinically. Antiepileptic therapy is initiated and discontinued after 3–6 months, if awake and sleep EEG records are normal.

Prehospital management during a seizure includes calming down the family, placing the patient in lateral face down position (recovery position) and protecting from injury. Rectal diazepam 0.5 mg/kg or intranasal midazolam spray 0.2 mg/kg may be given to abort the seizure.

*Competencies:* **PE27.6; PE30.9**

### Status Epilepticus

Any seizure persisting for more than 30 minutes or multiple seizures, irrespective of duration, without regaining of consciousness in between, is termed status epilepticus. A single convulsion usually lasts for less than 5 minutes. There is a growing opinion that if a convulsion lasts beyond that time, it should be treated as status epilepticus. As a corollary, if any child is brought convulsing to the emergency, he should be treated as status. In over 50% of cases, status epilepticus occurs as the patient's first seizure. Status epilepticus is caused by the same entities that cause isolated seizures. The condition can cause multiorgan dysfunction, neurodevelopmental sequelae, and, in 10% cases, death. **Figure 19.6** summarizes the management of status epilepticus. The term refractory status epilepticus is used for seizures that persist despite the use of benzodiazepine and one anticonvulsant in appropriate doses. Seizures that

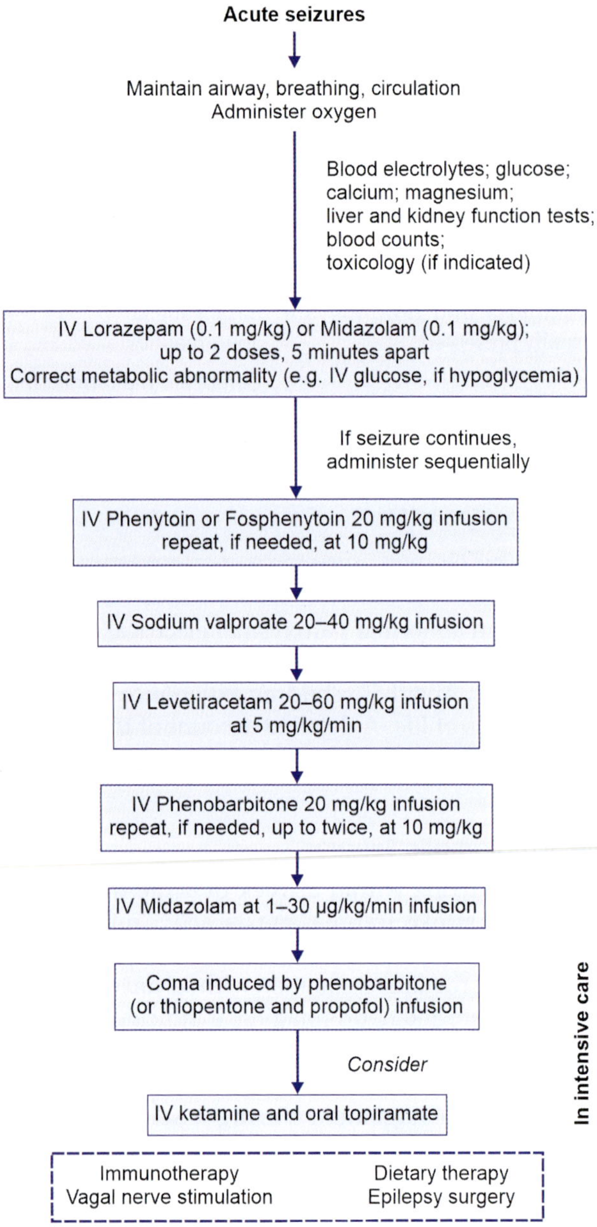


**Fig. 19.6:** Sequential drug therapy in the management of status epilepticus

do not respond despite 24 hours of anesthesia are termed super-refractory.

*Competency:* **PE30.7**

### Febrile Seizures

Febrile seizures refer to seizures associated with fever (>38°C) occurring in neurologically healthy children between 6 months and 5 years of age, without underlying intracranial infection or prior unprovoked seizures. Febrile seizures affect 3–8% children up to 7 years of age. About 25–40% have a positive family history. Fever may be caused by minor upper respiratory tract infection, gastroenteritis, viral exanthem, bacterial infection, malaria or immunization. Febrile seizures must be differentiated from acute symptomatic seizures due to intracranial infection and those triggered by fever in children with underlying epilepsy.

#### *Types*

A simple febrile seizure is a generalized seizure that lasts less than 15 minutes and occurs only once within a 24 hours period of fever in a neurologically normal child. Complex febrile seizure, which account for 15–20% cases are characterized by one or more of the following: (i) Focal signs or symptoms; (ii) duration >15 minutes; or (iii) recurrent seizures within the same febrile illness.

About one-third of patients experience a recurrent febrile seizure and 1/6th have multiple febrile seizures. Risk factors for recurrence are: (i) Age <18 months; (ii) family history of febrile seizures; (iii) multiple seizures in first episode and (iv) seizure at low temperature (<40°C).

#### *Outcome*

After an initial febrile seizure, 3–12% children develop epilepsy by adolescence. The risk of epilepsy is 1.5–2.4% for simple febrile seizures and increases in children with: (i) Pre-existing neurodevelopmental abnormality; (ii) complex febrile seizure; and (iii) family history of epilepsy. It was suggested that a prolonged febrile seizure in infancy can cause hippocampal injury and mesial temporal sclerosis, leading to subsequent temporal lobe epilepsy. However, this cause-effect relationship has not been established.

#### *Management*

An acute episode of seizure at home is terminated by nasal midazolam or rectal diazepam. In case the patient presents to the hospital in status, standard protocol for management of status epilepticus is followed.

In first episode of febrile seizure, lumbar puncture is indicated in clinically suspected meningitis. The threshold for lumbar puncture should be lower in: (i) Younger children, (ii) those who cannot be observed, (iii) those who have already received antibiotics, or (iv) those in whom immunization against Hib/pneumococcus has not been given or status is unknown.

#### *Prophylaxis*

In children with risk factors for recurrence or those with frequent recurrences (≥3 in 6 months or ≥4 in one year), intermittent prophylaxis reduces recurrences by 80%. Oral benzodiazepines (diazepam 0.6–0.8 mg/kg/day in 3 divided doses or clobazam 0.8–1 mg/kg/day in 2 divided doses) should be started at the first sign of any fever and continued for first 48 hours.

*Competency:* **PE30.8**

## EPILEPSY

Epilepsy is defined as occurrence of two unprovoked seizures more than a day apart beyond the neonatal period. Patients with one unprovoked seizure and a high probability of further seizures in the next decade, similar to the recurrence risk (over 60%) following two unprovoked seizures, are also termed having epilepsy. A multilevel classification with five components: (i) Seizure type,

(ii) epilepsy type, (iii) epilepsy syndrome, (iv) etiology, and (v) comorbidities, is also proposed. Some of the important types are discussed.

### Generalized Onset Seizure

*Tonic-clonic:* A tonic phase lasting at least 30 seconds and associated with uprolling of eyeballs, frothing from mouth, with or without perioral cyanosis, tongue bite and/or incontinence of stool and urine, is followed by clonic movement of all limbs. This phase is succeeded by post-convulsive drowsiness or sleep.

*Myoclonic:* Sudden, jerky shock-like violent contractions involve axial and appendicular muscles.

*Atonic:* Sudden loss of tone involving axial and appendicular muscles.

*Epileptic spasm:* These generally occur in infants and may look like 'startling' episodes. Flexion or extension movements of head, neck and extremities, especially on awaking from sleep occur in clusters or singly, several times a day.

*Tonic:* Only tonic phase, as described in tonic-clonic seizure, occurring without the clonic component.

*Absence:* Brief periods of lapses in awareness lasting 10–15 seconds occur without associated loss of tone, so the patient does not fall. They may appear like staring spells with few blinking movements. Rapid recovery of awareness occurs and many attacks may occur in a day. They are often precipitated by hyperventilation. The EEG typically shows 3/sec spike and wave activity.

### Focal Onset Seizures

These may be motor, sensory or autonomic. They account for 60% of epilepsies in childhood. They more often have a structural cause. Important causes are atrophic lesions, scars, inflammatory granulomas, strokes and vascular insults, head trauma, abscess and neoplasms. In our country, neurocysticercus granulomas are a common cause, which classically produce a ring or disc-like enhancing lesion on neuroimaging.

A focal seizure may or may not be associated with impaired awareness. A transient paralysis of the affected limb of up to 24 hours may result, and is known as Todd's palsy. Focal seizures may spread to become bilateral tonic-clonic.

Focal seizures may also be associated with automatisms. Focal seizures with impaired awareness arising from the temporal lobe are also called psychomotor epilepsy. Patients may have a 'déjà vu' feeling, visual, olfactory or visceral aura and peculiar posturing or automatisms which are usually repetitive. There is no memory for the event.

### Etiology

Table 19.6 lists the chief causes of seizures and epilepsy. The International League Against Epilepsy lists etiology under genetic, structural, metabolic, infectious, autoimmune and unknown causes. Many single gene disorders are now known to cause epilepsy. These genetic epilepsies may lend themselves to targeted 'precision' therapy.

**Table 19.6:** Etiology of seizures and epilepsy

**Neonatal seizures**

- Birth asphyxia and trauma
- Intracranial hemorrhage
- Hypoglycemia
- Hypocalcemia, hypomagnesemia
- Pyridoxine dependent seizures
- Inborn errors of metabolism
- Developmental malformations of the brain
- *Infections:* Meningitis, septicemia, tetanus neonatorum, intra-uterine infections
- Maternal withdrawal of medications
- Accidental antenatal injection of local anesthetic into fetal scalp

**Beyond newborn period**

- Simple febrile seizures
- Genetic epilepsies
- Infectious and postinfectious
- Traumatic and post-traumatic
- Vascular and post-vascular event
- Asphyxia and post-asphyxia
- Hypoglycemia and post-hypoglycemic injury
- Autoimmune disorders
- Space occupying lesions: Tumors, abscess, granulomas
- Malformations of the brain and neuronal migration disorders
- Neurocutaneous syndromes
- Degenerative brain disorders
- Metabolic disorders: Hypo- or hypernatremia, hypocalcemia, hypomagnesemia, inborn errors of metabolism
- Drugs and toxins: Phenothiazines, lead, camphor, salicylates, strychnine, amphetamines, carbon monoxide, organophosphorus compounds, baclofen, phenytoin
- Miscellaneous: Hypertension, Reye syndrome

### Differential Diagnosis

Various paroxysmal events mimic epilepsy. Entities seen commonly in children are discussed.

*Benign neonatal sleep myoclonus:* A well infant presents with bursts of myoclonic or clonic movements only during sleep in the first week of life. The movements abort as soon as the child awakens. The condition lasts for a few weeks to months. Only reassurance is required.

*Breath holding spells:* This behavioral problem usually affects boys between 6 months and 3 years of age. The sequence of events is typical. The child first has a long cry, usually after being denied some demand. Then he holds his breath and turns blue and limp. This may be followed by tonic and a few clonic movements. Parents must be reassured and advised about consistent parenting practices. They should refrain from giving into the child's demand or giving him undue attention just after the episode. Iron deficiency should be treated.

*Syncope:* This usually occurs in the upright position. The patient may have been standing immobile for some time or have suffered sudden fear or emotion. The fall to the ground is usually not as sudden as in a convulsion. The patient is pale and pulse is slow. The attack is aborted by lying flat or with legs elevated as this improves the cerebral blood flow.

*Psychogenic seizures:* These occur more commonly in older girls. The patient subconsciously tends to gain something. There are bizarre body movements with eyes tightly shut and pelvic thrusts. Very often the child does it when there is an audience around.

### Epileptic Encephalopathies

These are conditions in which epileptiform abnormalities themselves contribute to progressive cognitive decline.

#### West Syndrome

This is the most common epileptic encephalopathy in infancy, and is characterized by the triad of epileptic spasms, psychomotor retardation or regression and hypsarrhythmic (high voltage chaotic multifocal spike waves) EEG. Etiology is diverse. Almost any type of brain insult in early life can lead to this syndrome. About two-thirds patients are symptomatic and one-third cryptogenic. The treatment of choice is either ACTH or corticosteroids; vigabatrin is drug of choice for West syndrome associated with tuberous sclerosis. Prognosis for neurodevelopment is variable and depends on seizure control and underlying etiology, being better in the cryptogenic category.

#### Lennox-Gastaut Syndrome

This is one of the most difficult epilepsies to treat. Onset occurs in late infancy or early childhood. Multiple seizure types, including tonic, atonic, myoclonic, atypical absence and/or generalized tonic-clonic seizures, are characteristic. Etiology is diverse. Intellectual regression invariably occurs. Drugs used include valproate, lamotrigine, benzodiazepines, topiramate, levetirecetam and zonisamide. Refractory cases may require dietary therapy or epilepsy surgery.

*Competencies:* **PE30.21; PE30.22**

### Investigations

A video EEG is indicated in all cases of unprovoked seizure. While a normal EEG does not rule out seizure, it is useful in diagnosing epilepsy syndromes and pseudoseizures and in enabling decisions regarding antiepileptic drug withdrawal. Some salient EEG findings are summarized in Table 19.7. In tropical countries, neuroimaging (preferably MRI brain with contrast) is recommended in all cases with unprovoked seizure as neurocysticercosis is very common.

### Principles of Therapy

*General advice:* This includes counseling against unsupervised swimming, cycling or crossing a road. The family and even school authorities should be educated about what to do during an acute seizure. Decision to start long-term AED has to be tailored to the patient based on risk factors for recurrence such as abnormal neurological examination, neuroimaging or EEG, or presentation in status. Without risk factors, AED are usually started after two unprovoked episodes.

Initial therapy is monotherapy, initially in low dose that is gradually increased to maximum pharmacologically tolerated dose (Table 19.8). Polytherapy is indicated, if there are multiple seizure types or failure to respond to monotherapy. Rational combination should be used; drugs with the same mechanism of action and similar adverse effect profile should be avoided. The duration of therapy has to be individualized but is usually tapered after at least 2 years of seizure free period.

Up to one-third of epilepsies are drug refractory or medically intractable, which is defined as a failure of

**Table 19.7:** Diagnostic utility of electroencephalography in epilepsy

| *Finding* | *Likely diagnosis* |
|---|---|
| Spike followed by slow waves | Interictal pattern of epilepsy |
| 3 Hz spike and wave discharges; provoked by hyperventilation | Absence epilepsy |
| Chaotic high voltage record with multifocal spikes (hypsarrhythmia) | West syndrome |
| Brief bursts of polyspikes with photosensitivity | Juvenile myoclonic epilepsy |
| Spike wave complexes in Rolandic areas | Benign epilepsy with centrotemporal spikes |
| Generalized periodic epileptiform discharges | Subacute sclerosing panencephalitis |
| Lateralized periodic epileptiform discharges | Herpes simplex encephalitis |

**Table 19.8:** Choice of therapies for epilepsy

| *Seizure* | *First choice* | *Second choice* |
|---|---|---|
| Focal seizure | Oxcarbamazepine; carbamazepine | Valproate; phenytoin |
| Generalized tonic-clonic | Valproate; phenytoin | Levetiracetam; lamotrigine |
| Absence | Valproate; lamotrigine | Levetiracetam; topiramate; zonisamide |
| Epileptic spasms | ACTH or steroids | Vigabatrine |
| Myoclonic | Valproate | Levetiracetam; topiramate; zonisamide |
| Tonic | Valproate; lamotrigine | Levetiracetam; topiramate; zonisamide |
| Atonic | Valproate; lamotrigine | Levetiracetam; topiramate; zonisamide |

adequate trial of two tolerated and appropriately chosen AED schedules. Therapeutic options include dietary therapy, vagal nerve stimulation, immunotherapy and epilepsy surgery.

### Suggested Reading


1. Fenichel GM. Paroxysmal disorders. In: Pina-Garza JE, James KC. Elsevier (eds). Clinical Pediatric Neurology, 8th edn. 2020; pp 1–48.
3. Fisher RS, Cross JH, French JA, et al. Operational classification of seizure types by the International League Against Epilepsy: Position paper of the ILAE Commission for Classification and Terminology. Epilepsia 2017; 58: 522–30.
2. Scheffer IE, Berkovic S, Capovilla G, et al, ILAE classification of the epilepsies: Position paper of the ILAE Commission for Classification and Terminology. Epilepsia 2017; 58: 512–21.
4. Swanson LC, Ahmed R. Epilepsy syndromes: Current classification and future directions. Neurosurg Clin N Am 2022; 33: 113–34.


*Competency:* **PE30.16**

## HEADACHE

Headache is a common reason for neurological consultation in children. Headaches may be acute, recurrent or chronic and primary (e.g. migraine) or secondary to an intracranial or systemic cause.

### Pathophysiology

The brain and most of the dura and ependyma are pain insensitive. Pain sensitive intracranial structures are vascular sinuses, large arteries and dura mater at the base of the brain, and extracranial structures are skin, subcutaneous tissue, cranial nerves, arteries, muscles, periosteum, sinuses and teeth. Inflammation, injury, displacement or traction of these structures may cause headache. The trigeminal and upper cervical nerves mediate the pain sensations.

### Evaluation of a Child with Headache

Evaluation is primarily clinical and investigations to rule out serious underlying intracranial lesions are required infrequently. A detailed history about the pattern of headache should include description of episodes, frequency, duration, location and associated symptoms. Severe progressive recent onset headache may suggest intracranial pathology such a brain tumor.

### Migraine

Migraine presents as acute recurrent headache occurring in episodes lasting 2–72 hours. Migraine accounts for 75% of consultations for headache, affecting about 10% children aged 5–15 years. Below the age of 7 years, both sexes are equally affected. At older age, girls are affected more often. Typical features include unilateral localization (in two-thirds of patients), throbbing character, moderate to severe intensity, nausea, vomiting, photophobia and phonophobia. Triggers include stress, exercise, trauma and menstruation.

Migraine is classified as migraine with aura (classic migraine), migraine without aura (common migraine) and migraine equivalents. Migraine without aura is twice as common among school age children as migraine with aura, but both may occur in the same person. Usual features of aura are visual aberrations, flashing lights, colored lines, blind spots, blurred vision, hemianopia or visual hallucinations. Dysesthesias of limbs and perioral region, focal motor deficits like hemiplegia, ophthalmoplegia and aphasia may also occur. Aura is transient and usually lasts less than a day. Migraine equivalents are transitory disturbance in neurologic function, including benign paroxysmal vertigo, cyclic vomiting, paroxysmal torticollis, acute confusional migraine, hemiplegic migraine and ophthalmoplegic migraine.

Family history is present in 90% cases, especially in classic migraine. Inheritance is believed to be multifactorial.

Known triggers of migraine should be avoided. During the attack, the child should be given an analgesic and asked to rest. Nonsteroidal anti-inflammatory drugs like ibuprofen, are usually effective. Sleep is also effective; the attack is usually over by the time the child awakens. Selective serotonin agonists, like sumatriptan, available as oral, sublingual preparations and nasal sprays, are effective and non-sedative. A severe attack may benefit from intravenous prochlorperazine maleate, dihydroergotamine or sodium valproate. Prophylactic therapy is indicated, if there is significant school absenteeism. Flunarizine, amitriptyline, propranolol, topiramate and valproate may be used. Maintaining a headache dairy is useful.

### Tension Type Headache

This is a common type of headache, affecting 10–25% of children, with a lifetime prevalence of 70%. Headache could be episodic or chronic, persisting for weeks or months. Episodic tension type headache affects all ages and both sexes and is related to fatigue and stress. The pain is a constant ache usually localized to the back of head and neck. It is probably mediated by sustained contraction of muscles attached to the skull. Nausea and vomiting, photophobia and phonophobia are absent.

### Suggested Reading


1. Koken OY, Danis A, Yukel D, et al. Pediatric headache: Are the red flags misleading or prognostic? Brain Dev 2021;43:372–79.
2. Merison K, Victorio MCC. Approach to the diagnosis of pediatric headache. Semin Pediatr Neurol 2021;40:100920.
3. Szperka C. Headache in children and adolescents. Continuum (Minneap Minn) 2021;27:703–31.


*Competencies:* **PE27.7; PE30.1; PE30.2; PE30.20**

## INFECTIONS AND ACUTE ENCEPHALITIS SYNDROME

A wide variety of infectious agents can invade the central nervous system and produce a range of manifestations. The most common manifestations is meningoencephalitis, which literally means inflammation of the brain parenchyma and meninges. Pathologically, the inflammation of brain and meninges goes side by side although clinically one may get a picture of predominant meningitis or encephalitis. Other manifestations of central nervous system infection are granulomas, brain abscess and spinal arachnoiditis. Brain infections have the potential for increased risk of mortality and disabling permanent sequelae.

The term acute encephalitis syndrome (AES) was coined by the WHO in 2006 for the purpose of surveillance for Japanese encephalitis. It is defined as an illness characterized by acute onset of fever and a change in mental status manifesting as confusion, disorientation, coma, inability to talk and/or new onset seizures, except simple febrile seizures. Causes of acute encephalitis syndrome are listed in Table 19.9. Although the most important causes are infections of the brain, noninfectious causes include chemicals and toxins.

**Table 19.9:** Etiology of acute encephalitis syndrome

**Viral infections**
- Mosquito borne, flaviviruses (Japanese B encephalitis, St. Louis encephalitis, West Nile, Murray valley encephalitis, dengue)
- Arthropod borne, equine encephalitis viruses (Western, Eastern, Venezuelan)
- Herpes viruses (herpes simplex 1 and 2, varicella zoster, cytomegalovirus, Epstein-Barr, HHV-6)
- Enteroviruses (polio, Coxsackie, echoviruses, enteroviruses 70 and 71)
- *Others:* Rhabdovirus (rabies), orthomyxovirus (influenza), paramyxoviruses (mumps, measles, parainfluenza, Nipah), adenoviruses, parvoviruses, Bunyavirus (California encephalitis); reovirus (Colorado tick fever), HIV, lymphocytic choriomeningitis, prion infection, slow infections

**Bacteria**
- Pyogenic meningitis
- Tuberculous meningitis
- *Others: Shigella, Salmonella typhi*, sepsis; leptospirosis, syphilis, *Mycoplasma pneumoniae, Listeria monocytogenes*, Lyme disease, brucellosis, *Legionella*, Cat-scratch disease

**Other infections**
- Rickettsia (Rocky mountain spotted fever, endemic and epidemic typhus, *Coxiella burnetii*, Ehrlichiosis)
- Fungi (*Cryptococcus, Histoplasma, Aspergillus*, mucormycosis, *Candida*, coccidioidomycosis)
- Protozoa (*Plasmodium, Trypanosoma, Naeglaria, Acanthameba, Toxoplasma gondii*, schistosomiasis, *Echinococcus granulosus*)

**Non-infectious inflammation of the brain**
- Acute disseminated encephalomyelitis
- Antibody associated encephalitis

**Postinfectious**

Typhoid, shigella, Reye syndrome

**Other causes**
- Hypoxic encephalopathy, heat hyperpyrexia
- Hypertensive encephalopathy*
- *Metabolic causes*:* Diabetic acidosis, uremic coma, hepatic coma, neonatal hyperbilirubinemia, lactic acidosis, mitochondrial disorders, inborn errors of metabolism
- *Fluid and electrolyte disturbances*:* Hypernatremia, hyponatremia, alkalosis, acidosis
- *Toxins*:* Heavy metals (lead, mercury, arsenic), insecticides, *Cannabis indica*, carbon monoxide
- Post-vaccination
- *Structural causes*:* Tumor, vascular event, head injury, other space occupying lesion

HHV human herpes virus; *Associated fever might be due to another cause

## Viral Meningoencephalitis

Brain infections may be caused by primary neurotropic viruses (arboviruses, herpesviruses and rabies) and, less often, by 'incidental' CNS pathogens (enteroviruses, orthomyxoviruses, paramyxoviruses and adenoviruses). Sudden onset of fever with or without nonspecific symptoms is followed within hours to days by convulsions, coma, focal deficits and signs of raised intracranial tension. Presentation and outcomes vary between individuals, particularly if the host is immunocompromised. The patient may die in the acute phase or recover completely or partially.

Lumbar puncture shows up to 1000 cells/mm$^3$ in the cerebrospinal fluid (CSF) that are chiefly lymphocytes. Protein is mildly increased and sugar is normal. Identification of the specific viral etiology is possible in only a small proportion. Diagnosis is usually made by specific antibodies or viral detection through CSF polymerase chain reaction (PCR). Multiplex PCR are being developed.

Supportive management of sick patients includes careful monitoring in an intensive care unit, maintenance of vital functions and nutrition, asepsis, good nursing care and physiotherapy. Antipyretics, anticonvulsants and measures to reduce intracranial tension are instituted as needed. Specific antiviral treatment is available for herpes simplex encephalitis.

## Japanese Encephalitis (JE)

JE virus is the leading cause of viral encephalitis in India, Asia and worldwide. In India, most cases are reported from southern and eastern states with outbreaks during and after monsoons.

### *Etiology and Transmission*

JE virus is a single stranded neurotropic RNA virus belonging to family Flaviviridae. The chief vector across Asia is *Culex tritaenirrhynchus*, a zoophilic mosquito that breeds in rice fields. The infection is zoonotic, with pigs and Ardeid birds being the chief hosts that harbour, amplify and transmit the infection without developing illness. Man is an incidental dead-end host in whom the brief viremia deters further transmission.

### *Clinical Features*

JE tends to occur in epidemics and outbreaks, chiefly affecting children between 5 and 15 years of age or young adults. A prodrome of fever, headache, vomiting and diarrhea, lasting a few hours to days, is followed by an acute encephalitic stage lasting 7–10 days, with persistent fever, seizures, coma, focal deficits and signs of raised intracranial tension. Shock and death may ensue in severe cases. Survivors recover rapidly or gradually over weeks to months, but a significant proportion have prominent extrapyramidal sequelae.

### *Diagnosis*

CSF shows nil to moderate pleocytosis with elevated protein and normal sugar. MRI shows characteristic changes in

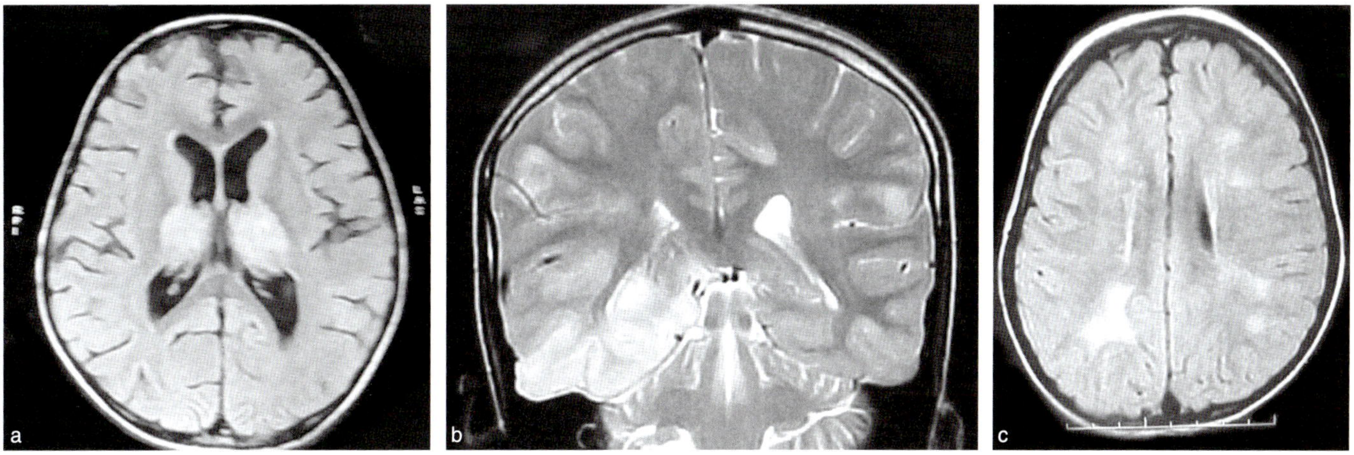

Fig. 19.7: Magnetic resonance imaging in acute encephalitis: (a) Axial FLAIR images showing bilateral thalamic involvement in Japanese B encephalitis; (b) Coronal T2-weighted images showing right temporal involvement in herpes encephalitis; (c) Axial FLAIR images showing bilateral subcortical and periventricular patchy asymmetrical white matter signal changes in acute disseminated encephalomyelitis

bilateral thalami, basal ganglia and midbrain (Fig. 19.7a). JE virus specific IgM can be detected by ELISA in CSF and serum. CSF IgM has 95% sensitivity and specificity by 10 days of illness. Viral isolation and detection by PCR in CSF or brain during early illness has low yield.

#### Management

Management is essentially supportive, as outlined above.

#### Prevention

JE can be controlled by reducing contact with mosquitoes (using insecticide spray, larvicides, bed nets and repellents), vaccination of pigs and location of pigsties away from human dwelling. The mainstay of prevention is vaccination of humans, which however, does not interrupt the natural cycle of JE virus nor provide herd immunity. JE vaccination is now part of the National Immunization Program in endemic states.

***Mouse brain killed vaccine:*** This was the first vaccine manufactured against JE, but is no longer used.

***Live attenuated SA-14-14-2 strain vaccine:*** This is the only live attenuated JE vaccine currently available. It is produced by Chengdu Biologicals and is being used in the public sector in China since 1998, Nepal (since 1999) and India (since 2006). Studies conducted in Nepal reported efficacy of 99.3% in the same year, 98.5% after one year and 96.2% after 5 years. Dose is 0.5 mL given subcutaneous.

***IC51 Vaccine–Ixiaro:*** This is a new generation formalin inactivated vaccine prepared from the SA-14-14-2 strain grown in Vero cells. This is the only JE vaccine to have received US Food and Drug Administration (FDA) approval for use in adults and children beyond 2 months of age. This vaccine produced with Austrian collaboration is available in India as JEEV (Biological E). Schedule is 2 doses 28 days apart followed by a booster after one year. Dose is 0.25 mL below 3 years and 0.5 mL beyond.

***Indian strain vaccine:*** Another Vero cell-derived purified inactivated JE vaccine is developed from an Indian strain of the virus (821564 XZ) isolated in Kolar, Karnataka. It has received approval from the Drug Controller General of India and is being marketed by the name, JENVAC.

### Herpes Simplex Virus Encephalitis (HSVE)

This is the leading cause of sporadic encephalitis and has a severe fulminant presentation with high rates of mortality and disabling sequelae. A non-specific prodrome of headache, malaise, fever and vomiting is followed by altered consciousness, focal or generalized seizures and characteristically, focal neurologic deficits. Presentations include movement disorders, stroke, behavioral disturbances, hallucinations and memory loss.

Examination of the CSF reveals pleocytosis, mild protein elevation and occasionally, red blood cells. EEG shows periodic lateralized epileptiform discharges in 35% cases. Neuroimaging shows characteristic temporal lobe signal changes, with MRI (Fig. 19.7b) being more sensitive than CT. PCR for herpes simplex virus type 1 in the CSF has 75% sensitivity and 100% specificity and is considered the gold standard for diagnosis.

Management includes supportive care and specific therapy with acyclovir at 20 mg/kg intravenously every 8 hr for 14–21 days. However, despite early therapy, less than 40% patients survive without disability and 5% may relapse.

### Acute Bacterial Meningitis

This is a relatively common and potentially fatal condition. A high index of suspicion is essential to enable timely diagnosis and treatment.

#### Risk Factors and Pathogenesis

Infections are most common in the first 5 years of life. Risk factors include bacterial colonization of nasopharynx, overcrowding, poverty and male sex. Anatomic defects such as fracture base of skull, pilonidal sinus and immunodeficiencies predispose to meningitis. Bacteremia is followed by lodging of bacteria in choroid plexus and the meninges. An intense inflammation leads to meningeal exudates, ventriculitis, perivascular inflammatory exudates, venous occlusion, infarction, necrosis and/or raised intracranial pressure.

### Etiology

The causative organisms vary with age. In the first 2 months of life, the most common pathogens include gram-negative bacteria, followed by *Staphylococcus aureus*, group B streptococci and *Listeria monocytogenes*. Between 2–24 months, *Hemophilus influenzae* type b infections are most common, followed by *Streptococcus pneumoniae* and meningococcus. Beyond 2 years of age, pneumococcus and meningococcus are the most common organisms, followed by *Hemophilus influenzae* type b.



### Clinical Features

Clinical features vary with age. Newborn and young infants present with lethargy, poor feeding, shrill cry and seizures. Older infants present with fever, poor feeding, irritability and photophobia. A tense bulging anterior fontanelle in a febrile infant suggests meningitis. Older children present with abrupt onset of high fever, severe unrelenting headache, anorexia, myalgia, photophobia and meningeal signs, and may develop convulsions and coma.

Meningeal signs are often lacking till 2 years of age. Signs of raised intracranial pressure include hypertension, bradycardia, bulging fontanelle, third or sixth cranial nerve palsy, posturing or breathing abnormalities. Papilledema is unusual, especially in infants. A search should be made for septic foci elsewhere. Purpuric rash suggests meningococcemia.

### Differential Diagnosis

Viral and tuberculous meningoencephalitis are the chief differential diagnoses. The latter is particularly difficult to differentiate from partially treated bacterial meningitis

### Diagnosis

Diagnosis is confirmed by CSF examination. However, lumbar puncture must be deferred, if there are signs suggesting raised intracranial pressure, due to risk of herniation and death. CSF examination reveals raised pressure, turbid fluid, markedly increased cell count (often in thousands per $mm^3$) chiefly comprised of polymorphonuclear cells, increased protein and low sugar (less than 40% of the concomitant blood sugar) . Gram stain and bacterial culture may enable diagnosis. However, PCR to detect bacterial DNA is more sensitive. If partially treated with antibiotics, CSF cell count is lower, has predominance of lymphocytes and culture is sterile.

Imaging in bacterial meningitis may be normal or show intense meningeal enhancement or intracranial complications such as subdural effusion **(Fig. 19.8a)** or empyema, ventriculitis, brain abscess, hydrocephalus or infarcts. Sequelae include deafness, epilepsy, intellectual disability and neurological deficits.

### Treatment

Empirical IV therapy with a third-generation cephalosporin is initiated without delay. Below 3 months of age, gram-negative coverage is also given. Antibiotics are revised based on results of culture. Therapy is usually administered for 3 weeks in neonates and for 7–10 days in older children. Dexamethasone, administered intravenously at 0.15 mg/kg/dose every 6 hours for two days, beginning with the first dose of antibiotic is considered useful in preventing sequelae. Repeat lumbar puncture and imaging is indicated, if clinical response is poor.

### Prevention

The risk of bacterial meningitis is reduced considerably by vaccination against *Hemophilus*, pneumococci and meningococci. Close contacts of patients with meningococcal meningitis should receive chemoprophylaxis with rifampicin at 10 mg/kg/dose twice daily for two days.

## Tuberculous Meningitis

This is the most severe form of tuberculosis. Predisposing factors are young age, household contact, recent measles and protein energy malnutrition.

### Pathophysiology

Primary pulmonary infection is followed by intermittent bacillemia and seeding of meninges, termed Rich foci. During stress and lowered immunity, these foci rupture to cause tuberculous meningitis, with characteristic thick exudates in the basal cisterns and endarteritis.

### Clinical Features

The first or prodromal phase of the illness, which lasts 1–4 weeks, is characterized by nonspecific irregular fever, anorexia, irritability and occasional vomiting. Stage 2 has neurological manifestations like seizures, focal deficits and meningeal signs. Stage 3 is one of coma and sequelae. Hydrocephalus (communicating or obstructive), decerebrate posturing, cranial nerve palsies, optic atrophy, extrapyramidal signs and focal deficits are more common in tuberculous than other CNS infections. The chief differential diagnosis is partially treated bacterial meningitis.

### Diagnosis

Diagnosis is based on clinical features and investigations. CSF typically shows raised pressure, up to 500 cells per $mm^3$ with lymphocytic predominance, increased protein and low sugar (level about half the concomitant blood sugar level). However, CSF may mimic bacterial meningitis or be normal in about 10–15% cases each.

Neuroimaging often shows hydrocephalus and basal exudates **(Fig. 19.8b)**. The diagnosis is supported by prolonged history of symptoms, family history of tuberculosis, positive Mantoux (tuberculin) test, chest radiographic evidence of tuberculosis and findings on CSF examination and neuroimaging. The diagnosis is confirmed if CSF culture or PCR is positive for *Mycobacterium tuberculosis* or acid-fast bacilli are present. GeneXpert is a quick cartridge based test for *M. tuberculosis* genome and drug resistance to rifampicin.

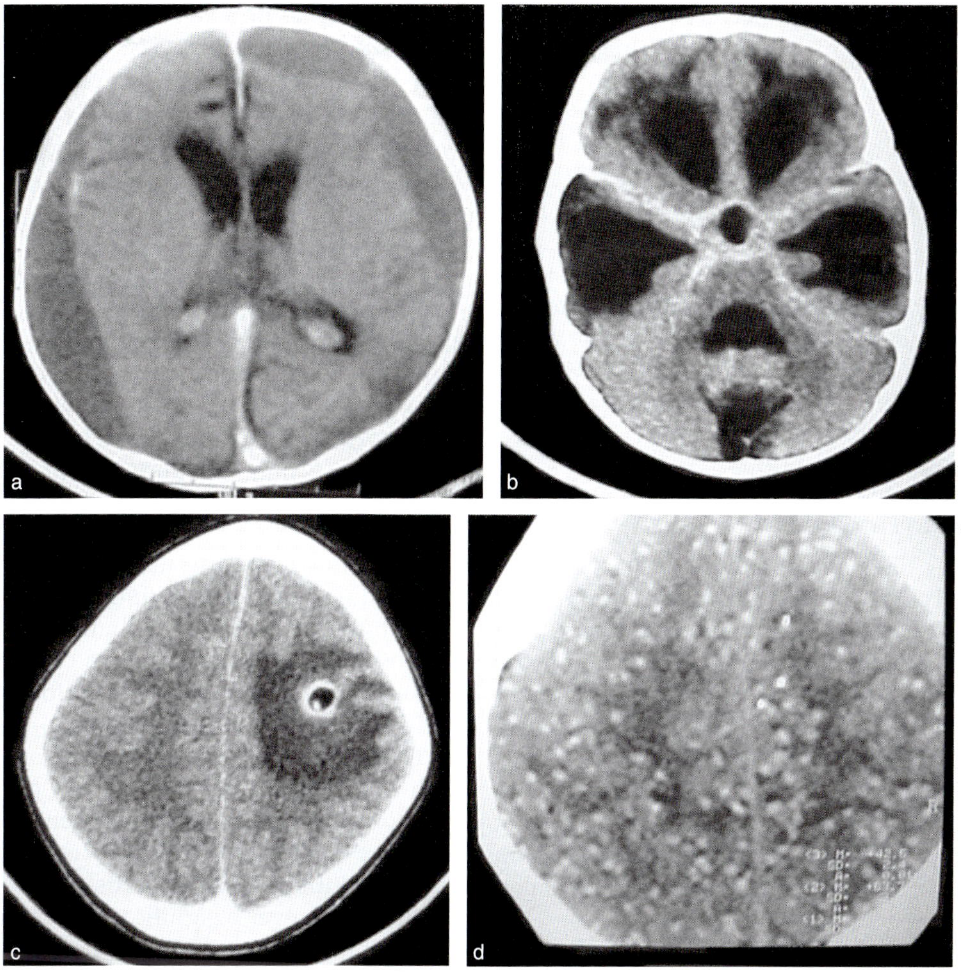

Fig. 19.8: Computed tomography in acute encephalitis. Contrast enhanced images showing: (a) Bilateral subdural effusion in a child with acute bacterial meningitis; (b) Communicating hydrocephalus with basal meningeal enhancement in a child with tubercular meningitis; (c) Ring enhancing lesion with eccentric dot in left parietal lobe suggestive of neurocysticercosis; (d) Non-contrast image shows multiple calcified neurocysticerci lesions, described as 'starry sky'

*Treatment*

Antitubercular treatment includes 2 months of four-drug (intensive) therapy and 7–10 months of two-drug (maintenance) therapy (Chapter 11). Intravenous dexamethasone is followed by oral steroids for 6–8 weeks to prevent sequelae. Patients with obstructive hydrocephalus require CSF diversion by shunt or third ventriculostomy.

*Prognosis*

Prognosis is related to patient age and stage of disease at diagnosis. Early treatment (stage 1) results in complete cure, while 80% of patients treated in stage 2 survive and 50% show sequelae. Only 50% of patients treated in stage 3 survive of which 80% show sequelae. Complications include hydrocephalus, optic neuritis, infarction and spinal block due to arachnoiditis. Sequelae include focal neurological deficits, epilepsy, intellectual disability, blindness and occasionally, endocrinopathies.

## Scrub Typhus Meningoencephalitis

Scrub typhus caused by *Orientia tsutsugamushi* is the commonest rickettsial infection in India.

Over the last decade, studies have shown that scrub typhus infections are widely distributed all over the country. About 15–20% of scrub typhus infections are associated with meningoencephalitis. Studies on acute encephalitis syndrome have shown a significant proportion to be caused by scrub typhus. Transmission to humans occurs by exposure to infected larval mites or chiggers.

Acute fever is the most common presenting symptom often associated with breathlessness, cough, nausea, vomiting, myalgia and headache. An eschar at the site of chigger bite can be seen in early disease and is a useful diagnostic clue. Other features are rash, thrombocytopenia, deranged liver and kidney function. Meningoencephalitis clinically resembles tuberculous meningitis with relatively long history. Focal deficits are uncommon. Diagnosis is made by detection of IgM by ELISA, immunofluorescence assay or polymerase chain reaction in serum. Doxycycline 100 mg twice daily for 7–14 days is the treatment of choice.

## Neurocysticercosis

Parasitic infestation of the brain by encysted larvae of pork tapeworm *Taenia solium* is a public health problem in many developing regions including Southeast Asia, Latin America and sub-Saharan Africa. A point prevalence of 4.5 per 1,000 population has been noted in rural Northwest India.Humans acquire the infection by consuming undercooked pork containing cysticerci or by eating food contaminated with feces containing tapeworm eggs. The eggs form larvae that cross into the bloodstream to seed the brain.

### Pathogenesis

Parenchymal or cerebral infection is more common than extraparenchymal. Cysts may be single or multiple, and usually form at the gray-white matter interface. Four stages are recognised—vescicular, colloidal, granular-nodular and nodular-calcified lesions. The first two are active stages, carry low risk of seizures and do not enhance on neuroimaging. Cysticerci usually cause seizures in the degenerating or granular-nodular stage, which are detected as enhancing lesions on CT or MRI.

### Clinical Features and Diagnosis

Patients are usually older than 3 years and present with recent onset of focal or generalized epilepsy. Neuro-imaging reveals one or multiple ring-enhancing lesions with perifocal edema (Fig. 19.8c) with or without an asymmetric scolex within the ring. Patients may occasionally present with encephalitis and raised intracranial pressure with or without seizures. Neuroimaging in these cases reveals cerebral edema in a brain studded with cysts in various stages, including enhancing and nonenhancing cysticerci, termed a 'starry sky' appearance (Fig. 19.8d). Extraparenchymal disease manifests as intraventricular, spinal or ocular cysts or arachnoiditis.

The combination of clinical and radiological findings is usually diagnostic. Radiological differential diagnoses include tubercular and *Toxoplasma* granulomas. Clinicoradiologic features favoring tuberculoma over neurocysticercosis are: (i) Size of CT lesion >20 mm, (ii) location at the base of the brain/posterior fossa (NCC lesions are often seen at the gray–white matter junction), (iii) lobulated irregular shape or conglomerate lesions, (iv) marked edema causing midline shift, (v) presence of raised intracranial pressure, (vi) progressive focal neurodeficits, and (vii) presence of a lactate peak, and choline/creatine ratio >1 on MR spectroscopy. Serology by enzyme linked immunoelectrotransfer blot assay has high sensitivity (100%) and specificity (83–100%) for multiple and extraparenchymal neurocysticercosis, but has poor diagnostic utility for one or few cysticerci or calcified lesions.

### Management

Symptomatic treatment of seizures is essential. Anti-epileptic therapy is continued for at least 6 months and until the lesions disappear. Albendazole is the preferred cysticidal agent and is administered at 15–20 mg/kg/day in two divided doses for 10–14 days in patient with 1–2 viable cysts. Additional therapy with praziquantel is advised for >2 viable cysts. Cysticidal therapy is contraindicated in ocular neurocysticercosis and cysticercal encephalitis since degenerating cysts may evoke intense inflammatory response. Steroids are used to reduce symptomatic edema in cysticercal encephalitis.

## Acute Disseminated Encephalomyelitis

Immune-mediated cerebral inflammation may follow viral exanthem or vaccination. While measles is the most common cause, causative infections include rubella, mumps, varicella zoster, influenza A and B, Rickettsia and *Mycoplasma pneumoniae*. Vaccines that may precipitate the syndrome are rabies, vaccinia, measles and yellow fever. Patients present with altered consciousness, convulsions and multifocal neurological signs affecting cerebellum, optic nerves, long tracts and spinal cord. Fever may be absent at onset. CSF may reveal mild pleocytosis. MRI shows characteristic scattered lesions in the white matter, at times affecting the deep gray matter and other areas (Fig. 19.7c). Treatment options include pulse corticosteroids, intravenous immunoglobulin and plasmapheresis.

## Autoimmune Encephalitis

This is considered the most common single cause of encephalitis in western countries, being commoner than any single infectious encephalitis. Serum and/or CSF antibodies are found against ion channels, receptors and associated proteins. Twenty three to forty percent of patients present in childhood. There are two types of antibodies: (i) Those directed towards surface or synaptic antigens such as NMDA receptor, which are often reversible, and (ii) those directed towards intracellular antigens, which are more commonly neoplasia associated. Anti-NMDA receptor antibody encephalitis is the most common in children. However, a significant proportion of children do not exhibit known antibodies. These children may have as yet unidentified antibodies or other mechanisms. Presenting symptoms include neuropsychiatric features, mutism, movement disorders, seizures and cognitive decline. Treatment options include pulse methylprednisolone, intravenous immunoglobulin, plasma exchanges and IV rituximab.

## Encephalopathies

The term encephalopathy is used for diffuse cerebral dysfunction due to a non-inflammatory pathology, as against encephalitis which is characterized by inflammation. However, the two are often difficult to distinguish clinically. Fever cannot discriminate between the two entities as encephalopathy may be precipitated by systemic infection, and fever may have an alternative cause.

### Dengue Encephalopathy

Neurological manifestations, including encephalopathy, are common with dengue infections and may be caused by vasculitis, cerebral edema, hypoperfusion or hyponatremia. However, virus invasion of the brain producing encephalitis has also been documented. Thrombocytopenia, rash and liver dysfunction are commonly seen.

### Reye Syndrome

This acute encephalopathy may follow a viral upper respiratory tract infection (90% cases) or varicella (5–7%). History of salicylate ingestion is common. The onset is abrupt with protracted vomiting followed by delirium, combative behavior and stupor. While most children have a mild course, there may be rapid worsening with seizures, coma and death. Common findings include mild hepatomegaly, hypoglycemia, elevated serum transaminases (>3-fold), hyperammonemia and coagulopathy with normal levels of serum bilirubin. Liver biopsy reveals diffuse microvesicular fatty infiltration without any inflammation or necrosis.

### Suggested Reading


1. Cherian A, Ajitha KC, Iype T, Divya KP. Neurotuberculosis: an update. Acta Neurol Belg 2021;121:11–21.
2. Co DO, Kwon JM. Autoimmune encephalitis: Distinguishing features and specific therapies. Crit Care Clin 2022;38:393–412.
3. Srivastava N, Deval H, Mittal M, et al. The outbreaks of acute encephalitis syndrome in Uttar Pradesh, India (1978-2020) and its effective management. Front Public Health 2022; 9: 793268.
4. Young SM, Sagull A. Bacterial meningitis in children. Am Fam Physician 2022;105:311–12.
5. White AC, Coyle CM, Rajshekhar V, et al. Diagnosis and treatment of neurocysticercosis. Clin Infectious Dis 2018;66:e49–e75.


*Competency:* **PE30.3**

## RAISED INTRACRANIAL PRESSURE, SPACE OCCUPYING LESIONS AND HYDROCEPHALUS

Intracranial pressure refers to the pressure of CSF within the cranium. It is normally pulsatile and less than 5 mm Hg in newborns, 6–15 mm Hg in infants and 10–15 mm Hg in older children. Intracranial pressure is considered severely elevated, if raised above 40 mm Hg.

### Pathophysiology

Raised intracranial pressure results in decreased cerebral blood flow and/or herniation of brain tissue. Cerebral blood flow is normally about 50 mL per 100 g of brain tissue per minute and depends on cerebral perfusion pressure, which equals the difference between mean arterial pressure and intracranial pressure. Various myogenic, metabolic and neurogenic autoregulatory mechanisms help maintain cerebral blood flow. Decrease in cerebral blood flow to below 40% leads to progressive ischemia, neuronal death, cerebral edema and further increase in intracranial pressure, leading to diffuse bilateral cortical dysfunction and coma. Causes of raised intracranial pressure are listed in Table 19.10.

**Table 19.10:** Causes of raised intracranial pressure

| |
|---|
| Hydrocephalus (for details, *see* Table 19.13) |
| Central nervous system infections |
| Intracranial hemorrhage |
| *Space occupying lesions:* Tumors, granulomas, abscesses |
| *Metabolic causes:* Reye syndrome; inborn errors of metabolism, acute encephalopathy |
| Arterial, venous stroke |
| Hypertensive encephalopathy |
| Idiopathic |

### Clinical Features

Symptoms of raised intracranial pressure are headache, vomiting and visual disturbances, progressing to focal neurological deficits and coma. Chronically raised intracranial pressure before closure of sutures results in increased head size and hydrocephalus, presenting as bilateral sunset sign, tense bulging anterior fontanelle, hypertension and bradycardia. Sixth cranial nerve palsy presenting as squint and diplopia can occur as a 'false localizing sign' of raised intracranial pressure. In older patients with closed fontanelles, separation of sutures produces a sound like a cracked pot, on percussion of the skull, termed positive MacEwen sign. Herniation of brain tissue causes various clinical syndromes (Table 19.11), compression of the brainstem, coma and death.

### Management

Invasive methods to monitor intracranial pressure with intracranial catheters and transducers should be used only in intensive care setting with strict aseptic precautions and are contraindicated in presence of coagulopathy. Measures to manage raised intracranial pressure are listed in Table 19.12.

### Hydrocephalus

This term refers to abnormal accumulation of CSF in the brain, leading to increased pressure and increased

**Table 19.11:** Herniation syndromes

| *Location/type* | *Abnormality* | *Clinical features* |
|---|---|---|
| Lateral transtentorial | Downward and medial displacement of uncus and parahippocampal gyrus | Unilateral dilated pupil with ptosis (third nerve palsy); impaired consciousness; abnormal respiration; hemiparesis |
| Upward transtentorial | Upward displacement of cerebellar vermis and midbrain | Prominent brainstem signs; downward gaze deviation; decerebrate posturing |
| Transforaminal | Downward displacement of cerebellar tonsils and medulla | Neck rigidity; impaired consciousness; ophisthotonus; decerebrate rigidity; vomiting; irregular respiration; apnea; bradycardia |
| Central transtentorial | Downward displacement of diencephalic structures | Impaired consciousness; abnormal respiration; symmetrical small reactive or midposition fixed reactive pupils; decorticate followed by decerebrate posturing |
| Subfalcine | Medial displacement of the cingulate gyrus | Impaired consciousness; monoparesis of the contralateral lower limb |

Table 19.12: Management of raised intracranial pressure

| Management of raised intracranial pressure |
|---|
| Raise head end by 30°; keep head in midline |
| Hyperventilate to maintain $PCO_2$ at 30–35 mm Hg |
| Administer mannitol at 0.25–1 g/kg (1.25–5 mL/kg of 20% solution) as intravenous (IV) bolus; repeat every 8 hours for 48–72 hours |
| Administer hypertonic (3%) saline at 0.1–1 mL/kg/hr to maintain serum sodium at 145–155 mEq/L |
| Administer IV furosemide at 1–2 mg/kg/dose |
| Switch to oral acetazolamide (30–50 mg/kg/day) or glycerol when stable |
| Consider corticosteroids (oral or IV) for vasogenic edema |
| Consider decompressive craniectomy |

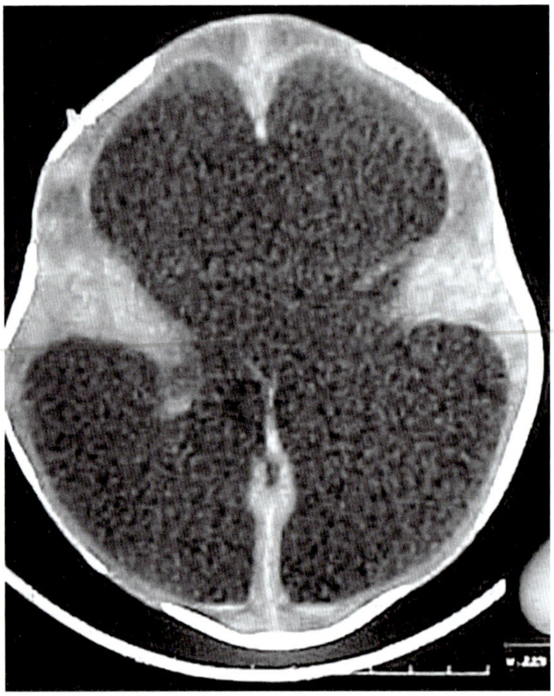

Fig. 19.9: Computed tomography of the brain in a child with gross hydrocephalus

ventricular size (Fig. 19.9), and if occurring before sutural fusion, an increase in head size.

*Pathophysiology*

CSF is produced by the ventricular choroid plexus by ultrafiltration and active secretion at a rate of 20 mL/hr and passes through the ventricular system to be absorbed by arachnoid granulations into venous sinuses. Hydrocephalus may be congenital or acquired. Hydrocephalus is also termed 'obstructive' when there is obstruction to flow of CSF within the ventricular system and 'communicating' when there is increased production or defective absorption of CSF due to non-obstructive causes. Chief causes are listed in Table 19.13.

*Clinical Features*

After sutural fusion, children usually present with symptoms of raised intracranial pressure. A positive MacEwen or crack pot sound on skull percussion suggests sutural separation. The 'setting sun sign' indicates upward gaze palsy due to pressure on the quadrigeminal plate.

Table 19.13: Causes of hydrocephalus in children

**Congenital**
- Aqueductal stenosis, X-linked
- Dandy-Walker malformation (cystic malformation of cerebellum and 4th ventricle)
- Arnold-Chiari malformation (elongation and downward displacement of cerebellum with distortion of CSF pathways)
- Intrauterine infections (toxoplasmosis, rubella, cytomegalovirus)
- Malformation of the vein of Galen
- Genetic dysplasias

**Acquired**
- Intraventricular hemorrhage
- Meningitis: Bacterial, tuberculous, mumps
- Tumors and other space occupying lesions, especially of the posterior fossa
- Posterior fossa subdural collection

Differential diagnoses of a large head include rickets, hemolytic anemia, achondroplasia, familial macrocephaly, megalencephaly and neurometabolic disorders (mucopolysaccharidoses, Tay-Sachs, glutaric acidemia, Canavan and Alexander diseases). Where fontanelle is open, cranial ultrasound can be done and reveals increased ventricular size. CT scan and MRI provide details on severity and etiology. Mildly enlarged ventricles may be seen in cerebral atrophy and should not be confused with hydrocephalus.

*Management*

Untreated hydrocephalus before sutural fusion results in grossly increased head size and cortical thinning. After sutural fusion, untreated cases usually succumb to raised intracranial pressure. While medical measures may temporarily reduce intracranial pressure, CSF diversion, most commonly by a shunt, is more useful. Usually valved tubing is placed between the ventricle and peritoneal cavity. The ventriculoperitoneal shunt usually requires multiple revisions as the child grows older. Complications of shunt surgery include infection leading to meningitis, shunt displacement, block or kinking leading to chronic shunt dysfunction, and abdominal complications such as peritonitis or abscess. Another CSF diversion procedure is endoscopic third ventriculostomy that allows CSF to pass directly into the basal cisterns.

*Prognosis*

Outcomes of hydrocephalus are guarded. Almost two-thirds of children have variable mental and motor disabilities, even with appropriate treatment.

## Space Occupying Lesions

### *Brain Tumors*

Primary brain tumors are a common malignancy in childhood, and may be malignant or benign. Their incidence is increased in neurocutaneous syndromes like tuberous sclerosis and neurofibromatosis. Tumors present chiefly with focal neurological deficits and symptoms of raised intracranial pressure. Two-thirds of pediatric brain tumors are infratentorial. Of these, medulloblastoma and cerebellar astrocytomas account for a third each while brainstem gliomas and ependymomas constitute the majority of the rest. Since the posterior fossa is tightly encased with narrow CSF pathways, infratentorial tumors present with early raised intracranial pressure and hydrocephalus. Common supratentorial tumors include astrocytomas, craniopharyngioma, ependymomas, choroid plexus papillomas and pineal body tumors. Neuroimaging by MRI helps define the nature and extent of tumor.

*Medulloblastoma:* These midline cerebellar tumors usually affect young children, accounting for 30–40% of pediatric posterior fossa tumors. Boys are affected 2–4 times as often than girls. These rapidly growing, malignant tumors present with cerebellar signs and features of raised intracranial pressure. Neuroimaging reveals a midline mass arising from the vermis, effacing the fourth ventricle and basal cisterns, causing obstructive hydrocephalus (Fig. 19.10a). The tumors are usually hyperdense with prominent enhancement (90%) and associated with cysts (40–50%) or calcification (10–20%). Forty percent of patients have evidence of CSF seeding at diagnosis. The prognosis is poor.

*Cerebellar astrocytoma:* These arise from either cerebellar hemispheres, and present with ataxia, incoordination and nystagmus. Most tumors are low-grade and slow-growing and carry a satisfactory prognosis as they can usually be excised completely.

*Brainstem glioma:* These usually present between 5 and 10 years of age with lower cranial nerve palsies, long tract signs, cerebellar signs and signs of raised intracranial pressure. Both focal brainstem gliomas and diffuse intrinsic pontine glioma carry grave prognosis.

*Ependymoma of the fourth ventricle:* These arise from cells lining the ventricle. Tumors arising from the floor of the fourth ventricle present with torticollis and ataxia, while those arising from the side of the ventricle affect cranial nerves, presenting with impaired hearing, dysphagia and clumsiness.

*Craniopharyngioma:* These are cystic benign supratentorial tumors arising from the squamous epithelial rest cells of the Rathke pouch. Clinical features include growth failure, visual field defects (bitemporal hemianopia or unilateral or asymmetric field defects), signs of raised intracranial pressure and endocrine abnormalities like diabetes insipidus and delayed puberty. X-ray skull may reveal calcifications. Treatment includes cyst aspiration and radiotherapy.

*Glioma of cerebral hemispheres:* These usually present with seizures and hemiparesis; features of raised intracranial pressure are usually delayed. Histologically, these may be astrocytoma, oligodendroglioma or glioblastoma.

*Glioma of optic nerve:* These relatively uncommon tumors usually occur in a setting of neurofibromatosis 1 and present with decreased vision, progressing to proptosis, symptoms of raised intracranial pressure, focal neurological deficits and hydrocephalus. Hypothalamic involvement may result in polyuria and polydipsia. Imaging indicates an enlarged optic nerve.

### Brain Abscess

Infection within the brain parenchyma leads to brain abscess formation, usually in the setting of a predisposing condition. Congenital cyanotic heart disease is an important risk factor. Infected sinuses, middle ear or tooth infection, bacterial meningitis, compound skull fractures, penetrating skull injury, neurosurgery and immunodeficiencies are other predisposing conditions. Microorganisms implicated include streptococci (both aerobic and anerobic), gram-negative anaerobic bacilli, *Enterobacteriaceae* and *Staphylococcus aureus*. Fungi and mycobacterial infection may occur in immunocompromised patients.

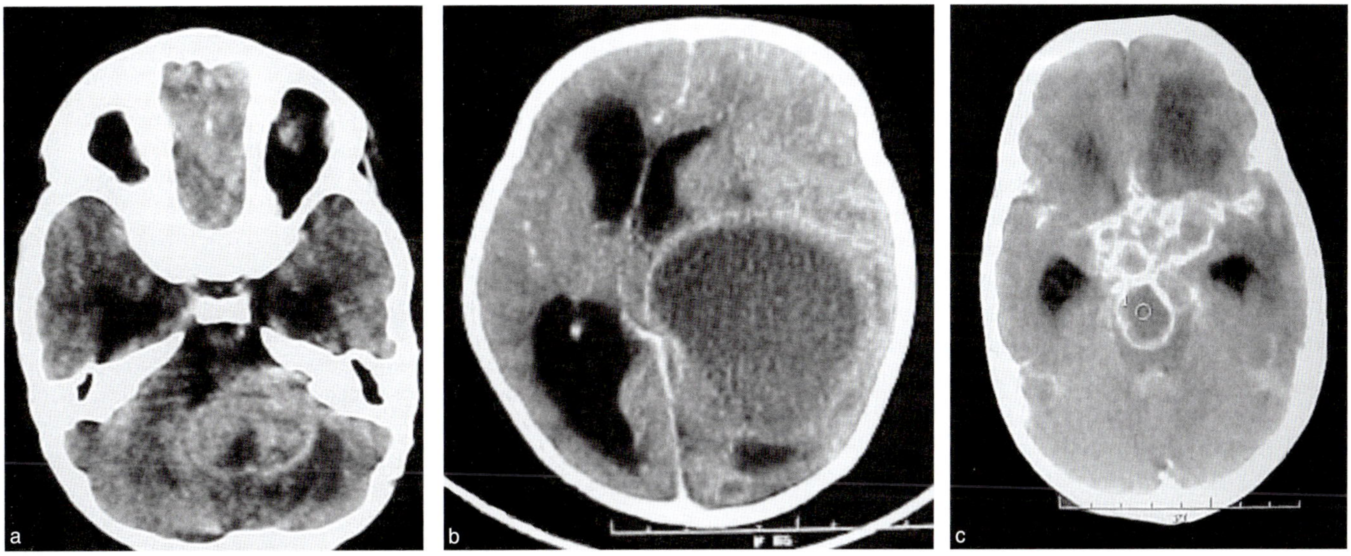


**Fig. 19.10:** Contrast enhanced tomography in the setting of raised intracranial tension showing: (a) Enhancing heterogenous mass arising from vermis suggesting medulloblastoma; (b) Left parietal enhancing lesion with midline shift in a case of brain abscess; (c) Multiple basal ring enhancing lesions and meningeal enhancement in a patient with tubercular meningitis

Classically, the presentation is subacute with a triad of fever, focal neurological deficits and signs of raised intracranial pressure. However, fever may be lacking in 20–50% patients or may be low grade. Intense inflammation and edema produce severe mass effect, leading to herniation and death. MRI helps identify early cerebritis, microabscesses and posterior fossa collection. The abscess appears as a ring-enhancing lesion with surrounding edema. Large lesions show distortion of surrounding structures and midline shift **(Fig. 19.10b)**. CSF may show mild pleocytosis due to meningeal reaction; however, lumbar puncture is usually contraindicated because of risk of herniation. Management includes administration of intravenous antibiotics with good penetration into the CSF for 4–8 weeks. Anaerobic coverage must be ensured. A third-generation cephalosporin with vancomycin and metronidazole provides satisfactory empiric coverage. Drainage of the abscess must be done through burr hole, craniectomy, craniotomy or by stereotactic aspiration.





#### *Subdural Collections*

Subdural collections usually occur as a complication of bacterial meningitis, chiefly in infancy. Subdural effusions are usually sterile and resolve spontaneously; drainage is only necessary, if associated with pressure effect. They may, however, be associated with prolonged fever. Subdural empyemas are collections of pus in subdural spaces and are detected on imaging by an enhancing capsule. They usually require drainage but may refill. Subdural hematomas are usually traumatic and present with features of chronically raised intracranial pressure. A vascular membrane forms around the hematoma. As blood cells get absorbed, the fluid's protein content increases, thus increasing oncotic pressure that draws fluid into the hematoma. The collection grows, tearing small bridging veins within the hematoma, further increasing bleeding. The sequence of bleeding, increased pressure and growth repeats itself. The skull may show positive transillumination. Imaging reveals a biconvex collection, as compared to the crescent shape seen with epidural collections.

#### *Granulomas*

These lesions are more common in developing countries, and include tubercular, parasitic, and less commonly, fungal granulomas.

***Tuberculoma:*** Tuberculoma is a common space occupying lesion, occurring alone or with tuberculous meningitis. Symptoms include seizures, focal neurological deficits and raised intracranial pressure. Imaging shows large (>20 mm) conglomerate ring-enhancing lesions in the supratentorial compartment **(Fig.19.10c)**. Tuberculomas are more irregular in outline than cysticercal lesions and may cause mass effect and midline shift. There may be intense perifocal edema. A hypodense center suggests a tubercular abscess. Tuberculomas may appear or increase in size even while the patient is on antitubercular treatment, probably due to immune reconstitution. Treatment involves antitubercular treatment, including 2 months of intensive (four-drug) therapy and 7–10 months of maintenance (isoniazid and rifampicin) therapy.

### Idiopathic Intracranial Hypertension

Previously termed benign intracranial hypertension or pseudotumor cerebri, the condition is characterized by normal or reduced ventricular size and normal CSF chemistry. Idiopathic intracranial hypertension usually affects adults or adolescents, chiefly female, and is associated with obesity. Its pathophysiology remains unclear. Suggested mechanisms include increased CSF production, decreased CSF absorption or increased cerebral venous pressure, in a setting of endocrinopathy, anemia or use of vitamin A derivatives, tetracyclines, steroids or hormonal contraceptives.

Patients present with symptoms of increased intracranial pressure, such as headache, diplopia, squint or blurred vision. Sixth cranial nerve palsy may occur as a false localizing sign. If present, papilledema and visual deficits require prompt evaluation and treatment. Options in management include oral acetazolamide, glycerol or corticosteroids, repeated lumbar puncture and surgical decompression (optic nerve sheath decompression and shunt surgery).

### Suggested Reading


1. Brun BN, Aylward SC. Pediatric intracranial hypertension. Semin Pediatr Neurol 2021;40:100922.
2. Koleva M. Hydrocephalus, 2021. www.statpearls.com
3. Pollack IF, Agnihotri S, Broniscer A. Childhood brain tumors: Current management, biological insights, and future directions. JNS 2019;23:261–73.


*Competencies:* **PE27.7**

## COMA

The word coma, derived from the Greek word *'koma'* or deep sleep, represents a state of sustained severe alteration of consciousness. Normal consciousness is maintained by integrity of cerebral cortex, thalamus and brainstem and regulated by the ascending reticular activating system, located in upper pons, midbrain and diencephalon. Altered consciousness or coma results from diffuse lesions of bilateral cerebral cortex or focal lesions of the ascending reticular activating system **(Table 19.14)**.

| **Table 19.14:** Causes of coma |
|---|
| Infections of the central nervous system (*see* **Table 19.9**) |
| Seizures, status epilepticus |
| Mass lesions, head trauma, stroke |
| Hypoxic ischemic injury |
| Demyelinating disorder |
| *Metabolic:* Shock, hypo- or hypernatremia, hypoglycemia, diabetic coma, hepatic coma, uremia, Reye syndrome, hypothyroidism, respiratory failure, acidosis, alkalosis, hyperosmolality, inborn errors of metabolism |
| *Drugs:* Barbiturates, benzodiazepines, opioids, tricyclic antidepressants, antihistaminics, iron, salicylates, acetaminophen, heavy metals |
| *Toxins:* Lead, carbon monoxide, pesticides, alcohol, ethylene glycol |
| *Miscellaneous:* Hypertensive encephalopathy, heat stroke, hypothermia |

### Causes of Coma

These can be divided into structural and functional coma. Structural coma is due to causes within the brain like CNS infections, mass lesions, trauma, hypoxic-ischemic injury and vascular causes. Functional coma results from diffuse bilateral cortical dysfunction due to metabolic and toxic causes (Table 19.14). Raised intracranial pressure causes herniation of brain structures, compressing the brainstem and lowering cerebral perfusion pressure leading to ischemia. The most common causes of coma in children in India are trauma and CNS infections.

### Evaluation

It is important to assess, if resuscitation is required. The onset and duration of coma, history of trauma or poisoning should be ascertained.

The respiratory pattern may indicate the level of the lesion. Cheyne-Stokes breathing is observed in diencephalic involvement, while apneustic and ataxic breathing patterns suggest progressive brainstem compression. Clues to etiology include evidence of injury and tongue bite (trauma); jaundice and fetor hepaticus (liver disease); petechiae (coagulopathy); ketotic breath (diabetic ketoacidosis), other unusual odor (metabolic disease); dry flushed skin (belladonna poisoning) and moist skin with increased salivation (organophosphorus poisoning).

The severity of coma is assessed by Glasgow Coma Scale which is modified for use in children below 2 years (Table 19.15). Alternatively, the alert, response to verbal, response to pain, unresponsive (AVPU) scale is administered, using a deep painful stimulus by a strong pinch or pressure on the nailbed or supraorbital area. Meningeal signs, tone and posturing are looked for. Decerebrate posturing suggests injury to upper pons, while decorticate posturing indicates bilateral cortical lesion with preserved brainstem function. Flaccid areflexia indicates loss of all cortical and brainstem functions up to the pontomedullary junction.

The retinal fundus examination may indicate papilledema, hemorrhage or signs of hypertension. Pupils are pinpoint in pontine lesions and morphine poisoning, and small, equal and reactive in coma due to metabolic or toxic causes. Bilateral fixed dilated pupils are seen preterminally, in severe ischemia or with atropine or belladonna poisoning. Unilateral unreactive pupil indicates impending transtentorial herniation. Sixth cranial nerve palsy is often a false localizing sign.

Focal neurological deficits suggest a structural lesion. Papilledema, hypertension, bradycardia, abnormal breathing pattern, posturing and third and sixth cranial nerve palsies suggest raised intracranial pressure. Brainstem reflexes including doll's eye, oculovestibular and corneal reflexes provide information on the integrity of the brainstem.

### Investigations

Complete blood counts, glucose, electrolytes, pH and bicarbonate, kidney and liver function tests, and blood ammonia and lactate help in determining the underlying cause. Where indicated, screening for toxins should be performed. Lumbar puncture should be done, if brain infection is suspected, but only after excluding raised intracranial pressure. Blood and CSF cultures should be obtained, if suspecting an infectious etiology. Neuroimaging helps assess for structural causes or brain injury.

### Management

The first priority in managing coma is ensuring that airway, breathing and circulation are maintained. Specific therapy is administered where available. Supportive treatment includes antipyretics for fever, anticonvulsants for seizures, and measures to manage raised intracranial pressure (Table 19.12). Sedative anticonvulsants are avoided to prevent interference with evaluation of depth of coma. Appropriate nursing is essential in improving outcomes during prolonged coma, and includes chest physiotherapy to prevent hypostatic pneumonia, adequate nutrition, care of the skin and eyes to prevent bedsores, corneal ulceration and exposure keratitis, care of the bowel and bladder to prevent constipation, fecal impaction and urinary tract infection, and physiotherapy to prevent deep vein thrombosis and contractures.

The patient should be placed in lateral head down position with frequent change from side-to-side. This position, also called the 'recovery' (from anesthesia) position, reduces obstruction to breathing from tongue falling back, protects against hypostatic pneumonia by facilitating drainage from lungs and guards against aspiration.

#### *Persistent Vegetative State*

This term refers to a state after recovery from coma when the patient returns to a wakeful state with preserved sleep wake cycle but without any awareness.

**Table 19.15:** Glasgow Coma Scale modified for children below 2 years of age

| Score | *Best motor response* | *Best verbal response* | *Eye opening* |
|---|---|---|---|
| 1 | None | None | None |
| 2 | Extension to pain | Moaning to pain | To pain |
| 3 | Flexion to pain | Crying to pain | To call |
| 4 | Withdrawal to pain | Irritable cry | Spontaneous |
| 5 | Localizes | Cooing and babbling | |
| 6 | Moves on command | | |

### Brain Death

This term refers to complete cessation of all brain function including the brainstem. Criteria for brain death are listed in Table 19.16. The criteria and laws pertaining to brain death differ between countries. The proximate cause of brain death should be known and the condition should be irreversible, with potentially reversible causes excluded, including use of CNS depressants, hypothermia, shock, and metabolic and endocrine disturbances. All brainstem reflexes should be absent with apnea. Since brains of young infants have increased resistance to damage, longer observation periods and ancillary tests are recommended in this group. Two independent physicians must conduct a full examination twice at the recommended time interval. The apnea test should be performed by disconnecting the patient from the ventilator after achieving normal blood gas, allowing arterial carbon dioxide to rise to 60 mm Hg or 20 mm Hg above baseline; absence of respiratory effort (positive apnea test) is consistent with brain death.

**Table 19.16:** Guidelines to determine brain death*

| |
|---|
| **Clinical criteria:** Complete loss of conciousness, vocalization and volitional activity |
| **Absent brainstem reflexes:** Absence of all of the following:<br>• Pupillary responses to light (with pupils midposition, 4–6 mm)<br>• Oculocephalic reflex<br>• Oculovestibular (caloric) responses<br>• Corneal reflex<br>• Jaw reflex<br>• Facial grimacing to deep pressure on supraorbital ridge or temporomandibular joint<br>• Pharyngeal gag reflex<br>• Coughing in response to tracheal suctioning<br>• Sucking and rooting reflexes |
| **Apnea:** Absence of respiratory drive at $PaCO_2$ of 60 mm Hg or 20 mm Hg above baseline<br>*Prerequisites*<br>• Clinical and/or neuroimaging evidence of acute CNS catastrophe severe enough to explain the condition<br>• Core temperature more than 32°C^<br>• No drug (sedatives, narcotics) or alcohol intoxication poisoning or neuromuscular blockade<br>• Normal blood pressure<br>• No confounding conditions such as severe electrolyte, acid–base, metabolic or endocrine disturbances<br>Two evaluations, separated by a time interval of 48 hours, if <2 months old; 24 hours, if 2–12 months old; 12 hours, if 1–18 years old; and at any interval, if >18 years old |
| **Ancilliary tests:** Two tests required, if <2-month-old; one test if 2–12-month-old; tests optional, if >1-year-old^^<br>• Cerebral angiography<br>• Electroencephalography<br>• Transcranial Doppler ultrasonography<br>• Cerebral scintigraphy |

*Adapted from American Academy of Pediatrics, Task Force on Brain Death in Children 2011, and the American Academy of Neurology, Practice Parameters for the Clinical Diagnosis of Brain Death; and consistent with the Indian Transplant of Human Organs (THO) Act, 2014
^35°C according to the THO Act
^^Two tests 6 hours apart at all ages according to the THO Act

It is possible to sustain life on life support systems sometimes indefinitely even after brain death but the individual can never return to a functional state. The diagnosis of brain death is important in deciding to discontinue the life support systems and also for organ transplantation.

Different countries have their own laws and criteria for diagnosis of brain death.

### Suggested Reading


1. Ganapathy K. Brain death revisited. Neurol India 2018;66: 308–15.
2. Karpenko A, Keegan J. Diagnosis of coma. Emerg Med Clin North Am 2021;39:155–72.
3. Sharma S, Kochar GS, Sankhyan N, Gulati S. Approach to the child with coma. Indian J Pediatr 2010; 77:1279–87.
4. Transplantation of human organs and tissues rules, 2014. Ministry of Health and Family Welfare.


*Competencies:* **PE30.6**

## HEMIPLEGIA

Neurological weakness of one-half of the body (upper and lower limbs) is termed hemiplegia. Hemiplegia can be caused by lesions in cervical spinal cord and above. Monoplegia refers to weakness of one limb. It may need to be differentiated from refusal to move a limb because of rheumatologic or orthopedic causes. Monoplegia can be caused by stroke involving the cerebral cortex or peripheral causes such as plexopathy or neuropathy. An apparent monoplegia may actually be a hemiplegia affecting one limb more than the other.

The most common cause of acute onset hemiplegia is stroke and other causes include transient ischemic attack, Todd palsy, granuloma, tumor, abscess, trauma, encephalitis, demyelinating disorders, and migraine.

### Stroke

A stroke is defined as rapidly developing focal or global disturbance of brain function lasting more than 24 hours with no obvious nonvascular cause.

Stroke may be broadly classified as ischemic or hemorrhagic, which account for 55% and 45% of cases in childhood, respectively. Ischemic stroke may be caused by arterial thrombi or embolism. A third type of stroke is cerebral venous sinus thrombosis. Weakness due to stroke is typically sudden, worst at the onset and improves gradually over days to months. Almost 20% of childhood stroke is recurrent.

### Acute Ischemic Stroke

One or more risk factors are present in two-thirds of patients with acute ischemic stroke (Table 19.17). In the remaining, no cause for stroke can be found despite extensive evaluation. Patients with arterial thrombi may have prodromal symptoms, stuttering course and history of transient ischemic attacks, while those with embolism usually present more suddenly. The precise neurological deficit depends on the site of infarction. The most common (90%) presentation

**Table 19.17:** Risk factors and etiology of stroke

| **Cardiac disease** |
|---|
| • Complex cyanotic heart disease; patent foramen ovale<br>• Infective endocarditis<br>• Valvular heart disease, prosthetic valves<br>• Cardiomyopathy<br>• Atrial myxoma; rhabdomyoma<br>• Fibrillation; sick sinus syndrome; heart block |
| **Hematological** |
| • Iron deficiency anemia; polycythemia; sickle cell disease<br>• Leukemias<br>• Thrombotic thrombocytopenic purpura, hemolytic uremic syndrome<br>• Disseminated intravascular coagulation |
| **Prothrombotic disorders** |
| • Protein C or S deficiency; activated protein C resistance<br>• Antithrombin III deficiency; prothrombin gene mutation *G20210A*<br>• Factor V Leiden mutation<br>• Hyperhomocysteinemia<br>• Antiphospholipid syndrome: Primary, secondary (e.g. with lupus) |
| **Vascular causes; trauma** |
| • Cervicocephalic or craniocervical arterial dissection<br>• Moyamoya disease; other primary or secondary vasculitides<br>• Fibromuscular dysplasia<br>• Cerebral venous sinus thrombosis<br>• Arterial rupture or thrombosis; pseudoaneurysm<br>• *Miscellaneous:* Neurofibromatosis; diabetes; tuberculosis; varicella; arteriovenous fistula |
| **Inherited metabolic disorders** |
| • Homocystinuria<br>• Mitochondrial encephalomyopathy, lactic acidosis and stroke<br>• Organic acidemias<br>• Ornithine transcarbamylase deficiency; pyruvate dehydrogenase deficiency<br>• Fabry disease |
| **Drugs and toxins** |
| • Cocaine; sympathomimetics; amphetamines<br>• Oral contraceptives; anabolic steroids<br>• L-asparaginase |

is with hemiparesis, hemisensory signs, aphasia and/or visual field defects. Cortical strokes may cause convulsions, contralateral hemiparesis or monoparesis, cortical sensory loss and aphasia. Internal capsule infarction may cause contralateral dense hemiplegia, upper motor neuron type of facial palsy, hemianesthesia and homonymous hemianopia. Altered sensorium may occur with posterior fossa stroke. Brainstem infarction causes ipsilateral cranial nerve palsies with contralateral limb palsy (crossed paralysis).

Initial stabilization includes attention to airway, breathing and circulation, supportive treatment for hypoxemia, hypoglycemia, dehydration, seizures and fever. Thrombolysis with tissue plasminogen activator (tPA), administered intravenously within 3 hours and intra-arterial within 6 hours of the event, are recommended in adults; however, no clear guidelines are available for children. Pending investigations for cause, unfractionated or low molecular weight heparin may be administered.

**Table 19.18:** Investigation for stroke

| Investigation |
|---|
| Complete blood count with erythrocyte sedimentation rate |
| Hemoglobin electrophoresis |
| Complete lipid profile |
| Imaging: Carotid Doppler; computed tomography, if hemorrhage suspected; MR imaging, arteriography and venography; carotid angiography, if indicated |
| Echocardiography and electrocardiography |
| Evaluation for procoagulant state<br>• *During acute phase:* Serum homocysteine levels; genetic testing for mutations (factor V Leiden, prothrombin gene); activated protein C resistance; lupus anticoagulant, anticardiolipin and $\beta_2$ glycoprotein-1 antibody<br>• *After 8–12 weeks:* Levels of protein C, S and antithrombin III |
| Antinuclear and anti-neutrophil cytoplasmic antibody; rheumatoid factor |

Evaluation for a patient with stroke is listed in Table 19.18. Neuroimaging should be done as soon as possible. Ultrasound is useful, if fontanelle is open. Transcranial Doppler shows changes in cerebral blood flow velocity in moderate to severe ischemia. CT is preferred in unstable patients or when intracranial hemorrhage is suspected. It may be normal in early ischemic stroke for up to 72 hours after onset, after which there is edema in the affected area (Fig.19.11a). MRI can identify ischemia within hours and diffusion weighted imaging within 45 minutes. Four vessel carotid angiogram is most accurate for distal arteries. MR angiography is a satisfactory alternative for lesions of internal carotid artery, Moyamoya disease, arteriovenous malformations and aneurysms. One or more prothrombotic states may be found in 20–50% patients with acute ischemic strokes. Long-term low dose aspirin is administered. Conditions with a high risk of recurrence (e.g. cardiac or prothrombotic disorders) require long-term oral anticoagulants. Treatment of the underlying cause is also important to prevent recurrence. Appropriate rehabilitation should be planned.

### Intracranial Hemorrhage

The clinical presentation is more dramatic than with ischemic stroke, with severe headache and vomiting due to raised intracranial pressure, and meningeal signs due to leaking of blood into the CSF. Causes of intracranial hemorrhage are listed in Table 19.19. Various connective tissue disorders, e.g., Ehlers-Danlos syndrome type IV, polycystic kidneys, pseudoxanthoma elasticum and fibromuscular dysplasia, may be associated with intracranial aneurysm. A thorough evaluation is warranted as a potential cause is found in about 90% cases. Occasionally cerebral venous sinus thrombosis can result in intracranial hemorrhage because of back pressure.

CT scan is preferred to MRI for the diagnosis of hemorrhage (Fig. 19.11b). MR, CT or 4-vessel carotid angiography is required to delineate arteriovenous malformations and aneurysms. Complete blood counts,

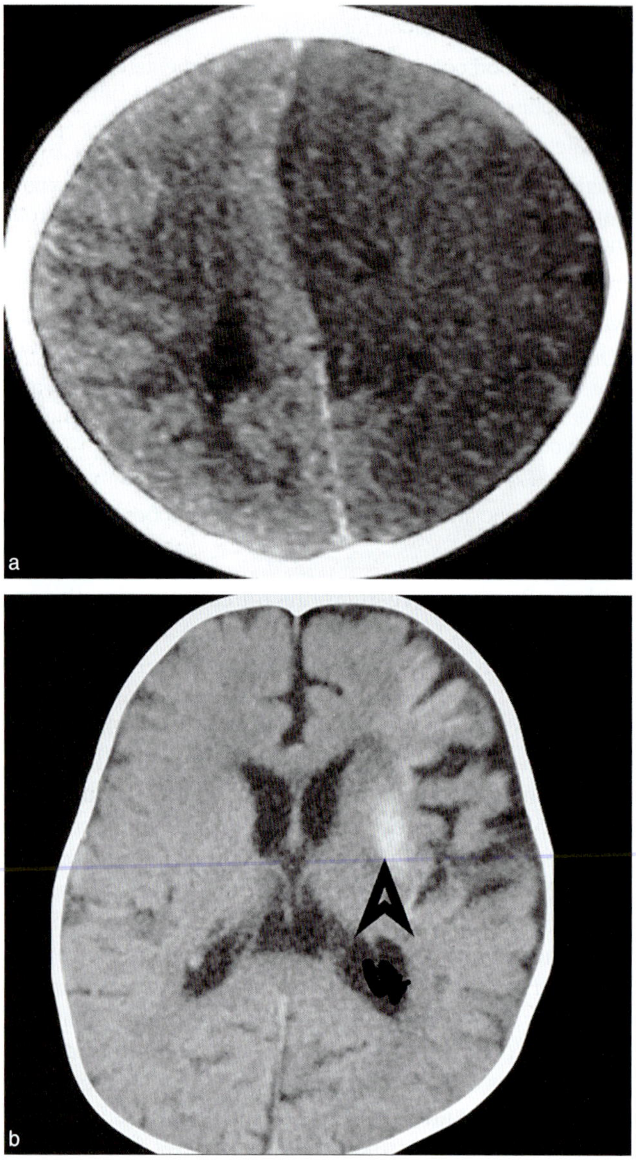

Fig. 19.11: Computed tomography images of the brain showing two types of stroke: (a) Diffuse hypodensity and midline shift in a patient with acute middle cerebral artery infarct; (b) Intracranial hemorrhage (arrow)

| Table 19.19: Causes of intracranial hemorrhage |
|---|
| *Arteriovenous malformation:* Sporadic; hereditary hemorrhagic telangiectasia |
| Capillary telangiectasias |
| Cavernous malformations |
| Aneurysms |
| Bleeding and clotting diathesis (including vitamin K deficiency) |
| Vasculitis |
| Hypertension |
| Trauma |
| Drugs: Anticoagulants, thrombolytic therapy, L- asparaginase, phencyclidine, ephedrine, phenylpropanolamine |

including platelet count, clotting factor assays (von Willebrand factor antigen, factor VIII, factor XII) and liver function tests are required. The management consists of resuscitation and supportive care. Identification of the cause should be followed by definitive treatment, in addition to rehabilitative measures.

### Cerebral Venous Sinus Thrombosis

Risk factors for thrombosis are listed in Table 19.20. Thrombosis of cerebral veins presents with dilated scalp veins, features of raised intracranial pressure and altered sensorium in addition to focal neurologic signs. Unenhanced CT scan may show linear densities (dense cord) in the sinuses. Later, enhanced CT scan may reveal a filling defect or 'empty delta' sign. CT or MR venography is more definitive. Diffusion and perfusion MRI and digital subtraction angiography are needed in equivocal cases. A detailed evaluation for prothrombotic states is essential as one or more may be found in up to 60% of cases.

Initial treatment is supportive. Antibiotics are given, if bacterial infection is suspected. Unfractionated heparin or low molecular weight heparin followed by warfarin for 3–6 months is the treatment of choice. Thrombolytic treatment is recommended only in selected cases.

### Hemiplegic Cerebral Palsy

The origin of hemiplegic cerebral palsy is usually a perinatal ischemic stroke. Presentation is nonspecific with lethargy, irritability or seizures. Hemiplega may be missed until early hand preference in infancy is noted. Facial palsy is absent, probably because of bilateral innervation of the lower face at this age. Neuroimaging often reveals porencephaly. Apart from hemiplegia, outcomes include developmental delay, intellectual disability and epilepsy.

### Suggested Reading


1. Bosch A, Albisetti M. Management of venous thromboembolism in children. Ther Clin Risk Manag 2020;16:673–79.
2. Ferreiro DM, Fullerton HJ, Bernard TJ, et al. Management of stroke in neonates and children. A scientific statement from the AHA/American Stroke Association. Stroke 2019;50:e51–e96.
3. Oborska Z, Urban P, Wychowaniec K. Pediatric stroke: Review of current guidelines. Neurol Neurochir Pol 2020;54:116–24.
4. Tsze DS, Valente JH. Pediatric stroke: A review. Emer Med Int 2011;734506.


| Table 19.20: Risk factors for cerebral venous sinus thrombosis |
|---|
| Dehydration, hypoxia |
| Cardiac disease: *Congenital, postoperative, post-catheterization* |
| Anemias: Sickle cell disease, iron deficiency anemia, thalassemia |
| Head and neck infections |
| Metabolic: Homocystinuria; prothrombotic disorders |
| Nephrotic syndrome |
| Malignancy: Leukemia, lymphoma |
| Systemic diseases: Systemic lupus erythematosus, Behçet disease, inflammatory bowel disease |
| Drugs: L-asparaginase, oral contraceptives, steroids |
| Other structural conditions: Head injury, brain tumor, hydrocephalus, Sturge-Weber syndrome |

## PARAPLEGIA AND QUADRIPLEGIA

Paraplegia refers to weakness of trunk and both lower limbs, while quadriplegia denotes weakness of all four limbs. Paraplegia or quadriplegia may occur due to disorders of cerebrum, spinal cord, peripheral nerves, neuromuscular junction or muscles (Table 19.21). Cerebral disorders are upper motor neuron type, spinal cord lesions may cause either upper or lower motor neuron weakness and disorders of peripheral nerves, neuromuscular junction and muscles show lower motor neuron signs.

### Cerebral Disorders

Lesions involving parasagittal and periventricular areas, in particular, cause paraplegia or quadriplegia. Spastic quadriplegic cerebral palsy is an example. Common causes include perinatal asphyxia, structural malformations and sequelae of CNS infections.

**Table 19.21:** Causes of paraplegia and hemiplegia

| |
|---|
| **Cerebral paraplegia or quadriplegia** |
| • Degenerative brain disorders |
| • Cerebral palsy: Spastic quadriplegia, spastic diplegia |
| • Hydrocephalus |
| **Spinal cord disorders** |
| *Acute spinal cord lesions* |
| • Trauma, hematomyelia |
| • Transverse myelitis |
| • Encephalomyelitis, herpes zoster myelitis |
| • Poliomyelitis |
| • Epidural abscess |
| • Acute infarction of the cord |
| • Lupus myelopathy |
| *Chronic progressive cord lesions* |
| • Malformations: Atlantoaxial dislocation, arteriovenous malformations, vascular anomalies of the spinal cord |
| • Chiari malformation; meningomyelocele |
| • Tethered cord (diastematomyelia) |
| • Arachnoid cyst, syringomyelia |
| • Tumors: Astrocytoma, ependymoma, Ewing sarcoma, neuroblastoma, metastasis |
| • Spinal muscular atrophy |
| • Tuberculosis of the spine |
| • Familial spastic paraplegia |
| • Adrenomyeloneuropathy |
| **Peripheral nerve disorders** |
| • Guillain-Barre syndrome |
| • Hereditary motor sensory neuropathies, other polyneuropathies |
| **Neuromuscular junction disorders** |
| • Myasthenia gravis |
| • Botulism |
| **Muscular weakness** |
| • Muscular dystrophies |
| • Myopathy |
| **Pseudoparalysis** |
| Surgery, osteomyelitis, fractures, myositis |

### Spinal Cord Disorders

These may cause acute or chronic progressive paraplegia or quadriplegia. Cervical cord lesions present as quadriplegia, whereas lower lesions present as paraplegia. Spinal paraplegia/quadriplegia may be asymmetric at first, giving the impression of monoplegia/hemiplegia. Lower motor neuron signs are present at the level of the cord lesion and upper motor neuron signs are noted below the lesion, along with bladder dysfunction. Acute transverse lesions of the cord may cause spinal shock with loss of all motor, sensory, autonomic and reflex functions below the level of lesion for a few weeks, after which upper motor neuron signs may supervene.

Patients with chronic spinal cord lesions present with clumsy gait, foot deformity, bladder dysfunction, or stunted limb growth. Malformations like meningocele and meningomyelocele are obvious at birth. The skin overlying spinal dysraphism may show abnormalities like pigmentation, tuft of hair, lipoma or a sinus. Congenital atlantoaxial dislocation may cause acute or slowly progressive quadriplegia at any age, and is usually caused by odontoid hypoplasia, occurring either in isolation or as part of Down syndrome, mucopolysaccharidosis (e.g. Morquio syndrome) or Klippel-Feil syndrome (decreased number and abnormal fusion of cervical vertebrae).

#### *Transverse Myelitis*

Transverse myelitis is an acute demyelinating condition characterized by sudden onset of symmetrical leg weakness with loss of reflexes, movements and sensation below a certain level with bladder and bowel dysfunction over 1–2 days. It may occur alone or along with demyelination in other locations in the nervous system. The exact cause is not known but believed to be related to infectious or autoimmune processes. Longitudinally extensive transverse myelitis involving 3 or more segments associated with optic neuritis sequentially or concomitantly, is termed neuromyelitis optica or Devic disease. Diagnosis is enabled by contrast enhanced magnetic resonance imaging of the cord. High dose intravenous steroids are the treatment of choice.

#### *Spinal Muscular Atrophy*

Spinal muscular atrophy is a hereditary disorder characterized by degeneration of the anterior horn cells of the spinal cord. Generalized weakness and hypotonia are present. Type 1 presents soon after birth with flaccid quadriplegia. Tongue fasciculations are seen. Extraocular muscles are spared and the baby appears alert. Type 2 presents between 6 and 18 months of age and type 3 presents after 18 months of age with motor delay. Diagnosis is by molecular testing (Chapter 20).

#### *Spinal Cord Compression*

Spinal cord compression may be caused by congenital lesions, tumors, tuberculosis and disc prolapse. Root pains may be an initial symptom. It is important to remember that early symptoms of a compressive cord lesion may be missed especially in a young child, and they may present suddenly like an acute noncompressive cord lesion. Cord compression due to any cause is a medical emergency. Early diagnosis and treatment are required to prevent permanent disability.

### Polyneuropathy

The most common polyneuropathy presenting as quadriplegia is acute inflammatory demyelinating polyneuropathy or Guillain-Barré syndrome. This postinfectious immune-mediated disorder presents acutely with symmetrical ascending paralysis, early and complete loss of deep tendon reflexes with or without sensory changes like pain, paresthesias and loss of position and vibration sense. Autonomic disturbances and bladder dysfunction may occur. Involvement of thoracic muscles may cause respiratory insufficiency, which is important to recognize. Treatment options include intravenous immunoglobulin and plasmapheresis.

Other neuropathies include the hereditary sensorimotor neuropathies or Charcot-Marie-Tooth disease which are slowly progressive with chronic symptoms.

### Neuromuscular Junction Disorders

Myasthenia gravis usually presents with ptosis and weakness of extraocular muscles worsening in the later part of the day. It may occasionally cause generalized weakness. Repetitive nerve stimulation test shows a decremental response. Antibodies against acetylcholine receptors are found in up to 85% of generalized immune-mediated myasthenia.

### Muscle Disorders

These cause proximal weakness, usually with preserved deep tendon reflexes (Chapter 20).

### Suggested Reading


1. Lechner C, Breu M, Wendel EM. Epidemiology of pediatric NMOSD in Germany and Austria. Front Neurol 2020;11:415.
2. Borchers AT, Gershwin ME. Transverse myelitis. Autoimmun Rev 2012;11:231–48.
3. Boutry M, Morais S, Stevanin G. Update on the genetics of spastic paraplegias. Curr Neurol Neurosci Rep 2019;19:18.


*Competencies:* **PE30.15**

## ATAXIA

The term 'ataxia' refers to disturbance of fine control of posture and movement. This control is provided by the cerebellum along with its input tracts from the frontal lobes and posterior columns of the spinal cord. Ataxic gait is wide-based, lurching and staggering, and the patient appears to be in the danger of falling down. Tandem walking is not possible. Patients may also show other signs of cerebellar involvement, including nystagmus, hypotonia dysmetria and pendular jerks. Lesions of the posterior tracts cause sensory ataxia. The patient constantly looks at the ground while walking and has a stamping gait. Gait and stability are much worse with the eyes closed (Romberg sign). Clinical findings provide clues to indicate the anatomical site affected (Table 19.22). Causes of ataxia can be divided into (i) acute or recurrent and (ii) chronic and progressive (Table 19.23).

### Acute or Recurrent Ataxia

The most common causes in children are acute postinfectious cerebellitis and drug toxicity, followed by migraine, brain stem encephalitis and underlying neuroblastoma.

#### *Brainstem Encephalitis*

Ataxia along with cranial nerve palsies may be the initial feature of viral encephalitis. Cerebrospinal fluid pleocytosis and abnormal brainstem auditory evoked potentials may be found.

#### *Brain Tumors*

The chief brain tumors in childhood that may present with ataxia are cerebellar astrocytoma, medulloblastoma and brainstem glioma.

#### *Migraine*

Basilar migraine may present as recurrent episodes of cerebellar or brainstem dysfunction. Peak occurrence is in adolescent girls. Gait ataxia, visual loss, vertigo, paresthesias, tinnitus and occasional loss of consciousness may occur, followed by throbbing occipital headache.

#### *Benign Paroxysmal Vertigo*

Benign paroxysmal vertigo is a migraine variant mainly seen in infants and preschool children. The predominant symptom is recurrent attacks of vertigo with pallor, nystagmus and fright lasting a few minutes. Consciousness is maintained. With time, these attacks decrease and stop altogether and typical migraine may develop.

**Table 19.22:** Anatomical localization of ataxia

| *Feature* | *Cerebellar* | *Sensory* | *Vestibular* |
|---|---|---|---|
| Ataxia | Limb or truncal | Limb | Truncal |
| Dysarthria | Present | Absent | Absent |
| Nystagmus | Present | Absent | Present |
| Vertigo | Absent | Absent | Present |
| Hypotonia | Present | Absent | Absent |
| Deep tendon reflexes | Pendular | Absent | Normal |
| Romberg sign | Absent | Present | Absent |
| Vibration and position sense | Normal | Decreased | Normal |

**Table 19.23:** Causes of ataxia

| |
|---|
| **Acute or recurrent** |
| • Postinfectious and autoimmune: Acute postinfectious cerebellitis, Miller-Fisher syndrome, opsoclonus myoclonus ataxia (occult neuroblastoma)<br>• Drugs: Phenytoin, psychotropic drugs, antihistaminics<br>• Brainstem encephalitis<br>• Migraine: Basilar migraine, benign paroxysmal vertigo<br>• Inherited disorders: Hartnup disease, maple syrup urine disease, pyruvate dehydrogenase deficiency, episodic ataxia types 1 and 2<br>• Trauma: Concussion; hematoma |
| **Chronic** |
| *Static*<br>• Malformations and inherited defects: Arnold-Chiari, Dandy-Walker and Joubert syndromes<br>• Stroke<br>• Post-traumatic<br>*Progressive*<br>• Inherited degenerative: Spinocerebellar ataxia, abetalipoproteinemia, ataxia telangiectasia, Friedreich ataxia, Refsum disease, Hartnup disease<br>• Brain tumors: Cerebellar astrocytoma, medulloblastoma, ependymoma<br>• Acquired: Multiple sclerosis, vitamin $B_{12}$ deficiency |

### *Conversion Reaction*

Hysterical ataxia is relatively common in older girls and occurs as a means to handle stress. Although the hysteria is involuntary, there is some secondary gain. The child does not have difficulty sitting but when made to stand there is severe swaying from the waist, so that she lurches and staggers from one object to the other. Diagnosis is by observation only.

### *Inborn Errors of Metabolism*

Some aminoacidurias and mitochondrial disorders present with intermittent ataxia and lethargy, or decreased consciousness during periods of stress or infections. Development is borderline or delayed. Pellagrous skin rash may suggest Hartnup disease. Metabolic acidosis and increased pyruvate to lactate ratio in blood suggest maple syrup urine disease and pyruvate dehydrogenase deficiency, respectively.

### *Episodic Ataxias (EA)*

These are autosomal dominant disorders due to ion channel mutations. EA type 1 results from a mutation of potassium channel *KCNA1*. Attacks of ataxia and myokymia of the face and limbs, 10 minutes to 6 hours in duration usually start after 5–7 years of age. EA type 2 is due to mutation in voltage dependent calcium channel gene, *CACNA1A*. Episodes of ataxia, vertigo, jerk nystagmus with vomiting lasting one hour to a day occur 1–3 times per month. Onset is in school age. Most patients are normal between attacks but some may have slowly progressive truncal ataxia and nystagmus. Acetazolamide is a commonly used medication in the treatment of EA1 and EA2. Alternate medications for EA1 include carbamazepine and valproic acid.

### *Acute Postinfectious Cerebellitis*

This most commonly affects children between 2 and 7 years of age after an attack of varicella. Ataxia starts suddenly and is worst at the onset. It varies from mild unsteadiness to complete inability to stand. Recovery occurs spontaneously over 3 to 20 weeks. No treatment is required.

### *Acute Disseminated Encephalomyelitis*

Acute disseminated encephalomyelitis is a parainfectious disorder that may initially present with ataxia, long tract signs and seizures. A monophasic course and encephalopathy are characteristic.

### *Miller-Fisher Syndrome*

This condition is considered a variant of Guillain-Barre syndrome characterized by acute onset of ataxia, ophthalmoplegia and areflexia. Cerebrospinal fluid shows findings similar to Guillain-Barre syndrome. The course is self-limited and complete recovery occurs within 6 months.

### *Multiple Sclerosis*

About 3–5% of patients of multiple sclerosis present before 6 years of age. Female to male ratio varies from 1.5:1 to 3:1. Ataxia is a common initial feature, along with seizures, long tract signs, optic neuritis, transverse myelitis, lethargy, nausea and vomiting. A polyphasic course is characteristic. Repeated episodes of demyelination occur in noncontiguous areas of the nervous system.

Cerebrospinal fluid during episodes show mild pleocytosis with raised protein and oligoclonal bands. MRI showing three or more white matter lesions, especially if one is perpendicular to the corpus callosum, is a sensitive predictor of the diagnosis.

### *Opsoclonus Myoclonus Ataxia Syndrome*

This syndrome is characterized by chaotic eye movements (opsoclonus), myoclonus, ataxia and encephalopathy. Occurrence is between one month and 4 years. Encephalopathy manifests as personality change or irritability. Opsoclonus persists even during sleep. Careful investigation reveals occult neuroblastoma in half the cases. A relapsing and remitting course is seen.

## Chronic Progressive Ataxia

### *Brain Tumors*

Progressive ataxia starting in a previously well child should raise the possibility of a brain tumor. Headache, vomiting and papilledema may also occur.

### *Abetalipoproteinemia*

This is an autosomal recessive disorder caused by defect in the gene for microsomal triglyceride transfer protein (*MTTP*). Manifestations are fat malabsorption, failure to thrive, acanthocytosis, severe anemia, ataxia and retinitis pigmentosa with night blindness. Ataxia results from severe vitamin E deficiency. Plasma cholesterol and triglycerides are low and apolipoprotein B is absent. Treatment includes dietary fat restriction and large doses of vitamin E.

### Ataxia Telangiectasia

Described in Chapter 25.

### Friedreich Ataxia

This is the most common autosomal recessive ataxia, localized to chromosome 9q13. The condition is caused by an unstable triplet repeat of *FXN*, which encodes frataxin. Onset of symptoms usually occurs between 2 and 15 years with slowly progressive ataxia. Dysarthria, absent tendon reflexes, extensor plantar responses, pes cavus, scoliosis, loss of position and vibration sense, hypertrophic cardiomyopathy and diabetes are associated features.

### Refsum Disease

This rare autosomal recessive disorder, due to variations in *PHYH* or *AEX7* is characterized by peripheral polyneuropathy, cerebellar ataxia, retinitis pigmentosa and ichthyosis. Symptoms evolve slowly and insidiously from childhood through adolescence and early adulthood. Blood levels of phytanic acid are increased.

### Joubert Syndrome

This is a rare brain malformation characterized by hypoplasia of the cerebellar vermis and malformed brainstem. The most common features in infancy include ataxia, hyperpnea, hypotonia, abnormal eye movements, seizures and impaired intellectual development. The condition may be associated with kidney disease (including nephronophthisis), liver disease and skeletal abnormalities. Most cases are autosomal recessive in inheritance but some appear to be sporadic. The 'molar tooth' appearance on transverse CT and MR images of the midbrain is characteristic. A large number of genes, which are known or suspected to play roles in the primary cilia, are considered causative.

## Suggested Reading

1. Brandsma R, van Egmond ME, Tijssen MAJ. Diagnostic approach to pediatric movement disorders. Dev Med Child Neurol 2021;63:252–58.
2. Garone G, Capuano A, Travaglini L, et al. Clinical and genetic overview of paroxysmal movement disorders and episodic ataxias. Int J Mol Sci 2020;21:3603.

## MOVEMENT DISORDERS

Disorders of movement that impact the smoothness and accuracy of movement are seen with many neurological conditions like hypo- or hypertonia, weakness and ataxia. This chapter will focus on involuntary abnormal movements, due to disorders of the basal ganglia.

Abnormal movements need to be differentiated from convulsions. Convulsions are usually paroxysmal, occur during sleep or wakefulness and are associated with altered consciousness and abnormal EEG. Abnormal movements are usually non-paroxysmal, tend to occur in awake state and disappear during sleep. They are unlikely to be associated with loss of consciousness or EEG abnormality.

### Chorea

This is a rapid, random, non-rhythmic, non-stereotyped and quasipurposive movement, often superimposed on a voluntary movement. Chorea may move from limb-to-limb or one side of body to another, giving the impression of restlessness. Describing chorea may be difficult as the movement is not stereotyped. The movements are often elicitable by asking the patient to raise both arms above the head or stretched out in front. The examiner may feel alternating 'milkmaid' movements, if the patient holds his hand. 'Jack in the box' movements may be seen in the protruded tongue. The most common conditions presenting with chorea in India are Sydenham chorea, sequelae of meningoencephalitis and Wilson disease (Table 19.24).

#### Sydenham Chorea (Rheumatic Chorea)

This is an immune-mediated late manifestation of rheumatic fever. Onset is insidious or subacute, often with unilateral chorea. Hypotonia, dysarthria and emotional lability may be present. The condition improves gradually over 3–4 months. T2-weighted MRI brain images may show increased signal intensity in the putamen and globus pallidus, which resolve with recovery. Patients should receive prophylaxis against group A streptococcal infection. Pimozide, valproate, haloperidol, benzodiazepines or phenothiazines may be used to control abnormal movements.

Chorea and other abnormal movements may be seen during recovery from tubercular or viral (especially Japanese) meningoencephalitis. Movements usually last several weeks to months and may be incapacitating.

### Athetosis

These are slow, writhing, distal movements of the limbs. It may occur alone, usually after perinatal brain injury (perinatal asphyxia, kernicterus), or along with chorea, as choreoathetosis.

### Dystonia

This refers to abnormal posture due to sustained muscle contraction. Focal dystonias, such as blepharospasm, orofacial or hemifacial spasm and writer's cramp are rare in childhood. However, generalized dystonias in children may begin as focal dystonia.

**Table 19.24:** Causes of chorea

**Chorea as predominant symptom**

- *Inherited defects:* Glutaric aciduria, benign familial chorea, Wilson disease, Fahr disease, abetalipoproteinemia, Huntington chorea, ataxia telangiectasia, Lesch-Nyhan syndrome
- *Systemic disorders:* Sydenham chorea, hyperthyroidism, systemic lupus erythematosus
- *CNS infections*
- *Tumors*
- *Drugs:* Anticonvulsants, oral contraceptives, antiemetics, theophylline

**Chorea as one of the symptoms**

- Perinatal brain insult
- Postinfectious
- *Vascular disease:* Stroke, Moyamoya disease

### Torticollis

Sustained turning of the head to one side may be caused by dystonia, benign paroxysmal torticollis, cervicomedullary malformations, syringomyelia, diplopia, juvenile rheumatoid arthritis, posterior fossa or cervical cord tumors and sternocleidomastoid injury or tumor.

### Benign Paroxysmal Torticollis

Benign paroxysmal torticollis is believed to be a migraine variant. Episodes of head tilting and rotation to one or other side begin in the first year. Pallor, irritability, malaise and vomiting may be associated. Attacks last 1–3 days, remit spontaneously and recur 3–6 times per year.

### Sandifer Syndrome

This is a paroxysmal dystonic movement disorder with arching of the back and rigid opisthotonic posturing. It occurs in association with gastroesophageal reflux and, in some cases, hiatal hernia. Onset is in infancy or early childhood. Management of the hernia alleviates symptoms.

### Dopa Responsive Dystonia

Dopa responsive dystonia or Segawa disease is inherited in an autosomal dominant or recessive manner. Children present between 4 and 8 years of age with gait disturbance, toe walking and/or posturing of arms. A diurnal pattern is observed in more than half, with symptoms worsening by the evening. Small doses of levodopa provide immediate and complete relief. Untreated patients may progress to parkinsonism with cogwheel rigidity and bradykinesia.

### Idiopathic Torsion Dystonia

Idiopathic torsion dystonia is an autosomal dominant condition with variable penetrance, occurring most commonly in Ashkenazi Jews. Presentation peaks bimodally at 9 years and 45 years. Dystonia begins in the legs to become generalized. Dysarthria, dysphagia, orofacial movements, postural tremor and blepharospasm may be present.

Botulinum toxin helps in focal problems. Trihexiphenidyl, baclofen, carbamazepine, benzodiazepines or levodopa may be tried. Outcomes vary from functional independence to complete disability. Deep brain stimulation may be useful.

### Wilson Disease

This is an autosomal recessive disorder due to *ATP7B* mutation, characterized by copper accumulation in liver, brain and cornea. The disease presents variably at 3–50 years. Children usually present with acute or chronic hepatitis or hepatic failure in the first decade of life. Neurological symptoms predominate in the second decade, and include disturbance of speech or gait, often unchanged for years. This is followed by dysarthria, dystonia, rigidity, abnormalities of gait and posture, tremor and drooling. Dementia and psychiatric symptoms may ensue. Almost all cases with neurological involvement show golden-brown pericorneal discoloration, termed Kayser-Fleischer rings. Diagnosis is suggested by reduced serum ceruloplasmin levels (<20 mg/dL in 96%), increased urinary copper excretion and increased hepatic copper content on biopsy.

A proportion of patients show features of renal tubular acidosis, more often proximal than distal. Patients require lifelong chelation with oral D-penicillamine or trientine, titrated to maintain urinary copper excretion at 5–10 times normal. Pyridoxine, zinc and vitamin E are given. Alkali and phosphate supplements are occasionally necessary. Patients slowly recover over months. However, some patients progress to liver failure despite therapy, necessitating liver transplantation.

### Pantothenate Kinase associated Neurodegeneration

This is an autosomal recessive disorder associated with iron deposition in basal ganglia. Patients present between 2 and 10 years of age with progressive dystonia, initially affecting feet, leading to equinovarus deformity, followed by rigidity in hands. Two-thirds patients have retinitis pigmentosa while one-fourth develop seizures. MRI is characterized by 'eye of tiger' appearance of the basal ganglia on T2-weighted images. Management is symptomatic.

### Symptomatic Generalized Dystonias

Symptomatic generalized dystonia may follow various types of brain injury. Progressively severe dystonia is observed beginning 2–3 years after kernicterus or perinatal asphyxia. Patients with stroke, head trauma, tumor of basal ganglia, antiphospholipid syndrome and neuronal storage disease may show hemidystonia.

## Myoclonus

These are sudden, brief, jerky, involuntary movements that are focal, multifocal or generalized. Generalized myoclonus is not stereotyped. Myoclonus is more common when awake but may not disappear completely during sleep. It may occur in isolation, as part of myoclonic epilepsy, where EEG shows epileptiform discharges, or as part of systemic or CNS disorders. Myoclonus cannot be voluntarily suppressed. A very wide variety of systemic and central nervous system disorders can cause myoclonus. Essential myoclonus refers to focal or generalized myoclonus that occurs chiefly during action or stress. Onset is in first or second decade of life. Face, trunk or proximal muscles are involved. EEG and neuroimaging are normal. Therapy with nitrazepam or clonazepam may be useful.

## Tics

These are sudden, brief, purposeless, complex stereotyped movements or utterances, which are exacerbated by stress. They are suppressible and disappear during sleep. Examples include clearing the throat, eye blinking, grimacing, lip smacking and shrugging of shoulders.

Tourette syndrome is characterized by motor and verbal tics, attention deficit and obsessive compulsive disorder. Verbal tics include snorting, sniffing, grunting or hissing. The disease course waxes and wanes over a prolonged period. It is believed that Tourette syndrome is a form of pediatric autoimmune neuropsychiatric disorders associated with *Streptococcus* infections (PANDAS).

Pimozide, haloperidol or fluphenazine may be used, if the tics are bothersome.

### Tremor

These are involuntary oscillating, rhythmic and usually distal movements of low amplitude on both sides of an axis. Tremors may be physiological, precipitated by anxiety, fatigue, stress or drugs such as xanthines, adrenergic agonists, nicotine, thyroid hormone and amphetamines. Tremors may be secondary to injury to basal ganglia following meningoencephalitis and neurodegenerative diseases.

#### *Infantile Tremor Syndrome*

Infantile tremor syndrome was described in exclusively breastfed Indian infants, presenting at 8–18 months of age with listlessness, developmental delay or regression, pallor, depigmented sparse hair and hyperpigmented knuckles. Megaloblastic anemia is usually present. Subsequent symptoms include progressive limb tremors, bleating cry, and arms positioned like a 'bird about to take flight'. Tremor is self-limited over 2–3 months but developmental problems may persist. The condition is linked to cobalamin deficiency and responds to therapy with cobalamin and propranolol.

### Suggested Reading

1. Goraya JS, Kaur S. Infantile tremor syndrome: A review and critical appraisal of its etiology. J Pediatr Neurosci 2016;11: 298–304.
2. Silveira-Moriyama L, Kovac S, Kurian MA, et al. Phenotypes, genotypes, and the management of paroxysmal movement disorders. Dev Med Child Neurol 2018;60:559–65.
3. van den Heuvel CNAM, Tijssen MAJ, van de Warrenburg BPC. The symptomatic treatment of acquired dystonia: A systematic review. Mov Disord Clin Pract 2016;3:548–58.

*Competencies:* **PE30.10**

## NEUROLOGICAL REGRESSION

Various disorders present with progressive deterioration in mental and motor functions, causing loss of acquired milestones. Many of these are inherited disorders called inborn errors of metabolism involving single genes and enzymes and causing a 'biochemical block'. Lack of enzyme causes absence or lack of an essential product or accumulation of toxic metabolites. When the molecule involved is small, manifestations are acute (with complete enzyme deficiency) or intermittent (with partial enzyme deficiency). The latter may have an ultimate downhill course thereby appearing like progressive deterioration. Examples are aminoacidopathies, urea cycle disorders, organic acidemias and fatty acid oxidation defects. When the defect involves a large molecule, the manifestations are chronic, e.g. lysosomal storage disorders, glycogen storage disorders and mucopolysaccharidoses. Table 19.25 lists disorders based on age of onset.

**Table 19.25:** Inherited causes of psychomotor regression

| | |
|---|---|
| **Onset in early infancy** | |
| *With hepatosplenomegaly* | |
| Gaucher type 2 | GM1 gangliosidosis |
| Niemann-Pick type A | Mucopolysaccharidosis types 1 and 2 |
| Sandhoff disease | Sialidosis type 1 |
| *Without hepatosplenomegaly* | |
| Maple syrup urine disease | Pelizaeus-Merzbacher disease |
| Classic phenylketonuria | Krabbe disease |
| Leigh disease | Canavan disease |
| Menkes kinky hair disease | GM2 Tay-Sachs disease |
| Biotinidase deficiency | Alexander disease |
| Glutaric aciduria | Early infantile neuronal ceroid lipofuscinoses |
| Zellweger syndrome | Lesch-Nyhan disease |
| **Onset at 1–2 years** | |
| Homocystinuria | Metachromatic leukodystrophy |
| Rett syndrome | Megalencephalic leukoencephalopathy with subcortical cysts |
| Late infantile neuronal ceroid lipofuscinosis | |
| **Onset after 2 years** | |
| *With hepatosplenomegaly* | |
| Gaucher type 3 | Niemann-Pick type C |
| Mucopolysaccharidosis type 2 (Hunter) | Mucopolysaccharidosis type 7 (Sly) |
| *Without hepatosplenomegaly* | |
| Juvenile neuronal lipofuscinosis | Adrenoleukodystrophy |
| Juvenile Tay-Sachs | Juvenile onset metachromatic leukodystrophy |
| Late onset Krabbe disease | Huntington disease |
| Myoclonic epilepsy with ragged red fibres | Subacute sclerosing panencephalitis |
| Wilson disease | Pantothenate kinase associated neurodegeneration |
| Cerebrotendinous xanthomatosis | |

Other causes include infections (e.g. HIV encephalopathy, subacute sclerosing panencephalitis and progressive rubella panencephalitis), hydrocephalus, hypothyroidism and vitamin $B_{12}$ deficiency. Epileptic encephalopathies also cause neuroregression. Static but evolving disorders such as cerebral palsy may appear to regress due to formation of contractures, epilepsy, movement disorders or emotional problems. Acute deterioration following illness, trauma or brain infections after which the child remains static or improves need to be differentiated. The neurocutaneous disorders also have progressive downhill course. Diseases like lupus erythematosus and multiple sclerosis and repeated strokes can also appear like a progressive degeneration.

### Evaluation

A detailed history should elicit the age at onset, course and evolution of illness, history of consanguinity and family history. Progressive deterioration may be difficult to detect in patients with infantile onset. Other features include feeding difficulties, vomiting, failure to thrive, lethargy, irritability and lack of visual fixation and social interaction. Attempt should be made to delineate whether the early symptoms are more suggestive of a gray matter disorder (cognitive decline, seizures) or white matter (gait abnormality, spasticity) (Table 19.26). Physical examination should focus on appearance (Fig. 19.12a and b), detailed neurological examination including fundoscopy (Fig. 19.13), hepatosplenomegaly, and specific findings in eye, skin and skeleton that may indicate the underlying etiology.

Biochemical tests are targeted towards detecting the suspected defect and include blood levels of ammonia, arterial and CSF lactate, sugar, tandem mass spectrometry, and urinary aminoacidogram, urine gas chromatography and mass spectroscopy (GCMS) and glycosaminoglycans. MRI of the brain may suggest the diagnosis in some cases, e.g., Leigh syndrome, glutaric aciduria, leukodystrophies (Fig. 19.14), pantothenate kinase associated neurodegeneration, megalencephalic leukoencephalopathy with subcortical cysts Specific diagnosis relies on enzyme analysis in leukocytes or skin fibroblasts and specific genetic testing. These are discussed in Chapter 24.

**Table 19.26:** Features that differentiate between gray and white matter degenerative disorders

| Feature | Gray matter | White matter |
|---|---|---|
| Seizures | Early | Late |
| Loss of cognitive abilities | Early | Late |
| Retinitis pigmentosa | May be seen | Rare |
| Peripheral neuropathy | Rare | May be present |
| Optic atrophy | Rare | May be present |
| Neuroimaging (MRI brain) | May show cortical atrophy | Shows white matter changes |

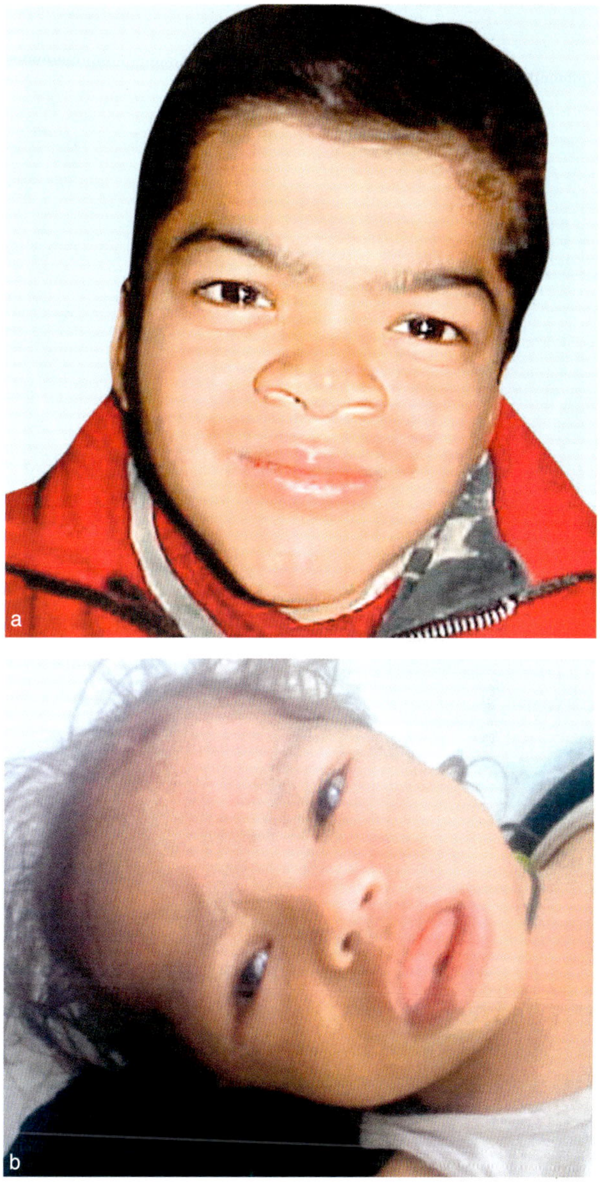

**Fig. 19.12:** Coarse facial features with psychomotor retardation in a child with (a) Mucopolysaccharidosis type 2; and (b) Cretinism (congenital endemic hypothyroidism)

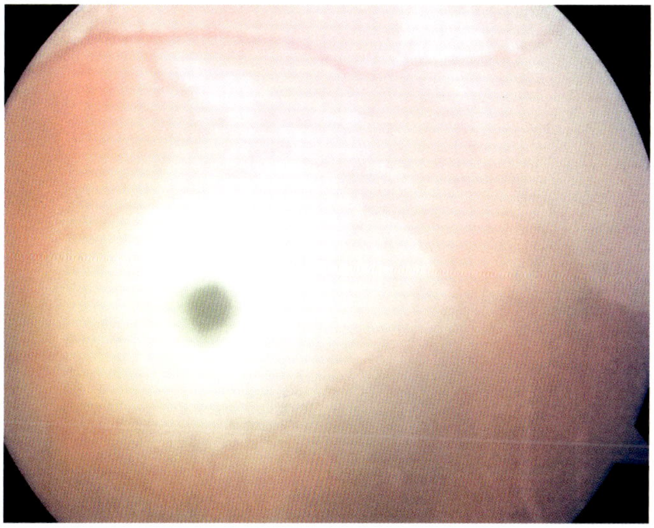

**Fig. 19.13:** Fundoscopy in a child with Tay-Sachs disease showing cherry red spot

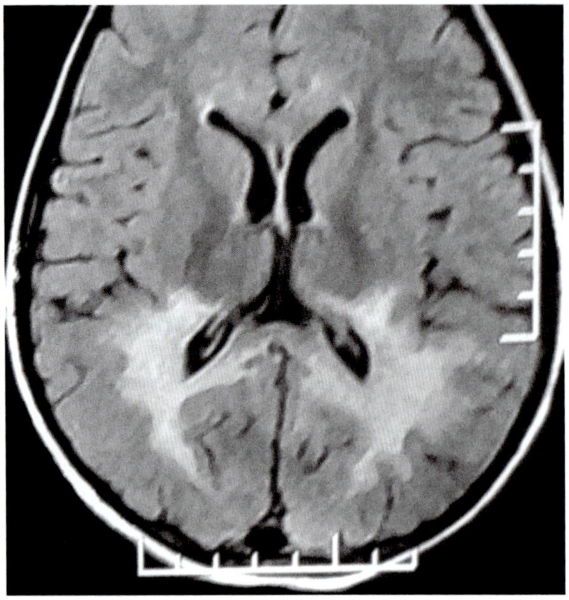

Fig. 19.14: Characteristic predominantly posterior white matter involvement in a patient with adrenoleukodystrophy

## Treatment

The first priority is to evaluate for and manage conditions for which specific therapy is available, such as hypothyroidism, hydrocephalus, vitamin $B_{12}$ deficiency, lead poisoning, Wilson disease, adrenoleukodystrophy, and biotinidase deficiency. Specific diets are useful in conditions such as galactosemia, fructose intolerance and phenylketonuria. Enzyme replacement therapy is available for Gaucher disease, milder variant of mucopolysaccharidosis type 1, glycogen storage disease type 2 (Pompe disease) and Fabry disease. Transplantation of the bone marrow and liver may be useful in patients with Hurler disease and glycogen storage disease, respectively.

## Prevention

Several disorders are already screened for as part of newborn screening programs in many countries. While most conditions have a poor outcome, specific diagnosis enables prenatal counseling and antenatal diagnosis in subsequent pregnancies.

## Suggested Reading

1. Adang LA, Sherbini O, Ball L, et al. Revised consensus statement on the preventive and symptomatic care of patients with leukodystrophies. Mol Genet Metab 2017;122:18–32.
2. Augustine EF, Adams HR, de Los Reys E, et al. Management of CLN1 disease. International clinical consensus. Pediatr Neurol 2021;120:38–51.

Chapter

20

# Neuromuscular Disorders

❍ Sheffali Gulati

A motor unit comprises one anterior horn cell and all the muscle fibers that it innervates. Neuromuscular disorders may be due to lesions anywhere along the motor unit (Fig. 20.1). These include neuronopathies (disorders of anterior horn cell), neuropathies (disorders of nerve axon or myelin), neuromuscular junction disorders and myopathies (disorders of muscle).

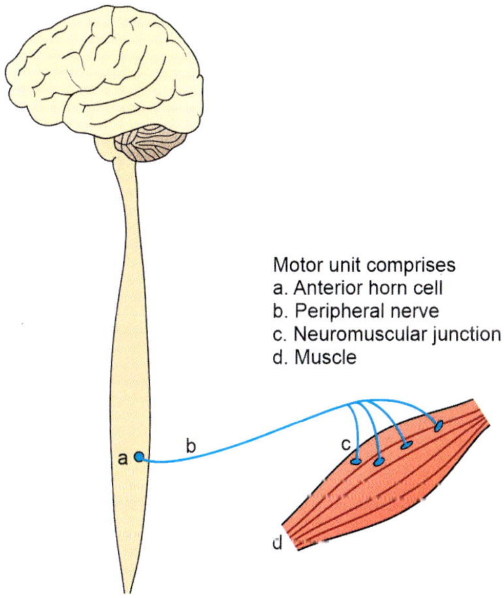


Fig. 20.1: Parts of a motor unit

## APPROACH TO EVALUATION

The predominant presenting complaint of a patient with a neuromuscular disorder is weakness. Weakness may also result from disorders of the upper motor neuron. Figure 20.2 demonstrates an approach to anatomical localization of lesion along the neuraxis in a child presenting with weakness.

Children with neuromuscular disorders are usually alert. Spinal muscular atrophy (SMA) type 0 and I, congenital myopathies, congenital myasthenia syndrome and metabolic disorders present at birth or in infancy. Muscular

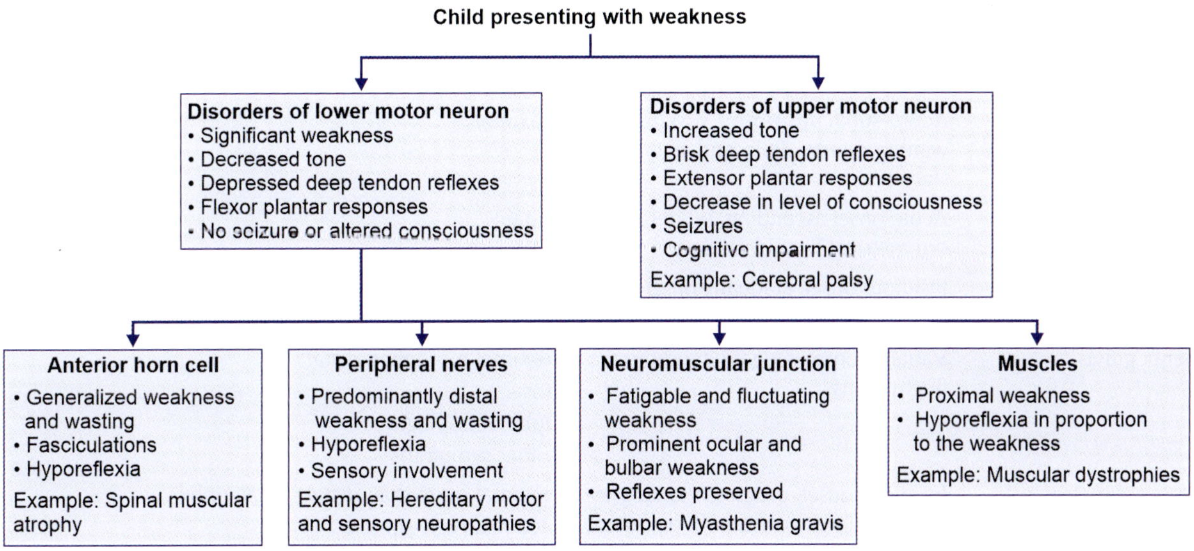


Fig. 20.2: Approach to anatomical localization in a child presenting with weakness

dystrophies, less severe forms of SMA, neuropathies, myasthenia gravis and inflammatory muscle disorders often present later.

Pattern of weakness can be identified on history by taking into account the points mentioned in Table 20.1. Further clinical clues to help a clinician reach a diagnosis are tabulated in Table 20.2. Chronic inflammatory demyelinating polyneuropathy (CIDP) shows both proximal and distal weakness.

Cardiac disease often accompanies Duchenne muscular dystrophy, Pompe disease and myotonic dystrophy. Skin rash is seen in dermatomyositis; eyes are involved in myotonic dystrophy, congenital muscle dystrophies and mitochondrial diseases. Liver involvement may be seen with mitochondrial disorders, acid maltase deficiency and carnitine deficiency. Feet deformity and callosities are seen in some hereditary neuropathies.

The neuromuscular disorders can be acquired or hereditary. The mode of inheritance in the hereditary disorders is variable. Most of the hereditary neuromuscular disorders are autosomal recessive, except Duchenne muscular dystrophy and Becker muscular dystrophy (both X-linked recessive), and fascioscapulohumeral dystrophy (autosomal dominant).

### Evaluation

Serum creatine kinase (CK), a muscle enzyme, is elevated in conditions with breakdown of muscles, typically seen in muscular dystrophies. Muscle biopsy aids in diagnosis based on specific morphological features, immunohistochemistry (absent or reduced staining for specific proteins) and enzyme histochemistry (absent or reduced enzyme function). Electrophysiological tests, including nerve conduction studies and electromyography, help to localize the lesion. Muscle imaging (ultrasound and MRI) is useful in certain cases. Molecular genetic testing is available for many disorders.

### Hypotonia

Hypotonia, decreased muscle tone, is a common sign of neuromuscular disorders. Hypotonia can be central,

**Table 20.1:** Eliciting history to identify the pattern of weakness

| *Points to be enquired on history* | *Pattern of weakness* |
|---|---|
| Difficulty in rising from the chair, going up and down the stairs, raising his/her arms above head or combing hair | Proximal limb weakness |
| Difficulty in buttoning, unbuttoning, holding objects in hands, and wearing slippers. Cannot clear his/her feet off the ground while walking due to foot drop | Distal limb weakness |
| Difficulty in blowing balloons, sipping through straw and inability to close eyes completely | Facial muscle weakness |
| Difficulty in swallowing, soft cry, nasal regurgitation, choking while feeding, recurrent aspiration pneumonia | Bulbar weakness |
| Turns to one side and takes support while getting up from supine position | Truncal weakness |

**Table 20.2:** Clinical clues to diagnosis of common childhood neuromuscular disorders

| | *Onset, duration and progression* | *Pattern of weakness* | *Muscle atrophy or hypertrophy* |
|---|---|---|---|
| Muscular dystrophies | Insidious onset, gradually progressive weakness over months to years | Proximal more than distal | Atrophy as well as hypertrophy of different muscles |
| Congenital myopathies | Early, insidious onset, static to slowly progressive course | Proximal more than distal<br>Facial weakness<br>Bulbar weakness ± | Atrophy |
| Metabolic myopathy, channelopathies (periodic paralysis) | Acute onset, progression over hours to days, episodic course | Proximal | — |
| Inflammatory disorders (dermatomyositis) | Acute-subacute onset, waxing and waning course. Pain and cutaneous signs present | Proximal | Atrophy ± |
| Guillain-Barre syndrome | Acute onset ascending, bilaterally symmetrical flaccid weakness | Distal | — |
| Hereditary neuropathies | Insidious onset, gradually progressive over years | Distal more than proximal<br>Feet deformities | Atrophy present |
| Myasthenia gravis | Variable onset, fatigability; diurnal fluctuations | Proximal more than distal<br>Ptosis<br>Ophthalmoplegia<br>Bulbar symptoms | — |
| Spinal muscular atrophy | Insidious onset, progressive; tongue fasciculations, polyminimyoclonus | Proximal more than distal<br>Face relatively spared<br>Bulbar symptoms ± | Atrophy |

**Table 20.3:** Characteristic differences between central and peripheral hypotonia

| | *Central hypotonia* | *Peripheral hypotonia* |
|---|---|---|
| Level of lesion | Proximal to anterior horn cell | Motor unit |
| Tone of muscle | Reduced | Reduced |
| Deep tendon reflexes | Normal or brisk | Depressed or absent |
| Weakness | + | ++ |
| Antigravity movement of limbs | Present | Absent |
| Contractures/foot deformities | Absent | Usually present |
| Seizures/dysmorphism | May be present | Absent |

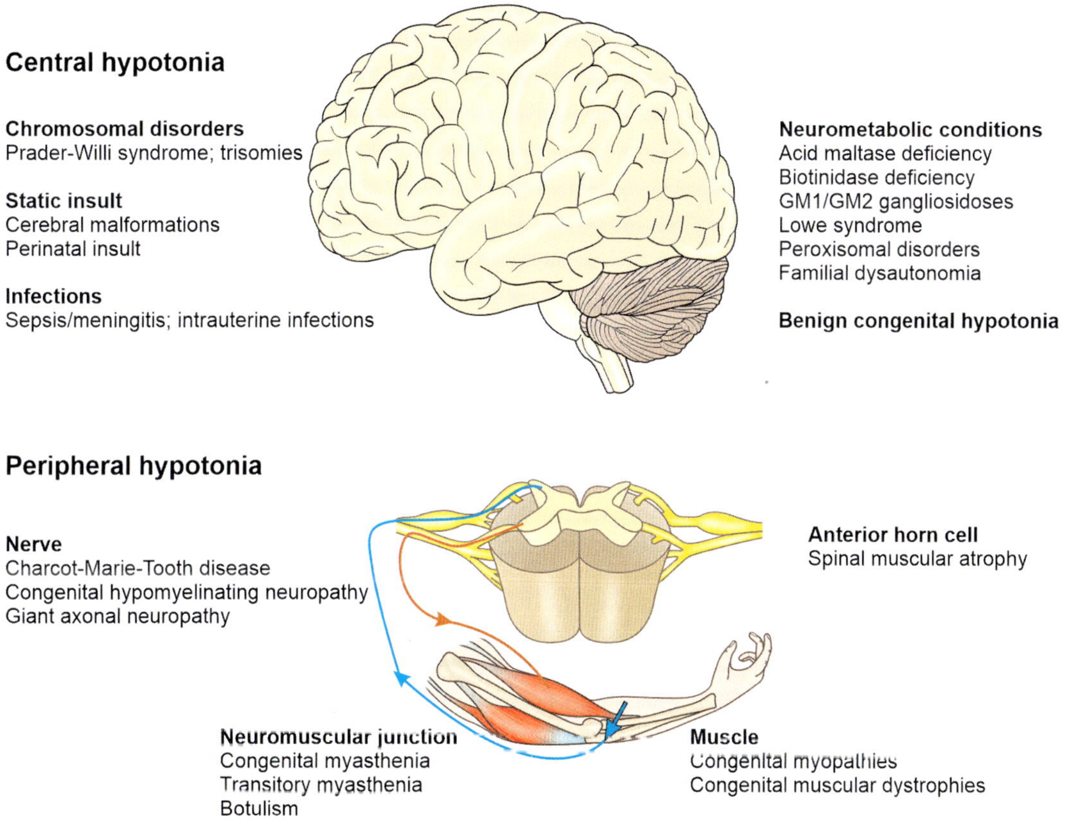


**Fig. 20.3:** Common causes of floppy infant. Maintenance of normal tone requires an intact central and peripheral nervous system

peripheral (Table 20.3) or mixed. The common causes of floppiness in infants are shown in Fig. 20.3. History of reduced fetal movements, polyhydramnios, hip dislocation and multiple contractures (arthrogryposis) in the child suggest *in utero* hypotonia and weakness.

Sometimes patients may have features of both central and peripheral hypotonia. Common causes of *mixed hypotonia* include motor unit disorders with superimposed hypoxia, acid maltase deficiency, mitochondrial disorders and infantile neuronal degeneration.

### Suggested Reading

1. Ahmed MI, Iqbal M, Hussain N. A structured approach to the assessment of a floppy neonate. J Pediatr Neurosc 2016;11(1): 2–6.
2. McDonald CM. Clinical approach to the diagnostic evaluation of hereditary and acquired neuromuscular diseases. Physical Med Rehab Clin N Am 2012;23:495–563.

*Competency:* **PE30.12**

## DISORDERS AFFECTING ANTERIOR HORN CELLS

Spinal muscular atrophy (SMA) is the most common genetic disorder affecting anterior horn cell in children. Among the acquired causes, infection by non-polio enteroviruses (e.g. coxsackie virus and echovirus) is common. Besides these, juvenile form of amyotrophic lateral sclerosis, and neurometabolic disorders like Tay-Sach disease and Pompe disease may also involve anterior horn cells.

### Spinal Muscular Atrophy

This is an autosomal recessive disease caused by a mutation in the survival motor neuron 1 (*SMN1*) gene at chromosome 5q13.2. This region also carries *SMN2* gene, the copy number of which acts as a main modifier of the various clinical phenotypes. Both genes encode the SMN protein

**Table 20.4:** Clinical classification of SMA

| *SMA type* | *Age of onset* | *Motor milestones* | *Lifespan* |
|---|---|---|---|
| 0 | Prenatal | None | Few weeks; <6 months |
| 1 (Werdnig-Hoffmann disease) | <6 months | Head held unaided | <2 years |
| 2 (Dubowitz disease) | <18 months | Sits independently, cannot stand | 2nd-3rd decade |
| 3 (Kugelberg-Welander disease) | >18 months | Stand and walk independently | Normal life expectancy |
| 4 | Adolescent or adult onset | Ambulatory, may complain of muscle pain and fatigue | Normal life expectancy |

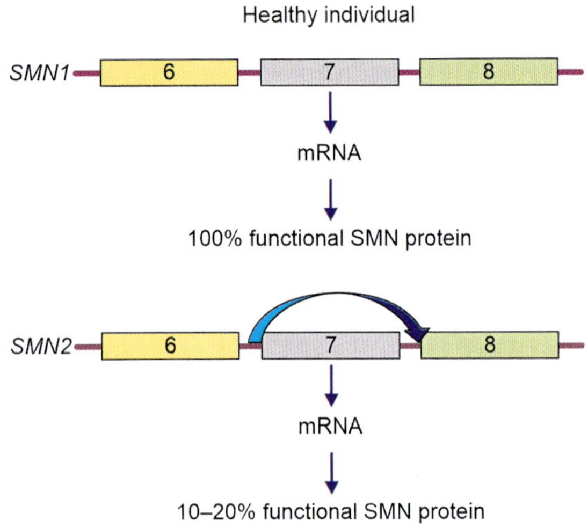


**Fig. 20.4:** Due to a minor change of C→T base change in exon 7 of *SMN2*, final product of SMN2 is mostly non-functional

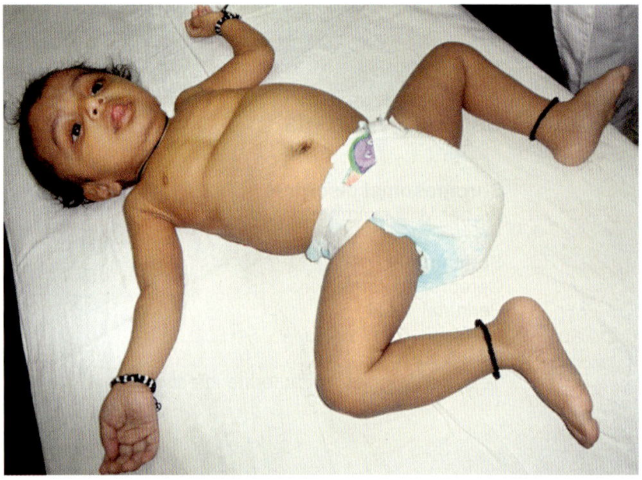

**Fig. 20.5:** A 5-month-old boy with motor delay and repeated chest infections shows generalized hypotonia, absent deep tendon reflexes, poor muscle power and tongue fasciculations. Note the 'frog-like' posture and subcostal retractions due to respiratory muscle weakness. A diagnosis of SMA type 1 was made

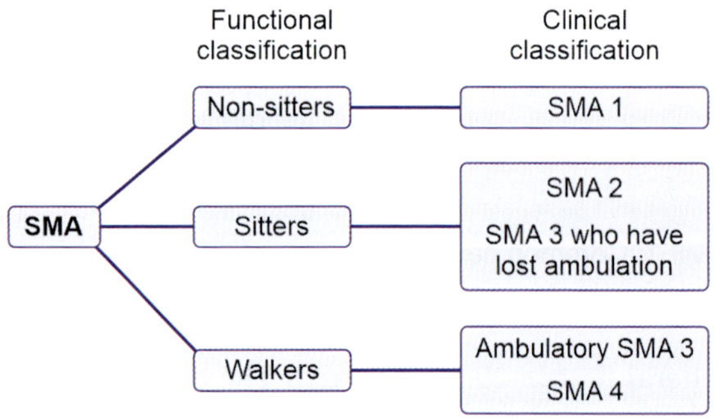


**Fig. 20.6:** Functional classification of spinal muscular atrophy

**Table 20.5:** Newer FDA approved therapies for SMA

| *Drugs* | *Route* | *Mechanism* |
|---|---|---|
| Zolgensma | Intravenous | Gene enhancing therapy |
| Nusinersen | Intrathecal | Antisense oligonucleotide directed to *SMN2* |
| Risdiplam | Oral | mRNA splicing modifier of *SMN2* |

of anterior motor horn cells. In healthy individuals, the *SMN1* is responsible for the functional SMN protein, while *SMN2* produces 10–20% of the full length SMN protein and ~80% of a non-functional product that lacks exon 7 (Fig. 20.4). In ptients with SMA, the *SMN1* is lost due to pathogenic variations or deletions. *SMN2* remains and the small amount of full length SMN protein is sufficient for survival. The number of *SMN2* copies correlates with disease severity, with a lower copy number being linked to more severe types of SMA.

Following clinical types are recognized depending on age of onset of symptoms and course of illness (Table 20.4)

SMA type 1 is a severe form, which presents early with profound hypotonia, flaccid weakness and global areflexia (Fig. 20.5). Respiratory weakness, poor swallowing are common in this form, which is less prominent in type 2 and absent in types 3 and 4. Tongue fasciculations are found in younger children, while polyminimyoclonus (irregular, small amplitude jerky movements of hands and fingers of an outstretched hand) is found in older children. Aspiration pneumonia is an important cause of morbidity and mortality. Children with SMA type 2 may develop kyphoscoliosis. Patients with type 3 disease are often misdiagnosed as limb girdle muscular dystrophy. A functional classification has recently been introduced (Fig. 20.6).

Treatment is supportive and includes respiratory care, management of problems in feeding and swallowing, ensuring nutrition, treatment for gastro-esophageal reflux, orthopedic care and rehabilitation, appropriate immunization, and family education and counseling. Newer gene-based therapies are listed in Table 20.5.

These medications are promising, but expensive. Supportive multidisciplinary care is the standard of therapy for SMA. Genetic counseling should be offered to families with an affected child.

## Suggested Reading


1. Finkel RS, Mercuri E, Meyer OH, et al. Diagnosis and management of spinal muscular atrophy: Pulmonary and acute care; medications, supplements and immunizations; other organ systems; and ethics. Neuromuscul Disord 2018;28:197–207.
2. Mercuri E, Finkel RS, Muntoni F, et al. Diagnosis and management of spinal muscular atrophy: Recommendations for diagnosis, rehabilitation, orthopedic and nutritional care. Neuromuscul Disord 2018;28:103–15.
3. Patient Education Leaflets on SMA; available at www.pedneuroaiims.org/parents_information-material.html
4. Scoto M, Finkel RS, Mercuri E, Muntoni F. Therapeutic approaches for spinal muscular atrophy. Gene Ther. 2017; 24:514–19.


## PERIPHERAL NEUROPATHIES

Neuropathies can be hereditary or acquired. Hereditary neuropathies are common in childhood and usually have a chronic course. The commonest acquired neuropathy which presents acutely is Guillain-Barré syndrome. Clinical features, presentation, electrophysiological characteristics and laboratory studies help in evaluating the patient (Fig. 20.7). Neuropathy can be due to damage to the axons (axonal) or damage to the myelin covering the axons (demyelinating).

*Type of neuropathy:* Most hereditary and acquired neuropathies are primarily axonal. Demyelinating pattern is seen in very few neuropathies. Classical distal predominant weakness is a feature of axonal neuropathies, while demyelinating neuropathies can have proximal as well as distal involvement. The differentiation between axonal and demyelinating neuropathies is mainly electrophysiological. (Table 20.6).

**Table 20.6:** Electrophysiological characteristics of demyelinating and axonal neuropathies

| *Compound muscle action potential properties* | *Demyelinating* | *Axonal* |
|---|---|---|
| Distal latency | Increased | Normal |
| Conduction velocity | Increased | Normal |
| Amplitude | Normal | Decreased |
| Conduction block | Present (acquired causes) | Absent |
| Temporal dispersion | Present (acquired causes) | Absent |

*Pattern of neuropathy:* Most polyneuropathies show distal-to-proximal gradient of symptoms and signs (length dependent or dying back pattern). Proximal weakness is seen in inflammatory demyelinating polyneuropathy and porphyria. The presence of asymmetry and a stepwise progression is seen in mononeuritis multiplex. Mononeuritis multiplex refers to the involvement of multiple separate non-contiguous peripheral nerves, either simultaneously or serially. Mononeuropathies are rare in children.

*Type of nerve fibers involved:* Large fiber neuropathies typically affect the motor nerves and sensory fibers of posterior column, hence result in impaired touch, vibration, weakness and loss of deep tendon reflexes. Small fiber neuropathies present with distal sensory deficit, burning dysesthesias and autonomic dysfunction. Pure sensory neuropathies are unusual.

### Hereditary Neuropathies

An insidious onset, slowly progressive course, prominent sensory signs in absence of sensory symptoms, foot deformities and a family history point suggest an inherited neuropathy (Table 20.7). Charcot-Marie-Tooth disease is the most common hereditary neuropathy, and the most common peripheral neuropathy in children (Fig. 20.8).

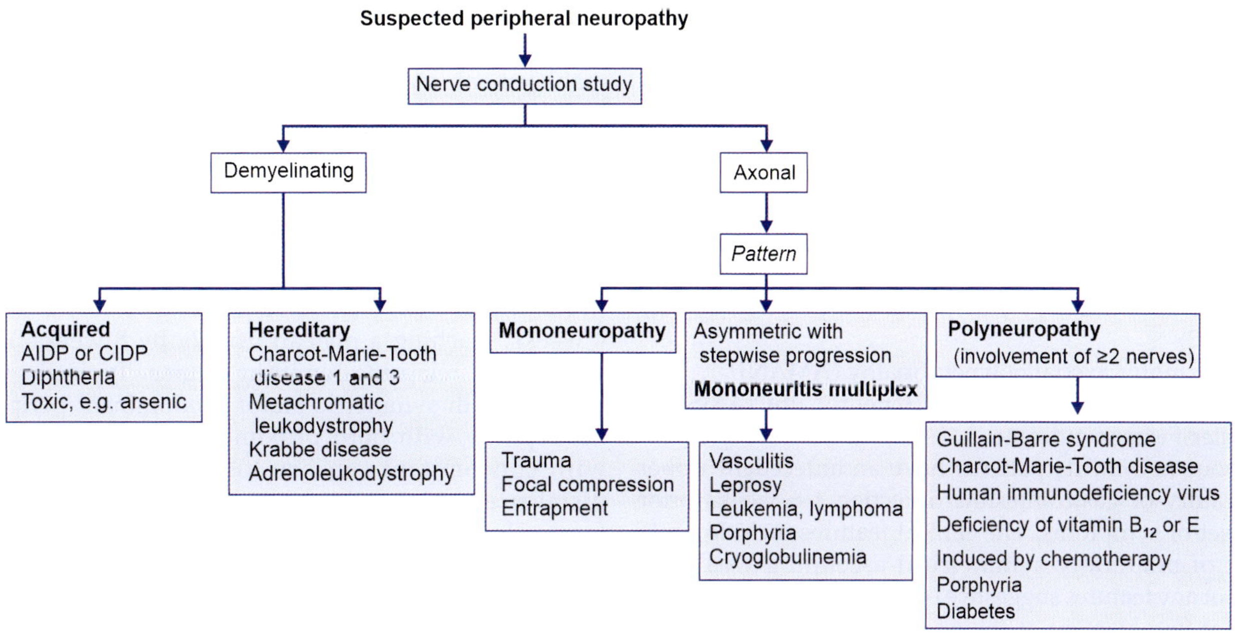


**Fig. 20.7:** Approach to peripheral neuropathies in childhood. AIDP acute inflammatory demyelinating polyneuropathy; CIDP chronic inflammatory demyelinating polyneuropathy

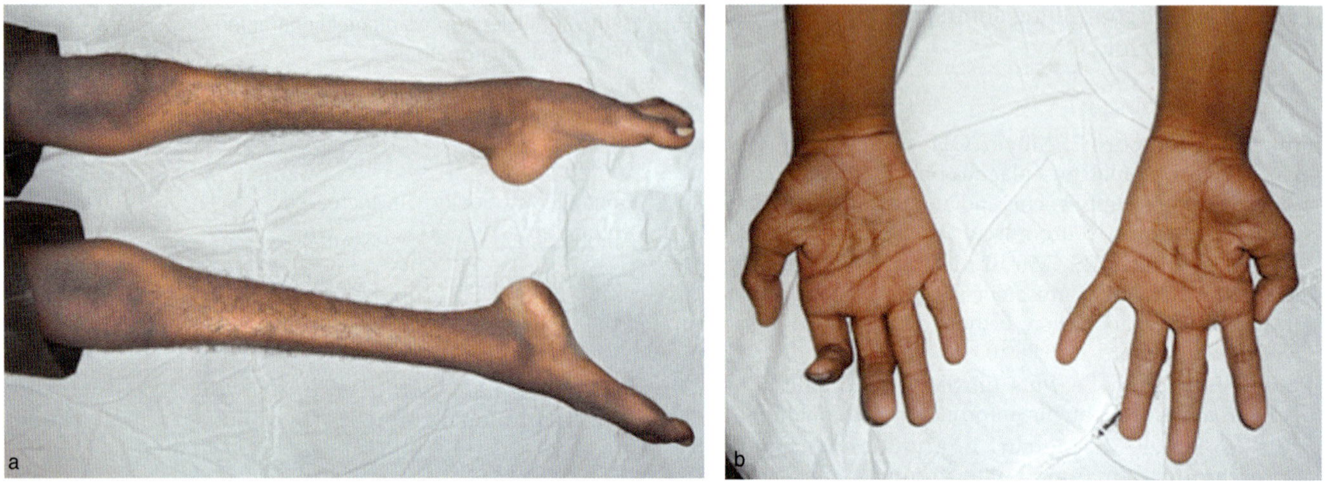


**Fig. 20.8:** Charcot-Marie-Tooth disease in a 7-year-old boy with progressive gait difficulties, frequent falls due to twisting of ankles, foot deformities and thinning of legs: (a) Note the 'stork leg' appearance of legs with foot deformities; (b) Atrophy of thenar and hypothenar muscles along with clawing of fingers, better appreciated in the right hand

**Table 20.7:** Hereditary neuropathies

| |
|---|
| **Primary disease**<br>• Charcot-Marie-Tooth disease<br>• Hereditary neuropathy with liability to pressure palsies<br>• Hereditary sensory and autonomic neuropathies<br>• Distal hereditary motor neuropathies<br>• Hereditary neuralgic amyotrophy |
| **Multisystem disorder**<br>*Lipid metabolism:* Leukodystrophies, phytanic acid storage disorder, sphingomyelin lipidoses<br>Porphyria<br>*Defective DNA repair:* Ataxia telangiectasia, xeroderma pigmentosa<br>*Hereditary ataxias:* Friedrich ataxia, spinocerebellar ataxia<br>*Miscellaneous:* Neuroacanthocytosis, mitochondrial disorders |

Clinical features and electrophysiology help in the diagnosis. Genetic tests are useful for confirming the diagnosis. Supportive care is the standard of therapy. Genetic counseling should be offered to the patient's family.

## Guillain-Barré Syndrome

This is a common cause of acute flaccid paralysis (AFP) in children with variable age of onset, relatively rapid course and predominantly motor symmetric polyradiculoneuropathy that leads to bulbar and respiratory compromise. Four subtypes are described:

- Acute inflammatory demyelinating polyneuropathy (AIDP)
- Acute motor axonal polyneuropathy (AMAN)
- Acute motor and sensory axonal neuropathy (AMSAN)
- Miller-Fisher syndrome

About two-thirds patients have an antecedent upper respiratory or gastrointestinal infection 1–6 weeks prior to onset of symptoms. The clinical features include acute onset of bilaterally symmetrical ascending weakness without any features suggestive of CNS involvement. Bowel bladder involvement at the onset of illness goes against the diagnosis of GBS. Facial weakness is frequent, and involvement of respiratory muscles occurs in 20–60% cases. Dysautonomia is common. The disease is progressive and reaches its nadir within 2 weeks. If the maximum disability is reached within 24 hours or continues to progress beyond 4 weeks, an alternative diagnosis should be sought. The illness is usually monophasic, but 6–10% patients may suffer from therapy-related fluctuations, and another 2–5% may have relapses after an initial improvement. Axonal form of Guillain-Barré syndrome has a more rapid and severe course. The Miller-Fisher syndrome is characterized by the triad of ophthalmological abnormalities, ataxia and areflexia. Diagnostic criteria of Guillain-Barre syndrome are summarized in Table 20.8.

Intravenous immunoglobulin (IVIG, 2 g/kg over 5 days) is the first line of treatment. Alternatively, plasma exchange (200–250 mL/kg for 5 sessions) can be performed. Treatment is indicated in non-ambulatory and critically sick patients. Patients who do not respond to initial treatment with IVIG may benefit from a second course of therapy, which is usually given after 2–4 weeks. Supportive care includes cardiorespiratory care, physical therapy, nutritional management, management of neuropathic pain, care of bladder and bowel and prevention of deep vein thrombosis. Rehabilitation should begin early, and patients should be followed closely after discharge.

## Chronic Inflammatory Demyelinating Polyradiculoneuropathy (CIDP)

In contrast to GBS, CIDP has a progressive course beyond 4 weeks, reaching a plateau usually by 8 weeks. It can also have a relapsing-remitting course. Typically, CIDP presents with symmetric motor predominant peripheral neuropathy with both proximal and distal weakness with concomitant sensory loss. Asymmetric forms, distal predominant forms and sensory predominant forms also occur. Electrophysiology and nerve biopsy help in diagnosis. Treatment modalities for chronic inflammatory demyelinating polyradiculoneuropathy include corticosteroid, IVIG, and plasma exchange. Spontaneous remissions are uncommon, and most patients require long-term immunomodulating therapy.

**Table 20.8:** Diagnostic criteria for Guillain-Barré syndrome

| |
|---|
| **Features required for diagnosis** |
| • Progressive weakness in more than 1 limb (usually starts in legs)<br>• Areflexia (or decreased tendon reflexes) in weak limbs |
| **Features that strongly support diagnosis** |
| • Progression of symptoms over days to 4 weeks<br>• Relative symmetry of symptoms<br>• Mild sensory symptoms or signs<br>• Autonomic dysfunction<br>• Cranial nerve involvement, most common bilateral weakness of facial muscles<br>• Absence of fever at the onset of neurological symptom<br>• Typical electrophysiological findings<br>Abnormal or absent F wave, and H reflex<br>Reduced motor with or without sensory nerve action potentials (axonal variant: AMAN)<br>Prolonged distal latencies, reduced conduction velocities, presence of conduction block or increased temporal dispersion (demyelinating variant: AIDP)<br>• Albuminocytologic dissociation on CSF: High concentration of protein in CSF; mononuclear cell counts <50/mm$^3$ |
| **Features that raised doubt about the diagnosis** |
| • Bladder or bowel dysfunction at onset and/or persistent bladder or bowel dysfunction<br>• Fever at onset<br>• Sharp sensory level<br>• Marked persistent asymmetry of weakness<br>• Severe pulmonary dysfunction with limited limb weakness at onset<br>• Marked sensory signs with limited weakness at onset<br>• CSF showing increased number of mononuclear cells (>50 cells/mm$^3$) or polymorphonuclear cells |

## Suggested Reading


1. Korinthanberg R, Trollman R, Plecko B, et al. Differential diagnosis of acquired and hereditary neuropathies. Concensus guidelines. Child (Basel) 2021;8(8):687.
2. Leonhard SE, Mandarakas MR, Gondim FAA, et al. Diagnosis and management of Guillain–Barré syndrome in ten steps. Nat Rev Neurol. 2019;15(11):671–83.
3. Shang P, Feng J, Wu W, Zhang HL. Intensive care and treatment of severe Guillain-Barré syndrome. Front Pharmacol 2021;12:608130.
4. Wilmshurst JM, Ouvrier R. Hereditary peripheral neuropathies of childhood: a brief overview for clinicians. Neuromuscul Disord 2011;21:763–67.


*Competency:* **PE30.13**

# ACUTE FLACCID PARALYSIS

Acute flaccid paralysis (AFP) is a clinical syndrome characterized by rapid onset of weakness, progressing to maximum severity within several days to weeks. The term 'flaccid' refers to the absence of spasticity or other upper motor neuron signs. In the Global Polio Eradication Initiative, AFP is defined as any case of flaccid weakness in children <15-year-old, or any paralytic illness at any age when polio is suspected. Common causes of AFP are Guillain-Barré syndrome, transverse myelitis, traumatic neuritis, post-diphtheric neuropathy and non-polio enteroviral illnesses. The differential diagnosis varies with age **(Table 20.9)**; distinguishing features are summarized in **Table 20.10**.

**Table 20.9:** Differential diagnoses of acute flaccid paralysis

| | |
|---|---|
| Muscle disorders | • Inflammatory myopathy<br>• Periodic paralysis<br>• Hypokalemia<br>• Infections |
| Neuromuscular junction disorders | • Myasthenia gravis<br>• Botulism<br>• Eaton-Lambert syndrome |
| Neuropathies | • Guillain-Barré syndrome<br>• Traumatic neuritis<br>• Post-diphtheric neuropathy<br>• Porphyria<br>• Vasculitis<br>• Bell's palsy |
| Anterior horn cell disorders | • Poliomyelitis<br>• Non-polio enteroviruses |
| Spinal cord disease | • Transverse myelitis<br>• Spinal cord compression<br>• Trauma |

Major immunization initiatives have resulted in sharp decline in poliomyelitis across the world. The last case of confirmed wild poliovirus (P1 type) in India was reported from West Bengal in January 2011. On 27 March 2014, the WHO declared India a polio-free country, since no cases of wild polio were reported in preceding three years. Currently polio remains endemic to two countries—Afghanistan and Pakistan.

## Acute Flaccid Paralysis (AFP) Surveillance

AFP surveillance underpins the polio eradication initiative and is the chief strategy to screen for circulating wild poliovirus in the post-polio eradication era. All patients with AFP within the last 6 months should be reported to Surveillance Medical Officer of the World Health Organization.

Surveillance is done in major four steps: (i) Finding and reporting children with AFP, (ii) transporting stool samples for analysis, (iii) isolating and identifying poliovirus in laboratory, and (iv) mapping the virus to determine its origin.

These cases are immediately investigated, within 48 hours of notification, by a trained medical officer. After confirming the case as AFP, the investigator takes medical history and conducts examination, and proceeds with other aspects of case investigation including collection and transportation of stool specimens for laboratory testing, search for additional cases and outbreak investigation in the affected community, 60 days follow-up examination, analysis of laboratory results and case classification.

Collection of stool specimens from every patient is an important aspect of the eradication strategy. From every case of AFP, two stool specimens are collected, ideally within 14 days of onset of paralysis and at least 24 hours

**Table 20.10:** Differentiating common causes of acute flaccid paralysis

| | *Poliomyelitis* | *Guillain-Barré syndrome* | *Transverse myelitis* | *Traumatic neuritis* |
|---|---|---|---|---|
| Fever | Present; may be biphasic | May have a prodromal | May have a prodromal illness | Absent |
| Symmetry | Asymmetric | Symmetrical | Symmetrical | Asymmetric |
| Sensations | Intact; may have diffuse myalgias | Variable | Impaired below the level of the lesion | Impaired in distribution of the affected nerve |
| Respiratory insufficiency | May be present | May be present | May be present | Absent |
| Cranial nerves | Affected in bulbar and bulbospinal variants | Usually affected | Absent | Absent |
| Radicular signs | May be present | Present | Absent | Absent |
| Bladder, bowel complaints | Absent | Transient, late; due to autonomic dysfunction | Present, early | Absent |
| Nerve conduction | May be abnormal | Abnormal | Normal | Abnormal |
| Cerebrospinal fluid | Lymphocytic pleocytosis; normal or increased protein | Albuminocytologic dissociation | Variable | Normal |
| MRI spine | Usually normal | Usually normal | Characteristic changes | Normal |





apart. While the optimal period for detection of polio virus in the stool is within 14 days of onset of paralysis, specimens may be collected from any late reported case up to 60 days from the onset of paralysis. Beyond 60 days after paralysis, the likelihood of detecting poliovirus is very low. Voided stool sample is preferred. In cases where it is not possible, other methods include digital extraction (when child is constipated or dies), postmortem stool collection (contents of large intestine) and use of rectal tube. Enema or purgatives are not recommended. Each specimen should be 8 g each (about the size of one adult thumb), collected in a clean, dry screw-capped container. The specimens are collected, labeled and then transported in the 'cold chain'.

Two types of cell lines are used for polio virus isolation. The human rhabdomyosarcoma (RD) cell lines favor growth of all enteroviruses, and L20B cell lines favor the growth of only polioviruses. If cytopathic effects appear in L20B cell line, the isolate then goes for neutralization test to determine the serotype (type 1, 2 or 3) using appropriate antisera. Intratypic differentiation is done to determine, if the isolate is wild or vaccine poliovirus; the former isolates undergo genetic sequencing.

A case is classified as polio, if wild polio virus is isolated from the stool specimen. Cases with inadequate stool specimens and having residual weakness who have died or are lost to follow-up undergo additional review by the National Expert Review Committee. This committee classifies the case as compatible with polio or discarded as non-polio AFP. Experience indicates that at least 1 case of non-polio AFP occurs for every 100 000 children aged <15 years per year (background AFP rate). As per National Polio Surveillance Project, the non-polio AFP rate, which is an indicator of surveillance sensitivity, should be equal or to ≥1:100,000.

### Suggested Reading


1. Reach project. Polio eradication in India. March 2020;www.reachprojectuoft.com
2. Surveillance of acute flaccid paralysis, 3rd edn. New Delhi: Ministry of Health & Family Welfare, Government of India; 2005.
3. Thacker N, Vashishtha VM, Thacker D. Polio eradication in India: The lessons learned. Pediatrics 2016;138(4): e 20160461.


## NEUROMUSCULAR JUNCTION DISORDERS

Disorders affecting the neuromuscular junction can be acquired or inherited (Table 20.11). They are usually pure motor syndromes affecting proximal, bulbar or extraocular muscles.

### Myasthenia Gravis

About 20% patients with myasthenia have onset in childhood or adolescence. Fatigable weakness is the hallmark. Most patients have ptosis or ophthalmoplegia (ocular form) which may be asymmetric and variable over time. Pupillary reactions are normal. Children may

**Table 20.11:** Neuromuscular junction disorders in children

| *Immune mediated* | *Metabolic toxins* |
|---|---|
| • Myasthenia gravis<br>• Lambert-Eaton myasthenic syndrome | • Botulism<br>• Organophosphates<br>• Snake envenomation<br>• Tick paralysis<br>• Hypermagnesemia |
| ***Congenital myasthenic syndromes***<br>• Choline acetyltransferase<br>• Paucity of synaptic vesicles<br>• Endplate acetylcholinesterase deficiency<br>• Acetylcholine receptor defects<br>• Mutations in *RAPSN, PLEC1, DOK7* | ***Drugs***<br>• Aminoglycosides<br>• Erythromycin<br>• Tetracycline<br>• Fluoroquinolones<br>• Neuromuscular blocking agents<br>• Phenytoin<br>• D-penicillamine<br>• Lithium<br>• Interferon α |

develop diplopia on sustained gaze or continuous activity like reading. On attempting to tightly close the eyes, after a few minutes, the cornea may get exposed due to inability to sustain contraction of orbicularis oculi (peep sign).

About half of the children with ocular findings may develop bulbar or limb girdle weakness within 2 years (generalized form). Limb weakness is usually symmetric and proximal. Deep tendon reflexes are either normal or reduced in proportion to the degree of muscle weakness. Respiratory muscles may also get involved and may lead to *myasthenic crises*. Myasthenia gravis may be associated with thyroid disorders, systemic lupus erythematosus, diabetes mellitus and rheumatoid arthritis. Thymomas are found chiefly in adolescent onset myasthenia gravis and are rare (<5%) in early childhood

***Transitory neonatal myasthenia*** occurs in about 15% of babies born to myasthenic mothers. Maternal antibodies cross placenta to reach fetus and causes transient symptoms. Symptoms start within a few hours after birth but may be delayed till the third day. These include difficulty in feeding, weak cry, hypotonia, lack of facial expression and respiratory insufficiency. Supportive care suffices in most cases. Oral or intramuscular pyridostigmine, usually for 4–6 weeks, may be warranted in severe cases.

***Edrophonium testing*** is usually the first test performed in a suspected case of myasthenia gravis. The dose used is 0.1–0.2 mg/kg; may be repeated every minute to a total dose of 5 mg (weight <34 kg) or 10 mg (weight >34 kg). Effects are seen within 10 seconds and persist till 120 seconds. A positive result consists of transient resolution of the clinical sign (ptosis, ophthalmoplegia, dysarthria) under observation. Edrophonium is not recommended for use in infants due to high risk of arrhythmias and short duration of action which precludes objective assessment.

***Neostigmine*** may also be used as a diagnostic test. The dose used is 0.125 mg/kg in an infant and 0.04 mg/kg IM in an older child. It is slower in action, with anticipated response in 10–15 min and maximum in 30 min **(Fig. 20.9)**. If the result is equivocal or negative, the dose may be repeated in 4 hours.

***Repetitive nerve stimulation studies*** are abnormal in 50–70% cases with generalized myasthenia gravis. A decrement of >10% is characteristic. Electromyography may be normal or may show unstable or myopathic muscle unit action potentials. Single fiber electromyography is more sensitive and may show increased jitter or blocking.

***Acetylcholine receptor (AChR) antibodies*** may be positive in children with myasthenia gravis; the rates are lower in peri- and prepubertal children (50–60%). ***Antibodies to muscle-specific kinase*** (anti-MuSK) are seen in 40% seronegative patients. X-ray chest or CT of anterior mediastinum may show thymoma or thymic hyperplasia.

### Congenital Myasthenia Syndromes

Congenital myasthenia syndromes are exceptionally rare. They may present at birth or during infancy. In almost all cases, onset of symptoms is within the first two years of life. They should be suspected in seronegative myasthenia gravis, floppy infant with underdeveloped muscles, and in adults with childhood history of difficulties affecting cranial, respiratory, truncal or limb muscles. Common features include hypotonia, limb weakness, feeding and respiratory difficulties, arthrogryposis, ptosis, ophthalmoparesis, dysphagia and dysarthria. Unlike myasthenia gravis, these do not respond to steroids and other immunosuppressants. Certain syndromes like endplate acetylcholinesterase deficiency and slow channel congenital myasthenia may worsen with pyridostigmine.

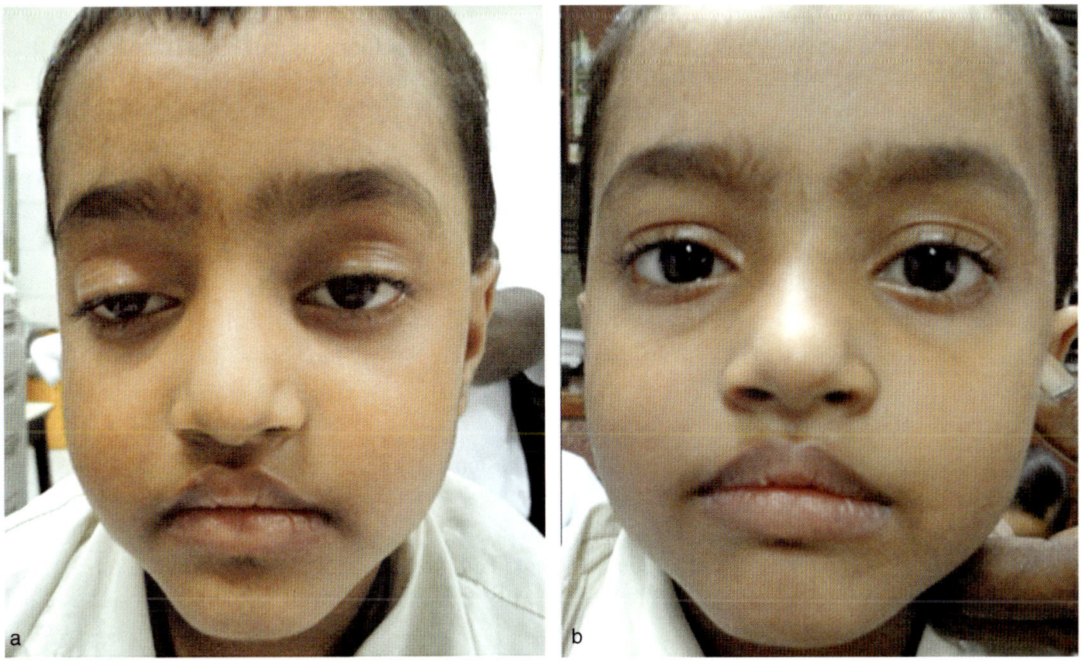


**Fig. 20.9:** Juvenile myasthenia gravis: A 9-year-old boy presented with drooping of eyelids, more in the evening than morning, and restricted eye movements. Examination revealed asymmetric ptosis, external ophthalmoplegia, normal pupils and normal motor examination. Note the improved ptosis (a) before and (b) after administration of neostigmine

### Treatment

Cholinesterase inhibitors are the initial treatment for myasthenia gravis. Pyridostigmine is commonly used at doses of 1–7 mg/kg/day in 4 divided doses. Prednisolone, at low doses (0.5 mg/kg/d), may be used in a nonacute setting. Azathioprine, cyclosporine, cyclophosphamide and mycophenolate mofetil are used as steroid sparing drugs or for refractory cases. Drugs that interfere with neuromuscular transmission (Table 20.11) should be used with caution. Thymectomy is beneficial in seropositive patients.

Myasthenic crisis necessitates cardiorespiratory monitoring and support. It should be differentiated from cholinergic crises due to overdosage of acetylcholinesterase inhibitors. Antecedent events, predominance of cholinergic symptoms, ice pack test and edrophonium challenge test help differentiate the two entities. IVIG or plasmapheresis may be required in patients with myasthenic crisis.

#### Suggested Reading


1. Finsterer J. Congenital myasthenic syndromes. Orphanet J Rare Dis 2019;14:57.
2. Narayanaswami P, Sanders DB, Wolfe G, et al. International consensus guidance for management of myasthenia gravis. Neurology 2021;96(3):114–22.


## MUSCLE DISORDERS

### Congenital Myopathies

The congenital myopathies are a diverse group of muscle disorders caused by genetic defects in the contractile apparatus of the muscle and defined by distinctive histochemical or ultrastructural changes on muscle biopsy. Majority of these disorders present as 'floppy infant' syndrome. The common presenting features include hypotonia, static or non-progressive muscle weakness and normal or decreased deep tendon reflexes. Respiratory insufficiency, feeding difficulties, contractures and skeletal deformities may be present. They may also present in late childhood or adulthood (Table 20.12).

Serum creatine kinase is either normal or mildly raised. Electromyography reveals a myopathic pattern. The disorders are clinically indistinguishable; distinction is possible by characteristic features on skeletal muscle biopsy incorporating new immunohistochemical techniques and electron microscopy. Advances in molecular genetics have improved our understanding of congenital myopathies.

#### Suggested Reading


1. Cassandrini D, Trovato R, Rubegni A, et al. Congenital myopathies: Clinical phenotypes and new diagnostic tools. Italian J Pediatr 2017;43:101.
2. Domingo-Horne RM, Salajegheh MK. An approach to myopathy for a primary care clinician. Am J Med 2018;131:237–43.
3. Wang HC, Dowling JM, North K, et al. Consensus statement on standard of care for congenital myopathies. J Child Neurol 2012;27:363.


*Competency:* **PE30.14**

### Muscle Dystrophies

The muscular dystrophies are diseases leading to breakdown of muscles. Histopathology shows evidence of ongoing muscle degeneration and regeneration. Diagnosis of these disorders is based on clinical features, muscle imaging, muscle biopsy and genetic studies. Clinical approach to common muscular dystrophies is demonstrated in Fig. 20.10. Important clues on history and examination include age at onset, differential weakness of muscles like hip adductors, abductors, face, neck extensors, neck flexors, scapular stabilizing muscles, and abdominal muscles.

*Competency:* **PE30.14**

#### Dystrophinopathies

Dystrophinopathies are a group of disorders resulting from mutations in the dystrophin gene (located on short arm of X chromosome, Xp21). The dystrophin protein is responsible for stabilization of membrane. Duchenne muscular dystrophy (DMD) is the most common dystrophinopathy with an incidence of 1 in 3500 live male births and present before 5 years of age. Its allelic variant, Becker muscular dystrophy (BMD), differs by a later onset (usually >6 years old), and slower progression, a higher incidence of myalgias, occasional rhabdomyolysis following exercise and early cardiomyopathy.

**Table 20.12:** Classification of congenital myopathies

| *Subtype* | *Inheritance, genes* | *Histology* | *Clinical features* |
|---|---|---|---|
| Core myopathies (central core disease; multiminicore disease) | AD, AR<br>*RYR1, SEPN1*<br>*ACTA1, MYH7* | Poorly defined fibers with short cores | *RYR1* mutation is most common<br>High risk of malignant hyperthermia |
| Nemaline myopathy | AD, AR, sporadic<br>*ACTA1, NEB, TPM2, TPM3, TNNT1* | Nemaline bodies on Trichrome Gomori stain | Nebulin (*NEB*) mutation most common<br>Onset congenital; muscles of face, ocular and neck; chest deformity, scoliosis |
| Centronuclear myopathies | AD, sporadic, X-linked<br>*MTM1, DNM2, BIN1, RYR1, DM1* | Central nuclei in all muscle fibers | Onset: Newborn to adult<br>Facial weakness, ptosis, external ophthalmoplegia, weakness of neck flexors |
| Congenital fiber type disproportion | AD, AR, X-linked<br>*ACTA1, TPM3, TPM2, RYR1, SEPN1* | Predominant type 1 fibers; small type 2 fibers | *ACTA1* mutation most common<br>Majority have less severe phenotype |

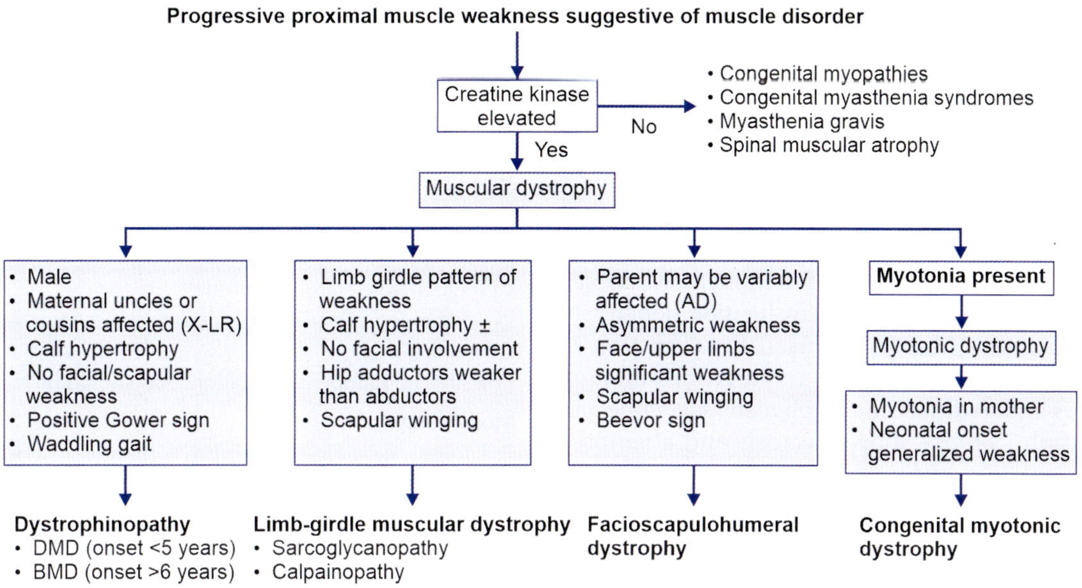


**Fig. 20.10:** Approach to common childhood muscular dystrophies. DMD Duchenne muscular dystrophy; BMD Becker muscular dystropy; LGMD limb girdle muscular dystrophy

The phenotypic variation is explained by the reading frame hypothesis. In >90% of cases, mutations that disrupt the reading frame (frameshift) lead to dystrophin deficiency and cause DMD. In BMD, mutations maintain the reading frame (in frame mutations) and result in abnormal but partly functional dystrophin.

Children with DMD have history of delayed walking, difficulty in climbing stairs and getting up from sitting position. Gait disturbances become apparent at 3–4 years of age. Waddling gait (due to hip abductors weakness), Gower sign and calf muscle pseudohypertrophy (hypertrophied appearance due to deposition of fat and connective tissue) (Fig. 20.11) are classical findings. Weakness of neck flexors is early. Other muscles that show hypertrophy include infraspinatus, deltoid, tongue and masseter. The progression of weakness may plateau between 3 and 6 years of age, followed by increasing gait difficulty, development of contractures, scoliosis and lumbar lordosis. The age at loss of independent ambulation in untreated patients is between 8.8 and 10.5 years. After loss of ambulation, there is worsening kyphoscoliosis, increasing upper limb weakness and bulbar dysfunction.

Weakness of intercostal and diaphragmatic muscles with spinal deformity affects respiratory function. Dropping of vital capacity <20% of normal leads to nocturnal hypoventilation. Children with deletion of exons 48, 48–49 and 45–53 are especially prone to cardiac complications, including cardiomyopathy and arrhythmias. The cause of death is a combination of respiratory insufficiency and cardiomyopathy. Other features include variable degree of intellectual disability and impaired gastric motility.

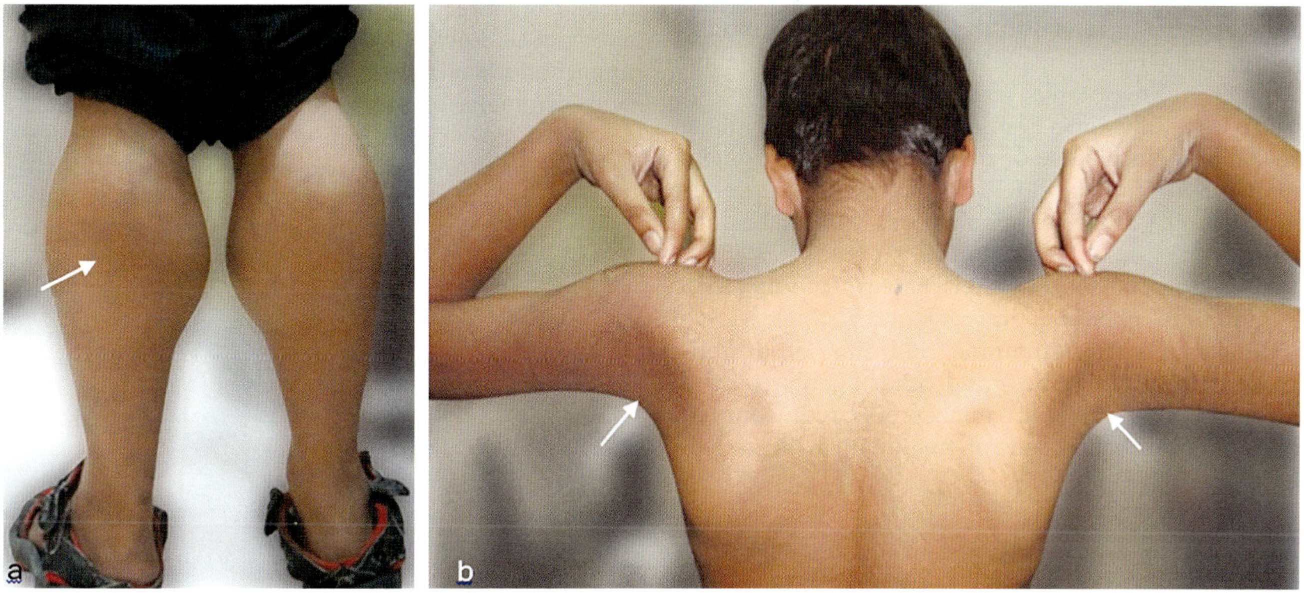


**Fig. 20.11:** (a) Duchenne muscular dystrophy. The child presented with waddling gait and lumbar lordosis. He had proximal muscle weakness, more in the lower limbs, calf hypertrophy and positive Gower sign; (b) Examination in another child shows hypertrophy of deltoid and infraspinatus muscles with wasting of posterior axillary fold muscles (valley sign)

Around 10% of female carriers show variable degree of weakness with elevated levels of creatine kinase, calf hypertrophy, myalgias and cramps and risk of dilated cardiomyopathy. Rarely, the full Duchenne phenotype may present in girls with complete inactivation of normal X chromosome.

Serum creatine kinase levels are highly elevated (>10 times upper limit of normal), but do not correlate with severity of the disease or response to treatment. Multiplex PCR and the more sensitive multiplex ligation dependent probe amplification (MLPA) are used for detection of mutations. Muscle biopsy may be required in mutation negative cases and to differentiate between Duchenne and Becker dystrophy. Biopsy shows necrosis and attempted regeneration of individual muscle fibers, variable muscle fiber diameter with both hypertrophic and small fibers, and central nuclei. Later, almost the entire muscle is replaced by fibrofatty tissue. On immunohistochemistry, absence of dystrophin (1,2,3) staining is seen in Duchenne dystrophy; dystrophin staining is reduced and patchy in Becker dystrophy.

*Management:* Patients with Duchenne dystrophy require multidisciplinary management, maintenance of muscle strength and range of motion of joints by exercise, physiotherapy and avoidance of prolonged immobility. Corticosteroids (prednisone, deflazacort) are the current standard of care, and increase muscle strength. Other newly approved drugs are mentioned in Table 20.13.

**Table 20.13:** Management of Duchenne muscular dystrophy

| Management of Duchenne muscular dystrophy |
|---|
| **Corticosteroids** |
| *Indication:* Children >2 years with declining function |
| *Dose:* Prednisone 0.75 mg/kg/day (initially 0.3–0.5 mg/kg/day, if non-ambulatory) |
| Deflazacort 0.9 mg/kg/day (preferred in children with excessive weight gain or behavioral problems) |
| Ensure immunization against pneumococcus, influenza and varicella before starting steroids |
| Weekly blood pressure and random blood sugar for monitoring side effects |
| Obesity can hamper ambulation, and should be avoided |
| **Monitoring** |
| *Pulmonary function tests:* Every 6 months, if non-ambulatory; annually in ambulatory patients |
| *Echocardiography:* Once in 2 yr for <10 yr of age; annually if >10 years |
| Serum calcium, phosphate, 25(OH) vitamin $D_3$ (biannually), DEXA scan annually |
| **Physical therapy** |
| Effective stretching and appropriate positioning at various joints, assistive devices to prevent contractures, avoid high resistance strength training |
| *Surgery:* For fixed contractures and spinal deformities |
| **Other components** |
| • Respiratory and cardiac care<br>• Ensure nutrition; manage gastrointestinal problems<br>• Psychosocial management<br>• Family education and genetic counseling |
| **Newer therapies** |
| • Exon skipping: Exon 45, 51, 53 (antisense oligonucleotides)<br>• Stop codon read through: Ataluren<br>• Gene therapy<br>• Others: Utrophin regulators, myostatin inhibitors |

### *Myotonic Dystrophy Type 1*

This disorder transmitted in an autosomal dominant manner, is caused by an abnormal expansion (>80) of trinucleotide [CTG] repeats in the *DMPK* gene on chromosome 19. The classic form presents in childhood with myotonia, facial weakness, distal limb weakness, cataracts (iridescent spoke-like posterior capsular cataract), frontal baldness, endocrinopathies (testicular atrophy, hyperinsulinism, adrenal atrophy and growth hormone disturbances), cardiac arrhythmias and disturbed gastrointestinal motility. The congenital form may present with respiratory failure, poor feeding, hypotonia, facial diplegia, club foot and gastroparesis. Myotonia is absent in neonates and infants. There may be a history of decreased fetal movements and polyhydramnios. EMG shows amyopathic pattern and myotonia ('revving engine' sound). Genetic testing is confirmatory.

Medications that block sodium channels (procainamide, disopyramide, phenytoin, quinine, mexiletine); tricyclic antidepressants (clomipramine, imipramine); diuretics (acetazolamide, thiazides) and other agents (taurine, nifedipine, diazepam, carbamazepine, prednisone and albuterol) have been used for treatment, with variable results.

### *Facioscapulohumeral Muscular Dystrophy*

The clinical spectrum of this autosomal dominant disorder ranges from asymptomatic children to wheelchair bound patients. The age at onset is variable. The disease may start with asymmetric facial weakness followed, sequentially, by scapular fixator, humeral, truncal and lower limb weakness. Biceps and triceps are typically involved with sparing of deltoid and forearm muscles resulting in the "Popeye" arm appearance. Lower abdominal muscles are weaker than upper abdominal muscles resulting in Beevor sign. Side-to-side asymmetry of muscle weakness is typical (Fig. 20.12).

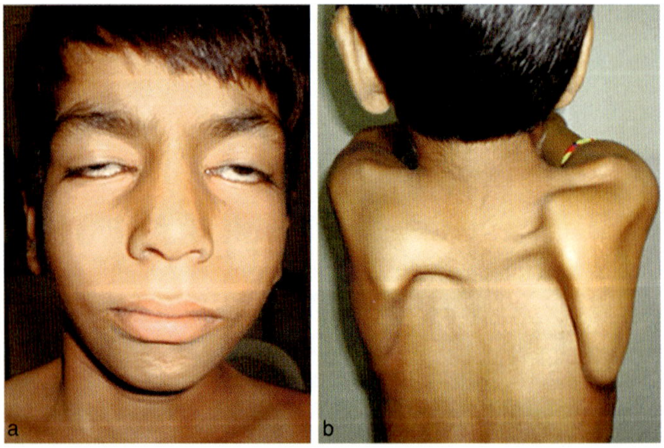


**Fig. 20.12:** Facioscapulohumeral dystrophy: (a) Note the facial weakness and inability to completely close the eyes; (b) Asymmetric scapular winging

Other features include high frequency hearing loss, Coats disease (retinal telangiectasia, exudation and detachment), atrial arrhythmias and restrictive respiratory disease. The diagnosis is confirmed by demonstrating the shortening of the macrosatellite repeat D4Z4 which is normally in one allele of 4q35. Treatment is supportive.

#### *Limb Girdle Muscular Dystrophies*

Limb girdle muscular dystrophies are a group of clinically heterogeneous syndromes with autosomal dominant or recessive inheritance. Most childhood onset limb girdle dystrophies are associated with predominant lower extremity weakness. Cardiac or other systemic involvement is variable. Serum creatine kinase is modestly elevated, but can be high in the sarcoglycanopathies, dysferlinopathy and caveolinopathy. Autosomal recessive limb girdle dystrophies have early onset, rapid progression and higher creatine kinase values. Treatment is symptomatic.

#### *Congenital Muscular Dystrophies*

These patients usually present at birth or in first year of life. Infants show hypotonia, weakness, arthrogryposis, bulbar dysfunction or respiratory insufficiency. Weakness is static or slowly progressive. Diagnosis is supported by dystrophic myopathic features on muscle biopsy, elevated creatine kinase levels and exclusion of common myopathies of newborn.

### Suggested Reading


1. Birnkrant DJ, Bushby K, Bann CM, et al. Diagnosis and management of Duchenne muscular dystrophy. Lancet Neurol 2018 Feb1;pii:S1474-4422(18)30026-7.
2. Duan D, Goemans N, Takeda S, et al. Duchenne muscular dystophy. Nat Rev Dis Primers 2021;7:31.
3. Kamsteeg EJ, Kress W, Catalli C, et al. Best practice guidelines on myotonic dystrophy. Eur J Hum Genetics 2012;20:1203–08.
4. Patient education leaflets are available at www.pedneuroaiims.org/parents_infromation_materials.html


### Inflammatory Myopathies

The inflammatory myopathies are a diverse group of disorders in which muscle appears to be injured by the immune system. Dermatomyositis is the most common pediatric inflammatory myopathy, which typically affects skin and muscle but may involve joints, gut, lung, heart and other internal organs (*see* Chapter 22).

### Metabolic Myopathies

The metabolic myopathies are a group of muscle disorders resulting from failed energy production related to defects in glycogen, lipid, or mitochondrial metabolism. The symptoms arise due to a mismatch between the rate of ATP utilization and the capacity of muscle metabolic pathways to regenerate ATP. Affected children and adults present with exercise intolerance, weakness and myoglobinuria. Newborns and infants present with severe multisystem disorders. Most metabolic myopathies have intermittent rather than static findings. Some children present with progressive proximal muscle weakness mimicking a dystrophy or an inflammatory myopathy.

In patients with glycolytic or glycogenolytic defects, symptoms are induced by either brief isometric exercise, such as lifting heavy weights, or by less intense but sustained dynamic exercise. In disorders of lipid metabolism, the abnormalities are induced by prolonged exercise and fasting. Investigations include serum creatine kinase and ammonia, urine myoglobulin, electrophysiologic studies, forearm ischemia test and muscle biopsy. Tandem mass spectroscopy, gas chromatography, mass spectrometry and molecular studies help confirm the diagnosis.

### Suggested Reading


1. Berardo A, Di Mauro S, Hirano M. A diagnostic algorithm for metabolic myopathies. Curr Neural neuroscience Rep 2010Mar;10(2):118–26.
2. Lilleker JB, Keh YS, Roncaroli F, et al. Metabolic myopathies: a practical approach. Practical Neurology 2018;18:14–26.

Chapter

21

# Childhood Malignancies

Rachna Seth

Advances in diagnosis, multimodal therapy, rational use of chemotherapy and radiation, increasing availability of hematopoietic stem cell transplantation, emergence of targeted therapy and improved supportive care have improved survival of children with cancer. Over 70% of childhood cancers are considered curable. The clinical features of childhood cancers are often nonspecific and mimic many routine childhood illnesses (Table 21.1). Cancers in children are different compared to adults (**Box 21.1**).

**Box 21.1: Childhood Cancers are Different from Adult Cancers**

- Childhood cancers are less common than cancers in adults.
- Many adult cancers are related to lifestyle risk factors (tobacco use, alcohol consumption,inappropriate diet, sedentary lifestyle), while the causes of most childhood cancers are not known.
- Association with genetic syndromes is reported.
- Most common childhood cancers are leukemias, lymphomas, brain tumors, and bone cancer. Adult cancers are more likely to occur in the lung, colon, breast, prostate, and pancreas.
- Treatment is more likely to be successful in childhood than adult cancers.
- Long-term and late effects are a significant concern.

Common childhood malignancies include leukemia (30–40%), lymphoma (12%), brain tumors (20%), neuroblastoma (7%), and Wilms tumor (7%) (Fig. 21.1). There are regional variations with higher proportion of T cell lineage acute lymphoblastic leukemia (ALL) in India as compared to the West. Brain tumors are less frequent and retinoblastoma more commonly reported in India, compared to developed countries.

## Suggested Reading


1. Arora RS, Bagai P, Bhakta N. Estimated national and state level incidence of childhood and adolescent cancer in India. Indian Pediatrics 2021;58(5):417–23.
2. Sung H, Ferlay J, Siegel RL, et al. Global Cancer Statistics 2020: GLOBOCAN estimates of incidence and mortality worldwide for 36 cancers in 185 countries. CA: Cancer J Clin 2021;71(3):209–49.


**Table 21.1:** Clinical features of cancers mimicking common illnesses

| *Features* | *Possible malignancy* |
|---|---|
| Fever, enlarged lymph nodes, malaise | Leukemia, lymphoma, Ewing sarcoma, neuroblastoma, LCH |
| Pallor, anemia | Leukemia, lymphoma, neuroblastoma |
| Headache, nausea, vomiting, fever associated with seizures | Brain tumors, leukemia |
| Earache, rhinitis, pharyngitis | Soft tissue sarcoma |
| Epistaxis | Leukemia |
| Diarrhea, vomiting, hepatosplenomegaly | Neuroblastoma, lymphoma, hepatic tumors, leukemia |
| Hematuria | Wilms tumor |
| Jaundice | Lymphoma, liver tumors, LCH |
| Failure to thrive | Common to many cancers, LCH |
| Bony pains, bone masses | Any tumors; more often with leukemia, osteosarcoma, LCH |
| Squint, epiphora, red eye | Retinoblastoma |

LCH Langerhans cell histiocytosis

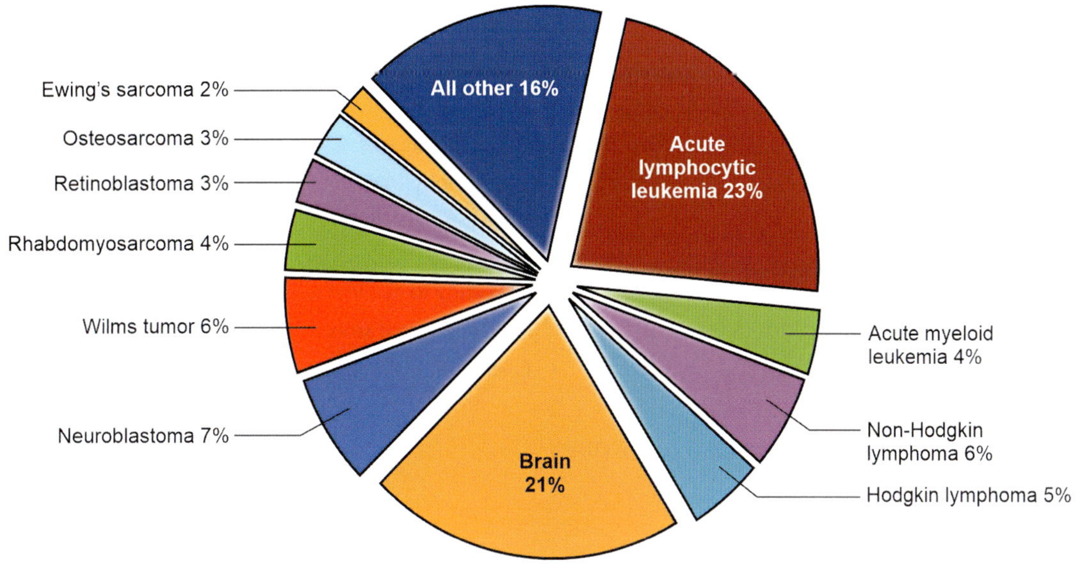


**Fig. 21.1:** Distribution of childhood cancers. One-third of childhood cancers comprise acute lymphocytic leukemia, acute myeloid leukemia, non-Hodgkin lymphoma, and Hodgkin lymphoma. Brain tumors account for approximately 20% of all childhood tumors

*Competencies:* **PE29.8; PE29.11; PE29.12; PE29.13**

## ACUTE LEUKEMIA

Acute leukemias are the most common cancers in children. They arise as a clonal proliferation of abnormal hematopoietic cells, with disruption of normal marrow function and marrow failure. The clinical manifestations of leukemia are the result of the unregulated proliferation of the malignant clone and bone marrow failure. They can be lymphoid or myeloid depending on the lineage of the progenitor stem cell and as acute or chronic depending on their natural history. Among the acute leukemias, ALL (73%) is commoner than AML (18%).

*Acute lymphoblastic leukemia (ALL)* is the commonest childhood malignancy accounting for one-fourth of all childhood cancers and three-fourths of all newly diagnosed patients with acute leukemia. Its incidence is approximately 3–4 cases per 100,000 children below 15 years of age. There is a peak in incidence of childhood ALL between 2 and 5 years. Boys have higher rates than girls, especially in adolescents with T cell ALL.

The cure rates for pediatric ALL have improved significantly approaching 90% in most high income and a few centers in middle and low income countries. This is attributed to advanced molecular and genetic testing techniques, development of effective chemotherapeutic agents, optimization of individual agent dosing and multiagent combination regimens.

*Acute myeloid leukemia (AML)* is the second most common type of leukemia in children, accounts for 15–20% of leukemia and results from clonal proliferation of hematopoietic precursors of myeloid, erythroid and megakaryocytic lineage. AML is much more complex and difficult to treat as only 40–50% patients achieve long-term survival in India. AML can occur at any age, more during adolescence; males are affected as frequently as females.

### Genetic Risk Factors for ALL

The etiology of acute leukemia is unknown in the majority. However, there is a possibility that ALL arises from a combination of susceptible ALL loci and a subsequent somatic mutation in genes involved in normal lymphoid development. With the availability and understanding of genome-wide association studies, several germ line single-nucleotide polymorphisms (SNPs) have been identified to be associated with higher risk of developing ALL . Genes that have been identified to be associated with occurrence of ALL include *ARID5B, IKZF1, CDKN2A, GATA3, CEBPE, ERG,* and *BMI1-PIP4K2A*. Several constitutional chromosomal abnormalities are associated with an increased incidence of childhood leukemia (Table 21.2).

### Classification

#### Acute Lymphoblastic Leukemia

*Morphology:* The classification of ALL has evolved from one that was primarily morphology and cytochemistry based to one that is based on immunophenotyping, karyotyping and molecular biology. Prior to use of immunophenotyping, a system proposed by the French-American-British (FAB) Cooperative Working Group was applied for morphologic classification of ALL (Table 21.3). The single most important utility of morphologic classification is to identify, if Auer rods are present, confirms the myeloid origin of blasts (Figs 21.2 and 21.3).

*Cytochemistry:* Cytochemical stains are useful in patients where the lineage is unclear or highly undifferentiated. Myeloperoxidase is useful for identification of myeloid lineage of blasts. Terminal deoxynucleotidyl transferase (TdT) is a DNA-polymerizing enzyme that is useful for identification of B or T lymphoblastic leukemia in contrast to mature B cell leukemia.

*Immunophenotype:* ALL is broadly divided into two major immunophenotypes—B-lineage and T-lineage (B-ALL and T-ALL), which are characterized by their surface

**Table 21.2:** Genetic and environmental risk factors for childhood leukemia

| *Genetic* | *Environmental* |
|---|---|
| Down syndrome | Ionizing radiation |
| Fanconi anemia, Diamond-Blackfan anemia, Kostmann syndrome | Alkylating agents: Cyclophosphamide, ifosphamide, carboplatin |
| Shwachman-Diamond syndrome | Epipodophyllotoxins: Etoposide, tenoposide |
| Bloom syndrome, Li-Fraumeni syndrome | Nitrosourea: Nitrogen mustard |
| Certain chromosomal abnormalities | Exposure to paint, benzene, pest control treatments, air pollution, proximity to nuclear facilities, low-frequency magnetic fields |
| *PAX5* deficiency caused by constitutional PAX5 p.Gly183Ser | Heavy paternal smoking in periconception period |
| Ataxia telangiectasia | Epstein–Barr virus (EBV) linked to endemic Burkitt lymphoma |
| *ETV6* mutations affecting regulation of DNA binding | |
| Constitutional Robertsonian translocation rob (15;21) (q10;q10)c | |
| Severe combined immune deficiency | |
| Paroxysmal nocturnal hemoglobinuria | |
| Neurofibromatosis type-I | |

**Table 21.3:** French-American-British (FAB) classification of acute lymphoblastic leukemia

| *Cytologic features* | *L1 (80–85%)* | *L2 (15%)* | *L3 (1–2%)* |
|---|---|---|---|
| Cell size | Small cells predominate, homogenous | Large, heterogeneous | Large, homogenous |
| Amount of cytoplasm | Scanty | Variable; often moderately abundant | Moderately abundant |
| Nucleoli | Small, inconspicuous | One or more, often large | One or more, prominent |
| Nuclear chromatin | Homogenous | Variable, heterogeneous | Stippled, homogenous |
| Nuclear shape | Regular, occasional clefts | Irregular clefts, indentation | Regular, oval to round |
| Cytoplasmic basophilia | Variable | Variable | Intensely basophilic |
| Cytoplasmic vacuolation | Variable | Variable | Prominent |

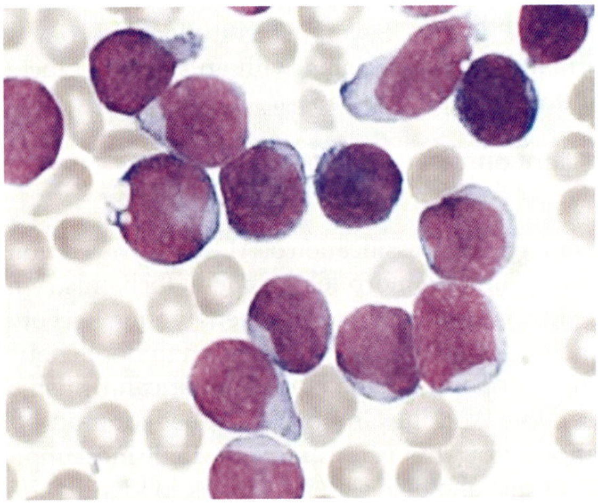

**Fig. 21.2:** Bone marrow from a child with acute lymphoblastic leukemia shows reduced normal marrow elements, which are replaced by lymphoblasts. The neoplastic lymphoblasts are slightly larger than lymphocytes and have round or convoluted nuclei, fine chromatin, often with a smudged appearance, inconspicuous nucleoli and scant, faintly basophilic cytoplasm

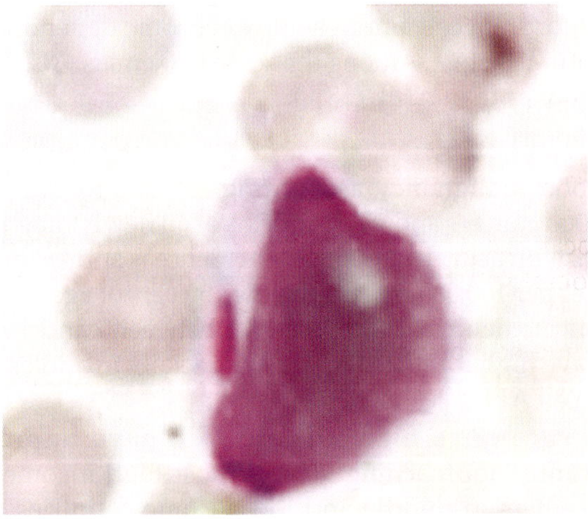

**Fig. 21.3:** Peripheral smear of a 6-year-old child diagnosed with acute myeloid leukemia (AML-M2) showing a myeloblast containing an Auer rod (pink-colored-aggregated lysosome)

markers. B-ALL comprises approximately 85% of ALL, whereas T-ALL makes up the remaining 15%. Several distinct subtypes of ALL have been described by the World Health Organization (WHO). A comprehensive panel of immunophenotypic markers, most commonly performed using flow cytometry, is the most definitive method for distinguishing B- and T-lineage lymphoblasts. The specific immunophenotype determined by these markers is useful in monitoring the minimal disease throughout the course of therapy (Table 21.4).

*Cytogenetics:* Genetic abnormalities in the leukemic clone greatly impact therapy and prognosis. Cytogenetic analysis may be done by karyotype, fluorescent *in situ* hybridization (FISH), newer technologies like array-based analysis

Table 21.4: Immune phenotypelineage markers

| *Lineage* | *Markers* | |
|---|---|---|
| B cells | CD10, CD19, CD20, CD45, kappa, lambda | Presence of CD10 and CD19 represent favorable prognosis Absence of CD10 associated with mixed lineage leukemia (MLL) translocations, particularly t(4;11) and poor outcome |
| Mature B cell ALL | CD19,CD20,CD21, sIg+ | L3 (Burkitt) leukemia; needs intensified therapy |
| T cells | CD2, CD3, CD4, CD5, CD7, CD8, CD45 | Older age, high initial leukocyte count, mediastinal mass, risk of CNS leukemia |
| Myelomonocytic cells | CD11b, CD13, CD14, CD15, CD16, CD33, CD34, CD45, CD117, HLA-DR | |

Table 21.5: Genetic abnormalities in acute lymphoblastic leukemia (ALL)

| *Chromosomal abnormality, translocation, affected gene* | *Subtype* | *Frequency (%)* | *Implication* |
|---|---|---|---|
| Hyperdiploidy (>50 chromosomes) | Pre-B | 20–30 | Excellent prognosis |
| t(12;21)(p13;q22) *ETV6-RUNX1* *TEL AML 1* | Pre-B | 15–25 | Excellent prognosis, needs minimal therapy |
| Trisomy 4 and 10 | Pre-B | 20–25 | Excellent prognosis |
| t(1;19)(q23;p13) *TCF3-PBX1* | Pre-B | 2–6 | High risk, probable CNS relapse |
| t(4;11)(q21;q23) *MLL-AF4* | Pre-B | 1–2 | Infant ALL, poor prognosis |
| High tumor burden, drug resistant | | | |
| t(9;22)(q34;q11.2) *BCR-ABL1* | | | |
| Philadelphia chromosome | Pre-B | 2–4 | Very high risk; improved outcome with imatinib and chemotherapy |
| t(8;14)(q23;q32.3) *MYC IgL* | Mature B cell | 2 | Burkitt leukemia, need intensive therapy, favorable outcome |
| Hypodiploidy (<44 chromosomes) | Pre-B | 1–2 | Unsatisfactory outcome |
| *HOX 11* rearrangement by t(5;14)(q35;q32) | T | 7–8 | Good prognosis |
| Early Tcell precursor | T | 12 | Poor prognosis |

of global gene expression, DNA copy number, SNPs, methylation, and genome-wide sequencing. Chromosomal analysis and banding are essential for the identification of aneuploidy, microscopic chromosomal anomalies, and some translocations. High hyperdiploidy (>50 chromosomes) is associated with favorable outcomes. In contrast, hypodiploidy (<45 chromosomes) has poor outcomes, the commonest being frequently recurring translocations, t(9;22)(q34.1;q11.2) *BCR-ABL1*, *KMT2A* (formerly MLL) rearrangements, t(12;21)(p13.2;q22.1) *ETV6-RUNX1*, t(1;19)(q23; p13.3) *TCF3-PBX1*, and t(5;14)(q31.1;q32.3) *IL3-IGH* (Table 21.5).

### *Acute Myeloid Leukemia*

Risk stratification of AML based on genetic variations. It is useful in planning therapy and prognosticating regarding the disease. The decision to do a hematopoietic stem cell transplantation (HSCT) in pediatric AML are primarily driven by genetic risk classification which is evolving. Favorable-risk genetics such as inv(16), t(8;21), and *CEBPA* and *NPM1* mutations may be cured with chemotherapy alone. In contrast, monosomy 7 and monosomy 5 or 5q deletions are high-risk features which require HSCT in first remission for the best outcomes.The classification is summarized in Tables 21.6 and 21.7.

Table 21.6: Classification of acute myeloid leukemia (AML)

| French-American-British (FAB) classification | |
|---|---|
| Mo | Minimal differentiation |
| M1 | Myeloblastic leukemia without maturation |
| M2 | Myeloblastic leukemia with maturation |
| M3 | Promyelocytic leukemia |
| M4 | Myelomonocytic leukemia |
| M5 | Monocytic leukemia |
| M6 | Erythroleukemia |
| M7 | Megakaryocytic leukemia |

## Clinical Features

The duration of symptoms in a patient with ALL varies from days to weeks and in some cases few months. The clinical features of ALL are attributed to bone marrow infiltration with leukemic cells (bone marrow failure) and extramedullary involvement. Common clinical features include pallor and fatigue, petechiae, purpura or bleeding, and infections. Lymphadenopathy, hepatomegaly and splenomegaly are present in more than 60% (Fig. 21.4). Malignant lymph node enlargement is characterized by being non-tender, firm, rubbery, rapid enlargement, confluent, fixed and at supraclavicular location.

**Table 21.7:** Risk stratification of acute myeloid leukemia by genetics

| *Risk category* | *Genetic abnormality* |
|---|---|
| Favorable | • t(8;21)(q22;q22.1); *RUNX1-RUNX1T1*<br>• inv(16)(p13.1q22) or t(16;16)(p13.1;q22); *CBFB-MYH11*<br>• Mutated NPM1 without *FLT3-ITD* or with *FLT3-ITD*$^{low}$<br>• Biallelic mutated *CEBPA* |
| Intermediate | • Mutated *NPM1* and *FLT3-ITD*$^{high}$<br>• Wild-type *NPM1* without *FLT3-ITD* or with *FLT3-ITD*$^{low}$ (without adverse-risk genetic lesions)<br>• t(9;11)(p21.3;q23.3); *MLLT3-KMT2A*<br>• Cytogenetic abnormalities not classified as favorable or adverse |
| Adverse | • t(6;9)(p23;q34.1); *DEK-NUP214*<br>• t(v;11q23.3); *KMT2A* rearranged<br>• t(9;22)(q34.1;q11.2); *BCR-ABL1*<br>• inv(3)(q21.3q26.2) or t(3;3)(q21.3;q26.2); variations in *GATA2, MECOM;* monosomy 5 or del(5q); monosomy 7; (17p)<br>• Complex karyotype, monosomal karyotype<br>• Wild-type *NPM1* and *FLT3-ITD*$^{high}$<br>• Mutated *RUNX1*<br>• Mutated *ASXL1*<br>• Mutated *TP53* |

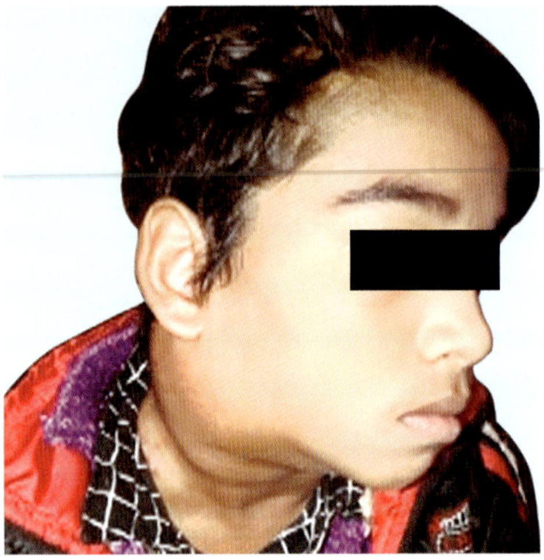

**Fig. 21.4:** An 8-year-old child presented with prolonged fever and generalized lymphadenopathy; was diagnosed with acute lymphoblastic leukemia (ALL)

Bone or joint pain and tenderness may occur due to leukemic involvement of periosteum of bones or joints; skin rash/eruption may occur due to cutaneous involvement. Infants and young children may present with a limp or refusal to walk. Tachypnea and respiratory distress may be present secondary to severe anemia leading to congestive heart failure or to the presence of mediastinal mass leading to tracheal compression (superior mediastinal syndrome). A large mediastinal mass may sometimes cause superior vena cava syndrome with facial edema and plethora, throbbing headache, conjunctiva congestion and dilated neck veins.

Patients with high tumor burden can present with very high total white cell (TLC) count (hyperleukocytosis, TLC >100000/cu mm) or tumor lysis syndrome with reduced urine output and azotemia secondary to uric acid nephropathy.

Involvement of the central nervous system at diagnosis is present in 5–10% cases. These patients present with cranial nerve palsies, seizures and occasionally raised intracranial pressure (headache, vomiting, irritability, papilledema). The diagnosis of CNS leukemia is made in presence of cranial nerve palsies, blasts in cerebrospinal fluid or imaging abnormalities. Overt testicular leukemia is seen in about 1% boys, when it presents with firm, painless, unilateral or bilateral swelling of the testes; the diagnosis is confirmed on biopsy. Rare sites of extramedullary involvement include heart, lungs, kidneys, ovaries, skin, eye or the gastrointestinal tract. Rarely, ALL may present with signs and symptoms of unusual extramedullary site involvement (i.e. ocular, urinary bladder, breast, pancreas) or uncommon endocrinologic manifestations or metabolic derangements.

The clinical features of AML are similar to ALL but more likely to have higher TLC with accompanying symptoms of leukostasis and higher incidence of systemic infections. (**Box 21.2**). Most patients with AML present with pallor, fatigue, bleeding and fever **(Fig. 21.5)**. As compared to ALL, lymphadenopathy and massive hepatosplenomegaly are not very common in AML. However, infants and toddlers with M4 and M5AML subtypes show organomegaly, high leukocyte counts and CNS disease at diagnosis. Gum hypertrophy is a common feature of AML, especially M4

**Box 21.2: Distinguishing Features between ALL and AML**

- AML is likely to have higher leukocyte counts
- Higher incidence of infections at presentation
- Less incidence of lymphadenopathy
- Bleeding tendencies more common with AML
- Gum hypertrophy and splenomegaly common
- Skin deposits, soft tissue mass: Extramedullary myeloid cell tumor (chloromas) common
- Features of hyperleukocytosis (100,000/cu mm) may be present at lower counts
- Central nervous system involvement may occur in up to 15% patients
- DIC is commonly seen in acute promyelocytic leukemia

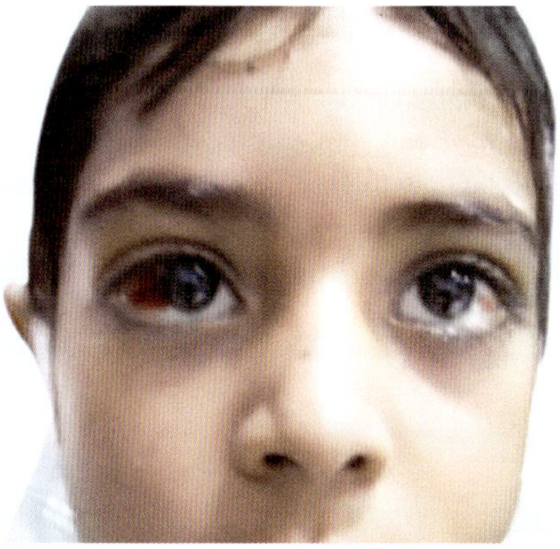

Fig. 21.5: A 6-year-old child with acute myeloid leukemia showing bilateral subconjunctival bleeds

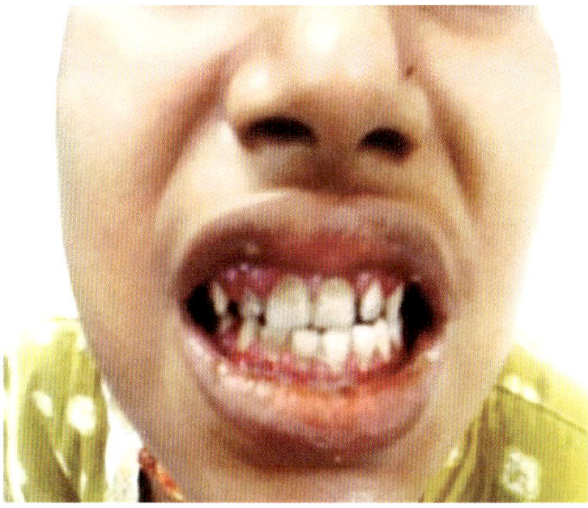

Fig. 21.6: An 8-year-old child with AML showing gum hypertrophy

subtype (Fig. 21.6). Similarly disseminated intravascular coagulation (DIC) may occur in all forms of AML, most commonly in acute promyelocytic leukemia (M3). Myeloid sarcoma (chloromas) is an extramedullary mass of myeloid blasts associated with effacement of normal tissue architecture. It may occur independently of, concomitant with, or subsequent to AML in the bone marrow. Approximately 10% of children with AML have a myeloid sarcoma, most commonly involving the skin and orbit (Fig. 21.7a and b). Patients with high leucocyte counts may present with signs of leukostasis such as pulmonary infiltrates causing respiratory distress or stroke. Central nervous system involvement may occur in up to 15% of patients.

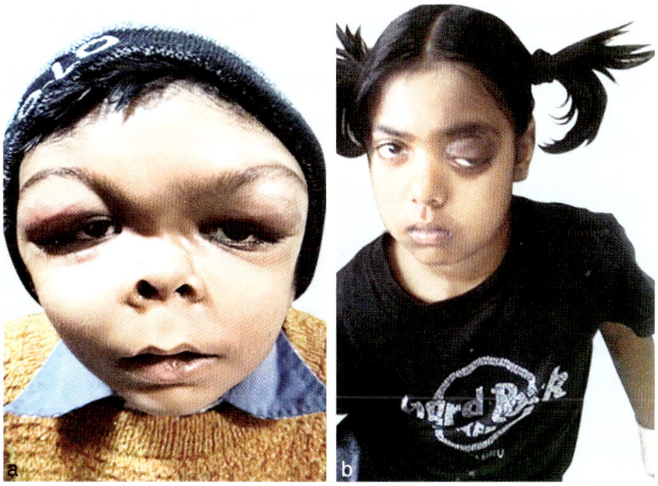

Fig. 21.7a and b: An 8- and a 10-year-old children diagnosed with AML. They presented with proptosis (chloroma orbit)

### Differential Diagnosis

The clinical profile of ALL may mimic other conditions like infectious mononucleosis, acute infectious lymphocytosis, other causes of generalized lymphadenopathy, idiopathic thrombocytopenic purpura, aplastic anemia and viral infections (e.g. cytomegalovirus) that result in leukemoid reactions and pancytopenia. Idiopathic thrombocytopenic purpura is the most common cause of acute onset of petechiae and purpura in children. Ordinarily, children with ITP have no evidence of anemia and have a normal TLC and differential count. Bone marrow smear reveals normal hematopoiesis and normal or increased number of megakaryocytes. A bone marrow examination is recommended prior to initiation of steroid treatment for presumed ITP, in order to exclude leukemia. ALL must be differentiated from aplastic anemia, which may present with pancytopenia. The condition may also be mistaken for juvenile rheumatoid arthritis in patients presenting with fever, joint symptoms (limp, arthralgia or arthritis), pallor, splenomegaly and leukocytosis. ALL should be distinguished from other malignancies (neuroblastoma, non-Hodgkin lymphoma, rhabdomyosarcoma, Ewing sarcoma and retinoblastoma) that present with bone marrow involvement. Occasionally patient with ALL may present with hypereosinophilia or as an emergency with very high leukocyte count, life-threatening infections, hemorrhage, organ dysfunction secondary to leukostasis, or features of superior vena cava/superior mediastinal syndrome.

### Laboratory Features and Diagnosis

Clinical presentation, peripheral blood counts and morphology are often indicative of the diagnosis of ALL. Children may present with pancytopenia or hyperleukocytosis (TLC more than 100000/cu mm). Age less than one year or greater than 10 years and white cell count greater than 50000/cu mm is associated with a poor outcome. The diagnosis is confirmed by peripheral smear examination and or bone marrow aspirate and biopsy. It is necessary to perform an aspirate as well as biopsy at time of initial diagnosis. Very rarely leukemic cells are seen only in the biopsy specimen and not in the aspirate. Higher leukocyte (TLC) counts are more common with T cell ALL. The bone marrow where >25% of bone marrow cells are leukemic blasts is diagnostic for ALL (20% in case of AML). While morphology of the leukemic blasts can give important clues to the diagnosis, it needs to be confirmed by immunophenotyping of the bone marrow (Box 21.3).

Immunophenotype differentiates the cellular lineages of ALL into pre-B, T cell and mature B cell. This distinction is important as there are therapeutic implications of the cellular origin of ALL. ALL patients may broadly be risk stratified into standard and high risk (Table 21.8). Evaluation of a suspected case of leukemia is shown in Table 21.9.

**Box 21.3: Distinguishing Features of Lymphoblast and Myeloblast**

| Cytopathology | Lymphoblast | Myeloblast |
|---|---|---|
| Size | Two to three times size of a lymphocyte diameter | Three to five times the size of a lymphocyte diameter |
| Nucleus | High nuclear/cytoplasmic ratio | Relatively lower nuclear/cytoplasmic ratio |
| Chromatin | Uniform coarse | Uniform fine chromatin |
| Nucleoli | Inconspicuous nucleoli | Twice or more prominent nucleoli |
| Cytoplasm | Scant blue cytoplasm | Moderate gray cytoplasm |
| Auer rods | Auer rods absent | Auer rods usually present |

**Table 21.8:** Risk stratification of ALL

| *Feature* | *Standard risk* | *High risk* |
|---|---|---|
| Age | 2–10 years | <1 year; >10 years |
| Sex | Female | Male |
| Initial leukocyte count | <50000/cu mm | >50000/cu mm |
| CNS leukemia | Absent | Present |
| Phenotype | Pre-B | Mature B cell<br>T cell lineage |
| Ploidy | Hyperdiploidy | Hypodiploidy |
| Cytogenetics | t(12;21), trisomy 4 and 10 | t(9;22), t(4;11),t(8;14) |
| Response to prednisolone (day 8) | Good early response<br>(absolute blast count less than 1000) | Poor early response<br>(absolute blast count greater than 1000) |
| Minimal residual disease after 1st induction | Negative | Positive |

**Table 21.9:** Evaluation of a child with suspected leukemia

| |
|---|
| History and physical examination |
| Complete blood count and differential count |
| Peripheral smear examination (morphology of cells); leukocyte and platelet count; immunophenotype |
| Chest X-ray (include lateral view, if mediastinal mass present) |
| Blood electrolytes, urea, creatinine, uric acid, lactate dehydrogenase, calcium, phosphate, bilirubin, oxaloacetate and pyruvate transaminases<br>Prothrombin time, coagulation profile |
| Bone marrow aspirate: Morphology, immunophenotype, karyotyping, cytogenetics, FISH/PCR for specific translocations<br>Bone marrow biopsy, if dry tap |
| Serology: HIV, hepatitis B surface antigen and antibody, hepatitis C antibody |
| CSF cytology (give first dose of methotrexate with diagnostic tap) |

The diagnosis for AML is also ascertained by peripheral smear and bone marrow examination, with determination of morphologic, cytochemical, immunophenotypic and genetic characteristics of blast cells.

Occasionally, the diagnosis of AML is preceded by a prolonged preleukemic phase lasting several weeks or months. Usually this is characterized by a lack of one of the normal blood cell lineages, resulting in refractory anemia, a moderate neutropenia or thrombocytopenia. The condition is referred to as a myelodysplastic syndrome; some patients show hypoplastic bone marrow that may develop later into acute leukemia.

## Management

The management of acute leukemia needs the combined effort of pediatric oncologist, laboratory oncologist, radiation oncologist, geneticist, nursing team, psychologist, medical social worker and dietician. Improved supportive care and use of combination chemotherapy has led to an overall survival greater than 80% and greater than 95% children in low risk ALL.

Treatment is determined by the risk of relapse in each patient. The *risk-based approach* allows use of modest therapy for children who have historically had very good outcomes, avoiding the adverse effects of high intensity therapy. Children with historically poor survival are treated with high intensity therapy to improve cure rates.

Successful treatment of ALL requires the control of bone marrow or systemic disease, and treatment (or prevention) of extramedullary disease in sanctuary sites, particularly the central nervous system (CNS). The cornerstone of this strategy is systemic combination chemotherapy with CNS prophylaxis.

Therapy for ALL is divided into 4 stages: (i) Induction therapy to attain remission; (ii) CNS prophylaxis or CNS preventive therapy; (iii) Intensification or consolidation phase; and (iv) Maintenance or continuation therapy **(Box 21.4)**. The average duration of treatment in ALL is 24–30 months, with no advantage of extending treatment beyond 3 years.

Patients who relapse or do not respond to treatment have unfavorable outcomes. The treatment options for relapsed ALL depends on time to relapse after remission induction, sites of relapse and presence/absence cytogenetic prognostic markers.

**Box 21.4: Treatment Phases of Acute Lymphoblastic Leukemia**

| Phase of therapy | Objective | Treatment details |
|---|---|---|
| Induction therapy | Eradicate leukemia from the bone marrow at end of induction cycle (<5% leukemic blasts in the bone marrow)<br>Patients who achieve rapid early remission (<5% blasts in marrow) by day 7 or 14 of induction have a better prognosis than slow responders.<br>Failure to achieve this at end of induction is associated with high risk of relapse. | Chemotherapeutic drugs used in induction regimens include vincristine, prednisolone, L-asparaginase and anthracycline. Remission is usually seen in 95–98% of cases by 4–6 weeks |
| CNS preventive therapy | To take care of subclinical CNS involvement at diagnosis (CNS sanctuary site)<br>Early institution of CNS prophylaxis to eradicate blasts that have passed the blood–brain barrier is necessary | High dose systemic chemotherapy (high dose methotrexate, cytarabine). Cranial radiation (CRT) is reserved only for CNS positive cases (CNS leukemia) and in few relapse settings |
| Intensification (consolidation) therapy | Period of intensified treatment soon after induction of remission to tackle the problem of drug resistance | High dose methotrexate, L-asparaginase, epipodophyllotoxin, cyclophosphamide and cytarabine<br>Highly myelotoxic and needs supportive care |
| Maintenance (continuing) therapy | Approximately 2–3 logs of leukemic blasts are killed during the induction therapy, leaving a cell burden in the range of $10^9$–$10^{10}$<br>Additional therapy is necessary to prevent a relapse. Once remission is achieved, maintenance therapy is continued for an additional 2 years. | Most commonly used are 6-mercaptopurine daily and methotrexate once a week.<br>It is important to monitor children for drug toxicity and compliance. |

Compared to ALL, cure rates in AML are hampered by lower remission and increased relapse rates due to resistance to multiple medications, and higher risk of death in remission due to infections and hemorrhage. Intensification of therapy and improved supportive care has resulted in improved long-term survival for AML from <10% to about 50%.

A *risk-based approach* is also used for treatment of AML. Patients with favorable features or normal cytogenetics are treated with chemotherapy alone. Patients with unfavorable genetic alterations undergo stem cell transplantation in the first remission. The induction regimen used commonly is cytosine arabinoside (100 mg/m²/day given as continuous infusion for 7 days) and daunorubicin (45 mg/m²/day for 3 days) with or without additional agents (etoposide). While remission is induced in about 70–80%, most children relapse within 1-year. Consolidation therapy includes high dose chemotherapy with cytosine arabinoside and etoposide. Allogeneic bone marrow transplantation during early remission is associated with a better long-term survival. Since patients with AML are at high risk for myelosuppression following chemotherapy, they require intensive blood component support including platelet transfusions and broad-spectrum antibiotics.

### Infant ALL

Outcome of ALL remains poor in infants, even with intense therapy including hematopoietic stem cell transplant (HSCT). Only 30–40% of children with MLL t(4;11) gene rearrangement are cured. Age and total leukocyte count at presentation are other important determinants. Therapy usually includes high dose cytarabine and methotrexate in addition to standard ALL therapy. Most children require HSCT.

### Philadelphia Chromosome Positive ALL

ALL with t(9;22), known as the Philadelphia chromosome positive ALL, was conventionally considered very high risk due to chemoresistance and need for bone marrow transplantation. It continues to be classified as high risk but long-term therapy with tyrosine kinase inhibitors (imatinib, dasatinib) has significantly improved the 3-yr survival to 80%.

### Down Syndrome and Acute Leukemia

Children with Down syndrome have a 15–20-fold higher risk of acute leukemia, compared to the general population with a cumulative risk of leukemia of approximately 2.1%. One-half to two-third patients with acute leukemia in Down syndrome are ALL, the exception being the first 3 years of life when AML predominates and exhibits a distinctive biology. Blast in these patients have high sensitivity to medications, they require less intense chemotherapy and show better outcomes than AML in those without trisomy 21. Outcome of ALL in trisomy 21 is inferior to those without Down syndrome and ALL.

Approximately 10% children with Down syndrome develop a preleukemic clone, transient myeloproliferative disorder (TMD) with somatic mutations in hematopoietic transcription factor *GATA1*. These children present with high leukocyte count, circulating blasts in peripheral blood, hepatosplenomegaly, effusions, anemia and thrombocytopenia in the neonatal period, which resolves by 3 months. About 20% patients with the transient myeloproliferative disorder develop AML.

***Acute promyelocytic leukemia (APML)*** is a subtype (M3) of acute myeloid leukemia (AML) and constitutes 10–15% patients of AML **(Fig. 21.8a and b)**.

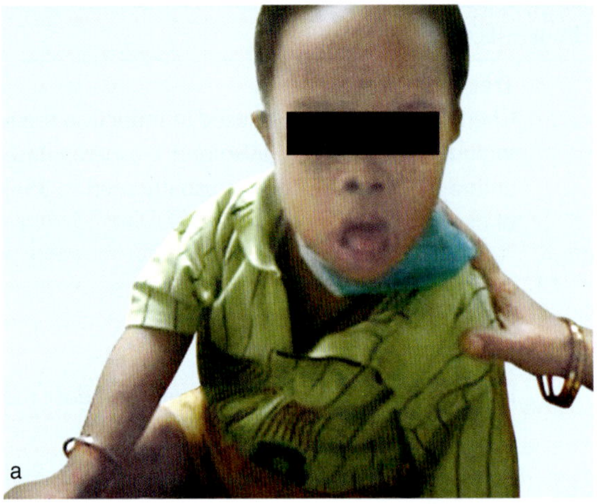

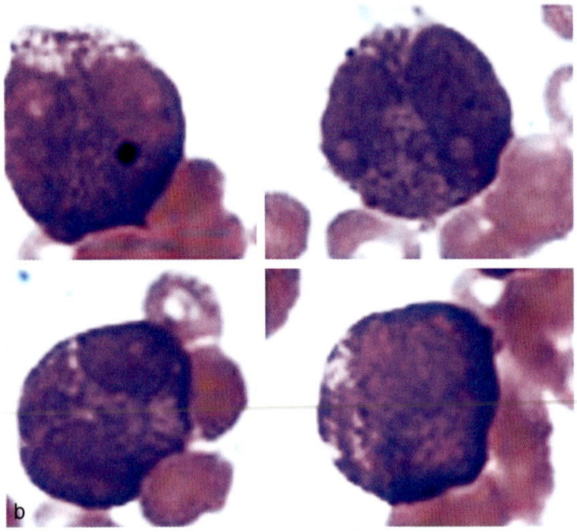

Fig. 21.8: (a) An 18-month-old child with Down syndrome was diagnosed with acute promyelocytic leukemia (APML); (b) Peripheral blood smear showing abnormal promyelocytes

Acute promyelocytic leukemia can be distinguished from other types of AML based on microscopic examination of the blood film or bone marrow aspirate. The presence of promyelocytes containing multiple Auer rods (faggot cells) on the peripheral blood smear is highly suggestive of acute promyelocytic leukemia. Definitive diagnosis requires testing for the *PML/RARA* fusion gene which is present in 95% cases of APML. This may be done by PCR, FISH, or conventional cytogenetics of peripheral blood or bone marrow. The *PML/RARA* fusion gene is sensitive to ATRA. Other rare gene rearrangements described in APML fusing with RARA include *PLZF, NPM1, NUMA1,* and *STAT5B.* Some of these rearrangements are ATRA-sensitive or have unknown sensitivity to ATRA because they are so rare; *STAT5B/RARA* and *PLZF/RARA* are known to be resistant to all *trans* retinoic acid (ATRA). Thrombocytopenia and coagulopathy resulting in minor and/or major bleeds are the commonest life threatening manifestations of APML and important cause of mortality.

APML is unique among leukemia due to its sensitivity to ATRA (tretinoin). ATRA does not directly kill the malignant cells. ATRA induces the terminal differentiation of the leukemic promyelocytes, after which these differentiated malignant cells undergo spontaneous apoptosis. ATRA has been combined with arsenic trioxide for better outcomes. Supportive care in the form of management of bleeding with blood component therapy forms an important component of therapy.

ATRA therapy is sometimes associated with the unique side effect of differentiation, the differentiation syndrome. This is associated with the development of dyspnea, fever, weight gain, peripheral edema and is treated with dexamethasone. The etiology of retinoic acid syndrome has been attributed to capillary leak syndrome from cytokine release from the differentiating promyelocytes. APL differentiation syndrome must be diagnosed promptly and differentiated from sepsis.

### Prognosis

Prognostic markers of ALL include initial leukocyte count, age at diagnosis, sex, CNS disease status, genetic alterations, immunophenotype characterization, extramedullary disease, genetic abnormalities (ploidy, Ph positive status mixed lineage leukemia, *CRLF2, IKZF-1* gene deletion, etc.), response to treatment (day 8 blast count, minimal residual disease at end of induction) and nutritional status. Prognosis in AML is determined by cytogenetics based risk stratification.

### Relapse and Refractory ALL

Despite improving treatment outcomes of pediatric ALL, unfortunately about 15–20% of children will relapse during or after the end of treatment. Relapse most commonly occurs in the bone marrow and followed by CNS and testis (Fig. 21.9). The prognosis for patients who relapse depends on the site, time of relapse, molecular/cytogenetic characteristics and treatment response.

Managing patients with relapse is more resource intense and needs aggressive salvage therapy and supportive care for a favorable outcome. Relapsed ALL children becomes the second most common cancer in children. More than half of these patients require a bone marrow transplant to ensure long-term cure.

### Late Effects of Treatment

Long-term effects of treatment are of concern. Thus, prolonged evaluation of these patients is necessary. Patients who have received cranial irradiation at a young

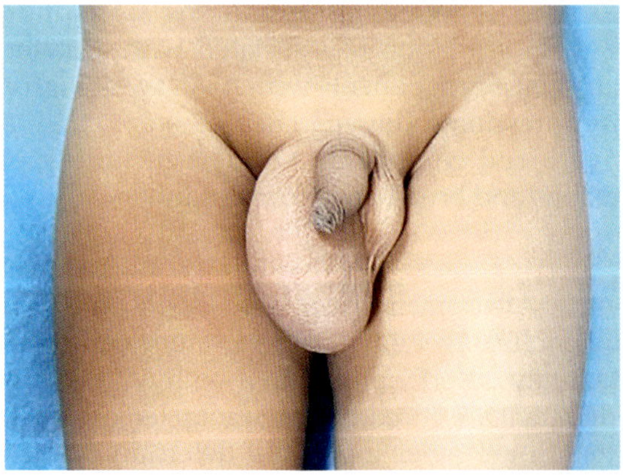

Fig. 21.9: Unilateral testicular enlargement confirmed as testicular relapse on biopsy in a 6-year-old survivor of acute lymphoblastic leukemia

age are at risk for cognitive and intellectual impairment and development of CNS neoplasms. There is a risk of secondary AML after intensive use of epipodophyllotoxins (etoposide, teniposide). Endocrine dysfunction leads to short stature, obesity, precocious puberty, osteoporosis, thyroid dysfunction and growth hormone deficiency. Patients with prior therapy with an anthracycline are at risk of cardiac toxicity.

### Suggested Reading


1. Agarwal M, Seth R, Chatterjee T. Recent advances in molecular diagnosis and prognosis of childhood B cell lineage acute lymphoblastic leukemia (B-ALL). Indian J Hematol Blood Transfus 2021;37(1):10–20.
2. Pui CH, Nichols KE, Yang JJ. Somatic and germline genomics in paediatric acute lymphoblastic leukaemia. Nat Rev Clin Oncol 2019;16:227–40.
3. Swerdlow S. WHO classification of tumours of haematopoietic and lymphoid tissues. 4th edn. 2017. http://publications.iarc.fr/Book-And-Report-Series/Who-Iarc-Classification-Of-Tumours/Who-Classification-Of-Tumours-Of-Haematopoietic-And-Lymphoid-Tissues-2017.


## CHRONIC MYELOID LEUKEMIA

Chronic leukemias are rare in childhood, constituting 3% of leukemias. Chronic myeloid leukemia (CML), the commonest myeloproliferative disorder, is a clonal disorder that originates in a pluripotent hematopoietic stem cell and is characterized by myeloid hyperplasia of the bone marrow, extramedullary hematopoiesis, elevation of white blood cell (WBC) count (with appearance of the complete range of granulocyte precursors in the peripheral blood). CML is consistently associated with the *BCR-ABL1* fusion gene, and is the product of the t(9;22)(q34;q11) reciprocal translocation that results in the Philadelphia (Ph1) chromosome.

The constitutively active *BCR-ABL1* tyrosine kinase, found in t(9;22)(q34;q11) chromosomal translocation-derived leukemia, initiates a comlex signaling transduction cascade that induces a strong state of resistance to chemotherapy. Targeted therapies based on tyrosine kinase inhibitors (TKI), such as imatinib, dasatinib, nilotinib, bosutinib, and ponatinib, have revolutionized the treatment of *BCR-ABL1* associated CML.

Incidence of CML is similar across the world. It is chiefly a disease of adults, with increasing diagnosis with advancing age (fourth and fifth decades). The environmental factor implicated in the etiology of CML is ionizing radiation. Two main forms are recognized.

*Adult CML:* The condition is clinically and hematologically comparable to the adult form of chronic myelogenous leukemia and occurs in children above the age of 4 years **(Fig. 21.10)**.

*Juvenile CML/JMML:* This form presents in infancy and early childhood, usually below the age of 4 years, and has a more rapid course **(Fig. 21.11)**.

### Adult Variety of CML

Though the adult variety of CML is a common leukemia in adults, it is rare in children accounting for 3–5% cases.

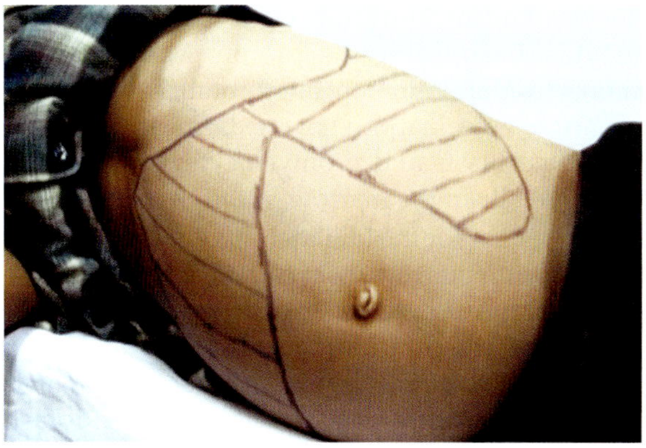

**Fig. 21.10:** A 6-year-old boy presented with fever, anemia, significant splenomegaly and hepatomegaly of 6 months duration. He was diagnosed with chronic myeloid leukemia

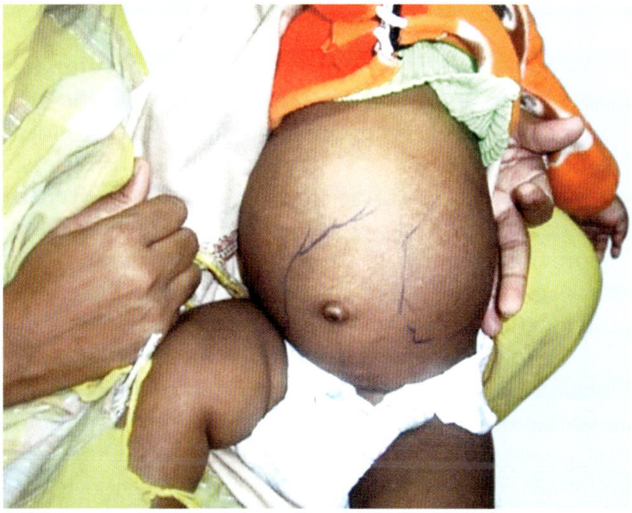

**Fig. 21.11:** A 1-year-old boy presented with fever, rashes, anemia, significant splenomegaly and hepatomegaly. He was diagnosed as JMML

CML patients show a triphasic course: The usual phase at diagnosis (~85% patients) is the *chronic phase*, which may progress to the *accelerated phase* and *blast crisis*. These phases represent the progressive shift in the nature of the disorder from one of hyperproliferation, with production of mainly mature hemic elements, to one characterized by differentiation arrest, with hyperproduction of predominantly immature (blast) cells characterized by reversion to a stem cell phenotype, lack of apoptosis, and therapeutic resistance. The blast crisis may be lymphoid/myeloid.

Children present in the chronic phase with fatigue, malaise, weight loss, excessive sweating, abdominal fullness, and bleeding due to platelet dysfunction; splenomegaly is usually massive. Symptoms of leukostasis such as headache, dizziness and visual disturbances may occur rarely. Symptoms in the accelerated phase or blast crisis include fever, night sweats, rapid weight loss, splenic pain, lymphadenopathy, cutaneous infiltration, bleeding or infection.

Leukocytosis is present in all cases and 80% patients have leukocyte counts >100,000/cu mm. The differential count shows all forms of myeloid cells from promyelocytes,

myelocytes and metamyelocytes to polymorphonuclear leukocytes; basophilia is common. Mild anemia and thrombocytosis are common, but thrombocytopenia is rare. Bone marrow examination shows extreme hypercellularity, with myeloid blasts and promyelocytes constituting less than 20% of cells in the marrow in the chronic phase.

Genetic testing for the Philadelphia (Ph) chromosome in conjunction with marrow morphology allows confirmation of the diagnosis. Cytogenetic analysis of 20 marrow metaphases is the standard method to detect the Ph chromosome, and can diagnose 95% patients. The remaining 5% with strong suspicion can be diagnosed by fluorescence *in situ* hybridization (FISH) analysis, or by reverse transcription polymerase chain reaction. Factors adversely affecting the prognosis are age 50 years or older, increasing spleen size, increased percentage of blasts in the peripheral blood, and eosinophilia, basophilia (3% or more) and thrombocytosis (greater than 1500000/cu mm).

Any deviation from the stable pattern development or new symptoms signals transformation into the acute phase or blast crisis. Features of the acute phase include: (i) Anemia, thrombocytopenia, granulocytopenia, progressive basophilia, rising LAP score, or rapidly increasing granulocytosis or erythroblastosis in a patient whose disease was previously under control; (ii) blasts involving 10% of marrow cells or peripheral blood; (iii) extramedullary blast formation (osteolytic bone lesions, lymphadenopathy); and (iv) large foci or clusters of blasts in bone marrow.

Blast crisis/blast phase is frequently associated with new molecular and cytogenetic abnormalities. *TP53* mutations and *CDKN2A* homozygous deletions are seen. Other genes potentially involved in phenotypic progression include *JUNB, FOS, PRAME, MXF1, EF1δ*, and *WNT/β-catenin*. These changes are seen to promote genomic instability and/or dysregulation of cell-cycle progression. The most commonly identifiable karyotypic alterations are +Ph1, +8, +19, i17q, and, rarely, a reciprocal t(3;21)(q26;q22).

#### *Treatment*

In the pre-imatinib era, stem cell transplant was the only treatment available for cure of CML. The aim of treatment during chronic phase is to control increasing white cell counts. With the advent of first and second-generation oral tyrosine kinase inhibitors (TKI), the treatment of choice is imatinib that targets the constitutively active tyrosine kinase and achieves long-term control of CML in majority of patients. Majority of patients achieve complete hematologic and cytogenetic response with therapy and the rate of progression to accelerated or blast crisis is reduced. The starting dose of imatinib is 340 mg/m$^2$/day. Dasatinib and nilotinib are more potent TKI. Dasatinib is gaining popularity as the median time to confirmed complete cytogenetic response was 3.1 months versus 5.8 months with imatinib.

Bone marrow cytogenetics should be monitored every 6 months until a complete cytogenetic response is obtained. Quantitative RT-PCR for *BCR-ABL* fusion gene is sensitive for assessment of residual disease/relapse. RT-PCR is monitored every 3 to 6 months using marrow or peripheral blood. Based on the PCR levels, dosage may need to be escalated. Survival after development of accelerated phase is usually less than a year and after blast transformation only a few months. Allogeneic stem cell transplantation is now used for patients who do not respond to TKI/ transform to blast crisis and sometimes in accelerated phase.

### Juvenile Chronic Myeloid Leukemia (JCML)

JCML, also termed as juvenile myelomonocytic leukemia (JMML), is an uncommon hematological malignancy accounting for less than 2% leukemias in children. The World Health Organization (WHO) has recently revised the French-American-British classification of myeloid neoplasms to list JMML as a mixed myelodysplastic/myeloproliferative neoplasm. Patients with neurofibromatosis type-1, Noonan syndrome and RASopathy are at high risk for development of JCML. JCML is a disease of infancy and early childhood below the age of 5 years, has more acute and severe course with relatively more frequent lymphadenopathy, anemia, hepatosplenomegaly, skin involvement (eczema, xanthoma and café-au-lait spots), infection and thrombocytopenia. It is important to distinguish JMML from chronic viral infections (especially cytomegalovirus, Epstein-Barr virus and human herpesvirus-6) that can also produce hepatosplenomegaly, lymphadenopathy, leukocytosis, thrombocytopenia, and elevated HbF levels.

Peripheral smear shows leukocytosis (usually less than 1000000/cu mm) with the full spectrum of granulocyte precursors and increased normoblasts; monocytosis is striking. Thrombocytopenia and anemia are common. The leukocyte alkaline phosphatase score is normal or low and fetal hemoglobin levels are elevated. Bone marrow aspirates show increased cellularity with predominance of granulocytic cells in all stages of maturation; megakaryocytes are normal or decreased. Nearly 100% of patients have an identifiable genetic lesion. Philadelphia chromosome is negative; monosomy 7 is found in 30% patients.

JMML has a fulminant and rapidly fatal course. Management involves supportive care including packed red cell and platelet transfusions, treatment of infections and allogenic stem cell transplant if a matched sibling donor is present. Even with transplant, there is 30–50% event-free survival rate at 3 years. *Cis* retinoic acid has been tried with some benefit in JMML. Azacytadine or cytosine-based protocols may be tried as a bridge to chemotherapy.

### Suggested Reading


1. Akihiko Tanizawa. Optimal management for pediatric chronic myeloid leukemia. Pediatr Int 2016;58:171–79.
2. Gupta AK, Meena JP, Chopra A, et al. Juvenile myelomonocytic leukemia—a comprehensive review and recent advances in management. Am J Blood Res 2021;11(1):1–21.


*Competencies:* **PE29.9; PE29.11; PE29.12; PE29.13**

## LYMPHOMA

Lymphomas are the third most common malignancy, comprising 10–15% of newly diagnosed childhood cancers. About 60% are non-Hodgkin lymphoma and 40% are

**Table 21.10:** Clinical features of Hodgkin and non-Hodgkin lymphoma

| *Clinical feature* | *Hodgkin lymphoma* | *Non-Hodgkin lymphoma* |
|---|---|---|
| Nodal spread | Continuous | Discontinuous |
| Localized | Yes | Rare |
| Extranodal disease | Rare | Common |
| CNS disease | Rare | Common |
| Bone marrow | Rare | Common |
| Class B symptoms | Common | Uncommon |
| Abdominal disease | Uncommon | Common |
| Subtype based therapy | Not important | Crucial |
| Cure rates | 85–90% | 70–80% |

Hodgkin lymphoma. Lymphomas are uncommon below the age of 5 years and the incidence increases with age. Both the major lymphoma subtypes are distinct in origin, clinical presentations, biology, treatment approaches and outcome (Table 21.10).

## Hodgkin Lymphoma

Hodgkin lymphoma, a lymphoreticular neoplasm primarily of B cell lineage involving lymph nodes and the lymphatic system, has unique molecular, histologic, immune phenotypic and clinical features. Its incidence ranges from 5–7/100000 population; the condition is uncommon below the age of 5 years and exhibits three distinct forms in developing countries—the childhood form (younger than 14 years), a young adult form (15–44 years) and older adult form (55–74 years). There is a male preponderance in children affected below 7 years of age, with equal sex distribution beyond 12 years of age. The vast majority achieve disease remission with multiagent chemotherapy without radiotherapy. Hodgkin lymphoma is cured in >80% of patients and in >90% with limited stage disease. Therapy is based on risk stratified approach based on disease stage and presence of adverse prognostic factors (B symptoms). The improved cure rates for the disease have increased so extensively that there is an emerging concern relating to long-term toxicity of chemotherapy and radiotherapy.

### *Epidemiology*

The etiology of Hodgkin lymphoma is considered multifactorial with a role for infectious agents, genetic susceptibility, socioeconomic factors and environment and immune dysregulation. Siblings have a 7-fold increase in risk and multiple studies confirm a gender concordance of sibling pairs. A strong evidence of genetic susceptibility further comes from a 100-fold increased risk in monozygotic twins compared with dizygotic twins. Epidemiologic studies have suggested links between Hodgkin lymphoma and viral illnesses like Epstein-Barr virus (EBV). EBV viral DNA can be found in Hodgkin-Reed-Sternberg cells, suggesting monoclonal proliferation of the neoplastic clone following infection. EBV-positive classic Hodgkin lymphoma tumors differ geographically and are more common in developing countries. EBV infection is commonly seen in young children with mixed cellularity disease. Immune deficiency (congenital/acquired) and autoimmune conditions (rheumatoid arthritis, SLE, sarcoidosis, ITP) are associated with increased risk of Hodgkin lymphoma.

### *Pathology*

Lymph nodes are the most common tissue on which the diagnosis of Hodgkin lymphoma is made. However, liver, spleen, bone marrow or lung may provide the material for histological examination. It is necessary to obtain the entire node by excision biopsy for proper examination. Fine needle aspiration biopsy and frozen section material are not optimal for histology.

The WHO classification of Hodgkin lymphoma recognizes two subtypes—nodular lymphocytic predominant Hodgkin lymphoma (NLPHL) and the commoner classical Hodgkin lymphoma (cHL). Both share a common histologic pattern where the neoplastic cells are very large and are relatively few in number. The main tumor mass consists predominantly of non-neoplastic cells. The underlying biology of cHL and NLPHL is distinct. The neoplastic lymphocyte cells have different immunophenotypes, and the appearance of the background tissue is also different. NLPHL subtype is characterized by large cells with multilobed nuclei referred to as popcorn cells. These patients are generally asymptomatic and present with localized non-bulky mediastinal disease. The hallmark of classic Hodgkin lymphoma is the Reed-Sternberg (R-S) cell. This is a binucleated or multinucleated giant cell that is characterized by a bilobed nucleus with two large nucleoli, giving an owl eye appearance to the cells. There are four varieties of this subgroup, characterized by the number of RS cells, characteristics of inflammatory milieu and presence or absence of fibrosis (nodular sclerosing, mixed cellularity, lymphocyte rich and lymphocyte depleted). Nodular sclerosing is the most common type in developed countries, whereas in developing countries including India, the mixed cellularity type is common, accounting for ~60% cases (Table 21.11). On immunophenotyping, the classic subtypes are positive for CD15 (60%) and CD30 (100%) and may be positive for CD20, whereas NLPHL is negative for CD15 and CD30 but positive for CD20 and CD45.

### *Clinical Features*

Children with Hodgkin lymphoma present with painless cervical or supraclavicular lymphadenopathy; the nodes are firm and rubbery in consistency (Fig. 21.12a and b)

Table 21.11: Histological subtypes of Hodgkin lymphoma

| Histology | Frequency | Prognosis |
|---|---|---|
| Nodular lymphocyte predominant | 10% | Excellent |
| Classical Hodgkin lymphoma | | |
| Nodular sclerosis | 20–50% | Very good |
| Mixed cellularity | 20–40%; most common in developing countries and in children | Good |
| Lymphocyte rich | 10–15% | Excellent |
| Lymphocyte depletion | 5–15% | Poor |

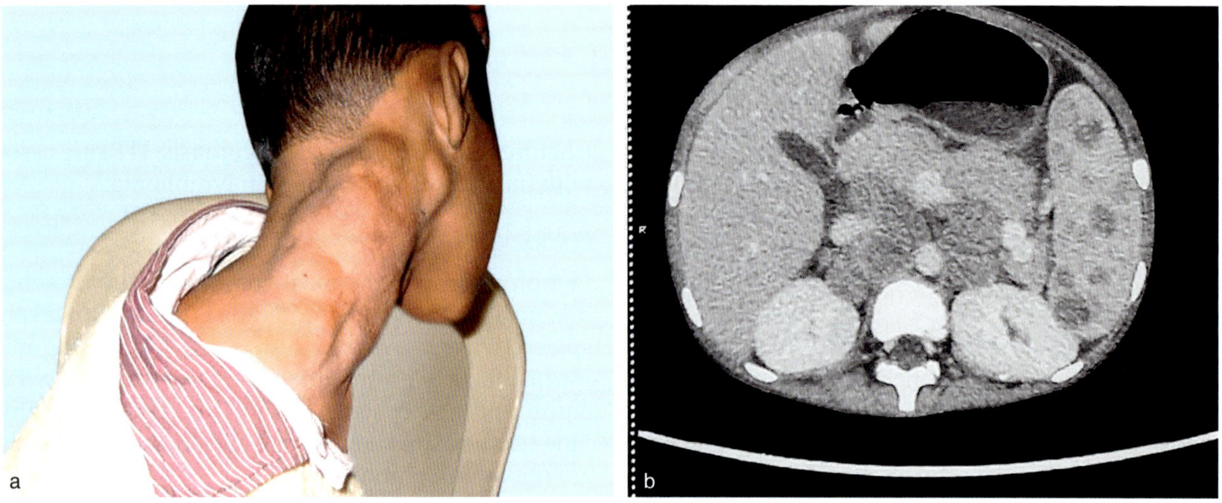

Fig. 21.12: (a) A 10-year-old boy presented with periodic fever and significant bilateral cervical lymphadenopathy. Lymph node biopsy showed features of Hodgkin lymphoma; (b) Multiple hypoechoic lesions in spleen due to lymphomatous involvement

Cervical lymph nodes are the most frequent (80%) site of primary involvement; 50% patients also have mediastinal adenopathy and superior mediastinal syndrome. Less commonly, axillary or inguinal lymphadenopathy is the presenting feature. About 20–30% of children present with systemic (B) symptoms, as defined by the Ann Arbor staging criteria, with fever over 38°C, night sweats and unexplained weight loss of >10% body weight at presentation. The frequency of these symptoms increases with advanced disease and indicate an unfavorable prognosis.

Besides 'B' symptoms, other prognostic factors include stage of disease, histopathogical subtype (risk increases from lymphocyte predominant to nodular sclerosis to mixed cellularity to lymphocyte depletion), bulky mediastinal disease, extensive splenic involvement and more than 5 nodal sites in stage III. Bone involvement by classical HL may cause pain. Bone marrow involvement rarely results in cytopenias and has been associated with a variety of paraneoplastic syndromes that may be the presenting feature of the disease. Splenic involvement occurs in 30–40% patients.

### Diagnostic Workup and Staging

Evaluation includes careful examination with assessment of all lymph node bearing areas and relevant investigations. The diagnostic workup and staging are outlined in Tables 21.12 and 21.13.

### Management

Treatment modalities have varied from total nodal radiation therapy to chemotherapy to combination of chemotherapy and radiotherapy with significant improvement in survival rate throughout the last three decades.

Most children are treated with combination chemotherapy alone or in combination with radiotherapy. Superior efficacy and absence of significant toxicity have made ABVD the preferred front line regimen for Hodgkin lymphoma; however, the concerns of this protocol include cardiomyopathy and pulmonary fibrosis. The

Table 21.12: Diagnostic evaluation for children with Hodgkin lymphoma

- Physical examination with measurement of size and number of lymph nodes
- Complete blood counts, ESR, CRP, liver and kidney functions, alkaline phosphatase, LDH
- Lymph node or involved extranodal site biopsy
- Chest X-ray posteroanterior and lateral views; measure mediastinal mass thoracic cavity ratio
- CT scan of neck, chest and abdomen (may be avoided, if PET CT is available)
- Bone marrow biopsy (all children except stages IA, IIA). Not required in centers with PET-CT facility
- CT scan brain, cerebrospinal fluid examination (if indicated by clinical profile)
- PET-CT is used to detect bone marrow involvement. It also identifies more sites of initial disease than conventional imaging and is more accurate indetecting tumor tissue in post-therapy masses. *Rapid early response* (significant reduction in disease volume and PET negativity within 1–2 chemotherapy cycles) has favorable outcome. PET-CT is advised >3 weeks following completion of chemotherapy, and 8–12 weeks post radiation

**Table 21.13:** Modified Ann Arbor staging for Hodgkin lymphoma

| *Stage* | *Involvement* |
|---|---|
| I | Single lymph node region (I) or one extralymphatic site/ organ (IE) by direct extension |
| II | Two or more lymph node regions on same side of diaphragm (II) or one or more lymph node regions on same side of diaphragm plus local extralymphatic extension (IIE) |
| III | Lymph node regions on both sides of the diaphragm (III) which may be accompanied by local extralymphatic extension (IIIE)<br>• III1 Abdomen disease is limited to the upper abdomen: spleen or its hilar nodes, celiac nodes, porta hepatis nodes<br>• III2 Abdomen disease includes paraortic, mesenteric and iliac nodes, with or without disease in upper abdomen |
| IV | Diffuse involvement of one/more extralymphatic organ/sites with or without associated lymph node involvement |
| A | No B symptoms |
| B | Presence of at least one of the following:<br>• Unexplained weight loss >10% baseline during 6 months before staging<br>• Recurrent unexplained fever >38°C<br>• Recurrent night sweats |
| X | Bulky tumor |

**X** Bulky tumor is either a single mass of tumor tissue exceeding 10 cm in largest diameter, or a mediastinal mass extending one-third of the maximum transverse intrathoracic diameter measured to the inside of the ribs on a standard posteroanterior chest radiograph

**E lesion** Localized extranodal extension of Hodgkin lymphoma from a contiguous/nearby nodal site

dose of radiation therapy ranges between 15 and 25 Gy with modifications based on patient age, response to chemotherapy and presence of bulky/residual tumor. Several studies have demonstrated that chemotherapy alone is effective therapy for pediatric Hodgkin lymphoma. The advantage of this approach is elimination of radiation associated adverse effects like myocardial dysfunction, musculoskeletal growth deficits and second malignancy.

Treatment for patients with favorable clinical presentation (localized node involvement: stage I, II, IIIA; absence of B symptoms; no evidence of bulky disease) consists of 2–4 cycles of chemotherapy (ABVD/others) and low dose involved field radiation. Several studies have reduced the dose of radiation in patients achieving a favorable response to chemotherapy. There is a possible role of chemotherapy alone without radiotherapy in early stage Hodgkin lymphoma. Patients with unfavorable clinical presentation (B symptoms; bulky mediastinal/ peripheral lymphadenopathy; extranodal extension of disease; advanced disease—stage IIIB–IV) are treated with 4–6 cycles of ABVD with/without radiotherapy. Other combinations include OPPA: Vincristine (oncovin), procarbazine, prednisone, and doxorubicin (adriamycin); OEPA: Vincristine (oncovin), etoposide, prednisone, and doxorubicin (adriamycin); and BEACOPP: Bleomycin, etoposide, adriamycin, cyclophosphamide, oncovin, procarbazine, prednisolone. The role of additional radiotherapy in stage III and IV lymphoma remains controversial. While better local tumor control is obtained, adjuvant radiotherapy presents no survival advantage. Hematopoietic stem cell transplantation (HSCT) and immune therapy is offered to patients who relapse or for those who are refractory to primary therapy.

### *Prognostic Factors*

Factors affecting outcome in pediatric Hodgkin lymphoma include pretreatment factors (advanced stage of disease, presence of 'B' symptoms, bulky disease, extranodal extension, male sex and elevated ESR) and treatment related factors such as rapidity of response to initial cycles of chemotherapy based on PET-CT (Table 21.15). Hodgkin lymphoma is one of the most curable cancers of childhood, especially if detected in early stages. Appropriate staging, availability of advanced techniques of investigation and use of risk adapted treatment protocols have resulted in excellent overall survival. The current protocols focus on maintaining high cure rates with minimal chemo- and radiotherapy and minimization of late effects of treatment.

### Suggested Reading

1. Radhakrishnan V, Kapoor G, Arora B, et al. Management of Hodgkins lymphoma: ICMR consensus document. Indian J Pediatr 2017;84:371–81.
2. Swerdlow SH, Campo E, Pileri SA, et al. The 2016 revision of the World Health Organization classification of lymphoid neoplasms. Blood 2016;127:2375–90.

## Non-Hodgkin Lymphoma

Non-Hodgkin lymphoma (NHL) comprises a heterogeneous group of neoplasms of low to high grade tumors of varied histology that arise from malignant proliferation of lymphoid cells (B/T lineage in various stages of maturation) seen in lymph nodes or lymphatic tissue elsewhere in the body. Together with Hodgkin disease, NHL comprises the third most common childhood malignancy. The reported incidence of NHL is 7–10% in West and in India, the incidence varies from 12 to 25%. NHL occurs most commonly in the second decade of life.

### *Epidemiology*

The relative frequency and incidence of NHL show geographic variations. There is male preponderance, with male to female ratio of 3:1 in children less than 15-yr-old. NHL are uncommon before 3 years of age. The four major types of NHL in children include Burkitt (BL) and Burkitt-like lymphoma, lymphoblastic lymphoma(LL), diffuse large B cell lymphoma (DLBCL) and anaplastic large cell lymphoma (ALCL). Age specific trends of incidence of NHL may correlate with histologic subtype. Burkitt and Burkitt-like lymphomas occur in children between 5 and 15 years, while the incidence of lymphoblastic lymphoma and diffuse large B cell lymphoma (DLBCL) is commonly seen in older children and adolescents. Burkitt lymphoma, the commonest subtype, is a highly aggressive tumor and has three subtypes. The endemic type seen in patients in sub-Saharan Africa, typically causes jaw or orbital lesions, is usually associated with EBV infection. The immunodeficiency-associated subtype is associated with HIV infection and is frequently EBV positive and is associated with high CNS involvement. The sporadic subtype, which is the most common form, frequently presents as rapidly expanding abdominal masses.

Scant Indian literature reports an equal distribution of B and T cell tumors. Of B cell, DLBCL was the commonest (22.9%) followed by BL (15.3%) and in T cell, LL was the commonest (31.5%) followed by ALCL in 11.1% cases. Overall, there seemed to be a higher prevalence of DLBCL and LL and lower frequency of BL in India compared to western countries. NHL may follow previous chemotherapy for Hodgkin disease, or be associated with immunodeficiency and DNA repair deficiency syndromes (Wiskott-Aldrich syndrome, X-linked lymphoproliferative disorders and ataxia telangiectasia), acquired immunodeficiency syndrome and organ transplantation (post-transplant lymphoproliferative disease). Infections with malaria and EB virus are considered risk factors for Burkitt lymphoma. With current treatment protocols, ~80% children and adolescents with NHL survive at least 5 years.

### Pathology

The major histological types of NHL are Burkitt/Burkitt-like lymphoma (BL), lymphoblastic lymphoma (LL), diffuse large B cell lymphoma (DLBL) and anaplastic large cell lymphoma (ALCL) (Table 21.14).

### Clinical Features

NHL in children has distinct clinical and behavior properties when compared to adults. Lymphomas in adults are commonly low or intermediate grade and are dominantly nodal, have variable growth fraction with poor long-term outcome. NHL in children is high grade, extranodal with high growth fraction and good outcome. They may have varied clinical presentation. Pyrexia of unknown origin may be the only symptom. Children usually present with extranodal disease involving the mediastinum, abdomen, or head and neck region (Fig. 21.13a). Intrathoracic NHL, most often T cell, may have features of superior mediastinal or superior vena caval syndrome. There may be associated pleural/pericardial effusion (Fig. 21.13b). Cervical adenopathy, abdominal pain, ascites, palpable abdominal mass, intestinal obstruction or intussusception, cranial nerve palsy, bone or jaw swelling, bony pains and cytopenias due to marrow involvement are other features. Sometimes the NHL subtypes may present as oncological

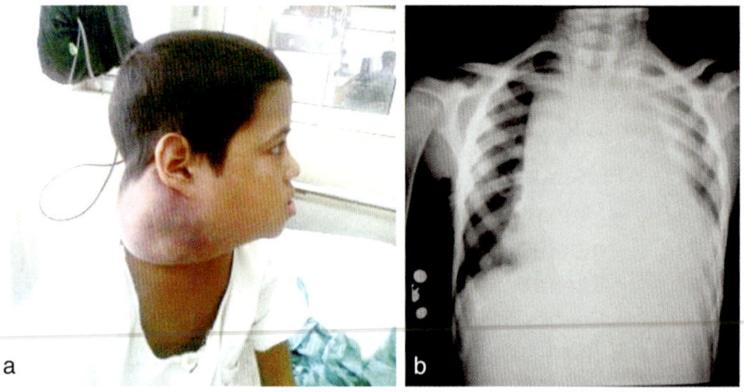


Fig. 21.13: (a) A 10-year-old child with fever, significant right cervical lymphadenopathy: diagnosed as Burkitt lymphoma; (b) Chest X-ray of a 7-yr-old boy with mediastinal mass and shift with left-sided pleural effusion. He was diagnosed as non-Hodgkin lymphoma (T lymphoblastic lymphoma) on lymph node biopsy

Table 21.14: Types of non-Hodgkin lymphoma (NHL)

| *Type* | *Immune type* | *Features* | *Translocation* | *Remarks* |
|---|---|---|---|---|
| **Burkitt, Burkitt-like lymphoma**<br>50% of NHL<br>("starry-sky" appearance on histopathology) | Mature B cell (surface IgG + IgM)<br>PAX5, CD10, 19, 20; kappa and lambda<br>Ki-67 proliferation index is very high | Intra-abdominal, head, neck; jaw (Waldeyer ring)<br>Less common: CNS, testes, marrow | t(8:14)(q24;q32)<br>t(2;8)(p11;q24)<br>t(8;22)(q23;q23) | India: Sporadic form is common and with abdominal presentation<br>Africa: Endemic form common with jaw mass |
| **Diffuse large B cell lymphoma (DLBCL)**<br>10–20% of NHL | Mature B cell (CD19, 20, 22, 38, 79a) | Nodal, abdomen, bone<br>Less common: CNS, marrow, mediastinum | t(8:14)(q24;q32)<br>t(2;17)(p11;q24) | 10–20% of NHL; often localized<br>20% present as primary mediastinal disease; poor prognosis |
| **Lymphomatous lymphoma (LL)**<br>20% of NHL | Immature T cell lymphoma<br>TdT and CD34 are positive | Mediastinal, bone marrow, skin, bone | t(1;14)(p32;q11)<br>t(11;14)(p13;q11)<br>t(11;14)(p15;q11)<br>t(10;14)(q24;q11)<br>t(7;19;)(q35;p13) | Majority (70% ) are T lineage with mediastinal mass >25% blasts: managed as leukemia |
| **Anaplastic large cell lymphoma (ALCL)**<br>10% of NHL | Mature T cell lymphoma<br>CD30; anaplastic lymphoma kinase (ALK, CD246), epithelial membrane antigen (EMA) positive | Lymph node, skin, bones, visceral, soft tissues | t(2;5)(p23;q35)<br>t(1;2)(q21;23)<br>t(2;3)(p23;q21)<br>t(2;17)(p23;q23)<br>t(X;2)(q11-12;p23)<br>Inv 2(p23;q35) | Varied presentation; extranodal involvement<br>Systemic symptoms present<br>Prolonged waxing/waning course<br>Diagnosis delayed and difficult |

emergencies like mediastinal mass causing superior mediastinal/vena caval syndrome, acute kidney injury due to tumor lysis syndrome, acute onset paraparesis, etc.

### Diagnosis

NHL are rapidly growing tumors and require prompt diagnosis; two-thirds have widespread disease at diagnosis, involving bone marrow, central nervous system or both. Selection of the appropriate lymph node or mass for histological diagnosis is necessary. Histology is supplemented, where possible, with immunophenotypic and cytogenetic studies. If the clinical condition is not suitable for biopsy, due to a large mediastinal mass causing superior vena cava syndrome, the diagnosis may be made with less invasive procedures including percutaneous needle aspiration, examination of body fluids (e.g. pleural fluid) or bone marrow. The St. Jude staging system and workup for non-Hodgkin lymphoma are described in Tables 21.15 and 21.16.

### Management

Improvement in survival has been possible due to use of highly effective chemotherapy and strong supportive care. Surgery has very limited role in treatment, other than for diagnosis or during emergencies like compressive myelopathy. Radiotherapy is restricted to emergencies, e.g spinal cord compression due to paraspinal disease.

*Emergency management:* Life-threatening complications in NHL include:

- Superior vena cava obstruction and esophageal compression from mediastinal masses with lymphoblastic lymphoma
- Airway obstruction from pharyngeal or intrathoracic mass
- Tumor lysis syndrome seen with lymphoblastic lymphoma and Burkitt lymphoma
- Respiratory/cardiac compromise due to massive pleural/pericardial fluid
- Paraplegia from epidural tumor or raised intracranial pressure, and neurological deficit from intracranial lymphoma or CNS involvement
- Obstructive jaundice and pancreatitis from compression of bile or pancreatic ducts
- Gastrointestinal bleeding, obstruction, intussusception and rarely perforation

These complications need to be recognized early and treated appropriately. Patients with superior mediastinal or vena caval syndrome require therapy with high dose IV dexamethasone. Tumor lysis syndrome must be anticipated and prevented by ensuring hydration, and use of rasburicase or allopurinol; those with acute kidney injury or metabolic aberrations require hemodialysis.

The cornerstone for treatment of pediatric NHL is multiagent chemotherapy. Different chemotherapeutic regimens are used for treatment of B and T cell lymphomas. The chemotherapy protocol varies based on the sub-type of NHL and stage of disease at diagnosis. Lymphoblastic lymphoma is treated on leukemia-like protocols which are based on the principle of continual exposure to cytostatics over a long period of time, in comparison to protocols used for mature-NHL.

Therapy for mature B cell (Burkitt, non-Burkitt, DLBCL) lymphomas is different. Most protocols consist of short duration (6 months) intensive alkylating high dose methotrexate, vincristine, anthracyclines, etoposide and cytarabine. The principle used is a pulse-intensive short-duration multi-agent chemotherapy given in courses of 3–5 d with a schedule characterized by fractionation or continuous infusion of alkylators and antimetabolites. CNS prophylaxis is provided with intrathecal chemotherapy. The use of anti-CD20 monoclonal antibodies (rituximab) directed against B cell antigens has been combined with standard chemotherapy to improve survival. Long-term survival is highly satisfactory with survival in more than 90% patients with limited disease and 75–85% in patients with extensive disease.

**Table 21.15:** St Jude staging system for childhood non-Hodgkin lymphoma

| Stage | Description |
|---|---|
| **Low risk (localized)** | |
| I | Single tumor (extranodal), single anatomic area (nodal) excluding mediastinum or abdomen |
| II | • Single tumor (extranodal) with regional node involvement<br>• Primary gastrointestinal tumor (completely resected with or without involvement of mesenteric nodes)<br>• Two/more tumors/nodal areas on one side of the diaphragm |
| **High risk (advanced)** | |
| III | • All primary intrathoracic (mediastinal, pleural and thymic) tumors<br>• All extensive primary intra-abdominal disease<br>• All paraspinal or epidural tumors regardless of other tumor sites<br>• Two/more nodal or extranodal areas on both sides of diaphragm |
| IV | Any of the above with CNS and or bone marrow involvement |

**Table 21.16:** Evaluation of a patient with non-Hodgkin lymphoma

- History and physical examination
- Complete blood count and peripheral smear examination
- Liver and renal function tests, electrolytes, LDH, uric acid
- Biopsy for histology; cytochemical, immunologic, cytogenetics and molecular studies
- Pleural, pericardial or peritoneal fluid: Cytomorphology, immunophenotype characterization
- Bone marrow aspiration and biopsy: Cytomorphology and immunophenotype characterization
- Chest radiograph (include lateral view, if mediastinal widening)
- Ultrasonography chest and/or abdomen
- CT scan/MRI of neck, chest and abdomen
- Positron emission tomography-CT (optional)
- Echocardiography

## Suggested Reading


1. Ehrhardt MJ, Hochberg J, Bjornard KL, et al. Long-term survivors of childhood, adolescent and young adult non-Hodgkin lymphoma. Br J Haematol 2019;185:1099–1110.
2. Thacker N, Bakhshi S, Chinnaswamy G, et al. Management of Non-Hodgkin lymphoma: ICMR Consensus Document. Indian J Pediatr 2017;84(5):382–92.

## RETINOBLASTOMA

### Epidemiology

Retinoblastoma is the most common primary intraocular tumor of infancy and childhood with an incidence of 1 in every 20,000 live births. About 90% cases are diagnosed by the age 3–4 years and 98% by 5 years. One-third patients have bilateral disease, which is often multifocal and diagnosed at a younger age. Burden of the disease is more in developing countries, especially Latin America, Africa and Asia including India. The tumor is highly sensitive to chemotherapy and survival rates in developed countries are greater than 90%. There is disparity in mortality in developing and developed countries; 40–70% children with retinoblastoma in the former die compared to 3–5% in the former, which is attributed chiefly to late diagnosis and advanced disease at presentation.



### Genetics

The retinoblastoma gene (*RB1*), encoded on chromosome 13q14, was the first described tumor suppressor gene. Loss of one *RB1* allele predisposes to cancer, while loss of the second allele, in developing retinal cells, leads to retinoblastoma.

Retinoblastoma can be sporadic or inherited. Sporadic tumors are unilateral, unifocal and occur at an older age, while inherited tumors occur earlier usually before two years of age and are often bilateral and multifocal. The "two hit" model of oncogenesis proposes that two mutational events are required for development of retinoblastoma, the first hit being an inherited mutation in *RB1* and the second is acquired in the somatic retinal cell. In sporadic retinoblastoma, both mutations occur in the somatic retinal cell. Most cases of hereditary retinoblastoma have a spontaneous new germline mutation while their parents have wild type *RB1* alleles. The risk of an offspring inheriting an *RB1* mutation from a parent with germline mutation is 50%; 97% with the inherited mutation is at risk of retinoblastoma. Germline mutations of *RB1* also cause an increased risk of a second malignancy of the lung, soft tissue, bladder, skin, bone and brain; the risk is higher when these patients receive radiation therapy for retinoblastoma. A small proportion (5–10%) of unilateral tumors is hereditary **(Box 21.5)**.

### Clinical Features

Retinoblastoma is an intraocular disease in the initial stages wherein it confines within the globe which, if untreated, most often progresses to extraocular form of the disease. The tumor arises from retina and grows towards the vitreous. Its progression results in involvement of ocular coats and optic nerve leading to scleral, orbit and central nervous system involvement. Hematogenous dissemination may lead to distant metastasis. Leukocoria (white pupillary reflex) is the most common presentation **(Fig. 21.14a)**. Strabismus, poor visual tracking and glaucoma are other presenting features **(Fig. 21.14b)**. Orbital inflammation, hyphema and irregular pupil, phthisis bulbi and a fungating ocular mass suggest advanced disease **(Fig. 21.14c)**. Pain may be present secondary to glaucoma. In developing countries, retinoblastoma presents late in its extraocular stage, either with an orbital mass (proptosis) or with distant metastasis to the bones, bone marrow, lymph nodes and central nervous system. Differential diagnosis include Coats' disease, persistent fetal vasculature, toxocariasis, cellulitis, metastasis, cataract, retinopathy of prematurity and retinal detachment.

**Box 21.5: Hereditary and Non-Hereditary Retinoblastoma**

Hereditary: One-third *RB1* gene mutation is present in all cells of body including gonads

- Altered *RB1* gene may be inherited from one parent, or be the result of a new mutation that occurred in an egg or sperm cell or just after fertilization.
- Mutation in *RB1* is inherited in AD pattern
- Increased risk of passing on the mutated *RB1* gene to the next generation, if family history of retinoblastoma is present

→ **Multifocal, bilateral tumors**

Non-hereditary: Two-thirds *RB1* gene mutation is present only in cells of eye

- Typically only one eye is affected and there is no family history of the disease
- Affected individuals are born with two normal copies of the *RB1* gene
- People with non-hereditary retinoblastoma are not at risk of passing these *RB1* gene mutations to their children

→ **Unifocal, unilateral tumors**

In hereditary retinoblastoma, a mutation involving the other copy of the *RB1* gene must occur in retinal cells during the person's lifetime. This second mutation usually occurs in childhood, typically leading to the development of retinoblastoma in both eyes.
In non-hereditary form, retinoblastoma develops in early childhood as a result of acquired mutation in both copies of the *RB1* gene.

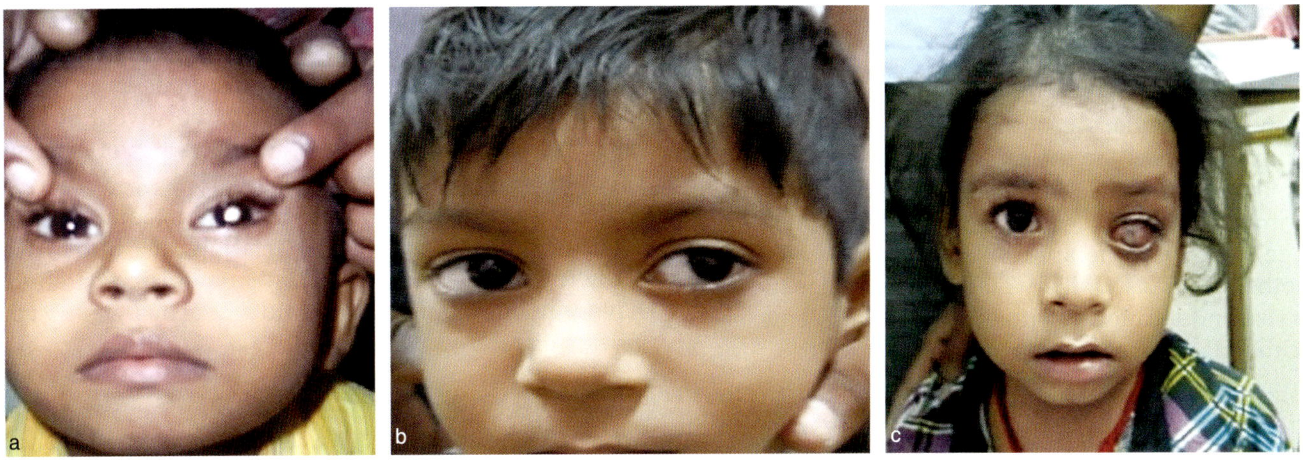


**Fig. 21.14:** Presenting features of retinoblastoma: (a) 3-yr-old with leukocoria; (b) 4-yr-old with squint; (c) 3-yr-old with phthisis bulbi



## Diagnosis

The diagnosis is based on history, clinical examination and imaging. Ocular examination of both eyes should be done under anesthesia. Imaging studies such as ultrasound and contrast enhanced MRI scans are used to assess the orbital, optic nerve and for intracranial extension. Rarely children with hereditary retinoblastoma show a pineal tumor (trilateral retinoblastoma) that is detected on imaging. CSF and bone marrow examination are done, only if indicated on clinical examination or imaging. Biopsy or aspiration cytology is not routinely required unless the diagnosis is in doubt. Occasionally, an adjacent lymph node needs to be aspirated for metastasis. Screening for *RB1* mutations on peripheral blood or tumor tissue, helps differentiate somatic from germline mutations.

## Staging

Retinoblastoma may be intraocular or extraocular. Intraocular retinoblastoma denotes that the disease is limited to the eye, and is confined to the retina or extends to the choroid, ciliary body, anterior chamber and optic nerve head (Tables 21.17 and 21.18). The term extraocular retinoblastoma refers to extension of the illness beyond the eye, including tissues around the eye (orbital retinoblastoma) or spread to the central nervous system, bone marrow or lymph nodes (metastatic retinoblastoma). The International Classification of Intraocular Retinoblastoma has developed a grouping system for intraocular disease with Groups A-E of increasing severity which helps to assess the vision prognosis uniformly and plan treatment.

There is a staging system for extraocular disease which prognosticates survival. The aim in the treatment of retinoblastoma is first to improve survival, then salvage globe, finally vision.

**Table 21.17:** International classification of intraocular retinoblastoma

| | |
|---|---|
| **Group A**<br>Very low risk | No tumor greater than 3 mm in dimension; away from fovea and optic nerve |
| **Group B**<br>Low risk | Any eye with tumor not in group A with no vitreous seeding, subretinal fluid <5 mm from base of tumor |
| **Group C**<br>Moderate risk, focal seeds | Tumors with focal fine vitreous seeding or subretinal fluid (<1 quadrant) |
| **Group D**<br>High risk | Massive/diffuse vitreous seeding, extensive subretinal masses |
| **Group E**<br>Very high risk, extensive retinoblastoma | • **Unsalvageable eyes**<br>• Tumor involving >50% globe, touching the lens, involves anterior segment<br>• Diffuse infiltrating retinoblastoma, neovascular glaucoma<br>• Opaque media from hemorrhage<br>• Tumor necrosis, aseptic orbital cellulitis, phthisis bulbi |

**Table 21.18:** International Retinoblastoma Staging System (IRSS)

| *Stage* | *Description* | |
|---|---|---|
| Stage 0 | Eye has not been enucleated and no dissemination of disease<br>Conservative treatment | |
| Stage I | Eye enucleated, completely resected histologically | |
| Stage II | Eye enucleated, microscopic residual tumor in form of<br>i. Tumor invasion into extrascleral space<br>ii. Tumor invasion into cut end of optic nerve | |
| Stage III | Regional extension | a. Overt orbital disease<br>b. Preauricular or cervical lymph node extension |
| Stage IV | Metastatic disease | a. Hematogenous metastasis (without CNS involvement): single or multiple lesions<br>b. CNS extension (with or without regional or metastatic disease) |

## Treatment

The aim of treatment is survival with eradication of disease; maintenance of vision and preservation of globe and vision are secondary goals. Treatment depends on size, location, extent of the tumor and whether it is hereditary or sporadic. Retinoblastoma is curable when the disease is intraocular. The various treatment modalities for RB range from focal therapies like laser photocoagulation, cryotherapy, transpupillary thermotherapy depending on the size and location of intraocular tumor to enucleation in Group E disease.

*Laser therapy:* Argon or diode laser is the primary treatment for smaller tumors, but is also sometimes used after chemoreduction.

*Cryotherapy:* A special probe applied through the sclera to produce low temperatures (–60 to –80°C) is suitable for tumors smaller than 4 disc diameters close to the retina.

*Chemotherapy:* Chemotherapy enables salvaging the affected eye, avoiding enucleation or external beam radiotherapy and risk of second malignancies. Systemic chemotherapy most often comprises a combination of vincristine, carboplatin and etoposide. Chemotherapy may also be used for chemoreduction, as an adjunct modality or for therapy of metastasis. Newer routes of drug (melphalan, carboplatin) administration by periocular, intravitreal and intraophthalmic artery injection have improved outcomes in intraocular retinoblastoma. Newer agents include topotecan, 2-deoxy-D-glucose, bevacizumab.

*Enucleation:* In cases of unilateral disease with large tumors where no useful vision can be preserved, enucleation is performed early. Survival from metastatic disease is poor. In children with bilateral disease, systemic chemotherapy is used initially, followed by local treatment with laser photocoagulation or cryotherapy in order to preserve vision. The eye with the no useful vision should be enucleated in these cases.

*Radiotherapy:* External beam radiotherapy (RT) should be considered only if chemotherapy and focal therapy fail. RT leads to orbital deformity, sicca syndrome, cataracts, radiation retinopathy, neovascular glaucoma and risk of second malignancy. Brachytherapy and episcleral plaque RT have less side effects.

*Hematopoietic stem cell transplantation (HSCT):* Patients with extraocular disease have poor prognosis with respect to survival. Those with regional extraocular disease (involving orbit, optic nerve or preauricular region) may be treated with a combination of conventional chemotherapy and external beam RT. Patients with distant metastasis require high dose chemotherapy, external beam RT and HSCT.

Newer and popular modalities in the treatment of RB, especially for eyes with diffuse vitreous seeds and aiming at vision and globe salvage include intra-arterial chemotherapy and intravitreal chemotherapy.

## Prognosis

Most tumors that are confined to the eye are cured. Focal therapy or enucleation is curative in more than 95% of patients with unilateral disease. Cures are infrequent when extensive orbital or optic nerve extension has occurred or the patient has distant metastasis. Patients with CNS metastasis have high mortality. With the advent of HSCT and aggressive chemotherapy, the outcomes of extensive diseases are showing improvement.

Genetic counseling is an important component of management. All first degree relatives of children with known or suspected hereditary retinoblastoma should have regular examination for evidence of malignancy until 7 years of age.

## Suggested Reading

1. Chawla B, Seth R, Moksha L. Chemotherapy for ocular cancers. In: Velpandian T. Pharmacology of Ocular Therapeutics. Adis Springer, 2016:333–58.
2. Chawla B, Hasan F, Azad R, et al. Clinical presentation and survival of retinoblastoma in Indian children. British J Ophthal 2016;100:172–78.

*Competency:* **PE21.7**

# WILMS TUMOR

Renal tumors constitute 7% of all childhood malignancies. They include the commonest nephroblastoma [Wilms tumor or WT (6%)], clear cell sarcoma of the kidney (CCSK), malignant rhabdoid tumor (MRT), renal cell carcinoma (RCC), and congenital mesoblastic nephroma (CMN). The peak incidence of WT is 2–3 years. Individuals with horseshoe kidney have a higher risk of Wilms tumor. Identification of clinical and biologic prognostic features and a risk stratified approach to multimodal treatment of WT has improved outcomes.

## Genetics

While a vast majority of Wilms tumors are sporadic, 1–2% may be familial. Familial tumors occur at an earlier age and have a high propensity for being bilateral. The tumor is thought to develop in the foci of embryonal kidney tissue called nephrogenic rests. *WT1* is the best characterized Wilms tumor gene, with mutations of this gene observed in approximately 20% of Wilms tumors, occasionally in association with mutations in *CTNNB1* (catenin beta 1; 3p22.1) and *WTX* (gene on the X-chromosome). Most cases do not have mutations in any of these genes.

The *WT1* gene is located on chromosome 11p13 and encodes for a transcription factor that is critical for normal development of kidneys and gonads. *WT2* is localized to a cluster of genes at 11p15. Patients with *WT1* mutations have a higher risk of recurrence and bilateral disease. Children with some genetic syndromes are predisposed to Wilms tumor. These include WAGR (Wilms tumor, aniridia, genitourinary abnormalities and mental retardation, del11p13), Denys-Drash syndrome (renal failure, mesangial sclerosis, male hermaphroditism, *WT1* missense mutation) Frasier, Li–Fraumeni, Bloom, and Beckwith-Wiedemann syndromes (hemihypertrophy, macroglossia, omphalocele, organomegaly, del11p15.5; *WT2*). Loss of heterozygosity of 1p and/or 16q and high expression of telomerase are associated with poorer outcome in children with Wilms tumor.

### Pathology

The histologic subtype varies with age at presentation. For children less than 3 months of age, CMN is the most common histologic diagnosis. MRT is commonly seen in infants, CCSK is rare after age 4, and by adolescence, RCC surpasses WT as the most common renal malignancy.

The histopathology of WT may be favorable (differentiated blastemal, stromal and epithelial cells) or unfavorable types (diffuse or focal anaplasia, clear cell sarcoma, rhabdoid tumor). Most tumors are unicentric; 11% are multicentric.

### Diagnosis

Most patients present with an asymptomatic abdominal mass detected by their parents or physician during routine examination. Other features at diagnosis include hematuria (10–25%), hypertension (25%), abdominal pain (30%), fever (20%), anorexia and vomiting. Wilms tumor should be considered in any child with abdominal mass (Fig. 21.15). Tumor thrombus extending into the inferior vena cava is found in 4–10%. Other features at presentation include anemia, thrombocytosis, acquired deficiency of von Willebrand factor and factor VII, and polycythemia. The differential diagnosis includes neuroblastoma and other flank masses, including hydronephrosis, multicystic kidney, and rarely abdominal lymphoma and retroperitoneal rhabdomyosarcoma. Features of associated syndromes may be present in 10–20%. Evaluation and staging of Wilms tumor are discussed in Tables 21.19 and 21.20.

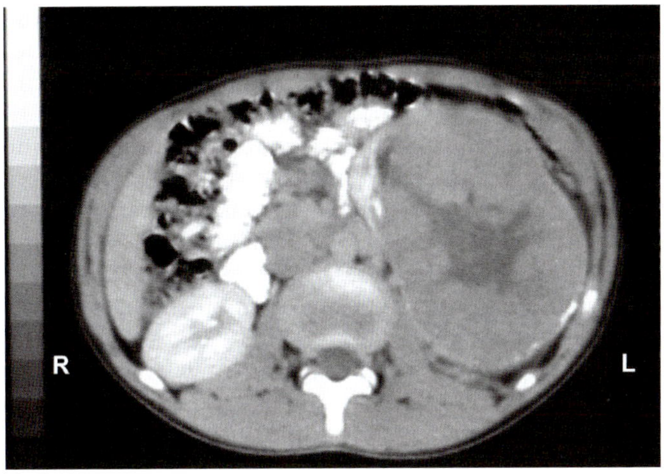


**Fig. 21.15:** 6-yr-old with hematuria and abdominal mass. CT abdomen suggestive of Wilms tumor

### Treatment

The approach to treatment differs across the world. While the Children's Oncology Group (US) recommends upfront resection of the tumor, the International Society of Pediatric Oncology (SIOP) recommends preoperative chemotherapy without biopsy. The outcome with both approaches is similar. Upfront surgery provides accurate diagnosis prior to starting chemotherapy while preoperative chemotherapy shrinks the tumors, making surgery easier and decreasing the risk of spillage and rupture. Radiation has limited role in the management.

Patients less than 2-year-old with tumors weighing less than 550 g with favorable histology are at low risk and

**Table 21.19:** Evaluation of Wilms tumor

| *Investigation* | *Purpose* |
|---|---|
| Abdominal ultrasound | Organ of origin, identify contralateral kidney<br>Location of tumor thrombus in vena cava |
| CT scan | Localization of tumor and extent of spread |
| Chest X-ray | Pulmonary metastasis |
| Bone scan, skeletal survey | Bone metastasis, especially in clear cell sarcoma |
| Brain imaging (MRI, CT scan) | Brain metastasis in rhabdoid tumor and clear cell sarcoma |
| Fine needle aspiration cytology | Cytological confirmation of tumor prior to chemotherapy |

**Table 21.20:** Staging for Wilms Tumor (National Wilms Tumor Study Group)

| | |
|---|---|
| Stage I | Tumor confined to the kidney and completely resected<br>Renal capsule and sinus vessels not involved beyond 2 mm<br>Regional lymph nodes dissected and negative |
| Stage II | Tumor extends beyond the kidney but is completely resected with negative margins and lymph nodes<br>At least one of the following has occurred: (i) Penetration of renal capsules, (ii) invasion of renal sinus vessels |
| Stage III | • Residual tumor abdomen following surgery confined to abdomen<br>• Lymph nodes (renal hilum, para-aortic chain, beyond) show tumor<br>• Diffuse peritoneal contamination by tumor<br>• Implants on peritoneal surface<br>• Tumor extends beyond surgical margins (microscopy, gross examination)<br>• Tumor not completely resected because of infiltration of vital structures |
| Stage IV | Hematogenous metastasis, metastasis to distant lymph nodes |
| Stage V | Bilateral renal involvement at time of initial diagnosis |

may be treated with nephrectomy alone followed by close observation. Chemotherapy for stage I or II patients includes vincristine and actinomycin for 18 weeks. Doxorubicin and abdominal radiation are additional therapies for stage III illness. Cyclophosphamide, carboplatin and etoposide are used for anaplasia and metastatic disease. Pulmonary radiation is used for pulmonary metastasis. Patients with bilateral Wilms tumor should undergo nephron sparing surgery, when feasible. Wilms tumor is a very radiosensitive tumor. The discovery of effective chemotherapeutic agents and their incorporation into multimodality regimens has profoundly impacted the management of RT. Newer drugs that have been used in management include: Topotecan, irinotecan, ixabepilone, cixutumumab, sorafenib, Aurora A kinase inhibitor.

Overall, approximately 90% of children with Wilms tumor are long-term survivors. Young age, lower stage and low weight (<550 g) are favorable prognostic factors. Presence of anaplasia and loss of heterozygosity of 1p or 16q increase the risk of recurrence. Survivors of Wilms tumor have relatively few late effects. However, cardiotoxicity, renal failure, fertility concerns, second malignancy and pulmonary toxicity are reported in survivors of advanced stage disease who receive intensive chemotherapy and radiation.

### Suggested Reading

1. Geller E, Kochan PS. Renal neoplasms of childhood. Radiol Clin N Am 2011; 49:689–709.
2. Prasad M, Vora T, Agarwala S, et al. Management of Wilms tumor: ICMR consensus document. Indian J Pediatr 2017; 84(6):437–45.

## NEUROBLASTOMA

Neuroblastoma, derived from the neural crest, is the most common intra-abdominal and extracranial solid tumor in children, accounting for 7–8% of all cancers. It is the most common cancer diagnosed in the first year of life, and the median age at diagnosis is approximately 19 months. This is a disease of early childhood with approximately 90% patients presenting before 5-yr of age and almost 50% within the first 2-yr of life. The etiology is not known but familial cases occur, and there is association with neurofibromatosis, Hirschsprung disease, heterochromia, fetal hydantoin and fetal alcohol syndromes and Friedreich ataxia. Rearrangement or deletion of the short arm of chromosome 1 is present in 80% patients. Neuroblastoma is one of the very few cancers that may undergo spontaneous regression.

The pathology varies from extremely undifferentiated small round blue cell tumors (neuroblastoma) to tumors with mature Schwannian stroma with ganglion cells (ganglioneuroblastoma and ganglioneuroma). The characteristic histopathologic feature is the Homer-Wright pseudorosette, which are circular groupings of dark tumor cells surrounding pale neurofibrils. Neuroblastoma can resemble other small round blue cell tumors such as rhabdomyosarcoma, Ewing sarcoma and non-Hodgkin lymphoma, but are differentiated by characteristic immunohistochemistry. Neuroblastomas are typically positive for synaptophysin, tyrosine hydroxylase, PHOX2B, neuron-specific enolase, and NB84 and negative for hematopoietic markers, desmin, myogenin, keratin, and CD99. PHOX2B has also been shown to be both specific and sensitive for detection of neuroblastic tumors. The pathology is closely correlated with prognosis, and tumors that show better differentiation, more Schwannian stroma and low mitosis-karyorrhexis index have favorable outcome.

### Genetics

The most common somatic genomic alterations in neuroblastomas are recurrent chromosomal copy number alterations. These can be gains and losses of whole chromosomes, gains and losses of chromosomal segments, focal gene amplification events, or, more rarely, focal homozygous deletions.

In addition, exome-wide and whole-genome sequencing have identified various driver genes like *MYCN* and *MYC*, *ALK*, and downstream *RAS/MAPK* pathway genes, telomerase reverse transcriptase (TERT) and chromatin remodeling genes (*ATRX*, *ARID1A* and *ARID1B*. The definition of *MYCN* amplification is defined by consensus as greater than fourfold *MYCN* copies (FISH signals) as compared with a control 2p probe, and in most tumors with *MYCN* amplification, the *MYCN* copy number greatly exceeds this threshold. The overall prevalence of *MYCN* amplification is approximately 20% in most series. The *MYCN* oncogene, which encodes the *N-myc* proto-oncogene protein, is used as a biomarker for risk stratification and is associated with more aggressive disease. Hyperdiploidy in the tumor tissue is associated with a favorable prognosis in children <2-yr-old. Loss of heterozygosity of 1p, 11q, 14q and gain of 17q are associated with worse prognosis. A family history of neuroblastic tumors is found in about 1 to 2% of newly diagnosed cases.

### Clinical Features

The tumor may occur at any site where sympathetic tissue is found: Abdomen 65% (adrenal medulla 46%, rest 19%), posterior mediastinum (25%), pelvis (4%), head and neck (3%) and others (3%). Chief systemic symptoms include pallor, fatigue, weight loss, abdominal distension and pain, fever, irritability and bone pains. Local symptoms include periorbital edema and ecchymosis, raccoon eyes (Fig. 21.16), proptosis, exophthalmos, squint, retinal hemorrhage and optic atrophy; cervical lymphadenopathy, Horner syndrome, supraclavicular mass; superior mediastinal syndrome; vertebral nerve compression causing gait disturbances, bowel and bladder dysfunction; abdominal mass, hepatomegaly; skin nodules and features of bone marrow involvement. Secretion of catecholamines might result in paroxysmal episodes of sweating, pallor, flushing, headache, palpitations and hypertension. The opsoclonus-myoclonus-ataxia (OMA) syndrome is uncommon and characterized by rapid eye movements, ataxia and irregular muscle movements. This syndrome is correlated with an immune-mediated antitumor host

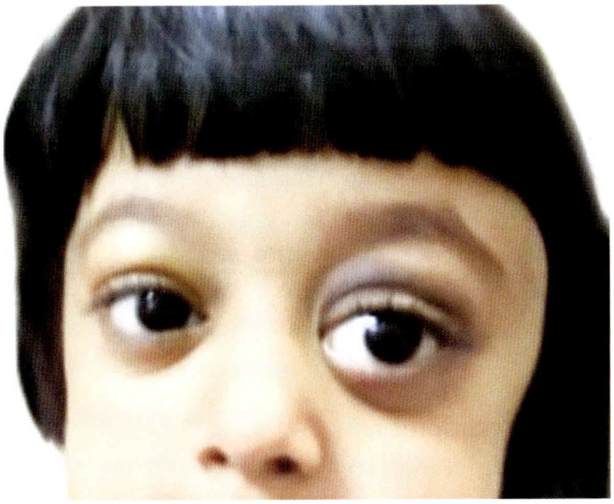

Fig. 21.16: 'Raccoon's eye' (left eyelid) in a child diagnosed with metastatic neuroblastoma

response. Most children with this syndrome have a localized disease and a favorable tumor-related outcome. However, majority of such children have long-term neurologic sequelae. Secretion of the vasoactive intestinal peptide may result in watery diarrhea and hypokalemia. Metastatic spread occurs via lymphatics and blood.

### Diagnosis

The gold standard for diagnosis is an examination of tumor tissue histopathology and immunohistochemistry. Key investigations include blood counts, urinary catecholamine excretion, bone marrow aspiration and biopsy, liver function tests and abdominal ultrasound. Nuclear scanning with $^{123}$I or $^{131}$I MIBG detects tumors and metastasis accurately. CT scan of chest, abdomen and pelvis are indicated to assess extent of disease (Fig. 21.17). MRI is preferred for paraspinal tumors to assess spinal cord compression.

Patients with neuroblastoma can be divided into those with favorable and unfavorable features. The former, characterized by young age (<1.5 yr), favorable stage (I, II and IV-S), normal levels of ferritin and favorable histology, has a survival expectancy of 90% or more. Older patients

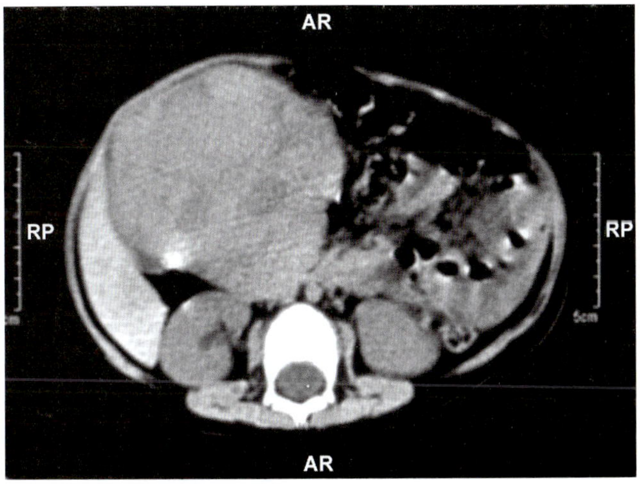


Fig. 21.17: CT image of abdomen showing a suprarenal mass suggestive of neuroblastoma

**Table 21.21:** International neuroblastoma staging system

| |
|---|
| **Stage I:** Localized tumor confined to the area of origin; complete excision, with or without microscopic residual disease; identifiable ipsilateral and contralateral lymph nodes negative microscopically |
| **Stage IIA:** Localized tumor with incomplete gross excision; identifiable ipsilateral and contralateral lymph nodes negative microscopically |
| **Stage IIB:** Localized tumor with complete or incomplete gross excision, with positive ipsilateral regional lymph nodes; identifiable contralateral lymph nodes negative microscopically |
| **Stage III:** Tumor infiltrating across the midline with or without regional lymph node involvement; or unilateral tumor with contralateral regional lymph node involvement; or midline tumor with bilateral regional lymph node involvement |
| **Stage IV:** Tumor disseminated to distant lymph nodes, bone, bone marrow, liver or other organs (except stage IV-S). |
| **Stage IV-S:** Localized primary tumor as defined for stage I or II with dissemination limited to liver, skin, and / or bone marrow (limited to infants less than one year of age). |

with stage III or IV disease, serum ferritin >150 ng/mL and tumors of unfavorable histology have survival rates of 20% or less (Table 21.21).

The prognosis is dependent on disease stage, age at diagnosis, tumor pathology (stromal component, the degree of differentiation, MKI), tumor cell ploidy, *MYCN* amplification status and additional genomic factors (segmental chromosomal aberrations).

### Treatment

Age and clinical stage are the two most important independent prognostic factors. Perinatal neuroblastoma tumors are similar both clinically and biologically to those identified by screening, and the vast majority do well with little or no therapy. Even with advanced disease, children less than 18 months at diagnosis have better outcome than those diagnosed later.

Treatment modalities most commonly include chemotherapy, surgery and radiation therapy. Localized neuroblastoma can be treated by surgery alone and does not require chemotherapy (Table 21.22). Patients with stage IV-S just require careful observation. Chemotherapy is the mainstay of treatment for advanced neuroblastoma. The regimens used include OPEC (vincristine, cyclophosphamide, cisplatin, teniposide (VM-26), CADO (vincristine, cyclophosphamide, doxorubicin) and PECADO (vincristine, cyclophosphamide, doxorubicin, cisplatin, teniposide). Other modalities include surgery, radiotherapy and autologous bone marrow transplantation. Addition of *cis*-retinoic acid to autologous stem cell transplantation has been shown to improve survival in patients with high-risk neuroblastoma. In all treatments, good remissions are often reached, but the recurrence rate is high.

### Suggested Reading

1. Swift CC, Eklund MJ, Kraveka JM, Alazraki AL. Updates in diagnosis, management, and treatment of neuroblastoma. Radiographics 2018;38(2):566–80.

**Table 21.22:** Management of neuroblastoma

| *Risk category* | *Stage* | *Age (months)* | *MYCN* | *Therapy* | *Survival* |
|---|---|---|---|---|---|
| Low | I | Any | No | Surgery | >90% |
| | IIA /IIB | Any | No | Surgery low dose chemotherapy | >80% |
| | IV-S | <12 | No | Observation/chemotherapy/radiation | |
| Intermediate | III | <18 | No | CT | >75% |
| | IV | Any | No | RT to tumor bed if residual disease present +/ second look surgery | |
| | IV-S | Any | No | | |
| High | II, III, IV, IV-S | >12 | Amplification | Multiagent chemotherapy+ autologous BMT + maintenance with 13-*cis*-retinoic acid | 50% |

2. Wienke J, Dierselhuis MP, Tytgat GA, et al. The immune landscape of neuroblastoma: Challenges and opportunities for novel therapeutic strategies in pediatric oncology. European Journal of Cancer 2021;144:123–50.



*Competency:* **PE29.12**



## MALIGNANT TUMORS OF THE LIVER

Primary tumors of the liver are rare and account for approximately 1% of all childhood malignancies. Over two-thirds of these tumors are malignant chiefly hepatoblastoma, which present by 5 years of age. Hepatocellular carcinoma is the second commonest liver malignancy and is seen at a median age of 12 years. Other less common malignant liver neoplasms include embryonal/undifferentiated sarcoma, rhabdomyosarcoma, angiosarcoma and germ cell-yolk sac tumors. Benign neoplasms of liver include mesenchymal hamartoma, hemangioma, hemangioendothelioma, adenoma and teratoma. For details, *see* Chapter 12.

## SOFT TISSUE SARCOMA

Pediatric soft tissue sarcomas are a group of malignant tumors that originate from primitive mesenchymal tissue and account for 6–7% of all childhood tumors. Rhabdomyosarcomas account for about one-half of all patients with soft tissue sarcoma in children. Other soft tissue sarcomas include fibrosarcoma, synovial sarcoma and malignant peripheral nerve sheath tumors.

### Rhabdomyosarcoma

Rhabdomyosarcoma (RMS), the commonest soft tissue sarcoma, is a malignant tumor of skeletal muscle, accounting for 3–4% of cancer in children. Almost half of these cases are diagnosed by 5 years of age and two-thirds by 10 years.

The chief sites are the head and neck (commonest), the genitourinary tract and the extremities (Fig. 21.18a and b). Tumors of the hand and foot occur in older patients, have an alveolar histology, with risk of metastasis. Orbital rhabdomyosarcoma presents in young children with proptosis or swelling of the eyelid. Parameningeal tumors (nose, nasopharynx, middle ear, mastoid and paranasal sinuses) may show intracranial extension. Genitourinary tumors may present as a pelvic mass, bladder and prostate enlargement or polypoid mass in the vagina. A unique form of RMS arising from the bladder or vagina, the botryoid variant (so named because of its resemblance to a protruding cluster of grapes), is seen almost exclusively in younger children. Almost one-fourth patients present with metastasis at diagnosis commonly in lungs, bone marrow and bone. The major histologic types are: (i) embryonal (60%); it is the commonest variant presents with tumors of head, neck and genitourinary tract, and has favorable prognosis; (ii) alveolar (20%) is more common in older children, at the extremities and perineal region and has unfavorable outcome. Most cases of RMS are sporadic, however, certain familial syndromes, such as neurofibromatosis and the Li–Fraumeni syndrome (LFS).

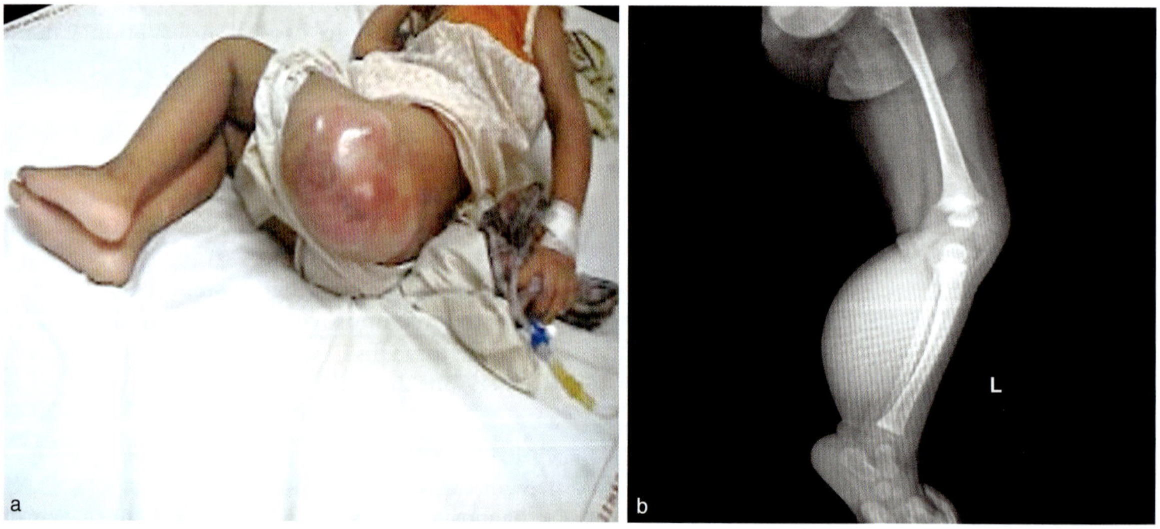


**Fig. 21.18:** Rhabdomyosarcoma in (a) 4-yr-old with gluteal mass; (b) 2-yr-old with calf swelling

RMS tumor cells resemble cells arrested in the early stages of skeletal muscle development. It is curable in most children with localized disease who receive combined therapy with chemotherapy, radiotherapy and surgery with more than 70% surviving 5-year after the diagnosis. Between 15% and 25% of newly diagnosed patients have distant metastases, lungs being the commonest site for metastasis.

### Suggested Reading

1. Skapek SX, Ferrari A, Gupta AA, et al. Rhabdomyosarcoma. Nat Rev Dis Primers 2019;5(1):1.

## BONE TUMORS

Osteogenic sarcoma and Ewing sarcoma are two major bone tumors in children and adolescents. Both tumors occur commonly during the second decade of life and show male predominance.

### Osteogenic Sarcoma

Its peak incidence is during adolescence, correlating with rapid bone growth. The distal femur and proximal tibia are the most frequent sites followed by proximal humerus and middle and proximal femur. Flat bones, e.g. vertebrae, pelvic bones and mandible are rarely affected. Patients present with a localized painful swelling that may be attributed to traumatic or infective conditions, delaying the diagnosis by months. Metastasis occurs early to the lungs and other bones.

Germline mutations of tumor suppressor genes, including the retinoblastoma (*RB1*) gene are associated with increased incidence of osteogenic sarcoma. Li-Fraumeni syndrome, associated with germline mutations of the tumor suppressor p53 gene, is characterized by increased incidence of breast cancer, soft tissue sarcoma, osteosarcoma, adrenocortical carcinoma and leukemia in first degree relatives. High dose radiation therapy, such as that for Ewing sarcoma or brain tumors, predisposes to development of osteosarcoma, either in or at sites distant from the radiation field. Benign bone lesions such as Paget disease, multiple hereditary exostoses, fibrous dysplasia and enchondromatosis may occasionally undergo malignant transformation to osteosarcoma.

Diagnostic imaging plays a major role in the management of patients with osteosarcoma. In most cases, conventional radiographs suggest the presence of a malignant bone tumor. Radiographic examination shows sclerotic or lytic bone lesions and periosteal new bone formation over the metaphyseal region. Further imaging, magnetic resonance imaging (MRI) or computed tomography (CT) of the involved area, is performed to evaluate the extent of local disease. MRI is preferred and provides an accurate assessment of tumor extent. Chest CT scan and 18FDG-PET are also performed to determine the presence and extent of metastatic disease. The differential diagnosis includes osteomyelitis and other bone tumors. A biopsy must be done to confirm the diagnosis that is characterized by highly malignant pleomorphic spindle cells with malignant osteoid formation.

Successful treatment requires complete surgical resection followed by multiagent chemotherapy. Limb sparing surgery by wide resection of the primary tumor is followed by replacement of missing bone by prosthesis. Chemotherapeutic agents include doxorubicin, cisplatin, ifosfamide, cyclophosphamide and high dose methotrexate. The tumor is unresponsive to radiotherapy. With current regimens, more than two-thirds of patients without metastasis are cured.

### Ewing Sarcoma

Ewing sarcoma most often arises from flat bones, such as pelvis, chest wall and vertebrae and the diaphyseal region of long bones (Fig. 21.19). Patients present with localized disease or clinically overt metastases. Common sites of metastasis are lungs and other bones; bone marrow metastasis is not uncommon. Osteomyelitis and Langerhans cell histiocytosis particularly eosinophilic granuloma are the chief differential diagnosis. Plain radiographs show destructive lesions of the diaphysis with multilayered or lamellated (onion skin) periosteal reaction (Fig. 21.19).

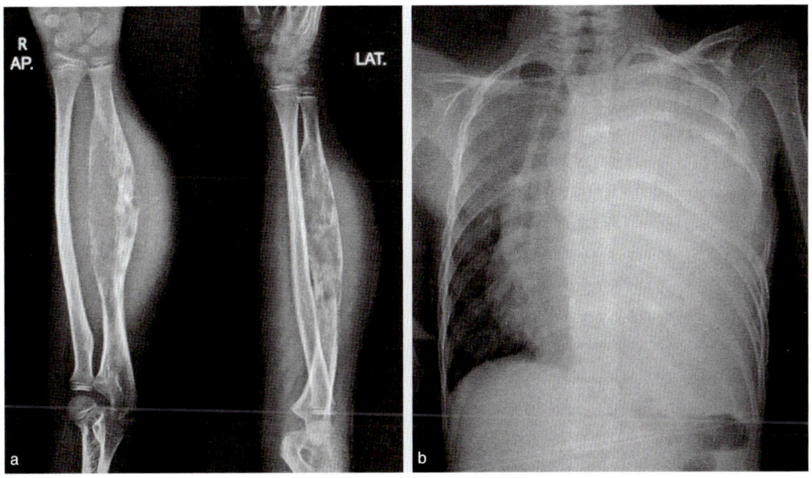


Fig. 21.19: (a) Radiograph of leg showing permeative lytic lesion with a prominent soft-tissue mass extending from the bone. Periosteal reaction is seen. The onion-skin or sunburst pattern indicates an aggressive process suggestive of Ewing sarcoma; (b) Chest wall Ewing sarcoma showing rib destruction

Biopsy is necessary for confirmation, which shows monotonous population of small round blue cells that is differentiated from other round cell tumors by immunohistochemistry. Ewing sarcoma shows strong expression of surface glycoprotein CD99 and vimentin; reciprocal chromosomal translocation t(11;22)(q24;q12) is pathognomonic and present in 85% cases. Chest CT, PET-CT and bone marrow biopsy are performed to evaluate for metastasis.

These tumors are responsive to both chemotherapy and radiotherapy. Local surgery is also an effective way to treat Ewing sarcoma, however, surgical amputation is rarely indicated. Tumor control with radiotherapy requires moderately high doses ranging from 5500 to 6000 cGy. Multiagent combination chemotherapy includes medications like vincristine, dactinomycin, cyclophosphamide, doxorubicin, ifosfamide and etoposide. In localized disease, without metastasis, the cure rate is nearly 60–70%, while in metastatic disease it is less satisfactory.

### Suggested Reading

1. Eaton BR, Claude L, Indelicato DJ, et al. Ewing sarcoma. Pediatr Blood Cancer 2021; 68:e28355.

## GERM CELL TUMORS

Gonadal and extragonadal germ cell tumors are infrequent in childhood, and constitute approximately 2 to 3% of cancers diagnosed in children and adolescents younger than 15 years. They are a varied group of benign and malignant neoplasms derived from primordial germ cells and occur in a variety of sites, both gonadal and extragonadal, the latter in midline locations as the sacrococcygeal, retroperitoneal, mediastinal, cervical, and pineal regions. Most germ cell tumors of the fetus and infant are histologically benign and are diagnosed as either mature or immature teratomas. Yolk sac tumor, second in frequency, occurs alone or in combination with a teratoma. Serum tumor markers, the "onco"-fetoproteins (AFP and β-hCG), aid in the diagnosis, as well as in the detection of residual or progressive disease.

Mature or immature teratomas are treated with surgery. For tumors with a malignant component, the use of platinum-based chemotherapy has dramatically increased survival. The role of radiotherapy for established for seminomas/germinomas.

### Suggested Reading

1. Fonseca A, Frazier AL, Shaikh F. Germ cell tumors in adolescents and young adults. J Oncol Pract 2019;15(8):433–41.

## BRAIN TUMORS

Central nervous system (CNS) tumors are one of the most common solid tumors in pediatrics, accounting for approximately 25% of all childhood cancers, and the second most common pediatric malignancy after leukemia. CNS tumors can be associated with significant morbidity and mortality irrespective of the grade of malignancy. The common tumors seen include: **S**upratentorial astrocytoma (low grade: 15–25% and high grade: 10–15%), cerebellar astrocytoma (10–20%), brainstem glioma (10–15%), medulloblastoma (10–15%), ependymona (5–10%), craniopharyngioma (6–9%), pineal and other tumors (12–15%) (Fig. 21.20a and b).

The vast majority of pediatric CNS tumors are sporadic, with no known cause. Exposure of CNS to significant doses of radiation and presence of certain genetic syndromes increase the risk of developing brain tumors. Meningiomas and malignant gliomas arise within the radiation field several years or decades after radiation therapy. Children who have received cranial or craniospinal radiation for treatment of ALL are at risk. Several genetic syndromes are associated with occurrence of tumors (Table 21.23). Approximately 15% patients with neurofibromatosis (NF1) develop optic gliomas during their lifetime; these usually have a benign course and may even regress spontaneously.

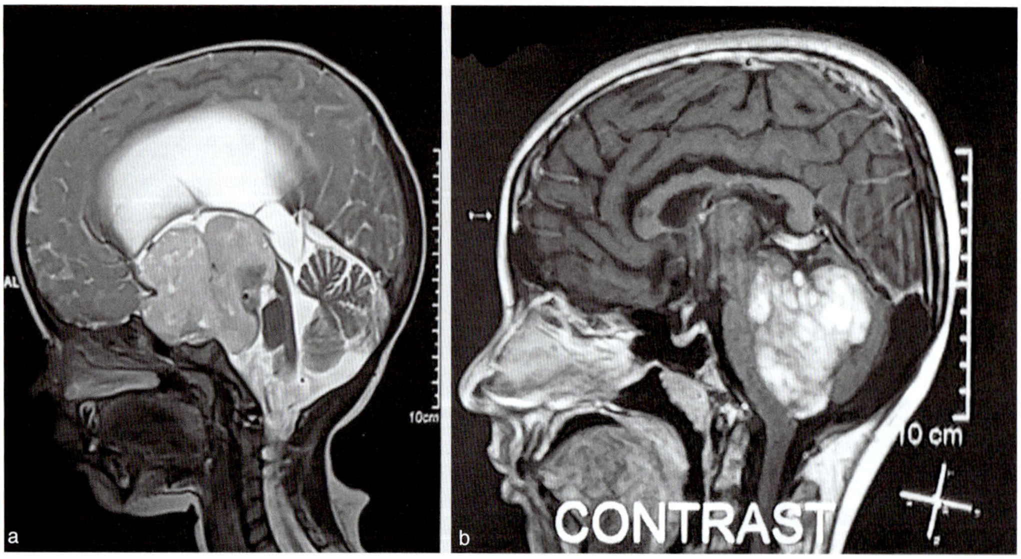


**Fig. 21.20:** MRI brain showing: (a) Heterogenous mass in the sellar and suprasellar area on T2-weighted segittal section, suggesting craniopharyngioma; (b) Hyperintense lobulated mass in the posterior fossa on T1-weighted segittal section, suggestive of medulloblastoma

**Table 21.23:** Genetic disorders associated with brain tumors

| *Disorder* | *Brain tumor* | *Other features* |
|---|---|---|
| Neurofibromatosis type 1 | Optic glioma | Autosomal dominant |
| Neurofibromatosis type 2 | Acoustic neuromas, Schwannoma | Peripheral nerve sheath tumors, cardiac sarcoma |
| Li-Fraumeni syndrome | Choroid plexus carcinoma | Sarcoma, adrenocortical cancer, breast cancer |
| Bilateral retinoblastoma | Pineal tumor (trilateral retinoblastoma) | Sarcoma |
| Tuberous sclerosis | Subependymal cell astrocytoma, malignant glioma | Autosomal dominant |
| von Hipplel-Lindau | Hemangioblastoma | Renal, adrenal and pancreatic tumors |
| Gorlin syndrome | Medulloblastoma | Very sensitive to radiation, basal cell carcinoma |
| Turcot syndrome | Medulloblastoma, malignant glioma | Adenomatous polyps in colon |

***Pediatric astrocytomas*** comprised a heterogenous group of pediatric tumors including juvenile pilocytic astrocytomas (JPAs), low grade diffuse astrocytomas, gangliogliomas, oligodendrogliomas and mixed oligoastrocytomas.

***Medulloblastomas*** are malignant, invasive tumors of cerebellum with over 70% of tumors occurring in children less than 16 years and are stratified into standard and high risk depending on age at presentation, extent of disease, histopathology, molecular characteristics and response to treatment.

***Ependymomas*** are generally slow growing well circumscribed tumors that arise predominantly infratentorially in children with a peak incidence at 6 years of age.

## Clinical Features

Clinical presentation of these tumors depends on location of the tumor and their rate of growth. The main symptoms are as follows.

### *Symptoms from Raised Intracranial Pressure (ICP)*

Infratentorial tumors are more common than supratentorial tumors in children and hence more likely to develop acute or chronic hydrocephalus. Recurrent headaches that are worse at night or early morning and worsen with lying down, early morning vomiting, vision loss or features of VI nerve palsy and 'sunset sign' indicate raised ICP. An acute increase in ICP may present with the Cushing triad of hypertension, bradycardia and altered pattern of respiration.

### *Symptoms from Compression or Infiltration*

Headache can occur from direct compression of the skull and meninges. *Vomiting* may be due to raised ICP but may occur due to direct infiltration of the vomiting centers at the base of fourth ventricle. Head tilt may occur as correction for diplopia arising from cranial nerve palsy. The *diencephalic syndrome* comprising of emaciation, euphoria and emesis is associated with tumors in the diencephalon. *Parinaud syndrome* of supranuclear vertical gaze palsy, with pupils that are reactive to accommodation but not to light is seen with tumors of the pineal region or upper brainstem.

*Frontal lobe tumors* may present with personality changes, seizures and headaches and tumors in the temporal lobe cause seizures and change in speech. *Suprasellar tumors* may be associated with endocrinopathies and visual changes. Multiple cranial nerve deficits are the classic presentation of *brainstem gliomas*, while nystagmus, ataxia and vomiting are present with *cerebellar tumors*. *Spinal tumors* may cause back pain, scoliosis, numbness, weakness and impaired bladder or bowel function.

## Diagnosis

MRI is the imaging modality of choice. CT scan is necessary in an acute presentation. The distinction between benign and malignant tumors is critical but location of the tumor is even more important. A benign tumor in an unresectable location may have as poor outcome as a malignant tumor in a surgically accessible area of the brain.

## Treatment

Treatment requires a multidisciplinary approach, with adequate use of surgery, chemotherapy and radiation. Complete surgical resection without damaging critical structures is the goal, but may be difficult to achieve depending on location of the tumor. The overall five-year survival of brain tumors in Western countries approaches more than 70%.

Modern technology has greatly impacted the practice of pediatric neurooncology. Neurosurgical procedure have become highly sophisticated and advanced: These include computer-guided stereotaxis, laser dissection and intraoperative physiologic monitoring and imaging. Radiation therapy is commonly used. Chemotherapy may be used concurrently with radiation therapy, including as a radiation sensitizer. Often high dose chemotherapy with autologous stem cell rescue is used for optimum treatment results. The efficacy of anti-angiogenic therapy (bevacizumab), vascular endothelial growth factor (VEGF), in combination of chemotherapy for childhood is emerging as a promising modality for management of high grade gliomas.

While survival and cure rates have improved, treatment–related morbidity remains high and significant long-term sequelae are common.

## Suggested Reading

1. Fleming AJ, Chi SN. Brain tumors in children. Curr Probl Pediatr Adolesc Health Care 2012;42:80–103.
2. Louis DN, Perry A, Reifenberger G, et al. The 2016 World Health Organization Classification of Tumors of the Central Nervous System: a summary. Acta Neuropathol 2016;131:803–20.

## HISTIOCYTOSES

The childhood histiocytoses are a rare and diverse group of proliferative disorders characterized by infiltration and accumulation of histiocytes within various tissues. The International Histiocyte Society has proposed a classification for these disorders as given in Table 21.24.

### Langerhans Cell Histiocytosis (LCH)

LCH is a rare non-malignant disease of unknown etiology characterized by a clonal proliferation of pathologic cells with the characteristics of Langerhans cells in single/multiple sites and an unpredictable course. This is usually a sporadic and non-hereditary condition. The clinical presentation is heterogeneous ranging from single-system involvement to a multisystem life-threatening disease (Table 21.25). The hallmark of LCH is the presence of Birbeck granules on electron microscopy and positivity for S-100 protein and CD1a positivity. The number of Langerhans cells with Birbeck granules can vary in different lesions with limited numbers seen in tissues taken from liver, spleen, gastrointestinal tract or central nervous system. Langerin (CD207) is a relatively new monoclonal antibody directed against a type II transmembrane protein associated with Birbeck granules and is presumed to be more sensitive and specific for LC than CD1a.

The spectrum of LCH (eosinophilic granuloma, Hand-Schuller-Christian disease, Letterer-Siwe disease) reflects varying extents of the disease. The course of disease is unpredictable, varying from rapid progression and death, to repeated recurrence and recrudescence with chronic sequelae, to spontaneous regression and resolution. Patients with disease that is localized (skin or bone) have a good prognosis and need minimum or even no treatment. In contrast, multiple organ involvement, particularly in young children (under 2-year-old), carries relatively poor prognosis.

The most common involvement is of the skeleton (80%). Bone lesions can be single or multiple affecting skull bones, long bones, vertebrae, mastoid and mandible. The lesions may be painless or present with pain and local swelling; X-rays show sharp lytic lesions (clinical manifestation includes vertebral collapse and spinal compression, pathological fractures in long bones, chronic draining ears and early eruption of teeth. Other manifestations include seborrheic skin rash in scalp area and back (60%), lymphadenopathy (33%), hepatosplenomegaly (20%) tachypnea, air leaks, parenchymal lung infiltrates (15%), jaundice, abdominal distension, neurodegenerative symptoms, features of malabsorption (Figs 21.21a–d). Bilateral infiltration of retro-orbital area may cause exophthalmos. Gingival mucous membrane may be involved with lesions, which look like candidiasis. Pituitary dysfunction may result in growth retardation and/or diabetes insipidus. Severe disease is characterized by fever, weight loss, malaise, failure to thrive and liver dysfunction. Liver involvement may

**Table 21.24:** Classification of histiocyte disorders

| | |
|---|---|
| Dendritic cell disorders | Langerhans cell histiocytosis (LCH)<br>Secondary dendritic cell processes<br>Juvenile xanthogranuloma<br>Solitary histiocytoma with dendritic phenotype |
| Macrophage-related disorders | Hemophagocytosis syndromes (primary and secondary)<br>Rosai-Dorfman disease<br>Solitary histiocytoma with macrophage phenotype |
| Malignant histiocyte disorders | Monocyte related leukemias<br>Extramedullary monocytic tumors<br>Dendritic cell/macrophage related histiocytic sarcoma |

**Table 21.25:** Clinical presentation of Langerhans cell histiocytosis

| | |
|---|---|
| Non-specific symptoms | Fever, lethargy, weight loss, diarrhea |
| Bone lytic lesions/deformity | Unifocal/multifocal; commonest site—skull, long bones, flat bones |
| Skin | Scaly erythematous lesions—red papules |
| Soft tissue | Scalp (commonest site) |
| Lymph node | Lymphadenopathy in 50% |
| Endocrine glands (hypothalamic pituitary axis) | Diabetes insipidus |
| Lungs | Asymptomatic<br>Radiologic involvement<br>Cough, respiratory distress |
| Spleen | Splenomegaly in 30% |
| Liver | Hepatomegaly, jaundice in 20%<br>Liver failure, sclerosing cholangitis |
| Bone marrow involvement | Pallor/anemia, petechial rash, superadded infection, pancytopenia |

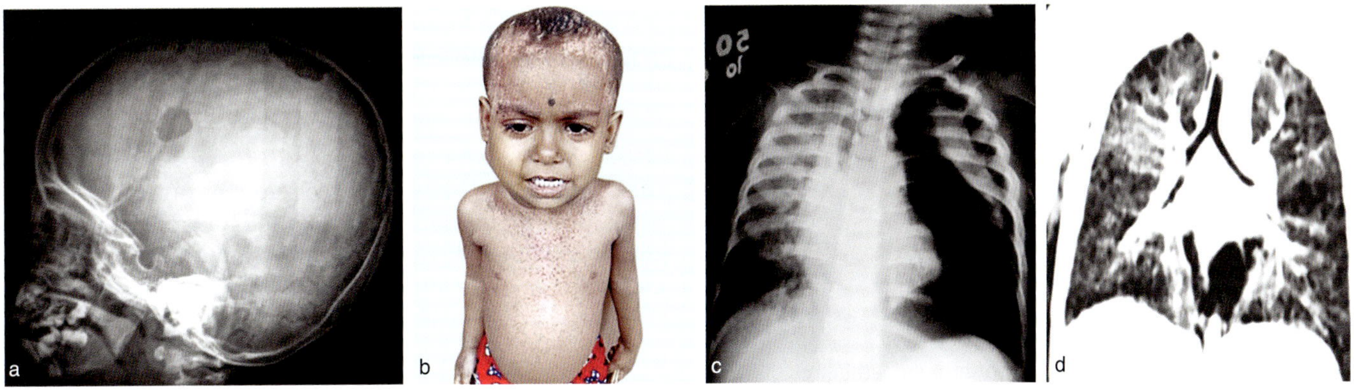


**Fig. 21.21:** Langerhans cell histiocytosis: (a) Radiograph skull showing lytic lesions; (b) Note the seborrhea, skin lesions and lymphadenopathy; (c) Radiograph of the chest shows bilateral pneumothorax; (d) Chest CECT showing bilateral cystic spaces and air leaks



result in sclerosing cholangitis and cirrhosis. Bone marrow involvement may lead to anemia and thrombocytopenia.

#### Diagnosis

The classical histopathologic feature of LCH is the presence of lesional histiocytes of LC phenotype, with varying proportion of macrophages, T lymphocytes, eosinophils and multinucleated giant cells. A definitive diagnosis requires that lesional cells show positivity to S-100 and CD1a, identification of Birbeck granules on electron microscopy (gold standard) or by Langerin (CD207), a relative new monoclonal antibody directed against a type II transmembrane protein associated with the granules. Diagnostic workup should include biopsy from most appropriate site, complete blood count, liver function tests, coagulation studies, skeletal survey, chest X-ray and urine specific gravity. In addition, evaluation of involved organ system should be under taken. These include ultrasound abdomen, CT chest and/or abdomen and MRI brain. Bone marrow biopsies are required to exclude infiltration.

#### Therapy

Treatment for localized disease or single bony lesion varies from observation, curettage, indomethacin, bisphosphonates low dose radiation or systemic chemotherapy. Multisystem disease is treated with chemotherapy, combining vinblastine, prednisone and 6 mercaptopurine. If there is response based on clinical evaluation and investigations, these children are treated for a total duration of 12 months. If there is no response, then they are shifted to the salvage protocol [systemic chemotherapy based on 2-chlorodeoxyadenosine (2-CDA) and or cytosine arabinoside, or bone marrow transplantation].

Multiorgan dysfunction is associated with poor prognosis. About 10–15% patients develop diabetes insipidus and require appropriate screening and follow-up. Childhood LCH may have long-term sequelae, some of which occur many years after completion of treatment. Patients of LCH require long-term follow-up not only to identify disease recurrence but also to follow for occurrence of long-term complications. These patients are at risk for second malignancies including solid tumors and hematopoietic malignancies. Long-term sequelae of LCH include neurodegenerative changes, gait abnormality, ataxia, dysarthria, intellectual impairment and hypothalamic-pituitary dysfunction.

Bone (vertebral collapse, orthopedic defects/scoliosis), facial asymmetry, limb asymmetry, tooth loss, hair loss, proptosis, lung (pneumothorax, pulmonary fibrosis, pulmonary hypertension), liver (sclerosing cholangitis, liver failure) and secondary malignancy (hematological) are seen in follow-up.

### Hemophagocytic Lymphohistiocytoses (HLH)

HLH is an aggressive and potentially fatal syndrome which results from an inappropriate prolonged activation of lymphocytes and macrophages, which lack Birbeck granules and CD1a positivity. Young children with HLH and known gene mutations, or a family history of HLH are described as having primary HLH. Older children with HLH or children without identifiable mutations are described to have secondary/acquired HLH.

HLH is attributed to defects in function of natural killer (NK) cells and cytotoxic cells with production of proinflammatory cytokines (interferon gamma, tumor necrosis factor alpha and interleukins). Hypercytokinemia results in multiorgan dysfunction leading to death. A number of genetic mutations have been found to be responsible for NK and cytotoxic T cell mediated killing of target cells. Associated immune deficiencies include Chediak-Higashi syndrome.

Clinical features include hepatomegaly (90%), splenomegaly (84%), neurological symptoms (47%), rash (43%) and lymphadenopathy (42%). Patients often develop liver failure with hyperbilirubinemia, pancytopenia, coagulopathy, acute kidney injury, ARDS and encephalopathy.

#### Diagnosis

In the absence of a known gene mutation, a diagnosis of HLH can be made when at least 5 of the 8 criteria are identified (Table 21.26).

#### Therapy

Standard treatment comprises dexamethasone and etoposide. Cyclosporine may be added. Treatment of any underlying infection should be undertaken. Patients require

Table 21.26: Diagnostic criteria for HLH

| HLH diagnosis established, if one of the two is fulfilled |
|---|
| A molecular diagnosis of HLH (e.g. *PERF, SAP, MUNC* mutations) OR 5 of the following 8 criteria are fulfilled<br>• Fever<br>• Splenomegaly<br>• Cytopenias in at least two cell lines<br>– Hemoglobin <90 g/L<br>– Platelets <100 × $10^9$/L<br>– Neutrophils <1 × $10^9$/L<br>• Hypertriglyceridemia and/or hypofibrinogenemia<br>– Fasting triglycerides >3 mmol/L (>265 mg/dL)<br>– Fibrinogen <1.5 g/L<br>• Hemophagocytosis in bone marrow or spleen or lymph nodes<br>• Low or absent activity of natural killer cells<br>• Ferritin >500 µg/L<br>• Soluble CD25 (soluble interleukin-2 receptor) >2400 units/mL |





multiple transfusions of blood components and prophylaxis against *P. jirovecii* (sulfamethoxazole-trimethoprim) and fungus (fluconazole). Other modalities having a role particularly for familial HLH include antithymocyte globulin (ATG) and stem cell transplantation.

### Suggested Reading


1. Allen CE, Ladisch S, McClain KL. How I treat Langerhans cell histicytosis. Blood 2015;126:26–35.
2. Canna SW, Marsh RA. Pediatric hemophagocytic lymphohistiocytosis blood 2020;135:1332–43.


## ONCOLOGIC EMERGENCIES

Oncologic emergencies may come as initial presentation of the malignancy, during course of the disease or as a consequence of therapy. A solid tumor may invade or compress vital organs like trachea, esophagus or superior vena cava. Effusions into the pleural space or pericardium may compromise functions of heart and lung. Metastasis into the brain may lead to cerebral edema and features of raised intracranial tension. Spinal cord tumor involvement by malignancy may lead to cord compression. Bone marrow involvement results in anemia, bleeding due to thrombocytopenia or coagulation abnormalities (disease/chemotherapy), leukostasis, thrombosis, cerebrovascular episodes and infections. Hormonal problems can occur because of paraneoplastic secretions. Finally, therapy-related complications include myocardial dysfunction (anthracyclines), extravasation of drugs (anthracyclines, vinca alkaloids), hemorrhagic cystitis (cyclophosphamide), cerebrovascular accidents (methotrexate, l-asparaginase) and pancreatitis (l-asparaginase, corticosteroids).

Common oncologic emergencies include tumor lysis syndrome, hyperleukocytosis, superior vena cava syndrome and febrile neutropenia (Table 21.27).

Other emergencies include:

*1. Cardiac tamponade:* This occurs due to massive pericardial effusion, constrictive pericarditis from radiation, intracardiac thrombus or tumors. Symptoms of tamponade include chest pain, cough, and dyspnea while signs include tachycardia, cyanosis, hypotension and pulsus paradoxus. Treatment includes provision of oxygen, hydration and percutaneous pericardial drainage. The fluid must be sent for relevant diagnostic investigations.

*2. Syndrome of inappropriate antidiuresis (SIAD)* may occur due to various chemotherapeutic agents (cyclophosphamide, vinca alkaloids, cisplatin) or with certain malignancies (craniopharyngioma, nasopharyngeal carcinoma). The management consists primarily of treatment of cause, if possible.

*3. Gastrointestinal emergencies:* The main acute gastrointestinal complications include acute abdomen, ileus, neutropenic enterocolitis, massive hepatomegaly and typhlitis. These conditions need early diagnosis; usually conservative management is preferred over surgical intervention. Infants with stage IV neuroblastoma may present with massive hepatomegaly sufficient to cause respiratory compromise. This needs urgent diagnosis and initiation of chemotherapy or irradiation. Typhlitis presents usually with fever, neutropenia and acute abdominal pain. It is a necrotizing colitis caused by bacterial invasion of the cecum that may progress to bowel infarction and perforation. Typhlitis requires IV antibiotics and aggressive supportive care. Hemorrhagic pancreatitis, due to l-asparaginase or other cause, is treated with IV antibiotics, providing parenteral fluids and nutrition, and management of pain.

*4. Urologic emergencies:* Priapism occurs mostly in chronic myeloid leukemia, and is treated with ensuring adequate hydration, and treatment with allopurinol and hydroxyurea. If leukocytosis and electrolyte problems persist, leukapheresis is recommended. If priapism does not respond to treatment within 48–72 hours, the child may be left with persistent deformity. Obstructive uropathy is seen in patients with bladder rhabdomyosarcomas, large retroperitoneal sarcomas or bulky retroperitoneal lymphomas. A CT scan helps to confirm the diagnosis. Placement of urinary catheter or stents may be helpful, until definitive therapy of the malignancy results in resolution of the obstruction.

### Suggested Reading


1. Handa A, Nozaki T, Makidono A, et al. Pediatric oncologic emergencies: Clinical and imaging review. Pediatr Int 2019; 61:122–39.
2. Seth R, Singh P, Puri K, et al. Morbidity profile and outcome of hyperleukocytosis in childhood acute leukemia. Int J Hematol Res 2015;1:90–94.


## LATE EFFECTS AND SURVIVORSHIP

With refinements in diagnostics and advances in therapeutics and supportive care, the overall survival of childhood malignancy has increased significantly over the past few decades. Over 80% children and adolescents with cancer survive 5 or more years from diagnosis in many centers and are effectively cured of the disease. This is, however, at the cost of increased morbidity in the form of various late effects of cancer treatment.

Table 21.27: Common oncologic emergencies: Clinical presentation and treatment

| *Oncologic emergency* | *Manifestation* | *Underlying disease* | *Treatment* |
|---|---|---|---|
| Tumor lysis syndrome (TLS) (biochemical syndrome which occurs from breakdown of malignant cells) | Laboratory-TLS is defined as ≥25% increase from baseline (or an absolute value exceeding the cut-offs) in ≥2 of the following serum biochemical parameters: Uric acid (>8 mg/dL), potassium (>6 mEq/L), phosphorus (>6.5 mg/dL), corrected serum calcium (<7 mg/dL). If biochemical derangements are accompanied by seizures, arrhythmias and acute kidney injury,it is known as clinical TLS | At high risk: ALL or AML with leukocytes ≥100000/cu mm<br>Stage III/IV Burkitt lymphoma (BL), or lymphoblastic lymphoma (LL) | Prevention by hydration, allopurinol/rasburicase<br>Treatment by hydration, allopurinol, rasburicase; dialysis for renal failure and correction of metabolic disturbances |
| Hyperleukocytosis (>100,000/cu mm) | Thrombosis, stroke, pulmonary infiltrate, hemorrhage, hypoxia | Leukemia | Hydration, hydroxyurea leukopharesis, chemotherapy |
| Superior vena caval/ mediastinal syndrome | Swelling of face and neck, difficulty in lying flat, difficulty in breathing and swallowing, hoarse voice, proptosis, Horner syndrome, chest pain, facial edema, wheezing, pleural effusion, pericardial effusion, features of carbon dioxide retention (anxiety, confusion, lethargy, headache, distorted vision, syncope) | Non-Hodgkin lymphoma (NHL) , acute lymphoblastic leukemia (ALL) and germ cell tumor | Chemotherapy, steroids<br>Intravenous lines in lower limb<br>Monitor for tumor lysis |
| Spinal cord compression | Paraplegia, back pain, urinary retention, loss of deep tendon reflexes | Neuroblastoma, Ewing sarcoma, lymphoma involving vertebral body | Dexamethasone<br>Surgery of the tumor |
| Increased intracranial pressure | Headache, emesis, hypertension, bradycardia, III and VI nerve palsy, seizures | Primary brain tumor, medulloblastoma, astrocytoma, brainstem glioma | Dexamethasone, surgical intervention<br>Phenytoin |
| Febrile neutropenia* | Sepsis, shock, pneumonia, typhlitis, DIC | Any immunosuppressed child | Broad-spectrum antibiotics and antifungals |

*Single oral/axillary or equivalent temperature of >38.3°C (101°F), or two consecutive temperature greater than 38.0°C (100°F) in a 12-hour period lasting at least 1 hour.
Neutropenia is defined as absolute neutrophil count (ANC) <500/mm³ or <1,000/mm³ with an expected decline

The main goals of the Cancer Survivorship Program are to improve the health and well-being of childhood cancer survivors by promoting adherence to a schedule of follow-up appointments and routine screening tests, educate patients, parents and healthcare professionals about the long-term effects of cancer treatment, integrate them appropriately into society, provide referrals to specialists as needed, offer psychological counseling and transition of patients to adult care when ready.

### Spectrum of Late Effects Associated with Childhood Cancer

The common late effects of pediatric cancer comprise deficits in growth and development, organ function, reproductive capacity and health of offspring and development of subsequent neoplasms.

*Growth and development:* The components affected within this domain include linear growth, sexual maturation, musculoskeletal development, skeletal maturation, intellectual function, emotional and social maturation (Table 21.28).

*Organ function:* Exposure to higher cumulative chemotherapy and radiation doses required for more biologically aggressive refractory disease increases the risk of both vital and non-vital organ toxicity (e.g. anthracycline related cardiotoxicity, pulmonary function abnormalities, chronic liver disease, etc) (Table 21.29).

*Reproductive capacity and pregnancy outcomes:* Reproductive functioning may be affected by various anticancer modalities (surgery, chemotherapy and radiation). Alkylating chemotherapy produces a dose-related gonadal germ cell injury. In boys, alkylators damage germ cells leading to infertility. Compared to boys, girls maintain an ovarian function at higher cumulative doses of alkylating agents, and if dysfunction occurs it is often reversible. Combined modality therapy including alkylating agents and abdominal or pelvic radiation may adversely affect fertility.

21

Essential Pediatrics

Table 21.28: Spectrum of effects on growth and development associated with pediatric cancer therapy

| *General domain* | *Specific late effect* | *Predisposing therapy* | *Modifying host factors* |
|---|---|---|---|
| Linear growth | Delayed/accelerated growth<br>Short stature<br>Growth failure | Radiation of hypothalamic-pituitary-growth hormone axis | Younger age poses higher risk |
| Sexual maturation | Delayed puberty, hypogonadism<br>Precocious puberty | Alkylating agents<br>Radiation of hypothalamic-pituitary-growth hormone axis | Boys at higher risk for alkylating agent gonadal injury; girls at higher risk for precocious puberty |
| Musculoskeletal development | Hypoplasia; fibrosis<br>Uneven/reduced skeletal growth | Radiation impacting bones and soft tissues | Younger age at irradiation |
| Skeletal maturation | Osteopenia<br>Osteoporosis<br>Osteonecrosis | Corticosteroids<br>Methotrexate<br>Radiation >40 Gy; corticosteroids | Younger age at irradiation<br><br>Older age (>10 yr) |
| Intellectual function | Neurocognitive deficits; learning deficits<br>Behavioral problems | High dose methotrexate, cytarabine, cranial irradiation | Younger age at irradiation |
| Emotional and social maturation | Mental health disorders Educational problems<br>Vocational limitations, unemployment<br>Psychosocial issues | Any cancer experience | Girls and CNS tumor survivors at increased risk |

Table 21.29: Organ/system affected, related effect, risk factor and evaluation

| *Late adverse effect* | *Therapeutic exposure* | *Risk factors* | *Evaluation* |
|---|---|---|---|
| Neurocognitive deficits | Cranial radiation, total body radiation, high dose systemic methotrexate, intrathecal methotrexate | Age <3 years, radiation dose >24 Gy, whole brain radiation, females | Psychometric evaluation |
| Sensorineural deafness | Cisplatin, carboplatin infratemporal and nasopharyngeal radiation | High cumulative dose of cisplatin (>360 mg/m$^2$), radiation >30 Gy | ENT evaluation, auditometry, BERA |
| Peripheral nervous system | Vinca alkaloids, carboplatin, paclitaxel | | Electromyography |
| Cataracts | Glucocorticoids, cranial or orbital radiation | Higher dose | Ophthalmological examination |
| Retinopathy | Cranial or orbital radiation | Higher dose | Ophthalmological examination |
| Growth hormone deficiency, precocious puberty | Cranial and orbital radiation | Radiation dose >18 Gy to hypothalamic pituitary axis, female gender | Provocative tests for growth hormone deficiency, LH, FSH |
| Primary hypothyroidism | Neck or mantle radiation | Radiation >20 Gy to thyroid | Thyroid function tests |
| Cardiomyopathy | Daunorubicin, doxorubicin, idarubicin, mediastinal radiation | Cumulative anthracycline dose >250 mg/m$^2$, age <5 years, cardiac radiation >30 Gy, female gender | ECG, ECHO, MUGA, angiography |
| Valvular and atherosclerotic heart disease, pericardial fibrosis | Mediastinal and abdominal radiation affecting the heart | Radiation dose to heart >30 Gy | |
| Pulmonary fibrosis, interstitial and restrictive lung disease | Busulphan, bleomycin, radiation to lungs | Higher dose of chemotherapy and radiation | Pulmonary function tests |
| Chronic kidney disease, renal tubular dysfunction | Cisplatin, carboplatin, ifosfamide, abdominal radiation | High dose of chemotherapy, radiation, surgical removal of one kidney | Urinalysis, kidney function tests, ultrasonography, cystometric evaluation |
| Delayed puberty, premature menopause, infertility | Cyclophosphamide, ifosfamide, busulphan, melphalan, procarbazine<br>Abdominal, pelvic, spinal and testicular radiation | Radiation dose >15 Gy to gonads in prepubertal and >10 Gy in pubertal girls<br>High dose of chemotherapy and pelvic radiation in boys (20–30 Gy) | Semen examination, FSH, LH, testosterone, estrogen estimation |
| Musculoskeletal problems | Radiation therapy corticosteroids | | Radiographs of affected bone and soft tissues |
| Second malignant neoplasm | Alkylating agents, procarbazine, etoposide, radiation | History of retinoblastoma, family history of Li-Fraumeni syndrome Hepatitis B /C infection | Tests as indicated by clinical features |

There is dose dependent reduction in sperm production following radiation. It is reversible at doses of 1–3 Gy but irreversible at higher doses above >3 Gy. Abdominal, pelvic and spinal radiation contributes to germ cell depletion in girls. Ovaries of younger girls are more resistant to radiation damage. Prepubertal status does not protect from germ cell injury. Very high radiation doses >20 Gy cause irreversible ovarian failure while doses between 20 and 30 Gy delay puberty.

***Second malignant neoplasm (SMN):*** Pediatric cancer survivors are at an increased risk for development of second cancers. Common malignancies that occur as second neoplasms include acute myeloid leukemia (AML), including myelodysplastic syndrome and solid tumors. Secondary AML commonly develops in association with use of alkylating agents or topoisomerase II inhibitor therapy. Radiation therapy is also implicated in the occurrence of second neoplasms, e.g. acute leukemia and solid tumors involving the breast, thyroid, CNS, bones, and soft tissues. Breast cancer is the most frequently reported secondary solid tumor in childhood cancer survivors with incidence varying from 10–20%, by 20 years from radiation.

### Recommendations for Clinical Care

Family practitioners, pediatricians, internists and nurses should be aware of the problems that may occur in survivors of childhood cancers. Follow-up care of child cancer survivors requires: (i) Measurement of height and weight and maintaining growth charts; (ii) assessment of pubertal development and fertility counseling; (iii) measurement of blood pressure; (iv) cardiac monitoring; (v) evaluation of viral markers; (vi) assessment of thyroid function and/or other endocrine evaluation as indicated; (vii) monitoring for relapse, second malignancies; and (viii) genetic counseling when indicated.

### Suggested Reading


1. Arora RS, Arora PR, Seth R, et al. Childhood cancer survivorship and late effects: The landscape in India in 2020. Pediatr Blood Cancer 2020;67:e28556.
2. Seth R, Singh A, Seth S, Sapra S. Late effects of treatment in survivors of childhood cancers: Indian J Med Res 2017;146:216–23.


## BONE MARROW TRANSPLANTATION (BMT)

BMT is the term used to describe the collection of hematopoietic stem cells from bone marrow, peripheral blood or umbilical cord blood. Bone marrow transplantation (BMT) is now called blood and marrow transplantation or hematopoietic stem cell transplantation (HSCT). This is the established therapy for congenital or acquired disorders of the hematopoietic system and for hematologic malignancies and few solid tumors. Details are given in Chapter 13.

Chapter

22

# Rheumatological Disorders

❍ Rakesh Kumar Pilania ❍ Surjit Singh

*Competency:* **PE22.1**

## ARTHRITIS

### Approach to Diagnosis

Arthritis is a common complaint in children. It is defined as swelling or effusion in a joint or if there are any two of the following four features: (i) Limitation of range of motion, (ii) pain, (iii) tenderness, and (iv) increased local temperature. Arthritis can be secondary to an underlying illness (infectious or noninfectious) or may be a primary disease in itself. Clinical assessment based on a good history and physical examination often provides more diagnostic clues than a battery of laboratory tests. A convenient way to classify arthritis is based on duration of illness at presentation (Table 22.1).

#### *Transient Synovitis*

This is a common condition in young children and is characterized by sudden onset of pain in hips, thighs, or knees following an upper respiratory catarrh. It is a self-limiting disorder, lasts only 2–4 days, and should not be confused with septic arthritis or acute osteomyelitis. Skin traction and a short course of nonsteroidal anti-inflammatory drugs (NSAIDs) bring prompt relief.

#### *Septic Arthritis*

This is usually seen in neonates and infants. It presents almost always as a monoarthritis and is accompanied by fever, tenderness, and limitation of joint movement. Causes include gram-negative bacilli, group B streptococci (in neonates), *Hemophilus influenzae* type b and *Streptococcus pneumoniae* in infants, and *Staphylococcus aureus* in older children. Ultrasonography, magnetic resonance imaging, and radionuclide scans provide useful clues to the diagnosis. A diagnostic arthrocentesis is necessary to confirm the diagnosis (Table 22.2). Appropriate antimicrobials, aspiration, and, in some cases (e.g. the hip joint), arthrocentesis are required for treatment.

**Table 22.1:** Classification of arthritis

| Classification of arthritis |
|---|
| **Acute arthritis (usually <2 weeks)** |
| • Acute rheumatic fever |
| • Transient ('toxic') synovitis |
| • Kawasaki disease, IgA vasculitis (Henoch-Schönlein purpura) |
| • Septic arthritis (*S. aureus, H. influenzae, N. meningitidis*) |
| **Subacute arthritis (2–6 weeks)** |
| • Reactive arthritis |
| • Systemic lupus erythematosus, dermatomyositis, polyarteritis nodosa |
| • Associated with leukemia or neuroblastoma |
| • Associated with Lyme disease, brucellosis |
| • Sickle cell disease |
| • Associated with hypogammaglobulinemia |
| **Chronic arthritis (>6 weeks)** |
| • Juvenile idiopathic arthritis |
| • Tubercular arthritis |
| • *Mimics of chronic arthritis* (non-inflammatory arthropathy): Progressive pseudorheumatoid arthropathy, idiopathic multicentric osteolysis, camptodactyly-arthropathy-coxa vara-pericarditis (CACP syndrome) |
| • Legg-Calvé-Perthes disease |

#### *Tubercular Arthritis*

It can result from infection with *M. tuberculosis* or from an allergic phenomenon secondary to a systemic focus (Poncet disease). The former usually presents as monoarthritis (e.g. hip or ankle joint), while the latter presents as polyarthritis with a strongly positive tuberculin reaction. Arthrocentesis or synovial biopsy may be diagnostic (Table 22.2).

#### *Reactive Arthritis*

This is not as common in children as in adults. Diagnosis is based on Berlin criteria: (i) Peripheral arthritis (usually

**Table 22.2:** Synovial fluid characteristics in childhood arthritides

| *Type of arthritis* | *Physical characteristics* | *Cytology* | *Biochemistry* | *Comments* |
|---|---|---|---|---|
| Septic arthritis | Turbid; serosanguineous | Polymorphonuclear cells present; Gram stain may be positive | Glucose reduced; protein elevated | Synovial fluid culture may be positive; synovial fluid, if inoculated in blood culture bottles, increases the yield |
| Tuberculous arthritis | Opaque | Lymphocytes present; stain for acid-fast bacilli may be positive | Glucose may be normal; protein elevated | Polymerase chain reaction may be positive |
| Juvenile inflammatory arthritis | Cloudy | Polymorphonuclear cells present; Gram stain negative | Glucose low; protein elevated | Fluid characteristics often mimic those of septic arthritis |
| Systemic lupus erythematosus | Clear | Lymphocytes present | Protein normal or elevated; glucose may be normal | Synovial fluid complement C3 may be low |

lower limb, asymmetric oligoarthritis); (ii) evidence of preceding gastrointestinal or genitourinary infection (usually by *Shigella*, *Chlamydia*, or *Yersinia*), in the absence of clinical symptoms, and (iii) exclusion of other arthritides.

### *Miscellaneous Causes of Joint Involvement*

A small proportion of children with acute lymphocytic leukemia show bone and joint pains. Bone pain, which is more marked at night, is the predominant complaint in affected children. Hemogram shows lymphocytic predominance and thrombocytopenia, in contrast to a polymorphonuclear predominance and thrombocytosis characteristic of juvenile idiopathic arthritis (JIA). Bone marrow examination is required to confirm the diagnosis. X-linked agammaglobulinemia (Bruton disease) may sometimes present as an unusual aseptic 'arthritis' (due to *Mycoplasma* infection); accompanying sinopulmonary infection is usual. Arthritis can, at times, be the presenting complaint of hemophilia or human immunodeficiency virus infection.

Legg Calvé-Perthes disease is characterized by avascular necrosis of femoral head and usually affects children (boys: girls 5:1) between 5 and 10 years of age. It may be a manifestation of an underlying hypercoagulable state (hypofibrinolysis or deficiency of protein C or S). Familial occurrence is common, and condition is bilateral in 10% of patients. Affected children present with a painful limp. Initial X-rays may be normal. Isotope bone scans and magnetic resonance imaging are required to confirm the diagnosis. Subsequent X-rays show a characteristic sequential progression: (i) Widening of joint space, (ii) fragmentation of epiphysis with patchy areas of increased lucency or density, (iii) abnormalities of shape of femoral head and neck, and (iv) deformed head. Treatment options include femoral varus osteotomies or containment splints.

### *Non-inflammatory Arthropathy*

Several congenital disorders can have joint involvement and may be mistaken as arthritis. Affected children usually present with non-specific musculoskeletal features such as joint discomfort, contractures, or deformity of joints without any signs of inflammation. Common conditions include progressive pseudorheumatoid arthropathy, camptodactyly-arthropathy-coxa vara-pericarditis (CACP) syndrome, idiopathic multicentric osteolysis, and mucopolysaccharidoses. These disorders should be considered when there is symmetrical joint involvement without signs of inflammation, a history of similar illness in multiple family members, early onset of disease, progressive restriction of movement, joint contractures, and, at times, involvement of other organ systems.

## Juvenile Idiopathic Arthritis (JIA)

This term was proposed by the International League of Associations for Rheumatology (ILAR, 1995) to refer to a group of conditions characterized by chronic inflammatory changes of joints. The condition is defined as arthritis of one or more joints with onset <16 years of age and persisting for at least 6 weeks. It has the following subtypes.

i. Systemic
ii. Oligoarthritis: (a) persistent, (b) extended
iii. Polyarthritis: Rheumatoid factor negative
iv. Polyarthritis: Rheumatoid factor positive
v. Psoriatic arthritis
vi. Enthesitis-related arthritis
vii. Undifferentiated arthritis that (a) fits no other category; or (b) fits more than one category

JIA is not rare; the estimated pooled prevalence in Caucasian population is 32.6 (31.3–33.9)/100,000 population at risk. School based survey from North India has reported a prevalence of 48/100,000 children below 14 years. It is the commonest rheumatological disorder of childhood and one of the most common causes of disability, chronic morbidity, and school absenteeism. While Western studies suggest that JIA is more common in girls, female predominance is not marked in India.

Systemic JIA (sJIA) is now considered a separate disease altogether. It is classified as an autoinflammatory disorder in which the innate immune system is primarily affected, unlike other JIA types, which represent adaptive immunity defects. The ILAR definition for sJIA requires that fever be present for at least 2 weeks and should be accompanied by one or more of the following: Evanescent rash, generalized lymphadenopathy, hepatosplenomegaly, or serositis.

### Etiology

The immune system is intimately involved in evolution of JIA. HLA DR5 and DR8 are linked to early-onset oligoarthritis (seen more often in girls), B27 to late-onset oligoarthritis (seen more commonly in boys), and DR4, Dw4 and DR1 to rheumatoid factor positive polyarthritis. JIA is not a homogeneous disease, and the different subtypes may represent separate clinical conditions.

Etiopathogenesis of JIA remains an enigma. Several environmental triggers (e.g. infection with rubella virus, parvovirus B19, *M. tuberculosis*, *Mycoplasma pneumoniae* and enteric organisms, physical trauma or psychological stress) are linked to onset of JIA, but their exact role is not clear. Cytokines like tumor necrosis factor-α (TNF-α), IL-6, and IL-1 play an important role in pathogenesis of the disease. A number of autoantibodies (for instance, antinuclear antibody) may be seen in sera of patients. The classical IgM rheumatoid factor (RF) is almost never detectable in preschool children with JIA. Older girls with polyarticular small joint disease of the hands (especially involving the metacarpophalangeal and proximal interphalangeal joints) may, however, be RF positive.

### Clinical Subtypes

Three major types of onset are described according to the presentation during the first 6 months of disease, namely systemic JIA (with fever and rash), oligoarthritis (4 or fewer joints involved), and polyarthritis (more than 4 joints involved).

***Systemic JIA (sJIA):*** About 5–15% of patients with JIA may have an acute onset with systemic features. These systemic features may precede joint manifestations by weeks or months. Therefore, this condition should be considered in differential diagnosis of any child with prolonged fever. The illness can occur at any age (peak 1–5 years) and is more common in boys.

It begins as an intermittent fever with a characteristic twice-daily peak; fever is prominent in the evening. It is accompanied by an evanescent maculopapular truncal rash. The rash may be difficult to recognize in individuals with dark complexion. Affected children show marked irritability that decreases with subsidence of fever. Serosal involvement (in form of pericarditis or pleuritis) may be present. Hepatosplenomegaly and lymphadenopathy are common at presentation and can lead to diagnostic confusion. There is moderate neutrophilic leukocytosis, elevated ESR, and thrombocytosis. Rheumatoid factor is negative.

***Oligoarthritis:*** This is the most frequent type of JIA, accounting for approximately 60–70% of patients. Four or fewer joints (usually large) are affected during the first 6 months of disease. Joint swelling, rather than joint pain, is the usual complaint. Two subtypes are described:

i. ***Persistent:*** If number of affected joints continues to be 4.
ii. ***Extended:*** If number of affected joints exceeds 4 during the disease course.

Oligoarthritis is more common in young girls, typically 3–5 years. Asymmetric involvement of knee or ankle is characteristic. Small joints of hands and feet are usually not involved. Asymptomatic and potentially blinding, iridocyclitis can be seen in up to 25% of patients with early-onset oligoarthritis and is especially common in girls with antinuclear antibody (ANA) positivity.

***Polyarthritis:*** Polyarthritis occurs in 25–30% of patients and is more common in girls. Joint pain, out of proportion to the degree of joint swelling, is the usual complaint. Fever and malaise can be significant. Two subtypes are known:

i. ***Rheumatoid factor negative:*** This subtype may occur at any age in childhood and usually involves the knees, wrists, and hips. Small joints of hands and feet are less commonly affected, and rheumatoid nodules are not seen. Joint disease in this subtype of JIA is far less severe than that seen in rheumatoid factor positive patients.
ii. ***Rheumatoid factor positive:*** Age at onset is late childhood or early adolescence, and arthritis is symmetrical, additive, severe, and deforming. Typically it involves small joints of hands, especially the metacarpophalangeal and the proximal interphalangeal. Cervical spine and temporomandibular joints can also be affected. This subtype of JIA is somewhat similar phenotypically to adult-onset rheumatoid arthritis. Rheumatoid nodules are present in some patients and are a marker of potentially severe disease.

***Psoriatic arthritis:*** Psoriatic arthritis is said to be present when there is arthritis in association with either psoriasis or any two of the following features: Dactylitis, nail pitting, and psoriasis in a first-degree relative. Arthritis may precede, accompany or follow occurrence of psoriasis in children. Clinical features include simultaneous occurrence of small and large joint arthritis or involvement of distal interphalangeal joints.

***Enthesitis-related arthritis (ERA):*** ERA is more common in boys, typically older than 8 years. Asymmetric large joint (e.g., knee, ankle, hip) involvement of lower extremity is characteristic.

Several children are HLA B27 positive, and a proportion of these may go on to develop ankylosing spondylitis later in life. However, sacroiliitis and spondylitis are usually not significant until late adolescence. Self-limiting acute symptomatic iritis may occur in some patients, but it does not progress onto chronic iridocyclitis, characteristic of oligoarthritis in young girls. A family history of ankylosing spondylitis, psoriasis, Reiter disease, and low back pain may be present.

### Laboratory Investigations

It is important to recognize the differing patterns of joint involvement in various types of JIA (Table 22.3).

Synovial fluid aspiration for microscopy and culture is indicated in children with monoarthritis because septic arthritis might need to be excluded (Table 22.2). Complete blood counts should be requested, along with ESR. Children with acute lymphocytic leukemia may have an arthritic presentation. Bone marrow aspiration may be required, if

**Table 22.3:** Pattern of joint involvement with juvenile idiopathic arthritis (JIA)

| *JIA subtype* | *Clinical presentation* | *Remarks* |
|---|---|---|
| Oligoarticular JIA | Young girls (3–5 years)<br>≤4 joints<br>Lower limb predominance (usually knee) | ANA positivity<br>High risk for chronic asymptomatic uveitis<br>Need regular slit-lamp examinations |
| RF–ve polyarthritis | Young girls<br>Symmetric or asymmetric polyarthritis | ANA positivity associated with high risk of chronic asymptomatic uveitis<br>Genetic similarities to oligoarticular JIA |
| RF+ve polyarthritis | Adolescent girls<br>Multiple small and large joints; often symmetric; deforming arthritis | Prognosis poor in comparison to RF –ve polyarthritis<br>Phenotypic similarities to adult-onset rheumatoid arthritis<br>Uveitis is not common |
| Systemic JIA | No age and sex predilection<br>High grade fever, evanescent rash, generalized lymphadenopathy, hepatosplenomegaly, serositis | Fever is typically quotidian (touches baseline)<br>Monoarthritis is uncommon; knee, wrist and ankle are involved usually<br>Change in pattern of fever (continuous high-grade fever) along with rise in CRP and decline in ESR may herald the onset of macrophage activation syndrome |
| Enthesitis (HLA B27) related arthritis | Older boys (9–10 years)<br>Lower limb large joint asymmetric arthritis<br>Evidence of enthesitis | May present with acute symptomatic uveitis |
| Psoriatic arthritis | Bimodal age of presentation<br>Usually start as lower limb monoarthritis<br>Distal interphalangeal joint involvement | Dactylitis<br>Family history of psoriasis<br>Arthritis often precedes cutaneous manifestations<br>DIP involvement is a characteristic feature; seen in approximately 30–50% patients |

ANA antinuclear antibodies; DIP distal interphalangeal joint; RF rheumatoid factor

use of glucocorticoids is being contemplated for treatment of JIA.

C-reactive protein (CRP) measurement is a marker of disease activity. Plain radiographs of affected joints are obtained at the time of initial diagnosis and may be repeated to assess erosive disease. Screening for rheumatoid factor is not a useful test for diagnosis of arthritis in young children, but is an important prognostic factor when it is positive. Joint ultrasound is a point of care test to assess the disease activity, monitor the response to therapy, and ultrasound-guided intra-articular corticosteroid injections. MRI is useful in detection for synovitis, bone marrow edema, and damage to bone, cartilage, tendon, and ligaments. MRI is helpful in diagnosis, assessment of disease activity, and response to therapy.

### *Treatment*

Management of JIA is multidisciplinary. Physiotherapy and occupational therapy should be tailored to specific needs of an individual child in order to prevent deformities and facilitate 'mainstreaming' and rehabilitation. Physical therapy helps in relieving pain, maintenance of posture and joint mobility, improves muscle strength, and prevents fixed flexion deformities. All patients with JIA need to be assessed by an ophthalmologist so that uveitis is detected early and treated appropriately. Children with oligoarthritis need regular ophthalmological follow-up as uveitis can develop later. NSAIDs are required for symptomatic treatment. Conventional NSAIDs inhibit both isoforms of the enzyme cyclo-oxygenase, i.e. COX-1 (constitutive; mediates physiologic prostaglandin production necessary for gastrointestinal mucosal integrity and adequacy of renal blood flow) and COX-2 (inducible; mediates pathologic prostaglandin production, especially at sites of inflammation).

NSAIDs commonly used in children are naproxen and ibuprofen. Indomethacin is believed to be of particular use in ERA. Doses of commonly used NSAIDs are given in Table 22.4. All children with NSAIDs must be monitored for gastrointestinal adverse effects. Selective COX-2 inhibitors (e.g. rofecoxib, valdecoxib) have fewer gastrointestinal adverse effects but are not commonly used in children. Although the mechanism of action of all NSAIDs is the same, idiosyncratic responses are well known, and a given patient may respond to one agent and not to the other. Response to therapy is usually slow, and treatment must continue for at least 2–3 weeks before a decision to switch over to another agent is made.

**Table 22.4:** Anti-inflammatory doses of commonly used NSAIDs*

| | *Dose, mg/kg/day* | *Maximum dose, mg/day* | *Frequency of administration* |
|---|---|---|---|
| Naproxen | 15–20 | 750 | Twice daily |
| Ibuprofen | 35–45 | 2400 | Four times daily |
| Indomethacin | 1–2 | 150 | Three times daily |
| Diclofenac | 2–3 | 150 | Four times daily |

*The analgesic dose is usually half the anti-inflammatory dose

Disease-modifying anti-rheumatic drugs (DMARDs) need to be started in almost all children with polyarthritis. Weekly methotrexate (15–25 mg/$m^2$/week given subcutaneously or orally) is the mainstay of management of severe arthritis. Children tolerate methotrexate better than adults and have fewer adverse effects. Once the child is in stable remission (usually achieved after several months), the drug can be tapered to the minimum effective dose and then stopped. Methotrexate should always be given under close medical supervision. Periodic testing of liver functions is mandatory. Development of hepatic fibrosis, a dreaded adverse effect, is uncommon in children. Sulfasalazine (40–50 mg/kg/day) is effective in patients with ERA. Hydroxychloroquine is a useful adjunct and is often used along with methotrexate. Leflunomide, an inhibitor of pyrimidine synthesis, has also been used in patients with polyarthritis.



Intra-articular injections of glucocorticoids (usually triamcinolone) are the preferred therapy for children with oligoarthritis who do not respond to an initial trial of NSAIDs. Systemic glucocorticoids (usually oral prednisolone 1–2 mg/kg/day; occasionally intravenous methylprednisolone 10–30 mg/kg) in tapering doses are necessary for severe unremitting arthritis, systemic manifestations (e.g. pericarditis, myocarditis, vasculitis), and rapidly progressive disease. Prednisolone, when used in this manner, is usually given as bridge therapy for a few weeks while awaiting the clinical response to methotrexate.

Iridocyclitis warrants therapy with local steroid instillation and mydriatic eye drops. Weekly methotrexate therapy may be required for patients with severe uveitis.

Newer modalities of treatment include biological agents like anakinra (IL-1 receptor antagonist); canakinumab (monoclonal antibody to IL-1); tocilizumab (monoclonal antibody to IL6 receptor); infliximab, golimumab, and adalimumab (monoclonal antibodies to TNF-α); etanercept (recombinant soluble TNF receptor p75 fusion protein) and abatacept (inhibitor of T cell activation). Etanercept, infliximab, and adalimumab are powerful biological agents against TNF-α. While etanercept has been used in children with polyarthritis not responding to methotrexate, infliximab has been more commonly used in adults with spondyloarthropathy. Adalimumab is frequently used for progressive arthritis and is also useful for severe uveitis refractory to methotrexate. Tocilizumab and anakinra have found favor in children with severe forms of sJIA. While these biologics are now being increasingly used as first-line therapy in children with JIA, long-term safety of these products in children remains a matter of concern.

### *Course*

- Oligoarthritis usually has a good prognosis, but localized deformities can develop due to asymmetric growth of limbs. Children with ERA can develop spondylitis and sacroiliitis later, especially if they are HLA B27 positive.
- Children with rheumatoid factor positive polyarthritis have a disease pattern similar to adults and show erosive and deforming arthritis. Prognosis is better for seronegative polyarthritis as remissions are obtained more often, and residual joint lesions may be minimal.
- The course of sJIA can be extremely variable, and response to therapy is not always satisfactory.
- Inappropriately treated or untreated patients with JIA may develop flexion contractures of hips, knees, and elbows, resulting in permanent disability. Neck stiffness is an especially debilitating problem and can result in torticollis. Temporomandibular joint involvement results in restricted opening of the mouth and may require surgical intervention.

### *Complications*

Due to ongoing chronic inflammation, anemia is almost always present in children with persistent active arthritis, and serial hemoglobin levels mirror disease activity. Blood loss induced by NSAIDs can also be a contributory factor for anemia. Chronic anterior uveitis may be clinically silent and potentially blinding. Girls below 6 years with oligoarthritis and who have ANA positivity are at the highest risk of developing this complication.

Children with sJIA are especially prone to develop macrophage activation syndrome (MAS). This potentially fatal complication presents with unremitting fever, sudden onset icterus, bleeding tendency, leukopenia, thrombocytopenia, hypofibrinogenemia, elevated triglycerides, and raised ferritin levels. Prompt administration of intravenous methylprednisolone pulses can be life-saving. Use of cyclosporine along with pulse steroids is associated with early resolution of features of MAS.

Growth disturbances, limb length discrepancies, and joint contractures can be seen in children with long-standing disease. Growth failure may occur secondary to severe inflammation or treatment with glucocorticoids. Treatment with recombinant human growth hormone may be considered. Secondary amyloidosis is a rare complication that presents with asymptomatic proteinuria and hypoalbuminemia.

*Competencies:* **PE22.1; PE22.3**

## SYSTEMIC LUPUS ERYTHEMATOSUS

Systemic lupus erythematosus (SLE) is a multisystem autoimmune connective disorder, characterized by the presence of antinuclear antibodies (ANA). Clinical features are variable, and the course unpredictable. Childhood SLE is more severe and has a poorer prognosis than adult SLE. Marked female predominance characteristic of adult SLE may not be seen in young children.

### Diagnosis

Diagnosis of SLE is facilitated by classification criteria developed by both the European League Against Rheumatism (EULAR) and the American College of Rheumatology (ACR). The 2019 EULAR/ACR classification criteria for SLE include positive ANA as an obligatory entry criterion **(Box 22.1)**. Patients can be classified as lupus, if entry criterion is fulfilled and score is 10.

It is important to note that SLE remains a clinical diagnosis, and the criteria merely provide helpful

**Box 22.1: 2019 European League Against Rheumatism/American College of Rheumatology Classification Criteria for Systemic Lupus Erythematosus (SLE)**

Entry criterion of ANA positive at a titer of >1:80 on Hep2 cells or equivalent positive test essential

**Additive criteria**

- Do not count a criterion, if there is a more likely explanation than SLE
- Occurrence of criteria on at least one occasion is sufficient
- SLE classification requires at least one clinical criterion and >10 points
- Criteria need not to be present simultaneously
- Within each domain, only the highest weighted criterion is counted towards the total score

| Clinical domain and criteria | Score | Immunological domain and criteria | Score |
|---|---|---|---|
| *Constitutional* | 2 | *Antiphospholipid antibodies (any)* | 2 |
| Fever | | Anticardiolipin | |
| | | anti-$\beta_2$ glycoprotein 1 | |
| | | Lupus anticoagulant | |
| *Hematologic* | | *Complement proteins* | |
| Leukopenia | 3 | Low C3 or C4 | 3 |
| Thrombocytopenia | 4 | Low C3 and C4 | 4 |
| Autoimmune hemolysis | 4 | | |
| *Neuropsychiatric* | | *SLE-specific antibodies* | |
| Delirium | 2 | Anti-dsDNA, or | 6 |
| Psychosis | 3 | Anti-Smith antibody | |
| Seizures | 5 | | |
| *Mucocutaneous* | | | |
| Non-scarring alopecia | 2 | | |
| Oral ulcers | 2 | | |
| Subacute cutaneous or discoid lupus | 4 | | |
| Acute cutaneous lupus | 6 | | |
| *Serosal* | | | |
| Pleural or pericardial effusion | 5 | | |
| Acute pericarditis | 6 | | |
| *Musculoskeletal* | | | |
| Joint involvement | 6 | | |
| *Renal* | | | |
| Proteinuria 0.5 g/24 hours | 4 | | |
| Renal biopsy class II or V lupus nephritis | 8 | | |
| Renal biopsy class III or IV lupus nephritis | 10 | | |

guidelines for arriving at a diagnosis. In many patients, especially children, treatment may be initiated even when they do not fulfil the requisite criteria.

The malar rash, which is virtually pathognomonic of SLE, may not be apparent initially. It involves the cheek, bridge of nose, and lower eyelids but characteristically spares the nasolabial folds (Fig. 22.1a). Discoid lesions are rare in childhood-onset SLE. Oral ulcerations may involve the buccal mucosa or palate and are usually painless. Some children may have prominent frontal alopecia (Fig. 22.1b). Arthritis is generally mild and always non-erosive.

Renal involvement is a dreaded complication of SLE and one of the chief causes of mortality in children. Approximately 50% children with SLE can have renal involvement. As per 2003 criteria of the International Society of Nephrology/Renal Pathology Society (ISN/RPS) lupus nephritis is classified as follows: **Class I:** minimal

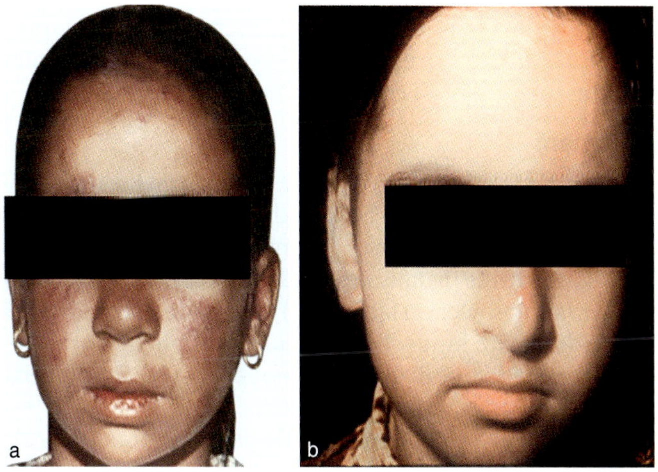


Fig. 22.1: Systemic lupus erythematosus. Note (a) Malar rash; (b) Frontal alopecia

mesangial; **Class II:** mesangial proliferative; **Class III:** focal proliferative; **Class IV:** diffuse proliferative; **Class V:** membranous; **Class VI:** advanced sclerosing. Renal biopsy is essential for therapeutic decision making. Class III and Class IV lesions (i.e. proliferative glomerulonephritis) require the most aggressive forms of therapy. The 2018 revision of the ISN/RPN classification for lupus nephritis has included the modified NIH lupus nephritis activity and chronicity scoring indices for better description of activity and chronicity of the disease.

Neurological features include psychosis, seizures, alterations in sensorium, focal deficits, and chorea. There may be no correlation between severity of clinical involvement and findings on neuroimaging. Hematologic abnormalities include Coombs positive hemolytic anemia, leukopenia, lymphopenia and thrombocytopenia. In addition, there may be coagulation abnormalities due to presence of antiphospholipid antibodies. Cardiac manifestations include pericarditis, myocarditis, or verrucous (Libman-Sacks) endocarditis. Other autoimmune diseases (e.g. autoimmune thyroid disease, celiac disease, and overlap syndromes) may coexist with lupus.

Early-onset lupus (<5 years age of onset) may have an underlying monogenic cause [e.g. deficiency of early complement components (C1q, C4), type I interferonopathies]. Clinical phenotype is characterized by more prominent skin and nervous system involvement. Affected children may be ANA positive and anti-double standard (ds) DNA negative.

### Laboratory Investigations

Acute phase reactants are usually elevated during disease activity. Typically, in patients with acute lupus ESR is increased, and CRP remains normal except in cases with infection, serositis, and arthritis where CRP levels can also be raised. Complements (C3 and C4) are usually low during disease activity.

#### *Serology*

Almost all patients with SLE have demonstrable ANA. Presence of anti-double stranded (anti-ds) DNA antibodies and anti-Smith (Sm) antibodies are highly specific of SLE; anti-dsDNA levels also correlate with disease activity. Antihistone antibodies are associated with drug-induced lupus. Anti-Ro antibodies are present in neonatal lupus especially those associated with congenital heart block.

### Treatment

Glucocorticoids and hydroxychloroquine form the mainstay of therapy. Prednisolone is started at doses of 1–2 mg/kg/day and tapered over several months, according to disease activity. Arthritis usually responds to NSAIDs. Sunscreens lotions (sun protection factor ≥30) need to be prescribed for all children with lupus. These should be applied 3–4 times/day at least 30 minutes prior to sun exposure. Sunscreens are necessary even on cloudy days.

Life-threatening complications (e.g. class III/IV lupus nephritis, myocarditis, encephalopathy) require intravenous pulses of methylprednisolone (30 mg/kg/day) for 3–5 days.

Induction therapy with monthly pulses of IV cyclophosphamide (500 mg/m$^2$) has improved the long-term outcome in children with severe forms of lupus nephritis. Once remission is achieved, the patient can be maintained on mycophenolate mofetil (MMF) or azathioprine. MMF is being increasingly used for induction therapy of severe forms of lupus nephritis in children. Rituximab, a monoclonal antibody to CD20, has also been found to be effective in some situations.

Low-dose prednisolone (2.5–5 mg/day) and hydroxychloroquine (5–6 mg/kg/day) may need to be continued for several years, depending on the clinical response. Infections must be treated aggressively with appropriate antimicrobials, and steroid doses increased during such episodes. With appropriate therapy, long-term outlook of SLE in children is encouraging.

### Antiphospholipid Syndrome

Antiphospholipid syndrome is a common accompaniment of SLE but can be seen in association with other rheumatological disorders as well. The syndrome can, at times, arise *de novo* when it is known as primary antiphospholipid syndrome. It is a common cause of acquired hypercoagulable states in children and presents with venous and arterial thrombosis, livedo reticularis, and thrombocytopenia. The presentation is sometimes 'catastrophic' and may result in rapid deterioration. Laboratory diagnosis may be suggested by a typical coagulation profile (normal prothrombin and prolonged partial thromboplastin times) and confirmed by detection of anticardiolipin antibodies (IgM and IgG), anti-β2 glycoprotein 1 antibodies (IgM and IgG) and lupus anticoagulant test. Treatment is with long-term oral anticoagulation. All patients with childhood onset of lupus should be screened for antiphospholipid antibodies at baseline and annually thereafter.

*Competency:* **PE22.1**

## JUVENILE DERMATOMYOSITIS

Juvenile dermatomyositis (JDM) is not merely a disorder of muscle and skin but a multisystem disease characterized by nonsuppurative inflammation of striated muscle and skin and systemic vasculopathy. Unlike adults, pure polymyositis (i.e. with no accompanying skin involvement) is uncommon in children. The diagnosis of JDM can be made on basis of the following criteria (1975):

i. Characteristic heliotrope discoloration over the upper eyelids **(Fig. 22.2a)** or a scaly, erythematous rash over dorsal aspects of metacarpophalangeal and proximal interphalangeal joints (Gottron papules; **Fig. 22.2b**)
ii. Symmetrical proximal muscle weakness
iii. Elevated levels of muscle enzymes (creatine kinase, alanine and aspartate aminotransferases, aldolase)
iv. Electromyographic evidence of myopathy
v. Muscle biopsy showing myonecrosis, myophagocytosis, and perifascicular atrophy

A 'definite' diagnosis of JDM can be made, if a child fulfils the first criterion along with any 3 of the remaining

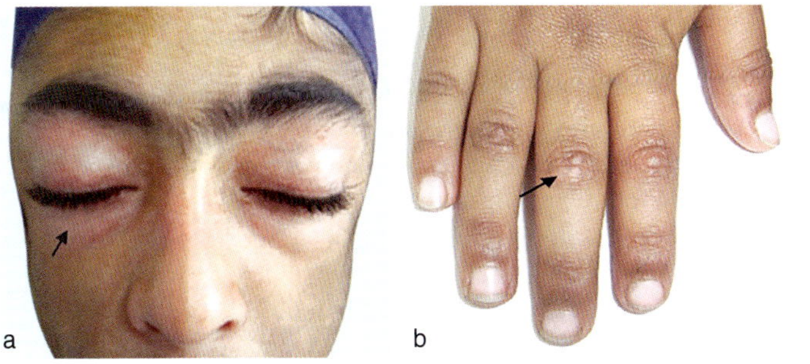

Fig. 22.2: Juvenile dermatomyositis. Note: (a) Heliotrope rash; (b) Gottron papules

4 and it is considered 'probable' if two of the four criteria are met. Other dermatological changes include edema over eyelids, photosensitivity, truncal rash, and calcinosis.

Muscle biopsy and electromyography are invasive procedures and are rarely required for diagnosis. Magnetic resonance imaging (MRI) shows characteristic hyperintense signals on T2-weighted images suggestive of muscle edema and inflammation, while T1-weighted images may show fibrosis, atrophy, and fatty infiltration. Although MRI is not a part of criteria, in clinical practice, it is widely used for assessment of muscle inflammation and extent of disease.

The EULAR/ACR (2017) have recently provided classification criteria for adult and juvenile idiopathic inflammatory myopathies (IIM). The criteria provide a score based upon: Age of onset (age <18 for juvenile IIM), cutaneous manifestations, muscle weakness, dysphagia, laboratory features (elevated muscle enzymes, presence of anti-Jo-1 autoantibodies), and muscle biopsy characteristics.

Detection of myositis-specific autoantibodies (e.g. anti-TIF-1γ, anti-NXP2, anti-MDA5, anti-Mi-2, antisynthetase) is helpful in prediction of clinical phenotypes and prognostication in these patients. Nail fold capillaroscopy is useful adjunct to assess the disease activity (Fig. 22.3a and b).

Treatment is with pulse intravenous methylprednisolone (30 mg/kg/day) for 3–5 days followed by gradually tapering doses of oral prednisolone (1.5–2 mg/kg/day). Weekly methotrexate (15–25 mg/m$^2$/week given subcutaneously or orally) is the standard maintenance therapy. Usual duration of therapy is 18–24 months. Rapid tapering of steroids may result in disease relapse. Calcinosis and lipodystrophy are important complications in children with JDM and usually develop during the course of the disease. The long-term prognosis is excellent, if treatment is started early.

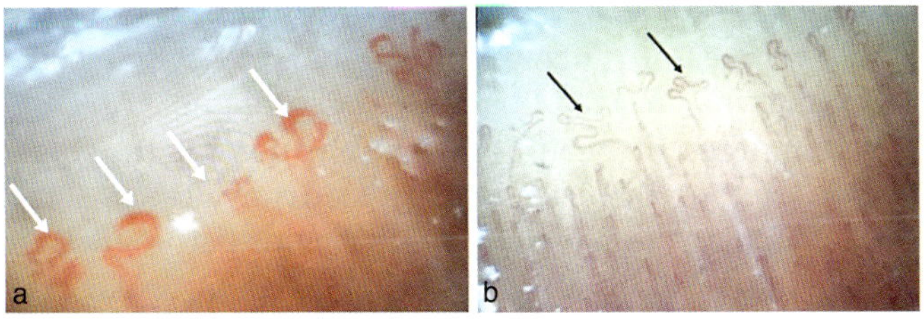

Fig. 22.3: Nailfold capillaroscopy findings in a patient with juvenile dermatomyositis showing: (a) Dilated capillaries; (b) Architectural disorganization of capillaries

## SCLERODERMA

Scleroderma is a complex rare connective tissue disorder associated with hardening and tightening of skin. Scleroderma in children can be classified as follows:

i. Juvenile systemic sclerosis (JSSc) (e.g. diffuse cutaneous, limited cutaneous)
ii. Juvenile localized scleroderma (JLS) (e.g. morphea, linear scleroderma, eosinophilic fasciitis)

While localized scleroderma is typically confined to the cutaneous manifestations, systemic sclerosis can have widespread involvement. Diffuse cutaneous systemic scleroderma is usually associated with widespread visceral involvement, including the gastrointestinal tract, heart, lungs, and kidneys. It is believed that fetomaternal graft-versus-host reactions are involved in pathogenesis of this condition. Onset of disease is insidious and may be difficult to recognize in initial stages. The child presents with skin tightening (edema, atrophy, and acrosclerosis), Raynaud phenomenon (i.e. blanching, cyanosis, and erythema), soft tissue contractures, arthralgias and myalgias, dysphagia (regurgitation, reflux, and aspiration), dyspnea (interstitial fibrosis, low diffusing capacity) and characteristic subcutaneous calcifications. Many children have abnormalities of nailfold capillaries that can be seen as capillary dropouts and dilated loops with a nail-bed capillaroscope or +40 lens of an ophthalmoscope. Onset of hypertension and proteinuria usually indicates renal involvement and should be a cause for concern.

Investigations show presence of ANA (with nucleolar pattern on immunofluorescence) and antibodies to Scl70 (DNA-topoisomerase1) or centromere. Timely diagnosis and early identification of internal organ involvement leading to specific therapy results in better outcomes. Methotrexate, MMF, and low-dose corticosteroids can be used for skin disease. Monthly pulses of intravenous cyclophosphamide (followed by maintenance daily azathioprine or MMF or weekly methotrexate) can be life-saving in patients with interstitial lung disease. Nifedipine is useful for managing Raynaud phenomenon, while enalapril is useful for controlling blood pressure and stabilizing renal functions. The latter is also the drug of choice for scleroderma renal crises. Phosphodiesterase-5 inhibitors (e.g. sildenafil) and endothelin receptor antagonists (e.g. bosentan) can be used for digital ulcers and pulmonary hypertension. With appropriate management, 10-year survival rates of up to 90% have been reported in children.

### Differential Diagnoses

i. Overlap syndromes
ii. Localized scleroderma
iii. Chemically induced scleroderma (e.g. with polyvinyl chloride, pentazocine, bleomycin)
iv. Pseudosclerodermas (e.g. phenylketonuria, scleredema, progeria, porphyria cutanea tarda)

Scleredema is a benign, self-limiting condition characterized by non-pitting indurated edema over the face, neck, shoulders, and chest, excluding the hands and feet. It is clinically distinct from scleroderma.

## MIXED CONNECTIVE TISSUE DISEASE

This is a multisystemic overlap syndrome characterized by features of juvenile idiopathic arthritis, systemic scleroderma, SLE, and dermatomyositis occurring in conjunction with high titers of anti-ribonucleoprotein (RNP) antibodies (specific for U1 RNP). Nephritis is usually less common and less severe than in SLE. Patients show good response to low-dose glucocorticoids and NSAIDs. Oral weekly methotrexate is a useful therapeutic option. Treatment must be individualized and should focus on the disease component that predominates in a given child.

*Competencies:* **PE22.1; PE22.3**





## VASCULITIDES

Childhood vasculitis can be classified according to the size of the vessel involved:

i. Predominately large vessel (i.e. aorta and major branches) vasculitis, e.g. Takayasu arteritis
ii. Predominately medium vessel (i.e. coronary, renal, hepatic, mesenteric) vasculitis, e.g. Kawasaki disease, polyarteritis nodosa
iii. Predominately small vessel (i.e. arterioles, capillaries, venules) vasculitis
   a. ANCA associated vasculitis [granulomatosis with polyangiitis (GPA), microscopic polyangiitis (MPA), eosinophilic granulomatosis with polyangiitis (EGPA)]
   b. Immune complex small vessel vasculitis (IgA vasculitis, cryoglobulinemic vasculitis, antiglomerular basement membrane disease, hypocomplementemic urticarial vasculitis)
iv. Other vasculitides: Behcet disease, Cogan syndrome, vasculitis secondary to infections (e.g. hepatitis B, hepatitis C), vasculitis associated with connective tissue disease (e.g. lupus vasculitis), and single organ vasculitis (cutaneous leukocytoclastic angiitis, primary central nervous system vasculitis)

### Takayasu Arteritis

Takayasu arteritis (TA) is characterized by a segmental inflammatory panarteritis resulting in stenosis and aneurysms of aorta and its major branches, causing weak arterial pulses. Typically, these patients present with constitutional symptoms (fever, weight loss, early fatigue), hypertension, and elevated acute-phase inflammatory markers. It is classified according to the site of involvement: Type I: aortic arch; Type IIa: ascending aorta, aortic arch and its branches; Type IIb: ascending aorta, aortic arch and its branches, descending thoracic aorta; Type III: descending thoracic aorta, abdominal aorta, and/or renal arteries; Type IV: abdominal aorta and/or renal arteries; Type V: a combination of type IIb and IV. Children with TA often show a strongly positive tuberculin reaction. The classification criteria for childhood TA are given in **Box 22.2**.

**Box 22.2: Classification Criteria for Childhood Takayasu Arteritis**

Angiographic abnormalities (conventional, CT, or MRI) of the aorta or its main branches and pulmonary arteries, plus at least one of the following 5 features:

- Decreased peripheral artery pulse(s) and/or claudication of extremities
- Blood pressure difference between four limbs >10 mm Hg
- Bruits over aorta and/or its major branches
- Hypertension
- Acute phase reactants (ESR >20 mm/hr or CRP more than upper limit of normal)

Diagnosis of TA is confirmed by CT angiography. Management of patients with TA includes immunosuppression, antihypertensive, antiplatelet agents, and surgical vascular interventions. Long-term immunosuppression with prednisolone and methotrexate (used in weekly doses) is warranted. Cyclophosphamide or azathioprine may be required in children who fail to show an adequate response to steroids. MMF has also been found to be useful. Angioplasty procedures are increasingly being performed, even in small children and show promising results. Biologics (e.g. IL-6 blocker: tocilizumab) are frequently used in severe or refractory disease. Hypertension needs to be managed appropriately.

### Kawasaki Disease

Kawasaki disease (KD) is an acute febrile mucocutaneous lymph node syndrome mainly affecting infants and young children. More than 80% of cases are seen in children under 5 years. It is the commonest vasculitic disorder of childhood and has replaced acute rheumatic fever as the leading cause of acquired heart disease in children in many countries. The basic lesion is a necrotizing vasculitis of medium-sized muscular arteries (especially coronaries), which may result in aneurysms, dilatations, and stenoses in untreated patients. In Japan, 1% of all children would develop KD before they reach 10 years of age. In India, this condition is now being increasingly recognized, but the vast majority of patients continue to remain undiagnosed, probably because of lack of awareness.

It is important to remember that the diagnosis of KD is based entirely on recognition of a temporal sequence of characteristic clinical findings **(Fig. 22.4)** and that there is no specific laboratory test. The diagnostic criteria for KD are as follows:

a. Fever lasting for at least 5 days
b. Presence of any 4 of the following 5 conditions:
   i. Bilateral nonpurulent conjunctival injection (without discharge)
   ii. Changes of mucosae of oropharynx (e.g. injected pharynx, injected lips, strawberry tongue)
   iii. Changes of peripheral extremities (acute stage: edema, erythema of hands or feet; convalescent stage: desquamation, which usually begins periungual)
   iv. Polymorphous rash (never bullous or vesicular)
   v. Cervical lymphadenopathy (at least 1 node 1.5 cm; usually unilateral)
c. Illness not explained by any other known disease process.

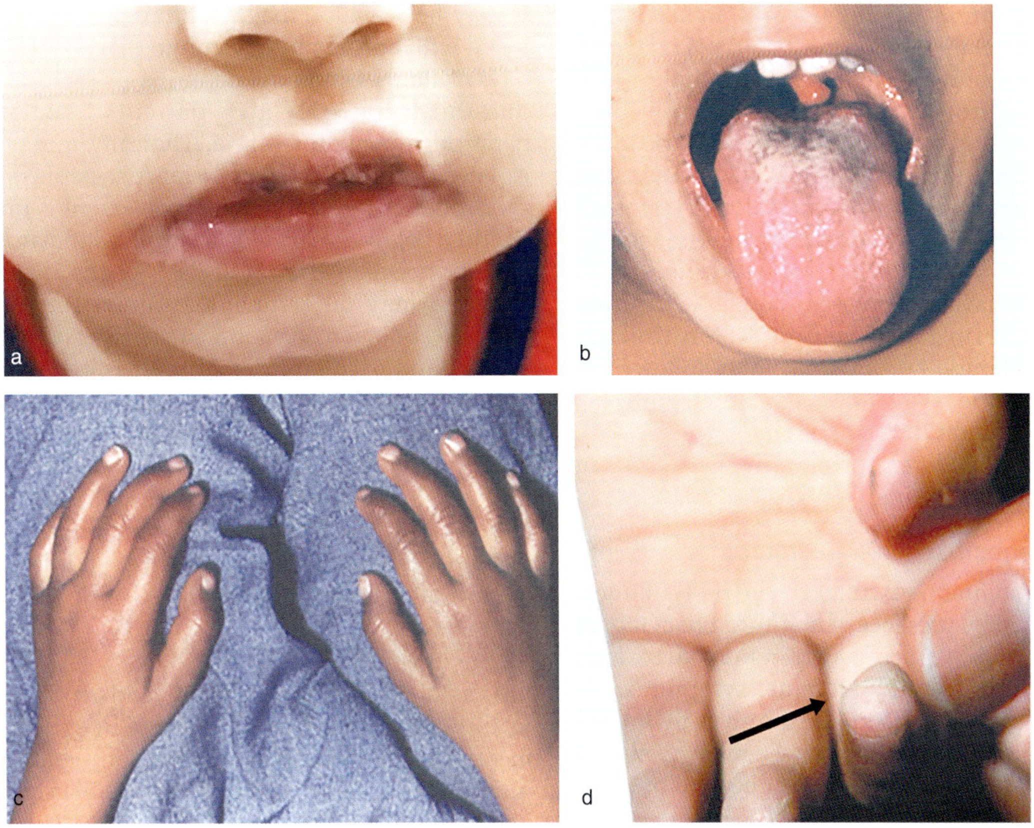

**Fig. 22.4:** Findings in acute phase of Kawasaki disease, showing: (a) Red cracked lips; (b) Strawberry tongue; (c) Swelling on dorsum of hands; (d) Periungual desquamation

These clinical features evolve sequentially over a period of days, and all need not be present together at a given point of time. This partly explains the difficulty that the clinician experiences in arriving at a correct diagnosis. The 2017 American Heart Association guidelines for KD have highlighted that presence of one or more principal clinical manifestations of disease that can be revealed on history but have disappeared by the time of presentation to the hospital should be considered for diagnosis. Most children have high grade fever and are extremely irritable. In fact, this irritability often provides the first clinical clue to diagnosis, especially in infants. Other characteristic findings include perianal desquamation (in first few days of fever) and reactivation of BCG scar, usually seen in infants). Arthritis is often seen in children with KD and may result in diagnostic confusion. Hydrops of gallbladder can also occur. Sterile pyuria is common and may lead to an erroneous diagnosis of urinary tract infection in presence of fever.

KD must be considered in differential diagnosis of all children, especially those below 5-year-old, who have fever without apparent focus lasting more than 5 days. Thrombocytosis with periungual peeling is characteristic of second week of illness. Beau lines may be seen during the convalescent phase (Fig. 22.5).

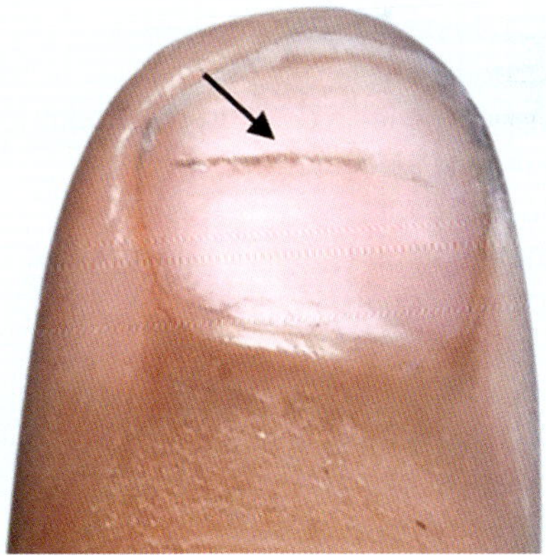

**Fig. 22.5:** Beau line in Kawasaki disease

Treatment is with a single dose of intravenous immunoglobulin (IVIg) (2 g/kg) and aspirin in anti-inflammatory doses (30–50 mg/kg) until the child becomes afebrile. Low dose aspirin (3–5 mg/kg/day) is then continued for 4–6 weeks for its antiplatelet activity. Approximately, 10–20% of patients with KD remains refractory to this treatment and may require second line treatment (second dose of IVIg, infliximab, or corticosteroids). Pre-emptive augmentation of therapy is required in children with severe forms of KD, evolving coronary artery abnormalities, and/or KD in infants. In appropriately treated children, the long-term prognosis is excellent. Coronary artery abnormalities may develop in 3–5% of children with KD even after treatment. Left untreated 15–25% children with KD develop coronary artery abnormalities.

## Polyarteritis Nodosa

Polyarteritis nodosa (PAN) is rare in childhood. Clinical manifestations can be extremely variable because of multisystem involvement and include fever, hypertension (seen in 80%), abdominal pain, arthritis, myalgia, skin involvement (especially livedo reticularis, Fig. 22.6a), neurological involvement (seizures, encephalopathy), and peripheral neuropathy (mononeuritis multiplex). Pathological diagnosis consists of demonstration of fibrinoid necrosis in medium-sized arteries with segmental involvement and a predilection for bifurcation of vessels. On angiography, aneurysms may be demonstrable in the renal arteries or celiac axis (Fig. 22.6b). The classification criteria for childhood PAN have been revised (Box 22.3). Treatment consists of long-term immunosuppression (initially with cyclophosphamide and prednisolone, followed by azathioprine, methotrexate, or MMF). Children with early onset PAN, vasculopathy, livedo reticularis, and recurrent stroke should be considered for underlying monogenic deficiency of adenosine deaminase type 2 (DADA2).

### IgA Vasculitis (Henoch-Schönlein Purpura)

IgA vasculitis is a common vasculitic disorder of childhood and is characterized by presence of non-thrombocytopenic and usually palpable purpura, transient arthralgia (occasionally, arthritis), and abdominal symptoms. The criteria for diagnosis of childhood HSP are given in Box 22.4.

The illness begins with a purpuric rash more prominent over the extensor aspects of lower extremities and buttocks. It may be macular, maculopapular, or even urticarial to begin with and can be difficult to diagnose in the first few days of illness. Glomerulonephritis is seen in approximately one-third, but only 10% patients have azotemia or nephrotic range proteinuria. Clinically, it may manifest as isolated hematuria, hypertension, or a nephritic/nephrotic syndrome. Significant renal involvement is uncommon in children below 6 years old. Gastrointestinal manifestations usually occur in first 7–10 days of the illness. Affected children may be erroneously diagnosed as having a 'surgical abdomen'. Abdominal pain is usually intermittent, colicky, and periumbilical. Vomiting occurs in about 60% of patients, but hematemesis and malena are less common. Intussusception (ileoileal or ileocolic) can be seen in the acute phase.

Most clinical features of IgA vasculitis are self-limiting and resolve in a few days. Rare manifestations include CNS vasculitis, coma, Guillain-Barré syndrome, pulmonary hemorrhage, carditis, and orchitis.

#### *Laboratory Investigations*

IgA vasculitis is a clinical diagnosis, and none of the laboratory features are pathognomonic. There may be a nonspecific increase in total serum IgA levels. Many children may have microscopic hematuria and proteinuria. Skin biopsy from the involved sites shows leukocytoclastic vasculitis. On direct immunofluorescence, there are deposits of IgA in skin as

**Box 22.3: Classification Criteria for Childhood Polyarteritis Nodosa**

A childhood illness characterized by the presence of either a biopsy showing small and midium-size artery necrotizing vasculitis or angiographic abnormalities (aneurysms or occlusions), plus at least one of the following:

- Skin involvement (livido reticularis, skin nodules, skin infarcts)
- Myalgia or muscle tenderness
- Systemic hypertension
- Abnormal urinalysis and/or impaired renal function
- Mononeuropathy or polyneuropathy

**Box 22.4: Classification Criteria for IgA Vasculitis**

Palpable purpura with at least one of the following:

- Diffuse abdominal pain
- Biopsy showing leukocytoclastic vasculitis with predominant IgA deposition
- Arthritis or arthralgia
- Renal involvement (any hematuria and/or proteinuria)

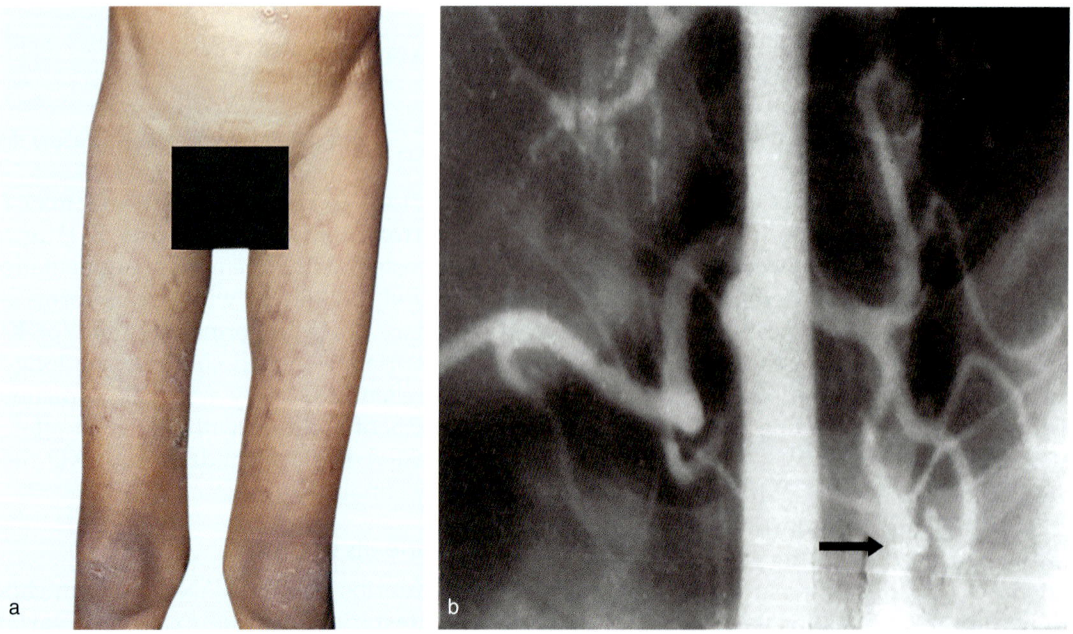


Fig. 22.6: Findings in polyarteritis nodosa include: (a) Livedo reticularis; (b) Microaneurysms (black arrow) on angiography

well as renal biopsies. Ultrasound examinations may need to be repeated for evolving abdominal findings.

#### *Treatment*

Management is generally supportive with maintenance of hydration and pain relief. Glucocorticoids are required in children with severe gastrointestinal involvement, orchitis, central nervous system involvement, and pulmonary hemorrhage. Oral prednisolone (1–1.5 mg/kg/day) is usually started and is continued for 2–3 weeks (in gradually tapering doses) depending on the clinical response. In severe cases, intravenous pulse steroids may be considered. There is, however, no clear evidence that steroids alter the natural course of disease. Nephritis due to IgA vasculitis may need aggressive management with immunosuppressants (prednisolone and azathioprine) (*see* Chapter 17).

#### *Prognosis*

The disease usually runs its entire course in 4 weeks, and majority of children have no permanent sequelae even when the short-term morbidity is quite significant. Children older than 6 years with significant kidney involvement (especially children with rapidly progressive glomerulonephritis and crescents) need to be closely followed up; their long-term prognosis may be unsatisfactory. Overall, 1–5% of children with nephritis due to IgA vasculitis show progressive kidney failure.

### Granulomatosis with Polyangiitis (Wegener Granulomatosis)

This condition is characterized by necrotizing granulomatous angiitis affecting the respiratory tract and kidneys. It is rare in children. Constitutional symptoms are quite prominent. Presence of anti-neutrophil cytoplasmic antibodies (ANCAs), especially c-ANCA, is virtually pathognomonic. With steroids and cyclophosphamide and occasionally IVIg, the long-term outlook is satisfactory. Intravenous rituximab has also been found useful.

### Behçet Disease

This is an uncommon condition with variable clinical manifestations.

i. *Major:* Aphthous stomatitis, genital ulceration, cutaneous manifestations, and ocular disease
ii. *Minor:* Gastrointestinal disease, thrombophlebitis, arthritis, family history and neurological involvement.

Behçet disease is characterized by multiple relapses with significant disability from ocular and neurological manifestations. Widespread thrombosis (venous and arterial) of large vessels may be life-threatening. Many patients show a positive pathergy test (cutaneous pustular reaction following needle pricks). HLAB5 and B51 haplotypes have been associated with this syndrome. Drug therapy involves use of colchicine and thalidomide. Methotrexate and chlorambucil have also been used.

### Autoinflammatory Disorders

These include a unique set of heterogeneous clinical conditions that results from defects of innate immunity. These disorders are characterized by recurrent or persistent generalized inflammation in the absence of infections or autoimmunity. Acute phase reactants are elevated during disease flares. In contrast to autoimmune diseases, high titer autoantibodies are usually absent. Common clinical manifestations include periodic or recurrent fever, rash, arthritis, abdominal pain, serositis, uveitis, and central nervous system involvement. Conditions that are categorized as autoinflammatory disorders include systemic JIA, familial Mediterranean fever, tumor necrosis factor receptor associated period syndrome (TRAPS), mevalonate kinase deficiency, NLRP3-associated autoinflammatory disease (also known as cryopyrin associated periodic syndrome), periodic fever–aphthous stomatitis–pharyngitis and adenitis (PFAPA) syndrome, hyper-IgD syndrome, deficiency of interleukin-1 receptor antagonist, Blau syndrome, deficiency of adenosine deaminase type 2, STING associated vasculopathy with onset in infancy (SAVI), and haploinsufficiency of A20. Diagnoses of these disorders are usually based on genetic sequencing. Treatment depends upon the specific cause.

### Suggested Reading


1. Aringer M, Costenbader K, Daikh D, et al. 2019 European League Against Rheumatism/American College of Rheumatology classification criteria for systemic lupus erythematosus. Ann Rheum Dis 2019;78(9):1151–59.
2. Lundberg IE, Tjarnlund A, Bottai M, et al. 2017 European League Against Rheumatism/American College of Rheumatology classification criteria for adult and juvenile idiopathic inflammatory myopathies and their major subgroups. Ann Rheum Dis 2017;76(12):1955–64.
3. Ozen S, Ruperto N, Dillon MJ, et al. EULAR/PRES endorsed consensus criteria for the classification of childhood vasculitis. Ann Rheum Dis 2006; 65:936–41.
4. Pilania RK, Bhattarai D, Singh S. Controversies in diagnosis and management of Kawasaki disease. World J Clin Pediatr 2018;7(1):27–35.
5. Pilania RK, Singh S. Rheumatology panel in pediatric practice. Indian Pediatr 2019; 56(5): 407–14.
6. Ravelli A, Consolaro A, Horneff G, et al. Treating juvenile idiopathic arthritis to target: recommendations of an international task force. Ann Rheum Dis 2018;77(6):819–28.
7. Singh S, Vignesh P, Burgner D. The epidemiology of Kawasaki disease: A global update. Arch Dis Child 2015; 100:1084–88.

Chapter 23

# Genetic Disorders

❍ Neerja Gupta ❍ Madhulika Kabra

## CHROMOSOMES AND GENES

Of 23 pairs of human chromosomes, the two members of 22 pairs that are apparently alike (or homologous) are called autosomes. The 23rd pair is homologous only in females with two X chromosomes. In males, the 23rd pair has one X chromosome and a much smaller Y chromosome. Each chromosome has a short arm (p) and a long arm (q) joined by a centromere (Fig. 23.1). Based on the position of the centromere, chromosomes are categorized as metacentric (centromere in the middle), submetacentric (centromere distant from center) and acrocentric (centromere at the end). Chromosomes are numbered based on their size and position of the centromere.

Chemically, the chromosomes are made up of deoxyribonucleic acid (DNA) and histones. Only about 3% of DNA in the human genome symbolizes genes; the rest does not have a clear-cut function (often termed junk DNA) though it is increasingly becoming evident that many regions of noncoding DNA play a role in controlling the gene function. There are about 20000–25000 genes in the human genome, each gene being the functional unit of heredity. Gene is a sequence of several nucleotides, and its position on a chromosome is called its locus. Each individual has two

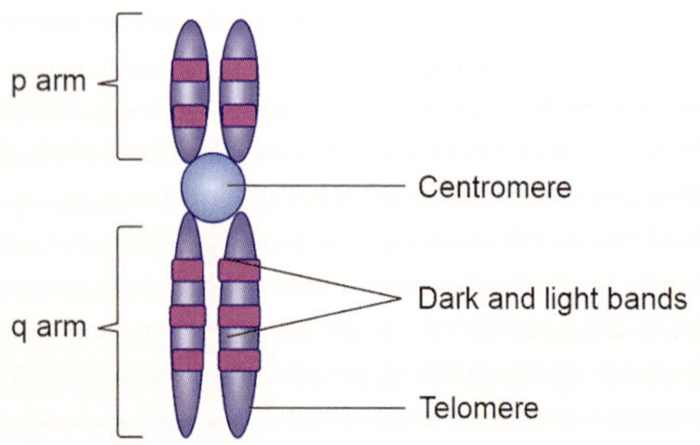


Fig. 23.1: Schematic structure of a chromosome

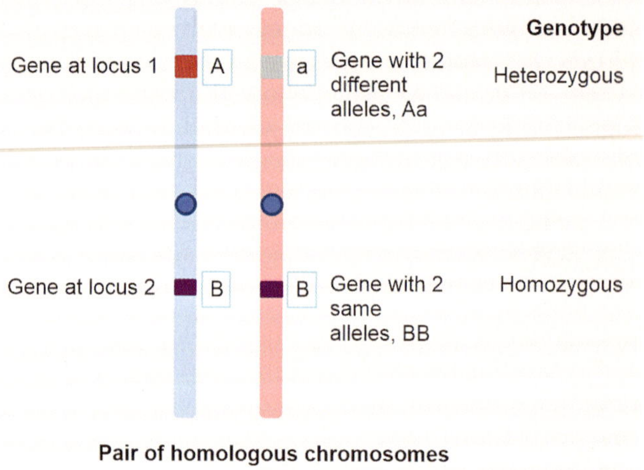


Fig. 23.2: Concept of locus, gene, allele and genotype

copies of genes on the two parental chromosomes (one each from mother and father). Alternative forms of a gene are known as alleles (Fig. 23.2). Presence of a pair of identical alleles for a particular gene is known as homozygous; if they are nonidentical, then it is a heterozygous state. If an allele clinically manifests itself even in the heterozygous state, it is called *dominant*, however, if it exerts its phenotypic effect only in homozygous state, then it is called *recessive*. The genetic makeup of an individual is called the genotype and the sum of observable characteristics is termed as phenotype. Occurrence of more than one allele at a locus each having a frequency of at least 1% is known as genetic polymorphism.

### Genetics and Disease

Most diseases have probable genetic and environmental basis. The genetic component may be the major or the only factor leading to manifestation(s) of the disease, or it may merely predispose the individual to get a disease in response to environmental stresses. Based on genetic mechanism, genetic disorders may be of five types: (i) Chromosomal disorders, (ii) single gene/monogenic disorders, (iii) polygenic disorders, (iv) mitochondrial disorders, and (v) somatic cell disorders.

*Competency:* **PE32.3**

## CHROMOSOMAL DISORDERS

Surveys in still-born or abortuses show chromosomal anomalies in a large proportion. Five of 1000 live newborns have chromosomal anomaly. There are two types of chromosomal abnormalities—numerical (aneuploidies) and structural.

### Mechanisms of Chromosomal Anomalies

Chromosomes contain a large number of genes. Loss or gain of a whole chromosome due to abnormalities in cell division may cause profound disturbances in the genetic constitution of the fetus and affect its survival. Depending upon the type of abnormality, the chromosome involved and the type of imbalance, there may be an early pregnancy loss, stillbirth, neonatal death, malformations or intellectual disability. At times, only a part of the chromosome may be deleted, causing less severe genetic disturbances. Generally, loss of a whole chromosome, except the X chromosome (as in Turner syndrome), is lethal.

Aneuploidies result from failure of chromosomes to separate normally during cell division. This phenomenon is known as nondisjunction. Nondisjunction during meiosis I leads to formation of disomic or nullisomic gametes, resulting in trisomic and monosomic zygotes, respectively; nondisjunction during meiosis II results in monosomic, disomic and nullisomic gametes, leading to disomic (46 chromosomes), trisomic (47 chromosomes) and monosomic (45 chromosomes) zygotes, respectively, as shown in Fig. 23.3. Nondisjunction may occur in maternal or paternal germ cells, but is more common in the former and with increasing age. Common aneuploidies in live born babies include Down syndrome (trisomy 21), Edward syndrome (trisomy 18), Patau syndrome (trisomy 13, Fig. 23.4) and Turner syndrome (monosomy X).

***Mosaicism:*** If nondisjunction occurs in the first mitotic division instead of meiosis, of the two new cells formed, one has 47 chromosomes and the other has 45 chromosomes. The error is perpetuated by repeated mitotic divisions. Thus, two cell lines with 47 and 45 chromosomes are observed in the same individual. If the nondisjunction occurs after a few mitotic divisions have already occurred, more than two cell lines are observed, some with normal and others with abnormal complement of chromosomes.

### Structural Chromosome Abnormalities

Chief types of structural chromosome abnormalities are: (i) Translocation, (ii) inversion, (iii) deletion, (iv) duplication, (v) ring chromosome, and (vi) isochromosomes.

***Translocation* (Fig. 23.5):** A chromosome or segment of a chromosome may break off from the parent chromosome and join another chromosome, in a process called translocation. One chromosome may appear shortened in this process. If no loss or gain of the genetic material occurs, the translocation is balanced and the person is phenotypically normal. Translocated chromosome may be transmitted to either gamete during meiosis, such that when it mates with a normal gamete, the resulting zygote may have either excess or deficiency of the genetic material. Such an offspring is abnormal. Viability of such zygotes would depend on the essentiality of the genes carried on translocated portion of the chromosome.

***Deletion* (Fig. 23.6):** A segment of chromosome may break off and be lost. Loss of a portion of chromosomal material large enough to be seen by light microscope is often lethal or poorly tolerated. Smaller deletions which are not visible under the microscope are referred to as microdeletions. Gene deletion syndromes are characterized

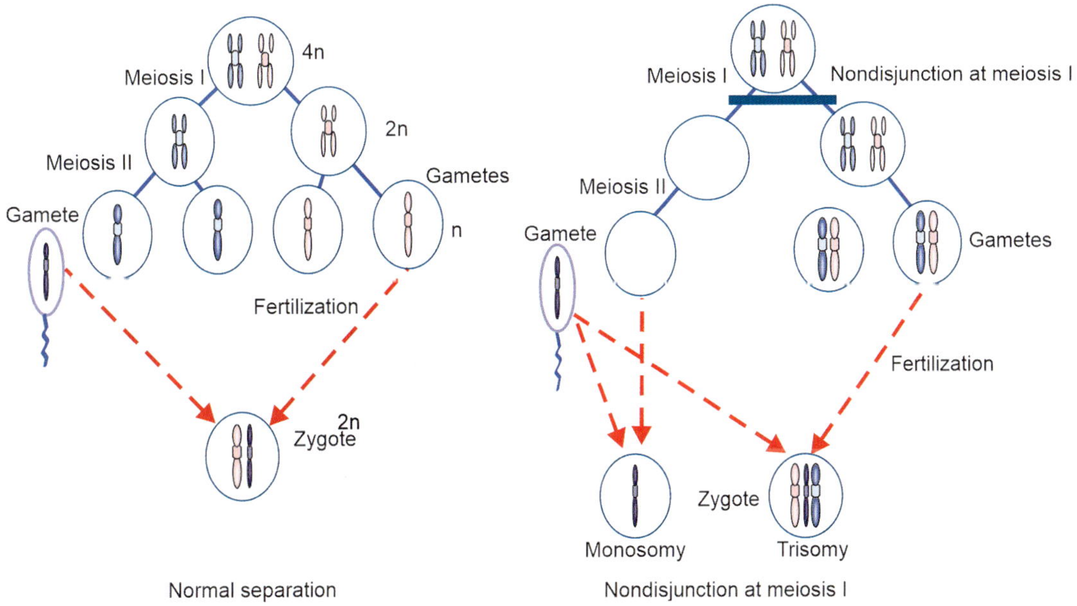


**Fig. 23.3:** (a) Normal separation; (b) Nondisjunction of chromosomes

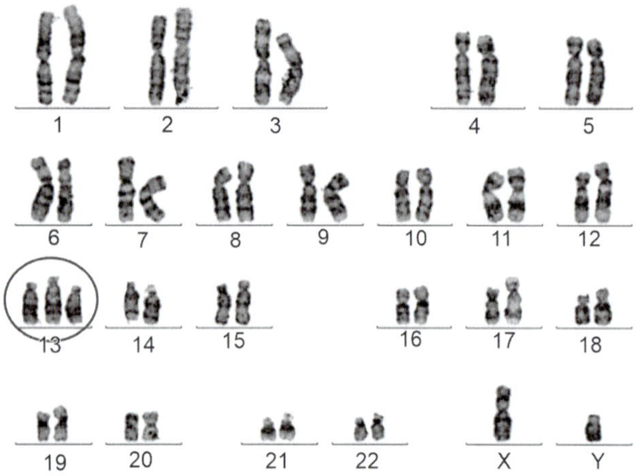


**Fig. 23.4:** Aneuploidy of chromosome 13 (trisomy 13)

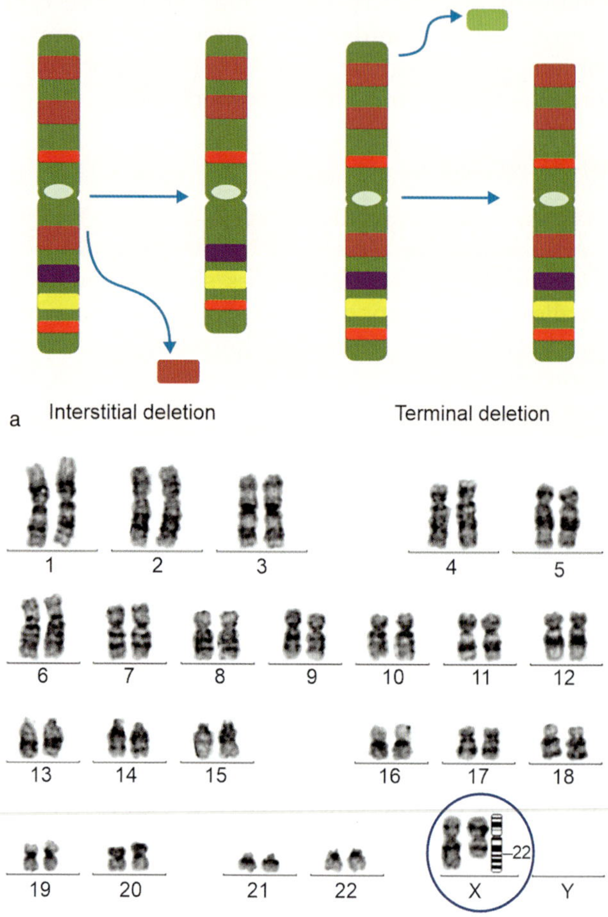


**Fig. 23.6:** (a) Schematic diagram of deletion; (b) Karyotype with deletion of long arm of X chromosome (Turner syndrome)

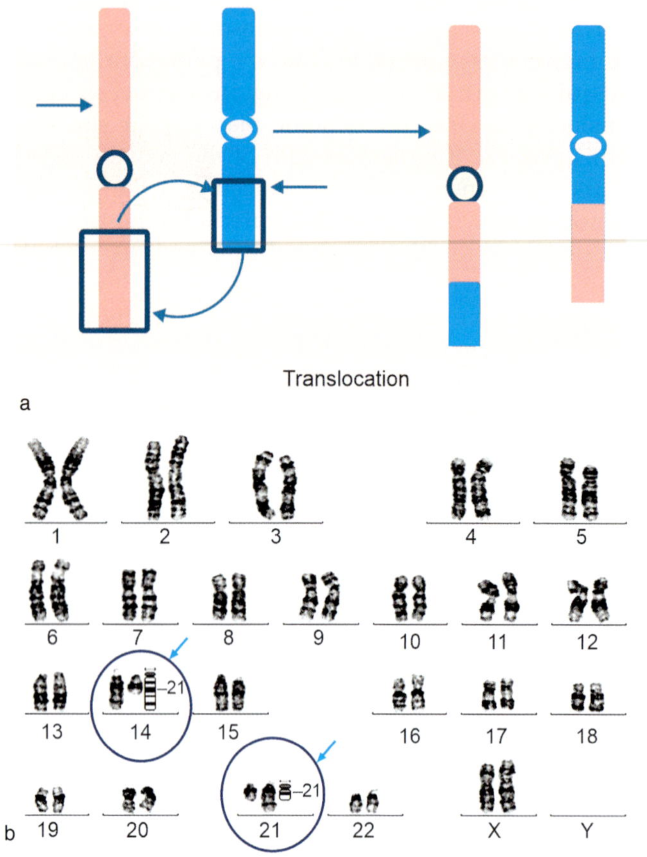


**Fig. 23.5:** Translocation: (a) Cartoon indicating exchange of parts of chromosomes; (b) Karyotype showing translocation between chromosome 14 and 21 [t(14;21)]. Arrows show the corresponding idiogram for a normal chromosome 14 and 21

by loss of a cluster of genes, giving rise to a consistent pattern of anomalies and developmental problems. A few common examples are William syndrome (7q11.23); retinoblastoma with mental retardation and dysmorphic facies (13q14.1); Prader-Willi syndrome (hypotonia, hyperphagia, hypomentia, intellectual disability and obesity, 15q11); and DiGeorge syndrome (congenital heart defect, hypoplasia of parathyroid and thymus, facial and palate anomalies; 22q11). Submicroscopic deletions are detected on special chromosomal staining or fluorescent *in situ* hybridization (FISH) (Fig. 23.7). DNA probes make it possible for FISH to be used for diagnosis for aneuploidies and microdeletion syndromes.

***Duplications*** are abnormal duplication or copy of part of a particular chromosome that result in extra genetic material.

***Ring chromosome*** (Fig. 23.8) occurs due to a two-breakpoint event involving the ends of the p and q arm which leaves two sticky chromosomal ends that join to form a ring.

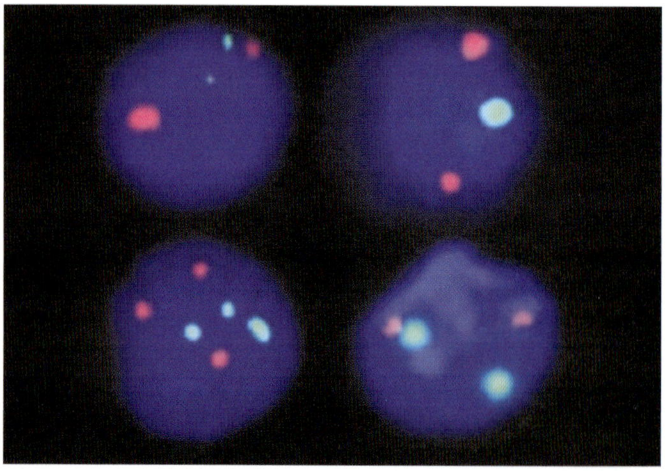

**Fig. 23.7:** Signals on fluorescent *in situ* hybridization (FISH) testing. Reduced or increased number of signals indicates aneuploidy

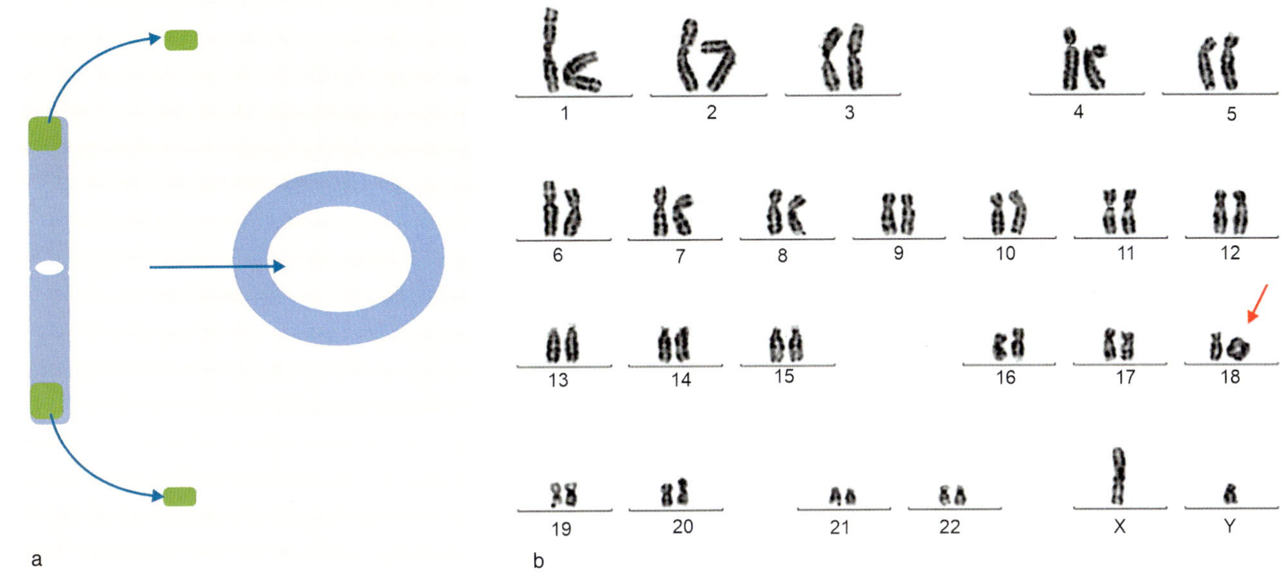


**Fig. 23.8:** (a) Schematic representation; and (b) Karyotype showing ring chromosome 18 in a child with developmental delay and seizures (red arrow)

*Inversion* (Fig. 23.9a) results from one or two breaks along the length of the chromosome arm. The broken pieces rotate by 180° and reinsert in a novel way. If there is no loss or gain of genetic material, there may be no significant clinical manifestations. Break point is important, if it disrupts a vital gene.

*Isochromosome* (Fig. 23.9b). During mitotic cell division, the chromosome divides longitudinally. Rarely it divides transversely across the centromere, with half of the chromosome replicating to form its complement. Thus, instead of normal chromosomes, two new types of chromosomes are formed, one having both the long arms and the other with both the short arms. These are known as isochromosomes. Each isochromosome has excess of some genetic material and deficiency of other genetic material. For example, isochromosomes cause some cases of Turner syndrome.

*Genomic imprinting:* Maternal and paternal sets of genes are not always functionally equal. Some genes are preferentially expressed from maternal or paternal side. Examples include Prader-Willi syndrome (microdeletion on paternal side or inheritance of both copies from maternal side) and Angelman syndrome (microdeletion on maternal side or inheritance of both copies from paternal side).

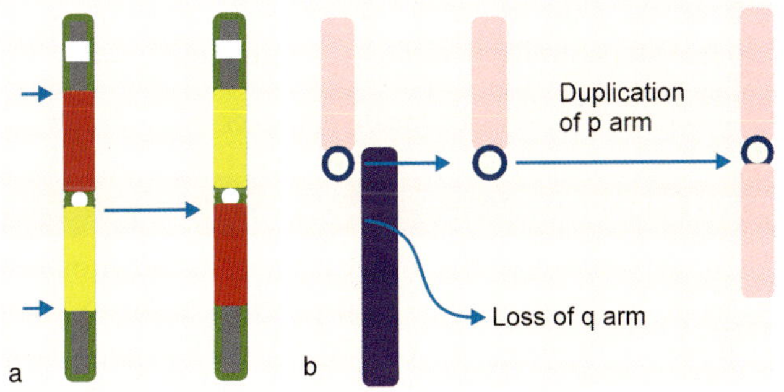


**Fig. 23.9:** (a) Inversion; (b) Isochromosome

Chromosomal abnormalities are generally sporadic and, therefore, the risk of recurrence in offsprings is low, except when either parent is carrying a balanced trans-location.

### Testing for Chromosomal Disorders

Laboratory testing for chromosomal disorders includes conventional karyotyping, fluorescent *in situ* hybridization (FISH), quantitative PCR (qPCR), multiplex ligation probe amplification (MLPA) and chromosomal microarray (CMA). Indicatios for chromosomal analysis are shown in Table 23.1.

Chromosomes are always prepared from dividing cells. Karyotyping can be performed on peripheral blood lymphocytes, skin biopsies, testicular biopsies, bone marrow aspirate, tumor biopsy, chorionic villi, and amniotic fluid. The process is labor intensive and involves culture, followed by harvesting chromosomes after the cells are arrested in mitosis by adding colecimid. After preparation of slides, staining (usually Giemsa stain) is done to produce a banding pattern unique for each chromosome (Fig. 23.10). This enables detection of numerical and structural abnormalities through the genome at a limited resolution of approximately 5 Mb. The chromosomes from one metaphase figure (a single cell) are classified according to their length (chromosome 1 is the longest) and banding pattern at 550 band level into a digital

| Table 23.1: Indications for chromosomal analysis |
|---|
| Suspected chromosomal disorders such as Down syndrome, Turner syndrome |
| Intellectual disability and autism with or without dysmorphism* |
| Family history of balanced chromosomal rearrangement |
| Disorder of sexual differentiation, primary amenorrhea, recurrent pregnancy losses, infertility |
| Multiple malformation syndrome* |

*Chromosomal microarray is preferred

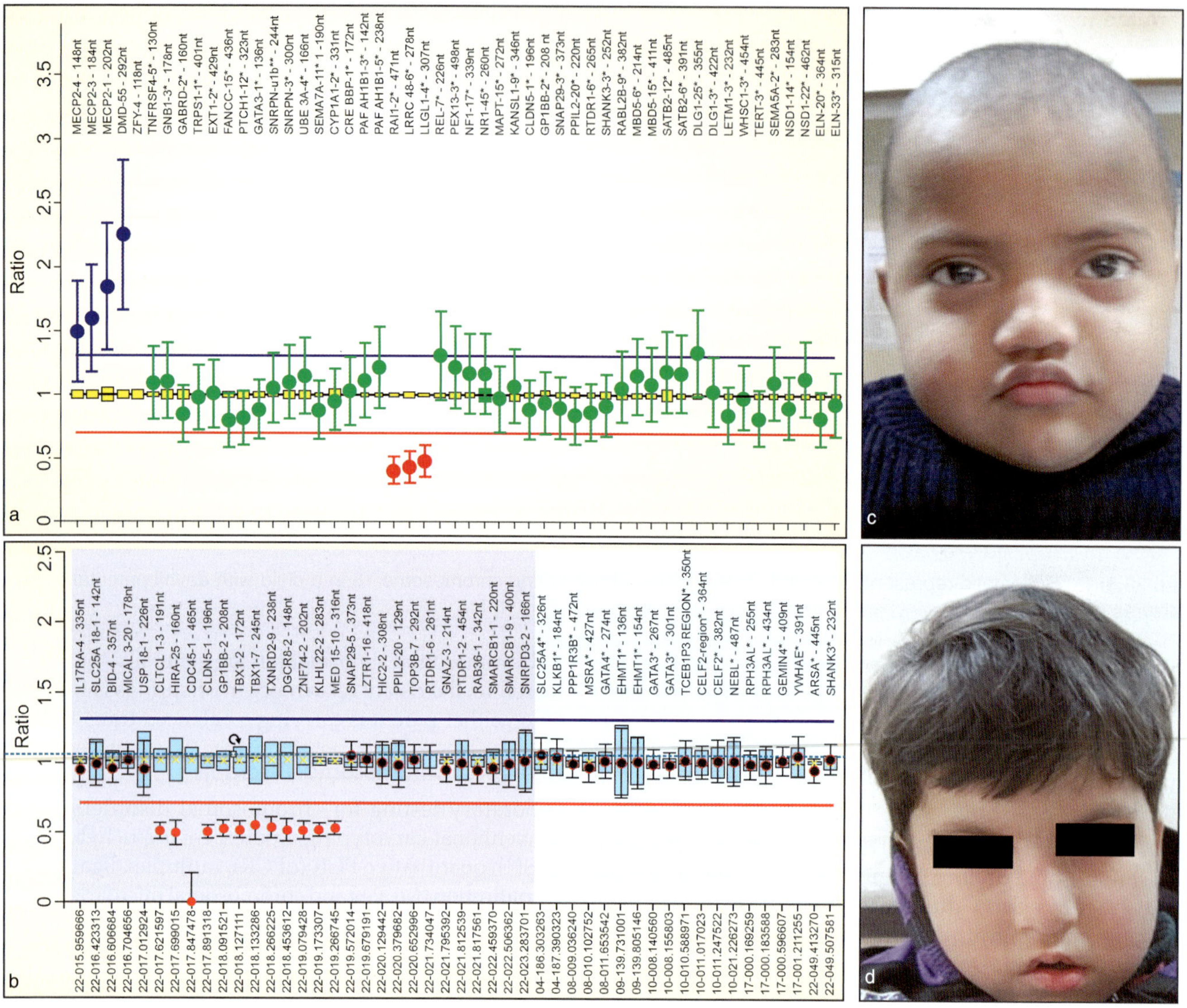


**Fig. 23.10:** MLPA analyses showing: (a) 17p11.2 deletion; (b) 22q11.2 deletion in patients with (c) Smith-Magenis syndrome and (d) DiGeorge syndrome, respectively

image which is usually called a karyotype or karyogram (Fig. 23.4). This also represents the entire genome for evaluating any numerical or structural chromosomal abnormality. Conventional karyotyping is still an important investigation for known recognizable aneuploidies and understanding the mechanism of structural chromosomal rearrangements.

Molecular cytogenetic techniques include FISH, quantitative polymerase chain reaction (qPCR) and multiplex ligation dependent probe amplification (MLPA) (Fig. 23.10). These detect chromosomal abnormalities in a targeted manner, since fluorescent probes (in case of FISH) and specific markers (qPCR and MLPA) are designed for a specific chromosome or region of chromosome, and can be used for submicroscopic abnormalities. All these tests are rapid (results within 1–2 days) but are expensive and will detect abnormalities only in the desired chromosome(s) or regions. These are highly useful for rapid aneuploidy detection in prenatal diagnosis and for microdeletion syndromes.

Chromosomal microarray is based on the principle of complementary DNA hybridization to screen entire genome for copy number variations, both losses (deletions) and gains (duplications). The genomic DNA is labelled and hybridized onto an array. Based on the relative fluorescence emitted at each target site, deletion and duplications are classified. It provides better diagnostic yield than conventional karyotype; it does not require dividing cells and the resolution is almost 50-fold higher. Chromosomal microarray is recommended for unexplained intellectual disability, multiple congenital anomalies and autistic spectrum disorders. DNA microarrays can be used to measure the expression of several genes simultaneously or to genotype multiple regions of a genome.

*Competencies:* **PE32.1; PE32.2; PE32.3; PE32.4; PE32.5**

## DOWN SYNDROME

Down syndrome is the most common chromosomal disorder, occurring with a frequency of 1:800 to 1:1000 newborns. Chromosome 21 is present in triplicate, usually because of meiotic nondisjunction in either maternal or parental gamete. In most cases, the extra chromosome is from the mother. Down syndrome occurs more often in offspring of mothers conceiving at older age; the risk in the newborn is 1:1550, if maternal age is 15–29 years, 1:800 at 30–34 years, 1:270 at 35–39 years, 1:100 at 40–44 years and 1:50 after 45 years.

## Cytogenetics

Trisomy 21 is found in 95% cases. Approximately 1% cases are mosaic and the rest (4%) are due to translocations, most commonly involving chromosomes 21 and 14 (Figs 23.5b, 23.11). Karyotype of the parents is only required, if the affected child has translocation causing Down syndrome.

## Clinical Features and Diagnosis

Patients with Down syndrome have intellectual disability, physical retardation, flat facial profile, an upward slant of eyes and epicanthic folds (Fig. 23.12). Oblique palpebral fissure is obvious only when the eyes are open. The nose is small with flat nasal bridge. Mouth shows a narrow short palate with small teeth and furrowed protruding tongue. There is significant hypotonia. The skull appears small and brachycephalic with flat occiput. Ears are small and dysplastic. There is a characteristic facial grimace on crying. Hands are short and broad. Clinodactyly (hypoplasia of middle phalanx of fifth finger) and simian crease are usual.

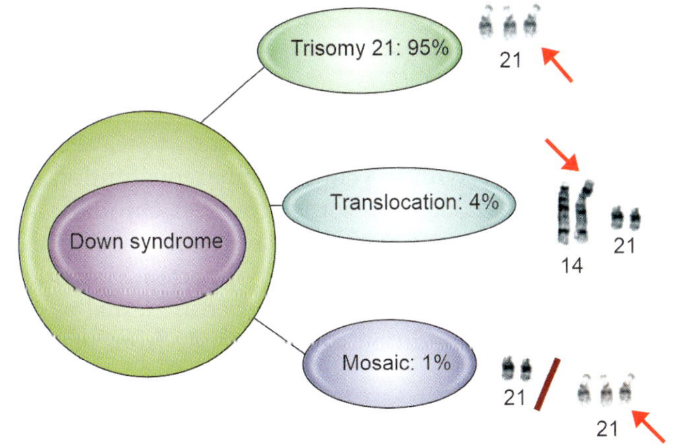


**Fig. 23.11:** Three types of chromosomal abnormalities found in children with Down syndrome. Arrows indicate the additional genetic material that results in the characteristic features

There is a wide gap between the first and the second toes (sandle gap).

### Comorbidities

*Congenital heart disease:* Approximately 40% children have congenital heart disease. Endocardial cushion defects account for 40–60% cases. Presence of heart disease is the chief factor in determining survival. All children should have a cardiac evaluation before 9 months of age, or at first contact by echocardiography.

*Gastrointestinal malformations:* Atresias are present in 12% of cases, especially duodenal atresia. There is an increased risk of annular pancreas and Hirschsprung disease.

*Ophthalmic problems:* There is an increased risk of cataract, nystagmus, squint and abnormalities of visual acuity. Routine evaluation is performed in infancy and then yearly.

*Hearing defects:* 40–60% patients have conductive hearing loss and are prone to serous otitis media (commonly during the first year). Routine evaluation is done before 6 months of age and then every year.

*Thyroid dysfunction:* About 13–54% patients with Down syndrome have hypothyroidism. Thyroid function tests (T4 and TSH) are recommended once in the neonatal period or at first contact, every six months in infancy and then every year. This should ideally include antithyroid antibodies, especially in older children, as etiology is usually autoimmune.

*Atlanto-occipital subluxation:* The incidence is variable, reported in 10–30%. Lateral neck radiograph is recommended once at 3–5 years, before surgery, for participation in special games, or earlier, if signs and symptoms suggest cord compression.

*Physical growth:* Regular follow up for height and weight is necessary. Linear growth is retarded as compared to normal; children tend to become obese with age. Muscle tone tends to improve with age.

*Malignancies:* Patients with Down syndrome are at increased risk of lymphoproliferative disorders, including acute lymphoblastic leukemia, acute myeloid leukemia, myelodysplasia and transient lymphoproliferative syndrome.

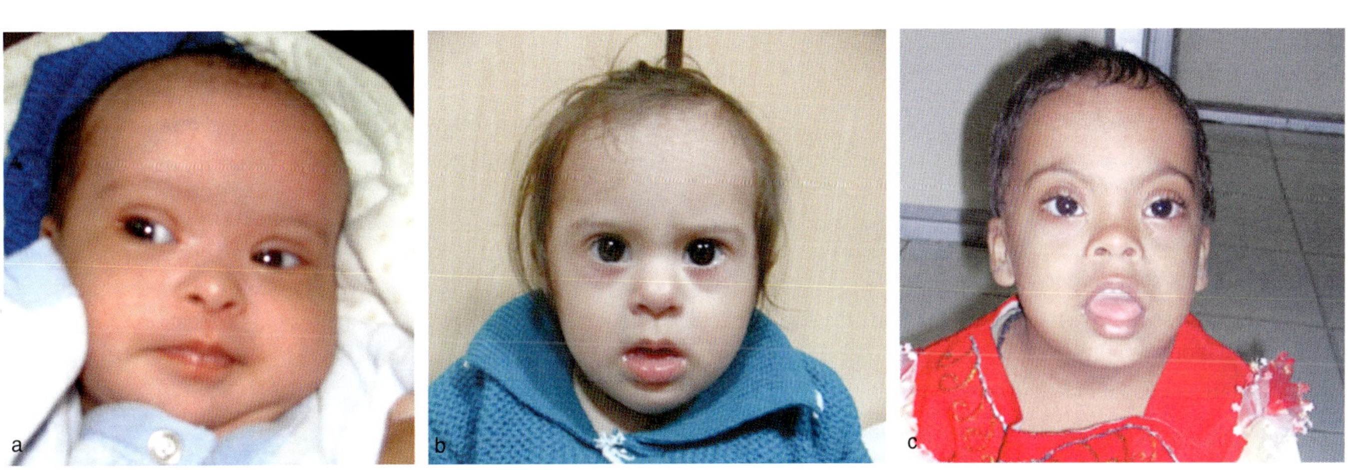


**Fig. 23.12:** Children with Down syndrome at (a) 3 months; (b) 15 months; and (c) 2 years of age. Note the flat facies, upward eye slant and open mouth appearance

## Management and Prognosis

The principles of management are early stimulation, physiotherapy and speech therapy. Associated problems need to be treated as required. Social performance is usually achieved beyond that expected for mental age. Generally, they behave as happy children, like mimicry, are friendly, have good sense of rhythm and enjoy music.

The chief cause for early mortality is congenital heart disease; almost 50% with cardiac anomalies die in infancy. Chronic rhinitis, conjunctivitis and periodontal disease are common. Lower respiratory tract infections pose a threat to life. Hematological malignancies are another cause of mortality. Table 23.2 outlines the protocol for care of children with Down syndrome.

## Counseling

Parents of a child with Down syndrome should be counseled with tact, compassion and truthfulness. Briefly, one should: (i) Inform about the disorder as early as possible after diagnosis is confirmed; (ii) counsel in presence of both the parents in privacy; (iii) talk in simple and positive language giving hope and allow sufficient time to the parents to ask questions; (iv) discuss known problems and associated disorders; (v) highlight the importance of early stimulation; (vi) not discuss institutionalization and adoption, unless asked, and discourage both the options; (vii) ask parents to contact the local Down syndrome parent association, if one exists; (viii) talk about genetics only after chromosomal analysis; (ix) inform about recurrence risks and possibilities of prenatal diagnosis; and (x) schedule future appointments.

It is important to note that parents should know about "what children with Down syndrome can do" not only about the intellectual disability and comorbidities. Most children are trainable, adjust very well, are caring and affectionate and many are employed.

*Risk of recurrence:* Women 35 years of age or less who have a child with trisomy 21 have a 1% risk of having another, which is significantly greater than the general population. The risk is little increased, if any, over the usual maternal age dependent frequency if the mother at risk is 35 years or older. For translocations inherited from the mother, the risk is about 10%, whereas it is about 4–5% when father is the carrier. Balanced translocation 21; 21, t (21q; 21q) is the only situation where all viable fetuses will have Down syndrome.

*Prenatal screening and diagnosis* (*see* section: Prevention of Genetic Disorders): Parents who wish to get a prenatal diagnosis have a number of options. They can directly get a fetal karyotype either by chorionic villus sampling (by transcervical or transabdominal route) or amniocentesis. Alternatively, an initial screening may be performed with maternal serum markers and ultrasonography and non-invasive prenatal screening (NIPS), as discussed below.

Options for couples who come late or opt for initial screening with serum markers and ultrasonography are karyotyping by amniocentesis at 16–18 weeks, trans-abdominal chorionic villus sampling (11–12 weeks earliest) and cordocentesis after 18 weeks (rarely performed). Karyotype results are available within a week with cord blood samples. The results of amniotic fluid cultures take about two weeks. Rapid testing using FISH and quantitative PCR is very reliable and results are available in 24–48 hours.

*Competencies:* **PE32.6; PE32.7; PE32.8; PE32.9; PE32.10**

## TURNER SYNDROME

Turner syndrome, with 45X chromosomal constitution, has an incidence of ~1:3000 newborns. However, chromosomal studies of spontaneous abortions have clearly shown that majority of 45X fetuses are likely to be aborted. Since there is no apparent relationship to advanced maternal age, it is likely that the condition does not arise from gametic nondisjunction.

Table 23.2: Evaluation in patients with Down syndrome

| *Evaluation* | *Frequency of assessment* |
|---|---|
| Growth | Twice a year in first year; annually till 5 years |
| Auditory (screen for hearing loss, otitis media) | |
| Ocular | |
| Thyroid profile | |
| Cardiac evaluation | At initial contact; follow up if congenital heart disease |
| Hematology | Screen for leukemia, twice a year in first year; monitor as per need |
| Dental | Annually |
| *Additional evaluations* | |
| Routine immunization as per schedule | |
| Vigilance about signs of gastroesophageal reflux disease, celiac disease, obstructive sleep apnea, atlantoaxial dislocation<br>Early stimulation therapy | |
| Physiotherapy, occupational and speech therapy | |
| Guidance regarding vocational training, hygiene and self-care | |
| Discuss behavioral issues | |
| Counseling regarding future pregnancies and prenatal diagnosis | |

## Cytogenetics

Majority of patients with Turner syndrome have 45X karyotype. Other chromosomal abnormalities include a variable degree of chromosomal mosaicism, i.e. 45, X/46, XX or Xp (short arm) deletion or isochromosome 46,X,i(Xq). Figure 23.6b shows a karyotype of a child with Turner syndrome with deletion of long arm of X chromosome. A small proportions of girls also have y-chromosome material (TS + Y).

## Clinical Features

Turner syndrome may be recognizable at birth. Lymphedema of the dorsum of hands and feet and loose skin folds at the nape of neck may be present. Other manifestations include short stature, short neck with webbing and low posterior hair line. Anomalous ears, prominent narrow and high-arched palate, small mandible and epicanthic folds may be noted. Chest is broad shield-like with widely spaced hypoplastic nipples (Fig. 23.13a and b). There is increased carrying angle at elbow. Bony anomalies include medial tibial exostosis, and short fourth metacarpals and metatarsals. Pigmented nevi may appear in older patients. At puberty, sexual maturation fails to occur. The phenotype is highly variable. It has been recommended that the diagnosis of Turner syndrome should be considered in all girls with short stature.

Ultrasound may show streak ovaries and hypoplastic uterus. Levels of FSH and LH are increased (hypergonadotropic hypogonadism). Adult stature is usually below 145 cm. Associated congenital defects are common in kidneys (horseshoe kidney, double or cleft renal pelvis), heart (coarctation aorta) and ears (perceptive hearing defect). Congenital lymphedema recedes in early infancy, leaving puffiness over dorsum of fingers and toes. Hypothyroidism occurs in about 15–30% adults with Turner syndrome. The clinical features are milder in Turner syndrome with mosaicism; patients may have normal stature and present with secondary amenorrhea.

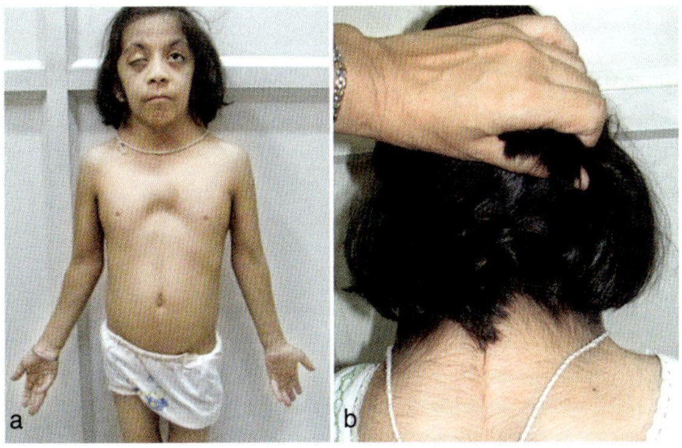


Fig. 23.13: Turner syndrome. Note: (a) Ptosis in right eye, shield chest, increased carrying angle, webbed and short neck; (b) Low posterior hair line

## Management

Height monitoring should be done using growth charts for Turner syndrome. Cardiac evaluation and measurement of blood pressure are recommended at baseline and every year. Treatment with growth hormone is recommended. While therapy may increase the final height by 8–10 cm, the cost is high. Thyroid testing should be done in infancy or early childhood, if the child is lagging in growth.

Routine evaluation is required after 10 years of age. Counseling regarding behavioral problems due to short stature, amenorrhea and sterility is an integral part of management. Ovarian hormone replacement is advised around 14 years. Conjugated estrogen (0.3 mg/day) or ethinyl estradiol (5–10 μg/day) are given for 3–6 months; the dose of medications may be increased. After 6–12 months, cyclical therapy with estrogen and progesterone is started.

Regular audiometry is advised in adulthood or earlier, if indicated. Ultrasonography is done for renal malformations. Prophylactic gonadectomy is advised for patients with Y chromosome due to the risk of gonadoblastoma.

Table 23.3 lists the clinical features of some other common aneuploidies.

Table 23.3: Clinical features of common aneuploidies

| | *Clinical features* | *Management* |
|---|---|---|
| Trisomy 18<br>Edward syndrome | Failure to thrive, developmental delay, hypertonia, micrognathia (Fig. 23.14a), shield-shaped chest, short sternum, joint abnormalities including flexion deformity of fingers (Fig. 23.14b and c), limited hip abduction and short dorsiflexed hallux, rocker bottom feet. Congenital heart disease is common | Symptomatic, supportive |
| Trisomy 13<br>Patau syndrome | Development delay and failure to thrive, microcephaly, sloping forehead; cleft lip with/without cleft palate common<br>Holoprosencephaly; varying degree of incomplete development of forebrain, olfactory and optic nerves<br>Microphthalmia, iris coloboma, retinal dysplasia and cataract; deafness<br>Capillary hemangiomata (Fig. 23.15); polydactyly, flexion deformities, rocker bottom feet<br>Congenital heart disease (80%); most die by 6 months of life | Symptomatic, supportive |
| Klinefelter syndrome<br>47,XXY | Hypergonadotropic hypogonadism, small testes, lack of secondary sex characters; tall stature, gynecomastia<br>Borderline intellectual disability, behavioral problems<br>Consider diagnosis in boys with intellectual disability, psychosocial or learning disability, or problems in school adjustment | Behavioral and psychosocial rehabilitation<br>Testosterone therapy in middle-late adolescence |

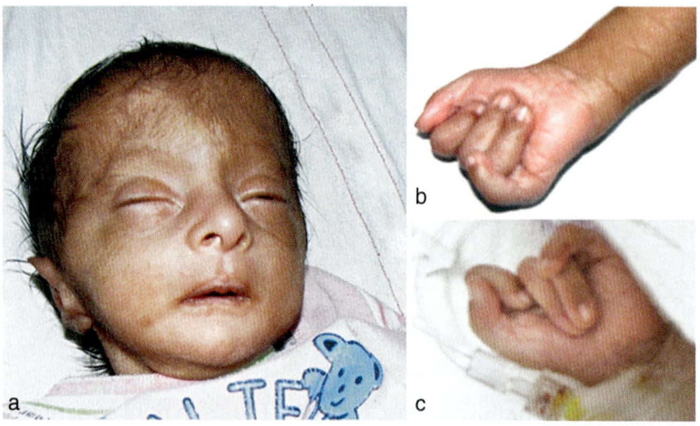


Fig. 23.14: Note the (a) Facial dysmorphism; (b and c) Overlapping of fingers in an infant with trisomy 18

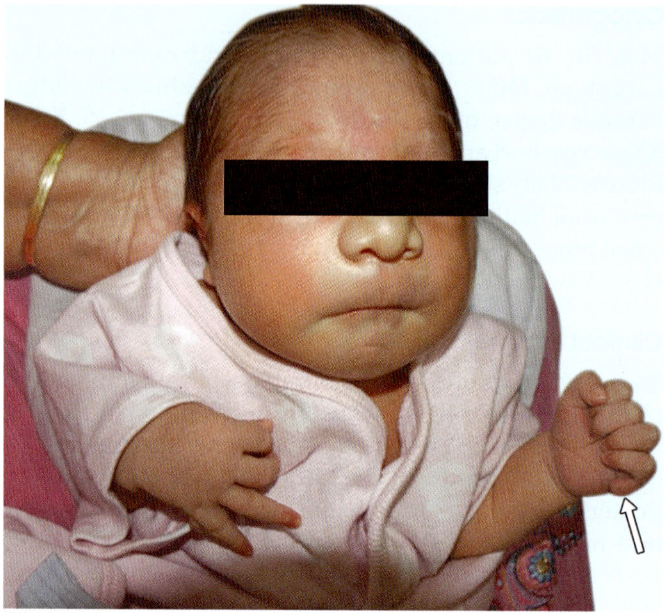

Fig. 23.15: Note postaxial polydactyly (white arrow) and forehead hemangioma in an infant with trisomy 13



## SINGLE GENE DISORDERS

Single gene disorders are inherited as autosomal dominant, autosomal recessive or X-linked disorders, due to mutation(s) in disease specific genes. Drawing and interpreting a pedigree is an inexpensive tool and integral part of diagnosis of single gene disorders (Fig. 23.16a and b).

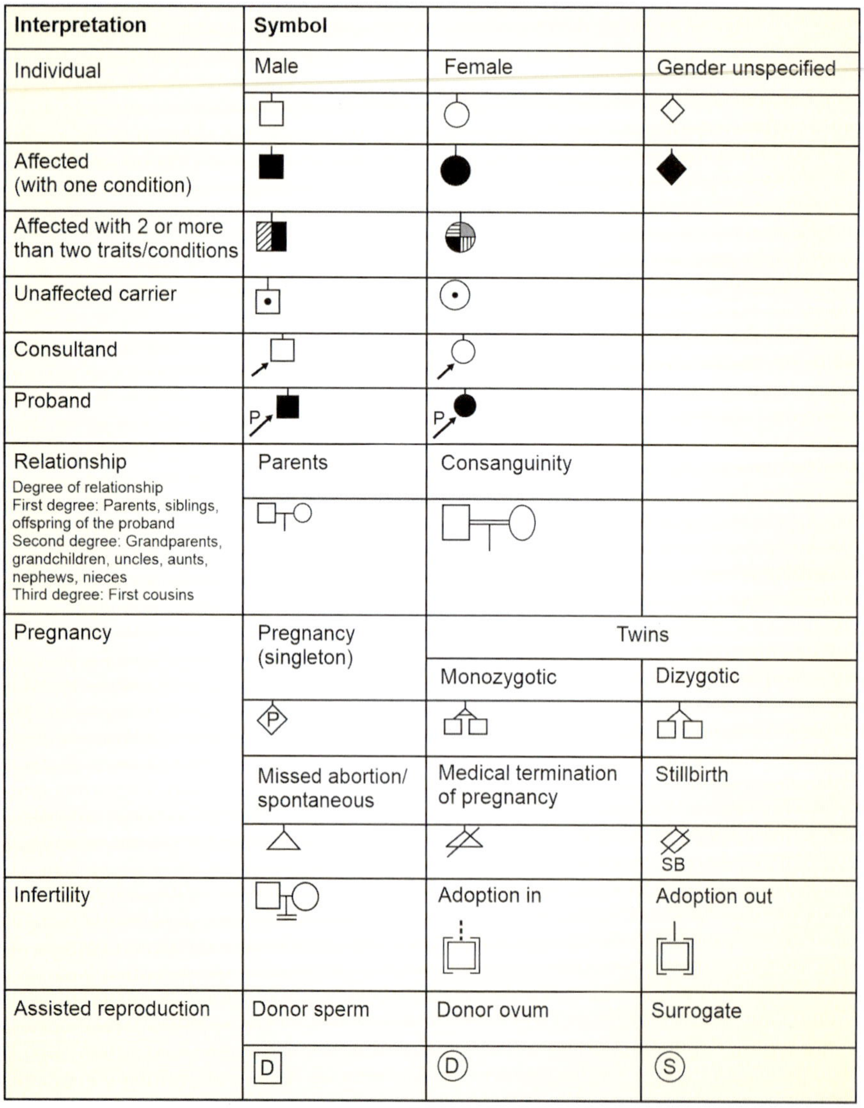


Fig. 23.16a: Standard symbols used for drawing pedigree

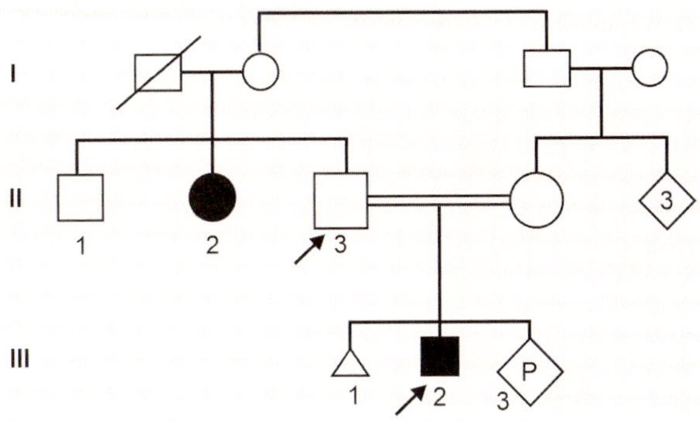


Fig. 23.16b: A three generation pedigree showing third degree consanguinity with two affected persons (proband) (II-2 and III-2 in generation II and III respectively). II-3 is the consultand who has come for seeking genetic counselling in current pregnancy (III-3) in view of a prior family history

A heritable change in the DNA sequence is referred to as mutation (the present preferred term is pathogenic variant) that consequently results in perturbed protein structure and function. DNA sequence variants can range from a single nucleotide to whole chromosome. Numerical and structural chromosomal abnormalities have been explained in the above section. Germline mutations affect all the cells including germ cells and are heritable resulting in monogenic conditions, whereas somatic mutations are confined to somatic cells and cause cancers. There are three types of mutations: Single base substitution, deletions and insertions.

*Substitution or point mutations,* the most common type, result in replacement of a single nucleotide by another that results in formation of altered amino acid (missense mutation). It may also generate a stop codon (nonsense mutation). If the change in nucleotide does not alter the amino acid, it is called a silent mutation.

*Deletion mutations* involve the loss of one or more nucleotides in a gene. If the deletion is a multiple of three base pair deletion, then it is an in-frame deletion, whereas if the deleted nucleotides are not the multiple of three, it results in disruption of the reading frame, known as frameshift mutation (out-of-frame deletions). Large deletions cause partial or whole gene deletion.

*Insertion* involves addition of one or more nucleotides into a gene. Frame shift mutations can also occur due to insertion of a nucleotide.

Triplet repeat expansions are dynamic mutations that expand over generations and become unstable on expansion, e.g. fragile X syndrome, myotonic dystrophy.

Currently, variants are classified as benign, likely benign, variant of unknown significance, likely pathogenic and pathogenic based on the possible effect of the variant on the phenotype.

## Autosomal Dominant Inheritance

Autosomal dominant (AD) disorders manifest even if only one of the alleles of the abnormal gene is affected. These disorders often affect several generations (vertical transmission). Homozygotes for the dominant mutant genes usually die prenatally, as in the case of achondroplasia. If the child is the only affected member, it is very likely that the observed mutation has occurred *de novo* and is not inherited. New dominant gene mutations are more likely to occur, if the paternal age is high. In AD inheritance, the chances of recurrence in next pregnancy is 1 in 2 unless the disorder is *de novo*. Examples include neurofibromatosis, achondroplasia, and Marfan syndrome. A typical pedigree and its characteristic features are shown in Fig. 23.17.

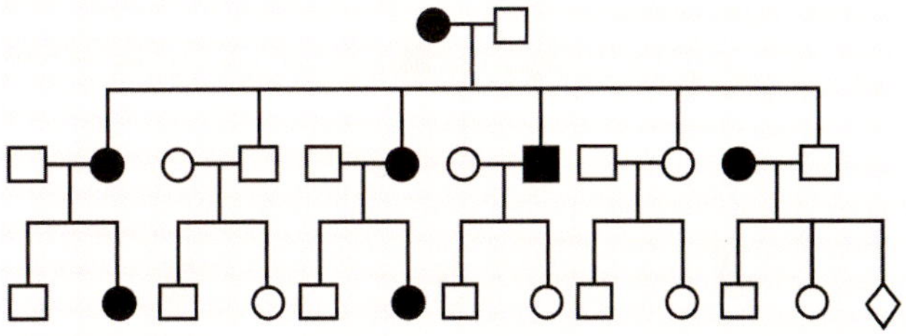

Fig. 23.17: Autosomal dominant inheritance and its characteristics

In some dominantly inherited conditions such as neurofibromatosis, there may be a variable phenotypic expression (ranging from few café au lait spots in one to plexiform neurofibroma in other) of the disease, even within the same family. This is known as variable expressivity. Similarly, few patients do not show any manifestations despite having disease causing variant (incomplete or reduced penetrance). A careful physical examination of other siblings and parents is necessary to uncover milder forms of the disorder.

## Autosomal Recessive Inheritance

Autosomal recessive disorders manifest only in homozygous state, i.e. both the alleles are mutant genes. Generally, autosomal recessive mutations affect synthesis of enzyme, leading to inborn errors of metabolism. The parents of the affected individuals are apparently normal but carry the mutant genes. As they are heterozygous, the mutant recessive gene does not express itself in the phenotype. In such matings, one-fourth of the offspring are affected (homozygous for the mutant genes), one-fourth are normal (both normal alleles) and half are carriers (heterozygote with one mutant allele and one normal allele). A classical pedigree is shown in Fig. 23.18. Recessive disorders are common in consanguineous marriage or in closed communities. It is possible to detect carrier status by hematological and molecular techniques in a number of autosomal recessive disorders. Common examples of autosomal recessive disorders are beta-thalassemia, sickle cell disease, spinal muscular atrophy, phenylketonuria and galactosemia.

## X-Linked Recessive Inheritance

Since in males there is only one X chromosome, X-linked recessive disorders manifest in male individuals. In the female, the disorder does not manifest (usually) clinically since the mutant gene is compensated for by the normal allele on the other X chromosome. Females thus act as carriers of the mutant allele. Half of their

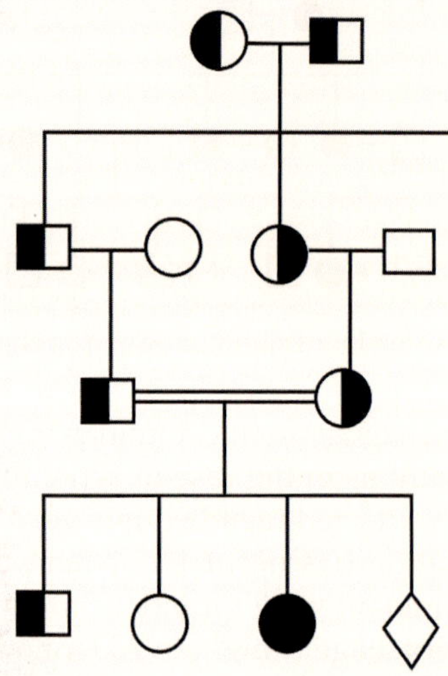

Fig. 23.18: Autosomal recessive inheritance and its characteristics. Carriers are indicated by partly shaded symbols

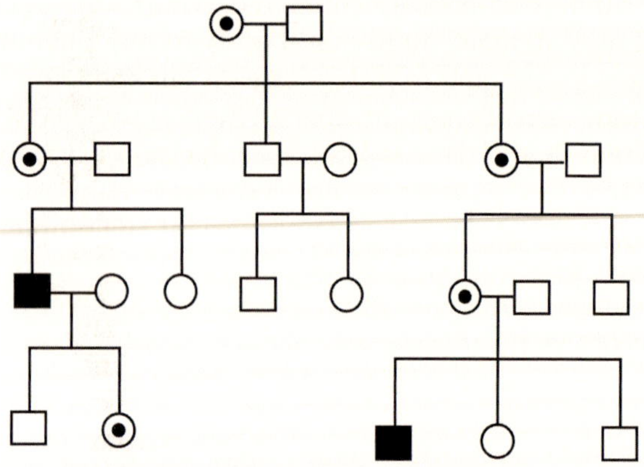

Fig. 23.19: X-linked recessive inheritance and its characteristics. Carriers are indicated by bold dot in the center

male children inherit the mutant allele and are affected. Figure 23.19 shows a family with X-linked recessive inheritance. It is now possible to detect carrier state in females in some disorders, e.g. hemophilia, Duchenne muscular dystrophy and mucopolysaccharidosis type II (Hunter syndrome). Color blindness also has an X-linked recessive inheritance.

### X-Linked Dominant Inheritance

Dominant X-linked conditions are rare. Both heterozygous females and hemizygous males are affected. All the sons of the affected males are normal and all daughters are affected. The affected females transmit the disease to half of the sons and half of the daughters, e.g. hypophosphatemic vitamin D resistant rickets, orofaciodigital syndrome and incontinentia pigmenti. In some cases, the effect of the mutant gene on development is severe, and affected males are seldom born alive. Majority of patients are heterozygous females (Fig. 23.20).

### Mitochondrial Inheritance

Mutations within a mitochondrial gene can lead to phenotypic defects and show a pattern of maternal genetic

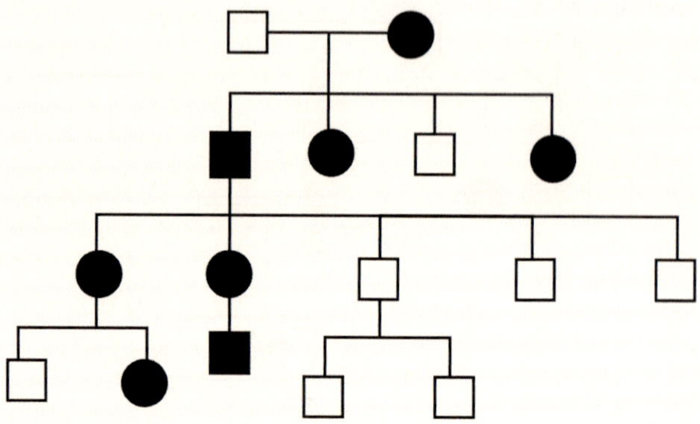

Fig. 23.20: X-linked dominant inheritance and its characteristics

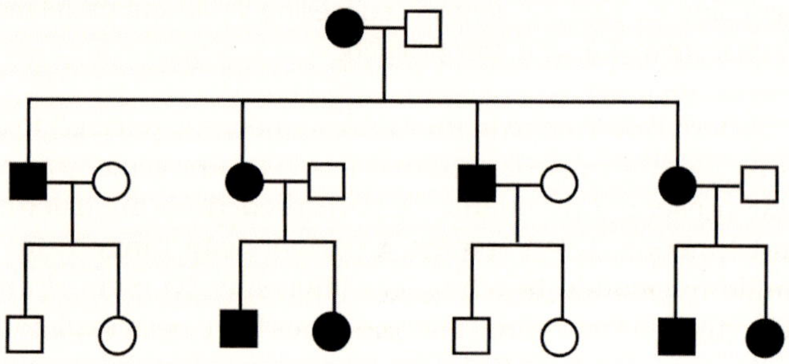

Fig. 23.21: Mitochondrial inheritance

transmission. Since mitochondria are only present in ovum and not sperms, the inheritance is maternal. All offsprings of an affected female are affected. All affected daughters transmit the disease. Sons are affected but do not transmit the disease (Fig. 23.21). Examples include Leigh disease, and mitochondrial encephalopathy, lactic acidosis and stroke (MELAS) like syndrome.

### Somatic Cell Genetic Disorders

In somatic cell disorders, the defects are restricted to specific somatic cells, in contrast to previous four types of genetic diseases (chromosomal, single gene, polygenic and mitochondrial) in which the abnormality is present in all cells, including germ line cells. These include cancers which can arise due to genetic changes in somatic cells alone.

### Molecular Genetic Testing

It involves evaluation of DNA that can be extracted from EDTA blood, saliva, dried blood spot or any tissue. DNA testing can be evaluated by the following approaches:

1. *Hybridizing* the test DNA (or RNA) to a labeled matching DNA or RNA molecule. These probes detect specific base sequences in the DNA. These assays include Southern blotting, fluorescence *in situ* hybridization (FISH), multiplex ligation-dependent probe amplification (MLPA), array-comparative genomic hybridization (aCGH) and microarrays. These are molecular cytogenetic techniques as discussed earlier in this chapter.
2. *Amplifying* the sequence of interest using polymerase chain reaction (PCR), wherein a large number of copies of DNA sequences are made in a short time. Various PCR-based methods for known mutations include size

analysis of PCR product for cystic fibrosis, restriction fragment length polymorphism (RFLP) for spinal muscular atrophy, amplification-refractory mutation system (ARMS) PCR for thalassemia. Real-time PCR is a rapid technique that uses special kits and can analyze results within 1 hr.

3. *Sequencing based methods:* Sequencing refers to evaluation of the sequence of the DNA which is then compared to a reference population (normal population) to detect any genetic alterations. It can be done by Sanger sequencing and next generation sequencing. Sanger sequencing is a gold standard method of screening for mutations. It is based on the selective incorporation of chain-terminating dideoxynucleotides by DNA polymerase during *in vitro* DNA replication. It can sequence only part of a gene at a time. **Figure 23.22a** shows the electropherogram of a child with common mutation (320insC) in megalencephalic leukodystrophy.

Next generation sequencing technology is a high throughput technique that can run thousands or millions of sequences in parallel at a comparatively lower cost and higher speed. Only 1% of DNA of the 3 billion base pairs of DNA is protein coding. The exonic sequence of the genome is called "exome". Genome includes both the coding and noncoding regions. NGS includes whole exome sequencing (WES), whole genome sequencing (WGS) and targeted gene panel testing for a specific disorder (e.g. nonsyndromic deafness, retinitis pigmentosa) or a group of disorders with overlapping phenotypes (e.g. neuromuscular disorders). WES includes sequencing of exomes whereas WGS includes sequencing of both coding and noncoding regions (exon and introns) or regulatory regions. Analyzing a smaller subset of genes derived from sources such as Online Mendelian Inheritance in Man (OMIM) that have an established association with disease is referred to as clinical or medical exome. NGS involves fragmentation of DNA into multiple fragments followed by capturing the selected specific regions (e.g. only the exonic regions of genome in WES or targeted sequences in the panel). Entire fragmented DNA is processed for sequencing in WGS.

The diagnostic yield of NGS is variable depending upon the disorder, platform used, capture kit and the gene coverage. The bioinformatics analysis utilizes a number of population databases and disease-causing databases to filter variants from several thousands to very few variants which are then correlated with the phenotype. The variants are classified as pathogenic, likely pathogenic, variant of unknown significance, benign and likely benign as per American College of Medical Genetics and Genomics and the Association for Molecular Pathology (ACMG-



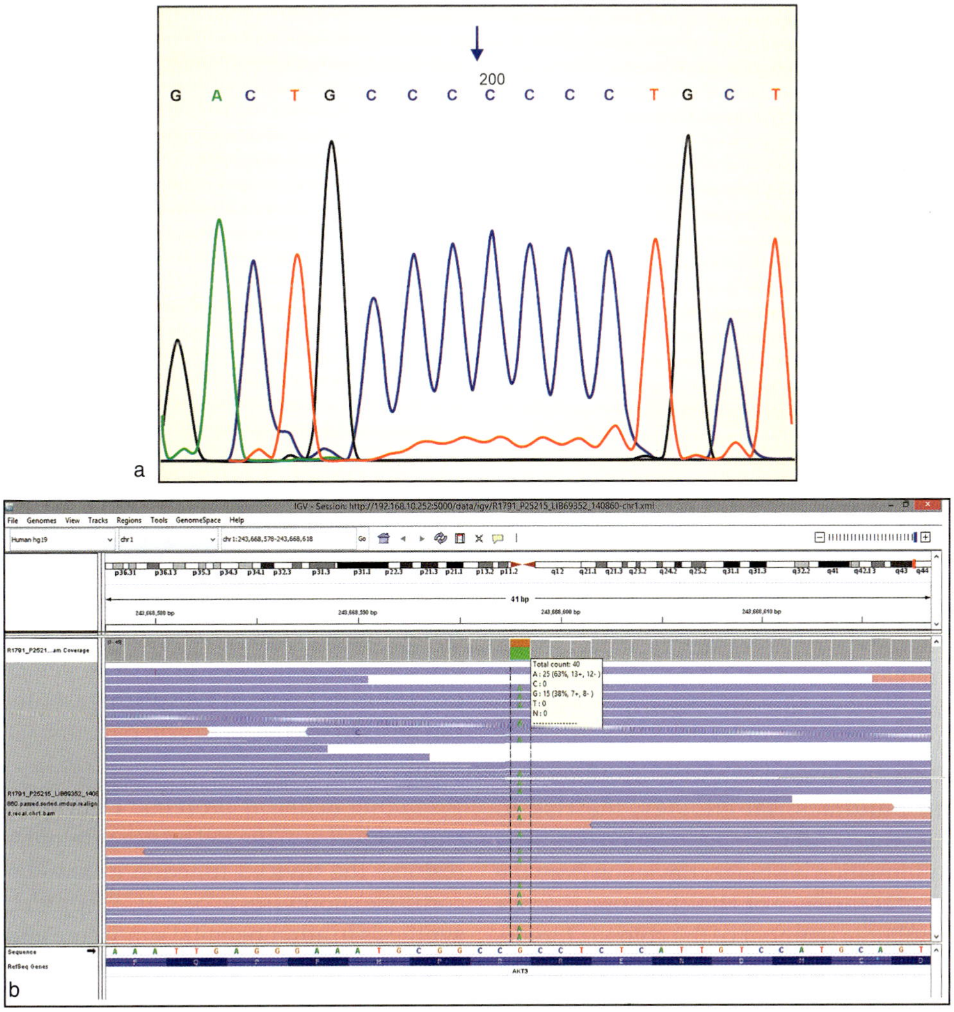


**Fig. 23.22:** (a) Insertion of cytosine "C" at 320 position (arrow) in exon 2 of *MLC1*; (b) Integrative genomic viewer (IGV) snapshot showing a heterozygous missense variation in exon 14 of *AKT3*

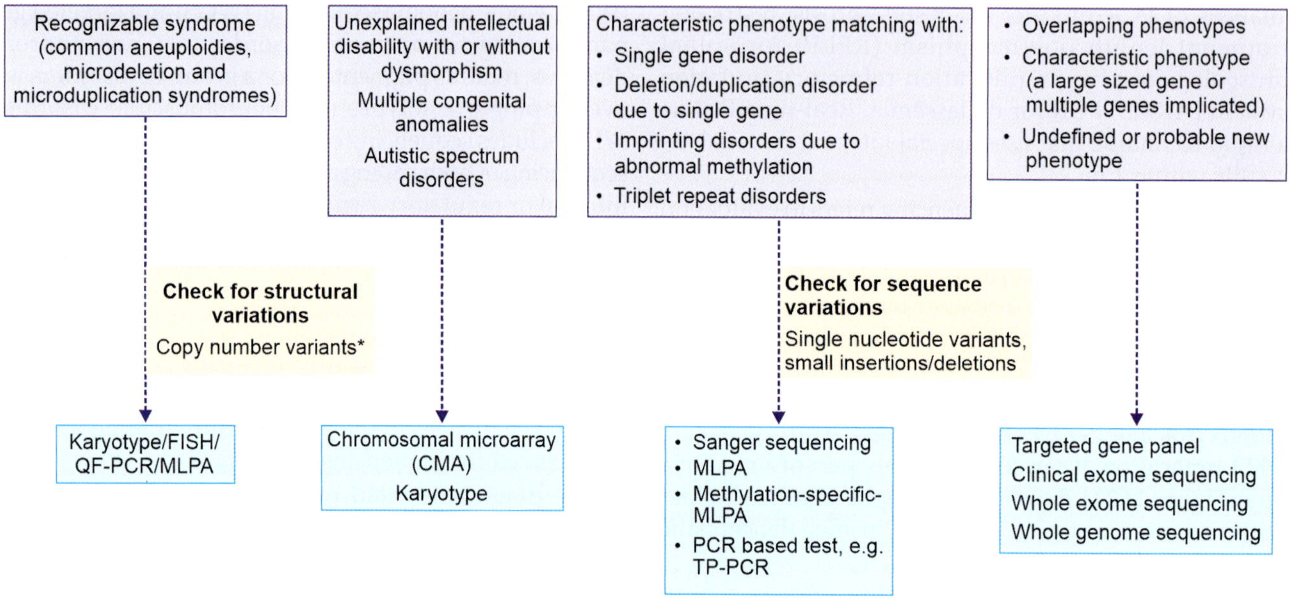


*Genomic alterations that involve segments of DNA larger than 1 kb
FISH fluorescence *in situ* hybridization; MLPA multiplex ligation-dependent probe amplification;
QF-PCR quantitative fluorescent PCR; TP-PCR triplet repeat primed PCR

**Fig. 23.23:** Choice of tests for various genetic disorders

AMP) guidelines. Correlation with the clinical phenotype, pedigree and other relevant investigations based on the presentation helps determine the effect of the variant. An opinion from a geneticist is helpful for interpretation of NGS data.

NGS technique is not useful for methylation disorders, triplet repeat disorders, chromosomal rearrangement and large deletions. Figure 23.22b shows a heterozygous missense variation in exon 14 of the *AKT3* (chr1:243668598G>A; depth: 39x) that results in the amino acid substitution of tryptophan for arginine at codon 465. Figure 23.23 shows the various indications and appropriate choice of a genetic test.

## POLYGENIC INHERITANCE

In several conditions, the affected individuals do not have a sharp division between the normal and the abnormal, but merely represent a spectrum of a continuously varying attribute. Such conditions are likely to be inherited by alterations in many gene loci, each of them individually having only a small effect. Many of these conditions are also affected by numerous environmental factors, individually of small effect. Examples of polygenic disorders are neural tube defect, cleft lip, cleft palate, Hirschsprung disease, congenital hypertrophic pyloric stenosis, diabetes mellitus, ischemic heart disease, hypertension and schizophrenia.

In diseases with multifactorial etiology, the risk to progeny and siblings is higher, if the malformation is severe, because a severe malformation is a bigger deviation from the normal, e.g. the risk of recurrence of Hirschsprung disease is higher, if the aganglionic segment of the colon is longer. For diseases with sex predilection, the risk of recurrence in the family is higher, if the index patient belongs to the less often affected sex. This is so, because the mutant genes are likely to be more severe so as to produce the disease in the sex with inherent resistance to the disease. The usual risk of recurrence for malformations caused by a polygenic or multifactorial cause is 2–5%.

## THERAPY FOR GENETIC DISORDERS

While genetic disorders cannot be cured completely, symptoms may be ameliorated and irreversible damage or handicap prevented or reduced through several therapeutic approaches (Table 23.4).

***Metabolic manipulation*** involves diet modification with or without drugs to reduce the substrate and is used mainly for inborn errors of metabolism involving small molecules. The intake of substances which cannot be metabolized by the body should be reduced, especially if their accumulation is potentially toxic, e.g. in galactosemia. Milk in the diet is substituted by lactose free dietary formulae to obviate damage due to excess galactose. Infants with phenylketonuria are placed on restricted phenylalanine in the diet, to prevent neurological damage.

***Promoting excretion of toxic substances:*** The excretion of certain metabolites can be promoted by agents, e.g. sodium benzoate in urea cycle disorders, penicillamine promotes excretion of copper in Wilson disease, and desferrioxamine can be used to chelate iron in patients with thalassemia and hemochromatosis.

***Providing deficient proteins:*** Deficiency of the metabolic end product is managed by its replacement. Thus, thyroxine restores the thyroid function in familial hypothyroidism; cortisone suppresses excess ACTH production and androgen synthesis in adrenogenital syndrome and administration of factor VIII/IX prevents bleeding in cases of hemophilia. Enzyme replacement therapy, although expensive, has become feasible with the availability of deficient enzymes for Gaucher disease, Hurler syndrome, Hunter syndrome,

Table 23.4: Strategies for the therapy of genetic disorders

| Intervention | Examples |
|---|---|
| Metabolic manipulation | Diet to reduced substrate accumulation (most inborn errors of metabolism); substrate reduction (lysosomal storage disorders) |
| Provide deficient protein | Hemophilia A and B; alpha-1 antitrypsin deficiency; growth hormone deficiency; lysosomal storage disorders |
| Avoid precipitating factors, drugs | Oxidants (glucose-6-phosphate dehydrogenase deficiency); avoid fasting in fatty acid oxidation defects and glycogen storage disorders |
| Promote excretion or removal of toxic substances | Penicillamine (Wilson disease); deferiprone (thalassemia); sodium benzoate (hyperammonemia); nitisinone (tyrosinemia) |
| Augmenting enzymes | Phenobarbitone (Crigler-Najjar syndrome); pyridoxine (homocystinuria) |
| Stem cell transplantation | Thalassemia major; severe form of Hurler syndrome; primary immunodeficiencies |
| Organ transplantation | Specific malformations; maple syrup urine disease (liver or liver–kidney); polycystic kidney or Remove diseased organ disease (kidney); cardiomyopathies (heart) |
| Remove diseased organ | Multiple endocrine neoplasia type II (thyroid); hereditary spherocytosis (spleen) |
| Molecular targeted therapies | Cystic fibrosis, spinal muscular atrophy, chronic myeloid leukemia |
| Supportive, symptomatic care | Osteogenesis imperfecta and hemophilia (avoiding trauma); xeroderma pigmentosa (avoid sun exposure); cardiac conduction defects (pacemaker) |
| Gene therapy | Spinal muscular atrophy, adenosine deaminase deficiency |

mucopolysaccharidosis type VI, Fabry disease, MPS IV, Pompe disease and Niemann-Pick disease type B.

*Augmenting enzymes:* Certain enzyme systems, which may be immature or reduced at certain phases of life may be induced or stabilized by the use of chemical agents. Phenobarbitone is used to induce hepatic microsomal enzymes like glucuronyl transferase in cases of neonatal hyperbilirubinemia or Crigler-Najjar syndrome. In some disorders, enzymatic block can be bypassed by administration of large quantities of the coenzyme, e.g. pyridoxine in homocystinuria.

*Avoid precipitating factors and drugs:* Certain drugs, which precipitate adverse symptoms in metabolic disorders, such as barbiturates in porphyria and oxidating agents in glucose-6-phosphate dehydrogenase deficiency, should not be given to affected patients.

*Stem cell transplantation* is recommended for many genetic disorders like thalassemia major, severe Hurler syndrome and some primary immunodeficiencies.

*Molecular targeted therapies* for certain disorders like cystic fibrosis with specific mutations (Ivacaftor for G551D and lumacaftor for F508del CFTR mutations), nusinersen and risdiplam for spinal muscular atrophy, exon skipping therapies and premature stop codon therapies for Duchenne muscular dystrophy, and imatinib for chronic myeloid leukemia have paved the way for future therapeutics for other genetic and somatic disorders.

*Gene therapy* is possible in patients with some disorders, e.g. spinal muscular atrophy, adenosine deaminase deficiency, familial hypercholesterolemia, metachromatic leukodystrophy, and some cancers. The normal gene is introduced in affected individuals using viral or nonviral vectors. As the regulation of function of single gene disorders is complex, the implementation of gene therapy is complicated.

*Surgery* helps to reduce the functional or cosmetic disability in some structural defects, e.g. removing the spleen in hereditary spherocytosis.

*Solid organ transplantation,* of liver, kidney and heart, is available across India. Conditions where transplantation may be useful include ornithine transcarbamylase deficiency, maple syrup urine disease, cardiomyopathies and polycystic kidney disease.

*Supportive care* is the mainstay of therapies for genetic disorders in the absence of specific therapies. Patients with hemophilia and osteogenesis imperfecta should be protected from trauma and other environmental hazards to prevent excessive bleeding and fractures, respectively. Supportive care also includes physical therapy, stimulation and rehabilitation. Bisphosphonate therapy has been found useful in cases of osteogenesis imperfecta by reducing osteoclastic activity.

## PREVENTION OF GENETIC DISORDERS

### Carrier Screening

It is now possible to detect the carrier state in a large number of autosomal recessive or X-linked recessive disorders. HbA2 levels are highly useful in identifying carriers of thalassemia trait pre-pregnancy or early in pregnancy. In India, ideally all partners should be tested for beta-thalassemia carrier status as the condition is very common. Female carriers of Duchenne muscular dystrophy may show high serum levels of the enzyme creatinine phosphokinase, but can be tested more precisely using MLPA.

Carrier screening, using NGS-approach, can be offered in couples with a family history suggestive of a monogenic disorder in previous offspring who died without a confirmed diagnosis.

## Newborn Screening

This is an example of secondary prevention by early diagnosis and treatment. Newborn infants are screened routinely for some endocrine disorders and inborn errors of metabolism in developed countries. This is of special value for detecting affected cases in the newborn period, so that handicap can be prevented or minimized by early treatment, examples include congenital hypothyroidism, congenital adrenal hyperplasia, biotinidase deficiency, G6PD deficiency, phenylketonuria and galactosemia. Newborn screening is also recommended for functional defects such as hearing and critical congenital heart disease.

## Prevention of Neural Tube Defects

Folic acid supplementation is recommended at a dose of 0.4 mg daily from 1 month before to 3 months after conception (periconception) to prevent neural tube defects. Expectant mothers at high-risk of such defects (e.g. previous fetus with neural tube defects) should consume 4 mg of folic acid daily periconceptionally to prevent recurrence.

## Maternal Serum Screening

Estimation of pregnancy associated plasma protein A (PAPP-A) and free human chorionic gonadotropin (hCG) in the first trimester, and serum alpha-fetoprotein, hCG, unconjugated estriol and inhibin A in second trimester are useful biochemical markers to detect high-risk mothers for having babies with aneuploidies. If the risk of bearing a child with Down syndrome is more than 1:250, prenatal fetal karyotyping can be offered. Fetal ultrasonography helps to detect fetuses at high-risk for chromosomal abnormalities. In the first trimester, increased nuchal translucency and absence of nasal bone are robust markers. Findings in the second trimester, which suggest Down syndrome, are increased nuchal fold thickness, short femur and humerus, and duodenal atresia.

Alpha-fetoprotein and estriol are low, whereas hCG is high, in pregnancies with Down syndrome fetuses. The detection rate of Down syndrome by triple test and quadruple test in the second trimester is about 65% and 75%, respectively with a false positive rate of 5%. All three markers are reduced in fetuses with trisomy 18. Ultrasound findings help in counseling, particularly if the parents have opted for initial screening with maternal serum markers. First trimester screening (dual test) when combined with ultrasound markers has high detection rates (85–90%). Elevated maternal serum alpha-fetoprotein level is also a sensitive marker for fetuses with open neural tube defects. Non-invasive prenatal screening (NIPS) is also being used for screening high risk pregnancies for aneuploidies (involving chromosomes 13, 18, 21, X and Y). This NGS-based technique evaluates mother's blood for common fetal aneuploidies after 10 weeks of gestation and has a negative predictive value of 98–99%. Positive tests would need confirmation by invasive testing.

## Invasive Prenatal Testing

This includes chorionic villus biopsy (at or after 11–12 weeks gestation), amniocentesis (16–20 weeks) and cord blood sampling (after 18 weeks). Procedure-related risk in experienced hands with amniocentesis and chorionic villus sampling is very low (0.2–0.3%). These samples can be used for chromosomal studies, DNA based tests or enzyme assays. Amniotic fluid is the preferred sample for chromosomal studies, and chorionic tissue for DNA based tests and enzyme assays.

## Genetic Counseling

Genetic counseling is a process of helping people understand and adapt to the medical, psychological and familial implications of genetic contributions to disease, which integrates:

- Interpretation of family and medical histories to assess the chance of disease occurrence/recurrence
- Education about inheritance, testing, management, prevention, resources and research
- Counseling to promote informed choices and adaptation to the risk or condition

Genetic counseling is an important component of management of genetic disorders.

Indications for genetic counseling include: (i) Known or suspected hereditary disease in a patient/family; (ii) birth defects in previous children; (iii) unexplained intellectual disability, dysmorphism, multiple malformations; (iv) consanguinity; (v) exposure to a teratogen during pregnancy; and (vi) identification of malformation(s) by ultrasonography during pregnancy. Ideally, genetic couselling should be provided by trained genetic counsellors, or clinicians trained in medical genetics.

## Suggested Reading


1. Carbone L, Cariati F, Sarno L, et al. Non-invasive prenatal testing: Current perspectives and future challenges. Genes 2020;12:15.
2. Cassidy SB, Allanson JE. Management of genetic syndromes, 4th edn. Wiley Blackwell, USA, 2021.
3. Harper PS. Practical Genetic Counseling, 8th edn. Wright Publishers, Bristol, 2019.
4. Manickam K, McClain MR, Demmer LA, et al. Exome and genome sequencing for pediatric patients with Congenital anomalies or intellectual disability: an evidence-based clinical guideline of the American College of Medical Genetics and Genomics. Genet Med 2021;23:2029–37.
5. Miller DT, Adam MP, Aradhya S, et al. Consensus statement: chromosomal microarray is a first-tier clinical diagnostic test for individuals with developmental disabilities or congenital anomalies. Am J Hum Genet 2010; 86, 749–64.

Chapter 24

# Inborn Errors of Metabolism

❍ Neerja Gupta ❍ Madhulika Kabra

Inborn errors of metabolism (IEM) usually occur due to abnormality or absence of an enzyme or its cofactor that results in the accumulation or deficiency of a specific metabolite. Most IEMs are inherited in an autosomal recessive manner although dominant, X-linked and maternally transmitted disorders are also known. These disorders are individually rare, but collectively common and can manifest at any time from the fetal life to old age. Early recognition of signs and symptoms, prompt evaluation and management result in optimal outcome.

## Classification

*Disorders of intoxication* include IEMs that lead to accumulation of toxic compounds proximal to the metabolic block resulting in acute (vomiting, lethargy, encephalopathy, seizures), progressive or chronic (developmental delay, failure to thrive, seizures) symptoms. Symptoms can be precipitated by catabolic states such as fever, infections, immunization, dehydration or fasting). Aminoacidopathies (e.g. phenylketonuria, maple syrup urine disease), organic acidurias, urea cycle defects, carbohydrate intolerance disorders (galactosemia, hereditary fructose intolerance), disorders of copper/iron metabolism, and porphyrias belong to this category. Neurotransmitter disorders and amino acid synthesis defects are also included in this category. The course may be recurrent and episodic, and response to supportive therapy is rapid. Majority of these disorders are easily diagnosed by measuring various plasma/urine metabolites and most are treatable.

*Disorders of energy metabolism* include conditions with deficient energy production or utilization within liver, muscle, heart and brain. These are classified as mitochondrial energy defects (congenital lactic acidosis, mitochondrial respiratory chain defects, fatty acid oxidation defects, and ketone body defects), cytoplasmic energy defects (disorders of glycogen metabolism, and gluconeogenesis), hyperinsulinism and creatine metabolism. Failure to thrive, hypoglycemia with high lactate, hepatomegaly, hypotonia, cardiac and skeletal myopathies, neurological symptoms, sudden death and circulatory collapse may occur. Mitochondrial disorders are most severe, phenotypically heterogeneous and do not have any definitive treatment. Cytoplasmic energy defects are less severe and majority have a treatment. Lactic acidosis is a prominent feature of mitochondrial disorders whereas cytoplasmic energy defects usually have less tolerance to fasting.

*Disorders of complex molecules* include disorders involving cellular organelles such as lysosomal storage disorders, peroxisomal disorders, α1-antitrypsin deficiency and congenital disorders of glycosylation. Symptoms are slowly progressive and permanent and do not have precipitating factors. Most disorders have multisystem involvement. They usually have characteristic findings such as developmental delay, organomegaly, coarse facies, ocular involvement and arthropathy that enable a specific clinical diagnosis. Treatment is available for a few conditions.

## Clinical Suspicion

The diagnosis of IEM requires a high index of suspicion and is often delayed. Symptoms are often nonspecific, leading to evaluation for other disorders. Various presentations and their clinical clues that suggest the presence of IEMs are shown in **Box 24.1**. Figures 24.1 and 24.2 show the initial approach in patients with acute IEM and chronic encephalopathy. Differentiating between predominant involvement of gray and white matter helps in narrowing the diagnosis (Table 24.1).

## Laboratory Investigations

Basic metabolic screening includes measurement of blood levels of glucose, electrolytes, lactate, acid base status (pH, bicarbonate), ammonia and ketones (GELAAK). Based on these abnormalities, IEMs can be characterized into various diagnostic groups as shown in Table 24.2 and Fig. 24.1. Pre-transfusion specimens are preferred. Blood samples should be promptly transported to the laboratory.

**Box 24.1: Clues Suggesting Inborn Errors of Metabolism (IEM)**

- **Neonates and young infants**
- Unexpected deterioration after normal initial period
- Nonspecific, unexplained features such as poor feeding, lethargy, vomiting, failure to thrive, respiratory abnormalities, apnea, bradycardia, hypothermia, tone abnormalities, seizures, and encephalopathy
- Conjugated or unconjugated jaundice, liver failure, hypoglycemia

**Older infants and children**

- Sudden and rapid illness in a previously well child, often precipitated by fever, infection or fasting
- Acute encephalopathy; previous similar episodes
- Recurrent coma, stroke, ataxia, cramps, myopathy
- Developmental delay, regression, tone abnormalities, abnormal movements, or seizures
- Facial dysmorphism, structural anomalies of brain, cataract, retinopathy
- Cardiomyopathy, arrhythmia, deafness
- Hepatomegaly,hypoglycemia, jaundice
- Peculiar urinary odor (musty in phenylketonuria; cabbage like in tyrosinemia; maple syrup like in maple syrup urine disease; sweaty feet in isovaleric acidemia or glutaric acidemia type II; cat urine in multiple carboxylase deficiency)
- Persistent or recurrent hypoglycemia, intractable metabolic acidosis, hyperammonemia, hyperkalemia
- Reye syndrome like illness
- *E. coli* sepsis
- History of aversion to sweets, high protein

**Others**

- Family history of similar illness, unexplained sib deaths, or progressive neurological disease
- Parental consanguinity: Most acutely presenting metabolic disorders are autosomal recessive.

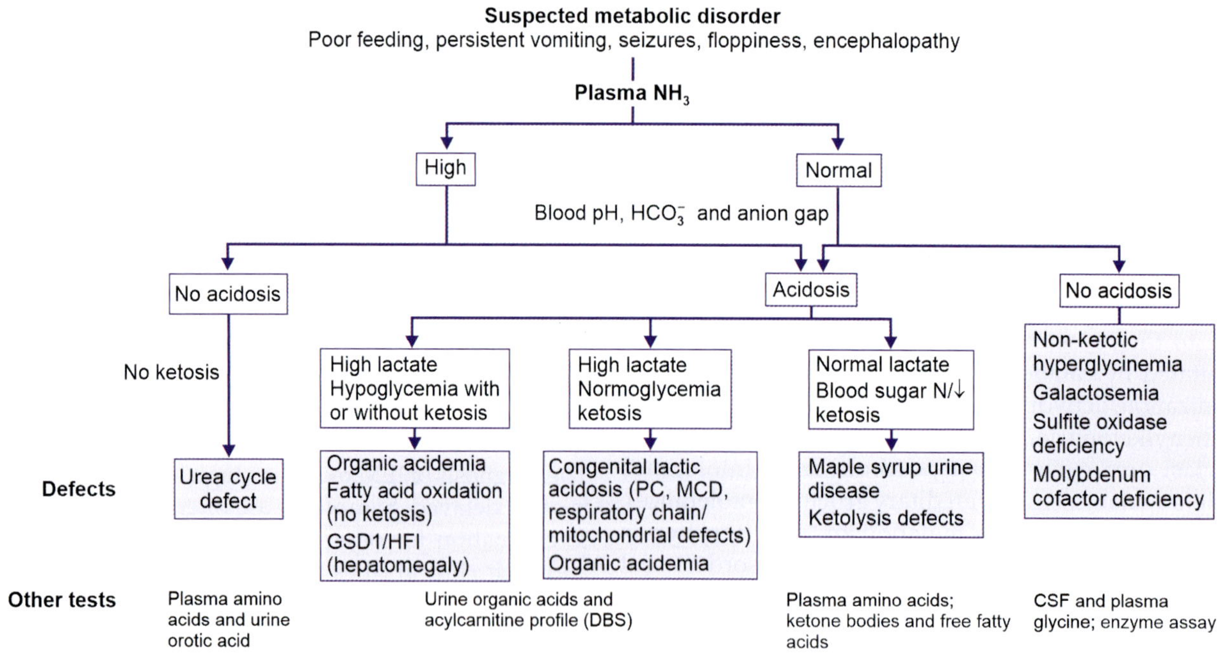


**Fig. 24.1.** Approach to a patient with acute IEM

N normal; DBS dried blood spot; HFI hereditary fructose intolerance; PC pyruvate carboxylase; MCD multiple carboxylase deficiency; MSUD maple syrup urine disease

*Blood ammonia:* During neonatal period, ammonia levels are <200 µg/dL; subsequently levels of <80 µg/dL are considered normal. In urea cycle disorders, ammonia levels usually exceed 1000 µg/dL and cause respiratory alkalosis with compensatory metabolic acidosis. Levels up to 500 µg/dL and 250 µg/dL are seen in organic acidurias, and fatty acid oxidation defects, respectively.

*Arterial lactate:* A free flowing sample is preferred. High lactate in the absence of shock, hypoxemia or cardiac disease are seen in organic acidemia, mitochondriopathies, glycogen storage disorder type 1 and fatty acid oxidation defects.

*Urine metabolic screen* includes pH, ketones and reducing substances. Urine is examined by ferric chloride,

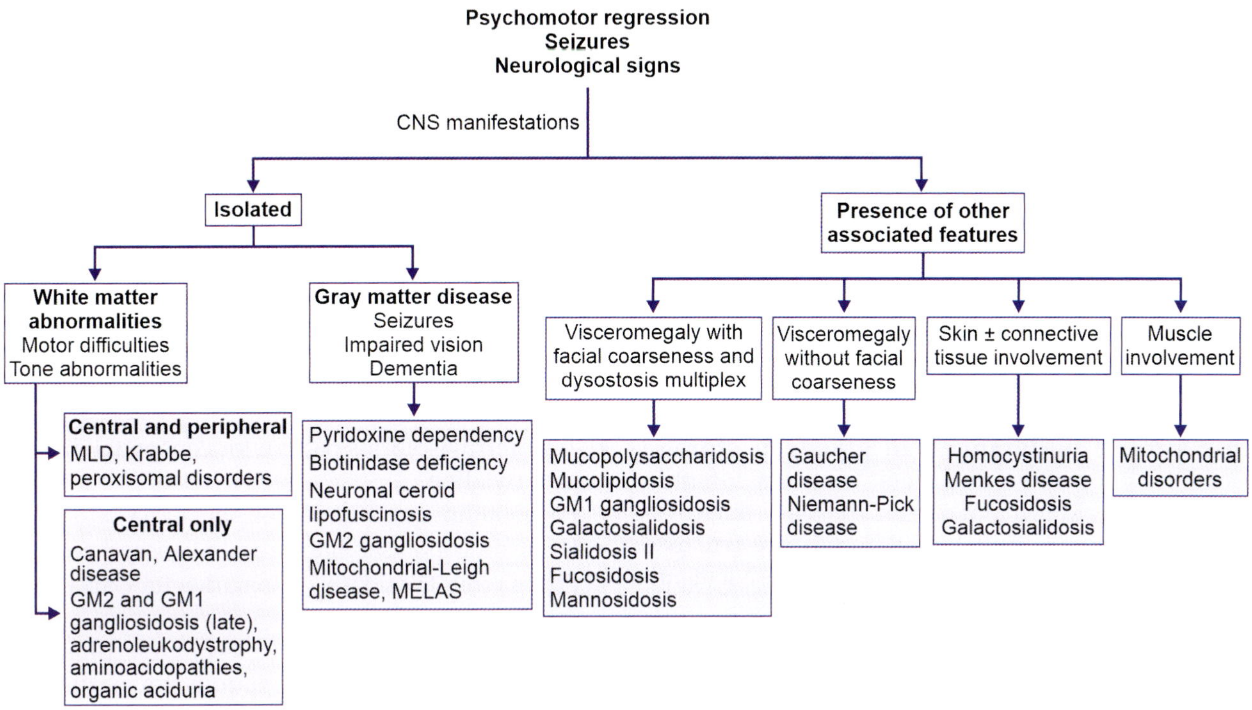


**Fig. 24.2:** Approach to child with chronic IEM

MLD metachromatic leukodystrophy; NCL neuronal ceroid lipofuscinosis; NPD Niemann-Pick disease; MPS mucopolysaccharidoses MELAS myopathy, encephalopathy, lactic acidosis and stroke like episodes; XLALD X-linked adrenoleukodystrophy

Modified from Clarke JTR. A Clinical Guide to Inherited Metabolic Disease (Reference 1)

**Table 24.1:** Differentiating features of gray matter and white matter disorders

| *Clinical features* | *Gray matter disease (poliodystrophy)* | *White matter disease (leukodystrophy)* |
|---|---|---|
| Age of onset | Early | Usually late (childhood) |
| Head size | Microcephaly (more common) | May have macrocephaly |
| Seizures | Early, severe | Late, uncommon |
| Cognitive functions | Affected early and progressive | May decline later in course |
| Spasticity | Late onset | Early, severe |
| Reflexes | Normal or brisk | Absent (neuropathy), brisk (long tracts involvement) |
| Eye | Retinal degeneration, cherry red spot | Optic atrophy, cataract |
| Peripheral neuropathy | Usually in late onset forms | Early demyelination |
| Electromyography | Usually normal | Slowed nerve conduction velocity |
| Visual evoked potentials | Usually normal | Prolonged or absent |
| Electroretinogram | Abnormal | Normal |
| MRI brain | Cerebral atrophy, basal ganglia involvement | White matter involvement (demyelination/dysmyelination) |
| Example | Tay-Sachs disease | Metachromatic leukodystrophy |

dinitrophenylhydrazine and nitroprusside tests for PKU, organic aciduria/maple syrup urine disease and homocystinuria, respectively. Biochemical screening may be normal during an asymptomatic state.

### *Other tests*

- Anemia and thrombocytopenia are important features of Gaucher disease; pancytopenia may be seen in propionic and methylmalonic acidemia. Peripheral smear may show vacuolated lymphocytes in neuronal ceroid lipofuscinosis, fucosidosis and sialidosis; acanthocytosis in abetalipoproteinemia and Hallervorden-Spatz disease.
- Liver function and renal function tests may be deranged in urea cycle defects, aminoacidopathies, organic acidemia, mitochondriopathies, peroxisomal, and lysosomal storage disorders. Metabolic acidosis with proximal tubular dysfunction is present in patients with Lowe syndrome, cystinosis, Wilson disease and galactosemia.
- Creatine phosphokinase may be elevated in disorders of glycogenolysis, gluconeogenesis, rhabdomyolysis, and fatty acid oxidation defects or mitochondrial disorders.
- Plasma uric acid is high in glycogen storage disorders type 1 and fatty acid oxidation defects; low in sulfite oxidase deficiency.
- Plasma vitamin $B_{12}$ and homocysteine levels may be deranged in cobalamin defects.

Table 24.2: Differential diagnosis of metabolic disorders with acute presentation

| | MSUD | Urea cycle defects | Organic acidemia | FAOD | Glycogen storage disorder | Mitochondrial disorders |
|---|---|---|---|---|---|---|
| Hypoglycemia | ± | – | ± | + | + | – |
| Lactic acidosis | ± | – | ± | ± | + | ++ |
| Metabolic acidosis | ± | –* | ++ | ± | ± | ± |
| Hyperammonemia | ± | ++ | + | ± | – | ± |
| Ketosis | ++ | – | ++ | – | ± | ± |

±may be present or absent; –absent; +present; ++always present
*respiratory alkalosis
FAOD fatty acid oxidation defect; MSUD maple syrup urine disease




- Lipid profile is deranged in glycogen storage disorders, lipoprotein disorders, transient infantile hypertriglyceridemia, Wolman disease, fructose-1,6-bisphosphatase deficiency, hereditary fructose intolerance and lipid storage disorders such as Niemann-Pick disease.
- Plasma copper levels are low in Wilson disease, Menkes disease and aceruloplasminemia. Serum iron levels are increased in hemochromatosis. Serum prolactin may be elevated in dopamine synthesis related neurotransmitter disorders.

*Special tests* detect abnormal metabolites in various body fluids.

- Acylcarnitine analysis using tandem mass spectrometry (MS/MS) or liquid chromatography LC-MS/MS (dried blood spot) for fatty acid oxidation defects and organic acidemia (methylmalonic acidemia/propionic acidemia) **(Box 24.2).**
- Organic acid analysis of urine samples by gas chromatography–mass spectrometry (GC-MS) for organic acidemia, fatty acid oxidation defects, mitochondrial disorders, urine orotic acid (urea cycle defects), and succinylacetone (tyrosinemia type 1).
- Quantitative amino acid analysis by U/HPLC (ultrahigh performance liquid chromatography) (plasma/cerebrospinal fluid) for maple syrup urine disease and PKU.
- Transferrin isoforms pattern for congenital disorders of glycosylation
- Porphobilinogen in urine for porphyria
- Urine mucopolysaccharide and oligosaccharide screen
- Plasma chitotriosidase: A biomarker for Gaucher disease and Niemann-Pick disease
- Specific enzyme assay (leukocytes, plasma, skin fibroblasts, liver biopsy) for various storage disorders are available and provide definitive diagnosis. Bone marrow aspirate is usually not required for making a diagnosis of specific storage disorders.
- Very long chain fatty acid analysis, phytanic and pristanic acids, plasmalogens for peroxisomal disorders.

Chest X-ray, echocardiography, and ultrasound abdomen are required in specific cases. Neuroimaging, electrophysiological studies, electroencephalogram (EEG) and skeletal survey are useful for various neurodegenerative and storage disorders.

### Molecular Testing

Although biochemical testing provides a quick diagnosis for acute IEM and helps in initiating quick management, a molecular diagnosis is necessary for the confirmation using either Sanger sequencing or next generation sequencing (NGS). Molecular testing using Sanger sequencing can be performed for common hotspot regions of a specific disorder. NGS is especially useful for the biochemical

**Box 24.2: Newborn Screening by Dried Blood Spot (DBS) Sampling**

Site of heel prick (shaded area) for newborn screening and a good dried blood spot. At least three spots are collected in full circle (15 mm) on S & S 903 (Schleicher and Schuell) on one side only and is thoroughly air dried. Clots and sample overlay should be avoided.

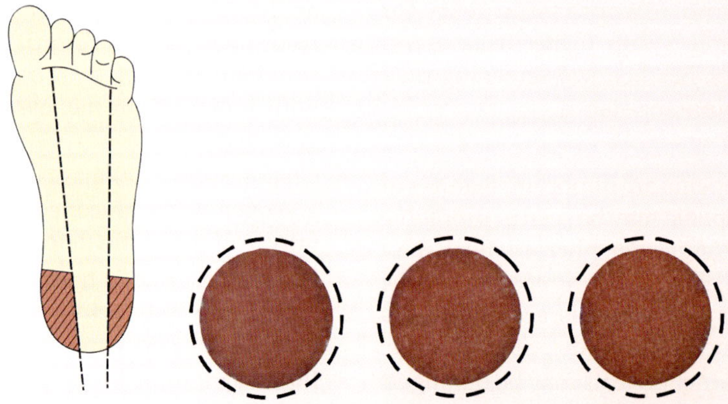

disorders lacking a specific biochemical test such as congenital disorder of glycosylation or for disorders involving large number or size of genes with a nonspecific clinical and biochemical phenotype such as organic acidemia, and mitochondriopathies. Molecular diagnosis is useful for prenatal diagnosis in subsequent pregnancies.

### *Biochemical Autopsy*

In a severely ill or dying child with suspected but undiagnosed IEM, parents should be advised about the need for a biochemical autopsy for confirmation of diagnosis. Following an informed written consent, the samples as given in Table 24.3 should be obtained before or within 1 to 2 hours of death to facilitate diagnosis.

## Principles of Management in Acute IEM

Treatment is symptomatic, supportive, prompt and often instituted empirically. Specific treatment is directed towards reversing the basic pathophysiological process causing the disease. It includes reduction of substrate accumulation for a deficient enzyme, reduce accumulated toxic metabolites, supplement metabolites, replace deficient enzyme or enhance residual enzyme activity (Fig. 24.3).

i. Eliminate dietary or parenteral intake of potentially toxic agents (e.g. protein, fat, galactose, fructose).

ii. Provide adequate calories (60–100 Cal/kg/day). Intravenous bolus of 2 mL/kg of 10% dextrose (200 mg/kg) followed by normal saline 10–20 mL/kg depending upon the perfusion, followed by 10% dextrose in 0.9% or 0.45% saline at 1.5 times the calculated maintenance. Add potassium chloride (1 cc per 100 cc fluids) when urinary output is established. Intralipids (2–3 g/kg/day) may be infused, if fatty acid oxidation defect is not suspected. In case of hyperglycemia (150–160 mg/dL), add insulin to prevent catabolism (0.05–0.1 units/kg/h).

iii. Correct metabolic acidosis (pH <7.30, bicarbonate <15 mEq/L, anion gap >16 mEq/L), dehydration and electrolyte imbalance.

iv. Treat intercurrent illness, if any.

v. Enhance excretion of toxic metabolites:

- Immediate measures to reduce blood ammonia are necessary as the risk for irreversible cerebral damage is related to its concentration. Intravenous phenylacetate and sodium benzoate with L-arginine are used as detoxifying agents in urea cycle defects and organic acidemias.
- In case of significant encephalopathy or ammonia levels persisting beyond 400 µg/dL (250 µmol/L), or if levels do not fall within 2 hr



**Table 24.3:** Workup in critically sick children with undiagnosed inborn error of metabolism

| *Investigations/sample/storage* | *Evaluate* |
|---|---|
| Clinical photograph; skeletal survey; infantogram (especially for peroxisomal/storage disorders) | Dysmorphism and skeletal abnormalities |
| *Blood:* | |
| 5 mL in heparin (plasma) at –20°C | Amino acids |
| 5–10 mL EDTA blood refrigerated; DNA frozen at –20°C | DNA |
| Dried blood spots on filter paper at room temperature | Acylcarnitines |
| EDTA blood 5 mL (for leukocytes) | Enzyme assays |
| *Urine:* 10–20 mL frozen in plain sterile tubes at –20° | Amino acids, organic acids |
| *Cerebrospinal fluid:* 3–5 mL in 1–2 aliquots frozen, at –70°C | Neurotransmitters, amino acids |
| *Tissue biopsy* | |
| *Skin biopsy:* ~3 mm diameter skin (include dermis) from the flexor aspect of the forearm or anterior aspect of thigh. Store at 37°C or refrigerate (not freeze) in culture medium or saline with glucose | Enzyme assays<br>DNA |
| *Liver, muscle, kidney, heart biopsy:* At least two tissue biopsies of about 1 mm$^3$; immediately frozen in liquid nitrogen and in glutaraldehyde | Enzyme assays<br>DNA |

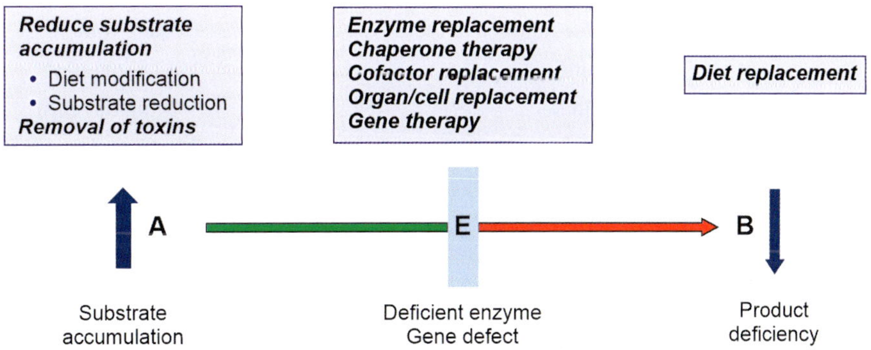


**Fig. 24.3:** Effect of deficient enzyme E on A and B of an affected pathway (lower panel) and the different therapeutic modalities (upper panel)

after initiation of IV treatment, dialysis is initiated. Hemodialysis is preferred to peritoneal dialysis and exchange transfusion. Oral carglumic acid (N-carbamylglutamate) is an adjunctive therapy for hyperammonemia and is used in N-acetylglutamate synthetase deficiency, propionic acidemia and methylmalonic acidemia.

- Carnitine eliminates organic acids as carnitine esters. Intravenous L-carnitine may be used in life-threatening situations associated with its deficiency, at a dose of 100 mg/kg over 30 minutes followed by a 100 mg/kg/day in 3–4 divided doses. L-carnitine should not be administered with sodium benzoate.
- In addition to above measures, intermittent oral therapy using metronidazole at 10 mg/kg/d is given in propionic acidemia.

vi. Empiric cofactor or coenzyme therapy may be administered in various metabolic disorders to maximize residual enzyme activity (Table 24.4). Oral anhydrous betaine (trimethylglycine) is given in cobalamin C deficiency (up to 250 mg/kg/day) and classical pyridoxine non-responsive homocystinuria (100 mg/kg/day) in divided doses.

vii. Empirically, daily higher doses of thiamine (300 mg), riboflavin (100 mg), biotin (10 mg) in addition to co-enzyme Q (5–15 mg/kg/day) are given for suspected mitochondriopathies.

viii. Intractable seizures without metabolic acidosis or hyperammonemia are treated with intravenous pyridoxine.

ix. Long-term adherence to dietary and pharmacologic regimen is recommended. Prompt recognition and avoidance of physiologic stresses (fever, infection, trauma, surgery, fasting) and changes in diet that may precipitate symptoms is important in preventing metabolic decompensation.

If clinical improvement is observed and a final diagnosis is not established, some amino acid intake should be provided after 2–3 days of complete protein restriction. Essential amino acids or total protein is provided orally or IV at an initial dose of 0.5 g/kg/day and gradually increased to 1.0–1.5 g/kg/day, until diagnostic evaluation is complete and plans are made for long-term therapy. Appropriate amino acid formula (free of precursor amino acids) or protein free infant formula with natural protein is gradually introduced with careful clinical and laboratory monitoring. In infants, expressed human milk is preferred as it can be measured and protein intake quantified.

### Principles of Management in Chronic IEM

A multidisciplinary team of metabolic specialists, pediatric neurologists, clinical geneticist, cardiologist, orthopedic surgeon and physiotherapist is required to maximize the supportive care in these patients. Supply of deficient enzyme (enzyme replacement), enhancing residual enzyme activity through cofactor and megavitamin therapy (enzyme enhancement/organ transplantation), or reduction of substrate accumulation (substrate reduction) are available for these disorders (Fig. 24.3).

Most IEMs are inherited in autosomal recessive manner and risk of recurrence in subsequent pregnancy is 25%. Few disorders are X-linked, autosomal dominant and mitochondrial in inheritance. Prenatal diagnosis is possible by enzyme assays or molecular testing on fetal DNA from chorionic villus biopsy or amniotic fluid at 11–13 weeks and 16–18 weeks' gestation, respectively (Chapter 23).

## SPECIFIC DISORDERS

### Aminoacidopathies

These result from abnormal breakdown of amino acids in the cytoplasm and do not involve coenzyme A (CoA) activated metabolites. Clinical symptoms occur due to accumulation of toxic metabolites that may cause specific organ damage. Dietary restriction of protein and the offending amino acid and avoidance and/or prompt treatment of catabolic states are main treatment modalities. Deficient absorption of essential amino acids such as tryptophan in Hartnup disease or increased urinary concentration of insoluble amino acids causing nephrolithiasis as seen in cystinuria are the disorders of intestinal and/or renal transport of amino acids.

#### *Tyrosinemia Type 1 (Hepatorenal Tyrosinemia)*

It is an autosomal recessive disorder of tyrosine metabolism that occurs due to deficient fumarylacetoacetate hydrolase (FAH), which is encoded by FAH.

**Table 24.4:** Cofactor therapy

| *Disorder* | *Cofactor/adjunctive therapy* | *Dosage (oral)* |
|---|---|---|
| Maple syrup urine disease | Thiamine | 10–15 mg/day |
| Methylmalonic acidemia | Vitamin $B_{12}$ | 1–2 mg/day (IM) |
| Glutaric aciduria type I | Riboflavin | 20–40 mg/day |
| Biotinidase<br>Propionic acidemia | Biotin | 5–10 mg/day |
| Multiple carboxylase deficiency | Biotin | 10–40 mg/day |
| Folinic acid responsive seizures | Folinic acid | 5–15 mg/day |
| Pyridoxine responsive seizures | Pyridoxine | 50–100 mg/day |
| Homocystinuria | Pyridoxine | 50–500 mg/day |

IM intramuscular

*Clinical features:* It classically presents as severe liver disease in young infants. Severe forms present during infancy with vomiting, diarrhea, bleeding diathesis, hepatomegaly, jaundice, hypoglycemia, ascites and coagulopathy. Children older than 6 months of age may come to medical attention with variable degree of renal dysfunction, hypophosphatemic rickets and aminoaciduria (Fig. 24.4). Untreated children may have repeated, often unrecognized, neurologic crises lasting 1–7 days that can include change in mental status, abdominal pain, peripheral neuropathy, autonomic dysfunction and/or respiratory failure requiring mechanical ventilation. Death in the untreated child usually occurs before age 10 years, typically from liver failure, neurologic crisis or hepatocellular carcinoma.

*Diagnosis:* Plasma amino acids show elevated tyrosine, methionine and phenylalanine in addition to markedly elevated alpha-fetoprotein (average 160,000 ng/mL) (normal: <1000 ng/mL for infants 1–3 months; <12 ng/mL for age 3 months to 18 yr). Presence of high succinylacetone in blood or urine is diagnostic. Molecular confirmation is done by Sanger sequencing or NGS.

*Treatment:* Initiation of oral nitisinone (NTBC) at 1 mg/kg/day along with dietary restriction of phenylalanine and tyrosine is the mainstay of treatment. NTBC blocks tyrosine degradation at an early step before the actual genetic defect to prevent the production of downstream damaging metabolites such as fumarylacetoacetate and succinylacetone. Liver transplant is indicated for liver failure, cancer, or failure to respond to NTBC.

### Maple Syrup Urine Disease (MSUD)

MSUD is due to decreased activity of branched chain alpha ketoacid dehydrogenase (BCKAD) complex, a mitochondrial enzyme involved in degradation of branched chain amino acids (leucine, isoleucine and valine). There are five different phenotypes based on clinical findings and response to thiamine. This enzyme has four subunits: E1$\alpha$, E1$\beta$, E2 and E3, deficiency of which causes MSUD type 1A (BCKDHA), MSUD type 1B (BCKDHB), MSUD type 2 (DBT) and MSUD type 3 (dihydrolipoamide dehydrogenase deficiency).

*Clinical features:* The first clinical sign of classic MSUD in untreated neonates is maple syrup odor in cerumen at 12–24 hours after birth. By the age of 2–3 days, ketonuria, irritability, and poor feeding develops followed by deepening encephalopathy manifesting as lethargy, intermittent apnea, opisthotonus, and stereotyped movements such as "fencing" and "bicycling" by age 4–5 days. Coma and central respiratory failure may occur by age 7–10 days. Individuals with intermediate or intermittent forms of MSUD show severe metabolic intoxication and encephalopathy under sufficient catabolic stress. In infants and toddlers, leucinosis causes altered level of consciousness, acute dystonia, and ataxia. Neurologic signs of intoxication in older individuals vary, and include cognitive impairment, hyperactivity, anorexia, sleep disturbances, hallucinations, mood swings, focal dystonia, choreoathetosis, and ataxia.

*Diagnosis:* Elevated plasma concentrations (5- to 10-fold greater than normal) of branched-chain amino acids (BCAAs) (leucine, isoleucine, and valine) and allo-isoleucine, as well as a generalized disturbance of plasma amino acid concentration ratios is detected by 12–24 hours of age.

Ketonuria can be detected by standard urine test strips. Dinitrophenylhydrazine (DNPH) added to urine produces a yellow-white precipitate due to presence of branched chain ketoacids. Molecular (DNA) testing is useful for confirming the diagnosis.

*Treatment:* Dietary leucine restriction, high-calorie BCAA-free formulas, judicious supplementation with isoleucine and valine, and frequent clinical and biochemical monitoring are necessary. Some patients with milder forms may respond to thiamine. Exchange transfusions, hemodialysis and hemofiltration reduce elevated levels of BCAAs in extremely sick children. Brain edema is a common complication. Orthotopic liver transplantation is an effective therapy for classic MSUD.

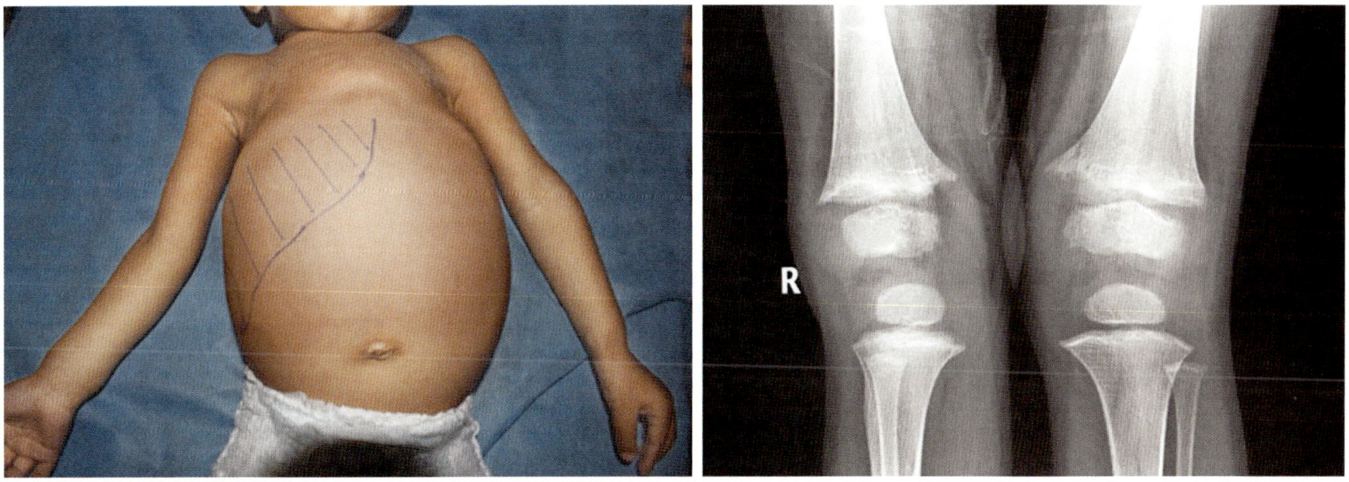


**Fig. 24.4:** A 3-year-old child with tyrosinemia type 1. Note the presence of hepatomegaly, wrist widening and rachitic changes at knees

### Alkaptonuria

This was the first inborn error of metabolism described by Garrod in 1902 and is caused by defect of the enzyme homogentisate 1,2-dioxygenase (homogentisic acid oxidase). It occurs worldwide.

*Clinical features:* The three cardinal features of alkaptonuria are darkening of urine on standing or dark urine (in infants staining of diapers), ochronosis and large joints arthritis involving shoulders and hips. Connective tissues and joints manifestions occur around third decade. A black pigment is deposited in the sclera (between the cornea and the canthi) and the ear and nose cartilage (ochronosis). The pigment in ochronosis is probably a polymer of homogentisic acid. Pigment deposits irritate the articular cartilage, resulting in degeneration and osteoarthritis like changes. Intervertebral disks are degenerated, spaces are narrowed and calcification occurs. Renal stones and cardiac valve involvement may occur after sixth decade. These patients may have associated hypothyroidism.

*Diagnosis:* The urine shows a black reaction with Fehling or Benedict reagents but no reaction with glucose oxidase. Urine GCMS detects homogentisic acid (HGA).

*Treatment:* Dietary restriction of tyrosine and phenylalanine and high dose of vitamin C are not efficacious. Nitisinone inhibits the enzyme that produces HGA and may be useful in decreasing progression of disease.

### Phenylketonuria

Phenylketonuria is an autosomal recessive disorder that occurs due to defect in phenylalanine hydroxylase (PAH) activity, encoded by PAH.

*Clinical features:* It is characterized by profound, irreversible intellectual disability, microcephaly, epilepsy, behavioral problems, and musty odor. Eczema, and skin and hair hypopigmentation occur due to low tyrosine levels (Fig. 24.5).

*Diagnosis:* A plasma phenylalanine concentration of >120 µmol/L (2 mg/dL), with a high (>3) ratio of phenylalanine to tyrosine (normal <1) is diagnostic. Untreated patients with classical PKU may show plasma phenylalanine levels >1,200 µmol/L. DNA testing is confirmatory.

*Treatment:* A low-protein diet and use of phenylalanine-free medical formula, as soon as possible after birth, to achieve plasma concentrations 120–360 µmol/L (2–6 mg/dL) up to 12 years of age and 120 to 600 µmol/L ≥12 years of age) is recommended. Sapropterin supplementation is given at a dose of 10–20 mg/kg/day based on the tetrahydrobiopterin ($BH_4$) responsiveness.

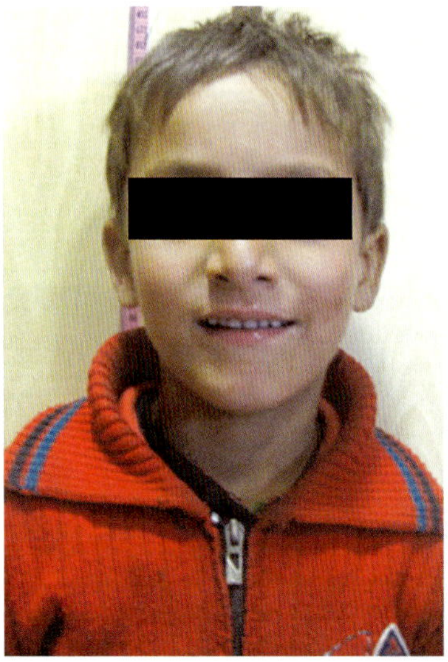

Fig. 24.5: Blond hair in a 6-year-old child with phenylketonuria

### Classic Homocystinuria

This occurs due to cystathionine β-synthase (CBS) deficiency leading to accumulation of plasma homocysteine, which has deleterious effects on the central nervous system, vessels, skin, joints and skeleton. Two clinical variants exist: B6 (pyridoxine)-responsive homocystinuria and B6-non-responsive homocystinuria. B6-responsive homocystinuria is typically, but not always, milder than the nonresponsive variant and has a better outcome than the nonresponsive ones.

*Clinical features:* The usual age of presentation is 3–4 years. Features include developmental delay/intellectual disability, ectopia lentis and/or severe myopia, skeletal abnormalities (tall stature and marfanoid habitus) (Fig. 24.6), and thromboembolism. They can also have seizures, psychiatric problems, extrapyramidal signs such

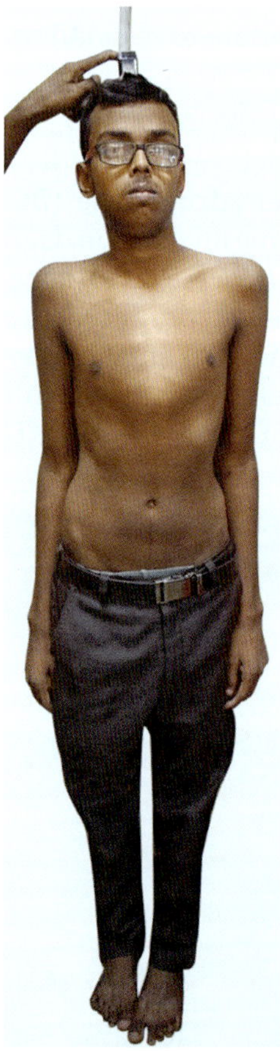

Fig. 24.6: A 15-year-old male child with classical homocystinuria with poor treatment compliance. Note the marfanoid habitus and pectus carinatum

as dystonia, hypopigmentation, and pancreatitis. Ectopia lentis occurs by 8 years of age. Thromboembolism is the major cause of early death and morbidity.

*Diagnosis*

i. Measurement of amino acids in plasma and urine: Markedly increased concentrations of plasma homocysteine >100 μmol/L; high levels of methionine >50 μmol/L; and increased concentration of urine homocysteine. Urine nitroprusside test is a good screening test. Plasma total homocysteine levels are important for monitoring the treatment (normal levels <15 μmol/L).
ii. Confirmation by CBS enzyme activity or molecular testing for variations in *CBS*.

*Treatment* is directed towards lowering the plasma homocysteine levels to as close to normal as possible, through lifelong methionine-restricted diet with frequent metabolic monitoring. Vitamin $B_6$ (pyridoxine) therapy at 200 mg/day is helpful for pyridoxine responsive forms. Oral folic acid (5 mg/day) and vitamin $B_{12}$ (1 mg IM once a month) are given for associated folate and vitamin $B_{12}$ deficiency. Oral betaine at 100 mg/kg/d (in two divided doses) is effective in lowering homocysteine levels and the vascular complications.

## Urea Cycle Defects

Large amounts of nitrogen is produced in the form of toxic ammonia after protein breakdown that normally gets converted to urea by urea cycle **(Fig. 24.7a)** and excreted in the urine.

Defects in any of these enzymes are characterized by encephalopathy and other symptoms of hyperammonemia and deranged amino acid metabolism requiring prompt management as mentioned above . A systematic approach to a case of hyperammonemia is illustrated **(Fig. 24.7b)**.

## Organic Aciduria

Organic aciduria are a group of disorders characterized by the excretion of non-amino organic acids in urine. These disorders result from enzyme deficiencies in the mitochondrial metabolism of CoA-activated carboxylic acids, most of which are derived from various amino acid degradation such as leucine, isoleucine, valine, methionine, threonine, lysine, hydroxylysine and tryptophan.

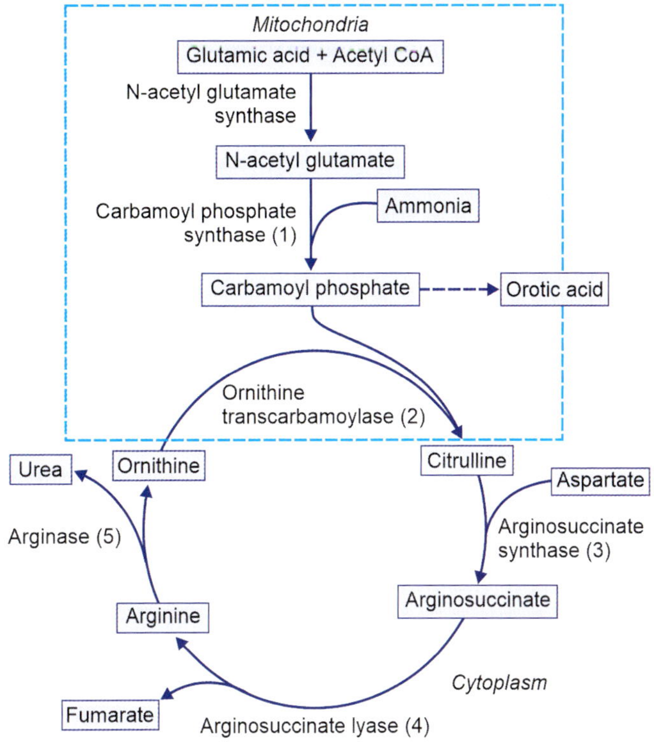


**Fig. 24.7a:** Pathways for ammonia disposal and ornithine metabolism. Deficiency of enzymes results in the following: (1) CPS deficiency, (2) OTC deficiency, (3) citrullinemia, (4) arginosuccinic aciduria and (5) argininemia

Clinical features such as encephalopathy and episodic metabolic acidosis occur as a result of accumulation of toxic intermediates and due to a disturbance of mitochondrial energy metabolism and carnitine homeostasis. As the defective enzymes are more distant, a complete return to normal metabolism may not be possible.

These disorders require avoidance of protein catabolism and dietary restriction of the relevant amino acid(s). Adjunctive therapy using carnitine or glycine (to form

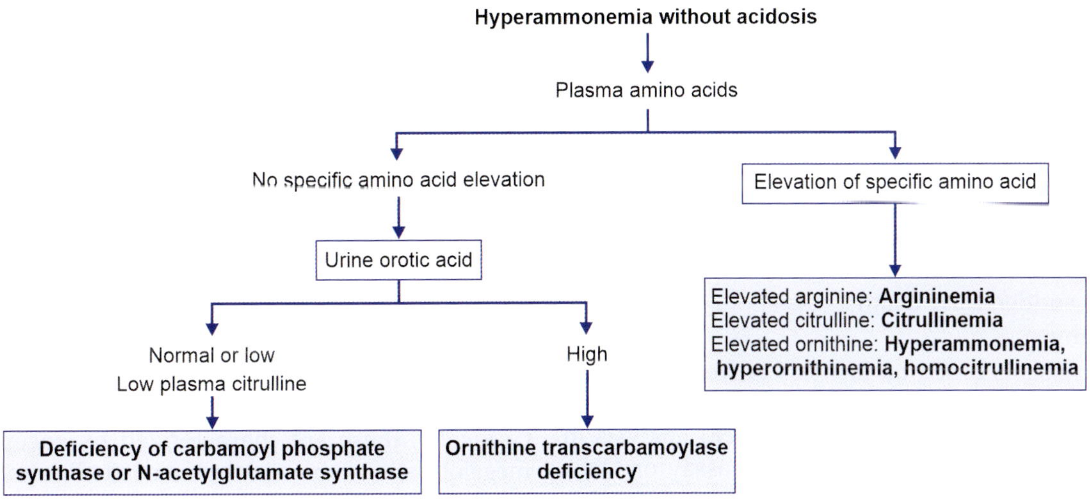


**Fig. 24.7b:** Algorithm to distinguish different urea cycle defects

isovalerylglycine in isovaleric aciduria) is useful. Biotin is a cofactor of the mitochondrial carboxylases. Disorders of biotin metabolism such as biotinidase deficiency or holocarboxylase synthetase deficiency (multiple carboxylase deficiencies) are often included among the organic acidurias as these usually diagnosed through urinary organic acid analysis. As biotinidase deficiency is treated by biotin supplementation, it has been included in newborn screening programs using dried blood spot.

### Fatty Acid Oxidation Defects

Mitochondrial fatty acid oxidation plays a major role in energy production during fasting or periods of high-energy demand either through complete oxidation or through ketone production in the liver, which serves as an alternative energy source for the brain. It involves three processes:

*Mobilization of fatty acids into mitochondria.* Long chain fatty acids (C14–20) undergo active transport through carnitine shuttle; whereas short (C4–C6) and medium chain (C8–C12) fatty acids enter independently of carnitine and are activated to coenzyme A (CoA) esters. Disorders of carnitine cycle includes carnitine palmitoyl transferase I and II deficiency.

*β-oxidation:* This involves removal of 2-carbon fragments (i.e. acetyl-CoA) from the transported saturated fatty acids via an enzymatic reaction. Each enzyme has different chain length specificity. Deficiency of various acyl-CoA dehydrogenases (AD) results in short chain AD (SCAD) deficiency, medium chain AD (MCAD) deficiency, long chain AD (LCHAD) and very long chain AD (VLCAD) deficiency.

*Electron transfer to the respiratory chain:* Acetyl-CoA is utilized as energy substrate in muscle and liver. Disorder includes glutaric aciduria type II (multiple acyl-CoA dehydrogenase or MAD deficiency).

#### Clinical Features

The illness may have varying severity and presents at any age. Symptoms are precipitated by fasting, exercise or intercurrent illness leading to episodes of metabolic decompensation. Accumulation of toxic metabolites can cause liver dysfunction or cardiomyopathy. These disorders usually present with:

i. Acute hypoketotic hypoglycemia and encephalopathy, precipitated by fasting, leading to coma or epileptic seizures (Reye-like illness)
ii. Hepatomegaly and liver dysfunction
iii. Cardiomyopathy (hypertrophic more common than dilated) and conduction defects including arrhythmias causing sudden early death
iv. Myopathy

The diagnosis is based on analysis of free fatty acids and ketone bodies (3-hydroxybutyrate and acetoacetate), acylcarnitine profile and urine organic acid analysis in acute state and is confirmed by enzyme assay or DNA analysis. Prolonged fasting should be avoided. Carnitine supplementation is mostly not required. Medium chain triglycerides rich formula can be used, but is not effective in MCAD and MAD deficiency.

### Mitochondrial Disorders

Mitochondria are mainly involved in the energy production pathway of oxidative phosphorylation. Mitochondrial disorders refer to defects that cause primary or secondary impairment of adenosine triphosphate (ATP) production. Affected proteins include components of respiratory chain complexes; components of the final pathways of pyruvate dehydrogenase complex and the Krebs cycle, mitochondrial deoxyribonucleic acid (DNA), ribonucleic acid (RNA) and various other components of mitochondrial homeostasis. Since mitochondria are mainly derived from the ovum, mitochondrial DNA (mtDNA) disorders are maternally inherited. Disorders that occur due to nuclear DNA (nDNA) mutations are autosomal recessive, autosomal dominant or X-linked.

A mitochondrial disorder is often suspected with multisystem involvement such as stroke, hearing loss, muscle weakness, cardiomyopathy, and variable degree of liver or endocrine dysfunction. Catabolic states such as intercurrent infections often trigger deterioration of clinical condition.

Disorders due to mtDNA deletion/duplication mutations are chronic progressive external ophthalmoplegia, Kearns-Sayre syndrome and Pearson syndrome. Disorders caused by mtDNA point mutations include Leber hereditary optic neuropathy, maternally inherited Leigh syndrome, mitochondrial encephalopathy, lactic acidosis and stroke (MELAS), myoclonic epilepsy with ragged red fibers (MERRF), neurogenic weakness, ataxia and retinitis pigmentosa (NARP), hypertrophic cardiomyopathy, mitochondrial myopathy and nonsyndromic aminoglycoside-induced sensorineural hearing loss.

Markedly elevated blood lactate and lactate-to-pyruvate ratio >30 suggests a defect in oxidative phosphorylation. Other biochemical features are elevated cerebrospinal fluid (CSF) lactate, altered plasma amino acids with elevated alanine, metabolic acidosis, hypoglycemia and ketosis. Muscle biopsy may show ragged red fibers as well as subsarcolemmal accumulation of mitochondria. Staining for succinate dehydrogenase and cytochrome C oxidase is useful. Brain magnetic resonance imaging and/or spectroscopy are helpful in diagnosis. Exome sequencing is useful in making a confirmatory diagnosis for the nuclear mitochondrial disorders.

No specific therapy is available. Supportive treatment includes supplementation with vitamins and cofactors such as riboflavin, coenzyme Q or thiamine. Sodium valproate and statins are avoided.

### Cobalamin and Folate Metabolism Disorders

Most disorders of cobalamin metabolism as well as nutritional deficiency of vitamin $B_{12}$ cause methylmalonic aciduria. Clinically, these are characterized by encephalopathy, megaloblastic anemia and thromboembolic complications of hyperhomocysteinemia. Diagnosis involves the analysis of urinary organic acids (methylmalonic aciduria in disorders of cobalamin metabolism, and vitamin $B_{12}$ nutritional deficiency), plasma amino acids (elevated homocysteine), and levels of folate. Treatment includes cobalamin and folate supplementation, betaine and methionine based on the underlying defect.

### Disorders of Metal Transport or Utilization

Altered copper metabolism due to defect in *ATP7B* and *ATP7A* genes results in Wilson disease and Menke disease, respectively. Wilson disease presents with hepatic, neurologic and psychiatric manifestations between early childhood till fifth decade, while patients with Menkes disease suffer from neurological and connective tissue related abnormalities. Presence of Kayser-Fleischer rings due to corneal copper deposition is pathognomonic of Wilson disease and is seen in half of patients with hepatic manifestations and in 90% of these with neurological features. Biochemical diagnosis involves the measurement of copper and ceruloplasmin in serum, urine, or liver tissue. Treatment in Wilson disease is aimed at reducing copper load, while copper should be parenterally substituted in Menkes disease.

Acrodermatitis enteropathica is an autosomal recessive disorder due to defects in *SLC39A4* characterized by zinc malabsorption. It manifests with chronic diarrhea, perioral and perianal vesicobullous skin lesions, alopecia and neurological problems. Diffuse hair loss and dystrophic changes in nails are frequent. It is treated with zinc supplementation.

### Defects of Carbohydrate Metabolism and Transport

These disorders include galactosemia, hereditary fructose intolerance and glycogen storage disorders. Major features include hypoglycemia, liver dysfunction with or without skeletal and/or cardiac muscle involvement due to toxicity, deficiency of energy or storage.

#### *Classical Galactosemia*

There are three disorders of galactose metabolism **(Fig. 24.8)**, but it is the deficiency of the enzyme galactose-1-phosphate uridylyltransferase (GALT), that is referred to as classical galactosemia. Deficiency of GALT results in accumulation of galactose-1-phosphate and other metabolites (e.g. galactitol) that have toxic effects on the liver and other organs.

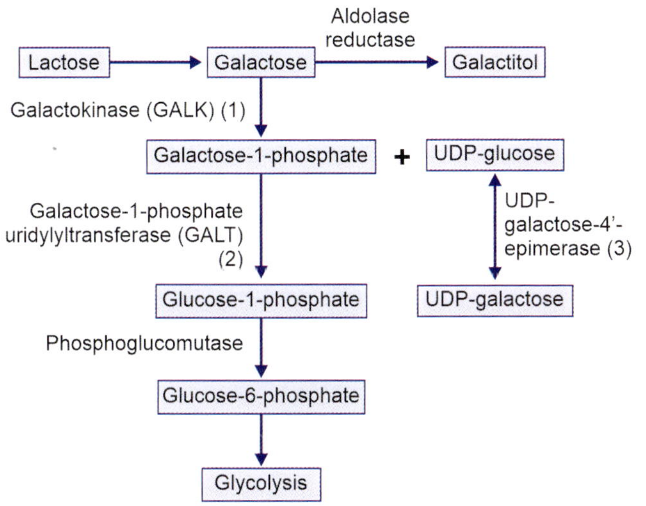


**Fig. 24.8:** Disorders of galactose metabolism. Deficiency of enzyme results in the following: (1) Galactokinase deficiency, (2) Classical galactosemia, (3) Epimerase deficiency galactosemia (GALE). UDP uridine diphosphate glucose

Patients are normal at birth, but by 3–4 days of breast milk or formula feeding show life-threatening disease with vomiting, diarrhea and poor weight gain. Jaundice, coagulopathy and liver dysfunction are progressive and appear at the end of first or second week of life. The disease may present initially with indirect hyperbilirubinemia due to hemolysis secondary to high levels of galactose-1-phosphate in erythrocytes. Many affected infants die of *E. coli* sepsis in the neonatal period. Untreated infants, if surviving the neonatal period, have persistent liver disease, cataracts and intellectual disability. Proximal renal tubular dysfunction may be present. Variable degree of growth abnormalities, intellectual disability, speech problems and hypergonadotrophic hypogonadism may be observed even in treated patients.

The diagnosis is confirmed by elevated RBC galactose-1-phosphate concentration (>10 mg/dL in classical galactosemia), reduced RBC GALT enzyme activity (absent or <1%) or DNA analysis. A negative urine dipstick by glucose oxidase method with positive Benedict reaction indicates presence of non-glucose reducing substances, such as galactose or fructose and is a useful bedside screening test. A negative test does not eliminate the possibility, especially if the patient has received IV glucose for more than a few hours.

***Management:*** If the diagnosis is suspected galactose-containing feedings should be discontinued immediately and replaced by soy based or lactose free formula pending results of confirmatory enzyme assay or genetic studies. Early and timely initiation of therapy results in resolution of symptoms and prevents complications. Galactose restricted diet is required throughout life. This disorder is being screened through newborn screening program in various states in India (Chapter 23).

#### *Glycogen Storage Diseases*

Glycogen is an extensively branched polysaccharide macromolecule formed by thousands of glucose units joined into chains by α-1–4 and α-1–6 bond. Ingested carbohydrate is absorbed as glucose via the portal system, phosphorylated to intermediate compounds (glucose-6-phosphate and glucose-1-phosphate) and stored as glycogen. Glycogen is stored predominantly in liver and muscle. and these are the tissues predominantly affected in the classic glycogenoses. Hepatic glycogen provides energy between meals or during fasting and is critical for glucose homeostasis whereas muscle glycogen is used to make adenosine triphosphate (ATP) for contraction. When peripheral glucose is utilized and its levels fall, glycogen is depolymerized, bonds at branch points are split and free glucose is released into blood by hydrolytic dephosphorylation (glycogenolysis) **(Fig. 24.9a)**. The glycogen storage diseases (GSDs) are an etiologically heterogenous group of disorders due to defect in the synthesis and degradation of glycogen, causing glycogen deposition in tissue cells. Hepatic glycogenoses

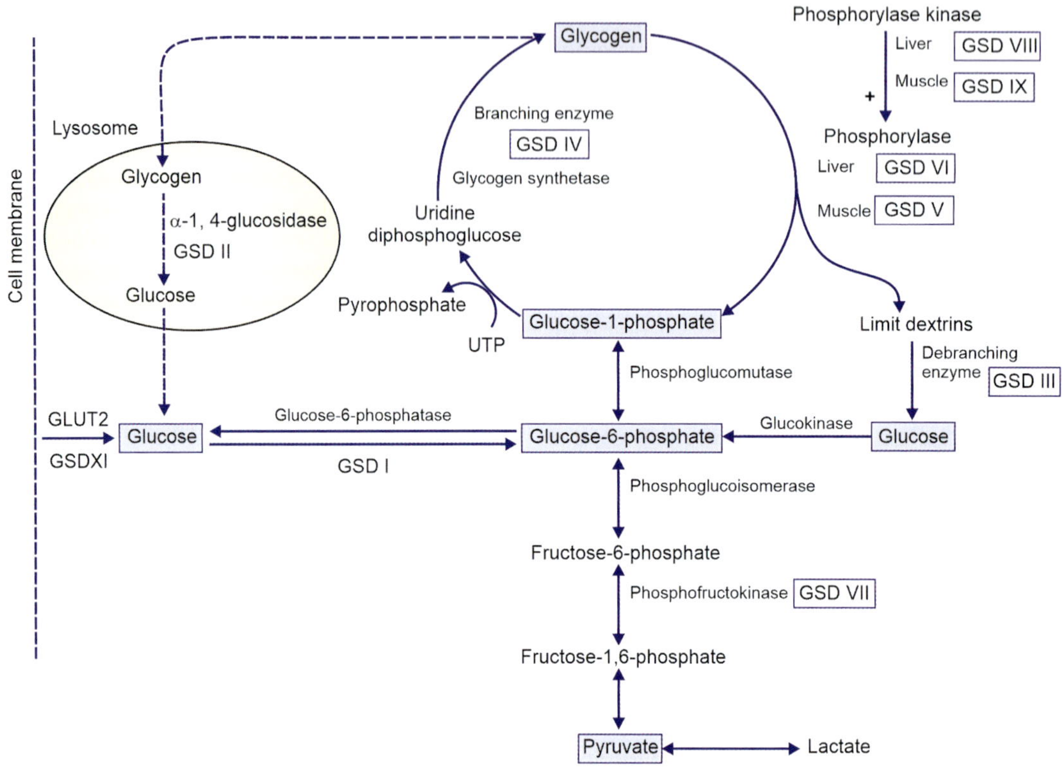


**Fig. 24.9a:** Schematic glucose and glycogen metabolism in liver and lysosomes. Common enzyme defects and corresponding glycogenoses are depicted

present classically with hypoglycemia after short periods of fasting, whereas muscle glycogenoses present with cramps, weakness, stiffness, or rhabdomyolysis.

***Hepatic glycogenoses*** GSD Ia (von Gierke disease), Ib, type IIIa (Cori/Forbes), IIIb, IV (Anderson), VI (Hers) and IX present with hepatomegaly and hypoglycemia. Figure 24.9b shows a child with GSD I with 'doll like facies' with protuberant abdomen due to marked hepatomegaly. Type 1 is classified as Ia, and Ib either due to deficiency of glucose-6-phosphatase (type 1a) or the translocase T1 deficiency that transports glucose-6-phosphate into microsomes (type 1b). Type 1b may resemble Crohn disease or ulcerative colitis as it is associated with chronic inflammatory bowel disease, neutropenia and/or neutrophil dysfunction.

Glycogenosis type IIIa is more common and may have associated high creatine phosphate kinase (CPK) and myopathy in addition to elevated transaminases. GSD IIIb has hepatic involvement only.

Patients with Fanconi-Bickel syndrome (GSD XI) present with features of type I GSD with hyperlipidemia and hyperuricemia along with renal tubular dysfunction (Fanconi syndrome). Patients have failure to thrive, hepatomegaly, fasting hypoglycemia and intolerance to galactose. It occurs due to defect in glucose/galactose transporter GLUT2.

In glycogen synthase deficiency (GSD 0) patients have fasting ketotic hypoglycemia, and ketosis with elevated lactate postprandially and on glucose tolerance test. There is no glycogen storage.

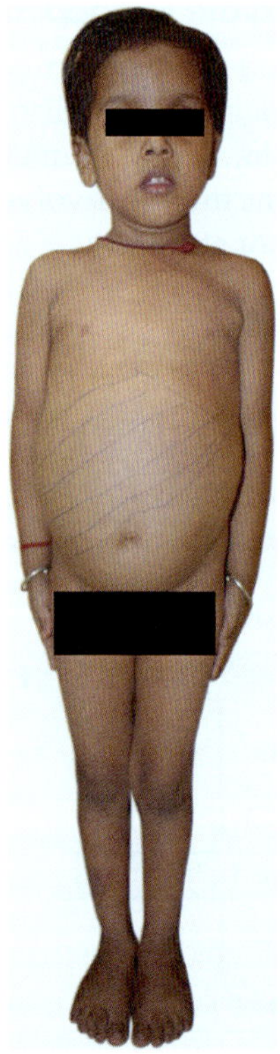

**Fig. 24.9b:** A 4–5-year-old child with GSD I on dietary therapy. Note massive hepatomegaly

The therapy of hepatic glycogenoses is targeted to maintain normoglycemia and is achieved by frequent feeds, uncooked corn-starch supplementation, or continuous overnight tube feeding. Uncooked starch at a dose of 1.6–2.6 g/kg body weight (depending on the age) acts as a slow release form of glucose. This is especially useful in type I, III and IV but most demanding in type I. Overtreatment with corn-starch should be avoided especially in type III as it can lead to excessive weight gain due to excess of glycogen formation. Medium chain triglycerides supplementation improves the growth and the metabolic control. A high carbohydrate and high protein diet is useful for GSD III, VI, IX. The intake of lactose, fructose and sucrose should be restricted, except fruits, vegetables and small amounts of milk products. Enough nutrients, vitamins and minerals should be given. If despite optimizing dietary treatment, serum triglyceride levels remain above 900 mg/dL, triglyceride-lowering drugs (nicotinic acid, fibrates) are advised to reduce risk of cholelithiasis and pancreatitis. Allopurinol (10 mg/kg/day, divided into 3 doses) should be given for hyperuricemia. Orthotopic liver transplant is an option for GSD I patients who have poor metabolic control or liver involvement in the form of multiple hepatic adenomas, hepatic failure or hepatocellular carcinoma.

*Muscle glycogenoses* GSD V (McArdle disease), VII (Tarui) and II (Pompe) primarily involve muscle. GSD V and VII often present in adolescence with exercise intolerance and myoglobinuria. These patients may have muscular hypotonia, weakness, easy fatigability and muscle cramps. Due to wider availability of DNA testing, a muscle biopsy is rarely necessary to confirm the diagnosis.

Glycogenosis type II or Pompe disease is a lysosomal storage disorder that results from lysosomal storage of glycogen in skeletal muscles, cardiac and smooth muscles due to deficiency of the enzyme acid alpha-glucosidase (GAA). It is characterized by relentlessly progressive motor, pulmonary, and cardiac dysfunction leading to high morbidity and mortality. The clinical spectrum of Pompe disease ranges from infantile onset Pompe disease with cardiomyopathy and muscle hypotonia in the first year of life to late onset Pompe disease, which can present from as early as the first year of life to as late as the 6th decade with proximal muscle weakness and respiratory insufficiency.

Infantile Pompe disease presents in the first few days to weeks of life with cardiomegaly and hypertrophic cardiomyopathy. Electrocardiogram shows left axis deviation, short PR interval and large QRS. Affected babies have macroglossia, feeding difficulties, failure to thrive, generalized hypotonia (Fig. 24.10), and respiratory distress. Without treatment, the disease is progressive; the majority fail to achieve motor milestones, become ventilator dependent by 4–5 months, and succumb before the age of 1 yr.

The diagnosis is established by either deficiency of acid alpha-glucosidase enzyme activity, and pathogenic variants in GAA.

Enzyme replacement therapy with recombinant human GAA (rhGAA, alglucosidase alfa) is available. It results in improvement in cardiomyopathy, and ventilator free and overall survival. The long-term outcome is not satisfactory.

### Lysosomal Storage Disorders

Lysosomes are one of the important cellular organelles responsible for degradation of complex cellular molecules using various acid hydrolases. Deficiency of these enzymes results in the accumulation or storage of an intermediate compound. Deposition of this stored material in several body tissues leads to cellular damage and disease symptoms.

Enzyme deficiencies in the degradation pathway of glycosaminoglycans cause *mucopolysaccharidoses*. In some glycolipid storage disorders, neurological functions are impaired due to abnormal deposition in the brain. The second category of *oligosaccharidoses* is the result of deficiencies of enzymes responsible for degradation of glycoproteins with a less complex polysaccharide (oligosaccharides) than glycosaminoglycans. The third category, *sphingolipidoses*, is caused by deficiency of sphingolipid degrading enzymes. Accumulation of lipid

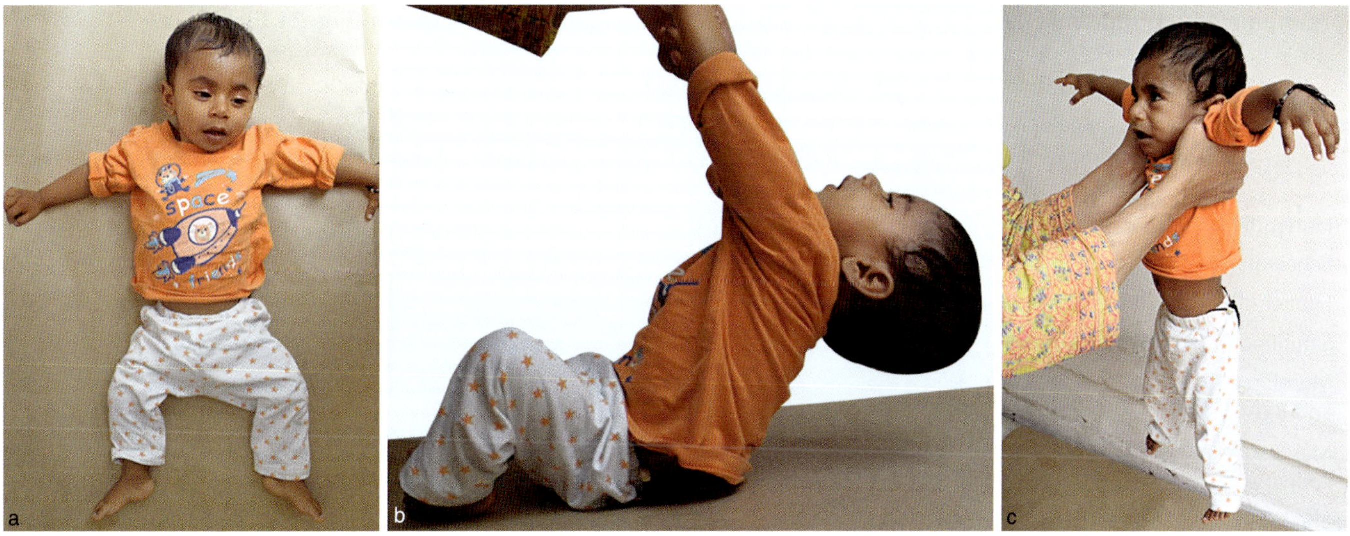

Fig. 24.10: A nine-month-old boy with infantile onset Pompe disease: (a) Note the frog leg position due to extreme floppiness; (b) Note the head lag on "pull to sit"; (c) Baby slips through at the shoulder when examiner grasps under the arms in an upright position

inside the cells gives them a foamy appearance, chiefly seen in liver, spleen, lungs and marrow, with enlargement of these organs. All conditions have autosomal recessive inheritance except mucopolysaccharidosis II and Fabry disease (X-linked). Common disorders are discussed below. Important clinical signs and the clinical approach is summarized in Fig. 24.2.

### *Mucopolysaccharidoses*

Mucopolysaccharides constitute a major part of connective tissue and consist of units of disaccharides, nitrogen and esters. In mucopolysaccharidoses, acid mucopolysaccharides are deposited in the tissues and excreted in the urine. Due to lack of degradation, mucopolysaccharides accumulate in the lysosomes causing disorganization of the cell structure and function. Partially degraded mucopolysaccharides are excreted in urine. Six different types of mucopolysaccharidoses with their subtypes are recognized. Their distinguishing features are described in Table 24.5 and are shown in Fig. 24.11.

Urinary excretion of glycosaminoglycans (GAG) by 2D electrophoresis is a useful screening test. Specific enzyme assays and DNA analyses confirm the diagnosis. Palliative care and multidisciplinary management are important. Enzyme replacement therapy is available for types I, II, IV, VI, and VII, but the cost is prohibitive. Early bone marrow transplantation has been found to be effective in MPS IH.

### *Sphingolipidoses and Lysosomal Lipid Storage Disorders*

It is a broad group of clinically heterogeneous disorders that occurs due to deficiency of a lysosomal hydrolase resulting in intralysosomal accumulation of a particular substrate. Sphingolipids are essential components of all the cell membranes and are derived from a lipid substrate that includes a common ceramide backbone (2 N-acylsphingosine). Inability to degrade these results in accumulation of glycosphingolipids in the brain causing neurodegeneration, and visceral organs resulting in organomegaly, pulmonary and skeletal manifestations.

Figure 24.12 shows the different sphingolipidoses due to defective enzymes in the sphingolipids degradation pathway. These disorders include:

- Mucolipidoses that combine features of mucopolysaccharidoses and sphingolipidosis due to defective enzyme processing causing multiple enzyme deficiencies.
- Sphingolipidoses such as GM1 and GM2 gangliosidoses, Gaucher disease, Niemann-Pick diseases A/B, Fabry disease, Farber disease, Krabbe disease and metachromatic leukodystrophy.
- Lipid storage disorders such as Niemann-Pick C disease, Wolman disease and neuronal ceroid lipofuscinosis (NCL).
- Oligosaccharidoses such as fucosidosis, sialidosis I and II and $\alpha/\beta$ mannosidosis.

The most consistent feature is enlarged liver and spleen, with or without neurological involvement (Gaucher disease I and III, Niemann-Pick disease A and B, and GM1 gangliosidosis). Metachromatic leukodystrophy and Krabbe disease are characterized by white matter involvement and demyelination without organomegaly.

***Gaucher disease:*** This is the commonest autosomal recessively inherited lysosomal storage disease. It occurs due to the deficiency of the tissue enzyme glucocerebrosidase that splits glucose from glucosylceramide, resulting in accumulation of the latter in cells of the reticuloendothelial system. Cerebroside-laden cells are large and have eccentric nuclei with vacuolated cytoplasm and 'wrinkled tissue paper' appearance (Gaucher cells). It is characterized by visceral (hepatosplenomegaly), and bone marrow involvement leading to anemia, thrombocytopenia, leukopenia, bone pains and fractures. There may be associated neurological symptoms like developmental delay, seizures and ocular involvement.

***Non-neuronopathic (type I)*** is the commonest form and characterized by absence of neurological symptoms. Signs and symptoms can develop at any age and include anemia, fatigue, poor growth, delayed puberty, easy bleeding and bruising, weak bones, bone and joint pain, fractures and enlarged liver and spleen (Fig. 24.13a).

**Table 24.5:** Distinguishing features of different mucopolysaccharidoses

| *MPS type* | *Developmental delay/intellectual disability* | *Coarse facies* | *Visceromegaly* | *Joint contractures* | *Dysostosis multiplex* | *Corneal clouding* | *Urine GAGs* |
|---|---|---|---|---|---|---|---|
| Hurler (IH) | + | + | + | + | + | + | Dermatan sulfate, keratan sulfate |
| Scheie (IS) | – | + | ± | + | ± | + | |
| Hunter (II) | + (mild to severe) | + | + | + | + | – | |
| Sanifilipo (III) | + | + | ± | – | ± | – | Heparan sulfate |
| Morquio A and B (IV) | – | + | – | – (laxity) | ++ | ± | Keratan sulfate, chondroitin sulfate |
| Maroteaux-Lamy (VI) | – | + | + | + | + | + | Dermatan sulfate |
| Sly (VII) | + (severe) | + | + | + | + | ± | All except keratan sulfate |

– absent; + present ; GAGs glycosaminoglycans

Coarse facies include depressed nasal bridge, thick lips and ala nasi, enlarged tongue and peg-shaped teeth. Dysostosis multiplex refers to thickening of skull, marked deformity of sella turcica, broad spatula-like ribs, beak-shaped vertebrae (around L1), and proximal tapering of metacarpals.

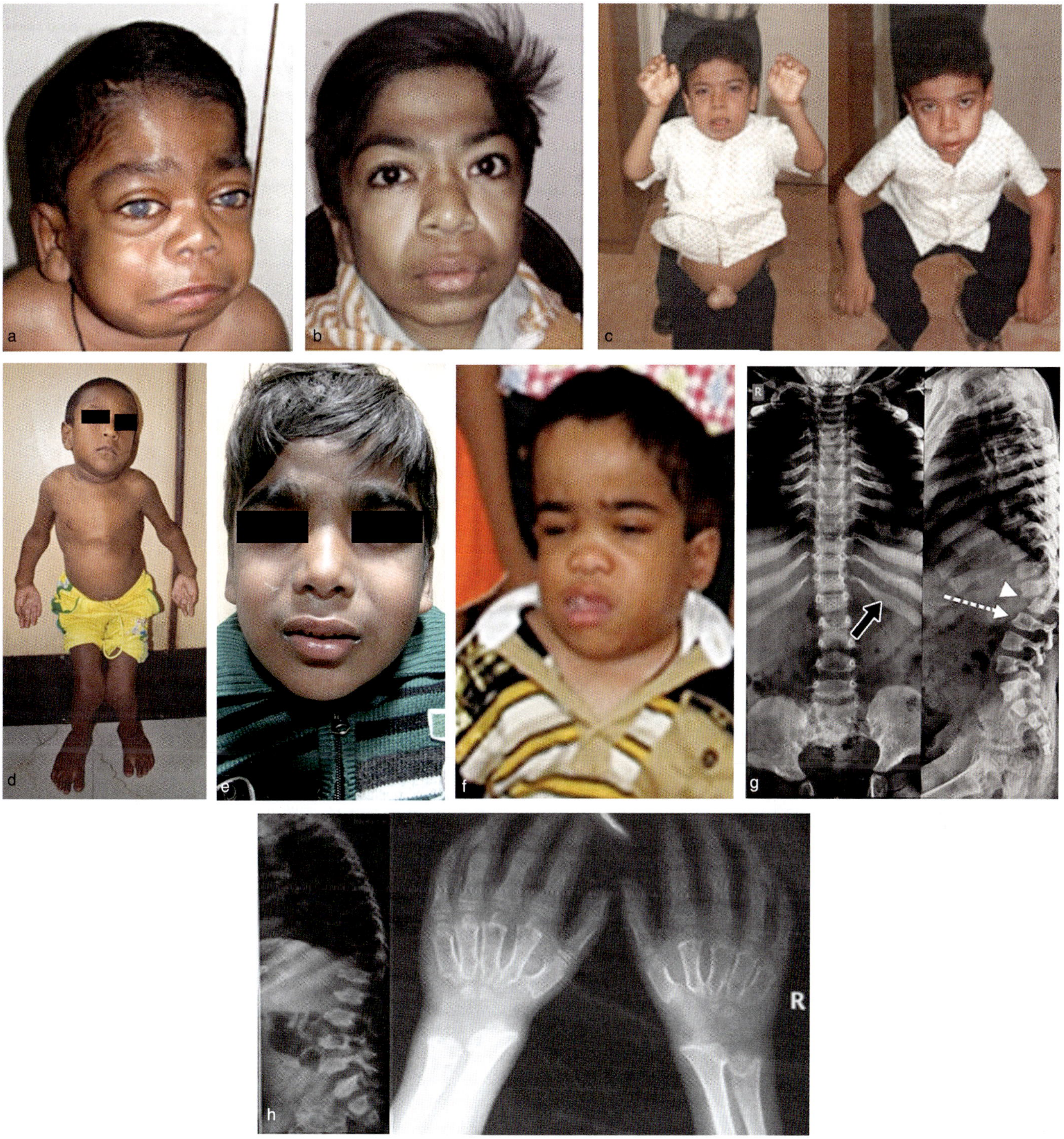

**Fig. 24.11:** Mucopolysaccharidoses: (a) Patient with type IH disease showing corneal clouding and coarse facial features; (b) MPS type II without corneal clouding but with facial coarseness; (c) MPS IHS (milder phenotype) with restriction of joint movements; (d) Short trunk with barrel-shaped chest, pectus carinatum and genu valgum in MPS IV (Morquio disease); (e) Mild facial coarseness in a child with MPS III; (f) MPS VI (Maroteaux-Lamy) with abnormal skull and facial coarseness; (g) Oar-shaped ribs (black arrow), localized angular kyphosis (arrow head), beaking of the inferior margins of vertebrae (dotted arrow) and proximal pointing of metacarpals in MPS type I; (h) Central beaking of the lumbar vertebrae with proximally pointed metacarpals and short ulnae in MPS IV

*Neuronopathic forms* show involvement of the central nervous system. Two types are distinguished by the rate of neurological progression. Type II (acute neuronopathic) presents early in fetal life as hydrops or in early infancy with neurological signs and involvement of spleen and liver. Course is rapidly progressive leading to early death by 2–4 years. Type III Gaucher disease (chronic neuronopathic, Fig. 24.13b) is a chronic form with indolent course and manifestations in early childhood. Signs and symptoms are same as in type 1 except that neurological involvement is slowly progressive and leads to death by second or third decade. Neurological symptoms include

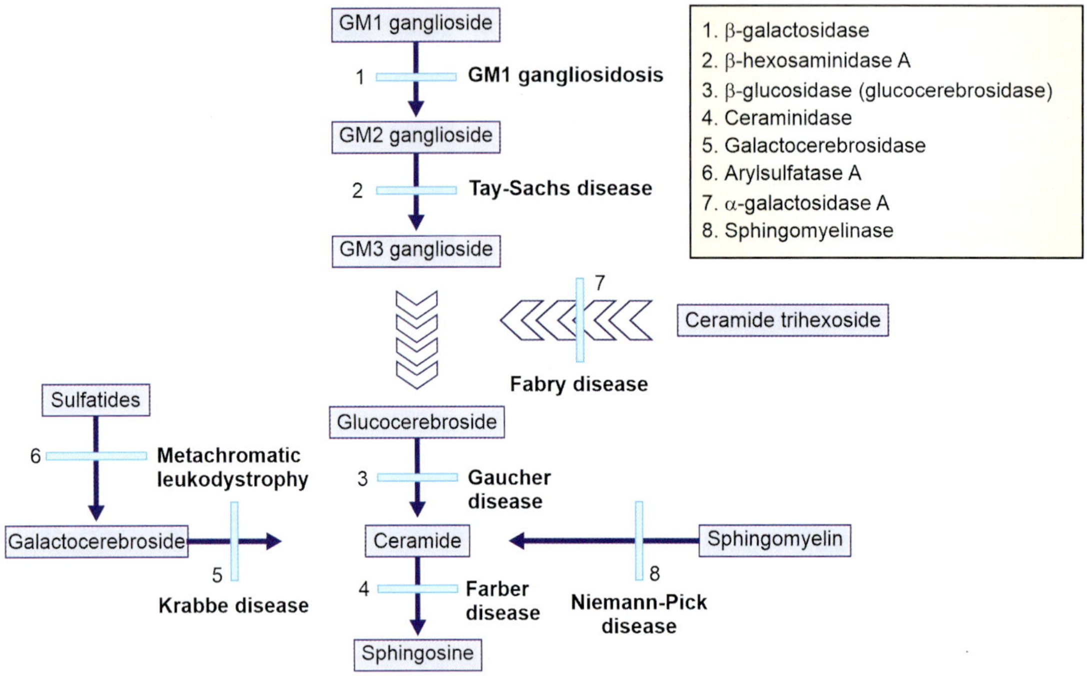


**Fig. 24.12:** Different sphingolipidoses due to defective enzymes in the sphingolipids degradation pathway

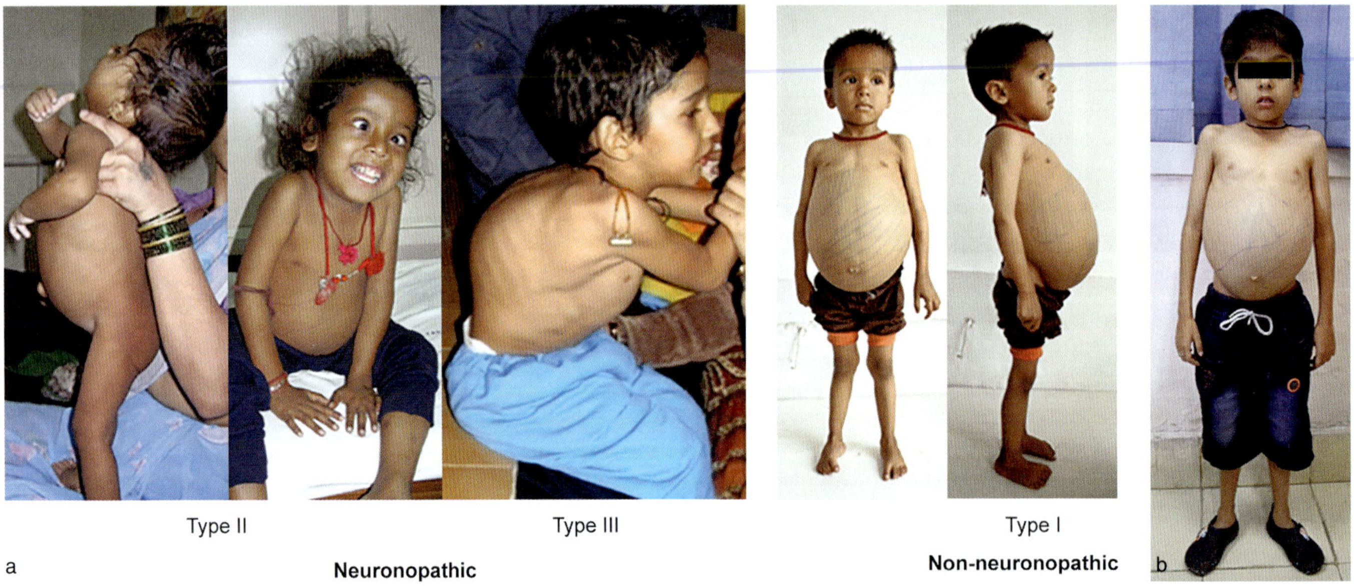


**Fig. 24.13:** (a) Children with neuronopathic and non-neuronopathic Gaucher disease. Note the retracted neck in type II, squint and gibbus in type III along with organomegaly. Massive splenohepatomegaly in type I; (b) A 9-year-old boy with Niemann-Pick disease A/B with splenohepatomegaly

developmental delay, stridor, squint and swallowing difficulty, opisthotonus, head retroflexion, spasticity and trismus, abnormal eye movements, oculomotor apraxia (trouble in moving eyes to look side-to-side, need to turn head to see things on the side), saccadic initiation failure (failure in starting fast eye movements) and optokinetic nystagmus, dementia and ataxia, generalized tonic-clonic seizures and progressive myoclonic epilepsy.

Diagnosis is made by measuring glucocerebrosidase levels in leukocytes or skin fibroblasts. Plasma biomarkers such as glucosylsphingosine (Lyso-GL1), chitotriosidase and, the chemokine PARC/CCL18 levels are elevated and correlate well with the disease severity and treatment. Neuro-ophthalmological investigations, hearing assessment by brain evoked response audiometry, EEG and neuropsychometry tests are required. DNA analysis is helpful in assessment of phenotype and prenatal diagnosis.

This was the first storage disorder for which treatment was available, chiefly as enzyme replacement therapy and substrate reduction therapy. The former provides deficient enzyme (imiglucerase, velaglucerase, taliglucerase) to allow breakdown of fat in cerebroside laden cells. The enzyme is provided intravenously at 60 units/kg every other week. It improves hematological parameters and reduces organomegaly and bone pain. It does not have much effect on neurons, thus the neurological manifestations are irreversible. Therapy is recommended in types I and III but not in type II. Substrate reduction therapy means reducing the production of fatty material, thereby avoiding cellular accumulation. Miglustat and eliglustat are the oral treatment for adult patients with type I Gaucher disease with mild to moderate manifestations for which enzyme therapy is not an option. Eliglustat is more effective substrate inhibitor. Splenectomy increases the risk of progressive skeletal and pulmonary disease. Stem cell transplantation is a potential option.

*Metachromatic leukodystrophy (MLD):* Sulfated glycosphingolipids accumulate in white matter of the central nervous system, stain them purple with a brown background, resulting in metachromatic staining. The disorder has infantile and juvenile forms. Early manifestations include disturbances of gait, incoordina tion and progressive mental deterioration in the second year of life. Knee jerk is brisk but ankle reflex and plantar response may be absent because of involvement of peripheral nerves. Diagnosis is confirmed by level of the enzyme, arylsulphatase A in white cells. There is no effective treatment; unrelated donor umbilical cord blood transplantation has been tried in some pediatric patients. Trials with recombinant arylsulfatase A enzyme are ongoing. Recent reports of autologous stem cell gene therapy with Libmeldy are promising.

*GM2 gangliosidoses:* Inborn errors of GM2 ganglioside metabolism result in accumulation of the metabolite within lysosomes of nerve cells. Most infants with Tay-Sachs form (type I) of the disease have severe deficiency of beta-N-acetylhexosaminidase A (hexosaminidase A). Hexosaminidase A and B are deficient in Sandhoff disease (type II).

*Tay-Sachs disease* is an autosomal recessively inherited defect, which results from deficiency of hexosaminidase enzyme leading to accumulation of GM2 ganglioside within ganglion cells of the nervous system. The disorder manifests by 6 months with loss of head control, ability to sit and an exaggerated startle response to sound. The head is disproportionately large. This is followed by progressive course with eventual spasticity, deafness and blindness. Fundus shows cherry-red spot. Death occurs within 4–5 years. In Sandhoff disease, visceral involvement is present in addition to features of Tay-Sachs disease.

*Niemann-Pick disease:* This is an autosomal recessive disorder of sphingomyelin and cholesterol in the lysosomes. In the classical form (type A), clinical features begin in early life with feeding difficulties, failure to thrive and developmental delay and later neuroregression. There is protuberant abdomen with hepatosplenomegaly. Cherry-red spot on fundus examination is seen in about half the cases. Diagnosis is confirmed by measurement of acid sphingomyelinase (ASM) levels. Type B disease is a milder form with hepatosplenomegaly but no neurological involvement (Fig. 24.13b). Niemann-Pick disease type C has variable age at onset manifesting as liver disease, organomegaly, developmental delay, vertical supranuclear gaze palsy, extrapyramidal manifestations and psychiatric features depending upon the age of onset. Enzyme replacement therapy with recombinant ASM is under clinical trials for type B. Miglustat is approved for type C in Europe. Liver transplantation and bone marrow transplantation are not useful for type A.

## Peroxisomal Disorders

Peroxisomes are involved in the oxidation (β-oxidation of phytanic acid and of very long-chain fatty acids, VLCFA) as well as synthesis of plasmalogens. Based upon their functioning, peroxisomal disorders can be divided into two major groups.

*Disorders of peroxisomal biogenesis or importation* are caused by defects in the transfer of proteins produced in the cytosol into the peroxisomes. This includes Zellweger syndrome, neonatal adrenoleukodystrophy and infantile Refsum disease, and rhizomelic chondrodysplasia punctata (Fig. 24.14). These disorders have autosomal recessive inheritance and are caused by defects in genes coding for peroxins (PEX). Defects interfere with peroxisomal biogenesis and import of proteins into peroxisome.

*Disorders of individual peroxisomal enzymes* include X-linked adrenoleukodystrophy and classical Refsum disease. *Adrenoleukodystrophy* (ALD) is an X-linked recessive disorder caused by tissue accumulation of VLCFA with a carbon chain length of 24 or more due to deficient peroxisomal degradation of fatty acids. The defective gene (*ABCD1*) is located on Xq28. The childhood cerebral form usually manifests between 4 and 8 years of age with subtle initial manifestations of worsening school performance and behavioral problems such as hyperactivity and emotional lability. Auditory and visual disturbances may be associated. Seizures are often the initial manifestation. In most patients, adrenal dysfunction is noticed after the cerebral symptoms. Rapid neurological progression ensues causing increasing spasticity, visual and hearing

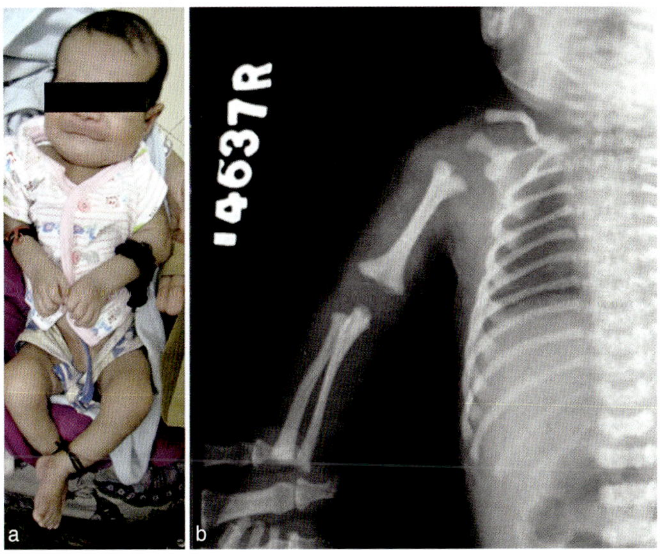


Fig. 24.14: (a) One-month-old child with rhizomelic chondrodysplasia punctata. Note the facial dysmorphism and contractures at elbow and knee; (b) X-ray showing rhizomelic shortening

**Table 24.6:** Modes of therapy for inborn errors of metabolism

| *Therapeutic strategy* | *Diseases (therapeutic product)* | *Advantages* | *Comments* |
|---|---|---|---|
| Dietary restriction and modification | Aminoacidopathies<br>Organic acidemias such as glutaric aciduria-I<br>Carbohydrate diseases, e.g. glycogen storage disorders, galactosemia, hereditary fructose intolerance<br>Fatty acid oxidation defects | Effective<br>Relatively low cost | Requires good compliance<br>Diets may be unpalatable<br>Monitor for nutritional deficiencies |
| Product replacement | Biotinidase deficiency (biotin) | Oral<br>Inexpensive | Excellent response if started early |
| Reduce production of toxic metabolites by enhancing the use of alternative metabolic pathways (diversion therapy) | Urea cycle defects (sodium benzoate and phenylbutyrate in urea cycle defect)<br>Organic acidemias (carnitine) | Effective in both acute and chronic setting | Intravenous sodium benzoate is not available in India |
| Deficient enzyme replacement | Gaucher disease (imiglucerase; velaglucerase, taliglucerase)<br>Fabry disease (agalsidase beta and alpha)<br>Pompe disease (alglucosidase alfa);<br>Mucopolysaccharidosis type I (laronidase); II (Idursulfase); IV-A (elosulphase alpha); VI (galsulfase); VII (vestronidase alpha)<br>Lysosomal acid lipase deficiency (Sebelipase alpha) | Provides the missing product | Immunogenic<br>Usually do not cross blood–brain barrier<br>Requires weekly/biweekly IV infusion<br>Expensive<br>Required lifelong |
| Substrate reduction therapy | Gaucher disease (miglustat, eliglustat)<br>Niemann-Pick C (miglustat)<br>Tyrosinemia type 1 (NTBC) | Oral<br>Non-immunogenic<br>Crosses blood–brain barrier | For few diseases only |
| Enhance residual enzyme activity using cofactor replacement | Biotinidase deficiency, cobalamin disorders, pyridoxine responsive homocystinuria | Oral<br>Widely available<br>Cost effective | IM injections for cobalamin disorders; for limited disorders |
| **Chaperone therapy** (enhancement of endogenous enzyme activity) | Fabry disease (Migalastat) | Oral; non-immunogenic cross blood-brain barrier acceptable safety | Mutation dependent<br>For a limited number of disorders |
| **Cell/organ transplantation** | Mucopolysaccharidosis IH#<br>X-linked adrenoleukodystrophy<br>#Metachromatic leukodystrophy, Krabbe disease, urea cycle defects, maple syrup urine disease<br>Methylmalonic acidemia*, propionic acidemia** | Permanent supply of deficient enzyme | Narrow therapeutic window<br>Cannot reverse irreversible damage<br>Post-procedure complications<br>Immunosuppression<br>Graft versus host disease |
| Gene therapy | Metachromatic leukodystrophy<br>X-linked adrenoleukodystrophy<br>Late infantile neuronal ceroid lipofuscinosis^ | Offers cure | Cost<br>Immune response<br>Toxicity<br>Possibility of oncogenesis |

Transplantation:
*liver
** liver and/or renal
#bone marrow
^Experimental

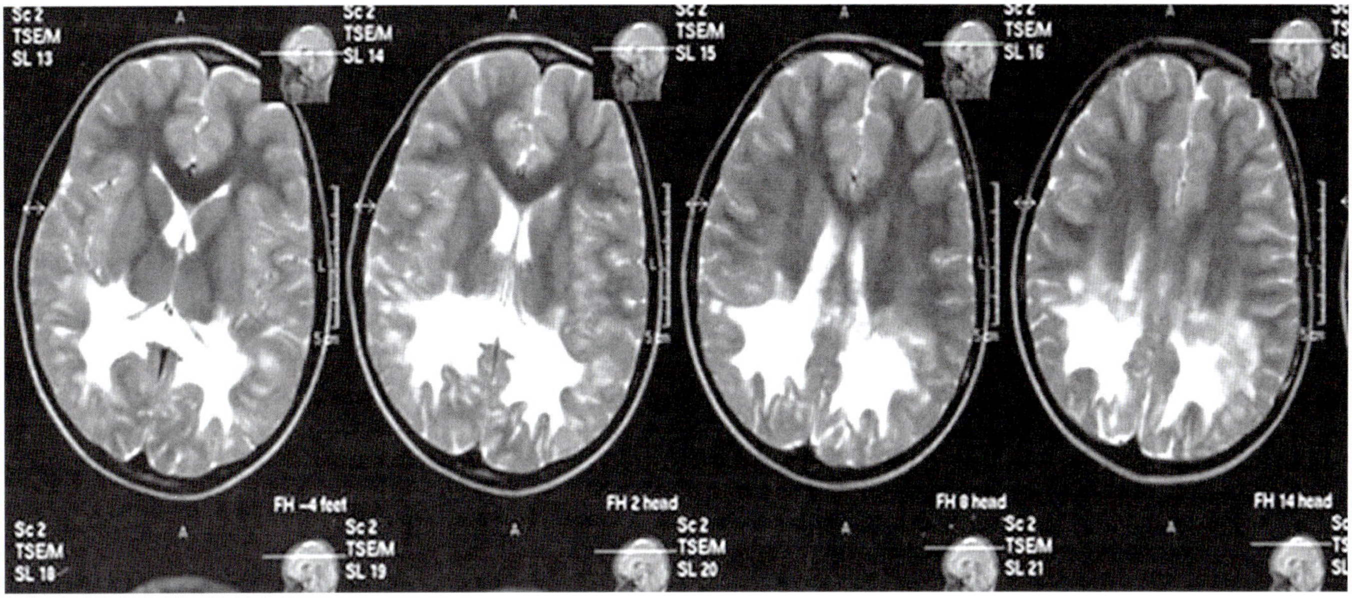


Fig. 24.15: Brain MRI findings in X-linked adrenoleukodystrophy. T2-weighted axial images show symmetrical hyperintense signal changes in bilateral perieto-occipital white matter and splenium of corpus callosum (*Courtesy:* Dr. Atin Kumar, AIIMS, New Delhi)

impairment. MRI brain typically shows demyelination in the parieto-occipital areas (Fig. 24.15).

*Adrenomyeloneuropathy* is a milder form with onset in late adolescence or adulthood and is characterized by progressive paraparesis due to long tract degeneration in the spinal cord.

Elevated plasma levels of VLCFA can identify patients and 85% of female carriers of X-adrenoleukodystrophy. As ALD cannot be distinguished from other forms of Addison disease, it is recommended to perform VLCFA analysis in all male patients with Addison disease. Mutation analysis is the most reliable method to identify carriers. Corticosteroid replacement should be given for adrenal insufficiency. Bone marrow transplantation (BMT) is curative and is most relevant in mildly affected patients, early in the course of disease. BMT is not indicated, if the MRI brain is normal. The role of Lorenzo oil is controversial.

To summarize, IEMs must be excluded in a sick child with an unexplained etiology. Treatment is possible for several IEMs using various modes of therapy (Fig. 24.3, Table 24.6). A high index of suspicion and early initiation of therapy prevents the morbidity and mortality.

## Suggested Reading


1. Clarke JTR. General principles. In: A clinical guide to inherited metabolic diseases, 3rd edn. New York: Cambridge University Press, 2006.
2. Hoffman GF, Zschocke J, Nyhan WL. Inherited metabolic diseases – A clinical approach. 2nd edn. Springer 2017.
3. Nyhan WL, Hoffman GF. Atlas of inherited metabolic diseases, 4th edn, CRC Press 2020.
4. Saudubray J-M, Baumgartner MR, Walter JH (editors). Inborn Metabolic Diseases. Diagnosis and Treatment. 6th edn. Springer 2016.

Chapter

25

# Inborn Errors of Immunity

❍ Rakesh Kumar Pilania ❍ Surjit Singh

## IMMUNITY

The immune system has two major components: Innate and adaptive. Innate immunity is nonspecific, has no memory and provides the first line of defense against infections. Adaptive immunity is highly evolved, antigen dependent and specific, has memory and is characterized by rapid immune response when exposed to the same microorganism. The innate and adaptive immune systems often work in tandem and are not mutually exclusive.

### Innate Immune System

Innate immune system is the first line defence of body. It consists of physical and physiologic barriers (skin, mucous membranes, temperature), and immune cells (neutrophils, monocytes, macrophages, natural killer cells) and proteins. Innate immunity basically relies on pattern recognition receptors (PRRs) on various microorganisms. These allow a limited range of immune cells to recognize pathogens/antigens through the pathogen-associated molecular patterns.

The complement system consists of multiple proteins circulating as inactive precursors. Once triggered, these proteins activate each other sequentially to generate active components. There are three pathways of activation of the complement cascade. The classical pathway is triggered by activation of C1q by antibody–antigen complexes or polyanions (heparin, protamine, nucleic acids from apoptotic cells). The alternative pathway is continuously active at low levels due to spontaneous C3 lysis, and amplified by binding of complement components to pathogen (bacterial lipopolysaccharide, endotoxin, yeast cell wall). The lectin pathway is activated by binding of mannose binding lectin to mannose residues on pathogen cell surface.

Activation of the classical pathway results in low levels of C4, C2 and C3; activation of alternative pathway is characterized by reduced levels of C3 with normal levels of C4 and C2. Activation of C3 by either pathway results in formation of the membrane attack complex, which binds to the surface of bacteria, fungi and viruses leading to their lysis. C3b component can opsonize immune complexes or foreign cell surfaces; anaphylatoxins (C3a, C4a, C5a) bind to receptors on mast cells and basophils, resulting in their degranulation and release of histamine and intracellular enzymes. C3a and C5a induce adherence of monocytes, macrophages and neutrophils to vascular endothelial cells causing extravasation and chemotaxis.

Cellular components of innate immunity consist of polymorphonuclear leukocytes, macrophages, dendritic cells, natural killer (NK) cells, and innate lymphoid cells. These ingest extracellular material by phagocytosis. Dendritic cells and macrophages are also involved in antigen presentation to T cells.

### Adaptive Immune System

Adaptive immune responses develop through synergy between lymphocytes and antigen-presenting cells following specific antigenic challenge, show tremendous diversity and exhibit immunological memory. The components of adaptive immune system are lymphocytes, macrophages and antigen-presenting cells.

Lymphocytes constitute 20–40% of white cells in peripheral blood and are classified using flow cytometry as B (CD19, CD20 positive), T (CD3 positive) and NK (CD16, CD56 positive) cells. T cell antigen receptor (TCR) is associated with CD3 to form the TCR–CD3 complex that remains unchanged during cell division. TCR recognizes antigen only when it is bound to MHC molecules on surface of antigen-presenting cells. Mature T lymphocytes are categorized into CD4 positive T helper (Th) cells, and CD8 positive T cytotoxic (Tc) cells based on membrane glycoprotein. The normal ratio of CD4+ and CD8+ cells in peripheral blood is 2:1. CD4+ cells recognize antigen only if bound to class II MHC molecules, whereas CD8+ cells recognize antigen bound to class I MHC molecules.

Th cells differentiate into Th1, Th2 and Th17 cells under influence of cytokines. Th1 immune response supports inflammation and activates Tc cells and macrophages (as in tuberculoid leprosy and rheumatoid arthritis), whereas Th2 responses induce antibody-mediated immunity (as in lepromatous leprosy and allergic disorders). Th17 cells contribute to host defense against extracellular bacteria and fungi and have a role in development of allergy and autoimmunity. Tc cells are important in eliminating intracellular pathogens like viruses, and in organ transplant rejection.

## INBORN ERRORS OF IMMUNITY

A small but significant proportion of children evaluated for frequent infections, autoimmunity and inflammation may have underlying immune defect. Immunodeficiency occurs when part of immune system is missing or not working properly. Immunodeficiency disorders can be secondary (Table 25.1) or primary, the former being far more common. Infection with the human immunodeficiency virus (HIV) is an example of secondary immunodeficiency.

The term primary immune deficiencies (PID) was used to describe genetic immune diseases leading to susceptibility to infection. However, autoimmunity, immune dysfunction and dysregulation are also an integral component of these monogenic immune diseases. Accordingly, the term inborn errors of immunity (IEI) is proposed by the International Union of Immunological Societies for disorders that were classified as PID. IEI are a heterogeneous group of inherited disorders associated with defects in one or more arms of immune system. Estimates suggest that the prevalence of IEI may be as high as 1 in 10,000 population.

An IEI should be suspected in patients presenting with ≥2 of the following 10 warning signs, proposed by the Jeffrey Modell Foundation: (i) ≥4 new infections in a year; (ii) ≥2 serious sinus infections in a year; (iii) ≥2 cases of pneumonia in a year; (iv) ≥2 months of antibiotics without effect; (v) failure of an infant to gain weight or grow normally, (vi) recurrent deep skin infections or organ abscesses; (vii) persistent oral thrush, or candidiasis elsewhere beyond infancy; (viii) need for intravenous antibiotics to clear infections; (ix) ≥2 deep-seated infections (e.g. meningitis, cellulitis); and (x) family history of immunodeficiency.

Diagnosis of IEI should also be considered in patients with autoimmune or chronic inflammatory disease and/or lymphoproliferation especially in context of atypical presentations or associated recurrent infections.

Table 25.2 shows the conditions included as IEI, based upon the phenotypically affected segment of the immune system and syndromic diagnosis. Table 25.3 outlines clinical clues that may point towards a specific IEI. **Box 25.1** outlines the laboratory workup for various disorders. Conditions that mimic IEI (e.g. gastroesophageal reflux, Kartagener syndrome, cystic fibrosis) should be excluded before investigations for IEIs are initiated.

### Cellular and/or Combined Immunodeficiency

#### *Severe Combined Immunodeficiency (SCID)*

Children with SCID present in early infancy with severe infections due to viruses, fungi (e.g. *Pneumocystis jirovecii*) or intracellular pathogens (e.g. mycobacteria), chronic

| Table 25.1: Common causes of secondary immunodeficiency |
|---|
| Human immunodeficiency virus infection |
| Following measles infection |
| Severe malnutrition |
| Nephrotic syndrome |
| Lymphoreticular malignancies |
| Severe burns |
| Severe, chronic infections |
| Medications: Glucocorticoids, cyclophosphamide, azathioprine, mycophenolate mofetil, phenytoin, monoclonal antibodies |

**Box 25.1: Laboratory Workup for Suspected Inborn Errors of Immunity**

**Initial workup**

- Total and differential leukocyte counts: Absolute lymphocyte count, neutrophil count and eosinophil count
- Leukocyte morphology; platelet count and size
- HIV serology; X-ray chest; ultrasonography for thymus

**Specific investigations**

- Quantitative immunoglobulin estimation: IgG, IgA, IgM, IgE and IgG subclasses
- Blood group isohemagglutinins (for functional IgM)
- Specific antibody response to protein (e.g. anti-diphtheria and anti-tetanus antibodies), or polysaccharide (anti-pneumococcal antibodies) antigens
- CD3, CD19, CD16, CD56 by flow cytometry
- B cell immunophenotyping, including class switch studies (for CVID)
- T cell immunophenotyping [CD4/CD8 ratio, memory (CD45RO), naïve (CD45RA), T cells, HLA-DR expression]
- Bruton tyrosine kinase protein expression (for XLA)
- Wiskott-Aldrich syndrome (WAS) protein expression
- Nitroblue tetrazolium dye reduction test, and dihydrorhodamine assay on flow cytometry (CGD)
- CD11/18 flow cytometry (for LAD)
- CH50, AH50 assays, and levels of complement component (complement pathway defects)
- CD62L shedding assay (for suspected TLR signaling defect)
- IL-12/23-IFN-γ pathway flow based studies (for MSMD)
- NK cell cytotoxicity, perforin expression and degranulation assay (for familial HLH)
- *STAT3* expression, Th17 cells enumeration (for *STAT3* hyper-IgE syndrome)
- Mannan binding lectin assay
- Delayed skin tests (*Candida*, tetanus toxoid)
- Mitogen stimulation tests (response to phytohemagglutinin)
- Enzyme assays, e.g. adenosine deaminase, purine nucleoside phosphorylase

**Molecular confirmation**

- Genetic sequencing: Sanger sequencing, next generation sequencing including targeted panels, whole exome sequencing

AH50 alternate pathway complement hemolytic assay; CD cluster differentiation; CGD chronic granulomatous disease; CH50 total hemolytic complement assay; CVID common variable immunodeficiency, HIV human immunodeficiency virus; HLH hemophagocytic lymphohistiocytosis; LAD leukocyte adhesion defects; MSMD mendelian susceptibility to mycobacterial disease; XLA X-linked agammaglobulinemia

**Table 25.2:** International Union of Immunological Societies (IUIS) classification of inborn errors of immunity (IEI)

| *Class* | *IUIS category* | *Representative disease* |
|---|---|---|
| I | Immunodeficiencies affecting cellular and humoral immunity | • Severe combined immunodeficiency (SCID) |
| II | Combined immunodeficiencies associated with syndromic features | • Wiskott-Aldrich syndrome<br>• Hyper-IgE syndrome<br>• DiGeorge syndrome<br>• Ataxia telangiectasia |
| III | Predominantly antibody deficiencies | • X-linked agammaglobulinemia (XLA)<br>• Common variable immunodeficiency (CVID)<br>• Selective IgA deficiency |
| IV | Diseases of immune dysregulation | • Familial hemophagocytic lymphohistiocytosis (HLH) syndromes<br>• Autoimmune lymphoproliferative syndrome (ALPS)<br>• Autoimmune polyendocrinopathy-candidiasis-ectodermal dystrophy |
| V | Congenital defects of phagocyte number, function, or both | • Chronic granulomatous disease (CGD)<br>• Severe congenital neutropenia, cyclical neutropenia<br>• Leukocyte adhesion deficiency (LAD) |
| VI | Defects in intrinsic and innate immunity | • Mendelian susceptibility to mycobacterial disease (MSMD)<br>• Chronic mucocutaneous candidiasis (CMC) |
| VII | Autoinflammatory disorders | • Type 1 interferonopathies<br>• Tumor necrosis factor receptor-1 associated periodic syndrome (TRAPS)<br>• Familial Mediterranean fever (FMF)<br>• Deficiency of adenosine deaminase type 2 (DADA2) |
| VIII | Complement deficiencies | • Early complement component deficiencies (e.g. C1q deficiency lupus)<br>• Hereditary angioedema |
| IX | Bone marrow failure | • Dyskeratosis congenita<br>• Fanconi anemia |
| X | Phenocopies of inborn errors of immunity | • ALPS like disorder due to somatic variants<br>• Good syndrome<br>• Adult-onset MSMD with autoantibodies to IFN-gamma<br>• Acquired angioedema with autoantibodies to C1 inhibitor |



diarrhea, failure to thrive or graft versus host disease like illness due to maternal engraftment. Classical SCID patients usually have absent tonsillar tissue and hypoplastic lymph nodes. Left untreated, such babies may not survive beyond a few weeks. Profound lymphopenia (absolute lymphocyte count $<3 \times 10^9$/L) is characteristic. SCID can be X-linked recessive (mutations in *IL2RG*, encoding the common γ chain of IL-2R) and autosomal recessive (adenosine deaminase deficiency) with associated chondro-osseous tissue abnormalities, scapular spurring, anterior rib cupping, and flared costochondral junctions, mesangial sclerosis, and adrenal gland cortical sclerosis, cognitive abnormalities and sensorineural deafness. SCID due to purine nucleoside phosphorylase deficiency is milder and usually presents later in childhood.

### *DiGeorge Syndrome*

This disorder arises from defects in embryogenesis of third and fourth pharyngeal pouches due to microdeletion on chromosome 22q11.2. It is characterized clinically by an unusual facies (hypertelorism, antimongoloid slant, low set ears, micrognathia, short philtrum, bifid uvula), hypocalcemic tetany, aortic arch anomalies and thymic hypoplasia or aplasia. In addition, 20–30% patients show a variable T cell defect ranging from mildly increased susceptibility to infections to severe disease requiring thymic or hematopoietic stem cell transplant.

### *Wiskott-Aldrich Syndrome (WAS)*

This X-linked recessive disorder is caused by mutations at Xp11.22–23, encoding WAS protein in cytoplasm of lymphocytes and platelets. WAS is characterized by microthrombocytopenia (reduced number and size of platelets), eczema, combined immunodeficiency and high incidence of autoimmunity and lymphoreticular malignancies. Eczema begins in early infancy and may mimic atopic dermatitis. Due to impaired responses to polysaccharide antigens, patients are susceptible to infections with encapsulated organisms (e.g. *S. pneumoniae, N. meningitides* and *H. influenzae*). However, infections with *P. jirovecii*, viruses (herpes simplex or molluscum contagiousm) and fungi (*Candida*) can also occur. The clinical phenotype varies—while, some children have a fulminant course with repeated severe infections (WAS spectrum), others present later, predominantly with bleeding manifestations (X-linked thrombocytopenia spectrum). A diagnosis of WAS should be considered in *boys presenting with congenital or early onset microthrombocytopenia.*

**Table 25.3:** Clinical clues to the diagnosis of inborn errors of immunity (IEI)

| *Type of infection* | *Age at presentation* | *Associated findings* | *Likely etiology* |
|---|---|---|---|
| Pneumonia or diarrhea; *P. jirovecii*, CMV, candidiasis, cryptosporidiosis, disseminated BCG infection | First few months of life | Failure to thrive; rash; atrophic tonsils and lymph nodes | Severe combined immunodeficiency (SCID) |
| Recurrent pneumonia or diarrhea; problems controlling viral infections, especially Epstein-Barr virus (EBV); Infection due to *Mycobacteria* spp, *P. jirovecii* or *Candida* spp | Late onset disease; >1 year of age | Autoimmunity, increased risk of malignancies, especially EBV lymphoma | Combined immunodeficiency (CID), hypomorphic/leaky SCID |
| Recurrent sinopulmonary infections; infections with encapsulated bacteria (*S. pneumoniae*, *H. influenzae*) and *Mycoplasma*; enteroviral infections; recurrent diarrhea (e.g. *G. lamblia*) | 4–6 months | Only boys affected; failure to thrive; arthritis | X-linked agammaglobulinemia (XLA) |
| Diarrhea (e.g. *G. lamblia*, *Salmonella*, *C. jejuni*); sinopulmonary infections, infections with encapsulated bacteria (*S. pneumoniae*, *H. influenzae*) | Later childhood (>5–10 years) | Cytopenias, autoimmune disorders; hepatosplenomegaly, lymphadenopathy; granulomatous diseases; B cell lymphoma | Common variable immunodeficiency (CVID) |
| Recurrent or persistent giardiasis | At any age | Often asymptomatic; autoimmune diseases | IgA deficiency |
| Recurrent staphylococcal cold abscesses; pneumonia; mucocutaneous candidiasis (particularly finger nails) | At any age | Eczema, coarse facial features, skeletal defects, persistent primary dentition | *STAT3* hyper-IgE syndrome |
| Recurrent skin viral infections (herpes simplex virus, molluscum contagiosum virus, papilloma virus) | At any age | Eczema, asthma, severe food allergies, | *DOCK-8* hyper-IgE syndrome |
| Recurrent staphylococcal infections; persistent fungal (*Aspergillus*) pneumonia; liver abscess | Usually early childhood | Lymphadenopathy; hepatosplenomegaly; granulomas | Chronic granulomatous disease |
| Severe bacterial infections; periodontitis; skin ulcers | Early infancy | Delayed umbilical cord separation; no pus formation; prominent leukocytosis | Leukocyte adhesion deficiency |
| Omphalitis; recurrent pneumonia; gingivitis; periodontitis | Infancy | Cardiac anomalies, developmental delay, epilepsy, bone marrow fibrosis | Severe congenital neutropenia |
| Disseminated BCG and other mycobacterial infections; recurrent salmonellosis; osteomyelitis caused by atypical mycobacteria | At any age | Risk for infections with mycobacteria, intracellular organisms (non-typhoidal salmonella, *Cryptococcus*, viruses, fungi) | Mendelian susceptibility to mycobacterial disease (MSMD) |
| Pyogenic encapsulated bacterial infections (*S. pneumoniae*, *H. influenzae*) | Any age | Systemic lupus, vasculitis, glomerulonephritis | Deficiency in early complement components (C1q, C1r, C1s, C4, C2, C3) |
| Recurrent *Neisseria* infections, e.g. meningitis | Any age | | Deficiency in late complement components (C5–C9) |
| Recurrent infections | Early infancy | Only boys affected; eczema; thrombocytopenia with small platelets | Wiskott-Aldrich syndrome |
| Varying spectrum of infections; a small proportion may have SCID | Any age | Hypocalcemia; conotruncal cardiac malformations, velopalatal insufficiency; abnormal facies; intellectual disability | DiGeorge syndrome |
| Recurrent bacterial infections, e.g. pneumonia | Early childhood | Progressive ataxia; precedes telangiectasia | Ataxia-telangiectasia |

Serum immunoglobulin assay may reveal elevated IgE and IgA, low IgM and, low or normal IgG. Flow cytometry may show abnormalities in T cell subsets, impaired T cell proliferation and defective T cell signaling, that is secondary to deficient expression of CD43 on lymphocytes.

### *Ataxia-Telangiectasia*

This autosomal recessive disorder is characterized by progressive ataxia (beginning during infancy), telangiectasia (initially on bulbar conjunctiva), sinopulmonary infections, chromosomal breakage and increased sensitivity to ionizing radiation. Immunodeficiency occurs in approximately two-thirds of patients. Recurrent sinopulmonary infections may occur. Serum IgA, IgG2 subclass and IgE levels are usually reduced, and IgM levels are normal or increased; lymphocyte proliferative responses are decreased and the number of γδ-positive T cells is increased.





### *Hyper-IgM Syndrome*

This syndrome can result from multiple causes, the most common being a CD40 ligand defect. Affected children have a profound immunodeficiency characterized by low levels of IgG but normal or raised IgM. There is increased susceptibility to infections with *P. jirovecii* and *C. parvum*. Some patients may have associated autoimmune disorders.

## Predominant Antibody Immunodeficiencies

### *X-linked (Bruton) Agammaglobulinemia (XLA)*

This X-linked recessive disorder is caused by mutation in the gene for tyrosine kinase, *BTK*. Affected boys present in second half of infancy with pyogenic infections; later presentation is also described. Recurrent bacterial respiratory and/or gastrointestinal infections are seen typically. Tonsils and lymph nodes are usually atrophic. These patients have severe reduction in all serum immunoglobulin levels along with absent B cells (CD19+) in peripheral blood; T cells (CD3+) are normal in number and function.

### *Common Variable Immunodeficiency (CVID)*

The term CVID refers to heterogeneous group of disorders characterized by hypogammaglobulinemia and variable defects in T cell number and function. Presentation is later in childhood and, unlike XLA, affected children show marked lymphadenopathy and hepatosplenomegaly. B cell number (CD19) is usually normal. Low levels of lymphocyte proliferation following mitogen stimulation may be seen. Autoimmune disorders (leukopenia, thrombocytopenia, hemolytic anemia and arthritis) are commonly associated with CVID. Patients are at risk of developing lymphoreticular malignancies later in life. With availability of high throughput genetic sequencing techniques, several monogenic forms of CVID have now been identified in about 20% patients (doi:10.3389/fimmu.2018.00636). Diagnosis of monogenic defects in patients with CVID is usually based on genetic sequencing. Treatment depends upon the molecular defect that is identified.

### *IgA Deficiency*

This is one of the most common causes of primary immunodeficiency. Affected individuals usually do not have a clinically significant immunodeficiency and may remain entirely asymptomatic or have recurrent mild respiratory infections, especially if IgG subclass deficiency is also present. These patients may occasionally evolve to CVID later.

### *IgG Subclass Deficiency*

IgG1 provides protection against bacterial pathogens (diphtheria, tetanus), IgG2 protects against capsular polysaccharide antigens (pneumococci, *Hemophilus influenzae*), IgG3 has antiviral properties, while IgG4 has antiparasitic activity. Children with deficiency of one of the subclasses may have normal, or sometimes elevated, total IgG levels.

### *Transient Hypogammaglobulinemia of Infancy*

Infants show physiological hypogammaglobulinemia between 3 and 6 months of age, when transplacentally acquired maternal IgG has been catabolized, and immunoglobulin production has not begun. In some infants, the physiological hypogammaglobulinemia is prolonged to 18–24 months, resulting in transient hypogammaglobulinemia of infancy. Serum IgG levels in infancy and early childhood should be interpreted in context of age-related nomograms. Unlike XLA, B cell numbers are normal. These children recover over time and long-term prognosis is excellent.

## Disorders of Innate Immunity

### *Phagocytic Defect*

Chronic granulomatous disease (CGD) refers to disorders with reduced activity of nicotinamide adenine dinucleotide phosphate (NADPH) oxidase leading to impaired generation of superoxide radical. CGD may be X-linked recessive (due to mutations in the gene encoding gp91-phox) or autosomal recessive (due to mutations in the gene encoding p47-phox, p67-phox, p22-phox or p40-phox; EROS). Children present with recurrent life-threatening infections, starting in early infancy. Infections are usually caused by catalase-positive bacteria (e.g. *Staphylococcus aureus*, *Serratia*) and fungi (e.g. *Aspergillus*). Clinical presentations include persistent smoldering pneumonia, prominent lymphadenitis, multiple liver abscesses and osteomyelitis of small bones of hands and feet. Diagnosis is suggested by screening on nitroblue tetrazolium dye reduction test (NBT) and confirmed by dihydrorhodamine assay on flow cytometry.

## Miscellaneous

### *Complement Component Deficiency*

Individuals with deficiencies of the early complement components (C1–C4) may present with recurrent infections with encapsulated bacteria. Those with deficiency of the later components (C5–C9) have predilection for neisserial infections. Early onset lupus may be associated with C2/C4 or C1q deficiency. C3 deficiency may be associated with glomerulonephritis. Deficiency of C1 esterase inhibitor (C1INH) is associated with hereditary angioedema, that is inherited as autosomal dominant trait, characterized by recurrent episodes of edema over face, trunk and extremities. These patients can have severe abdominal pain that mimic acute abdomen due to bowel wall edema and rarely life-threatening laryngeal edema.

#### Hyper-IgE Syndrome

The condition is characterized by elevated IgE, eczema and recurrent infections. Mutations in *STAT3* result in recurrent 'cold' staphylococcal abscesses, pneumonia with pneumatoceles, retained primary dentition and markedly elevated serum IgE levels (>2000 IU/mL). Inheritance is usually autosomal dominant. Autosomal recessive forms of the disease have also been identified (dedicator of cytokinesis 8—DOCK8, phosphoglucomutase 3—PGM3, and interleukin 6 signal transducer—IL6ST deficiencies).

#### Mendelian Susceptibility to Mycobacterial Diseases (MSMD)

MSMD is a group of monogenic disorders due to a defect in the interferon gamma/interleukin (IL)-12 axis. These patients are susceptible to infection with weakly virulent environmental mycobacteria, BCG vaccine strains, *M. tuberculosis*, other intramacrophagic bacteria (e.g. non-typhoidal *Salmonella*, *Listeria*), and fungi. The term MSMD is, therefore, a misnomer as patients remains susceptible to several organisms other than mycobacteria. In the 2022 IUIS classification, 18 genetic defects have been identified to result in MSMD. Diagnosis of MSMD rests on flow cytometry, functional assays and molecular confirmation. Children and adults with disseminated BCG infection and infections with atypical mycobacteria should be evaluated for MSMD.

## TREATMENT OF IEI

IEI are a heterogeneous group of disorders that can affect differentially impair components of immune systems. Therefore, treatment options are also equally diverse to address specific conditions.

Hematopoietic stem cell transplantation (HSCT) is the treatment of choice for most forms of significant cellular immunodeficiency (e.g. SCID, WAS, CD40L hyper-IgM syndrome). The procedure should be carried out in early infancy before serious infections have set in. Children with XLA, IgG2 subclass deficiency and CVID require *immunoglobulin replacement therapy* given either intravenously (IVIg) every 3–4 weeks or subcutaneously (SCIg) every week. Replacement therapy with IVIg/SCIg results in significant improvement in quality of life. Patients with IgA deficiency may not require any specific therapy initially if they remain well. *Prophylactic therapy with antimicrobials* (usually cotrimoxazole or azithromycin) is required for some children with IgG1 and IgG3 subclass deficiency. Long-term cotrimoxazole and itraconazole prophylaxis is required for patients while awaiting definitive therapy with HSCT. *Interferon-γ* may be useful for treatment of life-threatening infections in patients with chronic granulomatous disease.

*Plasma infusions* may be useful in patients with complement deficiencies. In C1 esterase inhibitor deficiency, prophylactic therapy with tranexamic acid, danazol or stanozolol results in significant improvement. Injections of synthetic C1 esterase inhibitor (25 units/kg infused over 1–2 minutes) are required, if there is laryngeal involvement with airway compromise. *Gene therapy* has been successfully used in patients with X-linked SCID, CGD and WAS.

### Immunoglobulin Therapy

Intravenous immunoglobulin (IVIg) is pooled normal intact polyspecific IgG derived from plasma of healthy donors that has been subjected to strict screening procedures. Each batch of IVIg represents a donor pool of several thousand individuals such that the repertoire of antibodies is representative of the population. Most preparations contain >90% monomeric IgG with only small amounts of IgA and IgM. The IgG subclass distribution depends on the manufacturing process; some IVIg preparations may not contain adequate proportions of IgG3.

Currently there are two types of immunoglobulin preparations, IVIg and the subcutaneous form, SCIg. IVIg preparations have a concentration of 5–10%. SCIg preparations have a concentration of 16–20%. SCIg can be given at home, has fewer side effects, provides more stable trough IgG levels and is more convenient for patients. SCIg is now being increasingly preferred to IVIg for replacement therapy in patients with IEI. While IVIg (dose 400–600 mg/kg) is administered every 3–4 weeks, SCIg (dose 100–200 mg/kg) is given at intervals of 7–10 days.

IVIg is therapy of choice for Kawasaki disease (2 g/kg single dose), idiopathic thrombocytopenic purpura (dose 0.8–1 g/kg/day single dose) and autoimmune demyelinating polyradiculoneuropathy (1 g/kg/day for 2 days). Use of IVIg may be considered in selected patients with severe myasthenia, lupus crisis, autoimmune neutropenia, neonatal alloimmune and autoimmune thrombocytopenia, dermatomyositis not responding to steroid therapy, and certain vasculitides.

Administration of IVIg may be associated with adverse effects, including anaphylactoid and anaphylactic (i.e. IgE-mediated) reactions. IVIg infusion must be started slowly and the child monitored closely; infusion rate is slowed or discontinued, if the child develops chills or rigors. Less than 1% may show features of aseptic meningitis. The risk of acute kidney injury is negligible with current iso-osmolar preparations. Rare long-term risks include transmission of blood-borne infections, including hepatitis C.

### Suggested Reading

1. Bousfiha A, Moundir A, Tangye SG, et al. The 2022 update of IUIS phenotypical classification for human inborn errors of immunity. J Clin Immunol 2022;42(7):1508–1520.
2. Meyts I, Bousfiha A, Duff C, Singh S, et al. Primary immunodeficiencies: A decade of progress and a promising future. Front Immunol. 2021;11:625753.
3. Pilania RK, Chaudhary H, Jindal AK, Rawat A, Singh S. Current status and prospects of primary immunodeficiency diseases in Asia. Genes Dis 2019 Sep 12;7(1):3–11.
4. Rawat A, Arora K, Shandilya J, et al. Flow cytometry for diagnosis of primary immune deficiencies. Front Immunol 2019;10:2111.

Chapter

26

# Ophthalmic Disorders

❍ Radhika Tandon

Adequate knowledge of ophthalmic disorders in children is important for a variety of reasons. Children may present with varied primary eye problems. Several systemic diseases have ocular manifestations, some of which are useful in making the correct diagnosis and instituting appropriate management. Also, therapies for some diseases are known to have ocular side effects, which need to be recognized. Rarely, medications for eye diseases can have systemic side effects. Finally, diseases beginning in the eyes and adnexa can have systemic complications.

## PEDIATRIC EYE SCREENING

The concept of screening children for eye diseases is based on the awareness that infants and young children cannot communicate their symptoms and visual difficulties. In addition, several potentially blinding diseases manifest in this age group; their early detection and treatment can limit ocular morbidity and prevent irreversible blindness.

The goal of pediatric eye screening is to detect eye and visual disorders in children or identify their risk factors so that the child can be referred for detailed ophthalmic evaluation, confirmation of diagnosis and appropriate medical management. The broad principles and priority areas at different levels based on common eye diseases in context of impact of early intervention and consequences of delay in management are outlined in Flowchart 26.1.

### Indications for Comprehensive Pediatric Eye Evaluation

Presence of any of the following risk factors is an indication for referral for comprehensive ophthalmic evaluation.

i. *General health condition, systemic disease or use of medications associated with eye disease:*
   - Extreme prematurity (gestational age ≤30 weeks); suspected retinopathy of prematurity
   - Intrauterine growth retardation
   - Perinatal complications
   - Neurological disorders
   - Juvenile rheumatoid arthritis
   - Thyroid disease

**Flowchart 26.1:** Principles of eye health care flow with priority areas

**Health education**
Health promotion
- Nutritional status
- Visual hygiene
- Vision screening
- Refractive error services

Preventive measures
- Protect from trauma
- Prevent infection

**Neonatal services**
Retinopathy of prematurity
- Prevention
- Screening
- Treatment

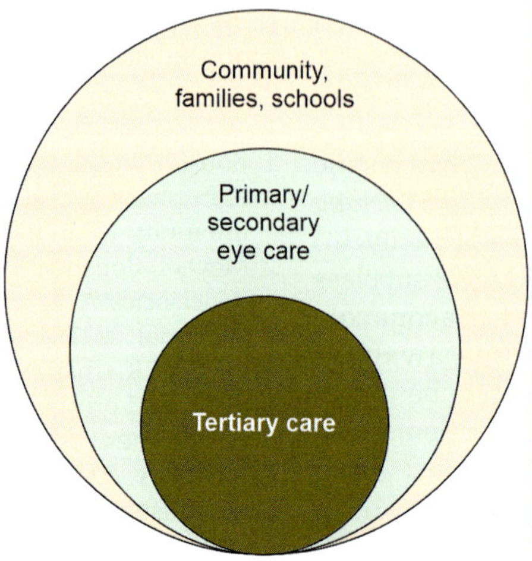


**Primary and secondary eye care**
Diagnosis and treatment of simple conditions
Refractive error services
Detection and referral/surgery
- Emergencies
- Cataract
- Visual impairment

Rehabilitation services

**Tertiary care**
Sub-speciality services
- Cataract
- Cornea
- Retina
- Squint
- Oncology
- Oculoplasty

- Craniofacial abnormalities
- Diabetes mellitus
- Syndromes with known ocular manifestations
- Chronic steroid therapy; use of hydroxychloroquine or other medications known to affect eyes
- Suspected child abuse

ii. *Family history of any of the following:*

- Retinoblastoma
- Childhood cataract
- Childhood glaucoma
- Refractive errors in early childhood
- Retinal dystrophy or degeneration
- Strabismus and/or amblyopia
- Sickle cell disease
- Syndromes with ocular manifestations
- Nontraumatic childhood blindness

iii. *Signs or symptoms reported by the family, health care provider or school teacher:*

- Defective ocular fixation or visual interactions
- Abnormal appearance of the eye(s)
- Squinting or tendency to close one eye
- Any obvious ocular alignment, movement abnormality, head tilt or nystagmus
- Large and/or cloudy eye(s)
- Drooping of the eyelid(s)
- Lumps or swelling around the eye(s)
- Persistent or recurrent tearing, sticky discharge, redness, itching or photophobia
- Learning disabilities or dyslexia

### Preliminary Assessment

An attempt should be made to gather as much background information before proceeding to actual examination. This will include information gathered from past records, referral notes, history taken from parents and observation of the child and his/her behaviour and responses. A few age appropriate questions can be asked from the child as well to determine the general and visual responses to the interaction. If there are any specific ocular or visual complaints, then suitable direct questions pertaining to the symptoms are indicated.

### Guidelines for Examination

Children are best examined in a comfortable and friendly environment. Very young children can remain in the lap of their mother, while older children can be distracted with toys and colorful objects. When the child first enters the room, simple observation of behavior, fixation, movement and general awareness of the surroundings indicate the child's visual status; gross abnormalities can often be detected.

Steady fixation and uniform steady alignment of the eyes develop in the first 4–6 weeks. Visual acuity assessment in children less than 6 months of age is limited to seeing, if the child attempts to fix and follow light. A child 6–12 months of age can follow and even reach out towards colorful objects, and this permits a very crude assessment of gross visual ability. A more objective assessment can be made with electrophysiological tests using a pattern-induced visual evoked response (pattern VER), using chequered patterns of varying degrees of resolution, or by observing the optokinetic response or nystagmus induced by the child's attempt to view a striped pattern on a moving drum (OKN). These tests are expensive and not readily available in routine clinics. For most preverbal children up to the age of 3 years, a simple observation of fixation pattern and behavior, ability to see, follow or pick-up small objects like toys or candy beads, preferential looking tests using Teller acuity cards or preferential looking cards are used to estimate the visual status. Unilateral loss is also tested for by observing, if the child resists closure or occlusion of one eye over the other.

Vision of children 3–5 years of age can be assessed using picture tests and symbols with matching cards such as the Kays symbols, tumbling E or HOTV card tests where one relies on the child's ability to recognize the shape and match the shape with a similar one on a card. Children 5 years or older can be tested with more conventional vision testing methods using a Snellen visual acuity chart with either alphabets or tumbling E or Landoldts C symbols (Fig. 26.1).

Ocular movements and external examination of the eye can be performed using adequate illumination with a torch and aided by toys or colorful pictures to capture the child's attention and interest to cooperate with the examiner. Pupillary reactions must be tested and fundus examination should be attempted with a direct ophthalmoscope through the undilated pupil to view the disc and macula. In case required, more detailed examination of the fundus and retinal periphery can be carried out after dilating the pupils with mydriatic eye drops such as 2.5% phenylephrine or short-acting cyloplegic-mydriatic drops such as 0.5% tropicamide or 1% cyclopentolate drops. The retina is best

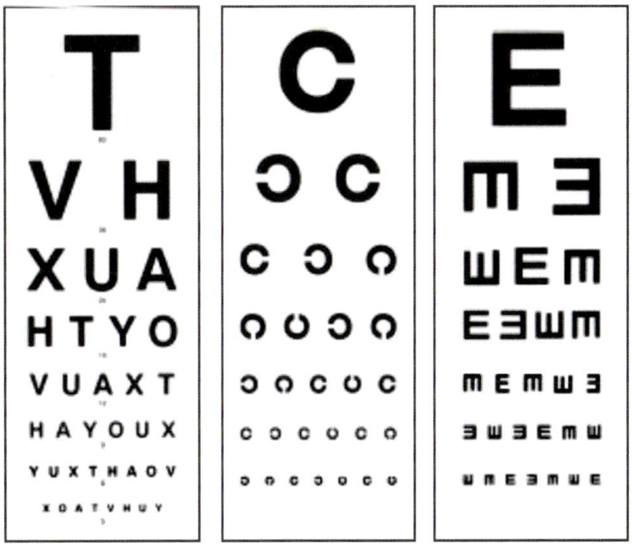


Fig. 26.1: Snellen visual acuity testing charts. The charts are printed on a semitransparent plastic sheet and mounted on an illuminated box. Vision is tested at a distance of 6 metres. The chart on left is in English, can be available in other languages and is used for children who are able to read. The chart in the middle is the C chart and on the right the E chart, both of which can be used for preschool children who can understand and communicate the directions

viewed with an indirect ophthalmoscope as this gives the maximum field of view and the examination can be completed efficiently. In general, as far as possible, most of the examination should be completed without touching or going too close to the child so that the child is comfortable and does not feel intimidated. Digital assessment of the intraocular pressure, eversion of the lids and slit-lamp examination are occasionally required. In certain situations, examination under anesthesia is required, following informed parental cosent.

## CONGENITAL AND DEVELOPMENTAL ABNORMALITIES

This group of diseases may or may not manifest at birth. If the disease is detected at birth, it is 'congenital' such as lid coloboma, severe corneal opacity or total cataract with a white opaque lens. Sometimes the disease is present at birth, but is detected later on, for example, a partial cataract or mild congenital glaucoma. Sometimes the disease is a defect of development but manifests later, such as developmental cataract or juvenile glaucoma.

### Globe Abnormalities

A child may be born with a small eye (microphthalmos or nanophthalmos), absent eyeball (anophthalmos) with or without an orbital cyst, or more complex abnormalities associated with craniofacial dysgenesis.

### Abnormalities of Development of the Orbit, Eyelids and Adnexa

Children are sometimes born with the eyes completely covered by the eyelids so that the globe is not apparent or visible (cryptophthalmos). A blocked nasolacrimal duct may manifest at birth as a dacryocystocele, or later as dacryocystitis. Lacrimal diverticulae or fistula are other abnormalities which may or may not be apparent at birth. Telangiectasias and vascular abnormalities such as capillary or cavernous hemangioma, lymphohemangioma, arteriovenous malformations and orbital varices may be present as isolated abnormalities or as part of syndromes such as the phakomatoses.

Other abnormalities of the lids include abnormal shape and position such as blepharophimosis, ptosis, prominent epicanthic folds, lid coloboma, congenital ichthyosis, entropion and ectropion. Early oculoplastic reconstruction needs to be undertaken, if the visual axis is covered or the cornea is at risk of exposure keratopathy due to lagophthalmos or inadequate lid closure.

### Diseases Affecting the Conjunctiva and Anterior Segment

Conditions that may be seen include conjunctival telangiectasia, hazy or opaque cornea (causes of which can be memorized using the mnemonic STUMPED, i.e. **s**clerocornea, birth **t**rauma, **u**lcer, **m**uco-polysaccharidosis, **P**eters anomaly, **e**ndothelial dystrophy or **e**ndothelial dysfunction secondary to congenital glaucoma, and **d**ermoid); flat cornea (cornea plana), anterior segment dysgenesis, aniridia, iris coloboma, primary congenital or juvenile developmental glaucoma, lens opacity or cataract, lens coloboma, displaced or subluxated lens or ectopia lentis, abnormal shape of lens such as microspherophakia, lens coloboma, lenticonus and persistent hyperplastic primary vitreous (Fig. 26.2).

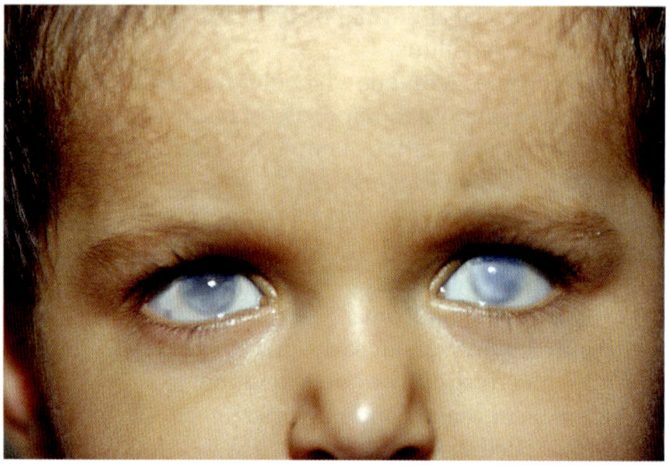

Fig. 26.2: Child with bilateral congenital corneal opacity due to anterior segment dysgenesis. Differential diagnoses include all causes of congenital corneal opacity, congenital glaucoma with buphthalmos, and corneal edema due to raised intraocular pressure

## ACQUIRED EYE DISEASES

### Nutritional Disorders

Vitamin A deficiency can be catastrophic in young children, if severe enough to produce keratomalacia. Up to the age of 6 months, children have adequate hepatic reserves of vitamin A. However, if the mother's nutrition is poor or the infant is not properly fed after birth, severe vitamin A deficiency may be precipitated by an attack of acute respiratory infection such as measles, pneumonia or acute gastroenteritis, which could lead to bilateral blindness due to severe keratomalacia (Fig. 26.3). Milder forms of vitamin A deficiency may manifest with xerosis of the conjunctiva, Bitot's spot and nyctalopia or night blindness.

Adequate nutritional advice to the pregnant and lactating mother, and proper weaning with a diet that is rich in vitamin A, fruits and vegetables is advised. Keratomalacia is treated with oral vitamin A 200,000 IU stat followed by a second dose after 24 hours and a third dose after 2 weeks. In case the child is vomiting and cannot retain oral supplement, an intramuscular injection of vitamin A may be given instead. For children less than 1 year of age and those weighing less than 10 kg, half the dose is given to avoid vitamin A toxicity, including intracranial hypertension.

### Infections

Preseptal cellulitis and orbital cellulitis manifest as swelling and inflammation of the eyelids, are differentiated clinically, and often occur due to spread of infection from the lids, adnexa or paranasal sinuses or following trauma. These are potentially dangerous infections as they involve the anatomical 'dangerous area of the face' and if not treated promptly and adequately, can spread intracranially,

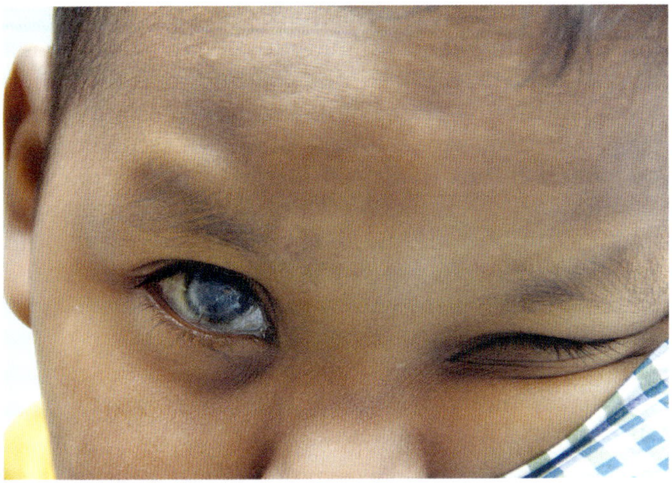

Fig. 26.3: Sequelae of keratomalacia causing corneal opacity right eye and phthisis bulbi left eye

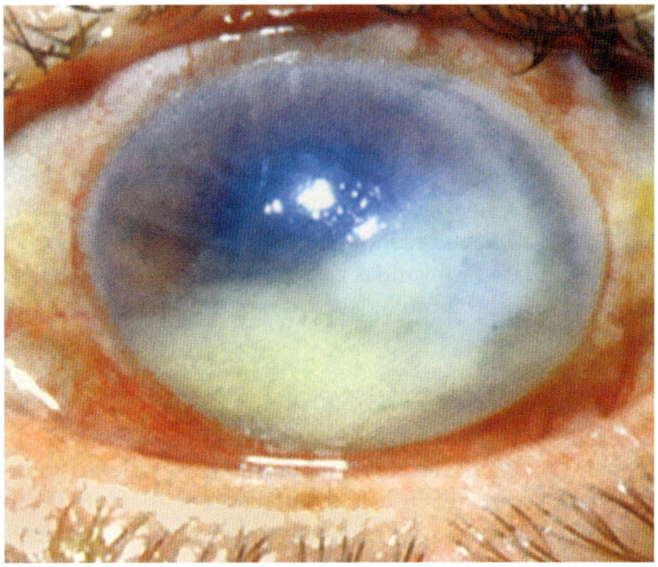

Fig. 26.4: A partially treated corneal ulcer. The overlying epithelial defect has healed, but there is a deep corneal abscess, corneal edema and purulent fluid, i.e. hypopyon in the anterior chamber

resulting in meningitis or cavernous sinus thrombosis. Ultrasonography is required to detect an orbital abscess, which has to be drained. CT scan or MRI is required, if involvement of adjacent paranasal sinuses or intracranial involvement is suspected. Treatment requires systemic antibiotics and anti-inflammatory agents, topical antibiotics, and supportive measures, including lubricating eyedrops to prevent corneal damage.

Other infections involving the eyelids include blepharitis, hordeolum externum (stye), hordeolum internum (infected chalazion), molluscum contagiosum and phthiriasis of the eyelashes. Lid hygiene, hot fomentation and local antibiotic ointments are useful along with instructions for personal hygiene. Phthiriasis will require mechanical removal of nits adhering to the eyelashes, local application of 20% fluorescein sodium to the lid margins and systemic ivermectin therapy for recalcitrant cases, along with advice on hygiene and treatment of other affected family members.

Common infections of the ocular surface include conjunctivitis which could be bacterial, viral or chlamydial. Conjunctivitis occurring within the first month after birth is called *ophthalmia neonatorum*. Every effort should be made to identify the etiologic agent, since gonococcal conjunctivitis can cause loss of vision in the newborn. Conjunctival smears and swabs can be sent for microbiological evaluation. Mucopurulent conjunctivitis is treated with topical antibiotic eyedrops and supportive measures such as cleansing the eye with clean water, lubricating eyedrops and cold compresses.

More severe infections include keratitis and corneal ulcers (Fig. 26.4). Trauma is the most common underlying predisposing factor, but poor hygiene and lowering of local immunity secondary to chronic inflammation, viral infections or use of topical steroids are other risk factors for bacterial and fungal infections of the cornea. Trauma with vegetative matter, such as a thorn, tree branch or wooden broomstick predisposes to fungal infections.

Corneal ulcers might require examination under anesthesia, and corneal scraping for microbiological analysis. Empirical therapy for bacterial corneal ulcers is started with a combination of freshly prepared fortified topical antibiotics such as 5% cephazolin and 1.3% tobramycin eye drops hourly and half hourly alternately round the clock for the first 48 hours. After 48 hours, the culture report and clinical response are reviewed. If there is no substantial clinical improvement, the antibiotic is changed based on microbiology results. If clinically responding to therapy, the frequency of antibiotics can be reduced to use during waking hours only, followed 2 days later by 2 hourly application, then reduced to 4 hourly or 6 hourly, and discontinued a week after the ulcer has healed. Supportive measures include topical cycloplegics, hot fomentation, analgesics, antiglaucoma medication, if secondary glaucoma is present, and antibiotic ointment at night. Fungal keratitis is treated with topical natamycin (5%) 1 hourly with supportive measures. Herpes simplex viral keratitis is treated with topical acyclovir 3% eye ointment for epithelial involvement and systemic acyclovir for herpetic keratouveitis or recurrent disease.

Other infections include endophthalmitis (traumatic, metastatic, or iatrogenic following intraocular surgery) and parasitic infestations, such as toxoplasmosis, toxocariasis, and cysticercosis of the eye, extraocular muscles or orbit.

### Allergic and Inflammatory Diseases

Children may develop allergic diseases of the skin around the eye and the ocular surface and conjunctiva. Dermatitis may be an allergic reaction to local ophthalmic medication or sometimes secondary to insect bite, application of traditional eye medicines or herbal remedies and use of local creams or lotions. In addition, a variety of environmental and hereditary factors may interplay to produce a variety of allergic conjunctival manifestations such as seasonal allergic conjunctivitis, hay fever conjunctivitis, perennial or chronic allergic conjunctivitis, atopic allergic conjunctivitis and vernal keratoconjunctivitis. Itching, redness, discomfort, gritty or foreign body sensation, watering, mucoid or thick ropy discharge, photophobia and blepharospasm are all seen in different combinations and varying degrees of severity. Treatment includes cold compresses, topical antihistaminic eyedrops for mild cases and counseling to avoid rubbing the eyes. Topical corticosteroid eyedrops give quick relief but are best avoided in mild cases because of the danger of self-medication and unsupervised chronic topical use complicated by steroid-induced glaucoma and secondary corneal infection and ulceration. More severe allergies may have secondary consequences in the form of dry eye, keratopathy and corneal ulceration. These are best referred to ophthalmologists for expert management and careful follow-up.

Other inflammatory diseases include phlyctenular conjunctivitis or keratoconjunctivitis (believed to be an 'allergic' immunological reaction to tubercular antigen); interstitial keratitis secondary to rubella, syphilis, leprosy and tuberculosis; and uveitis, either idiopathic or associated with juvenile chronic arthritis, psoriasis, tuberculosis, sarcoidosis and toxoplasmosis. Acute anterior uveitis (iritis, cyclitis and iridocyclitis) usually presents with a red inflamed eye with photophobia and reduced vision. Chronic uveitis may be less symptomatic with decreased vision due to complicated cataract. Intermediate and posterior uveitis (pars planitis, vitritis, retinitis, choroiditis and retinochoroiditis) are usually painless with symptoms of decreased vision (due to hazy media and retinal or optic nerve swelling and inflammation) and floaters (due to inflammatory cells in the vitreous). Treatment is with topical cycloplegic agents and steroids, supplemented with systemic steroids and specific therapy for any underlying disease, such as tuberculosis. Patients with uveitis need detailed examination with a slit lamp biomicroscope to identify the inflammatory response, ophthalmoscopy to view the fundus and specialist ophthalmic care and follow-up.

Intraocular (retinoblastoma or juvenile xanthogranuloma) or systemic malignant disorders may sometimes mimic the uveitis syndrome, due to malignant cells in the eye and vascular uveal tracts.

Optic neuritis is another important inflammatory disease which could be idiopathic, secondary to infections or associated with demyelinating disorders. Classical features include a rapid drop in vision, usually in one eye, which is accompanied by a relative afferent pupillary defect and normal fundus (retrobulbar neuritis) or inflammatory swelling of the optic disc (papillitis) and retinal edema and/or exudates (neuroretinitis). Patients need to be treated in consultation with a neuro-ophthalmologist after investigations to identify the cause.

### Metabolic and Endocrine Disorders

Homocystinuria is associated with subluxation of the lens, and secondary glaucoma can be seen as a complication. The lens is usually subluxated downwards, which causes poor vision due to displacement and astigmatism. Surgical lens removal has to be done under general anesthesia taking suitable precautions, as the patients are prone to thromboembolism. Optical rehabilitation is usually done with spectacles or contact lenses, though in some cases intraocular lenses can be fitted using scleral or bag fixation augmented with bag fixation devices.

Various storage disorders such as cerebral storage disease, lipidosis and gangliosidosis may be associated with a 'cherry red spot' due to abnormal deposition in the retina, corneal clouding as in some of the mucopolysaccharidoses, and Kayser-Fleischer ring in peripheral cornea in Wilson disease. Juvenile diabetes mellitus may be associated with cataract and diabetic retinopathy, and thyroid dysfunction with dysthyroid eye disease. Tyrosinase deficiency might be associated with ocular albinism with foveal hypoplasia and poor vision.

### Musculoskeletal and Neurodegenerative Diseases and Phakomatoses

Marfan and Ehlers-Danlos syndromes may be associated with subluxated lens and consequent secondary glaucoma. Marfan syndrome is usually associated with upward and outward displacement of the lenses and myopia with blurred vision. Retinal detachment is also common. Retinal detachment is also common. Surgical lens removal becomes necessary, if the vision is not corrected with spectacles or contact lenses. Leukodystrophies and demyelinating diseases may be associated with extraocular muscle weakness, ptosis and optic neuropathy. Phakomatoses like neurofibromatosis, Sturge-Weber syndrome and nevus of Ota may be associated with café au lait spots, plexiform neurofibromas of the lids and orbit, and Lisch nodules on the iris and glaucoma.

Muscular dystrophies or degenerations, such as chronic progressive external ophthalmoplegia, result in ptosis and restriction of eye movements. Duchenne muscular dystrophy may be associated with cataracts.

### Tumors and Neoplastic Diseases

Benign tumors include dermoids of orbit, lids or on cornea, hamartomas, osteoma, vascular malformations or hemangiomas of various types and neurofibromas. Malignant intraocular tumors are confined to retinoblastoma (Fig. 26.5), juvenile xanthogranuloma, medulloepithelioma and metastatic lesions from neuroblastomas, Ewing sarcoma, leukemias and lymphomas. Orbital tumors include rhabdomyosarcoma, Langerhans cell histiocytosis, extraocular spread of retinoblastoma, metastatic spread of Ewing sarcoma, neuroblastoma, leukemia and lymphoma.

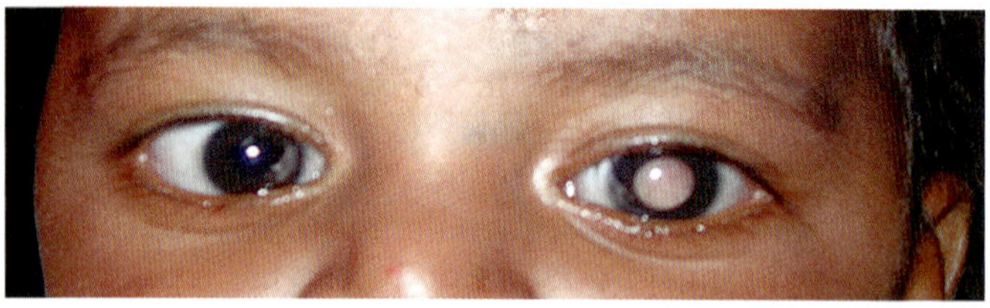

Fig. 26.5: 'Leukocoria' or white pupil in an infant secondary to retinoblastoma. Note the white appearance that appears to be from a structure located more posteriorly, has a slight yellowish pinkish tinge due to vascularization and has an appearance that is unlike that seen with a cataract. Ultrasonography of the orbits helps confirm the diagnosis

## Refractive Errors

An abnormality in the refractive and focusing apparatus makes it difficult for parallel rays of light from the distance to be accurately focused on the retina. This deviation from the normal emmetropic state is termed 'ametropia' or refractive error. This manifests as poor or blurred vision which may be noticed by parents, relatives, friends, school teachers or reported by the child as a difficulty in viewing clearly. Sometimes, indirect evidence is reported as eye rubbing, 'squinting', 'going too close to the television' or holding objects too close to the eyes. An assessment of visual acuity is followed by cycloplegic refraction; fundus evaluation is required in addition to routine ophthalmic evaluation.

Refractive errors include myopia, hypermetropia and astigmatism, and spectacles must be prescribed accordingly. Associated amblyopia or strabismus must be taken care of and any additional features like nystagmus or extraocular muscle imbalance ruled out. Patients need to be carefully counseled with respect to improvement of vision with spectacles and need for compliance with follow-up. Failure to show an improvement of vision warrants investigations to rule out any associated subtle pathology such as microstrabismus, retinal macular degeneration, retinitis pigmentosa, congenital hereditary cone dystrophy, delayed visual maturation, dyslexia or Leber amaurosis.

## Strabismus and Amblyopia

Strabismus is defined as the condition when the visual axes of the two eyes do not meet at the point of regard. In other words, the motor and sensory alignment of the two eyes and their images in the brain are not synchronized. The cause may be a basic abnormality of development as in essential esotropia or exotropia (concomitant squint when the angle of deviation or separation of the two eyes is uniform, irrespective of the direction or position of gaze) or secondary to extraocular muscle paralysis, e.g. paralytic squint, orbital space occupying lesion, myositis or orbital inflammation as in orbital pseudotumor syndrome, orbital musculofascial abnormality like Duane retraction syndrome or Brown's superior oblique tendon sheath syndrome.

An inward deviation of the eye is termed esotropia and outward deviation is termed exotropia. The child initially suffers diplopia due to the different images being presented to the visual cortex by the two eyes, but learns to suppress one image, eventually developing amblyopia or a 'lazy eye' with loss of binocularity and stereopsis. In very young children, the presence of an intermittent or constant squint or misalignment of the eyes should be indications for referral to an ophthalmologist.

Amblyopia or 'lazy eye' is a condition of subnormal vision defined as two lines less than normal or less than the fellow eye on the visual acuity chart with no anatomical cause detectable on examination, i.e. no media opacity and a normal fundus. Amblyogenic factors have their maximum impact on the immature developing visual system, i.e. during the first 6 yr of life and include sensory deprivation or abnormal binocular interaction. The former would refer to a corneal opacity or cataract which, even if taken care of surgically, do not indicate good chances of restoration of normal vision. Similarly, abnormal binocular interaction occurs in the presence of strabismus or anisometropia (difference in the refractive power of the two eyes), in which case one eye takes over and the visual cortical neurons meant to receive stimuli from the other eye are unable to develop normally, leading to a 'lazy eye'. These changes are potentially reversible with appropriate therapy in the first decade, but become irreversible and permanent later. Treatment involves restoration of vision with correction of refractive error, removal of media opacity if present (such as corneal opacity or cataract), patching therapy by part time patching of the 'good' eye to enable the 'lazy' eye to catch up, and strabismus surgery to restore ocular alignment, if required.

## Corneal Diseases

The spectrum of acquired corneal diseases in children is similar to adults in general. Degenerative non-inflammatory ectatic disorders include keratoconus and keratoglobus which are bilateral and are characterized by corneal thinning, ectasia, myopia and astigmatism. Treatment includes spectacles, contact lenses, collagen cross-linking to strengthen the cornea and later keratoplasty. Trauma or eye rubbing may lead to tears in Descemet membrane resulting in acute hydrops with pain, redness, corneal edema, photophobia and drop in vision which requires emergency care.

Another important category of non-inflammatory bilateral acquired corneal diseases are corneal dystrophies. Apart from congenital hereditary endothelial dystrophy which is present at birth, congenital hereditary stromal dystrophy and macular corneal dystrophy are associated with visibly hazy cornea and low vision manifesting in first decade of life. Lattice corneal dystrophy generally manifests later on, sometime in second decade and is associated with recurrent corneal erosions, hazy vision and characteristic stromal deposits in the form of translucent fine lattice lines visualized by slit lamp biomicroscopy.

## Cataract

A visible lenticular opacity in the eye is termed as a cataract. It is congenital, if present since birth; developmental, if appearing later on; and traumatic, if occurring after an episode of eye trauma. A central opacity is considered visually significant, if it impairs visual acuity, and on clinical assessment obstructs a clear view of the fundus. A cataract may be unilateral or bilateral and symmetric or asymmetric. In view of the risk of sensory deprivation amblyopia, visually significant cataract should be treated surgically as soon as possible after birth. Functional success is highest, if operated within the first few weeks after birth.

Unilateral cataracts must be supplemented with postoperative patching to take care of any amblyopic effect. Optical and visual rehabilitation for the aphakic state resulting from lens removal includes the implantation of an intraocular lens (IOL) for children above two years of age. Generally, intraocular lenses are avoided for children less than 2 years old as there are significant problems of change in lens power requirements as the maximum growth

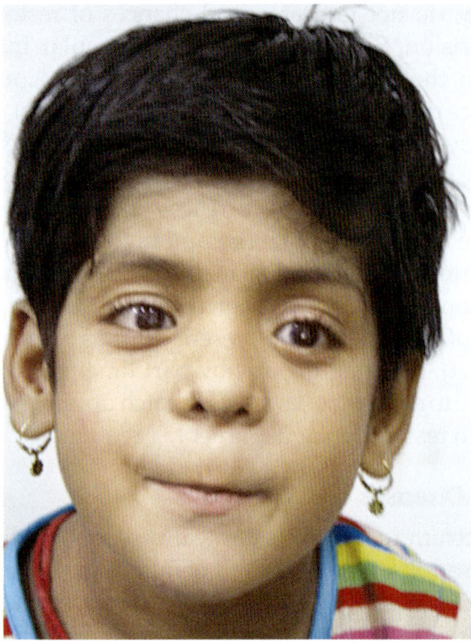

**Fig. 26.6:** A child with bilateral developmental cataract. The cataract is partial and the condition was detected late. Also note that the child has a convergent squint. The child also has impaired hearing and congenital heart disease, suspected to be due to congenital rubella syndrome

of the eyeball takes place during the first 2 years of life and the risk of complications of glaucoma and intraocular inflammation and fibrosis is higher. In very young children, therefore, a capsule rim is left for subsequent secondary IOL implantation, and temporary optical rehabilitation is provided with spectacles or contact lenses supplemented with patching for amblyopia in unilateral cases (Fig. 26.6).

### Glaucoma

Primary congenital and developmental juvenile glaucomas are recognized as inherited diseases. Primary congenital glaucoma is associated with mutations in *CYP1B1* (autosomal recessive inheritance) and juvenile galucoma with the myocillin (*MYOC*) gene (dominant inheritance). Photophobia, blepharospasm, watering and an enlarged eyeball are classic symptoms. Suspicion of glaucoma or buphthalmos warrants urgent referral to an ophthalmologist. Examination under anesthesia is required to measure the corneal diameter and intraocular pressure, and to visualize the optic disc. Once glaucoma is confirmed, medical therapy is started to lower the pressure and patient prepared for surgery. If the cornea is clear enough to allow visualization of the angle structures, a goniotomy is attempted. If the glaucoma is more severe or the cornea very edematous, a drainage procedure is undertaken to open alternative aqueous drainage channels such as trabeculectomy and trabeculotomy. If the cornea fails to clear after adequate control of the intraocular pressure, corneal transplantation is required to restore vision and prevent irreversible sensory deprivation amblyopia.

Children can also develop secondary glaucoma due to chronic use of topical corticosteroid eyedrops, following eye trauma particularly if associated with traumatic hyphema (blood in the anterior chamber) or angle recession, after surgery for developmental cataract and after chronic uveitis.

### Eye Trauma and Related Problems

Eye injuries are common in children (Fig. 26.7), and an important cause of preventable blindness. Effort must be made to educate the community in general, and mothers in particular, about the importance of not allowing children to play with sharp pointed toys like bows and arrows, firecrackers, chemicals including colors during Holi festival or other chemicals like edible 'chuna'. Dangerous household objects like knives, scissors and needles, and chemicals like cleaning liquid, acid, whitewash paint and edible 'chuna' should be out of reach of children.

In case an injury is sustained, the eyes should be immediately washed thoroughly with locally available

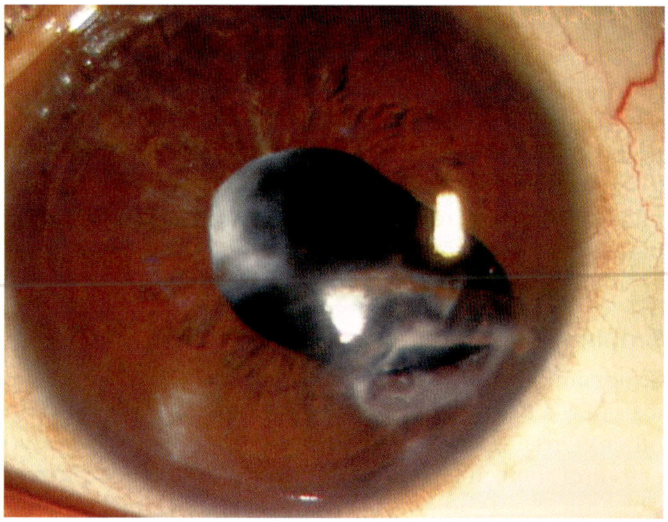

**Fig. 26.7a:** The sequelae of ocular trauma. Following injury with a wooden stick, the child had corneal perforation, which was repaired. Traumatic cataract was surgically removed. Note the irreversible anatomical damage with corneal scar, distorted iris and pupil and lens capsular opacification

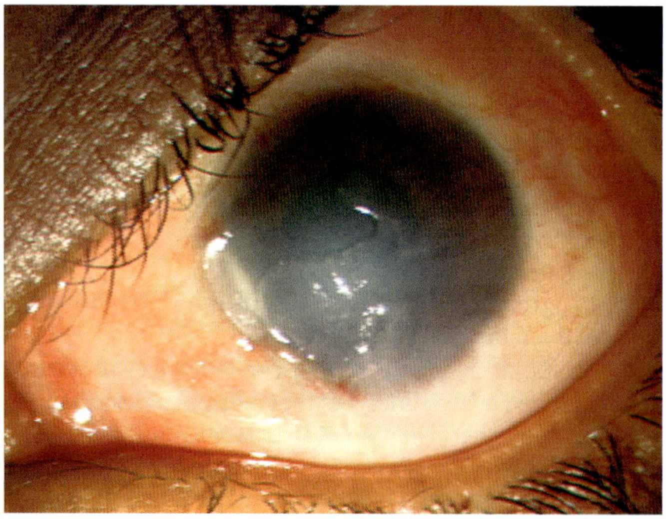

**Fig. 26.7b:** The sequelae of chemical injury, due to edible 'chuna'. Despite aggressive management, long-term sequelae include residual conjunctival inflammation with limbal stem cell deficiency and a scarred, irregular and opacified corneal surface

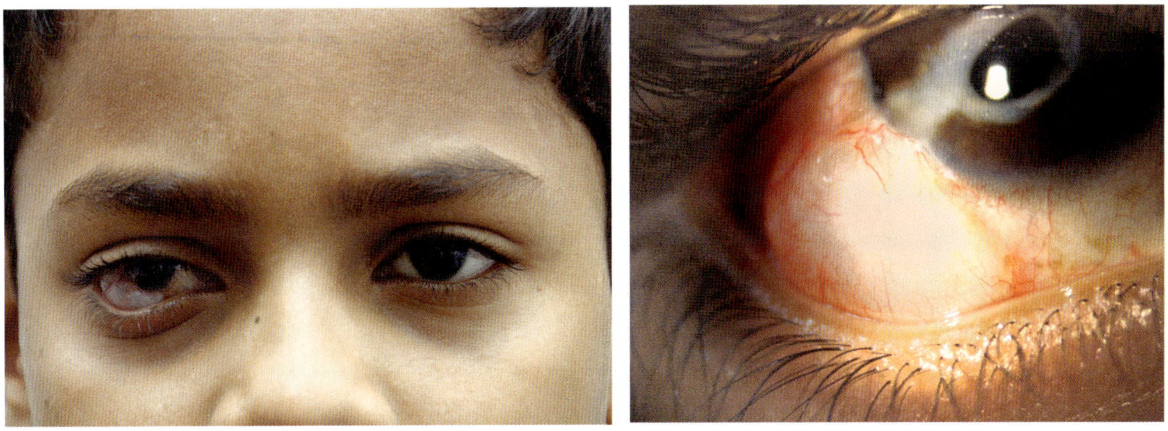

Fig. 26.7c: Following trauma with a compass, this young teenager had to be operated for trauma-induced cataract and retinal detachment and subsequently developed a conjunctival inclusion cyst



drinkable water, and the child should be rushed to the nearest hospital.

Perforating injuries of the globe require surgical repair under general anesthesia along with administration of systemic and topical antibiotics and tetanus prophylaxis. The child should be told not to rub the eyes and given only fluids while rushing the child to hospital so that there is no unnecessary delay in preparing the patient for general anesthesia and planning surgery. Meticulous repair of the wounds is undertaken as soon as possible to minimize the risk of secondary complications such as endophthalmitis, expulsion of intraocular contents and later risk of sympathetic ophthalmitis or an inflammatory panuveitis in the normal eye due to sensitization of the immune system to the sequestered antigens in the exposed uveal tissue.

### Retinal Diseases

Children may be affected by a wide variety of retinal diseases. Retinal detachment can occur secondary to trauma or spontaneously in cases with high or pathological myopia. Classical symptoms such as sudden loss of vision with floaters and photopsia may not be reported by children and the detachment may not be detected till much later. Retinal detachment requires surgical treatment and the sooner the surgery is performed, the greater are the chances of functional recovery of vision. Other diseases that can affect the retina in childhood include degenerative and hereditary conditions like retinitis pigmentosa and different forms of macular degeneration such as Stargardt disease. These diseases lead to gradual, painless, bilateral diminution of vision in the first or second decade of life which may be accompanied by defective dark adaptation or abnormal color vision. No specific treatment modalities are available, but refractive correction, low vision aids, visual rehabilitation and genetic counseling are ancillary measures.

Vascular abnormalities of the retina such as hemangiomas, arteriovenous malformations and exudative vitreoretinopathies like Coats disease may be seen. Retinal vasculitis may be seen in Eales disease and other inflammatory disorders. Diabetic retinopathy and hypertensive retinopathy can occur if these systemic disorders are present in sufficient grade of severity and for an adequate duration of time.

### Retinopathy of Prematurity

This condition, unique to children, is seen in preterm babies due to early exposure to oxygen and other environmental factors by a premature, underdeveloped retinal vascular system. The chief risk factors are prematurity, especially birth before 32 weeks of gestation, birth weight less than 1500 g and presence of other contributory risk factors such as supplemental oxygen therapy, hypoxemia, hypercarbia and concurrent illnesses like septicemia. Clinical features are graded in stages of severity depending on the retinal signs and the zone of retina involved. Children at risk should be screened periodically to look for evidence of developing what is considered as 'threshold' disease, i.e. requiring ablative laser treatment of the avascular zone of the retina to check further progression and prevent blinding stages of the disease, which would then require surgical intervention to treat the ensuing retinal detachment and other complications.

### Blindness and Low Vision in Children

The World Health Organization (WHO) has categorized blindness in different levels based on the extent of vision loss (Table 26.1).

*Vision 2020: The Right to Sight* is a global initiative for the elimination of avoidable blindness, a program jointly run by the WHO and the International Agency for Prevention of Blindness. Priority diseases identified include cataract, trachoma, onchocerciasis, childhood blindness and refractive errors and low vision. The Government of India through the National Programme for Control of Blindness (NPCB), Ministry of Health and Family Welfare and the Ministry of Social Justice and Empowerment, arranges for periodic surveys and surveillance to monitor the progress in controlling the problem and also offers financial and technical assistance for treatment and rehabilitation. Integrating children into society even if blind is being recognized as important and efforts are being made to help with education, training and preparation for future employment. Various agencies are involved in developing measures to help the visually challenged negotiate activities of daily living with help of visual aids and navigational devices (Fig. 26.8).

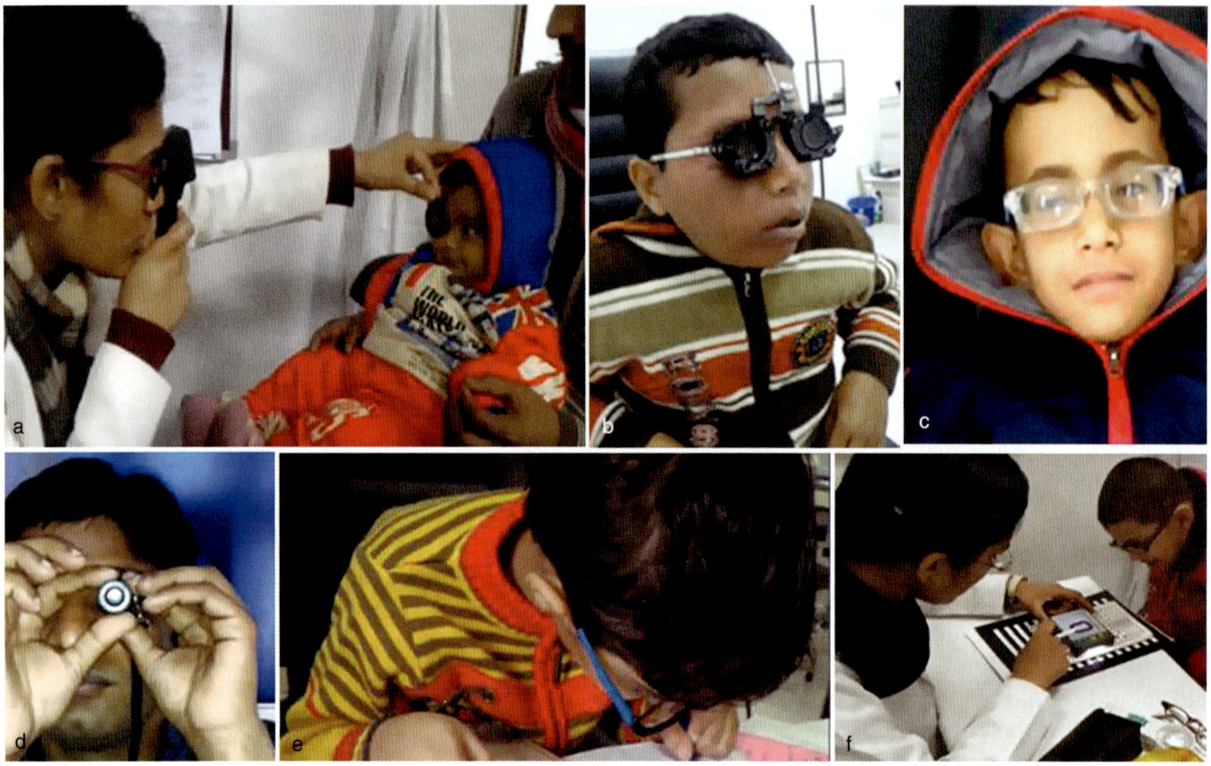

Fig. 26.8: Low vision and rehabilitation services: (a) Retinoscopy for refraction; (b) Checking acceptance; (c) Child wearing prescribed glasses; (d) Teenager using telescope; (e and f) Helping for near vision




**Table 26.1:** WHO categories of visual acuity

| *Better eye* | *Worse eye* | *Disability category* |
|---|---|---|
| 6/6 –6/18 | <6/18–6/60 | 0 |
| 6/6–6/18 | <6/60–3/60 | I |
| 6/6–6/18 | <3/60 | II (one-eyed person) |
| <6/18–6/60 or field* | <6/18–6/60 | IIIa (low vision) |
| 6/24–6/60 or field* | <6/60–3/60 | IIIb (low vision) |
| 6/24–6/60 or field* | <3/60 | IIIc (low vision) |
| 6/36–3/60 or field† | <6/60–3/60 | IIId (low vision) |
| 6/36–3/60 or field† | <3/60 | IIIe (low vision) |
| <3/60 or field‡ | <3/60 | IVa (blindness) |
| Only HMCF | Only HMCF | IVb (blindness) |
| Only light perception | Light perception | |
| No light perception | No light perception | |

*Visual field <40° up to 20° across, around centre of fixation or hemianopia involving macula

†Visual field <20° up to 10° across, around centre of fixation

‡Visual field <10° across, around centre of fixation

HMCF: Hand movement close to face

## Suggested Reading


1. AOA Evidence-Based Optometry Guideline Development Group. Comprehensive pediatric eye and vision examination. Evidence-based clinical practice guideline. 2017. https://www.aoa.org/AOA/Documents/Practice%20 Management/Clinical% 20Guidelines/EBO%20Guidelines/ Comprehensive% 20Pediatric%20Eye%20and%20Vision%20 Exam.pdf
2. Azari AA, Barney NP. Conjunctivitis: A systematic review of diagnosis and treatment. JAMA 2013; 310:1721–29.
3. Fanella S, Singer A, Embree J. Presentation and management of pediatric orbital cellulitis. Can J Infect Dis Med Microbiol 2011; 22: 97–100.
4. Malik A, Hu V. Childhood eye disease and ocular infections. Module 3403. London School of Hygiene and Tropical Medicine, 2021-22.
5. Retinopathy of prematurity: An update on screening and management. March 2017. Published by Canadian Pediatric Society. Available from http://www.cps.ca/documents/ position/retinopathy-of-prematurity-screening
6. Shukla R, Murthy GVS, Gilbert C, et al. Operational guidelines for ROP in India. Indian J Ophthal 2020;68:S108–114.

Chapter

27

# Skin Disorders

Neena Khanna ○ Neetu Bhari

Skin disorders account for a high proportion of ailments in children.

## BASIC PRINCIPLES

### Morphology of Lesions

#### *Macules*

Macule is a circumscribed area of change in skin color without any change in consistency (Fig. 27.1). A macule may be hyperpigmented (e.g. café au lait macule), hypopigmented (e.g. leprosy), depigmented (e.g. vitiligo), or erythematous (e.g. drug rash).

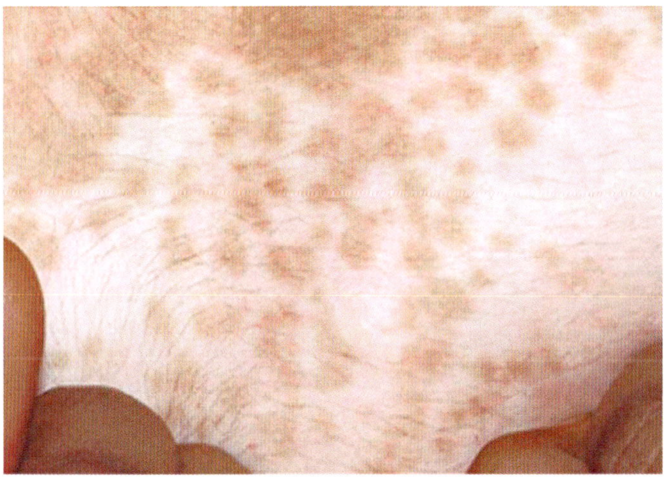

Fig. 27.1: Macule: Circumscribed area of change in skin color without any change in consistency

#### *Papules and Nodules*

Papule is a solid lesion <0.5 cm in diameter with major part projecting above the skin (Fig. 27.2a). Papules may be dome-shaped (e.g. trichoepithelioma), flat-topped (e.g. verruca plana), conical (e.g. condyloma acuminata), filiform (e.g. filiform warts), umbilicated (with crater on surface, e.g. molluscum contagiosum) or verrucous (with multiple closely packed firm elevations, e.g. verrucous warts). A papule which is >0.5 cm in size with the major part in the skin is called a nodule (Fig. 27.2b).

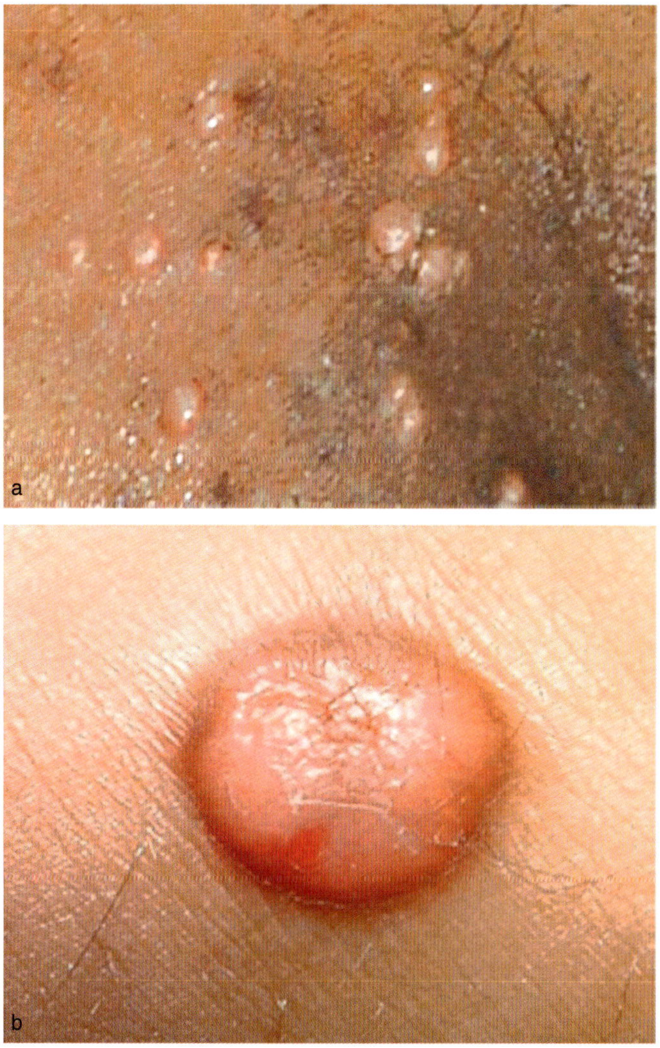


Fig. 27.2: (a) Papule: Solid lesion, ≤0.5 cm; (b) Nodule: Solid lesion, >0.5 cm

### Plaque

Plaque is an area of altered skin consistency, the surface area of which is greater than its depth (Fig. 27.3). A plaque can be elevated, depressed or flat.

### Wheal

Wheal, the characteristic lesion in urticaria, is an evanescent, pale or erythematous raised lesion which disappears within 24–48 hours (Fig. 27.4). Wheals are due to dermal edema, and when the edema extends into subcutis, it is called *angioedema*. When the wheals are linear, the phenomenon is called *dermographism*.

### Blisters

Blister is a circumscribed elevated, superficial fluid filled cavity (Fig. 27.5). If ≤0.5 cm, it is a vesicle and if >0.5 cm, a bulla.

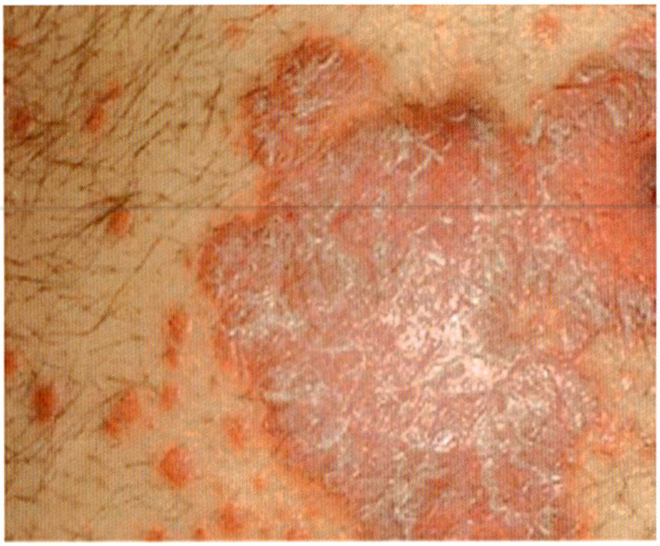

Fig. 27.3: Plaque: Area of altered skin consistency with a surface area greater than its depth

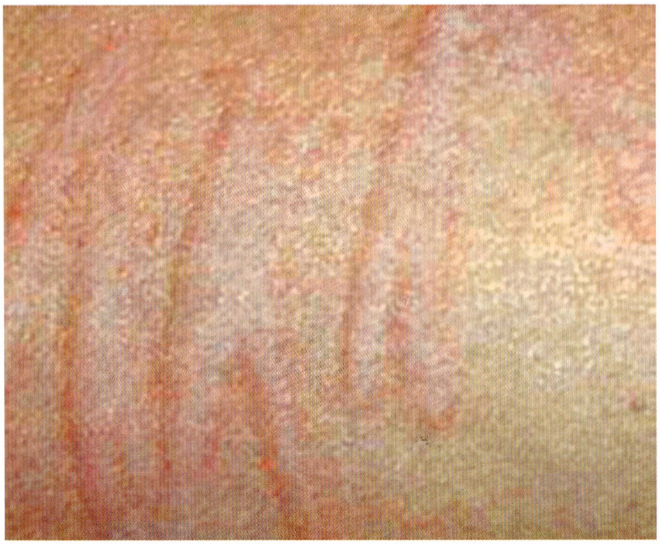

Fig. 27.4: Wheal: Evanescent, pale/erythematous raised lesion which disappears within 24–48 hours

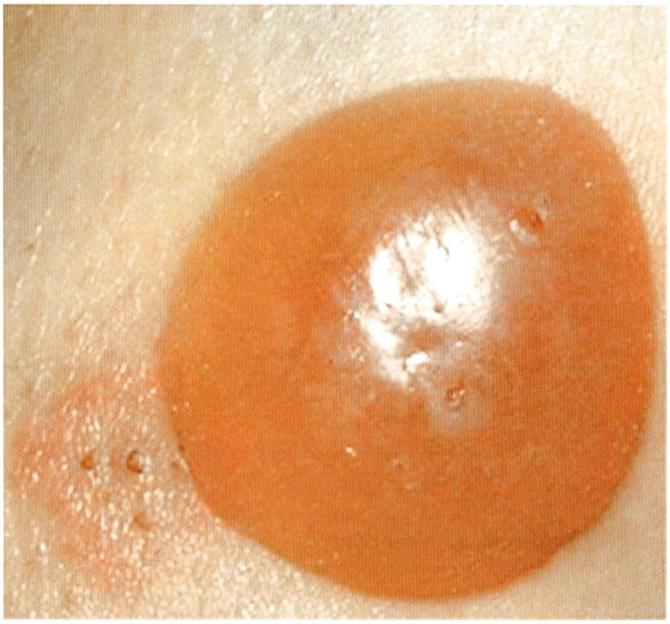

Fig. 27.5: Blister: Circumscribed, elevated, superficial fluid-filled lesion

### Scales

Scales are flakes of stratum corneum (Fig. 27.6) and are diagnostic in certain dermatoses, e.g. silver easily detachable flakes in psoriasis, branny scars in pityriasis versicolor and fish-like scales in ichthyosis.

### Crusts

Crusts are formed when serum, blood or pus dries on the skin surface (Fig. 27.7).

### Erosions and Ulcers

A defect, which involves only the epidermis and heals without a scar (Fig. 27.8a) is called an erosion, while an ulcer is a defect in the skin which extends into the dermis or deeper, and heals with scarring (Fig. 27.8b).

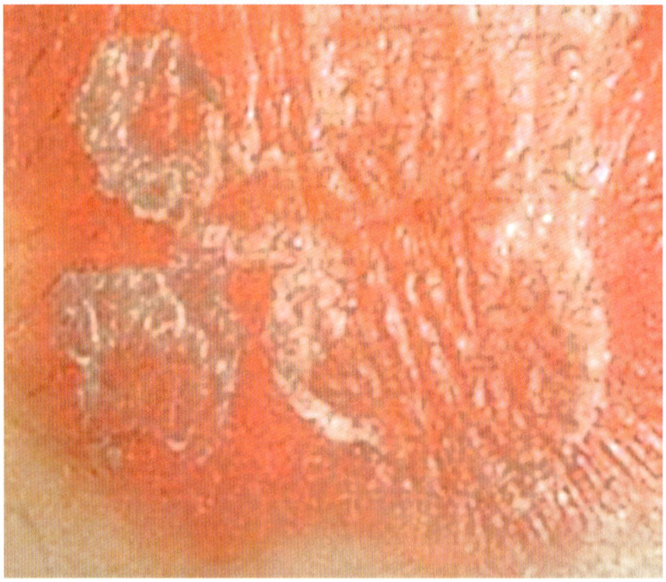

Fig. 27.6: Scale: Appears as flakes of stratum corneum

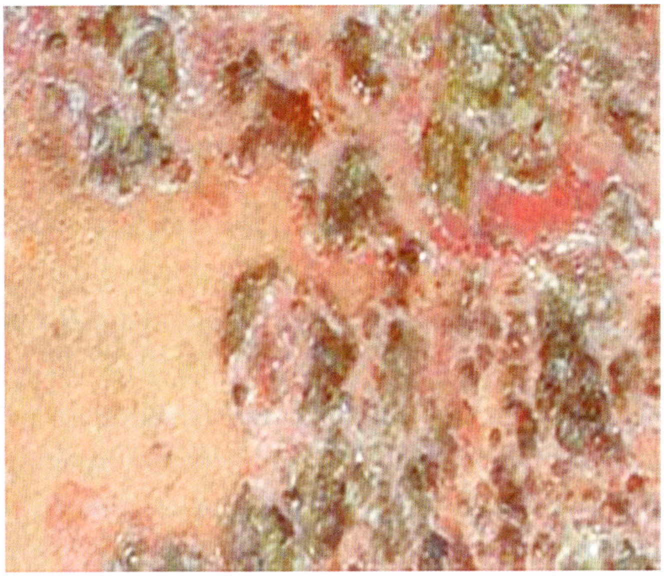

Fig. 27.7: Crust: Yellow brown collection of keratin and serum

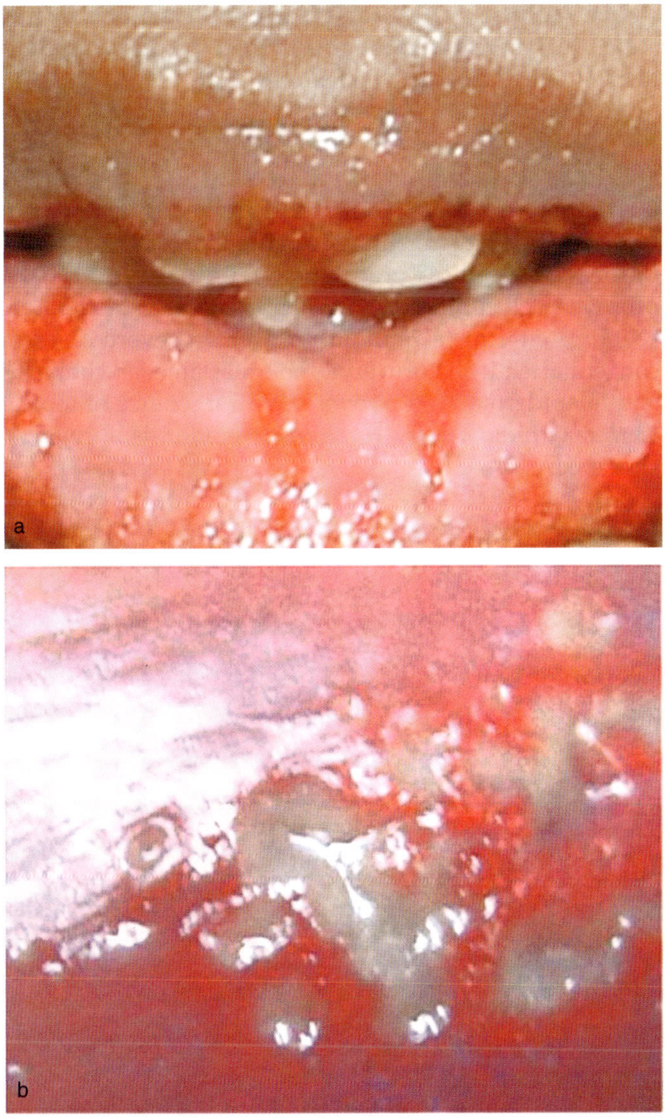


Fig. 27.8: Erosions and ulcers: (a) Erosions are due to complete or partial loss of epidermis with no loss of dermis; (b) Ulcer is a defect in the skin which extends into the dermis or deeper and heals with scarring

*Atrophy*

Atrophy is the reduction of some or all layers of skin. In epidermal atrophy, thinning of the epidermis leads to loss of skin texture and cigarette-paper like wrinkling without depression. In dermal atrophy, loss of connective tissue of the dermis leads to depression of the lesion.

*Lichenification*

Lichenification, which is caused by repeated scratching, consists of a triad of skin thickening, hyperpigmentation and increased skin markings (Fig. 27.9).

*Burrow*

Burrow is a dark serpentine, curvilinear lesion with a minute papule at one end and is diagnostic of scabies (Fig. 27.10).



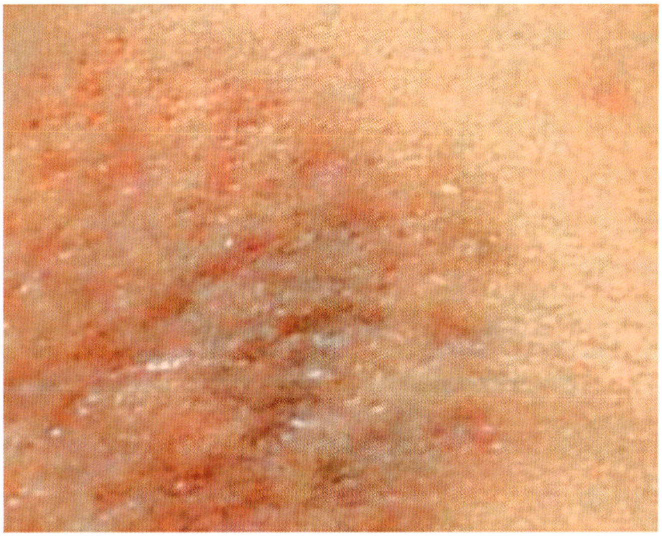

Fig. 27.9: Lichenification: Thickening and hyperpigmentation of skin with increased skin markings

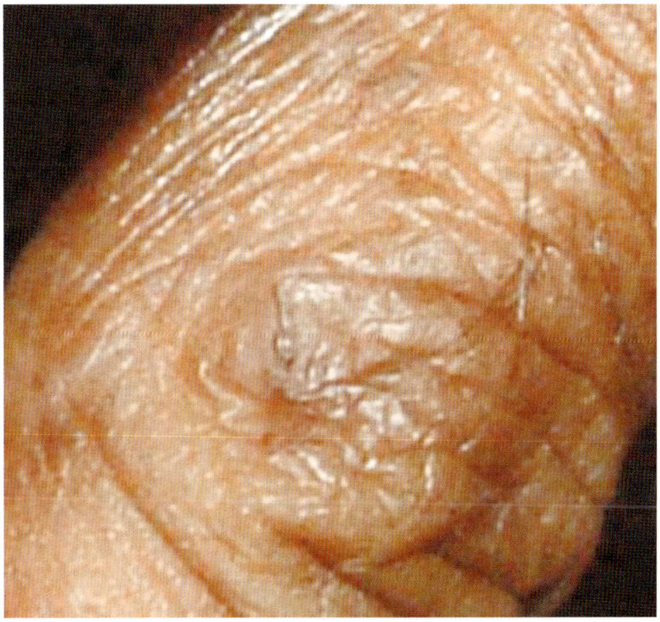

Fig. 27.10: Burrow: Serpentine, thread-like, grayish curvilinear lesion, diagnostic of scabies

### *Comedones*

Comedones are due to keratin plugs that form within pilosebaceous apparatus. Comedones can be open or closed **(Fig. 27.11)** and are pathognomonic of acne.

### Patterns Formed

Arrangement and configuration of skin lesions can help in diagnosis **(Table 27.1)**.

### Sites of Predilection

Sites of involvement often give important clues to the diagnosis **(Fig. 27.12)**.

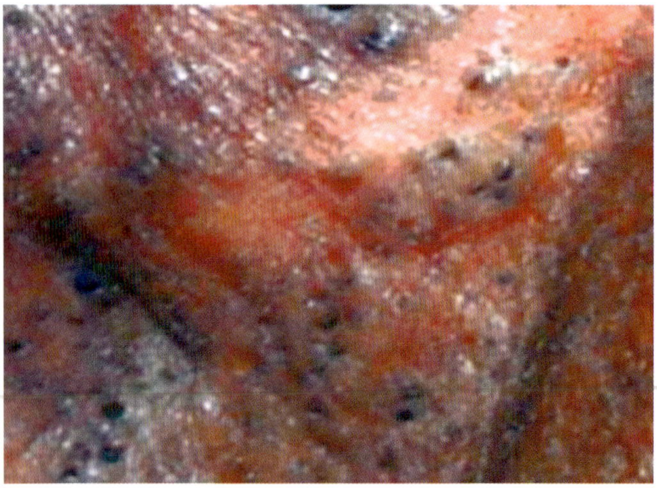

**Fig. 27.11:** Comedones: Keratin plugs that form within follicular

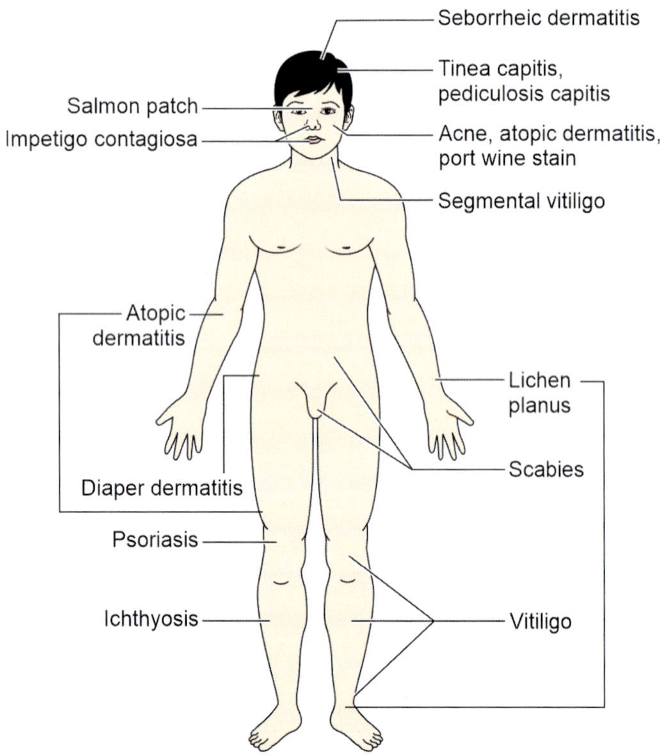



**Fig. 27.12:** Sites of predilection of common skin disease

**Table 27.1:** Arrangement and configuration of skin lesions

| *Arrangement* | *Example* |
|---|---|
| Linear | Verrucous epidermal nevus |
| Grouped | Herpes simplex |
| Dermatomal | Herpes zoster |
| Arcuate | Granuloma annulare |

## GENODERMATOSES

Genodermatoses are a group of inherited single gene cutaneous disorders that manifest themselves wholly or in part in skin, mucous membranes, hair and nails.

### Ichthyoses

Ichthyoses are a heterogeneous group of disorders characterized by the presence of fish-like scales. Several variants of ichthyoses are recognized, based on inheritance, gene defects and clinical features **(Table 27.2)**.

The hallmark of the disease is presence of fish-like scales, but there are variations in the type of scales, their distribution and associated features **(Table 27.2, Figs 27.13 to 27.17)**.

#### *Treatment*

Hydration (immersing in water) followed by immediate lubrication with petroleum jelly or urea containing creams/ lotions are useful. Keratolytic agents (hydroxy acids, propylene glycol) are used when lesions are moderately severe. Acitretin (a retinoid) is used in severe cases of congenital ichthyosiform erythroderma, lamellar ichthyosis and in epidermolytic ichthyosis. A short course of topical corticosteroids and antibiotic combination is applied, if skin is eczematized.

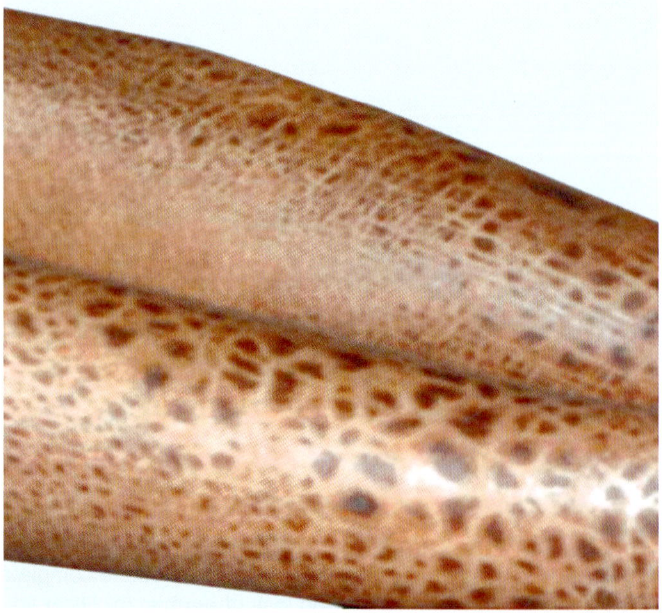

**Fig. 27.13:** Ichthyosis vulgaris: Large scales on extremities that are attached at the center and turned up at the edge

Table 27.2: Clinical features of ichthyoses

| | *Ichthyosis vulgaris* | *X-linked ichthyosis* | *Lamellar ichthyosis* | *Congenital ichthyosiform erythroderma* | *Epidermolytic ichthyosis* |
|---|---|---|---|---|---|
| Inheritance | Autosomal dominant | X-linked recessive | Autosomal recessive | Autosomal recessive | Autosomal recessive |
| Defect | Reduced or absent filaggrin | Deficiency of steroid sulfatase enzyme | Defect/deficiency of transglutaminase | Mutation of *ABCA12, ALOX12B* | Keratin 1 and 10 defect |
| Age of onset | 3–12 months | Birth | Birth | Birth | Birth |
| Sex | Equal in both sexes | Only males | Equal in both sexes | Equal both sexes | Equal both sexes |
| Incidence | Common | Rare | Very rare | Rare | Rare |
| Clinical features | Fine white scales on most parts of body; attached at center and upturned at edges on extensors of lower extremities (Fig. 27.13) | Large dark brown adherent scales (Fig. 27.14) | Collodion baby at birth, ensheathed in shiny lacquer-like membrane which on shedding reveals diffuse large thick brown plate-like scales (Fig. 27.15); erythema minimal | Collodion baby at birth; followed by fine branny scales and marked erythema (Fig. 27.16) | Generalized erythema with blistering at birth. Followed by brown, warty, broad linear plaques (Fig. 27.17). Scales may fall off leaving skip areas |
| Sites of predilection | Extensors of limbs; major flexures always spared; face usually spared | Generalized involvement; encroachment of flexures; palms and soles spared | Generalized involvement; accentuation on lower limbs and flexures | Generalized erythema and scaling | Generalized involvement; accentuation in flexures |
| Associated features | Hyperlinear palms and soles; keratosis pilaris; atopic diathesis | Corneal opacities; cryptorchidism | Ectropion and eclabium; crumpled ears; palmoplantar keratoderma | Palmoplantar keratoderma less frequent | Palmoplantar keratoderma in >60% |

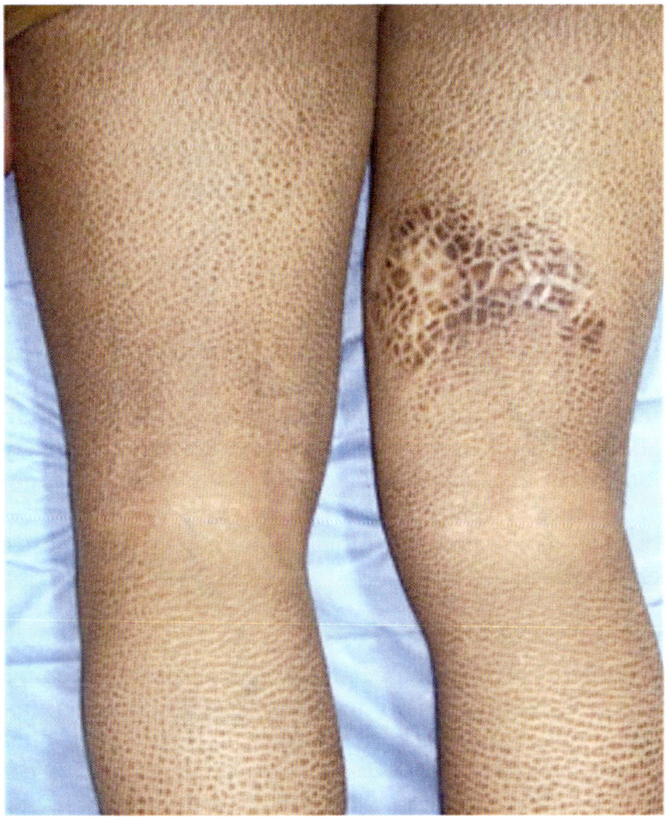

Fig. 27.14: X-linked ichthyosis: Large dark brown adherent scales encroaching flexures

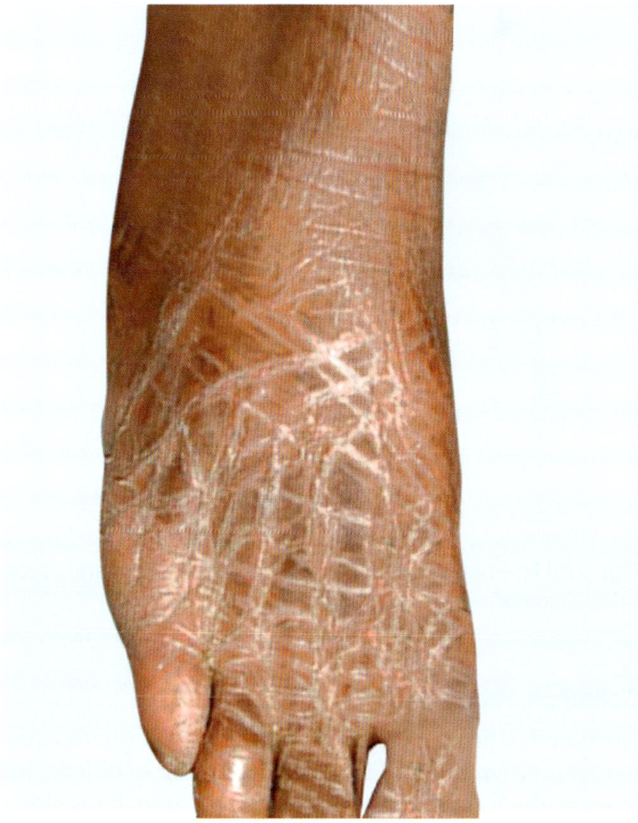

Fig. 27.15: Lamellar ichthyosis: Large plate-like scales

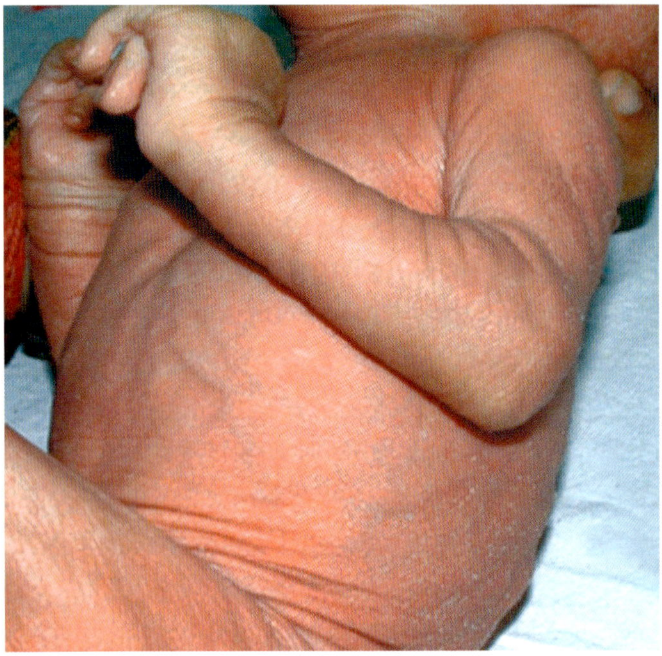

Fig. 27.16: Congenital ichthyosiform erythroderma: Diffuse erythema with fine scales

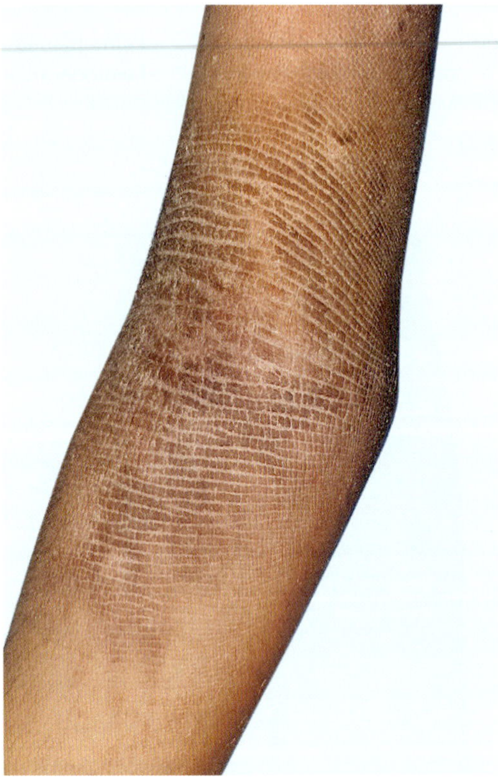

Fig. 27.17: Epidermolytic ichthyosis: Brownish, warty, broad linear plaques

### Collodion Baby

Neonate is born completely covered with shiny (lacquer-like), taut membrane (Fig. 27.18), resulting in obliteration of normal skin markings. Ectropion, eclabium, flattening of nose and ears, and sausage-shaped swelling of the digits are common. Over 1–2 weeks, the collodion membrane desiccates and is gradually shed, revealing underlying congenital ichthyosiform erythroderma or lamellar ichthyosis or sometimes normal skin.

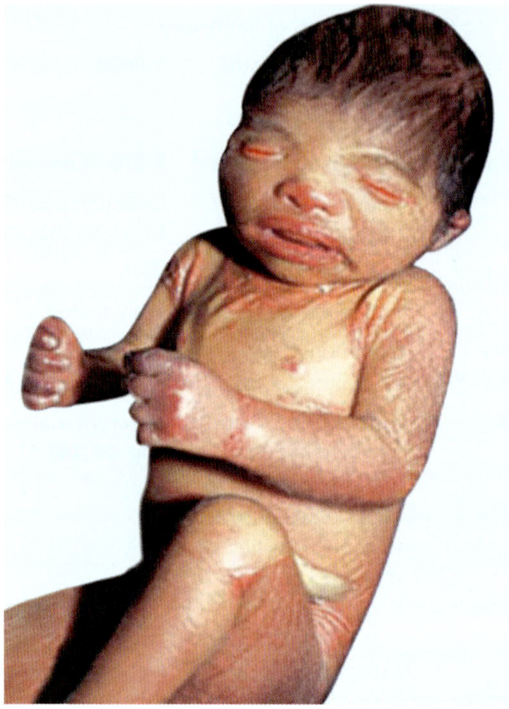

Fig. 27.18: Collodion baby: Baby is ensheathed in a shiny lacquer-like membrane

Collodion babies are at risk of thermoinstability, hypernatremic dehydration, skin infections, pneumonia and sepsis.

#### *Treatment*

Since collodion babies are frequently at risk of several complications, they are best managed in a controlled, humidified environment, carefully monitoring for fluid and electrolyte imbalance. Skin care (frequent application of emollients) and eye care are paramount. Oral acitretin is often needed.

### Palmoplantar Keratoderma (PPKD)

PPKD may be inherited or acquired. Hereditary keratodermas are a heterogeneous group of disorders with AD or AR inheritance. While diffuse and focal types of PPKD inherited in an ausomal dominant manner, the mutilating and transgradiens variants have an AR inheritance. They may occur in isolation or be part of a syndrome. Acquired PPKD may develop due to friction (corns and callosities) or be a manifestation of other inflammatory dermatoses, e.g. psoriasis.

#### *Clinical Features*

Inherited PPKD is characterized by thickening of palms and soles which usually manifest at birth or in the first few months of life. The thickening may vary from mild to moderate (Fig. 27.19) or may be severe, in which case it may be mutilating (Fig. 27.20). The keratoderma may be restricted to palms and soles or spill on to dorsae of hands and feet (keratoderma transgradiens; Fig. 27.21).

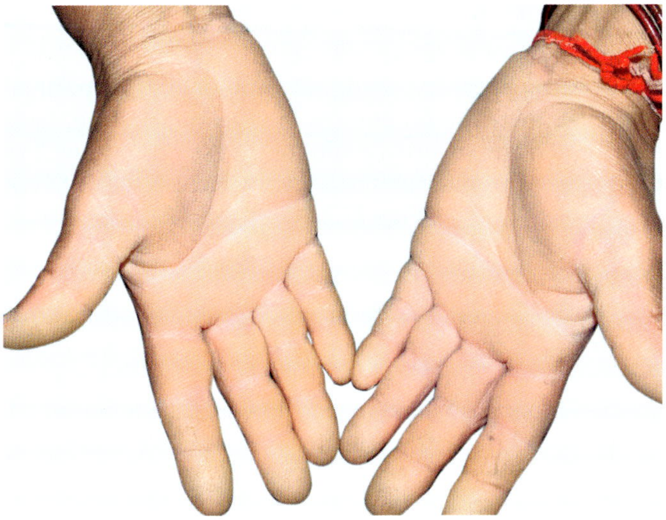

Fig. 27.19: Palmoplantar keratoderma: Autosomal dominant variant, with thickening of palms

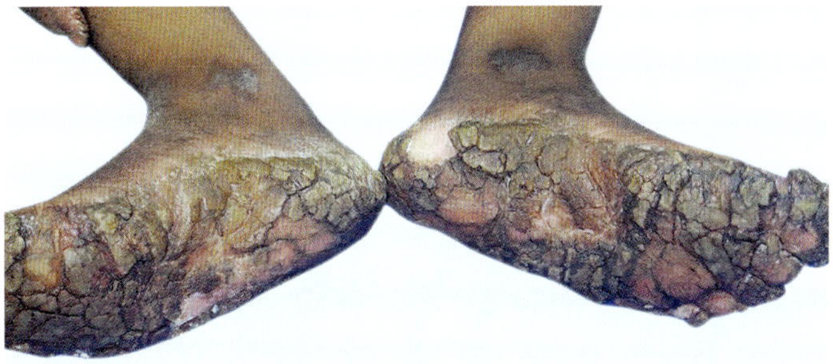

Fig. 27.20: Palmoplantar keratoderma: Autosomal recessive, massive thickening and mutilation

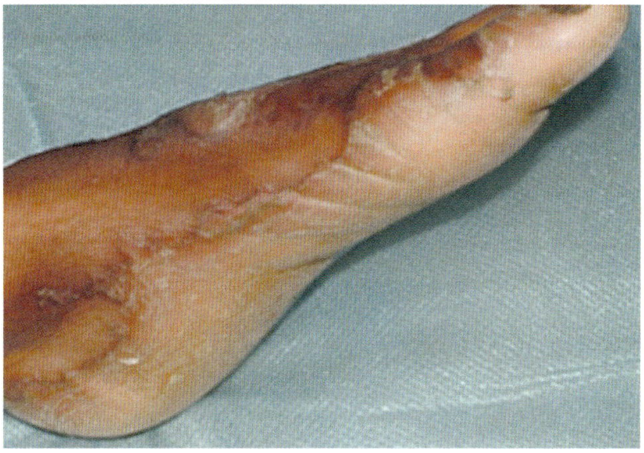

Fig. 27.21: Palmoplantar keratoderma: Transgradiens variant, with keratoderma spilling onto dorsae of feet

*Treatment*

Therapy for PPKD includes use of emollients, keratolytics (salicylic acid 6%, urea 30–40%), topical retinoids and vitamin D (calcipotriol), all used after soaking in water. In mutilating variants, treatment with oral acitretin may be warranted.

### Epidermolysis Bullosa

Epidermolysis bullosa are a heterogeneous group of disorders defined by a tendency to develop blisters even on trivial trauma. Several variants of EB are recognized based on inheritance, gene defects and clinical features (Table 27.3). EB simplex and dominant dystrophic EB have an AD inheritance, while junctional EB, recessive dystrophic EB, and Kindler syndrome have an AR inheritance.

Table 27.3: Clinical features of epidermolysis bullosa (EB)

| | *EB simplex* | *Junctional EB* | *Dominant dystrophic EB* | *Recessive dystrophic EB* | *Kindler syndrome* |
|---|---|---|---|---|---|
| Age of onset | Early childhood | At birth | At birth, infancy | At birth | At birth or early infancy |
| Skin lesions | Nonhemorrhagic bullae which heal without scarring (Fig. 27.22) | Large flaccid bullae which heal slowly (Fig. 27.23) | Hemorrhagic blisters which heal with some scarring and milia (Fig. 27.24) | Hemorrhagic blisters which heal with scarring (Fig. 27.25) | Aceral blisters, photosensitivity, poikiloderma (Fig. 27.26) |
| Sites | Hands and feet | Trunk and sites of trauma (knees, elbows, fingers). Periorificial granulation tissue | Sites of trauma | Generalized | Dorsum of hands and feet |
| Mucosal lesions | None | Involved | Minimal | Severe | Periodonitis, gingivitis |
| Nail involvement | Absent | Present | Present | Present | Long thick cuticle |
| Complications | Heal without scarring | One variant lethal | Scarring and milia formation | Severe scarring; development of contractures, fusion of digits and esophageal strictures | Skin atrophy, pseudosyndactyly, stricture involving esophageal, urogenital and ocular mucosa |
| Level of split | Intraepidermal | Lamina lucida | Sublamina densa | Sublamina densa | Multiple |
| Protein defect | Keratin 5 and 14 | Laminin, collagen XVII | Collagen VII | Collagen VII | Kindlin-1 |

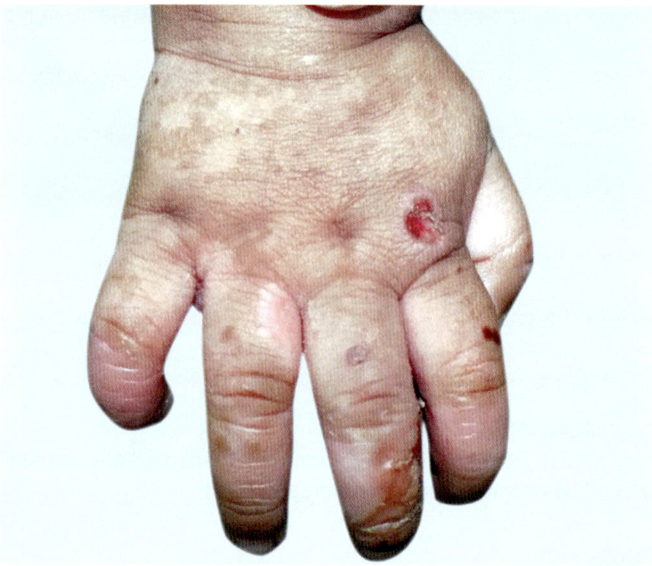

Fig. 27.22: Epidermolysis bullosa simplex: Bullae heal with minimal scarring

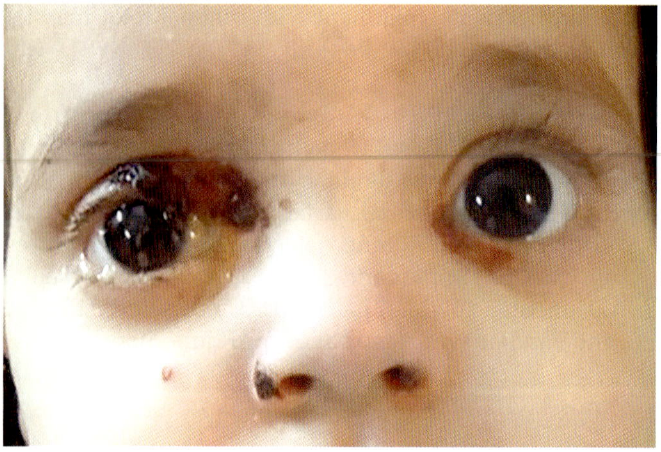

Fig. 27.23: Junctional epidermolysis bullosa: Periorificial granulation tissue

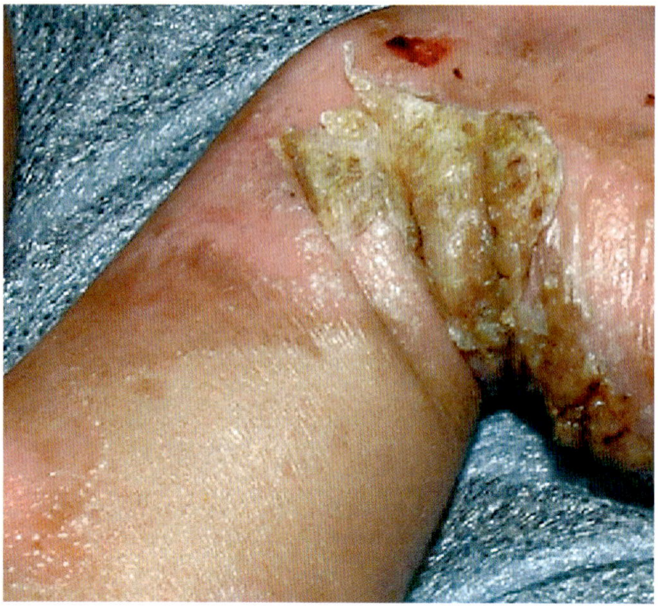

Fig. 27.24: Dominant dystrophic epidermolysis bullosa: Localized involvement of trauma prone site, bullae heal with milia formation

*Clinical Features*

The hallmark of the disease is tendency to develop blisters even on trivial injury, predominantly at sites of trauma. However, there are differences in type of blistering, their distribution and severity, evolution and sequelae as well as the degree of mucosal and nail involvement in the different variants (Table 27.3, Figs 27.22 to 27.26).

*Treatment*

General measures include avoiding friction and trauma, wearing soft, well-ventilated shoes and gentle handling. Prompt and appropriate use of antibiotics for blisters and infected lesions is necessary. Surgery may be required for release of fused digits, correction of limb contractures and esophageal strictures.

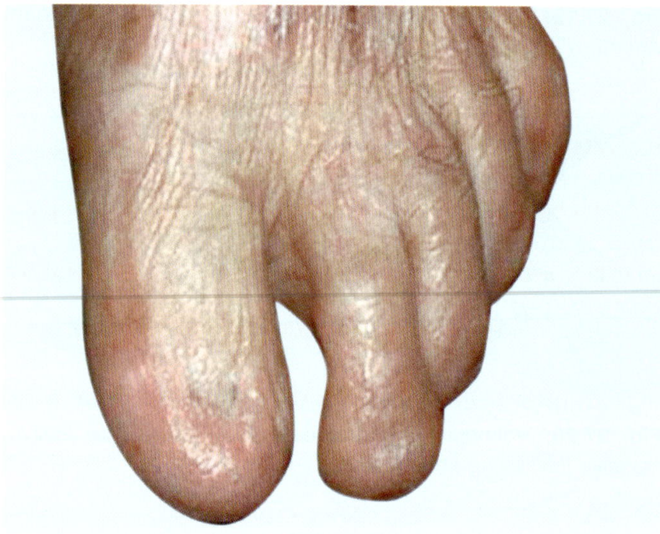

Fig. 27.25: Recessive dystrophic epidermolysis bullosa: Generalized involvement with bullae which heal with scarring. Note loss of nails

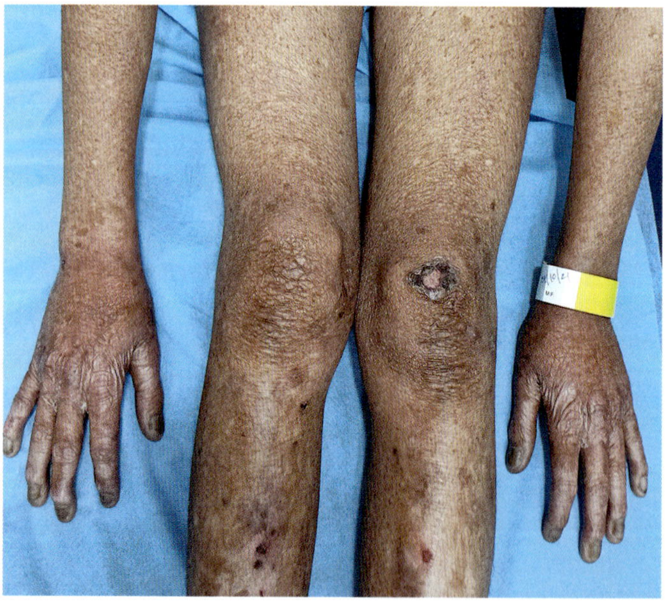

Fig. 27.26: Kindler syndrome: Predominant acral involvement, nail dystrophy and poikiloderma

Gene therapy, intradermal collagen 7 injections and stem cell transplantation are being evaluated.

## Ectodermal Dysplasias

Ectodermal dysplasias comprise a large, heterogeneous group of inherited disorders that are characterized by defects in development of two or more tissues derived from embryonic ectoderm. The disorders are classified based on either inheritance (AD, AR and XLR) or by structures involved (hair, teeth, nails, sweat glands).

### Anhidrotic Ectodermal Hypoplasia

The condition is inherited in an XLR manner. Child presents with intolerance to heat and episodes of high fever due to reduced sweating (hypohidrosis) because of presence of only a few sweat glands. The facies is distinctive with prominent forehead, thick lips and a flat nose. Additional features include thin, wrinkled, dark-colored periorbital skin. The hairs are sparse, light-colored, brittle and slow growing. The teeth may be absent (Fig. 27.27) or are peg-shaped.

***Treatment:*** There is no specific treatment, but quality of life can be improved by maintenance of cool ambient temperature and managing fever by tepid sponging. Dental restoration and use of artificial tears to prevent drying of eyes is often necessary.

### Hidrotic Ectodermal Dysplasia

This autosomal dominant disorder presents with patchy alopecia with sparse wiry hair, progressive palmar and plantar hyperkeratosis and dystrophic nails. Sweating and teeth are normal.

## Neurocutaneous Syndromes

### Neurofibromatoses

Neurofibromatoses encompass eight inherited disorders, of which neurofibromatosis type 1 (NF1) is most common. NF1 is an autosomal dominant disorder with 100% penetrance. The defect is mutation/deletion of NF1.

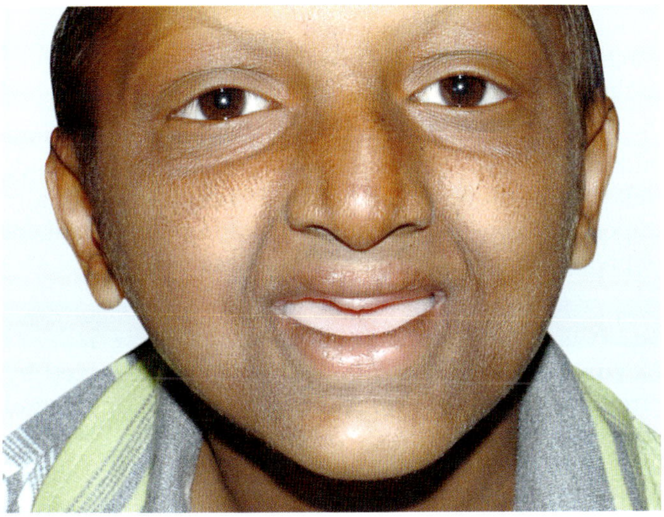

**Fig. 27.27:** Anhidrotic ectodermal hypoplasia: Typical facies, sparse hair and absence of teeth

***Clinical features:*** At least two of the following criteria should be met to reach a diagnosis of NF1:

1. Six or more café au lait macules (Fig. 27.28) which are >5 mm in prepubertal age group or >15 mm in post-pubertal age group
2. Two or more neurofibromas (Fig. 27.28) of any type, or one or more plexiform neurofibromas
3. Freckling in axillae or groin
4. Optic glioma
5. Two or more Lisch nodules on slit lamp examination
6. Dysplasia of the sphenoid; dysplasia or thinning of long bone cortex
7. First degree relative with NF1

Neurofibromas which are symptomatic or have turned malignant need to be excised.

### Tuberous Sclerosis Complex (TSC)

TSC is an AD inherited disorder with variable expressivity, even within the same family.

TSC may have protean manifestations involving several organ systems (Table 27.4, Fig. 27.29).

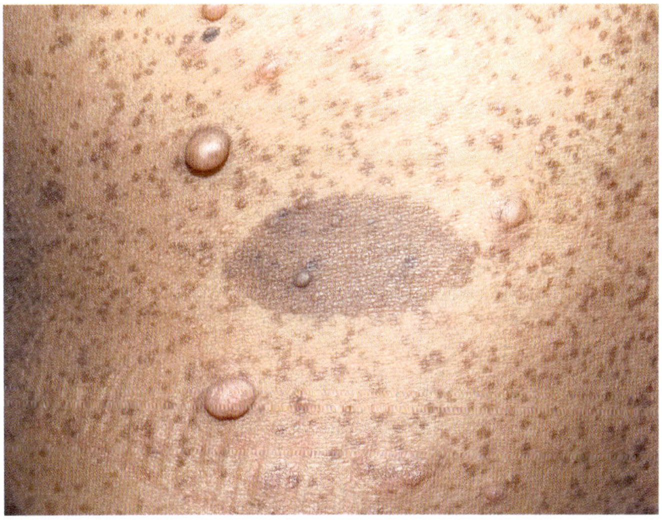

**Fig. 27.28:** Neurofibromatosis type 1: Presence of skin-colored soft papulonodular lesions associated with café au lait macules and lentigines

**Table 27.4:** Criteria for diagnosis of tuberous sclerosis complex

| *Major features* | *Minor features* |
|---|---|
| Facial angiofibromas (Fig. 27.29a) | Confetti skin lesions |
| Forehead plaque | Gingival fibromas |
| Periungual fibromas | Multiple dental pits |
| Ash leaf macules (Fig. 27.29b) | Rectal polyps |
| Shagreen patch | Bone cysts |
| Multiple retinal hamartomas | Multiple renal cysts |
| Cerebral tumors | Retinal achromic patch |
| Renal angiomyolipoma | |
| Cardiac rhabdomyoma | |

Definite TSC: Presence of either 2 major OR 1 major + 2 minor criteria
Probable TSC: Presence of 1 major + 1 minor criteria
Possible TSC: Presence of 1 major OR 2 minor criteria

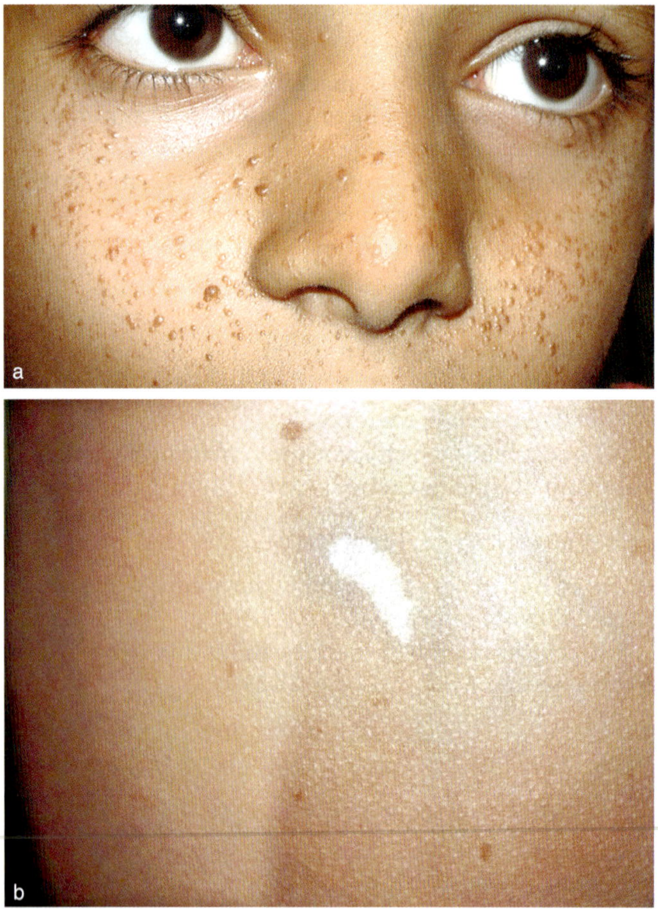

Fig. 27.29: Tuberous sclerosis: (a) Angiofibromas: Multiple small discrete erythematous papular lesions with irregular surface over bilateral cheeks and dorsum of nose; (b) Ash leaf macule: Well defined, oval, hypopigmented macule over the trunk

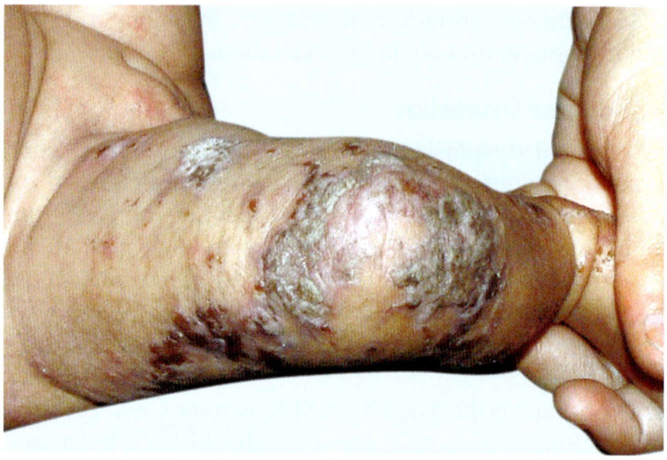

Fig. 27.30: Incontinentia pigmenti, vesicular phase: Multiple crusted vesicular lesions over the right lower limb of a female child

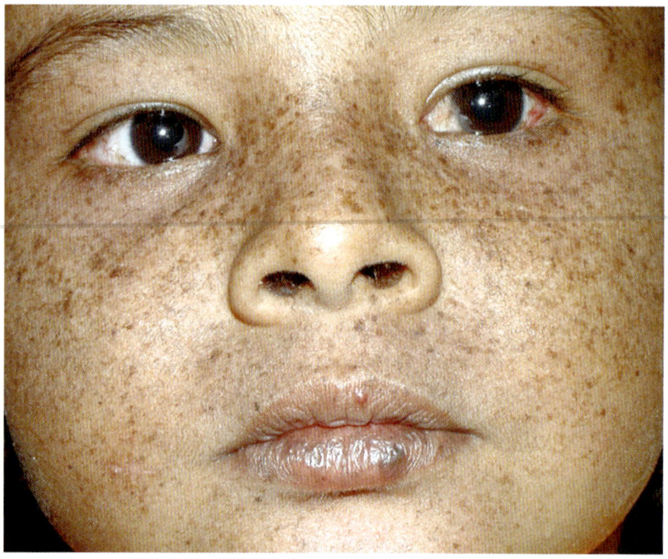

Fig. 27.31: Xeroderma pigmentosa: Multiple, brown to black freckle-like lesions over the face and lips, associated with conjunctival congestion

*Treatment:* Children with seizures need symptomatic treatment with anticonvulsants. Angiofibromas can be radiofrequency ablated. Rapamycin, administered by topical route for facial lesions and orally for cerebral lesions, has been used successfully.

### Incontinentia Pigmenti

This is an X-linked dominant multisystem disorder, predominantly affecting females. Characteristic cutaneous manifestations occur in four stages: The vesicular (Fig. 27.30), verrucous, hyperpigmented and hypopigmented stages. There can be associated dental, ocular, neurological and developmental anomalies. Management includes genetic counseling of the parents and symptomatic care.

### Xeroderma Pigmentosum

This is an AR condition, due to defective nucleotide excision repair of photodamaged DNA, and characterized by extreme photosensitivity (manifesting as acute sun burn) with onset in infancy. Over next 2–3 years, the child develops hyperpigmented (freckle-like) and hypopigmented lesions predominantly on the photoexposed skin on a background of xerosis (Fig. 27.31). Over time, most children develop actinic keratoses (a premalignant condition), basal cell carcinoma, squamous cell carcinoma and melanomas. Most children also have photophobia, conjunctivitis, keratitis, corneal opacities and develop malignancies of eyelids and conjunctiva. Neurological involvement is seen in one-third of the patients.

*Treatment:* Rigorous sun protection (lifestyle modifications and sunscreens) and use of topical and systemic retinoids delay and reduce development of neoplasias. Equally important is oncosurveillance and appropriate treatment of premalignant and malignant skin lesions.

## NEVI

Nevus is a developmental disorder characterized by circumscribed hyperplasia of epidermal or dermal structures.

### Melanocytic Nevi (MN)

MN are composed of nests of melanocytic nevus cells and may be congenital or acquired. Acquired MN may be

**Table 27.5:** Clinical features of melanocytic nevi in children

| | *Congenital nevus* | *Junctional nevus* | *Compound nevus* |
|---|---|---|---|
| Age of onset | Birth | Early childhood | Childhood |
| Morphology | Macules, papulonodules or plaques at birth; dark brown or black lesions | Macules with smooth margin; brown to dark brown-black with color variation | Dome-shaped, smooth papules; brown-black with color variation |
| Hair | Usually have coarse hair which may appear whorled (Fig. 27.32) | No hair | May have hair |
| Site | Any part of the body | Palms, soles or genitals | Face |
| Complications | Malignant transformation in giant lesions; meningeal involvement; spina bifida, if on midline on back | Malignant transformation rare | Inflammation; malignant transformation rare |

junctional (with nevus cells at dermoepidermal junction), compound (with nevus cells at dermoepidermal junction and in dermis) and dermal (with nevus cells only in dermis). Of these, first two are seen in children while the dermal variant is seen only in adults.

The clinical presentation depends on the type of MN (Table 27.5, Fig. 27.32).

### *Treatment*

Congenital MN especially those larger than 20 cm, need to be observed for malignant transformation. Acquired MN can be left alone.

## Dermal Melanocytosis

### *Mongolian Spot*

Mongolian spot is a dermal melanocytosis, due to entrapment of melanocytes in dermis during their migration from the neural crest into the epidermis. These spots present at birth (or soon thereafter) as gray blue macules, in the lumbosacral region and disappear spontaneously by early childhood.

### *Nevus of Ota*

Presents at birth or infancy (sometimes in adolescence) and consists of mottled slate-gray and brown hyperpigmented macules in the distribution of the maxillary division of

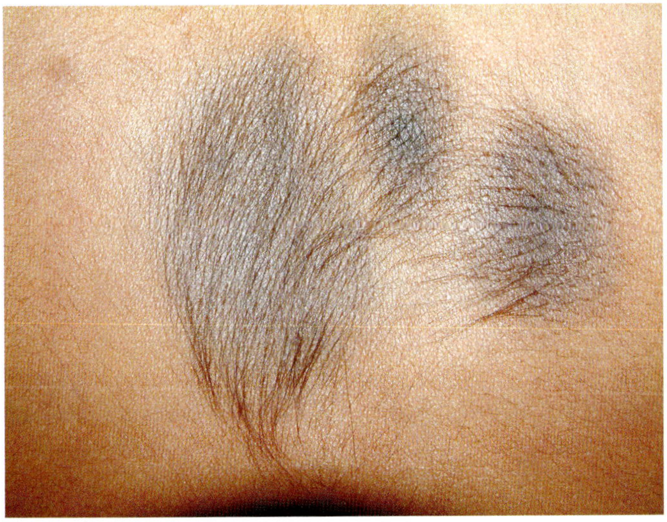

**Fig. 27.32:** Congenital melanocytic nevus: Dark brown black plaques surmounted with coarse black hair which appear whorled

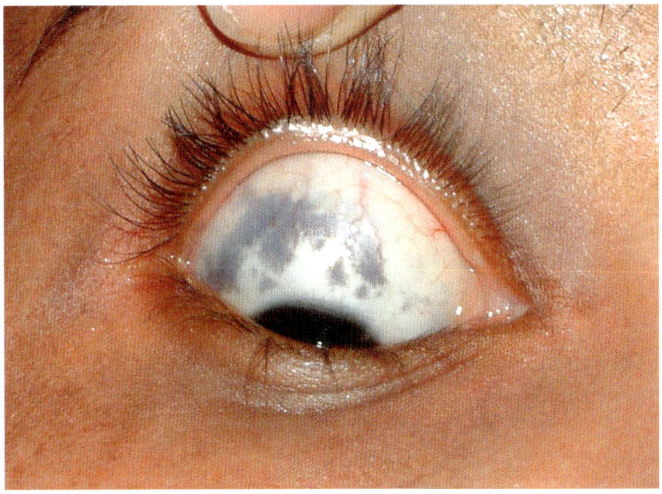

**Fig. 27.33:** Nevus of Ota: Slate-gray, mottled hyperpigmentation of skin of periorbital skin with slate-gray pigmentation of sclera

trigeminal nerve (Fig. 27.33). Lesion persists for life and is frequently associated with pigmentation of sclera (slate-gray) and conjunctiva (brown). Pigmentation of nevus of Ota frequently impacts child's psychosocial development and can be reduced by treating with Nd:YAG laser.

## Epidermal Nevi

These nevi usually present at birth, as multiple brown papules arranged linearly (Fig. 27.34). Several variants are described, including verrucous epidermal nevus,

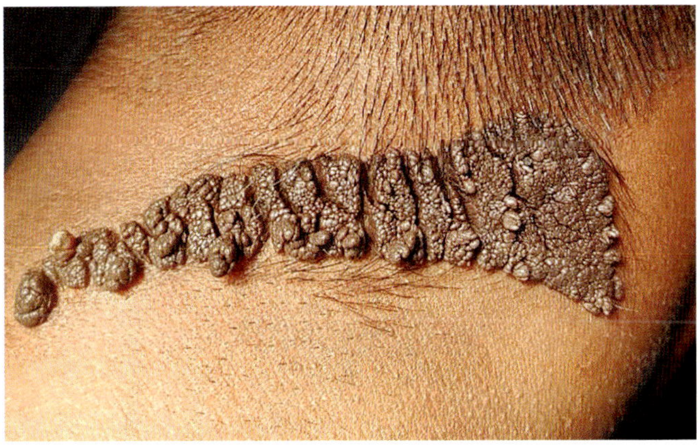

**Fig. 27.34:** Verrucous epidermal nevus: Multiple, brown papular lesions, arranged linearly

inflammatory linear verrucous epidermal nevus, naevus comedonicus and nevus sebaceous.

Topical retinoic acid and dermabrasion are helpful.

### Vascular 'Birthmarks'

Vascular 'birthmarks' are classified based on the pathogenesis, evolution, clinical manifestations and on the presence of associations into vascular tumors and vascular malformations (Table 27.6).

#### Clinical Features

The lesions could have one vascular component (simple) or have more than one component (combined malformations). Diagnosis is based on morphology and progression of lesion(s) (Table 27.7, Figs 27.35–27.37).

Combined malformations are characterized by presence of several vascular components (capillaries, veins and lymphatics) along with other nevi and are often associated with underlying skeletal abnormalities:

- **Klippel-Trénaunay syndrome** is characterized by presence of capillary malformations on the limbs in association with soft tissue swellings, venous varicosities with or without bony hypertrophy.
- **Proteus syndrome** is characterized by asymmetrical overgrowth (sometimes massive) of a part of the body (Fig. 27.38), associated with presence of epidermal nevi,



**Table 27.6:** Study of vascular anomalies according to International Society for the Study of Vascular Anomalies (ISSVA), 2018

| *Vascular tumors* | *Vascular malformations* |
|---|---|
| **Benign**<br>• Congenital hemangioma<br>• Pyogenic granuloma | **Simple**<br>• Capillary<br>• Lymphatics<br>• Venous<br>• Arteriovenous |
| **Locally aggressive**<br>• Kaposiform hemangioendothelioma<br>• Kaposi sarcoma | **Combined**<br>Associated with other anomalies of major vessels |
| **Malignant**<br>Angiosarcoma | |

**Table 27.7:** Clinical features of vascular 'birthmarks'

| | *Infantile hemangioma* | *Salmon patch* | *Port-wine stain* | *Lymphangioma* |
|---|---|---|---|---|
| Onset | After birth | At birth | At birth | At birth |
| Morphology | Soft, bright nodule with pale stippling (Fig. 27.35) | Telangiectatic macules | Light pink-deep red macules (Fig. 27.36); bosselated with age | Cluster of thin-walled vesicles (Fig. 27.37) |
| Site | Face forehead, eyelids and neck | Nape of neck | Face | Trunk |
| Complications | Interfere with function; bleeding or ulceration | None | Sturge-Weber syndrome associated with hamartomas; seizures, eye deficits | |
| Course | Grows for a few months; later regresses | Involutes by one year | Persists throughout life | Persists |

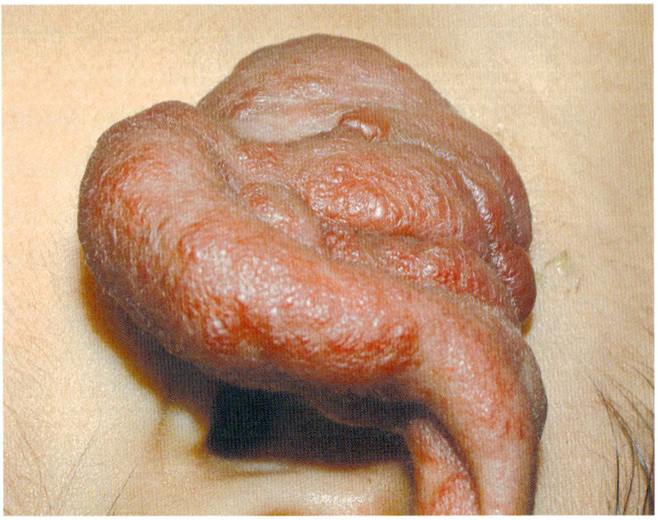

**Fig. 27.35:** Infantile hemangioma: Soft bright red nodule with pale stippling

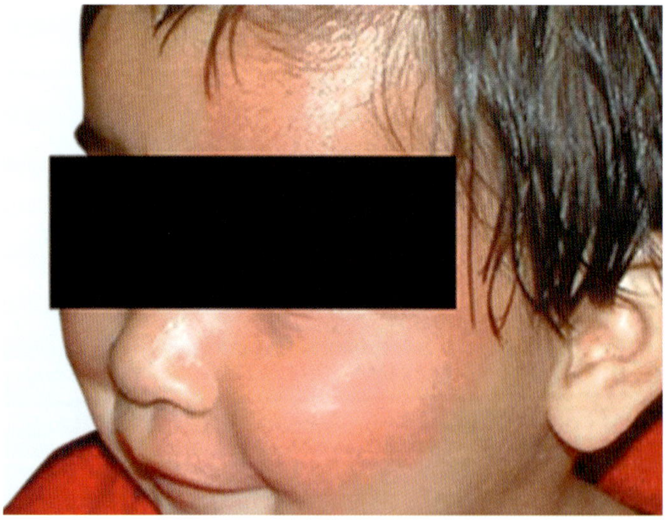

**Fig. 27.36:** Port-wine stain: Light pink to deep red macule often developing bosselation as child grows

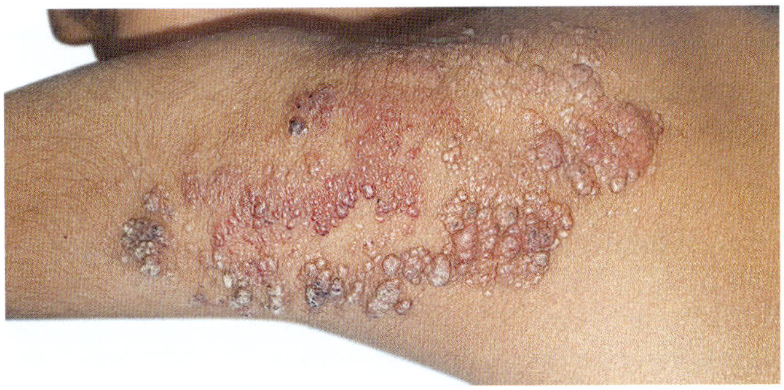

Fig. 27.37: Lymphangioma: Cluster of thin-walled vesicles, many of them contain hemorrhagic fluid

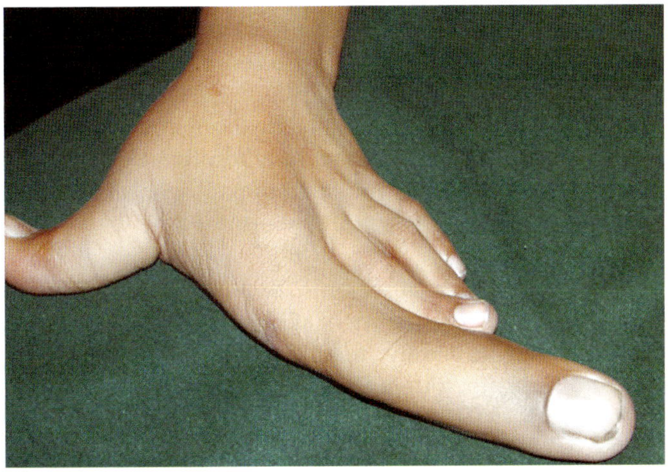

Fig. 27.38: Proteus syndrome: Asymmetrical, disproportionate soft tissue overgrowth of left index finger associated with misalignment

hemangiomas, vascular malformations and lipoma-like hamartomas. Extracutaneous findings include lung and renal cysts, skeletal and dental abnormalities, seizures and ocular complications.

#### Treatment

*Salmon patch:* No treatment required.

*Infantile hemangioma:* Small lesions resolve spontaneously. Large symptomatic lesions need treatment with systemic corticosteroids in the proliferative phase. Propranolol used under supervision shows dramatic result. Pulsed–tunable dye laser is useful for cosmetic results.

*Port-wine stain:* Cosmetic camouflage; laser ablation with pulsed–tunable dye laser.

*Lymphangioma:* Surgery, carbon dioxide laser, radio-frequency ablation.

## DERMATITIS

Dermatitis manifests in acute phase as papulovesicular lesions, and in chronic phase as thickened, dry sometimes lichenified skin.

*Competencies:* **PE31.3; PE31.4**

### Atopic Dermatitis

Atopic dermatitis is an acute, subacute or chronic relapsing, endogenous eczema, characterized by dry skin and recurrent, pruritic, symmetric dermatitic lesions.

The condition is due to a complex interaction between genetic susceptibility and immunological changes with heightened IgE response.

#### Clinical Features

Lesions develop in infancy, any time after 3 months of age. In children, two distinct patterns are recognized.

*Infantile pattern:* Manifests as itchy, erythematous papulovesicles, on the face (Fig. 27.39), but may become generalized. The lesions clear by 18 months of age in 40% and evolve into childhood pattern in the rest.

*Childhood pattern:* Childhood pattern is characterized by dry, lichenified and crusted plaques, seen mainly on antecubital (Fig. 27.40) and popliteal fossa, the neck and face. Most (70%) clear by 10 years of age.

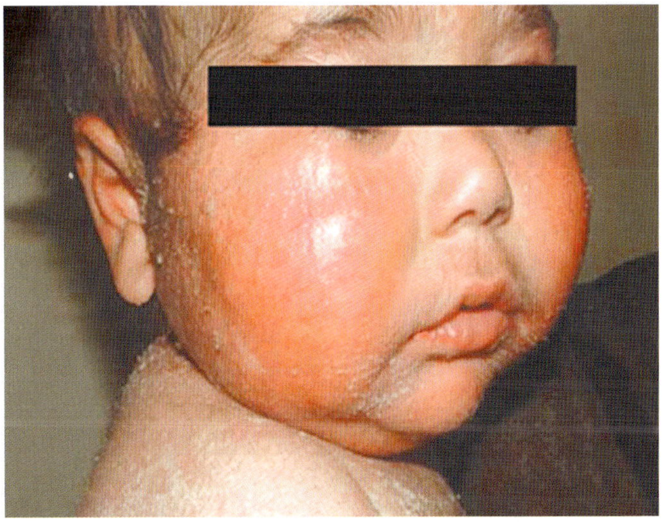

Fig. 27.39: Infantile pattern of atopic dermatitis. Crusted erythematous plaques on the face

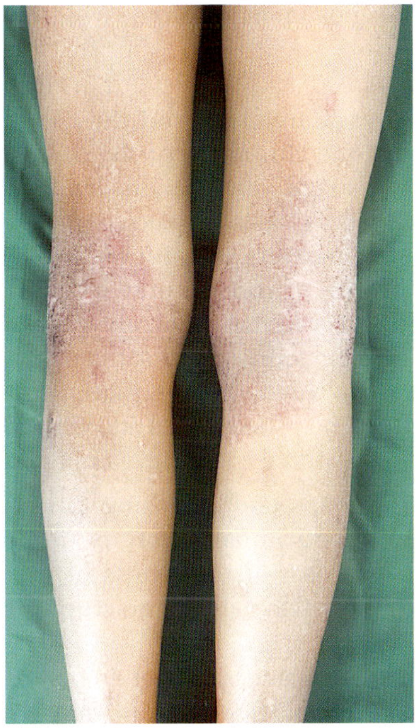

Fig. 27.40: Childhood pattern of atopic dermatitis. Dry excoriated plaques in the flexures

**Table 27.8:** Hanifin and Rajka criteria for atopic dermatitis

| |
|---|
| **Major features** (must have ≥3) |
| Pruritus |
| Typical morphology and distribution (facial and extensor involvement in infants and children; flexural lichenification in adults) |
| Dermatitis, chronic or chronically relapsing |
| Personal or family history of atopy (asthma, allergic rhinitis, atopic dermatitis) |
| **Minor features** (must have ≥3) |
| Cataracts (anterior subcapsular) |
| Cheilitis |
| Conjunctivitis, recurrent |
| Facial pallor or erythema |
| Food intolerance |
| Hand dermatitis: Nonallergic, irritant |
| Ichthyosis |
| Elevated levels of IgE |
| Immediate (type I) skin test reactivity |
| Infections |
| Itching, when sweating |
| Keratoconus |
| Keratosis pilaris |
| Nipple dermatitis |
| Orbital darkening |
| Palmar hyperlinearity |
| Perifollicular accentuation |
| Pityriasis alba |
| White dermographism |
| Wool intolerance |
| Xerosis |

The diagnosis is based on Hanifin and Rajka criteria (Table 27.8). Secondary bacterial and fungal infections are frequent. Viral infections like herpes simplex and molluscum contagiosum may become widespread.

#### Treatment

***General measures:*** Caretakers and the child should be counseled about the chronicity of the disease and that the child should avoid contact with irritants (woolens and chemicals). Measures to reduce exposure to house dust mite (using barriers on pillows and mattresses, regular vacuuming of rooms) may help. There is no contraindications to vaccination except in children specifically allergic to eggs, in whom influenza and yellow fever vaccines are avoided. Dietary restrictions are usually not warranted and breastfeeding is encouraged as it may decrease the chance of the infant developing the disease.

***Skin care:*** Mild soaps and cleansing lotions are used for bathing followed immediately by application of moisturizers. The cost-effectiveness of moisturizers, which claim to replenish natural moisturizing factors is debatable.

Acute lesions are treated with wet dressing and topical corticosteroids. Antibiotics and antifungals (topical/systemic) are used when indicated. Oral antihistaminics are often prescribed.

Chronic lichenified lesions are managed by hydration followed by application of emollients (like petrolatum) and a short course of topical corticosteroids. It is preferred to use the least potent corticosteroids which reduce symptoms; potent corticosteroids are avoided on face and genitalia. Topical immunomodulators (tacrolimus and pimecrolimus) are useful because of their steroid-sparing and antipruritic action. Oral antihistaminics are used to break the itch-scratch cycle. Narrowband UVB and systemic immunosuppressives (corticosteroids, cyclosporine and azathioprine) may be needed in extensive/resistant disease.

### Infantile Seborrheic Dermatitis

The onset is usually in the first 4 weeks of life, manifesting as erythema and yellow-orange scales and crusts (Fig. 27.41) on the scalp (cradle cap). Eczematous lesions may also develop in the major flexures and trunk. The illness is self-limiting and generally resolves by 12 weeks. Malassezia furfur is incriminated in pathogenesis.

#### Treatment

The crusts of cradle cap should be removed and this can be facilitated by pretreatment with an oil. Application of 2% ketoconazole shampoo, mild topical corticosteroid or pimecrolimus/tacrolimus hastens subsidence.

### Diaper Dermatitis

#### Etiology

Diaper dermatitis is irritant dermatitis in infants due to prolonged contact with feces and ammonia (produced by the action of urea-splitting organisms in urine), often complicated by superadded candidal infection. Area in contact with diapers (convexity of buttocks) shows moist, glazed erythematous lesions with sparing of depth of flexures (Fig. 27.42).

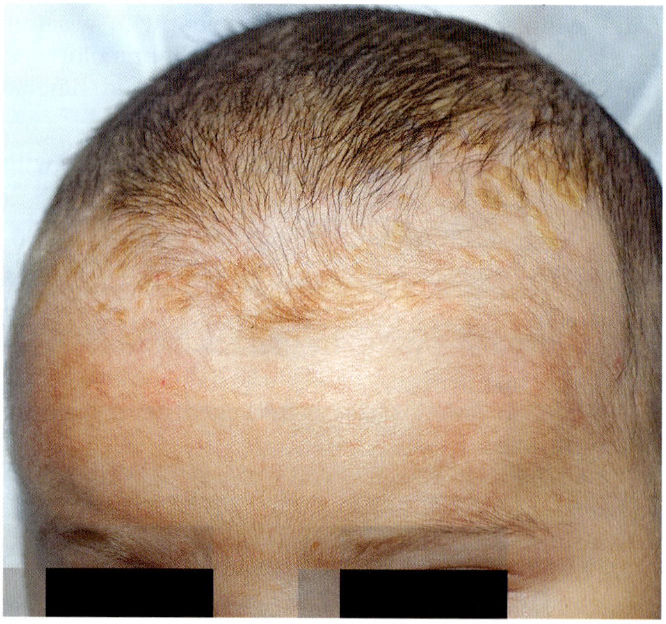

**Fig. 27.41:** Infantile seborrheic dermatitis: Erythema with yellow-orange scales on the scalp

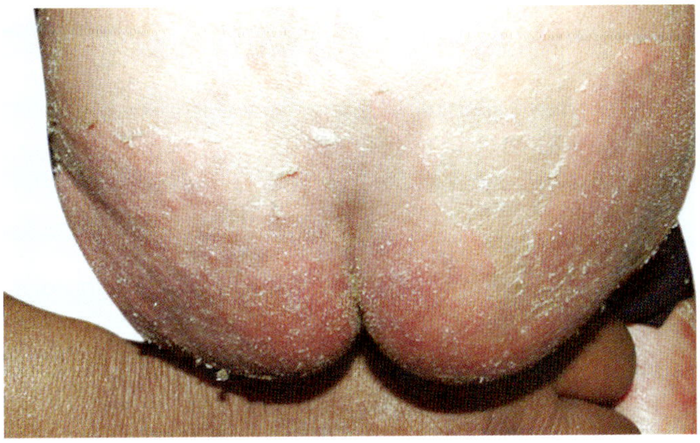

Fig. 27.42: Diaper dermatitis: Moist, glazed erythematous lesions. Depth of folds typically spared

### Treatment

Diaper dermatitis is prevented by keeping area clean and dry and avoiding the use of disposable semiabsorbent occlusive diapers. Washed cotton diapers should be rinsed in dilute lemon juice/vinegar. Emollients and mild topical corticosteroids with antifungal agents are useful in the acute phase.

## Pityriasis Alba

Asymptomatic, ill-defined, hypopigmented macules with fine scales are seen on face, in children 2–6 years of age. The lesions are self-limiting, clearing spontaneously in a few months to couple of years.

### Treatment

The family is reassured regarding the benign nature of the illness and that it is not vitiligo. Mild emollients may be used.

# DISORDERS OF SKIN APPENDAGES

## Acne Vulgaris

Acne vulgaris occurs in almost all peripubertal children. The age of onset is 12–14 years, being earlier in females and in about 70% of subjects, the lesions subside by third decade. It affects both sexes equally, but nodulocystic acne is more frequent in males.

### Etiology and Pathogenesis

Lesions develop due to inflammation of the pilosebaceous units and etiology is multifactorial.

*Increased sebum secretion:* Sebaceous glands in these patients show enhanced sensitivity to circulating androgens leading to increased sebum secretion.

*Microbial colonization:* Propionibacterium acne (a normal commensal) is most commonly implicated.

*Occlusion of pilosebaceous orifice:* Pilosebaceous orifice is occluded by keratin plugs leading to retention of sebum and consequent growth of microbes, setting up a vicious cycle.

*Release of inflammatory mediators:* Distended follicle ruptures, releasing inflammatory chemicals into dermis, stimulating intense inflammation.

### Clinical Features

Patients present with a polymorphic eruption of open and closed comedones, papules, pustules and nodules, on a background of oily skin (Fig. 27.43). The lesions usually heal with pitted scars. The lesions typically occur on face and upper trunk.

*Infantile acne* is caused by maternal hormones and presents at birth, lasting up to 3 years. It is common in males and lesions are similar to adolescent acne.

*Acne conglobata* is a severe form of acne characterized by abscesses, cysts and intercommunicating sinuses.

*Drug-induced acne:* Drugs causing acne include corticosteroids, androgens, antituberculous and anticonvulsant drugs. The eruption consists of monomorphic lesions of papules or pustules.

### Therapy

*General measures:* Though there is no restriction on use of cleansers, it is best to use pH-balanced syndets and avoid oil and oil-based skin care products. No dietary restrictions are usually needed. Specific therapy depends on the severity of the disease (Table 27.9).

**Table 27.9:** Management of acne

| *Severity* | *Subtype* | *Drug of choice* |
|---|---|---|
| Mild | Comedonal | Topical retinoids like retinoic acid and adapalene |
| | Papulopustular | Topical retinoids/benzoyl peroxide. Oral antibiotics, if necessary |
| Moderate | Papulopustular | Oral antibiotics + topical retinoids and/or benzoyl peroxide |
| | Nodular | Oral antibiotics + topical retinoids and/or benzoyl peroxide<br>In girls: Oral antiandrogens + topical retinoids |
| Severe | Nodular/acne conglobata | Oral retinoids*<br>In girls: Oral antiandrogens + topical retinoids |

*Oral retinoids may be used in females with moderate or severe lesions under supervision

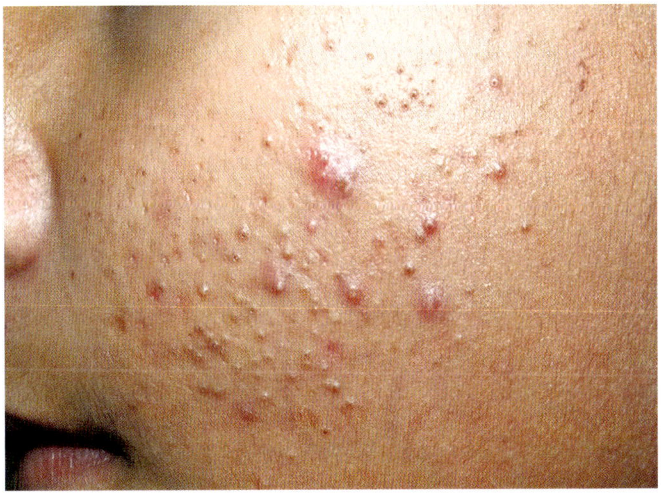

Fig. 27.43: Acne vulgaris: Polymorphic eruption with comedones, papules and pustules

## Alopecia Areata

### Etiology

This is a skin-specific autoimmune disease, due to inappropriate immune response to hair follicle associated antigens.

The condition affects children and young adults, who present with discoid areas of non-inflammatory, non-cicatricial alopecia with exclamation mark hair at periphery (Fig. 27.44a). The common sites of involvement are scalp, eyelashes and eye brows. In ophiasis, there is a band-like alopecia in the periphery of the scalp; in alopecia totalis, there is total alopecia in the scalp; while in alopecia universalis, there is total loss of terminal hair from scalp, eyebrows, eyelashes, beard and body (Fig. 27.44b). Nails may occasionally show fine pitting and thinning of the nail plate.

Spontaneous remission is common. Initially, the regrowing hairs are grey, but regain color over period of time. Poor prognostic features include onset in childhood, ophiasis, association with atopy and widespread alopecia.

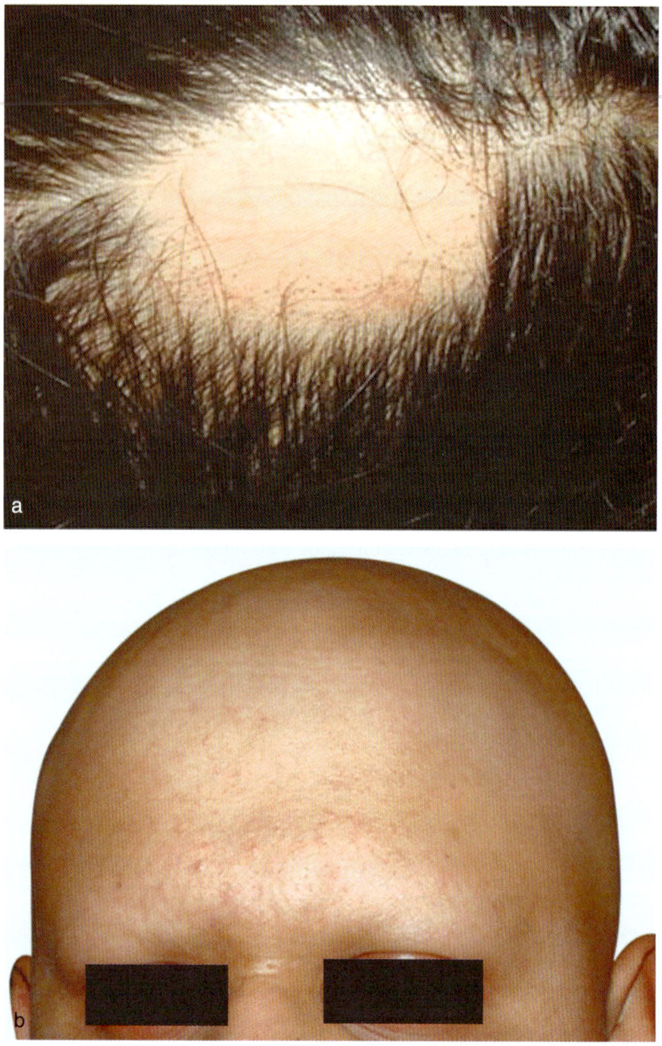


Fig. 27.44: (a) Alopecia areata: Noncicatricial, non-inflammatory, discoid lesions with exclamation mark hair at periphery; (b) Alopecia totalis: Total loss of terminal hair from scalp, face and body

**Table 27.10:** Treatment of alopecia areata

| *Clinical severity* | *Management* |
|---|---|
| Single or a few lesions of <6 months duration | Observe; spontaneous recovery common |
| Single or a few lesions of >6 months duration; rapid progression | • Topical corticosteroids<br>• Intralesional triamcinolone<br>• Topical minoxidil, 2–5%<br>• Topical psoralens and ultraviolet A (PUVA/PUVA sol) |
| Extensive lesions | Oral corticosteroids |
| Rapid progress | • Oral PUVA/PUVA sol<br>• Induction of allergic contact dermatitis with diphencyprone |

### Treatment

Treatment depends on extent and course of disease (Table 27.10).

## Miliaria

### Etiology

Miliaria is due to obstruction and rupture of eccrine sweat ducts resulting in spillage of sweat into adjacent epidermis/dermis. Depending on the level of rupture, miliaria is classified as follows.

*Miliaria crystallina:* Usually seen during high fever, miliaria crystallina is characterized by tiny, non-inflamed, superficial vesicles (Fig. 27.45).

*Miliaria rubra:* Usually seen in hot, humid climates, miliaria rubra is characterized by small erythematous papules, commonly surmounted by vesicles.

*Miliaria profunda:* Characterized by erythematous papules.

Therapy is symptomatic. Patients should avoid humidity and wear cotton clothes. Itching/burning can be reduced with calamine lotion and topical corticosteroids.

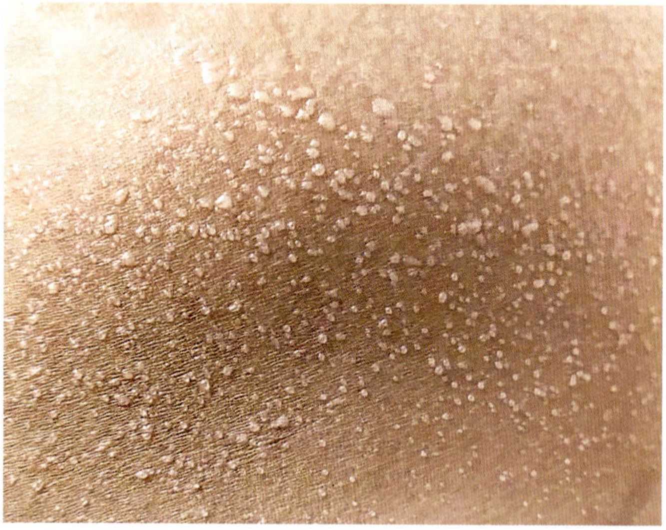

Fig. 27.45: Miliaria crystallina: Tiny, non-inflamed superficial vesicles

### Trachyonychia

Most common associations are alopecia areata, psoriasis, and lichen planus. It is characterized by the presence of gray rough surface due to multiple, longitudinal, linear striations affecting all nail plates (hence also called 20-nail dystrophy; Fig. 27.46). In children, it is a self-limiting condition.

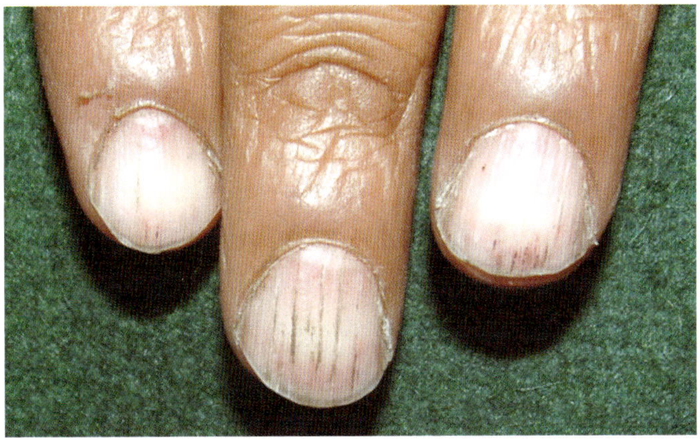

Fig. 27.46: Trachyonychia: Multiple, longitudinal, linear striations over the fingernails associated with roughness of nail surface

### Pachyonychia Congenita

It is a rare autosomal dominant disorder, characterized by gross thickening (tenting) of nail plates (Fig. 27.47a), oral lesions in form of leukoplakia (Fig. 27.47b) and keratoderma of palms and soles.

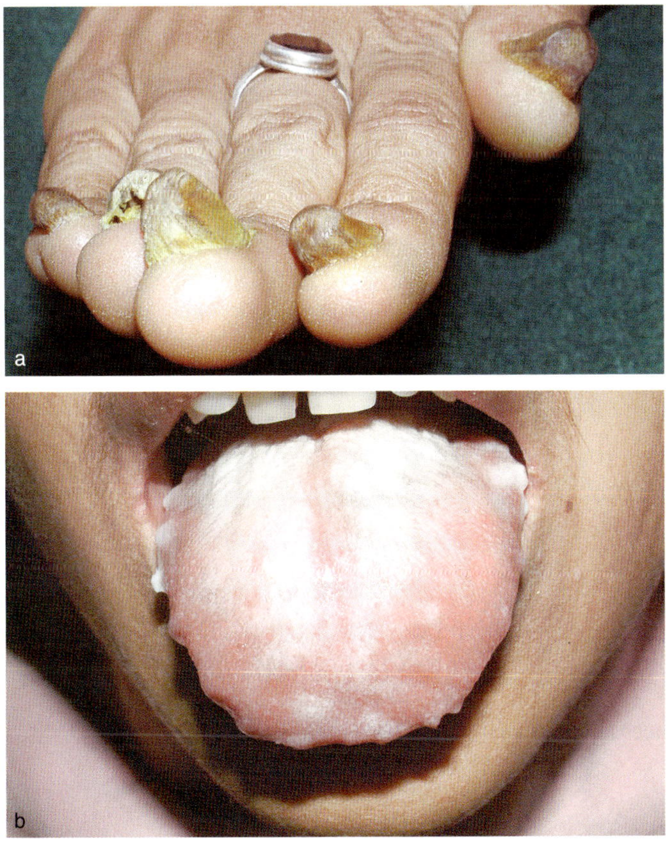

Fig. 27.47: (a) Pachyonychia congenita: Massive thickening of the nail plates resulting in tenting of nails; (b) Leukoplakia of the tongue

## PAPULOSQUAMOUS DISORDERS

### Psoriasis

#### *Etiology*

Psoriasis is a disease of T cells, with interplay of genetic factors (*PSORS1–8* genes, and several others) and environmental influences (physical trauma, infections and drugs).

Based on morphology of lesions, psoriasis is classified as chronic plaque psoriasis, guttate psoriasis and pustular psoriasis. Based on age of onset, chronic plaque psoriasis is classified into type I (onset in childhood or adolescence, positive family history, association with HLA-CW6, severe disease, prominent Koebner phenomenon and prolonged course, requiring aggressive therapy) and type II psoriasis (onset in adults).

#### *Clinical Features*

***Chronic plaque psoriasis (CPP):*** CPP is characterized by well-demarcated, indurated, erythematous, plaques surmounted by silvery scales (Fig. 27.48), which are accentuated on grating the lesion with a glass slide (Grattage test). Removal of the scales by further scraping reveals a glistening white membrane and on removing the membrane, punctate bleeding points become visible (Auspitz sign). Symmetrical involvement of knees, elbows and extensors, lower back, scalp and sites of trauma (Koebner or isomorphic phenomenon) is seen.

***Guttate psoriasis:*** It typically occurs in children and adolescents and is characterized by crops of small, erythematous scaly papules, predominantly on trunk. Guttate psoriasis is often triggered by streptococcal tonsillitis.

***Pustular psoriasis:*** Though pustular psoriasis is rare in children, several variants are described. Annular pustular psoriasis, the variant typically seen in children, is characterized by subacute onset of fiery red erythema surmounted by cluster of very superficial creamy white pustules, which form circinate or annular lesions

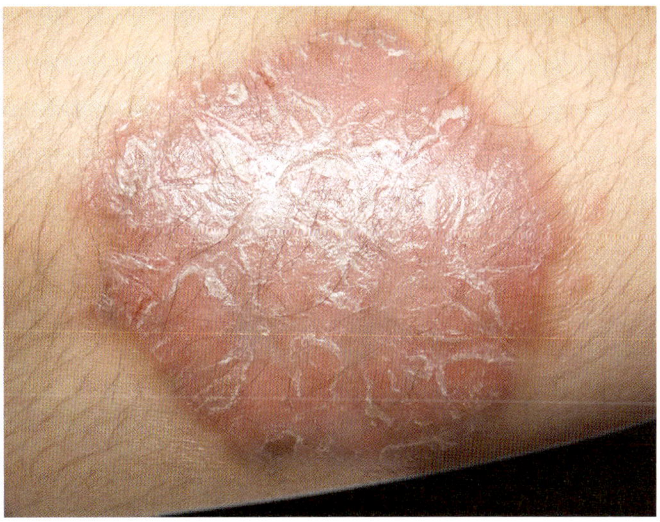

Fig. 27.48: Chronic plaque psoriasis: Well-demarcated, indurated, erythematous plaques surmounted by silvery scales

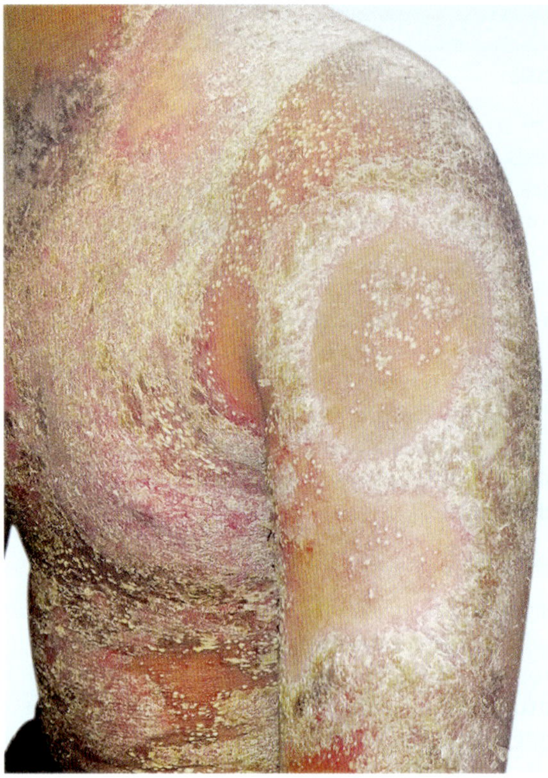

**Fig. 27.49:** Annular pustular psoriasis: Superficial pustules which coalesce to form annular lesions

(Fig. 27.49). Infantile and juvenile pustular psoriasis is seen in infants and has a benign course. It is often confused with seborrheic and napkin dermatitis.

***Nail changes:*** Include coarse irregular pits, thickening of nail plate, subungual hyperkeratosis, onycholysis, oil spots and discoloration of nail plates.

***Joints:*** Ten percent of patients have joint involvement.

#### *Treatment*

It is important to counsel the parents and the child about the chronic nature of the disease and the likelihood of relapses. Several options are available for treatment depending on the type and extent of disease (Table 27.11).

### Lichen Planus

The etiology is unknown. A lichenoid eruption may be triggered by drugs like chloroquine and as a manifestation of graft versus host disease.

Lichen planus is characterized by presence of pruritic, polygonal, purple (violaceous) plane (flat) topped papules (Fig. 27.50) with white streaks (Wickham striae) on the surface. They are seen on wrists, around ankles and may appear at sites of trauma (Koebner phenomenon). Mucosal involvement is seen in 25% patients in form of reticulate lacey pattern on buccal mucosa and gingiva or superficial erosions on tongue and buccal mucosa. Annular lesions may be seen on genitalia. Rarely scarring alopecia is present. Nail changes are infrequent in children.

#### *Treatment*

Therapy depends on the severity of the disease (Table 27.12).

### Lichen Nitidus

Lichen nitidus most commonly presents in children and young adults. Classically, tiny 1–2 mm, monomorphic,

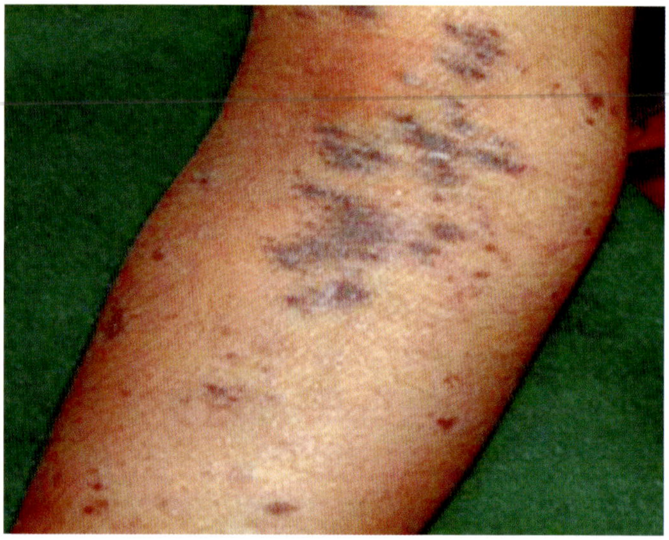

**Fig. 27.50:** Lichen planus: Polygonal, flat-topped, violaceous papules

**Table 27.11:** Treatment of psoriasis

| | *Treatment of choice* | *Alternative modalities* |
|---|---|---|
| Psoriasis vulgaris<br>*Localised (<10% BSA)*<br>*Extensive (>10% BSA)* | <br>Topical coal tar 1 + 1 salicylic acid<br>Narrowband UVB | <br>Topical corticosteroids + salicylic acid<br>Methotrexate<br>Acitretin<br>Cyclosporine A<br>PUVA/PUVA sol* |
| *Facial lesions*<br>Guttate psoriasis<br>Pustular psoriasis | <br>Topical tacrolimus, pimecrolimus<br>Antibiotics and emollients<br>Narrow band UVB<br>PUVA/PUVA sol*<br>Methotrexate<br>Cyclosporine | <br>Coal tar<br>Tacrolimus<br>Mild topical corticosteroids<br>Acitretin |

*PUVA: Psoralen + UVA should not be used in children <10 years of age

**Table 27.12:** Treatment of lichen planus in children

| *Type of disease* | *Therapy** |
|---|---|
| Localized | Topical corticosteroids |
| Extensive | • Narrowband UVB<br>• Oral corticosteroids<br>• Acitretin |
| Scalp lichen planus | Oral corticosteroids |
| Mucosal lichen planus | • Dapsone and topical corticosteroids<br>• Oral corticosteroids<br>• Acitretin |

*Oral antihistamines to be added, if lesions itchy

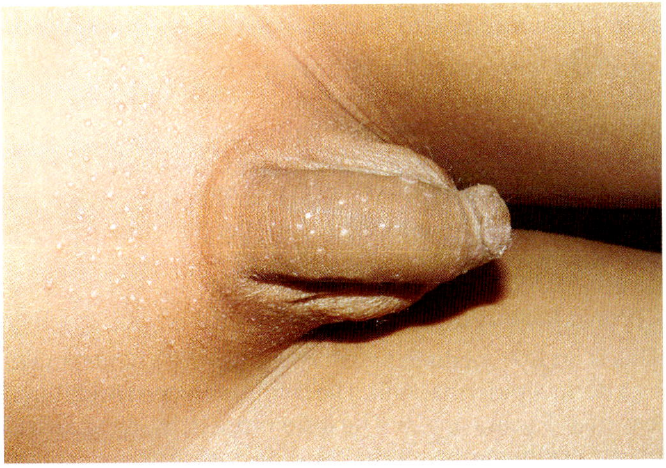

**Fig. 27.51:** Lichen nitidus: Multiple, small, monomorphic, hypopigmented papules over the lower abdomen and shaft of penis

hypopigmented/flesh-colored papules with a shiny surface are seen on the arms, chest and abdomen. The penile shaft is often involved (Fig. 27.51). Koebnerization with a linear arrangement of papules is a common finding. Lichen nitidus is a chronic, self-limiting disease, with an average course of about 1 year.

Mid-potent topical corticosteroid or topical tacrolimus can be used in children to relieve the pruritus. Phototherapy has been tried in refractory cases.

## Lichen Striatus

Lichen striatus is characterized by presence of hypopigmented/erythematous papular lesions configured linearly usually on the limbs. Active lesions subside spontaneously, leaving behind atrophic, post-inflammatory hypopigmentation (Fig. 27.52). Counseling about the self-limiting nature, and that it is not vitiligo is often all that is required.

## Pityriasis Rosea

### *Etiology*

The condition may be triggered by reactivation of human herpes viruses (HHV-7, HHV-6).

### *Clinical Features*

PR begins with a 'herald patch' in 80% cases. Lesion is characteristically oval, wrinkled with a collarette of

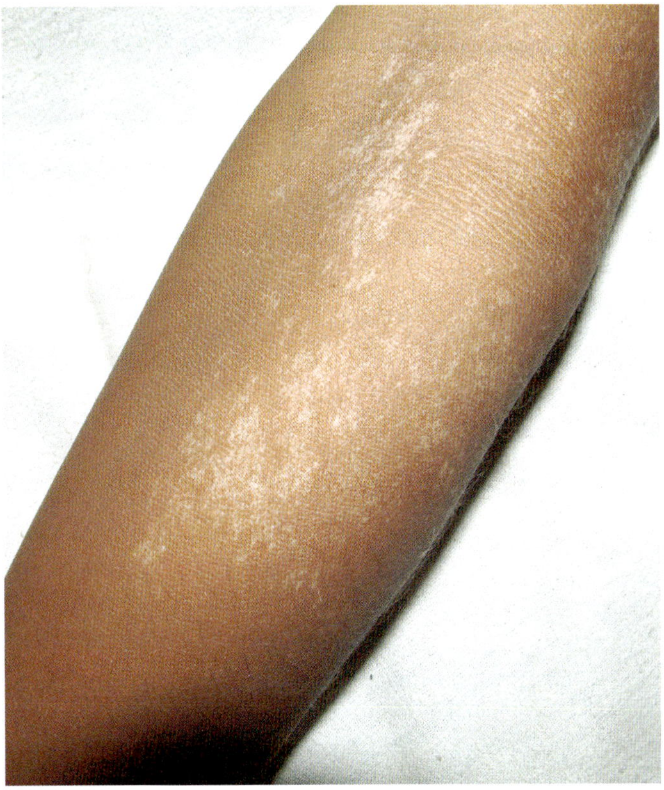

**Fig. 27.52:** Lichen striatus: Hypopigmented atrophic macules configured linearly over left forearm

scales at the periphery. This is followed by multiple, smaller, oval to round scaly secondary eruptions. Their arrangement is characteristic as lesions run downwards and outwards from the spine (Christmas tree appearance) along lines of cleavage. The condition is self-limiting, with the lesions resolving spontaneously within 2–10 weeks.

No treatment is usually required. Oral antihistamines, calamine lotion and topical corticosteroids may be used to decrease itching. Recalcitrant lesions may be treated with ultraviolet light.

## Erythroderma

Childhood erythroderma may be a manifestation of several dermatoses including ichthyoses (nonbullous ichthyosiform erythroderma), dermatitis (atopic dermatitis, seborrheic dermatitis) and papulosquamous dermatoses (psoriasis, pityriasis rubra pilaris) and as an adverse effect to drugs.

### *Clinical Features*

Erythroderma refers to a generalized erythema usually with, sometimes without, scaling that involves more than 90% of the child's body surface area (Fig. 27.53). Erythroderma is often complicated by thermodysregulation, sepsis and fluid, electrolyte and nutritional imbalance.

Treatment includes addressing the underlying disease and preventing complications. Treatment should be initiated with bland applications and antihistamines but oral corticosteroids and other immunosuppressives may be needed in recalcitrant disease.

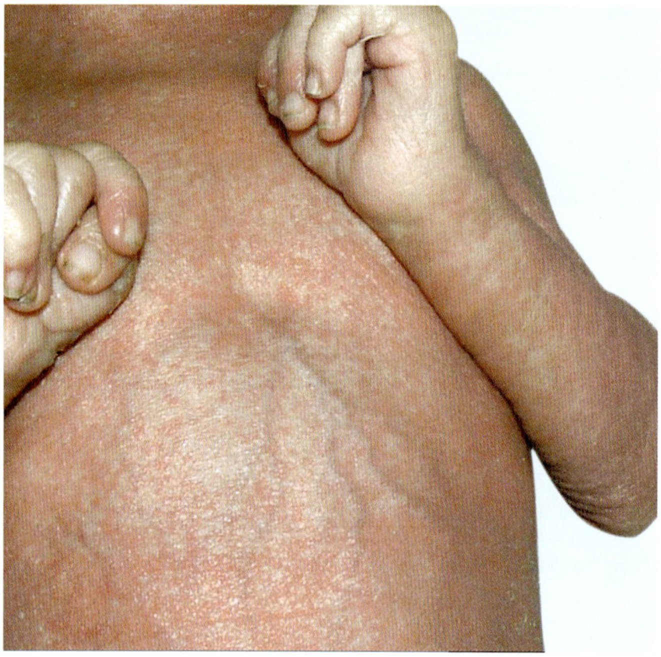

Fig. 27.53: Erythroderma: Generalized erythema associated with mild scaling in a newborn

## BULLOUS DISORDERS

### Pemphigus Vulgaris

This is the most common variant of pemphigus, accounting for over 80% cases.

Pemphigus vulgaris is an autoimmune disease, characterized by acantholysis, induced by deposition of IgG autoantibodies against desmogleins 3 and 1 present in desmosomes, which are cell-to-cell adhesion molecules in epidermis.

#### Clinical Features

Patients develop flaccid bullae on non-erythematous skin (Fig. 27.54). The bulla spreads on tangential pressure (bulla spread sign) and can be induced (Nickolsky sign). These rupture easily to form crusted erosions. The usual sites are scalp, face, flexures and trunk. Oral lesions might antedate skin lesions in 50% of patients and eventually 80–90% of patients develop oral lesions. Mucosal lesions are characteristically painful erosions with ragged margins.

#### Treatment

*General measures:* Counseling the caretakers about course of disease and necessity of continuing therapy during asymptomatic maintenance phase is important. Supportive measures including barrier nursing, skin and mucosal care (measures to augment healing, prevent and treat skin infections), maintaining fluid and electrolyte balance help to improve response to therapy.

*Specific measures:* Immunosuppressives including corticosteroids systemically (daily doses or as monthly bolus) along with steroid-sparing immunosuppressive adjuvants (azathioprine, methotrexate, cyclosporine) form the basis therapy. Maintenance therapy needs to be continued for several months. Intravenous rituximab has also been used successfully.

### Chronic Bullous Disease of Childhood

This is an IgA-mediated blistering disorder, characterized by a dermoepidermal split. The condition is seen in children less than 5 years of age. The lesions are itchy, tense bullae on an erythematous skin. New lesions appear around previous lesions resulting in a 'string of pearl' appearance (Fig. 27.55). The lesions are usually grouped around the orifices (perioral, perinasal, perigenital or perianal). They are also frequently seen on lower abdomen, buttocks, knees and elbows. Oral mucosal involvement is seen in 50% of patients. The illness is self-limiting, with lesions generally resolving within 2 years of onset.

Patients with mild disease are treated with dapsone (1–2 mg/kg) while in those with extensive disease, oral corticosteroids are administered.

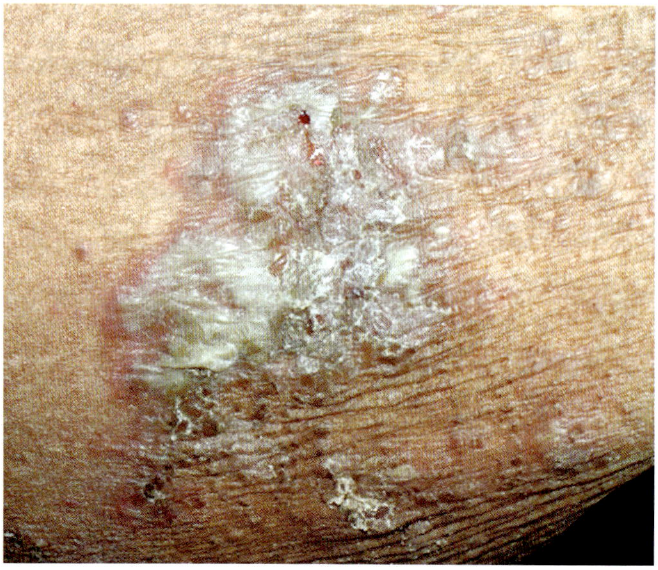

Fig. 27.54: Pemphigus vulgaris: Flaccid bullae on nonerythematous skin

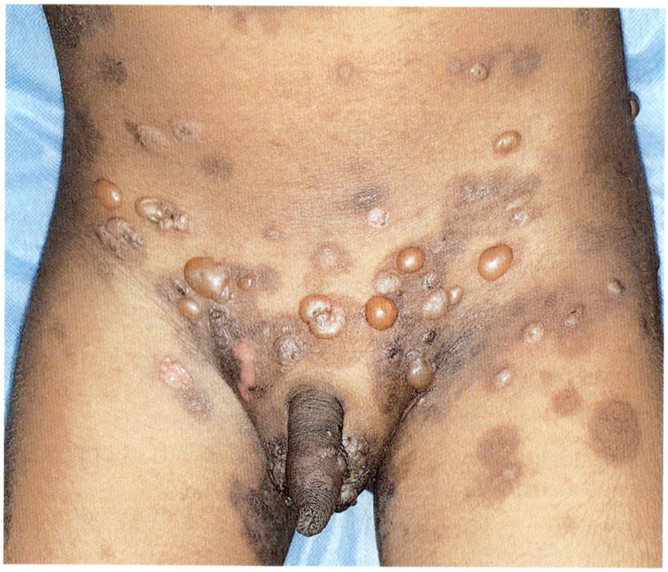

Fig. 27.55: Chronic bullous disease of childhood: Tense bullae on erythematous skin in perigenital area

## DISORDERS OF PIGMENTATION

### Vitiligo

Vitiligo affects both sexes equally with peak incidence being between 10 and 30 years. A positive family history is present in 20–30% of patients. Vitiligo is classified into:

- Segmental vitiligo.
- Nonsegmental vitiligo: Includes localized variants (focal and mucosal) and generalized variants (vulgaris, acrofacial and universalis).

#### *Etiology*

Nonsegmental vitiligo probably has an autoimmune pathogenesis with a polygenic predisposition. Segmental vitiligo has a neurogenic pathogenesis.

#### *Clinical Features*

The lesions are characterized by depigmented (chalky white or pale white) macules with sharp scalloped margins, which might coalesce to form geographical patterns (Fig. 27.56). Lesional hair may be depigmented (leukotrichia). Lesions may be present anywhere on the body, but areas prone to trauma are most susceptible. The lesion may be focal (1 macule at a single site), segmental (unilateral, dermatomal usually along distribution of mandibular division of the facial nerve), acrofacial (periorificial and acral) and universalis (extensive, generalized due to confluence of patches).

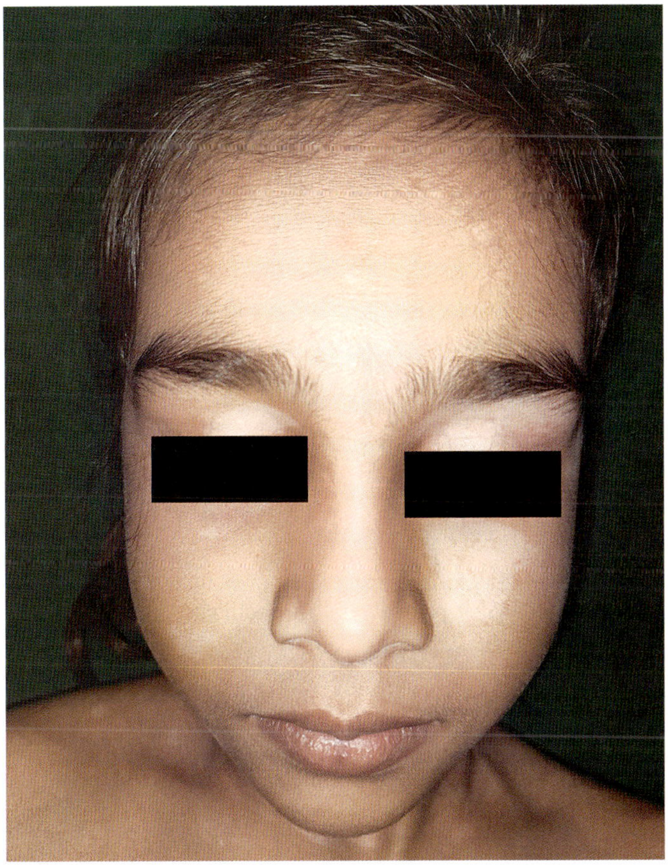

Fig. 27.56: Acrofacial vitiligo: Depigmented, scalloped macules on face and acral parts

**Table 27.13:** Treatment of vitiligo

| | Localized disease |
|---|---|
| New lesions | Topical corticosteroids<br>Topical calcineurin inhibitors |
| Old lesions | Topical PUVA*/PUVA sol |
| | **Extensive disease** |
| New lesions | Oral corticosteroids + PUVA*/PUVA* sol or NB-UVB** |
| Rapid increase | Oral corticosteroids + PUVA*/PUVA* sol or NB-UVB** |
| Old lesions | Oral PUVA*/ PUVA* sol or NB-UVB ** |
| Intolerance to PUVA | Oral corticosteroids |

*Oral PUVA/PUVA sol: Psoralen + UVA/psoralens + sunlight: not to be used in children <10 yr of age
**NB-UVB: Narrowband UVB

#### *Associations*

Segmental vitiligo progresses initially for about 6 months and then stabilizes. Patients with vitiligo should be examined for cutaneous associations (alopecia areata, atopic dermatitis), endocrine disorders (diabetes mellitus, Addison disease, hypoparathyroidism and thyroid disorders) and pernicious anemia.

#### *Course*

Non-segmental vitiligo is slowly progressive, though it can sometimes progress rapidly. Spontaneous pigmentation is seen in 10% of patients. Predictors of poor prognosis include long-standing disease, leukotrichia and lesions on resistant areas (bony prominences, nonhairy, nonfleshy areas and mucosae).

#### *Treatment*

Patient and family need to be reassured. Sunscreens and cosmetic cover up may be needed. The treatment depends on the extent of involvement (Table 27.13). In patients whose disease is refractory but not progressing and in patients with segmental vitiligo, surgical techniques like blister grafting and melanocytes transfer can be tried.

### Freckles and Lentigines

Both are characterized by presence of discrete hyperpigmented macules. Lesions of freckles are seen in red haired, very fair children. Lentigines show no such predilection. Lesions of freckles are seen in light exposed parts of body (face, V of neck and dorsolateral aspect of forearms) with conspicuous absence on covered skin. Lentigines do not show such a predilection and may be present even on mucosae (Peutz-Jeghers syndrome). Freckles (Fig. 27.57a) are lighter, with less delineated edges and show variegation in color including darkening on sun exposure. Lentigines are darker, sharply defined and do not darken on sun exposure. They may be a cutaneous marker of multisystem syndromes (Fig. 27.57b).

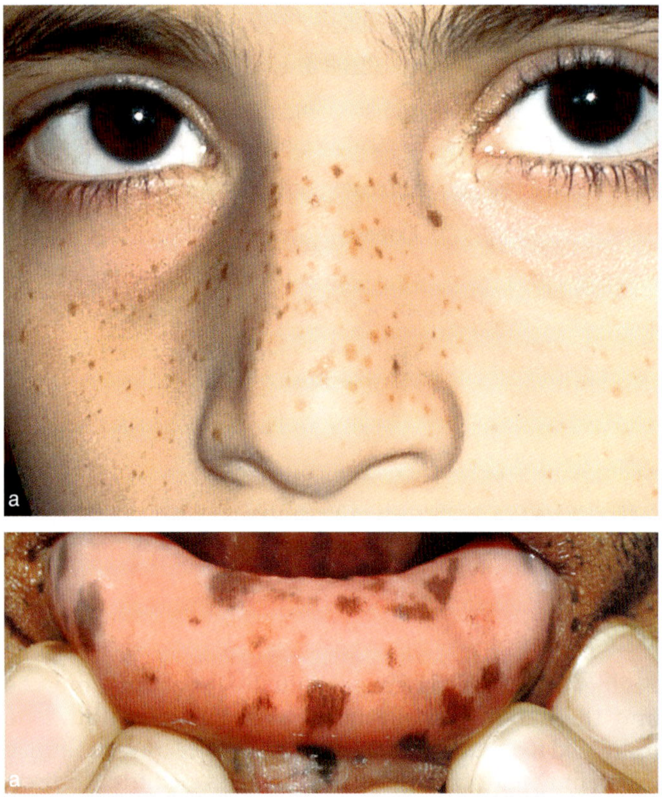

Fig. 27.57: (a) Freckles: Discrete, light brown, ill-defined macules with variegation in color, on the face of a fair child; (b) Lentigines: Discrete, dark brown, sharply defined macules on mucosal surface of lips in a patient with Peutz-Jeghers syndrome

## ABNORMAL VASCULAR RESPONSES

### Drug Eruptions

Drug eruptions are adverse events that occur after systemic or topical administration of a drug (Table 27.14).

Diagnosis is based on clinical features and temporal relation to drug use. Though any drug can cause a reaction after any length of treatment, some drugs are more suspect and the most recent introduction is the most likely cause. The role of drug provocation test is controversial but may be needed to find the culprit drug in patients on multiple drugs as well as to provide a list of safe alternative drugs.

#### Treatment

*General measures:* Withdrawal of drug is most effective approach but may not be easy as the child may be taking several drugs or the suspected drug may be essential and a chemically unrelated substitute may not be available. In severe reactions, maintenance of fluid-electrolyte balance, thermoregulation and skin care are very important. Symptomatic therapy is provided using antihistamines.

*Specific treatment:* In patients with erythroderma, local calamine lotion and topical corticosteroids are instituted initially. Oral corticosteroids may be required in recalcitrant patients. In Stevens-Johnson syndrome–toxic epidermal necrolysis complex, role of systemic corticosteroids is only established in the early stage. Intravenous immunoglobulins and cyclosporine have also been used successfully.

*Competency:* **PE31.12**

### Urticaria and Angioedema

Urticaria and angioedema are characterized by evanescent wheals which last 24–72 hours. Urticaria is due to edema of dermis while angioedema is due to edema of dermis and subcutis. Both conditions are mediated by chemicals (especially histamine) released from mast cells, triggered either immunologically (via IgE/autoimmune/complement pathways) or non-immunologically (by drugs/chemicals). Often urticaria is idiopathic.

**Table 27.14:** Common drug eruptions

| *Pattern* | *Morphology* | *Drugs implicated* |
|---|---|---|
| Exanthematous | Symmetric erythematous macules and papules | Antibacterials (penicillins, sulfonamides, cephalosporins), antitubercular drugs, anticonvulsants (barbiturates, carbamazepine, phenytoin, lamotrigene) |
| Erythroderma (exfoliative dermatitis) | Entire skin (>90%) is erythematous, scaly and edematous | Antibacterials, anticonvulsants, isoniazid, griseofulvin |
| Stevens-Johnson syndrome–toxic epidermal necrolysis (SJS–TEN) complex | Initial lesions often targetoid, followed by diffuse, intense erythema. Flaccid blisters, followed by large areas of skin denudation; mucosae always involved | Antibacterials (penicillins, sulfonamides quinolones, cephalosporins), anticonvulsants, frusemide, hydralazine, NSAIDs (oxicam derivatives and COX-2 inhibitors), antifungal agents (terbinafine, griseofulvin) |
| Fixed drug eruption | Well demarcated, erythematous plaques; subside with hyperpigmentation; recur at same site each time the implicated drug is taken | Antibacterials (dapsone, tetracyclines, penicillin, erythromycin), NSAIDs (salicylates, paracetamol), griseofulvin |
| Photosensitive eruption | Pruritic papules and plaques on sun-exposed areas | Antibacterials (sulphonamides, tetracyclines, quinolones), thiazides, phenothiazines, psoralens, NSAIDs, amiodarone |
| Vasculitis | Palpable purpura, urticarial vasculitis, necrotic ulcers, nodular vasculitis | Antibacterials (tetracyclines, ampicillin, erythromycin), NSAIDs, anticonvulsants, griseofulvin, levamisole |
| Urticaria and angioedema | Occur independently or along with bronchospasm and circulatory collapse (anaphylaxis) | Aspirin, penicillin, vaccines with egg proteins, ACE inhibitors, indomethacin, opiates, antifungals |

Urticaria is characterized by development of itchy, evanescent wheals (Fig. 27.58a), while the wheals in angioedema are less evanescent and not itchy (Fig. 27.58b). In dermographism, the wheals are linear (Fig. 25.58c) and in cholinergic urticaria, they are small.

Though removal of triggers seems a logical strategy of treatment, triggers are often difficult to identify. Antihistamines (preferably newer non-sedating ones), even in escalated doses (up to 4-times) are the mainstay of treatment. Oral corticosteroids are used in anaphylaxis while immunosuppressives (methotrexate, azathioprine and cyclosporine) are used in resistant (autoimmune) urticaria. Montelukast (leukotriene receptor antagonist) and omalizumab (anti-IgE monoclonal antibody) are also used in recalcitrant patients.

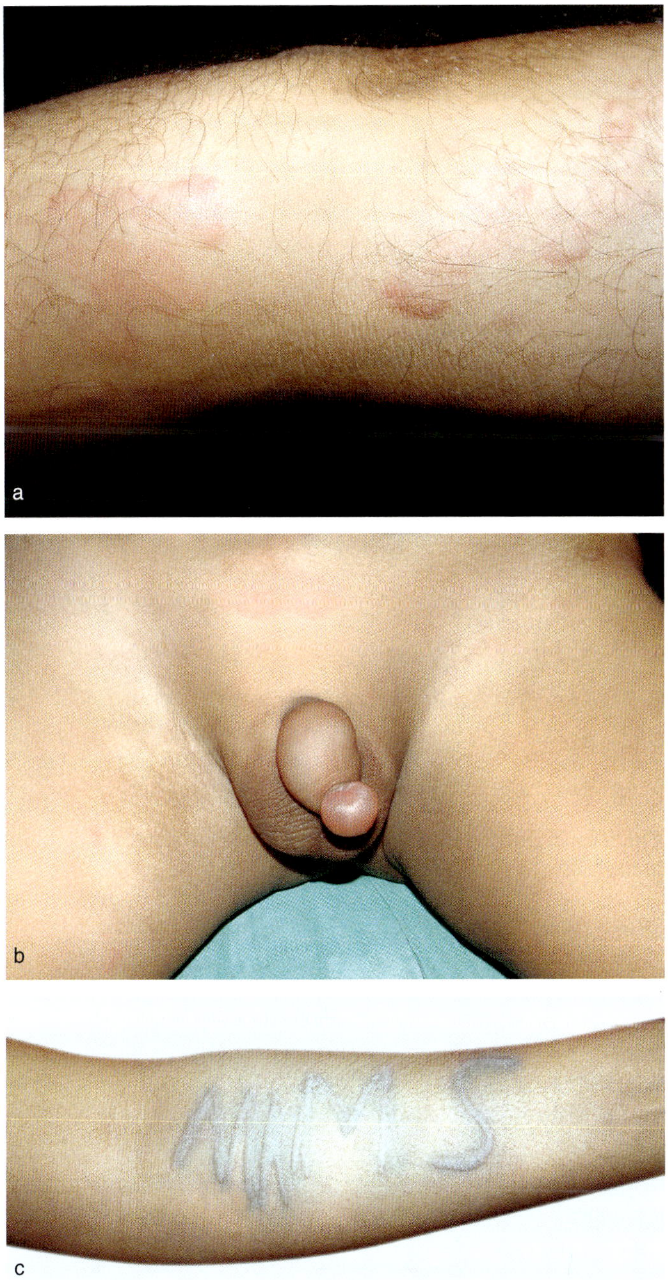


**Fig. 27.58:** (a) Urticaria: Pale pink edematous wheals with a surrounding flare; (b) Angioedema: Pale pink swelling of genitals; (c) Dermographism: Linear wheals

## Erythema Multiforme

Erythema multiforme has two main subtypes: Erythema multiforme (EM) minor, and EM major.

### *Etiology*

Infections like herpes simplex virus, mostly, and less commonly, *Mycoplasma pneumoniae* may trigger EM.

### *Clinical Features*

- *Cutaneous lesions:* Lesions usually appear in a single crop. Target lesions which consist of 3 concentric areas of varying degrees of erythema are characteristic (Fig. 27.59). Central bullous lesions are characteristic in EM major. Lesions are seen symmetrically on acral parts especially of upper extremities and on the face.
- *Mucosal lesions* are conspicuous in EM major (buccal erosions and hemorrhagic crusts of lips).
- *Constitutional symptoms* are present in EM major.

Most patients are managed symptomatically. In patients with recurrent EM, suppressive therapy with acyclovir may be instituted.

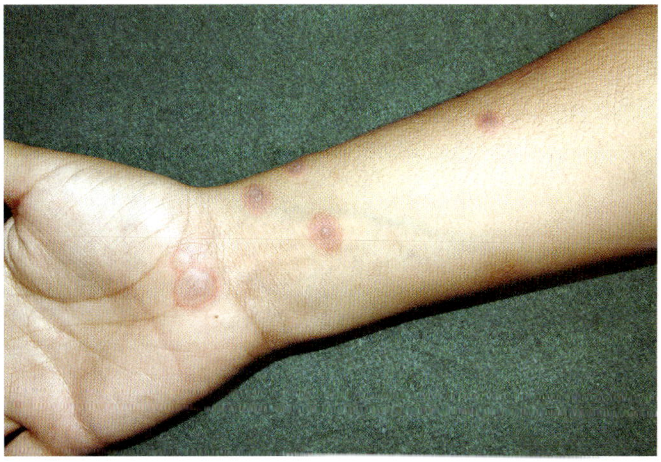

**Fig. 27.59:** Cutaneous lesions: Target lesions in acral parts. Target lesion consists of three concentric rings composed of central dusky erythema, sometimes surmounted with vesicle/bulla, surrounded by a pale edematous ring which is in turn surrounded by an erythematous halo

# INFECTIONS

## Pyodermas

Pyodermas are classified depending on whether they are follicular or non-follicular, and whether they are spreading or localized and the depth and extent of involvement (Table 27.15).

The chief causative organisms are *S. aureus* for folliculitis and furuncles, bullous impetigo, and some impetigo contagiosa and ecthyma.

*S. pyogenes* is causative for cellulitis and erysipelas and some impetigo contagiosa and ecthyma.

### *Clinical Features*

Manifestations depend on type of pyoderma (Tables 27.16 to 27.18, Figs 27.60–27.62).

**Table 27.15:** Classification of pyodermas

| | *Superficial* | *Deep* |
|---|---|---|
| | **Follicular** | |
| Folliculitis<br>Perifolliculitis | Superficial folliculitis<br>Furuncle | Deep folliculitis<br>Carbuncle |
| | **Nonfollicular** | |
| Spreading | Erysipelas | Cellulitis |
| Localized | Impetigo contagiosa<br>Bullous impetigo | Ecthyma |

**Table 27.16:** Clinical features of follicular pyodermas

| | *Folliculitis* | *Furuncle* |
|---|---|---|
| Clinical features | Erythematous follicular papules, often surmounted by pustules | Firm red follicular nodules which discharge pus and heal with minimal scarring (Fig. 27.60) |
| Sites of predilection | Face, lower extremities | Buttocks, lower extremities |

**Table 27.17:** Clinical features of spreading pyodermas

| | *Erysipelas* | *Cellulitis* |
|---|---|---|
| Clinical features | Tender, warm, erythematous rapidly spreading plaques; superficial vesiculation. Sharply demarcated border | Tender, warm erythematous; no distinct margins |
| Sites of predilection | Face | Lower extremities |

### *Treatment*

General measures include local hygiene, removal of crusts (in ecthyma), rest and limb elevation (for cellulitis). NSAIDs are used, if pain and constitutional symptoms are present.

Topical antibiotics like mupirocin, sodium fusidate and nadifloxacin are used for localized lesions. Systemic therapy is required in patients with extensive lesions, in spreading lesions (erysipelas and cellulitis), and in presence of constitutional symptoms and lymphadenopathy.

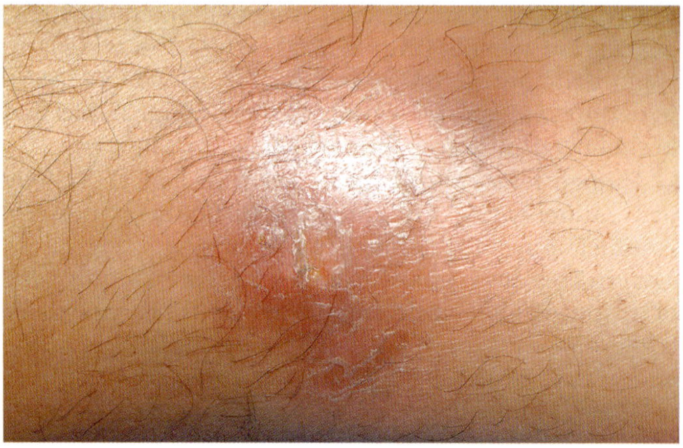

**Fig. 27.60:** Furuncle: Firm, red follicular nodules which discharge pus and heal with minimal scarring

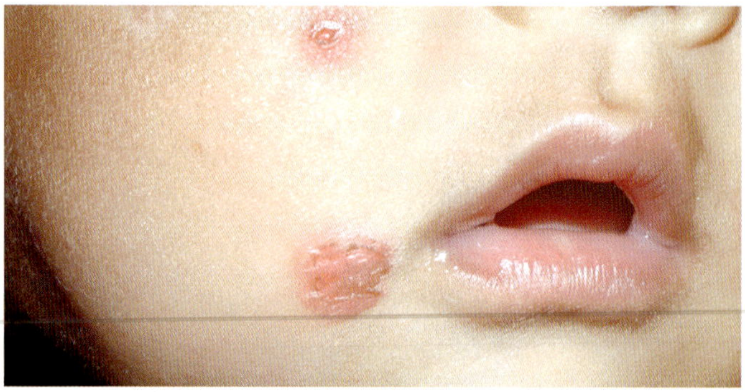

**Fig. 27.61:** Impetigo contagiosa: Honey-colored crusted lesions around mouth

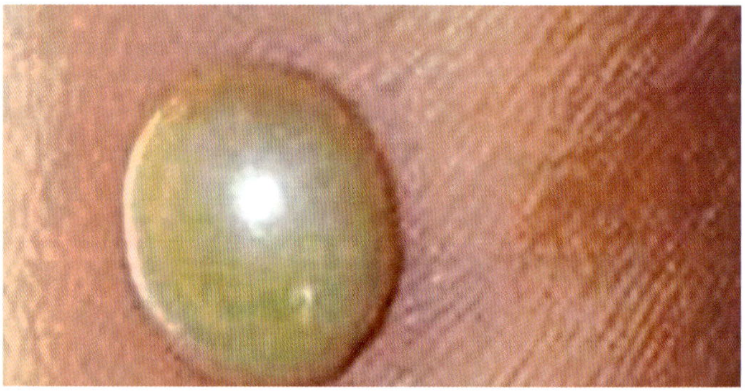

**Fig. 27.62:** Bullous impetigo: Thick-walled, persistent blisters on bland skin

**Table 27.18:** Clinical features of nonfollicular pyoderma

| | *Impetigo contagiosa* | *Bullous impetigo* | *Ecthyma* |
|---|---|---|---|
| Age | Children | Infants | Any age |
| Clinical features | Thin-walled blisters with erythematous halo; rupture to form honey colored crusts (Fig. 27.61) | Thick-walled, persistent blisters on bland skin; rupture only after a few days to leave thin varnish like crusts (Fig. 27.62) | Crusted, tender erythematous indurated plaque with thick adherent crusts |
| | Lesions spread without central clearing | Lesions heal in center to form annular plaques | Lesions heal with scarring |
| | Lymphadenopathy frequent | Lymphadenopathy rare | Frequent |
| Sites of predilection | Face, especially mouth and nose | Face, other parts of body | Thighs, legs |
| Complications | Post-streptococcal glomerulonephritis, eczematization | Staphylococcal scalded skin syndrome | Glomerulonephritis, eczematization, scarring |

Follicular pyodermas and bullous impetigo warrant use of antistaphylococcal antibiotics (cloxacillin or coamoxiclav) or macrolides. Spreading pyodermas should be treated with injectable penicillins.

### Staphylococcal Scalded Skin Syndrome

This condition is mediated by hematogenous spread of exotoxin produced by *S. aureus*, present usually in extracutaneous infections (e.g. otitis media, pneumonitis).

The illness is usually seen in newborns and infants younger than 2 years of age. Erythema and tenderness are followed by superficial peeling of skin in thin sheets, giving the appearance of scalding (Fig. 27.63). Constitutional symptoms are minimal.

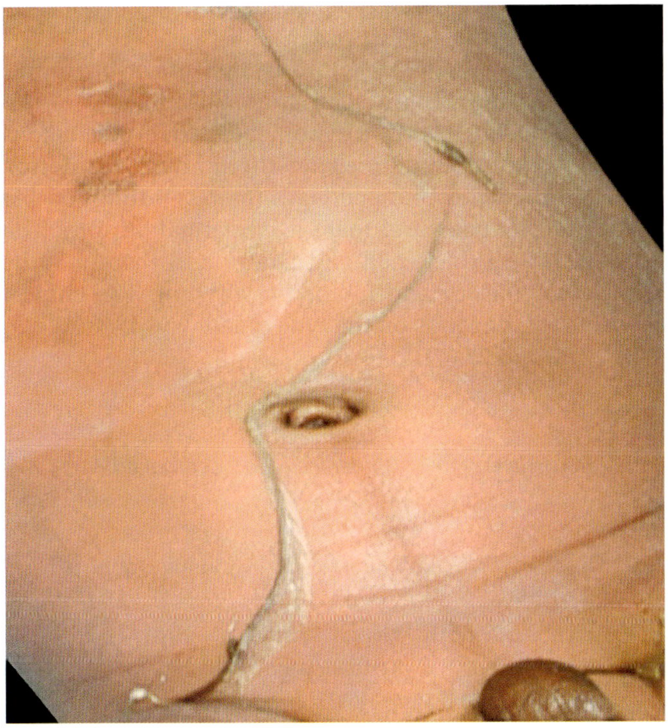

**Fig. 27.63:** Staphylococcal scalded skin syndrome: Erythema and superficial peeling of skin in thin sheets

Treatment is mainly supportive. Antistaphylococcal antibiotics are administered initially parenterally then orally. Fluid and electrolyte balance should be maintained.

### Cutaneous Tuberculosis

Cutaneous tuberculosis caused by *M. tuberculosis* is classified based on host's immune status as well as route of inoculation into (Table 27.19):

- Lupus vulgaris (Fig. 27.64)
- Scrofuloderma (Fig. 27.65)
- Tuberculosis verrucosa cutis
- Tuberculids

The diagnosis is confirmed by histopathology. Patients should be evaluated for systemic tuberculosis. Therapy of cutaneous tuberculosis comprises use of four antitubercular medications (isoniazid, rifampicin, ethambutol and pyrazinamide) for 8 weeks followed by three agents (isoniazid, rifampicin and ethambutol) for the next 16 weeks.

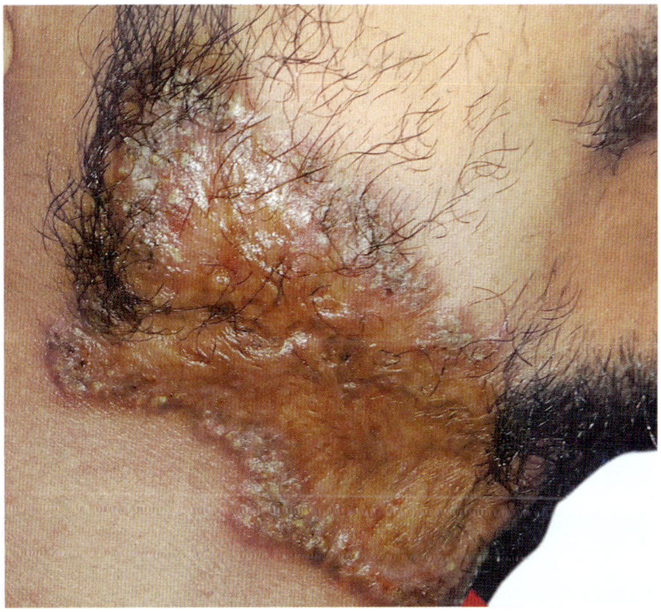

**Fig. 27.64:** Lupus vulgaris: Solitary, well-defined annular plaque with central scarring

**Table 27.19:** Clinical features of tuberculosis

| | *Lupus vulgaris* | *Scrofuloderma* | *Tuberculosis verrucosa cutis* | *Tuberculids* |
|---|---|---|---|---|
| Immune status of host | Moderate | Poor | Excellent | Excellent |
| Route of spread | Hematogenous/ contiguous | Contiguous from lymph nodes, bones or joints | Inoculation | Hypersensitivity reaction |
| Morphology | Solitary, well defined, annular/arcuate plaque with atrophic/scarred center (Fig. 27.64). Periphery shows pink-brown, deep-seated nodules which on diascopy may exhibit an apple-jelly appearance | Firm, subcutaneous nodules which break open to form sinuses. Mouth of sinus is serpiginous with undermined edges (Fig. 27.65) | Single, warty firm plaque with a violaceous halo. The surface has clefts and fissures that discharge pus. There may be scarring at the center | Papular or papulonecrotic lesions |
| Sites of predilection | Head, neck and buttocks | Cervical lymph nodes most frequently, tibia and sternoclavicular joints | Sites of trauma | Trunk |

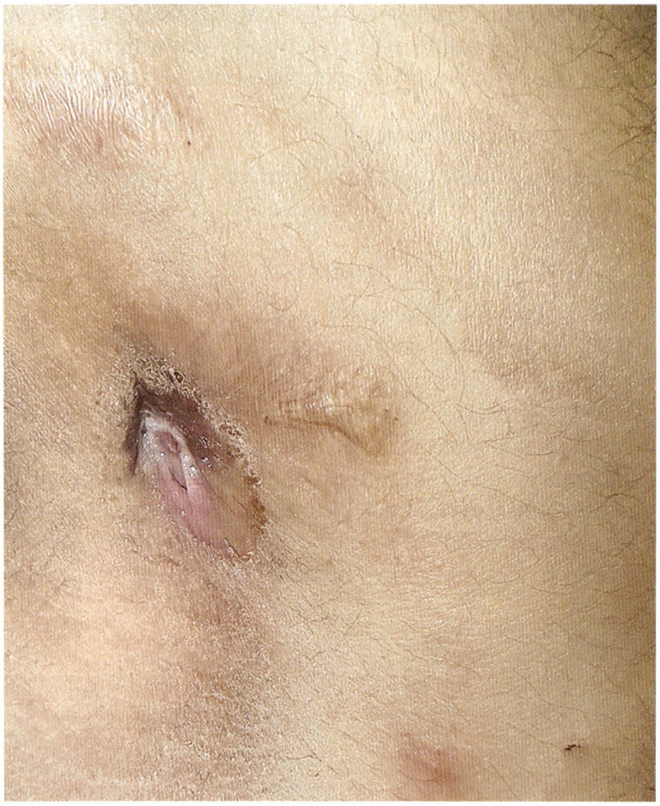

Fig. 27.65: Scrofuloderma: Sinus with mouth showing undermined edge and fixed to underlying lymph node

### Leprosy

The mode of transmission of *M. leprae* is uncertain but possibly nasal droplet infection is important. The clinical manifestations depend on the host immunological response. If the host mounts good cell-mediated immunity (CMI), the infection is localized (tuberculoid pole) while if the CMI is poor, the infection is extensive with visceral involvement (lepromatous pole). The Ridley-Jopling classification, based on clinical, pathological, immunological and bacteriological parameters, classifies leprosy into:

- Indeterminate leprosy
- Determinate leprosy
  - Tuberculoid
  - Borderline tuberculoid
  - Borderline
  - Borderline lepromatous
  - Lepromatous

Tuberculoid and lepromatous leprosy are stable forms, while borderline forms of leprosy are unstable.

Prototype skin lesion is a hypopigmented/erythematous macule/plaque, which is anesthetic/hypoaesthetic/normoaesthetic. Skin appendages (hair, sweating) on the lesions are reduced and there is epidermal atrophy. The nerves may be thickened and tender and there may be associated sensory and motor impairment. The clinical presentation depends on the type of leprosy (Table 27.20, Figs 27.66 and 27.67).

Table 27.20: Clinical features of leprosy

| | *Indeterminate* | *Tuberculoid* | *Borderline tuberculoid* | *Borderline* | *Borderline lepromatous* | *Lepromatous* |
|---|---|---|---|---|---|---|
| **Skin lesions** | | | | | | |
| Number | Single | Single/few | Few | Several | Numerous | Innumerable |
| Size | Variable | Variable | May be large | Variable | Small | Small |
| Sensations | Variable | Anesthetic | Hypoaesthetic | Hypoaesthetic | Hypoaesthetic | Normal |
| Symmetry | Asymmetrical | Asymmetrical | Asymmetrical | Bilateral, but asymmetrical | Tendency to symmetry | Symmetrical |
| Morphology | Hypopigmented macule; usually ill-defined hypoaesthetic; on face of child (Fig. 27.66) | Macule, plaque; well defined | Plaques; well defined; satellite lesions + (Fig. 27.67) | Macules, plaque; sloping edge (inverted saucer appearance) | Macules/ papules, nodules, plaques; ill-defined | Macules, papules, nodules, plaques; ill-defined; diffuse infiltration of face |
| **Nerves** | +/– | Single trunk/ feeder nerve related to lesion; thickened | Asymmetrical; few nerves thickened; anesthesia in its distribution | Asymmetrical; several nerves thickened | Several nerves, almost symmetrical, thickened; glove and stocking anesthesia | Several nerves asymmetrically thickened; glove and stocking anesthesia |
| **Systemic involvement** | None | None | None | None | May be present | Lymphadenopathy, hepatosplenomegaly, ocular and testicular involvement |
| **Reactions** | – | – | T1R | T1R | T1R, T2R | T2R |
| Lepromin reaction | +/– | + | +/– | – | – | – |
| **Presence of acid-fast bacilli** | +/– | – | – | +/– | ++ | +++ |

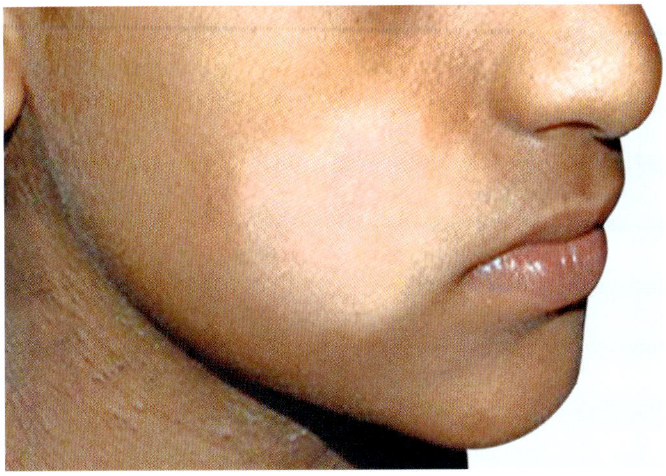

**Fig. 27.66:** Indeterminate leprosy: Ill-defined hypopigmented, hypoesthetic lesion on the face

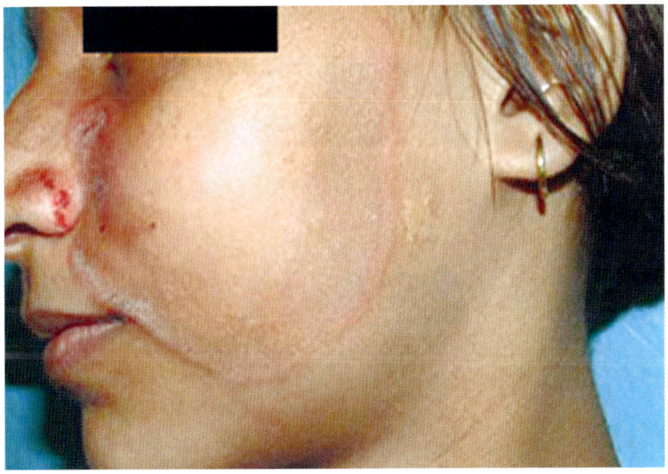

**Fig. 27.67:** Borderline tuberculoid: Well-defined erythematous plaque with satellite lesions

### Lepra Reactions

Two types of acute episodes (lepra reactions) are recognized in leprosy. Type 1 reaction (T1R), which develops in patients with borderline leprosy (BT, BB, BL) is due to alteration in host CMI. T1R manifests as edema and erythema of pre-existing lesions along with neuritis that may result in development of new sensory and motor impairment. Type 2 lepra reaction (T2R, erythema nodosum leprosum, ENL), which occurs in highly bacillated patients (BL and LL) is an immune complex reaction and manifests as several tender, erythematous, transient nodules on face, flexures and legs. Patients may show neuritis, orchitis, iridocyclitis, arthralgia and fever.

### Complications

Patients may show the following complications:

- Trophic ulcers
- *Deformities:* Claw hand, clawing of toes, foot drop and saddle nose deformity
- *Ophthalmologic complications:* Diminished corneal sensation, lagophthalmos, recurrent iridocyclitis
- Kidney involvement

### Investigations

***Slit skin smears:*** Slit skin smears, from the lesions and ear lobules, are stained with modified Ziehl-Neelsen method for acid-fast bacilli (AFB). The smears are usually negative in TT/BT/most BB leprosy and usually positive in LL, BL and some BB.

***Skin biopsy:*** Presence of granuloma (epithelioid cells in tuberculoid leprosy and foamy cells in lepromatous leprosy) and nerve involvement are typical.

### Treatment

Patient and parents are reassured and counseled regarding treatment compliance and care of hands, feet and eyes. For the purpose of treatment, leprosy is classified into paucibacillary (PB) and multibacillary (MB) leprosy (Table 27.21) and based on this multidrug therapy (MDT) is instituted (Table 27.21).

Treatment of lepra reactions requires specific treatment (Table 27.22).

**Table 27.21:** WHO recommendations for treatment of leprosy in children aged 10–15 years

| | *Paucibacillary* | *Multibacillary* |
|---|---|---|
| Definition | 5 or less lesions | >5 lesions |
| Duration of therapy | 6 months; to be completed in 9 months | 12 months; to be completed in 18 months |
| Supervised (monthly) | Rifampicin 450 mg | Rifampicin 450 mg + clofazimine 150 mg |
| Unsupervised (daily) | Dapsone 50 mg + clofazimine 25 mg | Dapsone 50 mg + clofazimine 25 mg |

Rifampicin 10 mg/kg; clofazimine 1 mg/kg daily, 6 mg/kg monthly; dapsone 2 mg/kg

**Table 27.22:** Treatment of reactions in leprosy

| | *Type 1 reaction* | *Type 2 reaction* |
|---|---|---|
| Mild | NSAIDs | NSAIDs |
| Moderate | NSAIDs | NSAIDs |
| | Oral corticosteroids | Thalidomide*<br>Chloroquine<br>Clofazimine |
| Severe | NSAIDs | Thalidomide* |
| | Oral corticosteroids | Oral corticosteroids |

NSAIDs–nonsteroidal anti-inflammatory drugs

*Thalidomide is a teratogenic agent and avoided in girls in the reproductive age

## Verruca (Warts)

Warts are caused by human papillomavirus, of which there are more than 100 types. They are transmitted by close contacts and autoinoculation. In children, non-genital warts are common, with an incidence of up to 10%. The clinical features differ in various types of warts (Table 27.23, Figs 27.68 and 27.69).

Modalities for treatment include cryotherapy, mechanical removal, radiofrequency ablation (RFA) and chemical cauterization (Table 27.23).

Table 27.23: Clinical features and therapy of warts

| | *Verruca vulgaris* (common warts) | *Verruca plana* (plane warts) | *Palmoplantar warts* | *Filiform warts* |
|---|---|---|---|---|
| Clinical features | Single or multiple firm papules with hyperkeratotic, clefted surface (Fig. 27.68) | Skin colored, flat smooth palpable papules (Fig. 27.69); Koebner phenomenon due to autoinoculation | Superficial (mosaic): Painless, hyperkeratotic papules and plaques<br>Deep (myrmecia): Painful, deep seated papules with a horny collar | Thin elongated, firm projections on a horny base |
| Site | Any part of body, most commonly on back of hands, fingers and knees | Face and back of hands | Soles and less often palms | Face |
| Therapy | Cryotherapy, mechanical removal and radio-frequency ablation (RFA) | Trichloroacetic acid touches; retinoic acid (0.025–0.05%) at night | Wart paint; cryotherapy; formalin soaks | RFA |





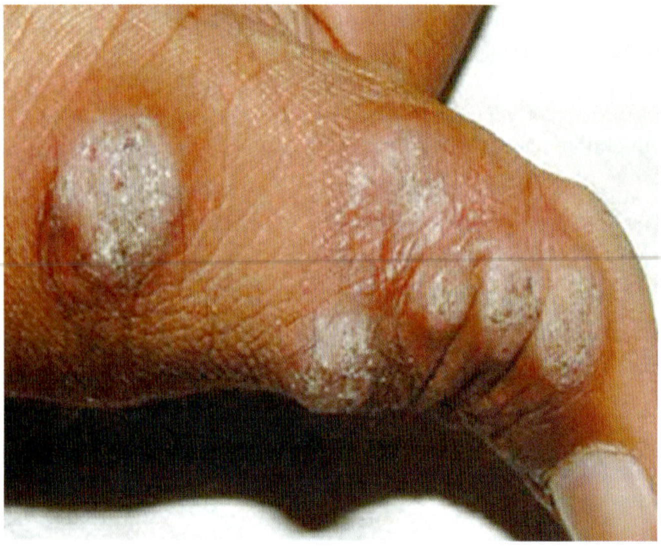

Fig. 27.68: Verruca vulgaris: Firm papules with hyperkeratotic, clefted surface

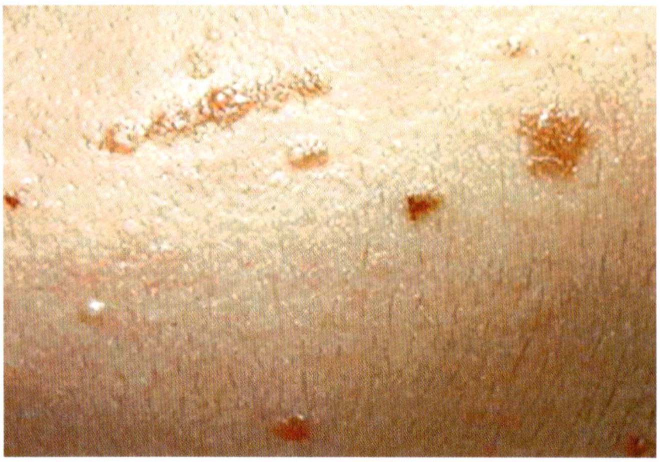

Fig. 27.69: Verruca plana: Multiple, skin-colored papules

## Molluscum Contagiosum

Caused by a poxvirus, patients show multiple, pearly white, dome-shaped papules with central umbilication (Fig. 27.70). The lesions are seen on any part of the body. The condition

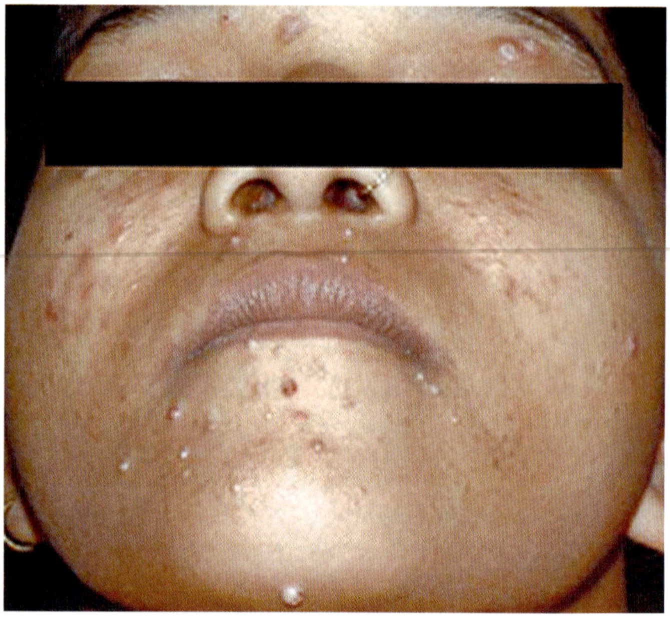

Fig. 27.70: Molluscum contagiosum: Pearly white dome-shaped papules with central umbilication

is self-limiting and lesions usually clear within a year, but widespread lesions are seen in patients with atopic dermatitis and in those who are immunocompromised.

Treatment modalities used include wart paint or mechanical extirpation.

## Hand-Foot-and-Mouth Disease

The illness is caused by coxsackie virus A16 infection, with feco-oral route being the predominant mode of transmission.

It most often affects children between 1 and 10 years of age during the summer and autumn months. The incubation period is 3–6 days. It manifests as an enanthem over the tongue and buccal mucosa, followed by painful vesicular exanthem involving lateral aspects of hands and feet (Fig. 27.71).

The disease usually runs a self-limiting course of 7–10 days, with a very rare incidence of cardiac and neurological complications.

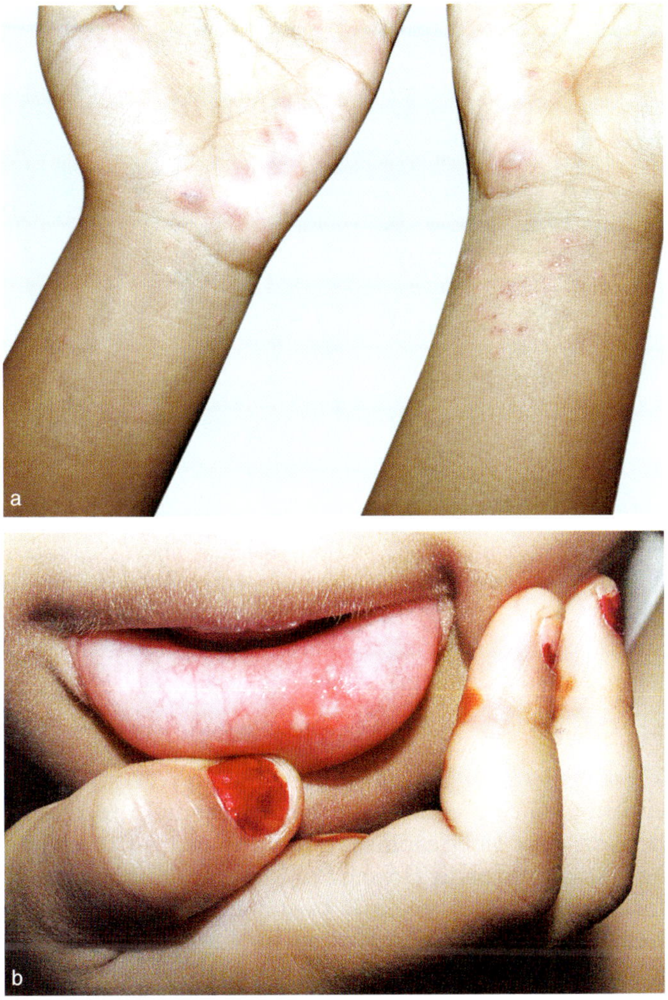


**Fig. 27.71:** (a) Hand-foot-and-mouth disease: Skin lesions—oblong vesicles with erythematous halo on palms; (b) Mucosal lesions: Oval, vesicular lesions with erythematous halo

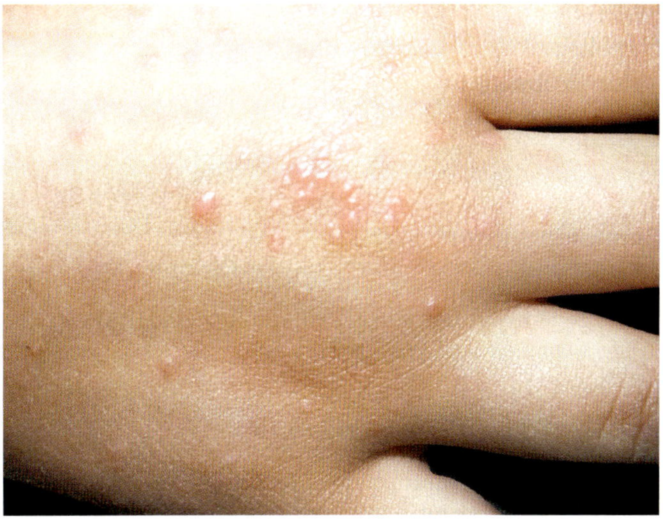

**Fig. 27.72:** Gianotti-Crosti syndrome: Multiple, monomorphic, flat/umbilicated erythematous papules present symmetrically over the dorsae of hands

### Gianotti-Crosti Syndrome

Also known as papular acrodermatitis of childhood, the condition is associated with hepatitis B virus and Epstein-Barr virus.

It presents as characteristic lesions (Fig. 27.72) on the face, buttocks and limbs, associated with mild constitutional symptoms. The mucous membranes are not affected. The eruption fades with mild desquamation in 3–4 weeks.

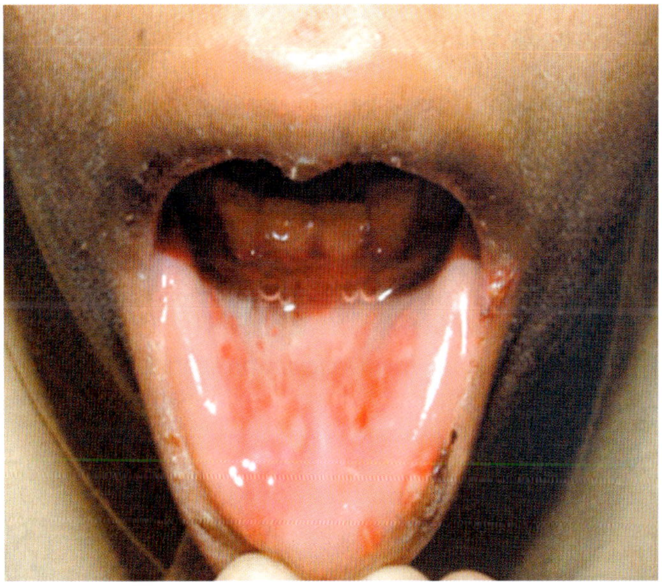

**Fig. 27.73:** Herpes gingivostomatitis: Closed grouped vesicles on an edematous base which coalesce to form polycyclic erosions

### Herpes Simplex Virus (HSV) Infections

HSV type 1 infection is often asymptomatic but when symptomatic, the manifestations depend on whether the infection is primary or recurrent. Primary HSV infection presents as acute gingivostomatitis with tightly grouped vesicles on an edematous base which rupture to form polycyclic erosions (Fig. 27.73). There may be associated malaise, fever and lymphadenopathy. Patients with recurrent herpes labialis have a prodrome of burning and stinging followed by appearance of grouped vesicular lesions (Fig. 27.74) with background of slight erythema. These lesions show polycyclic depigmentation after healing.

In patients with underlying dermatoses like atopic dermatitis and ichthyoses, HSV infection may become

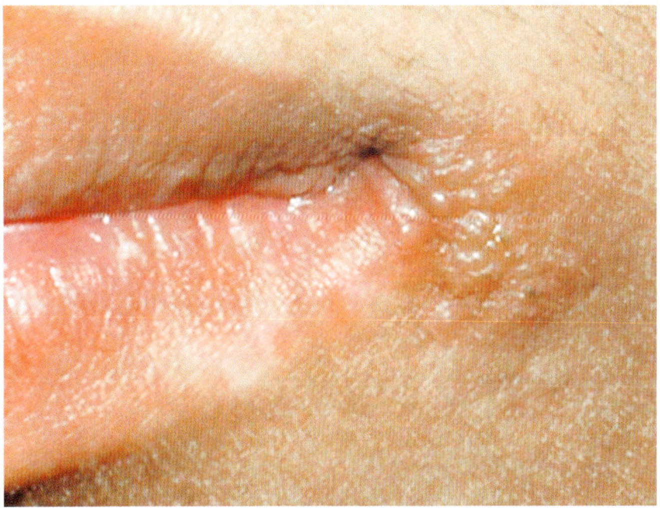

**Fig. 27.74:** Herpes labialis: Polycyclic area of hypopigmentation and vesicular lesions

generalized (Kaposi varicelliform eruption or eczema herpeticum).

No treatment is required, except in primary infection, severe recurrent infection or in immunocompromised patients where treatment with oral acyclovir is given for 5–7 days.

## Dermatophytoses

### Etiology

Three genera of fungi cause dermatophytoses: *Trichophyton*, *Epidermophyton* and *Microsporum*.

### Clinical Features

The infection is given different names depending on the site affected. Dermatophyte infection of skin is known as tinea corporis, of groin as tinea cruris, of hands as tinea manuum, of feet as tinea pedis and of nails as tinea unguium. The classical lesion is an annular/arcuate/polycyclic plaque with a clear center and an active edge showing papulovesiculation and scaling.

***Tinea capitis:*** Three patterns are recognized:

- *Non-inflammatory or epidemic type* caused by anthropophilic organisms and so is responsible for epidemics. It presents as alopecic patch, in which hairs break off easily **(Fig. 27.75)**.
- *Inflammatory or kerion:* Caused by zoophilic organisms and so does not cause epidemics. It presents as a boggy swelling **(Fig. 27.76)** from which hair is easily pluckable without pain. Usually associated with occipital lymphadenopathy.
- *Favus:* Caused by *T. schoenleinii*, presents as yellowish, foul smelling cup-shaped crusts with matting of hair.

### Investigations

The diagnosis is confirmed by the KOH test that shows fungal hyphae. Culture helps in identification of species

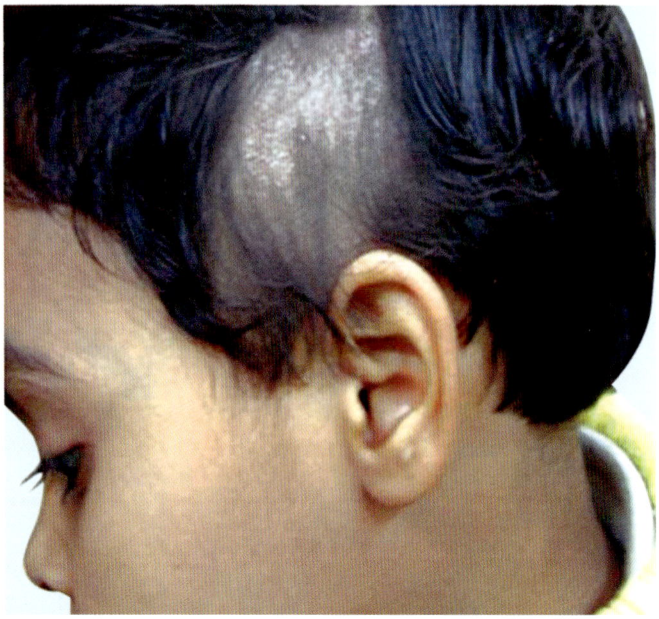

**Fig. 27.75:** Tinea capitis: Area of non-scarring alopecia with minimal inflammation with scaling at periphery

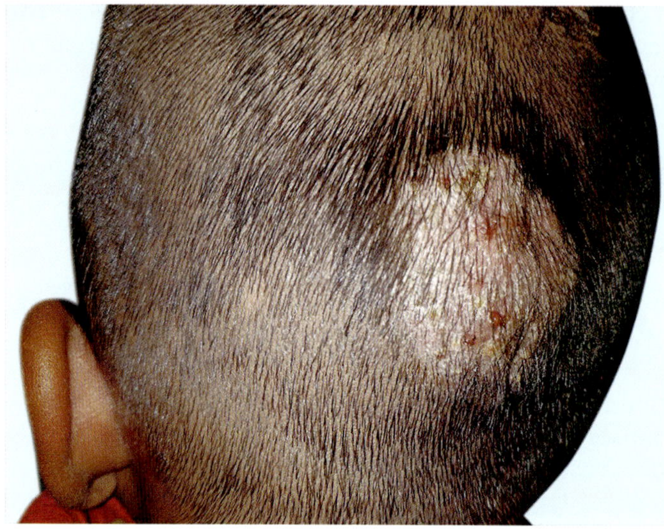

**Fig. 27.76:** Kerion: Boggy swelling of scalp which drains pus from multiple openings

and this is important in patients with tinea capitis. Wood's lamp may help in diagnosis during epidemics.

### Treatment

***Tinea capitis:*** Washing with ketoconazole shampoo and not sharing combs and head wear help to reduce transmission. Tinea capitis is always treated with systemic agents; griseofulvin (15 mg/kg/day of ultramicronized formulation) for 6 weeks is treatment of choice. Longer treatment (8 weeks) is needed for kerion. Terbinafine (5 mg/kg/day for 4–8 weeks) is effective in trichophyton (noninflammatory) but not in microsporum tinea capitis. Moroever, use of terbinafine in children is hindered by its unpleasant after taste.

***Tinea corporis:*** Localized lesions of tinea corporis are managed by topical therapy (azoles available as clotrimazole, miconazole or ketoconazole in lotion, gel and cream formulations). Widespread lesions require systemic antifungal therapy with terbinafine (2–6 weeks) or griseofulvin (4–8 weeks). Due to resistance to terbinafine, itraconazole is being used frequently.

## Candidiasis

*Candida albicans*, a normal commensal, becomes pathogenic in the presence of predisposing factors including obesity, diabetes and immunocompromised states. Less frequently other species like *C. glabrata* may be involved.

Candidiasis presents as oral thrush, vulvovaginitis, intertrigo, candidal diaper dermatitis or paronychia. Oral thrush presents as soft, creamy white to yellow, elevated plaques, that are easily wiped off to leave an erythematous, eroded or ulcerated surface. The lesions are seen on buccal mucosa, tongue, palate and gingiva.

Candidal intertrigo presents as erythematous, moist, macerated lesions with a frayed irregular edge with satellite pustules, present mainly in major skin folds, like axillae, groins and neck.

Candidal diaper dermatitis is characterized by well-defined weeping/eroded lesions with scalloped border and a collar of overhanging scales and satellite pustules. The lesion begins in the perianal region, spreading to perineum, upper thighs, lower abdomen and lower back.

### Diagnosis

KOH mount shows budding yeasts and pseudohyphae. Culture is done in unresponsive cases to speciate the candida.

### Treatment

Predisposing factors should be addressed and the area kept dry. Topical therapy includes imidazoles (clotrimazole, miconazole and ketoconazole), nystatin cream for folds and lotions for oral mucosa. Systemic therapy with weekly fluconazole is given in patients with extensive disease.

## Pityriasis Versicolor

The condition is cuased by *Malasezzia furfur*, a commensal yeast. Patient presents with scaly, perifollicular macules with variable pigmentation (hypopigmented, erythematous or hyperpigmented). The fine branny scales are accentuated by gentle abrasion with a glass slide. The lesions are frequently seen on upper trunk (both anterior and posterior), neck and sometimes also on proximal part of upper extremities.

### Diagnosis

KOH mount shows a mixture of short branched hyphae and spores (spaghetti and meatball appearance).

### Treatment

Topical therapy with imidazoles (ketoconazole, 2%) for 3 consecutive days is sufficient in most cases. Systemic therapy with fluconazole or itraconazole is occasionally required in extensive and recurrent disease.

# DISEASES CAUSED BY ARTHROPODS

## Scabies

Scabies is caused by *Sarcoptes scabei var hominis* and transmitted by close contact with infested humans.

Patient presents with itchy (worse at night) lesions, present in a characteristic distribution. The primary lesion is a burrow, a grey thread-like serpentine line with a minute papule at the end; papules and papulovesicles may also be seen. Secondary lesions consist of pustules, eczematized lesions and nodules. Lesions are seen in webs of hands, on wrists, ulnar aspects of forearms, elbows, axillae, umbilical area, genitalia, feet and buttocks. Face is usually spared, except in infants in whom face, scalp, palms and soles **(Fig. 27.77a)** are also involved. Nodular lesions are seen on genitalia **(Fig. 27.77b)**.

Secondary infections common. Secondary streptococcal infection may result in acute glomerulonephritis.

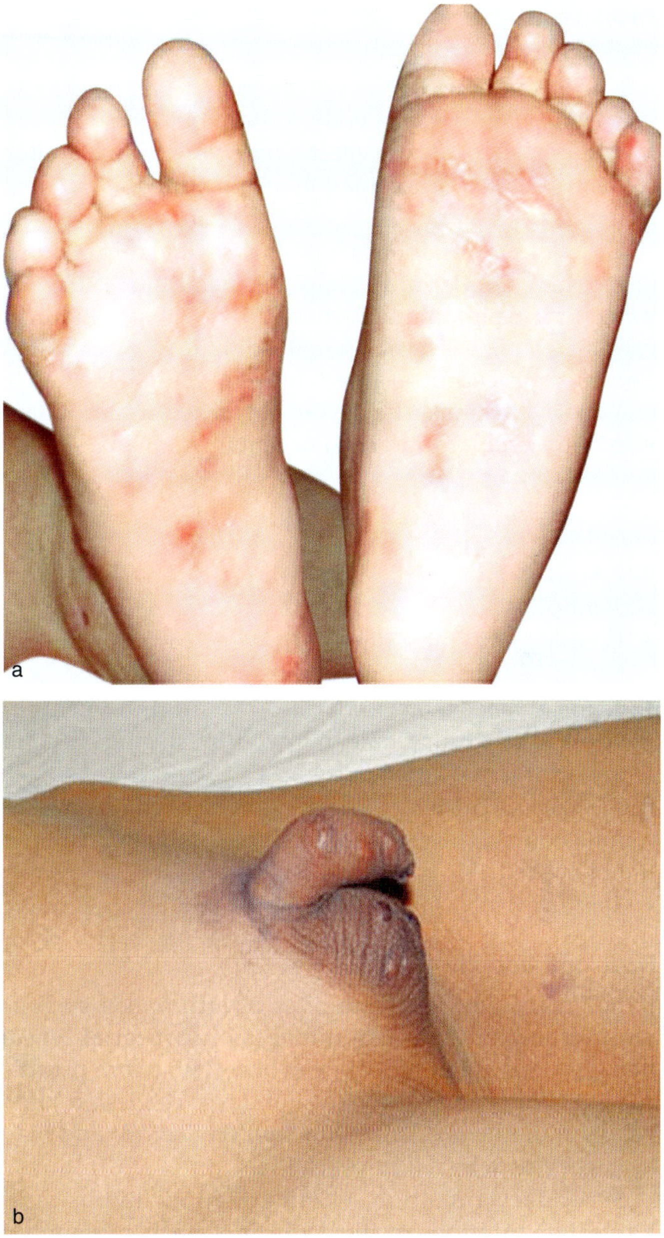


**Fig. 27.77:** (a) Infantile scabies: Multiple papulovesicular lesions on soles; (b) Infantile scabies: Nodular lesions of genitalia

### Treatment

***General measures:*** All close contacts of the patient, even if asymptomatic, should be treated. Overzealous laundering of bed linen and clothes is not warranted.

***Specific measure:*** Antibiotics are given, if secondary infection is present. Antihistamines are given for 1–2 weeks to reduce pruritus. The topical scabicide should be applied all over body below the neck, including on the free edge of nails, genitals, soles of feet after hydration of body with a bath. Scabicides available include:

***Permethrin 5%:*** Overnight single application is treatment of choice in children older than 2 months of age.

***Crotamiton 10%:*** Two applications daily for 14 days is recommended for infants less than 2 months.

***Benzyl benzoate 25%:*** Three applications at 12 hourly intervals.

***Ivermectin,*** single oral dose of 200 µg/kg body weight, in children older than 5 years is the treatment of choice for epidemics (as in orphanages). Moxidectin is under clinical trials as a new therapeutic oral agent for scabies.

### Pediculosis

Louse is an obligate ectoparasite and two species infest humans: *Pediculosis humanus* (*P. humanus capitis*, head louse and *P. humanus corporis*, body louse), and *Phthirus pubis* (pubic louse). Head louse infestation is transmitted by close contact and pubic louse infestation is acquired by children from infested parents.

Head louse infestation manifests as severe scalp pruritus or recurrent pyoderma of scalp. Pubic louse infestation is infrequent in children but when it occurs it also involves eyelashes and eyebrows. Though adult lice are difficult to find, nits (egg capsules) are easily seen, firmly cemented to hair on which they can be slid but not flicked off. Secondary infection, eczematization and occipital lymphadenopathy are frequent.

#### Treatment

All family members should be treated. The chief pediculicides are:

- *Permethrin*, 1% lotion, single 10 minutes application to wet hair followed by rinsing. Repeat application after 7 days.
- *Gamma benzene hexachloride*, 1% single overnight application to dry hair followed by rinsing. Second application used after 7 days.
- *Malathion*, 0.5% water-based lotion, applied on dry hair for 6 hours. Has residual effect, so second application is not needed.
- *Spinosad*, 0.9% suspension, single 10 minutes application.

### Papular Urticaria

Papular urticaria is due to bites of arthropods such as mosquitoes and fleas. An initial itchy, urticarial wheal that develops at the site of bite evolves into a firm pruritic papule, which persists for several days. The lesion often has a central hemorrhagic punctum (Fig. 27.78) and may be surmounted by a tiny vesicle.

Secondary infection, eczematization, hyper- and hypopigmentation, particularly in darkly pigmented individuals are not uncommon. New bites by the same species often cause a recrudescence of activity in existing and even healed lesions.

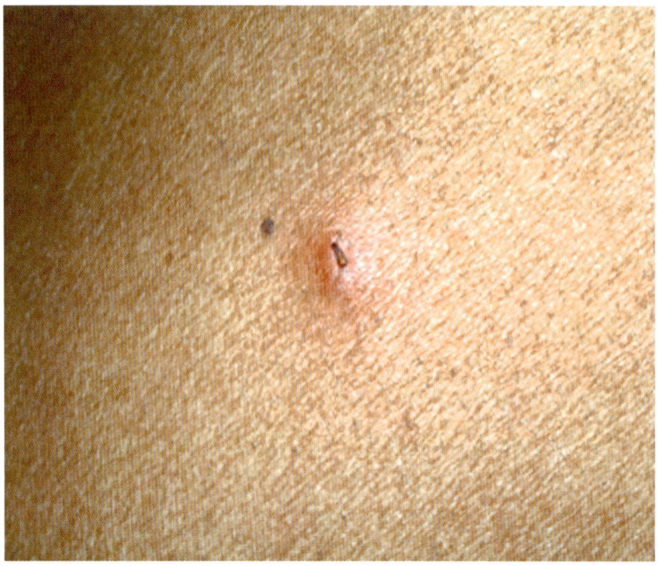

**Fig. 27.78:** Papular urticaria: Papule with a central hemorrhagic punctum

#### Treatment

Prevention of repeated insect bites through use of protective clothings, judicious use of insect repellents and treatment of pets with infestation is recommended. Topical steroid-antibiotic combination, and oral antihistamines help in reducing pruritus and hypersensitivity reaction.

## MISCELLANEOUS DERMATOSES

### Protein-Energy Malnutrition

Marasmus is characterized by emaciation and dry, thin, pale, wrinkled skin while kwashiorkor manifests as generalized edema and areas of hyperpigmentation and occasional desquamation (flaky paint appearance) predominantly at sites of pressure and friction (Fig. 27.79). Hairs may show alternate areas of discoloration (flag sign).

### Acrodermatitis Enteropathica

This is an autosomal recessively inherited disorder resulting in deficiency of zinc transporter protein and resultant defective zinc absorption. The condition is characterized by the dermatitis, diarrhea, alopecia and irritability. Characteristic skin lesions include periorificial sharply demarcated, erythematous crusted plaques with fissured margins (Fig. 27.80).

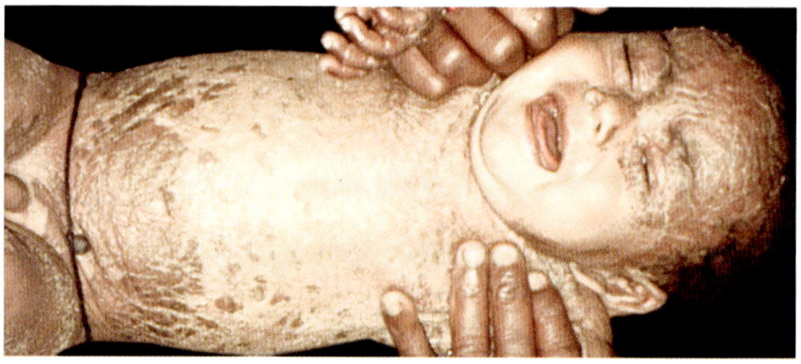

**Fig. 27.79:** Protein-energy malnutrition: Generalized, areas of hyperpigmentation and occasional desquamation ('flaky paint appearance') in an irritable child

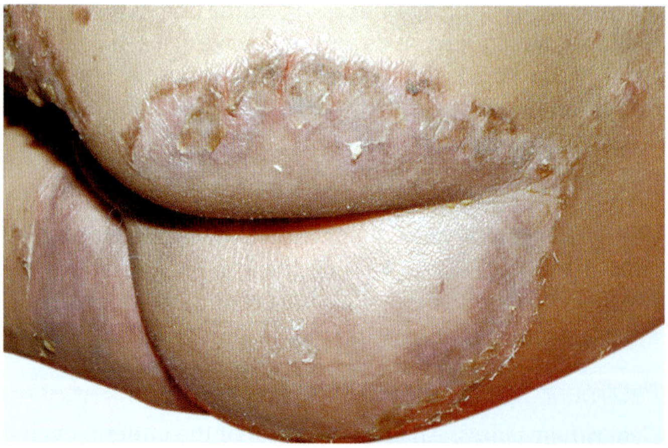

**Fig. 27.80:** Acrodermatitis enteropathica: Sharply demarcated erythematous plaque over the perianal area with fissured margins

*Treatment*

Oral administration of zinc sulfate or zinc gluconate (1–3 mg/kg).

## Porphyria

Porphyrias are a group of diseases characterized by genetic or acquired enzyme deficiencies in the pathway of heme-synthesis, resulting in accumulation of heme precursors: 5-aminolaevulinic acid (ALA), porphobilinogen and porphyrins. Based on clinical and biochemical parameters, porphyrias are classified into:

1. *Erythropoietic porphyria:* Congenital erythropoietic porphyria (CEP), erythropoietic protoporphyria (EPP)
2. *Hepatic porphyria:* Porphyria cutanea tarda (PCT), variegate porphyria (VP), acute intermittent porphyria.

Porphyrias are characterized by extreme photosensitivity and blistering and scarring of photo exposed areas (Fig. 27.81).

Treatment for all porphyrias includes genetic counseling, strict photoprotection and some specific measures (Table 27.24).

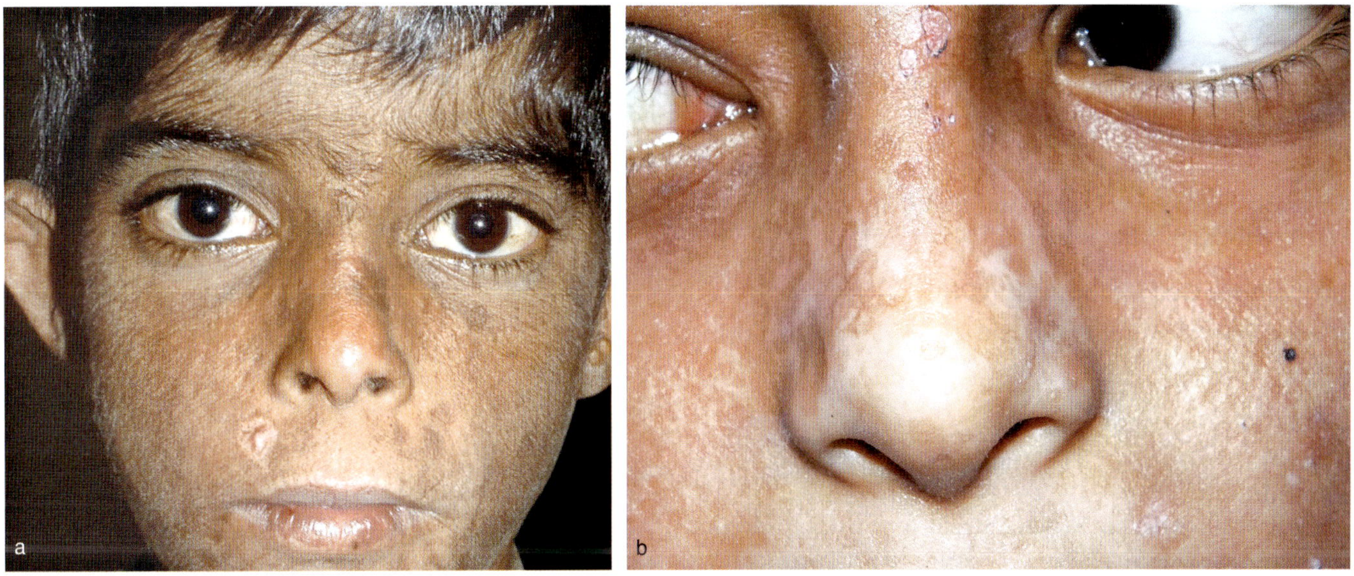

**Fig. 27.81:** Congenital erythropoietic porphyria: (a) Hypertrichosis over the face; (b) Hyperpigmentation, mutilating scarring

**Table 27.24:** Manifestations and treatment of porphyrias

| | *Congenital erythropoietic porphyria* | *Erythropoietic protoporphyria* | *Porphyria cutanea tarda (PCT)* | *Variegate porphyria* |
|---|---|---|---|---|
| Enzyme defect | Uroporphyrinogen synthase III | Ferrochelatase | Uroporphyrinogen decarboxylase | Protoporphyrinogen oxidase |
| Inheritance | Autosomal recessive | Autosomal dominant | Autosomal dominant, if early onset | Autosomal dominant |
| Onset | Soon after birth | Infancy or early childhood | Childhood | Post-pubertal |
| Cutaneous manifestations | Severe photo-sensitivity. Blisters on photo exposed areas, mutilation. Hypertrichosis conspicuous | Burning, edema and urticaria on sun exposure. Thickening of skin and superficial scarring | Blisters and fragility of skin on photo exposed areas. Skin thickened, sclerodermoid and scarred. Hypertrichosis conspicuous | Some patients asymptomatic, others have only cutaneous manifestations, while some have both manifestations. Skin involvement like that in PCT |
| Associated features | Brown teeth, show fluorescence under Wood's lamp<br>Hemolytic anemia | Gallstones<br>Liver disease, sometime fatal | | Abdominal pain<br>Neuropsychiatric symptoms |
| Urine | Red colored urine (also fluorescent) | Normal color | Pink (also fluorescent) | Red colored urine during acute attacks |
| Investigations | Estimation of porphyrins in blood, urine and stool | | | |
| Treatment | Bone marrow transplantation | Beta carotene | Blood letting and small dose of chloroquine | Avoiding triggers |

*The skin is not affected in patients with acute intermittent porphyria

### Mastocytoses

#### *Etiology*

Mastocytoses are a heterogeneous group of diseases characterized by localized or diffuse accumulation of clonal mast cells in the skin and/or in internal organs.

Urticaria pigmentosa is the most common variant (70–90%) of childhood mastocytosis. It may be seen at birth or appear in the first year of life and is characterized by itchy multiple, discrete, yellowish-brown hyperpigmented macules and slightly elevated plaques in a generalized distribution with a truncal predominance (Fig. 27.82). Dermographism is present in one-third of patients and in the first 2 years, pathognomonic Darier's sign may be present.

Diagnosis is confirmed with histological and immunohistochemical evaluation of skin biopsy.

Treatment is directed at alleviation of symptoms (pruritus) with antihistamines and/or disodium cromoglycate. Systemic corticosteroid and oral PUVA are helpful in the cases with systemic symptoms.

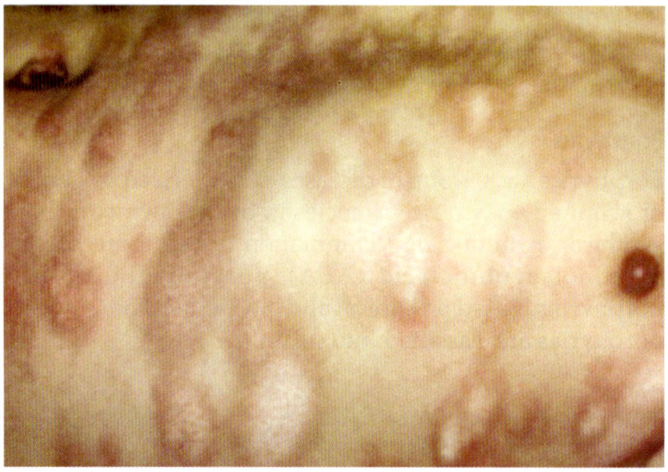

**Fig. 27.82:** Urticaria pigmentosa: Multiple, discrete, yellow-brown hyperpigmented plaques over the chest and abdomen

### Langerhans Cell Histiocytosis (LCH)

It is a multi-system infiltration with proliferating Langerhans cells.

#### *Classification*

Several subsets of LCH with overlapping features are recognized:

- *Letterer-Siwe disease* is generalized form, which occurs predominantly in children <2 years.
- *Hand-Schüller-Christian syndrome* is chronic, multifocal form, with peak onset in children aged 2–10 years.
- *Eosinophilic granuloma* is localized form, seen in children aged 5–15 years.

Letterer-Siwe disease is characterized by intractable 'seborrheic dermatitis-like' lesions with scaly/crusted yellowish reddish-brown (sometimes hemorrhagic) infiltrated papules over scalp and trunk (Fig. 27.83). Systemic manifestations include fever, anemia, diarrhea, thrombocytopenia, hepatosplenomegaly, lymphadenopathy and skeletal lesions.

Skin biopsy confirms the diagnosis. Systemic chemotherapy is indicated in children with disseminated multi-system involvement.

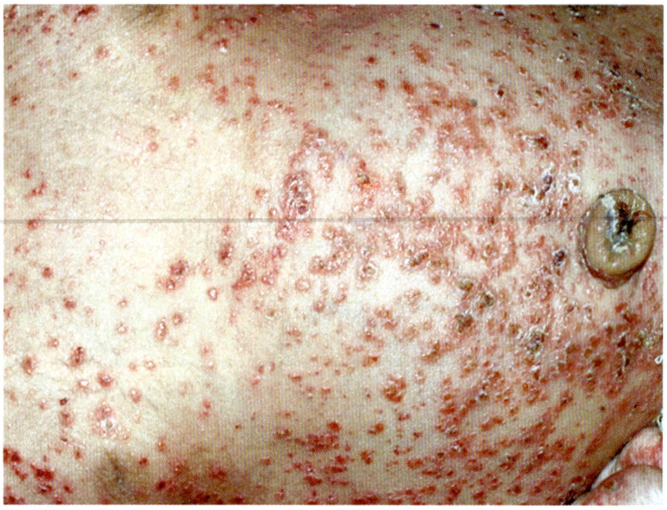

**Fig. 27.83:** Langerhans cell histiocytosis: Multiple, small, erythematous, discrete, crusted papules over the chest and abdomen

### Suggested Reading


1. Khanna N. Illustrated Synopsis of Dermatology and Sexually Transmitted Diseases. 5th edn. Elsevier, New Delhi, 2016.
2. Khanna N, Saurabh S. Bhutani's Color Atlas of Dermatology, 6th edn. Jaypee, New Delhi, 2015.

Chapter

28

# Poisonings, Injuries and Accidents

❍ Jhuma Sankar

Nearly 90% of childhood injuries are unintentional or accidental. Injuries account for 6–10% of all childhood deaths. A significant proportion of these children could be saved, if appropriate injury prevention measures were applied. Road traffic crashes, falls, drowning, burns and poisoning are the leading causes of child death from injuries. Firearm-related injuries and motor vehicle crashes are one of the chief causes of child mortality in North America. The following is a global resource on intentional and unintentional injury and its prevention: *www.who.int/news-room/fact-sheets/detail/injuries-and-violence*

## ROAD TRAFFIC ACCIDENTS AND FALLS

Road traffic crashes are the leading cause of death among children aged 10 to 19 years and account for about 30% of all injury-related deaths among children. Falls account for a significant proportion of visits by children to hospital emergencies. Seat-belts and child-restraints, helmets, pedestrian lanes, daytime running lights for vehicles, speed limits, laws against drinking alcohol and driving are among the successful interventions to prevent road traffic injuries. Severe falls can be avoided by changes in architectural designs, and specially designed child products and playground equipment.

### Factors Predisposing Children to Trauma

Factors including small physical size, less developed characteristics including sensory abilities, inability to identify danger signs and risk-taking impulsive behavior predispose children to road traffic accidents.

Children have a pliable skeleton with less fat and more elastic connective tissue, protecting tightly packed abdominal and thoracic structures. The impact of trauma is transmitted widely through the body resulting in multisystem injuries. Early recognition and aggressive management of emergencies like airway obstruction, hemorrhage including intra-abdominal and intracranial hemorrhages improve survival rates after major trauma. Subtle changes in heart rate and peripheral perfusion must be looked for, as these are signs of impending cardiorespiratory failure. Hypotension is a late sign of shock and blood pressure may remain normal despite 25–30% blood loss (Table 28.1).

Blunt injury is common compared to penetrating injury. Common visceral injuries include contusions, laceration or hematoma of liver, spleen, lungs as well as pneumothorax, rib fractures and gastrointestinal tract injury. Head injuries, alone alone or in association with multiple system injuries, are the most severe and cause most deaths.

**Table 28.1:** Systemic response to blood loss in children

| *System* | *Mild blood loss (<30%)* | *Moderate blood loss (30–45%)* | *Severe blood loss (>45%)* |
|---|---|---|---|
| Cardiovascular | Increased heart rate, weak peripheral pulses, normal systolic blood pressure, normal pulse pressure | Markedly increased heart rate, weak central pulses, absent peripheral pulses, low normal systolic pressure, narrow pulse pressure | Tachycardia followed by bradycardia, weak or absent central pulses, hypotension, narrow pulse pressure |
| CNS | Anxiety, irritability, confusion | Lethargy, minimal response to pain | Coma |
| Skin | Cool, mottled, prolonged capillary refill | Cyanotic, markedly prolonged capillary refill | Pale and cold |
| Urine output | Low | Negligible | None |

### Management

Children need to be managed in a calm, child-friendly environment, preferably in the presence of a parent or guardian. Initial management during 'the golden hour' in pediatric emergency includes primary survey and resuscitation by a well-organized team. The goal of the primary survey is to find and attend to immediate life- threatening conditions. It starts at the injury scene and aims to maintain a patent airway, provide adequate breathing, circulatory support, and to assess major neurologic disability. All patients should receive supplemental oxygen preferably with non-rebreathing mask (*see* Chapter 29).

*Disability:* A rapid neurological examination is carried out to assess level of sensorium with Glasgow Coma Scale and pupillary responses, alteration of which may indicate traumatic brain injury, hypoxemia or cerebral hypoperfusion. Various scores have been used to identify children at high risk of mortality of which the Pediatric Trauma Score is widely used; score ≤6 significantly predicts mortality and morbidity (Table 28.2).

*Secondary survey* includes assessment as per the mnemonic, "SAMPLE" (symptoms, allergies, medications, past illness, last meal, and events leading to the illness) and head to toe examination to identify intrathoracic, intra-abdominal, and skeletal or skull injuries. Continued resuscitation and reassessment should proceed simultaneously. Radiologic examination involves use of X-ray, ultrasonography and CT scan to define anatomy and abnormalities. Focused assessment by sonography in trauma (FAST) may be useful in detecting intra-abdominal bleeding that can be performed serially at the bedside.

*Management* of injuries requires a multidisciplinary team involving pediatric emergency physicians, anesthetists, surgeons, orthopedician, pediatric intensivists and trained nursing personnel. Life-threatening chest injuries, e.g. tension pneumothorax, flail chest, massive hemothorax and cardiac tamponade should be rapidly identified and managed. Abdominal blunt injury may result in contusions, hematomas or laceration of solid organs. Suitable analgesic medication is titrated to alleviate pain and anxiety. Availability of emergency medical services, transport systems and advanced trauma facilities has resulted in significant reduction in accident-related mortality.

## BURNS, ELECTRICAL AND INHALATIONAL INJURIES

Approximately 10% of all unintentional injury-related deaths are due to fire-related burns as per a WHO estimation. Compared to adults, children are at higher risk of death from burns. Skin, the largest organ of the body, insulates and prevents heat and moisture loss and protects from invasion by harmful environmental microbes. Loss of integrity of the skin exposes the body to microorganisms, hypothermia and loss of body fluids. Of all types of burns, fire-related burns are the commonest, followed by scalds and electrical burns. Fireworks are a seasonal injury and over 40% of those injured by fireworks are children younger than 15 years. Prevention of child labor in firearm manufacturing units and strict legislative action have helped prevent firework-related injury in our country. Parental supervision of use of fireworks and community restriction on certain types of fireworks may further reduce these injuries. Children should use flame retardant or nonflammable fabrics to prevent burns.

Children with severe burns often have associated traumatic injuries which might be missed because of edema and charring nature of the burn. Electrical injuries can occur from direct contact or by an arc such as a lightning strike. Direct contact often has entry and exit site wound. The extent of injury depends on the voltage of current, and course through the body. Current passing in the region of the heart can cause arrhythmias and death. Tissues with high resistance like bone and tendons convert electrical energy into thermal energy and sustain more damage. Inhalation injury, associated with large burns, includes upper airway direct thermal injury, chemical pneumonitis from harmful chemicals and systemic poisoning from inhalation of cyanide and carbon monoxide.

### Classification of Burns

Thermal burns may be scalds (caused by hot liquid or steam), contact burns (contact with hot objects), flame burns, chemical burns (exposed to strong acids or alkalis) or electrical. Based on depth, burns are classified as:

1. *First degree or superficial burns* is confined to the epidermis. Characterized as erythematous, painful and dry burns. They heal within a week without scar.
2. *Second degree or partial thickness burns* involve part of the dermis, and are characterized by erythematous, moist and painful burns. (a) *Superficial:* Takes less than 3 weeks

**Table 28.2:** Pediatric Trauma Score

| *Component* | *+2* | *+1* | *–1* |
|---|---|---|---|
| Size | >20 kg | 10–20 kg | <10 kg |
| Airway | Normal | Maintainable | Not maintainable |
| Systolic BP | ≤90 mm Hg | 50–90 mm Hg | <50 mm Hg |
| Central nervous system | Awake | Obtunded, coma | Coma, decerebrate |
| Skeletal | None | Close fracture | Open or multiple fractures |
| Cutaneous | None visible | Contusion, abrasion, laceration <7 cm not through fascia | Tissue loss, any gunshot wound or stab wound through fascia |

to heal; (b) *Deep:* Takes more than 3 weeks to heal and leaves scar.

3. *Third degree or full thickness burns* damage the full thickness of dermis. These are characterized as leathery, dry and insensate burn. They cannot regenerate themselves without grafting.

The "rule of nines" for calculating the surface area of burn is not applicable to children <15-year-old. The *Lund and Browder chart* can be used for the same. A practical approach is to consider the child's palm together with fingers as 1% of total body surface area (TBSA). The risk of mortality from burns involving 30% of body surface area is ~50% which increases to ~100% when more than 50% BSA is involved (Fig. 28.1).

### First Aid

*Fire injuries:* At the scene of fire, the child should be wrapped with a blanket or coat; attempt should be made to extinguish the flames by rolling the victim on the ground. Running with clothes on fire should be avoided. The victim is rescued to a safe airy place away from the fire to prevent exposure to gases like carbon monoxide and cyanide. In the case of minor burns or scalds, pour cold water, apply cold-water soaks or submerge the burned portion immediately in cold water. Application of grease, soda, oil, powder, butter, toothpaste or herbs should be avoided. The wound should be covered with clean sheets of sterile dressing and the patient wrapped in a blanket or foil. Management requires an assessment of the extent of injury, including surface area, depth and cause of burn.

*Electrical injuries:* The power supply should be switched off. Using a nonconductor material (dry wooden stick or dry cotton clothes), the victim is pulled from the electric source. The surface injury may be smaller and is often not indicative of the extent of injury to deeper tissues. Children should be monitored for arrhythmias, ongoing myolysis, and secondary organ dysfunction.

*Inhalational injury:* Children with inhalation injury may require to be intubated and provided supportive ventilation. Pneumonitis peaks after 3–5 days of injury. High blood levels of carboxyhemoglobin suggest carbon monoxide poisoning. Inhalation of 100% oxygen shortens the elimination half life of carbon monoxide from 4 hours to 40 minutes, and is thus recommended. Cyanide poisoning can occur when significant quantities of plastics are burned. The antidote, hydroxycobalamin, infused at a dose of 70 mg/kg IV, binds with cyanide forming cyanocobalamin that is stable and excreted in urine. *Amyl nitrite and sodium nitrite may induce methemoglobinemia and are not recommended.*

### Hospitalization

Minor burns can be treated at home with topical ointments. Indications for inpatient care include: (i) Third-degree burns at any age group; (ii) second-degree burns involving more than 10% TBSA; (iii) burn injuries involving the face, hands



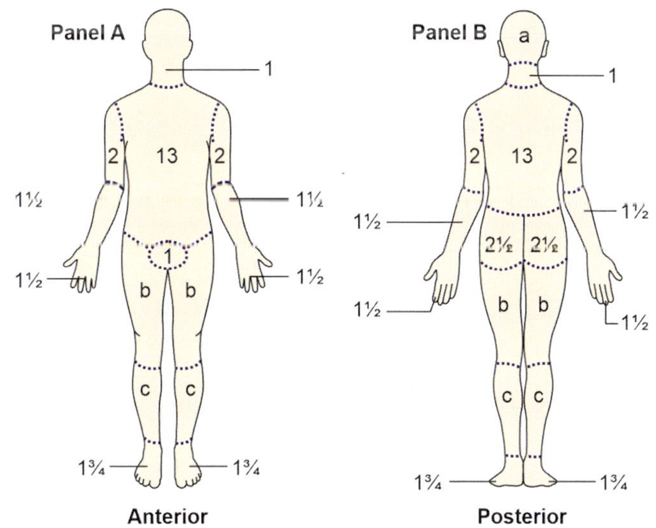


**Fig. 28.1:** Lund and Browder diagram for estimating burns. Panel A and Panel B may be used to calculate relative percentage of body surface areas (%BSA) affected by burns. The numbers indicate the percentage BSA contributed by the body part except for areas indicated by the letters a, b and c, indicating areas of head, thighs, and legs, respectively. The calculation for burn areas involving areas a, b and c are provided in Table 28.3 below.

**Table 28.3:** Guide to calculate the percentage BSA of burn when burns involve head (a), thigh (b) and leg (c)

| *Age* | *0 yr* | *1 yr* | *5 yr* | *10 yr* | *15 yr* |
|---|---|---|---|---|---|
| Front or back half | % | % | % | % | % |
| 'a' (1/ 2 of head) | 9½ | 8½ | 6½ | 5½ | 4½ |
| 'b' ( 1/2 of thigh) | 2¾ | 3¼ | 4 | 4¼ | 4½ |
| 'c' (1/2 of leg) | 2½ | 2½ | 2¾ | 3 | 3¼ |

**Example of calculation of % burns:** If a 5-year-old child has facial burns, burns in front of right thigh and leg, the % burns would be calculated as follows: 6½% for face + 4% for half of thigh +2¾% for half of leg = 13.25%

or genital areas; (iv) electrical burns, chemical burns and inhalational injury; and (v) burn patients with concomitant trauma.

The goals of resuscitation and early management are: (i) Adequate fluid replacement; (ii) correction of hypoxia and ventilatory disturbances; (iii) prevention of hypothermia; (iv) adequate control of pain and anxiety; (v) wound care; (vi) nutrition; and (vii) supportive care. IV access is established with the peripheral cannula and may be performed through burn-injured tissue, if required. Children with >10% burns should have urinary catheterization to titrate fluid resuscitation.

***Fluid replacement:*** The goal of fluid resuscitation is to replenish the fluid loss and to restore and maintain perfusion, tissue oxygen delivery at optimal levels in order to protect the zone of ischemia in burnt tissues without overloading the circulation. Monitoring urine output and a nasogastric tube for continuous suction to prevent emesis and aspiration are essential. The adequacy of fluid resuscitation is based on urine output, which should be maintained above 1 mL/kg/hr in infants and young children. The Parkland formula estimates the amount of fluid to be replaced over 24 hours as follows:

Volume of Ringer lactate (mL) = 4 mL × weight (kg) × % TBSA burn

In addition, maintenance fluid therapy is required. Half of the resuscitation volume should be given in initial 8 hours and the other half in following 16 hours. Potassium is administered after normal kidney function is confirmed. Subsequent fluid management should account for ongoing fluid losses (Fig. 28.2).

***Analgesia:*** Adequate control of pain is an essential component of burn management; opioids are commonly prescribed.

***Wound care and topical therapy:*** Adequate wound care and topical therapy results in healing of first and second-degree burns, without need for skin grafting. The most commonly used topical agents are 0.5% silver sulfadiazine, 0.5% silver nitrate and mafenide acetate. Application of silver sulfadiazine is painless, has a soothing effect and it restricts fluid and heat loss from burn surface. However, it can cause skin rash, leukopenia, and thrombocytopenia.

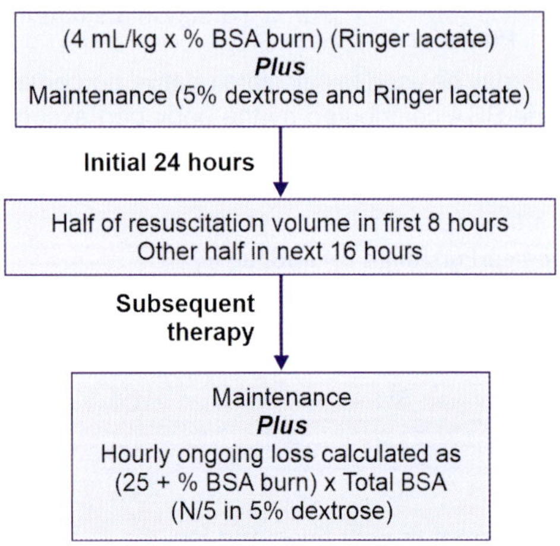


**Fig. 28.2:** Outline of fluid resuscitation in burns

Silver nitrate is not an effective antibacterial agent because of poor penetration of the burn eschar. The medication can cause hyponatremia, hypokalemia, hypochloremia and hypocalcemia. Mafenide acetate penetrates the burn eschar effectively, however, its application may be painful and is associated with skin reaction and metabolic acidosis.

Daily dressing changes are required; moist exposed burn ointment (MEBO; an oil-based herbal paste) is promising. Treatment for small, deep second-degree burns has two components: Excising the burn wound before it is infected and covering the excised wound with synthetic or biological wound dressings. For circumferential burns of the chest, abdomen and extremities, decompressive escharotomy need to be performed.

***Nutrition:*** Children with burns have a hypermetabolic state and need high calorie and protein intake for optimal wound healing and survival. Caloric requirement in children with burns is estimated as follows:

- *Infants:* 2100 Cal/m$^2$ + 1000 Cal/m$^2$ burn surface area
- *Children:* 1800 Cal/m$^2$ + 1300 Cal/m$^2$ burn surface area
- *Adolescents:* 1500 Cal/m$^2$ surface area and burn surface area

Adequate protein intake (2–4 g/kg body weight) and supplementation of trace vitamins and minerals are necessary. Whenever feasible, particularly in children with less than 15–20% burns, nutrients are given enterally. Tube feeding is started on the first day of admission with rapid advancement towards intake goals. Parenteral nutrition is considered in children with extensive burns, inhalation injury or prolonged paralytic ileus.

***Supportive measures:*** Assessment of physical abilities and enabling a full range of joint movements by physical and occupational therapy and play therapy is encouraged.

## DROWNING AND NEAR DROWNING

Drowning is an asphyxial death from submersion or immersion in liquid. It is the leading cause of injury-related death for young children under 5 years of age. Drowning rates in low-middle income countries are 6-times higher than in high-income countries. Risk factors for drowning include residence in densely populated areas with large amount of open water, young age, male gender and those with conditions such as epilepsy and autism. While drowning is most frequent in natural bodies like ponds, lakes and rivers, drowning in swimming pools and bathtubs is increasing.

Management includes immediate resuscitation and transfer to a tertiary care facility. In case of death due to drowning, parents need to be provided with psychosocial support, as it is difficult to cope with the unexpected death. Successful interventions to prevent drowning include the use of life jackets, fencing around swimming pools, covering water hazards and prompt first aid.

## CHOKING AND SUFFOCATION

Choking, suffocation and strangulation are important causes of unintentional injuries, especially in infants. Complications include anoxic brain damage and esophageal perforations. Food (chiefly nuts), latex balloons, toys, lids and small containers are commonly involved in choking, while suffocation is commonly seen in a crib, waterbed or with playground equipment.

Ingestion or inhalation of button batteries is dangerous. Most batteries pass through the alimentary tract, but occasionally are impacted in the esophagus or cause gastric erosion. Batteries have also been inserted into the nose. Ingested small coins are usually passed safely but may became impacted and require surgical intervention. Prevention strategies include enforcing regulatory standards for baby and child product design and manufacture, appropriate labeling and parental education.

*Competencies:* **PE27.8; PE27.11; PE27.12; PE27.13; PE27.14; PE27.15**

## POISONING

Children are susceptible to poisoning because of their curious and exploring nature, and propensity to put virtually everything in their mouths. Common poisoning agents in high-income countries include pharmaceuticals, household products and chemicals; in low and middle-income countries, pesticides, kerosene, cleaning agents and pharmaceuticals are commonly involved. Majority of poisonings in children <5 years of age are accidental, while in older children and teenagers, these are largely intentional.

### Clinical Approach to Child with Suspected Poisoning

The initial approach includes stabilization and rapid assessment of the airway, breathing, circulation and mental status. After initial assessment and stabilization of vital signs, general physical and neurological examination is done. Physical examination may show pallor (hemolysis), cyanosis (methemoglobinemia) or icterus (hepatotoxic agents, hemolytic agents). Acidotic breathing suggests poisoning due to alcohols, salicylates or agents causing hypotension, hypoxia or seizures. Tachycardia or tachyarrhythmia suggests overdose of sympathomimetic and anticholinergic agents, while bradycardia and bradyarrhythmia suggest toxicity with digitalis and cholinergic agents. Oral cavity examination may reveal signs of caustic ingestion such as excessive salivation and swallowing difficulties, or indicate a poison by its odor. Characteristic features with commonly reported poisoning agents are shown in Table 28.4.

Often a particular poison produces a constellation of features (toxidromes) involving various organ systems that confirm the likely diagnosis (Table 28.5).

**Table 28.4:** Key clinical features in poisoning

| *Signs and symptoms* | *Toxin* |
|---|---|
| ***Central nervous system*** | |
| Ataxia | Anticonvulsants (phenytoin), alcohols, sedative-hypnotics |
| Coma | Opioids, sedative-hypnotics, anti-convulsants, antidepressants, antipsychotics |
| Seizures | Sympathomimetics, *Ecstasy*, anti-cholinergics |
| ***Eyes*** | |
| Miosis | Opioids, organophosphates |
| Mydriasis | Anticholinergics, sympathomimetics |
| Nystagmus | Phenytoin, alcohol, ketamine, sedative-hypnotics |
| ***Cardiovascular system*** | |
| Tachycardia | Sympathomimetics, anticholinergics, antipsychotics, antidepressants, serotonin syndrome |
| Bradycardia | Beta-blockers, digoxin, organophos-phates, opioids |
| Hypertension | Sympathomimetics, anticholinergics |
| Hypotension | Beta blockers, calcium channel blockers |
| ***Respiratory system*** | |
| Respiratory depression | Opioids, sedative-hypnotics |
| Tachypnea | Salicylates, sympathomimetics |
| ***Gastrointestinal tract*** | |
| Diarrhea | Opioid withdrawal, cholinergics |
| Constipation | Lead intoxication |
| Jaundice | Acetaminophen, carbon tetrachloride |
| ***Cutaneous manifestations*** | |
| Diaphoresis | Cholinergics, sympathomimetics |
| Cyanosis | Methemoglobinemia |
| Alopecia | Arsenic, thallium poisoning |
| ***Oral cavity*** | |
| Salivation | Organophosphates, salicylates |
| Oral burns | Corrosives |
| Gum lines | Lead, mercury, arsenic, bismuth |
| ***Odor*** | |
| Bitter almond | Cyanide |
| Acetone | Isopropyl alcohol, methanol, salicylates |
| Alcohol | Ethanol |
| Garlic | Organophosphates, arsenic, kerosene |

### Laboratory Evaluation

Diagnosis of poisoning is chiefly clinical as quantitative estimation of most toxins is usually not possible or delayed. Laboratory evaluation is used to support the clinical diagnosis. Quantitative estimation of selected agents, such as heavy metals, salicylates, some anticonvulsants, digoxin and paracetamol, is available at the toxicology laboratory at the All India Institute of Medical Sciences, New Delhi as well as a few private centers in the country. Samples for quantitative assessment in a child with suspected poisoning should include vomitus or gastric aspirate, and urine and blood specimens. Simple bedside tests help in management and monitoring of these patients (Table 28.6).

### Management

Emergency cardiorespiratory stabilization is the priority and should precede diagnostic tests. While the patient is being stabilized, a member of the team should contact the *National Poisons Information Centre* (NPIC) at AIIMS, New Delhi which has an emergency helpline available 24 × 7. Based on the information provided, advice on diagnosis and

**Table 28.5:** Common toxidromes

| *Toxin* | *Toxidrome* |
|---|---|
| *Cholinergics* (organophosphates, carbamates) | *Muscarinic effects* (DUMBBELS): Diarrhea; urinary incontinence; miosis; bradycardia; bronchorrhea; emesis; lacrimation; salivation<br>*Nicotinic effects:* Fasciculations, weakness, paralysis; tachycardia, hypertension<br>*Central nervous system effects:* Lethargy, coma; agitation, seizures |
| *Anticholinergics* (atropine, tricyclic antidepressants, antihistaminics) | Delirium, agitation (mad as a hatter)<br>Mydriasis (blind as a bat)<br>Flushing (red as a beet)<br>Hyperthermia (hot as a hare)<br>Dry skin and oral mucosa (dry as bone)<br>Tachycardia, hypertension, urinary incontinence, ileus |
| *Sympathomimetics* (amphetamines, cocaine, ADHD medications) | Agitation, seizures<br>Mydriasis<br>Tachycardia, hypertension<br>Fever, diaphoresis<br>Pallor, cool skin |
| *Opioids* (methadone, morphine, heroin) | Coma, respiratory depression<br>Miosis<br>Bradycardia, hypotension, hypothermia |
| *Sedative hypnotics* (barbiturates, benzodiazepines) | Coma, respiratory depression<br>Arrhythmias, QT prolongation |
| *Serotonin syndrome* (SSRI, lithium, monoamine oxidase inhibitor, linezolid) | Agitation, confusion, coma<br>Hyperthermia, tachycardia, hypertension or hypotension<br>Mydriasis, diaphoresis, neuromuscular excitability |

SSRI selective serotonin receptor inhibitor; ADHD attention deficit hyperactivity disorder

**Table 28.6:** Laboratory clues in poisoning

| *Laboratory abnormality* | *Causative agents* |
|---|---|
| High anion gap metabolic acidosis | Methanol, metformin<br>Uremia<br>Diabetic ketoacidosis<br>Paraldehyde, propylene glycol<br>Isoniazid, iron<br>Lactic acidosis<br>Ethanol, ethylene glycol<br>Salicylates |
| Elevated osmolar gap | Alcohols: Ethanol, methanol, isopropranolol; ethylene glycol |
| Hypoglycemia | Oral hypoglycemics: Sulfonylurea, meglitinides<br>Quinine, unripe Ackee fruit<br>Beta blockers, insulin, ethanol, salicylates |
| Hyperglycemia | Salicylates (early)<br>Calcium channel blockers, caffeine |
| Hypocalcemia | Ethylene glycol, fluoride |
| Rhabdomyolysis | Neuroleptic malignant syndrome, serotonin syndrome, statins |
| Hyperkalemia | Digoxin, beta blockers, alpha agonists |
| *Urine color* | |
| Orange to red-orange | Rifampin, deferoxamine, phenazopyridine, lead and mercury poisoning |
| Pink | Cephalosporins or ampicillin |
| Brown | Chloroquine or carbon tetrachloride |
| Green to blue | Amitriptyline |
| *ECG changes* | |
| Prolonged PR interval | Digoxin, lithium |
| Prolonged QRS complex | Membrane active agents like tricyclic antidepressants |
| Prolonged QTc interval | Some macrolides and antifungals, amiodarone, antipsychotics |
| Radiopaque density | Chloral hydrate, calcium carbonate, heavy metals, iron<br>Phenothiazines, potassium chloride, enteric-coated tablets<br>Dental amalgam |

management is given and the poisoning is recorded in the National Database. Helpline numbers are 1800-116-117; 011-26589391; and 011-26593677.

*http://www.aiims.edu/aiims/departments/pharmacology/NPIC/home.htm*

Principles of management of patients with poisoning include: (i) Initial assessment and rapid stabilization of airway, breathing and circulation (basic life support) and supportive care, (ii) decontamination, (iii) enhancement of excretion, and (iv) administration of antidotes. These are discussed below.

### Basic Life Support

***Airway and breathing:*** Early elective intubation is preferred in patients with high risk of aspiration and progression to respiratory failure. Rapid sequence intubation is preferred, due to potential loss of protective airway reflexes and expectation of a full stomach, with risk for aspiration. Specific indications for intubation include failure to maintain patent airway due to CNS depression or increased secretions; respiratory failure (hypoxemia or hypercapnia) and severe pulmonary edema (salicylates). Establishment of airway may be difficult in children with poisoning due to caustics and upper airway burns and/or angioedema. Adequacy of breathing should be assessed by respiratory efforts, chest excursions, air entry, and oxygen saturation. Mechanical ventilation should be optimized to maintain adequate gas exchange and hemodynamics, taking care to avoid nosocomial infections.

***Circulation:*** Causes for cardiovascular instability in poisoned patients include decreased systemic vascular resistance, myocardial depression (tricyclic antidepressants, calcium channel blockers) and arrhythmias (digoxin, tricyclic antidepressants). Priority is given towards optimization of preload before using vasoactive agents. In hypotensive patients, it should be remembered that patients are often not hypovolemic; aggressive fluid resuscitation can, therefore, lead to fluid overload. If hypotension persists after 1 or 2 standard crystalloid boluses, infusion of a direct acting vasopressor, such as epinephrine and norepinephrine, is preferred. Arrhythmias caused by agents that block fast sodium channels (tricyclic antidepressants) are managed with sodium bicarbonate therapy.

### Supportive Care

The goals of care include post-stabilization care and monitoring for complications and organ dysfunction.

Convulsions may occur due to hypoglycemia, hypoxia, cerebral edema, direct effect of toxin on the central nervous system, and hypo- or hypernatremia. Seizure control is achieved through administration of benzodiazepines (lorazepam 0.1 mg/kg IV, midazolam 0.15 mg/kg IV, rectal diazepam 0.2–0.5 mg/kg/dose). Status epilepticus is managed as per standard protocol.

***Acid–base abnormalities*** are commonly observed with alcohols, salicylates and iron toxicity. The emphasis is directed at the underlying etiology rather than excessive use of sodium bicarbonate.

***Electrolyte and metabolic abnormalities*** are anticipated in poisoning with drugs such as digoxin, beta-blockers, insulin and potassium chloride. Administration of antidotes, if applicable, and correction of the underlying abnormality is important.

***Hypothermia*** is observed in poisoning with narcoleptic agents such as chlorpromazine. Management comprises keeping the patient warm, administering pre-warmed IV/nasogastric fluids and monitoring for complications of hypothermia, e.g. hyperglycemia and disseminated intravascular coagulation.

***Pulmonary edema*** is non-cardiogenic and occurs with substance abuse (heroin, cocaine) or with aspirin overdose. Treatment comprises administration of 100% oxygen and positive pressure ventilation, if required. The use of frusemide and atropine (for organophosphate poisoning) may be helpful.

***Pain*** is common with snake or scorpion bites and with ingestion of corrosives. Analgesics, narcotics (if no respiratory/CNS depression) and local anesthetics are often required.

***Nausea, vomiting and upper GI bleeding*** may be observed with ingestion of corrosives or drugs causing gastric irritation, or due to stress of illness itself. The use of antiemetics, H2 receptor antagonists and proton pump inhibitors should be considered.

### Decontamination or Removal of Unabsorbed Poison

Decontamination is an important step that helps reduce further absorption of the poison. The method varies depending on the type and route of exposure, patient's age, general condition, and the time elapsed since poisoning. However, decontamination should not be routinely employed for every patient.

***Dermal and ocular decontamination:*** Dermal and ocular decontamination begin with removal of any contaminated clothing and particulate matter, followed by flushing of the affected area with tepid water or saline. A minimum of 10–20 minutes of flushing is recommended for most exposures, although some chemicals (e.g. alkaline corrosives) require longer periods of flushing. Dermal decontamination should include thorough cleansing with soap and water especially in case of organophosphate poisoning. Water should *not* be used for decontamination after exposure to highly reactive agents, such as elemental sodium, phosphorus, calcium oxide and titanium tetrachloride.

***Gastrointestinal decontamination:*** GI decontamination strategies are most likely to be effective, if employed within the first hour after an acute ingestion. However, even rapid decontamination with activated charcoal will, at best, bind ~30% of the ingested substance. Of the methods of GI decontamination, only activated charcoal and whole-bowel irrigation (WBI) are of clinical benefit.

***Gastric lavage*** may be employed for patients who arrive within 1-hour of toxin ingestion. Following insertion of a large-bore orogastric tube (preferably 28 Fr in infants and

36 Fr in older children) into the stomach, the gastric contents are aspirated and washed. Child is kept in lateral decubitus position with head end lowered. Contraindications to gastric lavage include unprotected airway, ingestion of corrosive substances or hydrocarbons, and patients at risk for GI perforation or hemorrhage. Complications include pulmonary aspiration, respiratory compromise, mechanical injury or perforation of esophagus, and electrolyte imbalances. There is limited evidence to suggest that its use improves clinical outcome, so gastric lavage should not be considered unless a patient has ingested a potentially life-threatening amount of poison.

***Activated charcoal*** is a potentially useful method of GI decontamination. Charcoal is activated by heating to extreme temperatures, which lead to creation of extensive network of pores, providing large surface area for absorption. Charcoal is most likely to be effective when given within 1 hour of toxin ingestion. It adsorbs almost all toxins, except *common electrolytes, iron, mineral acids or bases, alcohols, cyanide, most solvents, most water insoluble compounds (hydrocarbons), pesticides and lithium*. The dose of activated charcoal is 1 g/kg in children and 50–100 g in adolescents and adults. A patent and stable airway must be ensured before administering activated charcoal. Its use is contraindicated in patients with intestinal obstruction, ileus, peritonitis and corrosive ingestions.

***Whole bowel irrigation*** (WBI) involves instilling large volume of polyethylene glycol electrolyte solution (PEG-ES) rectally or orally to wash out the entire gut. Recommended doses of PEG-ES are 35 mL/kg/hr in children and approximately 1–2 L/hr in adolescents. WBI is particularly useful in decontamination of gut of a child with ingestion of heavy metals, iron, sustained release or enteric-coated tablets and drug packets. Careful attention should be paid to assessment of the airway and abdominal exam before initiating WBI, and it should never be done in a patient without bowel sounds and in those with signs of obstruction or ileus, or without a protected airway. WBI is administered via a nasogastric tube and is continued until the rectal effluent is clear.

***Syrup of ipecac or use of other emetics*** is no longer recommended as the amount of poison removed is highly variable and the outcomes do not seem to improve with administration. Induced emesis is also contraindicated in infants, comatose patients, and in children with corrosive and hydrocarbon ingestion.

***Surgical decontamination:*** Comprises endoscopic removal of toxins in case of ingestion of large quantities of the toxin or substance (body packers) or lethal amounts of heavy metals refractory to WBI.

### Enhancement of Excretion

Enhancing excretion is useful only for a few toxins where prolonged exposure can result in hemodynamic and respiratory compromise or organ failure.

***Urinary alkalinization*** is used for enhancing excretion of weak acids. Alkalinization is accomplished by continuous infusion of sodium bicarbonate, aiming for urine pH of 7.5–8. This procedure is used to enhance excretion of weak acids, e.g. salicylates, isoniazid, phenobarbitone and methotrexate. Sodium bicarbonate is given at a dose of 1–2 mL/kg in one liter of N/5 normal saline and infused at a rate of 0.5 to 1 liter per hour until desired pH is achieved. Serum pH should be closely monitored, since pH >7.5 is potentially dangerous for cellular function.

***Forced diuresis*** in order to ensure urine flow ~5 mL/kg/hr facilitates drug elimination. Brisk diuresis reduces drug concentration in distal tubules and decreases the concentration gradient, reducing chances of reabsorption and enhancing elimination. Diuresis is usually combined with urinary alkalinization.

***Hemodialysis*** is effective in removal of substances having the following properties: (i) Low volume of distribution (<1 L/kg), (ii) low molecular weight, (iii) low degree of protein binding, and (iv) high degree of water solubility. Toxins removed by hemodialysis include barbiturates, carbon tetrachloride, digitalis, ethanol, ethylene glycol, salicylates, theophylline, bromide, lithium and valproic acid. In addition to enhancing elimination, hemodialysis benefits by correcting metabolic and electrolyte abnormalities resulting from ingestion of toxic substances.

***Hemoperfusion*** involves circulating blood through a cartridge with large surface area coated with activated charcoal. Hemoperfusion enables removal of substances with: (i) Low water solubility, (ii) high affinity for the adsorbent, (iii) faster rate of equilibrium between peripheral tissues and blood, and (iv) low affinity for plasma proteins. Toxins eliminated by this technique are carbamazepine, barbiturates and theophylline.

***Hemofiltration*** removes compounds with molecular weight 500 to 40000 RMM, and is used for removal of aminoglycosides, theophylline, iron and lithium.

***Exchange transfusion*** removes poisons affecting the red blood cells, as in methemoglobinemia or arsenic-induced hemolysis.

***Multiple dose activated charcoal*** (MDAC) enhances elimination by two mechanisms, interruption of enterohepatic circulation and gastrointestinal dialysis where intestinal mucosa is used as the dialysis membrane. MDAC is given at a dose of 0.5 g/kg every 4–6 hours, until there is significant decline in serum drug concentrations. Chief complications include bowel obstruction and perforation. The technique is recommended for drugs like carbamazepine, dapsone, phenobarbital, quinine and theophylline.

*IV infusion of intralipid* may be used for sequestering fat-soluble drugs (beta-blockers, calcium channel blockers, tricyclic antidepressants) and reducing their impact on target organs. This therapy has also been used in the setting of local anesthetic toxicity.

### Administration of Specific Antidotes

Antidotes are substances that counteract the effect of poisons, and whenever available, are of immense utility.

However, effective antidotes are not available for majority of poisonings, and symptomatic and supportive

**Table 28.7:** Poisoning agents and their antidotes

| *Toxin* | *Antidote* | *Dosage* |
|---|---|---|
| Acetaminophen | N-acetylcysteine | Oral: 140 mg/kg loading; then 70 mg/kg q4h (for 17 doses) |
| | | IV: 150 mg/kg over 1 hr; then 50 mg/kg over 4 hr; followed by 100 mg/kg over 16 hr |
| Benzodiazepines | Flumazenil | IV: 0.2 mg over 30 sec; if response inadequate, repeat q1 minute to maximum dose of 1 mg |
| Anticholinergics | Physostigmine | IV, IM: 0.02 mg/kg over 5 minutes; may repeat q 5–10 minutes to 2 mg maximum |
| Carbon monoxide | Oxygen | 100% oxygen via non-rebreathing mask or endotracheal tube (if intubated) |
| β Blockers | Glucagon | IV: 0.15 mg/kg bolus; then 0.05–0.15 mg/kg/hr infusion |
| Calcium channel blockers | Insulin | IV: 1 U/kg bolus; followed by infusion 0.5–1 U/kg/hr |
| Digoxin | Digoxin-specific Fab antibodies (Digibind; DigiFab) | 1 vial binds 0.5 mg of digoxin<br>*No of vials required:*<br>• 0.8 × dose of digoxin ingested (mg) × 2; or<br>• Serum digoxin concentration (ng/mL) × body weight (kg)/100; or<br>• Empirically 1–2 vials (if hemodynamically unstable) or 5 vials (if hemodynamically stable) |
| Methemoglobinemia | Methylene blue, 1% solution | IV: 0.1–0.2 mL/kg (1–2 mg/kg) over 5–10 minutes; may repeat q30–60 minutes |
| Opioids | Naloxone | IV: 0.01–0.1 mg/kg<br>Adolescents, adults: 0.04–2 mg; repeat as needed; or infusion |
| Organophosphates | Atropine<br>Pralidoxime | *see* **Box 28.1** |
| Salicylates | Sodium bicarbonate | IV: 1–2 mEq/kg bolus; followed by continuous infusion |

treatment remains the mainstay of management. Table 28.7 lists antidotes used for management of various poisonings. A list of manufacturers of specific antidotes in India is maintained by the NPIC.

*http://www. aiims.edu/aiims/departments/pharmacology/ NPIC/ masspoisoning.htm*

*Competency:* **PE14.2**

## COMMON POISONINGS

### Hydrocarbon Poisoning

Hydrocarbon ingestions account for ~5% of accidental poisonings and ~25% of deaths related to ingestions in children <5 years globally. Children are often accidental victims as these products are inappropriately stored in unlabeled containers or drinking glasses and are often attractive in color or pleasant smelling, e.g. furniture polishes. Hydrocarbons are categorized into aliphatic (kerosene), aromatic (benzene), halogenated (carbon tetrachloride) and mixed compounds. Aromatic and halogenated compounds have predominant effect on the central nervous system, while aliphatic hydrocarbons predisposes to risk of aspiration and pulmonary symptoms. The chief manifestation of hydrocarbon toxicity is aspiration pneumonitis caused due to inactivation of type II pneumocytes and resulting surfactant deficiency. The propensity of a hydrocarbon to cause aspiration pneumonitis is inversely proportional to its viscosity, and directly proportional to its volatility. Compounds with high volatility, low viscosity and low surface tension (kerosene, gasoline, naphtha) are likely to be aspirated and cause severe lung injury.

#### *Clinical and Laboratory Manifestations*

- *Respiratory system:* Symptoms develop early (within 6 hours) due to aspiration during ingestion or following vomiting. Symptoms vary from mild cough and respiratory distress to ARDS and respiratory failure. The chest radiograph may be normal initially or show infiltrates, pleural effusion, ARDS and pneumatoceles.
- *CNS:* Restlessness, drowsiness, seizures and coma due to hypoxia and acidosis.
- *CVS:* Dysrhythmias with aromatic hydrocarbon abuse.
- Fever and leukocytosis are common, and do not necessarily imply bacterial superinfection.

Recovery usually takes 3 to 8 days, but may be prolonged due to superadded pneumonia.

#### *Treatment*

Treatment is mainly supportive. Evacuation of stomach by gastric lavage or induction of emesis is not recommended because of risk of aspiration. Cautious evacuation of gastric contents is recommended in patients with poisoning by products contaminated by pesticides, heavy metals or other toxins. All patients with history of hydrocarbon ingestion should be observed for at least 6 hours irrespective of their clinical status. An approach to a case of hydrocarbon poisoning is shown in Fig. 28.3.

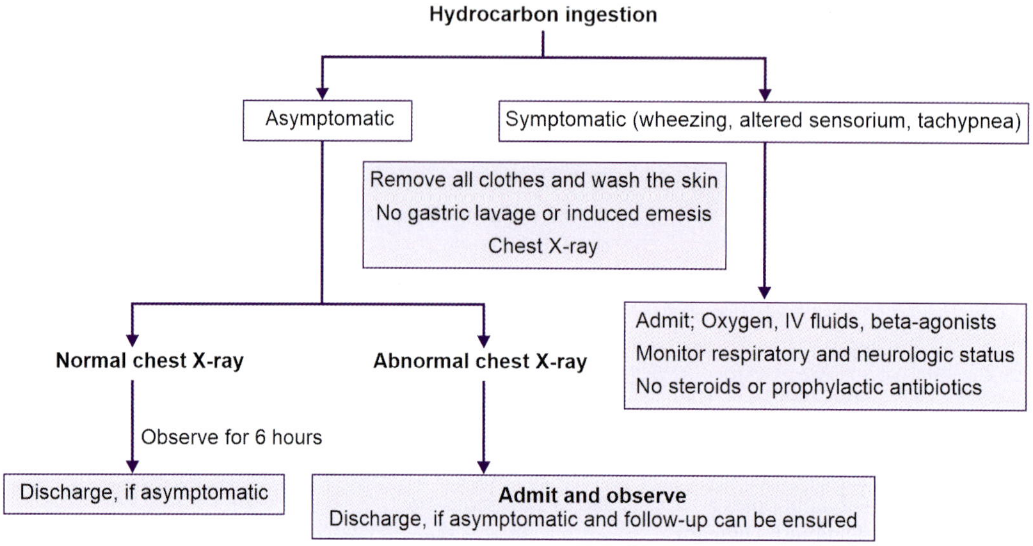


**Fig. 28.3:** Approach to a child with hydrocarbon poisoning

## Corrosive Ingestion

Corrosives are commonly reported agents of poisoning in children, especially in toddlers. Corrosives may be acidic or alkaline in nature. Acids are commonly found in various household or industrial products, batteries, and agents for cleaning purposes. Phenols are used as antiseptic and alkalis may be found in bleaching agents, paint removing agents (sodium hydroxide), soaps and household cleaning products. Alkalis cause liquefaction necrosis while acids cause coagulation necrosis, followed by fibrosis and stricture formation.

### *Clinical and Laboratory Manifestations*

Immediate effects may be burning pain at the site of ingestion or spill, and hoarseness of voice due to laryngeal edema. Excessive salivation, dysphagia, odynophagia, hematemesis and epigastric pain may be presenting features. There is risk of perforation of stomach and esophagus. Respiratory system involvement may manifest as dyspnea, pulmonary edema and chemical pneumonitis. Delayed effects include esophageal, laryngeal stricture and pulmonary fibrosis. Systemic effects include metabolic acidosis, hepatic and renal dysfunction.

Chest and abdominal radiographs or CT scan are done to screen for esophageal or intestinal perforation. Endoscopy is performed within 24-hour of ingestion to assess extent of esophageal injury. The procedure is contraindicated in patients with hemodynamic compromise, peritonitis, mediastinitis and in patients with mild ingestion. Zargar classification of corrosive injury helps grade the severity: Grade 0 normal mucosa; Grade 1 erythema, hyperemia; Grade 2a superficial ulceration, erosion, hemorrhage; Grade 2b findings in 2a plus deep discrete or circumferential ulcers; Grade 3a scattered necrosis; and Grade 3b extensive, circumferential necrosis of mucosa.

### *Management*

Management comprises emergency and supportive care (Fig. 28.4). Nasogastric tube should not be inserted and gastric lavage is contraindicated, as they increase the risk

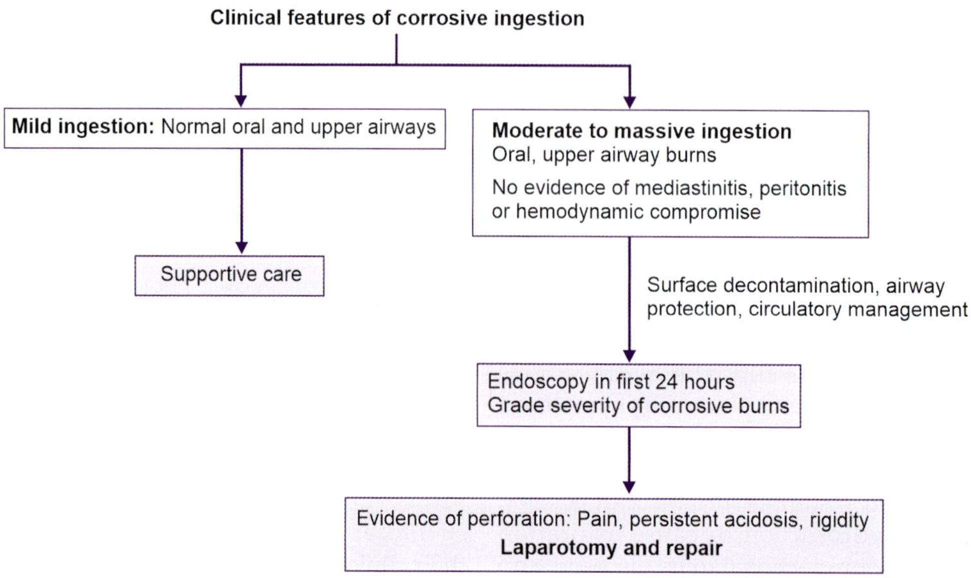


**Fig. 28.4:** Acute management in a child with corrosive ingestion

of injury and perforation. Exceptions are made in patients with mercury chloride, zinc chloride and phenol ingestion, as these compounds are associated with severe systemic toxicity and may be rapidly fatal. Airway protection is a priority as laryngeal edema may rapidly progress over minutes to hours and may cause airway obstruction and death. Elective intubation might be required in such cases, or in presence of respiratory distress or hoarseness of voice. Expertise to perform emergency tracheostomy or cricothyrotomy should be available at the time of elective intubation. There is no role for use of intravenous or nebulized corticosteroids or epinephrine in reducing the need for intubation.

*Long-term management* comprises ensuring nutrition and therapy for strictures. Patients are initially kept nil orally and managed with IV fluids. Endoscopic grading helps in planning nutritional support. While patients with grade 1 and 2a are allowed oral feeds, those with grade 2b or 3a are fed by nasogastric tube that is inserted by endoscopy. Patients with grade 3b injury receive enteral feeding through gastrostomy; some patients require total parenteral nutrition prior to gastrostomy.

Stricture formation is the most important complication. Dilatation therapy and surgery are recommended for prevention and treatment of strictures. Dilatation is done 3–6 weeks after injury, progressively increasing the size of bougies passed over endoscopically placed guidewires. The risk of perforation and aspiration are high. Esophageal strictures refractory to dilatation may be surgically corrected by resection and esophageal bypass.

*Competency:* **PE14.3**

## Organophosphate Poisoning

Organophosphates and carbamates are commonly used pesticide agents and a common cause of poisoning in developing nations. Organophosphates cause toxicity by inactivating acetylcholinesterase, resulting in excess of nicotinic and muscarinic activity in the peripheral and central nervous systems. These agents form an irreversible bond with and permanently inactivate the enzyme. On the other hand, carbamates reversibly bind with the enzyme.

### Clinical Features

The symptoms of organophosphate toxicity depend upon the route, duration of exposure, and the absorbed dose. Acute poisoning is characterized by three phases: Cholinergic crisis, intermediate syndrome and delayed neuropathy. The features of acute cholinergic crisis include diarrhea, urination, miosis, bronchorrhea/bronchospasm, bradycardia, emesis, lacrimation and salivation (DUMBBELS). Some patients show nicotinic features with hypertension, tachycardia and dysrhythmia, muscle weakness, fasciculations, tremors and hypoventilation. Patients with severe poisoning may present with coma and respiratory failure which may progress rapidly. While recovering from cholinergic crisis, some patients may develop respiratory failure (intermediate syndrome). Late complications include delayed polyneuropathy and a range of chronic neuropsychiatric symptoms.

### Laboratory Manifestations

The diagnosis of organophosphate poisoning is based on characteristic clinical signs, smell of the organophosphate compounds, and reduced butyrylcholinesterase in plasma or acetylcholinesterase activity in blood. The major differential diagnosis is carbamate poisoning, which is clinically indistinguishable.

*Cholinesterase assays:* There are two types of cholinesterases, acetylcholinesterase and butyrylcholinesterase; values <10% normal of either of the enzymes indicate severe poisoning. Emergency treatment should not be delayed while awaiting results of the enzyme assays.

### Treatment

Management of organophosphate toxicity involves dermal and ocular decontamination and expeditious administration of two available antidotes, atropine (reverses muscarinic effects) and pralidoxime aldoxime methiodide (PAM), which facilitates reactivation of acetylcholinesterase. A stepwise approach to treatment of organophosphate poisoning is described in **Box 28.1**.

Pralidoxime is not administered in patients with carbamate toxicity, since patients usually recover within 24-hour with or without treatment. Since organophosphate and carbamate poisoning are clinically indistinguishable, the initial therapy should be for the former poisoning. Since succinylcholine is metabolized by similar cholinesterase enzymes, its use should be avoided during rapid sequence intubation.

**Box 28.1: Treatment of Organophosphate Poisoning**

1. Check airway, breathing, circulation. Provide 100% oxygen and mechanical ventilation, as indicated.
2. IV access; administer IV fluids and atropine (0.02 mg/kg/dose as bolus). Record pupil size, sweat, pulse rate and blood pressure after first dose.
3. Pralidoxime (PAM, 25 mg/kg) IV over 20–30 minutes; then infusion at 10–20 mg/kg/hr in saline.
4. Repeat atropine (0.05 mg/kg/dose) after 5 minutes, if no improvement after first dose. Repeat boluses until heart rate is appropriate for age, systolic blood pressure >5th centile and chest is clear.
5. Once patient is stable, start infusion of atropine at 10–20% of the cumulative bolus doses administered.
6. Features of atropine toxicity: Stop infusion; wait 30 minutes; restart infusion at low doses.
7. Continue PAM infusion till atropine is no longer required for 12–24 hours and patient is extubated.
8. If tidal volume <6 mL/kg while weaning from mechanical ventilation (pressure support mode), continue to ventilate.
9. Sedation with benzodiazepines to combat atropine-induced agitation.
10. If features of cholinergic crisis recur, treat as above with PAM and atropine.

Competency: **PE14.4**

## Acetaminophen (Paracetamol)

Acetaminophen is a widely used analgesic and antipyretic agent. Acetaminophen toxicity is the most common cause of acute liver failure in the Western world. Acetaminophen toxicity results from formation of highly reactive metabolite, N-acetyl-p-benzoquinoneimine (NAPQI). NAPQI is normally detoxified by glutathione, but overdose of paracetamol leads to depletion of glutathione stores. Free NAPQI combines with hepatic macromolecules to produce hepatocellular necrosis. The toxic dose of acetaminophen in children is >200 mg/kg.

### Manifestations

The clinical manifestations of acetaminophen intoxication are described in four stages **(Table 28.8)**. Patients either recover completely or progress to fulminant hepatic failure.

### Treatment

The initial management of paracetamol overdose comprises gastric lavage within 4 hours of ingestion, and therapy with its antidote, *N-acetylcysteine* (NAC). NAC, a precursor for glutathione synthesis, reduces the incidence of hepatotoxicity, if administered promptly. A single acetaminophen blood level obtained after 4 hours of ingestion and 4 hourly thereafter plotted on the Rumack-Matthew nomogram **(Fig. 28.5)** is used to decide treatment. The normal therapeutic level is 10–20 μg/mL. The nomogram predicts the risk of hepatotoxicity at a single point in time, and thus cannot predict hepatic failure during the illness or patient death. It cannot be used for multiple doses of paracetamol or after 24 hours of ingestion, and is not useful for associated ingestion with opioid or anticholinergic agents. NAC can be administered orally or intravenously **(Table 28.7)**.

King's College criteria for acetaminophen toxicity are used for deciding referral for liver transplantation: (i) Acidemia (serum pH <7.3) after adequate fluid resuscitation, (ii) coagulopathy (INR >6), (iii) renal dysfunction (creatinine >3.4 mg/dL), and (iv) grade III or IV hepatic encephalopathy. The degree of transaminase elevation does not determine the need for liver transplantation.

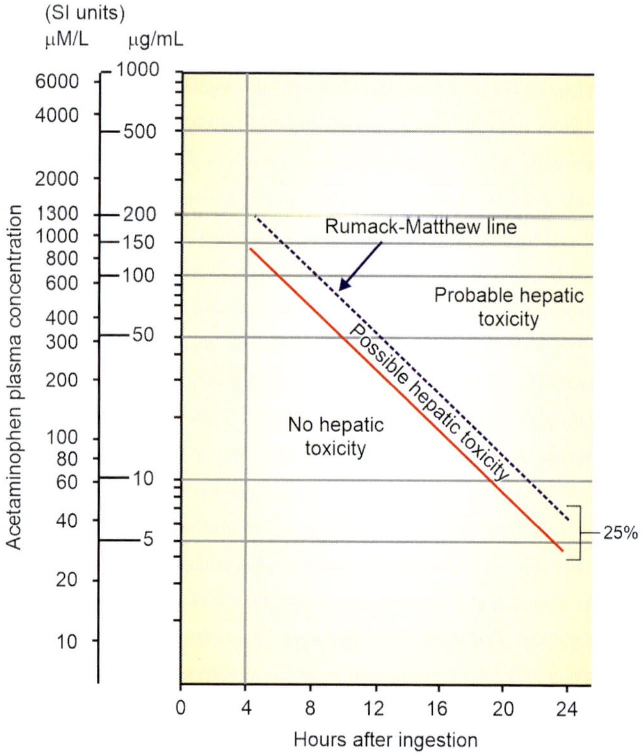


**Fig. 28.5:** Rumack-Matthew nomogram. The treatment-line is plotted 25% below the Rumack-Matthew line to allow for errors in blood assays and estimated time from ingestion of an overdose. N-acetylcysteine is administered if acetaminophen levels are above the solid line

## Methemoglobinemia

Methemoglobinemia is a condition where iron (within hemoglobin) is oxidized from ferrous ($Fe^{2+}$) to ferric ($Fe^{3+}$) state, resulting in inability to transport oxygen to the tissues. The physiologic level of MetHb is <1% of the total hemoglobin concentration. MetHb is reduced to hemoglobin by cytochrome b5, nicotinamide adenine dinucleotide, ascorbic acid, glucose-6-phosphate dehydrogenase (G6PD), and glutathione reduction enzymes. *Methemoglobinemia* occurs when the capacity of these mechanisms is overwhelmed by intake of various drugs and toxins that cause an oxidative stress (e.g. lidocaine, prilocaine, antimalarials, pyridium, sulfonamides and metoclopramide). It can be due to hereditary or acquired causes. *Acute methemoglobinemia* may be life-threatening when MetHb >50% of total circulating hemoglobin.

### Clinical and Laboratory Manifestations

Clinical features range from asymptomatic with cyanosis to severe anoxic symptoms like lethargy, stupor and seizures. The patient appears cyanosed, which does not respond to 100% oxygen. The severity of symptoms depends upon blood MetHb levels; levels >70% result in vascular collapse and death. Arterial blood gas reveals normal $PaO_2$ and low $SpO_2$. Bedside tests, such as the filter paper test, are useful for screening; blood is chocolate-colored and does not turn

**Table 28.8:** Clinical stages of acetaminophen toxicity

| *Stage* | *Time after ingestion* | *Characteristics* |
|---|---|---|
| 1 | 12–24 hours | Asymptomatic; nausea and vomiting |
| 2 | 24–48 hours | Resolution of earlier symptoms; evidence of elevated liver transaminases |
| 3 | 3–5 days | Anorexia, nausea, vomiting; multiorgan dysfunction; peak transaminase elevation |
| 4 | 4–14 days | Recovery phase with resolution of clinical symptoms and improvement in hepatic functions |

red on exposure to oxygen. The diagnosis is confirmed by multiple wavelength co-oximetry, which also gives MetHb levels in blood.

#### Treatment

Management comprises supportive care and administration of methylene blue, at a dose of 1–2 mg/kg followed by bolus of 25–30 mL normal saline. The dose can be repeated after 1 hr to a maximum of 7 mg/kg over 24 hours; at higher dosage, the oxidizing action of methylene blue exceeds the reducing action of leukomethylene blue. Even after resolution of symptoms, patients should be observed for recurrences. Patients with G6PD deficiency should not receive methylene blue. Other therapies include ascorbic acid, hyperbaric oxygen and exchange transfusions.

### Lead Poisoning

Lead poisoning is one of the most common diseases due to chronic exposure to an environmental toxin. Indian children account for one-third of the 800 million children suffering from lead poisoning globally. A blood lead level (BLL) >5 µg/dL is considered toxic; children in more than 23 states in our cuntry show average levels exceeding this cut-off.

Lead poisoning is characterized by fatigue, recurrent abdominal pain, vomiting, constipation or diarrhea, anorexia, anemia, a dark line along the gums, and weakness of limbs. Patients show anemia, hypertension, raised intracranial pressure, kidney dysfunction and toxicity to the immune and reproductive systems. Children below 6 years are especially vulnerable, with profound effects on intelligence, and mental and physical development. Exposure during pregnancy can cause miscarriage, stillbirth, premature birth and low birth weight.

Deaths due to lead poisoning have continued to rise in India, even though lead use in petrol was phased-out by 2000. Other sources of lead exposure include battery recycling, lead mining, smelting, welding, automobile repatriating, pigments, paints, lead crystal glassware, ammunition, ceramic glazes, jewellery and toys, and through some cosmetics, traditional medicines and water (from leaded pipes). The Ministry of Environment and Forest prohibits the manufacture and trade of household and decorative paints containing lead or lead compounds in excess of 90 parts per million.

#### Diagnosis

The diagnosis is made on venous BLL exceeding 5 µg/dL. Patients with BLL 10–20 µg/dL require removal from the exposure, repeat testing, and follow-up. There is microcytic anemia, and raised levels of free erythrocyte protoporphyrin, uric acid and transaminases; red cells show basophilic stippling. Dense metaphyseal bands may be seen in long bones with chronic poisoning.

#### Therapy

The most important step in treatment is to prevent further exposure to lead. Accurate assessment of environmental and occupational exposure is essential. Modifying children's behavior to decrease hand-to-mouth activity is also beneficial. The diet should be adequate in energy and replete in calcium, zinc, and iron.

Medical treatments vary depending on the BLL. Simply avoiding exposure to lead might be enough to reduce levels of lead in blood. In more severe cases (BLL >45 µg/dL), chelation therapy is recommended. Such levels also warrant urgent environmental assessment and remediation. BLL >70 µg/dL are considered medical emergencies, regardless of whether neurologic symptoms are present. The risk of encephalopathy is high and urgent treatment is required. Chelation agents contain sulfhydryl groups that bind or chelate lead, and the resulting complex is excreted either by the kidneys or liver. Succimer and penicillamine are given orally, whereas dimercaprol and edetate (EDTA) calcium disodium ($CaNa_2$ EDTA) are administered parenterally.



## ENVENOMATIONS

### Snake Bites

The highest burden of envenomations exists in south and southeast Asia and sub-Saharan Africa. India has the highest number (58,000 annually) of snake bite-related deaths in south Asia. More than one-quarter of these deaths occur in children 5–14-year-old, mostly in rural areas and during the monsoon season. The four most important venomous snakes in India are Indian cobra (*Naja naja*), Indian krait (*Bungarus caeruleus*), Russell viper (*Daboia russelii*) and saw-scaled viper (*Echis carinatus*).

#### Clinical Features

As per WHO, the diagnosis of envenomation is based on one or more of the following: (i) History of snake bite, (ii) presence of fang marks, (iii) local features such as pain and swelling at the site of bite, (iv) systemic manifestations such as spontaneous bleeding or neurotoxicity, or (v) if the dead snake is brought for identification. Systemic manifestations of snake bite depend on the species of snake.

- *Cardiovascular toxicity* is seen with cobra and viper bites and includes hypotension, bradycardia, arrhythmias and pulmonary edema.
- *Hemotoxic features* are seen with viper bites and include bleeding from the site of bite, spontaneous bleeding from gums, epistaxis, tears, intracranial bleeds, melena, hemoptysis, hematuria, and conjunctival and skin bleeds. Cerebral arterial thrombosis is seen with D. *russelii*.
- *Neurotoxic features* include ptosis, external ophthalmoplegia, mydriasis, bulbar and respiratory paralysis and seen with cobra and krait bites.
- *Nephrotoxicity* is a common manifestation of bites from vipers and sea snakes, and includes features of lower back pain, hematuria, hemoglobinuria, myoglobinuria, oliguria and uremia.
- *Endocrine features* may occur due to infarction of the anterior pituitary following bites of Russell viper.

#### Laboratory Findings

The diagnostic test used to confirm hemotoxic bites is the 20 minutes whole blood clotting time. Absence of clotting at 20 minutes confirms hemotoxic envenomation (Viperine species). Even though the test is useful to detect hemotoxic species, treatment with snake anti-venom (SAV) should be based on clinical assessment.

Other studies such as hemoglobin, hematocrit, platelet and leukocyte count, peripheral smear, muscle and liver enzymes, electrolytes and venous blood gases, and urinalysis are performed, if indicated.

### Management

The 'National Snakebite Protocol' was developed in 2006 to optimize the management of snake bite victims and to improve outcomes. There is emphasis on the Do's and Don'ts of snake bite (Table 28.9), especially with regard to tourniquet application, prehospital treatment, administration of SAV and management of adverse events associated with its use. Principles of management are as follows.

*Immobilization* of the bitten limb retards systemic venom absorption. Walking for >10 minutes is a risk factor for severe envenomation. A stretcher, bicycle, cart or any motor vehicle should be used for transport; if none available, the patient should be carried (e.g. fireman's lift method).

*Assessment:* Detailed clinical assessment and, if possible, species diagnosis should be carried out. One should look for the clues to severe systemic envenomation as described above. The bitten part is examined for edema, tenderness, pulses and the compartment syndrome. Systemic examination includes assessment for spontaneous bleeding from the skin, mucosa and internal organs, and neurologic examination for ptosis, trismus, ophthalmoplegia, pooling of oral secretions, and paradoxical breathing. Some children with neurological symptoms may be unresponsive to painful stimuli, areflexic and show fixed dilated pupils.

*Supportive care* of victims of snake bite is important and determines outcomes. Care comprises ventilation, inotropes, dialysis, administration of blood products, debridement as and when required, maintenance of asepsis, and prevention of nosocomial infections. Patients need to be monitored for complications such as respiratory failure, acute kidney injury, compartment syndrome, tissue necrosis, bleeding into internal organs, refractory shock, secondary infections and endocrine disturbances.

### Specific Management

Snake anti-venom (SAV) is recommended in patients with systemic symptoms and/or extensive local involvement. Local involvement is considered extensive if: (i) there is severe local swelling that crosses a joint, or involves more than half the bitten limb within 48 hours of bite in absence of a tourniquet; (ii) tourniquet is in place, the swelling continues after 1 hour of removal, or (iii) lymph node(s) in the drainage area are tender and enlarged. In patients with systemic envenomation, the clinical features and whole blood clotting time should guide SAV therapy. Contraindications to SAV administration are prior history of severe reaction to horse or sheep serum (TT or anti-rabies) and history of atopic diseases.

In India, polyvalent SAV raised in horses using venom of 4 snakes (Indian cobra; Indian krait; Russell and saw-scaled viper) is used. Since the average amount of venom injected by Russell viper is ~60 mg, and each vial of polyvalent anti-venom neutralizes ~6 mg viper venom, 8–10 vials are initially given irrespective of age. Further doses are based on sequential estimation of whole blood clotting time (persistence of blood incoagulability after 6 hours or bleeding after 1–2 hours), progression of weakness (repeat within 1–2 hours of first dose; no more than 2 doses required) and presence of cardiovascular signs (1–2 hours of first dose). SAV is administered, under supervision, as bolus (1 mL/ minute) without dilution, or IV infusion (diluted in 5–10 mL/kg isotonic fluid) over 1 hr.

Adverse reactions and the number of vials of SAV used should be recorded. All patients should be carefully monitored for two hours after administration of SAV. Early anaphylactoid reactions occur between 10 and 180 minutes of administration; life-threatening anaphylaxis is rare. Some patients show pyrogenic reactions (shaking chills, fever and hypotension) that occur 1–2 hours after infusion or serum sickness (fever, vomiting, diarrhea, lymphadenopathy, nephritis, and encephalopathy) 1–12 days following therapy.

At the earliest sign of a reaction, SAV administration is temporarily suspended. Epinephrine (0.01 mg/kg, 1 in 1000) is given intramuscularly for early anaphylactic and pyrogenic reactions. Subsequently patients should receive treatment with an antihistamine (chlorpheniramine maleate, 0.2 mg/kg IV) and hydrocortisone (2 mg/kg body weight IV). In patients with systemic envenomation, therapy with SAV might require to be given for several days until hemostatic abnormalities persist.

### Outcome

The mortality rates have varied between 5 and 15%. Among survivors, the main cause of permanent disability is local necrosis. Large areas of skin necrosis necessitate debridement and grafting whereas destruction of deep

**Table 28.9:** Do's and Don'ts of snake bite

| *Do's* | *Don'ts* |
|---|---|
| **RIGHT**<br>**R** Reassure patient (only 50% venomous snake bites actually envenomate)<br>**I** Immobilize as in a fractured limb; do not block blood supply<br>**GH** Get to Hospital immediately<br>**T** Tell the doctor of any systemic symptoms, such as ptosis | • Use traditional first aid measures, such as local incisions or pricks, punctures or tattooing at the site of bite, or in the bitten limb<br>• Attempt to suck the venom out of the wound<br>• Use (black) snake stones<br>• Tie tight bands (tourniquets) around bitten limb<br>• Give electric shock<br>• Apply or instill chemicals, herbs or ice packs |

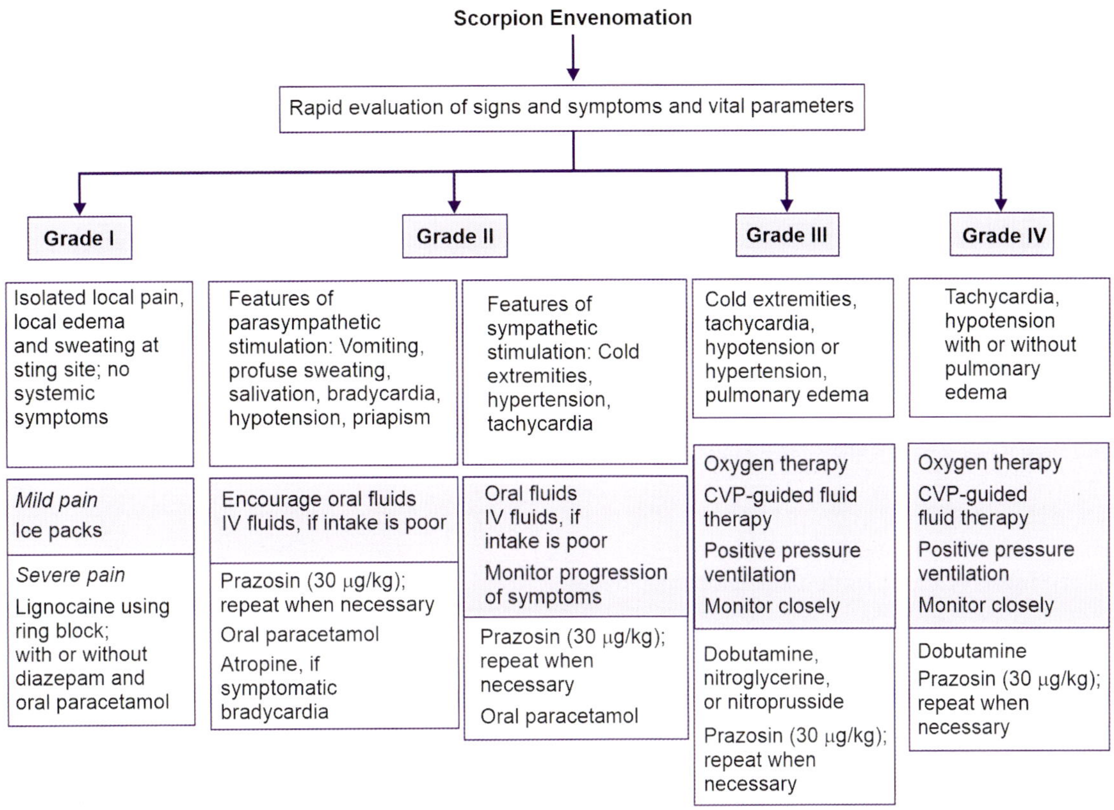


**Fig. 28.6:** Algorithm-based management of children with scorpion envenomation

tissues might require amputation. Cerebral hypoxia from delayed resuscitation and stroke may cause permanent neurological deficits. Some patients with marked hypotension and severe acute kidney injury may not recover and become dialysis dependent; others (Russell viper bite) may show acute hemorrhagic infarction of the pituitary and adrenal glands. Risk factors for adverse outcome in children include young age, vomiting, neurotoxicity, high creatinine, thrombocytopenia, ecchymosis at admission and delayed administration of SAV.

## Scorpion Sting

Scorpion envenomation is common in tropical and subtropical regions of the world. Most cases are reported from Maharashtra, Karnataka, Tamil Nadu, West Bengal and Pondicherry. Of 86 species in India, the *red* (*Mesobuthus tamulus*) and less poisonous *black scorpions* (*Palamnaeus swammerdami*) are implicated in most stings. Cardiac manifestations dominate clinical features in India, while neurologic symptoms are frequent in South Africa and USA. Stings are common during summer months and at night. scorpions sting when roughly handled or trodden. The case fatality rate before use of prazosin was 25–30% and with use of prazosin it has reduced to <1%.

### Clinical Features

The symptoms evolve over 30 minutes to 6 hours and subside within a day or two. Local features include severe pain and paresthesias. Systemic manifestations include a *cholinergic storm* with fever, shivering, sweating, salivation, vomiting, priapism, bradycardia and hypotension. This is followed by adrenergic stimulation, which start at 4 hours and last for 48 hours. Features include tachycardia, hypertension, myocardial dysfunction, arrhythmias, pulmonary edema, shock and hypotension. Complications include encephalopathy, convulsions, aphasia, hemiplegia, cerebral hemorrhage, DIC and respiratory failure (Fig. 28.6).

### Management

Management is directed towards providing symptomatic relief as specific therapy (antivenom) is not available, nor recommended for routine use. Blood samples are taken for electrolytes (hyperkalemia), lipid profile (low serum cholesterol and triglycerides with rise in free fatty acids), and amylase, LDH, and transaminases (all elevated).

Other investigations include chest X-ray, ECG and echocardiography. Myocardial perfusion and neurological abnormalities are identified on nuclear scintigraphy and CT scans, respectively.

***Local measures:*** The site of the sting is cleaned. Relief from pain allays anxiety and avoids myocardial stress. NSAIDs can be used for relief from severe pain. Local ice packs, xylocaine infiltration, dehydroemetine (counterirritant) and streptomycin (neuromuscular blockade) are reported to be useful.

***General measures*** include:

i. Oxygen administration by face mask or nasal cannula in case of respiratory distress, or impending shock.
ii. Frequent monitoring of vital signs, fluid balance, blood levels of electrolytes, pH, liver and kidney functions, and DIC profile.

**Table 28.10:** Do's and Don'ts of injury prevention

| *Do's* | *Don'ts* |
|---|---|
| • Use beds with rails for children aged <6 years<br>• Have safety gates at the top and bottom of the stairs, vertical bars on balconies; fire guard where required<br>• Teach older children how to cross the road safely<br>• Ensure that your child's bicycle is maintained in good condition<br>• Teach the child how to handle tools and mechanical instruments safely<br>• Keep children far away from the stove while cooking<br>• Always turn off the gas after use<br>• Check the temperature of milk before feeding the child<br>• Use electric points of the safe variety so that the child cannot insert a lead pencil or other object through the hole<br>• Keep all poisons in their original containers and not in fruit juice/ colored bottles; keep medicines out of reach<br>• Keep cleaning agents, kerosene and pesticides locked<br>• Keep plastic bags, scarves, ropes, cords out of reach of children | • Leave a small child alone in the house even for a few minutes<br>• Allow children to play on the stairs<br>• Keep the door open when the child is at home<br>• Allow young children to cross the streets alone<br>• Allow doubling on the bicycle<br>• Leave any sharp objects near the vicinity of the child<br>• Leave hot utensils or pans in the kitchen<br>• Allow him/her to ignite fireworks<br>• Drink, or pass hot tea or coffee while holding the infant<br>• Keep electric equipment plugged on when not in use<br>• Give nuts and seeds to infants<br>• Take medicines in front of your child<br>• Leave young children unattended in bath tubs or near swimming pools/ponds/beaches<br>• Leave cupboards, wardrobes, refrigerators unlocked |

28

Essential Pediatrics

iii. Sedation: Diazepam is recommended; long-acting sedatives are avoided.

***Drug therapy:*** Prazosin is the first-line agent in our country because of predominant cardiovascular manifestations. There is limited information on the efficacy and safety of *scorpion antivenom* in children. An algorithm based approach for management is given in Fig. 28.6.

Patients should be hemodynamically stable and show normal sensorium at discharge. Additional criteria for discharge include no respiratory distress and being free of complications.

## INJURY CONTROL

Principles that deserve emphasis in planning injury prevention strategies are as follows:

i. Passive injury prevention, such as automatic locks for medicine cabinets, is preferred over active strategies, e.g. "yuck" stickers on bottles.
ii. Specific instructions, e.g. keep water heater temperature lower than 120°F, are more likely to be followed than general advice, e.g. reduce temperature of hot water tap in your home.
iii. Reinforcement by community wide education programs is more effective than individual education sessions.

Targeted messages for prevention of injuries should be discussed with the parents (Table 28.10).

### Suggested Reading


1. CDC. National action plan for child injury prevention. https://www.cdc.gov/safechild/pdf/national_action_ plan_for_child_injury_prevention-a.pdf.
2. Katz A, Kluger Y. Caustic material ingestion injuries-Paradigm shift in diagnosis and treatment. Health Care Current Reviews 2015; 3:152.
3. World Health Organization. Children and poisoning. http://www.who.int/violence_injury_prevention/child/injury/world_report/Poisoning_english.pdf.
4. World Health Organization. World report on childhood injury prevention. http://apps.who.int/iris/bitstream/10665/43851/1/9789241563574_eng.pdf.

Chapter

29

# Pediatric Critical Care

❍ Nitin Dhochak ❍ Rakesh Lodha

Care for critically ill children has an important role in improving child survival. In tertiary care hospitals, 5–10% of pediatric beds are reserved for intensive care; higher numbers are required, if the hospital has surgical units. In order to optimize resource utilization in resource limited settings, it is useful to understand the indications of admission to PICU (Table 29.1).

The optimal number of beds in a PICU is 6–10. Attention is given to the layout, ensuring 200–250 square feet area per bed, with rapid access to head end for airway management. The unit should have uninterrupted power supply and preferably be air-conditioned. A crash cart having necessary drugs and resuscitation equipment should be available. The unit should have a central monitoring station and space for utilities and storage. The unit should have consistent supply of disposables and medications. The ICU should have access to laboratory facilities, including complete blood counts, glucose and electrolytes, and blood gas analysis that require small sample volumes. Portable X-ray and ultrasonography units are desirable. In addition to the treatment of the primary disorder, it is necessary to ensure nutrition, sedation and effective analgesia and infection control. Adequate communication with the parents is necessary to keep them informed about the condition of their child, and ensure their trust and cooperation.

**Table 29.1:** Indications for admission to the pediatric intensive care unit

| |
|---|
| Hemodynamic instability or shock requiring vasoactive drugs, e.g., septic shock, cardiac arrhythmias, cardiorespiratory arrest |
| Respiratory distress requiring oxygen therapy and/or impending or established respiratory failure requiring mechanical ventilation |
| Altered sensorium due to any cause, including encephalopathy, status epilepticus, raised intracranial pressure |
| Acute hepatic or renal failure and complications |
| Severe metabolic abnormalities, e.g., dyskalemia, dysnatremia, hypoglycemia, diabetic ketoacidosis; acute poisoning |
| Severe infections, e.g., severe malaria, severe pneumonia |
| Procedures: Peritoneal dialysis, exchange transfusion, central venous cannulation |
| Postoperative monitoring |

### Suggested Reading

1. Slusher TM, Kiragu AW, Day LT, et al. Pediatric critical care in resource-limited settings: Overview and lessons learned. Front Pediatr 2018;6:49.

*Competencies:* **PE27.1; PE27.2; PE27.3; PE27.4; PE27.11; PE27.12; PE27.13; PE27.14; PE27.15**

## ASSESSMENT OF A SERIOUSLY ILL CHILD

The initial evaluation of a sick child includes a hands-off assessment by checking appearance (tone, responsiveness), breathing (increased efforts or irregular/gasping), and circulation (pallor, bleeding). If a life-threatening condition is identified, emergency treatment is provided. A sick child who is non-responsive to verbal and physical stimuli should be immediately assessed for breathing efforts (gasping, apneic), and central pulses (present, absent) simultaneously. If the child has abnormal respiration (gasping or not breathing) or has absent central pulses, then child should receive CPR (cardiopulmonary resuscitation) immediately.

After initial evaluation, primary assessment is performed with ABCDE approach—**A:** 'airway assessment'; should categorize the airway as 'clear', 'maintainable' and 'not maintainable'. **B:** 'breathing assessment' and includes respiratory rate and effort, abnormal breath sounds on auscultation and pulse oximetry. **C:** 'circulation assessment' including skin color and temperature, heart rate and rhythm, blood pressure, central and peripheral pulses, capillary refill time and assessment of end organ perfusion by mental status (brain perfusion), and urine output (renal perfusion). **D:** 'disability' that establishes the level of consciousness by AVPU pediatric response scale or Glasgow Coma Scale and pupillary response to light. **E:** 'exposure'

| Table 29.2: Common danger signs |
|---|
| Seizure activity |
| Excessive, inconsolable cry |
| Decreased activity or drowsiness |
| Increased work of breathing |
| Abnormal sound on breathing |
| Apneic episodes or cyanosis |
| Cold extremities (particularly in absence of cold environment) |
| Decrease in the urine output |
| Decreased feeding, bilious vomiting |

where body parts are exposed to look for skin rashes or wounds. Features predictive of a serious illness, particularly in young infants are listed in Table 29.2. The history should focus on the underlying illness. Common investigations include complete blood counts, glucose, electrolytes and arterial blood gases.





## Monitoring

### *Respiratory*

The patient should be observed for respiratory rate and pattern, nasal flaring, use of accessory muscles and color (Table 29.3). Examination is done for symmetry of air entry, breath sounds and presence of stridor, rhonchi and crepitations. Respiratory rate is monitored continuously by monitors. Pulse oximetry allows non-invasive measurement of oxygen saturation. While reliable, some conditions lead to inaccuracies in pulse oximetry, e.g. dyshemoglobinemia (methemoglobin, carbon monoxide poisoning), dyes and pigments (methylene blue), poor peripheral perfusion, increased venous pulsations and interference with external light (phototherapy unit, fluorescent light). Chest radiography and arterial blood gas analyses are performed periodically.

### *Hemodynamic*

Hemodynamic monitoring provides information about circulatory status and perfusion of vital organs. The rate and character of pulse should be examined. Blood pressure can be monitored manually or by oscillometry. In children with shock in PICU, continuous arterial BP monitoring is preferred. The state of microcirculation is assessed by capillary refilling time. Pressure is applied with the index finger or ball of thumb over sternum or forehead in infants and pulp of fingers in older children for 5 seconds to cause blanching and then noting the time for the color to reappear. The normal capillary refill time is 3 seconds or lower; prolongation signifies impairment of microcirculation. Increased core-peripheral temperature gradient >5°C, also indicates hypoperfusion.

Table 29.3: Respiratory rates (RR) and heart rates (HR) at different ages, average (range)

| *Age, years* | *RR, breaths/min* | *HR, beats/min* |
|---|---|---|
| 1 | 30 (22–38) | 120 (80–160) |
| 2 | 25 (17–33) | 110 (80–130) |
| 4 | 23 (17–27) | 100 (80–120) |
| 6 | 21 (15–26) | 100 (75–115) |
| 8 | 20 (15–26) | 90 (70–110) |
| 10 | 18 (15–25) | 90 (70–110) |
| 12 | 18 (14–26) | 85 (65–105) |
| 14 | 17 (15–23) | 80 (60–100) |
| 16 | 17 (12–22) | 75 (55–95) |

Continuous ECG monitoring is necessary in children admitted to the PICU. Central venous pressure (CVP) is monitored by placing a catheter through a large vein into the right atrium; the pressure informs about venous return and preload. Normal right atrial pressure is less than 6 mm Hg. Low CVP in a child with hypotension signifies low intravascular fluid volume. CVP may be increased due to myocardial dysfunction, fluid overload or increased pulmonary artery pressures. Renal perfusion is assessed by monitoring urine output; output <0.5 mL/kg/hr in a child with normal kidneys signifies poor perfusion. Monitoring of the sensorium and neurologic status also gives information about brain perfusion.

## Suggested Reading

1. Bronicki RA, Spenceley NC. Hemodynamic monitoring. In: Nichols DG, Shaffner DH (eds). Roger's Textbook of Pediatric Intensive Care, 5th edn. Lippincott Williams and Wilkins 2016: pp 1120–36.
2. Cheifetz IM, Lee JH, Venkataraman ST. Respiratory monitoring. In: Nichols DG, Shaffner DH (eds). Roger's Textbook of Pediatric Intensive Care, 5th edn. Lippincott Williams and Wilkins 2016: pp 686–709.

*Competencies:* **PE27.16; PE27.17; PE27.18; PE27.19; PE27.28**

# PEDIATRIC BASIC AND ADVANCED LIFE SUPPORT

Cardiopulmonary arrest in children is much less common than adults and usually represents the terminal event of progressive shock or respiratory failure rather than a primary cardiac cause. The major causes in infants and children are respiratory failure, sepsis, neurologic diseases, submersion or drowning, injuries, and sudden infant death syndrome. In contrast to adults, sudden cardiac arrest in children is uncommon. Basic life support (BLS) refers to a protocol of procedures performed in cases of cardiopulmonary arrest to provide cardiopulmonary resuscitation (CPR) with or without devices and bag-mask ventilation till advanced life support (ALS) can be provided. The major objectives of CPR are to preserve vital organs, viability during cardiac arrest and to help return spontaneous circulation.

## Basic Life Support

To maximize survival and intact neurological status in post-resuscitation stage, early recognition of cardiac arrest and strict adherence to the BLS sequence is necessary. BLS includes a series of skills performed sequentially to assess and restore effective ventilation and circulation to the child with respiratory or cardiorespiratory arrest.

Evaluation and interventions in pediatric BLS are performed simultaneously, in the following sequence: (i) Assessment, (ii) circulation, (iii) airway, and (iv) breathing. The sequence Circulation–Airway–Breathing (C–A–B) has been recommended in 2015 update of Pediatric Basic Life Support.

### Assessment

Initial assessment is done to confirm cardiac arrest so that life-saving measures can be begun promptly to enable intact neurologic survival. The combination of unresponsiveness and absent or abnormal breathing most accurately identifies cardiac arrest. Palpation of the pulse for its absence is unreliable as the sole determinant of cardiac arrest. If the victim is unresponsive, not breathing normally, and there are no signs of life, lay rescuers should begin CPR; in such a setting, healthcare providers should begin CPR unless they definitely palpate a pulse within 10 seconds.

### Circulation

CPR should begin with chest compression. Chest compressions are serial rhythmic compressions of the chest that allow blood flow to vital organs (heart, lungs and brain) to keep them viable until ALS (advanced life support) is available. The victim should be laid supine on a hard and flat surface. Adequate chest compression is given by pushing hard to a depth of at least one-third of anteroposterior dimension or approximately 1½ inches (4 cm) in infants and 2 inches (5 cm) in children (but not more than 6 cm). The rate should be 100–120 compressions per minute, allowing full chest recoil and minimizing interruptions in chest compressions. Compression of the xiphoid process should be avoided.

*Chest compression in infants (<1 year)*

***Two-thumb technique:*** The infant's chest is encircled with both hands; fingers are spread around the thorax and the thumbs brought together over the lower half of the sternum (just below intermammary line), avoiding the xiphisternum. The sternum is compressed with the thumbs and the thorax with the fingers for counterpressure. The two-thumb-encircling hands technique is preferred because it produces higher coronary artery perfusion pressure, consistently appropriate depth and force of compression, and may generate higher systolic and diastolic pressures. While one provider should provide chest compressions, the other maintains the airway and provides ventilation at a ratio of 15:2 with as short a pause in compressions as possible. If the rescuer is unable to deliver breathes, the rescuer may continue with chest compressions only; however, one must remember that majority of pediatric cardiac arrests are secondary to hypoxia.

***Two-finger technique:*** If the rescuer is alone or unable to physically encircle the chest, the chest is compressed with two fingers, placing them vertically over the sternum just below the intermammary line ensuring that they are away from xiphoid process. One can use one hand to support the infant's body and head and the other hand to perform chest compression.

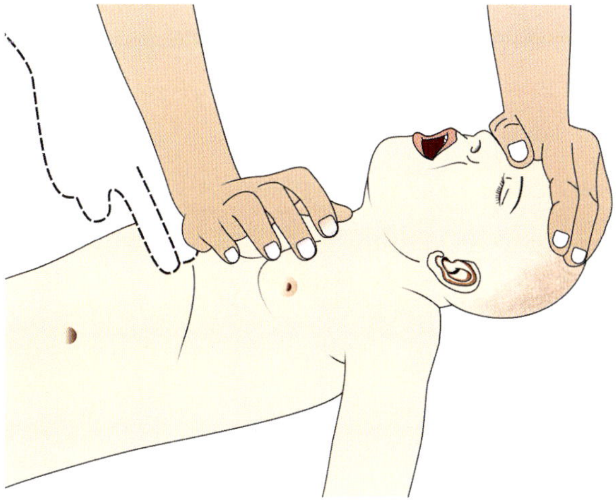

**Fig. 29.1:** Chest compression in a child (1–8-year-old)

*Chest compression technique in the child (1–8 years age):* Figure 29.1 indicates how the heel of one hand should be placed over lower half of sternum, avoiding pressure over xiphoid, and with fingers lifted above the chest wall to prevent compression of rib cage. Rescuer should position him/herself vertically above the victim's chest.

*Large children and >8 years of age:* The two-hand method for chest compression should be used to achieve an adequate depth of compression. This is achieved by placing the heel of one hand over the lower half of sternum and the heel of the other hand over the first hand, interlocking the fingers of both hands, with fingers lifted above the chest wall. External chest compression in children and infants should always be accompanied by rescue breathing. The lay rescuers should use a 30:2 compression-ventilation ratio for all (infant, child and adult) victims. For one healthcare provider, the compression-ventilation ratio should be 30:2 for all age groups and for two rescuers, the compression-ventilation ratio should be 30:2 in adults and 15:2 in infants and children. Once an advanced airway (tracheal tube) is placed, chest compressions should not be interrupted for ventilation. Breaths with advanced airway should be provided at rate range of 1 breath every 2–3 s (20–30 breaths/min).

The victim should be reassessed after 2 minutes. If signs of spontaneous circulation have reappeared, chest compression should be discontinued and only ventilation continued till return of spontaneous breathing.

### Airway

Infants and children are at increased risk of respiratory obstruction and failure compared to adults, for the following reasons: smaller upper airway in comparison to adults; large tongue in relation to oropharynx; smaller and compliant subglottic area more prone for collapse and/or obstruction; relatively compliant chest wall and rib cage; and limited oxygen reserve.

*Position of the victim:* If the child is unresponsive but breathing or signs of life are present, he should be placed on a hard surface in supine position. If head or neck trauma is suspected, head and torso should be moved as a unit, and the neck immobilized.

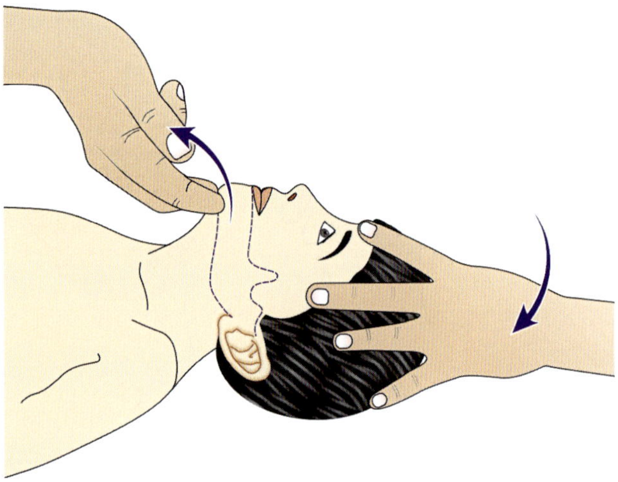

Fig. 29.2: Head-tilt chin-lift maneuver

***Open the airway:*** The tongue is lifted away from the posterior pharynx to keep the airway patent.

i. *Head-tilt chin-lift maneuver* (Fig. 29.2): If the victim is found unresponsive and has signs of life, the airway is opened by tilting the head back and lifting the chin. One hand is placed over the forehead and head is gently tilted back. Simultaneously, the fingers of the other hand are placed on the lower jaw to lift the chin to open the airway. This maneuver should not be used, if there is suspicion of trauma to cervical spine.
ii. *Jaw thrust* (Fig. 29.3): Two or three fingers are placed under each side of lower jaw at its angle to lift the jaw upwards and outwards. This method should be used in trauma patients with suspected cervical spinal injury. This method is not recommended for lay rescuer because it is difficult to learn and perform effectively and safely.

***Foreign body airway obstruction:*** The mouth is opened and examined for presence of foreign body, which is removed, if visible; blind sweeping is not recommended. If the victim is an infant who is responsive and has features of severe airway obstruction, back slap and chest thrust are performed till the foreign body comes out or till the infant becomes unresponsive. If the victim is an older child or adolescent, an abdominal thrust is given by standing behind the victim till the foreign body is expelled out or till the patient becomes unresponsive (Chapter 30).

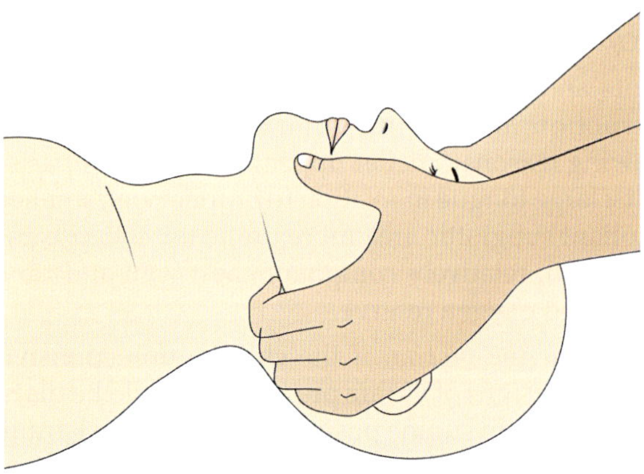

Fig. 29.3: Opening the airway with jaw thrust

If the victim becomes unresponsive, cardiopulmonary resuscitation should be begun with an additional maneuver of checking the airway for the foreign body after giving the chest compression and before breaths are given. Trained healthcare provider should perform a tongue-jaw lift to look for obstructing objects.

### *Breathing*

After opening the airway, one should check for breathing. Periodic gasping, also called *agonal gasps*, is not breathing. If there is effective spontaneous breathing without evidence of trauma, the child is turned to recovery position, which helps maintain a patent airway and prevents aspiration.

***Bag and mask ventilation (BMV):*** BMV remains the preferred technique for emergency ventilation during initial steps of resuscitation. In infants and children for whom BMV is unsuccessful, a laryngeal mask airway placed by appropriately trained providers may be considered for airway or support ventilation. Self-inflating bags are usually adequate in children. Flow inflating bags need oxygen flow and are used in hospitals. For term neonates, infants and children <8 years of age, ventilation bags of volume 450–500 mL should be used to deliver adequate amount of tidal volume. Neonatal size bags (250 mL) may be used in preterm neonates. An adequate amount of tidal volume should be used to cause visible chest rise. Excessive expansion may compromise cardiac output, increasing the chances of regurgitation and air leak. In patients with head injury or cardiac arrest, excessive ventilation may adversely affect neurological outcome.

The self-inflating bag delivers room air unless it is connected to an oxygen source. Pediatric bag-valve device, without a reservoir, if connected to an oxygen inflow of 10 L/min, delivers 30–80% of oxygen to the patient. If used with a reservoir, it may deliver 60–95% of oxygen, with an oxygen inflow of 15 L/min to provide adequate oxygen supply to the reservoir.

## Pediatric Advanced Life Support (PALS)

PALS refers to the assessment and support of pulmonary and circulatory function in the periods before, during and after an arrest. Pediatric chain of survival includes 6 components: (i) Early recognition and prevention of cardiac arrest, (ii) activation of emergency response, (iii) high-quality CPR, (iv) advanced resuscitation, (v) post-arrest care, and (vi) recovery. Algorithm for resuscitation of a child in cardiac arrest based on 2020 AHA guidelines is shown in Fig. 29.4.

***Components of PALS:*** (i) Basic life support; (ii) use of equipment and techniques to establish and maintain effective oxygenation, ventilation and perfusion; (iii) clinical and ECG monitoring with arrhythmia detection and management; (iv) establishing and maintaining vascular access; (v) identification and treatment of reversible causes of cardiopulmonary arrest; (vi) emergency treatment of patients with cardiac and respiratory arrest; and (vii) treating patients with trauma, shock, respiratory failure or other pre-arrest conditions.

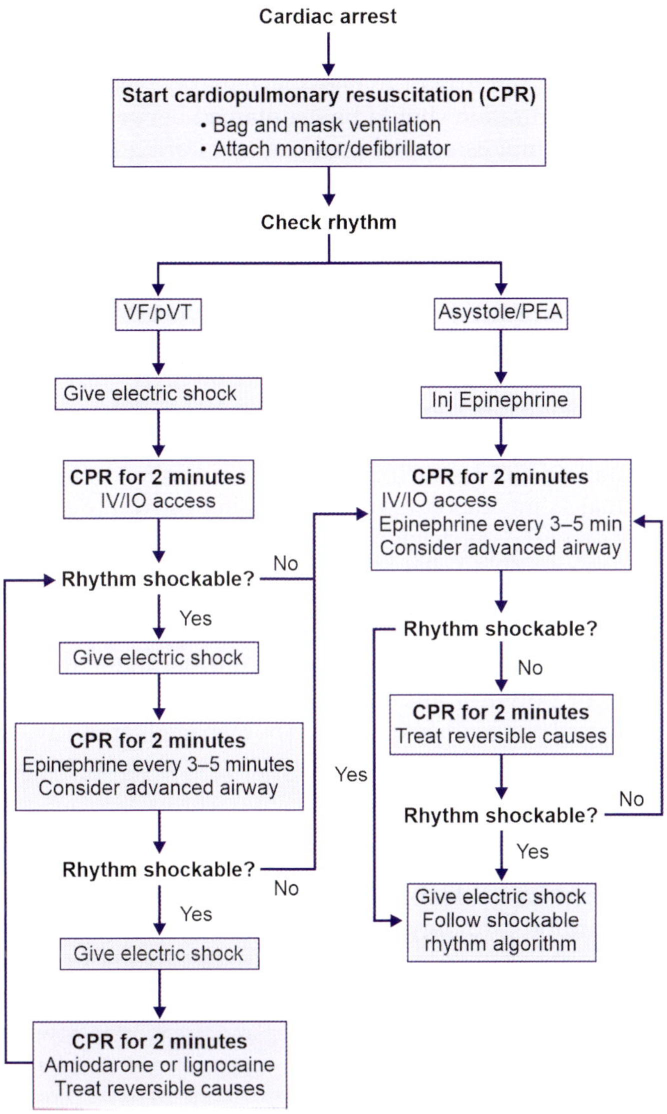


**Fig. 29.4:** Resuscitation of a child in cardiac arrest. VF/pVT ventricular fibrillation/pulseless ventricular tachycardia; PEA pulseless electrical activity; IV/IO intravenous/intraosseous

### *Adjuncts for Airway and Ventilation*

Oxygen should be given to all seriously ill or injured children with respiratory insufficiency, shock and trauma. During mouth-to-mouth rescue breathings, only 16–17% oxygen is delivered, with alveolar oxygen pressure of 80 mm Hg, and optimal external chest compressions provide only a fraction of the cardiac output, resulting in reduced tissue perfusion and oxygen delivery. Ventilation-perfusion mismatch during CPR and underlying respiratory disorders causes right-to-left shunting that reduces oxygenation.

### *Endotracheal Intubation*

If used properly, this is the most effective and reliable method of ventilation. The advantages of endotracheal intubation are: (i) It ensures adequate ventilation; (ii) reduced risk of aspiration of gastric contents; (iii) inspiratory time and peak inspiratory pressure can be controlled; (iv) suction can be done to keep airway patent; and (v) positive end-expiratory pressure can be provided. However, a skilled person is required for intubation. Hence, it is recommended that bag and mask ventilation should be continued in children who require ventilatory support in the out-of-hospital setting, when transport time is short or when an expert is not available for intubation. Indications for endotracheal intubation are listed in Table 29.4.

**Table 29.4:** Indications for endotracheal intubation

| |
|---|
| Excessive work of breathing leading to fatigue |
| Inadequate neurologic control of ventilation, and poor respiratory effort (GCS 8 or less) |
| Functional or anatomical airway obstruction |
| Need for high peak inspiratory pressure or positive end expiratory pressure |
| Lack of protective airway reflexes |
| For prolonged duration cardiopulmonary resuscitation |

An appropriate sized endotracheal tube is used (Table 29.5). Beyond 1 year, the size of the uncuffed tube is:

$$\text{Tracheal tube size (in mm)} = \frac{\text{(Age in years)}}{4} + 4$$

Size of cuffed endotracheal tube is usually 0.5–1 mm less than the uncuffed tube. Tubes 0.5 mm smaller and 0.5 mm larger than the estimated size should be available for use. The size of suction catheter is usually twice the internal diameter of the tracheal tube in mm, e.g. 8 Fr suction catheter for tracheal tube of size 4 mm. Cuffed tubes are preferred in all children beyond neonatal age as it is associated with better pressure delivery in patients with poor lung compliance, prevents peritubal leaks and aspirations without significant increased risk of subglottic stenosis. Cuffed endotracheal tubes help in decreasing ventilator associated pneumonia. Cuff pressure should be maintained at <20–25 cm $H_2O$ to prevent airway necrosis.

The depth of insertion of the tube is approximately three times its inner diameter. In neonates, the endotracheal tube is inserted to a depth of:

$$\text{Depth of insertion (cm)} = \text{birth weight (kg)} + 6$$

In children >2-year-old, the depth of insertion of the endotracheal tube is:

$$\text{Depth of insertion (cm)} = \frac{\text{(Age in years)}}{2} + 12$$

Tube placement is confirmed by looking for symmetrical chest rise and auscultating for air entry on both sides. Auscultation over upper abdomen is required to rule out esophageal intubation. Other markers of proper tube placement are condensation in ET tube, improving heart

**Table 29.5:** Size of ET tube and suction catheter in infants

| *Age; weight* | *Tracheal tube mm* | *Suction catheter Fr* |
|---|---|---|
| Premature newborn; <1 kg | 2.5 | 5 |
| Premature newborn; 1–2 kg | 3.0 | 5–6 |
| Newborn; 2–3 kg | 3.0–3.5 | 6–8 |
| Newborn; >3 kg | 3.5–4.0 | 8 |
| Infant | 3.5–4.0 | 8 |

rate, color, perfusion and oxygen saturation, and detection of end-tidal $CO_2$ by capnography. The position of the tube should be confirmed on chest radiograph.

### Vascular Access

During CPR, the preferred vascular access is the largest easily accessible vein (peripheral or central), cannulating which does not require interruption of resuscitation. All resuscitation drugs can be given through peripheral venous line. Agents with short half-life, such as adenosine, act better, if given through a proximal peripheral or central venous access.

If the central or peripheral venous assess is not achieved, intraosseous access should be secured. The usual site for intraosseous access is upper end of tibia medial to tibial tuberosity (Chapter 30). Other sites include the distal end of femur, lower end of tibia above medial malleolus and anterior superior iliac spine. All drugs and infusions which can be given by intravenous route can also be given by intraosseous line.

Tracheal route is not a preferred route of administration of medications even in emergencies. If intravenous or intraosseus access is not established, the tracheal route may be used for lipid-soluble agents like lidocaine, epinephrine, atropine and naloxone.

### Post-Arrest Care

Fever is common after cardiac arrest and should be controlled aggressively. Normothermia (36–37.5°C) should be maintained in all patients. In out-of-hospital cardiac arrest, therapeutic hypothermia (32–34°C) for 48 hours may be considered. After return of spontaneous circulation, hypoxia or hyperoxia should be avoided and oxygen saturation should be maintained between 94 and 99%. Continuous arterial pressure monitoring is done to maintain blood pressure above the 5th centile. **Table 29.6** shows doses for commonly used drugs during resuscitation.

### Fluid Therapy

Early restoration of the circulating blood volume is important to prevent progression to refractory shock or cardiac arrest. An initial fluid bolus of 10–20 mL/kg is recommended in shock, and after each bolus, the patient is reassessed. Volume expansion is best achieved with isotonic crystalloid fluids, such as Plasmalyte, Ringer lactate or normal saline. Blood replacement is indicated in patients with severe hemorrhagic shock who remain in shock despite infusing 40–60 mL/kg of crystalloids. Dextrose solutions should not be used for initial resuscitation as they do not expand the intravascular volume effectively and may cause hyperglycemia, leading to osmotic diuresis and a vicious cycle of polyuria and hypovolemia. Hypoglycemia, if suspected or documented, should be managed rapidly with intravenous glucose and measures to prevent recurrence.

### Arrhythmias

Most pediatric arrhythmias are the consequence of hypoxemia, acidosis or hypotension. Children with myocarditis, cardiomyopathy or following cardiac surgery are also at risk of arrhythmia. Drugs in therapeutic or toxic

**Table 29.6:** Drugs used during cardiopulmonary resuscitation

| *Drug* | *Indications* | *Dosage* | *Remarks* |
|---|---|---|---|
| Epinephrine | Symptomatic bradycardia, pulseless arrest | IV/IO: 0.01 mg/kg (1:10,000–0.1 mL/kg)<br>ET: 0.1 mg/kg (1:1000 flush with 1–2 mL of saline); repeat q3–5 minutes, if required | Tachyarrhythmia and hypertension may occur |
| Atropine | Bradyarrhythmias | 0.02 mg/kg | Tachycardia, pupil dilatation may occur |
| Calcium gluconate (10%, 9 mg/mL calcium) | Hypocalcemia, hypermagnesemia, hyperkalemia | 1 mL/kg IV or IO (slow push) | Monitor heart rate; flush line with saline before and after infusing calcium gluconate; avoid extravasation |
| Glucose | Suspected, documented hypoglycemia | 0.5–1 g/kg | Avoid hyperglycemia |
| Sodium bicarbonate | Severe metabolic acidosis, hyperkalemia | 1 mEq/ kg IV/IO slowly | Use once ventilation is adequate; dilute 1:1 with 5% dextrose |
| Adenosine | Supraventricular tachycardia | 0.1 mg/ kg; repeat dose 0.2 mg/kg; rapid bolus IV/IO | Monitor ECG during dose; give through vein close to heart |
| Amiodarone | Pulseless VF or VT | 5 mg/kg IV/IO | Monitor ECG during dose |
| Lidocaine | VF or VT | 1 mg/kg IV/IO; follow by infusion at 20–50 µg/kg/min | Monitor ECG during dose |
| Naloxone | Opioid intoxication | 0.1 mg/kg IV/IO/ET | Repeated doses may be required |
| Magnesium sulfate | Torsades, suspected hypomagnesemia, severe asthma | 25–50 mg/kg rapid push for Torsades; infusion over 20–30 min for hypomagnesemia and asthma | Watch for respiratory depression and hypotension |

ET endotracheal; IO intraosseous; IV intravenous; VF ventricular fibrillation; VT ventricular tachycardia

doses can cause arrhythmia. About 10% of pediatric cardiac arrest patients have ventricular fibrillation (VF) or pulseless ventricular tachycardia (VT).

***Bradyarrhythmia:*** Hypoxemia, hypothermia, acidosis, hypotension and hypoglycemia depress sinus node function and slow conduction through the myocardium. Excessive vagal stimulation, raised intracranial pressure or brainstem compression may cause bradycardia. Sinus bradycardia, sinus node arrest with junctional or idioventricular rhythm and AV blocks are usually preterminal rhythms. All slow rhythms resulting in hemodynamic instability require immediate treatment. Epinephrine is the most useful drug in treating symptomatic bradycardia, unless due to heart block or vagal overtone. For bradycardia due to vagal overtone, atropine is the drug of choice. If no positive or transient effect is observed after ventilation and oxygenation, continuous infusion of epinephrine should be considered.

***Pulseless electrical activity:*** It is a state of electrical activity observed on a monitor or ECG in absence of detectable cardiac activity. This is often a preterminal state preceding asystole, representing the electrical activity of a hypoxic and acidotic myocardium. Occasionally, pulseless electrical activity may be due to sudden impairment of cardiac output with normal ECG rhythm, with heart rate increased or rapidly decreasing. Pulses or other evidences of cardiac output are absent and child appears lifeless. This state is called electromechanical dissociation. Reversible causes of electromechanical dissociation are best remembered as **6Hs** and **5Ts**. The **6Hs** are severe **h**ypovolemia, **h**ypoxia, **h**ypothermia and **h**ypo-/**h**yperkalemia, hydrogen ion (acidosis), and hypoglycemia; while the **5Ts** are **t**ension pneumothorax, **t**oxins and drugs, **t**amponade (cardiac), pulmonary **t**hrombosis, and coronary **t**hrombosis. Treatment of pulseless electrical activity and electromechanical dissociation is the same as treatment of asystole; reversible causes should be identified and treated appropriately.

***Defibrillation:*** Defibrillation is the asynchronous depolarization of a critical mass of myocardium in order to terminate VF or pulseless VT. It is successful in cases of sudden onset VF having oxygenated normothermic myocardium without significant acidosis. Larger size defibrillator paddles, 8 to 10 cm in diameter, are recommended in children weighing more than 10 kg to maximize current flow. Smaller paddles are used in infants. One paddle is placed over the right side of the upper chest and the other over the apex of the heart. Alternatively, electrodes are placed in anterior-posterior position with one placed to the left of the sternum and the other one over the back.

The optimal electrical energy dose to defibrillate is not established in children. Available data suggest an initial dose of 2 J/kg, second dose of 4 J/kg and subsequent doses of >4 J/kg, to a maximum of 10 J/kg (adult dose). Children >8-year-old or those weighing >50 kg should receive adult doses of defibrillation. Single shock strategy followed by immediate CPR (beginning with chest compressions) is recommended for children with out-of-hospital or in-hospital VF/pulseless VT. After 5 cycles or 2 minutes of CPR, the rhythm is checked to look for reversion to sinus rhythm. If the rhythm is still VF or pulseless VF, another shock is given, followed by chest compressions, a dose of epinephrine and establishing an advanced airway, provided it does not interrupt the CPR. If after 2 minutes or 5 cycles of CPR, VF or pulseless VF persists, another shock may be given followed by chest compressions and administration of amiodarone or lidocaine. Simultaneous correction of hypoxia, acidosis and hypothermia is necessary to improve outcomes.

### Suggested Reading


1. Topjian AA, Raymond TT, Atkins D, et al. Pediatric Basic and Advanced Life Support: 2020 American Heart Association Guidelines for Cardiopulmonary Resuscitation and Emergency Cardiovascular Care. Circulation. 2020;142(16_suppl_2):S469–S523.


*Competencies:* **PE27.5; PE27.19**

## SHOCK

Shock is a state of cardiovascular dysfunction and inability of circulatory system to provide adequate oxygen and nutrients to meet the metabolic needs of vital organs. Shock can be normotensive or hypotensive. The chief types of shock are listed in Table 29.7.

### Blood Pressure Regulation

A host of neural and humoral reflexes maintain perfusion to vital vascular beds. Neural sympathetic reflexes act

**Table 29.7:** Types of shock

| *Type of shock* | *Clinical syndromes* |
|---|---|
| Hypovolemic | Hemorrhage<br>Dehydration due to diarrhea, vomiting, starvation, polyuria, burns, heat stroke |
| Cardiogenic | Congenital heart disease, myocarditis, cardiomyopathy, cardiac arrhythmias, tamponade, anoxia |
| Distributive | Anaphylaxis<br>Neurogenic<br>Drug toxicity<br>Burns<br>Toxic shock syndrome |
| Septic shock* | Bacterial, viral, fungal |

*This has components of distributive, cardiogenic and hypovolemic shock

29

Pediatric Critical Care

via the vasomotor center and include: (i) Baroreceptors in the carotid body and aortic arch; (ii) volume receptors in right atrium and pulmonary bed; (iii) chemoreceptors in aortic and carotid body; and (iv) cerebral ischemic response. Humoral responses are mediated by: (i) Adrenal medulla through catecholamines; (ii) hypothalamus and pituitary through ACTH and vasopressin; and (iii) renin–angiotensin–aldosterone system.

*Baroreceptors:* Reduction in mean arterial or pulse pressure results in decreased stimulation of carotid sinus and aortic arch baroreceptors, and vasoconstriction through inhibition of the vasomotor center. Vasoconstriction is severe in skeletal muscles, splanchnic and cutaneous vascular beds, while flow is preserved in cerebral, coronary and renal circulation.

*Chemoreceptors:* Hypotension and reduced perfusion cause local tissue hypoxia and acidosis, activating chemoreceptors that stimulate respiration, induce vasoconstriction and enhance cardiac function.

*Humoral receptors:* Hypotension-induced release of epinephrine and norepinephrine from adrenal medulla and systemic adrenergic nerve endings lead to vasoconstriction and inotropic and chronotropic effects. Release of vasopressin from neurohypophysis causes vasoconstriction and stimulates free water reabsorption in the distal nephron.

*Renin–angiotensin–aldosterone system:* Reduced renal perfusion results in release of renin from the juxtaglomerular apparatus, that helps convert angiotensinogen to angiotensin I and angiotensin II. Angiotensin II is a potent vasoconstrictor and stimulates release of aldosterone, enhancing sodium reabsorption.

### Diagnosis of Shock

An early diagnosis of shock or impending shock and its appropriate management improve outcomes. Early diagnosis of shock requires a high degree of suspicion and knowledge of predisposing conditions. Children who are febrile, have an identifiable source of infection or are hypovolemic due to any cause are at increased risk. Signs of early shock include tachycardia, mild tachypnea, prolonged capillary refill (>3 seconds), orthostatic change in blood pressure or pulse, and mild irritability. Decreased tissue perfusion is identified by change in body temperature (cold extremities) and decreased capillary refill. Vital organ hypoperfusion is assumed in presence of oliguria or altered mentation. Narrowing of pulse pressure is an early finding due to reduced systolic and mild increase in diastolic blood pressures. Patients with early septic shock may show bounding peripheral pulses, warm and over perfused extremities, wide pulse pressure and hyperdynamic precordium.

If shock continues, the compensatory mechanisms are insufficient to maintain the metabolic needs of tissues. This leads to multiorgan dysfunction. Cellular ischemia and inflammation affect brain, kidney and cardiac microcirculation. Tachypnea due to metabolic acidosis leads to respiratory alkalosis. Skin shows features of reduced capillary refill and mottling. Hypotension, oliguria and hypothermia set in. Mental changes include agitation, confusion, stupor and finally coma (Table 29.8).

**Table 29.8:** Stages of shock

| *Clinical parameter* | *Compensated* | *Decompensated* |
|---|---|---|
| Mental status | Agitation or confusion | Drowsiness |
| Heart rate | Tachycardia | Marked tachycardia |
| Respiration | Normal or mild tachypnea | Tachypnea |
| Skin and capillary refill time | Increased capillary refill time | Very slow capillary return with cold peripheral skin |
| Urinary output | Adequate | Oliguria or anuria |
| Blood pressure | Normal | Hypotension |

### Classification

Recognition and treatment of shock depends upon the etiology of shock.

*Hypovolemic shock* arises from loss of preload. Clues that suggest hypovolemic shock are: (i) fluid losses due to diarrhea, vomiting, blood loss, profuse and prolonged sweating, polyuria or a combination of these, or (ii) reduced intake due to vomiting, poor appetite or fluid deprivation. Third spacing can also lead to intravascular hypovolemia (seen in severe dengue). Physical examination shows dry mucous membranes, absence of tears, delayed capillary refill, diminished peripheral pulses and poor color. The CVP is low. Investigations show high blood urea and creatinine, elevated uric acid and small cardiac silhouette on chest X-ray.

*Cardiogenic shock* results from loss of cardiac contractility. Clues are history of congenital heart disease, recent cardiac surgery or diseases associated with cardiac disorders (e.g. Duchenne muscular dystrophy), presence of a murmur, S3, gallop or friction rub, elevated JVP and hepatomegaly. CVP is elevated and chest X-ray may show a large cardiac silhouette and pulmonary edema.

*Distributive shock* results from loss of afterload or systemic vascular resistance. Clues on history include recent allergies or spinal cord injury. Examination shows bounding pulses, well-perfused skin and low blood pressure requiring large volume of fluid.

*Septic shock* has components of all aforementioned types: Loss of preload, loss of afterload or systemic vascular resistance, and loss of contractility. Apart from fever and tachycardia, there may be features of decreased perfusion in form of altered sensorium, prolonged capillary refill >3 seconds (cold shock) or flash capillary refill (warm shock), diminished or bounding pulses, and/or decreased urine output. Hypotension is a late feature. A focus of infection should be looked for.

### Monitoring

Monitoring of patients, who are in shock or impending shock, is necessary. Parameters to be monitored are pulse rate and volume, respiratory rate and pattern, temperature, skin color, blood pressure, sensorium, urine output, ECG and pulse oximetry. Metabolic parameters include blood glucose, electrolytes, lactate and arterial gases.

## Therapy

Therapy depends on the type of shock. In hypovolemic shock, replacement of intravascular volume by isotonic fluids is necessary. In cardiogenic shock, inotropic support and reduction of afterload by use of vasodilators is beneficial.

### Fluid Therapy

***Vascular access:*** Large bore IV cannula or catheter is placed in a large peripheral vein initially. Later, central venous catheter placement in the internal jugular, subclavian or femoral veins can be considered.

***Fluids and blood products:*** The first choice of fluid for the acute stage is isotonic crystalloid solutions including balanced/ buffered solutions (Plasmalyte, Ringer lactate) or 0.9% normal saline. Large volumes of fluid have been used for acute stabilization in children without increasing the risk of acute respiratory distress syndrome or cerebral edema. When fluid requirement is high, colloids (e.g. 5% albumin) may be used. Packed red cells should be given at 10 mL/kg, to maintain hemoglobin ≥10 g/dL in the resuscitation phase.

***Volume of fluids:*** Normal saline or Ringer lactate, 10–20 mL/kg, is infused rapidly over 15–20 minutes (rapidly if hypotensive), and titrated with changes in heart rate, capillary refill and sensorium. If no significant improvement is noticed, repeat boluses of 20 mL/kg are given. Large volume fluid deficits require 40 to 60 mL/kg over first-hour for replenishing the deficit. In situations where intensive care support is not available, maintenance fluid rather than fluid boluses should be administered, if normotensive.

Patients who do not respond to boluses of 40–60 mL/kg in 1 hour are labeled as *fluid refractory* and should receive inotropic support. These patients require careful monitoring and are considered for intubation and mechanical ventilation.

### Vasoactive Drugs

***Vasopressors* (Table 29.9):** Adrenaline is the first-line inotrope for managing cold shock while noradrenaline is started in patients with warm shock. Use of vasopressors can be titrated to clinical features of peripheral perfusion, perfusion pressure, that refers to mean arterial pressure minus CVP, or systemic vascular resistance that ensures adequate urine output and creatinine clearance.

***Inotropes* (Table 29.10):** In patients with impaired cardiac contractility, inotropic agents are started. Epinephrine is the first-line inotropic agent in children.

Therapy with type III phosphodiesterase inhibitors is considered in patients who are normotensive with low output and high vascular resistance despite use of epinephrine and vasodilator. However, these agents have long half lives and should be discontinued at the first sign of tachyarrhythmia, hypotension or diminished systemic vascular resistance.

***Vasodilators* (Table 29.11):** Vasodilators are useful in children with normotensive shock with high systemic vascular resistance shock despite therapy with IV fluids and inotropes. Figure 29.5 outlines the management of a child with septic shock.

### Correction of Metabolic Abnormalities

Sodium bicarbonate may be infused to maintain arterial pH after optimizing perfusion and ventilation in patients with severe acidemia (pH <7.0). Hypoglycemia and hypocalcemia should be corrected.

**Table 29.9:** Vasoactive agents

| *Drug* | *Dose* | *Receptors* | *Use* | *Risk* |
|---|---|---|---|---|
| Dopamine | 10–20 µg/kg/min | $D_1/D_2 > \beta > \alpha$ | Renal effects, early inotropy needs, septic shock | Peripheral vasoconstriction |
| Epinephrine | 0.1–2 µg/kg/min* | $\beta_1 = \beta_2 > \alpha$ | Anaphylaxis, cardiogenic shock | Ischemia, hypertension |
| Norepinephrine | 0.1–1 µg/kg/min | $\alpha > \beta$ | Severe vasodilatation, hypotension | Acidosis from poor perfusion, ischemic injury |
| Phenylephrine | 0.1–0.5 µg/kg/min | α selective | Severe hypotension, hypercyanotic spells | Acidosis, ischemic injury |

*Vasoconstrictive dose >0.2 µg/kg/min

**Table 29.10:** Inotropic medications

| *Drug* | *Dosing* | *Receptors* | *Use* | *Risk* |
|---|---|---|---|---|
| Dopamine | 10–20 µg/kg/min | $D_1/D_2 > \beta > \alpha$ | Renal effects, early inotropy needs, septic shock | Peripheral vasoconstriction |
| Dobutamine | 10–20 µg/kg/min | $\beta_1 > \beta_2 > \alpha$ | Contractility | Tachycardia, vasodilation |
| Epinephrine | 0.1–2 µg/kg/min | $\beta_1 = \beta_2 > \alpha$, but both | Contractility, vasoconstriction (high dose) | Tachycardia, vasoconstriction |
| Milrinone | 0.3–0.7 µg/kg/min | Phosphodiesterase inhibitor | Inotropy, vasodilation | Tachycardia, vasodilation |
| Amrinone | 5–10 µg/kg/min | Phosphodiesterase inhibitor | Inotropy, vasodilation | |

**Table 29.11:** Vasodilator agents

| *Drug* | *Dosage* | *Site of action* | *Use* | *Risk* |
|---|---|---|---|---|
| Nitroprusside | 0.3–7 µg/kg/min | Arteries > veins | Afterload reduction | Cyanide toxicity, hypotension |
| Nitroglycerin | 0.5–5 µg/kg/min | Veins > arteries | Preload and afterload reduction | Hypotension, methemoglobinemia |



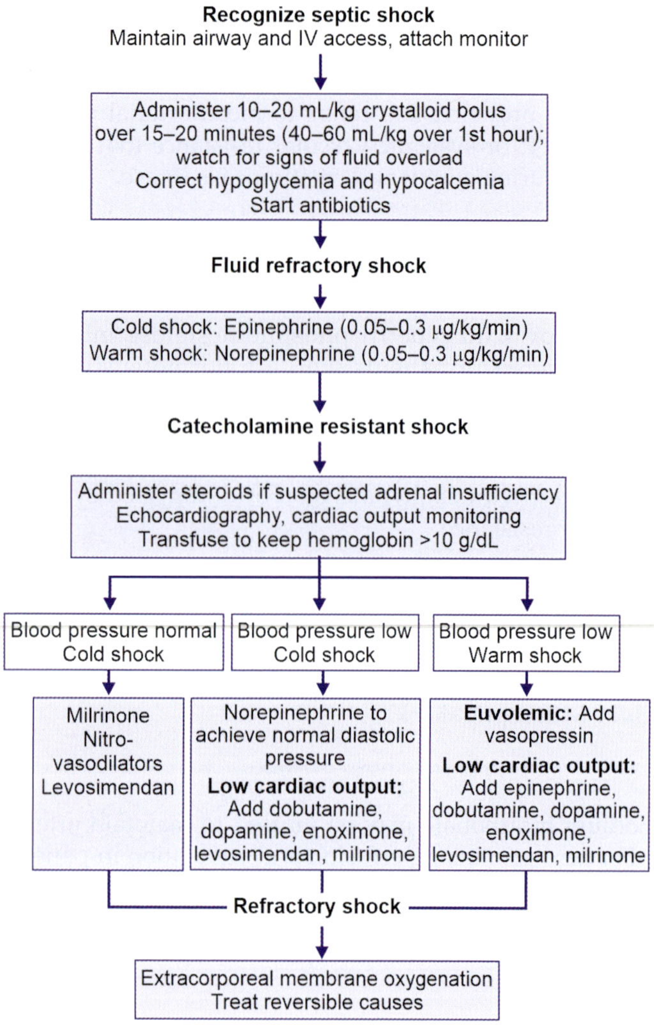


**Fig. 29.5:** Management of a child with septic shock

### *Control of Infection*

Patients with septic shock require prompt, appropriate and adequate antibiotic therapy. Even those without an obvious focus of infection must receive antibiotics that cover both gram-negative and gram-positive infections. Surgical drainage is ensured, if the child has pus collection (abscess, empyema, collection in soft tissues or abdomen).

Corticosteroids are reserved for catecholamine-resistant shock, and suspected or proven adrenal insufficiency. Adrenal insufficiency is perhaps more common in children with septic shock than previously thought. If available, extracorporeal membrane oxygenation may be offered to children with refractory shock.

### Suggested Reading

1. Khilnani P, Singhi S, Lodha R, et al. Pediatric sepsis guidelines: Summary for resource-limited countries. Indian J Crit Care Med 2010;14:41–52.
2. Weiss SL, Peters MJ, Alhazzani W, et al. Surviving Sepsis Campaign International Guidelines for the Management of Septic Shock and Sepsis-Associated Organ Dysfunction in Children. Pediatr Crit Care Med. 2020;21:e52–e106.

## NUTRITION IN THE CRITICALLY ILL

Critically ill children are prone to malnutrition, due to reduced intake and accelerated demands, increased resting energy expenditure, proteolysis, and glucose and insulin intolerance. It is essential to provide adequate nutrition early in the course of illness in order to improve outcomes. The enteral route is preferred, since it is safer and more cost-effective than total parenteral nutrition. Enteral nutrition helps maintain the gut barrier, preserves indigenous flora and prevents overgrowth of pathogens, reducing the risk of bacteremia and pneumonia. By preventing atrophy of gut mucosa, resumption of oral feeds is easier during recovery. Supplementation of vitamins and minerals is also best done by the enteral route.

Apart from milk-based feeds, commercial formulae are available to supplement nutrition. Elemental formulae contain carbohydrates as oligosaccharides, maltodextrins or hydrolyzed cornstarch; nitrogen as peptides or amino acids; and lipids as oils or medium chain triglycerides. Low lactose or lactose-free diets are available. Feeding is initiated at 50% of daily energy target and increased by 25% every second feed till targets are achieved. Initiation and hiking of feed can be more gradual in children at higher risk of intolerance. Feeds may be delivered directly into the stomach by naso- or orogastric routes. Bolus feeding is preferred over continuous feeding as it is physiological and requires less expertise to administer. Small bowel feeds are useful in gastroparesis. Continuous feeding is preferred for transpyloric feeding.

Conditions where enteral feeding is contraindicated are severe gastrointestinal hemorrhage, recent gastrointestinal surgery and intestinal obstruction. Complications of enteral feeding are intolerance, misplacement of the feeding tube, esophagitis and esophageal ulceration. Gastrointestinal reflux can lead to pulmonary aspiration. Diarrhea may occur because of hyperosmolar formulae, infection or malabsorption.

Parenteral nutrition refers to the delivery of nutrients directly into the bloodstream, including amino acid mixtures, lipids, glucose, trace minerals and vitamins. These are infused into a peripheral or central vein. A peripheral vein may be used, if the osmolality of infusate is less than 700 mOsm/kg. For delivery of adequate calories, central venous access is essential. For infants, glucose infusion is started at 5–6 mg/kg/min and increased gradually; insulin may be used, if there is hyperglycemia. Amino acids are begun at 1 g/kg/d and increased over 2–3 days to 2.5 g/kg/d. Lipids are given at 0.5 g/kg on day 1 and increased to 2–2.5 g/kg/d over 4–5 days. Appropriate combinations can be achieved by considering fluid requirements. Routine initiation of early parenteral nutrition (in first week) of PICU stay is not recommended. In a critically ill child, the energy requirement is lower, as metabolism may be decreased, there is decreased activity due to illness, sedation and analgesia, and growth is lacking. The energy goal in the initial phase of acute illness is less than for a normal child and revised regularly to avoid overfeeding and underfeeding.

Use of TPN requires monitoring of blood glucose 2–3 times a day; electrolytes and urea twice a week; and weekly biochemistry, triglycerides and blood counts. Complications include catheter-related infections, liver dysfunction, hyperglycemia, acidosis, hyperlipidemia and electrolyte imbalance.

### Suggested Reading


1. de Carvalho WB, Delgado AE, Leite HP. Nutritional support. In: Nichols DG, Shaffner DH (eds). Roger's Textbook of Pediatric Intensive Care, 5th edn. Lippincott Williams and Wilkins 2016: pp 1615–32.
2. Tume LN, Valla FV, Joosten K, et al. Nutritional support for children during critical illness: European Society of Pediatric and Neonatal Intensive Care (ESPNIC) metabolism, endocrine and nutrition section position statement and clinical recommendations. Intensive Care Med 2020;46:411–25.


## SEDATION, ANALGESIA, PARALYSIS

The goal of sedation is safe and effective control of pain, anxiety and motion, allowing necessary procedures to be performed and to provide appropriate amnesia or decreased awareness. The state of consciousness varies from mild to deep sedation to general anesthesia. In moderate sedation (conscious sedation), consciousness is depressed but protective airway reflexes are maintained and the child responds appropriately to verbal command or to light physical stimulation. Airway is maintained independently and spontaneous ventilation is adequate. Deep sedation refers to a medically controlled state of depressed consciousness from which the child is not easily aroused but responds purposefully to painful stimuli. The ability to maintain airway is impaired and requires assistance; spontaneous ventilation may be inadequate.

The child should be carefully assessed before sedation for underlying medical problems, medication use, allergies and time and nature of last oral intake. Monitoring is important during sedation and following procedures, including assessment of vital signs, movement of chest wall, ECG monitoring and pulse oximetry. Table 29.12 summarizes commonly used drugs for sedation and analgesia and Table 29.13 lists clinical scenarios requiring sedation and analgesia. For children on mechanical ventilation, continuous infusion of midazolam or diazepam is used for better control of ventilation. Intermittent doses or continuous infusion of fentanyl or morphine is used for pain control.

### Neuromuscular Blocking Drugs

The use of neuromuscular blocking drugs is common in patients with artificial airway who are undergoing mechanical ventilation. Succinylcholine is the only depolarizing muscle relaxant available. Non-depolarizing drugs are pancuronium, atracurium, vecuronium and rocuronium. Short-term indications for these drugs include airway instrumentation and invasive procedures. Long-term use facilitates: (i) Mechanical ventilation, overcoming patient ventilation dyssynchrony, and/or ensure high frequency ventilation; (ii) reduction of work of breathing and metabolic demands; (iii) treatment of agitation unresponsive to sedation and analgesia; and (iv) treatment of tetanus and status epilepticus, under continuous EEG monitoring. Children receiving these agents should be monitored carefully, particularly for position of artificial airway and adequate ventilation.

**Table 29.12:** Commonly used drugs for sedation and analgesia

| *Drug* | *Effects* | *Dose* | *Onset* | *Duration* |
|---|---|---|---|---|
| Chloral hydrate | Sedation, motion control, anxiolysis; no analgesia | 25–100 mg/kg PO | 15–30 min | 1–2 hours |
| Triclofos | Sedation, motion control; no analgesia | 20–100 mg/kg PO | 30–45 min | 4–6 hours |
| Midazolam | Sedation, motion control, anxiolysis; no analgesia | IV 0.05–0.1 mg/kg; up to 0.4–0.6 mg/kg<br>Infusion: 0.5–3.0 µg/kg/min | 2–3 min | 45–60 min |
| Diazepam | Sedation, motion control, anxiolysis; no analgesia | IV 0.2 0.3 mg/kg<br>Infusion: 0.1–0.5 mg/kg/hr | 2–5 min | 1–2 hours |
| Propofol | Sedation, motion control; no analgesia | IV 0.5–1 mg/kg; then 0.1–0.5 mg/kg every 3–10 min<br>Infusion: 5–10 mg/kg/hr | 1 min | 10 min |
| Morphine | Analgesia, sedation | IV 0.1 mg/kg | 2–3 min | 4–5 hours |
| Fentanyl | Analgesia, sedation | IV 1 µg/kg/dose; repeat every 3 min<br>Infusion: 1–5 µg/kg/hr | 2–3 min | 30–60 min |
| Ketamine | Analgesia, dissociation, amnesia, motion control | IV 1–1.5 mg/kg over 1–2 min<br>IM 3–5 mg/kg | 1 min<br>3–5 min | 15–60 min<br>15–150 min |

IM intramuscular; IV intravenous; PO per orally

**Table 29.13:** Clinical scenarios for sedation and analgesia

| *Clinical scenarios* | *Examples* | *Sedation strategy* |
|---|---|---|
| Non-invasive procedures | CT scan<br>Echocardiography<br>EEG<br>MRI<br>Ultrasonography | Comforting alone in older children<br>Chloral hydrate orally<br>Triclofos orally<br>Midazolam intravenous (IV)<br>Comforting alone |
| Procedures associated with low level of pain and high level of anxiety | IV cannulation<br>Phlebotomy<br>Lumbar puncture | Comforting and local anesthesia<br><br>Midazolam IV |
| Procedures associated with high level of pain and high level of anxiety | Central catheter placement<br>Bone marrow aspiration<br>Flexible bronchoscopy<br>Endoscopy<br>Abscess: Incision and drainage<br>Interventional radiology procedures<br>Intercostal drainage<br>Paracentesis | Midazolam and fentanyl or morphine IV<br>Ketamine IV or IM |



### Suggested Reading


1. Cote CC, Wilson S. American Academy of Pediatrics. Guidelines for monitoring and management of pediatric patients before, during and after sedation for dignostic and therapeutic procedures. Pediatrics 2019;143:e2019000.
2. McPherson C. Inder T. Perinatal and neonatal use of sedation and analgesia. Semin Fetal Neonatal Med 2017;22:314–20.


## HEALTHCARE-ASSOCIATED INFECTIONS

Healthcare-associated infections (HAI; earlier called nosocomial infections) are not present or incubating at admission, but occur during hospitalization. Infections diagnosed 48 hours after admission until 72 hours after discharge are considered as healthcare-associated (also *see* Chapter 11). Up to 6–10% patients admitted to PICUs develop HAI. Bloodstream infections are the most common (25–30%), followed by infections of lower respiratory (20–25%) and urinary tracts (15–20%). Important pathogens are coagulase negative and positive staphylococci, *Escherichia coli, Pseudomonas aeruginosa, Acinetobacter baumannii, Klebsiella*, enterococci and *Candida* spp.

The risk of HAI is related to the severity of underlying illness, length of PICU stay, invasive monitoring and diagnostic procedures, and indiscriminate use of antimicrobials. Almost 90% of bloodstream infections occur in children with central venous lines, 95% of pneumonia in those on mechanical ventilation and 75% of UTI in children with catheters. HAI may be caused by organisms that originate from exogenous sources in the hospital or from patient's own flora. Apart from increased duration of hospital stay and cost of therapy, mortality attributed to HAI ranges between 10 and 20%.

It is important for ICUs to have infection control programs to reduce the risk of HAI. A team of health professionals should ensure implementation and compliance on part of the PICU team. Infection control activities (Table 29.14) can reduce HAI rates by ~50%. The units should also have an *Antimicrobial Stewardship Program* to optimize the use of antimicrobials. It includes development of antibiotic policy, formulary restriction and adequate surveillance.

**Table 29.14:** Strategies to reduce HAI

| |
|---|
| Hand washing, hand hygiene, hand disinfection |
| Aseptic precautions during invasive procedures |
| Ensure nutrition: Prefer enteral to parenteral nutrition |
| Appropriate and rational prescription of antibiotics |
| Regular training: Infection control, procedure specific guidelines |
| **Surveillance for HAI** |
| *Health care associated pneumonia:* Avoid antacids and $H_2$ blockers; disinfect respiratory therapy equipment; use sterile fluids for nebulization and humidifiers; cuffed endotracheal tube; endotracheal tubes with subglottic continuous suction; do not routinely change ventilator circuit tubing unless soiled; care during suctioning; head end at 30–45° elevation |
| *Bloodstream infection:* Care of vascular access; use of Teflon or polyurethane catheters; avoid multilumen catheters; use transparent dressings; minimal "break in" into catheter and intravenous tubing; avoid TPN catheters for other infusions |
| *Urinary tract infections:* Minimal catheterization; asepsis during insertion; closed drainage; early removal of catheter |

### Suggested Reading


1. Joram N, de Saint Blanquat L, Stamm D, Launay E, Gras-Le Guen C. Healthcare-associated infection prevention in pediatric intensive care units: a review. Eur J Clin Microbiol Infect Dis 2012; 31:2481–90.
2. National guidelines for infections prevention and control in health care facilities: Ministry of Health and Family Welfare, India; 2002, pp 264.


## BLOOD TRANSFUSIONS

Blood component transfusion is an integral part of treatment for many patients cared for in PICU. Blood products are prepared from collected whole blood or apheresis donation. Whole blood units are separated into red cells

(RBC) and plasma and platelet components by differential centrifugation. Automated apheresis procedures are used to collect platelets, granulocytes or plasma. Cryoprecipitate is prepared from a plasma unit. Plasma proteins, e.g. albumin, anti-D immunoglobulins, IV immunoglobulins and concentrated coagulation factors are prepared by processing large pools of donor plasma obtained from whole blood or plasmapheresis.

Indications for red cell transfusion are listed in Table 29.15.

*Transfusion for acute blood loss:* If patient is not stabilized after 2 boluses of 20 mL/kg of isotonic crystalloids, it is likely that the blood loss is >30% and the patient should receive fresh blood.

*Transfusion for chronic anemia:* Children with chronic anemia usually tolerate hemoglobin levels as low as 4 g/dL. Investigations for the underlying cause of anemia should be sent, prior to instituting transfusions. Patients are screened for cardiovascular decompensation, an indication for emergency transfusion.

*Choice of blood group:* For red cell transfusions, the choices are based on the principle that the recipient plasma must not contain antibodies corresponding to donor A or B antigens. For plasma and platelet transfusion, donor plasma must not contain A or B antibodies corresponding to recipient A or B antigens (Table 29.16). Patients who are RhD negative should receive only RhD negative red cells. Ideally, the same blood group red cells that are compatible with the recipient plasma should be transfused.

*Quantity of transfusion:* The quantity of blood administered depends on hematocrit of the blood unit, pretransfusion hemoglobin level and patient weight. If the hemoglobin level is >5 g/dL and citrate phosphate dextrose red cells (hematocrit 70–75) are used, a transfusion of 10 mL/kg raises hemoglobin level by 2.5 g/dL. If anemia has developed slowly and hemoglobin is <5 g/dL, the transfusion should be given slowly or in small quantities to avoid precipitating cardiac failure.

**Table 29.15:** Indications for red blood cell transfusion in children

| |
|---|
| Hemoglobin level ≤4 g/dL (hematocrit ≤12) irrespective of clinical condition |
| Hemoglobin 4–6 g/dL (hematocrit 13–18) with features of hypoxia, acidosis, dyspnea or impaired consciousness |
| Malaria with hyperparasitemia >20% |
| Features of cardiac decompensation |
| Critically ill children with ARDS, septic shock (controlled), transfuse to keep Hb >7 g/dL |
| Septic shock, unstable children, keep Hb >10 g/dL |

**Table 29.16:** Choices of ABO blood groups for red cells, plasma and platelet transfusions

| *Recipient blood group* | *Acceptable ABO group of component* | | |
|---|---|---|---|
| | *Red blood cells* | *Plasma* | *Platelets* |
| O | O | O, A, B, AB | O, A, B, AB |
| A | A, O | A, AB | A, AB |
| B | B, O | B, AB | B, AB |
| AB | AB, A, B, O | AB | AB |

## Platelets

Platelet concentrates are prepared from whole blood donation, but may also be collected by apheresis. The usual platelet bag (random donor platelets, RDP) contains 7.0 × $10^{10}$ platelets, about 50 mL plasma, trace to 0.5 mL of red cells and varying number of leukocytes (up to $10^8$). Apheresis platelet units (single donor platelets, SDP) contain 3 × $10^{11}$ platelets, approximately 250–300 mL plasma, <5 mL of RBCs, and $10^6$–$10^9$ leukocytes. It can be stored for 5 days at 20–24°C. The need for platelet transfusions depends on the platelet count, bleeding tendency, etiology and setting of interventions like invasive procedures or surgery (Table 29.17). One unit of RDP per IU kg body weight increases platelet count by 20,000–50,000/mm³. One SDP collection is equivalent to 6 RDP units.

## Plasma

Plasma is prepared from a whole blood donation by centrifugation or automated apheresis. A unit of plasma contains 150–250 mL when prepared from whole blood donations. Immediately following collection, plasma contains approximately 1 unit/mL of each of coagulation factors. Coagulation factors V and VIII are labile and are not stable in plasma stored at 1–6°C. Plasma frozen within 8 hours of donation (fresh frozen plasma, FFP) contains 0.7 to 1.0 U/mL of factors II, V and VII to XIII. FFP may be stored for 12 months at –20°C. The use of FFP is limited to treatment or prevention of significant bleeding due to deficiency of one or more plasma coagulation factors (Table 29.18).

Compatibility tests before plasma transfusion are not necessary and plasma should be ABO compatible with recipients red cells. Usually, RhD group need not be considered unless in cases where large volume of FFP is

**Table 29.17:** Indications for platelet transfusion

| |
|---|
| Platelet count <10 × 10⁹/L due to any cause |
| Platelet count <20 × 10⁹/L and bone marrow infiltration, severe mucositis or anticoagulant use |
| Platelet count <30–40 × 10⁹/L and disseminated intravascular coagulation |
| Platelet count <50–60 × 10⁹/L and major surgical intervention |

**Table 29.18:** Indications for transfusion of fresh frozen plasma

| |
|---|
| Coagulation factor deficiency when individual factor replacement is not available |
| Anticoagulant (vitamin K antagonist) related bleeding |
| Severe liver disease with bleeding |
| Disseminated intravascular coagulation with active bleeding |
| C1 esterase deficiency in hereditary angioneurotic edema |
| Thrombotic thormbocytopenic purpura |

needed. FFP may be thawed in a water bath at 30–70°C or in microwaves designed for this purpose. The dose of FFP depends on the clinical situation and the underlying disease. If used at a dose 10–20 mL/kg (one bag per 10 kg body weight), it increases the level at coagulation factors by 20–30% immediately after infusion.

### Cryoprecipitate

Cryoprecipitate is the precipitate formed when FFP is thawed at 4°C. It is then refrozen within 1 hour in 10–15 mL of donor plasma and stored at –20°C for up to 1 year. This unit contains 80–120 units of factor VIII, 100–250 mg of fibrinogen, 40–60 mg of fibronectin, 100–150 units of vWF and 50–75 units of factor XIII. Cryoprecipitate does not contain factor IX. Indications for use include hemophilia A (factor VIII deficiency), von Willebrand disease and congenital deficiencies of fibrinogen or factor XIII. Compatibility testing of cryoprecipitate units is not necessary but ABO compatible units should be used. Cryoprecipitate infused at the rate of 1 unit per kg of recipient weight, over 2–4 hours, is expected to increase fibrinogen levels by 70 mg/dL.

### Risks of Transfusion

The chief risks of blood products include: (i) Transfusion reactions; (ii) transmission of infectious agents, including HIV, cytomegalovirus, hepatitis B and C viruses, syphilis and malaria; and (iii) bacterial contamination due to inappropriate collection or storage.

*Time limit for infusion:* There is risk of bacterial proliferation or loss of function in blood products once they are removed from storage.

i. Whole blood or packed red cell transfusion should begin within 30 minutes of removing from storage temperature (2–6°C) and completed within 4 hours, if ambient temperature is 22–25°C. In case of high ambient temperature, shorter 'out of refrigerator' times should be used.

**Table 29.19:** Adverse effects of use of blood and blood products

| *Category* | *Clinical features* | *Treatment* |
|---|---|---|
| Mild | Pruritus, urticaria, rash | • Slow transfusion<br>• Administer chlorpheniramine maleate 0.1 mg/kg<br>• If no improvement in 30 minutes, treat as next category |
| Moderately severe | Anxiety, itching, headache, mild dyspnea, palpitations, flushing, urticaria, rigors, tachycardia, fever, restlessness | • Stop infusion, replace IV set; notify blood bank<br>• Take sample from bag and patient for repeat crossmatching; urine sample for hemolysis<br>• Administer antihistaminic and antipyretic<br>• Give IV steroids and bronchodilator, if needed<br>• If improves, restart transfusion slowly<br>• If no improvement in 15 minutes, treat as next category |
| Life threatening | Anxiety, chest pain, pain at transfusion site, headache, dyspnea, respiratory distress, backache, rigors, fever, restlessness, hypotension, tachycardia, hemoglobinuria, bleeding from one or more sites | • Stop infusion, change IV set; notify blood bank<br>• Sample from bag and patient for repeat crossmatching; urine sample for hemolysis<br>• Ensure open airway; oxygen inhalation; elevate legs<br>• Normal saline 20 mL/kg; repeat, if needed<br>• Inotropes, if required; adrenaline (1:10000 for IM; 1:1000 for SC) 0.01 mg/kg IV/SC<br>• IV steroids and bronchodilator, if needed<br>• Bleeding (DIC): Consider use of platelets, FFP, factor concentrates, cryoprecipitate<br>• Acute kidney injury: Fluid balance; frusemide; dialysis<br>• Bacteremia: Send cultures; antibiotics |

**Table 29.20:** Delayed complications

| | | |
|---|---|---|
| Delayed hemolytic reaction | 5–10 days later<br>Fever, anemia, jaundice | No treatment; if hypotension, treat as acute intravascular hemolysis |
| Post-transfusion purpura | 5–10 days later<br>Bleeding tendency<br>Thrombocytopenia | High dose steroids<br>Intravenous immunoglobulins<br>Plasma exchange |
| Graft vs. host disease | 10–12 days later<br>Fever, rash, desquamation<br>Diarrhea, hepatitis, pancytopenia | Supportive care |
| Iron overload | Cardiac and liver failure in transfusion dependent patients | Desferioxamine (subcutaneous infusion)<br>Deferiprone (oral) |

ii. Platelets should be infused within 20–30 minutes of being received.
iii. Infusion of fresh frozen plasma should begin within 20–30 minutes of removal from refrigerator.

The products are infused through a sterile administration set containing a 170–200 µm filter. The set should be changed every 12 hours, if multiple transfusions are needed. For platelet transfusions, a fresh set primed with saline should be used.

*Transfusion reactions:* Tables 29.19 and 29.20 summarize adverse effects of transfusion of blood products. Hypersensitivity reactions cause mild and moderate reactions; life-threatening reactions can occur due to multiple causes, including intravascular hemolysis, bacterial contamination, fluid overload, anaphylaxis and transfusion associated lung injury.

*Massive transfusion:* This is the replacement of blood equivalent to or greater than the patient's total blood volume (70 mL/kg in adults; 80–90 mL/kg in children) with stored blood in less than 24 hours. Complications of massive transfusion are acidosis, hypothermia, hyperkalemia, citrate toxicity and hypocalcemia, depletion of fibrinogen and coagulation factors, depletion of platelets and disseminated intravascular coagulation.

## Suggested Reading

1. Karam O, Spinella PC, Wong ECC. Blood products and transfusion therapy. In: Nichols DG, Shaffner DH (eds). Roger's Textbook of Pediatric Intensive Care, 5th edn. Lippincott Williams and Wilkins 2016: pp 621–40.
2. Valentine SL, Cholette JM, Goobie S. Transfusion strategies for hemostatic blood products in critically ill children. Anesthesia Analgesia 2022;135:545–57.
3. Nellis ME, Karam O, Valentine SL, et al. Pediatric Critical Care Tranfusion and Anemia Expertise Initiative—Control/Avoidance of Bleeding (TAXI-CAB), Pediatric Critical Care Blood Research Network (BloodNet) and the pediatric. Actue Lung Injury and Sepsis Investigations (PALISI) Network. Pediatric Crit Care Med 2022;23:34–51.

Chapter

30

# Important Medical Procedures

❍ Nitin Dhochak ❍ Arvind Bagga

Medical procedures involved in care of children include diagnostic procedures and therapeutic interventions, some of which may be critical or life-saving. It is important to observe universal sterile precautions during medical procedure and dispose waste articles appropriately. Written informed consent should be obtained before all invasive procedures. Ultrasound and radiological guidance for invasive procedures is being used more frequently for better chances of success and enhanced safety.

## Removal of an Aspirated Foreign Body

Foreign body airway obstruction is a common medical emergency, especially in children younger than 5-year-old. Most events are witnessed and may be caused by choking on toy parts, seeds, nuts, grapes, pebbles or buttons. The usual presentation is with sudden onset of cough, gagging or stridor with or without respiratory distress. Degree of obstruction can be severe or mild. Signs of severe obstruction include universal choking sign (clutching the neck), weak or no cough, inability to make sound or talk, little or no breathing, and cyanosis. Mild obstruction is characterized by the ability to breathe, but may also have wheezing, coughing and stridor.

*Indication of immediate removal:* Severe obstruction.

*Procedure:* A choking infant younger than 1 year is placed face down over the rescuer's arm, with the head positioned below the trunk. Five measured back blows are delivered rapidly between the infant's scapulae using the heel of the hand (Fig. 30.1). If obstruction persists, the infant is rolled over and five rapid chest compressions are performed, similar to cardiopulmonary resuscitation. The sequence of back blows and chest compressions is repeated until the obstruction is relieved or infant becomes unconscious. Abdominal thrusts (Heimlich maneuver) may be performed in children older than 1 year (Fig. 30.2). When initial interventions fail, a jaw thrust is performed, since this may partially relieve the obstruction. If the foreign body can be

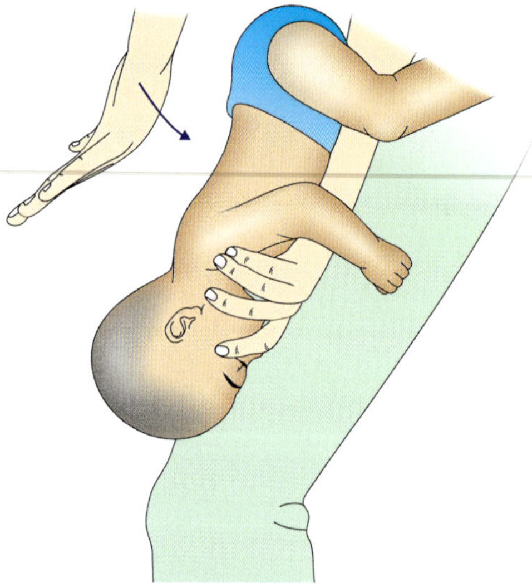

**Fig. 30.1:** Back blows in a choking infant

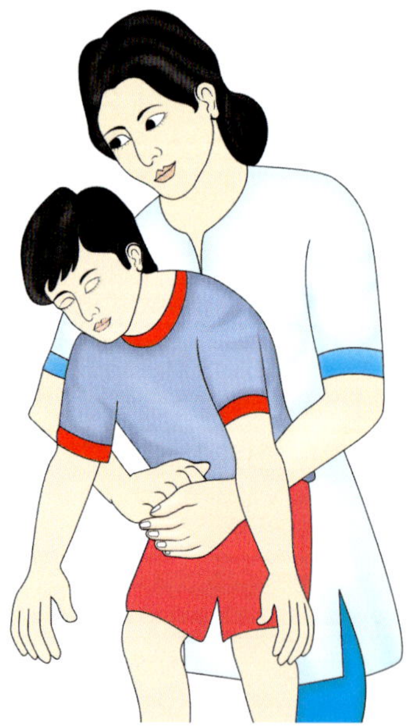

**Fig. 30.2:** Heimlich maneuver in a child

visualized, it should be removed manually using Magill or other large forceps. Any time child goes in cardiac arrest, CPR is performed.

Blind finger-sweeps are avoided in infants and young children because they may push the foreign body further back into the airway, worsening the obstruction. Children presenting with signs and symptoms of mild obstruction are referred to hospital and require further evaluation including bronchoscopy by experienced personnel.

*Complications:* Chest compressions may cause rib and cardiac damage in infants, but are rare, if performed by experienced personnel. Uncommon complications of the Heimlich maneuver, if performed incorrectly, include pneumomediastinum, rupture of spleen or stomach and injury to the aorta.

*Competency:* **PE24.5**

### Nasogastric Tube Insertion

*Indications:* Nasogastric intubation is usually performed for: (i) Administration of medications or nutrients in unconscious or anorexic children; (ii) gastrointestinal decompression in case of intestinal obstruction or trauma; and (iii) gastric lavage in a patient with upper gastrointestinal bleeding or toxin ingestion.

*Contraindication:* (i) Suspected basilar skull fracture, (ii) maxillofacial trauma.

*Procedure:* The largest size tube that does not cause undue discomfort to the child is chosen. Typically, a 5–8 Fr tube is used in neonates and infants, 10 Fr for a 1-year-old and increasing sizes in childhood up to 14–16 Fr tubes in teenagers. The length of tubing to be passed is estimated by measuring the distance from the nostrils to ear to the mid xiphoid-umbilicus point. The child is prepared by explaining the procedure as fully as possible; sedation is rarely needed.

Infants and obtunded children are placed supine with the head turned to one side. The curved tube is straightened and its patency checked with a syringe. Application of a lubricant facilitates atraumatic nasal passage. The tube is grasped 5–6 cm from the distal end and advanced posteriorly along the floor of the nose. It is inserted with its natural curve pointing downward in order to go past the bend of the posterior pharynx easily. The procedure is discontinued temporarily, if the child coughs or gags or if the tube emerges from the mouth. When the tube is passed successfully to the measured length, its position is checked. Using a 5 mL syringe filled with air attached to the proximal end, the plunger is depressed rapidly while one auscultates for gurgling over the stomach. The tube is taped securely to the nose.

*Complications:* The procedure may be associated with tracheal intubation, nasal or pharyngeal trauma, or vomiting.

### Central Venous Cannulation

*Indications:* Usual indications include: (i) Inability to establish venous access in the peripheral circulation; (ii) access for drugs and fluids that require central administration (e.g. vasopressors, hyperalimentation fluids, contrast medications); (iii) to monitor central venous pressure; and (iv) access for hemodialysis, plasmapheresis or continuous renal replacement therapies.

*Procedure:* Principles common to all central venous catheter procedures, regardless of site, include: (i) Strict attention to asepsis; (ii) use of the Seldinger technique (placement over a guidewire minimizes trauma and hematoma formation and enhances successful cannulation); (iii) adequate sedation to minimize movements; (iv) attention to appropriate location of catheter tip, avoiding high-risk sites such as ventricles and left atrium, verifying tip position with a radiograph; (v) use of ultrasound guidance whenever available; (vi) avoiding placement in presence of a bleeding diathesis; and (vii) continuous monitoring of vital signs and oxygen saturation.

*Sites:* The site of access depends on the indication (Table 30.1).

i. ***External jugular vein***: The external jugular vein can be identified easily. Complications are minimal because of the superficial position of the vein and the ability to compress the vein to prevent hemorrhage.
ii. ***Internal jugular vein:*** Internal jugular vein cannulation provides an excellent approach to the central circulation with a high success rate and minimal complications. Carotid artery puncture and pneumothorax are the most common complications. With left-sided cannulation, there is potential for injury to the thoracic duct and higher risk for pneumothorax because the apex of the left lung is higher than on the right.
iii. ***Subclavian vein cannulation:*** This vein is the preferred site in patients with long-term catheter requirements because of its relatively high level of patient comfort and ease of catheter maintenance. In patients with hypovolemia, the subclavian vein does not collapse

**Table 30.1:** Preferred choices for placement of central line

| *Indication* | *First choice* | *Second choice* |
|---|---|---|
| Emergency airway management or cardiopulmonary resuscitation | Femoral vein | Subclavian vein |
| Long-term parenteral nutrition | Subclavian vein | Internal jugular vein |
| Acute hemodialysis or plasmapheresis | Internal jugular vein | Femoral vein |
| Coagulopathy | Femoral vein | External jugular vein |
| Other purposes, e.g. access for surgery or medications | Internal jugular vein | Femoral or subclavian vein |

as readily as other major vessels. Major complications include pneumothorax, subclavian artery puncture, or occasionally, hemothorax. The chief long-term risk is subclavian vein stenosis.

iv. ***Femoral vein cannulation:*** Femoral vein cannulation is the most common site for central vein cannulation as it is easily accessible. Main complications are the risk of arterial puncture, infection, and rarely, deep vein thrombosis (more common with long-dwelling catheters in adolescents).

### Capillary Blood (Heel Prick)

*Indications:* Heel prick is a useful technique to obtain arterialized capillary blood for blood gas analysis, bilirubin, glucose, hematocrit and other parameters in newborns.

*Technique:* Figure 30.3 indicates the appropriate areas to use for heel punctures for blood collection. Prewarming the infant's heel (using a cotton wad soaked in sterile warm water at 40°C or a hot towel) is important to obtain capillary blood gas samples as it increases the flow of blood, allowing collection of blood specimen. Hot water should not be used since baby skin is thin and susceptible to thermal injury. After ensuring asepsis, a sterile blood lancet or a needle is punctured at the side of the heel in the appropriate regions as shown in Fig. 30.3. Wipe out the first drop of blood. The central portion of the heel is avoided as it might injure the underlying bone. Blood sample is obtained by alternate squeezing and releasing of calf muscles. Do not squeeze the heel.

*Complications:* The following complications may occur: (i) Puncture of the calcaneus, resulting in necrotizing chondritis or osteomyelitis; (ii) calcified nodules of the heel; (iii) hemolysis, resulting in falsely elevated bilirubin and potassium levels from mechanical trauma; (iv) erroneously high glucose values due to alcohol in the swab; and (v) inaccurate $pCO_2$ and $pO_2$ values from poor blood flow.

### Umbilical Vessel Catheterization

*Indications:* The umbilical vein is a convenient route for vascular access in newborns during the first 7–10 days of life. The route is used for administration of intravenous fluids or drugs during neonatal resuscitation, when establishing peripheral venous access is technically difficult. It is also employed as a route for central venous pressure monitoring and for performing exchange blood transfusion. Cannulation of the umbilical artery provides a route for arterial pressure monitoring or arterial blood sampling and alternative access for exchange transfusion.

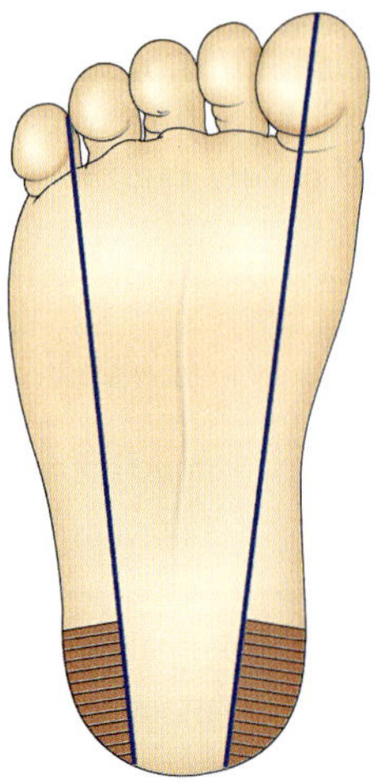

Fig. 30.3: Recommended sites for neonatal capillary blood sampling. Hatched areas indicate safe areas for puncture sites

*Contraindications:* Omphalitis is a contraindication; the procedure should also be avoided in presence of peritonitis or necrotizing enterocolitis.

*Equipment:* These include a 5 or 8 Fr catheter or feeding tube, 10 mL syringe, tape or silk suture to tie the base of the cord, normal saline for flushing, intravenous tubing and three-way connectors, a set of sterile drapes, sterile instruments (small iris forceps, needle holder and scalpel blade) and antiseptic for skin preparation.

*Procedure:* The neonate is placed beneath a radiant warmer. Anesthesia is not required; the limbs are restrained gently. The abdomen and umbilicus are cleaned with chlorhexidine gluconate or povidone-iodine and sterile drapes placed, leaving the umbilical area exposed. Vital signs are monitored continuously.

A suture is looped at the base of the cord with gentle constriction to anchor the cord and limit bleeding. The cord may need to be immobilized by two artery forceps grasping cord edges at 3 and 9 o'clock position. Using a scalpel blade, the cord is trimmed to 1–2 cm above the skin. The umbilical vessels are easily identified. The umbilical vein is a single, thin-walled, large diameter lumen, usually located at 12 o'clock position, while the two arteries have thicker walls with a small-diameter lumen (Fig. 30.4). The catheter or feeding tube is flushed with heparinized saline (1000 U/L) and attached to a three-way connector. A mark is placed at the length of insertion expected to place the catheter tip above the diaphragm but below the right atrium; this is calculated as 0.6 times the shoulder-to-umbilicus distance from the tip of the catheter. The closed ends of a pair of iris forceps are inserted into the lumen of the umbilical vein, and the lumen dilated by separating the ends of the forceps by opening it gently. Grasping the catheter with iris forceps 1 cm from its distal end, the catheter is inserted into the lumen of the umbilical vein and advanced gently inward until blood returns freely. Resistance to advancement of the catheter indicates that the tip is in the portal vein or the ductus venosus; the catheter should be withdrawn until free flow of blood is noted. The catheter is flushed with saline and secured with a purse string suture. An X- ray is ordered to ensure that the tip of the catheter is in the inferior vena cava and not the hepatic vein or right atrium.

A similar procedure is followed for insertion of catheter into the umbilical artery. Since the lumen is smaller, the vessel is dilated carefully 2–3 times using a curved iris forceps and the catheter inserted gently, taking care to avoid vascular spasm. The catheter is advanced to either the high position (above the diaphragm between thoracic vertebrae T6 and T9) or the low position (above the aortic bifurcation between lumbar vertebral bodies L3 and L4).

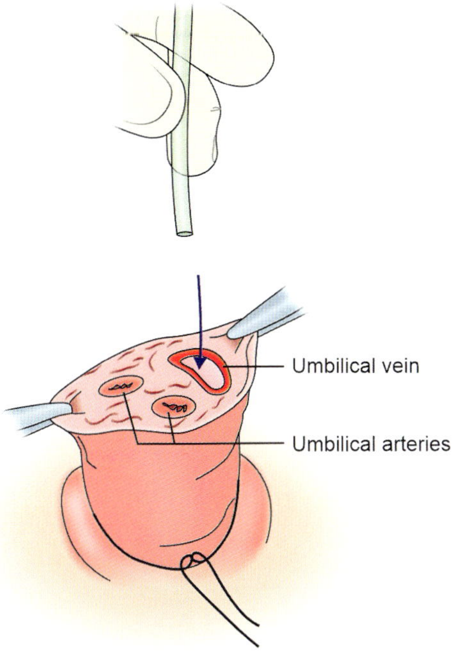


Fig. 30.4: Umbilical vein cannulation in a newborn. The umbilical vein is located at 12 o' clock position and is identified by its large lumen and thin walls

*Complications:* During insertion, vascular spasm, arterial injury or air embolism may occur and a false tract may get created. Other complications include bleeding due to accidental disconnection of IV tubing; catheter-related infection, thrombosis and embolism; and incorrect position of the catheter tip causing cardiac arrhythmias, hepatic necrosis or portal hypertension. Vascular complications are common with the umbilical artery catheter, particularly if placed in the low position.

## Arterial Catheterization

*Indications:* Arterial catheterization may be needed: (i) To monitor blood pressure continuously, especially in hemodynamically unstable patients; and (ii) to frequently monitor arterial blood gas.

*Sites and procedure:* Radial artery cannulation is a primary site of arterial cannulation in infants and children. Right radial artery cannulation is performed when preductal arterial oxygen tension is required for evaluating and treating infants with congenital heart disease. It is often helpful to stabilize the hand and wrist on an arm board, placing the wrist in approximately 30°–45° extension over several gauze pads. Adequacy of the palmar arterial arch should be assessed by the modified Allen test before radial arterial puncture.

*Complications*

i. Blood loss due to disconnection of the catheter from the IV infusion.
ii. *Ischemia:* The radial artery cannula should be withdrawn, if ischemic changes develop.
iii. *Emboli:* Blood clot or air may embolize to the digits or centrally, resulting in arteriolar spasm or ischemic necrosis.
iv. Infection may cause septicemia.

Competency: **PE24.17**

## Intraosseous Infusion

*Indications:* The bone marrow cavity is effectively a vascular space that does not collapse even in the setting of shock or cardiac arrest. Intraosseous access is usually the first line alternative when intravenous access is not feasible in collapsed veins due to severe hypotension such as cardiopulmonary arrest or decompensated shock. Almost any medication that can be administered into a central or peripheral vein can be safely infused into the bone marrow. Crystalloid solutions, colloids and blood products can be safely infused, as can hypertonic solutions.

*Procedure:* The technique of intraosseous infusion is rapid and simple. The most common sites are the proximal tibia, distal tibia and distal femur (Fig. 30.5). Due to differences in cortical thickness, the proximal tibia along the flat anteromedial surface of the shaft, 1–2 cm below and medial to the tibial tuberosity, is the preferred site in infants and young children. The distal tibia at the junction of the medial malleolus and the shaft of the tibia is preferred in older children.

*Technique:* Using aseptic technique, the site is prepared with an iodine solution. The skin is injected with 1% lidocaine for anesthesia in the awake patient. The needle is inserted at a 10° to 15° angle to the vertical, away from the joint space (caudal for the proximal tibia, cephalad for the distal tibia and femur). Pressure is applied in a 'to and fro' rotary motion. As the needle passes into the marrow, a 'give away' will be felt. Bone injection guns are also available for placement of intraosseous needles. The needle should stand without support. Evidence for successful entrance into the marrow include: (i) The lack of resistance (or a 'give away') after the needle passes through the cortex, (ii) the ability of the needle to remain upright without support, (iii) aspiration of bone marrow into a syringe, and

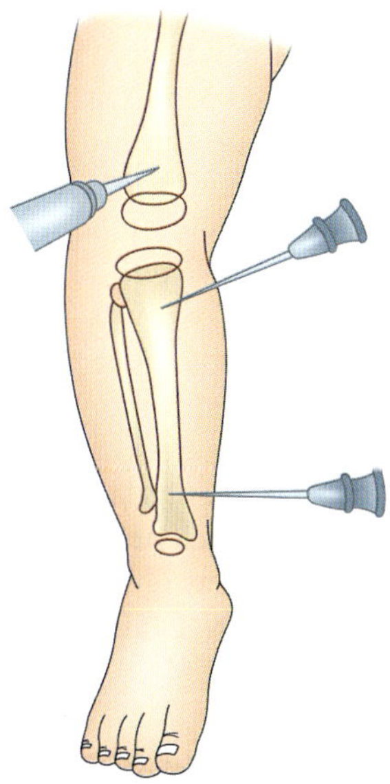

Fig. 30.5: Insertion sites for intraosseous infusion in the proximal tibia, 1–2 cm anteromedial from the tibial tuberosity, the distal tibia at the junction of medial malleolus and the shaft of the tibia, and the distal one-third of the femur

(iv) free flow of the infusion without significant subcutaneous infiltration. The stylet is removed. Proper placement is confirmed by aspiration of bone marrow into a 5 mL syringe and free flowing of a heparinized saline flush. The needle is connected to the desired intravenous tubing and solution. The site is observed for extravasation of fluids into the surrounding soft tissue.

***Complications:*** Potential complications include osteomyelitis, subcutaneous abscess, extravasation of fluid into subcutaneous tissue, compartment syndrome, epiphyseal trauma and fat embolism.

*Competencies:* **PE27.9; 27.10**



## Oxygen Therapy

Oxygen therapy devices are used to increase oxygen concentration of inspired gases with or without positive pressure. Oxygen supplementation is required in children with impaired lung gas exchange (pneumonia, bronchiolitis, interstitial lung diseases), impaired circulation (shock, congestive heart failure), and procedures requiring sedation. In pneumonia, impaired oxygenation is due to impaired diffusion across the alveolar capillary membrane, and shunting of deoxygenated blood passing through capillaries adjacent to unaerated alveoli (collapsed or flooded by secretions). Increasing oxygen concentration improves diffusion by increasing alveolar oxygen concentration, but does not improve hypoxemia due to shunting. Positive expiration pressure recruits the collapsed alveoli, and improves oxygenation by reducing shunting.

Oxygen therapy devices can be classified into devices that supplement oxygen without positive pressure (nasal cannula or prongs, face mask, oxygen hood, venturi mask, non-rebreathing mask) and with positive pressure (high flow nasal cannula—HFNC, continuous positive airway pressure—CPAP, non-invasive ventilation—NIV, and ventilator). Children with tachypnea/hypoxemia without significant respiratory distress may receive oxygen without positive pressure like nasal cannula, face mask or rebreathing mask. Children with hypoxemia with increased work of breathing should be administered oxygen through devices providing some positive pressure for recruitment of alveoli (e.g. HFNC, CPAP/NIV). Children with hypoxemia with poor respiratory efforts require invasive mechanical ventilation.

Oxygen therapy devices are also classified as low flow (device flow insufficient to provide all inspiratory gases, hence variable oxygen concentration depending on patient's respiratory effort; e.g. nasal cannula/ prong, face mask), and high flow devices (flow sufficient to provide all inspiratory gases, hence fixed oxygen concentration; e.g. venturi mask, non-rebreathing mask, HFNC, CPAP, NIV, ventilator).

### *Nasal Cannula*

Nasal cannula is a simple device with oxygen tubing and two small prongs, which are placed in the nostrils (Fig. 30.6a). Nasal prongs of different sizes from neonatal to adult are available and appropriate size should be selected such that it covers just less than 50% of the nostril area.

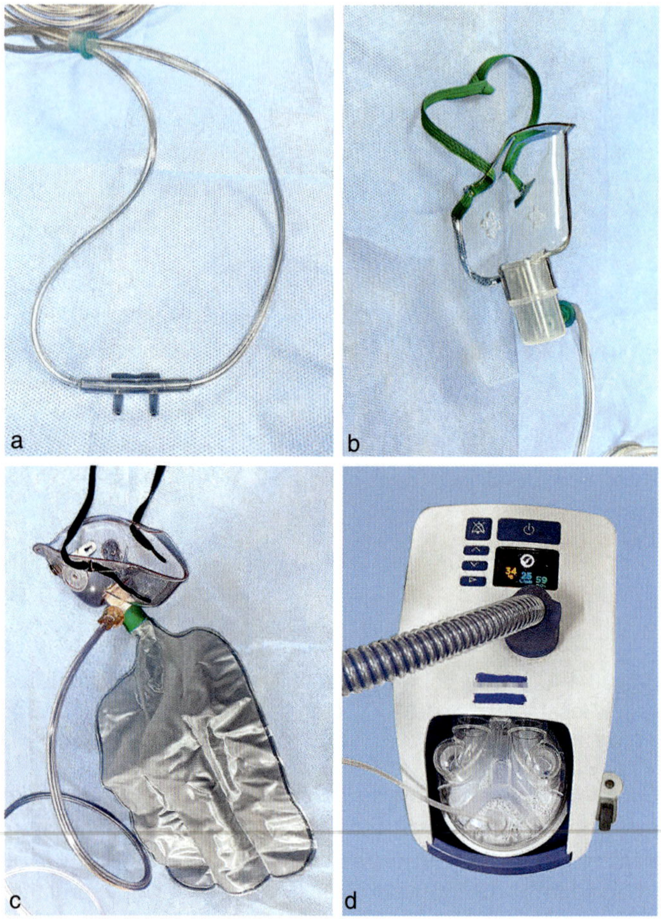

Fig. 30.6: (a) Nasal cannula with two prongs; (b) Face mask with side hole for exhalation; (c) Non-rebreathing mask with reservoir and valves; (d) High flow nasal cannula equipment with heated inspiratory tube

Maximum oxygen flow through nasal cannula is up to 2 L/min for infants and toddlers, up to 4 L/min for children and up to 6 L/min for adolescents and adults. Flow above this can lead to drying of nasal secretion and crusting. $FiO_2$ of up to 40% is delivered by nasal cannula (may reach up to 60% in small infants). Nasal cannula is well tolerated by children for longer periods, and feeding is possible while using nasal cannula. Nasal cannula may get displaced from nostrils in younger infants and may be taped gently to the cheeks.

### *Face Mask*

Face mask consists of a loosely fit mask applied over the face connected to an oxygen tubing (Fig. 30.6b). It has holes on the sides for exhaled air to evacuate. Appropriate size face mask should cover nose and mouth, but not eyes. Typically, oxygen flow of 6–10 L/min is set. For smaller face masks, lower flow of 3–4 L/min can also be used. Further lower flow may lead to rebreathing and $CO_2$ retention. $FiO_2$ delivered by face mask goes up to 60%. Face masks are generally well tolerated, but can interfere with feeding.

### *Non-Rebreathing Mask*

Non-rebreathing masks (NRM) are designed to provide high $FiO_2$ through a face mask assembly (Fig. 30.6c). NRM consists of a reservoir which can provide all the inspiratory gases. There are one way valves between mask and reservoir (opens during inspiration, closes during expiration) to prevent expiratory gases to enter the reservoir, and between mask and environment (opens during expiration, closes during inspiration) to prevent environmental air to be inspired. High $FiO_2$ above 90% can be delivered by NRM. Typically, 10–15 L/min of flow is set; flow is adjusted such that reservoir is not empty at any time during respiratory cycle. NRM are utilized for short periods, e.g. during resuscitation or severe respiratory distress, to provide high $FiO_2$, until measures like HFNC, NIV or ventilation is instituted.

### *High Flow Nasal Cannula*

HFNC provides heated humidified high flow gases of desired $FiO_2$. Most equipment consist of a heating chamber with heated tubing that deliver the gases to the patient though a nasal prong at ~34°C (Fig. 30.6d). The nasal prong is non-occlusive and should cover <50% of nostril areas. High flow up to 60 L/min and $FiO_2$ 21–100% can be administered. Typically 1–2 L/kg/min flow is administered in children. At such flow, a small positive expiratory pressure (2–4 cm $H_2O$) may develop in the pharynx. The benefits of HFNC include ability to administer high $FiO_2$, $CO_2$ washout from nasal and pharyngeal space, and decrease in work of breathing. Limitations of HFNC include patient discomfort, need for specialized equipment, and high per patient cost.

*Competency:* **PE30.23**

## Lumbar Puncture

*Indications:* The procedure is performed to obtain cerebrospinal fluid (CSF) for the diagnosis of meningitis, meningoencephalitis, subarachnoid hemorrhage, metastatic leukemia or benign intracranial hypertension. Intrathecal drugs can also be administered.

*Contraindications and caution:* Raised intracranial pressure, local infection at site of lumbar puncture, bleeding diathesis, hemodynamic instability.

*Procedure:* The spinal cord ends at approximately the level of the L1 and L2 vertebral bodies. Caudal to L2, only the filum terminale is present. The desired sites for lumbar puncture are the interspaces between the posterior elements of L3 and L4 or L4 and L5. These spaces are located by palpating the iliac crest. If one follows an imaginary 'plumb line' from the iliac crest to the spine, the interspace encountered is L4 to L5.

*Lateral decubitus position:* The patient is restrained in the lateral decubitus position as shown in Fig. 30.7a. The spine is maximally flexed without flexing the neck and compromising the upper airway.

The skin is cleaned with povidone-iodine solution and alcohol beginning at the intended puncture site and sponging in widening overlaping circles until an area of 10 cm in diameter has been cleaned. This is allowed to dry. Local anesthesia is used in children older than 1 year of age. The site is anesthetized by injecting 1% lidocaine intradermally to raise a wheal, then advancing the needle into the desired interspace and injecting the anesthetic, being careful not to inject it into a blood vessel or spinal canal.

The spinal needle is grasped firmly with the bevel facing 'up', parallel to the direction of the fibers of the ligamentum flavum. The needle is inserted into the skin over the selected interspace in the midline sagittal plane slowly, aiming slightly cephalad toward the umbilicus. When the ligamentum flavum and then the dura are punctured, a 'pop' and decreased resistance are felt. The stylet is removed to check for flow of spinal fluid.

About 1 mL of CSF is collected in sterile tubes for routine culture, glucose and protein determination and cell count. Additional samples are collected as indicated. The stylet is reinserted to remove the spinal needle with one quick motion. The back is cleaned and the puncture site covered.

*Sitting position:* The infant is restrained in the seated position with maximal spinal flexion (Fig. 30.7b). The assistant holds the infant's hands between his or her flexed legs with one hand and flexes the infant's head with the other hand. Drapes are placed underneath the child's buttocks and on the shoulders with an opening near the intended spinal puncture site. The interspace is chosen as noted earlier and the procedure follows steps as outlined for the lateral position. The needle is inserted so it runs parallel to the spinal cord.

*Complications:* Lumbar puncture may be associated with headache, local back pain or infection. Brainstem hernia-

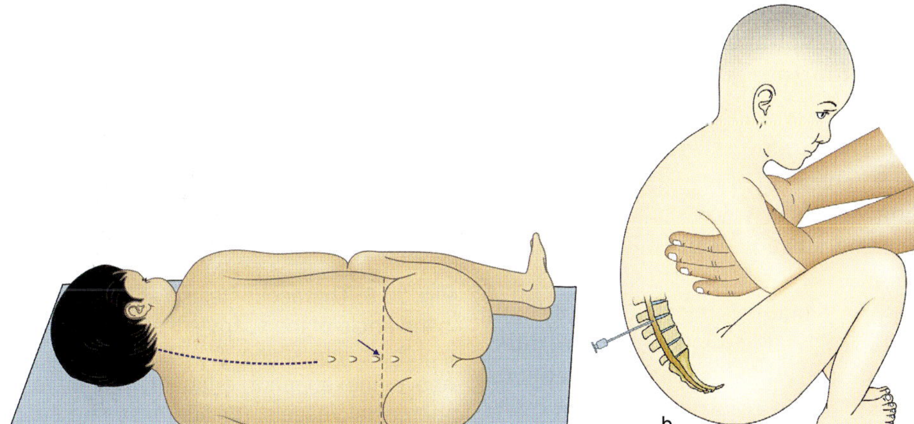


**Fig. 30.7:** Lumbar puncture with the child in: (a) Decubitus position; (b) Sitting position

tion may occur in the presence of symptomatic intracranial hypertension.

### Thoracocentesis (Pleural Tap)

*Indications:* Thoracocentesis is performed to evacuate fluid from the patient's pleural space for: (i) Diagnostic purpose, e.g. pleural effusion or empyema; or (ii) therapeutic purpose, e.g. when large collections of pleural fluid compromise ventilatory function.

*Contraindications:* These include: (i) Uncooperative child; (ii) uncorrected coagulopathy; and (iii) persistent inability to draw fluid (which suggests a loculated/organized effusion). The operator should consider withholding further attempts until the procedure can be performed under radiographic guidance (CT scan, ultrasound).

*Technique:* The first step in thoracocentesis is to ensure by clinical and radiological methods that fluid is present in the area tapped. Decubitus films are helpful in demonstrating free fluid that shifts with movement.

The procedure (Fig. 30.8) is carried out with the patient appropriately positioned upright and leaning forward. The site of entry is anesthetized with local anesthetic. The landmark for evacuation of the fluid is the angle of the scapula that corresponds approximately to the eighth rib interspace. An appropriate catheter is used over a needle. The needle is introduced immediately above the superior edge of the rib to avoid puncturing the intercostal artery and vein. Once the pleural space is entered and fluid is aspirated, the catheter is advanced as the needle is withdrawn. The catheter is connected to a three-way stopcock and syringe (10–20 mL). It is important to control the aspiration of fluid such that air is not allowed to enter the pleural space from the outside.

*Complications*

i. Intercostal artery puncture with severe hemorrhage
ii. Development of pneumo- or hemothorax
iii. Malposition of the thoracocentesis needle, with injury of abdominal viscera or lung parenchyma.

### Abdominal Paracentesis (Ascitic Tap)

*Indications:* Ascitic tap is performed for diagnostic purpose, e.g. to determine the etiology of the peritoneal fluid and to determine whether infiltration is present, or for therapeutic reason, i.e. to remove large volumes of abdominal fluid which impair respiratory function.

*Technique:* The patient is placed in a supine position and the bladder is emptied. The common sites for paracentesis are shown in Fig. 30.9. These sites are chosen to avoid puncture of underlying vessels or viscera. Usually, the left lower quadrant is preferred, since critically ill children may have cecal distension.

After the site is chosen, xylocaine is injected with a small needle to produce a skin wheal. The skin is then tilted anteriorly so that further infiltration into the subcutaneous tissue is in a different plane (Z tracking). A needle or over-the-needle catheter is then advanced using the Z tracking technique and at an angle perpendicular to the skin.

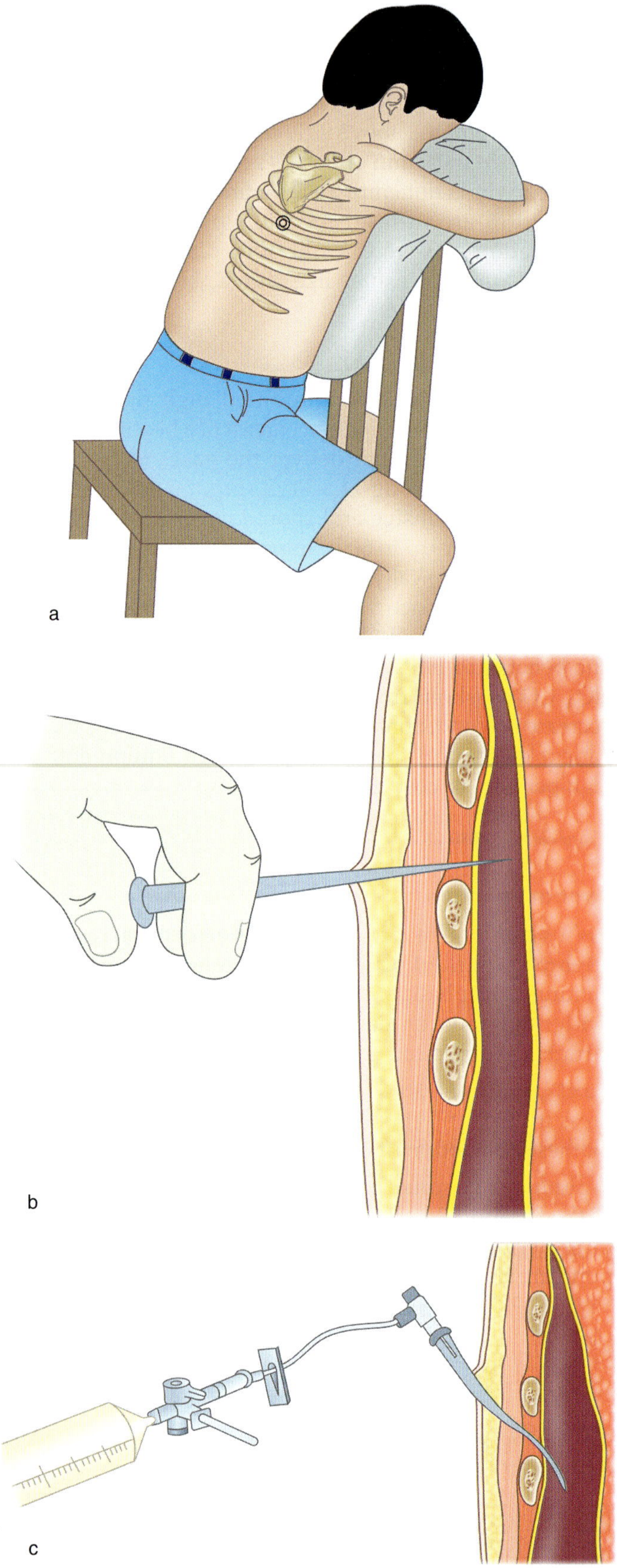


Fig. 30.8: Thoracocentesis: (a) The landmark for thoracocentesis is the angle of the scapula that corresponds approximately to the eighth rib interspace; (b) The needle is introduced immediately above the superior edge of the rib to avoid puncturing the intercostal vessels; (c) After inserting the catheter in the pleural space, the catheter is connected to a three-way stopcock and a syringe

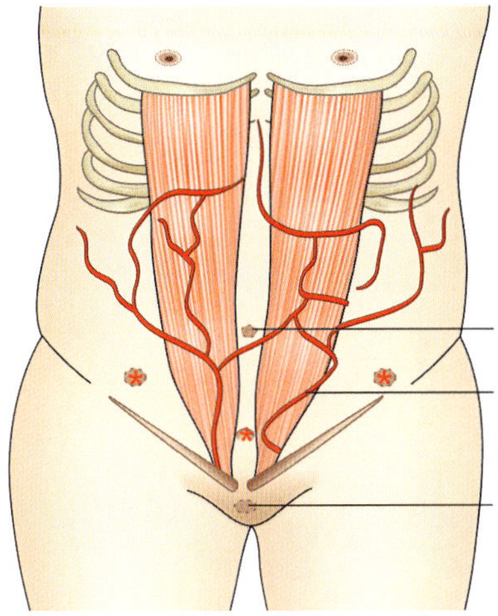


**Fig. 30.9:** Sites for abdominal paracentesis. The preferred sites are the linea alba (midway between the umbilicus and the pubic symphysis) and lateral to the rectus abdominis muscle

Continued aspiration of the needle is used until peritoneal fluid is aspirated. Approximately 10–15 mL of fluid is aspirated for studies. Appropriate studies may include cultures and Gram stain, cell count, cytology, amylase, LDH, bilirubin, albumin and protein. If the paracentesis is performed for therapeutic purposes, a catheter should be placed.

*Complications:* Complications include hemorrhage, fluid leak, intestinal or bladder perforation, and hypotension, if large volumes are removed.

### Catheterization of Bladder

*Indications:* Bladder catheterization is done in bedridden patients who need short-term assistance. It is also required in patients with (i) polytrauma, especially for evaluation of the urinary tract in an unconscious child; (ii) shock; (iii) acute urinary retention; (iv) to obtain a urine specimen for urinalysis; (v) in acute kidney injury, to monitor urine output; and (vi) for urodynamic studies.

*Procedure:* The patient is restrained as necessary. The urethral meatus, penis and the perineal area are cleaned thoroughly with a povidone-iodine solution. A Foley catheter of the appropriate size is selected (6–8 Fr in the newborn, 8–10 Fr in most children and 12 Fr in older children). The catheter tip should be lubricated with sterile lubricant to minimize local trauma.

***Boys:*** The penile shaft is gently grasped and extended. The catheter is held near the distal tip and advanced up the urethra unless resistance or an obstruction is encountered. If resistance is encountered, a smaller catheter is selected.

The full length of catheter should be inserted so that it passes into the bladder; this is important because urine may begin to flow while the catheter is in the proximal urethra and inflation of the balloon in the urethra may lead to urethral perforation. The balloon is then inflated. The catheter is taped to the child's leg.

***Girls:*** In girls, the principles of catheterization are similar to those in the male. An assistant carefully spreads the labia. A well-lubricated Foley catheter is introduced into the bladder. The catheter is advanced its entire length before inflating the balloon. A catheter that is passed in its entirety is unlikely to be inadvertently located in the small vagina of a young girl.

*Complications:* Injury to urethra or urinary bladder and inadvertent catheterization of the vagina may occur. Absence of aseptic precautions and prolonged catherization might result in urinary tract infection.

### Peritoneal Dialysis

This modality of dialytic support is used for renal replacement therapy both in acute kidney injury (AKI) and end-stage renal disease. Catheters placed surgically for chronic ambulatory peritoneal dialysis are not discussed here.

*Indications:* The modality is used in patients with AKI in whom dialysis is indicated (Chapter 17), and hemodialysis and continuous renal replacement therapies are not available, or contraindicated. The technique is widely available, inexpensive and technically easy to perform even in newborns.

*Contraindications:* Relative contraindications to peritoneal dialysis include recent abdominal and/or cardiothoracic surgery, diaphragmatic peritoneal-pleural fistula, fecal or fungal peritonitis and abdominal wall cellulitis.

*Procedure:* Access for peritoneal dialysis can be achieved by inserting a rigid catheter **(Fig. 30.10a)** or a single cuff soft Tenckhoff catheter at the bedside **(Fig. 30.10b)**. The double cuff Tenckhoff catheter, used for chronic peritoneal dialysis, is placed in the operating room by a surgeon. A rigid acute PD catheter is easily available, inexpensive and relatively simple to insert. However, the risks of peritonitis are high, particularly if used for more than 48 hours.

The abdomen is cleansed with chlorhexidine and betadine and draped. Following administration of sedation and local anesthesia, an 18–22 gauge cannula is inserted below the umbilicus in the midline or lateral to the rectus abdominis muscle at two-thirds the distance between the umbilicus and the anterior superior iliac spine **(Fig. 30.10c)**. About 20–30 mL/kg of peritoneal dialysis fluid is infused till the flanks appear full.

The cannula is removed and the stiff catheter is inserted using the trocar. Once a 'give away' sensation is felt, dialysis fluid flows freely back into the catheter lumen. The catheter is inserted carefully avoiding injury to viscus by the trocar and guiding the tip of the catheter into the left iliac fossa. The trocar is removed and the catheter attached to a three-way connection to the peritoneal dialysis fluid and the drain bag. Once easy inflow and outflow are confirmed, the catheter is secured with a purse-string suture and manual cycles of dialysis are initiated.

The soft single cuff catheter is inserted using an introducer kit using the modified Seldinger technique. A tunnel is created in the soft tissue so that the exit site is away from the entry point into the peritoneum and the cuff protects from bacterial migration. This catheter is associated with lower risk of peritonitis, particularly if used with an auto-

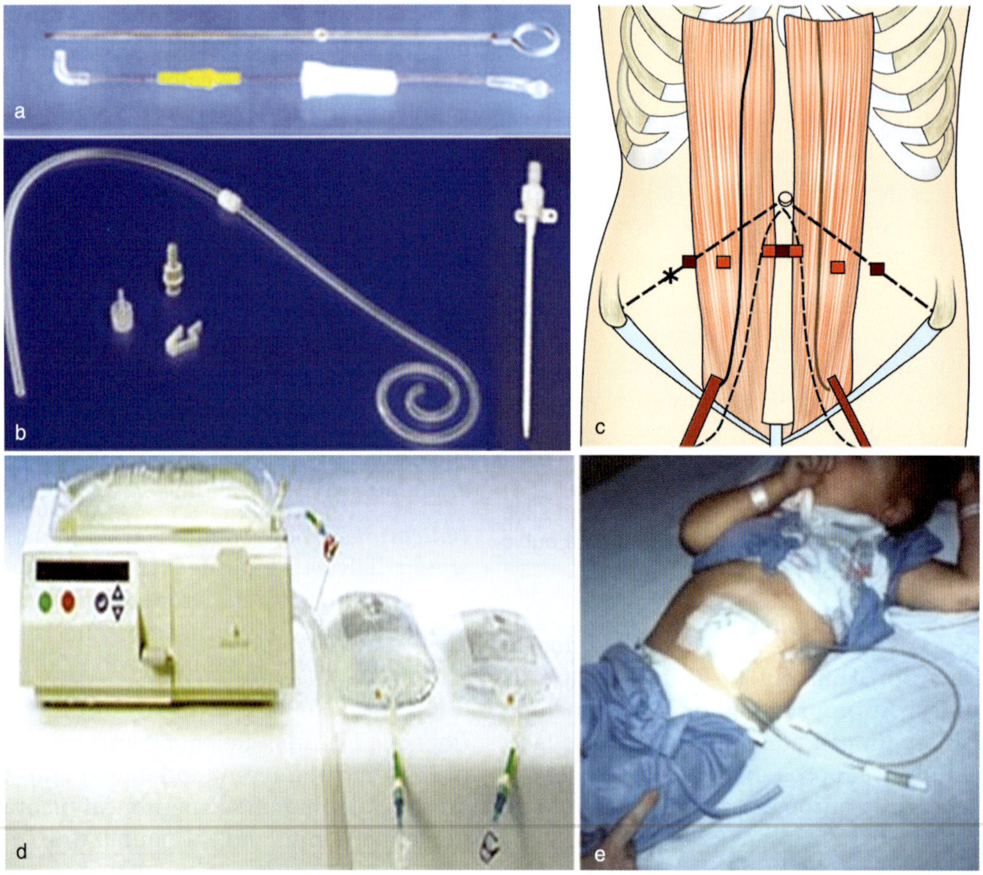


**Fig. 30.10:** Peritoneal dialysis: (a) Stiff uncuffed catheter used for acute peritoneal dialysis; (b) Soft single cuff Tenckhoff catheter inserted bedside for acute dialysis; (c) Usual site of catheter insertion is in midline below the umbilicus or two-thirds of the distance between umbilicus and anterior superior iliac spine; (d) Device for automated control of dialysis and aseptic handling; (e) Infant undergoing dialysis with soft Tenckhoff catheter

mated cycler device (Fig. 30.10d). It can be capped when not in use, allows ease of nursing, and can be used for several weeks (Fig. 30.10e).

*Prescription:* Acute PD can be performed intermittently or continuously depending upon the desired amount of fluid and solute removal, and either manually by nurses or via an automated device. About 20–30 mL/kg is infused over 5 min, kept in the abdomen for 20–40 min, and then drained out. Ultrafiltration should not exceed 5–10% of body weight over 24–48 hours. The prescription is modified every 6–12 hours based on clinical evaluation and laboratory parameters (serum electrolytes and blood sugar). Acute manual PD requires constant supervision to ensure accurate inflow, dwell and drain times and the maintenance of a record of exchange and drain volumes and net ultrafiltration. By comparison, the use of the automated cycler reduces need for constant supervision and record maintenance and decreases the number of manual interruptions and risk of peritonitis.

*Complications:* Abdominal pain or discomfort may occur due to abdominal distension, improper position of the catheter or peritonitis. Mild hemorrhage is frequent during catheter placement, particularly with rigid acute catheters. Leakage around the PD catheter site is managed by reducing the exchange volume or placing a suture at the exit site. Inadequate drainage is due to improper placement of the catheter tip or decreased bowel motility. Bowel perforations is rare but may be observed with placement of stiff catheters. Metabolic complications include hyperglycemia, hypokalemia, protein losses and hypernatremia.

### Bone Marrow Aspiration and Biopsy

A special bone marrow needle is introduced into the bone marrow space, and a sample aspirated for analysis. A marrow biopsy is taken to ascertain the cellularity and architecture of the marrow.

*Indications:* Bone marrow aspiration and biopsy are indicated in presence of pancytopenia, bicytopenia, unexplained thrombocytopenia or leukocytosis in order to rule out significant pathology such as lymphoreticular malignancy (acute lymphoblastic or myelogenous leukemia, Hodgkin or non-Hodgkin lymphoma, chronic myeloid leukemia, myelodysplasia, myelofibrosis); hypoplastic or aplastic anemia; megaloblastic anemia; sideroblastic anemia; Langerhans cell histiocytosis; hemophagocytosis syndrome; suspected metastasis (retinoblastoma, neuroblastoma); infiltrative storage diseases (Gaucher disease) or infections involving the bone marrow (kala-azar, tuberculosis).

*Sites:* The iliac crest is the most commonly used site. The sternum is not preferred in children because of associated pain and the risk of injuring underlying vital structures. Marrow may be aspirated from the proximal tibia medial to the tibial tuberosity in infants (<1-year-old). This site is preferred in infants since biopsy from the iliac site in young children is difficult as the iliac crest is small and carries risk of injuring pelvic viscera.

*Equipment:* Various types of bone marrow biopsy needles are available **(Fig. 30.11a and b)**. The Jamshidi needle and its modifications are used widely because of their light weight, sharp bevelled end that allows easy coring of bone, a tapering end that facilitates recovery of marrow specimen and suitability for both aspiration and biopsy.

*Procedure:* The child should be fasting for 6–8 hours before the procedure. The child is positioned prone with face turned to a side and the pelvis stabilized by folding a sheet below it. If tibia is to be aspirated, the leg is slightly flexed at the knee joint. Appropriate sedation (commonly with intravenous midazolam and ketamine) is administered with continuous monitoring of vital signs and oxygen saturation.

The site is cleaned with chlorhexidine and betadine to include the lumbar spine, iliac crests and posterior iliac spines (or for the tibial site, the entire leg up to the distal half of thigh) and draped. The posterior superior iliac spine is located by tracing the iliac crest backwards to its most prominent and elevated point. About 2 mL of 1% lidocaine is injected subcutaneously up to the periosteum. The bone marrow needle is held firmly in the dominant hand with the index finger placed over the needle to act as a guard. The needle is advanced perpendicularly into the identified area with twisting motion till bone is felt. On advancing further, a 'give way' is felt that indicates that the needle is in the bone marrow. The stylet is removed and a 20 mL syringe attached. The piston is pulled to create negative pressure and aspirate slowly around 0.5 mL of marrow. The syringe is disconnected and the marrow placed on slides. The marrow is spread on the slide by placing another glass slide so as to smear the marrow gently. Additional slides are prepared similar to a peripheral smear, using another glass slide at 30° angle to spread the marrow in a tongue shaped projection on the slide.

To perform marrow biopsy, the stylet is replaced and the needle withdrawn slightly. The needle is advanced through another site in the bone. Once the needle is lodged in the bone, the stylet is removed and the needle advanced in

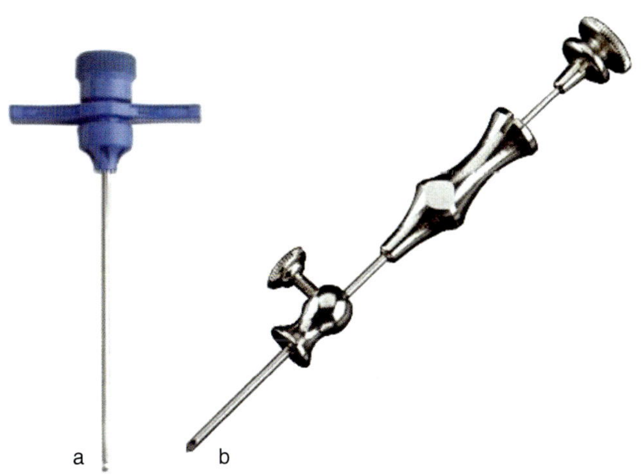

Fig. 30.11: Needles for bone marrow aspiration and biopsy: (a) Jamshidi needles; (b) Vim Silverman needle

rotatory motion through the marrow space. The needle is withdrawn and biopsy specimen is removed. The biopsy sample is rolled on a slide to prepare touch preparation. Then the tissue is placed in a vial containing formalin. Once the needle is removed, local pressure is applied to allow bleeding to stop. Drapes are removed, the skin is cleaned and pressure bandage applied.

Aspiration from the tibia is performed in a similar manner. The preferred site is medial to the tibial tubercle, one inch below the joint line to avoid the growth plate. The bone cortex is thinner and the marrow space is reached more quickly than with the pelvic site. Obtaining a biopsy is often difficult as the marrow is more spongy.

*Complications:* Bleeding and pain at the aspiration site are common. Bone injury with fractures of iliac bone and subcutaneous infections or osteomyelitis are rare.

### Liver Biopsy

*Indications:* Liver biopsy is used to evaluate hepatic histology in order to: (i) Diagnose parenchymal liver disease (e.g. neonatal hepatitis, suspected metabolic liver disease); (ii) understand the cause of persistently abnormal liver tests; (iii) determine the etiology of focal or diffuse abnormalities on imaging studies; (iv) assess the prognosis of known liver disease (e.g. extrahepatic biliary atresia, autoimmune hepatitis, chronic viral hepatitis); (v) determine response to therapeutic interventions; (vi) develop a treatment plan based on histology; and (vii) monitor effects of hepatotoxic drugs. Analysis of the biopsy specimen may include evaluation of histology, metal content, enzymatic assays and cultures for viral, bacterial, or fungal pathogen.

*Contraindications:* Absolute contraindications include coagulopathy, as suggested by low platelet count (<60,000/µL) or prolonged prothrombin time (international normalized ratio >1.5), and an inability to remain still (with or without sedation). Relative contraindications include anemia, peritonitis, marked ascites, high-grade biliary obstruction, and a subphrenic or right pleural infection or effusion.

*Procedure:* The biopsy may be performed percutaneously at bedside with or without ultrasound guidance. An ultrasound-guided biopsy carries lower risk of complications and allows visualization of the liver and any target lesions. Uncommonly, the biopsy is performed using the transjugular route, laparoscopically or by wedge resection during laparotomy. Transjugular venous biopsy is preferred in patients with severe coagulopathy.

The child should be fasting for 4–6 hours. An intravenous line is secured and the child made to lie supine. The abdominal girth is measured at the umbilicus to allow subsequent comparisons. The lower border of liver is localized by palpation or percussion, and its position on the midclavicular line marked.

During continuous monitoring of vital signs, sedation is administered. The site of biopsy is chosen based on the liver span. If the liver is palpable, a subcostal approach may be used. However, a right lateral transthoracic approach is most common, in which the needle is inserted in the tenth intercostal space in the midaxillary line, after confirming

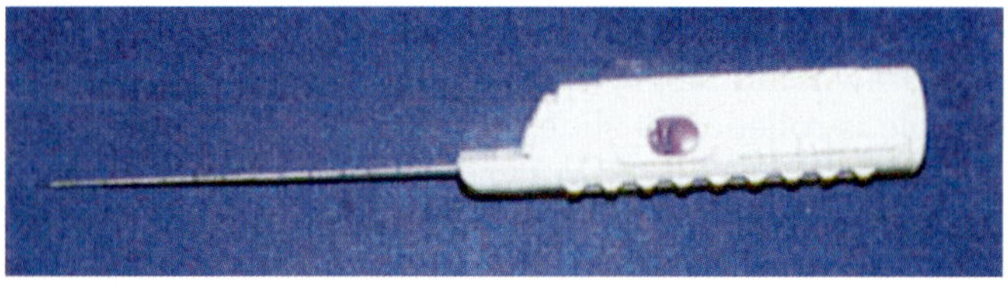

Fig. 30.12: Semiautomated gun for biopsy of liver and kidney

liver dullness. Local anesthesia is administered. The biopsy is usually performed using a spring-loaded semiautomatic biopsy gun (Fig. 30.12) of size 18 (infants) or 16 (children) gauge. The gun is loaded and its needle inserted through the marked intercostal site just above the border of the lower rib, so as to avoid injuring the neurovascular bundle running along the lower border of ribs. The needle is inserted carefully along a horizontal plane to a depth at which a 'give way' sensation is felt upon rupture of the liver capsule. The tip of the needle should rest just beyond the capsule and should move well with respiration. The gun is fired and the needle withdrawn quickly. The sample is transferred to vials, e.g. formalin for histopathology.

The biopsy site is sealed with tincture iodine and pressure dressing applied to prevent bleeding. The child is monitored over the next 6–8 hours for tachycardia, tachypnea, hypotension and increase in abdominal girth and excessive pain, which may suggest internal bleeding.

*Complications:* Complications include intra-abdominal hemorrhage, biliary peritonitis, hepatic laceration, hemothorax, hemobilia, pneumothorax, gallbladder or intestinal perforation and iatrogenic arteriovenous fistula.

## Suggested Reading


1. Percy A. Procedures. In: The Harriet Lane Handbook, 22nd edn. Elsevier, Philadelphia; 2021.
2. Relief of Choking For Adults, Children and Infants. Source: https://nhcps.com/lesson/relief-of-choking-for-adults-children-infants/

Chapter 31

# Rights of Children

Rajeev Seth

The Constitution of India guarantees equality before the law to all citizens, and has pledged special protection for children. In 1992, India accepted the obligations of the United Nations Convention on the Rights of the Child (UN CRC) and has taken several steps to advance child rights.

## UN Convention of Child Rights (UN CRC) and Child Health Care

The UN CRC has implications both at policy or decision-making level and at practice or healthcare provision level. There is sufficient evidence globally to acknowledge that the UN CRC has influenced child rights to health and well being. Every physician should have adequate knowledge of rights of every child in the area of child survival, identity, development, protection and participation. They should understand the broader social determinants of child health, become trained in the use of UN CRC, align themselves with child right organizations in advocacy efforts and lobby their local, state and national elected representatives to advance child rights **(Box 31.1)**.

**Box 31.1: Articles of the UN CRC that Apply to Child Health**

| Article | Purpose |
|---|---|
| Article 2 | Protection from discrimination |
| Article 3 | Best interests of the child a primary consideration: Institutions, services and facilities responsible for the care or protection of children shall conform to the standards established by competent authorities |
| Article 5 | Parents responsible for ensuring that child rights are protected |
| Article 6 | Right to survival and development |
| Article 9 | Right of the child who is separated from one or both parents to maintain personal relations and direct contact with both parents on a regular basis |
| Article 12 | Right of a child to express their views, considering the maturity of the child |
| Article 14 | Freedom of expression including seeking, receiving and imparting information |
| Article 16 | Protection of privacy |
| Article 17 | Access to information from mass media, with protection material injurious to child wellbeing |
| Article 18 | Assistance to parents with child rearing responsibilities |
| Article 19 | Protection from physical and mental violence, abuse or neglect |
| Article 20 | Special protection to children deprived of their families |
| Article 22 | Protection of children seeking refugee status |
| Article 23 | Rights of disabled children to special care |
| Article 24 | Right to health and access to healthcare |
| Article 27 | Right to an adequate standard of living |
| Article 28 | Right to education |
| Article 30 | Right to own culture and religion |
| Article 31 | Participation in leisure and play |
| Article 34 | Protection from sexual exploitation |

## The 2030 Agenda for Sustainable Development Goals (SDG)

The United Nations General Assembly formally adopted the 2030 Agenda for Sustainable Development Goals (SDG) in September 2015 (*sdgs.un.org/2030 agenda*). The SDGs are for universal, integrated and transformative vision for a better world. SDGs are composed of 17 goals and 169 targets to wipe out poverty, fight inequality and tackle climate change over the next 15 years.

## India's Approach to Promotion and Protection of Child Rights

The Ministry of Women and Child Development, Government of India addresses the issues of women and children. The National Commission for Protection of Child Rights (NCPCR) provides for protection and promotion of child rights in the country. Besides the institutional, administrative and legislative framework, India has a strong presence of non-governmental organizations, which along with media act as watch dogs to protect human and child rights.

### General Measurers of Implementation

To implement child rights commitment, several policies, laws and programs have been introduced:

- *National Policy for Children (2013) (www.india.gov.in/national-policy-children)*. The Government adopted this policy to reiterate its commitment to rights-based approach to children.
- *National Plan of Action for Children (2016) (www.india.gov.in/national-plan-action-children)*. The NAPC provides a road-map that links the policy objectives to actionable programs.
- *National Policy for Persons with Disabilities (2006) (www.nhp.gov.in/national-policy-for-persons-with-disabilities)*. The policy recognizes that a majority of persons with disabilities can lead a better quality of life, if they have access to equal opportunities and effective rehabilitation measures.



### National Legislations

The legislative framework for child rights is being strengthened with the formulations of new laws and amendments in old laws. These include the Food Security Bill (2011), Right to Free and Compulsory Education Act (2009), Prohibition of Child Marriage Act (2006), the Commissions for Protection of Child Rights Act (2005), Right to Information 2005, the Goa Children (amendment) Act 2005, the Child Labor (Prohibition & Regulation) Act, 1986 (two notifications in 2006 & 2008, expanded the list of banned and hazardous processes and occupation) & Information and Technology (Amendment) Act 2008. India adopted the Protection of Children from Sexual Offences Act (POSCO), 2012. This is the first comprehensive law on sexual abuse which expands the scope and range of forms of sexual offences, makes reporting of abuse mandatory and defines guidelines for child friendly police and procedures. Juvenile Justice (Care and Protection of Children) Act, 2015 is a proposed Act of the Parliament of India, under which juveniles involved in heinous offences in the age group of 16–18 years, will be tried as adults.

### National Programs

The Government of India is implementing several programs on social inclusion, gender sensitivity, child rights, participation and protection. The approach is based on UN CRC. These programs include: Integrated child development services (ICDS), *Kishori Shakti Yojana* and Nutrition program for adolescent girls, Rajiv Gandhi crèche scheme for children of working mother, scheme of assistance to home for children (*Sishu Griha*) to promote in country adoption, *Dhanalakshmi* conditional cash transfer schemes for girl child, Program for juvenile justice, Child Line (24-hr toll free no 1098 with outreach services for children in need of care and protection), Integrated Child Protection Scheme (ICPS), Integrated program for street children, Ujjawala (scheme for prevention of trafficking and rescue, rehabilitation, reintegration and repatriation), *Sarva Shiksha Abhiyan* (addresses the educational needs of 6–14 years and bridges social, gender and regional gaps with active participation of community), national program for education of girls at elementary level, *Kasturba Gandhi Balika Vidyalaya*, National Rural Health Mission, Mid-Day Meal scheme, Jawaharlal Nehru national urban renewal mission, Universal immunization program (UIP), and Integrated management of neonatal and childhood illness (IMNCI).

Competency: **PE35.1**

### Role of Physicians in Realizing Child Rights

The status and condition of children is the clearest indicator of whether nations and societies understand and respect human rights. Right to Education Act is now the law of the land. Physicians should work for adoption of the Right to Health legislation. They should advocate for evidence-based, proequity interventions; promote research, institute data collection, and monitor government programs. They should focus on the following activities:

a. Training on child rights, care and protection
b. Action on poverty, inequity, and the social determinants of health.
c. Addressing violence against children
d. Initiative for early child development
e. Inclusive care for children with disabilities.
f. Incorporating elements of child rights in clinical practice

Competencies: **PE27.29; PE27.30; PE27.31**

## CHILD MALTREATMENT (ABUSE AND NEGLECT)

The WHO defines child maltreatment to include all forms of physical and/or emotional ill-treatment, sexual abuse, neglect or negligent treatment or commercial or other exploitation, resulting in actual or potential harm to the child's health, survival, development or dignity, in the context of a relationship of responsibility, trust or power (Table 31.1).

### Extent of the Problem in India

Child maltreatment should be placed on the national agenda, both as a major child rights violation and public health problem. A Government of India, Ministry of Women and Child Development study (2007), among young children (5–12 years), revealed that (i) two of three (66%) children were physically abused, (ii) about 54% children

| Table 31.1: Types of child maltreatment |
|---|
| ***Physical abuse*** refers to any action that leads to physical harm. |
| ***Sexual abuse*** refers to any harm done to the child with the intention of sexual gratification. |
| ***Emotional abuse*** refers to the failure to provide a stable supportive emotional environment for the child. |
| ***Child neglect*** refers to the deprivation of the child in terms of health, education, emotional development, nutrition, shelter and safe living conditions in the presence and abundance of resources. The concept of child neglect occurs in context of availability of resources within the family and should not be confused with the provision of resources in context of poverty. |
| ***Child exploitation*** refers to profiting, in terms of monetary from children on account of their lack of power and vulnerability. |

reported having faced one of more forms of sexual abuse, (iii) 50% of the children were emotionally abused, (iv) 70.6% of girls reported having been neglected by family members, and (v) 48.4% of girls wished they were boys. Recently, India has been affected by a huge burden of COVID-19 pandemic infections in the world. The lockdown measures, losses of livelihood, and closure of schools has led to children experiencing heightened adversities within their homes. Children in marginalized communities are more vulnerable due to food insecurity, malnutrition, and limited access to health services, and routine immunizations.

## Short- and Long-Term Consequences of Child Abuse

Child abuse exerts a multitude of short- and long-term health effects on children, which may include serious and often lifelong adverse consequences to their mental, physical, and reproductive health, academic performance, and social functioning. Individuals across socioeconomic backgrounds and race had poor physical, mental and behavioral health on account of being exposed to violence and abuse during childhood. The adverse health effects in adult life include smoking, alcohol and drug abuse, promiscuity, and severe obesity, and also ill-health, such as depression, heart disease, cancer, chronic lung disease and shortened lifespan.

## Manifestations of Child Maltreatment

### *Physical Abuse*

Physical abuse is defined as "those acts of commission by a caregiver that cause actual physical harm or have the potential for harm". Corporal or physical punishment is the use of physical force to punish or discipline children. It is most commonly used to discipline a child in Indian schools. There is no evidence that corporal punishment leads to long-term positive outcomes; rather studies show negative outcomes such as child aggression and delinquent behavior.

Abusive head trauma or shaken baby syndrome usually occurs when a parent or caregiver severely shakes a child in frustration or anger, often because the child would not stop crying. The presenting symptoms can be mild and nonspecific. Retinal hemorrhage may be the only finding. Head trauma can cause permanent neurologic, cognitive or functional defects, and even death.

### *Clinical Assessment of Physical Abuse*

In addition to a disclosure of abuse from a child or parent, there are histories that raise a concern for physical abuse. Cases where no explanation is given for a significant injury, explicit denial of trauma in a child with obvious injury, inconsistency between the explanation (cause) of the injury with respect to the pattern, age, or severity of the injury or injuries, and notable delay in seeking medical care without explanation should raise concern for physical abuse. The responses from the parent and child should be documented verbatim. The child's developmental capabilities should receive critical consideration. Careful documentation of visible injuries by clear writing and/or body diagrams and medicolegal case reporting should be followed. Figure 31.1 demonstrates clinical response to a patient with child physical abuse.

### *Child Sexual Abuse*

Under the Protection of Children from Sexual Offences (POCSO) Act, any sexual activity with a child below 18 years, whether boy or girl, is a crime. As defined by the Act, sexual offences include penetrative sexual assault (section 3), sexual assault (i.e. non-penetrative) (section 7), sexual harassment (section 11) and use of a child for pornography (section 13). Figure 31.2 represents the clinical approach towards recognition and response to a patient with suspected sexual abuse.

### *Recognizing Child Sexual Abuse*

Children who have been sexually abused exhibit symptoms of infection, genital injury, abdominal pain, constipation, chronic or recurrent urinary tract infections or behavioral

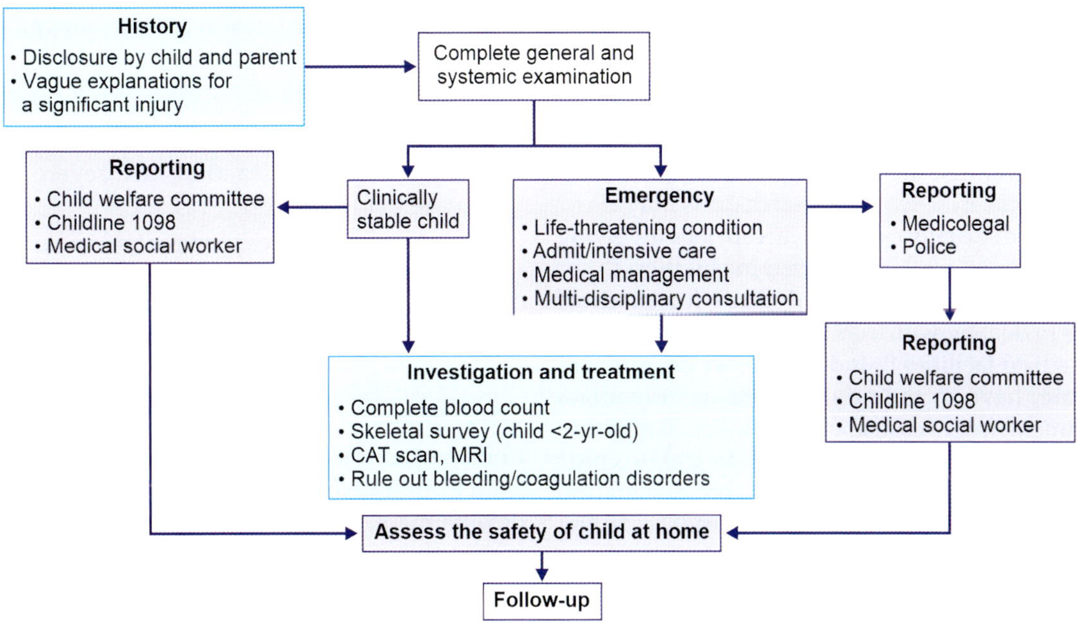


**Fig. 31.1:** Clinical response to chld physical abuse

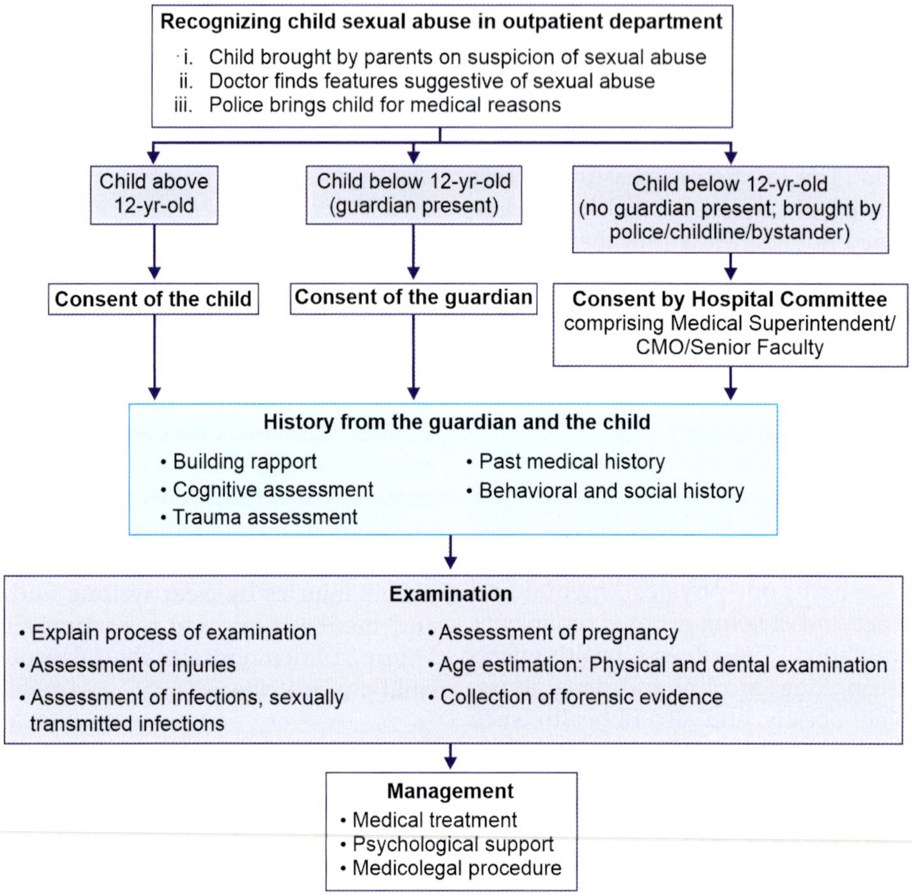


**Fig. 31.2:** Clinical approach towards recognition and response to child sexual abuse

problems. To be able to detect child sexual abuse requires a high index of suspicion and familiarity with the verbal, behavioral and physical indicators of abuse. Younger children do not have the vocabulary to express what is happening, feel embarrassed or ashamed to speak about sexual activity, or are unaware that they are experiencing sexual abuse. There are also social taboos on naming the genitals, or speaking within the family regarding sexuality. The cultural notions of "elders must be respected" and children's lack of power are other reasons for failure to disclose abuse.

Online child sexual abuse materials (formerly, child pornography) has increased many folds post-COVID in our country, as children are spending increased time on the internet. Parents in severe financial distress may allow their children to be sexually exploited, accept jobs involving hazardous labor or to get them married in childhood.

The POCSO Act provides guidelines for medical professionals in dealing with a child with suspected sexual abuse. All medical facilities in India, whether government run or private, have to provide first-aid or immediate medical treatment, free of cost, to victims of sexual offences. No hospital can refuse care or demand any legal records from the survivor. The doctor or healthcare professional are mandated to report all sexual offences to the police, failing which they may be punished with six months' imprisonment and/or fine. Clinical care, examination and collection of forensic evidence should be done as per the Ministry of Health and Welfare guidelines, Government of India.

### *Emotional Abuse*

Emotional abuse is defined as an act of causing various behavioral, cognitive, emotional, or mental traumas to a child by the caretakers or perpetrators. It is one of the most hidden form of maltreatment. Behaviors such as that of rejection, ignorance, shame, humiliation, terrorization, anxiety, depression and isolation have been broadly categorized as forms of emotional abuse. Early identification, mental health assessment and intervention should be initiated.

Children should be referred to a mental health professional in case of the following:

i. Traumatic stress reactions are severe or prolonged (more than a month)
ii. Traumatic stress reactions interfere with recovery or with returning to normal activities.
iii. Depression or suicidal risk
iv. Psychotic behavior

### *Child Neglect*

Child neglect is the failure to provide for the development of child in all spheres: Health, education, nutrition, emotional development, shelter and safe living conditions. Neglect may be distinguished from poverty in that culpable neglect is thought to occur only when there are resources available in the family, but caretakers are not providing them to the child.

*Specific subgroups at risk of neglect*

***Education and early child development:*** Failure to provide education or early stimulation for social, cognition and emotional needs.

***Medical neglect:*** Occurs when caregivers do not meet the child's basic healthcare needs, such as denial of immunizations, non-compliance with medicines, inadequate dental care.

***The girl child:*** Female infanticide, lack of birth registration, lack of social and legal protection, less likely to receive secondary education; or married early in childhood.

***Children with disabilities:*** Children with disabilities are 3–4 times more likely to be maltreated.

***Marginalized and vulnerable children:*** Examples include urban poor street children, child laborer, rural poor, tribal communities, scheduled and backward caste, children of construction workers, trafficked and sexually exploited children.

### Suggested Readings


1. Child maltreatment. World Health Organization. June 2020 www.who.int
2. Convention on the Rights of the Child, available from https://www.unicef.org/child-rights-convention, Accessed January 2022.
3. Seth R, Srivastava RN. Child sexual abuse: Management and prevention and protection of children from sexual offences (POCSO) Act. Indian Pediatrics, 2017; 54(11):949–53.
4. Seth R, Galagali P, Greenbaum J, et al. Child protection in context of COVID-19 pandemic: Practice guidelines for pediatricians. Asia Pacific Pediatr Child Health 2021;4:32–43.
5. The Protection of Children from Sexual Offences Act, 2012, available from https://legislative.gov.in/.../protection-children-sexual-offences-act-2012.


## ADOPTION

Adoption is an important alternative for the rehabilitation of children who are destitute and abandoned, or for social reasons cannot be brought up by their parents. Medical practitioners and pediatricians play a vital role in influencing health and social decisions of their adoptive patients and work closely with counselors and health professionals. 'Right to a family' is proposed as a fundamental right by the United Nations. Adoption agencies need to ensure that these rights are protected.

### Legal Aspects

In India, only specialized adoption agencies recognized by the State Government can deal with adoption placement. Direct adoption placement by hospitals, maternity and nursing homes is not permitted. Central Adoption Resource Authority (CARA) is an autonomous body under the Ministry of Women and Child Development, Government of India. It functions as a nodal body for adoption of Indian children and is mandated to monitor and regulate in-country and inter-country adoption. Prospective parents should be advised to read the guidelines from the CARA website and follow the due procedures. The Central Government has in July 2015 notified new guidelines issued by CARA, in pursuance of the Juvenile Justice (Care and Protection of Children) Act 2000. The Juvenile Justice Act enables citizens of all religions the freedom to adopt a minor child, irrespective whether he/she is a single parent and/or such adoptive parent/s adopt a child of the same sex, irrespective of the number of living biological sons or daughters. Prior to 2000, adoption was allowed to Hindus under the Hindu Adoption and Maintenance Act; other religious groups were governed by the Guardianship and Wards Act.

### Adoption Procedures

A child, who has been relinquished by his/her biological parents or found abandoned, must first be presented to the Child Welfare Committee. This committee has the sole authority to declare the child free for adoption under the current law. In case of an abandoned child, the committee, after due investigations, declares the child as destitute and free for adoption. In case the biological parents want to relinquish a child, they have to execute a document in favor of the adoption agency, duly witnessed by any authority of the hospital and a relative. A waiting period of 2 months is given to the biological parents to reconsider the decision, following which the child is free for adoption.

### Prospective Adoptive Parents

A child can be adopted by a married couple having infertility or voluntarily opting for adoption. Even single persons are eligible to adopt. Couples who have taken a decision to adopt should go to a registered agency, which is licensed to process adoption by both state government and the Central Adoption Resource Authority (an autonomous body under the Ministry of Women and Child Development, Government of India). Recognized placement agencies alone can process the application of abandoned children for in-country and inter-country adoptions of Indian children. Applications for inter-country adoption, of a child born in India, should be forwarded by an accredited agency of the country of the adoptive parents, to a recognized placement agency in India along with all documents to Central Adoption Resource Authority.

A social worker from the adoption agency provides guidelines and support to pre-adoptive parents, and helps them make informed decisions (pre-adoption counseling). A home study is conducted by the professional social worker. Additionally, parents are required to submit a document regarding their health, financial status; etc. Once their application is approved, a suitable child is shown to them. After they accept the child, placement is legalized. The placement is followed up to a period of 3 years or such time until legal adoption is complete. The adoptive parents are assured confidentiality and provided support as needed.

*Competency:* **PE35.1**

### Role of a Pediatrician

Pediatricians are in the position where families take them into confidence and seek their advice in many situations.

- All essential tests (HIV, hepatitis B), which have a window period may be repeated at 3 and 6 months, before placement.
- They can counsel and teach the potential families about the process of adoption.
- Parents who wish to relinquish their children due to any reason must be told about correct procedure; leaving young children in public places or in unhealthy surroundings is unsafe and traumatizing.
- Doctors should discourage private adoptions, since these are illegal.
- Babies in placement agencies are usually taken for a second opinion to a pediatrician, where the child should be examined carefully and a realistic diagnosis and prognosis should be explained to the adoptive parents.

## FOSTER CARE

Foster care is a system of alternative care in which children in need of care and protection are placed in temporary guardianship or custody of a caretaker, duly approved and certified by the State. The Ministry for Women and Child Development, Government of India has notified Model Guidelines for Foster Care in 2016. Children who are lost, abandoned, orphans, abused, trafficked, affected by conflicts, victims of natural disasters, addicted to substance abuse are all covered under the broad umbrella of children in need of care and protection and can benefit from placement in the foster care system. Foster care is a temporary solution until the time the child is united with its natural parents or given in adoption, which is a permanent placement.

### Role of Pediatrician

- The foster care is a non-institutional alternate care family arrangement, which might be temporary, but the impact on a child's life is forever.
- Pediatricians should recommend only formal alternative foster care arrangements directed by competent government bodies through child welfare committees.
- Pediatricians should ensure that foster parents protect the basic rights of the child including education, health, development, psychosocial support and protection.

### Suggested Reading

1. Concept of Foster Care in India. Int J Adv Legal Res 2020; ISSN: 2582-7340. https://wcd.nic.in/acts/model-guidelines-foster-care-2016.
2. Central Adoption Resource Agency (CARA). http://www.cara.nic.in/ accessed January 30, 2022.

Chapter

32

# Integrated Management of Neonatal and Childhood Illness

❍ P Ashok Babu ❍ Sumita Ghosh

Many well-known interventions like universal immunization, essential newborn care, exclusive breastfeeding during first 6 months of life, appropriate complementary feeding, oral rehydration therapy, and timely and appropriate use of antibiotics in pneumonia have proven to be effective in reducing child mortality. *While each of these interventions is successful, there is evidence to suggest that an integrated approach is needed to manage sick children.*

Sick children often present with overlapping signs and symptoms common to different illnesses and often suffer from more than one illness, which may necessitate different treatments. Another reason for integrated approach is the need for incorporating preventive strategies such as immunization and nutrition along with curative care.

*This chapter is an essential reading for students.* The core of normal and sick infant and child care is captured in the IMNCI strategy, content and algorithms. Several aspects of the key IMNCI themes have been covered in different chapters of the book, but the sections that follow here provide succinct, precise and structured information and guidance. Above all, the contents are aligned with the guidelines of our national programs.

*Competency:* **PE16.1**

## INTEGRATED MANAGEMENT OF NEONATAL AND CHILDHOOD ILLNESS STRATEGY

Integrated Management of Childhood Illness (IMCI) strategy, developed by World Health Organization in collaboration with UNICEF and many other agencies in mid-1990s, combines improved management of common childhood illnesses with prevention of diseases and promotion of health by including counseling on feeding and immunization. This strategy has been adapted and expanded in India to include neonatal care at home as well as in the health facilities and renamed as Integrated Management of Neonatal and Childhood Illness (IMNCI).

### Essential Components

The IMNCI strategy includes both preventive and curative interventions that aim to improve practices in health facilities, the health system and at home. At the core of the strategy is integrated case management of the most common neonatal and childhood problems with a focus on the most common causes of death in children <5 years of age.

The initial guidelines developed in 2003 were revised in 2009, and in 2022. *This chapter is based on the 2022 adaptation.* It elaborates the clinical guidelines for the treatment of sick children in an outpatient or primary care setting.

### Salient Adaptations in IMNCI (2022)

In general, the adaptations were undertaken to update as per global advancements and in line with the various guidelines of India released from time to time. The adaptation took into consideration revised WHO IMCI charts released in 2014 and antimicrobial therapy advancements. A major adaptation included incorporation of early child development messages along with nutritional counseling.

- Reduction of signs of possible severe bacterial infection (PSBI) in young infants
- Revised drug dosages for pre-referral treatment of possible severe bacterial infection
- Simplified classifications of diarrhea in young infants
- Mandatory assessment of breastfeeding in all young infants
- Revised immunization schedule and addition of deworming as per immunization and deworming policy of India
- Added classifying danger signs as severe disease with addition of convulsing now
- Added use of rapid acting bronchodilator before classifying wheeze with fast breathing/chest indrawing in children presenting with cough or difficult breathing
- Revised signs for classifying pneumonia as per WHO recommendations

- Added use of pulse oximetry for classifying pneumonia
- Revised classification of fever as per National Anti-Malaria Program guidelines including use of RDT and drugs for treating malaria and addition of additional classification of dengue in fever
- Signs for severe acute malnutrition revised
- Added early child development in the section on feeding counseling

### Clinical Guidelines

The clinical guidelines target children less than 5-year-old, the age group that bears the highest burden of morbidity and mortality. The guidelines represent an evidence-based syndromic approach to case management that includes rational, effective and affordable use of drugs. *Careful and systematic assessment of common symptoms, using selected reliable clinical signs, helps to guide rational and effective actions.*

An evidence-based syndromic approach can be used to determine:

i. Health problem(s) the child may have;
ii. Severity of the child's condition; and
iii. Actions that can be taken to care for the child (e.g. refer the child immediately, manage with available resources or manage at home). In addition, the guidelines suggest the adjustments required to manage with the capacity of health system and active involvement of family members in healthcare practices.

### Principles of Integrated Care

Depending on a child's age, various clinical signs and symptoms differ in their degrees of reliability and diagnostic value and importance. IMNCI clinical guidelines focus on children up to 5 years of age. The treatment guidelines have been broadly described under two age categories:

1. Young infants age up to 2 months
2. Children age 2 months up to 5 years

The IMNCI guidelines are based on the following principles:

1. All children under 5 years of age must be examined for conditions which indicate immediate referral.
2. Children must be routinely assessed for major symptoms, nutritional, quality of interaction with a child, immunization status, feeding problems and other problems.
3. Only a limited number of carefully selected clinical signs are used for assessment.
4. A combination of individual signs is used to classify the severity of illness which calls for specific action rather than a 'diagnosis'. Classifications are color-coded and suggest—referral (pink), initiation of treatment in health facility (yellow) or management at home (green).
5. IMNCI guidelines address most common, but not all, pediatric problems.
6. IMNCI management protocols use a limited number of essential drugs.
7. Caretakers are actively involved in the treatment of children.
8. IMNCI includes counseling of caretakers about home care including feeding, fluids and when to return to health facility.

The overall case management process is summarized in Fig. 32.1.

The case management of a sick child brought to a first-level health facility includes a number of important elements.

*Outpatient health facility:* Assessment; classification and identification of treatment; referral, treatment or counseling of the child's caretaker (depending on classification(s) identified); follow-up care.

*Referral health facility:* Emergency triage assessment and treatment (ETAT); diagnosis, treatment and monitoring of patient progress.

*Appropriate home management:* Teaching mothers or other caretakers how to give oral drugs and treat local infections at home; counseling mothers or other caretakers about food (feeding advice, feeding problems); development support care (playing and communication); fluids; when to return to the health facility; and the mother's own health.

### Classification Tables

IMNCI classification tables describe the steps of case management process: ASSESS, CLASSIFY and IDENTIFY TREATMENT. There are separate classification boxes for main symptoms, nutritional status and anemia.

IMNCI classifications are not necessarily specific diagnoses, but they indicate what action needs to be taken. All classifications are color-coded: Pink calls for hospital referral or admission, yellow for initiation of treatment, and green means that the child can be sent home with careful advice on when to return.

Classification tables are used starting with the pink rows. If the young infant or child does not have the severe classifications, look at the yellow rows. For the classification tables that have a green row, if the young infant or child does not have any of the signs in the pink or yellow rows, select the classification in the green row. If the young infant or child has signs from more than one row, the more severe classifications is selected. However, if the classification table has more than one arm (e.g. possible bacterial infection/jaundice, diarrhea in a sick child), one may have more than one classification from that box.

*Competencies:* **PE16.2; PE 20.18; PE 24.11**

## OUTPATIENT MANAGEMENT OF YOUNG INFANTS AGE UP TO 2 MONTHS

Young infants have special characteristics that must be considered when classifying their illnesses. They can become sick and die very quickly from serious bacterial infections. They frequently have only general signs such as few movements, fever or low body temperature. Mild chest indrawing is normal in young infants because their chest wall is soft. The assessment procedure for this age group includes a number of important steps that must be taken by the healthcare provider, which are given as follows.

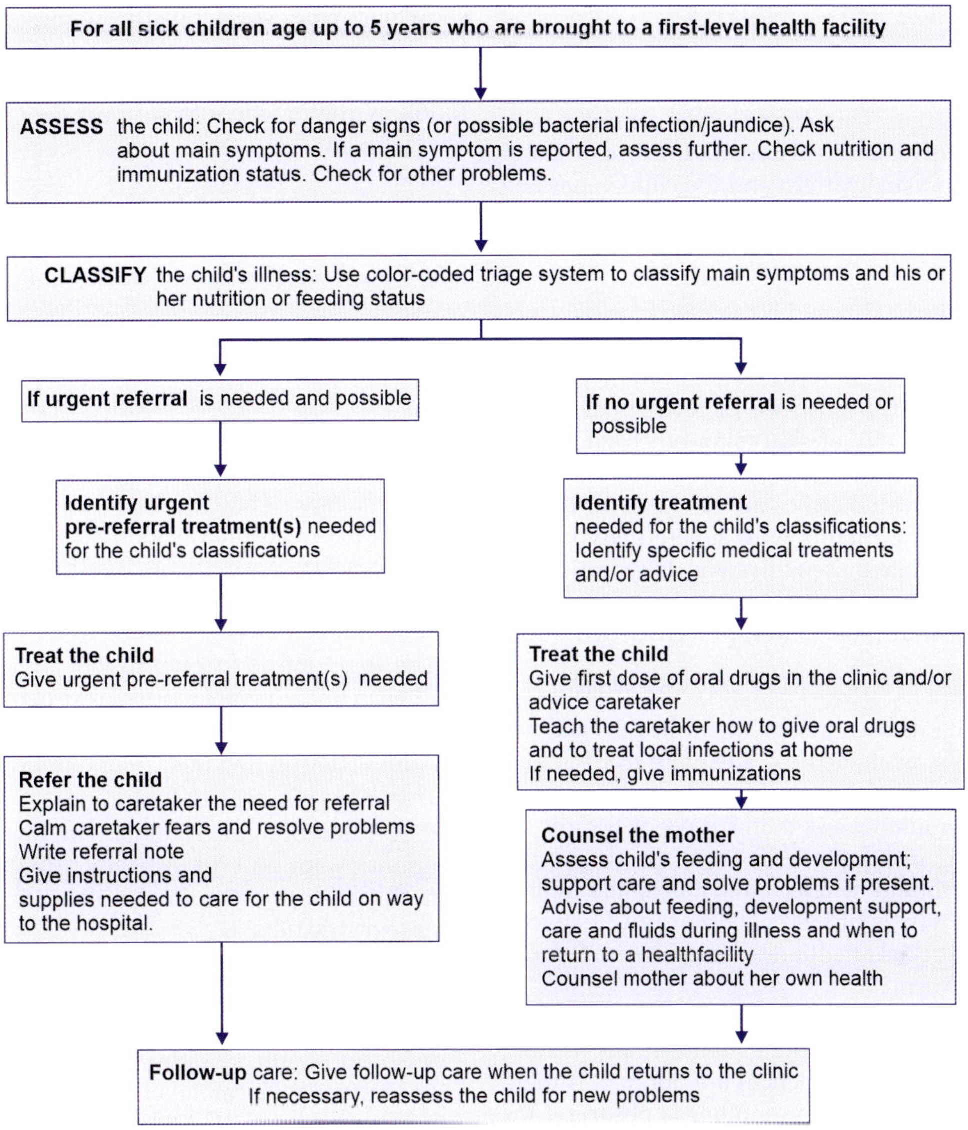


**Fig. 32.1:** Summary of the case management process

## Communicating with the Caretaker

It is critical to communicate effectively with the infant's mother or caretaker. Good communication techniques and an integrated assessment are required to ensure that common problems or signs of disease or malnutrition are not overlooked.

## Checking for Possible Bacterial Infection/Jaundice

A sick young infant with possible serious bacterial infection is one with any of the following signs: Not feeding well, convulsions, fast breathing, severe chest indrawing, fever, hypothermia, movement only when stimulated or no movement at all.

This infant should be referred urgently to the hospital after being given the first dose of intramuscular ampicillin/oral amoxycillin plus gentamicin, treatment to prevent hypoglycemia, and advice to the mother on keeping the young infant warm while arranging referral, and on the way to the hospital.

A sick young infant with local bacterial infection is the one with umbilicus red or draining pus or skin pustules. This infant may be treated at home with oral antibiotics but should be seen in follow-up after two days. For a sick young infant with no signs of possible serious bacterial infection and no signs of local bacterial infection, the classification should be infection unlikely.

Additionally, if the sick young infant has jaundice, classify for jaundice.

There are three possible classifications:

- A sick young infant with severe jaundice is one who has yellow palms and soles or has jaundice at age <24 hours or at age 14 days or more. This infant should be referred urgently to the hospital after being given treatment to prevent hypoglycemia and advice to the mother on keeping the young infant warm while arranging referral.
- A sick young infant with jaundice is one who has jaundice but the palms and soles are not yellow. This infant should be given home care, but mother should be advised when to return immediately and should be seen in follow-up in two days.
- A young infant with no signs of jaundice will be classified as no jaundice. The mothers or caretakers of such infants should be given advice to provide proper home care.

### Assessing for Diarrhea

Diarrhea is a main symptom, which is assessed if the mother says it is present. Exclusively breastfed infants normally pass frequent soft stools. This should not be confused with diarrhea. A young infant is said to have diarrhea, if the stools have changed from usual pattern and the child is passing many watery stools (more water than fecal matter).

#### *Clinical Assessment and Classification*

All infants with diarrhea should be assessed for presence of dehydration. A number of clinical signs are used to determine the level of dehydration: Infant's general condition (lethargic or unconscious or restless/irritable); sunken eyes and elasticity of skin (skin pinch goes back very slowly, slowly or immediately).

All young infants with diarrhea are classified for degree of dehydration. Young infants with severe dehydration will need IV fluids while those with some dehydration are treated as plan B with oral rehydration. Young infants with no dehydration will require more fluid to prevent dehydration.

### Checking for Feeding Problems or Very Low Weight

All sick young infants seen in outpatient health facilities should be routinely evaluated for adequate feeding and have their weight checked. Infants who are very low weight (weight <1800 g in infants less than 7 days or weight for age less than –3SD in infants 7–59 days) are given pink classification and should be referred to a hospital. Infants who are low weight (weight 1800–2500 g or WAZ between –2 to –3 SD) need special attention to how they are fed and on keeping them warm.

To assess the young infant for feeding problems, the mother is asked specific questions about infant feeding to determine, if the feeding practices are optimal. If there is no indication for referral, the mother is observed for breastfeeding. Breastfeeding is observed to see the signs of attachment and whether the infant is suckling effectively. Mothers of infants with problem in feeding are counseled appropriately. Infants who are not low weight for age and have no feeding problem are classified as 'no feeding problem' and counseled about home care of young infant.

### Checking Immunization Status

Immunization status should be checked in all sick young infants. A young infant who is not sick enough to be referred to a hospital should be given the necessary immunizations before he is sent home.

### Assessing other Problems

All sick young infants need to be assessed for other potential problems mentioned by the mother or observed during the examination. If a potentially serious problem is found or there are no means in the clinic to help the infant, he should be referred to hospital.

#### *Assessing the Mother/Caregiver's Development Supportive Practices*

All the mothers/caretakers should be asked, if they play with or talk to their infants. Observe them while comforting, showing love, or correcting the infants. These practices are feasible approaches for improving developmental outcomes in children. The mothers/caregivers should be counselled to follow the practices to support the child's growth and development.

### Identify Treatment and Treat

The next step is to identify treatment required for the young infant according to the classification (*see* Charts). All the treatments required are listed in the 'Identify Treatment' column of the ASSESS and CLASSIFY THE SICK YOUNG INFANT. If a sick infant has more than one classification, treatment required for all the classifications must be identified. The first step is to determine, if there is need to refer the child to hospital.

All infants and children with a severe classification (pink) are referred to a hospital as soon as assessment is completed and necessary pre-referral treatment is administered. Successful referral of severely ill infants to the hospital depends on effective counseling of the caretaker.

The first step is to give urgent prereferral treatment (written in bold font in Identify Treatment Section of Chart). This may be:

- Administering first dose of antibiotic
- Treatment of severe dehydration
- Prevention of hypoglycemia with breast milk; if young infant is not able to swallow, give expressed breast milk/appropriate animal milk with added sugar by nasogastric tube
- In young infants with diarrhea, giving frequent sips of ORS solution on the way to the hospital. Non-urgent treatments, e.g. applying gentian violet paint on skin pustules, should be deferred to avoid delaying referral or confusing the caretaker.
- If an infant does not need urgent referral, check to see if the infant needs non-urgent referral for further assessment. These referrals are not as urgent. Other necessary treatments may be done before referral.

### Treatment in Outpatient Clinic and at Home

Young infants who have local infection, feeding problem or low weight, or diarrhea with some dehydration should have treatment initiated in clinic, which is continued at home. Counseling a mother/caretaker is critical for home care. The health professional should use good communication skills while counseling the mother/caretaker for treatment **(Box 32.1)**.

### Advise when to Return

***Immediately:*** Return immediately, if the infant has any of these signs: Breastfeeding or drinking poorly, becomes sicker, develops a fever or feels cold to touch, fast breathing, difficult breathing, yellow palms and soles (if young infant has jaundice), diarrhea with blood in stool.

***For follow-up visit:*** Return not later than 2 days, if the infant has: Local bacterial infection, or jaundice or diarrhea or feeding problem or thrush; and not later than 14 days, if low weight.

**Box 32.1: Effective Communication and Counseling–APAC**

- *Ask and listen:* Ask the mother/caretaker and listen carefully to find out the young child's problems and what the mother/caretaker is already doing for the young infant
- *Praise:* Praise the mother/caretaker for what she has done well
- *Advise and teach:* Advise the mother/caretaker how to take care of young child at home (for tasks which require mother/caretaker to carry out treatment at home: Give information, show an example, and let her practice)
- *Check:* Before the mother/caretaker leaves, always check understanding by asking questions to find out what she understands and what needs further explanation

***Next well child visit:*** For immunization and feeding counseling.

### Counsel the Mother about her Own Health

During a sick infant visit, listen for any problems that the mother herself may be having. She may need treatment or referral for her own health problems. If the mother is sick, provide care for her, or refer her for help. Advise her to eat well to keep up her own strength and health. Check her immunization status and give tetanus toxoid, if needed. Give the mother iron folic acid tablets, if she is not taken them. Make sure she has access to family planning and counseling on STD and AIDS prevention.

*Competencies:* **PE10.4; PE16.3; PE28.15; PE24.11**

## OUTPATIENT MANAGEMENT OF SICK CHILD AGE 2 MONTHS TO 5 YEARS

The assessment procedure is similar to that of young infant including:

i. History taking and communicating with the caretaker about the child's problem;
ii. Checking for general danger signs;
iii. Checking main symptoms;
iv. Checking for malnutrition;
v. Checking for anemia;
vi. Assessing the child's feeding;
vii. Checking immunization status; and
viii. Assessing other problems.

### Communicating–History Taking

A sick child brought to an outpatient facility may have signs that clearly indicate a specific problem. However, some children may present with serious, nonspecific signs called *General Danger Signs* that do not point to a particular diagnosis. For example, a child who is lethargic or unconscious may have meningitis, severe pneumonia, cerebral malaria or any other severe disease. Great care should be taken to ensure that these general danger signs are not overlooked because they suggest that a child is severely ill and needs urgent attention.

### Assessing for General Danger Signs

The following signs should be routinely checked in all children: (i) History of convulsions during the present illness, (ii) unconsciousness or lethargy, inability to drink or breastfeed when mother tries to breastfeed, or to give child something to drink; (iii) child vomits everything; and (iv) child is presently having convulsions.

If a child has one or more of these signs, he must be considered seriously ill and will almost always need referral.

### Assessing for Main Symptoms

After checking for general danger signs, the healthcare provider must enquire about the following main symptoms: (i) Cough or difficult breathing; (ii) diarrhea; (iii) fever; and (iv) ear problems. If the symptom is present, the child is evaluated for that symptom.

#### *Cough or Difficult Breathing*

Four key clinical signs are used to assess a sick child with cough or difficult breathing:

- *Fast breathing:* Cut-off respiratory rate for fast breathing is >50 breaths per minute for a child 2–12 months and >40 breaths per minute for 12 months to 5 years
- Lower chest wall indrawing
- Stridor
- Wheeze

Patients with wheezing and either fast breathing or chest indrawing are given a trial of rapid acting inhaled bronchodilator for up to three times 15–20 minutes apart. The patient is observed again for respiratory rate and signs of chest indrawing, and reclassified as follows.

***Classification of cough or difficult breathing:*** Those requiring referral for possible **severe pneumonia or severe disease**. This group includes children with any general danger sign, or stridor when calm. Children with severe pneumonia or severe disease most likely have an invasive bacterial organisms and diseases that may be life-threatening. The patient needs urgent referral to a hospital for treatment, such as oxygen, a bronchodilator or injectable antibiotics. **Pulse oximeter is used to determine oxygen saturation and patient referred, if saturation is <90%.**

Those who require antibiotics as outpatients because they are highly likely to have **bacterial pneumonia**. A child with cough or difficult breathing who has fast breathing and/or chest indrawing is classified as having pneumonia. This child should not have a general danger signs, or stridor and his oxygen saturation is >90%.

Those who simply have a **cough or cold** and do not require antibiotics—such children may require a safe remedy to a relieve cough. A child with cough and cold normally improves in 1–2 weeks. However, a child with chronic cough (more than 14 days) needs to be further assessed (and, if needed, referred) to exclude tuberculosis, asthma, whooping cough or another problem.

#### *Diarrhea*

A child with diarrhea passes stools with more water than normal. A child with diarrhea may have (i) acute watery diarrhea (including cholera); (ii) dysentery (bloody diarrhea); or (iii) persistent diarrhea (diarrhea that lasts 14 days or more).

*Clinical assessment and classification:* All children with diarrhea should be assessed for dehydration based on the following clinical signs: General condition (lethargic or unconscious or restless/irritable); sunken eyes; child's reaction when offered to drink (not able to drink or drinking poorly or drinking eagerly/thirsty or drinking normally) and elasticity of skin (skin pinch goes back very slowly, slowly or immediately). In addition, a child with diarrhea should be asked how long the child has had diarrhea and if there is blood in the stool. This will allow identification of children with persistent diarrhea and dysentery.

### *Fever*

All cases with fever are suspected to have malaria after ruling out other common causes and should be investigated for confirmation of malaria by microscopy or rapid diagnostic kit (RDK) so as to ensure treatment with full therapeutic dose with appropriate drug to all confirmed cases.

History of duration of fever is important in evaluating fever. If fever has persisted daily for more than 7 days, the child needs to be referred to hospital for assessment and diagnostic tests. The other signs looked for in a child with fever include general danger signs (assessed earlier) and signs of meningitis, e.g. stiff neck. Besides these, signs of measles such as cough/difficult breathing, diarrhea, cornea clouding, mouth ulcers and ear infections. Before classifying fever, one should check for other obvious causes of fever such as malaria and dengue. A child with positive tourniquet test >20 petechiae per square inch area over forearm along with cold extremities with weak and fast pulse, or severe abdominal pain, or bleeding from any site or melena is classified as severe dengue/dengue with warning signs. Dengue should be suspected, if a child has fever lasting 2–7 days and residing in an area of dengue risk.

### *Ear Problems*

A child with an ear problem may have otitis. It may be acute or chronic infection. If the infection is not treated, the ear-drum may perforate. The mother is asked about history of ear pain and ear discharge or pus. The child is examined for tender swelling behind the ear. Based on these clinical findings, a child can be classified as mastoiditis, acute ear infection, chronic ear infection or no ear infection. Children with mastoiditis are classified as severe illness and referred urgently to hospital. Children with acute ear infection are given oral antibiotics and those with chronic ear infection are advised to keep the ear dry by wicking.

## Checking for Malnutrition

After assessing for general danger signs and the four main symptoms, all children should be assessed for malnutrition. There are two main reasons for routine assessment of nutritional status in sick children: (i) To identify children with severe malnutrition who are at increased risk of mortality and need urgent referral to provide active treatment; and (ii) to identify children with suboptimal nutritional status resulting from ongoing deficits in dietary intake plus repeated episodes of infection and who may benefit from nutritional counseling.

*Clinical assessment and classification:* Edema of both feet; weight for height; mid-upper arm circumference (only for children 6–59 months).

The child is classified as **complicated severe acute malnutrition** when they have severe acute malnutrition (edema of both feet, weight for height/length less than –3 SD scores, or mid-upper arm circumference less than 115 mm) and at **least one medical complication**, including any general danger sign, any severe classification, or pneumonia with chest indrawing or a feeding problem in children under 6 months. Children classified as having **complicated severe acute malnutrition** are at high risk of death from pneumonia, diarrhea, measles, and other severe diseases. These children need urgent referral to hospital where their treatment can be carefully monitored.

If the child has at least one sign of severe acute malnutrition, but does not have other signs of complication, they are classified as **uncomplicated severe acute malnutrition**. A child is classified as moderate acute malnutrition, if the weight-for-age is between –3 and –2 Z-scores or MUAC is between 115 and 125 mm. The child is classified as **no acute malnutrition,** if the child has a weight-for-age over –2 Z-scores, and has no other signs of malnutrition.

## Checking for Anemia

Palmar pallor can help to identify sick children with severe anemia. Wherever feasible, diagnosis of anemia can be supported by using a simple laboratory test for hemoglobin estimation. For clinical assessment of anemia, the color of the child's palm is compared with examiner's own palm. If the skin of the child's palm is pale, the child has some palmar pallor (Hb 7–10.9 g/dL). If the skin of the palm is very pale or so pale that it looks white, the child has severe palmar pallor (Hb <7 g/dL). Pallor is classified as severe anemia, anemia or no anemia.

## Assessing Child's Feeding and Development Support Care

All children less than 2 years old and all children classified as moderate acute malnutrition need to be assessed for feeding and development support care.

Feeding assessment includes questioning the mother or caretaker about: (i) Breastfeeding frequency and night feeds; (ii) types of complimentary foods or fluids, frequency of feeding and whether feeding is active; and (iii) feeding patterns during the current illness. The mother or caretaker should be given appropriate advice to help overcome any feeding problems found.

Assessment of development support care includes assessment of mother's sensitivity and responsiveness to the child's needs through questioning the mother or caretaker about: (i) Playing with the baby; (ii) talking to the baby, and (iii) making the baby smile and the learning pattern of the child. The mother or caretaker should be given appropriate advice to help overcome any playing and communication problems found (for more details, refer to the section on counselling the mother or caretaker).

#### Identify Feeding Problems

It is important to complete the assessment of feeding by referring to age appropriate feeding recommendations and identify all the feeding problems before giving advice. Other common feeding problems are: Difficulty breastfeeding, use of feeding bottle, lack of active feeding and not feeding well during illness.

#### Identify Developmentally Supportive (Family Interaction) Problems

It is important to complete the assessment of family interaction and identify all the problems before giving advice. Based on the mother's answers to the questions, identify any differences between the family's actual interaction (sensitivity and responsiveness) and the recommendations. These differences are problems. Some examples of interaction problems are listed in **Box 32.2**.

### Checking Immunization, Vitamin A and Folic Acid Supplementation and Deworming Status

The immunization status of every sick child brought to a health facility should be checked. After checking immunization status, determine if the child needs vitamin A supplementation and/or prophylactic iron folic acid supplementation or deworming administration.

### Assessing other Problems

The IMNCI clinical guidelines focus on five main symptoms. In addition, the assessment steps within each main symptom take into account several other common problems. For example, conditions such as meningitis, sepsis, tuberculosis, conjunctivitis, and different causes of fever such as ear infection and sore throat are routinely assessed within the IMNCI case management process.

### Identify Treatment and Treat

All the treatments required are listed in the Identify Treatment column of the Assess and Classify the Sick Child Age 2 months to 5 years (see Chart). All sick children with a severe classification (pink) are referred to a hospital as soon as assessment is completed and necessary pre-referral treatment is administered. If a child only has severe dehydration and no other severe classification, and IV infusion is available in the outpatient clinic, an attempt should be made to rehydrate the sick child. The principles of referral of a sick child are similar to those described for a sick young infant.

#### Referral of Children Age 2 Months to 5 Years

***For all children before referral***

1. Prevent low blood sugar by giving breast milk or sugar water.
2. For convulsions, give diazepam (10 mg/2 mL solution) in dose 0.2 mg/kg (0.05 mL/kg) IV or rectally; if convulsions continue after 10 minutes, give a second dose of diazepam.
3. For severe pneumonia or severe disease (as also for mastoiditis), give first dose of IV or intramuscular antibiotic. Options for an intramuscular antibiotic for pre-referral use include ampicillin plus gentamicin combination, or ceftriaxone.
4. For very severe febrile disease, give one dose of paracetamol for high fever (38.5°C or above). Give first dose of intramuscular quinine/artesunate for severe malaria in areas with high *Plasmodium falciparum*, and give first dose of an appropriate antibiotic.
5. For severe complicated measles, give first dose of appropriate antibiotic, give vitamin A, and if there is clouding of the cornea or pus draining from the eye, apply tetracycline eye ointment.
6. For severe dehydration, IV fluids should be given in the outpatient clinic according to WHO Treatment Plan C. Give 100 mL/kg IV fluids. Ringer's lactate solution is the preferred commercially available solution.
7. For severe persistent diarrhea, treat dehydration before referral using WHO Treatment Plan B for some dehydration and Plan C for severe dehydration.
8. For severe acute malnutrition, give first dose of intramuscular antibiotics. Options for an intramuscular antibiotic for pre-referral use include ampicillin plus gentamicin combination or ceftriaxone. Oral amoxicillin can be an option.

**Box 32.2: Examples of Interaction Problems**

| Family interaction | Recommended action |
|---|---|
| Mother reports, "she does not play with baby" | Discuss ways to help baby see, hear, feel and move, appropriate for age, ask caregiver to do play or communication activity, appropriate for age |
| Mother reports, "she does not talk to child or talks harshly to child" | If baby is less than 6 months, ask, caregiver to look into baby's eyes and talk to baby. For older children, give caregiver and child an activity to do together. Help mother interpret what child is doing and thinking and see child respond and smile. If the mother scolds child, help caregiver distract child from unwanted actions by giving alternative toy or activity. If the mother is not able to comfort child and child does not look at the mother for comfort: help mother look into child's eyes and gently talk to child and hold child. |
| Mother tries to force smile or is not responsive to baby | Ask mother to make large gestures and cooing sounds; copy baby's sounds and gestures and see baby's responses. |
| Mother says the child is slow to learn | Encourage more activity with the child, check hearing and seeing. Refer child with difficulties |

***Treatment in outpatient clinics and at home:*** Identify the treatment associated with each nonreferral classification (yellow and green) in the IMNCI chart. Treatment uses a minimum of affordable essential drugs **(Box 32.3)**.

## Counseling a Mother or Caretaker

A child who is seen at the clinic needs to continue treatment, feeding and fluids at home. The child's mother or caretaker also needs to recognize when the child is not improving, or is becoming sicker. The success of home treatment depends on how well the mother or caretaker knows how to give treatment, understands its importance and knows when to return to a healthcare provider. Table 32.1 lists the specific times to advise a mother or caretaker to return to a health facility.

**Table 32.1:** Follow-up visits

| **When to return** |
|---|
| *Immediately* |
| • Any sick child not able to drink or breastfeed, or becomes sicker or develops a fever<br>• If child has no pneumonia: Cough or cold, also return if fast breathing or difficult breathing<br>• If child has diarrhea, also return if blood in stool or drinking poorly |
| *For follow-up visit (not later than ...)* |
| **2 days:** Pneumonia, dysentery, malaria/suspected malaria/fever; malaria unlikely if fever persists; measles with eye or mouth complications.<br>**5 days:** Diarrhea, if not improving, persistent diarrhea, acute ear infection, chronic ear infection, uncomplicated acute malnutrition/feeding problem, any other illness, if not improving.<br>**14 days:** Anemia<br>**30 days:** Moderate acute malnutrition |

Advise when to return for the next immunization according to immunization schedule.

32

Essential Pediatrics

## Suggested Reading


1. IMCI: Global Survey report. World Health Organization; 2017
2. IMNCI: Ministry of Health and Family Welfare, Govt of India; 2022.
2. Integrated Management of Childhood Illness Chart Booklet. Geneva: World Health Organization; 2014
3. Oxygen therapy for children: a manual for health workers. Geneva: World Health Organization; 2016
4. Pediatric emergency triage, assessment and treatment: care of critically ill children: Updated guideline. Integrated Management of Child Illness. World Health Organization; 2016.

## Box 32.3: Treatment in Outpatient Clinics or at Home

| Classification | Treatment |
|---|---|
| Pneumonia | Oral amoxicillin for five days |
| No pneumonia–cough or cold | Soothe the throat and relieve the cough with a safe remedy |
| some dehydration | ***WHO Treatment Plan B*** <br> Give initial treatment with ORS over a period of four hours; a total of 75 mL/kg. If the child is breastfed, breastfeeding should continue. After four hours, the child is reassessed and reclassified for dehydration, and feeding should begin; resuming feeding early is important to provide required amounts of potassium and glucose. When there are no signs of dehydration, the child is put on Plan A. If there is still some dehydration, Plan B should be repeated. If the child now has severe dehydration, the child should be put on Plan C. <br> **Zinc supplements are given to children with acute diarrhea, persistent diarrhea and dysentery for 14 days** |
| No dehydration | ***WHO Treatment Plan A*** <br> Plan A focuses on the four rules of home treatment: Give extra fluids, zinc supplements, continue feeding, and advise the caretaker when to return to the doctor (if the child develops blood in the stool, drinks poorly, becomes sicker, or is not better in three days). Fluids should be given as soon as diarrhea starts; the child should take as much as she/he wants. Correct home therapy can prevent dehydration in many cases. ORS may be used at home to prevent dehydration. However, other fluids that are commonly available in the home may be less costly, more convenient and almost as effective. Most fluids that a child normally takes can also be used for home therapy especially when given with food. <br> **Zinc supplements are given to children with acute diarrhea, persistent diarrhea and dysentery for 14 days** |
| Persistent diarrhea | Encourage the mother to continue breastfeeding. <br> If yoghurt is available, give it in place of any animal milk usually taken by the child; yoghurt contains less lactose and is better tolerated. If animal milk must be given, limit it to 50 mL/kg/day; greater amounts may aggravate the diarrhea. <br> If milk is given, mix it with the child's cereal and do not dilute the milk. Food needs to be given in frequent, small meals, at least six times a day. All children with persistent diarrhea should receive supplementary multivitamins and minerals (copper, iron, magnesium, zinc) each day for two weeks. |
| Dysentery | The key elements of treatment are: Antibiotics, fluids, zinc supplements, feeding and follow-up. Selection of an antibiotic is based on sensitivity patterns of strains of *Shigella* isolated in the area (cefixime or ciprofloxacin is the drug of choice in many areas) for 5 days. |
| Malaria/suspected malaria | Use drugs recommended by the National Anti-Malaria Program in India |
| Fever–Malaria unlikely | Give one dose of paracetamol for high fever (38.5°C or above). Treat other obvious causes of fever. |
| Measles with eye or mouth complications | Give first dose of vitamin A. If clouding of cornea or pus draining from the eye, apply tetracycline eye ointment. If mouth ulcers, treat with gentian violet |
| Measles currently (or within the last 3 months) | Give first dose of vitamin A |
| Acute ear infection | Give appropriate antibiotic for five days; give one dose of paracetamol for pain; dry the ear by wicking. |
| Chronic ear infection | Dry the ear by wicking |
| Uncomplicated severe acute malnutrition | Counsel the mother on how to feed the child |
| Moderate acute malnutrition | Assess the child's feeding and counsel the mother accordingly on feeding |
| No acute malnutrition | If the child is less than 2 years old, assess the child's feeding and counsel the mother accordingly on feeding |
| Anemia | Give iron folic acid therapy as per national guidelines |
| No anemia | Give prophylactic iron folic acid as per national guidelines |

# ASSESS AND CLASSIFY THE SICK YOUNG INFANT AGE UPTO 2 MONTHS

## ASSESS

**ASK THE MOTHER WHAT THE YOUNG INFANT'S PROBLEMS ARE**
- Determine if this is an initial or follow-up visit for this problem.
  - if follow-up visit, use the follow-up instructions on the bottom of this chart.

**USE ALL BOXES THAT MATCH INFANT'S SYMPTOMS**

## CLASSIFY IDENTIFY TREATMENT

**A child with a pink classification needs URGENT attention, complete the assessment and pre- referral treatment immediately so that referral is not delayed**

## CHECK FOR POSSIBLE SERIOUS BACTERIAL INFECTION

***ASK:***

- Is the infant having difficulty in feeding?
- Has the infant had convulsions?

***LOOK, LISTEN, FEEL:***

- Count the breaths in one minute. Repeat the count if it is 60 or more breaths per minute.
- Look for severe chest indrawing.

} YOUNG INFANT MUST BE CALM

- Measure axillary temperature (if not possible, feel for fever or low body temperature).
- Look at the young infant's movements. *If infant is sleeping , ask the mother to wake him/her.*
  - Does the infant move on his/her own? -
  - Does the infant move only when stimulated but then stops ?
  - Does the infant not move at all?
- Look at the umbilicus. Is it red or draining pus?
- Look for skin pustules.

***Classify ALL YOUNG INFANTS***

| SIGNS | CLASSIFY AS | IDENTIFY TREATMENT (Urgent pre-referral treatments are in bold print.) |
|---|---|---|
| **Any one or more of the following signs:**<br>• Not able to feed at all or not feeding well <u>or</u><br>• Convulsions <u>or</u><br>• Fast breathing (60 breaths per minute or more in infants less than 7 days) <u>or</u><br>• Severe chest indrawing <u>or</u><br>• If axillary temperature 37.5°C or above (or feels hot to touch) <u>or</u><br>• Axillary temperature less than 35.5°C (or feels cold to touch) <u>or</u><br>• Movement only when stimulated or no movement at all | **POSSIBLE SERIOUS BACTERIAL INFECTION <u>OR</u> VERY SEVERE DISEASE** | ➢ ***Give first dose of intramuscular ampicillin and gentamicin.***<br>➢ ***Treat to prevent low blood sugar.***<br>➢ ***Advise the mother how to keep the infant warm on the way to the hospital.***<br>➢ ***Refer URGENTLY to hospital #*** |
| • Fast breathing ( 60 breaths per minute or more ) in infants 7-59 days old | **PNEUMONIA** | ➢ *If infant also has low weight for age or another severe classification:*<br>- ***Give first dose of intramuscular ampicillin and gentamicin***<br>- ***Refer URGENTLY to hospital***<br>➢ *If infant does not have low weight for age or another severe classification :*<br>***-Give oral amoxicillin for 7 days***<br>*-Advise the mother to give home care for the young infants*<br>-Advise mother when to return immediately<br>*- Follow up after 2 days* |
| • Umbilicus red or draining pus <u>or</u><br>• Skin pustules | **LOCAL BACTERIAL INFECTION** | ➢ **Give oral amoxicillin for 5 days**<br>➢ Teach the mother how to treat local infections at home.<br>➢ *Advise the mother to give home care for the young infants*<br>➢ Advise mother when to return immediately<br>➢ *Follow up after 2 days.* |
| • No Signs of bacterial infections or very severe disease | **INFECTION UNLIKELY** | ➢ *Advise the mother to give home care for the young infant* |

*# If referral is not possible, see the section* ***Where Referral Is Not Possible.***

## THEN, CHECK FOR JAUNDICE

**ASK:**

- When did jaundice first appear ?

**LOOK AND FEEL:**

- Look for jaundice (yellow skin) .
- Look at the young infant's palms and soles. Are they yellow ?

*Classify* **JAUNDICE**

| SIGNS | CLASSIFY AS | IDENTIFY TREATMENT (Urgent pre-referral treatments are in bold print.) |
|---|---|---|
| • Any jaundice in an infant aged less than 24 hours <u>or</u><br>• Yellow palms or soles at any age | **SEVERE JAUNDICE** | ➢ *Treat to prevent low blood sugar.*<br>➢ ***Refer URGENTLY to hospital*** #<br>➢ *Advise mother how to keep baby warm on the way to the hospital* |
| • Jaundice appearing after 24 hours of age <u>and</u><br>• Palms and soles not yellow | **JAUNDICE** | ➢ *Advise the mother to give home care for young infants*<br>➢ *Advise the mother to return immediately if the infant's palm or soles appear yellow .*<br>➢ *If the infant is older than 2weeks , refer to a hospital for assessment .*<br>➢ Follow up after 2 day. |
| • No jaundice | **NO JAUNDICE** | ➢ *Advise the mother to give home care to the young infant* |

\# *If referral is not possible, see the section* ***Where Referral Is Not Possible*** .

## THEN ASK:
## Does the young infant have diarrhoea?*

***IF YES LOOK AND FEEL:***

- Look at the young infant's general condition.
  - Look at Infant's movements :
    - Does the infant move on his/her own?
    - Does the infant move only when stimulated and then stops?
    - Does the infant not move at all?
  - Is the infant restless and irritable?
- Look for sunken eyes.
- Pinch the skin of the abdomen. Does it go back:
  - Very slowly (longer than 2 seconds)?
  - Slowly?

*Classify DIARRHOEA for DEHYDRATION*

| SIGNS | CLASSIFY | IDENTIFY TREATMENT (Urgent pre-referral treatment is shown in bold) |
|---|---|---|
| **Two of the following signs:**<br>• Movements only when stimulated or no movement at all<br>• Sunken eyes<br>• Skin pinch goes back very slowly. | **SEVERE DEHYDRATION** | ➢ ***Give first dose of intramuscular ampicillin and gentamicin.***<br>➢ *If infant also has another severe classification:*<br>- ***Refer URGENTLY to hospital*** *with the mother giving frequent sips of ORS on the way.*#<br>- *Advise mother to continue breastfeeding.*<br>- *Advise mother how to keep the young infant warm on the way to the hospital.*<br>*OR*<br>If infant does not have any other severe classification:<br>➢ Give fluid for severe dehydration (Plan C) and then refer to hospital after rehydration |
| **Two of the following signs:**<br>• Restless, irritable.<br>• Sunken eyes.<br>• Skin pinch goes back slowly. | **SOME DEHYDRATION** | ➢ *If infant also has low weight for age or another severe classification:*<br>- ***Give first dose of intramuscular ampicillin and gentamicin***<br>- ***Refer URGENTLY to hospital*** *with mother giving frequent sips of ORS on the way.*<br>- *Advise mother to continue breastfeeding.*<br>- *Advise mother how to keep the young infant warm on the way to the hospital.*<br>➢ *If infant does not have low weight or another severe classification:*<br>- Give fluids for some dehydration (Plan B). |
| • Not enough signs to classify as some or severe dehydration. | **NO DEHYDRATION** | ➢ *Give fluids and breastfeeds to treat diarrhea at home (Plan A).*<br>➢ *Advise mother when to return immediately.*<br>➢ *Follow up after 2 days if no improvement* |

**** What is diarrhoea in a young infant?***
If the stools have changed from usual pattern and are many and watery (more water than fecal matter). The normally frequent or loose stools of a breastfed baby are not diarrhoea.

*Blood in stool in young infant needs referral to a hospital to rule out surgical and medical causes*

# *If referral is not possible, see the section* ***Where Referral Is Not Possible*** .

# THEN CHECK FOR A FEEDING PROBLEM OR LOW WEIGHT FOR AGE

**ASK:**

- Is the infant having difficulty in feeding?
- Is the infant breastfed? If yes, how many times in 24 hours?
- Does the infant usually receive any other foods or drinks?
  - If yes, how often?
  - How is milk given ? Cup or bottle

**LOOK, FEEL:**

- Measure weight -
  - Is weight less than 1800gms ? Yes/ No
- Determine weight for age
  - Weight for age ≥ –2 SD score
  - Weight for age less than –2 SD score
  - Weight for age less than –3SD score
- Look for ulcers or white patches in the mouth (thrush)

*Classify FEEDING*

IF AN INFANT: **Has any difficulty feeding, or**
**Is breastfeeding less than 8 times in 24 hours, or**
**Is taking any other foods or drinks, or**
**Is low weight for age,**

ASSESS BREASTFEEDING:

- Has the infant breastfed in the previous hour?

If the infant has not fed in the previous hour, ask the mother to put her infant to the breast. Observe the breastfeed for 4 minutes.
(If the infant was fed during the previous hour, ask the mother if she can wait and tell you when the infant is willing to feed again.)

- Is the infant able to attach?

*no attachment at all* *not well attached* *good attachment*

*TO CHECK ATTACHMENT, LOOK FOR:*

- *Chin touching breast*
- *Mouth wide open*
- *Lower lip turned outward*
- *More areola visible above than below the mouth*

(All of these signs should be present if the attachment is good)

- Is the infant suckling effectively (that is, slow deep sucks, sometimes pausing)?

*not suckling at all* *not suckling effectively* *suckling effectively*

Clear a blocked nose if it interferes with breastfeeding.

- Does the mother have pain while breastfeeding?
  - If yes, look and feel for:
  - Flat or inverted nipples, or sore nipples
  - Engorged breasts or breast abscess

| SIGNS | CLASSIFY | PRE-REFERRAL TREATMENT |
|---|---|---|
| • Weight less than 1800 gm in infants less than 7 days<br>• Weight for age less than –3SD in infants 7-59days old | **VERY LOW WEIGHT** | ➢ ***Refer URGENTLY to hospital***[#]<br>➢ *Treat to prevent low blood sugar.*<br>➢ *Advise mother how to keep the young infant warm on the way to the hospital.* |
| • Not well attached to breast <u>or</u><br>• Not suckling effectively <u>or</u><br>• Less than 8 breastfeeds in 24 hours <u>or</u><br>• Receives other foods or drinks <u>or</u><br>• Thrush (ulcers or white patches in mouth) <u>or</u><br>• Low weight for age (Weight for age <-2 SD) <u>or</u><br>• Breast or nipple problems | **FEEDING PROBLEM <u>and/ or</u> LOW WEIGHT FOR AGE** | ➢ If receiving other foods or drinks, counsel mother about breastfeeding more, reducing other foods or drinks,<br>➢ If not well attached or not suckling effectively, teach correct positioning and attachment.<br>➢ If breastfeeding less than 8 times in 24 hours, advise to increase frequency of breastfeeding.<br>➢ If not breastfeeding at all -refer for breastfeeding counseling and relactation . -advise mother for about giving locally appropriate animal milk and teach the mother to feed with a cup and spoon<br>➢ If thrush, teach the mother to treat thrush at home.<br>➢ If low weight for age : - teach the mother how to keep the young infant warm at home. - advise to increase frequency of breastfeeding<br>➢ If breast or nipple problem, teach the mother to treat breast or nipple problems.<br>➢ Advise mother to give home care for the young infant.<br>➢ Advise mother when to return immediately.<br>➢ Follow-up any feeding problem or thrush after 2 days.<br>➢ Follow-up low weight for age after 14 days. |
| • Not low weight for age (≥ -2SD) and no other signs of inadequate feeding. | **NO FEEDING PROBLEM** | ➢ Praise the mother for feeding the infant well.<br>➢ Advise mother to give home care for the young infant.<br>➢ Advise mother when to return immediately. |

# *If referral is not possible, see the section* ***Where Referral Is Not Possible*** .

## THEN CHECK THE YOUNG INFANT'S IMMUNIZATION STATUS:

| IMMUNIZATION SCHEDULE *: | AGE | VACCINE |
|---|---|---|
| | Birth | BCG OPV 0 HEP-B 0 |
| | 6 weeks | Penta-1 OPV 1 Rotavirus-1 fIPV-1 PCV-1* |

* Rotavirus vaccine , f IPV , pneumococcal vaccine to be given wherever included in the immunization schedule

## ASSESS OTHER PROBLEMS

## ASSESS THE MOTHER/CAREGIVER'S DEVELOPMENT SUPPORTIVE PRACTICES AND COUNSEL FOR PRACTICES TO SUPPORT CHILD'S DEVELOPMENT

## COUNSEL THE MOTHER ABOUT HER OWN HEALTH

# TREAT THE YOUNG INFANT AND COUNSEL THE MOTHER

## GIVE THESE TREATMENTS IN CLINIC ONLY

- **Explain to the mother why the drug is given.**
- **Determine the dose appropriate for the infant's weight (or age).**
- **Use a sterile needle and sterile syringe. Measure the dose accurately.**
- **Give the drug as an intramuscular injection.**
- **Referral is the best option for a young infant classification with POSSIBLE SERIOUS BACTERIAL INFECTION, SEVERE DEHYDRATION, SOME DEHYDRATION WITH LOW WEIGHT & VERY LOW WEIGHT FOR AGE.**
- **If referral is not possible or refused, give oral amoxicillin ( 25-30 mg/kg) every 12 hours and intramuscular gentamicin once daily.**

♦ ***At each contact for injection of antibiotics, explain again to the caregiver that the infant is very sick and should urgently be referred for hospital care***

♦ ***If referral is still not possible, continue giving once-daily intramuscular gentamycin and twice – daily intramuscular ampicillin until referral is feasible or for 7 days.***

### ➢ *Give First Dose of Intramuscular Antibiotics*

➢ Give first dose of both ampicillin and gentamicin intramuscularly.

| Weight | **Ampicillin** Add 1.3 ml sterile water = 250 mg/1.5 ml or 166mg/ml | **Gentamicin** Undiluted 2 ml vial containing 20 mg = 2 ml at 10 mg/ml or Add 6 ml sterile water to 2 ml vial containing 80 mg* = 8 ml at 10 mg/ml | |
|---|---|---|---|
| | Dose : 50 mg per kg | Age <7 days Dose: 5 mg per kg | Age ≥7 days Dose : 7.5 mg/kg |
| <1.5kg | 0.4 ml | 0.6 ml | 0.9 ml |
| 1.5kg –up to 2.0 kg | 0.5 ml | 0.9 ml | 1.3 ml |
| 2kg– up to 3.0 kg | 0.8 ml | 1. 2 ml | 1.8 ml |
| 3kg- up to 4.0 kg | 1.0 ml | 1.6 ml | 2.4 ml |
| 4kg- up to 5.0 kg | 1.3 ml | 2.1 ml | 3. 0 ml |

**Avoid using undiluted 40 mg/ml gentamicin.*

### ➢ *Treat the Young Infant to Prevent Low Blood Sugar*

- ***If the child is able to breastfeed:***

  Ask the mother to breastfeed the child.

- ***If the child is not able to breastfeed but is able to swallow:***

  Give 20-50 ml (10 ml/kg) of expressed breastmilk or locally appropriate animal milk (with added sugar) before departure. If neither of these is available, give 20-50 ml (10 ml/kg) of sugar water.

  **To make sugar water: Dissolve 4 level teaspoons of sugar (20 grams) in a 200-ml cup of clean water.**

- ***If the child is not able to swallow:***

  Give 20-50 ml (10 ml/kg) of expressed breastmilk or locally appropriate animal milk (with added sugar) or sugar water by nasogastric tube.

# KEEP THE YOUNG INFANT WARM

## ➢ *Warm the young infant using Skin to Skin contact (Kangaroo Mother Care)*

- Provide privacy to the mother. If mother is not available, Skin to Skin contact may be provided by the father or any other adult.
- Request the mother to sit or recline comfortably.
- Undress the baby gently, except for cap, nappy and socks.
- Place the baby prone on mother's chest in an upright and extended posture, between her breasts, in Skin to Skin contact; turn baby's head to one side to keep airways clear .
- Cover the baby with mother's blouse, 'pallu' or gown; wrap the baby-mother duo with an added blanket or shawl.
- Breastfeed the baby frequently.
- If possible, warm the room (>25°C) with a heating device.

## ➢ *Skin to Skin contact is the most practical, preferred method of warming a hypothermic infant in a primary health care facility. If not possible:*

- Clothe the baby in 3-4 layers, cover head with a cap , put gloves, socks and cover body with a soft , dry cloth and then by a blanket or a shawl; hold baby close to caregiver's body.

## ➢ *Keep the young infant warm on the way to the hospital*

- By Skin to Skin contact OR
- Clothe the baby in 3-4 layers, cover head with a cap and body with a blanket or a shawl; hold baby close to caregiver's body.

# TREAT THE YOUNG INFANT FOR LOCAL INFECTIONS/ JAUNDICE AT HOME

## TEACH THE MOTHER TO GIVE ORAL DRUGS AT HOME

**Follow the instructions below for every oral drug to be given at home. Also follow the instructions listed with each drug's dosage table.**

- **Determine the appropriate drugs and dosage for the infant's age or weight.**
- **Tell the mother the reason for giving the drug to the infant.**
- **Demonstrate how to measure a dose.**
- **Watch the mother practise measuring a dose by herself.**
- **Ask the mother to give the first dose to her infant.**
- **Explain carefully how to give the drug, then label and package the drug.**
- **If more than one drug will be given, collect, count and package each drug separately.**
- **Explain that all the oral drug tablets or syrups must be used to finish the course of treatment, even if the infant gets better.**
- **Check the mother's understanding before she leaves the clinic**

## Give oral amoxicillin

- For pneumonia or when referral is not possible ,give twice daily for 7 days
- For local bacterial infection : Give twice daily for 5 days

| Weight (Kg) | Syrup ( 125 mg/5 ml) per dose in ml | Tab 125 mg ( per dose) | Tab 250 mg ( per dose) |
|---|---|---|---|
| 1.5– up to 2.0 | 2.0 | 1/2 | 1/4 |
| 2.0– up to 3.0 | 2.5 ml | 1/2 | 1/4 |
| 3.0- up to 4.0 | 3. 5 ml | 1 | 1/2 |
| 4.0– up to 5.0 | 5 ml | 1 | 1/2 |

## ➢ *Teach the Mother to Treat Local Infections at Home*

- Explain how the treatment is given.
- Watch her as she gives the first treatment in the clinic.
- She should return to the clinic if the infection worsens.
- Check the mother's understanding before she leaves the clinic.

## *To Treat Skin Pustules or Umbilical Infection*

➢ Apply gentian violet paint twice daily.

The mother should:

- Wash hands.
- Gently wash off pus and crusts with soap and water.
- Dry the area and paint with gentian violet 0.5% or antibacterial ointment.
- Wash hands.

## ➢ *Advise Mother to Give Home Care for the Young Infant*

- Immediately after birth , baby should be put on the mother's abdomen for skin to skin contact
- Initiate breastfeeding within one hour of birth
- Breastfeed day and night as often as your baby wants , at least 8 times in 24 hours . Frequent feeding produces more milk.
- If your baby is small ( low birth weight) , feed him or her at least every 2-3 hours . Wake the baby for feeding after 3 hours , if she or he does not wake self.
- Breastfeed as often as your child wants. Look for signs of hunger , such as beginning to fuss , sucking fingers , or moving lips.
- DO NOT give other foods or fluids. Breast milk is all your baby needs.
- Make sure the young infant stays warm at all times. In cool weather, cover the infant's head and feet and dress the infant with extra clothing.

➢ ***To Treat Diarrhoea, See TREAT THE CHILD Chart***

# TREAT THE YOUNG INFANT FOR FEEDING PROBLEMS

## ➢ *Teach Correct Positioning and Attachment for Breastfeeding*

- ➢ Show the mother how to hold her infant
  - with the infant's head and body straight
  - facing her breast, with infant's nose opposite her nipple
  - with infant's body close to her body
  - supporting infant's whole body, not just neck and shoulders.
- ➢ Show her how to help the infant to attach. She should:
  - touch her infant's lips with her nipple
  - wait until her infant's mouth is opening wide
  - move her infant quickly onto her breast, aiming the infant's lower lip well below the nipple.
- ➢ Look for signs of good attachment and effective suckling. If the attachment or suckling is not good, try again.

## ➢ *Teach the mother how to express breastmilk*

To express breast milk:

- The mother should wash hands, sit comfortably and hold a cup or 'katori' under the nipple and areola
- Place her finger on the top of the breast and the first finger on the underside of the breast so that they are opposite each other (at least 4 cm from the tip of the nipple )
- Compress and release the breast tissue between her finger and thumb a few times .
- If the milk does not appear , she should re-position her thumb and finger closer to the nipple and compress and release the breast as before compress and release all the way round the breast , keeping her fingers the same distance from the nipple .
- She should be careful not to squeeze the nipple , to rub the skin or move her thumb or finger on the skin .
- Express one breast until the milk just drips , and then express the other breast until the milk just drips
- Alternate 5 –6 times between breasts for at least 20-30 minutes

## ➢ Teach mother/caregiver where there is no prospects of breastfeeds or has to give replacement feeds temporarily

- Prepare milk correctly & hygienically

## ➢ *Teach the mother to feed with a cup and spoon*

- Place the young infant in upright posture (feeding him in lying position can cause aspiration)
- Keep a soft cloth napkin or cotton on the neck and upper trunk to mop the spilled milk.
- Gently stimulate the young infant to wake him up
- Put a measured amount of milk in the cup
- Hold the cup so that it rests lightly on young infant's lower lip
- Tilt the cup so that the milk just reaches the infant's lips
- Allow the infant to take the milk himself and swallows it. DO NOT pour the milk into the infant's mouth.

## ➢ *To Treat Thrush (ulcers or white patches in mouth)*

➢ Tell the mother to do the treatment twice daily.

The mother should:

- Wash hands.
- Wipe mouth with clean soft cloth wrapped around the finger and wet with salt water.
- Paint the mouth ( ulcers /patches) with gentian violet 0.25% or put two– three drops of clotrimazole mouth paint on white patches

# TREAT THE YOUNG INFANT FOR FEEDING PROBLEMS OR LOW WEIGHT

## ➢ *Teach the mother to treat breast or nipple problems*

- If the nipple is flat or inverted, evert the nipple several times with fingers before each feed and put the baby to the breast.
- If nipple is sore, apply breast milk for soothing effect and ensure correct positioning and attachment of the baby. If mother continues to have discomfort, feed expressed breast milk with a cup.
- If breasts are engorged, let the baby continue to suck if possible. If the baby cannot suckle effectively, help the mother to express milk and then put the young infant to the breast. Putting a warm compress on the breast may help.
- If breast abscess, advise mother to feed from the other breast and refer to a surgeon. If the young infant wants more milk, feed undiluted animal milk with added sugar by cup and spoon.

## ➢ *Teach the mother how to keep the young infant with low weight warm at home:*

- Do not bathe young infant with low weight or low body temperature; instead sponge with lukewarm water to clean.
- Provide Skin to Skin contact (Kangaroo mother care) as much as possible, day and night.
- When Skin to Skin contact not possible:
  - Keep the room warm (>25 °C) with a home heating device.
  - Clothe the baby in 3-4 layers; cover the head, hands and feet with cap, gloves and socks, respectively.
  - Let baby and mother lie together on a soft, thick bedding.
  - Cover the baby and the mother with additional quilt, blanket or shawl, especially in cold weather.

**FEEL THE FEET OF THE BABY PERIODICALLY– BABY'S FEET SHOULD BE ALWAYS WARM TO TOUCH**

## ➢ *Immunize Every Sick Young Infant, as Needed.*

## ➢ Assess the mother/caregiver's development supportive practices

**ASK -**

- ➢ How do you play with your baby ?
- ➢ How do you talk to your baby?

**LOOK -**

How does caregiver show he or she is aware of child's movements?

- ➢ How does caregiver comfort the child and show love?
- ➢ How does caregiver correct the child?

## Counsel the mother /caregiver for practices to support child's development

- ➢ **If the mother reports she does not** play with baby : Discuss ways to help baby see, hear, feel and move, appropriate for baby's age and Ask caregiver to do play or communication activity, appropriate for age.
- ➢ **If the mother reports she does not** talk to child or talks harshly to child: Ask caregiver to looks into baby's eye , gently hold and talk to the baby.

## ➢ Counsel the Mother About Her Own Health

- ➢ If the mother is sick , very thin or looking depressed , provide care for her, or refer her to hospital for help.
- ➢ If she has a breast problem (such as engorgement, sore nipples, breast infection), provide care for her or refer her for help.
- ➢ Advise her to eat well to keep up her own strength and health.Advise her to take one additional energy dense meal to meet requirements for good lactation.
- ➢ Give iron folic acid ( 1 tab 60 mg elemental iron daily + 500 microgram folic acid) & Calcium tablets ( 500 mg elemental calcium with 250 IU Vitamin D twice daily) . Advise her to continue it for a total of 180 days.
- ➢ Make sure she has access to:
  - Contraceptives
  - Counselling on STD and AIDS prevention

## Advise the Mother when to return to physician

| If the infant has: | Return for follow-up after: |
|---|---|
| PNEUMONIA<br>LOCAL BACTERIAL INFECTION<br>JAUNDICE<br>DIARRHOEA<br>ANY FEEDING PROBLEM<br>THRUSH | 2 days |
| LOW WEIGHT FOR AGE | 14 days |

**Advise the mother to return immediately if the young infant has any of these signs:**

Breastfeeding or drinking poorly
Becomes sicker
Develops a fever or feels cold to touch
Fast breathing
Difficult breathing
Yellow palms and soles ( if infant has jaundice)
Diarrhoea with blood in stool

# GIVE FOLLOW-UP CARE FOR THE SICK YOUNG INFANT

## ➢ PNEUMONIA after 2 days

- **Reassess the young infant for PSBI or PNEUMONIA as described on page –2**
- ***Refer URGENTLY to hospital* if the infant becomes worse or develops any new sign of POSSIBLE BACTERIAL INFECTION or VERY SEVERE DISEASE.**
- **If respiratory rate is less but still fast breathing , ask mother to continue amoxicillin twice daily and follow-up after 2 days**
- **If the young infant is improving , ask the mother to continue giving the oral amoxicillin twice daily and complete 7 days treatment**

## *LOCAL BACTERIAL INFECTION*

After 2 days:

➢ Look at the umbilicus. Is it red or draining pus?

➢ Look for skin pustules.

Treatment:

➢ If ***umbilical redness or pus remains or is worse***, refer to hospital. If ***umbilical pus and redness are improved***, tell the mother to continue giving the 5 days of antibiotic and continue treating the local infection at home.

➢ If skin pustules are the same or worse , refer the infant to hospital . If they are improved , tell the mother to complete 5 days of treatment and continue treating the local infection at home

## ➢ *LOW WEIGHT*

After 14 days:

Weigh the young infant and determine if the infant is still low weight for age.

Reassess feeding. > See "Then Check for Feeding Problem or Low Weight" above.

➢ If the infant is ***no longer low weight for age***, praise the mother and encourage her to continue feeding as advised.

➢ If the infant is ***still low weight for age but has gained weight and is feeding well***, praise the mother. Ask her to have her infant weighed again after 7 days.

➢ If the infant ***still has a feeding problem***, counsel the mother about the feeding problem. Ask the mother to return again in 2 days.

➢ If the young infant has ***lost weight*** in next follow-up visit or **there is static weight during two follow-ups** , refer to hospital for assessment.

## ➢ *JAUNDICE*

After 2 days:

Look for jaundice

- Are the palms and soles yellow?

➢ If palms and soles are yellow or age 14 days or more refer to hospital

➢ If palms and soles are not yellow and age less than 14 days, advise home care and when to return immediately

## ➢ *DIARRHOEA*

After 2 days:

Ask: Has the diarrhoea stopped?

➢ If diarrhoea persists, Assess the young infant for diarrhoea (> *See ASSESS & CLASSIFY chart)* and manage as per initial visit .

➢ If diarrhoea stopped—reinforce exclusive breastfeeding

## ➢ *FEEDING PROBLEM*

After 2 days:

Reassess feeding. > See "Then Check for Feeding Problem or Low Weight" above.

Ask about any feeding problems found on the initial visit.

➢ Counsel the mother about any new or continuing feeding problems. If you counsel the mother to make significant changes in feeding, ask her to bring the young infant back again in 2 days.

***Exception:*** If you do not think that feeding will improve, or if the young infant has ***lost weight***, refer to hospital

## ➢ *THRUSH*

After 2 days:

Look for ulcers or white patches in the mouth (thrush).

Reassess feeding. > See "Then Check for Feeding Problem or Low Weight"

➢ If ***thrush is worse***, or the infant has ***problems with attachment or suckling***, refer to hospital.

➢ If ***thrush is the same or better***, and if the infant is ***feeding well***, continue gentian violet 0.25% / clotrimazole for a total of 5 days.

# ASSESS AND CLASSIFY THE SICK CHILD AGE 2 MONTHS UP TO 5 YEARS

| ASSESS | CLASSIFY | IDENTIFY TREATMENT |
|---|---|---|

**ASK THE MOTHER WHAT THE CHILD'S PROBLEMS ARE**

- Determine if this is an initial or follow-up visit for this problem.
  - if follow-up visit, use the follow-up instructions on *TREAT THE CHILD* chart.
  - if initial visit, assess the child as follows:

## CHECK FOR GENERAL DANGER SIGNS

| ***ASK:*** | ***LOOK:*** |
|---|---|
| • Is the child not able to drink or breastfeed?<br>• Does the child vomit everything?<br>• Has the child had convulsions? | • See if the child is lethargic or unconscious.<br>• Is the child convulsing now ? |

URGENT ATTEN-TION

**USE ALL BOXES THAT MATCH THE CHILD'S SYMPTOMS AND PROBLEMS TO CLASSIFY THE ILLNESS.**

| SIGNS | CLASSIFY AS | IDENTIFY TREATMENT (Urgent pre-referral treatments are in bold print.) |
|---|---|---|
| • Not able to feed /drink <u>or</u><br>• Vomits everything <u>or</u><br>• Lethargy/unconscious <u>or</u><br>• Convulsion /Convulsing now | **VERY SEVERE DISEASE** | ➢ ***Give diazepam if convulsing now***<br>➢ ***Quickly complete the assessment***<br>➢ ***Give any pre-referral treatment immediately for other pink classification identified***<br>➢ ***Treat to prevent low blood sugar***<br>➢ ***Keep the child warm***<br>➢ ***Refer URGENTLY to hospital*** |

A child with any general danger signs needs URGENT attention; complete the assessment and any pre-referral treatment immediately so that referral is not delayed

# ASSESS AND CLASSIFY THE SICK CHILD AGE 2 MONTHS UP TO 5 YEARS

## THEN ASK ABOUT MAIN SYMPTOMS:

### Does the child have cough or difficult breathing?

**IF YES, ASK:** ***LOOK, LISTEN:***

- For how long?
- Count the breaths in one minute.
- Look for chest indrawing.
- Look and listen for stridor.
- Look and listen for wheezing

(CHILD MUST BE CALM)

- Check oxygen saturation ( Spo2)

***If wheezing with either fast breathing or chest indrawing***

Give a trial of rapid acting inhaled bronchodilator for up to three times 15-20 minutes apart. Count the breaths and look for chest indrawing again, and then classify.

| **If the child is:** | **Fast breathing is:** |
|---|---|
| 2 months upto 12 months | **50** breaths per minute or more |
| 12 months upto 5 years | **40** breaths per minute or more |

*Classify COUGH or DIFFICULT BREATHING*

| SIGNS | CLASSIFY AS | IDENTIFY TREATMENT (Urgent pre-referral treatments are in bold print.) |
|---|---|---|
| • Any general danger sign or<br>• Stridor in calm child or<br>• Spo2 < 90% | **SEVERE PNEUMONIA OR VERY SEVERE DISEASE** | ➢ *Give first dose of injectable ampicillin and gentamycin*<br>➢ ***Refer URGENTLY to hospital.***[#]<br>➢ *Provide oxygen to all children on the way to the hospital* |
| • Chest indrawing or<br>• Fast breathing. | **PNEUMONIA** | ➢ ***Give Amoxycillin for 5 days.***<br>➢ If wheezing ( or disappeared after rapidly acting bronchodilator) give an inhaled bronchodilator for 5 days*<br>➢ Soothe the throat and relieve the cough with a safe remedy if child is 6 months or older.<br>➢ Follow-up after 2 days. |
| No signs of pneumonia or very severe disease. | **NO PNEUMONIA** | ➢ If wheezing ( or disappeared after rapidly acting bronchodilator) give an inhaled bronchodilator for 5 days *<br>➢ Soothe the throat and relieve the cough with a safe home remedy if child is 6 months or older.<br>➢ If coughing more than 14 days ,refer for possible TB, or asthma assessment<br>➢ Advise mother when to return immediately.<br>➢ Follow-up after 5 days if not improving. |

*In settings where inhaled bronchodilator is not available, use oral salbutamol

# *If referral is not possible, see the section **Where Referral Is Not Possible***

## Does the child have diarrhoea?

**IF YES, ASK:**
- For how long?
- Is there blood in the stool?

**LOOK AND FEEL:**
- **Look at the child's general condition.**

Is the child:
Lethargic or unconscious?

Restless and irritable?

- **Look for sunken eyes.**
- **Offer the child fluid. Is the child:**
  - Not able to drink or drinking poorly?
  - Drinking eagerly, thirsty?
- **Pinch the skin of the abdomen.**
  Does it go back:
  - Slowly ?
  - Very slowly (longer than 2 seconds)?

***Classify DIARRHOEA***

***for DEHYDRATION***

| Signs | Classification | Treatment |
|---|---|---|
| **Two of the following signs**:<br>• Lethargic or unconscious<br>• Sunken eyes<br>• Not able to drink or drinking poorly<br>• Skin pinch goes back very slowly. | **SEVERE DEHYDRATION** | ➢ If child has no other severe classification:<br>- Give fluid for severe dehydration (Plan C).<br>➢ *If child also has another severe classification :* ***Refer URGENTLY to hospital#*** **with mother giving frequent sips of ORS on the way. Advise the mother to continue breastfeeding.**<br>➢ If child is 2 years or older and there is cholera in your area, give antibiotic for cholera. |
| **Two of the following signs:**<br>• Restless, irritable<br>• Sunken eyes<br>• Drinks eagerly, thirsty<br>• Skin pinch goes back slowly. | **SOME DEHYDRATION** | ➢Give fluid ,zinc supplements and food for some dehydration (Plan B).<br>➢*If child also has a severe classification:* ***Refer URGENTLY to hospital# with mother giving frequent sips of ORS on the way. Advise the mother to continue breastfeeding.***<br>➢Advise mother when to return immediately.<br>➢Follow-up after 5 days if not improving. |
| Not enough signs to classify as some or severe dehydration. | **NO DEHYDRATION** | ➢Give fluid, zinc supplements and food to treat diarrhoea at home (Plan A).<br>➢Advise mother when to return immediately.<br>➢Follow-up after 5 days if not improving. |

***and if diarrhoea 14 days or more***

| Signs | Classification | Treatment |
|---|---|---|
| • Dehydration present. | **SEVERE PERSISTENT DIARRHOEA** | ➢**Treat dehydration before referral unless the child has another severe classification.**<br>➢***Refer to hospital#*** |
| • No dehydration. | **PERSISTENT DIARRHOEA** | ➢Advise the mother on feeding a child who has PERSISTENT DIARRHOEA.<br>➢Give single dose of vitamin A.<br>➢Give zinc, multivitamin supplements daily for 14 days.<br>➢Follow –up after 5 days |

***and if blood in stool***

| Signs | Classification | Treatment |
|---|---|---|
| • Blood in the stool. | **DYSENTERY** | ➢**Treat with cefixime for 5 days**<br>➢Give zinc supplements for 14 days.<br>➢Follow-up after 2 days. |

# *If referral is not possible, see the section **Where Referral Is Not Possible** .*

## Does the child have fever?

(by history or feels hot or temperature 37.5°C* or above)

IF YES
Is it a PF (p. falciparum) predominant area? Yes/ No

| THEN ASK: | LOOK AND FEEL : |
|---|---|
| • Fever for how long?<br>-- If more than 7 days , has fever been present every day ?<br>• Is it a dengue season ? Yes/No<br>- If yes , is there a continuous fever of 2-7 days ? | • Look or feel for stiff neck<br>• Look for any bacterial focus /cause of fever |
| • Has the child had measles within last 3 months | • Look for signs of Measles<br>* Generalized rash and<br>* One of these : cough , runny nose or red eyes |

➢ Do RDT for malaria in all fever cases if it is PF predominant area and if no obvious cause of fever is present in other areas or malaria suspected

**Classify FEVER**

| Signs | Classify as | Treatment |
|---|---|---|
| • Any general danger sign or<br>• Stiff neck | **VERY SEVERE FEBRILE DISEASE** | ➢ ***Give first dose of appropriate IM antibiotics***<br>➢ ***Give first dose of artesunate or quinine if it is a PF predominant area or RDT is positive for malaria***<br>➢ ***Treat the child to prevent low blood sugar.***<br>➢ ***Give one dose of paracetamol in clinic for high fever (temp. 38.5°C or above).***<br>➢ ***Refer URGENTLY to hospital #.*** |
| • Positive RDT or<br>• RDT not available and no other obvious cause of fever | **MALARIA/ SUSPECTED MALARIA** | ➢ ***Give oral antimalarial as per national guidelines after making a smear***<br>➢ *Give one dose of paracetamol in clinic for high fever (temp. 38.5°C or above).*<br>➢ Advise mother when to return immediately.<br>➢ Follow-up after 2 days . |
| • Negative RDT and other causes of fever PRESENT** | **FEVER - MALARIA UNLIKELY** | ➢ *Give one dose of paracetamol in clinic for high fever (temp. 38.5°C or above)*<br>➢ *Give appropriate treatment for an identified cause of fever*<br>➢ Advise mother when to return immediately.<br>➢ Follow-up after 2 days if fever persists<br>➢ If fever is present every day for more than 7 days , refer for assessment |

➢ **Suspected dengue ( dengue season & has continuous fever of 2-7 days)**
Look for following warning signs :
• Cold extremities with weak and fast pulse
• Severe abdominal pain ( abdominal pain with restlessness /anxious look)
• Bleeding from any site ( skin , mucosal , hematemesis or melena)
• Positive Tourniquet test : >20 petechiae per square inch area over forearm)

***If Suspected Dengue, Classify***

| Signs | Classify as | Treatment |
|---|---|---|
| • Any general danger signs or<br>• Cold extremities with weak and fast pulse or<br>• Severe abdominal pain or<br>• Bleeding from any site or<br>• Positive Tourniquet test | **SEVERE DENGUE / DENGUE WITH WARNING SIGNS** | ➢ ***Give first dose of appropriate IM antibiotics***<br>➢ ***Refer URGENTLY to hospital***<br>➢ If accepting orally , advise mother to give frequent sips of ORS / fluids on the way to the hospital<br>➢ *Give one dose of paracetamol in clinic for high fever (temp. 38.5°C or above).* |
| • No warning signs | **DENGUE FEVER** | ➢ *Give one dose of paracetamol in clinic for high fever (temp. 38.5°C or above).*<br>➢ *Educate caregivers about care of a child with dengue fever*<br>➢ *Follow–up after 2 days* |

➢ **If the child has measles now or within the last 3 months:**
◆ Look for mouth ulcers – Are they deep and extensive ?
◆ Look for pus draining from the eye?

***If MEASLES Now or within last 3 months, Classify***

| Signs | Classify as | Treatment |
|---|---|---|
| • Any general danger sign or<br>• Clouding of cornea or<br>• Deep or extensive Mouth ulcers. | **SEVERE COMPLICATED MEASLES***** | ➢ ***Give first dose of Vitamin A.***<br>➢ ***Give first dose of IM ampicillin and gentamycin .***<br>➢ ***If clouding of the cornea or pus draining from the eye, apply antibiotic eye ointment.***<br>➢ ***Refer URGENTLY to hospital #*** |
| • Pus draining from the eye or<br>• Mouth ulcers. | **MEASLES WITH EYE OR MOUTH COMPLICATIONS** | ➢ ***Give first dose of Vitamin A.***<br>➢ *If pus draining from the eye, treat eye infection with antibiotic eye ointment.*<br>➢ If mouth ulcers, treat with gentian violet.<br>➢ Follow-up after 2 days. |
| • Measles now or within the last 3 months. | **MEASLES** | ➢ ***Give a dose of Vitamin A.*** |

**This cutoff is for axillary temperature*
*** Other causes of fever include no pneumonia: cough or cold, pneumonia, diarrhoea, dysentery, tonsillitis, skin infections , dengue , measles.*
**** Other important complications of measles - pneumonia, stridor, diarrhoea, ear infection, and malnutrition - are classified in other tables.*
*# If referral is not possible, see the section **Where Referral Is Not Possible** in the module **Treat the Child**.*

## Does the child have an ear problem?

**IF YES, ASK:**

- Is there ear pain?
- Is there ear discharge? If yes, for how long?

**LOOK AND FEEL:**

- Look for pus draining from the ear.
- Feel for tender swelling behind the ear.

***CLASSIFY EAR PROBLEM***

| Signs | Classify as | Treatment |
|---|---|---|
| • Tender swelling behind the ear. | **MASTOIDITIS** | ➢ ***Give first dose of injectable. Ampicillin and gentamycin***<br>➢ ***Give first dose of paracetamol for pain.***<br>➢ ***Refer URGENTLY to hospital [#].*** |
| • Pus is seen draining from the ear and discharge is reported for less than 14 days, <u>or</u><br>• Ear pain. | **ACUTE EAR INFECTION** | ➢ ***Give Amoxycillin for 5 days.***<br>➢ Give paracetamol for pain.<br>➢ Dry the ear by wicking.<br>➢ Follow-up after 5 days. |
| • Pus is seen draining from the ear and discharge is reported for 14 days or more. | **CHRONIC EAR INFECTION** | ➢ Dry the ear by wicking.<br>➢ Topical quinolone ear drops for 2 weeks.<br>➢ Follow-up in 5 days. |
| • No ear pain and No pus seen draining from the ear. | **NO EAR INFECTION** | No additional treatment. |

## THEN CHECK FOR MALNUTRITION

**LOOK AND FEEL:**

- Measure weight , length/height and determine WFL SD score
- Look for oedema of both feet.
- Measure MUAC if child is 6 months or older

Check for medical complications in children with Severe Acute Malnutrition

- Any general danger signs
- Any severe classification
- Pneumonia
- Diarrhea with dehydration
- Poor appetite

***Classify NUTRITIONAL STATUS***

| Signs | Classify as | Treatment |
|---|---|---|
| • WFL <-3 SD score <u>and /or</u><br>• MUAC <11.5 cm <u>and /or</u><br>• Oedema of both feet <u>and</u> Medical complications | **SEVERE ACUTE MALNUTRITION WITH MEDICAL COMPLICATION** | ➢ *Give injectable ampicillin and gentamycin*<br>➢ *Treat the child to prevent low blood sugar.*<br>➢ ***Refer URGENTLY to hospital[#]***<br>➢ *While referral is being organized, warm the child.*<br>➢ *Keep the child warm on the way to hospital.* |
| • WFL <-3 SD score <u>and /or</u><br>• MUAC <11.5 cm <u>and</u><br>• No medical complications | **SEVERE ACUTE MALNUTRITION WITHOUT MEDICAL COMPLICATION** | ➢ ***Give oral amoxicillin for 5 days***<br>➢ ***Give a dose of Vitamin A if not received in last one month***<br>➢ *Assess feeding & counsel the mother on how to feed the child*<br>➢ *Give multivitamins , zinc for 14 days*<br>➢ *Advise mother when to return immediately*<br>➢ *Follow-up after 7 days* |
| • WFL -3 SD score to <-2SD <u>and / or</u><br>• MUAC 11.5 –12.5 cm | **MODERATE ACUTE MALNUTRITION** | ➢ Assess feeding & counsel the mother on how to feed the child<br>➢ Advise mother when to return immediately<br>➢ Follow-up after 30 days |
| • WFL ≥ -2SD score and<br>• MUAC ≥ 12.5 cm and<br>• NO oedema of both feet. | **NO ACUTE MALNUTRITION** | ➢ If child is less than 2 years old, assess the child's feeding and counsel the mother on feeding according to the FOOD box on the *COUNSEL THE MOTHER* chart.<br>➢ If feeding problem, follow-up iafter 2 days.<br>➢ Advise mother when to return immediately. |

# *If referral is not possible, see the section **Where Referral Is Not Possible**.*

## THEN CHECK FOR ANAEMIA

**LOOK:**

- Look for palmar pallor. Is it
  Severe palmar pallor?
  Some palmar pallor?

- If there is no other pink classification and hemoglobin testing is available as outpatient services , test hemoglobin of all children with pallor and classify as per Hb level

***Classify ANAEMIA***

| Signs | Classify as | Treatment |
|---|---|---|
| • Severe palmar pallor ( Hb <7g/dl ) | **SEVERE ANAEMIA** | ➢ ***Refer URGENTLY to hospital*** |
| • Some palmar pallor ( Hb 7-10.9 g/dl) | **ANAEMIA** | ➢ *Give iron folic acid therapy for 14 days*<br>➢ Assess the child`s feeding and counsel the mother on feeding according to the FOOD box on the *COUNSEL THE MOTHER* chart. If feeding problem, follow-up iafter 5 days.<br>➢ Advise mother when to return immediately.<br>➢ Follow-up after 14 days. |
| • No palmar pallor ( Hb ≥ 11g/dl) | **NO ANAEMIA** | ➢ *Give prophylactic iron folic acid if child 6 months or older.* |

# *If referral is not possible, see the section* ***Where Referral Is Not Possible*** .

## THEN CHECK THE CHILD'S IMMUNIZATION *, PROPHYLACTIC VITAMIN A & IRON-FOLIC ACID SUPPLEMENTATION STATUS

**IMMUNIZATION SCHEDULE:**

| AGE | VACCINE |
|---|---|
| Birth | BCG + OPV-0 + Hep B 0 |
| 6 weeks | OPV-1 + Penta-1 +Rota Virus-1 + fIPV –1 + PCV –1 # |
| 10 weeks | OPV-2+ Penta-2+ Rota Virus –2* |
| 14 weeks | OPV-3+ Penta-3 +fIPV-2 + RVV-3 + PCV-2# |
| 9-12 months | Measles-rubella( MR-)1) + JE–1+ PCV booster |
| 16-24 months | MR-2, JE-2, DPT booster, OPV booster |
| 60 months | DT booster |

**PROPHYLACTIC IFA/ DEWORMING/ Prophylactic Vitamin A**

-Give IFA syrup ( 1ml 2 times a week with auto dispenser) containing 20 mg of elemental iron + 100 mcg of folic acid after the child has recovered from acute illness **if** the child 6 months of age or older*,

* Supplement IFA in LBW after 6weeks of age

-Give anthelminthic if child is one year or older and has not received deworming agents in last 6 months

- Give Vitamin A supplementation as per state guidelines

*** A child who needs to be immunized should be advised to go for immunization the day vaccines are available at AW/SC/PHC**
**# Rotavirus, fIPV, PCV, JE in States where it is included in their immunization schedule**

## ASSESS OTHER PROBLEMS

## ASSESS FEEDING IF *AGE IS LESS THAN 2 YEARS / HAS UNCOMPLICATED MODERATE/SEVERE ACUTE MALNUTRITION OR ANEMIA*

## *ASSESS THE MOTHER/CAREGIVER'S DEVELOPMENT SUPPORTIVE PRACTICES IF AGE IS LESS THAN 3 YEARS / HAS UNCOMPLICATED SEVERE ACUTE MALNUTRITION OR ANEMIA*

## COUNSEL THE MOTHER ABOUT HER OWN HEALTH

# TREAT THE CHILD

## GIVE THESE TREATMENTS IN CLINIC ONLY

### ➢ *Give Intramuscular Antibiotics*

- Explain to the mother why the drug is given.
- Determine the dose appropriate for the child's weight (or age).
- Use a sterile needle and sterile syringe. Measure the dose accurately.
- Give the drug as an intramuscular injection.
- Referral is the best option for a child classification with GENERAL DANGER SIGNS, SEVERE PNEUMONIA /VERY SEVERE DISEASE , SEVERE DEHYDRATION, VERY SEVERE FEBRILE DISEASE , SEVERE DEHYDRATION, SEVERE COMPLICATED MEASLES , SEVERE DENGUE , MASTOIDITIS , SEVERE ACUTE MALNUTRITION WITH MEDICAL COPLICATIONS AND SEVERE ANEMIA .
- If referral is not possible or refused, give oral amoxicillin ( 25-30 mg/kg) every 12 hours and intramuscular gentamicin once daily in cases requiring antibiotics .
- At each contact for injection of antibiotics , explain again to the caregiver that the child is very sick and should urgently be referred for hospital care

AMPICILLIN:
- Dilute 500 mg vial with 2.1 ml of sterile water ( 500mg/2.5ml)
- Give 50 mg/kg first dose ( repeat every 6 hours if referral not possible)

CEFTRIAXONE :
- If meningitis is strongly suspected give IM ceftriaxone if it is available (100mg/kg) in place of ampicillin ( repeat daily if referral not possible)

GENTAMYCIN:
- 7.5 mg/kg/day once daily( repeat daily if referral not possible)

| Age or Weight | Ampicillin ( 500mg/ 2.5 ml) | Gentamycin ( 40mg/ml) |
|---|---|---|
| 2—up to 4 m (4– up to 6 kg) | 1ml | 0.5-1.0 ml |
| 4—up to 12 m (6– up to 10 kg ) | 2ml | 1.1-1.8ml |
| 12– up to 3 y (10– up to 14 kg) | 3 ml | 1.9-2.7 ml |
| 3– up to 5 y (14-up to 19kg ) | 5 ml | 2.8-3.5ml |

Give Diazepam to stop Convulsions :
- ♦ Turn the child to his/her side and clear the airway .
- ♦ Give 0.5ml /kg diazepam injection solution per rectum using a small syringe ( tuberculin ) without needle or using a catheter
- ♦ Check for low blood sugar , treat and prevent
- ♦ Give oxygen and REFER
- ♦ If convulsions have not stopped after 10 minutes repeat diazepam dose

| AGE or WEIGHT | DIAZEPAM 10mg/2mls |
|---|---|
| 2 months up to 6 months (5 - 7 kg) | 0.5 ml |
| 6 months up to 12months (7 - <10 kg) | 1.0 ml |
| 12 months up to 3 years (10 - <14 kg) | 1.5 ml |
| 3 years up to 5 years (14-19 kg) | 2.0ml |

**Give Intramuscular Artesunate or Quinine for Severe Malaria :** FOR CHILDREN BEING REFERRED WITH VERY SEVERE FEBRILE DISEASE:
Intramuscular artesunate or quinine: Give first dose and refer child urgently to hospital.
IF REFERRAL IS NOT POSSIBLE:
For artesunate injection: Give first dose of artesunate intramuscular injection
Repeat dose after 12 hrs and daily until the child can take orally
Give full dose of oral antimalarial as soon as the child is able to take orally.
**For quinine**:
Give first dose of intramuscular quinine. The child should remain lying down for one hour. Repeat the quinine injection at 4 and 8 hours later, and then every 12 hours until the child is able to take an oral antimalarial. Do not continue quinine injections for more than 1 week. If low risk of malaria, do not give quinine to a child less than 4 months of age.

| AGE or WEIGHT | IM ARTESUNATE 60 mg vial (20mg/ ml) 2.4 mg/kg | IM QUININE 150 mg/ml* (in 2 ml ampoules) |
|---|---|---|
| 2 months up to 4 months (4 - <6 kg) | 0.5 ml | 0.4 ml |
| 4 months up to 12 months (6 - <10 kg) | 1.0 ml | 0.6 ml |
| 12 months up to 2 years (10 - <12 kg) | 1.5 ml | 0.8 ml |
| 2 years up to 3 years (12 - <14 kg) | 2.0 ml | 1.0 ml |
| 3 years up to 5 years (14 - 19 kg) | 2.5 ml | 1.2 ml |

* Quinine salt

# TREAT THE CHILD

## GIVE THESE TREATMENTS IN CLINIC ONLY

### ➢ Give Inhaled Salbutamol for Wheezing

Give 3 doses of nebulised Salbutamol OR 2-4 puffs (100 µgm/puff) of Salbutamol by MDI with spacer

**USE OF A SPACER* :** A spacer is a way of delivering the bronchodilator drugs effectively into the lungs. No child under 5 years should be given an inhaler without a spacer. A spacer works as well as a nebuliser if correctly used.

- Repeat up to 3 times every 15 minutes before classifying pneumonia.

**Spacers can be made in the following way:**

- Use a 500ml drink bottle or similar. Cut a hole in the bottle base in the same shape as the mouthpiece of the inhaler. This can be done using a sharp knife.
- Cut the bottle between the upper quarter and the lower 3/4 and disregard the upper quarter of the bottle. Cut a small V in the border of the large open part of the bottle to fit to the child's nose and be used as a mask. Flame the edge of the cut bottle with a candle or a lighter to soften it.
- In a small baby, a mask can be made by making a similar hole in a plastic (not polystyrene) cup.
- Alternatively commercial spacers can be used if available.

**To use an inhaler with a spacer:**

- Remove the inhaler cap. Shake the inhaler well.
- Insert mouthpiece of the inhaler through the hole in the bottle or plastic cup.
- The child should put the opening of the bottle into his mouth and breath in and out through the mouth.
- A carer then presses down the inhaler and sprays into the bottle while the child continues to breath normally.
- Wait for three to four breaths and repeat.
- For younger children place the cup over the child's mouth and use as a spacer in the same way.

* *If a spacer is being used for the first time, it should be primed by 4-5 extra puffs from the inhaler.*

### ➢ Treat the Child to Prevent Low Blood Sugar:

***If the child is able to breastfeed:*** Ask the mother to breastfeed the child

***If the child is not able to breastfeed but is able to swallow:*** Give 20-50 ml (10 ml/kg) of expressed breastmilk or locally appropriate animal milk (with added sugar) before departure. If neither of these is available, give 20-50 ml (10 ml/kg) of sugar water.

***If the child is not able to swallow:*** Give 20-50 ml (10 ml/kg) of expressed breastmilk or locally appropriate animal milk (with added sugar) or sugar water by nasogastric tube.

### ➢ Plan C: Treat Severe Dehydration Quickly

➢ **FOLLOW THE ARROWS. IF ANSWER IS "YES", GO ACROSS. IF "NO", GO DOWN.**

START HERE

**Can you give intravenous (IV) fluid immediately?**

YES →

- Start IV fluid immediately. If the child can drink, give ORS by mouth while the drip is set up. Give 100 ml/kg Ringer's Lactate Solution (or, if not available, normal saline), divided as follows:

* *Repeat once if radial pulse is still very weak or not detectable.*

| AGE | First give 30 ml/kg in: | Then give 70 ml/kg in: |
|---|---|---|
| Infants (under 12 months) | 1 hour* | 5 hours |
| Children (12 months up to 5 years) | 30 minutes* | 2 1/2 hours |

- Reassess the child every 1- 2 hours. If hydration status is not improving, give the IV drip more rapidly.
- Also give ORS (about 5 ml/kg/hour) as soon as the child can drink: usually after 3-4 hours (infants) or 1-2 hours (children).
- Reassess an infant after 6 hours and a child after 3 hours. Classify dehydration. Then choose the appropriate plan (A, B, or C) to continue treatment.

NO ↓

**Is IV treatment available nearby (within 30 minutes)?**

YES →

- Refer URGENTLY to hospital for IV treatment.
- If the child can drink, provide the mother with ORS solution and show her how to give frequent sips during the trip.

NO ↓

**Are you trained to use a naso-gastric (NG) tube for rehydration?**

NO ↓

**Can the child drink?**

YES (to both) →

- Start rehydration by tube (or mouth) with ORS solution: give 20 ml/kg/hour for 6 hours (total of 120 ml/kg).
- Reassess the child every 1-2 hours:
  - If there is repeated vomiting or increasing abdominal distension, give the fluid more slowly.
  - If hydration status is not improving after 3 hours, send the child for IV therapy.
- After 6 hours, reassess the child. Classify dehydration. Then choose the appropriate plan (A, B, or C) to continue treatment.

NO ↓

**Refer URGENTLY to hospital for IV or NG treatment**

**NOTE:**

- If possible, observe the child at least 6 hours after rehydration to be sure the mother can maintain hydration giving the child ORS solution by mouth.

# TEACH THE MOTHER TO GIVE ORAL DRUGS AT HOME

**Follow the instructions below for every oral drug to be given at home. Also follow the instructions listed with each drug's dosage table.**

## ➢ Give an Appropriate Oral Antibiotic

➢ **FOR PNEUMONIA, ACUTE EAR INFECTION , SEVERE ACUTE MALNUTRITION WITHOUT MEDICAL COMPLICATIONS (OR FOR VERY SEVERE DISEASE IF INJECTABLE AMPICILLIN IS NOT AVAILABLE )**

| | AMOXICILLIN* ➢ Give two times daily for 5 days | |
|---|---|---|
| **AGE or WEIGHT** | **TABLET** 250 mg | **SYRUP** 250 mg per 5 ml |
| 2 months up to 12 months (4 - <10 kg) | 1 | 5 ml |
| 12 months up to 3 years (10 - <14 kg) | 2 | 10 ml |
| 3 years up 5 years ( 14-19 kg) | 3 | 15 |

➢ **FOR DYSENTERY: Give Cefixime (10 mg /kg in two divided doses ) for 5 days**

| **AGE or WEIGHT** | Tablet ( 100 mg) Two times | Syrup 50 mg per 5 ml Two times |
|---|---|---|
| 2 months up to 8 months (4 - < 10 kg) | 1/ 2 | 5 ml |
| 12 months up to 3 years (10- <1 4kg) | 3/4 | 7.5 |
| 3 years up to 5 years (15- <20 kg) | 1 | 10 ml |

➢ **FOR CHOLERA:** Give single dose DOXYCYCLINE

| | **DOXYCYCLINE** ➢Single dose | |
|---|---|---|
| **AGE or WEIGHT** | **TABLET** 100 mg | **CAPSULE** 50 mg |
| 2 years up to 4 years (10 - 14 kg) | 1/2 | 1 |
| 4 years to 5 years (15-19 Kg) | 1 | 2 |

## ➢ Give Zinc

➢ For acute diarrhea, persistent diarrhea and dysentery. Give zinc supplements for 14 days.

| **AGE** | **ZINC TABLET** (20 mg) |
|---|---|
| 2 months upto 6 months | 1/2 |
| 6 months upto 5 years | 1 |

## ➢ Give Paracetamol for High Fever (≥ 38.5°C) or Ear Pain

➢ Give a single dose of paracetamol in the clinic
➢ Give 3 additional doses of paracetamol for use at home every 6 hours until high fever or ear pain is gone.

| | **PARACETAMOL** | |
|---|---|---|
| **AGE or WEIGHT** | **TABLET** (100 mg) | **TABLET** (500 mg) |
| 2 months up to 1years (4 - | 1 | 1/4 |
| 1 years up to 3 years (10- | 1 1/2 | 1/3 |
| 3 years up to 5 years ( 15-20 | 2 tab | 1/2 |
| | | |

## ➢ Give Vitamin A

➢ Give single dose in the clinic in Persistent Diarrhoea & Severe Malnutrition
➢ Give two doses in Measles ( Give first dose in clinic and give mother one dose to give at home the next day.).

| **AGE** | **VITAMIN A SYRUP** |
|---|---|
| | 100,000 IU/ml |
| Up to 6 months | 0.5 ml |
| 6 months up to 12 months | 1 ml |
| 12 months up to 5 years | 2 ml |

## ➢ Give Iron & Folic Acid therapy

➢ Give one dose daily for 60 days

| **AGE or WEIGHT** | **IFA PEDIATRIC TABLET** (20 mg elemental | **IFA SYRUP** (20 elemental iron + 100 mcg Folic acid per ml) | **IFA DROPS** 20 mg of elemental iron per 1 ml |
|---|---|---|---|
| 2 months up to 4 months (4 - <6 kg) | | 0.5 ml | 0.5 ml |
| 4 months up to 12 months (6 - <10kg) | 1 tablet | 1ml | 1 ml |
| 12 months up to 3 years months (10 - 14 kg) | 1.5 tablets | 1.5 ml | 1.5 ml |
| 2 years up to 5 years (14 -19 kg) | 2 tablets | 2 ml | |

# TEACH THE MOTHER TO TREAT LOCAL INFECTIONS AT HOME

## ➢ *Soothe the Throat, Relieve the Cough with a Safe Remedy if the infant is 6 months or older*

- Safe remedies to recommend:
  - Continue Breastfeeding
  - Honey, tulsi, ginger, herbal teas and other safe local home remedies
- Harmful remedies to discourage:
  - Preparations containing opiates, codeine, ephedrine and atropine

## ➢ *Treat Eye Infection with Antibiotic Eye Ointment* (Tetracycline or Chloramphenicol etc.)

➢ Clean both eyes 3 times daily.

- Wash hands.
- Ask child to close the eye.
- Use clean cloth and water to gently wipe away pus.

➢ Then apply antibiotic eye ointment ( in both eyes 3 times daily.

- Ask the child to look up.
- Squirt a small amount of ointment on the inside of the lower lid.
- Wash hands again.

➢ Treat until redness is gone.

➢ Do not use other eye ointments or drops, or put anything else in the eye.

## ➢ *Clear the Ear by Dry Wicking and Give Eardrops*

➢ **Dry the ear at least 3 times daily**

- Roll clean absorbent cloth or soft, strong tissue paper into a wick
- Place the wick in the child's ear
- Remove the wick when wet
- Replace the wick with a clean one and repeat these steps until the ear is dry
- Instil ciprofloxacin ear drops after dry wicking three times daily for two weeks

# GIVE EXTRA FLUID FOR DIARRHOEA

## ➢ *Plan B: Treat Some Dehydration with ORS*

***Give in clinic recommended amount of ORS over 4-hour period***

➢ DETERMINE AMOUNT OF ORS TO GIVE DURING FIRST 4 HOURS

| AGE* | Up to 4 months | 4 months up to 12 months | 12 months up to 2 years | 2 years up to 5 years |
|---|---|---|---|---|
| **WEIGHT** | < 6 kg | 6 - < 10 kg | 10 - < 12 kg | 12 - 19 kg |
| **In ml** | 200 - 400 | 400 - 700 | 700 - 900 | 900 - 1400 |

- *Use the child's age only when you do not know the weight. The approximate amount of ORS required (in ml) can also be calculated by multiplying the child's weight (in kg) times 75.*

- If the child wants more ORS than shown, give more.
- For infants under 6 months who are not breastfed, also give 100-200 ml clean water during this period.

➢ **SHOW THE MOTHER HOW TO GIVE ORS SOLUTION.**

- Give frequent small sips from a cup.
- If the child vomits, wait 10 minutes. Then continue, but more slowly.
- Continue breastfeeding whenever the child wants.

➢ **AFTER 4 HOURS:**

- Reassess the child and classify the child for dehydration.
- Select the appropriate plan to continue treatment.
- Begin feeding the child in clinic.

} **See Plan A for recommended fluids and See *COUNSEL THE MOTHER* chart**

➢ **IF THE MOTHER MUST LEAVE BEFORE COMPLETING TREATMENT:**

- Show her how to prepare ORS solution at home.
- Show her how much ORS to give to finish 4-hour treatment at home.
- Give her enough ORS packets to complete rehydration. Also give her 2 packets as recommended in Plan A.
- Explain the 4 Rules of Home Treatment:
  1. ***GIVE EXTRA FLUID***
  2. **GIVE ZINC SUPPLEMENT**
  3. ***CONTINUE FEEDING***
  4. ***WHEN TO RETURN***

# TEACH THE MOTHER TO GIVE ORAL DRUGS AT HOME

**Follow the instructions below for every oral drug to be given at home. Also follow the instructions listed with each drug's dosage table.**

## ➤ *Give Oral Antimalarials as per NAMP guidelines (other than NE-States)*

**➤ FALCIPARUM MALARIA: If RDT or blood smear Pf positive**

| Age group (years) | Day 1 | | Day 2 | | Day 3 |
|---|---|---|---|---|---|
| | Artesunate (AS) | Sulphadoxine Pyramethamine (SP) | Artesunate (AS) | Primaquine (PQ) | Aetesunate (AS) |
| 0-1* Pink Blister | 1 (25 mg) | 1 (250+12.5 mg) | 1 (25 mg) | Nil | 1 (25 mg) |
| 1-4 Yellow Blister | 1 (50 mg) | 1 (500+25 mg) | 1 (50 mg) | 1 (7.5 mg base) | 1 (50 mg) |

**NOTE:** ACT-SP (Artesunate based combination therapy) Artesunate 4 mg per pg daily for 3 days and Sulfadoxine (25 mg/kg)-Pyremethamine 1.25 mg per kg on first day.
Primaquine 0.75 mg per kg on day-2
SP is not to be prescribed for children <5 months of age and should be treated with alternate Artesunate Combination Therapy (ACT)
**-Vivax malaria: If blood smear positive for PV, give Chloroquine for 3 days and Primaquine for 14 days**
Chloroquine for P. Vivax: 25 mg/kg divided over 3 days i.e. 10mg/kg on day 1 and 2 and 5 mg/kg on day 3
Primaquine: 0.25 mg/kg daily for 14 days

| Age group | Chloroquine | | | | | | Primaquine |
|---|---|---|---|---|---|---|---|
| | Day 1 | | Day 2 | | Day 3 | | Give daily for 14 |
| | Tablet (150 mg) | Syrup 50 mg base | Tablet | Syrup | Tablet | Syrup | Tablet (2.5 mg) |
| 2 months upto 12 months | 1/2 | 7.5 ml | 1/2 | 7.5 ml | 1/4 | 4 ml | 0 |
| 12 months upto 5 years | 1 | 15 ml | 1 | 15 ml | 1/2 | 7.5 ml | 1 |

## ➤ *Give Oral Antimalarials as per NAMP guidelines (for NE-States)*

**➤ FALCIPARUM MALARIA: If blood smear positive for PF, give ACT-AL (ARTEMETHER AND LUMEFANTRINE) Co-formulated tablet**

| Age group | Co-formulated ACT-AL | | | | |
|---|---|---|---|---|---|
| | Dose | Times | No of days | Total dose | Availability under National prograe |
| > 5 months to < 3 years (5-14 kg ) | 1 tab (20 mg) | Twice/day | 3 | 120 mg | Yellow colored pack with 6 tablets |
| > =3 years to < 8 years (15 -24 kg) | 2 tab (40 mg) | Twice/day | 3 | 240 mg | Green colored pack with 12 tablets |

**NOTE: If blood smear or RDT positive for both P. Vivax + P. falciparum, give ACT-AL as above and Primaquine.**

➢ **EDUCATE CAREGIVERS TO PROVIDE CARE IN DENGUE FEVER**

**Control the fever**

- Give acetaminophen every 6 hours if high fever (maximum 4 doses per day).
- Do not give ibuprofen, aspirin, or aspirin containing drugs.

- **Prevent spread of dengue within your house**
- Use bed nets for the patient as well as for others to prevent mosquito bite.
- Kill all mosquitoes in house.
- Empty open water containers

**Prevent dehydration**:

Dehydration occurs when a person loses too much fluid (from high fever, vomiting, or poor oral intake). Give plenty of fluids (not only water).

**Watch for warning signs :**

-Look for cold extremities , pain abdomen with restlessness , bleeding from any site .

-Many patient develops warning signs when temperature declines usually 3 to 8 days after onset of fever .

➢ ***GIVE MULTIVITAMINS AND MICRONUTRIENTS TO CHILDREN WITH SEVERE ACUTE MALNUTRITION WITHOUT MEDICAL COMPLICATIONS***

➢ ***Give multivitamin containing vitamin B complex along with Vitamin A, C,D E, B12.***

- ***Give 2.5 ml twice daily for children < 5 kg***
- ***Give 5 ml twice daily for children who are 5 kg or more***

➢ ***Give Zinc 2 mg /kg for 2 weeks***

***COUNSEL THE MOTHER ON HOW TO FEED THE CHILD WITH SEVERE ACUTE MALNUTRITION WITHOUT MEDICAL COMPLICATIONS & MODERATE ACUTE MALNUTRITION***

- Tell mother about child's nutritional status
- Tell them to avail nutritional services for severely malnourished children in that area through anganwadi centers .
- Tell mothers , young children have a small stomach size , which can accommodate limited quantity at a time , so each meal must be made energy dense and should be given at least 5-6 times daily.
- Meals may be made energy dense by preparing porridge in milk; adding butter/ghee/oil/adding sugar or jaggery which makes food item tasty and also helps in absorption of vitamins.
- Foods can also be enriches by adding flours of sprouted and roasted grains.
- Encourage them to use milk and milk products like curd, paneer which are good source of protein, calcium and also provide energy.
- Encourage mothers to give animal origin food items like egg , fish etc. wherever culturally acceptable which is also good source of protein.
- Easily available uncooked seasonal fruits and vegetables are useful source of vitamins and minerals. They should be given daily as snacks in between meals.

# GIVE EXTRA FLUID, ZINC SUPPLEMENT FOR DIARRHOEA AND CONTINUE FEEDING

*(See FOOD advice on COUNSEL THE MOTHER chart)*

## ➢*Plan A: Treat Diarrhoea at Home*

***Counsel the mother on the 4 Rules of Home Treatment: Give Extra Fluid, Zinc supplement, Continue Feeding, When to Return***

1. ***GIVE EXTRA FLUID*** (as much as the child will take)

➢ **TELL THE MOTHER:**

- **If the child is exclusively breastfed** : Breastfeed frequently and for longer at each feed. If passing frequent watery stools:
  - For less than 6 months age give ORS and clean water in addition to breast milk
  - If 6 months or older give one or more of the home fluids in addition to breast milk.
- **If the child is not exclusively breastfed:** Give one or more of the following home fluids; ORS solution, yoghurt drink, milk, lemon drink, rice or pulses-based drink, vegetable soup, green coconut water or plain clean water.

***It is especially important to give ORS at home when:***

- *the child has been treated with Plan B or Plan C during this visit.*
- *the child cannot return to a clinic if the diarrhoea gets worse.*

➢ **TEACH THE MOTHER HOW TO MIX AND GIVE ORS. GIVE THE MOTHER 2 PACKETS OF ORS TO USE AT HOME.**

➢ **SHOW THE MOTHER HOW MUCH FLUID TO GIVE IN ADDITION TO THE USUAL FLUID INTAKE:**

| | |
|---|---|
| Up to 2 years | 50 to 100 ml after each loose stool |
| 2 years or more | 100 to 200 ml after each loose stool |

**Tell the mother to:**

- Give frequent small sips from a cup.
- If the child vomits, wait 10 minutes. Then continue, but more slowly.
- Continue giving extra fluid until the diarrhoea stops.

2. **GIVE ZINC SUPPLEMENTS FOR 14 DAYS**
3. ***CONTINUE FEEDING***
4. ***WHEN TO RETURN***

} See *COUNSEL THE MOTHER* chart

**IMMUNIZE EVERY SICK CHILD, AS NEEDED**

# COUNSEL THE MOTHER

## ➢ *Assess the Child's Feeding ( If age is less than 2 years/ Has Uncomplicated severe acute malnutrition/Moderate acute malnutrition/ Anemia )*

Ask questions about the child's usual feeding and feeding during this illness. Compare the mother's answers to the ***Feeding Recommendations***
for the child's age in the box below.

### *ASK -*

- Do you breastfeed your child?
  - How many times during the day?
  - Do you also breastfeed during the night?

- Does the child take any other food or fluids?
  - What food or fluids?
  - How many times per day?
  - What do you use to feed the child?
  - How large are servings? Does the child receive his own serving? Who feeds the child and how?

- During this illness, has the child's feeding changed?
  If yes, how?

# COUNSEL THE MOTHER

## ➢ *Feeding Recommendations During Sickness and Health*

| **Birth up to 6 Months** 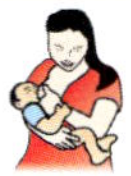 | **6 upto 9 Months** 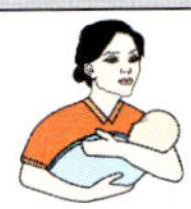 | **9 upto 12 Months** 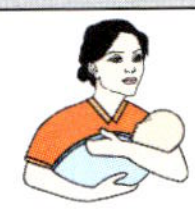 | **12 Months up to 2 Years** 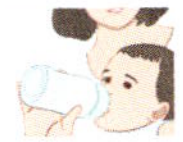 | **2 Years and Older** 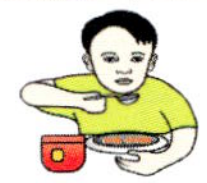 |
|---|---|---|---|---|
| • Immediately after birth , put your baby in skin to skin contact with you.<br>• Breastfeed as often as the child wants, day and night, at least 8 times in 24 hours.<br><br>• Do not give any other foods or fluids not even water<br>• If baby is small (low birth weight), feed at least every 2 to 3 hours. Wake the baby for feeding after 3 hours, if the baby does not wake self.<br><br>Remember:<br>• Continue breastfeeding if the child is sick | • Breastfeed as often as the child wants.<br>• **Start by giving 2 to 3 tablespoons of food. Gradually increase to 1/2 cups (1 cup = 250 ml)**<br>- Mashed roti/ rice /bread/biscuit mixed in sweetened undiluted milk OR<br>thick dal with added ghee/oil or khichri with added oil/ghee. Add cooked vegetables also in the servings OR<br>- Sevian/dalia/halwa/kheer prepared in milk or any cereal porridge cooked in milk OR<br>- Mashed boiled/fried potatoes.<br>Give 2 to 3 meals each day. Offer 1 or 2 snacks each day between<br>Remember:<br>• Keep the child in your lap and feed with your own hands<br>• Wash your own and child 's hands with soap and water every time before feeding | • Breastfeed as often as the child wants.<br>• Give at least 1½ katori serving* at a time of :<br>- Mashed roti/ rice /bread/biscuit mixed in sweetened undiluted milk OR<br>thick dal with added ghee/oil or khichri with added oil/ghee. Add cooked vegetables also in the servings OR<br>- Sevian/dalia/halwa/kheer prepared in milk or any cereal porridge cooked in milk OR<br>- Mashed boiled/fried potatoes .<br>*3 times per day if breastfed;<br>5 times per day if not breastfed.<br>Remember:<br>• Keep the child in your lap and feed with your own hands<br>• Wash your own and child 's hands with soap and water every time before feeding | • Breastfeed as often as the child wants.<br>• Offer food from the family pot<br>• Give at least 1½ katori serving* at a time of: Mashed roti/rice/bread mixed in thick dal with added ghee/oil or khichri with added oil/ ghee. Add cooked vegetables also in the servings OR<br>- Mashed roti/rice/bread/biscuit mixed in sweetened undiluted milk OR<br>- Sevian/dalia/halwa/kheer prepared in milk or any cereal porridge cooked in milk OR<br>- Mashed boiled/fried potatoes<br>- Offer banana/biscuit/cheeko/ mango/ papaya<br>*5 times per day.<br>Remember:<br>• Sit by the side of child and help him to finish the serving<br>• Wash your child's hands with soap and water every time before feeding | • Give a variety of family foods to your child, including animal source and vitamin A rich foods and vegetables<br>• Give family foods at 3–4 meals each day.<br>• Also, twice daily, give nutritious food between meals, such as: banana/biscuit/cheeko/ mango/papaya as snacks<br>• If child refuses a new food, offer "tastes "several times. Be patient.<br><br>Remember:<br>• Ensure that the child finishes the serving<br>• Teach your child wash his hands with soap and water every time before feeding |

* *A good daily diet should be adequate in quantity and include an energy-rich food (for example, thick cereal porridge with added oil); meat, fish, eggs, or pulses; and fruits and vegetables*

## ➢ Counsel the Mother About Feeding Problems

**If the child is not being fed as described in the above recommendations, counsel the mother accordingly. In addition:**

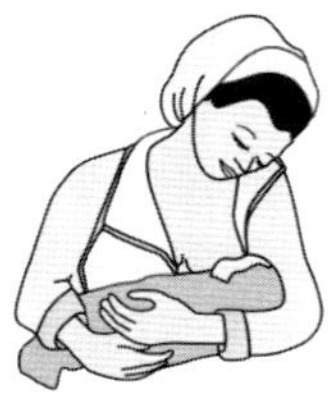

➢ **If the mother reports difficulty with breastfeeding, assess breastfeeding. (See *YOUNG INFANT* chart.)**
**As needed, show the mother correct positioning and attachment for breastfeeding.**

➢ **If the child is less than 6 months old and is taking other milk or foods:**

- Build mother's confidence that she can produce all the breastmilk that the child needs.
- Suggest giving more frequent, longer breastfeeds day or night, and gradually reducing other milk or foods.

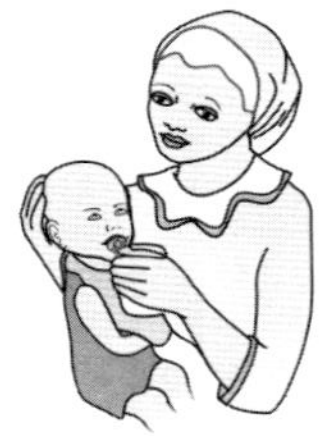

If other milk needs to be continued, counsel the mother to:

- Breastfeed as much as possible, including at night.
- Make sure that other milk is a locally appropriate dairy/animal milk .
- Make sure other milk is correctly and hygienically prepared and given in adequate amounts.
- Finish prepared milk within an hour.

➢ **If the mother is using a bottle to feed the child:**

- Recommend substituting a cup for bottle.
- Show the mother how to feed the child with a cup.

➢ **If the child is not being fed actively, counsel the mother to:**

- Sit with the child and encourage eating.
- Give the child an adequate serving in a separate plate or bowl.

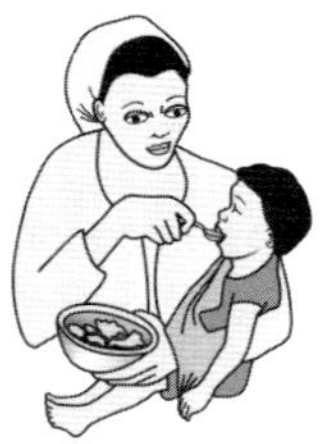

➢ **If the child is not feeding well during illness, counsel the mother to:**

- Breastfeed more frequently and for longer if possible.
- Use soft, varied, appetizing, favourite foods to encourage the child to eat as much as possible, and offer frequent small feedings.
- Clear a blocked nose if it interferes with feeding.

**Feeding Recommendations For a Child who Has PERSISTENT DIARRHOEA**

- If still breastfeeding, give more frequent, longer breastfeeds, day and night.
- If taking other milk:- replace with increased breastfeeding OR replace with fermented milk products, such as yoghurt OR replace half the milk with nutrient-rich semisolid food.
  - Add cereals to milk (Rice, Wheat, Semolina)
- For other foods, follow feeding recommendations for the child's age

# COUNSEL THE MOTHER

## ➢ *Assess the Mother/caregiver's practices to support Child's Development (If age is less than 3years / has Uncomplicated severe acute malnutrition/Anemia)*

Ask questions about the mother/caregiver's usual practices to support child's development. Compare the mother's answers to the ***Recommendations for*** *the child's development*

### *ASK* -

**Child age less than 6 months**

- How do you play with your baby?
- How do you talk to your baby?
- How do you get your baby to smile?

**Child age 6 months and older**

- How do you play with your child?
- How do you talk to your child?
- How do you get your child to smile?
- How do you think your child is learning?

### *LOOK– All children*

- *How does caregivers show he or she is aware of child's movements?*
- *How does caregiver comfort the child and show love?*
- *How does caregiver correct the child?*

# Recommendations for Care of Child Development

## NEWBORN, BIRTH UP TO 1 WEEK

**Your baby learns from birth**

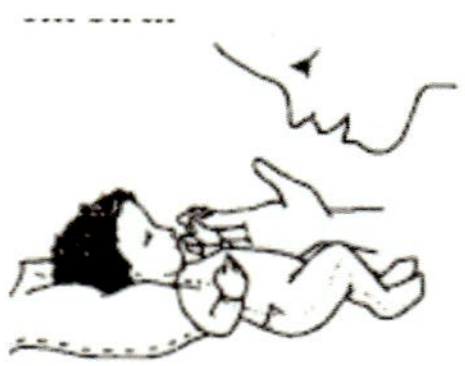

PLAY Provide ways for your baby to see, hear, move arms and legs freely, and touch you. Gently soothe, stroke and hold your child. Skin to skin is good.

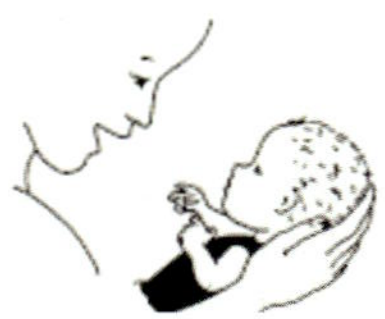

COMMUNICATE Look into baby's eyes and talk to your baby. When you are breastfeeding is a good time. Even a newborn baby sees your face and hears your voice.

## 1 WEEK UP TO 6 MONTHS

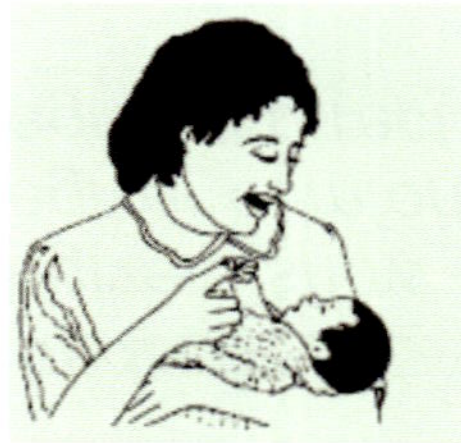

PLAY Provide ways for your child to see, hear, feel, move freely, and touch you. Slowly move colourful things for your child to see and reach for. Sample toys: shaker rattle, big ring on a string.

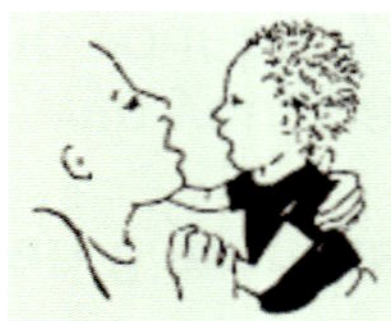

COMMUNICATE Smile and laugh with your child. Talk to your child. Get a conversation going by copying your child's sounds or gestures.

## 6 MONTHS UP TO 9 MONTHS

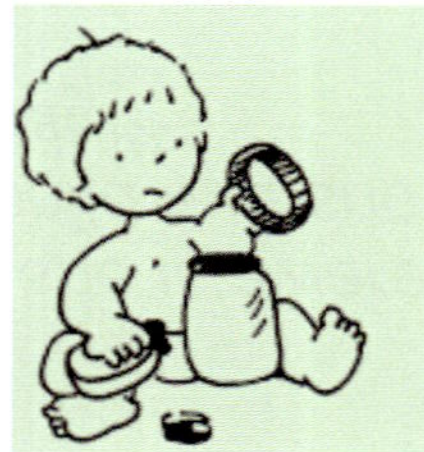

PLAY Give your child clean, safe household things to handle, bang, and drop. Sample toys: containers with lids, metal pot and spoon.

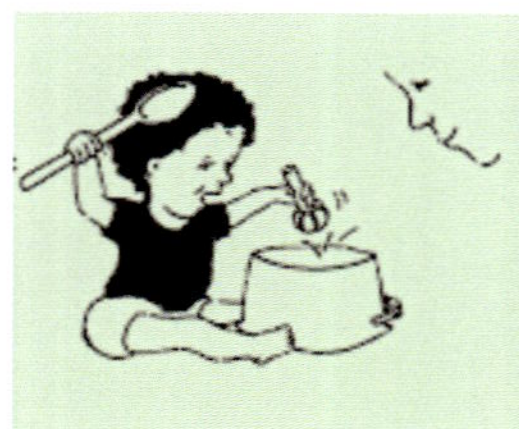

COMMUNICATE Respond to your child's sounds and interests. Call the child's name, and see your child respond.

## 9 MONTHS UP TO 12 MONTHS

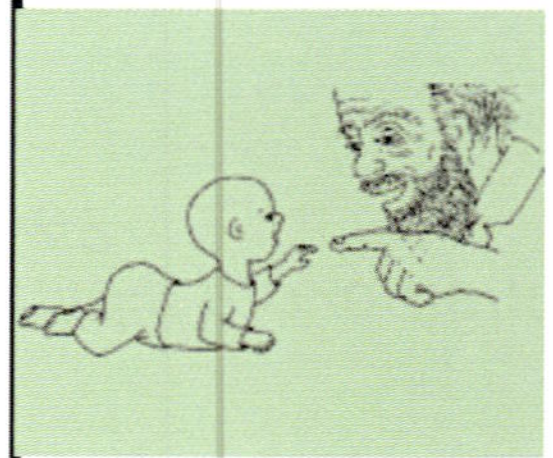

PLAY Hide a child's favourite toy under a cloth or box. See if the child can find it. Play peek-a-boo.

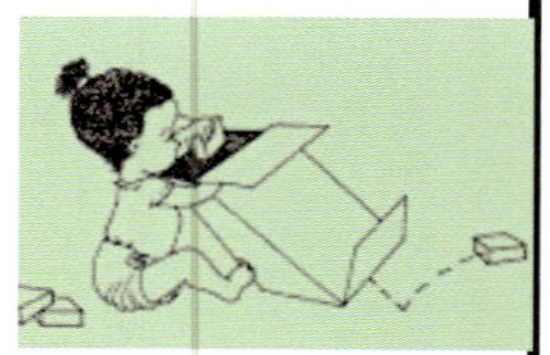

COMMUNICATE Tell your child the names of things and people. Show your child how to say things with hands, like "bye bye". Sample toy: doll with face.

## 12 MONTHS UP TO 2 YEARS

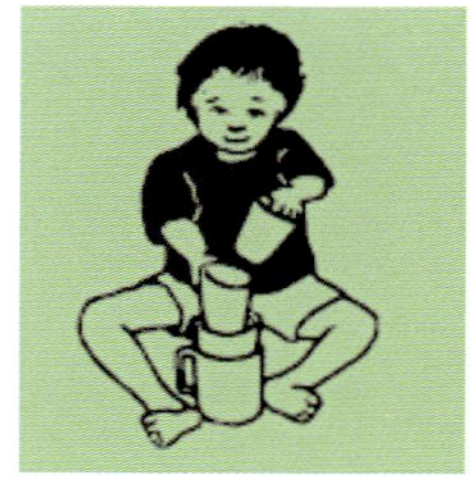

PLAY Give your child things to stack up, and to put into containers and take out. Sample toys: Nesting and stacking objects, container and clothes clips.

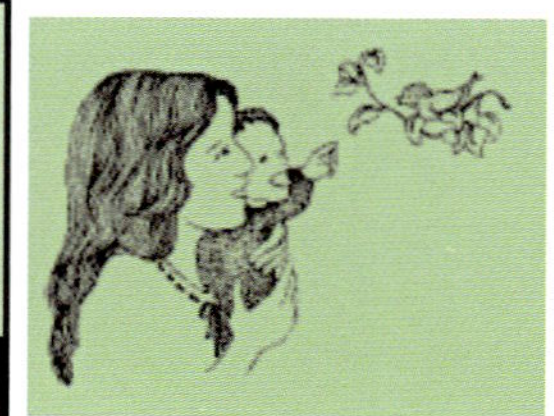

COMMUNICATE Ask your child simple questions. Respond to your child's attempts to talk. Show and talk about nature, pictures and things.

## 2 YEARS AND OLDER

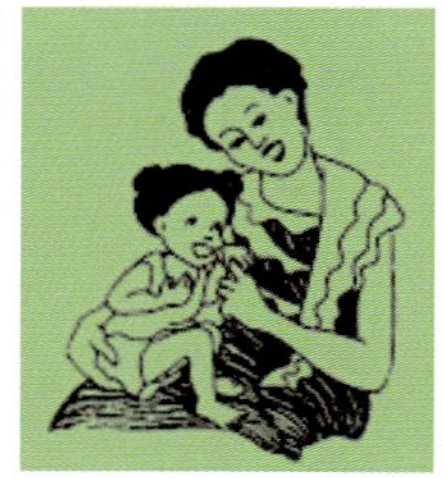

PLAY Help your child count, name and compare things. Make simple toys for your child. Sample toys: Objects of different colours and shapes to sort, stick or chalk board, puzzle.

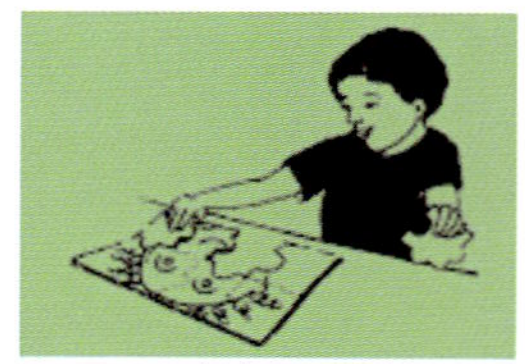

COMMUNICATE Encourage your child to talk and answer your child's questions. Teach your child stories, songs and games. Talk about pictures or books. Sample toy: book with pictures

## ➢ Counsel the Mother for practices to support child's development using MCP card

**If the mother does not breastfeed, counsel the mother to:**
- Hold the child close when feeding, look at the child, and talk or sing to the child.

**If caregivers do not know what the child does to play or communicate:**
- Remind caregivers that children play and communicate from birth.
- Demonstrate how the child responds to activities.

**If caregivers feel too burdened or stressed to play and communicate with the child:**
- Listen to the caregivers feelings, and help them identify a key person who can share their feelings and help them with their child.
- Build their confidence by demonstrating their ability to carry out a simple activity.
- Refer caregivers to a local service, if needed and available.

**If caregivers feel that they do not have time to play and communicate with the child:**
- Encourage them to combine play and communication activities
- with other care for the child.
- Ask other family members to help care for the child or help with chores.

**If caregivers have no toys for the child to play with, counsel them to:**
- Use any household objects that are clean and safe.
- Make simple toys.
- Play with the child. The child will learn by playing with the caregivers and other people.

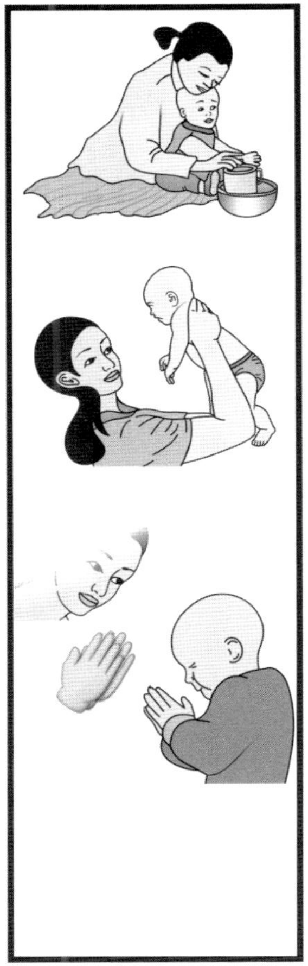

**If the child is not responding, or seems slow :**
- Encourage the family to do extra play and communication activities with the child.
- Check to see whether the child is able to see and to hear.
- Refer the child with difficulties to special services.
- Encourage the family to play and communicate with the child through touch and movement, as well as through language.

**If the mother or father has to leave the child with someone else for a period of time:**
- Identify at least one person who can care for the child regularly, and give the child love and attention.
- Get the child used to being with the new person gradually.
- Encourage the mother and father to spend time with the child when possible.

**If it seems that the child is being treated harshly:**
Recommend better ways of dealing with the child.
- Encourage the family to look for opportunities to praise the child for good behaviour.
- Respect the child's feelings.
  Try to understand why the child is sad or angry.
- Give the child choices about what to do, instead of saying "don't

## Advise the Mother to Increase Fluid During Illness

**FOR ANY SICK CHILD:**

- Breastfeed more frequently and for longer at each feed.
- Increase fluid. For example, give soup, rice water, yoghurt drinks or clean water.

**FOR CHILD WITH DIARRHOEA:**

- Giving extra fluid can be lifesaving. Give fluid according to Plan A or Plan B on *TREAT THE CHILD chart.*

## Advise the Mother When to Return to Health Worker

***FOLLOW-UP VISIT***

Advise the mother to come for follow-up at the earliest time listed for tthe child's problems.

| If the child has: | Return for follow-up |
|---|---|
| PNEUMONIA<br>DYSENTERY<br>MALARIA/SUSPECTED MALARIA<br>DENGUE FEVER<br>FEEDING PROBLEM<br>FEVER-MALARIA UNLIKELY (if fever persists),<br>MEASLES WITH EYE OR MOUTH | 2 days |
| DIARRHOEA, if not improving<br>PERSISTENT DIARRHOEA<br>ACUTE EAR INFECTION<br>CHRONIC EAR INFECTION<br>ANY OTHER ILLNESS , if not improving | 5 days |
| UNCOMPLICATED SEVERE ACUTE MALNUTRITION | 7 days |
| ANAEMIA | 14 days |
| Moderate acute malnutrition | 30 days |

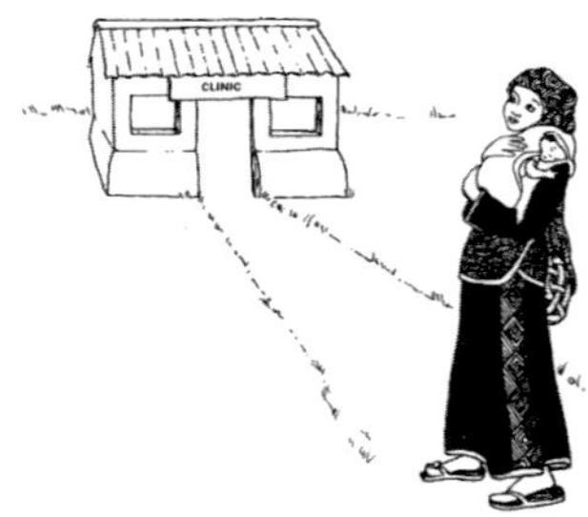

***WHEN TO RETURN***

| Advise mother to return immediately if the child has any of these signs: | |
|---|---|
| Any sick child | • Not able to drink or breastfeed<br>• Becomes sicker<br>• Develops a fever |
| If child has NO PNEUMONIA: COUGH OR COLD, also return if: | • Fast breathing<br>• Difficult breathing |
| If child has Diarrhoea, also return if: | • Blood in stool<br>• Drinking poorly |
| Dengue fever | • Any bleeding from any site<br>• Severe abdominal pain<br>• Cold hands and feet |

# GIVE FOLLOW-UP CARE FOR THE SICK CHILD

- **Care for the child who returns for follow-up using all the boxes that match the child's previous classifications.**
- **If the child has any new problem, assess, classify and treat the new problem as on the *ASSESS AND CLASSIFY* chart.**

## PNEUMONIA

After 2 days:

Check the child for general danger signs.
Assess the child for cough or difficult breathing.
Ask:
- Is the child breathing slower?
- Is there a chest indrawing?
- Is there less fever
- Is the child eating better?

} *See ASSESS & CLASSIFY chart.*

Treatment:

- If ***a general danger sign***, OR stridor refer URGENTLY to hospital.
- If ***breathing rate, chest indrawing, fever and eating are the same, or worse***, refer to hospital.
- If ***breathing slower, no chest indrawing, less fever, or eating better***, complete the 5 days of antibiotic.

## PERSISTENT DIARRHOEA

After 5 days:

Ask:
- Has the diarrhoea stopped?
- How many loose stools is the child having per day?

Treatment:

- If ***the diarrhoea has not stopped (child is still having 3 or more loose stools per day)***, do a full reassessment of the child. Give any treatment needed. Then refer to hospital.
- If ***the diarrhoea has stopped (child having less than 3 loose stools per day)***, tell the mother to follow the usual feeding recommendations for the child's age. Continue oral zinc for a total of 14 days.

## DIARRHOEA

After 5 days:
Ask:
- Has the diarrhoea stopped?
- How many loose stools is the child having per day ?

Treatment:
- If diarrhoea persists, Assess the child for diarrhoea (> *See ASSESS & CLASSIFY chart)* and manage as on initial visit .
- If diarrhoea has stopped *(child having less than 3 loose stools per day)*, tell the mother to follow the usual feeding recommendations for the child's age.

## DYSENTERY

After 2 days:

Assess the child for diarrhoea. > *See ASSESS & CLASSIFY chart.*
Ask:
- Are there fewer stools?
- Is there less blood in the stool?
- Is there less fever?
- Is there less abdominal pain?
- Is the child eating better?

Treatment:

- If the child is ***dehydrated***, treat dehydration.
- If ***fewer stools, less blood in the stools, less fever, less abdominal pain, and eating better,*** continue giving the same antibiotic until finished.
- If *number of* ***stools, amount of blood in stools, fever, abdominal pain or eating is the same or worst: Refer to hospital***
- If *fewer* ***stools, less blood in the stools, less fever, less abdominal pain and eating better, continue giving ciprofloxacin until finished***

**Ensure that mother understands the oral rehydration method fully and that she also understands the need for an extra meal each day for a week.**

# GIVE FOLLOW-UP CARE

- **Care for the child who returns for follow-up using all the boxes that match the child's previous classifications.**
- **If the child has any new problem, assess, classify and treat the new problem as on the *ASSESS AND CLASSIFY* chart.**

## MALARIA/SUSPECTED MALARIA

After two days :

Do a full reassessment of the child. > *See ASSESS & CLASSIFY chart. Review the test report .*
Assess for other causes of fever.

Treatment:

- If the child has ***any general danger sign or stiff neck***, treat as VERY SEVERE FEBRILE DISEASE.
- If the child has any ***cause of fever other than malaria***, provide treatment.
- If ***malaria is the only apparent cause of fever:***
  - Advise the mother to return again in 2 days if the fever persists. Continue Primaquine if P. vivax was positive for a total of 14 days.
  - If fever has been present for 7 days, refer for assessment.

## FEVER-MALARIA UNLIKELY

If fever persists after 2 days:
Do a full reassessment of the child. > *See ASSESS & CLASSIFY chart.*
Assess for other causes of fever.

Treatment:

- If the child has ***any general danger sign or stiff neck***, treat as VERY SEVERE FEBRILE DISEASE.
- If suspected dengue , assess for warning signs . Refer to hospital
- If the child has any ***cause of fever other than malaria***, provide treatment.
- If ***malaria is the only apparent cause of fever:***
  - Treat with the oral antimalarial. Advise the mother to return again in 2 days if the fever persists.
  - If fever has been present for 7 days, refer for assessment.

## DENGUE FEVER

Reassess for warning signs
-If any general danger signs or warning signs —Refer URGENTLY to hospital
- If no general danger sign / no warning signs—follow –up after 2 day
- If fever has been present for 7 days, refer for assessment.

## MEASLES WITH EYE OR MOUTH COMPLICATIONS

After 2 days:

Look for red eyes and pus draining from the eyes.
Look at mouth ulcers.
Check for foul smell from the mouth.

Treatment for Eye Infection:

- If ***pus is draining from the eye***, ask the mother to describe how she has treated the eye infection. If treatment has been correct, refer to hospital. If treatment has not been correct, teach mother correct treatment.
- If ***the pus is gone but redness remains***, continue the treatment.
- If ***no pus or redness***, stop the treatment.

Treatment for Mouth Ulcers:

- If ***mouth ulcers are worse, or there is a very foul smell from the mouth***, refer to hospital.
- If ***mouth ulcers are the same or better***, continue using half-strength gentian violet for a total of 5 days.

## EAR INFECTION

After 5 days:

Reassess for ear problem. > *See ASSESS & CLASSIFY chart.*
Measure the child's temperature.

Treatment:

- If there is ***tender swelling behind the ear or high fever (38.5°C or above)***, refer URGENTLY to hospital.
- ***Acute ear infection:*** if ***ear pain or discharge*** persists, treat with 5 more days of the same antibiotic. Continue wicking to dry the ear. Follow -up in 5 days.
- ***Chronic ear infection:*** Check that the mother is wicking the ear correctly and instilling ear drops. If ear discharge getting better encourage her to continue. If no improvement, refer to hospital for assessment
- If ***no ear pain or discharge***, praise the mother for her careful treatment. If she has not yet finished the 5 days of antibiotic, tell her to use all of it before stopping.

# GIVE FOLLOW-UP CARE

- **Care for the child who returns for follow-up using all the boxes that match the child's previous classifications.**
- **If the child has any new problem, assess, classify and treat the new problem as on the *ASSESS AND CLASSIFY* chart.**

## ➢ FEEDING PROBLEM

After 5 days:

Reassess feeding. > *See questions at the top of the COUNSEL chart.*
Ask about any feeding problems found on the initial visit.

- Counsel the mother about any new or continuing feeding problems. If you counsel the mother to make significant changes in feeding, ask her to bring the child back again.

## ➢ MODERATE ACUTE MALNUTRITION

After 30 days:

- Assess the child using the same measurement (WFH/L or MUAC) used on the initial visit:
- Check the child for oedema of both feet.
- Reassess feeding. See questions in the COUNSEL THE MOTHER chart

**Treatment:**

- If the child is no longer classified as **MODERATE ACUTE MALNUTRITION**, praise the mother and encourage her to continue.
- If the child is still classified as **MODERATE ACUTE MALNUTRITION**, counsel the mother about any feeding problem found. Ask the mother to return again in one month. Continue to see the child monthly until the child is feeding well and gaining weight regularly or his or her WFH/L is -2 z-scores or more or MUAC is 125 mm. or more.

**Exception:**
If you do not think that feeding will improve, or if the child has lost weight or his or her MUAC has diminished <11.5 cm , refer the child for assessment of medical causes like TB, HIV, etc.

## ➢ ANAEMIA: After 14 days:

- Check compliance and allay anxiety if black stools or minor side effects
- Do Hemoglobin estimation if possible
- If improvement ,give iron folic acid. Advise mother to return in 14 days for more iron folic acid. Continue giving iron folic acid every 14 days for 2 –3 months.
- If no improvement—check compliance . Refer to test for sickle cell anemia and hemoglobinopathies if family history present or common in that population.
- If there is anemia even after 2 months of supplementation , refer to hospital for assessment.

## ➢ UNCOMPLICATED SEVERE ACUTE MALNUTRITION

After 7 days:

- Do a full reassessment of the child. > See ASSESS & CLASSIFY chart. Assess child with the same measurements (WFH/L, MUAC) as on the initial visit and looking for oedema of both feet.

Treatment:

- If the child has **COMPLICATED SEVERE ACUTE MALNUTRITION** (WFH/L less than -3 z-scores or MUAC is less than 115 mm or oedema of both feet AND has developed a medical complication or oedema, refer URGENTLY to hospital. If static weight or weight loss at 2 FU visits –refer the child for assessment of medical causes like TB, HIV, etc..
- If the child has **UNCOMPLICATED SEVERE ACUTE MALNUTRITION** (WFH/L less than -3 z-scores or MUAC is less than 115 mm but NO medical complication, **counsel the mother and encourage her to continue with appropriate feeding. Ask mother to return again in 14 days.**
- If the child has **MODERATE ACUTE MALNUTRITION /NO ACUTE MALNUTRITION**, advise the mother to continue with appropriate feeding . **Continue to see the child monthly** until the child is feeding well and gaining weight regularly or his or her WFH/L is -2 z-scores or more or MUAC is 125 mm. or more.

**MANAGEMENT OF THE SICK YOUNG INFANT AGE UP TO 2 MONTHS**

Name:______________________________ Age:____ Sex: M____ F____ Weight:_____ kg Temperature:______ °C **Date:**

ASK: What are the infant's problems? ______________________________ Initial visit? _______ Follow-up Visit?______

**ASSESS** (Circle all signs present) — **CLASSIFY**

CHECK FOR POSSIBLE BACTERIAL INFECTION / JAUNDICE

- If the infant having difficulty in feeding?
- Has the infant had convulsions?

- Count the breaths in one minute._____breaths per minute
  Repeat if elevated ________ Fast breathing?
- Look for severe chest indrawing.
- Measure axillary temperature
(if not possible, feel for fever or low body temperature).
- Look at the young infant's movements.
- *If infant is sleeping , ask the mother to wake him/her.*
  - Does the infant move on his/her own? -
  - Does the infant move only when stimulated but then stops ?
  - Does the infant not move at all?
- Look at the umbilicus. Is it red or draining pus?
- Look for skin pustules.

**DOES THE YOUNG INFANT HAVE DIARRHOEA?** Yes ___ No ___

- Look at the young infant's general condition. Is the infant:
- - Lethargic or unconscious?
  - Restless and irritable?
- Look for sunken eyes.
- Pinch the skin of the abdomen. Does it go back:
  - Very slowly (longer than 2 seconds)?
  - Slowly

**THEN CHECK FOR FEEDING PROBLEM & VERY LOW WEIGHT**

- Is there any difficulty in feeding? Yes __ No ___

- Measure weight
- Determine weight for age
  - Weight for age ≥ –2 SD score
  - Weight for age less than –2 SD score
  - Weight for age less than –3SD score
- Look for ulcers or white patches in the mouth (thrush)

- Is the infant breastfed? Yes _____ No ___
  If Yes, how many times in 24 hours? ____ times
- Does the infant usually receive any other foods or drinks? Yes ___ No ___
  If Yes, how often?w is milk given? Cup or bottle

**If the infant has no indications to refer urgently to hospital:**

**ASSESS BREASTFEEDING:**

- Has the infant breastfed in the previous hour?

If infant has not fed in the previous hour, ask the mother to put her infant to the breast. Observe the breastfeed for 4 minutes.

- Is the infant able to attach? To check attachment, look for:
  - Chin touching breast Yes ___ No ___
  - Mouth wide open Yes _____ No ___
  - Lower lip turned outward Yes ____ No ___
  - More areola above than below the mouth Yes ___ No ___

  *no attachment at all* *not well attached* *good attachment*

- Is the infant suckling effectively (that is, slow deep sucks, sometimes pausing)?

  *not suckling at all* *not suckling effectively* *suckling effectively*

- Does the mother have pain while brteastfeeding? If yes, then look for:
  - Flat or inverted nipples, or sore nipples
  - Engorged breasts or breast abscess

**CHECK THE YOUNG INFANT'S IMMUNIZATION STATUS** Circle immunizations needed today. immunization

| | | | | | |
|---|---|---|---|---|---|
| Birth | BCG | OPV 0 | HEP-B 0 | | |
| 6 weeks | Penta-1 | OPV-1 | Rotavirus-1 | f IPV-1 | PCV-1* |

Circle needed todays, return for next immunization on:

Date

**ASSESS CAREGIVER'S PRACTICES TO SUPPORT CHILD'S DEVELOPMENT**

ASK : How do you play with your baby? Look how does caregiver show he/she is aware of child's movement?

How do you talk to h your baby?

How do you get your baby smile ? Look how does caregiver comfort the child and show love ?

Look how does caregiver correct the child ?

I

**ASSESS OTHER PROBLEMS**

## MANAGEMENT OF THE SICK CHIID AGE 2 MONTHS UP TO 5 YEARS

Name: ____________________ Age:_______ Sex: M____ F____ Weight: ____ kg Temperature: _____ $^0$C **Date**

**ASK:** What are the child's problems?______________________________________ Initial visit? ___ Follow-up Visit? ___

ASSESS (Circle all signs present) **CLASSIFY**

---

CHECK FOR GENERAL DANGER SIGNS

NOT ABLE TO DRINK OR BREASTFEED LETHARGIC OR UNCONSCIOUS

VOMITS EVERYTHING

CONVULSIONS

General danger sign present?

Yes___ No___

**Remember to use danger sign when selecting classifications**

---

**DOES THE CHILD HAVE COUGH OR DIFFICULT BREATHING?** Yes___ No___

- For how long ? _____ Days
- Check Spo2 <90%/≥ 90%
- Count the breaths in one minute
  _____ breaths per minute. Fast breathing?
- Look for chest indrawing.
- Look and listen for stridor.______
- Look and listen for wheezing

---

**DOES THE CHILD HAVE DIARRHOEA ?** Yes___ No___

- For how long ? _____ Days
- Is there blood in the stool?
- Look at the child's general condition. Is the child:
  Lethargic or unconscious?
  Restless and irritable
- Look for sunken eyes.
- Offer the child fluid. Is the child:
  Not able to drink or drinking poorly?
  Drinking eagerly, thirsty?
- Pinch the skin of the abdomen. Does it go back:
  Very slowly (longer than 2 seconds)?
  Slowly?

---

**DOES THE CHILD HAVE FEVER?** (by history/feels hot/ temperature 37.5$^0$C or above) Yes___ No___

Is it a PF( P. falciparum) predominant area ? Yes/no

- Fever for how long? ___Days
- Is there a sudden, continous fever of 2-7 days?
- If more than 7 days, has fever been present every day?
- Is there any rash/bleeding from any site ?
- Is there sever abdominal pain ?

RDT for P. falciparum /P vivax - Positive /Negative ?

- Look or feel for stiff neck.
- Look for any bacterial cause of fever
- Look for cold extremities with weak pulse

- Has the child had measles within the last 3 months?

Look for signs of MEASLES:

- Generalized rash
- One of these: cough, runny nose, or red eyes

**If the child has measles now or within the last 3 months:**

- Look for mouth ulcers
  If Yes, are they deep and extensive
- Look for pus draining from the eye.
- Look for clouding of the cornea.

---

**DOES THE CHILD HAVE AN EAR PROBLEM** Yes___ No___

- Is there ear pain?
- Is there ear discharge?
  If Yes, for how long? ____ Days
- Look for pus draining from the ear.
- Feel for tender swelling behind the ear.

---

THEN CHECK FOR ACUTE MALNUTRITION

- Look for oedema of both feet.
- Determine WFH/L SD score:
  Less than –3 SD/ between –3 and –2/ -2 SD or more
- If Child 6 months or older measure MUAC ____mm.

---

**THEN CHECK FOR ANAEMIA**

**Hemoglobin_____g/dl**

- Look for palmar pallor.
  Severe palmar pallor? Some palmar pallor? No pallor?

---

**CHECK THE CHILD'S IMMUNIZATION, PROPHYLACTIC VITAMIN A & IRON-FOLIC ACID STATUS**

Circle immunizations and Vitamin A or IFA supplements needed today.

| BCG | Penta 1 | Penta 2 | Penta 3 | MR-1/JE 1/PCV B | MR2 /JE2 |
|---|---|---|---|---|---|
| OPV 0 | OPV 1 | OPV 2 | OPV 3 +IPV 2 | VITAMIN A | DPT B-1+OPV B |
| | Rota-1 /PCV-1 | Rota-2 | Rota-3/PCV-2 | IFA | |

Return for next immunization or vitamin A or IFA

__________

(Date)

---

ASSESS CHILD'S FEEDING if child has UNCOMPLICATED SEVERE ACUTE MALNUTRITION / MODERATE ACUTE MALNUTRITION or ANAEMIA or is less than 2 years old

- Do you breastfeed your child? Yes___ No ___
  If Yes, how many times in 24 hours? ___ times. Do you breastfeed during the night? Yes__ No___
- Does the child take any other food or fluids? Yes___ No ___ If Yes, what foods or fluids?
  ow many times per day? ___ times. What do you use to feed the child and how? _____________
  How large are the servings? ___________________
  Does the child receive his own serving? _______ Who feeds the child and how? _____________
- During this illness has the child's feeding changed? Yes No

Chapter 33

# Rational Drug Therapy

❍ Anu Thukral ❍ Kana Ram Jat

## INTRODUCTION

Medications play an important role in protecting, maintaining and restoring health. Irrational and indiscriminate use may lead to toxicity and adverse reactions. It is better to use medications with which the physician is familiar. The expected benefits and side effects should always be kept in mind when prescribing. The principles of rational drug therapy can be summarized as:

i. There should be a genuine indication for use of the medication.
ii. Minimum number of appropriate, familiar and inexpensive agents of good quality should be used.
iii. Drugs should be prescribed by their generic name.
iv. Dosage should be optimum to achieve the desired benefits.
v. It is desirable to administer medication, as far as possible, through oral route.
vi. Adverse drug reactions should be anticipated, monitored and appropriately managed.

True synergism is rare; an exception is cotrimoxazole (trimethoprim and sulfamethoxazole). A combination of antibiotics may be necessary when the causative agent is not known. Multidrug therapy is indicated to prevent resistance to individual drugs, during long-term management of tuberculosis and leprosy and to reduce toxicity of individual drugs. Bactericidal drugs act best when the organism is actively multiplying and should ideally not be combined with bacteriostatic drugs.

Developmental and genetic factors affect the metabolism of drugs and thereby the response. Doses of drugs need to be modulated according to the individual responses. The dosages may vary in specific disease, e.g. pneumonia, meningitis, bacterial endocarditis and pyogenic arthritis.

The drugs, required dose and important side effects have been tabulated alphabetically below for easy reading and referral. Details on the following categories of drugs are provided elsewhere: Antiepileptic drugs (*Chapter 19*), antihypertensive agents (*Chapter 16*), antitubercular, antiretroviral and antileprosy drugs (*Chapter 11*).

The reader is advised to consult detailed prescribing information for each medication.

*Abbreviations:* g–gram; GI–gastrointestinal; hr–hour; IM–intramuscular; IV–intravenous; IO–intraosseus; kg–kilogram; $m^2$–square meter body surface; mg milligram; µg–microgram, PO–per oral; PR–per rectal; q–every; SC–subcutaneous; T–topical; wt–weight; yr–age in years; C/I–contraindication; GERD–gastroesophageal reflux disease.

## ANALGESICS, ANTIPYRETICS, NON-STEROIDAL ANTI-INFLAMMATORY DRUGS (NSAIDs)

### Non-Narcotic Analgesics

#### Aspirin

*Acute rheumatic fever:* 90–120 mg/kg/day PO q 4 hr
*Antipyretic dose:* 30–60 mg/kg/day PO q 4–6 hr; maximum 4 g/day
*Kawasaki disease:* 80–100 mg/kg/day PO q 6 hr till afebrile or for 2 weeks followed by 3–5 mg/kg/day PO q 24 hr for 6–8 weeks until platelet count and ESR are normal.
*Side effects:* Hypersensitivity, hypoprothrombinemia. There is epidemiologic association between salicylate use and Reye encephalopathy. Use of aspirin for upper respiratory tract infections and fever of undetermined origin in children is not advised. Salicylates should be avoided empty stomach.

#### Paracetamol

*Antipyretic/analgesic:* 40–60 mg/kg/day PO q 4–6 hr or 15 mg/kg/dose PO q 4–6 hr; maximum 90 mg/kg/day, 4 g/d; 5 mg/kg IM
IV <2 yr: 7.5–15 mg/kg q 6 hr
2–12 yr: 15 mg/kg q 6 hr
*Patent ductus arteriosus:* 15 mg/kg q 6 hr for 3 days
*Side effects:* Skin rashes, hepatotoxicity, renal damage

### Ibuprofen

*Antipyretic/analgesic:* 20–30 mg/kg/day PO q 6–8 hr or 10 mg/kg/dose PO q 4–6 hr; maximum dose 40–60 mg/kg/day
*Juvenile idiopathic arthritis:* 30–70 mg/kg/day PO q 4–6 hr
*Closure of ductus arteriosus in neonates:* 10 mg/kg/day PO followed by 5 mg/kg/day q 24 hr for 2 days
*Side effects:* Nausea, vomiting, rashes

### Naproxen

*Juvenile idiopathic arthritis:* 10–20 mg/kg/day PO q 12 hr; maximum 1 g/d
Analgesia 5–7 mg/kg/dose PO q 8–12 hr (after meals)
*Side effects:* Nausea, vomiting, rashes

### Diclofenac Sodium

1–3 mg/kg/day PO q 8 hr
*Side effects:* Gastric bleeding, ulcer

### Mefenamic Acid

25 mg/kg/day PO q 6–8 hr
*Antipyretic dose:* 5–8 mg/kg/dose
*Side effects:* Gastric bleeding, rash, seizures, colitis

### Indomethacin

1–3 mg/kg/day PO q 12–24 hr

Dose for ductal closure depends on the age of the neonate **(Table 33.1)**
*Side effects:* Oliguria, hypoglycemia, platelet dysfunction, necrotising enterocolitis.

### Tramadol

1–2 mg/kg q 4–6 hr up to maximum of 400 mg/day; avoid below 14 yr of age
*Side effect:* Seizures, renal and hepatic dysfunction

## Narcotic Analgesics (Opioids)

### Fentanyl

0.5–5 µg/kg/dose q 1–4 hr IV; may be administered as a continuous infusion 1–5 µg/kg/hr.
Potent narcotic analgesic; 0.1 mg dose possesses analgesic activity; equivalent to 10 mg of morphine.
*Side effects:* Rapid infusion may cause chest wall rigidity; respiratory distress and respiratory arrest.

### Morphine

0.1–0.2 mg/kg/dose q 4 hr (maximum 15 mg) IV/IM/SC
*Continuous infusion in neonates:* 0.01–0.02 mg/kg/hr
*Infants and children:* 0.01–0.04 mg/kg/hr

**Table 33.1:** Indomethacin dose (mg/kg) in neonates

| *Age at first dose* | *1st* | *2nd* | *3rd* |
|---|---|---|---|
| <48 hours | 0.2 | 0.1 | 0.1 |
| 2–7 days | 0.2 | 0.2 | 0.2 |
| >7 days | 0.2 | 0.25 | 0.25 |

Naloxone (0.01 mg/kg IV) is an antidote in case of respiratory depression.
*Side effects:* Respiratory distress, increased intracranial pressure, seizures.
*Contraindication:* Respiratory failure, obstructive airway disease.

## ANTIARRHYTHMICS

### Adenosine

0.1 mg/kg/dose (initial maximum dose 6 mg) rapid IV (over 1–3 sec); if no response in 1–2 min, 0.2 mg/kg bolus. To ensure that the drug reaches the circulation, administer directly into a vein with a three-way stop cock with 5–10 mL of saline flush ready to push immediately; maximum single dose 0.25 mg/kg or 12 mg
*Side effects:* Transient chest pain, dyspnea, flushing, bronchospasm. Carbamazepine and dipyramidole increase the toxicity/effect of adenosine.

### Atropine Sulfate

0.01 mg/kg/dose SC or IV
The dose can be repeated after 2 hr (maximum 4–6 times a day).
Organophosphorus poisoning: 0.02–0.05 mg/kg every 10–20 min until atropine effect, then q 1–4 hr for at least 24 hours.
*Side effects:* Dry mouth, blurred vision, tachycardia, urinary retention, constipation, dizziness, hallucinations, restlessness.

### Lidocaine Hydrochloride

0.5 to 1 mg/kg/dose (maximum dose: 100 mg) slowly IV; repeat in 10–15 min for two times; maximum total dose 5 mg/kg within the first hr; endotracheal dose is two to three times the IV dose.
Continuous infusion 20–50 µg/kg/min IV/IO (do not exceed 20 µg/kg/min for patients with shock or CHF); administer 1 mg/kg bolus when infusion is initiated (bolus not given within previous 15 min)
*Side effects:* Hypotension, seizures, asystole, respiratory arrest.

### Phenytoin Sodium

*Arrhythmia:* Loading 1.25 mg/kg IV over 3 min and repeat every 5–10 min to a maximum total dose of 15 mg/kg or until arrhythmia reverts or hypotension develops; maintenance 5–10 mg/kg/day PO q 12 hr
*Status epilepticus:* Loading 15–20 mg/kg IV, do not exceed 1–3 mg/kg/min, maintain with 5–8 mg/kg/day PO or IV q 12–24 hr.
*Side effects:* Gum hypertrophy, hirsutism, hypersensitivity, megaloblastic anemia, osteomalacia, vestibulocerebellar syndrome.

### Procainamide

*Arrhythmia:* 3–6 mg/kg/dose over 5 min, repeat q 5 min up to total of 15 mg/kg; IV infusion: 0.5 mg/kg/hr
Oral: 50 mg/kg/day PO q 3–4 hr

*Side effects:* Thrombocytopenia, Coombs positive hemolytic anemia, lupus-like syndrome
*Contraindication:* Heart block, myasthenia gravis

### Propranolol

*Arrhythmia:* 0.01–0.1 mg/kg/dose; given as IV bolus over 10 min (maximum 1 mg in infants; 3 mg in children), may repeat in 15 min and then q 6–8 hr.
*Antihypertensive:* 0.5–1 mg/kg/day PO q 6–8 hr
*Thyrotoxicosis:* 2–4 mg/kg/day PO q 6–8 hr
*Tetralogy spells:* 0.15–0.25 mg/kg/dose slow IV push, repeat q 15 min; 2–4 mg/kg/24 hr PO q 6–8 hr, increase to 4–8 mg/kg/day
*Infantile hemangioma:* 1 mg/kg/day PO q 8 hr. Increase to 2 mg/kg/day PO q 8 hr after 1 week, if well tolerated.
*Side effects:* Increase in pulmonary resistance, fatigue and bradycardia.

### Quinidine Sulfate

*Arrhythmia:* Test dose 2 mg/kg PO followed by 15 to 60 mg/kg/day PO q 6 hr
*Malaria:* Loading dose 10 mg/kg/day IV over 1–2 hr (maximum dose 600 mg) followed by 0.02 mg/kg/min (10 mg/kg/dose q 8 hr), 10 mg/kg/dose PO q 8 hr, infusion until oral dose can be tolerated. If more than 48 hours of intravenous therapy is required, decrease the dose by 30 to 50%
*Side effects:* Thrombocytopenia, anemia, tinnitus, hypotension, blood dyscrasias
*Contraindication:* Heart blocks, congestive heart failure

### Verapamil

*Arrhythmia:* 0.1–0.3 mg/kg IV over 2 min; repeat after 30 minutes
*Hypertension:* 4–8 mg/kg/day PO q 8 hr
*Contraindication:* Cardiogenic shock, AV block, children below 2 years of age

## AGENTS FOR MYASTHENIA

### Edrophonium Chloride

*Initial dose:* 0.04 mg/kg dose IV, IM (maximum 1 mg <30 kg); if no response after 1 min, may give 0.16 mg/kg/dose total of 0.2 mg/kg (maximum 5 mg for <30 kg)
*Side effects:* Arrhythmias, bronchospasm

### Neostigmine Bromide

*Myasthenia gravis*
Neonate: 0.05–0.1 mg IM/SC, then PO 1 mg 30 min before feed.
Children: 1–3 mg/kg/day PO q 4–6 hr; 0.01–0.04 mg/kg IV/IM/SC q 2–3 hr

Begin with lower dose and increase gradually till symptoms disappear.
*Side effects:* Cholinergic crisis, bronchospasm, respiratory depression, hypotension, seizures, salivation, vomiting, diarrhea and lacrimation.
*Contraindication:* Urinary and intestinal obstruction

### Pyridostigmine

*Infants of myasthenic mothers:* 0.05–0.15 mg/kg/dose; maximum dose 5 mg PO q 4–6 hr (benzyl alcohol-free formulation should be used for neonates).
*Children PO:* 7 mg/kg/day in 5–6 divided doses;
IM, IV: 0.05–0.15 mg/kg/dose (maximum dose 10 mg)
*Side effects:* Same as neostigmine

### Physostigmine

*Myasthenia:* 0.01–0.03 mg/kg/dose IM, SC, IV
Repeat q 15–20 min to desired effect or maximum dose of 2 mg
*Side effects:* Same as neostigmine

## ANTIMICROBIALSS

### Antibiotics (Tables 33.2 to 33.9)

#### Penicillins (Table 33.2)

Penicillin may cause hypersensitivity reactions in about 1% of individuals. Acute symptoms include urticaria, angioneurotic edema, anaphylactic shock, asthma, laryngeal edema and hypotension. Delayed reactions are fixed drug eruption, serum sickness, hemolytic anemia and recurrent arthralgia. Sodium and potassium content of penicillin G is 1.68 mEq per million units; large doses may cause seizures. Side effects specific to piperacillin additionally include impaired platelet aggregation and deranged liver function. The dosing for piperacillin needs to be adjusted in renal impairment.

#### Cephalosporins (Table 33.3)

Approximately 10% patients with penicillin hypersensitivity show allergy to cephalosporin; anaphylaxis may occur. Oral cephalosporins may cause loss of appetite, nausea, vomiting and diarrhea. Some parenteral cephalosporins cause serious renal toxicity. Ceftriaxone is contraindicated in neonates with hyperbilirubinemia because it may displace bilirubin from albumin.

#### Aminoglycosides (Table 33.4)

*Side effects:* Aminoglycosides cause variable degrees of auditory and vestibular toxicity, and reversible kidney dysfunction. Rashes and drug fevers occur in about 5% patients. Dosage should be reduced and interval between dosages increased in patients with impaired renal function. Administration of aminoglycoside dose once in 24 hours and as infusion reduces the risk of renal and auditory toxicity.

#### Chloramphenicol (Table 33.5)

*Side effects:* Idiosyncratic bone marrow depression. *Hypersensitivity:* Fever, rash, angioneurotic edema; GI disturbances. Neonates, especially premature, may show grey baby syndrome with abdominal distension, vomiting, refusal to suck and dyspnea; cyanosis, peripheral circulatory collapse and death.

Table 33.2: Penicillins

| Drug | Dose (mg/kg/day) | Route | Schedule |
|---|---|---|---|
| Penicillin G aqueous | Neonate: 50000–100000 U/kg/day (higher dose for meningitis) 100,000–400,000 U/kg<br>Meningitis and endocarditis: 200,000–400,000 U/kg | IV<br>IV/ IM | 8–12 hr<br>4–6 hr |
| Benzathine penicillin (acute rheumatic fever prophylaxis) | Less than 6 years: 0.6 million units <27 kg<br>6 years and above: 1.2 million units ≥27 kg | IM | 3–4 weekly |
| Procaine penicillin G | Neonates: 50,000 U<br>25,000–50,000 U | IM | 1–2 doses maximum |
| Phenoxymethyl penicillin V | Infants: 62.5–125 mg/ dose<br>Children less than 6 years: 125 mg/dose<br>6–12 years: 250 mg/dose<br>Rheumatic fever prophylaxis: 250 mg | PO | 12 hr |
| Methicillin sodium | 100 | IM or IV | 6 hr |
| Oxacillin | <2 kg: 50 mg/kg/day 12 hourly; ≥2 kg: 75 mg/kg/day 8 hourly | PO or IV | 6 hr |
| Cloxacillin | Child (<40 kg)<br>Mild/moderate infections: 12.5–50<br>Severe infections: 50–100<br>Child (≥40 kg) and adult: 125–500 mg/dose<br>Maximum dose: 2 g/24 hr | PO or IV<br><br><br>PO | 4–6 hr<br><br><br>6 hr |
| Ampicillin | 50–100<br>100–200<br>Meningitis and enteric fever: 200–400 | PO<br>IM or IV<br>IV | 6 hr<br>6 hr<br>4–6 hr |
| Amoxicillin | 25–50 | PO | 8–12 hr |
| Co-amoxiclav (amoxicillin + clavulanic acid) | 25–40<br>75 of Amoxicillin | PO<br>IV | 8–12 hr<br>8 hr |
| Ampicillin and sulbactam (100 mg ampicillin and 50 mg sulbactam) | 150 (Severe 200 to 300) | IM, IV | 6–8 hr |
| Carbenicillin | 400–600 | IV | 6 hr |
| Ticarcillin | 200–400 | IV | 6–8 hr |
| Ticarcillin (3 g) and clavulanate (100 mg) | 240–320 of ticarcillin | IV | 6–8 hr |
| Piperacillin | 200–300 | IV | 4–6 hr |
| Piperacillin and tazobactam | 300–400 of piperacillin; maximum 4 g/dose | IV | 6 hr |

### Macrolides (Table 33.6)

*Side effects:* Diarrhea, nausea and abnormal taste; raised transaminases and cholestatic jaundice. Drug interactions are less with azithromycin. Use with terfenadine, astemizole or cisapride may result in arrhythmias. Clarithromycin causes less abdominal discomfort.

### Quinolones (Table 33.7)

*Side effects:* GI upset, renal failure, insomnia, dizziness and seizures; no concerns of arthropathy. Inhibition of liver enzymes can result in elevated levels of theophylline.

*Other side effects include:* Rash, photosensitivity, raised transaminases, neutropenia.

### Sulfonamides (Table 33.8)

*Side effects:* Blood dyscrasias, exfoliative dermatitis, serum sickness and drug fever

## Antifungal Agents

### Amphotericin B

Test dose 0.1 mg/kg IV; then start 0.25 mg/kg/day; increase by 0.25 mg/kg daily, until dose of 1 mg/kg/day; dilute in 5% dextrose, saline; protect from light

Total dose should not exceed 30–35 mg/kg over 4–6 weeks

*Side effects:* Febrile reactions, nephrotoxicity, hypokalemia, blood dyscrasias.

### Liposomal Amphotericin B

*Systemic fungal infections:* 3–5 mg/kg/dose, infusion over 2 hours in 5% dextrose; 24 hr.

*Cryptococcal meningitis in HIV:* 6 mg/kg/day IV q 24 hr

*Side effects:* Fever, flushing, chills, loss of appetite, nausea, headache, shortness of breath

### Flucytosine

50–150 mg/kg/day PO q 6 hr; should not be used as monotherapy.

**Table 33.3:** Cephalosporins

| *Drug* | *Dose (mg/kg/day)* | *Route* | *Schedule* |
|---|---|---|---|
| **First generation cephalosporins** | | | |
| Cephalexin | 25–50 (recommended for community acquired pneumonia)<br>Severe infection 75–100 | PO | 6–8 hr |
| Cefazolin | 50–100 (maximum 600 mg/24 hr) | IM or IV | 6–8 hr |
| Cefadroxil | 30 to 50 (maximum 2 g/24 hr) | PO | 12 hr |
| **Second generation cephalosporins** | | | |
| Cefaclor | 20–40 (maximum 2 g/24 hr) | PO q | 6–8 hr |
| Cefuroxime | 50–100 | IM or IV | 6–8 hr |
| | 20–40 (enteric fever) | PO | 12hr |
| **Third generation cephalosporins** (high CSF concentrations; widely used in meningitis) | | | |
| Cefdinir | 14 600 (maximum mg/24 hr) | PO | 12 hr |
| Cefditoren | 3–10 | PO | 12 hr |
| Cefotaxime | 100–150<br>200 mg/kg/day IV q 6 hr in meningitis | IM, IV<br>IV | 8–12 hr<br>6 hr |
| Cefoperazone | 100–150 | IV | 8–12 hr |
| Cefoperazone, sulbactum | 40–80 | IV | 12 hr |
| Cefprozil | 15–30 | PO | 12 hr |
| Ceftriaxone | 125 mg single dose (prophylaxis for *Neisseria meningitidis*)<br>25–50 (ophthalmia neonatorum)<br>50–75 (mild/mod)<br>100 (meningitis) (maximum 4 g/d) | <br>IV<br>IV<br>IV | <br>12 hr<br>12–24 hr<br>12 hr |
| Ceftazidime | 100–150 (maximum + 6 g/d) | IV | 8–12 hr |
| Ceftizoxime | 100–200 | IV/ IM | 6–8 hr |
| Cefixime | 8–10; enteric fever: 20 (maximum 400 mg) | PO | 12 hr |
| **Fourth generation cephalosporins** | | | |
| Cefpirome | 30–60 | IM or IV | 12 hr |
| Cefpodoxime | 8–10 | PO | 12 hr |
| Cefepime | ≥2 wk: 100–150 mg/kg/day<br><2 wk: 60 mg/kg/d q 12 hr | IV | 12 hr; 8 hr in meningitis, febrile neutropenia, serious infections |
| **Fifth generation cephalosporins** | | | |
| Ceftaroline | 2–24 months: 24 mg/kg/day<br>>2 yr: 36 mg/kg/day<br>>33 kg: 400 mg q 8 hr | IV | 8–12 hr |

**Table 33.4:** Aminoglycosides

| *Drug* | *Dose (mg/kg/day)* | *Route* | *Schedule* |
|---|---|---|---|
| Streptomycin | 15–20 (maximum 1 g) | IM | 24 hr |
| Gentamicin | 5–7.5 | IM, IV | 8–24 hr |
| Amikacin | 15–20 | IM, IV | 24 hr |
| Tobramycin | 5–7.5 | IM, IV | 8–12 hr |
| Netilmicin | 5–7.5 | IM, IV | 12–24 hr |
| Kanamycin | 15–20 (infusion) | IM, IV | 8–12 hr |

**Table 33.5:** Chloramphenicol

| *Dose (mg/kg/day)* | *Common route* | *Schedule* |
|---|---|---|
| 50–75 | PO | 6 hr |
| 100 | IM or IV | 6 hr |

Ointment available as 0.5 and 1%

*Side effects:* Neutropenia, thrombocytopenia, colitis, hepatotoxicity.

### Griseofulvin

10 mg/kg/day; PO q 12 hr; double dose for extensive lesions.

*Microsize:* Children >2 yr: 20–25 mg/kg/day q 8–12 hr

*Ultramicrosize:* Children >2 yr: 15 mg/kg/day q 8–12 hr

*Side effects:* Urticaria, paresthesia, proteinuria, leukopenia, photosensitivity; multiple drug interactions

### Fluconazole

Loading dose 12 mg/kg IV/PO, then maintenance 6 mg/kg/day q 24 hr IV/ PO

*Neonate:* Loading dose 12–25 mg/kg; maintenance 6–12 mg/kg/day

*Side effects:* Dizziness, skin rash, hepatic dysfunction; drug interactions

**Table 33.6:** Macrolides

| *Drug* | *Dose (mg/kg/day)* | *Route* | *Schedule* |
|---|---|---|---|
| Erythromycin | 30–50 | PO | 6–8 hr |
| Azithromycin | Otitis media: 10 on day 1; then 5 on day 2–5<br>Enteric fever: 20 (7–14 days)<br>Cholera: 20 mg/kg single dose<br>Pertussis<br><6 months: 10 (5 days)<br>>6 months: 10 on day 1 then 5 on day 2–5 | PO | 24 hr |
| Clarithromycin | 15<br>Maximum dose: 1 g/24 hr | PO | 12 hr |

**Table 33.7:** Quinolones

| *Drug* | *Dose (mg/kg/day)* | *Route* | *Schedule* |
|---|---|---|---|
| Nalidixic acid | 50–60<br>UTI prophylaxis: 30 | PO<br>PO | 8 hr<br>12 hr |
| Ciprofloxacin | 20–40; max 1.5 g/day<br>10–20; max 800 mg/day<br>20 mg/kg single dose for contacts of *N. meningitidis* | PO<br>IV | 12 hr<br>12 hr |
| Gatifloxacin | 10 | PO | 24 hr |
| Norfloxacin | 10–15 | PO | 12 hr |
| Levofloxacin | 10–15<br>6 mo–<5 yr: 20<br>5–12 yr: 10; max 500 mg/24 hr | <br>PO/ IV<br>PO/ IV | <br>12hr<br>24 hr |
| Ofloxacin | 15<br>5–10 | PO<br>IV | 12 hr<br>12 hr |
| Sparfloxacin | 4 | PO | 24 hr |

**Table 33.8:** Sulfonamides

| | *Dose (mg/kg/day)* | *Route* | *Schedule* |
|---|---|---|---|
| Sulfonamide | 100–150 | PO, IV | 8 hr |
| Cotrimoxazole | Trimethoprim 5–8; sulfamethoxazole 25–40<br>Enteric fever: Trimethoprim 10<br>*Pneumocystis* pneumonia: Trimethoprim 20<br>**Prophylaxis**<br>*Pneumocystis:* Trimethoprim 5 mg/kg alternate day; 150 mg/m² alternate day)<br>Urinary infections: 1–2 | PO, IV<br><br><br><br>PO | 8–12 hr<br><br><br><br>OD |

### *Ketoconazole*

*Oral:* Child 2 yr: 3–6 mg/kg/day q 24 hr; maximum dose: 800 mg/day q 24 hr

*Topical:* 1–2 applications/24 hr

Shampoo (dandruff): Twice weekly with at least 3 days between applications for up to 8 weeks, thereafter, intermittently as needed to maintain control.

Suppressive therapy against mucocutaneous candidiasis in HIV: Child: 5–10 mg/kg/day PO q 12–24 hr; maximum dose: 800 mg/day q 12 hr.

*Side effects:* Abdominal pain, headache, dizziness, somnolence, photophobia, thrombocytopenia; gynecomastia; drug interactions.

### *Itraconazole*

3–5 mg/kg/day (oral thrush); 5–10 mg/kg/day (histoplasmosis); maximum 400 mg/day.

*Prophylaxis:* 2–5 mg/kg/dose; PO q 12–24 hr

*Side effects:* Hearing loss, arrhythmia, hepatotoxicity; use cautiously in patients with liver disease, cardiac dysfunction

### *Nystatin*

1–2 million units/day PO q 8 hr for diarrhea due to *Candida albicans*

*Mucosal application:* Dissolve 100,000 units nystatin per mL glycerine

*Side effects:* Gastrointestinal disturbance, Stevens-Johnson syndrome

**Table 33.9:** Miscellaneous antibiotics

| | Dose (mg/kg/day) | Route | Schedule | Major side effects |
|---|---|---|---|---|
| Aztreonam | 90–120<br>Cystic fibrosis: 150–200 | IV, IM | 6–8 hr | Low cross antigenicity with beta lactams, thrombophlebitis, leukopenia, eosinophilia, neutropenia, hypotension, seizures<br>*Adjust dose in renal impairment* |
| Clindamycin | 10–30; max 1.8 g/day<br>25–40; max 2.7 g/d | PO<br>IV<br>IV | 6 hr<br>6 hr<br>12 hr | Pseudomembranous colitis, rash, Stevens-Johnson syndrome, neutropenia, thrombocytopenia |
| Colistin sodium | 50,000 to 75,000 IU<br>2.5–5 mg/kg/day<br>1 mg colistin base = 30,000 IU<br>1 mg colistimethate sodium = 12500 IU | IV | 6 to 8 hr | Dizziness, paresthesia, nephrotoxicity and neurotoxicity |
| Imipenem | 0–4 wk old and <1.2 kg: 50<br><1 wk old and ≥1.2 kg: 50<br>1–4 wk: 75<br>Child (4 wk–3 mo): 100 mg/kg/ day IV q 6 hr<br>Child (>3 mo): 60–100; maximum 4 g/24 hr<br>Cystic fibrosis: 90; maximum 4 g/24 hr | IV | 12 hr<br>12 hr<br>8 hr<br>6 hr<br>6 hr<br>6 hr | Pruritus, urticaria, seizures, dizziness, hypotension, elevated liver enzymes |
| Meropenem | Neonatal sepsis: 20 mg/kg/dose<br>Meningitis: 40 mg/kg/dose | IV | 12 hr<br>8 hr | Nausea, vomiting, rarely seizures |
| Faropenem | 200 increased to 300 | PO | 8–12 hr | Diarrhea, abdominal pain, loose bowel movement, nausea, and rash; safety in infants not established |
| Ertapenem | 15–30 | IV/IM | 12 hr | Not approved for children less than 3 months, diarrhea, nausea, headache |
| Vancomycin | 30–45 in neonate (dosage and frequency varies with gestation age); 40–60 | IV | 6–8 hr | Ototoxicity and nephrotoxicity (exacerbated with concomitant aminoglycosides); adjust dose in renal failure |
| Linezolid | 10 mg/kg/dose | IV<br>PO | 12 hr<br>8–12 hr | Dysgeusia, constipation, diarrhea, dizziness, headache, anemia, leukopenia, thrombocytopenia |
| Teicoplanin | 10 mg/kg 12 hr for 3 doses; then 6–10 | IV, IM | 24 hr | Long half life; less nephrotoxic; less catheter-related phlebitis |
| Tigecycline | 1.2 mg/kg/dose (Maximum dose 50 mg) | IV | 12 hr | Hypersensitivity reactions, deranged liver function; use with caution below 8 yrs |
| Nitrofurantoin | 5–7<br>Prophylaxis: 1–2; Maximum 100 mg/day | PO | 6 hr | Dizziness, hypersensitivity, icterus, interstitial pneumonitis, nausea, vomiting |

### Voriconazole

*>12 yr:* 6 mg/kg/dose IV for 2 doses q 12 hr, then 3–4 mg/kg/dose IV q 12 hr; oral: 3–5 mg/kg/dose q 12 hr

*2–11 yr:* 9 mg/kg/dose IV 2 doses q 12 hr, then 8 mg/kg/dose IV q 12 hr

Prophylaxis in pediatric leukemia: 6 mg/kg/dose PO q 12 hr for 2 doses followed by maintenance of 4 mg/kg q 12 hr.
*Side effects:* Blurred vision, photophobia, photosensitivity; hepatic impairment; flu-like symptoms

### Caspofungin

*<3 months:* 25 mg/m$^2$/dose (maximum 50 mg) once daily; *Older children:* 70 mg/m$^2$ IV on day 1, followed by 50 mg/m$^2$ IV once daily (maximum 70 mg)
*Side effects:* Elevated transaminases; diarrhea, vomiting; flu-like symptoms; rash

To be used cautiously in patients with liver disease.

### Clotrimazole

Topical application for skin q 12 hr for 4–8 weeks
Thrush >3 yr: Dissolve slowly (15–30 min) one troche in the mouth 5 times/day × 14 days
*Side effects:* Erythema, blistering

## Anthelmintics

### Albendazole

1–2 yr 200 mg single dose; >2 yr and adults 400 mg single dose; repeat after two weeks for roundworm
*Strongyloides/H. nana/Taenia:* 300 mg PO q 24 hr for 3 days.
*Giardiasis:* 400 mg PO q 24 hr for 5 days
*Hydatidosis:* 400 mg PO q 12 hr for 28 days: Repeat every two weeks for 3 cycles
*Neurocysticercosis:* 15 mg/kg/day PO q 12 hr for 7 days (with corticosteroids)
*Side effects:* Anorexia, vomiting

### Diethylcarbamazine Citrate

*Filariasis:* 6 mg/kg/day q 8 hr for 2 weeks
*Tropical eosinophilia:* 10 mg/kg/day; PO q 8 hr for 1 month
*Loeffler syndrome:* 15 mg/kg single dose for 4 days
*Side effects:* Gastrointestinal upset, drowsiness

### Ivermectin

*Dose:* 200 µg/kg PO single dose.
*Contraindication:* In children <5 yr old

### Mebendazole

100 mg; PO q 12 hr for 3 days; repeat after two weeks
*Side effects:* Pain abdomen, vomiting, diarrhea, headache

### Praziquantel

*Neurocysticercosis:* 50 mg/kg/day q 8 hr; PO for 10–14 days.
*Tapeworms:* 10–20 mg/kg single dose
*Liver fluke infestation:* 75 mg/kg/day q 8 hr for 2 days
*Side effects:* Headache, vertigo, GI disturbance, urticaria, myalgia

### Pyrantel Pamoate

10 mg/kg of pyrantel base; PO single dose with a maximum of 1 g; repeat after one week

### Thiabendazole

50 mg/kg/day PO q 12 hr up to a maximum dose of 3 g/day

Duration of therapy for strongyloides: 2 days; intestinal nematodes: 2 days; cutaneous larva migrans: 2–5 days; visceral larva migrans: 5–7 days; and trichinosis: 2–4 days.
*Side effects:* GI disturbance, cholestasis, keratoconjunctivitis sicca, xerostomia, headache, giddiness.

## Antimalarials

Refer to Chapter 11.

## Antiprotozoal

### Chloroquine

10 mg/kg/day; PO q 8 hr for 14–21 days for extraintestinal amebiasis
*Malaria treatment:* Infant and child: 10 mg/kg/dose (maximum dose: 600 mg/dose) PO once; followed by 5 mg/kg/dose
*Maximum dose:* 300 mg/dose at 6 hr and then once daily for 2 days
*Side effects:* Nausea, vomiting, itching
IV administration has been reported to cause hypotension, arrhythmias, cardiac depression

### Diloxamide Furoate

Luminal amebic infection, cysts: 20 mg/kg/day PO q 8 hr for 10 days
*Side effects:* Nausea and flatulence

### Dehydroemetine Dihydrochloride

1–3 mg/kg/day; PO q 8 hr for 10–15 days or 1 mg/kg/day IM for 7–10 days
*Side effects:* Renal and cardiac toxicity

### Metronidazole

*Giardiasis:* 10 mg/kg/day; PO q 8 hr for 10 days
*Amebiasis:* 20 mg/kg/day; PO q 8 hr for 21 days or 50 mg/kg/day; PO q 8 hr for 7 days
*Side effects:* Diarrhea, leukopenia, metallic taste

### Pentamidine

*Leishmaniasis:* 4 mg/kg/day IM or slow IV infusion daily dose for 12–15 doses
A second course may be given after 2 weeks
*Side effects:* Breathlessness, tachycardia, dizziness, fainting, headache, vomiting

### Secnidazole

30 mg/kg; PO single dose; hepatic amebiasis treatment for 5 days
*Side effects:* Nausea, gastritis, metallic taste, rarely leukopenia and peripheral neuropathy

### Sodium Stibogluconate

*Cutaneous leishmaniasis:* 20 mg/kg/day IM/IV for 20 days, preferably for 28 days and even up to 40 days for systemic leishmaniasis in areas with high incidence of resistance,
*Mucocutaneous leishmaniasis and systemic infection:* Treat for 30 days
*Side effects:* Nausea, vomiting, prolonged QT interval

### Tinidazole

50 mg/kg/day PO for 2–3 days
*Giardiasis:* 50 mg/kg single dose
*Side effects:* Same as for metronidazole

### Nitazoxanide

*1–4 yr:* 100 mg; PO q 12 hr for 3 days
*4–12 yr:* 200 mg; PO q 12 hr for 3 days
*Side effects:* Gastrointestinal disturbance, discoloration of urine, headache

## Antiviral Agents

### Antiretroviral Drugs

Refer Chapter 11

### Aciclovir

HSV encephalitis >3 months, 20 mg/kg/dose IV q 8 hr; 21 days
*Neonatal herpes simplex:* <35 weeks-post-conceptional age 40 mg/kg/day IV q 12 hr 14–21 day
≥35 weeks post-conceptional age: 60 mg/kg/day IV q 8 hr 14–21 days
*Herpes simplex:* 1500 mg/m$^2$/day IV q 8 hr
*Varicella zoster:* (≥2 yr) 30 mg/kg/24 hr or 1500 mg/m$^2$/day q 8 hr IV × 7–10 days
(≥2 yr), 80 mg/kg/day q 6 hr PO for 5 days (benefit if within 24 hr of onset of rash) maximum dose 3200 mg/24 hr
*Adolescents:* 800 mg PO q 6 hr for 7 days
*Immunocompromised hosts:* 1500 mg/m$^2$/day IV q 8 hr for 7–10 days

*Side effects:* Seizures, congestive heart failure, urinary retention, leukopenia

#### Ganciclovir

10 mg/kg/day IV q 12 hr for 14–21 days; long term 6 mg/kg/dose once daily for 5 days in a week
*Side effects:* Bone marrow depression, rash, fever, vomiting

#### Valganciclovir

450 mg/m²/day or 30 mg/kg/day for 14–21 days
*Side effects:* Cytopenias, cholestasis, tremors, nausea, vomiting

#### Isoprinosine

Subacute sclerosing panencephalitis: 50–100 mg/kg/day PO q 12 hr
*Side effects:* Use cautiously in renal dysfunction

#### Oseltamivir

*Infants <3 months:* 12 mg q 24 hr
*3 to 5 months:* 20 mg q 24 hr
*6 to 11 months:* 25 mg q 24 hr for 5 days
<15 Kg: 30 mg; 15 to 23 kg: 45 mg; 23 to 40 kg: 60 mg; >40 kg: 75 mg 12 hr oral for 5 days
*Prophylaxis:* Same dose but once daily for 7 to 10 days after last known exposure
*Side effects:* Nausea, vomiting, insomnia, vertigo seizures, neuropsychiatric events, arrhythmia.

### Interferons

#### Interferon Alpha

*Chronic hepatitis B:* 3–10 million units/m² thrice a week SC for 24 weeks
*Chronic hepatitis C:* Same dose with oral ribavirin for 24 weeks for genotypes 2 and 3; for 48 weeks for genotypes 1 and 4
*Peg-IFN-2a:* 180 µg/m² weekly (may be used for children with hepatitis B although it is approved for use only for the treatment of children with chronic hepatitis C. Treatment duration is 48 weeks)
*Side effects:* Flu-like symptoms, headache, bodyache, malaise, fever and chills; Angioedema, urticaria, skin blistering or peeling; bone marrow depression; mood disorders; sepsis; seizures; arrhythmia; arthritis.

## ANTICANCER DRUGS

Refer Chapter 21

## ANTICOAGULANTS

#### Heparin

*Heparin IV:* 50 U/kg bolus; followed by 10–25 U/kg/hr as infusion or 50–100 U/kg/dose q 4 hr, 25–50 U/kg SC q 12 hr
*Antidote:* Protamine sulfate (1 mg neutralizes 1 mg heparin)
*Side effects:* Rash, alopecia, excessive bleeds, thrombocytopenia

#### Enoxaparin

*Infants <2 months:* Prophylaxis: 0.75 mg/kg/dose q 12 hr; Therapy: 1.5 mg/kg/dose q 12 hr
*Older children:* Prophylaxis: 0.5 mg/kg/dose q 12 hr; Therapy: 1 mg/kg/dose q 12 hr
Dosage titration with antifactor Xa level
*Side effects:* Bleeding, hypertension; use cautiously in patients with renal disease.

#### Warfarin

0.05–0.34 mg/kg/day; PO
Adjust dose to maintain international normalized ratio (INR) 2–3
*Side effects:* Bleeding, epistaxis, internal hemorrhage

## ANTICONVULSANTS

Refer Chapter 19

## ANTIDOTES

Table 33.10.
Ipecac syrup is used to induce vomiting.

## ANTIEMETICS AND GASTROINTESTINAL MEDICATIONS

#### Domperidone

0.2–0.5 mg/kg/dose PO q 6–8 hr; do not exceed 2.4 mg/kg/day or 80 mg
*Side effects:* Extrapyramidal disorders; angioedema, urticaria; rarely agitation, nervousness, arrhythmias, gynecomastia, amenorrhea

#### Metoclopramide

0.1–0.2 mg/kg/dose q 6–8 hr orally or IV; maximum dose 10 mg
*Side effects:* Extrapyramidal disorders including oculogyric crisis, tardive dyskinesia, dystonia, drowsiness

#### Ondansetron Hydrochloride

IV: 0.15–0.2 mg/kg/dose q 8–12 hr
Oral: 1.2–4 mg/dose q 8–12 hr
*Side effects:* Headache, diarrhea, constipation, fever, rash

#### Promethazine Hydrochloride

*Nausea, vomiting, sedation:* 0.25–1 mg/kg/dose PO/IM/IV/PR q 4–6 hr
*Motion sickness:* 0.5 mg/kg/dose PO q 12 hr. Maximum dose: 25 mg

#### Promethazine Theoclate

*Antiemetic:* Not approved for children below 2 yr
*Children 2–5 yr:* 5 mg q 6–8 hr; maximum daily dose 15 mg
*Children 6–12 yr:* 10 mg q 6–8 hr; maximum daily dose 25 mg
Motion sickness; administer 1–2 hr before travel
*Side effects:* Sedation, drowsiness, dry mouth, anorexia, blurred vision; rarely fever, jaundice, tremors, tinnitus, seizures, hallucinations and anxiety

**Table 33.10:** Antidotes

| *Drug* | *Dosage* | *Side effects* |
|---|---|---|
| Ipecac syrup | Infants 5–10 mL/dose; others 15–20 mL/dose<br>Do not use in semicomatose child or after charcoal administration | Diarrhea, vomiting, irregular heart beat, weakness, unusual tiredness |
| Deferoxamine | Acute iron poisoning<br>15 mg/kg/hr IV or 50 mg/kg/dose IM q 6 hr<br>Maximum dose: 6 g/24 hr<br>Chronic iron overload:<br>IV: 15 mg/kg/hr; maximum dose: 6 g/24 hr<br>SC: 20–40 mg/kg/dose once daily as infusion over 8–12 hr; maximum dose: 2 g/24 hr | Hypotension, shock, cramps, diarrhea<br>Contraindicated in renal failure |
| Dimercaprol | 2.5 mg/kg PO q 4 hr on first day, q 6 hr on next 2 days, q 12 hr for 10 days; and q 24 hr for 10 days | Burning sensation, muscle aches, fever, hemolysis in G6PD deficiency |
| Edetate calcium disodium | 12.5–30 mg/kg/dose IV q 12 hr for 5 days | Proteinuria and hematuria |
| Methylene blue | 1–2 mg/kg/dose IV (in 5 min), if needed then repeat after 1 hour | Abnormal urine or stool color<br>Dizziness, headache, increased sweating and nausea |
| Naloxone | 0.1 mg/kg/dose IM/IV; repeat if needed (maximum 2 mg) | May cause opioid withdrawal symptoms |
| Penicillamine | Wilson disease: 20–40 mg/kg/day PO q 6–12 hr; maximum dose 1 g/day | Nephrotic range proteinuria, hepatotoxic, leukopenia, thrombocytopenia |
| Pralidoxime | Organophosphate poisoning: 25–50 mg/kg IM or IV as 5% solution over 15–30 min<br>Dose may be repeated at 1–2 hr; then q 10–12 hr intervals, if cholinergic signs recur<br>Continuous infusion 10–20 mg/kg/hr following loading dose | Nausea, hypertension, dizziness |

### Ranitidine

2–5 mg/kg/day; PO, IM or IV q 12 hr
*Side effects:* Headache, renal impairment

### Famotidine

1–1.2 mg/kg/day, PO q 12 hr; maximum daily dose 40 mg

### Omeprazole

*5–10 kg:* 5 mg q 24 hr
*10–20 kg:* 10 mg q 24 hr
*≥20 kg:* 20 mg q 24 hr
*Side effects:* Headache, dizziness, confusion, light headedness, tiredness, hypomagnesemia

### Lansoprazole

1 mg/kg/day in a single dose empty stomach for GERD in infants
After infancy <30 kg: 15 mg; ≥30 kg: 30 mg once daily empty stomach
*Side effects:* Well tolerated, side effects as omeprazole

### Sucralfate

1 month–2 yr: 250 mg PO 4–6 hr; 2–12 yr: 500 mg 4–6 hr; 12–18 yr: 1 g 4–6 hr for 4–6 weeks
*Side effects:* Constipation, headache, dizziness, insomnia, vomiting

### Lactulose

*Constipation:* 1–3 mL/kg/day in 2 divided doses (maximum 60 mL/day)
*Hepatic coma:*
Infants: 2.5–10 mL daily, q 8 hr
Children: 30–50 mL daily, q 8 hr, adjust doses to produce 2–3 soft stools daily.
*Side effects:* Diarrhea

### Bisacodyl

5–10 mg bedtime; PO; Rectal suppository: 2–11 yr: 5–10 mg; >11 yr: 10 mg
*Side effects:* Abdominal pain, diarrhea, muscle pain, dizziness.

## ANTIHISTAMINICS

### Astemizole

0.2 mg/kg/day taken half-hr before meals; not recommended <6 yr
*Side effects:* Weight gain with prolonged use

### Cetrizine

6 months–2 yr: 2.5 mg PO once daily; 2–5 yr: 2.5 mg PO once daily, dose may be increased to 5 mg q 12–24 hr; 6 years: 5–10 mg; PO q 24 hr
*Side effects:* Drowsiness, dry mouth and nose

*Levocetrizine*

1–6 years: 1.25 mg/day PO in evening q 24 hr; >6 years: 2.5 mg/day PO q 24 hr, in evening
*Side effects:* Headache, muscle ache, sleepiness, sore throat

*Clemastine*

*1–3 yr:* 0.25–0.5 mg q 12 hr
*3–6 yr:* 0.5 mg q 12 hr
*6–12 yr:* 0.5–1 mg q 12 hr
*>12 yr:* 1 mg q 12 hr
*Contraindication:* Patients with ventilator failure, obstructive airway disease.

*Chlorpheniramine Maleate*

2–5 yr: 1 mg/dose PO q 4–6 hr; maximum dose: 6 mg/24 hr; 6–11 yr: 2 mg/dose PO q 4–6 hr; maximum dose: 12 mg/24 hr; *sustained release* (>12 yr): 8 mg/dose PO q 12 hr
*Side effects:* Hypotension, sedation, urinary retention, oculogyric spasms with high doses and after a few days of therapy

*Diphenhydramine Hydrochloride*

5 mg/kg/day q PO 6 hr oral; maximum daily dose 300 mg
*Anaphylaxis or phenothiazine overdose:* 1–2 mg/kg IV slowly
*Side effects:* Dizziness, drowsiness, loss of co-ordination, dry mouth, nose or throat

*Fexofenadine*

2–11 yr: 30 mg PO q 12 hr; ≥12 yr: 60 mg PO q 12 hr or 120 mg once daily
*Side effects:* Nausea, diarrhea, drowsiness, headache

*Hydroxyzine Hydrochloride*

2 mg/kg/day PO q 6 hr; 0.5–1 mg/kg/dose q 4–6 h IM
*Side effects:* Swelling over face, tremor, confusion, seizure

*Loratadine*

3–12 yr: 5 mg/day; >12 yr: 10 mg/day
*Side effects:* Diarrhea, epistaxis and flu-like symptoms

*Methdilazine Hydrochloride*

>3 yr: 4 mg q 6–12 hr
*Side effects:* Sedation, urinary retention, leukopenia, agranulocytosis, glaucoma

*Pseudoephedrine*

2–12 yr: 4 mg/kg/day PO q 6–8 hr oral; >12 yr: 30–60 mg/dose q 6–8 hr; maximum daily dose 240 mg
*Side effects:* Headache, tachycardia and tremor

## ANTIHYPERTENSIVES

*Amlodipine*

0.1–0.2 mg/kg/dose (maximum dose 5 mg) PO q 24 hr, increase to 0.6 mg/kg/dose up to 20 mg/24 hr
*Side effects:* Edema, dizziness, flushing, palpitations; reduce dose in hepatic insufficiency

*Atenolol*

0.5–2 mg/kg/day PO q 12–24 hr
*Side effects:* Dizziness, light headedness, tiredness, and nausea.
*Contraindicated:* Pulmonary edema, cardiogenic shock

*Captopril*

0.1–0.5 mg/kg/dose PO q 8–12 hr, maximum dose 6 mg/kg/24 hr
*Side effects:* Dizziness, lightheadedness, or loss of taste, dry cough

*Clonidine*

5–7 μg/kg/day q 6–12 hr, increase at 5–7 days interval to 5–25 μg/kg/day q 6 hr; maximum 0.9 mg/day
*Side effects:* Dry mouth, dizziness, drowsiness, fatigue, rebound hypertension

*Labetolol*

Begin at 3–5 mg/kg/day PO q 12 hr after meals; maximum 20 mg/kg/day up to 1200 mg/day
Hypertensive crisis: 0.25–1 mg/kg IV over 2 minutes, repeat after 5 minutes; may be administered as a continuous infusion (0.4–3 mg/kg/hr).
*Side effects:* Hypoglycemia, worsening asthma

*Nitroprusside Sodium* (solution is light sensitive)

0.3–0.5 μg/kg/min infusion with blood pressure monitoring, maximum dose 8–10 μg/kg/min; titrate dose to desired effect
*Side effects:* Tachycardia, hypotension, acidosis

## ANTITOXINS AND IMMUNOGLOBULINS

*Anti-RhD Immunoglobulin*

*Antenatal prophylaxis:* 300 μg IM single dose at 28 weeks and within 72 hr of delivery
*Twin pregnancy:* Double the dose.
*Other procedures:* Spontaneous/therapeutic abortion <12 weeks 50 μg; amniocentesis, percutaneous umbilical blood sampling 300 μg
*Side effects:* Local reactions (pain, discomfort, tenderness), fever, joint or muscle pain, headache, dizziness, weakness, tiredness, itching, skin rash, nausea, diarrhea, vomiting

*Anti-snake Venom*

Mixture of four enzyme-refined, lyophilized, polyvalent anti-snake venom (against Indian cobra, Indian krait, Russell viper, saw-scaled viper)
5 vials (50 mL) for mild, 5–15 vials for moderate, 15–20 vials (150–200 mL) for severe features.
*Exclude horse serum allergy (0.02 mL of 1:10 diluted antivenin intradermally); then infuse antivenin diluted in 5–10 mL/kg saline/5% dextrose and infuse over one hour or infuse slow IV (1–2 mL/min)

Use steroids and antihistamines in addition, if there is allergy to ASV.
*Side effects:* Serum sickness, anaphylaxis

### Diphtheria Antitoxin

(Antitoxin is diluted 1:20 in isotonic saline and administered at 1 mL/min)

Dose is not related to patient age and weight

Pharyngeal or laryngeal diphtheria of 48 hr duration: 20,000–40,000 units IV

*Nasopharyngeal diphtheria:* 40,000–60,000 units IV

Extensive disease of >3 days duration with neck swelling: 80,000–120,000 units IV

*Side effects:* Coagulopathy, thrombocytopenia; contra-indicated in IgA deficiency

### Human Normal Immunoglobulin

*Attenuation of disease among contacts of measles:* 0.25 mL/kg IM within 6 days of exposure

*Hepatitis A:* 0.02–0.04 mL/kg/IM

*Side effects:* Coagulopathy, thrombocytopenia; contraindicated in IgA deficiency

*Hepatitis B (hepatitis B immunoglobulin):* 0.06 mL/kg IM, maximum 3–5 mL within 7 days of exposure

### Human Rabies Specific Immunoglobulin

*If presents within 24 hr:* 20 units/kg; one-half infiltrated at site of bite, other half IM in gluteal region

*If presents between 1 and 7 days:* Total dose given IM

Rabies vaccine is administered simultaneously.

*Side effects:* Headache, vomiting, chills, rash

### Human Tetanus Specific Immunoglobulin

*Prophylactic:* 250 IU IM; therapeutic: 30–300 IU/kg IV; intrathecal: 250–500 IU single dose

*Side effects:* As above

### Intravenous Immunoglobulin (IVIG)

*Primary immunodeficiency:* 400 500 mg/kg IV infusion every 3–4 weekly

*Intravenous immunoglobulin (IVIG):* 0.4 g/kg IV infusion daily for 5 days; 1 g/kg/day for 2 days or 2 g/kg in one day as IV infusion over 10–12 hr as single dose

*Side effects:* Hypersensitivity reactions

### Tetanus Antitoxin

*Prophylactic:* 3000–5000 U SC, IM; Therapeutic: 10,000 U IM, IV

*Intrathecal:* 250–500 U q 24 hr for 3 days

*Side effects:* Serum sickness, anaphylaxis

### Varicella Zoster Immunoglobulin

125 U/kg IM within 48–72 hr of exposure to varicella

*Side effects:* Pain at injection side, hypersensitivity

## BRONCHODILATORS, RESPIRATORY STIMULANTS AND ANTI-ASTHMA AGENTS

### Adrenaline

*Anaphylaxis:* 0.01 mL/kg/dose (maximum 0.5 mL/dose) of 1:1000 solution SC, repeat after 15–20 min

*Resuscitation:* 0.1–0.3 mL/kg/dose (1:10000) IV

*Bronchiolitis:* 0.2 mL/kg of 1:1000 diluted in 3 mL saline

*Croup:* 0.5 mL/kg (maximum 5 ml), usually 3–5 mL of 1:1000 nebulization

*Side effects:* Tachycardia, palpitations and anxiety

### Aminophylline

*Status asthmaticus:* 5–7 mg/kg IV loading, followed by infusion at 0.5–1 mg/kg/hr

Do not use loading dose, if already giving aminophylline.

*Apneic spells in preterms:* 5 mg/kg IV loading, followed by 1–2 mg/kg PO/IV q 8 hr

*Side effects:* Tachycardia, tremors, irritability, convulsions

### Beclomethasone Dipropionate

*MDI 50, 100, 200, 250 μg/puff:* 100–1000 μg/day q 8 hr

*Rotacaps 100, 200, 400 μg/cap:* 100–1000 μg/day q 8 hr

*Side effects:* Dry/sore throat, hoarseness, a bad taste in the mouth, headache, and voice changes; not recommended for <5 yr children with oral inhalation and <6 yr with nasal administration due to unknown safety and efficacy.

### Budesonide

MDI 50, 100, 200 μg/puff, rotacaps 100, 200, 400 μg/cap: 200–800 μg/day q 12 hr

Raspules 0.5 mg/mL, 1 mg/mL: 0.25–1 mg q 12 hr

*Side effects:* Dry/irritated throat, hoarseness, voice changes, bad taste

### Caffeine

20 mg/kg (caffeine citrate); then 5–10 mg/kg as IV/PO q 24 hr, to begin 24 hr after loading dose

*Side effects:* Hyperglycemia, hypoglycemia, GI disturbances (nausea, vomiting, abdominal distension), irritability, sleeplessness, jitteriness, arrhythmias, hypertension, diuresis and dehydration.

### Ciclesonide

MDI 80, 160 μg/puff: 80–640 μg/day q 12 hr; not approved below 12 years of age

Benefit of less oropharyngeal candidiasis and HPA axis suppression

*Side effects:* Dry throat, hoarseness, altered taste

### Fluticasone Propionate

MDI 25, 50, 125 μg/puff; rotacaps: 50, 100, 200 μg/puff: 100–1000 μg/day q 12 hr

*Side effects:* Hoarseness, throat irritation, headache, dryness in mouth/nose/throat, cough

### Ipratropium Bromide

MDI 20 μg/puff: 2–4 puffs as needed

*Rotacap 40 μg/cap:* 1–2 cap as needed

Respules 0.5 mg/2 mL, <1 yr: 125 μg/dose; >1 yr: 250 μg/dose, repeat q 20 min for 1 hr (during exacerbation); then q 6–8 hr

*Side effects:* Sinusitis, exacerbation of chronic obstructive pulmonary disease.

### Montelukast Sodium

*1–5 yr:* 4 mg PO once a day in evening; 6–14 yr: 5 mg once daily; >14 yr: 10 mg once daily
*Side effects:* Fever, upper respiratory infection, headache, pharyngitis, cough, abdominal pain, diarrhea, otitis media

### Salbutamol

0.15 mg/kg/dose PO q 8 hr
*MDI 100 μg/dose:* 2–4 puffs as needed q 20 min for 1 hr (during exacerbation), then q 6–8 hr
*Nebulizer solution:* 0.15 mg/kg/dose (minimum 2.5 mg as needed), q 20 min for 1 hr, followed q 6–8 hr
*Side effects:* Headache, tremor, irritability, hypokalemia

33

### Levosalbutamol

MDI 50 μg/puff: 2–4 puffs as needed
*Side effects:* Tachycardia, tremors, headache and hypokalemia



### Terbutaline

0.1–0.15 mg/kg/day PO q 8 hr; 0.005–0.01 mg/kg SC q 6 hr; IV 0.4–1.0 μg/kg/min followed by infusion of 1–10 μg/kg/hr;
Nebulizer (10 mg/ml): 0.5–2 mg as needed.
MDI 250 μg/puff; 2–4 puffs as needed
*Side effects:* Same as salbutamol

### Magnesium Sulfate

Injection 25% (250 mg/mL), 50% (500 mg/mL)
IV 25–50 mg/kg diluted in saline infused over 30 minutes (maximum 2 g)
*Side effects:* Hypotension, respiratory depression, muscle weakness

*Note*

- Metered dose inhalers (MDI) should be used with large volume spacers. For infants, the spacer can be used with a face mask.
- Rotacap dose is double the inhaler dose; are administered using a Rotahaler.
- Nebulization: Final volume of 3–5 mL should be made by adding normal saline.

## INOTROPIC AGENTS

### Adrenaline

*Cardiac arrest:* 0.1 mL/kg/dose of 1:10,000 solution IV/intraosseous
*Endotracheal use:* 0.1 mL/kg/dose of 1:1000 solution (flush with 5 mL saline, followed by 5 ventilations) in case of non-response, repeat same dose q 3–5 min
*Side effects:* Tachycardia, palpitations, anxiety
*Inotrope:* 0.1–0.3 μg/kg/min IV infusion

### Dobutamine

(Available as 250 mg powdered form; reconstitute ampoule with 10 mL saline to make 25 mg/mL)
2–20 μg/kg/min IV
*Dosage (mg):* 15 mg × body weight dissolved in 24 mL of compatible solution (5% Dx/10% Dx/NS/DxNS), infusion @ 0.5 mL/hr delivers 5 μg/kg/min
*Side effects:* Hypotension, if there is hypovolemia, tachycardia

### Dopamine

(Available as 200 mg/5 mL ampoule)
2–20 μg/kg/min IV
*Dosage (mg):* 15 mg × body weight dissolved in 24 mL of compatible solution (5% Dx/10% Dx/NS/DxNS), infusion @ 0.5 mL/hr delivers 5 μg/kg/min
*Side effects:* Tachyarrhythmia, hypertension, vasoconstriction, vomiting. Extravasations may cause tissue necrosis.

### Digoxin

*Digitalizing dose:* Premature neonates 0.04 mg/kg/day; term neonates 0.06 mg/kg/day; infants 0.06–0.08 mg/kg/day; older children 0.04 mg/kg/day PO (parenteral dose is two-thirds of oral dose)
One-half of the digitalizing dose is given stat, followed by one-quarter each after 8 hr and 16 hr
Maintenance dose is one-quarter of digitalizing dose; given once a day
Digoxin specific fab antibody: IV infusion; 60 mg binds 1 mg of digoxin approximately
*Side effects:* Nausea, vomiting; bigeminy pulse, extrasystoles, partial or complete heart block, sinus arrhythmia, atrial or ventricular tachycardia

### Milrinone

50–75 μg/kg loading dose followed by 0.25–1.0 μg/kg/min.
*Side effects:* Extravasations may cause tissue necrosis, dizziness, headache, rarely severe allergic reactions

### Norepinephrine

0.05–0.1 μg/kg/min titrate dose to desired effect (maximum 2.0 μg/kg/min)
*Side effects:* Headache, bradycardia, hypertension

### Isoproterenol Hydrochloride

0.5–5.0 μg/kg/min
*Side effects:* Cardiac dysrhythmias, rarely cardiac arrest, wheezing, bronchospasm

### Vasopressin

Catecholamine refractory vasodilatory septic shock: 0.3–2.0 mU/kg/min IV infusion
*Side effects:* Hypertension, water intoxication, hyponatremia

## DIURETICS

### Acetazolamide

*Edema:* 5 mg/kg/day PO q 24 hr or every other day
*Epilepsy/glaucoma:* 8–30 mg/kg/day PO q 6–8 hr
*Hydrocephalus:* 25–100 mg/kg/day PO q 8 hr
*Seizures:* 8–30 mg/kg/day PO q 6–12 hr

*Pseudotumor cerebri:* Start with 25 mg/kg/day PO q 6–24 hr, increase by 25 mg/kg/day until clinical response or as tolerated up to maximum of 100 mg/kg/day
*Side effects:* Sodium and potassium depletion, acidosis, GI irritation, paresthesia and sedation
*C/I:* Marked hepatic and renal dysfunction

### Bumetanide

1–6 months: 0.01–0.05 mg/kg/dose PO q 24–48 hr; >6 months: 0.015–0.1 mg/kg/dose PO q 24–48 hr
Maximum dose 10 mg/24 hr
*Side effects:* Muscle cramps, nausea, vomiting, gynecomastia, leukopenia, thrombocytopenia

### Chlorthiazide

20 mg/kg/day q 12 hr
*Side effects:* Hyperglycemia, glucosuria, neutropenia, neonatal thrombocytopenia, hypokalemia, hypotension

### Frusemide

1–4 mg/kg/day in 1–2 divided doses; maximum 6 mg/kg/day. IV: 1–2 mg/kg/dose q 12 hr; infusion: 0.1–0.4 mg/kg/h
*Side effects:* Nausea, vomiting; hyponatremia, hypokalemia, metabolic alkalosis, hyperglycemia, hyperuricemia; pancreatitis, dizziness, vertigo, headache, tinnitus and hearing loss on prolonged use

### Hydrochlorthiazide

*Neonate and infant <6 mo:* 2–4 mg/kg/day PO q 12 hr maximum dose 37.5 mg/24 hr
*≥6 mo and child:* 2 mg/kg/day PO q 12hr; maximum dose 100 mg/24 hr
*Hypertension:* Infant and child: Start at 0.5–1 mg/kg/day PO q 24 hr; maximum dose of 3 mg/kg/24 hr up to 50 mg/24 hr
*Side effects:* Hyponatremia, hypokalemia, metabolic alkalosis, hyperuricemia

### Metolazone

0.2–0.4 mg/kg/day PO q 24 hr
*Side effects:* Hypotension, palpitations and hypovolemia, hypokalemia, hyponatremia

### Spironolactone

*Neonates:* 1–3 mg/kg/day q 12–24 hr
*Children:* 1.5–3 mg/kg/day or 60 mg/m$^2$/day q 12–24 hr; not to exceed 100 mg/day
*Side effects:* Dry mouth, dizziness, headache, irregular periods, gynecomastia, hirsutism, erectile dysfunction, hyperkalemia

### Triamterene

2–4 mg/kg/day q 12 hr
*Side effects:* Hyperkalemia, hyponatremia, dry mouth, headache

### Mannitol

0.5–1 g/kg/dose IV given over 30–60 min
*Side effects:* Hypotension, tachycardia, fluid and electrolyte imbalance.

## HORMONES

### Betamethasone

*Anti-inflammatory:* 0.0175–0.25 mg/kg/day or 0.5–7.5 mg/m$^2$/day PO q 6–8 hr; 0.0175–0.25 mg/kg/day or 0.5–7.5 mg/m$^2$/day IM q 6–12 hr
Fetal lung maturity (24–34 weeks); administer to mother 12 mg IM in 2 doses 24 hr apart
*Side effects (short term):* Sodium retention-related weight gain, glucose intolerance, hypokalemia, gastrointestinal upset and reversible depression of the hypothalamic–pituitary–adrenal axis
*Side effects (long term):* Hypothalamic–pituitary–adrenal activity suppression, cushingoid appearance, hirsutism or virilism, impotence, cataracts and increased intraocular pressure, myopathy, osteoporosis

### Cortisone Acetate

*Physiological requirement:* 0.7 mg/kg/day
*Therapeutic dose:* 2.5–10 mg/kg/day q 8 hr
*Side effects (immediate):* Moon facies, acne, increased appetite, reduced resistance to infections, headache, gastritis, hypertension, electrolyte disturbances, glaucoma, pseudotumor cerebri.
*Side effects (prolonged therapy):* Myopathy, osteoporosis, growth retardation, cataract, adrenal cortical atrophy.

### Fludrocortisone

*Infants:* 0.05–0.1 mg/day PO q 24 hr
*Children:* 0.05–0.2 mg/day PO q 24 hr
*Side effects:* Hypertension, hypokalemia, acne, rash

### Dexamethasone

0.05–0.5 mg/kg/day PO q 6 hr
*Congenital adrenal hyperplasia:* 0.5–1.5 mg/day
*Cerebral edema:* 0.5 mg/kg/dose IV/IM q 6 hr
*Pulse dexamethasone:* 5 mg/kg as slow infusion (maximum dose 100 mg)
*Croup:* 0.3–0.6 mg/kg IM/oral, single dose
*Side effects:* Weight gain, insomnia, mood changes, acne, dry skin, bruising or discoloration, slow wound healing, nausea

### Hydrocortisone

*Status asthmaticus:* 4–8 mg/kg/dose IV q 4–6 hr IV
*Endotoxic shock:* 50 mg/m$^2$ initial dose followed by 50–150 mg/m2/day q 6 hr IV for 48–72 hr
*Acute adrenal insufficiency:* 1–2 mg/kg/dose IV, then 25–150 mg/m$^2$/day IV or IM
*Side effects:* Hypertension, hyperglycemia, arrhythmias

### Prednisolone

(Prednisolone, 5 mg = 0.75 mg betamethasone or dexamethasone, 4 mg methylprednisolone or triamcinolone, 20 mg hydrocortisone and 25 mg cortisone acetate)

*Acute asthma:* 0.5–2 mg/kg/day PO q 12–24 hr (maximum. 40 mg/day)
*Anti-inflammatory:* 0.5–2 mg/kg/day PO q 8–12 hr

*Nephrotic syndrome:* 2 mg/kg/day, q 12–24 hr daily; then on alternate days (maximum. 60 mg/day)
*Congenital adrenal hyperplasia:* 2 mg/kg/day PO q 6–8 hr or single dose in the morning
*Side effects (immediate):* Moon facies, acne, increased appetite, gastritis, hypertension, electrolyte disturbances, glaucoma, pseudotumor cerebri
*Side effects (prolonged therapy):* Myopathy, osteoporosis, stunting, cataract, adrenal cortical suppression

### Methylprednisolone

1–2 mg/kg/dose IM or IV
*High dose (pulse) therapy:* 15–30 mg/kg daily for 3–5 days
*Side effects:* Hypertension, sweating, hyperglycemia, mood changes, dyselectrolytemia, rarely arrhythmias

### Triamcinolone

24 mg/day PO q 8–12 hr; deep IM 40 mg or intra-articular 2.5–15 mg; avoid <6 yr
*Side effects:* Fluid retention, hypokalemic alkalosis, aseptic necrosis of femoral heads, gastritis

### ACTH

*Infantile spasms:* 20–40 U/kg/day IM q 24 hr for 6 week or 150 U/m$^2$/day q 12 hr for 2 weeks followed by a gradual tapering
*Dynamic testing (short ACTH stimulation test) <6 months:* 62.5 µg; *6 months–2 years:* 125 µg; *>2 years:* 250 µg
*Side effects:* Acute psychosis, CHF, Cushing disease, peptic ulcer, fungal infections, recent surgery
C/I: Hepatic damage, recent surgery

### Vasopressin

*Catecholamine refractory septic shock:* 0.3–2.0 mU/kg/minute IV infusion
*Diabetes insipidus:* 2.5–10 U SC/IM q 6–12 hr; 0.5–10 mU/kg/hr IV infusion
*Bleeding esophageal varices:* 20 U IV over 15 min, then 0.2 U/min or 0.33 U/kg/hr
*Side effects:* Hypertension, water intoxication, hyponatremia

### Desmopressin

*Hemophilia: Infants >3 months of age and children:* 0.3 µg/kg IV by slow infusion over 15–30 min beginning 30 min before procedure; may repeat dose, if needed.
*Diabetes insipidus:* Intranasal 5–30 mg/day
*Side effects:* Water intoxication, hyponatremia

### Growth Hormone

0.09–0.2 unit/kg/day SC or IM till accepted height is achieved or bone fusion occurs
*Turner syndrome:* 0.11–0.14 unit/kg/day
*Side effects:* Abnormal bone growth, abnormal touch sensation, pseudotumor cerebri and hyperglycemia

### Insulin

Refer to Chapter 18

### Glucagon

*Hypoglycemia (neonates/infants):* 0.025–0.3 mg/kg/dose q 30 min IM/IV/SC
*Side effects:* Nausea, vomiting, urticaria, respiratory distress

### Diazoxide

*Hypertensive crisis:* 1–3 mg/kg/dose up to maximum of 150 mg/dose
*Hyperinsulinemic hypoglycemia:* 8–15 mg/kg/day PO q 8–12 hr
*Side effects:* Hyponatremia, salt and water retention, gastrointestinal disturbance, hyperuricemia

### Carbimazole

1–2 mg/kg/day q 8 hr
*Side effects:* Urticaria, ageusia, pigmentation, bone marrow depression

### Thyroxine

10–15 µg/kg/day in newborn babies, 5 µg/kg/day in children, single dose PO empty stomach in the morning
*Side effects:* Tachycardia, headache, insomnia, muscle cramps

### Potassium Iodide (SSKI) and Lugol's Iodine*

5 drops q 6 hr
*Side effects:* Hypo- or hyperthyroidism, GI disturbance, iododerma, hypersensitivity, interference with anion gap calculation
**SSKI (1 g/mL) contains 76.4% iodine. Five drops four times a day (assuming 20 drops/mL) contain about 764 mg iodine. Lugol's solution (125 mg/mL of total iodine) contains, in each 100 mL, 5 g of iodine and 10 g of potassium iodide. Four drops four times a day contain about 134 mg of iodine.*

### Propylthiouracil

*Neonate:* 5–10 mg/kg/day q 8 hr; <10 yr: 50–150 mg/day q 8 hr; >10 yr: 150–300 mg/day q 8 hr
*Maintenance:* 50 mg q 12 hr
*Side effects:* Hepatitis, vertigo, rash, interstitial pneumonitis

### Erythropoietin

*Anemia of prematurity:* 25–100 U/kg/dose SC or IV, 3 times a week
*Chronic kidney disease:* 50–150 U/kg/dose SC or IV, 2–3 times a week
SC route requires lower doses than IV; rotated through arm, thigh and anterior abdominal wall.
*Side effects:* Local swelling, dizziness, nausea, pain at the site of the injection, fever

### Darbepoetin Alpha

Prolonged half life; administered less frequently; 0.45 µg/kg IV/SC once a week; 0.75 µg IV/SC once a fortnight
*Side effects:* Hypertension, seizures, venous thrombosis

### Octreotide

1 µg/kg/hr (up to 50 µg/hr); given as continuous IV infusion

*Side effects:* Local pain, stinging, tingling at site of injection, hypothyroidism, conduction abnormalities, pancreatitis

### Vitamin D

Treatment doses of vitamin D for nutritional rickets (dose in IU).

| *Age* | *Daily dose for 90 days* | *Single dose* | *Maintenance daily dose* |
|---|---|---|---|
| <3 mo | 2000 | N/A | 400 |
| 3–12 mo | 2000 | 50,000 | 400 |
| >12 mo–12 y | 3000–6000 | 150,000 | 600 |
| >12 y | 6000 | 300,000 | 600 |

Dosing of 1, 25-dihydroxyvitamin D (calcitriol) in patients with chronic kidney disease: Chapter 17
*Side effects:* Hypercalcemia, nausea, vomiting, abdominal cramps

## MICRONUTRIENTS

### Magnesium Sulfate*

*Protein energy malnutrition:* 0.3 mL/kg (maximum 2 mL) of 50% magnesium sulfate on day 1, then 2–3 mEq/kg/day PO q 24 hr (maintenance requirement)
**Magnesium sulfate 50% solution provides 4 mEq/mL*
*Side effects:* Hypotension, respiratory depression, muscle weakness

### Zinc Sulfate

*Therapy of deficiency:* 0.5 mg/kg/day for infants; 10 mg/day for <6 months, 20 mg >6 months for two weeks
Acrodermatitis enteropathica 1–3 mg/kg/day of elemental zinc
*Side effects:* Uncommon and include gastritis and vomiting; excessive doses may cause copper deficiency.

### Parenteral Iron Therapy

*Parenteral:* Iron dextran: 4 mg/kg/dose (maximum 100 mg); slow IV push at 1 mL (50 mg) per minute. The first dose for iron dextran is 10 mg (weight <10 kg), 15 mg (weight 10–20 kg) or 20–25 mg for older children
*Polynuclear ferric hydroxide sucrose or iron sucrose:* 0.5–2 mg/kg (maximum 7 mg/kg or 100 mg); diluted 20-fold with normal saline; infused over 30 minutes
*Oral (ferrous sulfate):* Prophylaxis: 1–2 mg/kg/day; treatment: 3–6 mg/kg/day
*Side effects:* Hypersensitivity reactions (bronchospasm, angioedema, urticaria, hypotension); pain and muscle spasms. Severe or persistent symptoms require therapy with antihistaminics. Iron sucrose preparation has lesser side effects.

The dose required for correction of iron deficiency is calculated as:
Total iron deficit (mg) = Weight in kg × (target Hb – actual Hb in g/dL) × 2.4 + depot iron in mg
The depot iron is 15 mg/kg body weight for children <35 kg, and 500 mg for >35 kg.

### Calcium Gluconate (Elemental Calcium 9%)

1–2 mL/kg of 10% solution; slow IV infusion under cardiac monitoring
*Side effects:* Bradycardia, hypotension, local extravasation can cause tissue necrosis hence the patency of the line should be rechecked before every administration.
*Contraindication:* Ventricular fibrillation

### Potassium Chloride

1–2 mEq/kg/d PO q 8 hr; not to exceed 200 mEq/L in central line infusions
*Side effects:* Hyperkalemia, GI disturbances, phlebitis

### Sodium Bicarbonate

1–2 mEq/kg/dose

The dose is calculated as:
Base deficit × weight in kg × 0.6 = mEq, or mL of 7.5% solution of sodium bicarbonate

*Side effects:* Metabolic alkalosis, hypernatremia, hypokalemia, thrombophlebitis, intracranial hemorrhage in neonates.

### Calcium Carbonate

*Neonates:* 50–150 mg/kg/day PO q 4–6 hr (maximum dose 1 g/24 hr); children 45–65 mg/kg/day PO q 6 hr
*Side effects:* Constipation, hypercalcemia, vomiting, headache, confusion.

### Calcitriol

<1 yr: 0.04–0.08 µg/kg/dose PO q 24 hr; 1–5 yr: 0.25–0.75 µg/day PO q 24 hr; >6 yr: 0.5–2 µg/day PO q 24 hr; titrate in increments of 0.005–0.01 µg/kg/24 hr every 4–8 weeks based on clinical response
*Side effects:* Weakness, headache, vomiting, constipation, hypotonia, polydipsia, polyuria.

### Vitamin A

*Prophylaxis:* 100000 units at 9 months, then 200000 units every 6 months up to 3 yr; if measles: 100000 in <1 yr and 200000 in >2 yr at 0, 1 and 14 day
*Side effects:* Irritability, hypercalcemia, pseudotumor cerebri

### Folic Acid

0–6 months: 25–35 µg (PO q 24 hr)
6 months–2 years: 50 µg
4–6 years: 75 µg; 7–10 years: 100 µg; 11–14 years: 150 µg
Megaloblastic anemia: 0.5–1.0 mg for 4 weeks OD

### Vitamin $B_6$

*Pyridoxine:* $B_6$ dependent seizures: 50–100 mg/day, IV/IM/PO
*Isoniazid-induced neuritis:* 1 mg/kg/day, PO
*Side effect:* Nausea, deranged liver function tests.

## SEDATIVES, HYPNOTICS, ANTIDEPRESSANTS AND ANTIEPILEPTICS

### Diazepam

*Sedation and anxiolysis:* 0.2–0.3 mg/kg
*Anticonvulsant:* 0.2 mg/kg/dose IV (maximum 10 mg); repeat in 15 minutes. Per rectal: 1–3 yr, 5 mg; 3–12 yr, 5–10 mg; 12–18 yr, 10 mg.
*Contraindication:* Myasthenia gravis and acute narrow angle glaucoma

### Flumezanil

Reversal of benzodiazepine sedation (IV):
*Child:* Initial dose: 0.01 mg/kg (maximum dose: 0.2 mg) given over 15 sec; may repeat, q 1 min to a maximum total cumulative dose of 0.05 mg/kg or 1 mg, whichever is lower. Usual total dose: 0.08–1 mg (average 0.65 mg); as an alternative for repeat bolus doses, a continuous infusion of 0.005–0.01 mg/kg/hr has been used.
*Side effects:* Nausea, vomiting, dizziness, tremor, depression, euphoria, agitation, palpitations, dyspnea, hyperventilation

### Lorazepam

0.1 mg/kg IV; repeat at 5 minutes; longer duration of action than diazepam; 0.03–0.05 mg/kg/dose PO q 8–12 hr
*Side effects:* Confusion, depressed mood, hyperactivity, agitation, hostility

### Clonazepam

Infant and child <10 yr or <30 kg: initial: 0.01–0.03 mg/kg/day PO q 8 hr; increment: 0.25–0.5 mg/day q 72 hr, up to maximum maintenance dose of 0.1–0.2 mg/kg/day q 8 hr
Child 10 yr or 30 kg and adult: initial: 1.5 mg/24 hr PO q 8 hr; increment: 0.5–1 mg/day q 72 hr; maximum dose: 20 mg/24 hr
*Side effects:* Drowsiness, dizziness, muscle weakness, loss of balance or coordination

### Chloral Hydrate

5–10 mg/kg/dose for sedation; 20–75 mg/kg/dose for heavy sedation
*Side effects:* Nausea and vomiting are more common, diarrhea; dizziness and drowsiness are less common

### Chlorpromazine

2.5–6 mg/kg/day PO q 6 h
*Chorea:* Start with 50 mg/day PO; increase by 25 mg/day till controlled; maximum dose 300 mg/day
*Neonatal tetanus:* 1–2 mg/kg/dose q 2–4 hr
*Side effects:* Extrapyramidal reactions (e.g. Parkinson-like symptoms, dystonia, tardive dyskinesia), drowsiness, dizziness, skin reactions or rash, dry mouth, orthostatic hypotension, amenorrhea, galactorrhea, weight gain

### Fluoxetine Hydrochloride

5–10 mg/day; maximum 20 mg/day
*Side effects:* Insomnia, weakness, anxiety, drowsiness, tremor, diarrhea, dyspepsia, nausea, nervousness, headache, xerostomia

### Haloperidol

*Psychotic disorder:* 0.05–0.15 mg/kg/day PO q 8–12 hr; agitation: 0.01–0.03 mg/kg/day q 8–12 hr; chorea: 0.25 mg PO q 12 hr
*Side effects:* Extrapyramidal reactions, dyskinesia

### Ketamine

*IV induction:* 0.5–2 mg/kg at a rate not to exceed 0.5 mg/kg/min
*IM, oral, rectal:* 3–10 mg/kg/dose; *nasal and sublingual:* 3–5 mg/kg/dose
Minor procedures 0.5–1.0 mg/kg; sedative dose 2 mg/kg
The concomitant use of midazolam is beneficial.
*Side effects:* Hypertension, hypertonia, diplopia, increased intraocular pressure, salivary hypersecretion

### Midazolam

0.07–0.2 mg/kg/dose IM or IV
Preoperative sedation or conscious sedation (mechanical ventilation) above dose followed by 0.2–1 µg/kg/min for neonates and 0.5–3.0 µg/kg/min for infants and children
Status epilepticus 0.2 mg/kg IV or IM followed by 0.1–0.2 mg/kg/hr
Intranasal 0.2 mg/kg may be used for acute seizure control
*Side effects:* Respiratory depression, shock

### Triclofos

20 mg/kg/dose for sedation PO q 12 hr
*Side effects:* Gastrointestinal disturbance, mild rash

### Carbamazepine

*<6 yr:* 10–20 mg/kg/day PO q 8 hr, increment q 5–7 days up to maximum of 35 mg/kg/24 hr;
*6–12 yr:* 10 mg/kg/24 hr PO q 12 hr up to maximum 100 mg/dose q 12 hr; maintenance 20–30 mg/kg/day q 6–12 hr
*Side effects:* Dizziness, drowsiness, nausea, ataxia, and vomiting, pruritus, speech disturbance, xerostomia and amblyopia

### Clobazam

*<30 kg:* 5 mg PO q 24 hr, increase to 20 mg q 24 hr
*>30 kg:* 10 mg PO q 24 hr, increase to 40 mg q 24 hr
*Side effects:* Dizziness, drowsiness, anxiety, suicidal thoughts, withdrawal symptoms, lower doses in liver diseases

### Pentobarbital

Refractory status epilepticus: 10 mg/kg loading IV over 1 hr, maintenance 1–5 mg/kg/hr
*Side effects:* Hypotension, respiratory suppression, arrhythmia

### Phenobarbital

*Anticonvulsant:* 20 mg/kg loading IV; 3–5 mg/kg/day IV q 12–24 hr as maintenance
*Side effects:* Dizziness, respiratory depression, hypotension

**Table 33.11:** Miscellaneous drugs

| *Drug* | *Dosage* | *Side effects* |
|---|---|---|
| Acetylcysteine | Meconium ileus: 5–10 mL/kg (10% soln PR) q 6 hr<br>Nebulization: 3–5 mL/kg of 20% or 6–10 mL/kg (10%) q 6–8 hr<br>Acetaminophen poisoning (see Chapter 28) | Bronchospasm, stomatitis, drowsiness, rhinorrhea, nausea, vomiting, hemoptysis<br>Anaphylactic reactions with IV use |
| Albumin (20%) | 0.5–1 g/kg/dose over 30–120 minutes; coadministered with IV frusemide in patients with nephritic syndrome | Rapid infusion may lead to fluid overload; rarely hypersensitivity |
| Allopurinol | 10 mg/kg/day PO q 8 hr, max dose 800 mg/24 hr; IV dosage is alkaline and should be diluted to minimum concentration of 6 mg/mL and infused over 30 min | Rash (frequent); nausea, diarrhea; allergic liver toxicity (increased risk with renal impairment) |
| Alprostadil prostaglandin E1 | Initial: 0.05–0.2 µg/kg/min; advance to 0.2 µg/kg/min, if necessary<br>Maintenance: Decrease to lowest effective dose when increase in partial pressure of oxygen<br>Usual dose 0.01–0.4 µg/kg/min | Fever, apnea, flushing, bradycardia, hypotension, platelet aggregation defect |
| Amphetamine | 0.15–0.5 mg/kg/day<br>Children 3–5 years: 2.5 mg daily, increase by 2.5 mg q weekly<br>Children >6 years: 5 mg once daily; increase by 5 mg q weekly | Restlessness, excitability, tremor, headache, anxiety, agitation, insomnia, dry mouth, palpitations |
| Atropine | Cardiopulmonary resuscitation: 0.01–0.03 mg/kg/dose IV every 2–5 min for 2–3 doses; maximum 1.0 mg<br>Pre-anesthesia (30–60 min prior): 0.03–0.04 mg/kg/dose IV<br>Bronchospasm: 0.02–0.05 mg/kg/dose (maximum 2.5 mg/dose) | C/I: Thyrotoxicosis, tachycardia due to cardiac insufficiency; obstructive gastrointestinal lesions |
| Baclofen | 0.75–2 mg PO q 8 hr; maximum dose 40 mg for <8 years and 60 mg for >8 years | Drowsiness, weakness, tiredness, nausea, constipation, confusion |
| Lidocaine hydrochloride | Without epinephrine: Maximum dose 4.5 mg/kg/dose (up to 300 mg); do not repeat within 2 hr<br>With epinephrine: Maximum dose 7 mg/kg/dose (up to 500 mg); do not repeat within 2 hr<br>Topical: Apply cream to affected intact skin q 6–12 hr<br>Oral: 4.5 mg/kg/dose or 300 mg/dose swish and spit q 3 hr; maximum 4 doses per 12 hr | Hypotension, seizures, asystole, respiratory arrest |
| Oxyphenonium bromide | 0.8 mg/kg/day PO q 6 hr<br>Preschool children: 5–10 drops; older children: 10–20 drops q 6 hr | Dry mouth, blurred vision, retention of urine, dizziness, fatigue, tremors |
| Pethidine | Analgesic 1–2 mg/kg/dose IM/IV | Seizures |
| Ribavirin | 6 g in 300 mL sterile water; nebulize q 12–18 hr/day for 3–7 d<br>Oral: 10 mg/kg/day q 6–8 hr (max <10 yr: 150 mg/d; >10 yr; 200 mg/d) | Seizures, congestive heart failure, urinary retention, leukopenia |
| Senna | Constipation: 10–20 mg/kg/dose, PO q 12–24 hr | Loose stools, cramping |
| Sildenafil | 0.3–3 mg/kg/day PO q 8 hr, 0.3–2 mg/kg/ dose PO q 6–12 hr<br>IV bolus: 0.4 mg/ kg over 3 hr; followed by 1.6 mg/kg/d infusion | Dizziness, light headed |
| Sotalol | Arrhythmia: 2–8 mg/kg/day, PO q 8–12 hr | May cause arrhythmia |
| Succinylcholine | Neuromuscular blocking agent: 1–2 mg bolus, maintenance 0.04–0.07 mg/kg/dose IV q 5–10 min as per desired effect | Hypotension, bronchospasm, hyperkalemia, malignant hyperthermia |
| Sulfasalazine | Inflammatory bowel disease: Start at 40–75 mg/kg/day, PO q 6 hr; maintenance: 30–50 mg/kg/day PO q 8 hr | Headache, nausea, rash, neutropenia |
| Theophylline | Apnea in preterm: Loading 6–10 mg/kg; maintenance 2–4 mg/kg/dose PO q 12 hr<br>Bronchodilator: 10–20 mg/kg/day | GI disturbance, tachycardia, feeding intolerance, irritability |
| Tolazoline | 1–2 mg/kg IV over 10 min followed by 1–2 mg/kg/hr continuous infusion | Dizziness, faintness |

### Phenytoin Sodium

*Arrhythmia:* Loading 1.25 mg/kg IV over 3 min and repeat every 5–10 min to a maximum total dose of 15 mg/kg or until arrhythmia reverts or hypotension develops; maintenance 5–10 mg/kg/day PO q 12 hr

*Status epilepticus:* Loading 15–20 mg/kg IV, do not exceed 1–3 mg/kg/min. Maintain with 5–8 mg/kg/day PO or IV q 12–24 hr

*Side effects:* Gum hypertrophy, hirsutism, hypersensitivity, megaloblastic anemia, osteomalacia and vestibulocerebellar syndrome.

### Fosphenytoin Sodium

15–20 mg/kg/day; then 4–6 mg/kg/day

*Side effects:* Pruritus, dizziness, ataxia, nystagmus, contraindicated in porphyria

### Pentothal Sodium (Thiopental)

*Refractory status epilepticus:* 5–10 mg/kg loading dose IV over 2–5 minutes followed by 2–10 mg/kg/hr continuous infusion.

*Side effects:* Gastrointestinal disturbance, hypotension, respiratory depression, bronchospasm

### Valproic Acid

*Seizures (generalized, simple and complex partial):* Start with 10–15 mg/kg/day PO q 8–12 hr, increase by 5–10 each week if required to maximum 60 mg/kg/day

*Status epilepticus:* 20 mg/kg loading followed by 10 mg/kg IV q 12 hr

*Side effects:* Hepatotoxicity, irritability, hearing loss, nausea, vomiting, pyrexia

### Vigabatrin

*Infantile spasm:* 40–150 mg/kg/day PO q 12–24 hr

*Side effects:* Visual field defects, GI and psychiatric symptoms

## VASODILATORS

### Isosorbide Dinitrate

0.1 mg/kg/day PO q 6–8 hr

*Side effects:* Flushing, headache

### Nifedipine

0.3 mg/kg/dose oral q 6 hr

*Antihypertensive:* 0.25–0.5 mg/kg/dose (maximum10 mg) PO q 6 hr

*Vasodilator:* 0.3 mg/kg/dose PO q 6 hr

*Side effects:* Hypotension, dizziness

### Prazosin

*Antihypertensive:* 0.05–0.1 mg/kg/day q 8 hr (maximum 0.5 mg/kg/dose)

*Side effects:* Postural hypotension, dizziness, faintness, nasal stuffiness, priapism

## Suggested Reading


1. de Vries TPGM, Heming RH, Hogerzeil HV, Fresle DA. Guide to Good Prescribing–A Practical Manual. World Health Organisation 1994. Available at: https://apps.who.int/iris/bitstream/handle/10665/59001/WHO_DAP_94.11.pdf
2. https://www.drugs.com
3. Ritter JM, Lewis LD, Mant TGK, Ferro A. A Textbook of Clinical Pharmacology and Therapeutics, 5th edn, 2008. London, Hodder Arnold. Available at http://pharmaresearchlibrary.com/wp-content/uploads/2013/03/A-Textbook-of-Clinical-Pharmacology-and-Therapeutics-5th-edition.pdf
4. Singh MB, Deorari AK. Drug dosages in children, 10th edn. New Delhi, CBS Publishers & Distributors Pvt Ltd. 2020
5. Unni JC, Nair MKC, Menon PSN, Bansal CP. IAP Pediatric Drug Formulary, 3rd edn. Mumbai: Indian Academy of Pediatrics 2012.

# Annexures

## Annexure 1

### Weight-for-age (Girls) from birth to 5 years (z-scores)

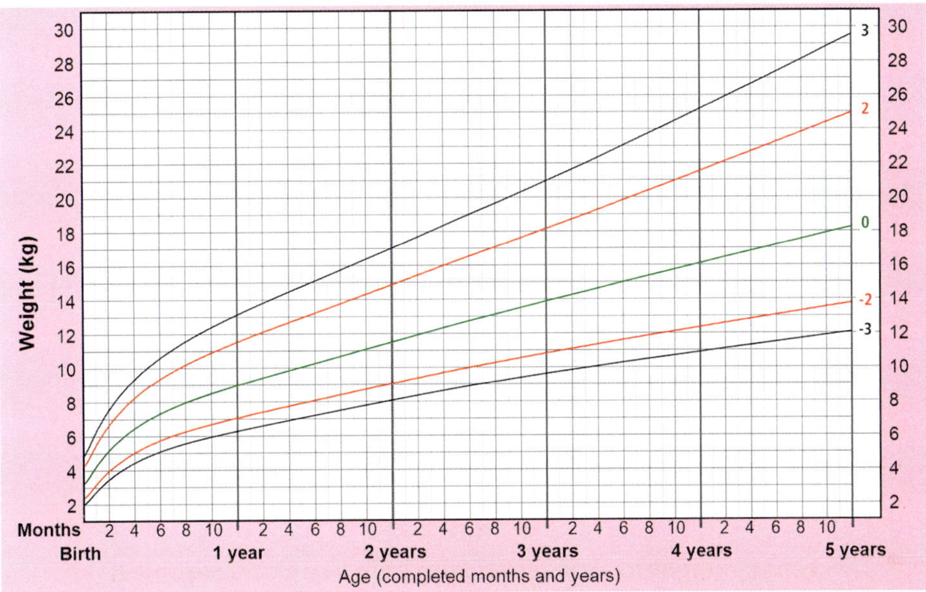


WHO Child Growth Standards

## Annexure 2

### Weight-for-age (Boys) from birth to 5 years (z-scores)

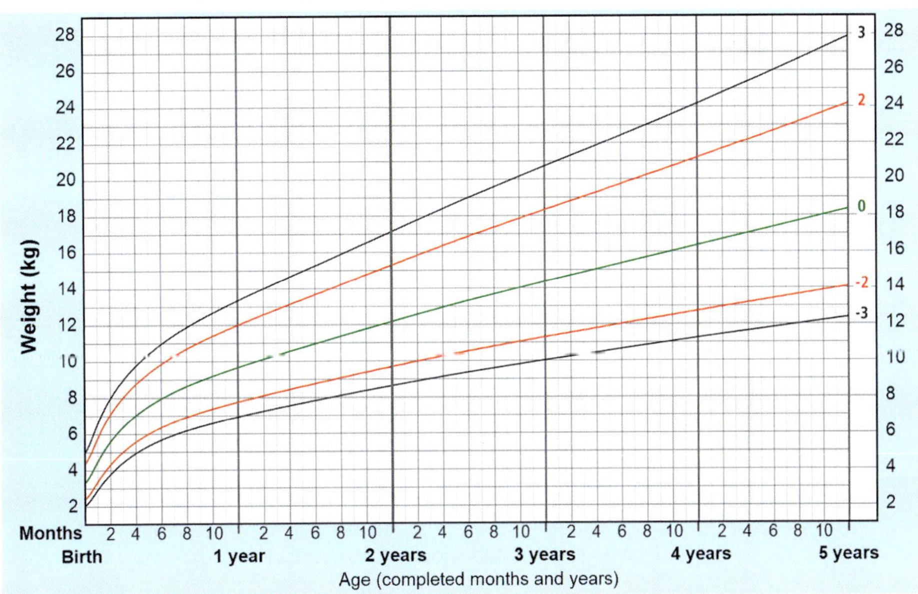


WHO Child Growth Standards

## Annexure 3

### Length/Height-for-age (Girls) from birth to 5 years (z-scores)

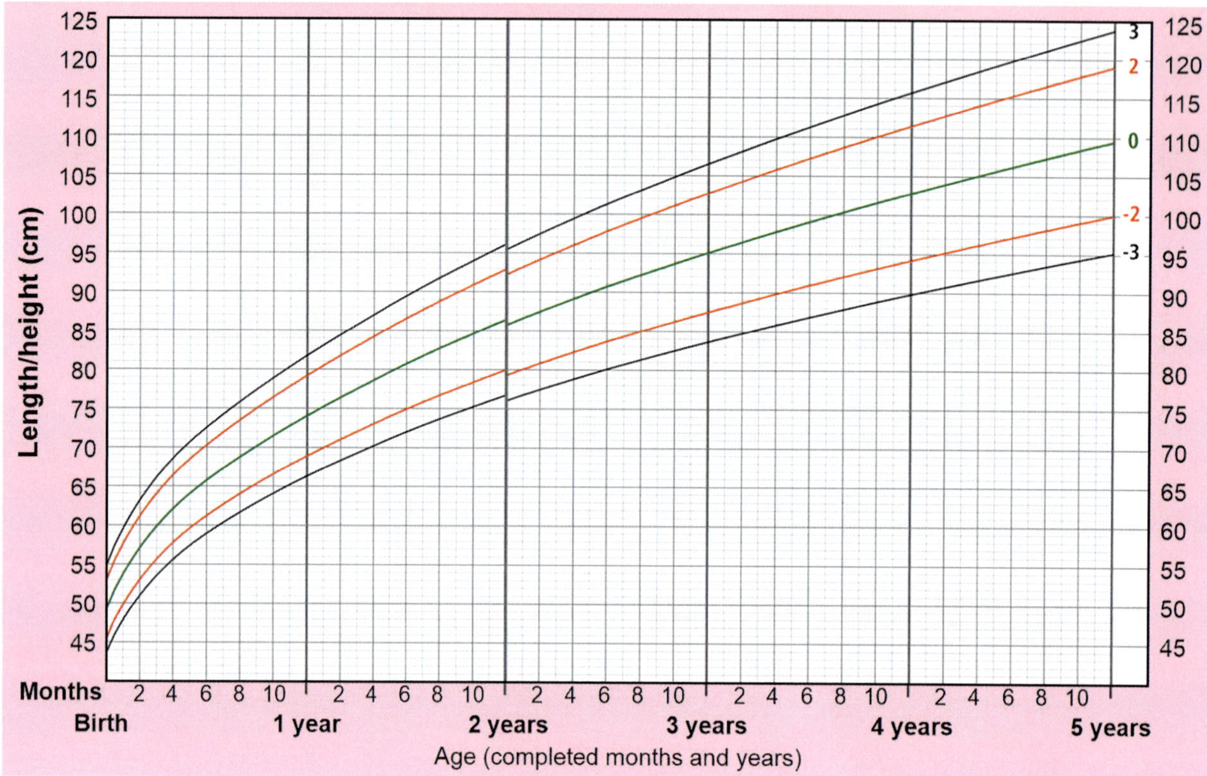


WHO Child Growth Standards

## Annexure 4

### Length/Height-for-age (Boys) from birth to 5 years (z-scores)

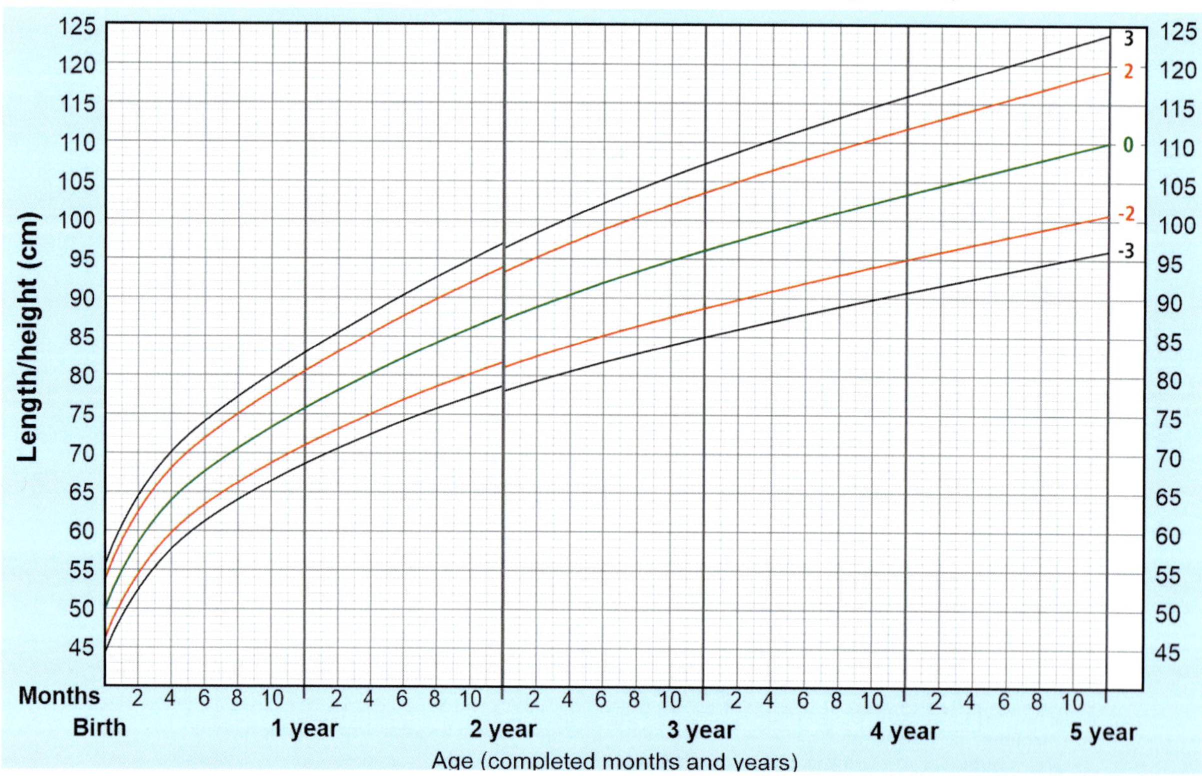


WHO Child Growth Standards

## Annexure 5

### Weight-for-length/height (Girls) from birth to 5 years (z-scores)

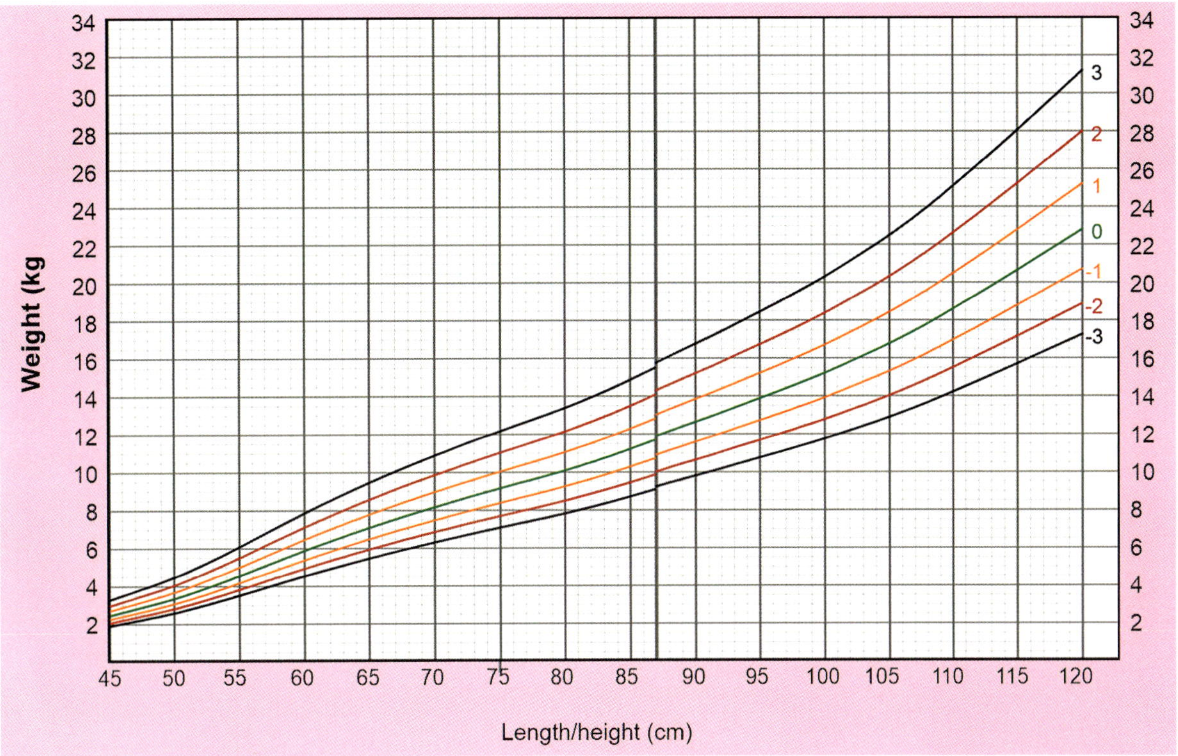


WHO Child Growth Standards

## Annexure 6

### Weight-for-length/height (Boys) from birth to 5 years (z-scores)

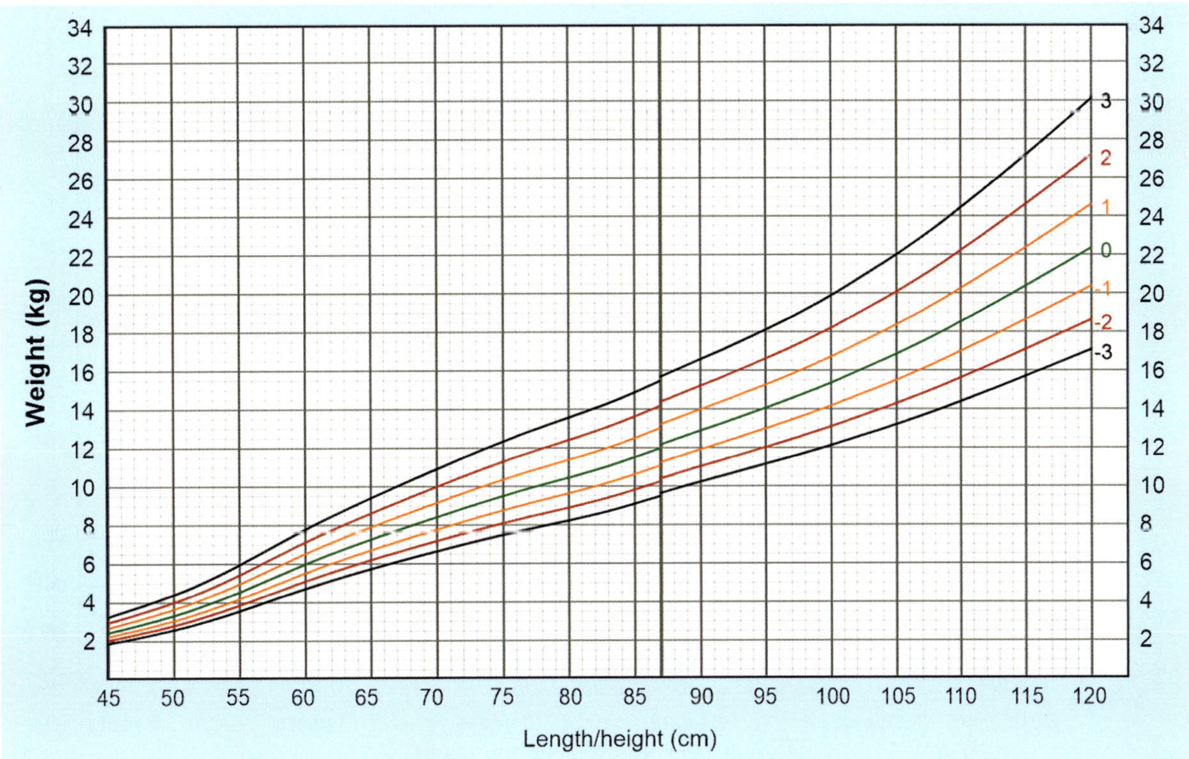


WHO Child Growth Standards

## Annexure 7

### Head circumference-for-age (Girls) from birth to 5 years (z-scores)

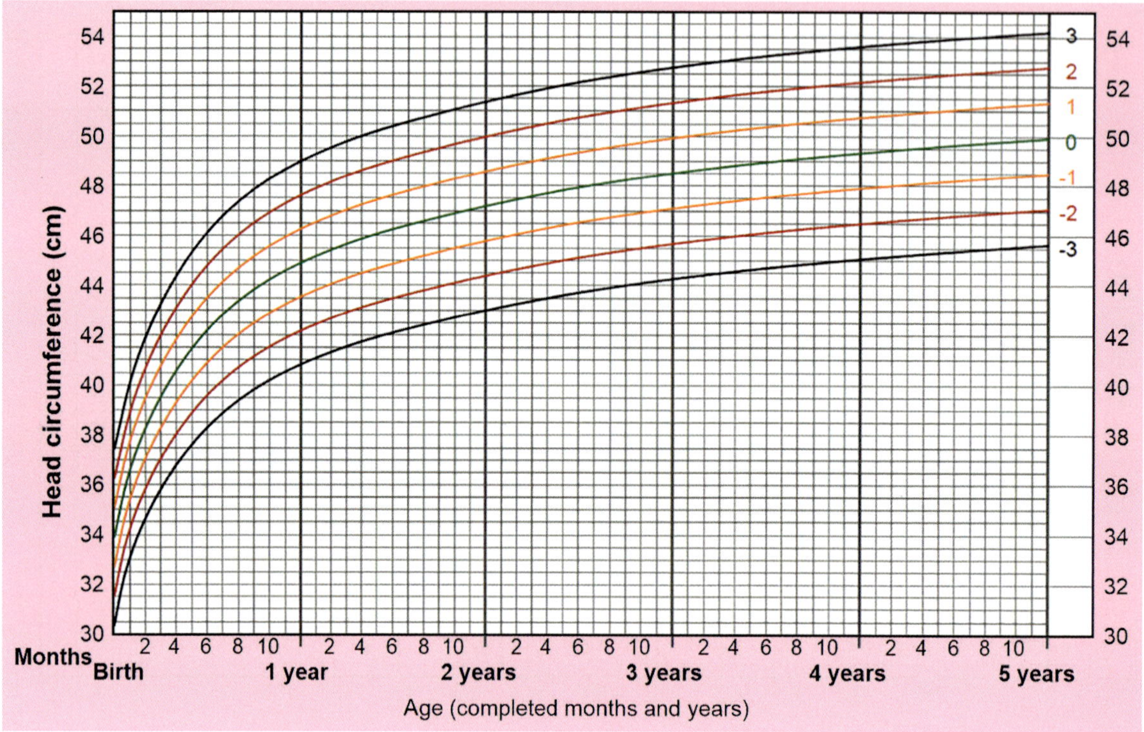


WHO Child Growth Standards

## Annexure 8

### Head circumference-for-age (Boys) from birth to 5 years (z-scores)

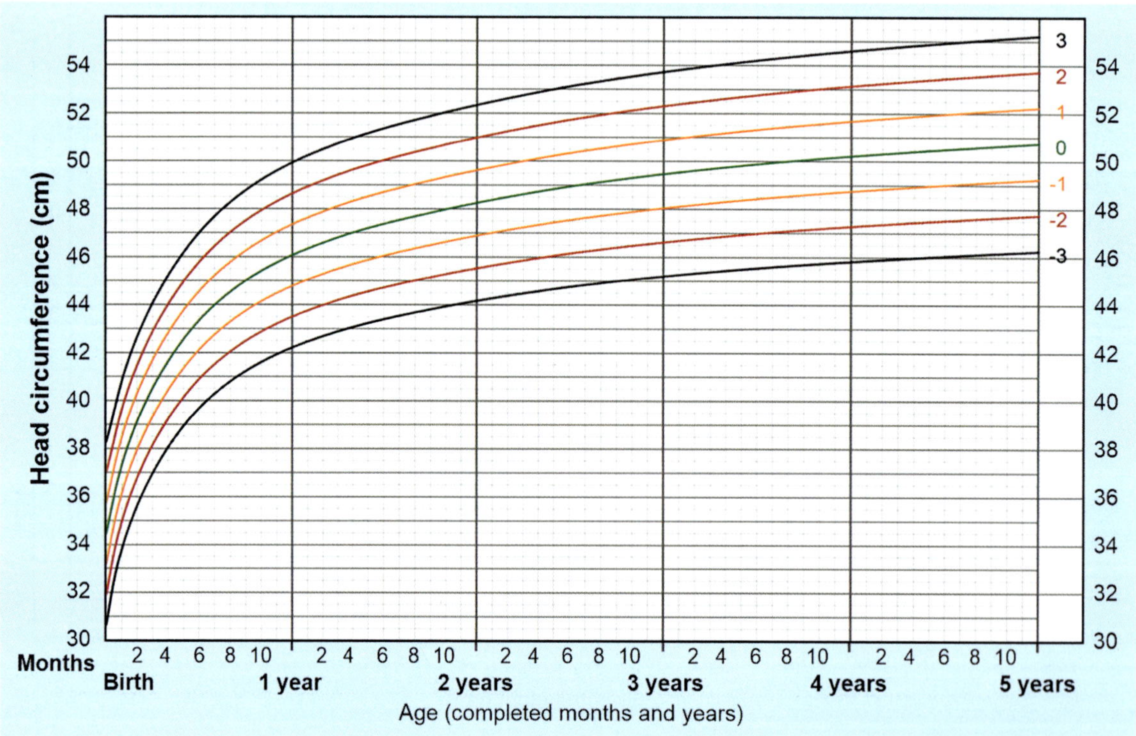


WHO Child Growth Standards

## Annexure 9

## IAP height and weight chart for Boys aged 5 to 18 years

**Father's Height ________, Mother's Height ________, Target Height________**

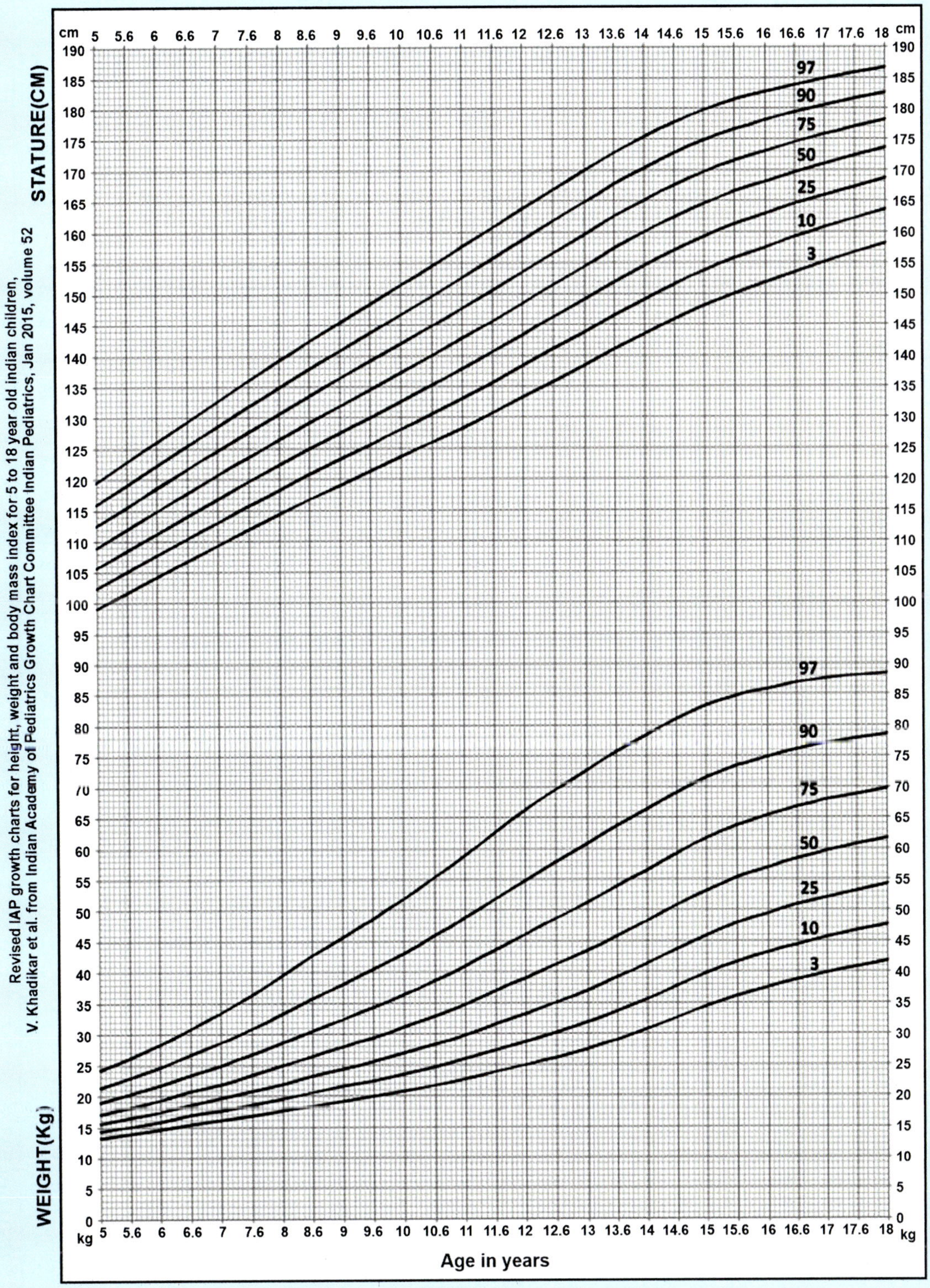

## Annexure 10

### IAP height and weight chart for Girls aged 5 to 18 years

Father's Height ________, Mother's Height ________, Target Height ________

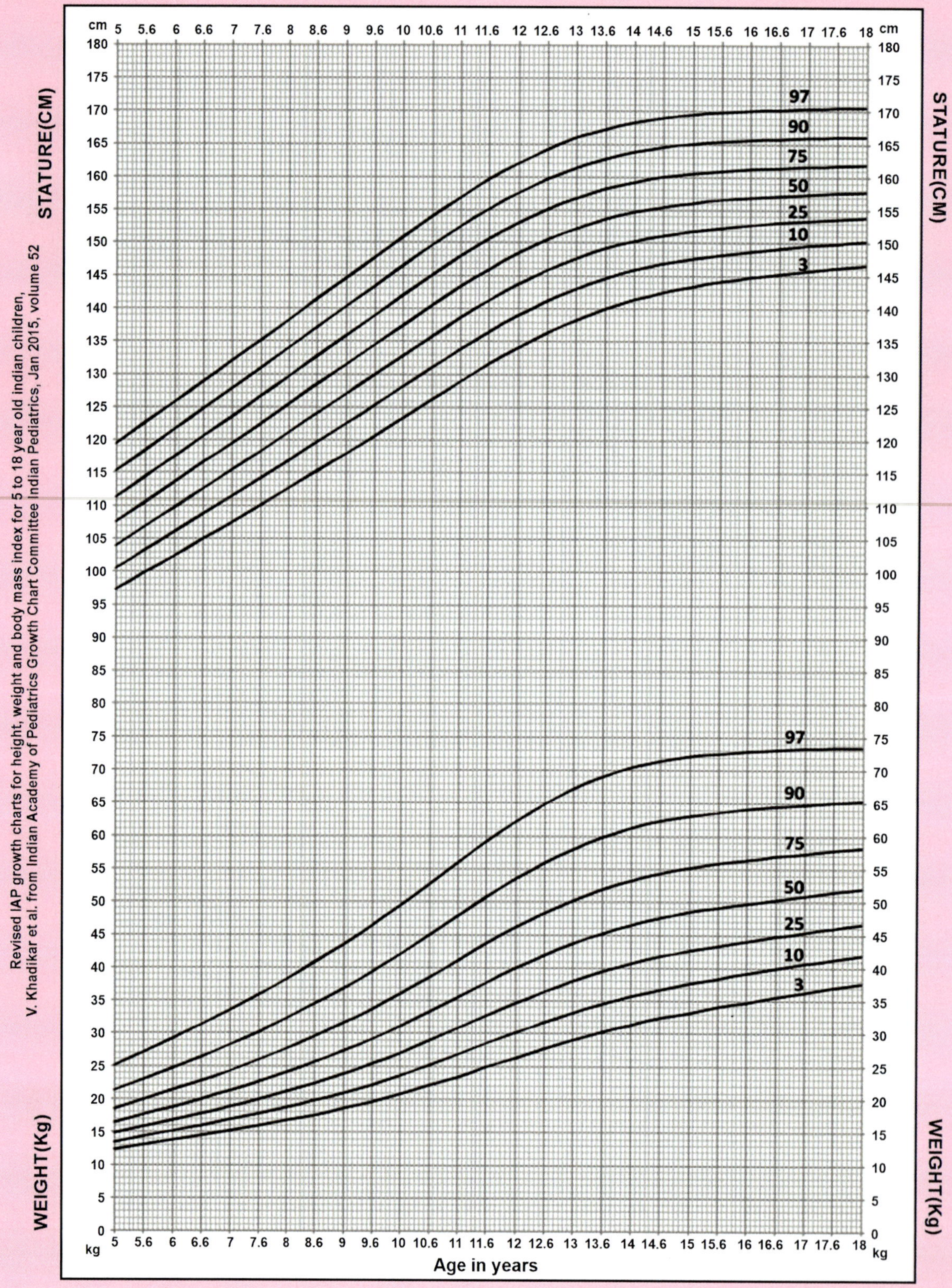

## Annexure 11

## IAP BMI chart for Boys aged 5 to 18 years

**Name** ______________________________

**DOB** ______________________________

Revised IAP growth charts for height, weight and body mass index for 5 to 18 year old indian children,
V. Khadikar et al. from Indian Academy of Pediatrics Growth Chart Committee Indian Pediatrics, Jan 2015, volume 52

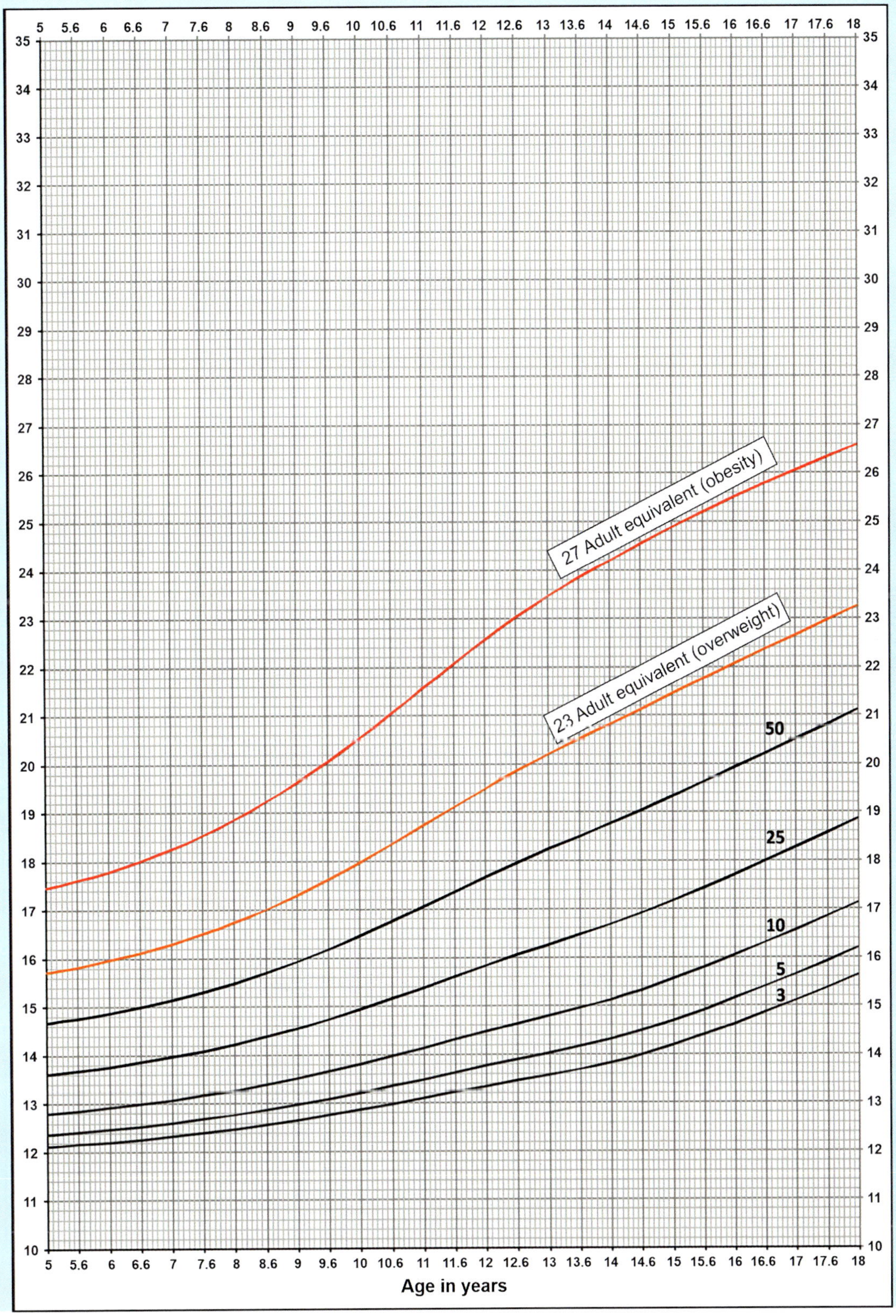

## Annexure 12

## IAP BMI chart for Girls aged 5 to 18 years

Name ____________________

DOB ____________________

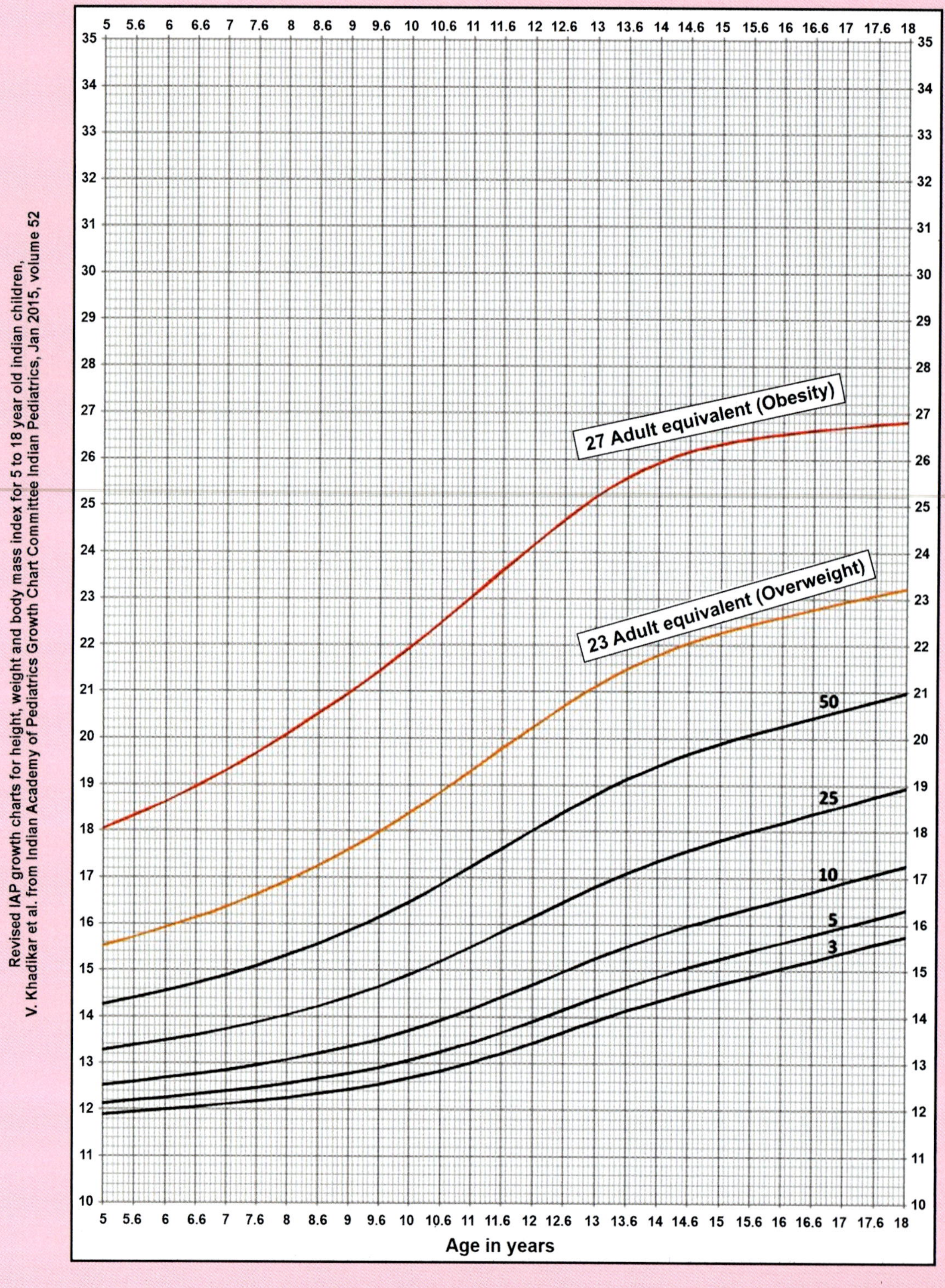

# Annexure 13

## Weight-for-age and length/height-for-age in girls 0–5 years of age

| *Months* | *Weight-for-age, kg* | | | | | | | *Length-for-age, cm* | | | | | | |
|---|---|---|---|---|---|---|---|---|---|---|---|---|---|---|
| | *−3 SD* | *−2 SD* | *−1 SD* | *Median* | *1 SD* | *2 SD* | *3 SD* | *−3 SD* | *−2 SD* | *−1 SD* | *Median* | *1 SD* | *2 SD* | *3 SD* |
| 0 | 2.0 | 2.4 | 2.8 | 3.2 | 3.7 | 4.2 | 4.8 | 43.6 | 45.4 | 47.3 | 49.1 | 51.0 | 52.9 | 54.7 |
| 1 | 2.7 | 3.2 | 3.6 | 4.2 | 4.8 | 5.5 | 6.2 | 47.8 | 49.8 | 51.7 | 53.7 | 55.6 | 57.6 | 59.5 |
| 2 | 3.4 | 3.9 | 4.5 | 5.1 | 5.8 | 6.6 | 7.5 | 51.0 | 53.0 | 55.0 | 57.1 | 59.1 | 61.1 | 63.2 |
| 3 | 4.0 | 4.5 | 5.2 | 5.8 | 6.6 | 7.5 | 8.5 | 53.5 | 55.6 | 57.7 | 59.8 | 61.9 | 64.0 | 66.1 |
| 4 | 4.4 | 5.0 | 5.7 | 6.4 | 7.3 | 8.2 | 9.3 | 55.6 | 57.8 | 59.9 | 62.1 | 64.3 | 66.4 | 68.6 |
| 5 | 4.8 | 5.4 | 6.1 | 6.9 | 7.8 | 8.8 | 10.0 | 57.4 | 59.6 | 61.8 | 64.0 | 66.2 | 68.5 | 70.7 |
| 6 | 5.1 | 5.7 | 6.5 | 7.3 | 8.2 | 9.3 | 10.6 | 58.9 | 61.2 | 63.5 | 65.7 | 68.0 | 70.3 | 72.5 |
| 7 | 5.3 | 6.0 | 6.8 | 7.6 | 8.6 | 9.8 | 11.1 | 60.3 | 62.7 | 65.0 | 67.3 | 69.6 | 71.9 | 74.2 |
| 8 | 5.6 | 6.3 | 7.0 | 7.9 | 9.0 | 10.2 | 11.6 | 61.7 | 64.0 | 66.4 | 68.7 | 71.1 | 73.5 | 75.8 |
| 9 | 5.8 | 6.5 | 7.3 | 8.2 | 9.3 | 10.5 | 12.0 | 62.9 | 65.3 | 67.7 | 70.1 | 72.6 | 75.0 | 77.4 |
| 10 | 5.9 | 6.7 | 7.5 | 8.5 | 9.6 | 10.9 | 12.4 | 64.1 | 66.5 | 69.0 | 71.5 | 73.9 | 76.4 | 78.9 |
| 11 | 6.1 | 6.9 | 7.7 | 8.7 | 9.9 | 11.2 | 12.8 | 65.2 | 67.7 | 70.3 | 72.8 | 75.3 | 77.8 | 80.3 |
| 12 | 6.3 | 7.0 | 7.9 | 8.9 | 10.1 | 11.5 | 13.1 | 66.3 | 68.9 | 71.4 | 74.0 | 76.6 | 79.2 | 81.7 |
| 13 | 6.4 | 7.2 | 8.1 | 9.2 | 10.4 | 11.8 | 13.5 | 67.3 | 70.0 | 72.6 | 75.2 | 77.8 | 80.5 | 83.1 |
| 14 | 6.6 | 7.4 | 8.3 | 9.4 | 10.6 | 12.1 | 13.8 | 68.3 | 71.0 | 73.7 | 76.4 | 79.1 | 81.7 | 84.4 |
| 15 | 6.7 | 7.6 | 8.5 | 9.6 | 10.9 | 12.4 | 14.1 | 69.3 | 72.0 | 74.8 | 77.5 | 80.2 | 83.0 | 85.7 |
| 16 | 6.9 | 7.7 | 8.7 | 9.8 | 11.1 | 12.6 | 14.5 | 70.2 | 73.0 | 75.8 | 78.6 | 81.4 | 84.2 | 87.0 |
| 17 | 7.0 | 7.9 | 8.9 | 10.0 | 11.4 | 12.9 | 14.8 | 71.1 | 74.0 | 76.8 | 79.7 | 82.5 | 85.4 | 88.2 |
| 18 | 7.2 | 8.1 | 9.1 | 10.2 | 11.6 | 13.2 | 15.1 | 72.0 | 74.9 | 77.8 | 80.7 | 83.6 | 86.5 | 89.4 |
| 19 | 7.3 | 8.2 | 9.2 | 10.4 | 11.8 | 13.5 | 15.4 | 72.8 | 75.8 | 78.8 | 81.7 | 84.7 | 87.6 | 90.6 |
| 20 | 7.5 | 8.4 | 9.4 | 10.6 | 12.1 | 13.7 | 15.7 | 73.7 | 76.7 | 79.7 | 82.7 | 85.7 | 88.7 | 91.7 |
| 21 | 7.6 | 8.6 | 9.6 | 10.9 | 12.3 | 14.0 | 16.0 | 74.5 | 77.5 | 80.6 | 83.7 | 86.7 | 89.8 | 92.9 |
| 22 | 7.8 | 8.7 | 9.8 | 11.1 | 12.5 | 14.3 | 16.4 | 75.2 | 78.4 | 81.5 | 84.6 | 87.7 | 90.8 | 94.0 |
| 23 | 7.9 | 8.9 | 10.0 | 11.3 | 12.8 | 14.6 | 16.7 | 76.0 | 79.2 | 82.3 | 85.5 | 88.7 | 91.9 | 95.0 |
| 24 | 8.1 | 9.0 | 10.2 | 11.5 | 13.0 | 14.8 | 17.0 | 76.7 | 80.0 | 83.2 | 86.4 | 89.6 | 92.9 | 96.1 |
| | *Weight-for-age, kg* | | | | | | | *Height-for-age, cm* | | | | | | |
| 24 | | | | | | | | 76.0 | 79.3 | 82.5 | 85.7 | 88.9 | 92.2 | 95.4 |
| 25 | 8.2 | 9.2 | 10.3 | 11.7 | 13.3 | 15.1 | 17.3 | 76.8 | 80.0 | 83.3 | 86.6 | 89.9 | 93.1 | 96.4 |
| 26 | 8.4 | 9.4 | 10.5 | 11.9 | 13.5 | 15.4 | 17.7 | 77.5 | 80.8 | 84.1 | 87.4 | 90.8 | 94.1 | 97.4 |
| 27 | 8.5 | 9.5 | 10.7 | 12.1 | 13.7 | 15.7 | 18.0 | 78.1 | 81.5 | 84.9 | 88.3 | 91.7 | 95.0 | 98.4 |
| 28 | 8.6 | 9.7 | 10.9 | 12.3 | 14.0 | 16.0 | 18.3 | 78.8 | 82.2 | 85.7 | 89.1 | 92.5 | 96.0 | 99.4 |
| 29 | 8.8 | 9.8 | 11.1 | 12.5 | 14.2 | 16.2 | 18.7 | 79.5 | 82.9 | 86.4 | 89.9 | 93.4 | 96.9 | 100.3 |
| 30 | 8.9 | 10.0 | 11.2 | 12.7 | 14.4 | 16.5 | 19.0 | 80.1 | 83.6 | 87.1 | 90.7 | 94.2 | 97.7 | 101.3 |
| 31 | 9.0 | 10.1 | 11.4 | 12.9 | 14.7 | 16.8 | 19.3 | 80.7 | 84.3 | 87.9 | 91.4 | 95.0 | 98.6 | 102.2 |
| 32 | 9.1 | 10.3 | 11.6 | 13.1 | 14.9 | 17.1 | 19.6 | 81.3 | 84.9 | 88.6 | 92.2 | 95.8 | 99.4 | 103.1 |
| 33 | 9.3 | 10.4 | 11.7 | 13.3 | 15.1 | 17.3 | 20.0 | 81.9 | 85.6 | 89.3 | 92.9 | 96.6 | 100.3 | 103.9 |
| 34 | 9.4 | 10.5 | 11.9 | 13.5 | 15.4 | 17.6 | 20.3 | 82.5 | 86.2 | 89.9 | 93.6 | 97.4 | 101.1 | 104.8 |
| 35 | 9.5 | 10.7 | 12.0 | 13.7 | 15.6 | 17.9 | 20.6 | 83.1 | 86.8 | 90.6 | 94.4 | 98.1 | 101.9 | 105.6 |
| 36 | 9.6 | 10.8 | 12.2 | 13.9 | 15.8 | 18.1 | 20.9 | 83.6 | 87.4 | 91.2 | 95.1 | 98.9 | 102.7 | 106.5 |
| 37 | 9.7 | 10.9 | 12.4 | 14.0 | 16.0 | 18.4 | 21.3 | 84.2 | 88.0 | 91.9 | 95.7 | 99.6 | 103.4 | 107.3 |
| 38 | 9.8 | 11.1 | 12.5 | 14.2 | 16.3 | 18.7 | 21.6 | 84.7 | 88.6 | 92.5 | 96.4 | 100.3 | 104.2 | 108.1 |
| 39 | 9.9 | 11.2 | 12.7 | 14.4 | 16.5 | 19.0 | 22.0 | 85.3 | 89.2 | 93.1 | 97.1 | 101.0 | 105.0 | 108.9 |
| 40 | 10.1 | 11.3 | 12.8 | 14.6 | 16.7 | 19.2 | 22.3 | 85.8 | 89.8 | 93.8 | 97.7 | 101.7 | 105.7 | 109.7 |
| 41 | 10.2 | 11.5 | 13.0 | 14.8 | 16.9 | 19.5 | 22.7 | 86.3 | 90.4 | 94.4 | 98.4 | 102.4 | 106.4 | 110.5 |
| 42 | 10.3 | 11.6 | 13.1 | 15.0 | 17.2 | 19.8 | 23.0 | 86.8 | 90.9 | 95.0 | 99.0 | 103.1 | 107.2 | 111.2 |
| 43 | 10.4 | 11.7 | 13.3 | 15.2 | 17.4 | 20.1 | 23.4 | 87.4 | 91.5 | 95.6 | 99.7 | 103.8 | 107.9 | 112.0 |
| 44 | 10.5 | 11.8 | 13.4 | 15.3 | 17.6 | 20.4 | 23.7 | 87.9 | 92.0 | 96.2 | 100.3 | 104.5 | 108.6 | 112.7 |
| 45 | 10.6 | 12.0 | 13.6 | 15.5 | 17.8 | 20.7 | 24.1 | 88.4 | 92.5 | 96.7 | 100.9 | 105.1 | 109.3 | 113.5 |
| 46 | 10.7 | 12.1 | 13.7 | 15.7 | 18.1 | 20.9 | 24.5 | 88.9 | 93.1 | 97.3 | 101.5 | 105.8 | 110.0 | 114.2 |
| 47 | 10.8 | 12.2 | 13.9 | 15.9 | 18.3 | 21.2 | 24.8 | 89.3 | 93.6 | 97.9 | 102.1 | 106.4 | 110.7 | 114.9 |
| 48 | 10.9 | 12.3 | 14.0 | 16.1 | 18.5 | 21.5 | 25.2 | 89.8 | 94.1 | 98.4 | 102.7 | 107.0 | 111.3 | 115.7 |
| 49 | 11.0 | 12.4 | 14.2 | 16.3 | 18.8 | 21.8 | 25.5 | 90.3 | 94.6 | 99.0 | 103.3 | 107.7 | 112.0 | 116.4 |
| 50 | 11.1 | 12.6 | 14.3 | 16.4 | 19.0 | 22.1 | 25.9 | 90.7 | 95.1 | 99.5 | 103.9 | 108.3 | 112.7 | 117.1 |
| 51 | 11.2 | 12.7 | 14.5 | 16.6 | 19.2 | 22.4 | 26.3 | 91.2 | 95.6 | 100.1 | 104.5 | 108.9 | 113.3 | 117.7 |
| 52 | 11.3 | 12.8 | 14.6 | 16.8 | 19.4 | 22.6 | 26.6 | 91.7 | 96.1 | 100.6 | 105.0 | 109.5 | 114.0 | 118.4 |
| 53 | 11.4 | 12.9 | 14.8 | 17.0 | 19.7 | 22.9 | 27.0 | 92.1 | 96.6 | 101.1 | 105.6 | 110.1 | 114.6 | 119.1 |
| 54 | 11.5 | 13.0 | 14.9 | 17.2 | 19.9 | 23.2 | 27.4 | 92.6 | 97.1 | 101.6 | 106.2 | 110.7 | 115.2 | 119.8 |
| 55 | 11.6 | 13.2 | 15.1 | 17.3 | 20.1 | 23.5 | 27.7 | 93.0 | 97.6 | 102.2 | 106.7 | 111.3 | 115.9 | 120.4 |
| 56 | 11.7 | 13.3 | 15.2 | 17.5 | 20.3 | 23.8 | 28.1 | 93.4 | 98.1 | 102.7 | 107.3 | 111.9 | 116.5 | 121.1 |
| 57 | 11.8 | 13.4 | 15.3 | 17.7 | 20.6 | 24.1 | 28.5 | 93.9 | 98.5 | 103.2 | 107.8 | 112.5 | 117.1 | 121.8 |
| 58 | 11.9 | 13.5 | 15.5 | 17.9 | 20.8 | 24.4 | 28.8 | 94.3 | 99.0 | 103.7 | 108.4 | 113.0 | 117.7 | 122.4 |
| 59 | 12.0 | 13.6 | 15.6 | 18.0 | 21.0 | 24.6 | 29.2 | 94.7 | 99.5 | 104.2 | 108.9 | 113.6 | 118.3 | 123.1 |
| 60 | 12.1 | 13.7 | 15.8 | 18.2 | 21.2 | 24.9 | 29.5 | 95.2 | 99.9 | 104.7 | 109.4 | 114.2 | 118.9 | 123.7 |

WHO: MGRS

## Annexure 14

### Weight-for-age and length/height-for-age in boys 0–5 years of age

| Months | Weight-for-age, kg | | | | | | | Length-for-age, cm | | | | | | |
|---|---|---|---|---|---|---|---|---|---|---|---|---|---|---|
| | –3 SD | –2 SD | –1 SD | Median | 1 SD | 2 SD | 3 SD | –3 SD | –2 SD | –1 SD | Median | 1 SD | 2 SD | 3 SD |
| 0 | 2.1 | 2.5 | 2.9 | 3.3 | 3.9 | 4.4 | 5.0 | 44.2 | 46.1 | 48.0 | 49.9 | 51.8 | 53.7 | 55.6 |
| 1 | 2.9 | 3.4 | 3.9 | 4.5 | 5.1 | 5.8 | 6.6 | 48.9 | 50.8 | 52.8 | 54.7 | 56.7 | 58.6 | 60.6 |
| 2 | 3.8 | 4.3 | 4.9 | 5.6 | 6.3 | 7.1 | 8.0 | 52.4 | 54.4 | 56.4 | 58.4 | 60.4 | 62.4 | 64.4 |
| 3 | 4.4 | 5.0 | 5.7 | 6.4 | 7.2 | 8.0 | 9.0 | 55.3 | 57.3 | 59.4 | 61.4 | 63.5 | 65.5 | 67.6 |
| 4 | 4.9 | 5.6 | 6.2 | 7.0 | 7.8 | 8.7 | 9.7 | 57.6 | 59.7 | 61.8 | 63.9 | 66.0 | 68.0 | 70.1 |
| 5 | 5.3 | 6.0 | 6.7 | 7.5 | 8.4 | 9.3 | 10.4 | 59.6 | 61.7 | 63.8 | 65.9 | 68.0 | 70.1 | 72.2 |
| 6 | 5.7 | 6.4 | 7.1 | 7.9 | 8.8 | 9.8 | 10.9 | 61.2 | 63.3 | 65.5 | 67.6 | 69.8 | 71.9 | 74.0 |
| 7 | 5.9 | 6.7 | 7.4 | 8.3 | 9.2 | 10.3 | 11.4 | 62.7 | 64.8 | 67.0 | 69.2 | 71.3 | 73.5 | 75.7 |
| 8 | 6.2 | 6.9 | 7.7 | 8.6 | 9.6 | 10.7 | 11.9 | 64.0 | 66.2 | 68.4 | 70.6 | 72.8 | 75.0 | 77.2 |
| 9 | 6.4 | 7.1 | 8.0 | 8.9 | 9.9 | 11.0 | 12.3 | 65.2 | 67.5 | 69.7 | 72.0 | 74.2 | 76.5 | 78.7 |
| 10 | 6.6 | 7.4 | 8.2 | 9.2 | 10.2 | 11.4 | 12.7 | 66.4 | 68.7 | 71.0 | 73.3 | 75.6 | 77.9 | 80.1 |
| 11 | 6.8 | 7.6 | 8.4 | 9.4 | 10.5 | 11.7 | 13.0 | 67.6 | 69.9 | 72.2 | 74.5 | 76.9 | 79.2 | 81.5 |
| 12 | 6.9 | 7.7 | 8.6 | 9.6 | 10.8 | 12.0 | 13.3 | 68.6 | 71.0 | 73.4 | 75.7 | 78.1 | 80.5 | 82.9 |
| 13 | 7.1 | 7.9 | 8.8 | 9.9 | 11.0 | 12.3 | 13.7 | 69.6 | 72.1 | 74.5 | 76.9 | 79.3 | 81.8 | 84.2 |
| 14 | 7.2 | 8.1 | 9.0 | 10.1 | 11.3 | 12.6 | 14.0 | 70.6 | 73.1 | 75.6 | 78.0 | 80.5 | 83.0 | 85.5 |
| 15 | 7.4 | 8.3 | 9.2 | 10.3 | 11.5 | 12.8 | 14.3 | 71.6 | 74.1 | 76.6 | 79.1 | 81.7 | 84.2 | 86.7 |
| 16 | 7.5 | 8.4 | 9.4 | 10.5 | 11.7 | 13.1 | 14.6 | 72.5 | 75.0 | 77.6 | 80.2 | 82.8 | 85.4 | 88.0 |
| 17 | 7.7 | 8.6 | 9.6 | 10.7 | 12.0 | 13.4 | 14.9 | 73.3 | 76.0 | 78.6 | 81.2 | 83.9 | 86.5 | 89.2 |
| 18 | 7.8 | 8.8 | 9.8 | 10.9 | 12.2 | 13.7 | 15.3 | 74.2 | 76.9 | 79.6 | 82.3 | 85.0 | 87.7 | 90.4 |
| 19 | 8.0 | 8.9 | 10.0 | 11.1 | 12.5 | 13.9 | 15.6 | 75.0 | 77.7 | 80.5 | 83.2 | 86.0 | 88.8 | 91.5 |
| 20 | 8.1 | 9.1 | 10.1 | 11.3 | 12.7 | 14.2 | 15.9 | 75.8 | 78.6 | 81.4 | 84.2 | 87.0 | 89.8 | 92.6 |
| 21 | 8.2 | 9.2 | 10.3 | 11.5 | 12.9 | 14.5 | 16.2 | 76.5 | 79.4 | 82.3 | 85.1 | 88.0 | 90.9 | 93.8 |
| 22 | 8.4 | 9.4 | 10.5 | 11.8 | 13.2 | 14.7 | 16.5 | 77.2 | 80.2 | 83.1 | 86.0 | 89.0 | 91.9 | 94.9 |
| 23 | 8.5 | 9.5 | 10.7 | 12.0 | 13.4 | 15.0 | 16.8 | 78.0 | 81.0 | 83.9 | 86.9 | 89.9 | 92.9 | 95.9 |
| 24 | 8.6 | 9.7 | 10.8 | 12.2 | 13.6 | 15.3 | 17.1 | 78.7 | 81.7 | 84.8 | 87.8 | 90.9 | 93.9 | 97.0 |
| | Weight-for-age, kg | | | | | | | Height-for-age, cm | | | | | | |
| 24 | | | | | | | | 78.0 | 81.0 | 84.1 | 87.1 | 90.2 | 93.2 | 96.3 |
| 25 | 8.8 | 9.8 | 11.0 | 12.4 | 13.9 | 15.5 | 17.5 | 78.6 | 81.7 | 84.9 | 88.0 | 91.1 | 94.2 | 97.3 |
| 26 | 8.9 | 10.0 | 11.2 | 12.5 | 14.1 | 15.8 | 17.8 | 79.3 | 82.5 | 85.6 | 88.8 | 92.0 | 95.2 | 98.3 |
| 27 | 9.0 | 10.1 | 11.3 | 12.7 | 14.3 | 16.1 | 18.1 | 79.9 | 83.1 | 86.4 | 89.6 | 92.9 | 96.1 | 99.3 |
| 28 | 9.1 | 10.2 | 11.5 | 12.9 | 14.5 | 16.3 | 18.4 | 80.5 | 83.8 | 87.1 | 90.4 | 93.7 | 97.0 | 100.3 |
| 29 | 9.2 | 10.4 | 11.7 | 13.1 | 14.8 | 16.6 | 18.7 | 81.1 | 84.5 | 87.8 | 91.2 | 94.5 | 97.9 | 101.2 |
| 30 | 9.4 | 10.5 | 11.8 | 13.3 | 15.0 | 16.9 | 19.0 | 81.7 | 85.1 | 88.5 | 91.9 | 95.3 | 98.7 | 102.1 |
| 31 | 9.5 | 10.7 | 12.0 | 13.5 | 15.2 | 17.1 | 19.3 | 82.3 | 85.7 | 89.2 | 92.7 | 96.1 | 99.6 | 103.0 |
| 32 | 9.6 | 10.8 | 12.1 | 13.7 | 15.4 | 17.4 | 19.6 | 82.8 | 86.4 | 89.9 | 93.4 | 96.9 | 100.4 | 103.9 |
| 33 | 9.7 | 10.9 | 12.3 | 13.8 | 15.6 | 17.6 | 19.9 | 83.4 | 86.9 | 90.5 | 94.1 | 97.6 | 101.2 | 104.8 |
| 34 | 9.8 | 11.0 | 12.4 | 14.0 | 15.8 | 17.8 | 20.2 | 83.9 | 87.5 | 91.1 | 94.8 | 98.4 | 102.0 | 105.6 |
| 35 | 9.9 | 11.2 | 12.6 | 14.2 | 16.0 | 18.1 | 20.4 | 84.4 | 88.1 | 91.8 | 95.4 | 99.1 | 102.7 | 106.4 |
| 36 | 10.0 | 11.3 | 12.7 | 14.3 | 16.2 | 18.3 | 20.7 | 85.0 | 88.7 | 92.4 | 96.1 | 99.8 | 103.5 | 107.2 |
| 37 | 10.1 | 11.4 | 12.9 | 14.5 | 16.4 | 18.6 | 21.0 | 85.5 | 89.2 | 93.0 | 96.7 | 100.5 | 104.2 | 108.0 |
| 38 | 10.2 | 11.5 | 13.0 | 14.7 | 16.6 | 18.8 | 21.3 | 86.0 | 89.8 | 93.6 | 97.4 | 101.2 | 105.0 | 108.8 |
| 39 | 10.3 | 11.6 | 13.1 | 14.8 | 16.8 | 19.0 | 21.6 | 86.5 | 90.3 | 94.2 | 98.0 | 101.8 | 105.7 | 109.5 |
| 40 | 10.4 | 11.8 | 13.3 | 15.0 | 17.0 | 19.3 | 21.9 | 87.0 | 90.9 | 94.7 | 98.6 | 102.5 | 106.4 | 110.3 |
| 41 | 10.5 | 11.9 | 13.4 | 15.2 | 17.2 | 19.5 | 22.1 | 87.5 | 91.4 | 95.3 | 99.2 | 103.2 | 107.1 | 111.0 |
| 42 | 10.6 | 12.0 | 13.6 | 15.3 | 17.4 | 19.7 | 22.4 | 88.0 | 91.9 | 95.9 | 99.9 | 103.8 | 107.8 | 111.7 |
| 43 | 10.7 | 12.1 | 13.7 | 15.5 | 17.6 | 20.0 | 22.7 | 88.4 | 92.4 | 96.4 | 100.4 | 104.5 | 108.5 | 112.5 |
| 44 | 10.8 | 12.2 | 13.8 | 15.7 | 17.8 | 20.2 | 23.0 | 88.9 | 93.0 | 97.0 | 101.0 | 105.1 | 109.1 | 113.2 |
| 45 | 10.9 | 12.4 | 14.0 | 15.8 | 18.0 | 20.5 | 23.3 | 89.4 | 93.5 | 97.5 | 101.6 | 105.7 | 109.8 | 113.9 |
| 46 | 11.0 | 12.5 | 14.1 | 16.0 | 18.2 | 20.7 | 23.6 | 89.8 | 94.0 | 98.1 | 102.2 | 106.3 | 110.4 | 114.6 |
| 47 | 11.1 | 12.6 | 14.3 | 16.2 | 18.4 | 20.9 | 23.9 | 90.3 | 94.4 | 98.6 | 102.8 | 106.9 | 111.1 | 115.2 |
| 48 | 11.2 | 12.7 | 14.4 | 16.3 | 18.6 | 21.2 | 24.2 | 90.7 | 94.9 | 99.1 | 103.3 | 107.5 | 111.7 | 115.9 |
| 49 | 11.3 | 12.8 | 14.5 | 16.5 | 18.8 | 21.4 | 24.5 | 91.2 | 95.4 | 99.7 | 103.9 | 108.1 | 112.4 | 116.6 |
| 50 | 11.4 | 12.9 | 14.7 | 16.7 | 19.0 | 21.7 | 24.8 | 91.6 | 95.9 | 100.2 | 104.4 | 108.7 | 113.0 | 117.3 |
| 51 | 11.5 | 13.1 | 14.8 | 16.8 | 19.2 | 21.9 | 25.1 | 92.1 | 96.4 | 100.7 | 105.0 | 109.3 | 113.6 | 117.9 |
| 52 | 11.6 | 13.2 | 15.0 | 17.0 | 19.4 | 22.2 | 25.4 | 92.5 | 96.9 | 101.2 | 105.6 | 109.9 | 114.2 | 118.6 |
| 53 | 11.7 | 13.3 | 15.1 | 17.2 | 19.6 | 22.4 | 25.7 | 93.0 | 97.4 | 101.7 | 106.1 | 110.5 | 114.9 | 119.2 |
| 54 | 11.8 | 13.4 | 15.2 | 17.3 | 19.8 | 22.7 | 26.0 | 93.4 | 97.8 | 102.3 | 106.7 | 111.1 | 115.5 | 119.9 |
| 55 | 11.9 | 13.5 | 15.4 | 17.5 | 20.0 | 22.9 | 26.3 | 93.9 | 98.3 | 102.8 | 107.2 | 111.7 | 116.1 | 120.6 |
| 56 | 12.0 | 13.6 | 15.5 | 17.7 | 20.2 | 23.2 | 26.6 | 94.3 | 98.8 | 103.3 | 107.8 | 112.3 | 116.7 | 121.2 |
| 57 | 12.1 | 13.7 | 15.6 | 17.8 | 20.4 | 23.4 | 26.9 | 94.7 | 99.3 | 103.8 | 108.3 | 112.8 | 117.4 | 121.9 |
| 58 | 12.2 | 13.8 | 15.8 | 18.0 | 20.6 | 23.7 | 27.2 | 95.2 | 99.7 | 104.3 | 108.9 | 113.4 | 118.0 | 122.6 |
| 59 | 12.3 | 14.0 | 15.9 | 18.2 | 20.8 | 23.9 | 27.6 | 95.6 | 100.2 | 104.8 | 109.4 | 114.0 | 118.6 | 123.2 |
| 60 | 12.4 | 14.1 | 16.0 | 18.3 | 21.0 | 24.2 | 27.9 | 96.1 | 100.7 | 105.3 | 110.0 | 114.6 | 119.2 | 123.9 |

WHO: MGRS

## Annexure 15

### Weight-for-length/height (kg) in girls and boys 0–5 years of age

| Length (cm) | Weight (kg) Girls | | | | | | | Length (cm) | Weight (kg) Boys | | | | | | |
|---|---|---|---|---|---|---|---|---|---|---|---|---|---|---|---|
| | −3 SD | −2 SD | −1 SD | Median | 1 SD | 2 SD | 3 SD | | −3 SD | −2 SD | −1 SD | Median | 1 SD | 2 SD | 3 SD |
| 45.0 | 1.9 | 2.1 | 2.3 | 2.5 | 2.7 | 3.0 | 3.3 | 45.0 | 1.9 | 2.0 | 2.2 | 2.4 | 2.7 | 3.0 | 3.3 |
| 45.5 | 2.0 | 2.1 | 2.3 | 2.5 | 2.8 | 3.1 | 3.4 | 45.5 | 1.9 | 2.1 | 2.3 | 2.5 | 2.8 | 3.1 | 3.4 |
| 46.0 | 2.0 | 2.2 | 2.4 | 2.6 | 2.9 | 3.2 | 3.5 | 46.0 | 2.0 | 2.2 | 2.4 | 2.6 | 2.9 | 3.1 | 3.5 |
| 46.5 | 2.1 | 2.3 | 2.5 | 2.7 | 3.0 | 3.3 | 3.6 | 46.5 | 2.1 | 2.3 | 2.5 | 2.7 | 3.0 | 3.2 | 3.6 |
| 47.0 | 2.2 | 2.4 | 2.6 | 2.8 | 3.1 | 3.4 | 3.7 | 47.0 | 2.1 | 2.3 | 2.5 | 2.8 | 3.0 | 3.3 | 3.7 |
| 47.5 | 2.2 | 2.4 | 2.6 | 2.9 | 3.2 | 3.5 | 3.8 | 47.5 | 2.2 | 2.4 | 2.6 | 2.9 | 3.1 | 3.4 | 3.8 |
| 48.0 | 2.3 | 2.5 | 2.7 | 3.0 | 3.3 | 3.6 | 4.0 | 48.0 | 2.3 | 2.5 | 2.7 | 2.9 | 3.2 | 3.6 | 3.9 |
| 48.5 | 2.4 | 2.6 | 2.8 | 3.1 | 3.4 | 3.7 | 4.1 | 48.5 | 2.3 | 2.6 | 2.8 | 3.0 | 3.3 | 3.7 | 4.0 |
| 49.0 | 2.4 | 2.6 | 2.9 | 3.2 | 3.5 | 3.8 | 4.2 | 49.0 | 2.4 | 2.6 | 2.9 | 3.1 | 3.4 | 3.8 | 4.2 |
| 49.5 | 2.5 | 2.7 | 3.0 | 3.3 | 3.6 | 3.9 | 4.3 | 49.5 | 2.5 | 2.7 | 3.0 | 3.2 | 3.5 | 3.9 | 4.3 |
| 50.0 | 2.6 | 2.8 | 3.1 | 3.4 | 3.7 | 4.0 | 4.5 | 50.0 | 2.6 | 2.8 | 3.0 | 3.3 | 3.6 | 4.0 | 4.4 |
| 50.5 | 2.7 | 2.9 | 3.2 | 3.5 | 3.8 | 4.2 | 4.6 | 50.5 | 2.7 | 2.9 | 3.1 | 3.4 | 3.8 | 4.1 | 4.5 |
| 51.0 | 2.8 | 3.0 | 3.3 | 3.6 | 3.9 | 4.3 | 4.8 | 51.0 | 2.7 | 3.0 | 3.2 | 3.5 | 3.9 | 4.2 | 4.7 |
| 51.5 | 2.8 | 3.1 | 3.4 | 3.7 | 4.0 | 4.4 | 4.9 | 51.5 | 2.8 | 3.1 | 3.3 | 3.6 | 4.0 | 4.4 | 4.8 |
| 52.0 | 2.9 | 3.2 | 3.5 | 3.8 | 4.2 | 4.6 | 5.1 | 52.0 | 2.9 | 3.2 | 3.5 | 3.8 | 4.1 | 4.5 | 5.0 |
| 52.5 | 3.0 | 3.3 | 3.6 | 3.9 | 4.3 | 4.7 | 5.2 | 52.5 | 3.0 | 3.3 | 3.6 | 3.9 | 4.2 | 4.6 | 5.1 |
| 53.0 | 3.1 | 3.4 | 3.7 | 4.0 | 4.4 | 4.9 | 5.4 | 53.0 | 3.1 | 3.4 | 3.7 | 4.0 | 4.4 | 4.8 | 5.3 |
| 53.5 | 3.2 | 3.5 | 3.8 | 4.2 | 4.6 | 5.0 | 5.5 | 53.5 | 3.2 | 3.5 | 3.8 | 4.1 | 4.5 | 4.9 | 5.4 |
| 54.0 | 3.3 | 3.6 | 3.9 | 4.3 | 4.7 | 5.2 | 5.7 | 54.0 | 3.3 | 3.6 | 3.9 | 4.3 | 4.7 | 5.1 | 5.6 |
| 54.5 | 3.4 | 3.7 | 4.0 | 4.4 | 4.8 | 5.3 | 5.9 | 54.5 | 3.4 | 3.7 | 4.0 | 4.4 | 4.8 | 5.3 | 5.8 |
| 55.0 | 3.5 | 3.8 | 4.2 | 4.5 | 5.0 | 5.5 | 6.1 | 55.0 | 3.6 | 3.8 | 4.2 | 4.5 | 5.0 | 5.4 | 6.0 |
| 55.5 | 3.6 | 3.9 | 4.3 | 4.7 | 5.1 | 5.7 | 6.3 | 55.5 | 3.7 | 4.0 | 4.3 | 4.7 | 5.1 | 5.6 | 6.1 |
| 56.0 | 3.7 | 4.0 | 4.4 | 4.8 | 5.3 | 5.8 | 6.4 | 56.0 | 3.8 | 4.1 | 4.4 | 4.8 | 5.3 | 5.8 | 6.3 |
| 56.5 | 3.8 | 4.1 | 4.5 | 5.0 | 5.4 | 6.0 | 6.6 | 56.5 | 3.9 | 4.2 | 4.6 | 5.0 | 5.4 | 5.9 | 6.5 |
| 57.0 | 3.9 | 4.3 | 4.6 | 5.1 | 5.6 | 6.1 | 6.8 | 57.0 | 4.0 | 4.3 | 4.7 | 5.1 | 5.6 | 6.1 | 6.7 |
| 57.5 | 4.0 | 4.4 | 4.8 | 5.2 | 5.7 | 6.3 | 7.0 | 57.5 | 4.1 | 4.5 | 4.9 | 5.3 | 5.7 | 6.3 | 6.9 |
| 58.0 | 4.1 | 4.5 | 4.9 | 5.4 | 5.9 | 6.5 | 7.1 | 58.0 | 4.3 | 4.6 | 5.0 | 5.4 | 5.9 | 6.4 | 7.1 |
| 58.5 | 4.2 | 4.6 | 5.0 | 5.5 | 6.0 | 6.6 | 7.3 | 58.5 | 4.4 | 4.7 | 5.1 | 5.6 | 6.1 | 6.6 | 7.2 |
| 59.0 | 4.3 | 4.7 | 5.1 | 5.6 | 6.2 | 6.8 | 7.5 | 59.0 | 4.5 | 4.8 | 5.3 | 5.7 | 6.2 | 6.8 | 7.4 |
| 59.5 | 4.4 | 4.8 | 5.3 | 5.7 | 6.3 | 6.9 | 7.7 | 59.5 | 4.6 | 5.0 | 5.4 | 5.9 | 6.4 | 7.0 | 7.6 |
| 60.0 | 4.5 | 4.9 | 5.4 | 5.9 | 6.4 | 7.1 | 7.8 | 60.0 | 4.7 | 5.1 | 5.5 | 6.0 | 6.5 | 7.1 | 7.8 |
| 60.5 | 4.6 | 5.0 | 5.5 | 6.0 | 6.6 | 7.3 | 8.0 | 60.5 | 4.8 | 5.2 | 5.6 | 6.1 | 6.7 | 7.3 | 8.0 |
| 61.0 | 4.7 | 5.1 | 5.6 | 6.1 | 6.7 | 7.4 | 8.2 | 61.0 | 4.9 | 5.3 | 5.8 | 6.3 | 6.8 | 7.4 | 8.1 |
| 61.5 | 4.8 | 5.2 | 5.7 | 6.3 | 6.9 | 7.6 | 8.4 | 61.5 | 5.0 | 5.4 | 5.9 | 6.4 | 7.0 | 7.6 | 8.3 |
| 62.0 | 4.9 | 5.3 | 5.8 | 6.4 | 7.0 | 7.7 | 8.5 | 62.0 | 5.1 | 5.6 | 6.0 | 6.5 | 7.1 | 7.7 | 8.5 |
| 62.5 | 5.0 | 5.4 | 5.9 | 6.5 | 7.1 | 7.8 | 8.7 | 62.5 | 5.2 | 5.7 | 6.1 | 6.7 | 7.2 | 7.9 | 8.6 |
| 63.0 | 5.1 | 5.5 | 6.0 | 6.6 | 7.3 | 8.0 | 8.8 | 63.0 | 5.3 | 5.8 | 6.2 | 6.8 | 7.4 | 8.0 | 8.8 |
| 63.5 | 5.2 | 5.6 | 6.2 | 6.7 | 7.4 | 8.1 | 9.0 | 63.5 | 5.4 | 5.9 | 6.4 | 6.9 | 7.5 | 8.2 | 8.9 |
| 64.0 | 5.3 | 5.7 | 6.3 | 6.9 | 7.5 | 8.3 | 9.1 | 64.0 | 5.5 | 6.0 | 6.5 | 7.0 | 7.6 | 8.3 | 9.1 |
| 64.5 | 5.4 | 5.8 | 6.4 | 7.0 | 7.6 | 8.4 | 9.3 | 64.5 | 5.6 | 6.1 | 6.6 | 7.1 | 7.8 | 8.5 | 9.3 |
| 65.0 | 5.5 | 5.9 | 6.5 | 7.1 | 7.8 | 8.6 | 9.5 | 65.0 | 5.7 | 6.2 | 6.7 | 7.3 | 7.9 | 8.6 | 9.4 |
| 65.5 | 5.5 | 6.0 | 6.6 | 7.2 | 7.9 | 8.7 | 9.6 | 65.5 | 5.8 | 6.3 | 6.8 | 7.4 | 8.0 | 8.7 | 9.6 |
| 66.0 | 5.6 | 6.1 | 6.7 | 7.3 | 8.0 | 8.8 | 9.8 | 66.0 | 5.9 | 6.4 | 6.9 | 7.5 | 8.2 | 8.9 | 9.7 |
| 66.5 | 5.7 | 6.2 | 6.8 | 7.4 | 8.1 | 9.0 | 9.9 | 66.5 | 6.0 | 6.5 | 7.0 | 7.6 | 8.3 | 9.0 | 9.9 |
| 67.0 | 5.8 | 6.3 | 6.9 | 7.5 | 8.3 | 9.1 | 10.0 | 67.0 | 6.1 | 6.6 | 7.1 | 7.7 | 8.4 | 9.2 | 10.0 |
| 67.5 | 5.9 | 6.4 | 7.0 | 7.6 | 8.4 | 9.2 | 10.2 | 67.5 | 6.2 | 6.7 | 7.2 | 7.9 | 8.5 | 9.3 | 10.2 |
| 68.0 | 6.0 | 6.5 | 7.1 | 7.7 | 8.5 | 9.4 | 10.3 | 68.0 | 6.3 | 6.8 | 7.3 | 8.0 | 8.7 | 9.4 | 10.3 |
| 68.5 | 6.1 | 6.6 | 7.2 | 7.9 | 8.6 | 9.5 | 10.5 | 68.5 | 6.4 | 6.9 | 7.5 | 8.1 | 8.8 | 9.6 | 10.5 |
| 69.0 | 6.1 | 6.7 | 7.3 | 8.0 | 8.7 | 9.6 | 10.6 | 69.0 | 6.5 | 7.0 | 7.6 | 8.2 | 8.9 | 9.7 | 10.6 |
| 69.5 | 6.2 | 6.8 | 7.4 | 8.1 | 8.8 | 9.7 | 10.7 | 69.5 | 6.6 | 7.1 | 7.7 | 8.3 | 9.0 | 9.8 | 10.8 |
| 70.0 | 6.3 | 6.9 | 7.5 | 8.2 | 9.0 | 9.9 | 10.9 | 70.0 | 6.6 | 7.2 | 7.8 | 8.4 | 9.2 | 10.0 | 10.9 |
| 70.5 | 6.4 | 6.9 | 7.6 | 8.3 | 9.1 | 10.0 | 11.0 | 70.5 | 6.7 | 7.3 | 7.9 | 8.5 | 9.3 | 10.1 | 11.1 |
| 71.0 | 6.5 | 7.0 | 7.7 | 8.4 | 9.2 | 10.1 | 11.1 | 71.0 | 6.8 | 7.4 | 8.0 | 8.6 | 9.4 | 10.2 | 11.2 |
| 71.5 | 6.5 | 7.1 | 7.7 | 8.5 | 9.3 | 10.2 | 11.3 | 71.5 | 6.9 | 7.5 | 8.1 | 8.8 | 9.5 | 10.4 | 11.3 |
| 72.0 | 6.6 | 7.2 | 7.8 | 8.6 | 9.4 | 10.3 | 11.4 | 72.0 | 7.0 | 7.6 | 8.2 | 8.9 | 9.6 | 10.5 | 11.5 |
| 72.5 | 6.7 | 7.3 | 7.9 | 8.7 | 9.5 | 10.5 | 11.5 | 72.5 | 7.1 | 7.6 | 8.3 | 9.0 | 9.8 | 10.6 | 11.6 |
| 73.0 | 6.8 | 7.4 | 8.0 | 8.8 | 9.6 | 10.6 | 11.7 | 73.0 | 7.2 | 7.7 | 8.4 | 9.1 | 9.9 | 10.8 | 11.8 |
| 73.5 | 6.9 | 7.4 | 8.1 | 8.9 | 9.7 | 10.7 | 11.8 | 73.5 | 7.2 | 7.8 | 8.5 | 9.2 | 10.0 | 10.9 | 11.9 |
| 74.0 | 6.9 | 7.5 | 8.2 | 9.0 | 9.8 | 10.8 | 11.9 | 74.0 | 7.3 | 7.9 | 8.6 | 9.3 | 10.1 | 11.0 | 12.1 |
| 74.5 | 7.0 | 7.6 | 8.3 | 9.1 | 9.9 | 10.9 | 12.0 | 74.5 | 7.4 | 8.0 | 8.7 | 9.4 | 10.2 | 11.2 | 12.2 |
| 75.0 | 7.1 | 7.7 | 8.4 | 9.1 | 10.0 | 11.0 | 12.2 | 75.0 | 7.5 | 8.1 | 8.8 | 9.5 | 10.3 | 11.3 | 12.3 |
| 75.5 | 7.1 | 7.8 | 8.5 | 9.2 | 10.1 | 11.1 | 12.3 | 75.5 | 7.6 | 8.2 | 8.8 | 9.6 | 10.4 | 11.4 | 12.5 |
| 76.0 | 7.2 | 7.8 | 8.5 | 9.3 | 10.2 | 11.2 | 12.4 | 76.0 | 7.6 | 8.3 | 8.9 | 9.7 | 10.6 | 11.5 | 12.6 |
| 76.5 | 7.3 | 7.9 | 8.6 | 9.4 | 10.3 | 11.4 | 12.5 | 76.5 | 7.7 | 8.3 | 9.0 | 9.8 | 10.7 | 11.6 | 12.7 |
| 77.0 | 7.4 | 8.0 | 8.7 | 9.5 | 10.4 | 11.5 | 12.6 | 77.0 | 7.8 | 8.4 | 9.1 | 9.9 | 10.8 | 11.7 | 12.8 |

*Contd.*

## Annexure 15 *(Contd...)*

Weight-for-length/height (kg) in girls and boys 0–5 years of age

| Length (cm) | Weight (kg) Girls −3 SD | −1 SD | −1 SD | Median | 1 SD | 2 SD | 3 SD | Length (cm) | Weight (kg) Boys −3 SD | −2 SD | −1 SD | Median | 1 SD | 2 SD | 3 SD |
|---|---|---|---|---|---|---|---|---|---|---|---|---|---|---|---|
| 77.5 | 7.4 | 8.1 | 8.8 | 9.6 | 10.5 | 11.6 | 12.8 | 77.5 | 7.9 | 8.5 | 9.2 | 10.0 | 10.9 | 11.9 | 13.0 |
| 78.0 | 7.5 | 8.2 | 8.9 | 9.7 | 10.6 | 11.7 | 12.9 | 78.0 | 7.9 | 8.6 | 9.3 | 10.1 | 11.0 | 12.0 | 13.1 |
| 78.5 | 7.6 | 8.2 | 9.0 | 9.8 | 10.7 | 11.8 | 13.0 | 78.5 | 8.0 | 8.7 | 9.4 | 10.2 | 11.1 | 12.1 | 13.2 |
| 79.0 | 7.7 | 8.3 | 9.1 | 9.9 | 10.8 | 11.9 | 13.1 | 79.0 | 8.1 | 8.7 | 9.5 | 10.3 | 11.2 | 12.2 | 13.3 |
| 79.5 | 7.7 | 8.4 | 9.1 | 10.0 | 10.9 | 12.0 | 13.3 | 79.5 | 8.2 | 8.8 | 9.5 | 10.4 | 11.3 | 12.3 | 13.4 |
| 80.0 | 7.8 | 8.5 | 9.2 | 10.1 | 11.0 | 12.1 | 13.4 | 80.0 | 8.2 | 8.9 | 9.6 | 10.4 | 11.4 | 12.4 | 13.6 |
| 80.5 | 7.9 | 8.6 | 9.3 | 10.2 | 11.2 | 12.3 | 13.5 | 80.5 | 8.3 | 9.0 | 9.7 | 10.5 | 11.5 | 12.5 | 13.7 |
| 81.0 | 8.0 | 8.7 | 9.4 | 10.3 | 11.3 | 12.4 | 13.7 | 81.0 | 8.4 | 9.1 | 9.8 | 10.6 | 11.6 | 12.6 | 13.8 |
| 81.5 | 8.1 | 8.8 | 9.5 | 10.4 | 11.4 | 12.5 | 13.8 | 81.5 | 8.5 | 9.1 | 9.9 | 10.7 | 11.7 | 12.7 | 13.9 |
| 82.0 | 8.1 | 8.8 | 9.6 | 10.5 | 11.5 | 12.6 | 13.9 | 82.0 | 8.5 | 9.2 | 10.0 | 10.8 | 11.8 | 12.8 | 14.0 |
| 82.5 | 8.2 | 8.9 | 9.7 | 10.6 | 11.6 | 12.8 | 14.1 | 82.5 | 8.6 | 9.3 | 10.1 | 10.9 | 11.9 | 13.0 | 14.2 |
| 83.0 | 8.3 | 9.0 | 9.8 | 10.7 | 11.8 | 12.9 | 14.2 | 83.0 | 8.7 | 9.4 | 10.2 | 11.0 | 12.0 | 13.1 | 14.3 |
| 83.5 | 8.4 | 9.1 | 9.9 | 10.9 | 11.9 | 13.1 | 14.4 | 83.5 | 8.8 | 9.5 | 10.3 | 11.2 | 12.1 | 13.2 | 14.4 |
| 84.0 | 8.5 | 9.2 | 10.1 | 11.0 | 12.0 | 13.2 | 14.5 | 84.0 | 8.9 | 9.6 | 10.4 | 11.3 | 12.2 | 13.3 | 14.6 |
| 84.5 | 8.6 | 9.3 | 10.2 | 11.1 | 12.1 | 13.3 | 14.7 | 84.5 | 9.0 | 9.7 | 10.5 | 11.4 | 12.4 | 13.5 | 14.7 |
| 85.0 | 8.7 | 9.4 | 10.3 | 11.2 | 12.3 | 13.5 | 14.9 | 85.0 | 9.1 | 9.8 | 10.6 | 11.5 | 12.5 | 13.6 | 14.9 |
| 85.5 | 8.8 | 9.5 | 10.4 | 11.3 | 12.4 | 13.6 | 15.0 | 85.5 | 9.2 | 9.9 | 10.7 | 11.6 | 12.6 | 13.7 | 15.0 |
| 86.0 | 8.9 | 9.7 | 10.5 | 11.5 | 12.6 | 13.8 | 15.2 | 86.0 | 9.3 | 10.0 | 10.8 | 11.7 | 12.8 | 13.9 | 15.2 |
| 86.5 | 9.0 | 9.8 | 10.6 | 11.6 | 12.7 | 13.9 | 15.4 | 86.5 | 9.4 | 10.1 | 11.0 | 11.9 | 12.9 | 14.0 | 15.3 |
| 87.0 | 9.1 | 9.9 | 10.7 | 11.7 | 12.8 | 14.1 | 15.5 | 87.0 | 9.5 | 10.2 | 11.1 | 12.0 | 13.0 | 14.2 | 15.5 |
| 87.5 | 9.2 | 10.0 | 10.9 | 11.8 | 13.0 | 14.2 | 15.7 | 87.5 | 9.6 | 10.4 | 11.2 | 12.1 | 13.2 | 14.3 | 15.6 |
| 88.0 | 9.3 | 10.1 | 11.0 | 12.0 | 13.1 | 14.4 | 15.9 | 88.0 | 9.7 | 10.5 | 11.3 | 12.2 | 13.3 | 14.5 | 15.8 |
| 88.5 | 9.4 | 10.2 | 11.1 | 12.1 | 13.2 | 14.5 | 16.0 | 88.5 | 9.8 | 10.6 | 11.4 | 12.4 | 13.4 | 14.6 | 15.9 |
| 89.0 | 9.5 | 10.3 | 11.2 | 12.2 | 13.4 | 14.7 | 16.2 | 89.0 | 9.9 | 10.7 | 11.5 | 12.5 | 13.5 | 14.7 | 16.1 |
| 89.5 | 9.6 | 10.4 | 11.3 | 12.3 | 13.5 | 14.8 | 16.4 | 89.5 | 10.0 | 10.8 | 11.6 | 12.6 | 13.7 | 14.9 | 16.2 |
| 90.0 | 9.7 | 10.5 | 11.4 | 12.5 | 13.7 | 15.0 | 16.5 | 90.0 | 10.1 | 10.9 | 11.8 | 12.7 | 13.8 | 15 | 16.4 |
| 90.5 | 9.8 | 10.6 | 11.5 | 12.6 | 13.8 | 15.1 | 16.7 | 90.5 | 10.2 | 11 | 11.9 | 12.8 | 13.9 | 15.1 | 16.5 |
| 91.0 | 9.9 | 10.7 | 11.7 | 12.7 | 13.9 | 15.3 | 16.9 | 91.0 | 10.3 | 11.1 | 12.0 | 13.0 | 14.1 | 15.3 | 16.7 |
| 91.5 | 10.0 | 10.8 | 11.8 | 12.8 | 14.1 | 15.5 | 17.0 | 91.5 | 10.4 | 11.2 | 12.1 | 13.1 | 14.2 | 15.4 | 16.8 |
| 92.0 | 10.1 | 10.9 | 11.9 | 13.0 | 14.2 | 15.6 | 17.2 | 92.0 | 10.5 | 11.3 | 12.2 | 13.2 | 14.3 | 15.6 | 17.0 |
| 92.5 | 10.1 | 11.0 | 12.0 | 13.1 | 14.3 | 15.8 | 17.4 | 92.5 | 10.6 | 11.4 | 12.3 | 13.3 | 14.4 | 15.7 | 17.1 |
| 93.0 | 10.2 | 11.1 | 12.1 | 13.2 | 14.5 | 15.9 | 17.5 | 93.0 | 10.7 | 11.5 | 12.4 | 13.4 | 14.6 | 15.8 | 17.3 |
| 93.5 | 10.3 | 11.2 | 12.2 | 13.3 | 14.6 | 16.1 | 17.7 | 93.5 | 10.7 | 11.6 | 12.5 | 13.5 | 14.7 | 16.0 | 17.4 |
| 94.0 | 10.4 | 11.3 | 12.3 | 13.5 | 14.7 | 16.2 | 17.9 | 94.0 | 10.8 | 11.7 | 12.6 | 13.7 | 14.8 | 16.1 | 17.6 |
| 94.5 | 10.5 | 11.4 | 12.4 | 13.6 | 14.9 | 16.4 | 18.0 | 94.5 | 10.9 | 11.8 | 12.7 | 13.8 | 14.9 | 16.3 | 17.7 |
| 95.0 | 10.6 | 11.5 | 12.6 | 13.7 | 15.0 | 16.5 | 18.2 | 95.0 | 11.0 | 11.9 | 12.8 | 13.9 | 15.1 | 16.4 | 17.9 |
| 95.5 | 10.7 | 11.6 | 12.7 | 13.8 | 15.2 | 16.7 | 18.4 | 95.5 | 11.1 | 12 | 12.9 | 14.0 | 15.2 | 16.5 | 18.0 |
| 96.0 | 10.8 | 11.7 | 12.8 | 14.0 | 15.3 | 16.8 | 18.6 | 96.0 | 11.2 | 12.1 | 13.1 | 14.1 | 15.3 | 16.7 | 18.2 |
| 96.5 | 10.9 | 11.8 | 12.9 | 14.1 | 15.4 | 17.0 | 18.7 | 96.5 | 11.3 | 12.2 | 13.2 | 14.3 | 15.5 | 16.8 | 18.4 |
| 97.0 | 11.0 | 12.0 | 13.0 | 14.2 | 15.6 | 17.1 | 18.9 | 97.0 | 11.4 | 12.3 | 13.3 | 14.4 | 15.6 | 17.0 | 18.5 |
| 97.5 | 11.1 | 12.1 | 13.1 | 14.4 | 15.7 | 17.3 | 19.1 | 97.5 | 11.5 | 12.4 | 13.4 | 14.5 | 15.7 | 17.1 | 18.7 |
| 98.0 | 11.2 | 12.2 | 13.3 | 14.5 | 15.9 | 17.5 | 19.3 | 98.0 | 11.6 | 12.5 | 13.5 | 14.6 | 15.9 | 17.3 | 18.9 |
| 98.5 | 11.3 | 12.3 | 13.4 | 14.6 | 16.0 | 17.6 | 19.5 | 98.5 | 11.7 | 12.6 | 13.6 | 14.8 | 16.0 | 17.5 | 19.1 |
| 99.0 | 11.4 | 12.4 | 13.5 | 14.8 | 16.2 | 17.8 | 19.6 | 99.0 | 11.8 | 12.7 | 13.7 | 14.9 | 16.2 | 17.6 | 19.2 |
| 99.5 | 11.5 | 12.5 | 13.6 | 14.9 | 16.3 | 18.0 | 19.8 | 99.5 | 11.9 | 12.8 | 13.9 | 15.0 | 16.3 | 17.8 | 19.4 |
| 100.0 | 11.6 | 12.6 | 13.7 | 15.0 | 16.5 | 18.1 | 20.0 | 100.0 | 12.0 | 12.9 | 14.0 | 15.2 | 16.5 | 18.0 | 19.6 |
| 100.5 | 11.7 | 12.7 | 13.9 | 15.2 | 16.6 | 18.3 | 20.2 | 100.5 | 12.1 | 13 | 14.1 | 15.3 | 16.6 | 18.1 | 19.8 |
| 101.0 | 11.8 | 12.8 | 14.0 | 15.3 | 16.8 | 18.5 | 20.4 | 101.0 | 12.2 | 13.2 | 14.2 | 15.4 | 16.8 | 18.3 | 20.0 |
| 101.5 | 11.9 | 13.0 | 14.1 | 15.5 | 17.0 | 18.7 | 20.6 | 101.5 | 12.3 | 13.3 | 14.4 | 15.6 | 16.9 | 18.5 | 20.2 |
| 102.0 | 12.0 | 13.1 | 14.3 | 15.6 | 17.1 | 18.9 | 20.8 | 102.0 | 12.4 | 13.4 | 14.5 | 15.7 | 17.1 | 18.7 | 20.4 |
| 102.5 | 12.1 | 13.2 | 14.4 | 15.8 | 17.3 | 19.0 | 21.0 | 102.5 | 12.5 | 13.5 | 14.6 | 15.9 | 17.3 | 18.8 | 20.6 |
| 103.0 | 12.3 | 13.3 | 14.5 | 15.9 | 17.5 | 19.2 | 21.3 | 103.0 | 12.6 | 13.6 | 14.8 | 16.0 | 17.4 | 19.0 | 20.8 |
| 103.5 | 12.4 | 13.5 | 14.7 | 16.1 | 17.6 | 19.4 | 21.5 | 103.5 | 12.7 | 13.7 | 14.9 | 16.2 | 17.6 | 19.2 | 21.0 |
| 104.0 | 12.5 | 13.6 | 14.8 | 16.2 | 17.8 | 19.6 | 21.7 | 104.0 | 12.8 | 13.9 | 15.0 | 16.3 | 17.8 | 19.4 | 21.2 |
| 104.5 | 12.6 | 13.7 | 15.0 | 16.4 | 18.0 | 19.8 | 21.9 | 104.5 | 12.9 | 14.0 | 15.2 | 16.5 | 17.9 | 19.6 | 21.5 |
| 105.0 | 12.7 | 13.8 | 15.1 | 16.5 | 18.2 | 20.0 | 22.2 | 105.0 | 13.0 | 14.1 | 15.3 | 16.6 | 18.1 | 19.8 | 21.7 |
| 105.5 | 12.8 | 14.0 | 15.3 | 16.7 | 18.4 | 20.2 | 22.4 | 105.5 | 13.2 | 14.2 | 15.4 | 16.8 | 18.3 | 20.0 | 21.9 |
| 106.0 | 13.0 | 14.1 | 15.4 | 16.9 | 18.5 | 20.5 | 22.6 | 106.0 | 13.3 | 14.4 | 15.6 | 16.9 | 18.5 | 20.2 | 22.1 |
| 106.5 | 13.1 | 14.3 | 15.6 | 17.1 | 18.7 | 20.7 | 22.9 | 106.5 | 13.4 | 14.5 | 15.7 | 17.1 | 18.6 | 20.4 | 22.4 |
| 107.0 | 13.2 | 14.4 | 15.7 | 17.2 | 18.9 | 20.9 | 23.1 | 107.0 | 13.5 | 14.6 | 15.9 | 17.3 | 18.8 | 20.6 | 22.6 |
| 107.5 | 13.3 | 14.5 | 15.9 | 17.4 | 19.1 | 21.1 | 23.4 | 107.5 | 13.6 | 14.7 | 16.0 | 17.4 | 19.0 | 20.8 | 22.8 |
| 108.0 | 13.5 | 14.7 | 16.0 | 17.6 | 19.3 | 21.3 | 23.6 | 108.0 | 13.7 | 14.9 | 16.2 | 17.6 | 19.2 | 21.0 | 23.1 |
| 108.5 | 13.6 | 14.8 | 16.2 | 17.8 | 19.5 | 21.6 | 23.9 | 108.5 | 13.8 | 15.0 | 16.3 | 17.8 | 19.4 | 21.2 | 23.3 |
| 109.0 | 13.7 | 15.0 | 16.4 | 18.0 | 19.7 | 21.8 | 24.2 | 109.0 | 14.0 | 15.1 | 16.5 | 17.9 | 19.6 | 21.4 | 23.6 |
| 109.5 | 13.9 | 15.1 | 16.5 | 18.1 | 20.0 | 22.0 | 24.4 | 109.5 | 14.1 | 15.3 | 16.6 | 18.1 | 19.8 | 21.7 | 23.8 |
| 110.0 | 14.0 | 15.3 | 16.7 | 18.3 | 20.2 | 22.3 | 24.7 | 110.0 | 14.2 | 15.4 | 16.8 | 18.3 | 20.0 | 21.9 | 24.1 |

WHO: MGRS

## Annexure 16

Weight-for-height/length (kg) in girls and boys 0–5 years of age

| Height (cm) | Weight (kg) Girls | | | | | | | Height (cm) | Weight (kg) Boys | | | | | | |
|---|---|---|---|---|---|---|---|---|---|---|---|---|---|---|---|
| | –3 SD | –2 SD | –1 SD | Median | 1 SD | 2 SD | 3 SD | | –3 SD | –2 SD | –1 SD | Median | 1 SD | 2 SD | 3 SD |
| 65.0 | 5.6 | 6.1 | 6.6 | 7.2 | 7.9 | 8.7 | 9.7 | 65 | 5.9 | 6.3 | 6.9 | 7.4 | 8.1 | 8.8 | 9.6 |
| 65.5 | 5.7 | 6.2 | 6.7 | 7.4 | 8.1 | 8.9 | 9.8 | 65.5 | 6.0 | 6.4 | 7.0 | 7.6 | 8.2 | 8.9 | 9.8 |
| 66.0 | 5.8 | 6.3 | 6.8 | 7.5 | 8.2 | 9.0 | 10.0 | 66 | 6.1 | 6.5 | 7.1 | 7.7 | 8.3 | 9.1 | 9.9 |
| 66.5 | 5.8 | 6.4 | 6.9 | 7.6 | 8.3 | 9.1 | 10.1 | 66.5 | 6.1 | 6.6 | 7.2 | 7.8 | 8.5 | 9.2 | 10.1 |
| 67.0 | 5.9 | 6.4 | 7.0 | 7.7 | 8.4 | 9.3 | 10.2 | 67 | 6.2 | 6.7 | 7.3 | 7.9 | 8.6 | 9.4 | 10.2 |
| 67.5 | 6.0 | 6.5 | 7.1 | 7.8 | 8.5 | 9.4 | 10.4 | 67.5 | 6.3 | 6.8 | 7.4 | 8.0 | 8.7 | 9.5 | 10.4 |
| 68.0 | 6.1 | 6.6 | 7.2 | 7.9 | 8.7 | 9.5 | 10.5 | 68 | 6.4 | 6.9 | 7.5 | 8.1 | 8.8 | 9.6 | 10.5 |
| 68.5 | 6.2 | 6.7 | 7.3 | 8.0 | 8.8 | 9.7 | 10.7 | 68.5 | 6.5 | 7.0 | 7.6 | 8.2 | 9.0 | 9.8 | 10.7 |
| 69.0 | 6.3 | 6.8 | 7.4 | 8.1 | 8.9 | 9.8 | 10.8 | 69 | 6.6 | 7.1 | 7.7 | 8.4 | 9.1 | 9.9 | 10.8 |
| 69.5 | 6.3 | 6.9 | 7.5 | 8.2 | 9.0 | 9.9 | 10.9 | 69.5 | 6.7 | 7.2 | 7.8 | 8.5 | 9.2 | 10.0 | 11.0 |
| 70.0 | 6.4 | 7.0 | 7.6 | 8.3 | 9.1 | 10.0 | 11.1 | 70 | 6.8 | 7.3 | 7.9 | 8.6 | 9.3 | 10.2 | 11.1 |
| 70.5 | 6.5 | 7.1 | 7.7 | 8.4 | 9.2 | 10.1 | 11.2 | 70.5 | 6.9 | 7.4 | 8.0 | 8.7 | 9.5 | 10.3 | 11.3 |
| 71.0 | 6.6 | 7.1 | 7.8 | 8.5 | 9.3 | 10.3 | 11.3 | 71 | 6.9 | 7.5 | 8.1 | 8.8 | 9.6 | 10.4 | 11.4 |
| 71.5 | 6.7 | 7.2 | 7.9 | 8.6 | 9.4 | 10.4 | 11.5 | 71.5 | 7.0 | 7.6 | 8.2 | 8.9 | 9.7 | 10.6 | 11.6 |
| 72.0 | 6.7 | 7.3 | 8.0 | 8.7 | 9.5 | 10.5 | 11.6 | 72 | 7.1 | 7.7 | 8.3 | 9.0 | 9.8 | 10.7 | 11.7 |
| 72.5 | 6.8 | 7.4 | 8.1 | 8.8 | 9.7 | 10.6 | 11.7 | 72.5 | 7.2 | 7.8 | 8.4 | 9.1 | 9.9 | 10.8 | 11.8 |
| 73.0 | 6.9 | 7.5 | 8.1 | 8.9 | 9.8 | 10.7 | 11.8 | 73 | 7.3 | 7.9 | 8.5 | 9.2 | 10.0 | 11.0 | 12.0 |
| 73.5 | 7.0 | 7.6 | 8.2 | 9.0 | 9.9 | 10.8 | 12.0 | 73.5 | 7.4 | 7.9 | 8.6 | 9.3 | 10.2 | 11.1 | 12.1 |
| 74.0 | 7.0 | 7.6 | 8.3 | 9.1 | 10.0 | 11.0 | 12.1 | 74 | 7.4 | 8.0 | 8.7 | 9.4 | 10.3 | 11.2 | 12.2 |
| 74.5 | 7.1 | 7.7 | 8.4 | 9.2 | 10.1 | 11.1 | 12.2 | 74.5 | 7.5 | 8.1 | 8.8 | 9.5 | 10.4 | 11.3 | 12.4 |
| 75.0 | 7.2 | 7.8 | 8.5 | 9.3 | 10.2 | 11.2 | 12.3 | 75 | 7.6 | 8.2 | 8.9 | 9.6 | 10.5 | 11.4 | 12.5 |
| 75.5 | 7.2 | 7.9 | 8.6 | 9.4 | 10.3 | 11.3 | 12.5 | 75.5 | 7.7 | 8.3 | 9.0 | 9.7 | 10.6 | 11.6 | 12.6 |
| 76.0 | 7.3 | 8.0 | 8.7 | 9.5 | 10.4 | 11.4 | 12.6 | 76 | 7.7 | 8.4 | 9.1 | 9.8 | 10.7 | 11.7 | 12.8 |
| 76.5 | 7.4 | 8.0 | 8.7 | 9.6 | 10.5 | 11.5 | 12.7 | 76.5 | 7.8 | 8.5 | 9.2 | 9.9 | 10.8 | 11.8 | 12.9 |
| 77.0 | 7.5 | 8.1 | 8.8 | 9.6 | 10.6 | 11.6 | 12.8 | 77 | 7.9 | 8.5 | 9.2 | 10.0 | 10.9 | 11.9 | 13.0 |
| 77.5 | 7.5 | 8.2 | 8.9 | 9.7 | 10.7 | 11.7 | 12.9 | 77.5 | 8.0 | 8.6 | 9.3 | 10.1 | 11.0 | 12.0 | 13.1 |
| 78.0 | 7.6 | 8.3 | 9.0 | 9.8 | 10.8 | 11.8 | 13.1 | 78 | 8.0 | 8.7 | 9.4 | 10.2 | 11.1 | 12.1 | 13.3 |
| 78.5 | 7.7 | 8.4 | 9.1 | 9.9 | 10.9 | 12.0 | 13.2 | 78.5 | 8.1 | 8.8 | 9.5 | 10.3 | 11.2 | 12.2 | 13.4 |
| 79.0 | 7.8 | 8.4 | 9.2 | 10.0 | 11.0 | 12.1 | 13.3 | 79 | 8.2 | 8.8 | 9.6 | 10.4 | 11.3 | 12.3 | 13.5 |
| 79.5 | 7.8 | 8.5 | 9.3 | 10.1 | 11.1 | 12.2 | 13.4 | 79.5 | 8.3 | 8.9 | 9.7 | 10.5 | 11.4 | 12.4 | 13.6 |
| 80.0 | 7.9 | 8.6 | 9.4 | 10.2 | 11.2 | 12.3 | 13.6 | 80 | 8.3 | 9.0 | 9.7 | 10.6 | 11.5 | 12.6 | 13.7 |
| 80.5 | 8.0 | 8.7 | 9.5 | 10.3 | 11.3 | 12.4 | 13.7 | 80.5 | 8.4 | 9.1 | 9.8 | 10.7 | 11.6 | 12.7 | 13.8 |
| 81.0 | 8.1 | 8.8 | 9.6 | 10.4 | 11.4 | 12.6 | 13.9 | 81 | 8.5 | 9.2 | 9.9 | 10.8 | 11.7 | 12.8 | 14.0 |
| 81.5 | 8.2 | 8.9 | 9.7 | 10.6 | 11.6 | 12.7 | 14.0 | 81.5 | 8.6 | 9.3 | 10.0 | 10.9 | 11.8 | 12.9 | 14.1 |
| 82.0 | 8.3 | 9.0 | 9.8 | 10.7 | 11.7 | 12.8 | 14.1 | 82 | 8.7 | 9.3 | 10.1 | 11.0 | 11.9 | 13.0 | 14.2 |
| 82.5 | 8.4 | 9.1 | 9.9 | 10.8 | 11.8 | 13.0 | 14.3 | 82.5 | 8.7 | 9.4 | 10.2 | 11.1 | 12.1 | 13.1 | 14.4 |
| 83.0 | 8.5 | 9.2 | 10.0 | 10.9 | 11.9 | 13.1 | 14.5 | 83 | 8.8 | 9.5 | 10.3 | 11.2 | 12.2 | 13.3 | 14.5 |
| 83.5 | 8.5 | 9.3 | 10.1 | 11.0 | 12.1 | 13.3 | 14.6 | 83.5 | 8.9 | 9.6 | 10.4 | 11.3 | 12.3 | 13.4 | 14.6 |
| 84.0 | 8.6 | 9.4 | 10.2 | 11.1 | 12.2 | 13.4 | 14.8 | 84 | 9.0 | 9.7 | 10.5 | 11.4 | 12.4 | 13.5 | 14.8 |
| 84.5 | 8.7 | 9.5 | 10.3 | 11.3 | 12.3 | 13.5 | 14.9 | 84.5 | 9.1 | 9.9 | 10.7 | 11.5 | 12.5 | 13.7 | 14.9 |
| 85.0 | 8.8 | 9.6 | 10.4 | 11.4 | 12.5 | 13.7 | 15.1 | 85 | 9.2 | 10.0 | 10.8 | 11.7 | 12.7 | 13.8 | 15.1 |
| 85.5 | 8.9 | 9.7 | 10.6 | 11.5 | 12.6 | 13.8 | 15.3 | 85.5 | 9.3 | 10.1 | 10.9 | 11.8 | 12.8 | 13.9 | 15.2 |
| 86.0 | 9.0 | 9.8 | 10.7 | 11.6 | 12.7 | 14.0 | 15.4 | 86 | 9.4 | 10.2 | 11.0 | 11.9 | 12.9 | 14.1 | 15.4 |
| 86.5 | 9.1 | 9.9 | 10.8 | 11.8 | 12.9 | 14.2 | 15.6 | 86.5 | 9.5 | 10.3 | 11.1 | 12.0 | 13.1 | 14.2 | 15.5 |
| 87.0 | 9.2 | 10.0 | 10.9 | 11.9 | 13.0 | 14.3 | 15.8 | 87 | 9.6 | 10.4 | 11.2 | 12.2 | 13.2 | 14.4 | 15.7 |
| 87.5 | 9.3 | 10.1 | 11.0 | 12.0 | 13.2 | 14.5 | 15.9 | 87.5 | 9.7 | 10.5 | 11.3 | 12.3 | 13.3 | 14.5 | 15.8 |
| 88.0 | 9.4 | 10.2 | 11.1 | 12.1 | 13.3 | 14.6 | 16.1 | 88 | 9.8 | 10.6 | 11.5 | 12.4 | 13.5 | 14.7 | 16.0 |
| 88.5 | 9.5 | 10.3 | 11.2 | 12.3 | 13.4 | 14.8 | 16.3 | 88.5 | 9.9 | 10.7 | 11.6 | 12.5 | 13.6 | 14.8 | 16.1 |
| 89.0 | 9.6 | 10.4 | 11.4 | 12.4 | 13.6 | 14.9 | 16.4 | 89 | 10.0 | 10.8 | 11.7 | 12.6 | 13.7 | 14.9 | 16.3 |
| 89.5 | 9.7 | 10.5 | 11.5 | 12.5 | 13.7 | 15.1 | 16.6 | 89.5 | 10.1 | 10.9 | 11.8 | 12.8 | 13.9 | 15.1 | 16.4 |
| 90.0 | 9.8 | 10.6 | 11.6 | 12.6 | 13.8 | 15.2 | 16.8 | 90 | 10.2 | 11.0 | 11.9 | 12.9 | 14.0 | 15.2 | 16.6 |
| 90.5 | 9.9 | 10.7 | 11.7 | 12.8 | 14.0 | 15.4 | 16.9 | 90.5 | 10.3 | 11.1 | 12.0 | 13.0 | 14.1 | 15.3 | 16.7 |
| 91.0 | 10.0 | 10.9 | 11.8 | 12.9 | 14.1 | 15.5 | 17.1 | 91 | 10.4 | 11.2 | 12.1 | 13.1 | 14.2 | 15.5 | 16.9 |
| 91.5 | 10.1 | 11.0 | 11.9 | 13.0 | 14.3 | 15.7 | 17.3 | 91.5 | 10.5 | 11.3 | 12.2 | 13.2 | 14.4 | 15.6 | 17.0 |

*Contd...*

## **Annexure 16** *(Contd...)*

Weight-for-height/length (kg) in girls and boys 0–5 years of age

| Height (cm) | Weight (kg) Girls | | | | | | | Height (cm) | Weight (kg) Boys | | | | | | |
|---|---|---|---|---|---|---|---|---|---|---|---|---|---|---|---|
| | –3 SD | –2 SD | –1 SD | Median | 1 SD | 2 SD | 3 SD | | –3 SD | –2 SD | –1 SD | Median | 1 SD | 2 SD | 3 SD |
| 92.0 | 10.2 | 11.1 | 12.0 | 13.1 | 14.4 | 15.8 | 17.4 | 92.0 | 10.6 | 11.4 | 12.3 | 13.4 | 14.5 | 15.8 | 17.2 |
| 92.5 | 10.3 | 11.2 | 12.1 | 13.3 | 14.5 | 16.0 | 17.6 | 92.5 | 10.7 | 11.5 | 12.4 | 13.5 | 14.6 | 15.9 | 17.3 |
| 93.0 | 10.4 | 11.3 | 12.3 | 13.4 | 14.7 | 16.1 | 17.8 | 93.0 | 10.8 | 11.6 | 12.6 | 13.6 | 14.7 | 16.0 | 17.5 |
| 93.5 | 10.5 | 11.4 | 12.4 | 13.5 | 14.8 | 16.3 | 17.9 | 93.5 | 10.9 | 11.7 | 12.7 | 13.7 | 14.9 | 16.2 | 17.6 |
| 94.0 | 10.6 | 11.5 | 12.5 | 13.6 | 14.9 | 16.4 | 18.1 | 94.0 | 11.0 | 11.8 | 12.8 | 13.8 | 15.0 | 16.3 | 17.8 |
| 94.5 | 10.7 | 11.6 | 12.6 | 13.8 | 15.1 | 16.6 | 18.3 | 94.5 | 11.1 | 11.9 | 12.9 | 13.9 | 15.1 | 16.5 | 17.9 |
| 95.0 | 10.8 | 11.7 | 12.7 | 13.9 | 15.2 | 16.7 | 18.5 | 95.0 | 11.1 | 12.0 | 13.0 | 14.1 | 15.3 | 16.6 | 18.1 |
| 95.5 | 10.8 | 11.8 | 12.8 | 14.0 | 15.4 | 16.9 | 18.6 | 95.5 | 11.2 | 12.1 | 13.1 | 14.2 | 15.4 | 16.7 | 18.3 |
| 96.0 | 10.9 | 11.9 | 12.9 | 14.1 | 15.5 | 17.0 | 18.8 | 96.0 | 11.3 | 12.2 | 13.2 | 14.3 | 15.5 | 16.9 | 18.4 |
| 96.5 | 11.0 | 12.0 | 13.1 | 14.3 | 15.6 | 17.2 | 19.0 | 96.5 | 11.4 | 12.3 | 13.3 | 14.4 | 15.7 | 17.0 | 18.6 |
| 97.0 | 11.1 | 12.1 | 13.2 | 14.4 | 15.8 | 17.4 | 19.2 | 97.0 | 11.5 | 12.4 | 13.4 | 14.6 | 15.8 | 17.2 | 18.8 |
| 97.5 | 11.2 | 12.2 | 13.3 | 14.5 | 15.9 | 17.5 | 19.3 | 97.5 | 11.6 | 12.5 | 13.6 | 14.7 | 15.9 | 17.4 | 18.9 |
| 98.0 | 11.3 | 12.3 | 13.4 | 14.7 | 16.1 | 17.7 | 19.5 | 98.0 | 11.7 | 12.6 | 13.7 | 14.8 | 16.1 | 17.5 | 19.1 |
| 98.5 | 11.4 | 12.4 | 13.5 | 14.8 | 16.2 | 17.9 | 19.7 | 98.5 | 11.8 | 12.8 | 13.8 | 14.9 | 16.2 | 17.7 | 19.3 |
| 99.0 | 11.5 | 12.5 | 13.7 | 14.9 | 16.4 | 18.0 | 19.9 | 99.0 | 11.9 | 12.9 | 13.9 | 15.1 | 16.4 | 17.9 | 19.5 |
| 99.5 | 11.6 | 12.7 | 13.8 | 15.1 | 16.5 | 18.2 | 20.1 | 99.5 | 12.0 | 13.0 | 14.0 | 15.2 | 16.5 | 18.0 | 19.7 |
| 100.0 | 11.7 | 12.8 | 13.9 | 15.2 | 16.7 | 18.4 | 20.3 | 100.0 | 12.1 | 13.1 | 14.2 | 15.4 | 16.7 | 18.2 | 19.9 |
| 100.5 | 11.9 | 12.9 | 14.1 | 15.4 | 16.9 | 18.6 | 20.5 | 100.5 | 12.2 | 13.2 | 14.3 | 15.5 | 16.9 | 18.4 | 20.1 |
| 101.0 | 12.0 | 13.0 | 14.2 | 15.5 | 17.0 | 18.7 | 20.7 | 101.0 | 12.3 | 13.3 | 14.4 | 15.6 | 17.0 | 18.5 | 20.3 |
| 101.5 | 12.1 | 13.1 | 14.3 | 15.7 | 17.2 | 18.9 | 20.9 | 101.5 | 12.4 | 13.4 | 14.5 | 15.8 | 17.2 | 18.7 | 20.5 |
| 102.0 | 12.2 | 13.3 | 14.5 | 15.8 | 17.4 | 19.1 | 21.1 | 102.0 | 12.5 | 13.6 | 14.7 | 15.9 | 17.3 | 18.9 | 20.7 |
| 102.5 | 12.3 | 13.4 | 14.6 | 16.0 | 17.5 | 19.3 | 21.4 | 102.5 | 12.6 | 13.7 | 14.8 | 16.1 | 17.5 | 19.1 | 20.9 |
| 103.0 | 12.4 | 13.5 | 14.7 | 16.1 | 17.7 | 19.5 | 21.6 | 103.0 | 12.8 | 13.8 | 14.9 | 16.2 | 17.7 | 19.3 | 21.1 |
| 103.5 | 12.5 | 13.6 | 14.9 | 16.3 | 17.9 | 19.7 | 21.8 | 103.5 | 12.9 | 13.9 | 15.1 | 16.4 | 17.8 | 19.5 | 21.3 |
| 104.0 | 12.6 | 13.8 | 15.0 | 16.4 | 18.1 | 19.9 | 22.0 | 104.0 | 13.0 | 14.0 | 15.2 | 16.5 | 18.0 | 19.7 | 21.6 |
| 104.5 | 12.8 | 13.9 | 15.2 | 16.6 | 18.2 | 20.1 | 22.3 | 104.5 | 13.1 | 14.2 | 15.4 | 16.7 | 18.2 | 19.9 | 21.8 |
| 105.0 | 12.9 | 14.0 | 15.3 | 16.8 | 18.4 | 20.3 | 22.5 | 105.0 | 13.2 | 14.3 | 15.5 | 16.8 | 18.4 | 20.1 | 22.0 |
| 105.5 | 13.0 | 14.2 | 15.5 | 16.9 | 18.6 | 20.5 | 22.7 | 105.5 | 13.3 | 14.4 | 15.6 | 17.0 | 18.5 | 20.3 | 22.2 |
| 106.0 | 13.1 | 14.3 | 15.6 | 17.1 | 18.8 | 20.8 | 23.0 | 106.0 | 13.4 | 14.5 | 15.8 | 17.2 | 18.7 | 20.5 | 22.5 |
| 106.5 | 13.3 | 14.5 | 15.8 | 17.3 | 19.0 | 21.0 | 23.2 | 106.5 | 13.5 | 14.7 | 15.9 | 17.3 | 18.9 | 20.7 | 22.7 |
| 107.0 | 13.4 | 14.6 | 15.9 | 17.5 | 19.2 | 21.2 | 23.5 | 107.0 | 13.7 | 14.8 | 16.1 | 17.5 | 19.1 | 20.9 | 22.9 |
| 107.5 | 13.5 | 14.7 | 16.1 | 17.7 | 19.4 | 21.4 | 23.7 | 107.5 | 13.8 | 14.9 | 16.2 | 17.7 | 19.3 | 21.1 | 23.2 |
| 108.0 | 13.7 | 14.9 | 16.3 | 17.8 | 19.6 | 21.7 | 24.0 | 108.0 | 13.9 | 15.1 | 16.4 | 17.8 | 19.5 | 21.3 | 23.4 |
| 108.5 | 13.8 | 15.0 | 16.4 | 18.0 | 19.8 | 21.9 | 24.3 | 108.5 | 14.0 | 15.2 | 16.5 | 18.0 | 19.7 | 21.5 | 23.7 |
| 109.0 | 13.9 | 15.2 | 16.6 | 18.2 | 20.0 | 22.1 | 24.5 | 109.0 | 14.1 | 15.3 | 16.7 | 18.2 | 19.8 | 21.8 | 23.9 |
| 109.5 | 14.1 | 15.4 | 16.8 | 18.4 | 20.3 | 22.4 | 24.8 | 109.5 | 14.3 | 15.5 | 16.8 | 18.3 | 20.0 | 22.0 | 24.2 |
| 110.0 | 14.2 | 15.5 | 17.0 | 18.6 | 20.5 | 22.6 | 25.1 | 110.0 | 14.4 | 15.6 | 17.0 | 18.5 | 20.2 | 22.2 | 24.4 |
| 110.5 | 14.4 | 15.7 | 17.1 | 18.8 | 20.7 | 22.9 | 25.4 | 110.5 | 14.5 | 15.8 | 17.1 | 18.7 | 20.4 | 22.4 | 24.7 |
| 111.0 | 14.5 | 15.8 | 17.3 | 19.0 | 20.9 | 23.1 | 25.7 | 111.0 | 14.6 | 15.9 | 17.3 | 18.9 | 20.7 | 22.7 | 25.0 |
| 111.5 | 14.7 | 16.0 | 17.5 | 19.2 | 21.2 | 23.4 | 26.0 | 111.5 | 14.8 | 16.0 | 17.5 | 19.1 | 20.9 | 22.9 | 25.2 |
| 112.0 | 14.8 | 16.2 | 17.7 | 19.4 | 21.4 | 23.6 | 26.2 | 112.0 | 14.9 | 16.2 | 17.6 | 19.2 | 21.1 | 23.1 | 25.5 |
| 112.5 | 15.0 | 16.3 | 17.9 | 19.6 | 21.6 | 23.9 | 26.5 | 112.5 | 15.0 | 16.3 | 17.8 | 19.4 | 21.3 | 23.4 | 25.8 |
| 113.0 | 15.1 | 16.5 | 18.0 | 19.8 | 21.8 | 24.2 | 26.8 | 113.0 | 15.2 | 16.5 | 18.0 | 19.6 | 21.5 | 23.6 | 26.0 |
| 113.5 | 15.3 | 16.7 | 18.2 | 20.0 | 22.1 | 24.4 | 27.1 | 113.5 | 15.3 | 16.6 | 18.1 | 19.8 | 21.7 | 23.9 | 26.3 |
| 114.0 | 15.4 | 16.8 | 18.4 | 20.2 | 22.3 | 24.7 | 27.4 | 114.0 | 15.4 | 16.8 | 18.3 | 20.0 | 21.9 | 24.1 | 26.6 |
| 114.5 | 15.6 | 17.0 | 18.6 | 20.5 | 22.6 | 25.0 | 27.8 | 114.5 | 15.6 | 16.9 | 18.5 | 20.2 | 22.1 | 24.4 | 26.9 |
| 115.0 | 15.7 | 17.2 | 18.8 | 20.7 | 22.8 | 25.2 | 28.1 | 115.0 | 15.7 | 17.1 | 18.6 | 20.4 | 22.4 | 24.6 | 27.2 |
| 115.5 | 15.9 | 17.3 | 19.0 | 20.9 | 23.0 | 25.5 | 28.4 | 115.5 | 15.8 | 17.2 | 18.8 | 20.6 | 22.6 | 24.9 | 27.5 |
| 116.0 | 16.0 | 17.5 | 19.2 | 21.1 | 23.3 | 25.8 | 28.7 | 116.0 | 16.0 | 17.4 | 19.0 | 20.8 | 22.8 | 25.1 | 27.8 |
| 116.5 | 16.2 | 17.7 | 19.4 | 21.3 | 23.5 | 26.1 | 29.0 | 116.5 | 16.1 | 17.5 | 19.2 | 21.0 | 23.0 | 25.4 | 28.0 |
| 117.0 | 16.3 | 17.8 | 19.6 | 21.5 | 23.8 | 26.3 | 29.3 | 117.0 | 16.2 | 17.7 | 19.3 | 21.2 | 23.3 | 25.6 | 28.3 |
| 117.5 | 16.5 | 18.0 | 19.8 | 21.7 | 24.0 | 26.6 | 29.6 | 117.5 | 16.4 | 17.9 | 19.5 | 21.4 | 23.5 | 25.9 | 28.6 |
| 118.0 | 16.6 | 18.2 | 19.9 | 22.0 | 24.2 | 26.9 | 29.9 | 118.0 | 16.5 | 18.0 | 19.7 | 21.6 | 23.7 | 26.1 | 28.9 |
| 118.5 | 16.8 | 18.4 | 20.1 | 22.2 | 24.5 | 27.2 | 30.3 | 118.5 | 16.7 | 18.2 | 19.9 | 21.8 | 23.9 | 26.4 | 29.2 |
| 119.0 | 16.9 | 18.5 | 20.3 | 22.4 | 24.7 | 27.4 | 30.6 | 119.0 | 16.8 | 18.3 | 20.0 | 22.0 | 24.1 | 26.6 | 29.5 |
| 119.5 | 17.1 | 18.7 | 20.5 | 22.6 | 25.0 | 27.7 | 30.9 | 119.5 | 16.9 | 18.5 | 20.2 | 22.2 | 24.4 | 26.9 | 29.8 |
| 120.0 | 17.3 | 18.9 | 20.7 | 22.8 | 25.2 | 28.0 | 31.2 | 120.0 | 17.1 | 18.6 | 20.4 | 22.4 | 24.6 | 27.2 | 30.1 |

WHO: MGRS

## Annexure 17

Body mass index (BMI) for age in girls and boys 0–5 years

| Age (mo) | BMI Girls | | | | | | | BMI Boys | | | | | | |
|---|---|---|---|---|---|---|---|---|---|---|---|---|---|---|
| | *−3 SD* | *−2 SD* | *−1 SD* | *Median* | *1 SD* | *2 SD* | *3 SD* | *−3 SD* | *−2 SD* | *−1 SD* | *Median* | *1 SD* | *2 SD* | *3 SD* |
| 0 | 10.1 | 11.1 | 12.2 | 13.3 | 14.6 | 16.1 | 17.7 | 10.2 | 11.1 | 12.2 | 13.4 | 14.8 | 16.3 | 18.1 |
| 1 | 10.8 | 12.0 | 13.2 | 14.6 | 16.0 | 17.5 | 19.1 | 11.3 | 12.4 | 13.6 | 14.9 | 16.3 | 17.8 | 19.4 |
| 2 | 11.8 | 13.0 | 14.3 | 15.8 | 17.3 | 19.0 | 20.7 | 12.5 | 13.7 | 15.0 | 16.3 | 17.8 | 19.4 | 21.1 |
| 3 | 12.4 | 13.6 | 14.9 | 16.4 | 17.9 | 19.7 | 21.5 | 13.1 | 14.3 | 15.5 | 16.9 | 18.4 | 20.0 | 21.8 |
| 4 | 12.7 | 13.9 | 15.2 | 16.7 | 18.3 | 20.0 | 22.0 | 13.4 | 14.5 | 15.8 | 17.2 | 18.7 | 20.3 | 22.1 |
| 5 | 12.9 | 14.1 | 15.4 | 16.8 | 18.4 | 20.2 | 22.2 | 13.5 | 14.7 | 15.9 | 17.3 | 18.8 | 20.5 | 22.3 |
| 6 | 13.0 | 14.1 | 15.5 | 16.9 | 18.5 | 20.3 | 22.3 | 13.6 | 14.7 | 16.0 | 17.3 | 18.8 | 20.5 | 22.3 |
| 7 | 13.0 | 14.2 | 15.5 | 16.9 | 18.5 | 20.3 | 22.3 | 13.7 | 14.8 | 16.0 | 17.3 | 18.8 | 20.5 | 22.3 |
| 8 | 13.0 | 14.1 | 15.4 | 16.8 | 18.4 | 20.2 | 22.2 | 13.6 | 14.7 | 15.9 | 17.3 | 18.7 | 20.4 | 22.2 |
| 9 | 12.9 | 14.1 | 15.3 | 16.7 | 18.3 | 20.1 | 22.1 | 13.6 | 14.7 | 15.8 | 17.2 | 18.6 | 20.3 | 22.1 |
| 10 | 12.9 | 14.0 | 15.2 | 16.6 | 18.2 | 19.9 | 21.9 | 13.5 | 14.6 | 15.7 | 17.0 | 18.5 | 20.1 | 22.0 |
| 11 | 12.8 | 13.9 | 15.1 | 16.5 | 18.0 | 19.8 | 21.8 | 13.4 | 14.5 | 15.6 | 16.9 | 18.4 | 20.0 | 21.8 |
| 12 | 12.7 | 13.8 | 15.0 | 16.4 | 17.9 | 19.6 | 21.6 | 13.4 | 14.4 | 15.5 | 16.8 | 18.2 | 19.8 | 21.6 |
| 13 | 12.6 | 13.7 | 14.9 | 16.2 | 17.7 | 19.5 | 21.4 | 13.3 | 14.3 | 15.4 | 16.7 | 18.1 | 19.7 | 21.5 |
| 14 | 12.6 | 13.6 | 14.8 | 16.1 | 17.6 | 19.3 | 21.3 | 13.2 | 14.2 | 15.3 | 16.6 | 18.0 | 19.5 | 21.3 |
| 15 | 12.5 | 13.5 | 14.7 | 16.0 | 17.5 | 19.2 | 21.1 | 13.1 | 14.1 | 15.2 | 16.4 | 17.8 | 19.4 | 21.2 |
| 16 | 12.4 | 13.5 | 14.6 | 15.9 | 17.4 | 19.1 | 21.0 | 13.1 | 14.0 | 15.1 | 16.3 | 17.7 | 19.3 | 21.0 |
| 17 | 12.4 | 13.4 | 14.5 | 15.8 | 17.3 | 18.9 | 20.9 | 13.0 | 13.9 | 15.0 | 16.2 | 17.6 | 19.1 | 20.9 |
| 18 | 12.3 | 13.3 | 14.4 | 15.7 | 17.2 | 18.8 | 20.8 | 12.9 | 13.9 | 14.9 | 16.1 | 17.5 | 19.0 | 20.8 |
| 19 | 12.3 | 13.3 | 14.4 | 15.7 | 17.1 | 18.8 | 20.7 | 12.9 | 13.8 | 14.9 | 16.1 | 17.4 | 18.9 | 20.7 |
| 20 | 12.2 | 13.2 | 14.3 | 15.6 | 17.0 | 18.7 | 20.6 | 12.8 | 13.7 | 14.8 | 16.0 | 17.3 | 18.8 | 20.6 |
| 21 | 12.2 | 13.2 | 14.3 | 15.5 | 17.0 | 18.6 | 20.5 | 12.8 | 13.7 | 14.7 | 15.9 | 17.2 | 18.7 | 20.5 |
| 22 | 12.2 | 13.1 | 14.2 | 15.5 | 16.9 | 18.5 | 20.4 | 12.7 | 13.6 | 14.7 | 15.8 | 17.2 | 18.7 | 20.4 |
| 23 | 12.2 | 13.1 | 14.2 | 15.4 | 16.9 | 18.5 | 20.4 | 12.7 | 13.6 | 14.6 | 15.8 | 17.1 | 18.6 | 20.3 |
| 24 | 12.1 | 13.1 | 14.2 | 15.4 | 16.8 | 18.4 | 20.3 | 12.7 | 13.6 | 14.6 | 15.7 | 17.0 | 18.5 | 20.3 |
| **Age (mo)** | *By height* | | | | | | | *By height* | | | | | | |
| | *−3 SD* | *−2 SD* | *−1 SD* | *Median* | *1 SD* | *2 SD* | *3 SD* | *−3 SD* | *−2 SD* | *−1 SD* | *Median* | *1 SD* | *2 SD* | *3 SD* |
| 24 | 12.4 | 13.3 | 14.4 | 15.7 | 17.1 | 18.7 | 20.6 | 12.9 | 13.8 | 14.8 | 16.0 | 17.3 | 18.9 | 20.6 |
| 25 | 12.4 | 13.3 | 14.4 | 15.7 | 17.1 | 18.7 | 20.6 | 12.8 | 13.8 | 14.8 | 16.0 | 17.3 | 18.8 | 20.5 |
| 26 | 12.3 | 13.3 | 14.4 | 15.6 | 17.0 | 18.7 | 20.6 | 12.8 | 13.7 | 14.8 | 15.9 | 17.3 | 18.8 | 20.5 |
| 27 | 12.3 | 13.3 | 14.4 | 15.6 | 17.0 | 18.6 | 20.5 | 12.7 | 13.7 | 14.7 | 15.9 | 17.2 | 18.7 | 20.4 |
| 28 | 12.3 | 13.3 | 14.3 | 15.6 | 17.0 | 18.6 | 20.5 | 12.7 | 13.6 | 14.7 | 15.9 | 17.2 | 18.7 | 20.4 |
| 29 | 12.3 | 13.2 | 14.3 | 15.6 | 17.0 | 18.6 | 20.4 | 12.7 | 13.6 | 14.7 | 15.8 | 17.1 | 18.6 | 20.3 |
| 30 | 12.3 | 13.2 | 14.3 | 15.5 | 16.9 | 18.5 | 20.4 | 12.6 | 13.6 | 14.6 | 15.8 | 17.1 | 18.6 | 20.2 |
| 31 | 12.2 | 13.2 | 14.3 | 15.5 | 16.9 | 18.5 | 20.4 | 12.6 | 13.5 | 14.6 | 15.8 | 17.1 | 18.5 | 20.2 |
| 32 | 12.2 | 13.2 | 14.3 | 15.5 | 16.9 | 18.5 | 20.4 | 12.5 | 13.5 | 14.6 | 15.7 | 17.0 | 18.5 | 20.1 |
| 33 | 12.2 | 13.1 | 14.2 | 15.5 | 16.9 | 18.5 | 20.3 | 12.5 | 13.5 | 14.5 | 15.7 | 17.0 | 18.5 | 20.1 |
| 34 | 12.2 | 13.1 | 14.2 | 15.4 | 16.8 | 18.5 | 20.3 | 12.5 | 13.4 | 14.5 | 15.7 | 17.0 | 18.4 | 20.0 |
| 35 | 12.1 | 13.1 | 14.2 | 15.4 | 16.8 | 18.4 | 20.3 | 12.4 | 13.4 | 14.5 | 15.6 | 16.9 | 18.4 | 20.0 |
| 36 | 12.1 | 13.1 | 14.2 | 15.4 | 16.8 | 18.4 | 20.3 | 12.4 | 13.4 | 14.4 | 15.6 | 16.9 | 18.4 | 20.0 |
| 37 | 12.1 | 13.1 | 14.1 | 15.4 | 16.8 | 18.4 | 20.3 | 12.4 | 13.3 | 14.4 | 15.6 | 16.9 | 18.3 | 19.9 |
| 38 | 12.1 | 13.0 | 14.1 | 15.4 | 16.8 | 18.4 | 20.3 | 12.3 | 13.3 | 14.4 | 15.5 | 16.8 | 18.3 | 19.9 |
| 39 | 12.0 | 13.0 | 14.1 | 15.3 | 16.8 | 18.4 | 20.3 | 12.3 | 13.3 | 14.3 | 15.5 | 16.8 | 18.3 | 19.9 |
| 40 | 12.0 | 13.0 | 14.1 | 15.3 | 16.8 | 18.4 | 20.3 | 12.3 | 13.2 | 14.3 | 15.5 | 16.8 | 18.2 | 19.9 |
| 41 | 12.0 | 13.0 | 14.1 | 15.3 | 16.8 | 18.4 | 20.4 | 12.2 | 13.2 | 14.3 | 15.5 | 16.8 | 18.2 | 19.9 |
| 42 | 12.0 | 12.9 | 14.0 | 15.3 | 16.8 | 18.4 | 20.4 | 12.2 | 13.2 | 14.3 | 15.4 | 16.8 | 18.2 | 19.8 |
| 43 | 11.9 | 12.9 | 14.0 | 15.3 | 16.8 | 18.4 | 20.4 | 12.2 | 13.2 | 14.2 | 15.4 | 16.7 | 18.2 | 19.8 |
| 44 | 11.9 | 12.9 | 14.0 | 15.3 | 16.8 | 18.5 | 20.4 | 12.2 | 13.1 | 14.2 | 15.4 | 16.7 | 18.2 | 19.8 |
| 45 | 11.9 | 12.9 | 14.0 | 15.3 | 16.8 | 18.5 | 20.5 | 12.2 | 13.1 | 14.2 | 15.4 | 16.7 | 18.2 | 19.8 |
| 46 | 11.9 | 12.9 | 14.0 | 15.3 | 16.8 | 18.5 | 20.5 | 12.1 | 13.1 | 14.2 | 15.4 | 16.7 | 18.2 | 19.8 |
| 47 | 11.8 | 12.8 | 14.0 | 15.3 | 16.8 | 18.5 | 20.5 | 12.1 | 13.1 | 14.2 | 15.3 | 16.7 | 18.2 | 19.9 |
| 48 | 11.8 | 12.8 | 14.0 | 15.3 | 16.8 | 18.5 | 20.6 | 12.1 | 13.1 | 14.1 | 15.3 | 16.7 | 18.2 | 19.9 |
| 49 | 11.8 | 12.8 | 13.9 | 15.3 | 16.8 | 18.5 | 20.6 | 12.1 | 13.0 | 14.1 | 15.3 | 16.7 | 18.2 | 19.9 |
| 50 | 11.8 | 12.8 | 13.9 | 15.3 | 16.8 | 18.6 | 20.7 | 12.1 | 13.0 | 14.1 | 15.3 | 16.7 | 18.2 | 19.9 |
| 51 | 11.8 | 12.8 | 13.9 | 15.3 | 16.8 | 18.6 | 20.7 | 12.1 | 13.0 | 14.1 | 15.3 | 16.6 | 18.2 | 19.9 |
| 52 | 11.7 | 12.8 | 13.9 | 15.2 | 16.8 | 18.6 | 20.7 | 12.0 | 13.0 | 14.1 | 15.3 | 16.6 | 18.2 | 19.9 |
| 53 | 11.7 | 12.7 | 13.9 | 15.3 | 16.8 | 18.6 | 20.8 | 12.0 | 13.0 | 14.1 | 15.3 | 16.6 | 18.2 | 20.0 |
| 54 | 11.7 | 12.7 | 13.9 | 15.3 | 16.8 | 18.7 | 20.8 | 12.0 | 13.0 | 14.0 | 15.3 | 16.6 | 18.2 | 20.0 |
| 55 | 11.7 | 12.7 | 13.9 | 15.3 | 16.8 | 18.7 | 20.9 | 12.0 | 13.0 | 14.0 | 15.2 | 16.6 | 18.2 | 20.0 |
| 56 | 11.7 | 12.7 | 13.9 | 15.3 | 16.8 | 18.7 | 20.9 | 12.0 | 12.9 | 14.0 | 15.2 | 16.6 | 18.2 | 20.1 |
| 57 | 11.7 | 12.7 | 13.9 | 15.3 | 16.9 | 18.7 | 21.0 | 12.0 | 12.9 | 14.0 | 15.2 | 16.6 | 18.2 | 20.1 |
| 58 | 11.7 | 12.7 | 13.9 | 15.3 | 16.9 | 18.8 | 21.0 | 12.0 | 12.9 | 14.0 | 15.2 | 16.6 | 18.3 | 20.2 |
| 59 | 11.6 | 12.7 | 13.9 | 15.3 | 16.9 | 18.8 | 21.0 | 12.0 | 12.9 | 14.0 | 15.2 | 16.6 | 18.3 | 20.2 |

WHO: MGRS

## Annexure 18

Head circumference for age (cm) in girls and boys 0–5 years of age

| Age (mo) | BMI Girls −3 SD | −2 SD | −1 SD | Median | 1 SD | 2 SD | 3 SD | BMI Boys −3 SD | −2 SD | −1 SD | Median | 1 SD | 2 SD | 3 SD |
|---|---|---|---|---|---|---|---|---|---|---|---|---|---|---|
| 0 | 30.3 | 31.5 | 32.7 | 33.9 | 35.1 | 36.2 | 37.4 | 30.7 | 31.9 | 33.2 | 34.5 | 35.7 | 37.0 | 38.3 |
| 1 | 33.0 | 34.2 | 35.4 | 36.5 | 37.7 | 38.9 | 40.1 | 33.8 | 34.9 | 36.1 | 37.3 | 38.4 | 39.6 | 40.8 |
| 2 | 34.6 | 35.8 | 37.0 | 38.3 | 39.5 | 40.7 | 41.9 | 35.6 | 36.8 | 38.0 | 39.1 | 40.3 | 41.5 | 42.6 |
| 3 | 35.8 | 37.1 | 38.3 | 39.5 | 40.8 | 42.0 | 43.3 | 37.0 | 38.1 | 39.3 | 40.5 | 41.7 | 42.9 | 44.1 |
| 4 | 36.8 | 38.1 | 39.3 | 40.6 | 41.8 | 43.1 | 44.4 | 38.0 | 39.2 | 40.4 | 41.6 | 42.8 | 44.0 | 45.2 |
| 5 | 37.6 | 38.9 | 40.2 | 41.5 | 42.7 | 44.0 | 45.3 | 38.9 | 40.1 | 41.4 | 42.6 | 43.8 | 45.0 | 46.2 |
| 6 | 38.3 | 39.6 | 40.9 | 42.2 | 43.5 | 44.8 | 46.1 | 39.7 | 40.9 | 42.1 | 43.3 | 44.6 | 45.8 | 47.0 |
| 7 | 38.9 | 40.2 | 41.5 | 42.8 | 44.1 | 45.5 | 46.8 | 40.3 | 41.5 | 42.7 | 44.0 | 45.2 | 46.4 | 47.7 |
| 8 | 39.4 | 40.7 | 42.0 | 43.4 | 44.7 | 46.0 | 47.4 | 40.8 | 42.0 | 43.3 | 44.5 | 45.8 | 47.0 | 48.3 |
| 9 | 39.8 | 41.2 | 42.5 | 43.8 | 45.2 | 46.5 | 47.8 | 41.2 | 42.5 | 43.7 | 45.0 | 46.3 | 47.5 | 48.8 |
| 10 | 40.2 | 41.5 | 42.9 | 44.2 | 45.6 | 46.9 | 48.3 | 41.6 | 42.9 | 44.1 | 45.4 | 46.7 | 47.9 | 49.2 |
| 11 | 40.5 | 41.9 | 43.2 | 44.6 | 45.9 | 47.3 | 48.6 | 41.9 | 43.2 | 44.5 | 45.8 | 47.0 | 48.3 | 49.6 |
| 12 | 40.8 | 42.2 | 43.5 | 44.9 | 46.3 | 47.6 | 49.0 | 42.2 | 43.5 | 44.8 | 46.1 | 47.4 | 48.6 | 49.9 |
| 13 | 41.1 | 42.4 | 43.8 | 45.2 | 46.5 | 47.9 | 49.3 | 42.5 | 43.8 | 45.0 | 46.3 | 47.6 | 48.9 | 50.2 |
| 14 | 41.3 | 42.7 | 44.1 | 45.4 | 46.8 | 48.2 | 49.5 | 42.7 | 44.0 | 45.3 | 46.6 | 47.9 | 49.2 | 50.5 |
| 15 | 41.5 | 42.9 | 44.3 | 45.7 | 47.0 | 48.4 | 49.8 | 42.9 | 44.2 | 45.5 | 46.8 | 48.1 | 49.4 | 50.7 |
| 16 | 41.7 | 43.1 | 44.5 | 45.9 | 47.2 | 48.6 | 50.0 | 43.1 | 44.4 | 45.7 | 47.0 | 48.3 | 49.6 | 51.0 |
| 17 | 41.9 | 43.3 | 44.7 | 46.1 | 47.4 | 48.8 | 50.2 | 43.2 | 44.6 | 45.9 | 47.2 | 48.5 | 49.8 | 51.2 |
| 18 | 42.1 | 43.5 | 44.9 | 46.2 | 47.6 | 49.0 | 50.4 | 43.4 | 44.7 | 46.0 | 47.4 | 48.7 | 50.0 | 51.4 |
| 19 | 42.3 | 43.6 | 45.0 | 46.4 | 47.8 | 49.2 | 50.6 | 43.5 | 44.9 | 46.2 | 47.5 | 48.9 | 50.2 | 51.5 |
| 20 | 42.4 | 43.8 | 45.2 | 46.6 | 48.0 | 49.4 | 50.7 | 43.7 | 45.0 | 46.4 | 47.7 | 49.0 | 50.4 | 51.7 |
| 21 | 42.6 | 44.0 | 45.3 | 46.7 | 48.1 | 49.5 | 50.9 | 43.8 | 45.2 | 46.5 | 47.8 | 49.2 | 50.5 | 51.9 |
| 22 | 42.7 | 44.1 | 45.5 | 46.9 | 48.3 | 49.7 | 51.1 | 43.9 | 45.3 | 46.6 | 48.0 | 49.3 | 50.7 | 52.0 |
| 23 | 42.9 | 44.3 | 45.6 | 47.0 | 48.4 | 49.8 | 51.2 | 44.1 | 45.4 | 46.8 | 48.1 | 49.5 | 50.8 | 52.2 |
| 24 | 43.0 | 44.4 | 45.8 | 47.2 | 48.6 | 50.0 | 51.4 | 44.2 | 45.5 | 46.9 | 48.3 | 49.6 | 51.0 | 52.3 |
| 25 | 43.1 | 44.5 | 45.9 | 47.3 | 48.7 | 50.1 | 51.5 | 44.3 | 45.6 | 47.0 | 48.4 | 49.7 | 51.1 | 52.5 |
| 26 | 43.3 | 44.7 | 46.1 | 47.5 | 48.9 | 50.3 | 51.7 | 44.4 | 45.8 | 47.1 | 48.5 | 49.9 | 51.2 | 52.6 |
| 27 | 43.4 | 44.8 | 46.2 | 47.6 | 49.0 | 50.4 | 51.8 | 44.5 | 45.9 | 47.2 | 48.6 | 50.0 | 51.4 | 52.7 |
| 28 | 43.5 | 44.9 | 46.3 | 47.7 | 49.1 | 50.5 | 51.9 | 44.6 | 46.0 | 47.3 | 48.7 | 50.1 | 51.5 | 52.9 |
| 29 | 43.6 | 45.0 | 46.4 | 47.8 | 49.2 | 50.6 | 52.0 | 44.7 | 46.1 | 47.4 | 48.8 | 50.2 | 51.6 | 53.0 |
| 30 | 43.7 | 45.1 | 46.5 | 47.9 | 49.3 | 50.7 | 52.2 | 44.8 | 46.1 | 47.5 | 48.9 | 50.3 | 51.7 | 53.1 |
| 31 | 43.8 | 45.2 | 46.6 | 48.0 | 49.4 | 50.9 | 52.3 | 44.8 | 46.2 | 47.6 | 49.0 | 50.4 | 51.8 | 53.2 |
| 32 | 43.9 | 45.3 | 46.7 | 48.1 | 49.6 | 51.0 | 52.4 | 44.9 | 46.3 | 47.7 | 49.1 | 50.5 | 51.9 | 53.3 |
| 33 | 44.0 | 45.4 | 46.8 | 48.2 | 49.7 | 51.1 | 52.5 | 45.0 | 46.4 | 47.8 | 49.2 | 50.6 | 52.0 | 53.4 |
| 34 | 44.1 | 45.5 | 46.9 | 48.3 | 49.7 | 51.2 | 52.6 | 45.1 | 46.5 | 47.9 | 49.3 | 50.7 | 52.1 | 53.5 |
| 35 | 44.2 | 45.6 | 47.0 | 48.4 | 49.8 | 51.2 | 52.7 | 45.1 | 46.6 | 48.0 | 49.4 | 50.8 | 52.2 | 53.6 |
| 36 | 44.3 | 45.7 | 47.1 | 48.5 | 49.9 | 51.3 | 52.7 | 45.2 | 46.6 | 48.0 | 49.5 | 50.9 | 52.3 | 53.7 |
| 37 | 44.4 | 45.8 | 47.2 | 48.6 | 50.0 | 51.4 | 52.8 | 45.3 | 46.7 | 48.1 | 49.5 | 51.0 | 52.4 | 53.8 |
| 38 | 44.4 | 45.8 | 47.3 | 48.7 | 50.1 | 51.5 | 52.9 | 45.3 | 46.8 | 48.2 | 49.6 | 51.0 | 52.5 | 53.9 |
| 39 | 44.5 | 45.9 | 47.3 | 48.7 | 50.2 | 51.6 | 53.0 | 45.4 | 46.8 | 48.2 | 49.7 | 51.1 | 52.5 | 54.0 |
| 40 | 44.6 | 46.0 | 47.4 | 48.8 | 50.2 | 51.7 | 53.1 | 45.4 | 46.9 | 48.3 | 49.7 | 51.2 | 52.6 | 54.1 |
| 41 | 44.6 | 46.1 | 47.5 | 48.9 | 50.3 | 51.7 | 53.1 | 45.5 | 46.9 | 48.4 | 49.8 | 51.3 | 52.7 | 54.1 |
| 42 | 44.7 | 46.1 | 47.5 | 49.0 | 50.4 | 51.8 | 53.2 | 45.5 | 47.0 | 48.4 | 49.9 | 51.3 | 52.8 | 54.2 |
| 43 | 44.8 | 46.2 | 47.6 | 49.0 | 50.4 | 51.9 | 53.3 | 45.6 | 47.0 | 48.5 | 49.9 | 51.4 | 52.8 | 54.3 |
| 44 | 44.8 | 46.3 | 47.7 | 49.1 | 50.5 | 51.9 | 53.3 | 45.6 | 47.1 | 48.5 | 50.0 | 51.4 | 52.9 | 54.3 |
| 45 | 44.9 | 46.3 | 47.7 | 49.2 | 50.6 | 52.0 | 53.4 | 45.7 | 47.1 | 48.6 | 50.1 | 51.5 | 53.0 | 54.4 |
| 46 | 45.0 | 46.4 | 47.8 | 49.2 | 50.6 | 52.1 | 53.5 | 45.7 | 47.2 | 48.7 | 50.1 | 51.6 | 53.0 | 54.5 |
| 47 | 45.0 | 46.4 | 47.9 | 49.3 | 50.7 | 52.1 | 53.5 | 45.8 | 47.2 | 48.7 | 50.2 | 51.6 | 53.1 | 54.5 |
| 48 | 45.1 | 46.5 | 47.9 | 49.3 | 50.8 | 52.2 | 53.6 | 45.8 | 47.3 | 48.7 | 50.2 | 51.7 | 53.1 | 54.6 |
| 49 | 45.1 | 46.5 | 48.0 | 49.4 | 50.8 | 52.2 | 53.6 | 45.9 | 47.3 | 48.8 | 50.3 | 51.7 | 53.2 | 54.7 |
| 50 | 45.2 | 46.6 | 48.0 | 49.4 | 50.9 | 52.3 | 53.7 | 45.9 | 47.4 | 48.8 | 50.3 | 51.8 | 53.2 | 54.7 |
| 51 | 45.2 | 46.7 | 48.1 | 49.5 | 50.9 | 52.3 | 53.8 | 45.9 | 47.4 | 48.9 | 50.4 | 51.8 | 53.3 | 54.8 |
| 52 | 45.3 | 46.7 | 48.1 | 49.5 | 51.0 | 52.4 | 53.8 | 46.0 | 47.5 | 48.9 | 50.4 | 51.9 | 53.4 | 54.8 |
| 53 | 45.3 | 46.8 | 48.2 | 49.6 | 51.0 | 52.4 | 53.9 | 46.0 | 47.5 | 49.0 | 50.4 | 51.9 | 53.4 | 54.9 |
| 54 | 45.4 | 46.8 | 48.2 | 49.6 | 51.1 | 52.5 | 53.9 | 46.1 | 47.5 | 49.0 | 50.5 | 52.0 | 53.5 | 54.9 |
| 55 | 45.4 | 46.9 | 48.3 | 49.7 | 51.1 | 52.5 | 54.0 | 46.1 | 47.6 | 49.1 | 50.5 | 52.0 | 53.5 | 55.0 |
| 56 | 45.5 | 46.9 | 48.3 | 49.7 | 51.2 | 52.6 | 54.0 | 46.1 | 47.6 | 49.1 | 50.6 | 52.1 | 53.5 | 55.0 |
| 57 | 45.5 | 46.9 | 48.4 | 49.8 | 51.2 | 52.6 | 54.1 | 46.2 | 47.6 | 49.1 | 50.6 | 52.1 | 53.6 | 55.1 |
| 58 | 45.6 | 47.0 | 48.4 | 49.8 | 51.3 | 52.7 | 54.1 | 46.2 | 47.7 | 49.2 | 50.7 | 52.1 | 53.6 | 55.1 |
| 59 | 45.6 | 47.0 | 48.5 | 49.9 | 51.3 | 52.7 | 54.1 | 46.2 | 47.7 | 49.2 | 50.7 | 52.2 | 53.7 | 55.2 |
| 60 | 45.7 | 47.1 | 48.5 | 49.9 | 51.3 | 52.8 | 54.2 | 46.3 | 47.7 | 49.2 | 50.7 | 52.2 | 53.7 | 55.2 |

WHO: MGRS

## Annexure 19

Boys aged 5 to 18 years old: IAP charts for weight, height, body mass index (percentiles) (reproduced with permission from Indian Pediatr 2015;52:47–55)

| Age (years) | Height (cm) | | | | | | Weight (kg) | | | | | | Body mass index | | | | | | |
|---|---|---|---|---|---|---|---|---|---|---|---|---|---|---|---|---|---|---|---|
| | 3rd | 10th | 50th | 90th | 97th | SD | 3rd | 10th | 50th | 90th | 97th | SD | 3th | 5th | 10th | 50th | 23rd AE | 27th AE | SD |
| 5.0 | 99.0 | 102.3 | 108.9 | 115.9 | 119.4 | 5.7 | 13.2 | 14.3 | 17.1 | 21.3 | 24.2 | 3.2 | 12.1 | 12.4 | 12.8 | 14.7 | 15.7 | 17.5 | 1.6 |
| 5.5 | 101.6 | 105.0 | 111.9 | 119.0 | 122.7 | 5.3 | 13.8 | 15.0 | 18.2 | 22.9 | 26.1 | 2.9 | 12.2 | 12.4 | 12.9 | 14.8 | 15.8 | 17.6 | 1.5 |
| 6.0 | 104.2 | 107.7 | 114.8 | 122.2 | 126.0 | 5.6 | 14.5 | 15.8 | 19.3 | 24.6 | 28.3 | 3.6 | 12.2 | 12.5 | 12.9 | 14.9 | 16.0 | 17.8 | 1.8 |
| 6.5 | 106.8 | 110.4 | 117.8 | 125.4 | 129.3 | 5.5 | 15.3 | 16.8 | 20.7 | 26.6 | 30.8 | 3.8 | 12.3 | 12.5 | 13.0 | 15.0 | 16.1 | 18.0 | 1.8 |
| 7.0 | 109.3 | 113.0 | 120.7 | 128.6 | 132.6 | 5.9 | 16.0 | 17.6 | 21.9 | 28.6 | 33.4 | 4.2 | 12.3 | 12.6 | 13.1 | 15.1 | 16.3 | 18.2 | 1.9 |
| 7.5 | 111.8 | 115.7 | 123.5 | 131.7 | 135.9 | 5.7 | 16.7 | 18.5 | 23.3 | 30.8 | 36.2 | 4.9 | 12.4 | 12.7 | 13.2 | 15.3 | 16.5 | 18.5 | 2.2 |
| 8.0 | 114.3 | 118.2 | 126.4 | 134.8 | 139.1 | 6.3 | 17.5 | 19.5 | 24.8 | 33.2 | 39.4 | 5.7 | 12.5 | 12.8 | 13.3 | 15.5 | 16.7 | 18.8 | 2.5 |
| 8.5 | 116.7 | 120.8 | 129.1 | 137.8 | 142.2 | 6.1 | 18.3 | 20.5 | 26.4 | 35.7 | 42.6 | 6.5 | 12.6 | 12.9 | 13.4 | 15.7 | 17.0 | 19.2 | 2.8 |
| 9.0 | 119.0 | 123.2 | 131.8 | 140.7 | 145.3 | 6.4 | 19.1 | 21.5 | 27.9 | 38.0 | 45.5 | 6.3 | 12.7 | 13.0 | 13.5 | 15.9 | 17.3 | 19.6 | 2.6 |
| 9.5 | 121.3 | 125.6 | 134.5 | 143.7 | 148.3 | 6.4 | 19.9 | 22.4 | 29.4 | 40.5 | 48.6 | 7.0 | 12.8 | 13.1 | 13.7 | 16.2 | 17.6 | 20.1 | 2.8 |
| 10.0 | 123.6 | 128.1 | 137.2 | 146.6 | 151.4 | 6.8 | 20.7 | 23.5 | 31.1 | 43.0 | 51.8 | 7.9 | 12.9 | 13.2 | 13.8 | 16.4 | 18.0 | 20.5 | 3.1 |
| 10.5 | 125.9 | 130.5 | 139.9 | 149.5 | 154.4 | 6.5 | 21.6 | 24.6 | 32.8 | 45.8 | 55.2 | 8.3 | 13.0 | 13.3 | 14.0 | 16.7 | 18.3 | 21.0 | 3.2 |
| 11.0 | 128.2 | 133.0 | 142.7 | 152.5 | 157.5 | 7.6 | 22.6 | 25.9 | 34.7 | 48.7 | 58.7 | 8.9 | 13.1 | 13.5 | 14.1 | 17.0 | 18.7 | 21.5 | 3.2 |
| 11.5 | 130.7 | 135.6 | 145.5 | 155.6 | 160.6 | 7.3 | 23.8 | 27.3 | 36.9 | 51.8 | 62.5 | 9.3 | 13.2 | 13.6 | 14.3 | 17.3 | 19.1 | 22.1 | 3.3 |
| 12.0 | 133.2 | 138.3 | 148.4 | 158.6 | 163.7 | 8.1 | 24.9 | 28.7 | 39.0 | 54.8 | 66.1 | 10.0 | 13.3 | 13.8 | 14.5 | 17.7 | 19.5 | 22.6 | 3.4 |
| 12.5 | 135.7 | 141.0 | 151.4 | 161.7 | 166.8 | 7.9 | 26.1 | 30.2 | 41.2 | 57.8 | 69.5 | 10.6 | 13.5 | 13.9 | 14.6 | 17.9 | 19.8 | 23.0 | 3.6 |
| 13.0 | 138.3 | 143.7 | 154.3 | 164.7 | 169.9 | 9.0 | 27.5 | 31.8 | 43.3 | 60.7 | 72.6 | 11.3 | 13.6 | 14.0 | 14.8 | 18.2 | 20.2 | 23.4 | 3.5 |
| 13.5 | 140.9 | 146.4 | 157.2 | 167.6 | 172.7 | 8.4 | 29.0 | 33.6 | 45.7 | 63.6 | 75.6 | 11.4 | 13.7 | 14.2 | 14.9 | 18.5 | 20.5 | 23.8 | 3.7 |
| 14.0 | 143.4 | 149.0 | 159.9 | 170.3 | 175.4 | 9.0 | 30.7 | 35.5 | 48.2 | 66.3 | 78.3 | 12.1 | 13.8 | 14.3 | 15.1 | 18.7 | 20.8 | 24.2 | 3.7 |
| 14.5 | 145.8 | 151.5 | 162.3 | 172.7 | 177.7 | 7.8 | 32.6 | 37.7 | 50.8 | 69.1 | 80.9 | 11.6 | 14.0 | 14.5 | 15.3 | 19.0 | 21.1 | 24.5 | 3.5 |
| 15.0 | 148.0 | 153.7 | 164.5 | 174.8 | 179.7 | 7.9 | 34.5 | 39.8 | 53.1 | 71.5 | 83.1 | 12.1 | 14.2 | 14.7 | 15.5 | 19.3 | 21.4 | 24.9 | 3.7 |
| 15.5 | 150.0 | 155.7 | 166.5 | 176.5 | 181.4 | 6.6 | 36.1 | 41.6 | 55.2 | 73.4 | 84.7 | 11.2 | 14.4 | 14.9 | 15.8 | 19.6 | 21.7 | 25.2 | 3.4 |
| 16.0 | 151.8 | 157.4 | 168.1 | 178.0 | 182.7 | 7.2 | 37.5 | 43.1 | 56.8 | 74.8 | 85.8 | 12.2 | 14.6 | 15.1 | 16.0 | 19.9 | 22.0 | 25.5 | 3.7 |
| 16.5 | 153.4 | 159.1 | 169.6 | 179.3 | 183.8 | 6.7 | 38.7 | 44.4 | 58.2 | 76.1 | 86.8 | 12.6 | 14.9 | 15.4 | 16.3 | 20.2 | 22.4 | 25.8 | 3.8 |
| 17.0 | 155.0 | 160.6 | 171.0 | 180.4 | 184.8 | 6.9 | 39.8 | 45.6 | 59.5 | 77.1 | 87.5 | 12.3 | 15.1 | 15.6 | 16.6 | 20.5 | 22.6 | 26.0 | 3.8 |
| 17.5 | 156.6 | 162.1 | 172.3 | 181.5 | 185.8 | 6.1 | 40.3 | 46.7 | 60.6 | 77.8 | 88.0 | 12.3 | 15.4 | 15.9 | 16.8 | 20.8 | 22.9 | 26.3 | 3.6 |
| 18.0 | 158.1 | 163.6 | 173.6 | 182.5 | 186.7 | 6.9 | 41.8 | 47.7 | 61.6 | 78.6 | 88.4 | 11.3 | 15.6 | 16.2 | 17.1 | 21.1 | 23.2 | 26.6 | 3.2 |

23rd AE: equivalent to BMI of 23 in adults (overweight); 27th AE: equivalent to BMI of 27 in adults (obesity)

IAP

## Annexure 20

Girls aged 5 to 18 years old: IAP charts for weight, height, body mass index (percentiles) (reproduced with permission from Indian Pediatr 2015;52:47–55)

| Age (years) | Height (cm) | | | | | | Weight (kg) | | | | | | Body Mass Index | | | | | | |
|---|---|---|---|---|---|---|---|---|---|---|---|---|---|---|---|---|---|---|---|
| | 3rd | 10th | 50th | 90th | 97th | SD | 3rd | 10th | 50th | 90th | 97th | SD | 3rd | 5th | 10th | 50th | 23rd AE | 27th AE | SD |
| 5.0 | 97.2 | 100.5 | 107.5 | 115.2 | 119.3 | 5.4 | 12.3 | 13.4 | 16.4 | 21.3 | 25.0 | 2.5 | 11.9 | 12.1 | 12.5 | 14.3 | 15.5 | 18.0 | 1.4 |
| 5.5 | 99.8 | 103.2 | 110.5 | 118.3 | 122.5 | 5.7 | 13.0 | 14.3 | 17.6 | 22.9 | 27.0 | 3.5 | 11.9 | 12.2 | 12.6 | 14.4 | 15.7 | 18.3 | 1.7 |
| 6.0 | 102.3 | 106.0 | 113.5 | 121.5 | 125.6 | 5.8 | 13.7 | 15.1 | 18.7 | 24.6 | 29.1 | 3.4 | 12.0 | 12.2 | 12.7 | 14.5 | 15.9 | 18.6 | 1.7 |
| 6.5 | 104.9 | 108.7 | 116.5 | 124.6 | 128.7 | 5.5 | 14.4 | 15.9 | 19.9 | 26.3 | 31.2 | 4.1 | 12.1 | 12.3 | 12.8 | 14.7 | 16.1 | 18.9 | 2.0 |
| 7.0 | 107.4 | 111.4 | 119.4 | 127.7 | 131.9 | 6.1 | 15.1 | 16.8 | 21.2 | 28.2 | 33.4 | 4.4 | 12.1 | 12.4 | 12.8 | 14.9 | 16.4 | 19.3 | 2.1 |
| 7.5 | 110.0 | 114.1 | 122.4 | 130.8 | 135.0 | 6.0 | 15.9 | 17.7 | 22.5 | 30.1 | 35.7 | 4.8 | 12.2 | 12.5 | 12.9 | 15.1 | 16.6 | 19.7 | 2.2 |
| 8.0 | 112.6 | 116.8 | 125.4 | 133.9 | 138.1 | 6.2 | 16.7 | 18.7 | 24.0 | 32.2 | 38.1 | 5.2 | 12.3 | 12.6 | 13.1 | 15.3 | 16.9 | 20.1 | 2.3 |
| 8.5 | 115.2 | 119.6 | 128.4 | 137.0 | 141.3 | 6.8 | 17.5 | 19.7 | 25.5 | 34.4 | 40.7 | 6.4 | 12.3 | 12.7 | 13.2 | 15.6 | 17.2 | 20.5 | 2.7 |
| 9.0 | 117.8 | 122.4 | 131.4 | 140.2 | 144.5 | 6.9 | 18.5 | 20.9 | 27.2 | 36.7 | 43.4 | 6.4 | 12.4 | 12.8 | 13.3 | 15.8 | 17.6 | 21.0 | 2.7 |
| 9.5 | 120.5 | 125.2 | 134.4 | 143.3 | 147.6 | 6.6 | 19.5 | 22.1 | 29.0 | 39.3 | 46.3 | 6.9 | 12.5 | 12.9 | 13.5 | 16.1 | 18.0 | 21.4 | 2.8 |
| 10.0 | 123.3 | 128.1 | 137.4 | 146.4 | 150.8 | 7.8 | 20.7 | 23.5 | 31.0 | 42.0 | 49.4 | 7.7 | 12.7 | 13.1 | 13.7 | 16.5 | 18.4 | 21.9 | 2.9 |
| 10.5 | 126.1 | 130.9 | 140.4 | 149.5 | 153.9 | 7.3 | 22.0 | 25.1 | 33.2 | 44.8 | 52.6 | 8.3 | 12.8 | 13.2 | 13.9 | 16.8 | 18.8 | 22.5 | 3.1 |
| 11.0 | 128.8 | 133.7 | 143.3 | 152.4 | 156.8 | 7.9 | 23.3 | 26.7 | 35.4 | 47.7 | 55.9 | 8.5 | 13.0 | 13.4 | 14.1 | 17.2 | 19.3 | 23.0 | 3.1 |
| 11.5 | 131.5 | 136.4 | 145.9 | 155.1 | 159.6 | 7.1 | 24.8 | 28.4 | 37.6 | 50.6 | 59.1 | 9.1 | 13.2 | 13.7 | 14.4 | 17.6 | 19.8 | 23.6 | 3.3 |
| 12.0 | 134.0 | 138.9 | 148.4 | 157.5 | 162.0 | 7.0 | 26.2 | 30.0 | 39.8 | 53.4 | 62.1 | 9.0 | 13.4 | 13.9 | 14.7 | 18.0 | 20.2 | 24.1 | 3.2 |
| 12.5 | 136.3 | 141.1 | 150.5 | 159.6 | 164.1 | 6.7 | 27.6 | 31.6 | 41.8 | 55.8 | 64.8 | 9.7 | 13.7 | 14.2 | 15.0 | 18.4 | 20.7 | 24.7 | 3.3 |
| 13.0 | 138.2 | 142.9 | 152.2 | 161.3 | 165.9 | 6.9 | 28.9 | 33.1 | 43.6 | 57.9 | 67.1 | 9.4 | 13.9 | 14.4 | 15.2 | 18.8 | 21.1 | 25.2 | 3.2 |
| 13.5 | 139.9 | 144.5 | 153.6 | 162.7 | 167.2 | 6.0 | 30.2 | 34.4 | 45.1 | 59.7 | 69.0 | 9.8 | 14.1 | 14.6 | 15.5 | 19.1 | 21.5 | 25.6 | 3.5 |
| 14.0 | 141.3 | 145.8 | 154.7 | 163.7 | 168.2 | 6.6 | 31.3 | 35.6 | 46.4 | 61.1 | 70.4 | 9.6 | 14.3 | 14.9 | 15.7 | 19.4 | 21.8 | 25.9 | 3.4 |
| 14.5 | 142.4 | 146.8 | 155.5 | 164.5 | 169.0 | 5.9 | 32.3 | 36.6 | 47.5 | 62.2 | 71.4 | 9.4 | 14.5 | 15.1 | 16.0 | 19.7 | 22.0 | 26.2 | 3.3 |
| 15.0 | 143.3 | 147.5 | 156.1 | 165.0 | 169.5 | 6.6 | 33.1 | 37.5 | 48.4 | 62.9 | 72.1 | 9.6 | 14.7 | 15.2 | 16.1 | 19.9 | 22.3 | 26.3 | 3.4 |
| 15.5 | 144.1 | 148.1 | 156.6 | 165.3 | 169.8 | 5.9 | 34.0 | 38.3 | 49.1 | 63.5 | 72.5 | 8.7 | 14.9 | 15.4 | 16.3 | 20.1 | 22.4 | 26.4 | 3.1 |
| 16.0 | 144.7 | 148.6 | 156.9 | 165.6 | 170.1 | 6.1 | 34.7 | 39.1 | 49.7 | 64.0 | 72.8 | 8.7 | 15.0 | 15.6 | 16.5 | 20.3 | 22.6 | 26.5 | 3.1 |
| 16.5 | 145.2 | 149.1 | 157.2 | 165.7 | 170.2 | 6.4 | 35.5 | 39.8 | 50.3 | 64.4 | 73.1 | 9.2 | 15.2 | 15.8 | 16.7 | 20.4 | 22.8 | 26.6 | 3.2 |
| 17.0 | 145.7 | 149.5 | 157.4 | 165.9 | 170.4 | 6.5 | 36.2 | 40.5 | 50.9 | 64.7 | 73.3 | 8.8 | 15.4 | 16.0 | 16.9 | 20.6 | 22.9 | 26.7 | 3.0 |
| 17.5 | 146.2 | 149.8 | 157.6 | 166.0 | 170.5 | 6.7 | 36.9 | 41.1 | 51.5 | 65.0 | 73.4 | 9.5 | 15.5 | 16.1 | 17.1 | 20.8 | 23.1 | 26.7 | 3.1 |

23rd AE: equivalent to BMI of 23 in adults (overweight); 27th AE: equivalent to BMI of 27 in adults (obesity)

IAP

# Index


Abdominal pain 303
causes of 304
chronic 308
Abdominal paracentesis 782
Abetalipoproteinemia 568
Acetaminophen poisoning 756
clinical stages 756
N-acetylcysteine 753
treatment 756
Acid–base equilibrium
buffers 70, 71
regulation of 69
Acne vulgaris 725
Acrodermatitis enteropathica 115, 742
Acute appendicitis 303
Acute diarrhea 309
assessment for dehydration 310
clinical findings 310
etiology 309
guidelines for treating 311
home available fluids 312
laboratory investigations 311
management 311, 313
prevention 314
WHO–ORS 312
Acute flaccid paralysis 611
surveillance 611
Acute kidney injury 511
continuous renal replacement therapies 515
definition and classification 511
dialysis 515
evaluation 512
hemodialysis 515
incidence and etiology 511
management 513
newborn 516
pathophysiology 511
peritoneal dialysis 515
slow low-efficiency dialysis 516
Acute pericarditis 473
Acute respiratory distress syndrome 418
clinical features 419
pathogenesis 418
Adolescent health care 53
adolescent-friendly health services 53
Adolescents 48, 50
contraception 54
environmental and social challenges 52
genital infections 51
health problems 50
immunization 54
infections 51
legal age definitions 52
lifestyle diseases 52
nutrition 50
problems specific to females 51
sexual violence 53
sexually transmitted infections 51
sleep disturbances 51
substance abuse 52
transition to adult care 54
vulnerability 52
Adoption 791
Adrenal insufficiency 546
Adrenoleukodystrophy 604
Advanced life support 764
cardiopulmonary resuscitation 766
Adverse events following immunization 212
Aldosterone excess 545
Alopecia areata 726
Amebiasis
clinical features 281
diagnosis 282
treatment 282
Amebic meningoencephalitis 283
granulomatous 284
primary 283
Anemia 350
approach to
macrocytic 353
microcytic 352
normocytic 353
clinical features 351
diagnosis 351
investigations 352
iron deficiency 354
megaloblastic 355
Angioedema 732
Anion gap 71
Anorectal malformations 177
Antenatal hydronephrosis 530
Anthelmintics 846
Antiarrhythmics 841
Antiasthma agents 851
Anticoagulants 848
Antidepressants 856
Antiemetics 848
Antiepileptics 856
Antifungal agents 843
Antihistaminics 849
Antihypertensives 850
Antimicrobials 842
Antiprotozoal 847
Antipyretics 840
Antitoxins 850
Antiviral agents 847
Aortic regurgitation 465
Aortic stenosis 453
Apgar score 120
Aplastic anemia
clinical features 365
congenital syndromes 366
differential diagnosis 365
evaluation 367
treatment 367
Apnea, newborn 160, 161
Arnold-Chiari malformations 575
Arterial catheterization 779
Arthritis 650
approach to diagnosis 650
DMARDs 654
iridocyclitis 654
juvenile idiopathic 651
Legg-Calvé-Perthes disease 651
reactive 650
septic 650
systemic JIA 652
transient synovitis 650
treatment 653
tubercular 650
Ascites
causes 337
evaluation 337
treatment 337
Aspergillosis 273
Asphyxia 119, 163
consequences 162
hypoxic ischemic encephalopathy 162
perinatal 161
Ataxia 598, 599
Ataxia-telangiectasia 578
Atopic dermatitis
clinical features 723
treatment 724
Atrial septal defect 437
Attention deficit hyperactivity disorder 43
Autism spectrum disorder 42
Autoimmune liver disease
diagnosis 340
management 340
Autoinflammatory diseases 225, 661
Ayushman Bharat initiative 3

Bartter syndrome 525
Basic life support 762
airway 762
assessment 762
bag and mask ventilation 764
chest compression 763
circulation 762
foreign body airway obstruction 764
BCG vaccine 190, 192
Biotin 112
Birth injury 175, 176
Blood transfusions 375, 772
adverse effects 774
choice of blood group 773
cryoprecipitate 375, 774
fresh frozen plasma 375, 773
platelet transfusion 375, 773
red cell transfusion 773
transfusion reactions 775
Bone age 7
Bone marrow aspiration, biopsy 784
Brain abscess 591
Brain tumors 590, 642

Breast milk 100, 142
banking 147
Breastfeeding 81, 142
benefits 142
composition of breast milk 144
exclusive 81
expressed breast milk 146, 153
physiology 143
problems 146, 147
techniques 145
Breath holding spells 46
Bronchial asthma 407
acute exacerbation 415
clinical features 408
differential diagnosis 408
grading severity 415
home management 414
inhalational devices 412
investigations 418
life-threatening 415
management 409, 411
monitoring therapy 413
pathophysiology 407
pharmacotherapy 409, 410
recurrent wheeze 416
triggers of attack 407
Bronchiectasis 416
Bronchiolitis 406
Brucellosis 261
Burns 746
classification 746
first aid 747
fluid replacement 748
Lund and Browder chart 747
wound care and topical therapy 748
Button batteries 749

Calcium 65, 114
hypercalcemia 67, 542
causes 68
clinical features 68
therapy 68
hypocalcemia 66, 541
causes 67
management 67
physiology 65
regulation of 66
Candidiasis 272, 389, 740
Capillary blood (heel prick) 778
Cardiomyopathies 470
anomalous left coronary artery from pulmonary artery 471
dilated 472
hypertrophic 472
restrictive 471
Cardiovascular disease, prevention 485
Catheterization of bladder 783
Celiac disease 318
diagnosis 319
presentation 318
treatment 320
Central venous cannulation 777
Cerebral palsy 578
Cestodes 289
echinococcosis (hydatid disease) 291
hymenolepiasis 291
taeniasis and cysticercosis 289, 563
treatment 290
Chikungunya
clinical features 241
diagnosis 241
epidemiology 240
Child guidance clinics 38
Child health 3, 4
Child mortality 2, 3
Choledochal cyst 305
Cholesteatoma 381
Chromosomal disorders 663
chromosomal microarray 666
Down syndrome 666
enzyme replacement therapy 674
genomic imprinting 665
karyotyping 665
maternal serum screening 676
mechanisms of chromosomal anomalies 663
mitochondrial inheritance 672
newborn screening 676
polygenic inheritance 674
prevention of genetic disorders 675
prevention of neural tube defects 676
single gene disorders 670
therapy for genetic disorders 674
Turner syndrome 668
Chronic bullous diseases of childhood 730
Chronic constrictive pericarditis 474
Chronic cough, causes 419
Chronic diarrhea 317
approach 317
causes of 317
celiac disease 318
drug induced 322
inflammatory bowel disease 322
Chronic kidney disease 518
anemia 519
clinical features 518
diet 519
growth 519
hypertension 519
investigations 518
long-term care 520
management 518
mineral bone disease 519
retarding progression 519
Chronic liver disease
clinical features 334
complications 336
etiology 334, 336
hepatic encephalopathy 336
hepatorenal syndrome 336
nutrition failure 336
Chronic myeloid leukemia 627
juvenile 628
Chronic otitis media 381
Cleft lip, palate 178, 389
Coarctation of aorta 455
Cobalamin (vitamin $B_{12}$) 112
deficiency 112
metabolism 112
requirements 112
sources 112
treatment 113
Coma 571, 592
AVPU scale 571
brain death 594
Glasgow Coma scale 571, 593
management 593
Combination vaccines 211, 212
Common respiratory symptoms
cough 396
dyspnea 398
epistaxis 398
expectoration 396
hemoptysis 396
stridor 397
wheezing 397
Complementary feeding 82
Conduct disorder 45
Congenital abnormalities of kidney and urinary tract 528
multicystic dysplastic kidney 528
posterior urethral valves 529
single kidney 528
Congenital adrenal hyperplasia 547
Congenital heart diseases 427
complications of 435
cyanotic spells 436
duct-dependent lesions 431
epidemiology and etiology 427
fetal circulation 428
hemodynamic classification of 429
Nadas criteria 432
natural history 437
physiology of 427
pre-tricuspid vs. post-tricuspid shunts 430
prevention of 437
second heart sound 432
single ventricle physiology 431
transitional circulation 429
unfavorable streaming and parallel circulation 432
VSD-PS (Fallot) physiology 430
Congenital infections 284
CMV 285
perinatal HSV 285
rubella 285
syphilis 286
toxoplasmosis 284
Congestive cardiac failure 423
Constipation 300
causes of 300
functional 300, 303
Hirschsprung disease 302
management 301
Copper 116
deficiency 116
Cord clamping 121
Coronavirus disease (COVID-19) 225
cardiovascular features 473
clinical features 226
complications 226
diagnosis 227
epidemiology and etiology 225
management 227
newborn 227
pathogenesis 226
Corrosive ingestion 754
clinical manifestations 754
management 754
Cow milk protein allergy 320
Cranial nerves 571
Croup 401
spasmodic 402

Cryptococcosis 273
Cushing syndrome 543
Cystic fibrosis 417
 clinical features 418
 diagnosis 418
 genetics 418
 management 418
Cystic kidney diseases 531
 glomerulocystic kidney disease 532
 nephronophthisis 532
 polycystic kidneys 531
Cystinosis 524

Dandy-Walker malformations 575
Dehydration 58
Delayed puberty 557
 in boys 557
 in girls 556
Dengue 224, 241
 clinical manifestations 242
 differential diagnosis 242
 epidemiology 241
 management 243
 pathophysiology 242
 prevention 245
 prognosis 245
 vaccine 211
Dermatophytoses 740
 tinea capitis 740
 tinea corporis 740
Development, factors affecting 22
 early childhood development 39
 early stimulation 37
 perinatal asphyxia 23
 protective 23
 psychosocial 23
Developmental assessment 24, 36
 developmental milestones 29, 32, 35, 41
 developmental quotient 36
 developmental surveillance 37
 domains of development 24
 screening tests 37, 38
Diabetes insipidus 524, 536
Diabetes mellitus 562
 classification 562
 complications 567, 569
 diabetic ketoacidosis 567
 diagnostic criteria 562
 education 566
 hypoglycemia 567
 insulin regimen 564
 management 565
 MODY 570
 monitoring 566
 neonatal 570
 type 1 diabetes mellitus 562
 type 2 diabetes mellitus 562, 570
Diaper dermatitis 724
Diet
 assessment 79
 balanced 81
 complementary feeding 82
 planning 84
 standards 77
Diphtheria
 clinical features 264
 diagnosis 264
 etiopathogenesis 264
 management 264
Diphtheria, pertussis and tetanus vaccine 195
 acellular pertussis vaccine 196
Disorders of calcium metabolism 541
 hypercalcemia 543
 hypocalcemia 541
 pseudohypoparathyrodism 542
Disorders of pituitary gland 533
 approach to short stature and GHD 534
 diabetes insipidus 536
 growth hormone deficiency 534
Disorders in sexual development 558
 cryptorchidism 561
 evaluation 560
 management 561
 physiology 558
Disseminated intravascular coagulopathy 373
 blood component therapy 375
 causes 373
 DIC score 374
 laboratory features 374
 pathophysiology 373
 treatment 375
Diuretics 852
Drooling 394
Drowning, near 748
Drug eruptions 732
Dysentery 314
Dysphagia 298
 achalasia cardia 299
 foreign bodies in esophagus 298
Dystonia 600

Eating disorders 45
Ebola virus 253
Ebstein anomaly 447
Eisenmenger syndrome 452
Emerging viruses 254
 Chandipura virus 254
 Crimean-Congo hemorrhagic fever 254
 hantaviruses 254
 Nipah virus 254
Empyema thoracis 417
Encephalitis
 acute 583
 autoimmune 588
 etiology 584
 herpes simplex 585
 Japanese 584
 scrub typhus 587
 viral 584
Encephalomyelitis 588
Encephalopathies 588
Encopresis 46
Endotracheal intubation, neonate 124
Enteric fever
 clinical features 266
 complications 266
 diagnosis 267
 treatment 267
Enuresis 46, 527
Epidermolysis bullosa 717
Epilepsy
 EEG 582
 epileptic encephalopathies 582
 etiology 581
 febrile seizures 580
 focal onset epilepsy 581
 generalized onset epilepsy 581
 Lennox-Gastaut syndrome 582
 localization of neurological lesion 573
 principles of drug therapy 582
 seizures 579
 status epilepticus 579
 West syndrome 582
Epistaxis 388
Erythema infectiosum 234
Erythema multiforme 733
Erythroderma 729
Ewing sarcoma 641
Exanthematous illnesses 224

Failure to thrive 21
Feeding of LBW babies 152, 154
Fetal growth 8
Fever 220
 evaluation 220, 222
 management 221
 of unknown origin 223
 recurrent 225
 short duration 221
 with rash 224
Filarial infections 287
Fluid and electrolyte management 55
 in neonates 151
Folic acid 113
Food
 carbohydrates 75
 energy 77
 fats 76
 proteins 76
Foreign body aspiration 392, 416, 776
Foster care 792
Functional gastrointestinal disorders 308

Gallstones 305
Gastroesophageal reflux disease 296
 clinical features 296
 evaluation 296
 management 297
Gastrointestinal bleeding 325
 lower GI bleeding 327
  evaluation 328
 upper GI bleeding 325
  common causes 325
  management 326
Germ cell tumors 642
Giardiasis 282
 clinical features 283
 diagnosis 283
 treatment 283
Glomerular filtration rate 491
Glomerulonephritis
 acute 496
 C3 glomerulopathy 499
 chronic 506
 IgA nephropathy 499
 infection related 496
 lupus nephritis 499
Glucose-6-phosphate dehydrogenase deficiency 359
Glycogen storage disorders 343
Growth 6
 assessment 9
 charts 12, 14
 factors affecting 8

Growth hormone deficiency 534
therapy 535
Growth hormone excess 535
Growth monitoring
of LBW infants 154
software and apps 13, 14
Growth standards 12
head circumference 12
height-for-age 13
Indian Academy of Pediatrics charts 13
Multicentre Growth Reference Study 12
secular trends 14
velocity 13
weight-for-age 15
weight-for-height 15
weight-for-length 15
Guillain-Barré syndrome 610

Hand-foot-and-mouth disease 237, 738
Headache
migraine 583
Healthcare associated infections 772
strategies to reduce 772
Hearing loss
cochlear implantation 385
conductive 383
management 384
screening for 384
sensorineural 384
Heart disease, epidemiology 422
Helminthic infestations 286
cestodes 289
nematodes 289
Hematopoietic stem cell transplantation 367
allogenic 367
autologous 368
complications 369
cord blood 368
indications 368
peripheral blood 368
Hematuria 493
Alport syndrome 495
renal biopsy 495
Hemiplegia 594
stroke 595
Hemolytic anemias
autoimmune 359
causes 357
clinical features 357
intravascular, extravascular hemolysis 358
laboratory manifestation 357
management 358
Hemolytic uremic syndrome 517
atypical 517
shigatoxin-associated 517
Hemophilia 372
management 373
Hemophilus vaccine 199
Hemorrhagic disease of the newborn 110
Hepatic manifestations of systemic diseases 344
Hepatitis A
clinical features 238
diagnosis 238
treatment 238
vaccine 207
Hepatitis B
clinical features 239, 332, 340
epidemiology 238
prevention 341
treatment 341
vaccine 198
Hepatitis C
clinical features 239, 341
diagnosis 240
epidemiology 239
evaluation 342
treatment 342
Hepatitis D 239
Hepatitis E 240
Hepatobiliary system
evaluation 328
Hepatomegaly 328
Hereditary spherocytosis 358
Herniation syndromes 589
Histiocytosis
bone marrow transplantation 649
hemophagocytic lymphohistiocytosis 645
Langerhans cell 744
HIV infection 245
clinical features 247
clinical staging in children 247
diagnosis 249
epidemiology 245
immunization 251
management 250
natural history 246
opportunistic infections 247
prevention of mother-to-child transmission 251
pulmonary features 420
Hoarseness 393
Home based young child program 40
Human papillomavirus vaccine 201
Hydrocephalus 574, 575, 589, 590
Hyperthyroidism 540
Hypocalcemia, newborn 181
Hypoglycemia 180
Hypothyroidism 538
Hypotonia 606

Ichthyoses 714
collodion baby 716
ichthyoses vulgaris 715
non-bullous ichthyosiform erythroderma 716
X-linked 715
Immune thrombocytopenic purpura 371
evaluation 370
management 372
Immunization
active immunity 185
passive immunity 185, 217, 218
principles 188
protective efficacy of vaccines 185
special circumstances 215, 217
types of vaccines 186
Immunization programs 187, 189
Immunodeficiency 321
acquired immunodeficiency syndrome 321
Inborn errors of immunity 696
ataxia-telangiectasia 700
cellular immunodeficiency 697
classification 698
clues to the diagnosis 699
common variable immunodeficiency 700
DiGeorge syndrome 698
hyper-IgM syndrome 700
hypogammaglobulinemia of infancy 700
IgA deficiency 700
IgG subclass deficiency 700
severe combined immunodeficiency 697
treatment 701
Wiskott-Aldrich syndrome 698
X-linked (Bruton) agammaglobulinemia 700
Inborn errors of metabolism 677
approach 678
defects of carbohydrate metabolism 687
fatty acid oxidation defects 686
galactosemia 687
glycogen storage diseases 687
laboratory investigations 677
lysosomal storage disorders 689
management 681
mitochondrial disorders 686
peroxisomal disorders 693
Incontinentia pigmenti 720
Infantile seborrheic dermatitis 724
Infectious mononucleosis 233
clinical features 233
diagnosis 234
Infective endocarditis 466
prophylaxis 469
treatment 468
Inflammatory bowel disease 322
clinical features 322
diagnosis 323
treatment 323
Influenza 251
clinical features 252
diagnosis 252
epidemiology 251
treatment 252
vaccine 205
Inotropic agents 852
Integrated Child Development Services 97, 98
Integrated Management of Neonatal and Childhood Illness (IMNCI) 793
charts 802
classification tables 794
effective communication 797, 799
outpatient management up to 2 months 794
outpatient management 2 months–5 years 797
principles of integrated care 794
Interstitial nephritis 507
Intestinal malrotation 306
Intestinal lymphangiectasia 321
Intracranial hypertension 592
Intraosseous infusion 779
Intrauterine growth curves 133
Intrauterine growth restriction 148
Intussusception 304
Iodine
deficiency 116, 117, 540
goiter 117, 539
neonatal hypothyroidism 117
recommended daily intake 116

Iron deficiency anemia 115, 354
diagnosis 354
non-response to hematinic therapy 355
treatment 355

Japanese B encephalitis vaccine 202, 203
Jaundice 155, 170, 331
approach to a neonate 155, 171
breast milk 170
breastfeeding 170
causes 171, 331
cholestasis 175
clinical estimation, Kramer 171
Crigler-Najjar syndrome 331
Dubin-Johnson syndrome 331
exchange transfusion 173
Gilbert syndrome 331
infant cholestasis 345
pathological 172
phototherapy 173, 174
physiological 170, 172
prolonged 174, 175
Juvenile dermatomyositis 656

Kangaroo mother care
eligibility 149
initiation 149
procedure 149
Kidney replacement therapy 520
chronic hemodialysis 521
chronic peritoneal dialysis 521
renal transplantation 521
Klinefelter syndrome 20

Lead poisoning 757
Learning disability 43, 44
Leishmaniasis 279
clinical features 279
diagnosis 280
prevention and control 281
treatment 280, 281
Lentigines 731
Leprosy 736
complications 737
investigations 737
lepra reactions 737
lepromatous 736
treatment 737
tuberculoid 736
Leptospirosis 268
clinical features 268
diagnosis 268
treatment 269
Leukemias
acute lymphoblastic 619
acute myeloid 619
Down syndrome 625
late effects of treatment 626
management 624
prognosis 626
Leukocytosis
eosinophilia 377
lymphocytosis 378
monocytosis 377
neutrophilia 377
Leukopenia 378
Level of newborn care
newborn care corner 126
newborn stabilization units 126
special newborn care units 126
Lichen nitidus 728
Lichen planus 728
Lichen striatus 729
Liver abscess 329
diagnosis 330
management 330
Liver biopsy 329, 785
Liver failure
acute 333
causes 333
clinical features 333
management 333
stages of hepatic encephalopathy 334
Liver transplantation 349
Liver tumors
hepatoblastoma 330
hepatocellular carcinoma 330
infantile hemangioendothelioma 330
Low birth weight 147
feeding 152, 153
growth monitoring 154
Lowe syndrome 524
Lumbar puncture 781
Lung abscess 416
Lymphoma 628
Hodgkin 629
non-Hodgkin 631

Macroglossia 389
Magnesium 68
hypermagnesemia 69
hypomagnesemia 68
physiology 68
Maintenance fluids 57
Malaria 274
clinical features 275
complicated malaria 277
control and prevention 279
diagnosis 275
epidemiology 274
life cycle of the parasite 274
National Vector-Borne Disease Control Program 279
severe 276
treatment failures, recrudescence and relapse 278
uncomplicated malaria 276
vaccine 211
Malnutrition 88
dehydration 93
electrolyte imbalance 94
hypoglycemia 92
hypothermia 92
infection 91, 94
management 89
micronutrient deficiencies 97
moderate acute malnutrition 88
nutrition rehabilitation centres 90
post-discharge care at home 96
prevention 97
refeeding 95
severe acute malnutrition 88–91
Maltreatment 788
extent of problem 788
features of 789
neglect 790
POCSO Act 789
types 788
Mastocytosis 744
Measles
clinical features 231
complications 231
diagnosis 232
Measles-containing vaccines 197
Meconium aspiration syndrome
clinical features and course 159
management 160
stained liquor 122
Meningitis
acute 585
diagnosis 586
treatment 586
Meningococcal vaccine 208
Meningomyelocele 574
Mental health 47, 51
Metabolic acidosis
causes 71
treatment 72
Metabolic alkalosis
causes 73
treatment 73
Metabolic liver disease 342
diagnosis 342
management 342
Methemoglobinemia
clinical manifestations 756
treatment 757
Microcephaly 575
Micrognathia 389
Micropenis 562
Miliaria 726
Mixed connective tissue disease 658
Molluscum contagiosum 738
Mother-child protection card 40
Mother-neonatal intensive care unit 127
Movement disorders 600
athetosis 600
chorea 600
dystonia 600
infantile tremor syndrome 602
myoclonus 601
Sydenham chorea 600
tics 601
tremors 602
Wilson disease 601
Mucormycosis 273
Multisystem inflammatory syndrome in children (MIS-C) 228
clinical features 229
diagnosis 229
epidemiology 228
management 230
Mumps 235
clinical features 235
diagnosis 235
treatment 235
Munchausen by proxy 45
Myasthenia, agents for 842
Mycoplasma infections
clinical features 272
diagnosis 272
epidemiology 271
treatment 272
Myocarditis 469

Nasal obstruction
  adenoid hypertrophy 387
  choanal atresia 388
  deviated nasal septum 387
Nasogastric tube insertion 777
Necrotising enterocolitis 170
Neonatal cholestasis 175
Neonatal seizures 164
Neonatal sepsis 166, 168
  prevention 169
Neonates, high risk 179
Nephrolithiasis, nephrocalcinosis 525
  cystinuria 526
  idiopathic hypercalciuria 526
  management of renal calculi 526
  primary hyperoxaluria 526
Nephrotic syndrome (*see* steroid sensitive, steroid resistant nephrotic syndrome) 500
  congenital 506
Neural tube defects 177, 574
Neuroblastoma 638
Neurocutaneous syndromes 576, 719
  ataxia-telangiectasia 578
  neurofibromatosis 576
  Sturge-Weber syndrome 577
  tuberous sclerosis 576, 719
Neurocysticercosis 587
Neurological regression 602
Neuronal migration defects 575
Neuropathy
  chronic inflammatory demyelinating polyradiculoneuropathy 610
  hereditary neuropathy 609
  peripheral neuropathy 609
Neuromuscular junction disorders 612
  Becker muscular dystrophy 614
  congenital myasthenia syndromes 613
  congenital myopathies 614
  Duchenne muscular dystrophy 614
  dystrophinopathies 614
  muscle dystrophies 614
  myasthenia gravis 612
  myotonic dystrophy 616
Nevi 720
  Klippel-Trenaunay syndrome 722
  melanocytic 720
  mongolian spot 721
  nervus of Ota 721
  Proteus syndrome 722
Newborn
  anthropometry 132
  asphyxia 161
  cephalhematoma 135
  cyanosis 160
  effect of maternal conditions 181
  evaluation 131
  gestational age assessment 133
  hypoglycemia 180
  infections 166
  intestinal obstruction 176
  screening 183
  seizures 164
Newborn care 188, 127
  common parental concerns 129
  danger signs 126
  definitions 118
  levels of 126
  low birth weight 147
  resuscitation 119
Niacin 111
Non-alcoholic fatty liver disease
  investigations 344
  treatment 344
Nurturing care 39, 41
Nutrition in critically ill 770
Nutritive value of common foods 80

Obesity 98, 547
  complications 550
  criteria for diagnosis 548, 550
  lifestyle measures 552
  management 549
Obstructive sleep apnea 391
Ophthalmic disorders
  acquired eye diseases 704
  blindness and low vision 709
  cataract 707
  congenital and developmental abnormalities 704
  glaucoma 708
  retinopathy of prematurity 709
Oppositional defiant disorder 45
Organophosphate poisoning 755
  clinical features 755
  treatment 755
Osmolality 56
Osteogenic sarcoma 641
Otitis externa 383
Otitis media
  acute 379
  chronic 381
  complications 382
  recurrent 381
Overnutrition 98
Oxygen therapy 780

Pachyonychia congenita 727
Palmoplantar keratoderma 716
Pancreatitis
  acute 307
  chronic 307
Pantothenic acid 112
Papular urticaria 742
Parasomnias 45
Parathyroid glands
  hyperparathyroidism 543
  hypoparathyroidism 542
Patent ductus arteriosus 442
Pediatrics 1
Pediatric eye screening 702
Pediculosis 742
Pemphigus vulgaris 730
Peptic ulcer disease 306
Peritoneal dialysis 783
  complications 784
Persistent diarrhea
  clinical features 315
  etiopathogenesis 315
  management 315
Pertussis 265
  complications 265
  diagnosis 266
  epidemiology 265
  management 266
Pheochromocytoma 545
Physical trauma 745
  prevention 760
Pica 46
Pityriasis alba 725
Pityriasis rosea 729
Pityriasis versicolor 741
Pneumococcal infections
  clinical features 263
  diagnosis 263
  treatment 264
Pneumococcal vaccine 199
Pneumonia 402
  aliphatic hydrocarbon associated 404
  etiology 402
  hemophilus 402
  Loeffler syndrome 405
  pneumococcal 402
  primary atypical 404
  staphylococcal 403
  streptococcal 404
  treatment 405
  viral 404
Poisoning
  clinical approach 749
  laboratory evaluation 749
  management 749
  National Poisons Information Center 749
Poliomyelitis 235
  diagnosis 236
  epidemiology 235
  residual paralysis 236
Polio vaccines
  oral 192
  bivalent oral 193
  immunization schedule 194
  inactivated 193
  polio eradication 194
Polycythemia, neonate 155
Polyuria 536
Porphyria 743
Portal hypertension 338
  Budd-Chiari syndrome 339
  clinical features 338
  complications 339
  extrahepatic portal venous obstruction 339
  management 339
Potassium 62
  hyperkalemia 64
  hypokalemia 63
Precocious puberty 553, 556
  etiology 553, 555
  evaluation 553, 555
Prematurity 155
  criteria for discharge 156
  growth charts 156
  hearing impairment 155
  intraventricular hemorrhage 155
  respiratory distress syndrome 156
  retinopathy of prematurity 155
Protection of Children from Sexual Offences Act 54, 789
Proteinuria 496
Psoriasis 727
Pumonary arterial hypertension 477
  persistent, newborn 479
Pulmonary function test 399

Pulmonic stenosis 456
Pyodermas 733
bullous impetigo 734
cellulitis 734
ecthyma 734
erysipelas 734
folliculitis 734
impetigo contagiosa 734
staphylococcal scalded skin syndrome 735
Pyridoxine (vitamin $B_6$) 112
Pyruvate kinase deficiency 359

Rabies vaccine 206
Radionuclide imaging 492
Rational drug therapy 840
Recommended dietary allowances 77
Renal anatomy 486
Renal physiology
development 488
renal acidification 487
tubular reabsorption 487
Renal tubular acidosis 521
distal 522
Fanconi syndrome 522
proximal 522
type 4 523
Respiratory acidosis 73
Respiratory alkalosis 74
Respiratory distress syndrome 156
Respiratory tract infection control program 405
Resuscitation of a newborn 119, 121, 125
algorithm 122
Retinoblastoma 634
Retinopathy of prematurity 155
Rhabdomyosarcoma 640
Rheumatic fever 457
clinical features 458
epidemiology 457
etiopathogenesis 458
laboratory manifestations 459
prevention 461
revised Jones criteria 459
treatment 461
Rheumatic heart disease 462
mitral regurgitation 462
mitral stenosis 463
Rhinitis 385, 400
Rhinosinusitis 386
Rhythm disorders 480
clinical features 480
diagnosis and management of tachyarrhythmias 481
stable narrow-QRS tachycardia 481
wide-QRS tachycardia 484
Riboflavin (vitamin $B_2$) 110
Rickets 104
chronic kidney disease 108
clinical features 104
etiology 104
familial hypophosphatemic 107
fluorosis 109
hypophosphatemic 107
metaphyseal dysplasia 109
nutritional 104, 106
oncogenous 108
refractory 107
renal tubular acidosis 108
vitamin D dependent 107
Rickettsial infections
clinical manifestations 270
diagnosis 270
epidemiology 270
Roseola infantum 234
Rotavirus vaccine 200

Salivary gland infections
bacterial 394
mumps 394
tuberculosis 394
SARS-CoV-2 vaccines 209
Scabies 741
Scleroderma 657
Scorpion sting
clinical features 759
management 759
Screen time 38
Sedation and analgesia 771
Seizures 579
Selenium 116
Sexual maturity rating 17, 48
Shock 767
classification 768
diagnosis 768
management 769
vasoactive drugs 769
Short stature
assessment 17
causes 17
constitutional growth delay 18
differential diagnosis 18
evaluation 18
familial 18
growth hormone deficiency 534
psychosocial dwarfism 20
small-for-gestational age 20
undernutrition 19
Sickle cell disease
clinical evaluation 364
hospital management 365
laboratory studies 365
preventive care 365
Snake bite
clinical features 757
laboratory findings 757
management 758
snake anti-venom 758
Sodium 59
hypernatremia 61
hyponatremia 59
Sore throat
acute bacterial pharyngotonsillitis 390
Centor score 390
diphtheria 390
infectious mononucleosis 390
viral pharyngitis 389
Spinal muscular atrophy 609
Splenomegaly 328
Spontaneous bacterial peritonitis 337
Staphylococcal infections
clinical features 262
toxic shock syndrome 263
treatment 263
Steroid resistant nephrotic syndrome 505
Steroid sensitive nephrotic syndrome 500, 502
complications 504
frequent relapses 503
long-term outcome 505
management of initial episode 502
management of relapse 503
steroid dependence 503
steroid-sparing agents 504
Stomatitis
herpetic 289
recurrent aphthous 389
Stridor 391, 397
acute epiglottitis 391
acute laryngotracheobronchitis 391
acquired subglottic stenosis 392
bacterial tracheitis 391
iatrogenic causes 391
laryngomalacia 392
retropharyngeal abscess 391
vocal cord paralysis 392
Stroke 594
acute ischemic 594
cerebral venous sinus thrombosis 596
intracranial hemorrhage 595
paraplegia and quadriplegia 597
Sturge-Weber syndrome 577
Stuttering 46, 389
Suppurative lung disease
bronchiectasis 416
empyema thoracis 417
lung abscess 416
Sustainable Development Goals 787
Systemic hypertension
clinical features 476
definition, staging 474
etiology 474
evaluation 476
guidelines on management 476
managing emergencies 477
measurement of blood pressure 475
Systemic lupus erythematosus 654
antiphospholipid syndrome 656
classification criteria 655
diagnosis 654
lupus nephritis 655

TABC of resuscitation 120
Tall stature 20
Tay-Sachs disease 603
Television viewing 38
Temper tantrums 46
Tetanus 269
clinical features 269
neonatal 269
prevention 270
treatment 270
Tetralogy of Fallot 494
Thalassemia 360
chelation therapy 363
curative therapy 363
iron overload 363
laboratory studies 362
management 362
pathophysiology 360
presentation 361
splenectomy 363
thalassemia intermedia 361
thalassemia major 361
thalassemia trait 361

Thermal protection 139
hypothermia 140
severe hypothermia 142
thermoneutral environment 141
Thiamine (vitamin $B_1$) 110
Thoracocentesis 782
Thrombocytopenia 369
bleeding child 369
Thrombotic disorders
clinical evaluation 375
laboratory evaluation 376
management 376
Thumb sucking 46
Tic disorder and stereotypies 44, 601
Tourette syndrome 45, 601
Tonsillectomy 390
Total anomalous pulmonary venous connection 451
Toxidromes 750
administration of antidotes 752
enhancement of excretion 752
removal of unabsorbed poison 751
Trace elements 115
Tracheoesophageal fistula 160, 175
Transient tachypnea of newborn 157
Transport of neonates 179
Transverse myelitis 597
Transposition of great vessels 449
corrected TGA 451
Tricuspid atresia 447
Tricuspid regurgitation 466
Tuberculoma 592
Tuberculosis
abdominal 324
antitubercular drugs 260
clinical categories for therapy 259
clinical features 255
cutaneous 735
diagnosis 256
drug-resistant 260
epidemiology 254
extrathoracic 256, 324
non-tuberculous mycobacteria (NTM) 261
Tuberculous meningitis 586
Turner syndrome 19
Typhoid vaccine 203

Umbilical vessel catheterization 778
UN Child Rights Convention 787
National Plan of Action for Children 788
National Policy for Children 788
National Policy for Persons with Disabilities 788
Undernutrition 85
clinical syndromes 85
determinants of 87
epidemiology 86
management 88
severe acute malnutrition 97
stunting 85
underweight 85
wasting 85
WHO Growth Reference Standards 85
Upper to lower segment 17
Urinalysis 489
Urinary tract infections 507
clinical features 507
diagnosis 508
imaging studies 509
microbiology 507
recurrent 509
treatment 508, 510
Urticaria 732

Vaccine storage and cold chain 213
heat sensitivity of various vaccines 214
vaccine vial monitor 214
Vaccines
combination 211
route of 187
subunit polysaccharide and conjugate 187
types 186
Varicella (chickenpox)
clinical features 232
complication 233
diagnosis 233
treatment 233
vaccine 204
Vasculitides 658
IgA vasculitis (Henoch-Schönlein purpura) 660
Behçet disease 661
granulomatosis with polyangiitis 661
Kawasaki disease 658
polyarteritis nodosa 659
Takayasu arteritis 658
Ventilation 123
positive pressure 123
Ventricular septal defect 439
Verruca (warts) 737
Vesicoureteric reflux
management 510
reflux nephropathy 511
Vitamin A 100
carotenemia 102
deficiency 101
hypervitaminosis A 102
physiologic functions 100
prevention 102
recommended daily allowance 100
sources 101
treatment of vitamin A deficiency 101
Vitamin B 111
Vitamin C 113
deficiency 114
metabolism 114
sources 114
therapy 114
Vitamin D
deficiency 104
hypervitaminosis D 103
mechanism of action 102
requirements 103
sources 103
Vitamin E
deficiency 109
hypervitaminosis E 109
nutritional requirement 109
sources 109
Vitamin K
deficiency 110, 183
nutritional requirements 109
sources 109
Vitiligo 731
Vomiting 294
causes 294
cyclic 295
evaluation 295
idiopathic hypertrophic pyloric stenosis 295

Water deprivation test 491
Wilms tumor 636
Wilson disease 342, 601

Xeroderma pigmentosum 720

Yellow fever vaccine 208

Zika virus 253
Zinc
deficiency 115
dietary sources 115
treatment 116